Rutter's Child and Adolescent Psychiatry and Psychology

Rutter's Child and Adolescent Psychiatry and Psychology

Seventh Edition

Edited by

Anita Thapar, MBBCh, PhD, FRCPsych, FMedSci, CBE

Professor of Child and Adolescent Psychiatry, Child and Adolescent Psychiatry Section, Division of Psychological Medicine and Clinical Neurosciences, Cardiff University School of Medicine, Cardiff, UK
Developmental Psychiatry Lead, Centre for Neuropsychiatric Genetics and Genomics, Division of Psychological Medicine and Clinical Neurosciences, Cardiff University School of Medicine, Cardiff, UK
Professor of Child and Adolescent Psychiatry, Wolfson Centre for Young People's Mental Health, Division of Psychological Medicine and Clinical Neurosciences, Cardiff University School of Medicine, Cardiff, UK

Daniel S. Pine, MD

Chief, Section on Development and Affective Neuroscience, National Institute of Mental Health (NIMH) Intramural Research Program, Bethesda, MD, USA

Samuele Cortese, MD, PhD

NIHR Research Professor and Professor of Child and Adolescent Psychiatry, University of Southampton, UK
Honorary Consultant Child and Adolescent Psychiatrist, Hampshire and Isle of Wight Healthcare NHS Foundation Trust, UK
Professor of Child and Adolescent Neuropsychiatry, University of Bari "Aldo Moro", Italy
Adjunct Professor, Department of Child and Adolescent Psychiatry, NYU Grossman School of Medicine, New York, USA

Cathy Creswell, BA (Ox Hons), DClinPsy, PhD

Professor of Developmental Clinical Psychology, Department of Experimental Psychology, University of Oxford, Oxford, UK
Professor of Developmental Clinical Psychology, Department of Psychiatry, University of Oxford, Oxford, UK

Tamsin J. Ford, PhD, FRCPsych, FMedSci, CBE

Professor of Child and Adolescent Psychiatry, Department of Psychiatry, University of Cambridge, Cambridge, UK

James F. Leckman, MD, PhD

Neison Harris Professor of Child Psychiatry, Child Study Center, Yale University, New Haven, CT, USA

Argyris Stringaris, MD, PhD, FRCPsych

Professor of Child and Adolescent Psychiatry, Faculty of Brain Sciences, University College London, London, UK
Professor, First Department of Psychiatry, Aiginiteio Hospital, National and Kapodistrian University of Athens, Athens, Greece

WILEY Blackwell

This edition first published 2025

Edition History
Wiley Blackwell (6e, 2015), Blackwell Publishing (5e, 2008), Blackwell Publishing (4e, 2002)

Registered Office(s)
John Wiley & Sons, Inc., 111 River Street, Hoboken, NJ 07030, USA
John Wiley & Sons Ltd, New Era House, 8 Oldlands Way, Bognor Regis, West Sussex, PO22 9NQ, UK

For details of our global editorial offices, customer services, and more information about Wiley products visit us at www.wiley.com.

The manufacturer's authorized representative according to the EU General Product Safety Regulation is Wiley-VCH GmbH, Boschstr. 12, 69469 Weinheim, Germany, e-mail: Product_Safety@wiley.com.

Wiley also publishes its books in a variety of electronic formats and by print-on-demand. Some content that appears in standard print versions of this book may not be available in other formats.

Library of Congress Cataloging-in-Publication Data Applied for:
Hardback ISBN: 9781119906063

Cover Design: Wiley
Cover Image: © Flashpop/Getty Images

Set in 9.5/12pt MinionPro by Straive, Pondicherry, India

SKY10157376_052226

Contents

List of contributors

Stephanie H. Ameis MD, MSc, FRCP(C)
Associate Professor, Child & Youth Mental Health, Department of Psychiatry and Institute of Medical Science, Temerty Faculty of Medicine, University of Toronto, Toronto, Ontario, Canada
Associate Director, Senior Scientist and Staff Psychiatrist, Cundill Centre for Child and Youth Depression, Campbell Family Mental Health Research Institute, Centre for Addiction and Mental Health, Toronto, Ontario, Canada
Staff Psychiatrist, Neurosciences & Mental Health and Department of Psychiatry, The Hospital for Sick Children, Toronto, Ontario, Canada

Louise Arseneault PhD
Professor of Developmental Psychology, Institute of Psychiatry, Psychology and Neuroscience, King's College London, London, UK

Duncan E. Astle PhD
Gnodde Goldman Sachs Professor of Neuroinformatics, Department of Psychiatry and MRC Cognition and Brain Science Unit, University of Cambridge, Cambridge, UK

Isang Awah PhD
Head of Advocacy, Global Parenting Initiative, Department of Social Policy and Intervention, University of Oxford, Oxford, UK

Christian Bachmann MD, PhD
Professor, Department of Child and Adolescent Psychiatry, Ulm University Medical School, Ulm, Germany

Skye Barbic PhD, MSc, BScOT, Reg. OT(BC)
Canada Research Chair (Tier 2) in Integrated Youth Services, Associate Professor, Department of Occupational Science and Occupational Therapy, The University of British Columbia, Vancouver, British Columbia, Canada

Fionna Bathgate MA, DClinPsy
Principal Clinical Psychologist, Psychological and Mental Health Services, Great Ormond Street Hospital NHS Foundation Trust, London, UK

Julian Baudinet BA (Hons), MSc, DClinPsy
Consultant Clinical Psychologist, Michael Rutter Centre, South London and Maudsley NHS Foundation Trust, London, UK

Jessica E. Becker MD, MPH
Clinical Assistant Professor, Department of Child and Adolescent Psychiatry, NYU Grossman School of Medicine and NYU Langone Health, New York, NY, USA

Rachael Bedford PhD
Professor in Biological and Experimental Psychology, Centre for Brain and Behaviour, Department of Psychology, Queen Mary University of London, London, UK

Kristin Bernard PhD
Associate Professor of Clinical Psychology, Department of Psychology, Stony Brook University, Stony Brook, NY, USA

Michael H. Bloch MD, MS
Professor, Child Study Center, Yale University, New Haven, CT, USA

Rohan Borschmann PhD, DPsych, BBSc, PG-Dip (Psych)
Professorial Fellow, The University of Melbourne (Centre for Mental Health and Community Wellbeing), Melbourne, Victoria, Australia
Visiting Academic, Department of Psychiatry, The University of Oxford, Oxford, UK
Research Facilitator, Oxford Health NHS Foundation Trust, Oxford, UK

Rachel Bryant-Waugh BSc, MSc, DPhil
Consultant Clinical Psychologist and Honorary Senior Lecturer, Michael Rutter Centre, South London and Maudsley NHS Foundation Trust, London, UK

Kristin A. Buss PhD
Tracy Winfree and Ted H. McCourtney Professor in Children, Work, and Families and Professor of Psychology & Human Development and Family Studies, Department of Psychology, The Pennsylvania State University, PA, USA

Gabrielle A. Carlson MD
Professor of Psychiatry and Pediatrics, Renaissance School of Medicine at Stony Brook University, Stony Brook, NY, USA

Dante Cicchetti PhD
Professor Emeritus, Institute of Child Development, University of Minneapolis, Minneapolis, MN, USA

Lucie Cluver D.Phil, DipSW
Professor of Child and Family Social Work, Department of Social Policy and Intervention, University of Oxford, Oxford, UK
Honorary Professor in Psychiatry and Mental Health, Department of Psychiatry and Mental Health, University of Cape Town, Cape Town, South Africa

David Coghill MB, ChB, MD
Professor, Departments of Paediatrics and Psychiatry, University of Melbourne, Melbourne, Victoria, Australia

Stephan Collishaw D.Phil
Professor, Wolfson Centre for Young People's Mental Health, Division of Psychological Medicine and Clinical Neurosciences, School of Medicine, Cardiff University, Cardiff, UK

Samuele Cortese MD, PhD
NIHR Research Professor, UK
Professor of Child and Adolescent Psychiatry, University of Southampton, UK
Honorary Consultant Child and Adolescent Psychiatrist, Hampshire and Isle of Wight Healthcare NHS Foundation Trust, UK
Professor of Child and Adolescent Neuropsychiatry, University of Bari "Aldo Moro", Italy
Adjunct Professor, Department of Child and Adolescent Psychiatry, NYU Grossman School of Medicine, New York, USA

Andy Cotgrove Mb, ChB, MSc, MRCPsych
Formerly Consultant in Adolescent Psychiatry, Cheshire and Wirral Partnership NHS Foundation Trust, UK

Cathy Creswell BA (Ox Hons), DClinPsy, PhD
Professor of Developmental Clinical Psychology, Department of Experimental Psychology, University of Oxford, Oxford, UK
Professor of Developmental Clinical Psychology, Department of Psychiatry, University of Oxford, Oxford, UK

Naomi Dale MA, PhD, CPsychol
Consultant Clinical Psychologist and Paediatric Neuropsychologist, Psychological and Mental Health Services, Great Ormond Street Hospital NHS Foundation Trust, London, UK
Professor of Paediatric Neurodisability, Developmental Neurosciences, UCL Great Ormond Street Institute of Child Health, London, UK

Andrea Danese MD, PhD
Professor of Child & Adolescent Psychiatry, Social, Genetic and Developmental Psychiatry Centre, Institute of Psychiatry, Psychology, and Neuroscience, King's College London, London, UK
Professor of Child & Adolescent Psychiatry, Department of Child and Adolescent Psychiatry, Institute of Psychiatry, Psychology, and Neuroscience, King's College London, London, UK
Honorary Consultant Child & Adolescent Psychiatrist, National and Specialist CAMHS Clinic for Trauma, Anxiety, and Depression, South London and Maudsley NHS Foundation Trust, London, UK

Stephane De Brito BSc, MPhil, PhD
Professor of Developmental Psychopathology and Neuroscience, School of Psychology, Centre for Human Brain Health, Institute for Mental Health, Centre for Developmental Science, Centre for Neurogenetics, University of Birmingham, Birmingham, UK

Daniel P. Dickstein MD
Chief, Simches Division of Child and Adolescent Psychiatry, McLean Hospital, Belmont, MA, USA
Professor of Psychiatry, Harvard Medical School, Boston, MA, USA

Enrica Donolato PhD
Researcher, Department of Special Needs Education and CREATE, University of Oslo, Oslo, Norway

Mary Dozier PhD
Amy E DuPont Chair of Child Development, Professor, Department of Psychological and Brain Sciences, University of Delaware, Newark, DE, USA

Bernadka Dubicka BSc, MBBs, MD, FRCPsych
Professor, Hull York Medical School, University of Hull/University of York, Kingston upon Hull/York, UK

Consultant Child and Adolescent Psychiatrist, Greater Manchester Mental Health NHS Foundation Trust, Prestwich, UK
Honorary Professor, Manchester Academic Health Science Centre, University of Manchester, Manchester, UK

Sara Evans-Lacko PhD
Associate Professorial Research Fellow, Care Policy and Evaluation Centre, London School of Economics and Political Science, London, UK

Mina Fazel MB, BCh, DM, FRCPsych
Professor of Child and Adolescent Psychiatry, Department of Psychiatry, University of Oxford, Oxford, UK

Seena Fazel BSc (Hons), MBChB, MD, FRCPsych
Professor of Forensic Psychiatry, Department of Psychiatry, University of Oxford, Oxford, UK
Consultant Forensic Psychiatrist, Oxford Health NHS Foundation Trust, Oxford, UK

Julianna Finelli MD
Assistant Professor of Psychiatry, Department of Psychiatry and Behavioral Sciences, Tulane University School of Medicine, New Orleans, LA, USA

Tamsin J. Ford PhD, FRCPsych, FMedSci, CBE
Professor of Child and Adolescent Psychiatry, Department of Psychiatry, University of Cambridge, Cambridge, UK

Brittnie Fowler MD
Assistant Professor of Psychiatry and Behavioral Sciences, Department of Psychiatry and Behavioral Sciences, Tulane University School of Medicine, New Orleans, LA, USA

Lauren Franz M.B., CH.B
Honorary Associate Professor, Department of Psychiatry and Mental Health, University of Cape Town, Cape Town, South Africa
Associate Professor of Psychiatry and Behavioral Sciences and Global Health, Duke University School of Medicine, Duke University, Durham, NC, USA

Frances Gardner MPhil, DPhil
Professor of Child and Family Psychology, Centre for Evidence-Based Intervention, Department of Social Policy and Intervention, University of Oxford, Oxford, UK

Eilish Gilvarry
Honorary Professor in Addiction Psychiatry, Faculty of Medical Sciences, Newcastle University, Newcastle-upon-Tyne, UK
Consultant Psychiatrist in Addictions, Addictions Unit, Cumbria, Northumberland, Tyne and Wear NHS Foundation Trust, Newcastle-upon-Tyne, UK

Danya Glaser MB, DCH, FRCPsych, Hon FRCPCH
Retired Consultant Child and Adolescent Psychiatrist, formerly at Great Ormond Street Hospital for Children NHS Foundation Trust, London, UK

Jonathan Green FRCPsych, FMedSci
Professor of Child and Adolescent Psychiatry, Division of Psychology and Mental Health, University of Manchester, Manchester, UK
Honorary Consultant, Royal Manchester Children's Hospital, Manchester, UK

Danella M. Hafeman MD, PhD
Associate Professor, Department of Psychiatry, University of Pittsburgh School of Medicine, Pittsburgh, PA, USA

Brenda Hale, Baroness Hale of Richmond, DBE, PC, MA (Cantab), FRCPsych (Hon), LL.D (Hon), DUniv (Hon), FBA
Formerly President, Supreme Court of the United Kingdom, London, UK

Charlotte L. Hall PhD
Principal Research Fellow, NIHR MindTech Health Research Centre, School of Medicine, Institute of Mental Health, University of Nottingham, Nottingham, UK

Francesca Happé PhD, FBA, FMedSci, CBE
Professor of Cognitive Neuroscience, Social, Genetic and Developmental Psychiatry Centre, Institute of Psychiatry, Psychology and Neuroscience, King's College London, London, UK

Gordon Harold BSc, MSc, PhD
Professor of the Psychology of Education and Mental Health, Faculty of Education, University of Cambridge, Cambridge, UK
Professor, Child and Adolescent Psychiatry Unit, School of Medicine, University College Dublin, Dublin, Ireland

Eric P. Hazen MD
Assistant Professor of Psychiatry, Harvard Medical School, Boston, MA, USA
Director, Pediatric Psychiatry Consultation-Liaison Service, Department of Psychiatry, Massachusetts General Hospital, Boston, MA, USA

J.L. Henderson PhD, CPsych
Scientific Director, Centre for Addiction and Mental Health; Professor Department of Psychiatry, University of Toronto, Toronto, Ontario, Canada

Jonathan Herring MA (Oxon), BLC
Professor of Law, Faculty of Law, University of Oxford, Oxford, UK
DM Wolfe-Clarendon Fellow, Exeter College, University of Oxford, Oxford, UK

Isobel Heyman MBE, MBBS, PhD, FRCPsych
Consultant Child and Adolescent Psychiatrist and Honorary Professor, Great Ormond Street Institute of Child Health, University College London, London, UK

Jonathan Hill BA, MBBChir, MRCP, FRCPsych
Professor of Child and Adolescent Psychiatry, School of Psychology and Clinical Language Sciences, University of Reading, Reading, UK
Honorary Consultant Psychiatrist, Oxford Health NHS Foundation Trust, Oxford, UK

Rachel Hiller PhD
Professor of Child and Adolescent Mental Health, Department of Clinical, Educational and Health Psychology, University College London, London, UK

Mauricio Scopel Hoffmann MD, MSc, PhD
Professor and Head of Department, Department of Neuropsychiatry, Universidade Federal de Santa Maria, Santa Maria, Rio Grande do Sul, Brazil

Chris Hollis PhD, FRCPsych
Professor of Child and Adolescent Psychiatry and Digital Mental Health, NIHR MindTech Health Research Centre, School of Medicine, Institute of Mental Health, University of Nottingham, Nottingham, UK

Jennifer L. Hudson BA (Hons), MClinPsych, PhD, FASSA
Child Mental Health Program Lead, Black Dog Institute, Faculty of Medicine and Health, University of New South Wales, Sydney, NSW, Australia

Charles Hulme MA, DPhil, FAcSS, FBA
Department of Experimental Psychology, University of Oxford, Oxford, UK
Professor of Psychology, School of Psychology, Social Work and Public Health, Oxford Brookes University, Oxford, UK

Aron Janssen MD
Vice Chair of Clinical Affairs, Pritzker Department of Psychiatry and Behavioral Health, Northwestern Feinberg School of Medicine, Ann and Robert H. Lurie Children's Hospital of Chicago, Chicago, IL, USA

Jennifer Jenkins PhD
Atkinson Chair of Early Child Development and Education/Director. Dr. Eric Jackman Institute of Child Study (JICS), Applied Psychology and Human Development, University of Toronto, Toronto, Ontario, Canada

Mark H. Johnson PhD, FBA
Professor of Experimental Psychology, Department of Psychology, University of Cambridge, Cambridge, UK
Associate Director, Centre for Brain and Cognitive Development, School of Psychology, Birkbeck College, University of London, London, UK

Michael Kaess MD
Professor of Child and Adolescent Psychiatry, University of Bern, Bern, Switzerland
Director, University Hospital of Child and Adolescent Psychiatry and Psychotherapy, Bern, Switzerland
Group Leader, Department of Child and Adolescent Psychiatry, Center for Psychosocial Medicine, University Hospital Heidelberg, Heidelberg, Germany

Martin Knapp CBE, PhD, FAcSS
Professor of Health and Care Policy, Care Policy and Evaluation Centre, London School of Economics and Political Science, London, UK

Helena Chmura Kraemer PhD
Professor of Biostatistics in Psychiatry, Emerita, Department of Psychiatry and Behavioral Sciences, Stanford University, Stanford, CA, USA

Georgina Krebs DClinPsy, PhD
Associate Professor, Research Department of Clinical, Educational and Health Psychology, University College London, London, UK
Honorary Consultant Clinical Psychologist, Anxiety, self-Image and Mood (AIM) Clinic, North London NHS Foundation Trust, London, UK

Marinos Kyriakopoulos PhD, FRCPsych
Assistant Professor in Child and Adolescent Psychiatry, 1st Department of Psychiatry, National and Kapodistrian University of Athens, Eginition Hospital, Athens, Greece
Visiting Senior Lecturer, Department of Child and Adolescent Psychiatry, Institute of Psychiatry, Psychology and Neuroscience, King's College London, London, UK
Consultant Child and Adolescent Psychiatrist, Kaleidoscope Child Development Centre, South London and Maudsley NHS Foundation Trust, London, UK

Meng-Chuan Lai MD, PhD
Associate Professor, Child & Youth Mental Health, Department of Psychiatry and Institute of Medical Science, Temerty Faculty of Medicine, University of Toronto, Toronto, Ontario, Canada
Senior Scientist and Staff Psychiatrist, The Margaret and Wallace McCain Centre for Child, Youth & Family Mental Health and Azrieli Adult Neurodevelopmental Centre, Campbell Family Mental Health Research Institute, Centre for Addiction and Mental Health, Toronto, Ontario, Canada
Project Investigator and Staff Psychiatrist, Neurosciences & Mental Health and Department of Psychiatry, The Hospital for Sick Children, Toronto, Ontario, Canada

James F. Leckman MD, PhD
Neison Harris Professor of Child Psychiatry, Child Study Center, Yale University, New Haven, CT, USA

Eleanor Leigh BSc (Hons), DClinPsy, DPhil
Associate Professor, Department of Experimental Psychology, University of Oxford, Oxford, UK

Alexandra Lewis BMSc, MBChB LLM, MBA, MRCPsych
Consultant Forensic and Child & Adolescent Psychiatrist, Cambridge & Peterborough NHS Foundation Trust, Cambridge, UK
Clinical Advisor, Health & Justice Team, NHS, England, London, UK

Ashley Liew MBChB, MSc, MRCPsych
Consultant Paediatric Neuropsychiatrist, South London and Maudsley NHS Foundation Trust, London, UK
Honorary Associate Professor, University of Warwick, Warwick, UK

Maria Loades DClinPsy, PhD
Clinical Psychologist and Reader, Department of Psychology, University of Bath, Bath, UK

Sheri Madigan PhD
Professor of Clinical Psychology, Canada Research Chair in Determinants of Child Development, Department of Psychology, University of Calgary, Calgary, Alberta, Canada

William Mandy
Professor of Neurodevelopmental Conditions, Department of Clinical, Educational and Health Psychology, University College London, London, UK

Laura Markley MD
Pediatrician/Division Director of Medical Coping and Addictions, Department of Pediatrics/Department of Psychiatry and Behavioral Health, Akron Children's Hospital, Akron, OH, USA
Associate Professor, Department of Pediatrics/Department of Psychiatry, Northeastern Ohio Medical University, Rootstown, OH, USA

David Mataix-Cols CPsychol, PhD
Professor, Centre for Psychiatry Research, Department of Clinical Neuroscience, Karolinska Institutet, Stockholm, Sweden
Consultant Clinical Psychologist, Stockholm Health Care Services, Region Stockholm, CAP Research Centre, Stockholm, Sweden
Visiting Professor, Department of Clinical Sciences, Lund University, Lund, Sweden

Eamon McCrory PhD, DClinPsy
Professor of Developmental Neuroscience and Psychopathology, Division of Psychology and Language Sciences, University College London, London, UK
Chief Executive, Anna Freud, London, UK

Eleanor L. McGlinchey PhD
Associate Professor of Psychology, School of Psychology and Counseling, Fairleigh Dickinson University, Teaneck, NJ, USA

Richard Meiser-Stedman PhD
Professor of Clinical Psychology, Department of Clinical Psychology & Psychological Therapies, Norwich Medical School, University of East Anglia, Norwich, UK

Monica Melby-Lervåg PhD
Professor, Department of Special Needs Education and CREATE, University of Oslo, Oslo, Norway

Sally Merry FRANZCP, CCAP
Emeritus Professor, Department of Psychological Medicine, The University of Auckland, Auckland, New Zealand

Nick Midgley PhD
Professor of Psychological Therapies for Children and Young People, Research Department of Clinical, Educational and Health Psychology, University College London, London, UK
Director, Child Attachment and Psychological Therapies Research Unit (ChAPTRe), Anna Freud, London, UK

Rick Miller PhD
Professor, School of Family Life, Brigham Young University, Provo, UT, USA

Helen Minnis
Professor of Child and Adolescent Psychiatry, School of Health and Wellbeing, University of Glasgow, Glasgow, UK

Tara Murphy BSc (Hons), MSc, DClinPsy, QiCN
Consultant Paediatric Neuropsychologist and Clinical Psychologist, Great Ormond Street Hospital for Children, London, UK

Tamsin Newlove-Delgado PhD, MRCPsych, FFPH
Associate Professor in Child Public Mental Health, Medical School, University of Exeter, Exeter, UK

Courtenay Norbury DPhil
Professor of Developmental Language and Communication Disorders, Division of Psychology and Language Sciences, University College London, London, UK

Dennis Ougrin MBBS, MRCPsych, PGDip(Oxon), PGCAPHE, PhD
Professor of Child and Adolescent Psychiatry and Global Mental Health, Youth Resilience Unit, Centre for Psychiatry and Mental Health, Wolfson Institute of Population Health, WHO Collaborating Centre for Mental Health Services Development, Queen Mary University of London, London, UK
East London NHS Foundation Trust, London, UK

Judith A. Owens MD, MPH
Senior Faculty/Professor of Neurology, Boston Children's Hospital, Harvard Medical School, Boston, MA, USA

Rebecca M. Pearson PhD, BSc
Professor of Developmental Psychology and Epidemiology, School of Psychology and Institute of Children's Futures, Manchester Metropolitan University, Manchester, UK

Koraly Pérez-Edgar PhD
McCourtney Professor of Child Studies, Professor of Psychology, Department of Psychology, The Pennsylvania State University, PA, USA

Daniel S. Pine MD
Chief, Section on Development and Affective Neuroscience, National Institute of Mental Health (NIMH) Intramural Research Program, Bethesda, MD, USA

Judith L. Rapoport, MD
Scientist Emeritus, National Institute of Mental Health (NIMH) Intramural Research Program, Bethesda, MD, USA

Charlotte Ulrikka Rask MD, PhD
Senior Consultant, Department of Child and Adolescent Psychiatry, Aarhus University Hospital Psychiatry, Aarhus, Denmark
Clinical Professor, Department for Clinical Medicine, Aarhus University, Aarhus, Denmark

Brittany Rhoades Cooper PhD
Associate Professor, Department of Human Development, Washington State University, Pullman, WA, USA

Frances Rice PhD
Professor of Developmental Psychopathology, Wolfson Centre for Young People's Mental Health, Division of Psychological Medicine and Clinical Neurosciences, School of Medicine, Cardiff University, Cardiff, UK

Nathaniel R. Riggs PhD
Professor, Department of Human Development and Family Studies, Colorado State University, Fort Collins, CO, USA

Mark Rivett
Systemic Family Psychotherapist, South Wales, UK
CEDAR, University of Exeter, Exeter, UK

Maria Rogdaki MRCPsych, PhD
Clinical Lecturer, Department of Psychosis Studies, Institute of Psychiatry, Psychology and Neuroscience, King's College London, London, UK

Luis Augusto Rohde LA, MD, PhD
Coordinator, ADHD Outpatient and Development Psychiatry Program, Hospital de Clinicas de Porto Alegre, Porto Alegre, Brazil
Professor of Psychiatry, Department of Psychiatry, Universidade Federal do Rio Grande do Sul, Porto Alegre, Brazil
Full Member, Advisory Council, Medical School, UNIEDUK, Indaiatuba, Brazil

Michelle Rozenman PhD
Associate Professor, College of Arts, Humanities, and Social Sciences, University of Denver, CO, USA

Giovanni Abrahão Salum MD, PhD
Professor of Psychiatry and Behavioral Sciences, Universidade Federal do Rio Grande do Sul, Porto Alegre, Rio Grande do Sul, Brazil
Child Mind Institute, Global Programs, NY, USA

Stephen Scott CBE, PhD, FRCPsych, FMedSci
Professor of Child Health and Behaviour, Department of Child and Adolescent Psychiatry, Institute of Psychiatry, Psychology and Neuroscience, King's College London, London, UK

Carla Sharp PhD
Professor of Clinical Psychology, Department of Psychiatry, University of Houston, Houston, TX, USA

Philip Shaw BM, BCh, PhD
Director and Head of Department, King's Maudsley Partnership for Children and Young People, Department of Child and Adolescent Psychiatry, Institute of Psychiatry, Psychology and Neuroscience, King's College London, London, UK

Tomer Shechner PhD
Professor, School of Psychological Sciences and the Integrated Brain and Behavior Research Center, University of Haifa, Haifa, Israel

Hannah Sherbersky DClinPrac
Associate Professor, CEDAR, University of Exeter, Exeter, UK
CEO, Association for Family Therapy and Systemic Practice, Warrington, UK

Emily Simonoff MD, FRCPsych
Professor of Child and Adolescent Psychiatry, Department of Child and Adolescent Psychiatry, Institute of Psychiatry, Psychology and Neuroscience, King's College London, London, UK

David Skuse MD, FRCP, FRCPsych, FRCPCH
Professor of Behavioural and Brain Sciences, Great Ormond Street Institute of Child Health, University College London, London, UK

Patrick Smith PhD
Professor of Clinical Psychology, Department of Psychology, Institute of Psychiatry, Psychology and Neuroscience, King's College London, London, UK

Margaret J. Snowling PhD, Dip Clin Psych, FBA, F Med Sci, FBPsS
Professor of Psychology, Department of Experimental Psychology, University of Oxford, Oxford, UK
President, St John's College, Oxford, UK

Daniel Stahl PhD
Professor in Medical Statistics and Statistical Learning, Department of Biostatistics and Health Informatics, Institute of Psychiatry, Psychology and Neuroscience, King's College London, London, UK

Matthew W. State MD, PhD
Oberndorf Family Distinguished Professor & Chair, Department of Psychiatry and Behavioral Sciences, Langley Porter Psychiatric Institute, Weill Institute for Neurosciences, University of California San Francisco, San Francisco, CA, USA

Alan Stein MB, BCh, MA, FRCPsych
Senior Research Fellow in Global Health and Public Policy, Blavatnik School of Government, and Emeritus Professor of Child and Adolescent Psychiatry, University of Oxford, Oxford, UK

Dan J. Stein
Professor, Head of Department, Department of Psychiatry and Mental Health, University of Cape Town, Cape Town, South Africa

Jeffrey R. Strawn MD
Professor of Psychiatry & Behavioral Neuroscience, Pediatric and Clinical & Translational Pharmacology, Department of Psychiatry, College of Medicine, University of Cincinnati, Cincinnati, OH, USA

Argyris Stringaris MD, PhD, FRCPsych
Professor of Child and Adolescent Psychiatry, Faculty of Brain Sciences, University College London, London, UK
Professor, First Department of Psychiatry, Aiginiteio Hospital, National and Kapodistrian University of Athens, Athens, Greece

Peter Szatmari MD, MSc, FRCP (C)
Emeritus Professor, Child & Youth Mental Health, Department of Psychiatry, Temerty Faculty of Medicine, University of Toronto, Toronto, Ontario, Canada
Scientific Director, Cundill Centre for Child and Youth Depression, Campbell Family Mental Health Research Institute, Centre for Addiction and Mental Health, Toronto, Ontario, Canada
Senior Scientist Emeritus, Neurosciences & Mental Health and Department of Psychiatry, The Hospital for Sick Children, Toronto, Ontario, Canada

Eva Szigethy MD, PhD
Chair of Psychiatry and Behavioral Health, Department of Psychiatry and Behavioral Health, Akron Children's Hospital, Akron, OH, USA
Professor of Psychiatry, Department of Psychiatry, Northeastern Ohio Medical University, Rootstown, OH, USA

Hiran Thabrew FRACP, FRANZCP
Senior Lecturer, Department of Psychological Medicine, The University of Auckland, Auckland, New Zealand

Anita Thapar MBBCH, PhD, FRCPsych, FMedSci, CBE
Professor of Child and Adolescent Psychiatry, Child and Adolescent Psychiatry Section, Division of Psychological Medicine and Clinical Neurosciences, Cardiff University School of Medicine, Cardiff, UK
Developmental Psychiatry Lead, Centre for Neuropsychiatric Genetics and Genomics, Division of Psychological Medicine and Clinical Neurosciences, Cardiff University School of Medicine, Cardiff, UK
Professor of Child and Adolescent Psychiatry, Wolfson Centre for Young People's Mental Health, Division of Psychological Medicine and Clinical Neurosciences, Cardiff University School of Medicine, Cardiff, UK

Kate Tilling BSc, MSc, PhD
Professor of Medical Statistics, Bristol Medical School, University of Bristol, Bristol, UK

Kenneth E. Towbin MD
Senior Research Physician, Emotion and Development Branch, National Institute of Mental Health, Intramural Research Program, Bethesda, MD, USA
Clinical Professor of Psychiatry and Behavioral Science, Department of Psychiatry and Behavioral Health, The George Washington University School of Medicine, Washington, DC, USA

Essi Viding PhD, FBA, FMedSci
Professor of Developmental Psychopathology, Division of Psychology and Language Sciences, University College London, London, UK

John T. Walkup MD
Margaret C. Osterman Professor of Psychiatry Chair, Pritzker Department of Psychiatry and Behavioral Health, Lurie Children's Hospital of Chicago & Northwestern University Feinberg School of Medicine, Chicago, IL, USA

V. Robin Weersing PhD
Professor of Psychology, Joint Doctoral Program in Clinical Psychology, San Diego State University, San Diego, CA, USA

Tonya White MD, PhD
Chief, Section on Social and Cognitive Developmental Neuroscience, National Institutes of Mental Health, Bethesda, MD, USA

William Yule PhD
Emeritus Professor of Applied Child Psychology, Department of Psychology, Institute of Psychiatry, Psychology and Neuroscience, King's College London, London, UK

Charles H. Zeanah MD
Mary Peters Sellars-Polchow Chair of Psychiatry, Professor of Psychiatry and Pediatrics, Department of Psychiatry and Behavioral Sciences, Tulane University School of Medicine, New Orleans, LA, USA

Foreword

Mike's mission to research child development began in the early 1960s. He commenced this journey with immense excitement, energy, and determination. This never wavered throughout his long career. He was greatly influenced by his mentor, Aubrey Lewis, the first child psychiatrist in the UK, who taught Mike to "think deeply, challenge accepted wisdom and never accept anything without careful scrutiny of the available empirical evidence." These words of wisdom guided Mike in all his endeavours and can clearly be seen in the rigour he applied to all the editions of the textbook. In addition, Mike always approached his work with humanity and kindness. Mike was committed to ensuring that younger generations of child psychiatrists and child psychologists continued to take the discipline forward and it was with this in mind that the 1st edition of the textbook was born. I know that Mike would be very proud of this 7th edition and delighted that his mission to bring together and create, with worldwide researchers and clinicians, an extraordinary body of knowledge and understanding of child psychiatry, which continues beyond his lifetime. I am so pleased and proud that his work has helped others to make a lasting and profound impact on the mental health of children around the world.

Marjorie Rutter

Preface

This textbook was the brainchild of Mike Rutter, the forefather of modern child and adolescent psychiatry who died in 2021, aged 88 years. The 1st edition was published in 1976, and subsequent editions were led by Mike, until we were entrusted with the 6th edition. However, Mike remained much involved in supporting us as we prepared the 6th edition; with his death, he asked that we continue the tradition of the textbook. We have felt enormously honored and privileged to take the volume forward with the 7th edition. The textbook is renowned for the high standards created by Mike, and we have retained many of the approaches he initiated in the hope of sustaining this tradition. We insisted that chapters continue to be written by the field's most brilliant minds with a conceptual focus and a skilled appraisal of the most current scientific evidence. For clinical chapters, these experts viewed their material through the lens of clinical wisdom.

To achieve excellence, Mike initiated a review process that would have been envied by the editors of many peer-reviewed journals. We have retained the process for editing chapters in this 7th edition. This has included a review of chapter outlines, followed by two stages of critical review for full chapters by the editorial team. Naturally, this has entailed an enormous amount of work for the editorial team and authors. We have been extremely fortunate in having such a wonderfully enthusiastic, kind, and responsive editorial team: Samuele Cortese, Cathy Creswell, Tamsin Ford, James Leckman, Argyris Stringaris. This has made a task that could have been arduous one to relish. Accordingly, both of us have greatly enjoyed working with the team. What has been striking to us is not only the extremely high quality of author contributions but also the willingness of senior researchers and clinicians to take on editor peer reviews and repeatedly revise their chapters. We are very grateful for their contributions and their graciousness in response to our repeated requests for different material and changes when there are so many demands on people's time.

We have also introduced a number of changes. The title of the textbook now has been changed to *Rutter's Child and Adolescent Psychiatry and Psychology* to reflect the readership and authorship of the book. This honors the multidimensional nature of our evolving field, where many professionals, including psychologists, have been instrumental for our growth. Mike would have been immensely pleased. Other changes were inspired by two notable issues: growing use of digital media, as well as increasing reliance on the textbook for teaching and training materials. For these reasons, authors provided short video clips to give a taste of their chapter, as well as slides for teaching and training. For this extra material, we did not insist on a standard approach so readers can expect much variation in author styles. Naturally, this represented even more work for the authors. Once again, we are very grateful and hope readers share our enthusiasm.

Other novel features of the edition mirror changes in science and the needs of children around the world. It contains several new chapters, including one on public health that covers global threats including the COVID-19 pandemic, wars, and natural disasters. We are also delighted to include a chapter on low-resource settings that is of relevance to clinicians in high- as well as low-income countries. Such material is vital since most of the world's children, young people, and their families live in resource-poor settings. Other new topics include: diversity in relation to gender and sexual orientation, as well as a chapter on digital technology, given the growing interest in digital approaches to assessment and intervention. Finally, our "Clinical Syndromes" section has changed with a new chapter, on body dysmorphic disorder, and new clinical highlights. We realize that some readers might peruse the textbook while working in the clinic. Hence, new highlights appear as assessment and treatment "at a glance boxes" to facilitate ready access to this information.

One of us (DSP) was supported by the Intramural Research Program of the National Institute of Mental Health to undertake editorial duties, and the work for this book (AT) was supported by the Wolfson Foundation.

Our final thanks are to Caroline Warren at Cardiff University who played the key role in coordinating much of the textbook process. It has taken us three years of weekly meetings and heavy reliance on Caroline's truly unique skill and commitment. Delivering a textbook of this complexity requires monumental organization and planning; all the editors are grateful for her hard work, perseverance, and stellar administrative and organizational support.

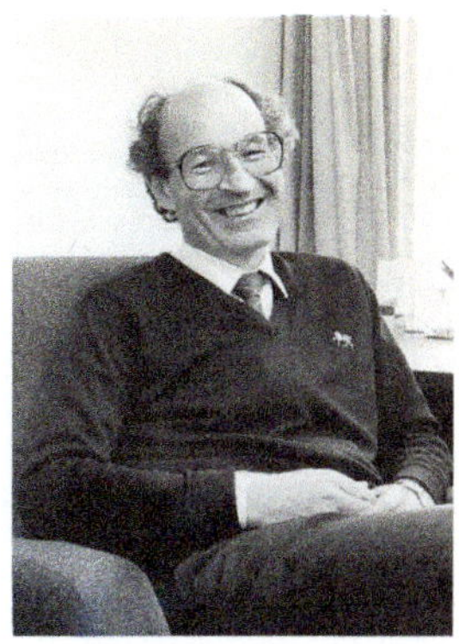

Anita Thapar and Daniel S. Pine

About the Companion Website

This book is accompanied by a companion website:

www.wiley.com/go/thapar/ruttersspsych7

This website includes:

- Videos
- PowerPoint slides

Scan this QR code to visit the companion website:

PART I

Conceptual issues and research approaches

A: Developmental psychopathology

CHAPTER 1

Development and psychopathology: a life course perspective

Stephan Collishaw and Frances Rice
Wolfson Centre for Young People's Mental Health, Division of Psychological Medicine and Clinical Neurosciences, School of Medicine, Cardiff University, UK

Why is a life course perspective to mental health important?

A developmental perspective is essential for understanding mental health at different stages of the life course. Childhood and adolescence are critical life stages where mental health problems can have profound impacts on young people's healthy development, including their education, relationships, and developing self-concept. Evidence shows that mental health problems in children and young people are common. More than 1 in 10 children and young people have a diagnosable condition at any given time (Sadler *et al.*, 2018).

Psychiatric conditions in childhood and adolescence often continue or recur across adult life, and they may also signal the emergence of new or additional forms of psychopathology. Indeed, an earlier onset often heralds a poorer long-term prognosis (de Girolamo *et al.*, 2012). Conversely, the majority of adult mental health problems have their origins earlier in life; prospective cohorts indicate that more than 50% of young adults with a psychiatric condition first met criteria for a psychiatric diagnosis before age 15 (Kim-Cohen *et al.*, 2003), while global epidemiological evidence indicates that the peak age of onset of most mental disorders ranges between 5 and 21 years (Solmi *et al.*, 2022).

At the same time, *longitudinal research* shows that recovery and improvement of childhood psychopathology are commonplace. Evidence suggests that around half of children and adolescents with a psychiatric condition experience no psychiatric disorder or major functional impairment in young adulthood (Costello & Maughan, 2015). A question of particular concern for young people and their families is what can be done to improve outcomes. A developmental perspective is essential for understanding the mechanisms that underlie *continuities and discontinuities* in psychopathology. Understanding modifiable risk and protective factors is a necessary first step for developing more effective prevention and early intervention. *Developmental transitions*, such as starting or changing school, puberty, or entering adulthood, are of particular interest, given that these are times of significant challenge as well as potential opportunities for intervention. This chapter sets out key principles that underpin theory and research of developmental psychopathology, together with examples that highlight the utility of a developmental approach. The chapter is structured as follows: (i) introduction to key concepts; (ii) longitudinal methods for studying developmental change; (iii) five brief snapshots to highlight developmental understanding for anxiety, depression, neurodevelopmental conditions, psychosis, and behavior problems; (iv) types of mechanisms that account for developmental continuity and discontinuity; and (v) early adversity, adverse outcomes, and resilience.

What is developmental psychopathology?

Developmental psychopathology is a scientific approach that focuses on the development of the person over time and aims to understand the processes underlying typical and atypical development including reasons for continuity and discontinuity in patterns of maladaptive thoughts, feelings, and behavior. There is a recognition that particular emotions and behaviors may be normative at certain stages of development (e.g., temper tantrums in toddlers, crying in infants) or in some situations (anxiety and fear in traumatic or stressful situations). However, where such symptoms are disproportionate, sustained over time, and out-of-keeping with children's developmental stage then these can impact on functioning and healthy development and thus represent psychopathology.

Rutter's Child and Adolescent Psychiatry and Psychology, Seventh Edition.
Edited by Anita Thapar, Daniel S. Pine, Samuele Cortese, Cathy Creswell, Tamsin J. Ford, James F. Leckman, and Argyris Stringaris.

Companion website: www.wiley.com/go/thapar/rutterspsych7

Developmental psychopathology considers adaptation and maladaptation to be the product of a series of multifaceted influences involving genes and biological factors, as well as both current and earlier environmental experiences. These *multifactorial influences* act together in complex ways, and many causal processes are thought to act as a series of chain reactions operating over time. Development is therefore viewed as a dynamic interplay between inherited/biological factors and environmental context with the person playing an active role in this process (Rutter & Sroufe, 2000; Figure 1.1). Longitudinal and genetically sensitive study designs have highlighted the active role of the person in development by illustrating that characteristics of the person, including their inherited tendencies, shape exposure to particular types of experience, which then impact on developmental outcomes. For example, antisocial behavior is moderately heritable (Burt, 2022) and children with antisocial behavior frequently evoke hostile reactions from other people with whom they interact, with these hostile interpersonal exchanges serving to further exacerbate those behaviors in the child (Burt, 2022). These types of "person effects" on environmental circumstances also apply to individual differences in personality; for example, a child concentrating on an academic task may elicit positive responses from adults (e.g., teachers, parents) that sustain that behavior (Caspi *et al.*, 2005). In summary, developmental psychopathology views development as the outcome of multiple factors operating over time and considers the person an active participant in this process.

Individuals add meaning to their experiences by cognitively and affectively processing them, which shapes how individuals respond to their experiences. For instance, children with a tendency toward antisocial behavior are more likely to attribute hostile intent to others, which over time can lead to the further development of antisocial behavior (Dodge, 2006). Another example relates to the development of working models of early attachment relationships that are posited to act as a template for later relationships and are "carried forward" into later development, via cognitive–affective representations (Waters & Waters, 2006).

Genetic and biological influences on development and sensitive periods

Many aspects of development are influenced by genetic and biological factors. Infancy is a period of profound cognitive and temperamental development and much of this development is driven by brain development and *maturational processes* that are under genetic control. Longitudinal studies over childhood, adolescence, and adult life show normative brain anatomical changes. These include increases in white matter volumes (myelinated axons) during childhood and adolescence as well as inverted U-shaped developmental changes of gray matter volumes (cell bodies of neurons) that are brain region specific (Lenroot & Giedd, 2006; Bethlehem *et al.*, 2022). Gray matter maturation occurs first in brain areas that support the primary functions of motor and sensory systems with association areas that integrate primary functions maturing later. These maturational changes are protracted with some changes, such as the remodeling of gray and white matter, continuing well into adult life (into the 30s). Other earlier maturational changes include the proliferation and organization of neurons and synapses during early prenatal life (Lenroot & Giedd, 2006).

Twin studies illustrate genetic influences on indices of white and gray matter volume and the stability of these measures in longitudinal studies during childhood and adolescence (Maggioni *et al.*, 2020). However, as with other traits, these

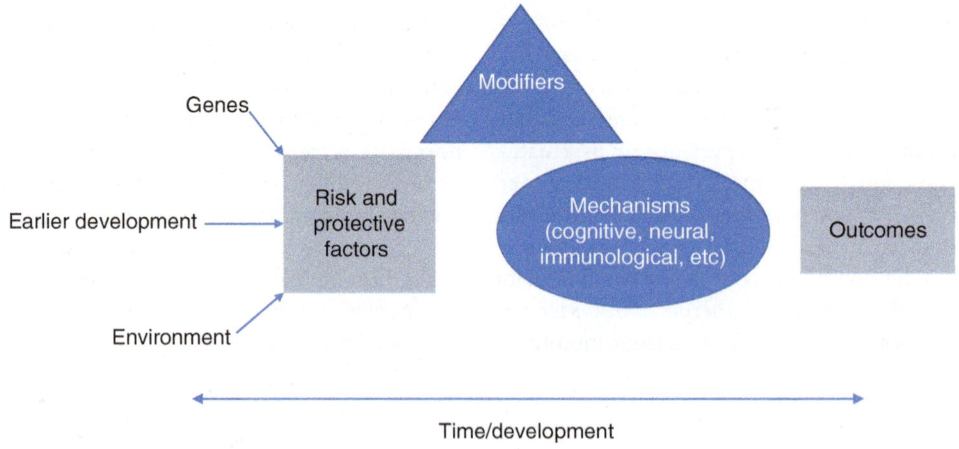

Figure 1.1 Development of the person in a multifactorial system. The time/development axis is double arrowed to represent the possibility of bidirectional influences where, for instance, one developmental outcome may influence factors, mechanisms, and/or modifiers at a later developmental point. Single arrows on risk and protective factors indicate a range of types of influence. *Source:* Adapted from Rutter & Sroufe (2000).

studies also indicate variability in changes of brain morphology over time with heritability measures changing depending on the brain region studied. This is consistent with longitudinal twin studies for a range of abilities and traits which highlight that new genetic influences can emerge at certain developmental stages—so called "genetic innovation"—and that the effect of earlier genetic influences can diminish over time; known as "genetic attenuation" (Bergen *et al.*, 2007). Sroufe *et al.* (2005) highlight three principles of development: (i) that the "organism develops as a whole;" (ii) that development is "characterized by emerging complexity;" and (iii) that differentiation and refinement can only operate on previous structures. The last principle highlights the fact that early damage can have profound effects on developmental outcomes. Examples of this are the *teratogenic effects* of thalidomide, rubella, high levels of alcohol, and Zika virus infection on the developing fetus (Thapar & Rutter, 2009; Rasmussen *et al.*, 2016). This principle of development also suggests the importance of the timing of certain exposures and that certain periods of development, often in early life, can act as *sensitive periods* of development where certain inputs are expected from the environment for normative development to occur (see the penultimate section on early adversity later in this chapter).

Important features of a life course approach

A fundamental aspect of developmental psychopathology is taking a *life course approach*. The central developmental challenges for an individual will include the primary concerns of the developing person or the most pressing capacities to be acquired, and these will vary across different developmental periods. For example, during the first year of life, establishing an effective attachment relationship with a caregiver may be a central concern whereas in early adult life this may be establishing a meaningful romantic relationship.

Several important features of the developmental psychopathology perspective emerge because of the life course approach. These include the concepts of *developmental snares*, *resilience* and/or *recovery*, and *turning points*. Developmental snares are events or experiences that "trap" people in particular circumstances which then further disadvantage individuals. As one example, Moffitt *et al.* (2011) examined self-control (the ability to control immediate urges or impulses in preference for longer-term goals) in a longitudinal cohort study. Children with lower self-control tended to do less well in terms of social and occupational outcomes in adult life compared to children higher on self-control. Although there was a main effect of childhood self-control on adult outcomes, the authors found that part of the effect of low childhood self-control on adult outcomes was due to children "making mistakes" as teenagers (e.g., unplanned pregnancy, leaving school early) which then impacted on adult outcomes such as earnings, health, and criminal convictions in adult life (Moffitt *et al.*, 2011). Children with the lowest self-control experienced more of these snares and were more likely than children with better self-control to show poor adult outcomes.

Resilience is often defined as a better-than-expected outcome following experience of adversity, and *recovery* as a period of adaptive development following a period of maladaptive development. The use of a life course perspective therefore allows resilience to be viewed as a developmental process and implies that development is not static, and that change is possible. Indeed, change is always possible in a developmental psychopathology perspective but becomes more or less likely depending on a range of factors including the characteristics of the individual, their environment, inherited and biological liabilities, and earlier experiences (Rutter & Sroufe, 2000). Concepts related to recovery and resilience are those of transition and turning points. Periods of transition can act as *turning points* (e.g., starting a new school, parenthood, marriage) by involving heightened susceptibility to either adaptive or maladaptive changes. For instance, in examining continuities between childhood and adult life, Rutter (1989) describes instances where negotiating transition points effectively can set in motion chains of events that have positive effects over extended periods of time. One classic example involved examining the adult outcomes of women who were raised in institutions as children following breakdown of parenting in the family (Rutter, 1989). A series of interrelated events were identified that were associated with good social functioning and parenting in adult life. Positive school experience, planning for work and marriage, marriage for positive reasons, and marital support were protective events associated with positive outcomes in this vulnerable group of young women who had experienced early adversity. Indeed, longitudinal research highlights the importance of planful behavior and problem-solving as well as interpersonal support in predicting positive outcomes following adversity (Rutter, 1989). More detailed examination, utilizing longitudinal and behavior genetic designs, supports the view that turning points such as marriage may have a causal effect on trajectories of psychopathology but that the nature of any protective (or indeed risk) effects is not uniform, with variation according to the characteristics of a partner (Kendler *et al.*, 2017). The normative educational transition from primary/elementary to secondary/high school can also act as a turning point. There are opportunities for some children to form new and more supportive friendships (Shell *et al.*, 2014; Ng-Knight *et al.*, 2019). Evidence that transition periods involve heightened susceptibility to change has led to suggestions that such periods are potentially useful points to introduce intervention programs (Vitaro & Tremblay, 2008).

Methods that are useful for the study of developmental psychopathology

Longitudinal studies with repeated assessments of psychopathology are critical for examining factors that shape children's development, as insights about developmental patterns and underpinning etiological processes are often misleading when based on cross-sectional data (Kraemer *et al.*, 2000). Longitudinal studies differ in the extent to which they aim to provide a picture for the whole population or for particular groups of interest, the length of follow-up, and number of assessments over the follow-up period, as well as the breadth and depth of assessments of psychopathology and associated aspects of children's development, biology, and social environment.

Population birth cohorts, in principle, provide a picture of normative development unaffected by clinical referral, diagnostic, or other selection biases. With assessments often starting at or before birth, population cohorts provide opportunities to observe how psychopathology first develops. They help identify groups of children most at risk of developing mental health difficulties and developmental periods when risk is most strongly observed. Comparisons *between* population cohorts can address questions related to population differences in mental health. This includes testing whether and why rates of psychopathology have changed over time or differ between countries, and whether outcomes for children with mental health problems have improved or worsened (Collishaw, 2015; Sellers *et al.*, 2019).

There are challenges and limitations to population cohort studies that are important to consider. Longitudinal population cohorts typically experience sample drop-out which can introduce bias due to factors related to the probability of participants staying in the study. A further challenge is that population cohorts are costly and often broad-ranging in focus, limiting detailed phenotyping and density of repeated measurement. Guarding against the exclusion of high-risk and typically disadvantaged groups is a particular concern. Children from ethnic minority backgrounds, with disabilities, who are LGBTQ+, and those educated in non-mainstream school settings are very often underrepresented in population cohorts. Where they are included, it is often not possible to draw reliable conclusions because sample sizes are small. New cohorts have begun to adapt their methods to overcome some of these difficulties; for example, by oversampling families from socioeconomically disadvantaged or ethnic minority groups and by ensuring that a diverse range of young people's voices is heard when designing study assessments. Inevitably, each population cohort represents a picture of life course development that is particular to one generation of children.

An important complement to population cohorts are longitudinal studies of patient samples or high-risk groups that allow for more focused investigation of specific groups of vulnerable children. An example of this approach is the prospective investigation of children at high familial risk where one aim is to better understand the emergence of conditions such as depression, bipolar disorder, or psychosis (Rice *et al.*, 2017). Other examples include in-depth clinical studies of children with rare conditions such as childhood-onset schizophrenia (Driver *et al.*, 2013), or children with genetic conditions such as carriers of copy number variations that confer increased susceptibility to a range of mental health problems (Chawner *et al.*, 2019).

Developmental "catch-up" studies are sometimes a more pragmatic way to investigate life course outcomes for children in high-risk groups. Examples include a study of maltreatment which used record-based data to identify a sample with documented childhood maltreatment together with a matched control group to investigate adult psychosocial outcomes (Widom *et al.*, 2007) and a very long-term follow-up (up to age 70 years) of a juvenile delinquency sample first studied in the 1940s (Laub & Sampson, 2006). Registry studies which include anonymous data from routine social, health, and educational records are another way in which historical data on certain exposures (e.g., death of a parent, perinatal complications, potential maltreatment) can be used to generate insights about a life course perspective.

Prospective studies provide contemporaneous assessments of experiences at each time point in a longitudinal study, whereas *retrospective assessment* refers to the measurement of experiences that occurred in the past. Prospective and retrospective studies present distinct challenges in study design, implementation, and interpretation. It is now clear that there is often little agreement between prospective and retrospective assessments of experiences such as childhood maltreatment, and prospective and retrospective data can lead to different conclusions, including the estimation of lifetime prevalence of disorder (Reuben *et al.*, 2016).

Prospective study designs are often essential for assessing the temporal ordering of events, and to assess developmental change in psychopathology and associated risk and prospective factors. However, retrospective data can provide an important complement, particularly in circumstances where there are ethical or practical challenges in assessing aspects of children's lives contemporaneously, or where it is likely that informants might underreport certain experiences such as child maltreatment. There is very little evidence that participants in research studies fabricate or exaggerate problematic childhood experiences. Instead, an important bias can be that adults who are functioning well often underreport adverse childhood experiences (Hardt & Rutter, 2004).

A critical consideration in observational studies of developmental psychopathology is the extent to which it is possible to make *causal inferences* (Chapter 13). It is always important to consider alternative explanations for findings, including the possibilities of reverse causation, measured or unmeasured confounding, and collider bias. *Triangulation* of findings using study designs and statistical approaches with different strengths, limitations, and underlying assumptions is strongly advised (Hammerton & Munafò, 2021).

Thinking to the future, there are important decisions for scientists and research funders in how to prioritize the development of research infrastructure and how to maximize the utility of available data for scientific and clinical discovery. There is a need to overcome common limitations of traditional research designs. For example, a recent study demonstrates how the utility of population-wide, cross-sectional school questionnaire data can be enhanced by linkage with national patient record data, enabling longitudinal analysis of clinically relevant outcomes at scale. The study showed that bullying and loneliness are common experiences and strongly predict subsequent clinical presentation for self-harm (John *et al.*, 2023).

Patterns of continuity across childhood, adolescence, and adulthood

Developmental life course studies involve tracking individuals over time and are crucial for understanding influences on continuity and discontinuity of psychopathology, as well as for describing the typical developmental sequences of different types of psychiatric disorder. Patterns of continuity can be described as *homotypic* (where the same disorder persists over different developmental periods) or *heterotypic* (where an earlier disorder is followed by a disorder of a different kind). Such patterns of continuity can reflect continuation of the same underlying illness/maladaptation process, one disorder acting as a risk factor for another disorder, or that manifestation of the same underlying illness/maladaptation looks different at different developmental stages. Sankey diagrams are a data visualization technique to show flow (e.g., of energy, material, individuals) through a series of stages, and these have been applied in psychopathology research to visualize patterns of continuity and discontinuity (Caspi *et al.*, 2020) or co-occurrence of disorders over time (Plana-Ripoll *et al.*, 2019). In Figure 1.2, we present a *Sankey diagram* based on data from the Early Prediction of Adolescent Depression study (Rice *et al.*, 2017) which is tracking the development of psychopathology in high-risk offspring of depressed parents. The figure illustrates patterns of continuity and discontinuity of disorder over time in that sample. This indicates a range of developmental pathways characterized by homotypic and heterotypic continuities, emergence of new difficulties, and recovery from earlier difficulties. Indeed, life course studies can identify influences on the 'persistence of' compared to 'recovery from' mental health disorders over time, whether etiological influences vary as a function of age of onset of a disorder, the childhood antecedents of adult-onset conditions, and the broader psychosocial and functional outcomes of psychopathology. Developmental life course studies have also highlighted the phenomena of *equifinality*, which refers to the fact that different sets of risk and protective factors can lead to the same outcome in different individuals, and *multifinality*, which refers to the fact that the same sets of risk and protective factors can lead to different outcomes in different individuals (Cicchetti & Rogosch, 1996; and see Figure 1.3).

In the next sections, we give a brief overview of studies focusing on different types of psychopathology to illustrate how a

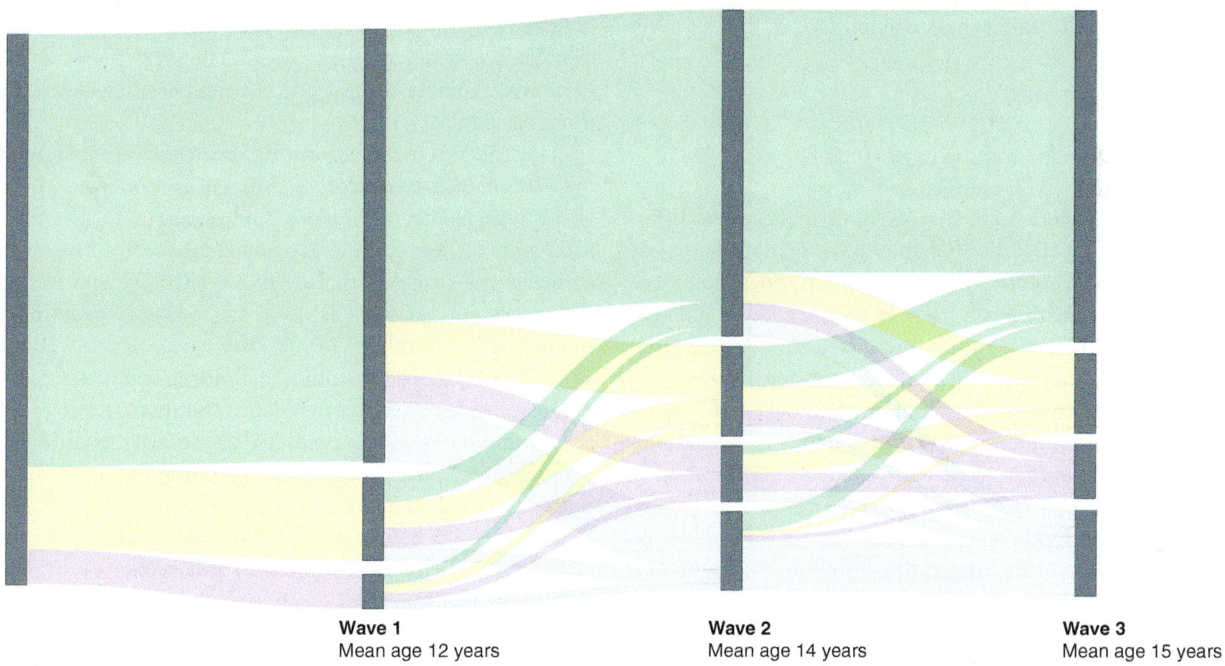

Figure 1.2 Homotypic and heterotypic continuity over time. Sankey diagram illustrating rates of anxiety (yellow), depressive (blue), behavioral (red), ADHD (purple), and no (green) disorders over a four-year follow-up period including three assessment waves in the Early Prediction of Adolescent Depression study (Rice et al., 2017). Homotypic continuity is demonstrated by the same-colored band over assessment wave (e.g., yellow to yellow shows continuity in anxiety; red to red shows continuity in behavioral disorders). Heterotypic continuity is demonstrated by changes in colors over assessment waves (e.g., red to blue shows behavioral to depression). Recovery is shown by offset of disorder (e.g., yellow to green shows recovery from earlier anxiety). Gray denotes missing data. *Source:* Diagram created by Dr Vicky Powell using information from the Early Prediction of Adolescent Depression study via a Sankey tool on this website http://sankey-diagram-generator.acquireprocure.com/.

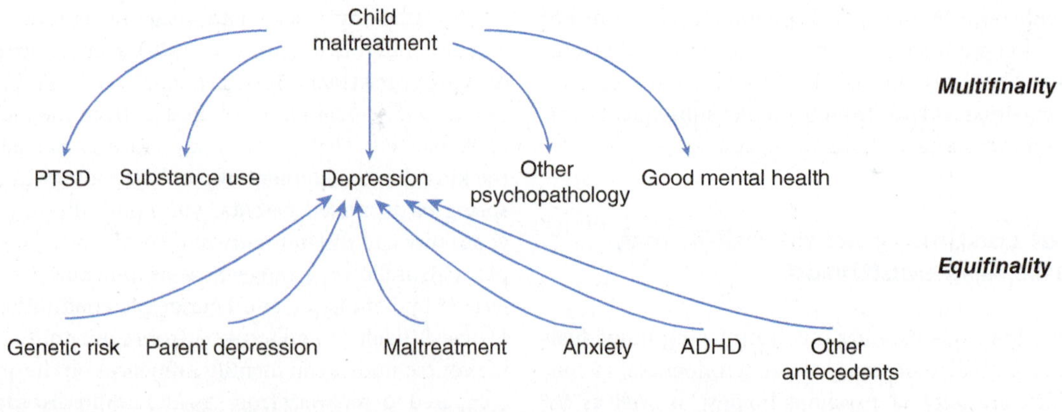

Figure 1.3 Multifinality and equifinality. Multifinality: a variety of endpoints are possible following the same beginning. Equifinality: the same endpoint can be reached through a variety of paths and from a variety of beginnings. *Source:* Adapted from Cicchetti & Rogosch (1996).

developmental approach can be helpful for understanding mental health, and to draw attention to some of the paradigmatic issues described earlier, as well as to commonalities and distinctions between different forms of psychopathology in terms of their developmental picture—age at onset, developmental course, and predictors of persistence and long-term outcomes. It is worth bearing in mind that psychopathology exists on a spectrum. While there is evidence for a dimensional approach for all of the disorders we consider, we focus primarily on disorder or clinically elevated symptoms in the examples provided.

Anxiety

There is marked heterogeneity in age of onset between different forms of anxiety disorder (Chapter 59). Separation anxiety and specific phobias typically begin in childhood, social anxiety has a median age of onset in early adolescence, while agoraphobia, panic disorder, and generalized anxiety disorder typically emerge in late adolescence or young adulthood (Beesdo-Baum & Knappe, 2012; Solmi *et al.*, 2022). It is noteworthy, that later onset anxiety disorders reflect more generalized forms of anxiety than those with a typical childhood onset which are characterized by circumscribed fears. It is important, however, not to view anxiety disorders in isolation from one another. Prospective longitudinal studies highlight that anxiety disorders in childhood or adolescence strongly predict anxiety disorders in adulthood. There is little specificity in continuities for particular anxiety disorders (with the exception of specific phobia), suggesting that continuities in anxiety reflect developmental change in the manifestation of anxiety (Gregory *et al.*, 2007).

Child and adolescent anxiety in the general population is associated with a broad range of problematic life course outcomes, notably depression, as well higher risk of substance use, behavioral problems, disrupted educational and occupational trajectories, impaired relationships, and poor physical health (Copeland *et al.*, 2014). Adolescent anxiety also contributes to long-term risk of suicide ideation and attempts, over and above other psychopathology such as depression (Pickles *et al.*, 2010). Anxiety may also be one developmental precursor of severe adult psychiatric disorders such as major depression, bipolar disorder, or schizophrenia, at least in children at already high familial risk of these conditions (Sandstrom *et al.*, 2019). However, the vast majority of children with anxiety do not go on to experience severe mental illness as adults.

There is heterogeneity in the persistence of anxiety and in broader life course outcomes. Anxiety is moderately heritable, and although current evidence is limited as to the role of genetic influences on homotypic and heterotypic continuities in anxiety, evidence does suggest that there are both age-specific genetic influences on anxiety, as well as common genetic factors predicting continuity in anxiety over time (Waszczuk *et al.*, 2016). Follow-up studies of children and adolescents with anxiety provide consistent evidence that persistence of anxiety across the life course is predicted by severity and duration of avoidance behaviors, degree of functional impairment, cognitive factors such as catastrophizing, and higher behavioral inhibition (Beesdo-Baum *et al.*, 2012; Hovenkamp-Hermelink *et al.*, 2021). Behavioral inhibition and avoidance likely shape children's environments, influencing parenting style and contributing to social risk exposures such as peer exclusion and victimization (Degnan *et al.*, 2010).

Finally, considerable progress has been made in understanding cognitive and neurobiological features of anxiety (Chapters 12 and 59; LeDoux & Pine, 2016). Developmental research holds the promise of elucidating their role as vulnerabilities, manifestations, or consequences of anxiety.

Depression

Several lines of evidence including from epidemiological, twin, and treatment studies suggest developmental differences in the etiology of depressive symptoms and depressive disorder between childhood and adolescence (Chapter 63). Indeed, twin studies suggest that depressive symptoms are moderately heritable in adolescence but that the influence of genetic factors is negligible in childhood. Thus, evidence for genetic innovation where "new" genetic influences become active during adolescence has been identified in longitudinal twin studies (Kendler *et al.*, 2008; Lau & Eley, 2010). It has been suggested that genetic innovation over the transition from childhood to adolescence may be partly due to genetic influence on hormonal changes associated with puberty, structural brain changes, and increased gene–environment correlation associated with increasing independence in selecting environments as children grow up. The correlation between changes in hormones associated with puberty leading to changes in the social environment has been highlighted as involved in the increase in depressive symptomatology seen in females around adolescence (Ge *et al.*, 1996). Thus, girls who began puberty earlier experienced greater psychological distress than on-time or later maturing peers and were more vulnerable to deviant peer pressure and paternal hostility. Several studies also highlight that females may experience increases in psychosocial stressors during adolescence, particularly interpersonal stressors, and may also be particularly sensitive to negative affect following these types of stressors (Oldehinkel & Bouma, 2011; Ordaz & Luna, 2012). Long-term studies highlight that the risk effects of early puberty for females are mostly time-limited and tend to dissipate by early adult life (Copeland *et al.*, 2010). It is also noteworthy that exposure to social stressors is correlated with genetic liability for depression (Rice *et al.*, 2003). This means that those with higher genetic liability are also more likely to be exposed to stressors.

Depression shows strong associations with anxiety (Copeland *et al.*, 2009). The finding that anxiety typically precedes depression in longitudinal studies is also consistent with the possibility that some forms of anxiety may be early developmental manifestations of depression (Rutter *et al.*, 2006). Consistent with the suggestion of common etiological influences for anxiety and depression, evidence from genetically sensitive family designs including twin studies shows considerable genetic overlap between depression and anxiety, particularly with generalized anxiety disorder (Silberg *et al.*, 2001; Kendler *et al.*, 2022). Thus, it is possible that these common genetic influences are expressed phenotypically in different ways at different stages of development.

An important feature of depression is whether it persists over time. Studies of adults (Eaton *et al.*, 2008) and adolescents (Patton *et al.*, 2014) in community studies suggest that one-off episodes of depressive disorder that do not recur are relatively common. Nevertheless, clinical follow-up studies of individuals treated for depressive disorder during childhood and adolescence report high recurrence rates of 70% within five years (Harrington *et al.*, 1997). This highlights depression as a condition that can desist or persist although it is worth noting that subthreshold symptomatology can be present between full-blown episodes (Judd *et al.*, 1998). When depression in young people does persist, it is associated with particularly poor mental health, educational, and functional outcomes (Weavers *et al.*, 2021). Systematic reviews indicate that approximately 5–12% of young people in the general population show persistently elevated depressive symptom trajectories (Musliner *et al.*, 2016; Schubert *et al.*, 2017). Persistent trajectories have been associated with an earlier age of onset, inherited vulnerabilities, and exposure to a range of stressors both chronic and acute, as well as female sex, minority status, and lower socioeconomic status (Musliner *et al.*, 2016; Schubert *et al.*, 2017; Rice *et al.*, 2019; Weavers *et al.*, 2021).

Neurodevelopmental disorders (NDDs)

The developmental course of NDDs (Chapters 51–57) can be distinguished from other forms of psychopathology in that most have an early onset of symptoms and demonstrate a steady stable course of symptoms. This points to the predominant importance of early etiological influences, whether genetic or environmental in nature (Nigg *et al.*, 2020).

The course of most NDDs is marked by apparent improvement in core symptoms, and rates of NDDs are higher in childhood than in adulthood. Estimates of diagnostic persistence vary considerably according to methods of assessment and whether clinical or population cohorts are considered (Thapar *et al.*, 2017). Specific symptoms also vary in the extent to which they show developmental change; for example, for children with attention deficit hyperactivity disorder (ADHD) symptoms of hyperactivity show greater attenuation with age than symptoms of inattention (Pingault *et al.*, 2015). Improvement in neurodevelopmental symptoms might reflect neurocognitive maturation, the development of adaptive mechanisms (or adaptation of environmental contexts to children's needs), and for some, the beneficial effects of treatment. Nevertheless, continuities in neurodevelopmental symptoms are observed from childhood into adulthood (Faraone *et al.*, 2006; Maughan *et al.*, 2009), and as discussed later in the chapter, impacts on psychosocial functioning and health persist across the life course. It is clear, that for most individuals with an NDD, this is not a childhood-limited condition that will naturally resolve with time.

Recent developmental research also demonstrates the possibility of late-emerging neurodevelopmental problems. Epidemiological studies with repeated assessments across development have shown that for some individuals symptoms of ADHD or autism spectrum disorder (ASD) are first reported in adolescence or in adulthood (Moffitt *et al.*, 2015; Caye *et al.*, 2016). It remains unclear how far the emergence of "late-onset" neurodevelopmental conditions reflects measurement artifacts such as variability in informant reports, the influence of adolescent- or adult-onset conditions such as depression, or "masking" of childhood symptoms due to earlier protective influences, nor is it clear whether late-onset neurodevelopmental problems are typical or atypical in terms of etiology (Livingston *et al.*, 2019; Riglin *et al.*, 2022).

Individuals with neurodevelopmental conditions are at increased risk of experiencing peer victimization, loneliness, and educational underachievement. They are also at substantially heightened risk of other mental health problems including anxiety, depression, substance-use disorders, conduct problems, and self-harm (Caye *et al.*, 2016), and risk of death by young adulthood (Dalsgaard *et al.*, 2015). Longer-term impacts on health are less well-established, and different mechanisms may account for morbidity associated with neurodevelopmental conditions in early and later life (e.g., accidents vs. cardiovascular health risks).

Psychosis

A developmental approach has been a crucial part of theories about the genesis of schizophrenia (Howes & Murray, 2014; see also Chapter 56). Schizophrenia is a highly heritable condition and hundreds of genetic variants have been identified as showing robust associations with schizophrenia (Trubetskoy *et al.*, 2022). Nonetheless, it has long been hypothesized that schizophrenia involves an important neurodevelopmental component (Weinberger, 1987). This is based on the following observations: that early prenatal and perinatal complications are associated with an increased risk for schizophrenia, that individuals who develop schizophrenia have elevated rates of neurological, cognitive, and social problems as children, and that structural brain differences can be observed when schizophrenia onsets in the absence of any evidence of neurodegenerative abnormalities in post-mortem studies (Howes & Murray, 2014). A prominent view of the development of schizophrenia is that multiple "hits" are required to generate the condition and that these involve genetic and environmental insults experienced throughout development (Davis *et al.*, 2016; Owen *et al.*, 2016). The role of a range of early adverse experiences has been highlighted including prenatal infection, perinatal complications, childhood adversity, and stress associated with migration and urban living (Howes & Murray, 2014). However, there is also strong evidence for disrupted brain development that is apparent early in life, and recent evidence highlights reduced neuronal connectivity in frontal cortex and hippocampal brain areas which begins *in utero* and continues through development (Hall & Bray, 2022). It is understood that such early neuronal developmental aberrations will involve genetic influences (Howes & Murray, 2014). It has been suggested that later maturational events in brain development such as synaptic pruning or environmental events or insults such as trauma exposure and cannabis use can elicit psychopathology because of the effects they have on an already vulnerable neuronal/cognitive system. Thus, exposures that are experienced during adolescence or young adulthood may lead to the onset of psychotic symptomatology because the exposure means that preexisting neuronal/cognitive vulnerabilities manifest themselves. Studies of childhood trauma have indicated that this may include potentially causal associations on psychosis (Heins *et al.*, 2011) as well as gene–environment correlation whereby genetic loading for schizophrenia is associated with an increased likelihood of experiencing particular traumatic events (Sallis *et al.*, 2021).

Studies of subclinical psychotic symptoms illustrated that these are relatively common during adolescence (Jones *et al.*, 2016). For many individuals these symptoms are transient and remit, but in others they are persistent and associated with an increased risk for psychosis and other psychiatric disorders (Catalan *et al.*, 2021). Psychotic symptoms in adolescents have shown strong association with co-occurring anxiety and depression (Jones *et al.*, 2016; Catalan *et al.*, 2021) and an inconsistent association with genetic risk for schizophrenia (Jones *et al.*, 2016).

Behavioral problems

Developmental models of antisocial behavior have played a major role in guiding policy and practice, including emphasis on early parenting interventions (Leijten *et al.*, 2019). Moffitt's (1993) model of antisocial behavior distinguishes two common developmental subtypes: early-onset life course persistent and adolescent-limited antisocial behavior. Studies of children's normative development in contrast illustrate that physical aggression is common among very young children and typically reduces by school entry (Tremblay, 2010). Longitudinal and intergenerational studies suggest multiple factors act as predictors of the onset and persistence of behavioral problems, including children's callous emotional traits, harsh parenting, parental antisocial behavior, maltreatment, poverty, and deviant peer relationships (Basto-Pereira & Farrington, 2022). Research highlights the importance of person–environment interplay. For example, adoption studies point to genetically influenced traits and behaviors evoking more hostile parenting (Harold *et al.*, 2017). In adolescence and young adulthood, assortative selection into more problematic peer and romantic relationships, as well as problematic substance use, act as potential "developmental snares" that reinforce antisocial behavior (Quinton *et al.*, 1993; Hussong *et al.*, 2004). Conversely, the transition to adulthood also offers opportunities for desistance of antisocial behavior, for example, due to changes in peer affiliations, establishing a supportive romantic relationship, or starting a new job (Laub & Sampson, 2006).

Behavioral problems are associated with a wide variety of adverse outcomes, including elevated risks of mental health problems, substance misuse, educational and occupational difficulties, and poor health (Colman *et al.*, 2009), but mechanisms of risk remain to be fully clarified. One complication is that traditional diagnostic specifications of behavioral disorders include a broad range of symptoms with differing developmental features and implications. Conduct disorder symptoms show stronger homotypic continuity than do symptoms of oppositional defiant disorder (ODD) which more strongly predict later emotional disorders (Rowe *et al.*, 2010). Research is increasingly considering individual "symptoms," for example, irritability is now viewed as an important transdiagnostic marker of mood dysregulation with links not just to behavioral disorders, but also neurodevelopmental conditions, anxiety, depression, and suicide/self-harm (Brotman *et al.*, 2017).

Different types of developmental association

As highlighted by these brief snapshots, a developmental approach has been instrumental in improving our understanding of psychopathology, highlighting early life, childhood, and adolescence as important developmental periods, and drawing attention to developmental connections that very often cross traditional diagnostic boundaries (Chapter 9). Developmental studies reveal different types of longitudinal associations between variables. One useful distinction is between associations that are "distal," i.e., have remote or indirect causal influence on a disorder and those that are "proximal" which have a more direct impact on causal chains of events (Rutter, 2009). *Distal associations* are often thought to influence behavior mainly via more proximal factors. For example, there is a strong association between low socioeconomic status and psychopathology in children, but these effects appear to be driven in part by more proximal features of children's family and social contexts such as parenting (Bifulco *et al.*, 2002). Understanding *proximal processes* is clearly important because they can explain how and why psychopathology arises. There has been much interest in identifying proximal explanatory mechanisms for psychopathology that transcend traditional diagnostic boundaries. Research to identify potentially *transdiagnostic mechanisms* influencing psychopathology has tended to focus on patterns of neural circuitry and cognitive–affective processing (Insel *et al.*, 2010). For instance, Harvey *et al.* (2004) asked which cognitive and behavioral processes (e.g., selective attention, overgeneral memory, repetitive negative thinking) were shared across a range of disorders. A number of models including the Research Domain Criteria (RDoC; Insel *et al.*, 2010) and the Hierarchical Taxonomy of Psychopathology (HiTOP; Kotov *et al.*, 2017) specify transdiagnostic processes (e.g., negative valence systems, positive valence systems, cognitive systems) and transdiagnostic structures (e.g., internalizing, externalizing, thought disorder, detachment) to psychopathology. While there are strengths and weaknesses of both a disorder-oriented and a transdiagnostic approach the hope is that identifying transdiagnostic risk and protective mechanisms can improve understanding about processes, contribute to knowledge about the taxonomy of psychopathology, and help develop treatments that are effective in targeting more than one primary problem (Dalgleish *et al.*, 2020).

Early life experience and long-term implications for mental health

Early life experiences, both negative and positive, are associated with potentially long-lasting consequences for development of psychopathology. Certain groups are at particularly elevated risk of developing mental health difficulties. These include children: with a parent with mental illness; exposed to parental conflict; growing up in poverty; who have experienced trauma, maltreatment, or peer victimization; and who experience discrimination due to race, religion, sexuality, or gender identity, as well as children with special educational needs, or chronic physical health conditions. Adverse childhood experiences are common, and both retrospective and prospective reports of adversity demonstrate strong associations with adult mental health (Newbury *et al.*, 2018). It is also clear that adverse childhood experiences often do not occur in isolation, that the cumulative burden of adversities is an important predictor of long-term outcomes, and that both chronic stress and severe acute events can have long-lasting consequences for children's development (Lacey *et al.*, 2020). Several important questions arise in the interpretation of long-term associations between early adversity and psychopathology.

First, it is important to understand whether identified childhood risk factors exert causal effects on children's outcomes (see Chapter 13). Alternative explanations such as confounding, reverse causation, and possibilities of collider bias need to be considered. A variety of research designs that approximate *"natural experiments"* can help tease apart alternative explanations (Thapar & Rutter, 2019). Examples of such designs include comparisons of children born through *in vitro* fertilization who are related or unrelated to their mothers to test the role of *in utero* exposures such as maternal smoking (Rice *et al.*, 2009), *regression discontinuity* designs to examine the role of factors that are quasi-randomly assigned to children in the population such as relative age in the school year (Broughton *et al.*, 2023), and the impact of *universal interventions* such as poverty reduction (Costello *et al.*, 2003).

Second, it is important to understand the developmental mechanisms by which particular early-life risk factors impact on children's mental health. For example, observational studies suggest an increased risk of emotional and behavioral difficulties among children who have experienced parental separation. While parental separation is often stressful for children, of particular relevance to children's psychosocial outcomes are the proximal features of children's family relationships that impact children prior to, during, and subsequent to the break-up of a parental relationship (Harold & Sellers, 2018). There are also important unresolved questions about the psychological and biological processes through which early adversity impacts children's development, including impacts on the set-points and functioning of neurophysiological reactivity, as well as consequences for children's development of emotion regulation, self-concept, and social information processing (Cicchetti, 2016).

Third, early-life adversities do not exert deterministic effects on psychopathology. Children exposed to even the most severe stressors show variability in outcomes, with resilience and recovery not uncommon (Rutter, 2006). Reducing risk exposure is important but not always possible. An additional priority therefore is identifying modifiable protective factors that can buffer risk and promote recovery. Multifactorial explanations for resilience are required, and research demonstrates that affective, cognitive, behavioral, social, and contextual factors act together to predict resilience in the context of adversity (Figure 1.4). An important conclusion is that specific protective factors on their own are rarely sufficient to promote resilience and recovery in the context of severe adversity. Furthermore, a developmental perspective holds that patterns of resilience will change over time, influenced by previous experiences of successfully (or unsuccessfully) negotiating similar challenges, as well as by maturation and the specific challenges facing an individual at different developmental stages. Furthermore, salient protective factors will vary between individuals and for differing developmental outcomes.

A developmental perspective is also useful for considering the importance of *timing of exposure* to stress. There are sensitive periods in development during which experience can have larger impacts on development of particular traits than during other periods. The English and Romanian Adoptees (ERA) study, for example, examined the development of children who experienced severe early institutional deprivation and were then adopted into socioeconomically advantaged families (Sonuga-Barke *et al.*, 2017). The study highlighted profound immediate impacts of early deprivation on social and cognitive development, as well as longer-term impacts on mental health. At the same time, many children showed evidence of recovery and catch up, especially those who were adopted early, suggesting that both the timing and the duration of exposure to early stress can be important.

Conclusion and priorities for the future

Developmental studies have improved our understanding of how common mental health conditions develop and progress, possible reasons for homotypic and heterotypic continuities over the life course, and of factors that promote resilience and recovery. A priority for the future is to ensure that this rich understanding of life course development can inform more effective approaches to both the prevention of mental health problems and the provision of tailored support for children with mental health and neurodevelopmental conditions as they grow up. Other priorities for the future include incorporating multiple approaches and measurements of important potential drivers of psychopathology into longitudinal studies in efficient and

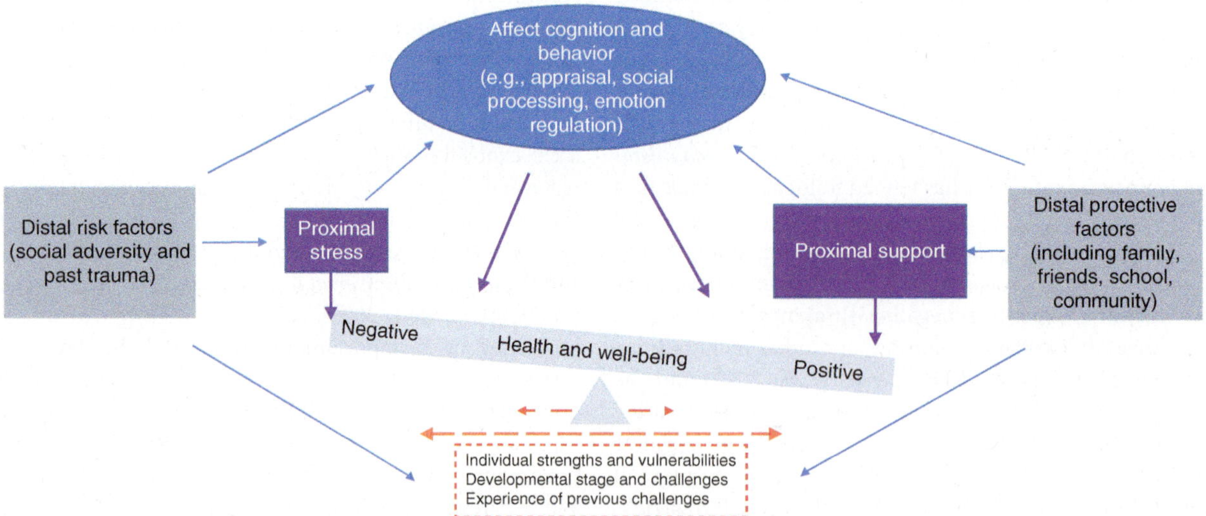

Figure 1.4 Resilience—dynamic interplay of person and context. Vulnerability and resilience in the context of stress varies according to children's underlying strengths and vulnerabilities, their developmental stage, and past (un)successful negotiation of stressful situations. In the context of greater vulnerability, greater levels of support are needed to promote resilience. The balance of proximal stressors and supports is influenced by contexts of adversity and available support systems, in interplay with children's own appraisal, emotional responses, and behaviors. *Source:* Adapted from National Scientific Council on the Developing Child (2015).

creative ways. Understanding routes to adaptive and maladaptive outcomes in vulnerable populations will also be important for the development of policies to support mental health. This includes developing an understanding of how psychopathology is shaped by society via a more in-depth understanding of population differences, cohort effects, and how socioeconomic and cultural influences impact psychopathology. Understanding long-term outcomes of psychopathology across multiple domains of functioning will be important for interventions that impact on the outcomes that matter most to those affected by psychopathology.

References

Basto-Pereira, M. & Farrington, D.P. (2022) Developmental predictors of offending and persistence in crime: a systematic review of meta-analyses. *Aggression and Violent Behavior* **65**, 101761.

Beesdo-Baum, K. & Knappe, S. (2012) Developmental epidemiology of anxiety disorders. *Child and Adolescent Psychiatric Clinics of North America* **21**(3), 457–478. doi:10.1016/j.chc.2012.05.001.

Beesdo-Baum, K. *et al.* (2012) The natural course of social anxiety disorder among adolescents and young adults. *Acta Psychiatrica Scandinavica* **126**(6), 411–425.

Bergen, S.E. *et al.* (2007) Age-related changes in heritability of behavioral phenotypes over adolescence and young adulthood: a meta-analysis. *Twin Research and Human Genetics: The Official Journal of the International Society for Twin Studies* **10**(3), 423–433. doi:10.1375/twin.10.3.423.

Bethlehem, R.A.I. *et al.* (2022) Brain charts for the human lifespan. *Nature* **604**(7906), 525–533. doi:10.1038/s41586-022-04554-y.

Bifulco, A. *et al.* (2002) Childhood adversity, parental vulnerability and disorder: examining inter-generational transmission of risk. *Journal of Child Psychology and Psychiatry* **43**(8), 1075–1086. doi:10.1111/1469-7610.00234.

Brotman, M.A. *et al.* (2017) Irritability in youths: a translational model. *The American Journal of Psychiatry* **174**(6), 520–532. doi:10.1176/appi.ajp.2016.16070839.

Broughton, T. *et al.* (2023) Relative age in the school year and risk of mental health problems in childhood, adolescence and young adulthood. *Journal of Child Psychology and Psychiatry* **64**(1), 185–196. doi:10.1111/jcpp.13684.

Burt, S.A. (2022) The genetic, environmental, and cultural forces influencing youth antisocial behavior are tightly intertwined. *Annual Review of Clinical Psychology* **18**, 155–178.

Caspi, A. *et al.* (2005) Personality development: stability and change. *Annual Review of Psychology* **56**, 453–484.

Caspi, A. *et al.* (2020) Longitudinal assessment of mental health disorders and comorbidities across 4 decades among participants in the Dunedin birth cohort study. *JAMA Network Open* **3**(4), e203221. doi:10.1001/jamanetworkopen.2020.3221.

Catalan, A. *et al.* (2021) Annual research review: prevention of psychosis in adolescents—systematic review and meta-analysis of advances in detection, prognosis and intervention. *Journal of Child Psychology and Psychiatry* **62**(5), 657–673. doi:10.1111/jcpp.13322.

Caye, A. *et al.* (2016) Predictors of persistence of ADHD into adulthood: a systematic review of the literature and meta-analysis. *European Child & Adolescent Psychiatry* **25**(11), 1151–1159. doi:10.1007/s00787-016-0831-8.

Chawner, S.J. *et al.* (2019) Genotype–phenotype associations in children with copy number variants associated with high neuropsychiatric risk in the UK (IMAGINE-ID): a case-control cohort study. *The Lancet Psychiatry* **6**(6), 493–505. doi:10.1016/S2215-0366(19)30123-3.

Cicchetti, D. (2016) Socioemotional, personality, and biological development: illustrations from a multilevel developmental psychopathology perspective on child maltreatment. *Annual Review of Psychology* **67**, 187–211. doi:10.1146/annurev-psych-122414-033259.

Cicchetti, D. & Rogosch, F.A. (1996) Equifinality and multifinality in developmental psychopathology. *Development and Psychopathology* **8**(4), 597–600.

Collishaw, S. (2015) Annual research review: secular trends in child and adolescent mental health. *Journal of Child Psychology and Psychiatry* **56**(3), 370–393.

Colman, I. *et al.* (2009) Outcomes of conduct problems in adolescence: 40 year follow-up of national cohort. *BMJ (Clinical Research Edition)* **338**, a2981. doi:10.1136/bmj.a2981.

Copeland, W. *et al.* (2010) Outcomes of early pubertal timing in young women: a prospective population-based study. *The American Journal of Psychiatry* **167**(10), 1218–1225. doi:10.1176/appi.ajp.2010.09081190.

Copeland, W.E. *et al.* (2009) Childhood and adolescent psychiatric disorders as predictors of young adult disorders. *Archives of General Psychiatry* **66**(7), 764–772. doi:10.1001/archgenpsychiatry.2009.85.

Copeland, W.E. *et al.* (2014) Longitudinal patterns of anxiety from childhood to adulthood: the Great Smoky Mountains study. *Journal of the American Academy of Child and Adolescent Psychiatry* **53**(1), 21–33. doi:10.1016/j.jaac.2013.09.017.

Costello, E.J. & Maughan, B. (2015) Annual research review: optimal outcomes of child and adolescent mental illness. *Journal of Child Psychology and Psychiatry* **56**(3), 324–341. doi:10.1111/jcpp.12371.

Costello, E.J. *et al.* (2003) Relationships between poverty and psychopathology: a natural experiment. *JAMA* **290**(15), 2023–2029. doi:10.1001/jama.290.15.2023.

Dalgleish, T. *et al.* (2020) Transdiagnostic approaches to mental health problems: current status and future directions. *Journal of Consulting and Clinical Psychology* **88**(3), 179–195. doi:10.1037/ccp0000482.

Dalsgaard, S. *et al.* (2015) Mortality in children, adolescents, and adults with attention deficit hyperactivity disorder: a nationwide cohort study. *The Lancet* **385**(9983), 2190–2196.

Davis, J. *et al.* (2016) A review of vulnerability and risks for schizophrenia: beyond the two hit hypothesis. *Neuroscience and Biobehavioral Reviews* **65**, 185–194. doi:10.1016/j.neubiorev.2016.03.017.

de Girolamo, G. *et al.* (2012) Age of onset of mental disorders and use of mental health services: needs, opportunities and obstacles. *Epidemiology and Psychiatric Sciences* **21**(1), 47–57. doi:10.1017/s2045796011000746.

Degnan, K.A. *et al.* (2010) Temperament and the environment in the etiology of childhood anxiety. *Journal of Child Psychology and Psychiatry* **51**(4), 497–517. doi:10.1111/j.1469-7610.2010.02228.x.

Dodge, K.A. (2006) Translational science in action: hostile attributional style and the development of aggressive behavior problems. *Development and Psychopathology* **18**(3), 791–814. doi:10.1017/s0954579406060391.

Driver, D.I. *et al.* (2013) Childhood onset schizophrenia and early onset schizophrenia spectrum disorders. *Child and Adolescent Psychiatric Clinics* **22**(4), 539–555.

Eaton, W.W. *et al.* (2008) Population-based study of first onset and chronicity in major depressive disorder. *Archives of General Psychiatry* **65**(5), 513–520.

Faraone, S.V. *et al.* (2006) The age-dependent decline of attention deficit hyperactivity disorder: a meta-analysis of follow-up studies. *Psychological Medicine* **36**(2), 159–165. doi:10.1017/S003329170500471X.

Ge, X. *et al.* (1996) Coming of age too early: pubertal influences on girls' vulnerability to psychological distress. *Child Development* **67**(6), 3386–3400. doi:10.1111/j.1467-8624.1996.tb01919.x.

Gregory, A.M. *et al.* (2007) Juvenile mental health histories of adults with anxiety disorders. *American Journal of Psychiatry* **164**(2), 301–308. doi:10.1176/ajp.2007.164.2.301.

Hall, J. & Bray, N.J. (2022) Schizophrenia genomics: convergence on synaptic development, adult synaptic plasticity, or both? *Biological Psychiatry* **91**(8), 709–717. doi:10.1016/j.biopsych.2021.10.018.

Hammerton, G. & Munafò, M.R. (2021) Causal inference with observational data: the need for triangulation of evidence. *Psychological Medicine* **51**(4), 563–578. doi:10.1017/S0033291720005127.

Hardt, J. & Rutter, M. (2004) Validity of adult retrospective reports of adverse childhood experiences: review of the evidence. *Journal of Child Psychology and Psychiatry* **45**(2), 260–273. doi:10.1111/j.1469-7610.2004.00218.x.

Harold, G.T. & Sellers, R. (2018) Annual research review: interparental conflict and youth psychopathology: an evidence review and practice focused update. *Journal of Child Psychology and Psychiatry* **59**(4), 374–402. doi:10.1111/jcpp.12893.

Harold, G.T. *et al.* (2017) How can genetically informed research help inform the next generation of interparental and parenting interventions? *Child Development* **88**(2), 446–458. doi:10.1111/cdev.12742.

Harrington, R. *et al.* (1997) Psychiatric disorders in the relatives of depressed probands. I. Comparison of prepubertal, adolescent and early adult onset cases. *Journal of Affective Disorders* **42**(1), 9–22. doi:10.1016/s0165-0327(96)00091-2.

Harvey, A. *et al.* (2004) *Cognitive Behavioral Processes Across Psychological Disorders: A Transdiagnostic Approach to Research and Treatment.* Oxford University Press, Oxford.

Heins, M. *et al.* (2011) Childhood trauma and psychosis: a case-control and case-sibling comparison across different levels of genetic liability, psychopathology, and type of trauma. *The American Journal of Psychiatry* **168**(12), 1286–1294. doi:10.1176/appi.ajp.2011.10101531.

Hovenkamp-Hermelink, J.H.M. *et al.* (2021) Predictors of persistence of anxiety disorders across the lifespan: a systematic review. *The Lancet Psychiatry* **8**(5), 428–443. doi:10.1016/S2215-0366(20)30433-8.

Howes, O.D. & Murray, R.M. (2014) Schizophrenia: an integrated sociodevelopmental-cognitive model. *The Lancet.* doi:10.1016/S0140-6736(13)62036-X.

Hussong, A.M. *et al.* (2004) Substance abuse hinders desistance in young adults' antisocial behavior. *Development and Psychopathology* **16**(4), 1029–1046. doi:10.1017/s095457940404012x.

Insel, T. *et al.* (2010) Research domain criteria (RDoC): toward a new classification framework for research on mental disorders. *The American Journal of Psychiatry* **167**(7), 748–751. doi:10.1176/appi.ajp.2010.09091379.

John, A. *et al.* (2023) Self-harm, in-person bullying and cyberbullying in secondary school-aged children: a data linkage study in Wales. *Journal of Adolescence* **95**(1), 97–114.

Jones, H.J. *et al.* (2016) Phenotypic manifestation of genetic risk for schizophrenia during adolescence in the general population. *JAMA Psychiatry* **73**(3), 221–228. doi:10.1001/jamapsychiatry.2015.3058.

Judd, L.L. *et al.* (1998) A prospective 12-year study of subsyndromal and syndromal depressive symptoms in unipolar major depressive disorders. *Archives of General Psychiatry* **55**(8), 694–700. doi:10.1001/archpsyc.55.8.694.

Kendler, K.S. *et al.* (2008) A developmental twin study of symptoms of anxiety and depression: evidence for genetic innovation and attenuation. *Psychological Medicine* **38**, 1567–1575.

Kendler, K.S. *et al.* (2017) The role of marriage in criminal recidivism: a longitudinal and co-relative analysis. *Epidemiology and Psychiatric Sciences* **26**(6), 655–663.

Kendler, K.S. *et al.* (2022) An extended Swedish adoption study of anxiety disorder and its cross-generational familial relationship with major depression. *The American Journal of Psychiatry* **179**(9), 640–649. doi:10.1176/appi.ajp.21111110.

Kim-Cohen, J. *et al.* (2003) Prior juvenile diagnoses in adults with mental disorder: developmental follow-back of a prospective-longitudinal cohort. *Archives of General Psychiatry* **60**(7), 709–717. doi:10.1001/archpsyc.60.7.709.

Kotov, R. *et al.* (2017) The hierarchical taxonomy of psychopathology (HiTOP): a dimensional alternative to traditional nosologies. *Journal of Abnormal Psychology* **126**(4), 454–477. doi:10.1037/abn0000258.

Kraemer, H.C. *et al.* (2000) How can we learn about developmental processes from cross-sectional studies, or can we? *American Journal of Psychiatry* **157**(2), 163–171. doi:10.1176/appi.ajp.157.2.163.

Lacey, R.E. *et al.* (2020) Adverse childhood experiences and adult inflammation: single adversity, cumulative risk and latent class approaches. *Brain, Behavior, and Immunity* **87**, 820–830.

Lau, J.Y.F. & Eley, T.C. (2010) The genetics of mood disorders. *Annual Review of Clinical Psychology* **6**, 313–337.

Laub, J.H. & Sampson, R.J. (2006) *Shared Beginnings, Divergent Lives: Delinquent Boys to Age 70.* Harvard University Press, Cambridge, MA.

LeDoux, J.E. & Pine, D.S. (2016) Using neuroscience to help understand fear and anxiety: a two-system framework. *The American Journal of Psychiatry* **173**(11), 1083–1093. doi:10.1176/appi.ajp.2016.16030353.

Leijten, P. *et al.* (2019) Meta-analyses: key parenting program components for disruptive child behavior. *Journal of the American Academy of Child and Adolescent Psychiatry* **58**(2), 180–190. doi:10.1016/j.jaac.2018.07.900.

Lenroot, R.K. & Giedd, J.N. (2006) Brain development in children and adolescents: insights from anatomical magnetic resonance imaging. *Neuroscience & Biobehavioural Reviews* **30**, 718–729.

Livingston, L.A. *et al.* (2019) Compensatory strategies below the behavioural surface in autism: a qualitative study. *The Lancet Psychiatry* **6**(9), 766–777. doi:10.1016/S2215-0366(19)30224-X.

Maggioni, E. *et al.* (2020) Twin MRI studies on genetic and environmental determinants of brain morphology and function in the early lifespan. *Neuroscience & Biobehavioural Reviews* **109**, 139–149.

Maughan, B. *et al.* (2009) Persistence of literacy problems: spelling in adolescence and at mid-life. *Journal of Child Psychology and Psychiatry, and Allied Disciplines* **50**(8), 893–901. doi:10.1111/j.1469-7610.2009.02079.x.

Moffitt, T.E. (1993) Adolescence-limited and life course-persistent antisocial behavior: a developmental taxonomy. *Psychological Review* **100**(4), 674.

Moffitt, T.E. *et al.* (2011) A gradient of childhood self-control predicts health, wealth, and public safety. *Proceedings of the National Academy of Sciences* **108**, 2693–2698.

Moffitt, T.E. *et al.* (2015) Is adult ADHD a childhood-onset neurodevelopmental disorder? Evidence from a four-decade longitudinal cohort study. *The American Journal of Psychiatry* **172**(10), 967–977. doi:10.1176/appi.ajp.2015.14101266.

Musliner, K.L. *et al.* (2016) Heterogeneity in long-term trajectories of depressive symptoms: patterns, predictors and outcomes. *Journal of Affective Disorders* **192**, 199–211. doi:10.1016/j.jad.2015.12.030.

National Scientific Council on the Developing Child (2015) *Supportive Relationships and Active Skill-Building Strengthen the Foundations of Resilience: Working Paper 13*. Available: https://developingchild.harvard.edu/resources/supportive-relationships-and-active-skill-building-strengthen-the-foundations-of-resilience/ [5 September 2024].

Newbury, J.B. *et al.* (2018) Measuring childhood maltreatment to predict early-adult psychopathology: comparison of prospective informant-reports and retrospective self-reports. *Journal of Psychiatric Research* **96**, 57–64. doi:10.1016/j.jpsychires.2017.09.020.

Ng-Knight, T. *et al.* (2019) 'Best friends forever'? Friendship stability across school transition and associations with mental health and educational attainment. *The British Journal of Educational Psychology* **89**(4), 585–599. doi:10.1111/bjep.12246.

Nigg, J.T. *et al.* (2020) Development of ADHD: etiology, heterogeneity, and early life course. *Annual Review of Developmental Psychology* **2**(1), 559–583. doi:10.1146/annurev-devpsych-060320-093413.

Oldehinkel, A.J. & Bouma, E.M. (2011) Sensitivity to the depressogenic effect of stress and HPA-axis reactivity in adolescence: a review of gender differences. *Neuroscience and Biobehavioral Reviews* **35**(8), 1757–1770. doi:10.1016/j.neubiorev.2010.10.013.

Ordaz, S. & Luna, B. (2012) Sex differences in physiological reactivity to acute psychosocial stress in adolescence. *Psychoneuroendocrinology* **37**(8), 1135–1157. doi:10.1016/j.psyneuen.2012.01.002.

Owen, M.J. *et al.* (2016) Schizophrenia. *The Lancet* **388**(10039), 86–97. doi:10.1016/S0140-6736(15)01121-6.

Patton, G.C. *et al.* (2014) The prognosis of common mental disorders in adolescents: a 14-year prospective cohort study. *The Lancet* **383**(9926), 1404–1411.

Pickles, A. *et al.* (2010) Predictors of suicidality across the life span: the Isle of Wight study. *Psychological Medicine* **40**(9), 1453–1466. doi:10.1017/S0033291709991905.

Pingault, J.B. *et al.* (2015) Genetic and environmental influences on the developmental course of attention-deficit/hyperactivity disorder symptoms from childhood to adolescence. *JAMA Psychiatry* **72**(7), 651–658. doi:10.1001/jamapsychiatry.2015.0469.

Plana-Ripoll, O. *et al.* (2019) Exploring comorbidity within mental disorders among a Danish national population. *JAMA Psychiatry* **76**(3), 259–270. doi:10.1001/jamapsychiatry.2018.3658.

Quinton, D. *et al.* (1993) Partners, peers, and pathways: assortative pairing and continuities in conduct disorder. *Development and Psychopathology* **5**(4), 763–783.

Rasmussen, S.A. *et al.* (2016) Zika virus and birth defects—reviewing the evidence for causality. *New England Journal of Medicine* **374**, 1981–1987. doi:10.1056/NEJMsr1604338.

Reuben, A. *et al.* (2016) Lest we forget: comparing retrospective and prospective assessments of adverse childhood experiences in the prediction of adult health. *Journal of Child Psychology and Psychiatry, and Allied Disciplines* **57**(10), 1103–1112. doi:10.1111/jcpp.12621.

Rice, F. *et al.* (2003) Negative life events as an account of age-related differences in the genetic aetiology of depression in childhood and adolescence. *Journal of Child Psychology and Psychiatry* **44**(7), 977–987. doi:10.1111/1469-7610.00182.

Rice, F. *et al.* (2009) Disentangling prenatal and inherited influences in humans with an experimental design. *Proceedings of the National Academy of Sciences of the United States of America* **106**(7), 2464–2467. doi:10.1073/pnas.0808798106.

Rice, F. *et al.* (2017) Antecedents of new-onset major depressive disorder in children and adolescents at high familial risk. *JAMA Psychiatry* **74**(2), 153–160. doi:10.1001/jamapsychiatry.2016.3140.

Rice, F. *et al.* (2019) Characterizing developmental trajectories and the role of neuropsychiatric genetic risk variants in early-onset depression. *JAMA Psychiatry* **76**(3), 306–313. doi:10.1001/jamapsychiatry.2018.3338.

Riglin, L. *et al.* (2022) "Late-onset" ADHD symptoms in young adulthood: is this the same as child-onset ADHD? *Journal of Attention Disorders* **26**(10), 1271–1282.

Rowe, R. *et al.* (2010) Developmental pathways in oppositional defiant disorder and conduct disorder. *Journal of Abnormal Psychology* **119**(4), 726–738. doi:10.1037/a0020798.

Rutter, M. (1989) Pathways from childhood to adult life. *Journal of Child Psychology and Psychiatry* **30**, 23–51.

Rutter, M. (2006) Implications of resilience concepts for scientific understanding. *Annals of the New York Academy of Sciences* **1094**, 1–12. doi:10.1196/annals.1376.002.

Rutter, M. (2009) Understanding and testing risk mechanisms for mental disorders. *Journal of Child Psychology and Psychiatry, and Allied Disciplines* **50**(1–2), 44–52. doi:10.1111/j.1469-7610.2008.01976.x.

Rutter, M. & Sroufe, L.A. (2000) Developmental psychopathology: concepts and challenges. *Development and Psychopathology* **12**, 265–296.

Rutter, M. *et al.* (2006) Continuities and discontinuities in psychopathology between childhood and adult life. *Journal of Child Psychology and Psychiatry* **47**(3–4), 276–295.

Sadler, K. *et al.* (2018) *Mental Health of Children and Young People in England, 2017*. NHS Digital.

Sallis, H.M. *et al.* (2021) Genetic liability to schizophrenia is associated with exposure to traumatic events in childhood. *Psychological Medicine* **51**(11), 1814–1821. doi:10.1017/S0033291720000537.

Sandstrom, A. *et al.* (2019) Offspring of parents with schizophrenia, bipolar disorder, and depression: a review of familial high-risk and molecular genetics studies. *Psychiatric Genetics* **29**(5), 160–169.

Schubert, K.O. *et al.* (2017) Depressive symptom trajectories in late adolescence and early adulthood: a systematic review. *The Australian and New Zealand Journal of Psychiatry* **51**(5), 477–499. doi:10.1177/0004867417700274.

Sellers, R. *et al.* (2019) Cross-cohort change in adolescent outcomes for children with mental health problems. *Journal of Child Psychology and Psychiatry* **60**(7), 813–821.

Shell, M.D. *et al.* (2014) Anxious solitude and the middle school transition: a diathesis × stress model of peer exclusion and victimization trajectories. *Developmental Psychology* **50**(5), 1569–1583. doi:10.1037/a0035528.

Silberg, J.L. *et al.* (2001) Genetic and environmental influences on the temporal association between earlier anxiety and later depression in girls. *Biological Psychiatry* **49**(12), 1040–1049. doi:10.1016/s0006-3223(01)01161-1.

Solmi, M. *et al.* (2022) Age at onset of mental disorders worldwide: large-scale meta analysis of 192 epidemiological studies. *Molecular Psychiatry* **27**, 281–295.

Sonuga-Barke, E.J.S. *et al.* (2017) Child-to-adult neurodevelopmental and mental health trajectories after early life deprivation: the young adult follow-up of the longitudinal English and Romanian Adoptees study. *The Lancet* **389**(10078), 1539–1548. doi:10.1016/S0140-6736(17)30045-4.

Sroufe, L.A. *et al.* (2005) *The Development of the Person: The Minnesota Study of Risk and Adaptation from Birth to Adulthood.* The Guilford Press, London.

Thapar, A. & Rutter, M. (2009) Do prenatal risk factors cause psychiatric disorder? Be wary of causal claims. *British Journal of Psychiatry* **195**, 100–101. doi:10.1192/bjp.bp.109.062828.

Thapar, A. & Rutter, M. (2019) Do natural experiments have an important future in the study of mental disorders? *Psychological Medicine* **49**(7), 1079–1088.

Thapar, A. *et al.* (2017) Neurodevelopmental disorders. *The Lancet Psychiatry* **4**(4), 339–346. doi:10.1016/S2215-0366(16)30376-5.

Tremblay, R.E. (2010) Developmental origins of disruptive behaviour problems: the 'original sin' hypothesis, epigenetics and their consequences for prevention. *Journal of Child Psychology and Psychiatry, and Allied Disciplines* **51**(4), 341–367. doi:10.1111/j.1469-7610.2010.02211.x.

Trubetskoy, V. *et al.* (2022) Mapping genomic loci implicates genes and synaptic biology in schizophrenia. *Nature* **604**(7906), 502–508. doi:10.1038/s41586-022-04434-5.

Vitaro, F. & Tremblay, R.E. (2008) Clarifying and maximising the usefulness of targeted preventive interventions. In: *Rutter's Child and Adolescent Psychiatry*. (eds M. Rutter, *et al.*), 5th edn. Blackwell, Oxford. pp. 989–1008.

Waszczuk, M.A. *et al.* (2016) The stability and change of etiological influences on depression, anxiety symptoms and their co-occurrence across adolescence and young adulthood. *Psychological Medicine* **46**(1), 161–175. doi:10.1017/S0033291715001634.

Waters, H.S. & Waters, E. (2006) The attachment working models concept: among other things, we build script-like representations of secure base experiences. *Attachment & Human Development* **8**(3), 185–197.

Weavers, B. *et al.* (2021) The antecedents and outcomes of persistent and remitting adolescent depressive symptom trajectories: a longitudinal, population-based English study. *The Lancet Psychiatry* **8**(12), 1053–1061. doi:10.1016/S2215-0366(21)00281-9.

Weinberger, D.R. (1987) Implications of normal brain development for the pathogenesis of schizophrenia. *Archives of General Psychiatry* **44**, 660–669.

Widom, C.S. *et al.* (2007) A prospective investigation of major depressive disorder and comorbidity in abused and neglected children grown up. *Archives of General Psychiatry* **64**(1), 49–56.

CHAPTER 2
Diagnosis, diagnostic formulation, and classification

Daniel S. Pine
Section on Development and Affective Neuroscience, National Institute of Mental Health (NIMH) Intramural Research Program, Bethesda, MD, USA

Introduction

This chapter includes four sections pertaining to diagnosis, formulation, and classification. The first section describes the purpose of classification and its application to patients. Moreover, a diagnosis is differentiated from a diagnostic formulation, and the clinical impact of classification is delineated. The second section reviews historical events related to classification and highlights complex issues impacting attempts to improve classifications. The section also describes how such complexities influence the diagnostic process for clinicians working in various scenarios. The third section describes research designed to validate placement of diagnoses within a classification scheme. Finally, ongoing issues are described that complicate attempts to improve classification and diagnosis. Such attempts seek improvements by leveraging the complimentary features of categorical and dimensional approaches as well as by capitalizing on discoveries in genetics and neuroscience.

Classification, diagnosis, and diagnostic formulation

Definitions

Classification refers to the process of grouping diagnoses into categories. While classification serves many purposes, none is more important than providing clinicians with a shared language, and the current chapter emphasizes this and other clinical applications. Shared language is codified in the placement of criteria and diagnoses in a classification scheme, which generates standard ways to describe phenomena that enable efficient, accurate communication among health professionals. Classification serves many additional functions, and conflicts can arise among these functions, as discussed in the section on complexities of the diagnostic process.

Classifications involve a subtle but important framing of clinical problems. This framing occurs by emphasizing the utility in a classifications scheme of "diagnoses," which are entities to be differentiated from "disorders" (Kraemer, 2007). The term "disorder" refers to the presence of a clinically meaningful perturbation that manifests within a person and that adversely affects their functioning. This definition views disorders as entities reflecting facets of biology. This contrasts with the term "diagnosis," which is less closely tied to biology. Rather, this term refers to the label that clinicians assign to certain problems observed in the patient. The diagnosis is a social convention agreed upon by health professionals; it represents the clinicians' "best guesses" about underlying disorders, as they are presumed to reflect biology.

Definitions of the term "mental disorder" impact this framing. While different definitions exist, Wakefield's exposition of "harmful dysfunction" informs many of the currently accepted definitions (Wakefield, 2007). The first part of this definition, pertaining to "harm," indicates that patients with a mental disorder experience excessive distress or impairment in function. This differentiates mental disorders from many unusual behaviors without such impact on function. For example, some individuals might possess far-below-average skill in an isolated area: they may be extremely slow runners. This extreme behavior is not part of a mental disorder because it fails to impact functioning or produce extreme distress. Moreover, even when behavior creates difficulty for some individuals, debate persists about the origin of these difficulties. For example, among some highly functional individuals who manifest symptoms of an autism spectrum disorder (ASD), difficulty could arise from intolerance exhibited by peers toward

Rutter's Child and Adolescent Psychiatry and Psychology, Seventh Edition.
Edited by Anita Thapar, Daniel S. Pine, Samuele Cortese, Cathy Creswell, Tamsin J. Ford, James F. Leckman, and Argyris Stringaris.

Companion website: www.wiley.com/go/thapar/ruttERSpsych7

the individual rather than directly due to these symptoms. Principles related to neurodiversity could impact the framing of such behavior, as discussed in depth in Chapter 3. Full discussions of the neurodiversity movement appear in Chapters 50 on ASD and 54 on attention deficit hyperactivity disorder.

The term "dysfunction," the second part of Wakefield's definition, implies that something malfunctions within the patient. The presence of dysfunction differentiates mental disorders from other entities associated with harm that are unconnected to problems with physiologic processes supporting health. For example, some individuals might possess hateful views about certain groups of people. These views can stimulate behaviors that produce substantial levels of harm, both in the person who holds the views and in the people who are targets of hate. However, this pattern is not considered a "mental disorder" because it does not relate to physiologic dysfunction. In this way, mental disorders differ from entities typically labeled by political or social movements when the entities lack such grounding in physiology.

Among individual patients, scholars struggle with precisely identifying physiological dysfunction, the second part of Wakefield's definition, as it applies to a mental disorder. Less clarity exists in this area, as compared to procedures for detecting the presence of harm. Harmfulness in an individual patient is rated with high levels of reliability using tools for assessing impairment, which are discussed in Chapter 28. At an abstract level, the views of many thinkers converge to consider dysfunction as relating to perturbation in physiology supporting successful cognitive or behavioral adaptation. However, difficulty arises when trying to concretely define levels of specific physiological functions to be ascertained in patients. No standards exist for using such levels to differentiate an individual who is affected from one who is not affected by a mental disorder. This contrasts with standards in many areas in medicine. For example, medicine typically defines precise values for measures such as blood pressure, levels of glucose control, or many other functions that alert the clinician to the presence of risk in the patient or the need for intervention. For mental disorders, this difficulty in defining physiologic dysfunction heavily informs attempts to revise classification, as discussed in the last section of the chapter. Of note, other branches of medicine face similar struggles when attempting to precisely define illnesses where physiologic dysfunction is difficult to quantify.

Finally, scholars also recognize the need to consider factors beyond physiology when weighing the impact of mental illnesses. Clearly, mental illnesses manifest strong, bidirectional relations with social factors and other features of the environment. In this way, social and environmental factors operate as risks for mental disorders; moreover, mental disorders often produce substantial harm through their effects on social and environmental factors. Discussions of mental disorders should recognize the impact of biology as well as nonbiological factors, such as factors in the environment or other aspects of context. An emphasis on physiology arises when attempting to define features of mental disorders that differentiates them from other phenomena with similarly intimate relations to social and environmental factors.

The philosophy of diagnosis

Emphasis on distinctions between disorders and diagnoses raises philosophical issues. These issues reflect essentialist and postmodern notions of diagnosis and the underlying problems they attempt to classify. Kendler describes notable issues affecting classification that follow from such philosophical considerations (Kendler, 2022). He suggests that views on diagnosis of mental illnesses relate to debates in the philosophy of science about the nature of difficult-to-measure constructs.

In philosophical debates highlighted by Kendler, one camp argues that phenomena such as mental disorders exist in ways that endure. Even when difficult to measure, these phenomena are seen as existing in nature, independent of any attempt to label them through the diagnostic process. Recalling discussions of physiologic dysfunction, members of this camp attempt to identify enduring biological features of the phenomena. Applied to mental disorders, these efforts seek procedures that would distinguish true instances of a mental disorder from phenocopies that bear only superficial resemblance based on overlapping clinical features.

The focus in this first camp encounters difficulties associated with defining physiologic dysfunction. Even with extensive effort, procedures to identify core features of mental disorders are likely to remain years away from being widely established. Considering such difficulties, Kendler emphasizes the advantages of the other camp. This camp adopts a more utilitarian view that leaves open questions about the essence of an entity. Rather, emphasis is placed on the usefulness of labeling the entity, which provides practical utility, independent of the labels' true relations to disorders. Assigning a diagnosis allows the accumulation of knowledge about prognosis and treatment, which clinicians can utilize to improve the quality of care.

Philosophical debates remain relatively abstract, but consideration of these issues might affect a practitioner's approach to a patient. Such consideration can imbue humility in clinicians engaged in the diagnostic process. Classification and diagnosis offer the best approach possible at the current time, but humility seems appropriate since knowledge on mental disorders is less definitive than for other health problems. The difficulty in precisely defining mental disorders in a specific patient complicates the life of the mental health professional. The diagnostic process for mental disorders is more prone to error than other biomedical syndromes. For these other syndromes, such as ischemic cardiovascular disease to take one example, diagnosis incorporates the greater biologic understandings of the conditions to reduce error. In mental illnesses, diagnosis almost entirely reflects clinical features, which refer to patterns of signs that are features directly observed by the clinician, and symptoms, which are features that the patient or their family members report to the clinician. When compared to the example of ischemic cardiovascular disease, this limitation reveals the complex ways that many factors shape risks for mental illnesses and affect the brain, an organ whose functions are more complex than the heart.

The formulation

The process of assigning a diagnosis involves other related considerations. The clinician must remember that a diagnosis refers to a narrow set of features in the life of an individual. Unlike a diagnosis, a diagnostic formulation provides a fuller description of a person. To highlight this fact, clinicians only describe a diagnosis as applying to a person but not as an intimate part of their identity. For example, in a patient suffering from major depressive disorder (MDD), clinicians describe the individual as "a person with MDD," and they should not label the person as "a depressive," which is viewed as offensive and dismissive of the person's many qualities that extend beyond their health. In similar ways, the term "cure" refers to the eradication of a disorder, and clinicians use this term sparingly. This is because it is difficult to confidently state that a disorder has been eliminated, which only happens rarely in many quarters of medicine.

A diagnostic formulation is prepared in a way that elucidates considerably more information than provided by a diagnosis (Hoyos & Cortese, 2022). The term "formulation" refers to a description of the circumstances leading a patient to seek care. This description attempts to explain the factors contributing to symptom onset and persistence. This includes a review of each clinical problem's unique features in the patient that may be irrelevant to many other people who carry the same diagnosis. Whereas a diagnosis rests primarily on the report of signs and symptoms, a formulation goes far beyond these features to also consider features of pathophysiology, descriptions of risk, and protective factors, as well as discussions of the diagnosis as it relates to the multiple nested contexts inhabited by the patient. This includes home, school, community, and groups related to other identities adopted by the patient.

Formulations record information related to causal webs of influences in the clinical presentation. They end by using this causal web to discuss prognosis and to provide entry points for treatments designed to alter causal influences. Formulations also describe plans for later evaluations of the treatment, often in a list of proposed treatments to be considered. This list can support discussions that outline the orderly series in which these treatments might be considered, based on the patient's response to each treatment. For example, Chapter 59 discusses treatment for anxiety disorders. Based on information in this chapter, a formulation for a child with separation anxiety disorder might recommend cognitive behavioral therapy (CBT). This formulation might stipulate consideration of a selective serotonin reuptake inhibitor (SSRI) if a child continues to show signs of significant impairment after 12 weeks of CBT.

Information is conveyed to patients and their families. In providing this information, some clinicians prefer a written format, others prefer verbal formats, and still others utilize both formats. Written material provides something concrete to which patients and families can return when they develop questions or forget aspects of clinical encounters. Verbal presentations are typically entered into the medical record to document the information conveyed to the patient and their family. Moreover, in some countries, patients have full access to their medical record. As a result, families can readily obtain the written summary of the diagnostic formulation that clinicians enter into the record. Of note, clinicians should enter information into the medical record in a format that they expect patients to read. Regardless, the main advantage of verbal presentation over written summaries is that it provides an immediate context to elicit and answer questions from patients and their families about the formulation. This is helpful since multiple questions often follow from a clinician's answer to an initial question. Similarly, presenting this materially verbally allows the clinician to immediately address unexpected reactions or confusion evoked in patients and family members from aspects of the formulation.

Classification complexities and contexts

The origins of current classifications

Areas of biomedical science concerned with mental disorders emphasize the importance of classification. This was not the case during much of the 20th century, and this shifting emphasis reflected a confluence of forces raising major concerns with conceptualizations of mental illness. These concerns related to observations on poor reliability of diagnosis and neglect of biomedical features (Wilson, 1993).

Publication of the *Diagnostic and Statistical Manual of Mental Disorders III* (DSM-III) in 1980 represented a watershed moment that punctuated this shifting emphasis. After this event, consensus grew both on the importance of classification and the need to ground diagnosis firmly on observable features of mental illnesses. Such a grounding offered an avenue for addressing concerns with unreliability. Classification schemes emphasizing these features rose to prominence throughout the remainder of the 20th century. Advocates of this change continued to prioritize observable features as anchors for a diagnosis, despite views of such features by some scholars as mere superficial reflections of events in the minds of patients. This focus on reliable criteria remains prominent in current classification schemes, including the DSM, 5th edition, text revision (DSM-5-TR) (American Psychiatric Association, 2022) and the 11th edition of the *International Classification of Diseases* (ICD-11) (World Health Organization, 2019). Both schemes' use of criteria-based definitions resembles DSM-III (American Psychiatric Association, 1980), as does the schemes' grouping of diagnoses into sections and avoidance of data on pathophysiology as a justification for a diagnosis.

Figure 2.1 depicts a timeline related to changes in nosology that conveys the vast impact of classification. The figure

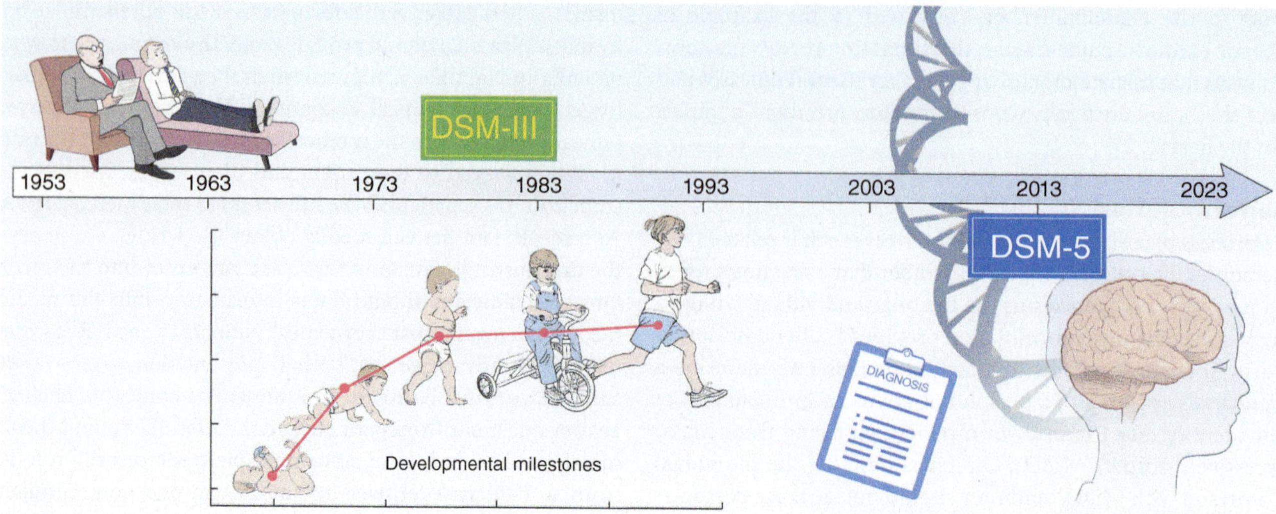

Figure 2.1 Displays a timeline during which major changes in classification occur. The timeline begins in the middle of the 20th century when a focus on psychodynamics was prominent. Events leading up to the publication of DSM-III, depicted in 1980, increased the focus on classification. As discoveries were applied to assessments of children and adolescents, developmental views of mental illness began to arise, and these views were emphasized in DSM-5, published in 2013. Future changes in classification might consider incorporating data from rating scales, as depicted by the clipboard, as well as data from genetics and imaging, as indicated by the other images on the right-hand end of the timeline.

highlights how research with children and adolescents shaped classification during the timeline. The publication of DSM-III prominently appears, given its impact, and the figure foreshadows other important features that allowed research with children and adolescents to influence the assessment and treatment of patients of all ages.

Parallel changes occurred in the ICD and the DSM. This produced greater similarity between the current versions as compared to earlier versions of the ICD and the DSM. Nevertheless, significant differences between these two classification schemes have existed throughout the past 50 years. Thus, schemes for classifying mental disorders in the ICD exist alongside parallel schemes for classifying diseases of body systems, including the immune, visual, circulatory, and respiratory systems. No such parallel schemes exist in the DSM. Similarly, earlier versions of the ICD used descriptive prototypes rather than individual lists of syndromes. While ICD-11 includes more extensive lists than earlier editions, the approach to diagnosis does not require the types of highly specified criteria and algorithms contained in all versions of the DSM since DSM-III.

Prior to 2013, mental disorders first identified during childhood appeared in a separate DSM section; similar placement occurred in the ICD prior to 2019. This served more as a reminder that such disorders exist than a reflection of their prominent effect on mental health (Pine, 2013). Beginning in the 1970s, as research with children and adolescents grew, the impact of this work gradually began to influence virtually all aspects of classification. Rutter's classic Isle of Wight Study laid the seeds for many of these influences, which unfolded through the first decade of the 21st century (Rutter, 1989).

Many key diagnostic facts were discerned in these early studies with children. One such example involved documenting high comorbidity for disorders classified as distinct. Initially, this was emphasized as a major factor affecting the health and treatment of children and adolescents before its presence was fully appreciated at other ages. Similarly, early studies with children stressed the importance of gathering information from multiple informants and conducting repeated interviews with a patient to maximize assessment reliability. Such procedures also began to be used at other ages. Finally, studies in children prioritized dimensional assessments and used longitudinal data to shape classifications, strategies also implemented at other ages.

A time arose with the publication of DSM-5 in 2013 (American Psychiatric Association, 2013) when scholars widely recognized the ubiquitous impact of research with children on understandings of mental illnesses at all ages. This led some leaders at the National Institute of Mental Health in the United States to proclaim mental illnesses to be "disorders of the young." Such impact also led DSM-5 and ICD-11 to remove the separate section dedicated to diagnosis in children and adolescents. Many current schemes, treat development as an essential component of mental illnesses at all ages. Otherwise, scholars worry that relegating diagnoses for children to a separate section would diminish a clinician's appreciation of development's importance at all ages.

Changing views on classification

Beyond removing the special section on diagnoses in children and adolescents, other notable changes have occurred with revisions in nosology during the past 10 years. These changes reflected uncertainties about many facets of diagnoses, including both features of individual diagnoses and broader features of classification. For many individual diagnoses, debate persists on the most appropriate definitions for classifications. This led to many changes between DSM-III and DSM-5-TR. Many major changes are described in individual chapters within this textbook, but three specific instances are described in this chapter to illustrate relatively broad themes impacting views on diagnosis.

One notable set of changes occurred for the diagnosis of ASD, which is discussed in Chapter 50. Major debates consider the advantages and disadvantages of relatively broad versus narrow groupings for sets of related diagnoses, which have been characterized as arguments about "lumping" or "splitting." For autism, earlier diagnoses had included multiple narrow entities, such as Asperger's Syndrome and childhood disintegrative disorder, which were combined into an overarching family of pervasive developmental disorders (PDDs). DSM-5 and ICD-11 eliminated the term PDD as well as many of the underlying narrow entities and replaced them with an overarching ASD category. While multiple factors informed this change, high reliability of the ASD diagnosis in the DSM-5 field trials played a key role (Regier *et al.*, 2013). Reliability for the broad category was better than reliability for narrower diagnoses in other studies.

While one major change for ASD occurred in DSM-5 and ICD-11, many other incremental changes occurred between DSM-III and DSM-5-TR for another neurodevelopmental disorder (NDD), ADHD, discussed in Chapter 54. Changes in ADHD provide the second example illustrative of broader themes in classification. Changes in the diagnosis of ADHD between 1980 and 2013 related to two major issues in classification. One issue involved the use of domains of psychopathology in assigning diagnoses and subtypes. Since DSM-III, ADHD has been viewed as a condition involving problems in three domains: attention, impulsivity, and hyperactivity. Across different versions of the DSM and the ICD published in the past 30 years, classification placed varying emphasis on these domains. This reflected ongoing debates about the appropriateness of resting equal weight on multiple domains as opposed to a single or narrow subset of domains. The other active issue illustrated by changes in ADHD related to the impact of research in children on diagnostic practices in adults. Greater emphasis appeared in DSM-5 on procedures for assigning an ADHD diagnosis after childhood, and Chapter 54 describes features of these changes. This illustrated one of the many growing ways in which criteria in children have impacted diagnostic criteria for adults.

A final set of notable changes illustrative of broad themes in classification occurred for post-traumatic stress disorder (PTSD), which is discussed in Chapter 58. At one level, major change occurred in the diagnosis among children, adolescents, and adults, where the same criteria applied to these age groups. This reflected problems with earlier diagnostic rules in many age groups. However, other changes had broader implications for many diagnoses. In this instance, a different set of criteria was created in DSM-5 for PTSD in young children as compared to older individuals, which reflected trends in other conditions. As discussed in Chapter 7 on mental health in young children, the utility of diagnosis in older-aged children and adolescents generated interest in applying novel criteria among young as opposed to older children, as exemplified by the new PTSD diagnosis in preschool children.

Beyond these three examples, other notable changes involved the creation of important new conditions, including conditions described in the chapter on depressive disorders (Chapter 63) and the chapter on suicidal behavior and self-harm (Chapter 64). A final set of changes affected overarching classification structure. The grouping of disorders is very similar in DSM-5 and ICD-11, which differs from the grouping in earlier versions of the DSM. For example, PTSD and obsessive–compulsive disorder (OCD) were once treated as anxiety disorders, as described in Chapter 59. Both diagnoses now appear in separate sections of the scheme for both DSM-5 and ICD-11. Similarly, the multiaxial classification scheme that existed for more than 30 years no longer appears in DSM-5.

Removing the multiaxial system affects impairment ratings. Prior to DSM-5, impairment was rated on an axis distinct from other axes where symptoms of individual diagnoses were rated. This placement reinforced the idea that impairment reflects unique factors, such as the environment where a child lives or the resources to which the child has access. These factors can vary in ways orthogonal to symptoms. DSM-5-TR continues the practice in earlier schemes that requires impairment to be part of the threshold for each individual diagnosis. This appears in criteria for each condition, which restricts diagnoses to clinically meaningful problems. However, removal of the separate impairment axis could reduce attention to the ways that symptoms severity can fluctuate orthogonally to levels of impairment.

While differences exist between current and earlier classification schemes, these differences may be minor, compared to changes in future schemes. Possible changes involve important long-standing issues. Proposals seeking a paradigm shift considered major changes that ultimately were not made in DSM-5 or ICD-11 (Regier *et al.*, 2009; Kupfer & Regier, 2011; Kendler, 2013; Zachar *et al.*, 2019).

Context and complexities in the diagnostic process

Classification affects views about mental illnesses in many ways that extend beyond the boundaries of clinical encounters. These include facilitating applications of the research literature and supporting communications among stakeholders who use classification schemes in multiple contexts outside of the clinic. Problems can occur when differing views arise related to these differing applications. Such problems relate at least partly to the fact that diagnoses apply to a group of individuals where there is enormous individual variability in clinical presentation.

Clinical and research classification

Close alignment between clinical and research classification creates both opportunities and problems. When the two systems relate in clear and understandable ways, advances in research can quickly impact the care of patients. Moreover, such alignment allows clinical classification to reflect the best-established views regarding mental illnesses. Nevertheless, close alignment can also burden the clinician. This is because many avenues pursued in research never impact clinical care, reflecting differences in factors influencing clinical care and research. The history of advances in medicine shows that research can advance understanding when it pursues a very wide array of questions. Many questions relate to relatively new features of a clinical problem. Hence, the number of new questions pursued in research creates risks of entering blind alleyways, which are tolerable given the possibility of future scientific breakthroughs. Clinical care focuses more narrowly than research on the here-and-now of the patient. As such, blind alleyways are less tolerable when providing care.

While classification informs both clinical endeavors and research, other differences exist. Clinical systems encompass all forms of mental illness presentations no matter how complex, whereas classification in research often targets only subsets of many possible presentations, applying to situations where questions can be answered with some definitiveness. Practicalities in assessment in these two contexts also often differ. Research classification typically involves greater standardization in both tools and training. On some occasions, an assessor's performance in research can be more closely scrutinized over time than an assessor's performance in the clinic.

Differences in the practicalities of research and clinical assessment may affect quality. Consistent with this possibility, the field trials for the creation of DSM-5 mirrored clinical practice, avoiding the more extensive levels of standardization, training, and monitoring typically utilized in research. This generated far lower reliabilities even for established conditions, such as MDD, as compared to reliabilities in clinical trials for MDD (Regier *et al.*, 2013). Interestingly, this effect on MDD and many other disorders appeared less profound for some conditions, such as ADHD and ASD, where reliabilities approached levels typically seen in research settings. This suggests that more acceptable standards exist for clinical approaches to the assessment of some disorders as compared to others. As such, clinical assessment may need greater improvement in some specific areas. This could relate to the considerable latitude clinicians use to evaluate diagnostic criteria.

Differences in clinical and research classification could lead clinicians to focus limited attention on research classification, but this would be unfortunate. Linking the two schemes supports treatment because many clinical trials enroll patients using research classifications. Understanding both schemes allow clinicians to remain confident that the treatment guidelines they follow apply to the patients they see. Understanding research classification also grants clinicians access to a wealth of other important information. Classification schemes group diagnoses, based on patterns of shared and distinguishing features, which helps shape expectations about comorbidity, prognosis, and treatment that meaningfully informs care delivery.

Classification in other contexts

The broad impact of classification on society speaks to the importance that mental health holds for people in multiple contexts. However, diversity of purpose can create problems when classification schemes prioritize different goals in distinct settings. For example, classifications utilized in health economics or legal settings may not apply to health care settings.

Many chapters in this textbook describe uses of classification. This includes discussions of legal settings, where classification can inform decisions about competence or child placement. Such material appears in Chapter 19, focused on legal issues, Chapter 25, focused on child abuse and neglect, Chapter 41, focused on issues related to displacement, and Chapter 42, focused on adoption and related issues. Individuals charged with regulating aspects of health care also often utilize aspects of classification, given mental illnesses' tremendous impact on health outcomes. Relevant issues appear in Chapter 17, focused on health economics, and Chapter 18, focused on public health challenges. This includes the marked impact on public health from the COVID-19 pandemic. Finally, classification and diagnosis influence access to resources in schools and other settings where children spend time. Readers can find discussions of these issues in Chapters 29, 30, 37, 38, 43, and 44. These chapters describe issues in educational and health care settings related to pediatric mental disorders.

Ideally, scientists and practitioners around the world would adopt a shared classification scheme to reduce the complexities that already exist, even within a single scheme. However, some countries have sought their own classifications to adapt them to fit in with local practice. While this is reasonable, such local classification also should be linked to more widely used schemes to maintain standards that are shared across countries. DSM-5-TR and ICD-11 are closely linked with the goal of providing such a widely used scheme. Similar issues confront attempts to create separate schemes to categorize culture-specific syndromes. As with local practices, differences in cultures readily create scenarios where features of cultures need to be handled in classification. Again, this also is reasonable but also creates a need to link such classifications with schemes shared in many countries.

Diagnostic validity

Scientifically meaningful and clinically useful diagnoses are ones that possess validity, an issue of growing importance with changes in classification (Robins & Guze, 1970; Kendler, 2013). The process of validation accumulates data that are arranged in multiple categories, and the current section reviews data in

Table 2.1 Validators of diagnoses.

	Epidemiology	Family genetics	Psychosocial	Medication response	Cognitive correlates	Biology	Long-term course
Autism	X	X	–	–	X	X	X
Schizophrenia	X	X	X	X	X	–	X
ADHD	X	X	–	X	X	–	X
Dyslexia	X	X	–	–	X	–	X
Eating disorders	X	X	–	–	–	–	–
Obsessive compulsive disorder	X	X	–	–	X	–	–
Bipolar disorder	X	X	–	X	–	–	X
PTSD	–	–	X	–	X	–	
Rett	X	X	–	–	–	X	X
Substance abuse	X		–	–	–		
Severe intellectual disability	X	X	–	–	–	X	X
Conduct disorder	X	–	X	–	–	–	X
Anxiety/depression	X	X	X	–	X	–	X

An X indicates the presence of some validating data in a column. Evidence is considered "present" when at least two studies exist that suggest the syndrome can be differentiated from at least two of the other syndromes given in the rows.

seven such categories. As these data accumulate, findings raise increasingly pressing questions about classification, because distinct validator categories support different classification schemes (Solomon & Kendler, 2021). The following seven sections provide a narrative review, and Table 2.1 summarizes, in an abbreviated format, data that support the validity of individual diagnoses. Readers should focus less attention on individual conditions in the text or table and more attention on the columns across all conditions. This suggests that some research on validation, as in family-genetic studies, provides relatively strong support for aspects of classification, whereas other research on validation, as for studies of treatment, provides relatively weak support.

Demography in epidemiology

Different groups of disorders are distinguished by patterns of demographic correlates in epidemiological studies. Here, the strongest, most consistent findings exist for relations with age and gender. Chapter 3 discusses the NDDs, which are grouped together in both DSM-5-TR and ICD-11. This placement reflects relations with demographics as well as other validators. NDDs are approximately three-to-four times more common in boys than girls. This differs from patterns in most emotional disorders described in Chapters 58 through 65, which are approximately two-times more common in girls than boys. Demography also relates to subdivisions for individual disorders. One such example is described in Chapter 65, where subtypes of conduct disorder (CD) differ for age-of-onset, with the early-onset form being more persistent and associated with other unique features.

Familial and genetic patterns

Many schemes emphasize data on family-genetic relations among disorders. As suggested by the research summarized in Table 2.1, these data are informative for classification (Kendler, 2013). This reflects evidence of familial aggregation for virtually all mental disorders in tandem with some evidence of disorder specificity in such patterns.

Other portions of the textbook devote considerable space to validation based on patterns of familial aggregation and genetics. Evidence in these areas is reviewed in Chapter 21 on genetics and in many chapters discussing pathophysiology of individual disorders. This chapter emphasizes the importance of pleiotropy and nonspecificity in genetic and familial risk. Some syndromes involving intellectual disability (ID) and severe problems in neurodevelopment can be defined entirely based on the presence of genetic anomalies, as described in Chapters 3, 21, 51, and 53. Rett syndrome, classified as a subtype of ASD in DSM-5-TR, provides one such illustrative example of a genetic syndrome. Features of these syndromes, particularly their long-term course, provide strong evidence of validity. For other disorders, genetics represents only one of many factors that inform classification by acting as validators.

Beyond genetic syndromes, other sections of the textbook describe many ways that data on familial aggregation distinguish groups of disorders. For example, different disorders express different overall rates of familial aggregation as well as differences in the genetic and environmental contributions to such aggregation. ADHD shows both stronger familial aggregation and stronger heritability than anxiety disorders. Material in other chapters describes other ways that data on familial aggregation influence groupings of disorders. For example, as noted above and discussed in Chapters 59 and 60, OCD was once categorized with anxiety disorders but is now classified with another group of disorders in DSM-5-TR. This at least partly reflects data on familial aggregation.

Data on this validator illustrate some of the problems in revising classifications based on accumulating evidence. For example, data on longitudinal outcome and treatment response provide some support for differentiations between bipolar disorder and nonaffective psychosis, as exists in current and earlier versions of nosology (Robins & Guze, 1970). However, data on genetic correlates suggest that these two sets of diagnoses might fall in more closely related groups (Smoller *et al.*, 2019). Different groupings based on different validators suggest the need for major changes in classification, as described in the final section of this chapter.

Psychosocial correlates

Compared to familial and genetic correlates, data summarized in Table 2.1 suggest that psychosocial correlates feature less prominently as validators in classification schemes. This difference reflects greater evidence of specificity for familial and genetic as compared to psychosocial correlates. Individual chapters describe various features of psychosocial factors that relate to mental disorders and their treatments. For example, anxiety disorders, described in Chapter 59, and conduct disorder, described in Chapter 65, both relate to psychosocial factors. Nevertheless, nonspecificity exists in such relations: psychosocial correlates of anxiety also relate to conduct problems. PTSD and attachment disorders represent the rare conditions where psychosocial factors uniquely relate to classification. In PTSD, exposure to trauma is considered a causal factor in the genesis of the disorder, much in the way that stressors are considered to cause adjustment disorders. This issue is discussed in Chapter 58. Similarly, the role of psychosocial factors in attachment disorders is discussed in Chapter 7.

Long-term course

Like data on familial aggregation and genetics, data on the long-term course of a condition powerfully influence classification. Indeed, some of the strongest data differentiating diagnoses arise in research that longitudinally tracks the outcomes of patients with various diagnoses. Again, Table 2.1 reflects this pattern. As described in Chapters 3, 21, 51–53, and 56 very high degrees of stability manifest in many forms of learning, psychotic, and NDDs. Slightly weaker but still quite strong stability, with some periodicity, also manifests for ADHD and certain behavioral disorders, as described in Chapters 54 and 65. These relatively stable patterns contrast with patterns in emotional disorders, described in Chapters 57 through 63. These conditions typically exhibit a more episodic course, with periods of exacerbation and relative quiescence. Moreover, compared to ADHD, larger proportions of children affected with an emotional disorder mature to become relatively symptom-free adolescents or adults. Indeed, the grouping of disorders into sections as part of Part IV of this textbook at least partially reflects these differences, which have also been a consistent feature of classifications.

Treatment response

On theoretical grounds, treatment response heavily shapes classification across medicine. For mental disorders, scholars grant priority for data on treatment response, in addition to familial aggregation and genetics, as well as long-term course, when attempting to validate diagnoses (Kendler, 2013; Solomon & Kendler, 2021). On empirical grounds, however, data for therapeutics less heavily influence current classifications than data in the other two areas. Concerns exist about the utility of treatment response as a validator, which can be criticized as *ex juvantibus* reasoning. Other chapters review details of these concerns. Chapters 58 through 64 discuss data on therapeutics for a diverse array of the emotional disorders, where the similarities in aspects of therapeutics are at least as great as the differences. Data on the responsiveness of bipolar disorder in adults to lithium provides one of the better examples of specificity in treatment response. However, even here other conditions exist, including diagnoses involving high levels of aggression discussed in Chapter 54, where lithium may have a role in treatment. In general, hopes that treatments heavily inform diagnostic classification remain unfulfilled. As noted in the last section of this chapter, hope has been renewed by recent imaging studies.

Cognition

Cognitive correlates provide varying levels of validation for diagnoses. For some disorders, cognition represents a defining feature of the diagnosis, to the point where it cannot be considered an independent validator. This applies to the learning disorders discussed in Chapter 52 and ID discussed in Chapter 53, where cognition is a criterion for many diagnoses. For these disorders, standardized instruments with population-based norms exist to facilitate assignment of appropriate diagnoses. Other diagnoses also have strong relations with cognitive variables, though the connection with normed instruments is more tenuous. ASD discussed in Chapter 50 provides a good example of such a diagnosis, where the relevant feature manifests on measures of social cognition. Still other diagnoses show some relation with cognition, but evidence of specificity is weaker than for ASD and its relations with social cognition. Cognitive capacities relate to many conditions described in Chapters 58 through 64 for the emotional disorders as well as for the diagnosis of ADHD described in Chapter 54 and behavioral disorders described in Chapter 65. Some of these conditions do show features of specificity. This includes the relation that anxiety disorders show with cognitive biases in the processing of threats, as described in Chapter 59. Nevertheless, classification schemes typically draw on cognition as a justification for diagnostic grouping less comprehensively than validators such as familial aggregation and genetics as well as longitudinal course.

Biology

Data on biological factors resemble data on cognition in terms of relations with classification. Examples of biological factors include measures of brain functioning, collected through imaging or electrophysiology, or measures of chemistry, as reflected in hormonal or neurochemical levels. Thus, some disorders relate closely to biological measures. Relevant examples include sleep disorders described in Chapter 68 and certain eating disorders described in Chapter 69. As with cognition, biological variables can serve as criteria in some of these conditions as well as in subtypes of other disorders such as forms of ASD associated with Rett or similar genetic syndromes. Other disorders relate to a biological factor, but the strength of the relation is insufficient to consider a biological measure a core feature of the diagnosis. The relation between ASD and epilepsy noted in Chapter 50 provides a relevant example. For most diagnoses, however, biology provides weak grounds to validate classification. As discussed in Chapters 11 and 12, brain imaging and other tools in neuroscience raise hopes for validation. However, neuroscience currently plays limited roles in clinical care for any mental disorder among most children and adolescents. The complexity of the brain coupled with the pace of progress in clinical translation of neuroscience suggest that this will likely be the case for many years.

The future of classification

The study of classification remains a lively research area, where effects on practice continue to unfold. Such effects are seen in the ongoing refinements in criteria for individual disorders and the movement of disorders from research classification into clinical schemes. Other sections of this chapter describe details of these changes. This final chapter section describes three broader areas of research that could exert more fundamental effects on future classification schemes.

The classification of risk

One fundamental issue relates to risk, exemplified in classifications of psychotic disorders discussed in Chapter 56. Considerable work describes the antecedents of psychosis, and this work informs the creation of a diagnosis for an attenuated psychosis syndrome used only in research classifications in DSM-5-TR (Carpenter, 2020). Adolescents affected by the attenuated psychosis syndrome face an approximate twofold increased risk for psychotic disorders. Thus, clinicians are encouraged to identify youth with these features. Continued research on the syndrome may ultimately shape clinical practice in more powerful ways. Similar issues appear in Chapter 59 concerning relations between early life temperament and risk for anxiety disorders. Much as in the attenuated psychosis syndrome, clinical trials target early-life temperament, where CBT has been shown to provide meaningful preventative benefit on the risk for anxiety disorders (Lau & Rapee, 2011). Finally, eating disorders described in Chapter 69 provide a third example of a risk syndrome. This involves adolescent instances of intermittent loss-of-control eating, which carries risk for progression to an eating disorder. All three patterns are reasonably common, involve a substantial risk for the development of conditions appearing in current nosology, and provide targets that are amenable to interventions designed to reduce the risk for progression to associated mental disorders.

Despite the public health importance of reducing premorbid risk, problems arise when applying a diagnostic label to risk syndromes. This relates to the differences that exist between early subclinical manifestations and diagnoses. Whereas diagnoses involve notable signs of distress or impairment, some early risk phenotypes involve no such features. Attempts to incorporate early manifestations must avoid combining current classes of mental disorders with these other syndromes associated only with risk for some mental disorder in the future. For example, it would be a mistake to combine individuals manifesting behaviors that place them at risk for schizophrenia into the same category as individuals who manifest overt symptoms of schizophrenia. Similarly, it would be a mistake to combine individuals with a temperament that places them at risk for anxiety disorders into the same category as individuals with overt expressions of an anxiety disorder. This is important since large proportions of individuals with early manifestations will remain free of distress or impairment; many such individuals will never warrant service provision.

The approach in DSM-5-TR for attenuated psychosis provides useful guides for handling these complications. This syndrome appears with explicit severity criteria in a section of the manual noting differences from other conditions in DSM-5-TR. Moreover, criteria explicitly describe symptoms of sufficient severity to warrant clinical attention. However, ICD-11 and DSM-5-TR do treat such syndromes differently. Unlike ICD-11, DSM-5-TR considers such syndromes as only appropriate for research as opposed to service provision. This acknowledges the risks associated with assigning a diagnostic label to a patient. Not only does this create opportunities for unearthing of stigma, but it could also lead to exposure to treatment-emergent adverse effects. Moreover, as the boundaries of classifications expand in these ways, scholars must remain vigilant for the medicalization of social problems. This risk remains high when features of mental disorders are limited to unusual behaviors, in the absence of impairment or dysfunction in physiology.

Dimensions and categories

The second set of fundamental issues relates to an increasing reliance on dimensions, as seen in DSM-5 and DSM-5-TR (Regier *et al.*, 2011). Disagreement persists on the best way to maximize the advantages of the two approaches while limiting their weaknesses. The timeline in Figure 2.1 and the earlier section on historical events in classification underlines influences from Rutter's early work (Rutter, 1989). This includes an emphasis on utilizing dimensional approaches to classification. Such emphasis embraces traditions in medicine for combining dimensions with diagnoses. Thus, endocrinologists regularly monitor a patient's compliance with dietary plans on a continuous scale or on continuous measures of physiology. Such monitoring occurs alongside categorical determinations concerning the presence or absence of conditions like diabetes. Similarly, physicians who treat pulmonary illnesses assess patients along multiple continuous dimensions through parameters from pulmonary function tests; these assessments also function alongside diagnostic determinations, such as the presence or absence of asthma. Such examples from many areas of medicine meaningfully inform attempts to achieve similar integration in the assessment of mental disorders.

Dimensions

Many factors support the use of dimensions. This includes statistical advantages when examining relations with validators. Dimensional approaches generate greater variation than categorical approaches, due to their use of a full range of values on a scale, which yields some advantages. As one example, clinical trials possess more statistical power when testing for effects on a symptom scale as opposed to a change in diagnostic status. In addition, the greater variability on a scale makes errors less costly than in categorical schemes.

Beyond statistics, dimensions more closely reflect the structure of psychopathology than categories based on studies of external validators. Research in these areas compares relations between a clinical measure and validating factors such as familial aggregation or long-term outcome. This work finds external validators to relate to symptoms across the full range of scores, as opposed to just the extremes. Moreover, these relations appear smooth and linear, without obvious break points across levels of severity, suggesting a dimensional structure.

Some might look to statistics to resolve the question of dimensions or categories. Can mathematics provide insights about discreteness in symptom scales? For example, can advanced techniques uncover signs of discontinuity in relations with validators not observable with more traditional techniques? Similarly, can statistics identify the number of curves underlying relations between dimensions and external factors? As with the broader emphasis on dimensions, the history of medicine provides clues to potential answers. Platt and Pickering engaged in a debate about hypertension, where statistics did not resolve questions about dimensions and categories (Swales, 1985). However, Kraemer notes that the field of statistics provides a standard approach to integrating dimensions and categories (Kraemer, 2007): with scale cut-points, categories can be modified to produce dimensions, and dimensions can be made into categories. In the psychopathological arena, one relevant example concerns ID, as discussed in Chapter 53.

Some suggest that current classifications remain ill-equipped to integrate categorical and dimensional approaches. From this perspective, scholars argue for a comprehensive change that leverages widely recognized advantages of dimensions. The Hierarchical Taxonomy of Psychopathology (HiTOP) represents one notable proposal for such a comprehensive change (Kotov *et al.*, 2021; Conway *et al.*, 2022). Moreover, with some of these approaches, dimensions can be combined across a range of psychopathological domains, to create transdiagnostic measures of psychopathology. Chapter 9 describes recent advances in this area. Many leading scientists work together as part of this process, which departs significantly from the categorical perspective informing most widely used classification schemes. Like other approaches emphasizing dimensional assessment, HiTOP deploys statistical techniques with multiple dimensions and multiple informants to create a structure that encompasses most forms of psychopathology. Co-occurring problems are classified based on correlations among dimensions, which offers more precise estimates of relations than categorical approaches.

A final advantage of dimensions relates to an outdated tradition that viewed diagnoses as syndromes wholly separate from one another, with rare mixed or overlapping patterns. As explicit criteria informed epidemiological studies in the 1980s and 1990s, this tradition led scientists to expect presentations of mental disorders involving predominant symptoms in one domain. However, much research demonstrates the incorrectness of these expectations. Approaches like HiTOP address the stronger than anticipated overlap among many dimensions.

Categories

Given the advantages, readers may appreciate calls for fundamental changes that incorporate dimensions. This could reflect the many strengths of continuous measures coupled with the newness of this approach, as compared to the long-established use of categorical approaches. However, despite the many advantages of dimensions, categorical distinctions are unavoidable for clinicians who deliver care to patients.

Clinicians must make decisions with patients. These decisions involve categorical choices, such as whether to provide treatment, whether to change the level of care, or even whether to ask the patient to return for another appointment. Like many decisions, these require categorical judgments concerning whether to act. Even choices that involve dimensions can be viewed as a series of categorical decisions. For example, therapists must often recommend numbers of psychotherapy sessions. However, when finishing the last session, the therapist must decide whether to end treatment or transition to a different treatment plan. Similar issues confront clinicians who consider medication prescriptions, where most data find weak relations between levels of medications prescribed and clinical response. Finally, clinical trials demonstrating efficacy of both psychotherapies and medications typically enroll patients using categories. Classifications based only on dimensions would relate less closely to such clinical trials research, providing limited justification for treatment. These considerations reveal the serious problems that would arise in a classification scheme free of categories.

Beyond clinical classification

The final major issue concerns the attempt to move beyond clinical features in the structure of classification. Figure 2.1 and associated sections of this chapter describe historical trends shaping a cycle of major changes and steady adaptation in classification schemes. Beyond a focus on dimensions, other efforts seek to address nagging problems reflecting classification's exclusive reliance on clinical features.

In some ways, these efforts have brought scientists full circle with respect to the events appearing in Figure 2.1. DSM-III moved classification away from theory and a focus on the causes of mental disorders, topics prominent at the origin of the Figure 2.1 timeline. Observable behaviors were prioritized to address problems at the time with the unreliability of diagnosis, shaping many events in Figure 2.1. Other portions of this chapter describe problems with a theoretical approach. Definitions of mental disorders are difficult to apply without better measures of physiologic dysfunction. Data on validity are difficult to understand when they fail to converge around the current categories. Some scholars suggest that these problems could be addressed by a movement "back to the future," which reincorporates ideas about the causes of mental disorders. Moreover, as compared to prevalent ideas abandoned in DSM-III, scholars argue that these newer theories possess much firmer grounding in science, as depicted in the images on the right-hand side of the timeline.

Many proposals exist for revising current classification schemes, based on theory and associated data on pathophysiology. These proposals appear in diverse formats with varying levels of detail. They range from isolated position papers to funded systematic efforts supported by dozens if not hundreds of publications (Insel, 2009; Insel *et al.*, 2010; Owen, 2014). Two relevant, relatively well-developed efforts comprise A Roadmap for Mental Health Research in Europe (ROAMER) (Haro *et al.*, 2014) and the Research Domain Criteria Initiative in the United States (RDoC) (Insel, 2009; Insel *et al.*, 2010). Like HiTOP, which focuses on utilization of dimensions, these proposals focus on other facets of diagnosis as part of arguments for major changes in many aspects of current classification schemes.

RDoC places particular emphasis on findings in genetics and neuroscience. Multiple chapters in this textbook describe major advances in methodologies related to this emphasis. These improvements generate greater consistency than during earlier times in relations between clinical and genetic or neuroscientific features of mental disorders. Such steady accumulation of findings is described for genetic research in Chapter 21, as well as for aspects of neuroscience research in Chapters 10–12. Despite a brisk pace of discovery, systematic, widespread clinical applications of either genetic or neuroscience research appear years away. This leaves proposals resembling RDoC as relatively removed from the daily life of the clinician. Before these new proposals can influence clinical care, two major hurdles must be cleared.

One hurdle relates to research advances. Discoveries are needed that impact decision-making based on strong associations with clinical variables. Some findings in genetics may move the field closer toward this goal; work finds large effects of rare gene variants on risk for neurodevelopmental syndromes, ID, and ASD. This work could inform predictions about long-term outcome and co-occurring medical problems, but it remains unclear how such discoveries could impact treatment, where other work suggests the need for caution. For example, patients in some countries seek treatment guidance through direct-to-consumer genetic reports, but research finds no benefits from these products (Vande Voort *et al.*, 2022).

The second hurdle relates to large-scale implementation. If genetic tests are to influence clinical care, as described in Chapter 21, standards for evaluating test results must reflect consensus views, systems must be implemented to train clinicians, and structures must exist to oversee quality control. Similar hurdles must be cleared for virtually all new neuroscientific tools. Moreover, new technologies incur costs related to training and maintenance that could limit availability.

ROAMER creates a research agenda based on systematic reviews completed by multidisciplinary experts. This research agenda attempts to ease the burden on health that mental disorders create in Europe. As a central goal, ROAMER attempts to integrate approaches to mental health across European countries. In some ways, ROAMER emphasizes similar themes highlighted in RDoC. These include a focus on new approaches to mental illness that recognizes the latest breakthroughs in biomedicine. In other ways, ROAMER goes beyond RDoC to consider impacts from mental illnesses that extend into many areas. These include a consideration of psychological treatment and economic issues in ways that might shape policy in the near term.

Proposals such as RDoC and ROAMER stimulate calls for wholesale change in classification, but piecemeal approaches seem more feasible, where changes in classification selectively incorporate the most clinically relevant findings. As noted above, genetics is moving toward clinical utility as part of the diagnostic work up for some neurodevelopmental problems. Beyond genetics, Chapter 68 discusses sleep disorders, where mobile technology may enable home-based assessments of physiology parameters typically assessed in sleep laboratories. This could inform changes in classification closely aligned to findings generated from novel technology.

Other new technologies appear tightly linked to novel therapies, which can provide strong justification for revising classification. Studies of transcranial magnetic stimulation (TMS) demonstrate one viable path for interrelated changes in classification and therapeutics. TMS is an established treatment for MDD in adults, which has yet to be successfully extended to large groups of youth. Moreover, even in adults, marked heterogeneity exists in treatment response levels, though active TMS therapy consistently produces stronger benefit than sham therapy. Recent work suggests that imaging technology can isolate a subset of patients with particularly robust responses to active forms of TMS (Cash *et al.*, 2021). If continued efforts in this area succeed, imaging data could be used in classification to identify subtypes of patients with MDD based on their anticipated response to TMS.

These efforts in genetics, sleep disorders, and TMS treatment of MDD represent isolated areas of progress. It appears likely that progress will continue in this fashion, with isolated areas of success. In the past, classification revisions have comprehensively updated entire schemes for all mental disorders. When seeking to incorporate data from genetics and neuroscience, more piecemeal approaches appear more feasible.

Conclusions

Classification organizes clinicians' activities by assembling diagnoses in a framework based on shared features. The current chapter describes the many purposes of classification, diagnosis, and formulations, as demonstrated in a rich history. The chapter summarizes data on the validity of diagnoses and describes findings suggesting the need for refinements in classification. The chapter closes by describing issues that inform such attempts at refinement. History suggests that classification shapes many aspects of care for mental disorders, including diagnosis and formulation. Hence, readers seeking to anticipate future changes in the care of mental disorders might attend to issues impacting proposed changes in classification.

Acknowledgment

The work for this chapter was supported by projects ZIA-MH002781 and ZIA-MH002782 in the Intramural Research Program of the National Institute of Mental Health.

References

American Psychiatric Association (1980) *Diagnostic and Statistical Manual of Mental Disorders*, 3rd edn. American Psychiatric Association, Washington, DC.

American Psychiatric Association (2013) *Diagnostic and Statistical Manual of Mental Disorders*, 5th edn. American Psychiatric Association, Washington, DC.

American Psychiatric Association (2022) *Diagnostic and Statistical Manual of Mental Disorders*, 5th edn. text revision edn. American Psychiatric Association, Washington, DC.

Carpenter, W.T. (2020) Classification is essential for the attenuated psychosis syndrome. *Biological Psychiatry* **88**, 289–290.

Cash, R.F.H. *et al.* (2021) Using brain imaging to improve spatial targeting of transcranial magnetic stimulation for depression. *Biological Psychiatry* **90**, 689–700.

Conway, C.C. *et al.* (2022) Translating the hierarchical taxonomy of psychopathology (HiTOP) from potential to practice: ten research questions. *American Psychologist* **78**, 873–885.

Haro, J.M. *et al.* (2014) ROAMER: roadmap for mental health research in Europe. *International Journal of Methods in Psychiatric Research* **23**(Suppl 1), 1–14.

Hoyos, C. & Cortese, S. (2022) Beyond diagnosis: formulation-storytelling and maps. *Journal of the American Academy of Child and Adolescent Psychiatry* **62**, 120–122.

Insel, T.R. (2009) Translating scientific opportunity into public health impact: a strategic plan for research on mental illness. *Archives of General Psychiatry* **66**, 128–133.

Insel, T. *et al.* (2010) Research domain criteria (RDoC): toward a new classification framework for research on mental disorders. *The American Journal of Psychiatry* **167**, 748–751.

Kendler, K.S. (2013) A history of the DSM-5 scientific review committee. *Psychological Medicine* **43**, 1793–1800.

Kendler, K.S. (2022) Potential lessons for DSM from contemporary philosophy of science. *JAMA Psychiatry* **79**, 99–100.

Kotov, R. *et al.* (2021) The hierarchical taxonomy of psychopathology (HiTOP): a quantitative nosology based on consensus of evidence. *Annual Review of Clinical Psychology* **17**, 83–108.

Kraemer, H.C. (2007) DSM categories and dimensions in clinical and research contexts. *International Journal of Methods in Psychiatric Research* **16**(Suppl 1), S8–S15.

Kupfer, D.J. & Regier, D.A. (2011) Neuroscience, clinical evidence, and the future of psychiatric classification in DSM-5. *The American Journal of Psychiatry* **168**, 672–674.

Lau, E.X. & Rapee, R.M. (2011) Prevention of anxiety disorders. *Current Psychiatry Reports* **13**, 258–266.

Owen, M.J. (2014) New approaches to psychiatric diagnostic classification. *Neuron* **84**, 564–571.

Pine, D.S. (2013) A 60-year climb on the mountain of nosology. *Journal of the American Academy of Child and Adolescent Psychiatry* **52**, 1251–1254.

Regier, D.A. *et al.* (2009) The conceptual development of DSM-V. *The American Journal of Psychiatry* **166**, 645–650.

Regier, D.A. *et al.* (eds) (2011) *The Conceptual Evolution of DSM-5*. American Psychiatric Publishing, Washington, DC.

Regier, D.A. *et al.* (2013) DSM-5 field trials in the United States and Canada, Part II: test-retest reliability of selected categorical diagnoses. *The American Journal of Psychiatry* **170**, 59–70.

Robins, E. & Guze, S.B. (1970) Establishment of diagnostic validity in psychiatric illness: its application to schizophrenia. *The American Journal of Psychiatry* **126**, 983–987.

Rutter, M. (1989) Isle of Wight revisited: twenty-five years of child psychiatric epidemiology. *Journal of the American Academy of Child and Adolescent Psychiatry* **28**, 633–653.

Smoller, J.W. *et al.* (2019) Psychiatric genetics and the structure of psychopathology. *Molecular Psychiatry* **24**, 409–420.

Solomon, M. & Kendler, K.S. (2021) The problem of aggregating validators for psychiatric disorders. *The Journal of Nervous and Mental Disease* **209**, 9–12.

Swales, J.D. (1985) *Platt Versus Pickering: An Episode in Recent Medical History*. Keynes Press, London.

Vande Voort, J.L. *et al.* (2022) A randomized controlled trial of combinatorial pharmacogenetics testing in adolescent depression. *Journal of the American Academy of Child and Adolescent Psychiatry* **61**, 46–55.

Wakefield, J.C. (2007) The concept of mental disorder: diagnostic implications of the harmful dysfunction analysis. *World Psychiatry* **6**, 149–156.

Wilson, M. (1993) DSM-III and the transformation of American psychiatry: a history. *The American Journal of Psychiatry* **150**, 399–410.

World Health Organization (2019) *International Statistical Classification of Disease and Related Health Problems*, 11th edn, Geneva, Switzerland.

Zachar, P. *et al.* (2019) The aspirations for a paradigm shift in DSM-5: an oral history. *The Journal of Nervous and Mental Disease* **207**, 778–784.

CHAPTER 3

Neurodevelopmental disorders

Anita Thapar[1,2,3] and Francesca Happé[4]

[1] Child and Adolescent Psychiatry Section, Division of Psychological Medicine and Clinical Neurosciences, Cardiff University School of Medicine, Cardiff, UK
[2] Centre for Neuropsychiatric Genetics and Genomics, Division of Psychological Medicine and Clinical Neurosciences, Cardiff University School of Medicine, Cardiff, UK
[3] Wolfson Centre for Young People's Mental Health, Division of Psychological Medicine and Clinical Neurosciences, Cardiff University School of Medicine, Cardiff, UK
[4] Social, Genetic and Developmental Psychiatry Centre, Institute of Psychiatry, Psychology, and Neuroscience, King's College, London, UK

What we mean by neurodevelopmental disorders

Neurodevelopmental disorders (NDDs) are a group of conditions that involve disruptions or differences in typical development and affect an individual's language, motor function, and ability to learn, socialize and preserve self-control. Although the concept of different developmental disabilities has been recognized for many centuries (Morris-Rosendahl & Crocq, 2020; Shoychet, 2021), it is only with the publication of the 5th edition of *Diagnostic and Statistical Manual of Mental Disorders* (DSM-5) (American Psychiatric Association, 2013), that the current grouping of NDDs was introduced. In this diagnostic classification, NDDs are defined as a group of conditions with onset in the developmental period, that typically first manifest early in development and result in impaired personal, social, occupational, or academic functioning (Box 3.1). The 11th and latest edition of the *International Classification of Diseases* (ICD-11) (World Health Organization, 2015) has adopted the same grouping but further emphasized the separation of neurodevelopmental conditions from psychiatric disorders with the chapter heading: "Mental, behavioural or neurodevelopmental disorders." Both DSM-5 and ICD-11, unlike preceding diagnostic classification systems, allow for co-diagnosis of autism spectrum disorder (ASD) and attention deficit hyperactivity disorder (ADHD) and between ASD and other disorders. Controversially, ICD-11 has not grouped Tourette's syndrome with NDDs but as a movement disorder (Müller-Vahl *et al*., 2022).

Early attitudes to neurodevelopmental disability are now viewed as largely, although not exclusively, negative (Morris-Rosendahl & Crocq, 2020; Shoychet, 2021). By the 18th century in Europe, societal views became more positive due to a greater emphasis on humanitarianism. However, this changed toward the end of the 19th century with industrialization and urbanization when many individuals with NDDs were viewed as being unable to successfully contribute. Furthermore, the idea of eugenics took hold; policies were taken to an extreme in Nazi Germany, first with sterilization and then extermination of children and adolescents with disabilities. Although a greater emphasis on human rights emerged after World War II, it was only in 2006 that the United Nations (UN) adopted the Convention on the Rights of Persons with Disabilities (CRPD). This was the first human rights treaty that included, but was not limited to, individuals with NDDs (Kanter, 2014). Thereafter, in many but not all countries,

Box 3.1 Neurodevelopmental disorders

DSM-5/DSM-5-TR	ICD-11
Intellectual disability (Intellectual developmental disorder in DSM-5-TR)	Disorders of intellectual development
Communication disorders	Developmental speech or language disorders
Autism spectrum disorder	Autism spectrum disorder
attention deficit hyperactivity disorder	Attention deficit hyperactivity disorder
Specific learning disorder	Developmental learning disorder
Motor disorders including: Developmental coordination disorder	Developmental motor coordination disorder
Tic disorders[a]	

[a] ICD-11 does not include tic disorders as NDDs—they are placed with movement disorders.

Rutter's Child and Adolescent Psychiatry and Psychology, Seventh Edition.
Edited by Anita Thapar, Daniel S. Pine, Samuele Cortese, Cathy Creswell, Tamsin J. Ford, James F. Leckman, and Argyris Stringaris.

Companion website: www.wiley.com/go/thapar/rutterspsych7

there has been a shift to inclusive education for those with NDDs and legislation protecting equal status in society, although civil rights and justice in relation to NDDs are still an issue today across much of the world.

In this chapter we will adopt the DSM-5 definition of NDDs although we recognize that the term NDD is used much more broadly by some. For example, early developmental difficulties such as motor, language, and cognitive impairments often precede the onset of psychosis in schizophrenia; they are also more common in those with early-onset conduct disorder. Thus, these disorders could also be viewed as neurodevelopmental in origin although they are not included in this grouping by DSM-5 or ICD-11. There is a rationale for this decision given their defining features (e.g., serious rule violations; hallucinations) typically do not manifest early in development. Genetic syndromes (e.g., Fragile X), conditions that are explained by an environmental insult, such as fetal alcohol syndrome (FAS), cerebral palsy, and neurological conditions, such as epilepsy, are also considered by some as NDDs. Many of these disorders may present with a DSM-5 or ICD-11 NDD (e.g., ASD), although typically they are also characterized by physical stigmata (as observed in many genetic syndromes and FAS) and neurological presentations such as seizures. The approach taken by DSM-5 (and maintained in DSM-5-TR; American Psychiatric Association, 2022) is that these specific causes or associated conditions can be used as NDD diagnostic specifiers (e.g., for ASD "Specify if: Associated with a known medical or genetic condition or environmental factor"). NDDs, as discussed in this chapter, are typically multifactorial in origin and defined by their observed manifestation and effects on functioning, not by presumed etiology.

Prevalence of neurodevelopmental disorders

Although DSM-5 was published in 2013, very few studies have examined the current grouping of NDDs, and the predominant research and clinical approach remains focused on single disorders, even if comorbidities and multimorbidities are now well-recognized (Francés et al., 2022). As a result, there are no large-scale, population-based epidemiological studies that have examined either the prevalence or disability-adjusted life years (DALYs) of all DSM-5/DSM-5-TR NDDs together using contemporary diagnostic criteria.

One Spanish, school-based study of 6834 students aged 5–17 years found that 18.3% met criteria for at least one NDD (using parent, teacher, and adolescent self-report on standard screening instruments followed by clinician full diagnostic assessment for those who screened positive) (Bosch *et al.*, 2022). The largest study of incidence relied on US clinical diagnostic record data from 2,070,541 publicly insured children and 1,309,900 privately insured children (Straub *et al.*, 2022), thus clinically recognized NDDs. The authors showed that by eight years of age, 23.9% of publicly insured children and 11.0% of privately insured children received a diagnosis of one or more NDDs. Another US investigation suggested a 9.5% increase in NDD prevalence from 2009 to 2017, driven primarily by increased rates of ADHD and ASD, a pattern that also has been shown in other countries. However, this study of secular changes in prevalence, broadened the concept of NDDs to encompass cerebral palsy, hearing loss, and seizures, although rates of those other disorders declined over the same period (Durkin, 2019). A limitation of diagnostic record data is that they do not capture all NDDs in the population and may be inaccurate. Taken together, the findings suggest that NDDs are common and that rates of referral and recognition, at least for ASD and ADHD, appear to be rising. However, research on the current grouping of NDDs is more limited and totally absent in low- and middle-income countries, to the best of our knowledge. That is because the focus remains on single diagnoses, with most research focusing on ASD and ADHD, and higher-income countries.

The rationale for grouping neurodevelopmental disorders

There are several arguments in favor of grouping NDDs although there is no evidence of there being a clear-cut boundary around this group (Box 3.2). The current definition of NDDs provides a concept rather than a clearly defined biological entity or set of entities (Thapar *et al.*, 2017). The first argument for grouping different NDDs together is that these disorders typically onset and manifest early in development. This makes them different from many psychiatric disorders, such as mood disorders and psychosis, that usually onset after puberty (although note that tic disorders do not necessarily present in the early developmental period). However, a recent challenge to this view is that for some individuals, at least with ADHD and possibly social communication deficits, symptoms appear to onset later (Asherson & Agnew-Blais, 2019; Riglin et al., 2021). It is unclear as to whether these later-onset forms are genuine variants of ADHD and ASD and can be considered neurodevelopmental in nature. Alternative explanations are that these late-onset cases are phenocopies, or that NDDs were present from early childhood but were not noticed/impairing due to environmental scaffolding or compensatory mechanisms, only becoming evident when demand outstripped capacity in later life.

Second, a well-recognized feature is that the core characteristics of NDDs show prominent developmental change with maturation; for example, communication and motor difficulties

Box 3.2 Some typical shared features of neurodevelopmental disorders

- Onset in early developmental period
- A steady-state rather than remitting and relapsing symptom course
- Developmental changes in presentation with maturation
- Early cognitive differences, challenges
- Male excess more evident in childhood
- Prominent clinical overlap: comorbidity

tend to improve with age, and motor hyperactivity declines in ADHD. So, do children with NDDs eventually catch-up developmentally? This is plausible given robust evidence that individual development shows enormous variation in its timing (e.g., eruption of teeth, language skills). The maturational lag hypothesis suggests NDDs represent delays in terms of brain development and developmental skills (e.g., language). However, although there is a general tendency for gains in function and less prominent brain differences with increasing age, longitudinal studies have generally failed to observe that NDDs represent a simple maturational lag from which those affected eventually "catch up" in terms of symptoms and functioning with their typically developing peers. Indeed, longer-term follow-up studies suggest that most individuals with any NDD show residual symptoms, differences, or difficulties in adult life (Faraone *et al.*, 2006; Maughan *et al.*, 2009; Tal Saban & Kirby, 2018; Mason *et al.*, 2021; Sibley *et al.*, 2021), although many still achieve good functional outcomes, such as gaining employment and forming meaningful romantic relationships.

A third characteristic relates to the developmental or symptom course of NDDs. NDDs have typically been considered to show a steady-state clinical course rather than one that is characterized by episodes of remission and relapse, like many psychiatric disorders. One exception however is tic disorders, especially Tourette's syndrome where it is well-recognized that waxing and waning with full episodes of remission are common. However, recent research suggests that other NDDs may also show a more fluctuating course than previously realized (Elias & Lord, 2022). For example, two studies from the United States (Sibley *et al.*, 2021; Norman *et al.*, 2023) that followed children with ADHD to adolescence and adult life, suggested that some individuals showed a fluctuating course of symptoms.

A fourth characteristic feature of NDDs is the well-recognized male excess, with a male:female ratio of up to 4:1. One exception is specific learning disorder related to mathematical skills (dyscalculia) (Devine *et al.*, 2013). For NDDs that require specialist assessment and intervention, the sex ratio is much more biased in clinically referred groups of children and adolescents than in the general population or adult clinics. This, taken together with other evidence, suggests that females, at least with ASD or ADHD, tend to present at an older age. Also, there is much greater awareness now that many NDDs in females are missed, misdiagnosed (e.g., as personality disorder, psychosis), or masked by new comorbidities (e.g., depression) that do not respond well to treatment (e.g., antidepressants) because the underlying NDD has not been recognized. Sex differences will be discussed later.

One of the strongest arguments for grouping NDDs, apart from their typical age of onset, is that they show prominent overlap with each other such that comorbidity is the rule rather than the exception (Figure 3.1) (Thapar *et al.*, 2017). The majority of those with one NDD will display features of or meet full diagnostic criteria for another NDD or multiple NDDs. Associated impairments and outcomes—such as learning, communication,

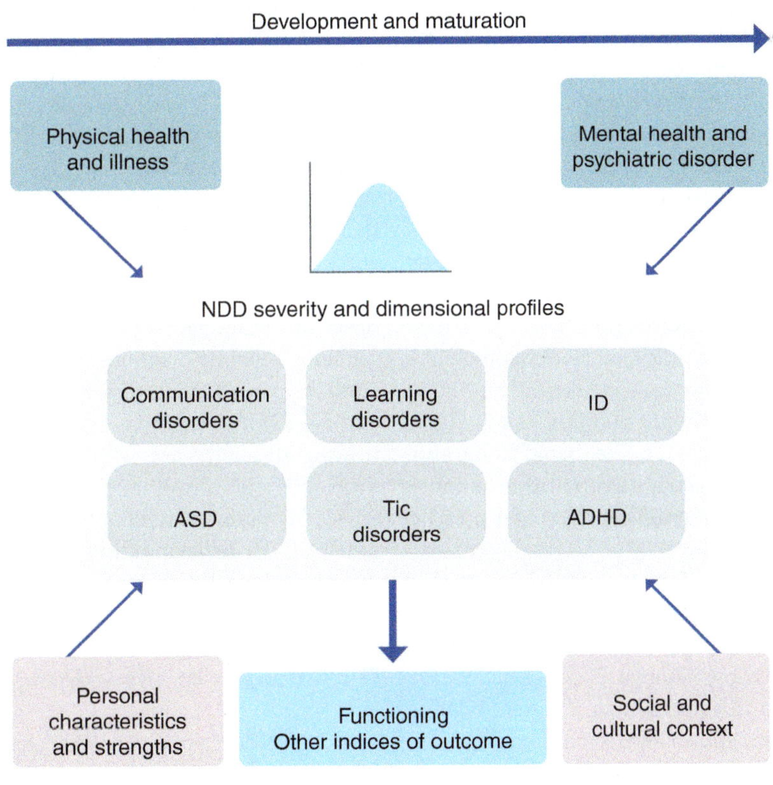

Figure 3.1 Overlaps and complexities of neurodevelopmental disorders (NDDs).

and social difficulties, and underachievement in education and employment—can also be shared across different NDDs. These overlaps suggest potential advantages of services that encompass all NDDs, especially as expertise in their core features and affected domains of functioning (e.g., learning) typically cross disciplinary boundaries (e.g., medical, speech and language, occupational therapy) and professional organizations (e.g., education, health). A shared neurodevelopmental service model has been adopted by some nations and areas of the UK (e.g., Wales, Scotland, and a few areas of England).

A final feature of NDDs that supports their grouping is that many of their risk factors are shared. NDDs are among the most highly heritable of all brain and psychiatric phenotypes (see Chapter 21 on genetics), with reported heritability estimates of between 60% and 95% (Bishop, 2015; Mataix-Cols *et al.*, 2015; Thapar, 2018; Thapar & Rutter, 2021; Lichtenstein *et al.*, 2022). Family and twin studies have shown that the same familial and genetic risks contribute across the different NDDs (Lichtenstein *et al.*, 2010; Faraone *et al.*, 2017; Thapar *et al.*, 2017; Ghirardi *et al.*, 2018). In addition, molecular genetic studies have yielded mainly convergent findings; for example, genome-wide association studies (GWAS) have revealed that small effect size, common gene variants associated with ADHD and ASD are strongly correlated with each other. A large factor analysis of common gene variants associated with multiple different psychiatric disorders and NDDs (ADHD, ASD), also showed that ASD and ADHD separate out into a childhood-onset neurodevelopmental factor (Grotzinger *et al.*, 2022). However, an underpowered GWAS of reading disability showed genetic correlation with ADHD but not with ASD, and also stronger genetic correlation with bipolar disorder and schizophrenia (Gialluisi *et al.*, 2021). It has also long been recognized that rare single gene disorders and syndromes, such as Fragile X syndrome and tuberous sclerosis (see Chapters 26 and 53), increase risk for different and multiple NDDs. More recent research advanced by new technologies (Chapter 21) further shows that other rare gene variants, including rare chromosomal deletions and duplications (copy number variants; CNVs) and damaging variants within genes, contribute risk for multiple different NDDs including intellectual disability (ID, termed intellectual developmental disorder in DSM-5-TR; American Psychiatric Association, 2022), ASD, ADHD, and Tourette's syndrome (Willsey et al., 2017; Maia *et al.*, 2021; Thapar & Rutter, 2021). The shared family and genetic risks not only contribute to comorbidity within an individual but also mean that different family members may present with different NDDs.

NDDs are multifactorial and are not explained by genetic factors alone. In some instances, the same early environmental toxins or stressors, such as preterm birth (Cha *et al.*, 2022) and extreme environmental privation (Sonuga-Barke *et al.*, 2017), appear to be associated with risk for multiple different NDDs. Although many risk factors are shared between different NDDs, thereby providing evidence in favor of grouping them, it is important to recognize that they also disrupt the NDD grouping. That is because risk factors associated with NDDs also contribute to increased risk of different psychiatric disorders, including depression and schizophrenia, as well as physical health conditions (Lee *et al.*, 2021).

In summary, there are empirical and to some extent potentially service-based reasons for grouping NDDs. The prominent clinical overlaps between different NDDs highlight the importance of clinicians, services, and scientists moving beyond a single diagnosis approach. However, we also highlight that, while the NDD grouping may be useful for some purposes, the concept is challenged by other research findings and there are also good reasons to consider NDDs separately for other purposes (e.g., selecting an evidence-based intervention).

The rationale for continuing to split neurodevelopmental disorders

Although there is a rationale for grouping NDDs, it would be premature to dispense with the separate diagnostic categories. First, the predominant and core clinical features of each NDD are very dissimilar (e.g., hyperactivity, tics, motor coordination difficulties, restricted repetitive behaviors, communication impairments). Second, although the main risk factors and correlates of the different NDDs appear to be mainly shared, there are also variations between the individual disorders. For example, a composite measure of ASD common gene risk variants (polygenic score—see Chapter 21) appears to be associated with higher cognitive ability (Clarke *et al.*, 2016), which is not the case for ADHD. There are other differences in risk factor profiles; for example, advanced parental age is associated with ASD (Wu *et al.*, 2017), whereas ADHD is associated with younger parental age (Min *et al.*, 2021). Associations of parental age with other NDDs are inconsistent. Third, as described in the individual disorder chapters (see Chapters 37 and 50–55), while there is some overlap in terms of cognitive and neuroimaging correlates of different NDDs, again these are not the same for each disorder (Tamon *et al.*, 2024). Finally, diagnoses need to have clinical utility, and one of the most important reasons for retaining separate diagnoses is that the same intervention is not effective for all NDDs (see individual disorder chapters 37 and 50–55). For example, educational strategies for those with reading disability are very different from interventions for developmental coordination disorder. Medications that reduce ADHD symptoms are not effective for core features of ASD or other NDDs. Behavioral interventions for tic disorders clearly would not be helpful for other NDDs.

Dimensions or disorders

Although NDDs are diagnosed categorically in DSM-5-TR and ICD-11, some children and adults will show many features of an NDD, yet fall short of the clinical cutoff. This pattern will often be seen in the parents or siblings of a child with a NDD diagnosis because these conditions are heritable. In relation to ASD, this subclinical pattern is sometimes referred to as the "broad autism phenotype." Thus, in terms of their clinical manifestation, most NDDs can be thought of as lying at the extreme of a normal distribution of traits or symptoms. It is important, of course, that a nuanced understanding of NDD is held in mind; not every child with social difficulties is "a bit autistic," and not every child whose mind wanders is "a bit ADHD." These, and other NDDs, encompass multiple facets and interfere with functioning; for example, in ASD, social-communicative difficulties must be accompanied by rigid/repetitive interests and behaviors. Both facets can be measured dimensionally, and will vary in the general population—with those receiving a diagnosis of ASD falling at the extreme on both.

NDDs also behave as dimensions in terms of associations with impairment and adverse outcomes such as poor educational attainment (Thapar *et al.*, 2017). As described in the specific disorder chapters, there is no clear-cut threshold at which impairment and adverse outcomes appear, for most NDDs. In this regard, NDD dimensions are akin to physical health dimensions, such as blood pressure or lipid levels, where there is no distinct, biologically-determined cut-point beyond which adverse consequences arise; hence, thresholds for treatment of high blood pressure and lipid levels have become lower over time and differ between countries.

The dimensional approach to NDDs is supported also by genetic research (see Chapter 21). Twin studies highlight that it is largely the same genetic liability that operates across the population continuum for ASD, ADHD, mild ID and learning problems, with the exception of those with profound and severe ID (Lichtenstein *et al.*, 2022). Although a proportion of those with ASD, ADHD, mild ID, and Tourette's syndrome carry rare genetic variants of high penetrance, for most people their NDDs are due to the contribution of thousands of common alleles, each of tiny effect. The common genetic influences that contribute to diagnosed ASD, ADHD, mild ID, and Tourette's syndrome also contribute to relevant traits in the general population. So, at the phenotypic, epidemiological, and genetic levels of analysis, in most instances NDDs can be seen as quantitatively rather than qualitatively differentiated from typical-range traits underlying these conditions.

However, at the cognitive level, there may be some qualitative distinctions, at least according to some theoretical approaches. For example, an influential account of ASD traces the defining social-communication difficulties to lack of an intuitive "theory of mind," that is the automatic ability to infer what others are thinking. Among the cognitive theories of dyscalculia, some postulate a specific impairment in cognitive systems used to process continuous and discrete magnitudes. However, other theoretical accounts of these conditions propose quantitative differences in, for example, local–global processing biases or visuospatial abilities, respectively. Other NDDs are primarily thought to represent extremes of individual differences in cognitive processing (e.g., phonological processing in dyslexia, executive functioning in ADHD), and some researchers have argued strongly that we should move away from a "core deficits" approach and toward a fully dimensional conception of NDDs (Astle & Fletcher-Watson, 2020).

Sex differences and explanations

As already highlighted, most NDDs are more commonly diagnosed in males than females, with male:female ratios ranging from 1.2:1 to 4:1 (for a useful review see Bölte *et al.*, 2023). For some NDDs, sex ratio changes with age; ADHD, for example, shows a male preponderance in childhood but an almost balanced sex ratio in adulthood (May *et al.*, 2019). As touched on above, this raises the possibility of later diagnosis for females, and indeed it should be considered whether the high male:female ratios reflect, in part, an underrecognition of these conditions in women and girls. This can be illustrated with the case of ASD, which is the NDD where sex differences in diagnosis have perhaps been most scrutinized to date.

Older estimates of the male:female ratio for classic autism were around 4–5:1, with even higher ratios for "Asperger's syndrome" or autism with average or higher IQ (now all encompassed as ASD). However, these were primarily from clinical or special educational needs registers, including only those diagnosed. More recent estimates from epidemiologically ascertained samples, estimate the ratio to be 3:1 (Loomes *et al.*, 2017). They also suggest that, counter to previous reports, this ratio holds across the IQ range; earlier studies suggested fewer females were autistic but that when they were, they were more likely to also have ID compared to males. Together, these changing figures suggest that a large number of autistic women and girls have been missed or misdiagnosed, particularly those with good intellectual functioning. It is possible that similar findings may apply for other NDDs; while communication disorders are more common in boys than girls, for example, they are also more often accompanied by behavioral difficulties in boys, perhaps bringing them to swifter clinical attention. A notable emerging finding in relation to sex/gender is the apparently raised prevalence of some NDDs (e.g., ASD) in gender identity clinics (Thrower *et al.*, 2020), and the greater rate of nonbinary, transgender, and other minority gender identities in NDD populations (see Chapter 40).

Biological explanations for male preponderance

The male preponderance in NDDs, has led to suggestions that males are more vulnerable to early developmental perturbations. Male excess has been hypothesized to reflect genetic, hormonal, and neurotransmitter sex differences during development, as well as the interplay with environmental stressors. The "female protective effect" posits that females require a larger "dose" of whatever etiological factor(s) cause an NDD (often assumed to be largely genetic), compared to males, to manifest

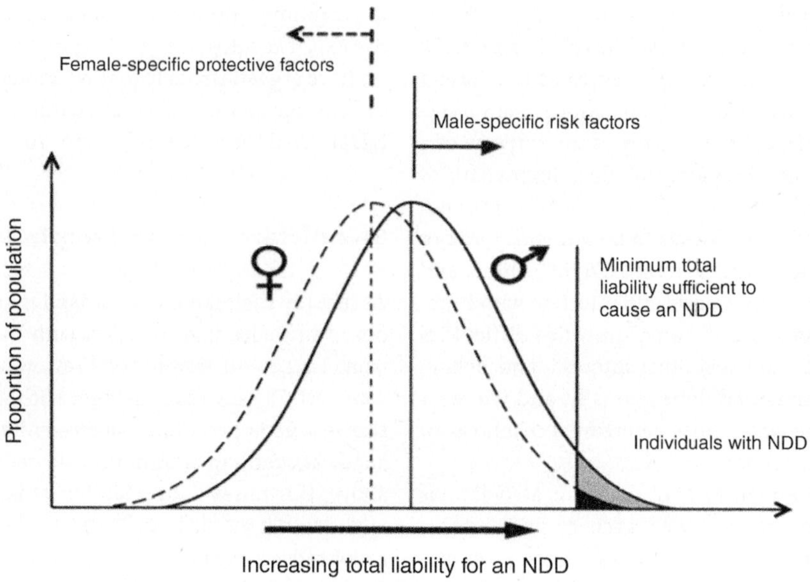

Figure 3.2 The hypothesized female protective effect: differential distribution of liability for a neurodevelopmental disorder (NDD) by sex.

the condition (Figure 3.2). This would provide one possible explanation for the so-called "gender paradox"; more marked symptoms of a disorder in the sex where the prevalence is lower. Evidence in support of this theory for ASD includes genomic findings of a greater burden of rare variants and higher ASD polygenic scores in females versus males diagnosed with ASD (Wigdor *et al.*, 2022). In addition, brothers or sisters of autistic females are more likely than siblings of autistic males to have high autistic trait levels/ASD diagnosis; suggesting a higher genetic burden in the former. The same does not appear to be true for ADHD. Although siblings of girls with ADHD were more likely than siblings of boys with ADHD to also have high ADHD traits/diagnosis in a large twin study (Taylor *et al.*, 2016), the burden of common genetic variants does not appear to be higher in females with ADHD than in males (Martin *et al.*, 2018). Other NDDs have yet to be examined in this way.

Societal and behavioral explanations for male preponderance

For many NDDs, under-recognition in girls and women may contribute to the male preponderance. There are at least five possible explanations for the historical underdiagnosis of NDDs in females. First, much research, at least on ASD and ADHD, has included predominantly or solely male participants—often based on exaggerated male:female estimates and anticipation of small numbers of female participants. This means that much of what we think we know about these disorders is actually what we know about them in boys and men. This research then feeds into diagnostic criteria, tools, and processes, potentially perpetuating the underdiagnosis of females.

Second, many NDDs have been seen as male conditions, and many clinicians, teachers, and even parents carry an implicit gender bias; seeing a boy who is socially awkward we spontaneously think "ASD?", but seeing a socially awkward girl we are more likely to think "social anxiety? Shyness?" This would affect recognition. Also, many teachers and parents may rate and identify NDDs more severely for boys than girls even when objective observations do not differ, at least for ADHD (Meyer *et al.*, 2017).

Third, and related to the former gender bias, "diagnostic overshadowing" happens when clinicians identify one (often sex-stereotype congruent) disorder but do not look beyond this to see the additional, underlying NDD. For example, anorexia nervosa is a commonly "overshadowing" diagnosis in autism; approximately 25% of women attending inpatient clinics for anorexia meet criteria for autism on standardized assessments but most have not received this diagnosis previously. Anxiety and depression are elevated in those with NDDs and can overshadow and delay the diagnosis of relevant NDDs, perhaps particularly for females.

A fourth factor underlying underdiagnosis of some NDDs in females is that some features of these conditions may look somewhat different in women and girls, on average, compared to men and boys. "On average" should be emphasized, as an individual girl may manifest her NDD with the "classic" signs, and an individual boy may show the more atypical manifestations often described in females. To take one example, while a boy's fascination with electricity pylons or vacuum cleaners may raise a red flag for ASD in a clinician's mind, a girl's fascination with a boy band, particular actress, or breed of pony may not seem unusual. However, closer questioning might well reveal that the girl obsessively collects facts about the band or actress, with less desire to see them perform; or is intensely interested in one breed of pony only. A meta-analysis suggests social-communication abilities are, on average, better in ASD girls than boys (mirroring a similar average effect in nonautistic young people) (Wood-Downie *et al.*, 2021). In ADHD, boys are on average more hyperactive than girls, but other differences in presentation are not consistently reported, or have yet to be explored (e.g., in mind-wandering).

Last, recognition of NDDs in females may be hampered by so called "camouflaging" or "masking." These refer to efforts, conscious or unconscious, to hide characteristic traits and behaviors and blend in with neurotypical norms, and have been highlighted first in relation to ASD. Autistic women and girls often describe copying the behavior, dress, and conversation of a neurotypical peer to blend in, or studying social behavior in films or books to practice, plan, and "script" their interactions. Often these efforts to camouflage, which are described as exhausting and eroding sense of self, are prompted by experiences of bullying and stigma. Camouflaging has been associated with poorer mental health and, in qualitative work, possible delayed or underdiagnosis. Whether camouflaging is common in other NDDs has yet to be investigated, although interest in masking and compensating in ADHD and in dyslexia is growing.

Maturation and development across the life span

NDDs are generally conceptualized as manifesting early in development, although recognition and diagnosis may not occur until later in life, or when demands outstrip capacity. ASD and ID have been thought of as lifelong conditions, whereas ADHD and many other NDDs have traditionally been thought to remit in adulthood. However, recent data from multiple follow-up timepoints suggests a fluctuating course in ADHD for most individuals, with only 10% showing sustained remission from ADHD symptoms (Sibley *et al.*, 2021). Long-term follow-up of ADHD and other NDDs, including literacy and language problems, and developmental coordination disorder, suggest signs also persist into adult life (Clegg *et al.*, 2005; Maughan *et al.*, 2009; Kirby *et al.*, 2010). However, NDDs may show changes in their predominant manifestations with maturation, and psychosocial impacts also vary across the life span. For example, a person with developmental coordination disorder may struggle as a child to dress themselves, but as an adult may find shaving or make-up a challenge.

The early developmental period is traditionally an important stage for manifestation of NDDs, but how should we understand the diminishing or even apparent disappearance of many features in later life; do some people "grow out" of their NDD? Or have they developed layers of compensatory strategies and behaviors, to "pass as neurotypical"? To date this has been examined most in ASD (Livingston *et al.*, 2019), where "high compensators" (autistic children who look more neurotypical than would be expected from their characteristic cognitive differences) not only have better executive functioning and intelligence than low compensators, but also self-report more anxiety. Other potential factors that may contribute to apparent improvements include finding suitable social and occupational niches that enable adults to avoid or overcome situations that are more challenging but unavoidable as children (e.g., writing with a pen or spelling correctly in school).

To date, the majority of research on NDDs has focused on children and young people, but with many Western countries having an increasingly aging population, the needs of older adults with NDDs deserve consideration. Recent evidence suggests ADHD symptoms and impairment reduce over the adulthood period from 18 to 60+ years (Vos & Hartman, 2022), while ASD appears to show a similar prevalence throughout adulthood. Both ADHD and ASD appear to be underdiagnosed in adults aged 50 or older (Dobrosavljevic *et al.*, 2020; O'Nions *et al.*, 2023). For example, a recent meta-analysis suggested ADHD diagnosis rates were as low as 0.23% in the over 50s, while prevalence was estimated at 2.2% in population-based studies using symptom scales. A number of NDDs have been linked to age-related cognitive decline; one large population-based study found ADHD was a risk factor for dementia and cognitive impairment, although the link was reduced when comorbid psychiatric disorders were taken into account (Dobrosavljevic *et al.*, 2021). A similar pattern has been reported for ASD (Vivanti *et al.*, 2021), and ID (with or without Down Syndrome) has been associated with earlier and steeper cognitive decline for some time (Strydom *et al.*, 2013). How the features of NDDs change in old age remains a neglected topic for most NDDs.

Challenges and new considerations for researchers and clinicians

Neurodiversity

Interpretation of the term neurodiversity varies considerably, although it is primarily a social justice movement (Sonuga-Barke & Thapar, 2021; Shah *et al.*, 2022). For many, the neurodiversity movement champions replacing the notion of disorder underpinned by dysfunction with the idea that individuals show normative differences in how they learn, interact, think, and behave, and that neurodivergent individuals differ on cognitive and brain dimensions that can be advantageous in some situations and not in others. The term "neurodiversity" was first coined by Australian sociologist Judy Singer (who is autistic and has autistic relatives) in the late 1990s (Singer, 2017). Her thesis focused on ASD with good intellectual functioning and highlighted neurological diversity (as a parallel to ecological diversity)—"neurodiversity"—emphasizing social justice and civil rights.

It is relevant that Singer's work was predated by strong psychoanalytic traditions in the 20th century, including a dominant view that ASD was caused by "refrigerator mothers" where lack of maternal warmth and maternal withdrawal were causes of ASD. Singer recommended a swing from "nurture" to "nature."

The notion that NDDs were psychogenic in origin was increasingly challenged in the later 20th century by research that benefitted from specific symptom criteria. For example, a pioneering twin study (Folstein & Rutter, 1977), showed the major contribution of genetic factors to autism and challenged the "refrigerator mother" psychogenic hypothesis. There followed an explosion of research into the genetic and neurobiological basis of NDDs, which continues to this day.

The social constructionist theory opposes the medical model of NDDs and other disabilities that takes a deficit or dysfunction approach and situates all difficulties in the individual. Instead, this theory proposes that disability is socially constructed entirely by societal barriers, negative attitudes, and exclusions. However, in her thesis, Judy Singer did not agree fully with this view. An important aspect of the neurodiversity movement is that it emphasizes civil rights and justice for individuals with NDDs and moves the clinician away from "curing" deficits to optimizing function. For schools, the workplace, services, and society as a whole, the emphasis shifts from medical or psychological solutions focused on changing the neurodivergent individual, to changing societal attitudes and public expectations, and adapting environments to ensure neurodivergent individuals are fully included and enabled to function optimally. It also changes the emphasis for individuals and their families to one of self-advocacy. This has led to some but not all individuals challenging the notion that they have a disorder, or self-identifying as being neurodivergent without clinical involvement. Our view is that the neurodiversity concept can be helpful for some purposes (e.g., policies, school and workplace, societal attitudes), especially for neurodivergent individuals with lower support needs (Sonuga-Barke & Thapar, 2021). However, we also believe that we cannot dispense with the notion of diagnosis of disorders where an individual's NDD characteristics cause them significant impairment. However, a diagnosis of an NDD should not carry stigma, and the inherent equal value of all human beings is an inalienable right.

Box 3.3 Advantages and limitations of a neurodevelopmental disorder diagnosis

Advantages	Limitations
Communication	Concepts not distinct categorical entities
Transparent definition to enable robust research and replication	Not underpinned by definitive biomarker
Transparent definition to aid decisions on likely effective treatment/intervention	NDDs lie on a continuum
Self-understanding for those with an NDD and their family	Ignores heterogeneity
Access to appropriate information for self-management	Emphasizes core symptoms more than functioning and quality of life
Access to appropriate support	Can be stigmatizing and increase exclusion
Enables connection with others who face similar challenges/feel different	Focuses on deficits rather than differences and strengths

Why we still need diagnoses

There are multiple reasons why we cannot remove the concept of diagnosis completely (Box 3.3). First, using a term that is explicitly defined is crucial for effective communication. Second, for research to be robust, findings require replication; in the absence of robust biomarkers for NDDs, operationalized diagnostic criteria mean that different scientists can attempt to include broadly similar groups of individuals. Third, clinical decisions are mainly categorical yes/no decisions, such as deciding what evidence-based intervention to use and applying clinical guidelines (e.g., medication for ADHD). Fourth, in many countries, a diagnosis often attracts helpful support (e.g., education), funding, and health insurance coverage. Finally, a diagnosis can be helpful toward gaining self-insight and promoting greater understanding in others. It is also needed for accessing appropriate support, reasonable adjustments in the workplace, information, and self-management ideas. Many individuals and families obtain practical and emotional help via support groups, and these currently tend to be focused on single diagnoses. For example, in the United Kingdom this would include organizations such as the Tourette's Association, the ADHD Foundation, and the National Autistic Society, among many others.

Limitations of diagnosis

Despite the advantages of retaining diagnostic terms, there is a wealth of research challenging the way we conceptualize NDDs. Epidemiological, clinical, and genetic studies have repeatedly shown that NDDs lie on a continuum, with disorder/diagnoses lying at one extreme. There appears to be no discontinuity in terms of risk factor profile or outcomes at the diagnostic threshold, with the exception of severe ID. Another key challenge is that every NDD shows marked heterogeneity across a variety of indices. These include the number and severity of core defining symptoms or difficulties, level of functioning, age-at-onset of symptom manifestation or clinical recognition, and comorbidity with other NDDs or mental health disorders. A further source of heterogeneity that may be overlooked is an individual's profile of strengths (Hoogman *et al.*, 2022) (e.g., attentional strengths, creativity) and social context (e.g., family support, social scaffolding) (Clegg *et al.*, 2013). This has led to calls to focus more on a strengths-based approach in research and practice (Astle & Fletcher-Watson, 2020). The multiple types of heterogeneity highlight a major challenge for researchers; results from one sample do not necessarily apply to others. It also highlights flaws where services and support (e.g., educational) are based exclusively on diagnosis rather than a broader profile of functioning and strengths; that is, a person-centered approach.

Overlap with mental health disorders

So far, we have argued the case for why it can be useful to group NDDs but highlighted that the boundaries between different NDDs are not clear-cut. A further challenge is the high rate of comorbidity with mental health conditions (Thapar *et al.*, 2017). It is well-recognized from community and large patient-registry data that individuals with NDDs are at increased risk of anxiety disorders, depression, eating disorders, substance misuse, bipolar disorder, and schizophrenia (Plana-Ripoll *et al.*, 2019; Solberg *et al.*, 2019). Typically, NDD onset predates the manifestation of these disorders, which most commonly manifest from adolescence onwards. Most of this research has focused on ASD, ADHD, and ID, with much less on learning, communication, and motor disorders. A full discussion of overlaps with mental health disorders is considered in each separate diagnosis chapter (see Chapters 57–70). Such prominent comorbidity in part arises from shared genetic factors (Grotzinger *et al.*, 2022). However, the types of environmental risks relevant to elevated mental health disorders (e.g., bullying, victimization) do not appear to be the same early risks thought to predispose to NDDs. Overlaps can also arise if NDDs increase risk for mental health disorders directly or indirectly via social and environmental mechanisms such as social isolation, socioeconomic disadvantage, substance misuse, bullying, and stigma (Thapar *et al.*, 2022).

Attachment, early trauma

A final challenge, especially for clinicians, is when NDD features are accompanied by a history of early trauma (e.g., maltreatment) and disrupted attachment (see Chapters 6, 25, 42, and 57). Is the pattern of current difficulties the result of developmental trauma or NDD? The profile of environmental exposures and relationship/attachment quality is clearly relevant to the package of clinical support and intervention. However, to date, research suggests that although rates of early adversities, including maltreatment, are much higher in children with NDDs, unlike very severe privation as experienced by the Romanian adopted-away orphans, they do not appear to be causal (Dinkler *et al.*, 2017) (see Chapter 13). There is also no evidence to suggest that the choice or effectiveness of an intervention for any NDD depends on presumed etiology (e.g., genetic syndrome, FAS, preterm birth). Although research here is lacking, it is interesting to note that one meta-analysis of adult depression found that depression symptoms improved with standard treatment for depression even where there was a history of childhood trauma (Kuzminskaite *et al.*, 2022). It is also important to note that the question should not be "trauma or NDD?" (since one does not rule out the other), but rather what role have early environment/experiences and in-built neurodivergent differences played in the observed clinical presentation, and what are the treatment implications? As described further in Chapter 42, there is no rationale for clinicians to ask the question—is this trauma/attachment or an NDD? The presence of one does not rule out the possibility of the other and the key tasks are to treat symptom presentations, not presumed etiology that often is unknown.

Conclusions

In this chapter we consider the grouping and concept of NDDs. Our view is that this is a useful grouping but that it is important for clinicians and scientists to recognize that there are no clear-cut biological or clinical boundaries for this grouping, between different NDDs, or between NDDs and mental health disorders.

Although NDDs share some common features, each also has its distinctive features and thus splitting is also required. Moreover, while NDDs lie at the extreme of continuous dimensions, we consider that for many purposes diagnostic categories can still be helpful. However, going forward, several challenges remain. How should clinicians deal with subthreshold diagnoses if NDDs are dimensional in nature? Given the high degree of heterogeneity, what are the optimal methods to capture case complexity and functioning, and inform appropriate interventions? As NDD clinicians and services become increasingly specialized, timely recognition and intervention for comorbid mental health disorders can be problematic (Ono *et al.*, 2019). Another issue is that NDD core symptoms, the profile of functioning, and mental health comorbidities all change with age and maturation. These developmental changes effectively mean that children with NDDs will require regular reassessment. Although persistence is more common than desistance in adult life, the transition to adult services remains a problem in many countries. Developmental change also means that assessment measures and diagnostic criteria for an NDD at one age may not be suitable at other ages; DSM-5/DSM 5-TR has explicitly recognized this for ADHD by requiring fewer symptoms in adult life. A further concern is that some diagnostic criteria may not necessarily be optimally suited for identifying females with NDDs. Finally, we recognize that at times researchers and clinicians may feel they face challenges from the neurodivergent community around attitudes and language used. However, working collaboratively and as equals with neurodivergent people is an important and helpful way forward (Fletcher-Watson *et al.*, 2021) for research and service design.

References

American Psychiatric Association (2013) *Diagnostic and Statistical Manual of Mental Disorders*, 5th edn. American Psychiatric Association, Washington, DC. doi:10.1037/10518-009.

American Psychiatric Association (2022) *Diagnostic and Statistical Manual of Mental Disorders*, 5th edn text revision edn. American

Psychiatric Association, Washington, DC. doi:10.1176/appi.books.9780890425787.

Asherson, P. & Agnew-Blais, J. (2019) Annual research review: does late-onset attention-deficit/hyperactivity disorder exist? *Journal of Child Psychology and Psychiatry* **60**(4), 333–352.

Astle, D.E. & Fletcher-Watson, S. (2020) Beyond the core-deficit hypothesis in developmental disorders. *Current Directions in Psychological Science* **29**, 431–437.

Bishop, D.V.M. (2015) The interface between genetics and psychology: lessons from developmental dyslexia. *Proceedings of the Royal Society. Biological Sciences* **282**, 20143139.

Bölte, S. *et al.* (2023) Sex and gender in neurodevelopmental conditions. *Nature Reviews. Neurology* **19**(3), 136–159.

Bosch, R. *et al.* (2022) Neurodevelopmental disorders among Spanish school-age children: prevalence and sociodemographic correlates. *Psychological Medicine* **52**(14), 3062–3072.

Cha, J.H. *et al.* (2022) Impact of preterm birth on neurodevelopmental disorders in South Korea: a nationwide population-based study. *Journal of Clinical Medicine* **11**, 2476.

Clarke, T.K. *et al.* (2016) Common polygenic risk for autism spectrum disorder (ASD) is associated with cognitive ability in the general population. *Molecular Psychiatry* **21**, 419–425.

Clegg, J. *et al.* (2005) Developmental language disorders—a follow-up in later adult life. Cognitive, language and psychosocial outcomes. *Journal of Child Psychology and Psychiatry* **46**, 128–149.

Clegg, J. *et al.* (2013) Conceptual issues in neurodevelopmental disorders: lives out of synch. *Current Opinion in Psychiatry* **26**(3), 289–294.

Devine, A. *et al.* (2013) Gender differences in developmental dyscalculia depend on diagnostic criteria. *Learning and Instruction* **27**, 31–39.

Dinkler, L. *et al.* (2017) Maltreatment-associated neurodevelopmental disorders: a co-twin control analysis. *The Journal of Child Psychology and Psychiatry and Allied Disciplines* **58**, 691–701.

Dobrosavljevic, M. *et al.* (2020) Prevalence of attention-deficit/hyperactivity disorder in older adults: a systematic review and meta-analysis. *Neuroscience and Biobehavioral Reviews* **118**, 282–289.

Dobrosavljevic, M. *et al.* (2021) Attention-deficit/hyperactivity disorder as a risk factor for dementia and mild cognitive impairment: a population-based register study. *European Psychiatry* **65**(1), 1–19.

Durkin, M.S. (2019) Increasing prevalence of developmental disabilities among children in the US: a sign of progress? *Pediatrics* **144**(4), e20192005.

Elias, R. & Lord, C. (2022) Diagnostic stability in individuals with autism spectrum disorder: insights from a longitudinal follow-up study. *The Journal of Child Psychology and Psychiatry and Allied Disciplines* **63**, 973–983.

Faraone, S.V. *et al.* (2006) The age-dependent decline of attention deficit hyperactivity disorder: a meta-analysis of follow-up studies. *Psychological Medicine* **36**(2), 159–165.

Faraone, S.V. *et al.* (2017) The familial co-aggregation of attention-deficit/hyperactivity disorder and intellectual disability: a register-based family study. *Journal of the American Academy of Child and Adolescent Psychiatry* **56**, 167–174.e1.

Fletcher-Watson, S. *et al.* (2021) Inclusive practices for neurodevelopmental research. *Current Developmental Disorders Reports* **8**. doi:10.1007/s40474-021-00227-z.

Folstein, S. & Rutter, M. (1977) Infantile autism: a genetic study of 21 twin pairs. *Journal of Child Psychology and Psychiatry* **18**, 297–321.

Francés, L. *et al.* (2022) Current state of knowledge on the prevalence of neurodevelopmental disorders in childhood according to the DSM-5: a systematic review in accordance with the PRISMA criteria. *Child and Adolescent Psychiatry and Mental Health* **16**(1), 27.

Ghirardi, L. *et al.* (2018) The familial co-aggregation of ASD and ADHD: a register-based cohort study. *Molecular Psychiatry* **23**, 257–262.

Gialluisi, A. *et al.* (2021) Genome-wide association study reveals new insights into the heritability and genetic correlates of developmental dyslexia. *Molecular Psychiatry* **26**(7), 3004–3017.

Grotzinger, A.D. *et al.* (2022) Genetic architecture of 11 major psychiatric disorders at biobehavioral, functional genomic and molecular genetic levels of analysis. *Nature Genetics* **54**, 548–559.

Hoogman, M. *et al.* (2022) Editorial: looking at it from a different angle: positive aspects and strengths associated with neurodevelopmental disorders. *Frontiers in Psychiatry* **13**, 1111086.

Kanter, A.S. (2014) *The Development of Disability Rights Under International Law: From Charity to Human Rights*, 1st edn. Routledge. doi:10.4324/9780203711712.

Kirby, A. *et al.* (2010) The development and standardization of the adult developmental co-ordination disorders/dyspraxia checklist (ADC). *Research in Developmental Disabilities* **31**, 131–139.

Kuzminskaite, E. *et al.* (2022) Treatment efficacy and effectiveness in adults with major depressive disorder and childhood trauma history: a systematic review and meta-analysis. *The Lancet Psychiatry* **9**, 860–873.

Lee, P.H. *et al.* (2021) Pleiotropy and cross-disorder genetics among psychiatric disorders. *Biological Psychiatry* **89**(1), 20–31.

Lichtenstein, P. *et al.* (2010) The genetics of autism spectrum disorders and related neuropsychiatric disorders in childhood. *The American Journal of Psychiatry* **167**, 1357–1363.

Lichtenstein, P. *et al.* (2022) Familial risk and heritability of intellectual disability: a population-based cohort study in Sweden. *The Journal of Child Psychology and Psychiatry and Allied Disciplines* **63**, 1092–1102.

Livingston, L.A. *et al.* (2019) Compensatory strategies below the behavioural surface in autism: a qualitative study. *The Lancet Psychiatry* **6**, 766–777.

Loomes, R. *et al.* (2017) What is the male-to-female ratio in autism spectrum disorder? A systematic review and meta-analysis. *Journal of the American Academy of Child and Adolescent Psychiatry* **56**(6), 466–474.

Maia, N. *et al.* (2021) Intellectual disability genomics: current state, pitfalls and future challenges. *BMC Genomics* **22**(1), 909.

Martin, J. *et al.* (2018) A genetic investigation of sex bias in the prevalence of attention-deficit/hyperactivity disorder. *Biological Psychiatry* **83**, 1044–1053.

Mason, D. *et al.* (2021) A meta-analysis of outcome studies of autistic adults: quantifying effect size, quality, and meta-regression. *Journal of Autism and Developmental Disorders* **51**, 3165–3179.

Mataix-Cols, D. *et al.* (2015) Familial risks of Tourette syndrome and chronic tic disorders a population-based cohort study. *JAMA Psychiatry* **72**, 787–793.

Maughan, B. *et al.* (2009) Persistence of literacy problems: spelling in adolescence and at mid-life. *Journal of Child Psychology and Psychiatry* **50**, 893–901.

May, T. *et al.* (2019) Sex differences in neurodevelopmental disorders. *Current Opinion in Neurology* **32**(4), 622–626.

Meyer, B.J. *et al.* (2017) Sex differences in the meaning of parent and teacher ratings of ADHD behaviors: an observational study. *Journal of Attention Disorders* **24**, 1847–1856.

Min, X. *et al.* (2021) Parental age and the risk of ADHD in offspring: a systematic review and meta-analysis. *International Journal of Environmental Research and Public Health* **18**(9), 4939.

Morris-Rosendahl, D.J. & Crocq, M.A. (2020) Neurodevelopmental disorders: the history and future of a diagnostic concept. *Dialogues in Clinical Neuroscience* **22**, 65–72.

Müller-Vahl, K.R. *et al.* (2022) European clinical guidelines for Tourette syndrome and other tic disorders: summary statement. *European Child & Adolescent Psychiatry* **31**, 377–382.

Norman, L.J. *et al.* (2023) Longitudinal trajectories of childhood and adolescent attention deficit hyperactivity disorder diagnoses in three cohorts. *eClinicalMedicine* **60**, 102021.

O'Nions, E. *et al.* (2023) Autism in England: assessing underdiagnosis in a population-based cohort study of prospectively collected primary care data. *The Lancet Regional Health Europe* **29**, 100626.

Ono, E. *et al.* (2019) Falling through the cracks: how service gaps leave children with neurodevelopmental disorders and mental health difficulties without the care they need. *British Columbia Medical Journal* **61**, 114–124.

Plana-Ripoll, O. *et al.* (2019) Exploring comorbidity within mental disorders among a Danish national population. *JAMA Psychiatry* **76**, 259–270.

Riglin, L. *et al.* (2021) Variable emergence of autism spectrum disorder symptoms from childhood to early adulthood. *The American Journal of Psychiatry* **178**, 752–760.

Shah, P.J. *et al.* (2022) Neurodevelopmental disorders and neurodiversity: definition of terms from Scotland's national autism implementation team. *The British Journal of Psychiatry* **221**(3), 577–579.

Shoychet, G. (2021) Historical perspectives on neurodevelopmental disorders: the merging of us and them. *Canadian Journal of Undergraduate Research* **6**, 6–10.

Sibley, M.H. *et al.* (2021) Variable patterns of remission from ADHD in the multimodal treatment study of ADHD. *The American Journal of Psychiatry* **179**, 142–151.

Singer, J. (2017) *Neurodiversity: The Birth of an Idea.* Faculty of Humanities and Social Science Sydney: University of Technology Sydney. ISBN 978-0-6481547-0-9

Solberg, B.S. *et al.* (2019) Patterns of psychiatric comorbidity and genetic correlations provide new insights into differences between attention-deficit/hyperactivity disorder and autism spectrum disorder. *Biological Psychiatry* **86**, 587–598.

Sonuga-Barke, E. & Thapar, A. (2021) The neurodiversity concept: is it helpful for clinicians and scientists? *The Lancet Psychiatry* **8**(7), 559–561.

Sonuga-Barke, E.J.S. *et al.* (2017) Child-to-adult neurodevelopmental and mental health trajectories after early life deprivation: the young adult follow-up of the longitudinal English and Romanian adoptees study. *The Lancet* **389**, 1539–1548.

Straub, L. *et al.* (2022) Neurodevelopmental disorders among publicly or privately insured children in the United States. *JAMA Psychiatry* **79**, 232–242.

Strydom, A. *et al.* (2013) Incidence of dementia in older adults with intellectual disabilities. *Research in Developmental Disabilities* **34**(6), 1881–1885.

Tal Saban, M. & Kirby, A. (2018) Adulthood in developmental coordination disorder (DCD): a review of current literature based on ICF perspective. *Current Developmental Disorders Reports* **5**. doi: 10.1007/s40474-018-0126-5

Tamon, H. *et al.* (2024) Shared and specific neural correlates in attention-deficit/hyperactivity disorder and autism spectrum disorder: a meta-analysis of 243 task-based functional MRI studies. *American Journal of Psychiatry* **181**, 541–552.

Taylor, M.J. *et al.* (2016) Is there a female protective effect against attention-deficit/hyperactivity disorder? Evidence from two representative twin samples. *Journal of the American Academy of Child and Adolescent Psychiatry* **55**, 504–512.e2.

Thapar, A. (2018) Discoveries on the genetics of ADHD in the 21st century: new findings and their implications. *The American Journal of Psychiatry* **175**(10), 943–950.

Thapar, A. & Rutter, M. (2021) Genetic advances in autism. *Journal of Autism and Developmental Disorders* **51**(12), 4321–4332.

Thapar, A. *et al.* (2017) Neurodevelopmental disorders. *The Lancet Psychiatry* **4**(4), 339–346.

Thapar, A. *et al.* (2022) Practitioner review: attention-deficit hyperactivity disorder and autism spectrum disorder—the importance of depression. *The Journal of Child Psychology and Psychiatry and Allied Disciplines* **64**(1), 4–15.

Thrower, E. *et al.* (2020) Prevalence of autism spectrum disorder and attention-deficit hyperactivity disorder amongst individuals with gender dysphoria: a systematic review. *Journal of Autism and Developmental Disorders* **50**, 695–706.

Vivanti, G. *et al.* (2021) The prevalence and incidence of early-onset dementia among adults with autism spectrum disorder. *Autism Research* **14**(10), 2189–2199.

Vos, M. & Hartman, C.A. (2022) The decreasing prevalence of ADHD across the adult lifespan confirmed. *Journal of Global Health* **12**, 03024.

Wigdor, E.M. *et al.* (2022) The female protective effect against autism spectrum disorder. *Cell Genomics* **2**(6), 100134.

Willsey, A.J. *et al.* (2017) De novo coding variants are strongly associated with Tourette disorder. *Neuron* **94**(3), 486–499.

Wood-Downie, H. *et al.* (2021) Research review: a systematic review and meta-analysis of sex/gender differences in social interaction and communication in autistic and nonautistic children and adolescents. *Journal of Child Psychology and Psychiatry* **62**(8), 922–936.

World Health Organization (2015) *The International Classification of Diseases 11th Revision* [online]. WHO, Geneva, Switzerland. Available: https://icd.who.int/en [20 July 2024].

Wu, S. *et al.* (2017) Advanced parental age and autism risk in children: a systematic review and meta-analysis. *Acta Psychiatrica Scandinavica* **135**, 29–41.

CHAPTER 4

Conceptual issues and empirical challenges in relation to disruptive and challenging behavior

Essi Viding[1] and Stephane De Brito[2]

[1] Division of Psychology and Language Sciences, University College London, UK

[2] School of Psychology, Centre for Human Brain Health, Institute for Mental Health, Centre for Developmental Science, Centre for Neurogenetics, University of Birmingham, UK

Introduction

Disruptive and challenging behavior (DCB) has been conceptualized in different ways across the fields of psychiatry, developmental psychopathology, and criminology in their attempts to understand its development and etiology. As a result, the measurement and outcome measures that have been used across those disciplines to research DCB have differed quite substantially (Loeber *et al.*, 2009).

In psychiatry, where the focus is on diagnoses, conceptualized as distinct categories or entities, DCB that persists and impacts a child's social and educational functioning is classified in the *Diagnostic and Statistical Manual of Mental Disorders* 5th edition, text revision (DSM-5-TR) under disruptive, impulse-control, and conduct disorders (CD) and under disruptive behavior or dissocial disorders in the *International Classification of Diseases* 11th edition (ICD-11). The most common of these disorders are oppositional defiant disorder (ODD) and CD and they have also received the most research attention. ODD and CD are characterized by an antagonistic and irritable disposition and behaviors that violate social norms and the rights of others (World Health Organization, 2018; American Psychiatric Association, 2022) (see Chapter 64).

In contrast to psychiatry, developmental psychopathology is not concerned with traditional diagnostic classification and instead posits that (i) there are individual differences in the qualitative and quantitative aspects of psychopathology, and that (ii) these differences may manifest and evolve over the course of development (Loeber *et al.*, 2009). For example, decades of research have examined the development of aggression and shown that it peaks in early childhood to then decrease over the course of development, but there are important interindividual differences in the quantity, as well as quality of aggressive behavior (e.g., reactive[1] versus instrumental[2] aggression) (Lansford, 2018; Girard *et al.*, 2019).

Finally, in criminology DCB is conceptualized as delinquent acts; that is behaviors that breach criminal laws. This includes various forms of property crime including theft and breaking and entering, as well as violent crime such as rape and sexual assault, robbery, assault, and murder (Liebling *et al.*, 2017). The primary methods employed to assess DCB in criminological studies involve using official records of criminal behavior and self-reported measures of delinquency (Liebling *et al.*, 2017). From a developmental perspective, it is important to highlight two different, yet related, robust findings in this field. First, the age–crime curve reflects the fact that the association between age and criminal DCB follows an asymmetrical bell-shaped pattern such that the prevalence of crime, represented by the percentage of offenders in a population, tends to rise from late childhood, reaches its highest point during the teenage years (around 15–19 years), and subsequently decreases from the early 20s until late adulthood (Tremblay & Nagin, 2005). Second, the peak of the age–crime curve is thought to reflect the presence of two subgroups of offenders with different developmental trajectories: life-course persistent offenders (whose antisocial behavior (ASB) has early-onset and persists) and adolescent-limited offenders (whose ASB begins during adolescence and often decreases after that period) (Moffitt, 1993).

In this chapter we will discuss DCB drawing primarily on the developmental psychopathology perspective as we take a life-course approach that does not rely on diagnosis or criminal

[1] Aggression underpinned by negative affect, in response to threat, frustration, or social provocation.

[2] Aggression that involves the planned execution of aggression for a particular goal (e.g., acquisition of goods).

Rutter's Child and Adolescent Psychiatry and Psychology, Seventh Edition.
Edited by Anita Thapar, Daniel S. Pine, Samuele Cortese, Cathy Creswell, Tamsin J. Ford, James F. Leckman, and Argyris Stringaris.

Companion website: www.wiley.com/go/thapar/rutterspsych7

records. Historically, there has been an emphasis on examining DCB as a sociological phenomenon, with focus on societal, socioeconomic, and family factors associated with DCB. Prominent examples of such research include seminal criminological theories positing that DCB is a normal response of individuals to abnormal conditions (Shaw & McKay, 1942) and influential work by Patterson and colleagues on social learning and "coercive cycles," emphasizing the role of family social environmental factors in maintaining DCB (Butler *et al.*, 2020). The sociological framework for examining DCB partly stems from the urge to consider DCB as a "societal problem," rather than a disorder, so as not to stigmatize the child or medicalize their behavior. This approach has led to the development of effective parenting programs that are the gold standard for addressing DCB in children, but although such programs have a strong evidence base in reducing DCB, they do not work equally well for every child and family. Moreover, some have argued that focusing on the role of the environment can make parents feel like they are being judged (Butler *et al.*, 2020; Beelmann *et al.*, 2023).

More recently, there have been calls to recognize the neurodevelopmental nature of DCB and to examine different neurodevelopmental risk presentations that have the potential to explain heterogeneity among children with DCB and to inform treatment approaches (Blair *et al.*, 2014; Wakschlag *et al.*, 2018; Viding & McCrory, 2020) (Box 4.1). The contribution of child and parent neurocognitive profiles to intervention success is being increasingly recognized and investigated (Fleming *et al.*, 2022; Zhang *et al.*, 2023). Although DCB is typically pitted against emotional disorders in developmental psychology research (comparison of "externalizing" and "internalizing" disorders), some of the neurodevelopmental vulnerabilities associated with DCB are also associated with emotional disorders (Wakschlag *et al.*, 2018; Viding & McCrory, 2020). Furthermore, at the behavioral level it is clear that DCB symptoms are not just a feature of disruptive, impulse-control, and conduct disorders, but are also a prominent feature of other childhood conditions, including neurodevelopmental disorders (NDDs) such as attention deficit hyperactivity disorder (ADHD) and autism spectrum disorder (ASD) (Kaat & Lecavalier, 2013; Demontis *et al.*, 2021). These findings highlight the need to situate research into DCB within a transdiagnostic, developmental, transactional framework. Within such a framework, we would expect DCB to be associated with transdiagnostic vulnerability mechanisms (both neurodevelopmental and social) that are shared with a number of disorders. We should also expect both equifinality and multifinality (the latter also known as heterotypic continuity in developmental psychopathology research) (Cicchetti & Rogosch, 1996) (see also Chapters 1 and 23 for an extensive discussion of these concepts). This means that similar behavioral profiles can be the product of different causal pathways (equifinality). It also means that similar neurodevelopmental vulnerabilities may lead to different outcomes over time (multifinality) (Figure 4.1). This ties in with what we know about seemingly different triggers for DCB in different individuals, different comorbidity profiles, and the fact that DCB may not only develop into persistent ASB, but may also be a precursor to other symptom profiles such as depressive symptomatology (heterotypic continuity) (Kim-Cohen *et al.*, 2003). In such a framework DCB should not be viewed as a product of something either intrinsic or extrinsic to the child, but instead as an emergent phenomenon that results from the iterative unfolding of neurodevelopment within a relational context (Viding & McCrory, 2020; Viding *et al.*, 2023).

Box 4.1 Neurodevelopmental risk for disruptive and challenging behavior

Neurodevelopmental disorders (NDDs) are conditions that begin in infancy or childhood, potentially even during prenatal life (Raine, 2018) (see also Chapter 3 for a detailed discussion on NDDs). They are characterized by abnormalities in brain development that can impact brain structure or function throughout an individual's life. Such disorders are associated with neurocognitive deficits, have an origin that is partly genetic, follow a relatively stable course across one's life span, and are associated with poorer adult outcomes across multiple domains.

Some individuals with DCB meet all these criteria for NDDs, while others may only experience problems in childhood, which they eventually "grow out" of. There is a compelling argument for childhood-onset, persistent CD, also known as "life course persistent antisocial behaviour," to be considered an NDD (Fairchild *et al.*, 2019). Further evidence supporting the view of CD as an NDD includes its moderate heritability (with higher heritability in cases with callous-unemotional (CU) traits), its overlap with other "neurodevelopmental" disorders in terms of genetic liability (e.g., ADHD and ASD), its association with abnormalities in brain structure and function, its strong links with neuropsychological deficits (especially in emotion processing), and its poor prognosis in adulthood (Fairchild *et al.*, 2019).

NDDs emerge because of diverse risk factors that can disrupt various phases of brain maturation (Khodosevich & Sellgren, 2023). The interplay of these risk factors shapes the phenotype seen in adulthood. Because of the intricate nature of human brain development and the wide range of potential disruptions, the resulting neurodevelopmental profiles of DCB and underlying mechanisms are likely to vary significantly across the spectrum of DCB (see Chapter 3 and Khodosevich and Sellgren (2023) for detailed discussions).

Disruptive and challenging behavior: the need for more funding and advocacy

DCB is concurrently and prospectively associated with enormous personal, societal, and economic costs across the life span (Fairchild *et al.*, 2019) (see also Chapter 64). For example, we know that untreated CD can develop into a full-blown diagnosis of antisocial personality disorder (ASPD) (what we would call homotypic continuity in developmental psychopathology). Indeed, a diagnosis of CD by age 15 is a prerequisite for receiving an ASPD diagnosis (American Psychiatric Association, 2013). Furthermore, CD in childhood also increases the risk of many other poor physical and mental health outcomes (Fairchild *et al.*, 2019). This calls for substantial efforts and funding for research, prevention, and treatment to mitigate the costs

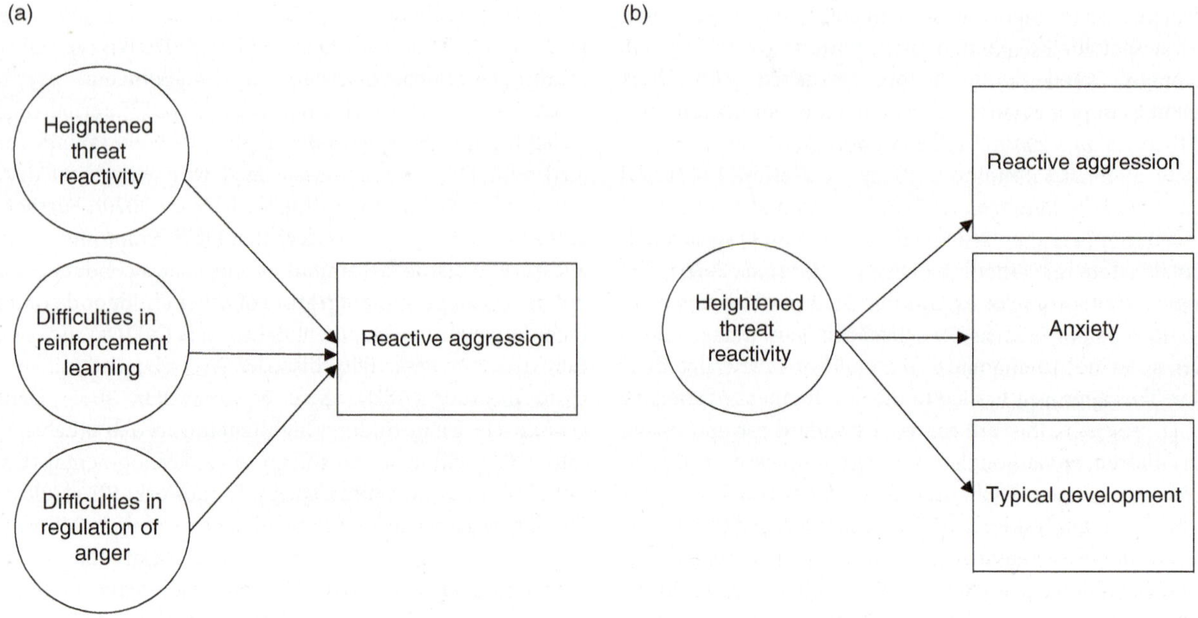

Figure 4.1 (a) A simplified representation of equifinal pathways to reactive aggression, a common form of disruptive and challenging behavior (DCB). Here three different types of cognitive–affective process are shown to underlie increased risk for reactive aggression. Heightened threat reactivity may lead to an aggressive "fight response" in individuals who interpret a particular situation as threatening. Difficulties in reinforcement learning may lead to errors in predicting outcomes and subsequent frustration can lead to aggression. Finally, difficulties in regulating anger can cause an individual to react aggressively. Some individuals may have difficulties in more than one of these cognitive–affective processes and they are thought to interact with other cognitive–affective features and social environmental inputs over development. (b) A simplified representation of multifinal pathways from "heightened threat reactivity" to different outcomes. Heightened threat reactivity has not only been linked with reactive aggression, but also with clinical levels of anxiety. There are also TD individuals who do have heightened threat reactivity, but who do not display DCB or other symptoms at clinically concerning levels. Other cognitive–affective features, as well as social environment, are likely to influence how heightened threat reactivity canalizes over time.

associated with DCB. Despite the high prevalence of DCB and the robust evidence supporting the association between DCB and poor outcomes, disruptive behavior disorders are not discussed in funding reports such as *The Anatomy of NIMH Funding* in the United States or *Mental Health Research Funding* in the United Kingdom (Fairchild *et al.*, 2019). This is baffling, as DCB are associated with the highest burden for mental health disorders in children aged 0–14 years and the fourth highest in youth aged 15–24 (GBD 2019 Mental Disorders Collaborators, 2022). As an example, a recent report from the International Alliance of Mental Health Research Funders showed that CD only receives 0.4% of the US$3.7 billion global mental health budget (Woelbert *et al.*, 2020). The underfunding of research and clinical provision for disruptive behavior disorders needs to be addressed if we are to reduce the societal impact of DCB and make progress in helping children and young people (CYP) who display these behaviors (Burt *et al.*, 2018; Fairchild *et al.*, 2019).

The reasons for the relative neglect of disruptive behavior disorders—even compared to already meager mental health funding for other conditions—are not clear. One possible explanation is the tendency to view DCB as a sociological phenomenon, a response to particular family and community circumstances—something that does not belong to the mental health sphere. Linked with this view is the reluctance to label children, to avoid any potential risk of stigmatizing them. This is a reasonable concern, but one that will not be addressed by simply not researching or treating CYP with DCB. Indeed, CYP with DCB who do not receive the support they need, almost invariably behave in ways that end up stigmatizing them among their peers and adults. There is also no doubt that CYP with DCB have not traditionally enjoyed the level of advocacy seen for other conditions, such as ASD or depression. This is likely due to several interlinked factors, including challenging family circumstances and perceived parenting blame attached to DCB, which may reduce the ability and willingness of family members to lobby for visibility and funding. Furthermore, CYP with DCB do not always elicit sympathy due to the very nature of their behavior and there has also been a tendency to view DCBs as a matter for the criminal justice system, rather than mental health services (Burt *et al.*, 2018; Fairchild *et al.*, 2019).

Current conceptualizations of disruptive and challenging behavior

DSM-5-TR recognizes several disruptive, impulse-control, and conduct disorders, including ODD, CD, and intermittent explosive disorder. ODD is characterized by resistance to authority figures and irritable disposition. CD is defined by disregard for social norms and the rights of others, including serious aggression. A child or adolescent may earn an ODD or CD diagnosis through many different symptom combinations and these need not be overlapping for two children who receive the same diagnosis (Nock *et al.*, 2006) (see a comprehensive overview of research related to ODD and CD diagnoses in Chapter 64). The heterogeneity seen among those diagnosed with CD and ODD likely partly reflects the many different trait dimensions that increase the risk of DCB. Two such dimensions, callous–unemotional (CU) traits and irritability, have received substantial attention in the past decades (Wakschlag *et al.*, 2018) and will be considered in some detail in this chapter. It is worth noting that both noncompliance (also known as defiance, or rule-breaking) and aggression have also been identified as dimensions of DCB (Loeber & Schmaling, 1985; Wakschlag *et al.*, 2018). However, there is currently a lack of evidence base at multiple levels of explanations for noncompliance, while aggression lacks clinical specificity and its different forms have been linked to both CU traits (proactive aggression and reactive aggression) and irritability (reactive aggression).

CU traits reflect a lack of empathy and guilt combined with a shallow affect, the callous use of others for one's own gain, and a lack of concern about one's own performance in important activities. Two decades of research have shown that elevated levels of CU traits in youth with CD or ODD designate a particularly severe subgroup of youth with a distinct etiology and a more severe, aggressive, and stable pattern of ASB (De Brito *et al.*, 2021). As a result, a CU traits-based "limited prosocial emotions" specifier for the diagnoses of CD (DSM-5 and ICD-11) and ODD (ICD-11) has been included in the most recent incarnation of the two major psychiatric classification systems (Frick *et al.*, 2014; De Brito *et al.*, 2021). It has been estimated that in community samples between 10–46% of youth with CD have high levels of CU traits, while in clinical samples it is thought that between 21–50% of youth with CD have elevated levels of CU traits (Rowe *et al.*, 2010; Kahn *et al.*, 2012; De Brito *et al.*, 2021). There is also evidence suggesting that CU traits might be useful for distinguishing subgroups of youth with DCB beyond CD and ODD, such as among those with ADHD and ASD (Rogers *et al.*, 2006; Frick *et al.*, 2014; Tye *et al.*, 2017; Zhang *et al.*, 2021a).

Irritability refers to interindividual differences in proneness to anger, which may reach a pathological extent if it causes significant impairment or distress in daily life (Vidal-Ribas *et al.*, 2016). Irritability can be elicited by abnormal reactions to frustration or perceived danger (Leibenluft, 2017) and includes both mood (i.e., tonic) and behavioral (i.e., phasic) components. In DSM-IV-TR (American Psychiatric Association, 2000), irritability was a core symptom of ODD, depression, and anger dysregulation disorders, such as intermittent explosive disorder (see Chapters 5, 62, and 64). In DSM-5 irritable presentation is included as a defining feature of disruptive mood dysregulation disorder (Vidal-Ribas *et al.*, 2016) and irritability symptoms also feature in the ODD diagnosis. Epidemiological data from community samples suggest a prevalence of up to 9% for extreme irritability (Althoff *et al.*, 2016; Mayes *et al.*, 2016).

CU and irritability appear to predispose to at least partly distinct types of DCB (Kaat *et al.*, 2015; Waschbusch *et al.*, 2020). CU traits are associated with both pre-mediated, instrumental aggression (i.e., aggression that is planned for a specific purpose/goal) and reactive aggression, whereas irritability has been more strongly associated with reactive aggression (Kaat *et al.*, 2015; Blair, 2018; Waschbusch *et al.*, 2020). Recent data also suggest that CU traits are uniquely linked to lower expectations of feeling remorse and empathy for victims following aggression, as well as reduced concern about being punished and causing harm to the victim (Elowsky *et al.*, 2022). In contrast, irritability is uniquely and positively associated with expectations and concerns about using aggression as a means of establishing dominance and gaining respect (Elowsky *et al.*, 2022). In line with the behavioral findings, DCBs coupled with CU traits versus irritability are associated with at least partly distinguishable neural and information processing atypicalities (see the section on 'The origins of DCB at different levels of explanation' in this chapter) (Elowsky *et al.*, 2022).

DCB and related traits (CU traits and irritability) often co-occur with depression, anxiety, ADHD, and ASD symptoms (Kaat & Lecavalier, 2013; Demontis *et al.*, 2021). This may be explained by particular features increasing the risk of DCB. For example, those with elevated levels of ADHD symptoms often make impulsive decisions, which may lead to unanticipated outcomes and cause frustration-based aggression. CYP with ASD may display substantial temper tantrums as a result of being intolerant to changes in routines. Common, transdiagnostic neurodevelopmental vulnerability factors may also explain comorbidity (e.g., threat reactivity can predispose to both reactive aggression and anxiety) (Bubier & Drabick, 2009). Finally, DCB itself can lead to development of other features, such as anxiety (Roza *et al.*, 2003; Bubier & Drabick, 2009). The accumulating evidence for shared etiological processes between what are traditionally considered to be distinct features or conditions (Caspi & Moffitt, 2018; Allegrini *et al.*, 2022) provides a strong case for a more dimensional approach to studying and treating DCB.

The origins of disruptive and challenging behavior at different levels of explanation

Genetic factors

Research using twin and adoption designs has demonstrated that genetics play a significant role in DCB, with heritability estimates ranging from 40–50% (Salvatore & Dick, 2018; Wesseldijk *et al.*, 2018). The traits associated with DCB (CU traits and irritability) are moderately to strongly heritable, with estimates ranging from 30% to nearly 80% (Vidal-Ribas *et al.*, 2016; Moore *et al.*, 2019). Evidence suggests that the heritability of DCB may vary depending on specific subtypes.

For instance, DCB in combination with high CU traits appears higher in heritability than DCB alone (Viding *et al.*, 2005, 2008). There is also evidence indicating that distinct genetic risk factors may influence the initial risk and developmental course of (ASB), and the same applies to CU traits and irritability (Pingault *et al.*, 2015; Roberson-Nay *et al.*, 2015; Takahashi *et al.*, 2021). Studies investigating the genetic overlap between DCB and CU traits have demonstrated both shared and unique genetic influences, with about half of the genetic variance shared between conduct problems and CU traits (Viding *et al.*, 2007; Saunders *et al.*, 2019). There is also some indication of over half of the genetic variance shared between delinquency and irritability, and conduct problems and anger/frustration—a construct related to irritability (Deater-Deckard *et al.*, 2007; Stringaris *et al.*, 2012). A meta-analysis examining genetic overlap between disruptive behavior and neurodevelopmental symptomatology found strong genetic overlap between disruptive behavior disorder features and ADHD symptoms (genetic correlation of 0.66), but a more modest genetic overlap with ASD symptoms (genetic correlation of 0.35) (Gidziela *et al.*, 2023). A recent empirical study that focused on the degree to which phenotypic correlations between variables were explained by genetic factors, reported that over half of the covariance between depression, conduct problems, and ADHD symptomatology was accounted for by shared genetic risk (Waszczuk *et al.*, 2021). Finally, a modest genetic overlap with DCB and anxiety has been reported (less than one-third shared genetic variance) (Gregory *et al.*, 2004). Overall, these findings point to genetic liability to DCB that is partly shared with other psychopathology, as well as some specific genetic liability, which may influence the precise phenotypic expression and the types of DCB someone engages in. The molecular genetic research into DCB is not as advanced as for other psychiatric phenotypes. However, a recent study utilizing multivariate genome-wide association meta-analyses implicated neurodevelopmental genes, that have also been associated with broader psychiatric risk, in the development of DCB (Baselmans *et al.*, 2021).

Environmental factors

Approximately half of the variability in DCB can be attributed to environmental factors. Studies have identified associations with prenatal factors, such as maternal smoking, alcohol use, drug use, and stress during pregnancy, as well as with perinatal factors, such as obstetric complications, parental psychopathology, malnutrition, and exposure to heavy metals (Raine *et al.*, 1997; Simonoff *et al.*, 2004; Liu, 2011; Barker *et al.*, 2012; Lukkari *et al.*, 2012). Maladaptive parenting (including harsh, coercive, and inconsistent discipline) and childhood maltreatment have also been linked to the development of DCB (Jaffee *et al.*, 2012; Johnson *et al.*, 2017). Neighborhood risk factors, such as exposure to deviant peers, low socioeconomic status, poverty, and community violence, are also significant distal environmental factors (Piotrowska *et al.*, 2015; Kersten *et al.*, 2017; Jennings *et al.*, 2018). Many of the same risk factors that contribute to DCB have also been linked to the development of CU traits and irritability (as well as other forms of psychiatric symptomatology), including prenatal maternal stress, child maltreatment, harsh parental discipline, negative parental emotions, maternal depression, disorganized parent–child attachment, and disrupted family functioning (Vidal-Ribas *et al.*, 2016; De Brito *et al.*, 2021). Environmental risk factors may operate differently in CYP with DCB and high versus low levels of CU traits. For instance, poor parental monitoring and supervision are more strongly associated with DCB coupled with high levels of CU traits, rather than DCB with low levels of CU traits (Roberts *et al.*, 2022), although the direction of causality is not clear.

Gene–environment interplay

Many of the risk factors that have traditionally been thought of as purely environmental are in part shaped by people's genetic propensities. For this reason, we cannot assume causality between particular environmental risk factors and child DCB and have to be mindful of potential genetic confounding (Moffitt 2005; Jaffee *et al.*, 2012). This has indeed been shown, for example, for the association between maternal smoking and child DCB—an example of passive gene–environment correlation (Rice *et al.*, 2009). Children with DCB may also evoke more harsh parenting (evocative gene–environment correlation) or may actively seek out particular environments, such as delinquent peers (active gene–environment correlation) (Moffitt 2005; Jaffee *et al.*, 2012). Children with different genetic risk factors can also react differently to specific environmental factors, a phenomenon known as gene–environment interaction (Knopik *et al.*, 2017). Studies on adoptees have shown that the effects of parental risks, such as having an adoptive parent who is a criminal, on the development of DCB were more pronounced in genetically vulnerable individuals (i.e., those with a criminal biological parent) than in adoptees without a genetic predisposition (Cloninger *et al.*, 1982). Additionally, warm parenting from adoptive mothers has been found to buffer the effects of heritable risk for DCB and CU traits (Hyde *et al.*, 2016).

Cognitive–affective processes

CYP with DCB exhibit deficits in facial and vocal emotion recognition, empathy, decision-making, and reinforcement learning compared to typically developing (TD) youth (Fairchild *et al.*, 2019). Three meta-analyses published over the past decade across preschool, child, and adolescent samples have further shown that CYP with DCB exhibit moderate impairment in executive functions (Ogilvie *et al.*, 2011; Schoemaker *et al.*, 2013; Bonham *et al.*, 2021), including inhibition, working memory, and cognitive flexibility and these deficits appear most pronounced in those individuals whose DCB start early and persist across the life course (Moffitt & Caspi, 2001).

Existing experimental work suggests that CU traits and irritability are each associated with distinct patterns of responses during emotion and reward processing tasks. Studies examining emotional processing in CYP with DCB have consistently found that CU traits are associated with reduced recognition and orientation toward visual and vocal emotional expressions, in particular fear, but also sadness and happiness (Dawel *et al.*, 2012; Fanti *et al.*, 2016). By contrast, irritability in CYP with DCB has been associated with abnormal threat processing, particularly in the form of attention-related bias (rapid and preferential orientation toward angry versus neutral faces) (Brotman *et al.*, 2017). Relatedly, irritability has also been associated with a hostile attributional bias in ambiguous situations (i.e., judging neutral faces as more hostile and reporting being more fearful of them) and superior ability to recognize anger in ambiguous facial stimuli (Brotman *et al.*, 2017). Both CU traits and irritability have been associated with atypicalities in motivational value attached to rewards and in reinforcement learning, although the precise nature of the atypicalities may vary between those with high levels of CU traits and those with high levels of irritability (Brotman *et al.*, 2017; De Brito *et al.*, 2021). DCB, coupled with high levels of CU traits, has been associated with lower motivational salience of rewards (Roose *et al.*, 2010, 2011; Byrd *et al.*, 2018) and difficulties integrating and utilizing punishment feedback to inform their future actions (Finger *et al.*, 2008; Byrd *et al.*, 2014). Irritability has been associated with increased sensitivity to the receipt of rewards (Brotman *et al.*, 2017) and with deficits in learning from both reward and punishment contingencies (Brotman *et al.*, 2017).

The pattern of cognitive–affective functioning seen in CYP with high levels of CU traits can offer clues as to what underlies their DCB. Atypical processing of other's distress is thought to underlie their lack of empathy and remorse. Atypical motivational value attached to rewards may help explain unconcern about performance (one of the criteria for the "limited prosocial emotions" specifier in DSM-5-TR Conduct Disorder diagnosis) and failure to integrate punishment feedback may lead to consequences that are unexpected by a child and result in frustration-based aggression. The hostile attributional bias and hypersensitivity to angry facial expression are thought to underpin the increased propensity for threat-based reactive aggression in individuals with irritability. Increased sensitivity to the receipt of rewards coupled with a compromised ability to shift attention control during the nonreceipt of rewards may increase the risk of frustration-based reactive aggression seen in this group of children with DCB.

Brain function and structure

The majority of functional magnetic resonance imaging (fMRI) studies on DCB have focused on CD and have examined emotion processing through tasks that involve viewing emotional images, facial expressions of emotion, or empathy-inducing stimuli. Meta-analyses on this body of evidence have shown that, compared to TD controls, CYP with DCB exhibit lower activation of the dorsal and rostral anterior cingulate cortex (ACC), medial prefrontal cortex, temporal cortex, insular cortex, ventral striatum, and amygdala in tasks indexing emotion processing and reinforcement-based decision-making (Figure 4.2) (Alegria *et al.*, 2016; Berluti *et al.*, 2023). Meta-analytical evidence also indicates that high levels of CU traits are associated with reduced activation in the amygdala and cortical regions (e.g., anterior insula and ventromedial prefrontal cortex, fusiform gyrus) in tasks indexing the processing of negative faces or pain (Dugré *et al.*, 2020; De Brito *et al.*, 2021; Aggensteiner *et al.*, 2022). By contrast, a recent meta-analysis of 28 fMRI studies examining irritability in CYP did not find clear functional brain correlates of irritability (Lee *et al.*, 2023). Finally, two recent fMRI studies that have considered simultaneously the influence of CU traits and irritability have shown that CU traits are associated with reduced brain response during both threat processing and reinforcement learning, while irritability is associated with increased brain response to threat, but

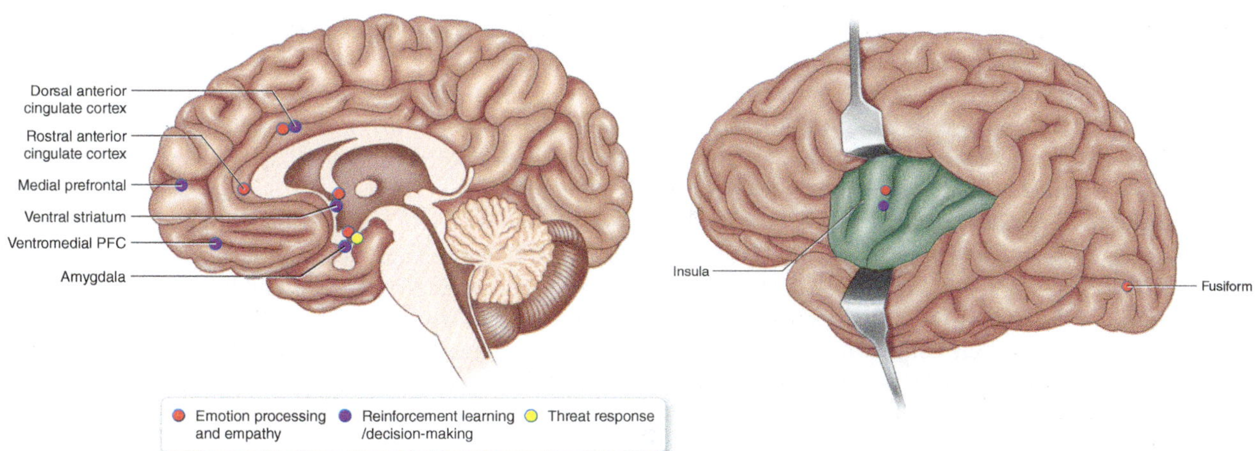

Figure 4.2 Functional brain abnormalities associated with disruptive and challenging behavior (DCB).

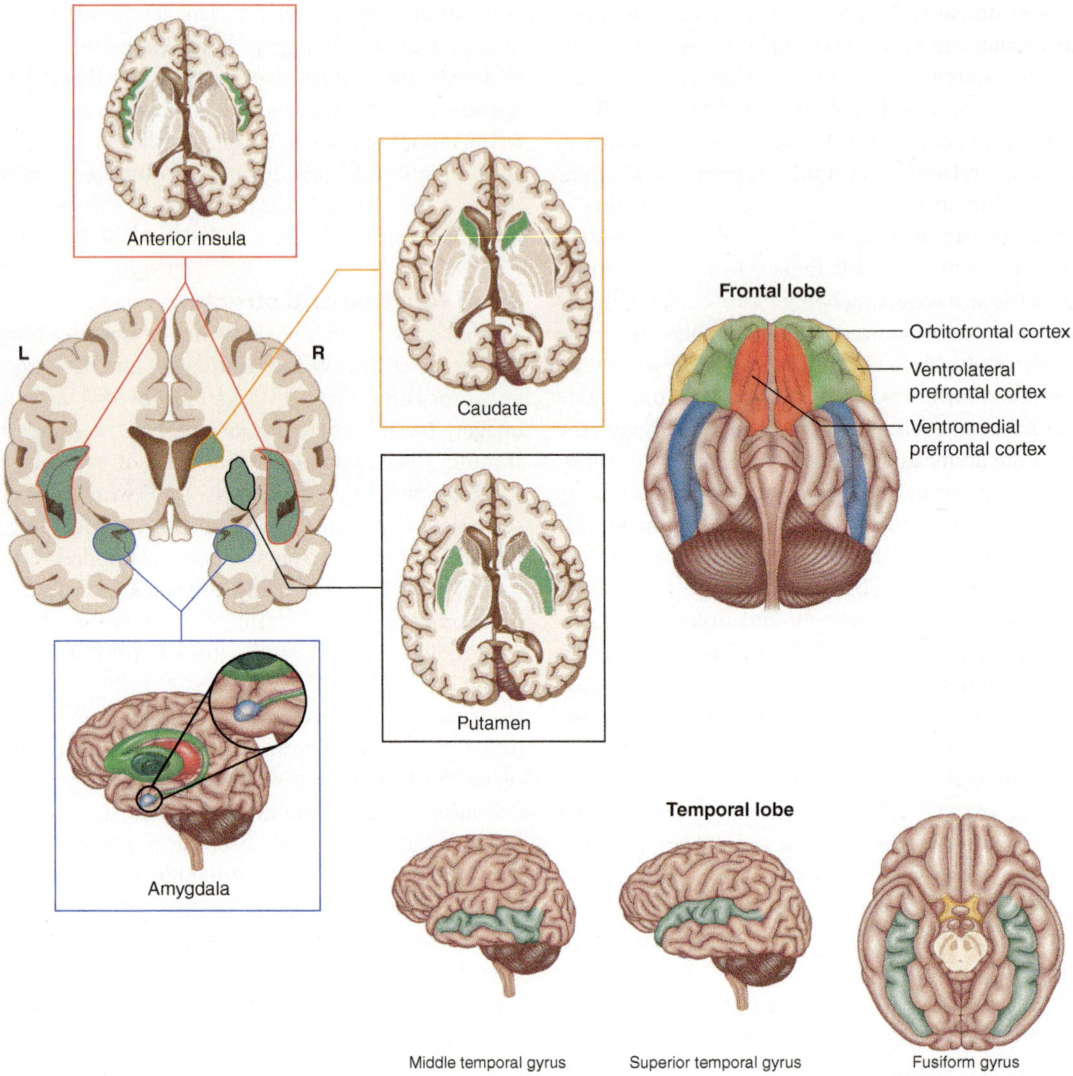

Figure 4.3 Structural brain abnormalities associated with disruptive and challenging behavior (DCB).

unrelated to brain response during reinforcement learning (Zhang *et al.*, 2021b; Zhang *et al.*, 2021c).

Several meta-analyses of structural MRI studies in youths with CD, ODD, conduct problems, and aggressive behavior (Raschle *et al.*, 2015; Noordermeer *et al.*, 2016; Rogers & De Brito, 2016) have consistently shown reductions in gray matter volume in areas implicated in emotion and reinforcement processing, including the ventrolateral, medial prefrontal, middle temporal, superior temporal, and anterior insular cortices, as well as in subcortical regions such as the amygdala, caudate, and putamen (Figure 4.3). Meta-analyses also indicate that the severity of CU traits is positively correlated with gray matter volume in the putamen and negatively correlated with gray matter volume in the amygdala (Rogers & De Brito, 2016; De Brito *et al.*, 2021). The evidence base for irritability is more limited with no consistent structural brain differences associated with irritability to date (Cardinale *et al.*, 2019; Dennis *et al.*, 2019; Jirsaraie *et al.*, 2019; Piguet *et al.*, 2021).

Disruptive and challenging behavior through a developmental lens

Studying the etiology and development of DCB is challenging for several reasons. First, it is not self-evident what behaviors/symptoms would be considered as most informative and discriminating across different developmental stages and consequently how we might best measure DCB over time (Wakschlag *et al.*, 2010). For example, while frequent antagonistic behaviors may be concerning in middle childhood, they may not be equally indicative of difficulties during toddlerhood or adolescence. An additional measurement challenge relates to potential rater biases, as different raters have different exposures to DCB and use different standards when rating severity and impact of the behavior. Second, the same underlying difficulties may manifest in different ways at different ages and age-relevant contexts. For example, callous lack of empathy may manifest as cruelty to younger siblings or animals at home during early to middle childhood, and as serious, premeditated violence toward peers in late adolescence. Third, children and adolescents develop DCB for different reasons and often have varying constellations of comorbid difficulties, all of which are likely to influence how DCB canalize over time. As we have discussed earlier in this chapter, two children may have very similar patterns of DCB, but the underlying reasons for their behavior, as well as the final developmental outcomes, can vary between them. Charting different traits (e.g., CU traits or irritability) or comorbidities can be used to subdivide children and adolescents with DCB to different subgroups, but as these co-occurring traits and diagnoses are also based on ratings of behavior, they are an imperfect tool for indexing heterogeneity.

The recognition of the problems of relying on behavioral ratings/diagnoses has contributed to initiatives such as the National Institute of Mental Health's Research Domain Criteria (RDoC) (Insel *et al.*, 2010). These initiatives have proposed that we should focus on basic domains of functioning (e.g., emotion processing) rather than diagnostic criteria. We might, for example, examine individual differences in a particular domain using different paradigms (e.g., experimental and neuroimaging tasks designed to engage emotion processing and the neural circuitry subserving it) and then test whether functioning in that domain explains risk for DCB. This line of work is important, but it has its own set of challenges. Difficulties in a particular domain can characterize two individuals who in fact qualify for different diagnoses, or may even be present in some individuals who appear largely free from mental health problems. This is in line with the notion of there being domains that confer transdiagnostic risk for different forms of psychopathology (Caspi & Moffitt, 2018; Astle *et al.*, 2022) (see Chapter 9 "Transdiagnostic perspectives" for a more detailed discussion). Cicchetti and Rogosch (1996) described the phenomenon of common mechanisms being associated with different outcomes as multifinality. They proposed the following: "The principle of multifinality (Wilden, 1980) suggests that any one component may function differently depending on the organization of the system in which it operates" (pp. 597–598). Individuals who share particular characteristics—for example, poorer emotion regulation—often differ in their genetic and environmental endowments in multiple ways. This is why developmental outcomes for people with similar emotion regulation difficulties in childhood may vary considerably, with only a subset of those who display difficulties developing persistent DCB. Both equifinality and multi-finality need to be considered as we seek to understand the development of DCB.

Since Cicchetti and Rogosch's article on equifinality and multifinality was published, we have not made as much progress in uncovering these phenomena as we might have hoped for. Perhaps one reason for this has been the tendency to study developmental risk for DCB in a fairly siloed way, with only a few studies attempting to combine different methodologies within a longitudinal framework (Carlisi *et al.*, 2020). Furthermore, many of the measures designed to probe cognitive–affective or neural functioning have not been psychometrically validated to robustly and reliably index individual differences in a single point in development, let alone across multiple developmental stages (Viding & McCrory 2020; Pezzoli *et al.*, 2023; Viding *et al.*, 2023). This limits our ability to examine how neurocognitive risk unfolds, how it relates to different dimensions/comorbidities associated with DCB (e.g., CU traits, irritability, or ADHD), and how it moderates or is moderated by the social environment across development.

Studying the "embedded brain": signposting future research into disruptive and challenging behavior

In order to make progress in our understanding of developmental risk for DCB, we need to find ways of studying the complex, transactional relationships between neurocognitive functioning and the social world (Viding & McCrory, 2020; Viding *et al.*, 2023). The suggestion that we should capture the interplay between child characteristics and the social environment, as it unfolds over time, is not new (Sameroff 1975; Bronfenbrenner 1977). Several studies have examined the reciprocal associations between DCB and social environmental factors and most have reported bidirectional influences (Lansford *et al.*, 2011; Rolon-Arroyo *et al.*, 2018). Furthermore, as alluded to above, genetically informative study designs have demonstrated both the impact of a child's genetic endowment on parenting, as well as parenting effects on child behavior that reflect both genetic and environmental processes (Moffitt, 2005; Larsson *et al.*, 2008; Klahr *et al.*, 2011). However, there has not been an effective integration of experimental and neuroimaging work into a transactional framework as we study development of DCB. We lack data that capture how particular patterns of neurocognitive processing in a child can influence their social interactions, as well as how social factors can influence the development and expression of neurocognitive vulnerabilities. We call this the study of the *"embedded brain"* (See Figure 4.4) (Viding & McCrory, 2020; Viding *et al.*, 2023). To advance the study of the "embedded brain" we need prospective, longitudinal, multilevel data from representative samples that allow us to study how genetic and environmental risk shape brain and social development over time. Ideally, such work would begin during the prenatal period to enable study of the earliest influences on behavior.

There are several key challenges to consider in this context. First, recruiting and retaining a representative sample of individuals with DCB is not trivial. The multiple difficulties faced with families of CYP with DCB means that they are often harder to reach and retain in studies (Hodgins *et al.*, 2018). Second, doing multilevel research that combines genetic, social/environmental, and neurocognitive measures is not straightforward. Genetically informative studies typically require sample sizes that vastly exceed those traditionally available for neuroimaging or experimental studies. Furthermore, there is a clear need to develop better measures of environmental risk and neural and cognitive–affective functioning that

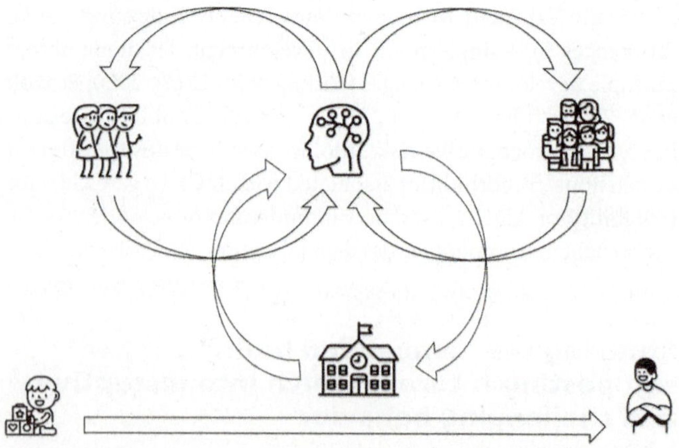

Figure 4.4 A schematic conceptualization of "The Embedded Brain." The relationships between neurocognitive functioning and the social world are complex. Much of the past research on disruptive and challenging behavior (DCB) has either focused on neurocognitive vulnerability, often conceptualized as "located within the child," or on social/environmental risk factors, often conceptualized as "external to the child." This separation is artificial and unhelpful and hampers our efforts to understand why DCB develops and how it is maintained. We need to adopt a developmental focus where the transactional mechanisms between intra- and extra-individual factors—and how these may differ between different individuals—are studied. We can consider, for example, the interplay between hypervigilance to threat and peer relationships, lack of empathy and family relationships, and poor executive functions and the learning environment. Threat-based reactive aggression is likely to lead to reduced social support from friends over time, which in turn can reinforce the threat bias. Reduced empathy is likely to result in weaker bonds with family members, which can, over time, contribute to poor family relationships and reinforce the lack of common feeling between family members. Poor executive functioning includes poor impulse control, which reduces opportunities to learn at school, which can in turn hamper future executive function development. *Source:* Viding & McCrory (2020); Viding *et al.* (2023).

sensitively capture individual differences and can be administered at scale (Viding & McCrory, 2020). Third, studying *development* within a multilevel, multidisciplinary framework adds a further layer of complexity. To date, we have a meager understanding of: (i) genetic risk for DCB and how this may vary across the development; (ii) the impact of particular environmental risk factors at different developmental junctures; and (iii) how different neural and cognitive–affective processes evolve over time and how they are best measured at different ages. These challenges are multiplied as we consider that individuals with DCB can have very different trait profiles, that DCB is often seen in conjunction with other disorders, and that DCB may canalize into other psychiatric conditions (e.g., depression) over time (heterotypic continuity). These challenges are not unique to the study of DCB, but given the historical underfunding of this area of enquiry (Woelbert *et al.*, 2020), less progress has been made than in investigating other conditions such as depression, autism, or ADHD.

We see, however, several opportunities for moving the field forward. First, the field should embrace working together with young people, parents, and professionals with lived experience of DCB. Genuine coproduction, listening to the concerns and needs of those affected by DCB, has the potential to: improve our ability to recruit and retain participants for studies, shape research questions in ways that enhance their translational potential, and achieve greater advocacy for the needs of those with DCB (Butler *et al.*, 2020; Gatera & Singh, 2023). Second, we need to form consortia that will pool data and collaborate to generate improved measures of environmental risk and neural/psychological function, harmonized across samples, and readily administered longitudinally and at scale (Viding & McCrory, 2020; Blair *et al.*, 2022; Griem *et al.*, 2022). Encouragingly this is already under way in relation to structural brain imaging data with the *ENIGMA Antisocial Behavior* working group. Third, embedding multilevel measures to longitudinal, transdiagnostic studies will be essential to improve our understanding of how DCB emerges and develops and to develop interventions that are less focused on disorder categories and more specifically target particular profiles of need. To achieve this, DCB researchers need to work together with consortia and samples focusing on other conditions or broader mental health risk. Finally, we need more agile ways of translating findings from empirical research into clinical benefit. This could include adapting randomized controlled trials to optimize treatment allocation to suit particular participant profiles (nested-precision randomized controlled trials) (Kappelmann *et al.*, 2021), as informed by findings from genetically informative, neuroscience, and environmental risk findings.

Conclusions

DCB are concurrently and prospectively associated with enormous personal, societal, and economic costs across the life span. Paradoxically, however, disruptive behavior disorders are among the least widely recognized and studied psychiatric disorders and often go untreated, despite the availability of evidence-based interventions. Prevention and early intervention should be a key priority, particularly as DCB can be identified from early childhood. The etiology underpinning DCB and its different profiles is complex and arises from the interplay of various individual (e.g., genetic) and environmental (e.g., parenting) risk factors shaping neurocognitive and social development. However, the precise timing and nature of the transactional processes between intrinsic and extrinsic factors related to DCB are not yet well-understood, primarily due to the limited prospective longitudinal multimethod research in this area. Nonetheless, we remain hopeful that improvements in the methodology of studying DCB, along with large-scale international and interdisciplinary collaborations, can revolutionize our understanding of DCB. These advances could subsequently contribute to further enhancement of diagnosis and treatment of DCB, ultimately reducing their public health impact, and delivering significant benefits for those with DCB, their families, and society. A key challenge will be to persuade policymakers and health care commissioners to embrace this long-term outlook (Burt *et al.*, 2018).

Acknowledgments

Essi Viding was supported by UKRI MRC grant MR/V033905/1. Stephane De Brito was supported by a grant from the Economic and Social Research Council (grant ES/V003526/1).

References

Aggensteiner, P.M. *et al.* (2022) The effects of callous-unemotional traits and aggression subtypes on amygdala activity in response to negative faces. *Psychological Medicine* **52**(3), 476–484. doi:10.1017/S0033291720002111.

Alegria, A.A. *et al.* (2016) Meta-analysis of fMRI studies of disruptive behavior disorders. *The American Journal of Psychiatry* **173**(11), 1119–1130. doi:10.1176/appi.ajp.2016.15081089.

Allegrini, A.G. *et al.* (2022) Developmental co-occurrence of psychopathology dimensions in childhood. *JCPP Advances* **2**(3), e12100. doi:10.1002/jcv2.12100.

Althoff, R.R. *et al.* (2016) Disruptive mood dysregulation disorder at ages 13–18: results from the national comorbidity survey—adolescent supplement. *Journal of Child and Adolescent Psychopharmacology* **26**(2), 107–113. doi:10.1089/cap.2015.0038.

American Psychiatric Association (2000) *Diagnostic and Statistical Manual of Mental Disorders (DSM-4-TR)*, 4th edn, text revision. edn. American Psychiatric Association, Washington, DC.

American Psychiatric Association (2013) *Diagnostic and Statistical Manual of Mental Disorders (DSM-5)*, 5th edn. American Psychiatric Association, Washington, DC.

American Psychiatric Association (2022) *Diagnostic and Statistical Manual of Mental Disorders (DSM-5-TR)*, 5th edn, text revision. edn. American Psychiatric Association, Washington, DC.

Astle, D.E. *et al.* (2022) Annual research review: the transdiagnostic revolution in neurodevelopmental disorders. *Journal of Child Psychology and Psychiatry* **63**(4), 397–417. doi:10.1111/jcpp.13481.

Barker, E.D. *et al.* (2012) Relative impact of maternal depression and associated risk factors on offspring psychopathology. *The British Journal of Psychiatry* **200**(2), 124–129. doi:10.1192/bjp.bp.111.092346.

Baselmans, B. *et al.* (2021) The genetic and neural substrates of externalizing behavior. *Biological Psychiatry Global Open Science* **2**(4), 389–399. doi:10.1016/j.bpsgos.2021.09.007.

Beelmann, A. *et al.* (2023) Parent training programs for preventing and treating antisocial behavior in children and adolescents: a comprehensive meta-analysis of international studies. *Aggression and Violent Behavior* **68**, 101798. doi:10.1016/j.avb.2022.101798.

Berluti, K. *et al.* (2023) Emotion processing in youths with conduct problems: an fMRI meta-analysis. *Translational Psychiatry* **13**(1), 1–10. doi:10.1038/s41398-023-02363-z.

Blair, R.J.R. (2018) Traits of empathy and anger: implications for psychopathy and other disorders associated with aggression. *Philosophical Transactions of the Royal Society, B: Biological Sciences* **373**(1744), 20170155. doi:10.1098/rstb.2017.0155.

Blair, R.J.R. *et al.* (2014) Conduct disorder and callous–unemotional traits in youth. *New England Journal of Medicine* **371**(23), 2207–2216. doi:10.1056/NEJMra1315612.

Blair, R.J.R. *et al.* (2022) Future directions for cognitive neuroscience in psychiatry: recommendations for biomarker design based on recent test re-test reliability work. *Current Opinion in Behavioral Sciences* **44**, 101102. doi:10.1016/j.cobeha.2022.101102.

Bonham, M.D. *et al.* (2021) Inhibitory control deficits in children with oppositional defiant disorder and conduct disorder compared to attention deficit/hyperactivity disorder: a systematic review and meta-analysis. *Research on Child and Adolescent Psychopathology* **49**(1), 39–62. doi:10.1007/s10802-020-00713-9.

Bronfenbrenner, U. (1977) Toward an experimental ecology of human development. *American Psychologist* **32**(7), 513–531. doi:10.1037/0003-066X.32.7.513.

Brotman, M.A. *et al.* (2017) Irritability in children and adolescents. *Annual Review of Clinical Psychology* **13**(1), 317–341. doi:10.1146/annurev-clinpsy-032816-044941.

Bubier, J.L. & Drabick, D.A.G. (2009) Co-occurring anxiety and disruptive behavior disorders: the roles of anxious symptoms, reactive aggression, and shared risk processes. *Clinical Psychology Review* **29**(7), 658–669. doi:10.1016/j.cpr.2009.08.005.

Burt, S.A. *et al.* (2018) Commentary: childhood conduct problems are a public health crisis and require resources: a commentary on Rivenbark et al. (2018). *Journal of Child Psychology and Psychiatry* **59**(6), 711–713. doi:10.1111/jcpp.12930.

Butler, J. *et al.* (2020) Parents' perceptions and experiences of parenting programmes: a systematic review and metasynthesis of the qualitative literature. *Clinical Child and Family Psychology Review* **23**, 176–204. doi:10.1007/s10567-019-00307-y.

Byrd, A.L. *et al.* (2014) Antisocial behavior, psychopathic features and abnormalities in reward and punishment processing in youth. *Clinical Child and Family Psychology Review* **17**(2), 125–156. doi:10.1007/s10567-013-0159-6.

Byrd, A.L. *et al.* (2018) Boys with conduct problems and callous-unemotional traits: neural response to reward and punishment and associations with treatment response. *Developmental Cognitive Neuroscience* **30**, 51–59. doi:10.1016/j.dcn.2017.12.004.

Cardinale, E.M. *et al.* (2019) Parsing neurodevelopmental features of irritability and anxiety: replication and validation of a latent variable approach. *Development and Psychopathology* **31**(3), 917–929. doi:10.1017/S095457941900035X.

Carlisi, C.O. *et al.* (2020) Associations between life-course-persistent antisocial behaviour and brain structure in a population-representative longitudinal birth cohort. *The Lancet Psychiatry* **7**(3), 245–253. doi:10.1016/S2215-0366(20)30002-X.

Caspi, A. & Moffitt, T.E. (2018) All for one and one for all: mental disorders in one dimension. *American Journal of Psychiatry* **175**(9), 831–844. doi:10.1176/appi.ajp.2018.17121383.

Cicchetti, D. & Rogosch, F.A. (1996) Equifinality and multifinality in developmental psychopathology. *Development and Psychopathology* **8**(4), 597–600. doi:10.1017/S0954579400007318.

Cloninger, C.R. *et al.* (1982) Predisposition to petty criminality in Swedish adoptees: II. Cross-fostering analysis of gene-environment interaction. *Archives of General Psychiatry* **39**(11), 1242–1247. doi:10.1001/archpsyc.1982.04290110010002.

Dawel, A. *et al.* (2012) Not just fear and sadness: meta-analytic evidence of pervasive emotion recognition deficits for facial and vocal expressions in psychopathy. *Neuroscience & Biobehavioral Reviews* **36**(10), 2288–2304. doi:10.1016/j.neubiorev.2012.08.006.

De Brito, S.A. *et al.* (2021) Psychopathy. *Nature Reviews. Disease Primers* **7**(49), 1–21. doi:10.1038/s41572-021-00282-1.

Deater-Deckard, K. *et al.* (2007) Anger/frustration, task persistence, and conduct problems in childhood: a behavioral genetic analysis. *Journal of Child Psychology and Psychiatry* **48**(1), 80–87. doi:10.1111/j.1469-7610.2006.01653.x.

Demontis, D. *et al.* (2021) Risk variants and polygenic architecture of disruptive behavior disorders in the context of attention-deficit/

hyperactivity disorder. *Nature Communications* **12**(576), 1–12. doi:10.1038/s41467-020-20443-2.

Dennis, E.L. *et al.* (2019) Irritability and brain volume in adolescents: cross-sectional and longitudinal associations. *Social Cognitive and Affective Neuroscience* **14**(7), 687–698. doi:10.1093/scan/nsz053.

Dugré, J.R. *et al.* (2020) Neurofunctional abnormalities in antisocial spectrum: a meta-analysis of fMRI studies on five distinct neurocognitive research domains. *Neuroscience & Biobehavioral Reviews* **119**, 168–183. doi:10.1016/j.neubiorev.2020.09.013.

Elowsky, J. *et al.* (2022) Differential associations of conduct disorder, callous-unemotional traits and irritability with outcome expectations and values regarding the consequences of aggression. *Child and Adolescent Psychiatry and Mental Health* **16**(1), 38. doi:10.1186/s13034-022-00466-x.

Fairchild, G. *et al.* (2019) Conduct disorder. *Nature Reviews. Disease Primers* **5**(43), 1–25. doi:10.1038/s41572-019-0095-y.

Fanti, K.A. *et al.* (2016) Unemotional on all counts: evidence of reduced affective responses in individuals with high callous-unemotional traits across emotion systems and valences. *Social Neuroscience* **11**(1), 72–87. doi:10.1080/17470919.2015.1034378.

Finger, E.C. *et al.* (2008) Abnormal ventromedial prefrontal cortex function in children with psychopathic traits during reversal learning. *Archives of General Psychiatry* **65**(5), 586–594. doi:10.1001/archpsyc.65.5.586.

Fleming, G.E. *et al.* (2022) Parent training adapted to the needs of children with callous–unemotional traits: a randomized controlled trial. *Behavior Therapy* **53**(6), 1265–1281. doi:10.1016/j.beth.2022.07.001.

Frick, P.J. *et al.* (2014) Can callous-unemotional traits enhance the understanding, diagnosis, and treatment of serious conduct problems in children and adolescents? A comprehensive review. *Psychological Bulletin* **140**(1), 1–57. doi:10.1037/a0033076.

Gatera, G. & Singh, S. (2023) Beyond tokenism: the influence of lived experience and its future possibilities in mental health science. *Nature Mental Health* **1**(3), 151–152. doi:10.1038/s44220-023-00027-x.

GBD 2019 Mental Disorders Collaborators (2022) Global, regional, and national burden of 12 mental disorders in 204 countries and territories, 1990–2019: a systematic analysis for the global burden of disease study 2019. *The Lancet Psychiatry* **9**(2), 137–150. doi:10.1016/S2215-0366(21)00395-3.

Gidziela, A. *et al.* (2023) A meta-analysis of genetic effects associated with neurodevelopmental disorders and co-occurring conditions. *Nature Human Behaviour* **7**(4), 642–656. doi:10.1038/s41562-023-01530-y.

Girard, L.C. *et al.* (2019) Development of aggression subtypes from childhood to adolescence: a group-based multi-trajectory modelling perspective. *Journal of Abnormal Child Psychology* **47**(5), 825–838. doi:10.1007/s10802-018-0488-5.

Gregory, A.M. *et al.* (2004) Exploring the association between anxiety and conduct problems in a large sample of twins aged 2-4. *Journal of Abnormal Child Psychology* **32**(2), 111–122. doi:10.1023/b:jacp.0000019765.29768.1c.

Griem, J. *et al.* (2022) Key challenges in neurocognitive assessment of individuals with antisocial personality disorder and psychopathy. *Frontiers in Behavioral Neuroscience* **16**. doi:10.3389/fnbeh.2022.1007121.

Hodgins, S. *et al.* (2018) Antisocial personality disorder. In: *The Wiley Blackwell Handbook of Forensic Neuroscience*. (eds A.R. Beech, *et al.*). Wiley Blackwell, Hoboken, NJ. pp. 229–271.

Hyde, L.W. *et al.* (2016) Heritable and nonheritable pathways to early callous-unemotional behaviors. *American Journal of Psychiatry* **173**(9), 903–910. doi:10.1176/appi.ajp.2016.15111381.

Insel, T. *et al.* (2010) Research domain criteria (RDoC): toward a new classification framework for research on mental disorders. *American Journal of Psychiatry* **167**(7), 748–751. doi:10.1176/appi.ajp.2010.09091379.

Jaffee, S.R. & et al. (2012) From correlates to causes: can quasi-experimental studies and statistical innovations bring us closer to identifying the causes of antisocial behavior? *Psychological Bulletin* **138**(2), 272–295. doi:10.1037/a0026020.

Jennings, W.G. *et al.* (2018) Conduct disorder and neighborhood effects. *Annual Review of Clinical Psychology* **14**(1), 317–341. doi:10.1146/annurev-clinpsy-050817-084911.

Jirsaraie, R.J. *et al.* (2019) Accelerated cortical thinning within structural brain networks is associated with irritability in youth. *Neuropsychopharmacology: Official Publication of the American College of Neuropsychopharmacology* **44**(13), 2254–2262. doi:10.1038/s41386-019-0508-3.

Johnson, A.M. *et al.* (2017) Emotion socialization and child conduct problems: a comprehensive review and meta-analysis. *Clinical Psychology Review* **54**, 65–80. doi:10.1016/j.cpr.2017.04.001.

Kaat, A.J. & Lecavalier, L. (2013) Disruptive behavior disorders in children and adolescents with autism spectrum disorders: a review of the prevalence, presentation, and treatment. *Research in Autism Spectrum Disorders* **7**(12), 1579–1594. doi:10.1016/j.rasd.2013.08.012.

Kaat, A. *et al.* (2015) Factor validity of a proactive and reactive aggression rating scale. *Journal of Child and Family Studies* **24**(9), 2734–2744. doi:10.1007/s10826-014-0075-5.

Kahn, R.E. *et al.* (2012) The effects of including a callous unemotional specifier for the diagnosis of conduct disorder. *Journal of Child Psychology and Psychiatry* **53**(3), 271–282. doi:10.1111/j.1469-7610.2011.02463.x.

Kappelmann, N. *et al.* (2021) Adapting the randomised controlled trial (RCT) for precision medicine: introducing the nested-precision RCT (npRCT). *Trials* **22**(1), 13. doi:10.1186/s13063-020-04965-0.

Kersten, L. *et al.* (2017) Community violence exposure and conduct problems in children and adolescents with conduct disorder and healthy controls. *Frontiers in Behavioral Neuroscience* **11**(219), 1–14. doi:10.3389/fnbeh.2017.00219.

Khodosevich, K. & Sellgren, C.M. (2023) Neurodevelopmental disorders: high-resolution rethinking of disease modeling. *Molecular Psychiatry* **28**(1), 34–43. doi:10.1038/s41380-022-01876-1.

Kim-Cohen, J. *et al.* (2003) Prior juvenile diagnoses in adults with mental disorder: developmental follow-back of a prospective-longitudinal cohort. *Archives of General Psychiatry* **60**(7), 709–717. doi:10.1001/archpsyc.60.7.709.

Klahr, A.M. *et al.* (2011) The association between parent-child conflict and adolescent conduct problems over time: results from a longitudinal adoption study. *Journal of Abnormal Psychology* **120**(1), 46–56. doi:10.1037/a0021350.

Knopik, V.S. *et al.* (2017) *Behavioral Genetics*, 7th edn. Worth Publishers, New York. pp. 93–110.

Lansford, J.E. (2018) Development of aggression. *Current Opinion in Psychology* **19**, 17–21. doi:10.1016/j.copsyc.2017.03.015.

Lansford, J.E. *et al.* (2011) Reciprocal relations between parents' physical discipline and children's externalizing behavior during middle childhood and adolescence. *Development and Psychopathology* **23**(1), 225–238. doi:10.1017/S0954579410000751.

Larsson, H. *et al.* (2008) Relationships between parental negativity and childhood antisocial behavior over time: a bidirectional effects model in a longitudinal genetically informative design. *Journal of Abnormal Child Psychology* **36**(5), 633–645. doi:10.1007/s10802-007-9151-2.

Lee, K.S. *et al.* (2023) Systematic review and meta-analysis: task-based fMRI studies in youths with irritability. *Journal of the American Academy of Child & Adolescent Psychiatry* **62**(2), 208–229. doi:10.1016/j.jaac.2022.05.014.

Leibenluft, E. (2017) Pediatric irritability: a systems neuroscience approach. *Trends in Cognitive Sciences* **21**(4), 277–289. doi:10.1016/j.tics.2017.02.002.

Liebling, A. *et al.* (2017) *The Oxford Handbook of Criminology*, 6th edn. Oxford University Press, Oxford.

Liu, J. (2011) Early health risk factors for violence: conceptualization, evidence, and implications. *Aggression and Violent Behavior* **16**(1), 63–73. doi:10.1016/j.avb.2010.12.003.

Loeber, R. & Schmaling, K.B. (1985) Empirical evidence for overt and covert patterns of antisocial conduct problems: a metaanalysis. *Journal of Abnormal Child Psychology* **13**(2), 337–353. doi:10.1007/BF00910652.

Loeber, R. *et al.* (2009) Development and etiology of disruptive and delinquent behavior. *Annual Review of Clinical Psychology* **5**(1), 291–310. doi:10.1146/annurev.clinpsy.032408.153631.

Lukkari, S. *et al.* (2012) Exposure to obstetric complications in relation to subsequent psychiatric disorders of adolescent inpatients: specific focus on gender differences. *Psychopathology* **45**(5), 317–326. doi:10.1159/000336073.

Mayes, S.D. *et al.* (2016) Disruptive mood dysregulation disorder symptoms and association with oppositional defiant and other disorders in a general population child sample. *Journal of Child and Adolescent Psychopharmacology* **26**(2), 101–106. doi:10.1089/cap.2015.0074.

Moffitt, T.E. (1993) "Life-course-persistent" and "adolescence-limited" antisocial behaviour: a developmental taxonomy. *Psychological Review* **100**, 674–701.

Moffitt, T.E. (2005) The new look of behavioral genetics in developmental psychopathology: gene-environment interplay in antisocial behaviors. *Psychological Bulletin* **131**, 533–554. doi:10.1037/0033-2909.131.4.533.

Moffitt, T.E. & Caspi, A. (2001) Childhood predictors differentiate life-course persistent and adolescence-limited antisocial pathways among males and females. *Development and Psychopathology* **13**(2), 355–375. doi:10.1017/S0954579401002097.

Moore, A.A. *et al.* (2019) The genetic underpinnings of callous-unemotional traits: a systematic research review. *Neuroscience and Biobehavioral Reviews* **100**, 85–97. doi:10.1016/j.neubiorev.2019.02.018.

Nock, M.K. *et al.* (2006) Prevalence, subtypes, and correlates of DSM-IV conduct disorder in the national comorbidity survey replication. *Psychological Medicine* **36**(5), 699–710. doi:10.1017/S0033291706007082.

Noordermeer, S.D.S. *et al.* (2016) A systematic review and meta-analysis of neuroimaging in oppositional defiant disorder (ODD) and conduct disorder (CD) taking attention-deficit hyperactivity disorder (ADHD) into account. *Neuropsychology Review* **26**(1), 44–72. doi:10.1007/s11065-015-9315-8.

Ogilvie, J.M. *et al.* (2011) Neuropsychological measures of executive function and antisocial behavior: a meta-analysis. *Criminology* **49**(4), 1063–1107. doi:10.1111/j.1745-9125.2011.00252.x.

Pezzoli, P. *et al.* (2023) Challenges and solutions to the measurement of neurocognitive mechanisms in developmental settings. *Biological Psychiatry: Cognitive Neuroscience and Neuroimaging*, 815–821. doi:10.1016/j.bpsc.2023.03.011.

Piguet, C. *et al.* (2021) Irritability is associated with decreased cortical surface area and anxiety with decreased gyrification during brain development. *Frontiers in Psychiatry* **12**. doi:10.3389/fpsyt.2021.744419.

Pingault, J.B. *et al.* (2015) Developmentally dynamic genome: evidence of genetic influences on increases and decreases in conduct problems from early childhood to adolescence. *Scientific Reports* **5**(1), 10053. doi:10.1038/srep10053.

Piotrowska, P.J. *et al.* (2015) Socioeconomic status and antisocial behaviour among children and adolescents: a systematic review and meta-analysis. *Clinical Psychology Review* **35**, 47–55. doi:10.1016/j.cpr.2014.11.003.

Raine, A. (2018) Antisocial personality as a neurodevelopmental disorder. *Annual Review of Clinical Psychology* **14**(1), 259–289. doi:10.1146/annurev-clinpsy-050817-084819.

Raine, A. *et al.* (1997) Interaction between birth complications and early maternal rejection in predisposing individuals to adult violence: specificity to serious, early-onset violence. *American Journal of Psychiatry* **154**(9), 1265–1271. doi:10.1176/ajp.154.9.1265.

Raschle, N.M. *et al.* (2015) Structural and functional alterations in right dorsomedial prefrontal and left insular cortex co-localize in adolescents with aggressive behaviour: an ALE meta-analysis. *PLoS One* **10**(9), e0136553. doi:10.1371/journal.pone.0136553.

Rice, F. *et al.* (2009) Disentangling prenatal and inherited influences in humans with an experimental design. *Proceedings of the National Academy of Sciences* **106**(7), 2464–2467. doi:10.1073/pnas.0808798106.

Roberson-Nay, R. *et al.* (2015) Longitudinal stability of genetic and environmental influences on irritability: from childhood to young adulthood. *The American Journal of Psychiatry* **172**(7), 657–664. doi:10.1176/appi.ajp.2015.14040509.

Roberts, R. *et al.* (2022) Parenting boys with conduct problems and callous-unemotional traits: parent and child perspectives. *European Child & Adolescent Psychiatry*, 1–9. doi:10.1007/s00787-022-02109-0.

Rogers, J.C. & De Brito, S.A. (2016) Cortical and subcortical gray matter volume in youths with conduct problems: a meta-analysis. *JAMA Psychiatry* **73**(1), 64–72. doi:10.1001/jamapsychiatry.2015.2423.

Rogers, J. *et al.* (2006) Autism spectrum disorder and psychopathy: shared cognitive underpinnings or double hit? *Psychological Medicine* **36**(12), 1789–1798. doi:10.1017/S0033291706008853.

Rolon-Arroyo, B. *et al.* (2018) Reciprocal relations between parenting behaviors and conduct disorder symptoms in preschool children. *Child Psychiatry & Human Development* **49**(5), 786–799. doi:10.1007/s10578-018-0794-8.

Roose, A. *et al.* (2010) Assessing the affective features of psychopathy in adolescence: a further validation of the inventory of callous and unemotional traits. *Assessment* **17**(1), 44–57. doi:10.1177/1073191109344153.

Roose, A. *et al.* (2011) Psychopathic traits in adolescence: associations with the revised reinforcement sensitivity theory systems. *Personality and Individual Differences* **50**(2), 201–205. doi:10.1016/j.paid.2010.09.028.

Rowe, R. *et al.* (2010) The role of callous and unemotional traits in the diagnosis of conduct disorder. *Journal of Child Psychology and Psychiatry* **51**(6), 688–695. doi:10.1111/j.1469-7610.2009.02199.x.

Roza, S.J. *et al.* (2003) Stable prediction of mood and anxiety disorders based on behavioral and emotional problems in childhood: a 14-year follow-up during childhood, adolescence, and young adulthood. *American Journal of Psychiatry* **160**(12), 2116–2121. doi:10.1176/appi.ajp.160.12.2116.

Salvatore, J.E. & Dick, D.M. (2018) Genetic influences on conduct disorder. *Neuroscience & Biobehavioral Reviews* **91**, 91–101. doi:10.1016/j.neubiorev.2016.06.034.

Sameroff, A. (1975) Transactional models in early social relations. *Human Development* **18**(1–2), 65–79. doi:10.1159/000271476.

Saunders, M.C. *et al.* (2019) The associations between callous-unemotional traits and symptoms of conduct problems, hyperactivity and emotional problems: a study of adolescent twins screened for neurodevelopmental problems. *Journal of Abnormal Child Psychology* **47**(3), 447–457. doi:10.1007/s10802-018-0439-1.

Schoemaker, K. *et al.* (2013) Executive functions in preschool children with externalizing behavior problems: a meta-analysis. *Journal of Abnormal Child Psychology* **41**(3), 457–471. doi:10.1007/s10802-012-9684-x.

Shaw, C.R. & McKay, H.D. (1942) Juvenile delinquency and urban areas. In: *Understanding Deviance: Connecting Classical and Contemporary Perspectives*. (ed T.L. Anderson). Routledge, New York. pp. 106–127.

Simonoff, E. *et al.* (2004) Predictors of antisocial personality: continuities from childhood to adult life. *The British Journal of Psychiatry* **184**(2), 118–127. doi:10.1192/bjp.184.2.118.

Stringaris, A. *et al.* (2012) Adolescent irritability: phenotypic associations and genetic links with depressed mood. *The American Journal of Psychiatry* **169**(1), 47–54. doi:10.1176/appi.ajp.2011.10101549.

Takahashi, Y. *et al.* (2021) Genetic and environmental influences on the developmental trajectory of callous-unemotional traits from childhood to adolescence. *Journal of Child Psychology and Psychiatry* **62**(4), 414–423. doi:10.1111/jcpp.13259.

Tremblay, R.E. & Nagin, D.S. (2005) The developmental origins of physical aggression in humans. In: *Developmental Origins of Aggression*. (eds R.E. Tremblay, *et al.*). Guildford Press, New York. pp. 83–106.

Tye, C. *et al.* (2017) Callous-unemotional traits moderate executive function in children with ASD and ADHD: a pilot event-related potential study. *Developmental Cognitive Neuroscience* **26**, 84–90. doi:10.1016/j.dcn.2017.06.002.

Vidal-Ribas, P. *et al.* (2016) The status of irritability in psychiatry: a conceptual and quantitative review. *Journal of the American Academy of Child and Adolescent Psychiatry* **55**(7), 556–570. doi:10.1016/j.jaac.2016.04.014.

Viding, E. & McCrory, E. (2020) Disruptive behavior disorders: the challenge of delineating mechanisms in the face of heterogeneity. *American Journal of Psychiatry* **177**(9), 811–817. doi:10.1176/appi.ajp.2020.20070998.

Viding, E. *et al.* (2005) Evidence for substantial genetic risk for psychopathy in 7-year-olds. *Journal of Child Psychology and Psychiatry* **46**(6), 592–597. doi:10.1111/j.1469-7610.2004.00393.x.

Viding, E. *et al.* (2007) Aetiology of the relationship between callous-unemotional traits and conduct problems in childhood. *The British Journal of Psychiatry* **190**(49), s33–s38. doi:10.1192/bjp.190.5.s33.

Viding, E. *et al.* (2008) Heritability of antisocial behaviour at 9: do callous-unemotional traits matter? *Developmental Science* **11**(1), 17–22. doi:10.1111/j.1467-7687.2007.00648.x.

Viding, E. *et al.* (2023) An "embedded brain" approach to understanding antisocial behaviour. *Trends in Cognitive Sciences* **28**, 159–171. doi:10.1016/j.tics.2023.08.013.

Wakschlag, L.S. *et al.* (2010) Research review: "Ain't misbehavin": towards a developmentally-specified nosology for preschool disruptive behavior. *Journal of Child Psychology and Psychiatry* **51**(1), 3–22. doi:10.1111/j.1469-7610.2009.02184.x.

Wakschlag, L.S. *et al.* (2018) The neurodevelopmental basis of early childhood disruptive behavior: irritable and callous phenotypes as exemplars. *American Journal of Psychiatry* **175**(2), 114–130. doi:10.1176/appi.ajp.2017.17010045.

Waschbusch, D.A. *et al.* (2020) Irritability and limited prosocial emotions/callous-unemotional traits in elementary-school-age children. *Behavior Therapy* **51**(2), 223–237. doi:10.1016/j.beth.2019.06.007.

Waszczuk, M.A. *et al.* (2021) Why do depression, conduct, and hyperactivity symptoms co-occur across adolescence? The role of stable and dynamic genetic and environmental influences. *European Child & Adolescent Psychiatry* **30**(7), 1013–1025. doi:10.1007/s00787-020-01515-6.

Wesseldijk, L.W. *et al.* (2018) Genetic and environmental influences on conduct and antisocial personality problems in childhood, adolescence, and adulthood. *European Child & Adolescent Psychiatry* **27**(9), 1123–1132. doi:10.1007/s00787-017-1014-y.

Wilden, A. (1980) *System and Structure*. Tavistock, London.

Woelbert, E. *et al.* (2020) *The Inequities of Mental Health Research (IAMHRF)*. Digital Science. doi: 10.6084/m9.figshare.13055897.v2.

World Health Organization (2018) *International Classification of Diseases 11th revision* [online]. WHO, Geneva, Switzerland. Available: https://icd.who.int/en [20 July 2024].

Zhang, J. *et al.* (2021a) Callous-unemotional traits in Chinese preschool children with attention-deficit/hyperactivity disorder. *Child and Adolescent Psychiatry and Mental Health* **15**(35), 1–9. doi:10.1186/s13034-021-00388-0.

Zhang, R. *et al.* (2021b) Dysfunction in differential reward-punishment responsiveness in conduct disorder relates to severity of callous-unemotional traits but not irritability. *Psychological Medicine* **53**(5), 1–11. doi:10.1017/S0033291721003500.

Zhang, R. *et al.* (2021c) Callous-unemotional traits moderate the relationship between irritability and threatening responding. *Frontiers in Psychiatry* **12**, 617052. doi:10.3389/fpsyt.2021.617052.

Zhang, J. *et al.* (2023) Emotion regulation difficulties in military fathers magnify their benefit from a parenting program. *Prevention Science* **24**(2), 237–248. doi:10.1007/s11121-021-01287-8.

CHAPTER 5

Emotion, emotion regulation and disorder: conceptual issues for clinicians and neuroscientists

Argyris Stringaris
[1] Faculty of Brain Sciences, University College London, London, UK
[2] First Department of Psychiatry, Aiginiteio Hospital, National and Kapodistrian University of Athens, Athens, Greece

Overview

In this chapter I attempt to convey some of the basic ideas about mood and emotions in a way that is relevant to practitioners and links clinical knowledge with progress in mechanistic understanding. I also aim to make clear to the reader the challenges in the field, particularly the uncertainties surrounding some fundamental claims about emotions, as well as the degree to which they are indeed relevant to practice.

I start by describing a simple experimental setup that also represents a simple and familiar problem to clinician—I will use this to highlight many of the concepts across the chapter.

Overall, the chapter is focused on what has come to be called mechanisms, that is, processes that are (typically assumed rather than proven to be) causal to emotions or emotional disorders. This is not least because of the promise—backed by progress in other areas of medicine—that understanding mechanisms will facilitate innovation in clinical practice.

A simple experiment

Think of an experiment where a young person is presented with a spider approaching them (the spider is behind thick glass and cannot reach the person). Think of condition A, the *control* condition, which is when the spider has not been presented yet, and condition B, the *threat* condition, where the spider is approaching. Such a setup helps us examine some of the following basic aspects of emotions. I purposely avoid providing a definition of emotion here for two main reasons. First, because there is simply not a universally agreed upon definition of emotion; indeed, there is a lot of debate and confusion about the various attempts at defining emotion and the interested reader can consult recent attempts at a typology of definitions (Moors, 2022). Second, because one of the main aims of the chapter is to help the reader appreciate the complexity of the matter and the implications this has for psychopathology. I do however, make the argument that for clinicians it is both reasonable and useful to rely on a working definition that regards emotions as things that their patients can express in words or gestures that are valenced, i.e., they have positive (e.g., pleasant) or negative (e.g., sad) connotations.

What sorts of differences are we interested in?

There are two main things one could discover from such a setup. First, how people change, on average, when a threat is presented to them. For example, one would expect that in condition B, when the threat stimulus is presented, more young people would experience some degree of fear than when presented with a control stimulus. This difference between condition A and condition B is what is described as an *intraindividual difference*. Second, how people vary between each other in how they respond to threats, termed *interindividual difference*. Obviously, one would expect a person with arachnophobia to respond with more fear to such a presentation than a zoologist with years of fieldwork on spiders.

Demonstrating and explaining such sources of intraindividual and interindividual differences is what emotion researchers

Rutter's Child and Adolescent Psychiatry and Psychology, Seventh Edition.
Edited by Anita Thapar, Daniel S. Pine, Samuele Cortese, Cathy Creswell, Tamsin J. Ford, James F. Leckman, and Argyris Stringaris.

Companion website: www.wiley.com/go/thapar/rutterspsych7

do. Assessing and treating interindividual differences in emotions is what clinicians do.

How do we know about emotions?

In the spider experiment setup, as in a clinic, there are several ways in which we try to find out about emotions. Clinicians will typically ask the patient or rely on their observation; experimentalists also use physiological measurement.

Self-knowledge of emotions and reports by others

We call *feelings* those emotional states that are conscious and are usually communicable through language. They are special in their epistemic value, the person who has them knows best about their own emotions and is able to speak about them. Self-report is not only the cornerstone of our knowledge about our own emotions, but also the way we most commonly learn about the emotions of others, including our patients (at least after a certain age). Self-report is typically the gold standard for most emotion research and clinical practice (see also Chapter 28 on assessment).

In the spider experiment, the experimenter would ask the participant to tell them how much fear they experienced during the presentation of the spider versus the control condition. The experimenter would typically ask the young person to rate their fear on a scale of 0–100 (or 0–10 or something similar). In a clinical setup, a psychiatrist would ask a patient similar questions about fear and any accompanying feelings.

If the child were very young, we might ask a parent to give us information on the child's state, or we could ask a peer about the adolescent's overall emotional expression (see Chapter 28 on assessment).

Observation

Observation of emotions in others has a long tradition in research and has its value in the clinic. It is standard in the assessment of emotional responses of young children, but it is also how *affect* is assessed during the mental state examination performed by clinicians: not only facial emotional expression and the volume, prosody, and rate of their speech, but also a patient's posture and speed of bodily movements are indicators of emotional state. Humans are endowed with the ability to recognize emotions in other humans and animals—we know our children's joy when they smile at us and know that they are in distress if they cry in the middle of the night. Scientists often refer to the ability to *decode* emotions in others and efforts have been made to understand how this is achieved and how to emulate it. As a result, elaborate systems of coding facial affect—the expression of emotion in faces—have been developed by Ekman and others (Ekman & Cordaro, 2011); more recently, artificial intelligence (AI) has been deployed to decode emotions from both faces and voices, so far with relatively modest success. The experiment described above would be typical of a setup where such measurement efforts would be applied in research.

Physiological and neural measurement

At least since the end of the 19th century, attempts have been made to measure emotions like other physical phenomena. Indeed, it is standard to think of emotions as encompassing specific physiological responses that are related to evolutionary survival (see Why Do We Have Emotions). For example, humans and several other animals have a standard response to acute threat that may include tachycardia, sweating, piloerection, and pupil dilation, all phenomena that are thought to facilitate fighting or fleeing (Ohman, 2007). This has led to decades of research devoted to measuring the physiology of emotions, including cardiovascular, immune, metabolic, and hormonal responses to acute and chronic stress. The advent of functional neuroimaging extended this work to the brain, highlighting anatomical regions, such as the amygdala, as being central to, for example, fear responses. Indeed, the experiment described above could be performed in a magnetic resonance imaging (MRI) scanner and the participant might have heart rate, skin conductance, and other devices attached to them. These measurements generated great expectations for psychiatry as they would help relate mental phenomena to physiological processes. However, so far, these measurements have been of limited value to clinicians, a problem on which we expand further in this chapter. Here it is important to note that there is only a relatively weak relationship between any set of physiological measures and self-report of emotions (Lench *et al.*, 2011), or even between different forms of physiological measurements (e.g., brain and hormones (Harrewijn *et al.*, 2020)), and the same is true for the relationship of observational measures with any of the other domains. It is therefore no surprise that physiological measurement has not yet had much influence on clinical practice.

Why do we have emotions?

Thinking about the introductory spider experiment, why would people respond with fear to spiders and why is there fear in the first place?

Darwinian origins

Questions about why we have emotions are mostly dealt with by evolutionary scientists and originate with Darwin's *Expression of Emotions in Man and Animals* (Darwin, 1872). There, Darwin makes several important claims which permeate the conceptions of emotions we have today. In particular, Darwin explicitly states that emotions have a material basis, which Darwin seeks to situate in his era's knowledge about reflex circuits and brain circulation.

He makes the central claim that emotions possess a *survival value*, for example, when he writes: "The movements of expression in the face and body, whatever their origin may have been, are in themselves of much importance for our welfare."

He also claims that they are *universal*: "the corners of the mouth are drawn downwards, which is so universally recognized as a sign of being out of spirits." He is probably the first to postulate that emotions have a common evolutionary descent: "the movements of the same facial muscles during laughter by man and by various monkeys, is rendered somewhat more intelligible, if we believe in their descent from a common progenitor."

Darwin also situates emotional responses in *different evolutionary periods*. "blushing originated at a very late period in the long line of our descent."

Finally, according to Darwin, emotions have *communicative value and are the basis for habit forming*: "They serve as the first means of communication between the mother and her infant; she smiles approval, and thus encourages her child on the right path, or frowns disapproval."

These pioneering thoughts by Darwin have formed the basis of evolutionary psychology, for example, as expressed in the work of Tooby and Cosmides.

Evolutionary psychology

A dominant evolution-based conceptualization of emotions sees them as detectors of situations in the environment that require a response, and which also put in motion the set of responses necessary; emotions are indeed described as "response programs." A brief outline of the argument follows. The idea is that humans, much like other organisms, are faced with adaptive problems that include fighting, evading predators, or suffering loss of relatives or of one's status. These problems are thought to have recurred in evolutionary history and to require the concerted action of various components of our cognition and physiology.

Cosmides and Tooby (2000) define emotions as a

> superordinate program whose function is to direct the activities and interactions of the subprograms governing perception; attention; inference; learning; memory; goal choice; motivational priorities; categorization and conceptual frameworks; physiological reactions (such as heart rate, endocrine function, immune function, gamete release); reflexes; behavioral decision rules; motor systems; communication processes; energy level and effort allocation; affective coloration of events and stimuli; recalibration of probability estimates, situation assessments, values, and regulatory variables (e.g., self-esteem, estimations of relative formidability, relative value of alternative goals, states, efficacy discount rate); and so on. An emotion is not reducible to any one category of effects, such as effects on physiology, behavioral inclinations, cognitive appraisals, or feeling states, because it involves evolved instructions for all of them together.

Perhaps most importantly : "We think it is perfectly possible that individuals sometimes remain unaware of their emotional states, which is one reason we do not use subjective experience as the *sine qua non* of emotion." according to Cosmides and Tooby (2000).

This account is recurring in other evolutionary accounts of emotions, for example, in Nettle and Bateson's (2012) widely cited account of mood, who also define emotions without reference to subjective feelings: "Why exactly there should be phenomenally experienced components of mood and emotion, and how these evolved from mechanisms we share with other vertebrates is—as the philosophers say—a hard problem. . ."

These evolutionary accounts are interesting but raise several questions about what emotions are. First, they raise the question about how differentiable emotions are from other phenomena, thoughts in particular. Second, there is the question of how superordinate such superordinate programs are meant to be—and how they are themselves set in motion or regulated. Third, the inability to account for the conscious aspect of emotions, namely feelings, makes it hard to relate the evolutionary account to what matters most to clinicians (and arguably most people), namely their own experiences of emotions. Finally, it should be borne in mind that evolutionary theories can often be hard to test, particularly when paleontological records are absent, as in the case of emotions.

How many emotions are there?

Returning to the spider experiment, is it justified to talk about a single emotion of fear and distinguish it from other emotions, such as sadness or anger, or should we think of emotions as coming in many different forms and be highly contextual and constructed in the situation?

The debate about basic emotions

In the examples above and in the experiment with the spider, we have used fear as a prototype of emotion which we would distinguish from other negative emotions such as sadness, mirroring the way we would distinguish between anxiety and depressive disorders. Some authorities claim that emotions are discrete entities, that they can be distinguished fundamentally from one another (Ekman & Cordaro, 2011). Yet, many researchers challenge this common-sense distinction between emotions (Ortony, 2022). The basic emotion view has certain affinities with Darwin's project of identifying universal and innate expressions in animals.

Basic emotions are said to be characterized by distinctive universal signals (for example, facial expressions), a distinctive physiology, distinctive subjective experience, and the fact that they are present in humans as well as other primates (Ekman & Cordaro, 2011) or are said to refer to "affective processes generated by evolutionarily old brain systems upon the sensing of an ecologically valid stimulus" (Izard, 2009). Typical examples, according to these authors, are anger, disgust, fear, joy, surprise, and sadness. The debate around basic emotions is neatly summarized in a meta-analysis on basic emotions (Lench *et al.*, 2011). The authors examined four so-called basic emotions—happiness, sadness, anger, and anxiety—and found that they can be distinguished from each other with moderate effect sizes and are correlated with changes in behavioral experience and physiology. However, the effect sizes of the differences between emotions of the same valence were very small. A good example is the distinction between sadness and anger: the best differentiation between these two emotions was through subjective experience ($d = 0.38$, $p < 0.001$); however, neither cognition ($d = 0.12$, $p > 0.05$), nor behavior ($d = -0.18$, $p > 0.05$), nor physiology ($d = 0.19$, $p > 0.05$) distinguished between anger and sadness. In a critique of this meta-analysis, Lindquist *et al.* (2012) suggest that valence and arousal explain most of the differences observed between so-called basic emotions. A meta-analysis of brain studies found little evidence that emotions can be consistently and specifically localized to particular brain areas. Yet more recent approaches suggest that there may be at least some support for distinguishable basic emotions: when strict 1:1 locationist approaches to emotions are abandoned (Celeghin *et al.*, 2017), support for basic emotions may be hard to dismiss. Indeed, when allowing for pluripotentiality of brain areas, i.e., allowing a neural location to subserve more than one function, depending on network coactivations displayed at any given moment, basic emotions can receive support (Celeghin *et al.*, 2017). Similarly, Saarimäki *et al.* (2016) also find support for concepts of basic emotions.

It should be clear that the question about how many emotions there are has not been resolved and may be ill-posed in the first place. The fact that a young person can reliably distinguish between feelings of fear and anger (or a mixture of the two) itself requires an understanding that has not been provided yet. There are also other unresolved practical and conceptual questions about whether, for example, pain or hunger ought to be classified as emotions or not, with diverse opinions expressed about the matter (Adolphs & Andler, 2018).

Emotion regulation

In our introductory spider experiment, the young person may indeed feel fear but make a conscious decision to control the expression of their emotion, for example, in order to avoid embarrassment. Another young person may be vocal about their distress and decide to respond with anger in order to protest being subjected to such a fearful stimulus. Emotions are thought to be regulated consciously or unconsciously in various ways.

How are emotions regulated?

If emotions are so powerful and important, then it should come as no surprise that mechanisms will have evolved that can modify them. Emotion regulation is defined in various different ways. A broad, yet concise definition is provided by Ross Thompson and will provide a useful background for the rest of this chapter:

> Emotion regulation consists of the extrinsic and intrinsic processes responsible for monitoring, evaluating, and modifying emotional reactions, especially their intensive and temporal features, to accomplish one's goals. (Thompson, 1994)

Given the uncertainties about how to define emotion it is no surprise that the compound derivatives "emotion regulation" or "emotion dysregulation" are also vaguely defined. Also, the word "regulation" can give rise to confusion. It is a naïve view that all negative emotion is a bad thing that ought to be regulated. Such a view ignores findings that children prone to negative affect may be more resilient under certain environmental circumstances (deVries, 1984). Similarly, it would ignore the idea that even very intense sadness or fear may be adaptive, as we will discuss.

Distinctions between emotion and emotion regulation

It has been rightly said that emotions are themselves partly defined as a means of evaluating and modifying experience. This suggests that emotions act to regulate other emotions in their own right (Cole *et al.*, 2004). For example, the teenager in the introduction's imaginary spider experiment may experience less fear if they were presented with pleasant emotional stimuli at the same time as they were presented with the spider images. Such an interaction between emotions could be automatic, rather than a deliberate act of regulation. This type of emotion regulation by emotion is rarely studied and therefore much less understood. Another problem with the distinction between emotion and emotion regulation is methodological. Does the teenager in our example in the introduction report intense fear because they have experienced a strong emotional reaction or because they have not been able to regulate their emotion?

Different forms of emotion regulation

One of the most influential ways of classifying emotion regulation is a model proposed by James Gross (Gross, 1998). It distinguishes between two major phases of emotion regulation: *antecedent-focused* and *response-focused*. The first of the antecedent-focused subphases is *situation selection*. This refers to approaching or avoiding people, places, or objects. In our spider experiment from the introduction, the teenager could effectively regulate his emotions by taking precautions to avoid spiders. The second of the antecedent-focused subphases of emotion regulation is *situation modification*. This act of attention deployment includes distraction, concentration, and rumination. As we will see, infants who are better able to distract themselves by shifting their gaze away from distressing stimuli, better regulate their emotion. Similarly, concentrating on pleasant tasks, such as playing a game, may regulate emotions. Rumination on negative emotions or feelings can have negative emotional consequences (Watkins & Roberts, 2020). Cognitive change refers to how people interpret an emotional experience and it includes cognitive appraisal of a situation. As we will see, this focus on reappraisal has been studied extensively in the emotion regulation literature, with meta-analyses reporting on consistent neural circuits underlying reappraisal (Buhle *et al.*, 2014), and is central to cognitive and behavior treatment approaches. *Response modulation* is listed as the only instance of response-focused emotion regulation strategy in Gross's model (Gross, 1998). This is a very wide category and includes taking drugs to decrease physiological responses, as well as exercise and relaxation.

Notwithstanding its heuristic value, this model has a number of shortcomings. First, the boundaries between the phases of emotion regulation are not always clear; for example, cognitive change can involve situation selection and modification and also have attention redeployment as a consequence. Second, the category of response modulation is quite wide and may obscure important differences between regulation processes as diverse as drug treatment or biofeedback. Third, many important physiological aspects of emotion regulation, such as sleep or food intake, do not fall neatly into any of these categories. Also, exposure and habituation are some of the best-known and clinically relevant strategies of emotion regulation, and do not fit well with these distinctions. Because of their relevance for research in practice, I discuss them separately here.

Emotion regulation through exposure and habituation involves the activation of a fear through successive exposures to a fear-evoking stimulus (Craske *et al.*, 2014). Habituation simply refers to the decreased response after repeated application of the stimulus. The principle is best illustrated through its clinical application in exposure therapy, such as when the teenager of our introduction's spider experiment is repeatedly, and gradually, presented with spider-related items (this could involve the very word "spider", then progressing with spider images through to plastic spiders and eventually the approach of living spiders); however, it is likely that emotion regulation in everyday life—the warming up in social situations, the improvement of performance by "facing one's fear"—relies on the same principles. The exposure and habituation experiments also make clear a more general principle relevant to emotion regulation, namely the often reciprocal relationship between emotions, actions, and the environment. In our spider experiment from the introduction, the young person could simply run away—or, if more aggressive and presented with a real spider, they might simply kill it. This is consistent with the definition of emotions as response tendencies and their postulated role in evolution. It is also important to recognize how actions themselves impact on emotions. It is the action of repeated exposure or of avoidance that regulates emotions in different ways. In keeping with this, one of the fundamental approaches of cognitive behavioral therapy (CBT) (Kendall *et al.*, 2014) to depressed mood is to postulate the primacy that action can have over thoughts and emotions. I will talk more about the relationships between psychological treatment and emotion regulation in the sections under "Emotion, mechanisms and treatment."

While it may be convenient for scientists to consider emotions as phenomena that are generated and regulated by the individual themselves, it is clinically evident that situational factors are very important. Returning to our spider experiment at the beginning of the chapter, the young person's response could be strongly moderated by the presence of a trusted other (parent) versus that of a competing peer. Similarly, a person may already be in a threat situation—a young person from a deprived socioeconomic background who experiences daily exclusion and bullying would reasonably be expected to respond differently to additional threat compared to someone from a supportive background.

Pleasure seeking and emotion regulation

One of the dominant theories of emotion regulation relates to the pursuit of pleasure. Our young person in the spider experiment will feel relief at the removal of the stimulus and distress if the fear stimulus becomes more real. Similarly, if they were presented with a pleasant stimulus (e.g., a favorite food when hungry or the sight of good friends) they would be both happy and willing to approach the stimulus.

Ed Rolls (2013a) expresses this view most clearly. As shown in Figure 5.1, emotions are responses to either positive or negative stimuli (denoted as S+ and S− respectively) and their omission (the underlining) or termination (denoted by !). These stimuli are described as reinforcers, and are defined in the following way: positive reinforcers (also termed rewards) are stimuli that people will work toward, negative reinforcers (also termed punishers) are stimuli that people will avoid. As such, emotions vary across the two axes of a Cartesian system giving rise to four quadrants. In such a scheme the presence of a positive stimulus would lead, depending on its intensity, to anything between pleasure and ecstasy. By contrast, a negative stimulus would lead to anything between apprehension and terror. The omission of a positive reinforcer would lead to anger or rage and the omission of a negative one to relief.

Such a conception of emotions is implicit in many approaches to mood and emotions that seek to explain clinical phenomena too. The critical element here is that humans (and organisms more generally) will avoid negative stimuli and pursue positive ones, and that the person's emotional valence will coincide with the stimulus, thus also implying that humans will generally pursue happiness (or positive emotions) and shun negative ones. This would give rise to a form of hedonic regulation, in which people choose activities that would increase their happiness.

There is also another related and equally important implication of such theories, namely that rewards and punishers (and the ensuing emotions) are ways in which humans can learn and adapt to their environment. Indeed, reinforcement learning models—of the types used by engineers Sutton and Barto (2018)—are deployed to describe the phenomenon that organisms will adjust their behavior so as to maximize rewards and reduce punishers, thus further increasing rewards. The first formalization of such models by Rescorla and Wagner (Rescorla & Wagner, 1972) indicated that learning about stimuli in the environment related to positive (or negative) surprises. Positive surprises (induced by stimuli that are better than expected on the basis of previous trials) increase the likelihood of choosing the

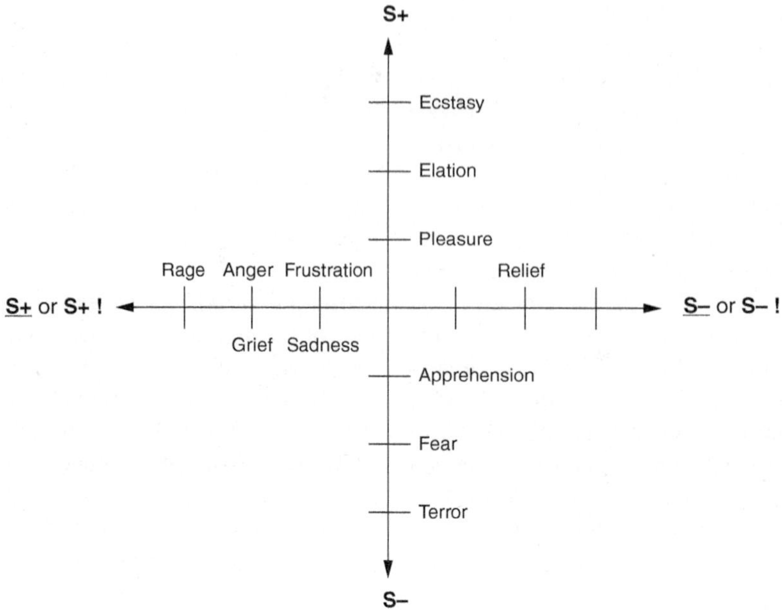

Figure 5.1 Emotions in response to reinforcers. Emotions generated in response to different reinforcers: presentation of reinforcers (S+), presentation of negative reinforcers (S–), omission of positive reinforcers (S+) termination of positive reinforcers (S+ !), and omission of negative reinforcers (S–) termination of a negative reinforcers (S– !). *Source:* Rolls, (2013a, 2013b)/with permission of SAGE Publications.

action that brought about these stimuli in subsequent trials; conversely, negative surprises will decrease the likelihood of choosing these stimuli.

The important point here is that because positive stimuli (rewards) are equated with pleasure, reward processing has achieved a prominent position in trying to understand the origins of mood disorders and their treatment. Indeed, as we will discuss in detail, depression has been variably described as an inability to recognize or enjoy pleasures, or an inability to learn from pleasant events in the environment. Conversely, a lot of effort has been expended in trying to influence people's ability to experience pleasure, for example, through changing their exposure to reinforcers, as we shall see in the section on "Emotion, mechanisms and treatment."

A particular attraction of reward-based conceptions is that there is a fairly clear understanding of brain systems underlying reward processing in the brain across organisms (Keren *et al.*, 2018). Indeed, experiments in rodents and other animals delineate dopamine-rich projections from the ventral tegmental area to the nucleus accumbens and the ventral prefrontal cortex (Ferenczi *et al.*, 2016) as key for the anticipation of rewards in the environment. Using neuroimaging, a similar network of areas has been highlighted for reward processing. As we will see, this has also influenced approaches to research, particularly in depression and bipolar disorder.

Instrumental emotion regulation

More recent systematic approaches to emotion regulation highlight instrumental motivation for regulating emotions, that is people may consciously or unconsciously choose emotions because they allow them to achieve a goal. Could the young person in our spider experiment display a particular emotion in anticipation of the fear stimulus or in order to achieve a goal?

Rather than simply pursuing happiness, humans also pursue what is useful. Tamir (2016) makes a useful distinction between hedonic and instrumental emotion regulation. An example of the former would be the reduction of unpleasant states, such as anxiety or depression; an example of instrumental regulation would be to feel in such way as to improve performance in a task. Instrumental regulation has been demonstrated in relation to anger: people are more likely to want to feel anger (by choosing appropriate mood induction studies) ahead of a competitive game (Tamir *et al.*, 2008). In that sense, people choose to feel in the way that they perceive best serves their needs. This view is contrary to concepts of happiness maximization that are often implicit in psychopathology and align with recent observations that humans may even seek to reduce positive affect so as to achieve mood homeostasis (Taquet *et al.*, 2020).

There can be many superordinate reasons for choosing to regulate emotions in a particular way. One relates to the regulation of emotions to be in accordance with the ideas one has of themselves. Prabhakar *et al.* (2022) recently proposed that emotions and even psychiatric symptoms, such as anhedonia (see section on " Reward and reinforcement as prototypical mechanisms of emotional disorders"), may represent an interactive relationship, unfolding over the course of development, between emotion knowledge (the set of emotion representations that a person remembers about themselves), autobiographical memory (a person's memory of their own past, personal experiences), and self-concept (a person's often implicit belief about who they are and who they will be). This interactive relationship is due to a person's desire to "make choices and decisions that allow them to maintain a coherent sense of self," that is, remain consistent with their own beliefs about who they are. For example, in a person with past experiences that reflect a high rate of negative experiences or a low rate of positive events those experiences may lead to self-concept representations that are negative. In another example, repeated experiences of bullying may result in an individual representing their own self as "a loser" or as "awkward." This self-concept representation is itself an explanatory framework for negative experiences and may be to "protect" the self against making choices, like attending social gatherings, that may cause distress. Continuing efforts to avoid these feelings lead to greater avoidance of social gatherings, strengthening self-concept representations as "shy" or "awkward."

More generally, there is an emerging recognition that people may regulate their emotions in order to serve particular goals including social ones (Hochschild, 1979, 2012).

What is mood?

Mood is one of the most commonly used terms in nosology. In the spider experiment, it is important to consider that the young person may not arrive in a neutral mood (if such a thing even exists), and that their emotional responses to fear stimuli may be increased or decreased depending on how they "feel on the day."

Mood is often defined as an emotional state that lasts longer. However, it is never clear how long such a longer-lasting emotion is supposed to be, e.g., milliseconds, seconds, minutes. This point is not trivial, as duration is central to psychopathology, where emotional states have to last weeks (e.g., two weeks in depression) in order to meet prespecified thresholds.

One of the most dominant conceptions of mood is that it integrates across events in the environment and thus "keeps tracks" of rewards and punishers in the longer term (Nesse, 2019). In such a model, mood represents a history of the environment one is in.

This integration of events in the environment finds support in computational models, where mood is expressed as a quantity that is proportional to an integral of recent events in the environment. In the simplest case, this integration can be thought of as a summation of rewards and punishers over a particular time. Most commonly, such models are fitted onto experimental data that come from variations of gambling games, with losses and wins representing negative and positive events, respectively (Rutledge *et al.*, 2014). The mood measurement is provided on a trial-by-trial basis by the individual (Jangraw *et al.*, 2023).

In such work, it has been found that mood expressed by individuals at any given moment is described well as a function of the running average of rewards in the environment. It also seems that events (wins or losses) experienced early in such an experiment weigh more in the moment-to-moment rating of mood, than do ones that occur later, giving rise to a primacy model of mood.

More recently, it has been shown that mood changes even in the absence of stimuli—in fact, most people's mood starts to drift downwards when asked to "rest," for example, by looking at a cross during an experiment. This is more likely to happen for people who are more sensitive to rewards, i.e., more likely to change their mood in response to rewards. This finding is important and suggests that humans represent not only the history of observed events, but also hold in mind a potential reward environment by generating an opportunity cost, a "what could have been".

Emotion and psychopathology

In our spider experiment, we would expect that different young people might react differently to one and the same stimulus. One only has to imagine how one's own clinic patients might take to any given potential threat, in terms of their emotional responses. Psychopathology is primarily concerned with studying this sort of variability and its sources—why and how individuals differ from each other in their emotions and responses to emotion-related stimuli.

Boundaries to normality

The boundaries between emotional disorder and normality are often unclear and currently debated (Stringaris, 2021). In our introductory spider experiment, the response of our young person may have been judged differently by different observers at different times and with different information available to them.

Classification systems typically take the pragmatic approach of using cutoffs that would restrict the prevalence of a disorder to a relatively small proportion of the population, trying to account for impairment (Stringaris, 2011) and whether the emotional reaction is proportional to the stimulus. A typical example is that of the boundaries between bereavement reaction and depression. Such decisions often involve an evaluative judgment about what constitutes an appropriate reaction, though in the case of bereavement certain symptoms (e.g., suicidal ideation) are said to predict the persistence of depression and impairment (American Psychiatric Association, 2022).

Genetic sources of interindividual variability

The sources of interindividual variability can be either genetic or environmental, or due to the interplay between both (see Chapter 21).

Most of the common emotional disorders, including depression, generalized anxiety, and social anxiety disorders, are moderately heritable at around $h = 0.3–0.4$, according to twin studies. The heritability of physiological markers of emotions, such as heart rate and blood pressure or neural activity, are also generally thought to be modest (Rappaport *et al.*, 2018; Tegegne *et al.*, 2020). Environmental effects seem to be quite important, but identifying factors that are purely due to the environment is difficult, as genetic effects can predispose to life events (a phenomenon termed gene–environment correlation) and genetic background can also create environments for the offspring that may increase the chances of psychopathology (passive gene–environment correlation) (Plomin *et al.*, 2012).

Overlap between emotional and disruptive disorders

Our young person in the introductory spider experiment may not only display fear, but also intense anger to the experimental setup. Indeed, he or she may go as far as to destroy the equipment. Emotional disorders co-occur with other emotional disorders and also with disruptive disorders more often than one might expect to happen by chance. For example, up to 70% of people with social phobia may have depression (Ohayon & Schatzberg, 2010) concurrently and symptoms of oppositionality are strongly related to future emotional problems such as depression (Stringaris & Goodman, 2009). This co-occurrence appears to be predominantly explained by the genes that these disorders share with each other, for example, the genetic covariance between depression and social phobia explains a lot of their phenotypic overlap (Mosing *et al.*, 2009).

Importantly, there is also a sequence to the occurrence of emotional disorders. Conditions such as separation anxiety disorder and phobias may occur early on, whereas panic disorder is rare before adolescence and depression rises sharply in incidence after the onset of puberty. It is more common than not to find that a depressed adolescent who presents in clinic to have experienced anxiety problems before. This form of longitudinal comorbidity (Costello *et al.*, 2005), where anxiety is antecedent to depression is also borne out in epidemiological samples with a clear anxiety pathway to depressive disorders (Rice *et al.*, 2017).

Emotion and development

Our young person in the introductory spider experiment might have responded differently as an adolescent as opposed to when they were a 5-year-old, not least because of changes in emotion regulation. Interest in mechanisms of development has grown in parallel with research efforts in developmental psychopathology and has highlighted challenges to developmental research in this area before appraising the existing evidence.

Emotion and development: challenges to its study

The first challenge concerns the *limits of reporting source* and descriptive phenomenology. Most of the research about mood and emotion in adults relies on self-report. Indeed, self-reported emotional states are validating outcomes for most research studies—including imaging and genetics—in adolescence and adults. However, research in newborns, infants, and young children must rely on parent report or on observation. The correlation between different informants and methods is at best modest (see Chapter 28 on assessment). The use of different informants or different methods of assessment at different age groups limits our ability to judge the continuity of emotional states.

A related challenge is that some experimental paradigms are often *age-specific.* Another challenge concerns the technology used to study mood and emotion. For example, functional magnetic resonance imaging (fMRI) is hard to use on toddlers. Finally, as is the case for most of psychiatric research, it is unclear how best to map findings from different methods and sources onto each other. A particular challenge for research in early development is to map functional findings onto a fairly rapidly changing brain structure (Goddings *et al.*, 2014; Gilmore *et al.*, 2018; Kaczkurkin *et al.*, 2019).

Emotional disorders and their developmental moderation

Certain symptoms and symptom-constellations are more likely to occur at certain developmental stages. For example, while anxiety, particularly in the form of separation from attachment figures, is very common in early life, panic and agoraphobia are very rarely present in prepubertal children (Beesdo *et al.*, 2009). Similarly, symptoms of social phobia and body dysmorphic disorder are far less common in children than they are in adolescents or adults (Krebs *et al.*, 2024). Also, depression is less common in childhood than in adolescence and it is only in puberty that the higher frequency in girls versus boys establishes itself (Thapar *et al.*, 2022). As discussed in Chapter 63, the prevalence of depression increases after puberty when the 2:1 female to male ratio in depression is established (Salk *et al.*, 2017). The reasons for this gender difference are unclear and it is plausible that biological, social, and cognitive factors interact to increase girls' vulnerability.

The reasons for these developmental moderations are unclear. It is notable though that adolescence is also a time of heightened reward sensitivity (van Duijvenvoorde *et al.*, 2014). Indeed, there appears to be an inverted U-shape (Figure 5.2) relationship between reward sensitivity and age, as evidenced in a study of over 200 adolescents across several years by Crone and her group in the Netherlands (Braams *et al.*, 2015).

They found that both fMRI-measured activity in the nucleus accumbens during reward processing, one of the key areas related to reward processing, and reward-sensitivity behavioral scores show a quadratic relationship with age, such that they peak during adolescence. Whether this relationship is specific to rewards, or whether it represents more general hypersensitivity to other stimuli remains unclear—there is evidence for such a generalized hypersensitivity in the social domain (Foulkes & Blakemore, 2016). Importantly, while heightened reward sensitivity has been linked to a series of negative outcomes, more recent interpretations suggest that it may underlie more general plasticity and enhance the ability to learn from stimuli in the environment, for example, via reinforcement learning (Crone & Dahl, 2012; Davidow *et al.*, 2016). In the following section,

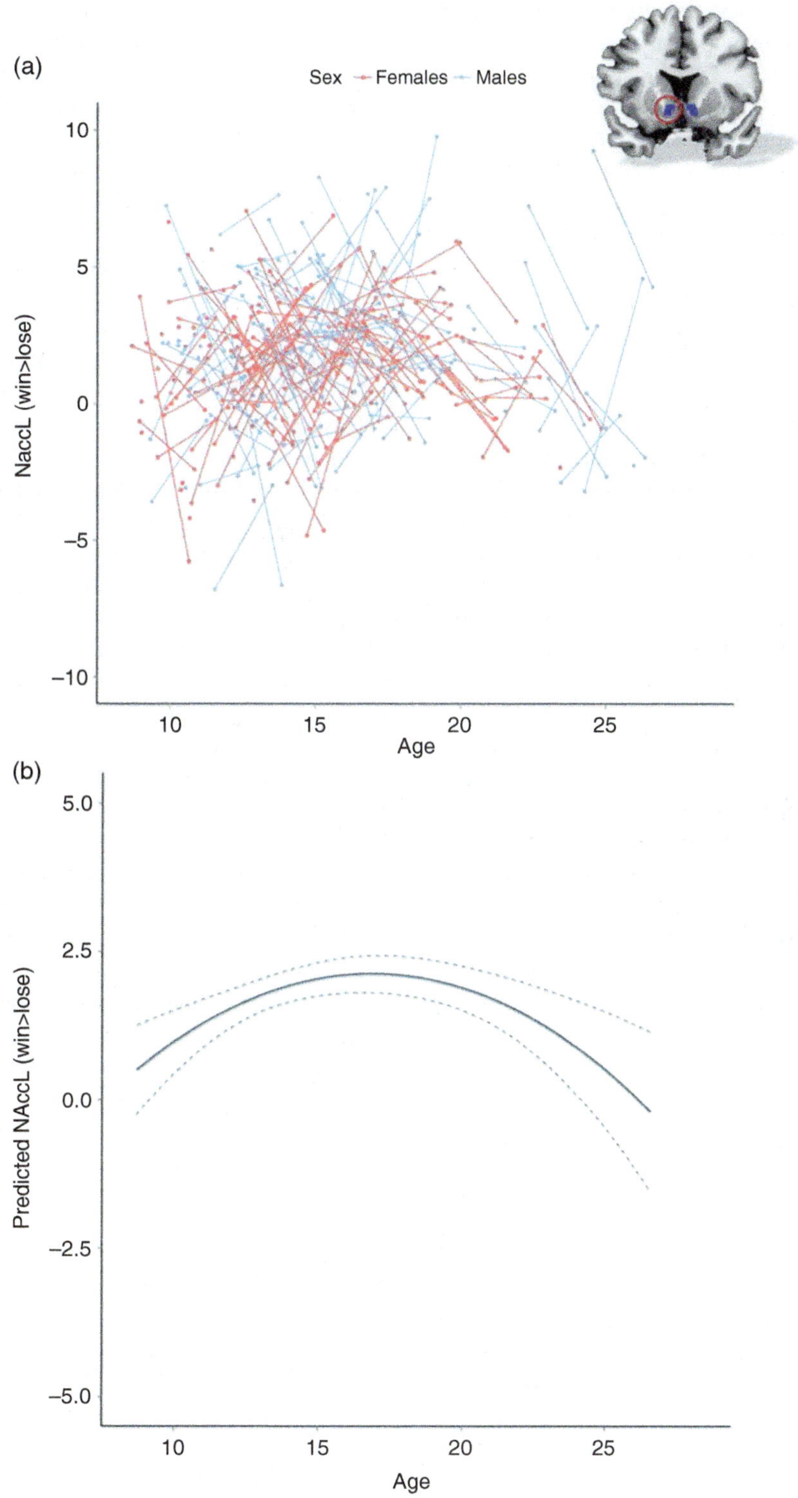

Figure 5.2 Depiction of the relationship between brain activity in the nucleus accumbens and age at two time points; on the *y*-axis are observed (upper panel a) and predicted (lower panel b) contrast values for win > lose in a reward-related task, with the dotted lines representing 95% confidence intervals. *Source:* Braams *et al.* (2015)/Society for Neuroscience/CC by 4.0.

I discuss the importance of reward-processing aberrations for depression and its possible developmental moderation.

Emotion, mechanisms, and treatment

In this section, I focus on reward processing as a prototype mechanism for emotion disorders and their treatment. There are several reasons for focusing on reward processing, including the fact that it has been widely studied in psychopathology, is theory driven, and that it has cross-species evidence. It also links with some key symptoms that clinicians encounter, such as irritability and anhedonia.

Reward and reinforcement as prototypical mechanisms of emotional disorders

Reward processing is one of the central themes in emotion regulation research and its developmental moderation. Its relevance for clinical mechanistic research in psychopathology is most obvious in the field of depression. The interest stems from understanding depression through the lens of disturbed hedonic processes. Indeed, anhedonia is typically defined as either anticipatory, referring to the reduction of interest in, or consummatory, referring to the difficulty in deriving pleasure from, previously pleasurable activities. Together with low mood, anhedonia is a cardinal symptom of depression (Thapar *et al.*, 2022). The lack of interest, termed anticipatory anhedonia, is mapped onto reward anticipation in the experimental literature; consummatory anhedonia is mapped onto the outcome phase (Keren *et al.*, 2018; Nielson *et al.*, 2021). Anticipating and experiencing rewards allows an individual to learn about their environment. Termed reward learning (Schultz & Dickinson, 2000), it updates their expectations about what might come next. Moreover, such learning allows an individual to allocate resources and effort. There is evidence that these reward-related processes are disturbed in people with depression, as evidenced by recent meta-analyses of reward-processing behavioral paradigms of close to 50 individual studies showing that the maximal difference between depressed and nondepressed participants was during reward-based decision-making (SMD = 0.644), indicating that reward-bias deficits are the strongest in depression (Halahakoon *et al.*, 2020). This also seems true in adolescents where a longitudinal sample, showed that lower reward seeking could predict depressive symptoms and new onset of depression in adolescents at high risk of depression (Rawal *et al.*, 2013). Convergent evidence for the importance of reward processing has been provided from early studies (Forbes & Dahl, 2012; Stringaris *et al.*, 2015), indicating a longitudinal relationship between reward and depression (and anhedonia in particular). This has been borne out by a meta-analysis of fMRI studies showing decreased brain fMRI activations in the caudate, the thalamus, and the globus pallidus during the outcome phase of reward (Keren *et al.*, 2018).

The findings emerging from these studies indicate that striatal hypoactivations are linked to depressive symptoms and, more specifically, anhedonia. However, a recent critical review of imaging studies of reward processing in depression (Nielson *et al.*, 2021) highlighted a number of conceptual and method-related problems that limit the clinical translation of these results.

Mechanism-based treatments of emotional disorders

Treatments for individual mood and anxiety disorders are discussed in the relevant chapters. Here I focus on mechanism-based treatments, in particular those that relate to reward processing in the broad sense, continuing with the theme from preceding section.

Treatments that are trying to make use of the principles of reward processing and, more generally, reinforcement learning are increasing in psychology and psychiatry. They are to be found in the field of anxiety (Craske *et al.*, 2014), as well as in disruptive mood dysregulation disorder (Kircanski *et al.*, 2018). Behavioral activation (BA) therapy features most prominently among psychological treatments that are based on reward processing and reinforcement principles, and it is also discussed in Chapter 63 as one of the treatments with evidence in adults (Ekers *et al.*, 2014) and in some adolescents (Jenness *et al.*, 2022). While there are many developments in BA (Jenness *et al.*, 2022), one of the early central ideas concerns the decreased access to rewards that people with depression have. These rewards are typically described as response-contingent positive reinforcement and are thought to be key in the onset and maintenance of clinical depression (Lewinsohn, 1974). Indeed, BA uses functional behavioral analysis to identify what is rewarding to a young person and highlights barriers to accessing these rewards; it also uses principles of operant conditioning to replace avoidant behaviors (that restrict access to reinforcing experiences), with approach-focused behaviors and goals. A summary of BA is provided in the Box 5.1.

Box 5.1 An example of a mechanism-inspired treatment for depression

Behavioral activation (BA) treatment

- is based on a functional analytic model of depression that utilizes the principles of operant conditioning to increase positive reinforcement and decrease barriers to engaging in positively reinforcing behaviors.
- addresses avoidant behaviors related to anhedonia and similar symptoms.
- takes an idiographic approach in order to identify what contributes to reduced positive reinforcement and maintains depression symptoms within the individual's context.
- aims at increasing engagement in positively reinforcing activities and at replacing avoidant behaviors with approach-focused goal setting.
- emphasizes goal-directed over mood-directed behavior and can be adapted to characterize approach and avoidance impairments stemming from conditions co-occurring with depression.

The central notion is that a change in mood is brought about by changes in goals. Indeed, BA therapists distinguish between mood-directed behavior (i.e., when a young person behaves in a particular way because of their mood, whether positive or negative) versus goal-directed behavior (when the behavior followed is due to goal setting congruent with the young person's values). One can see how regulation is thought to happen through the effects of action/behaviors on mood, rather than on mood directly. It should be emphasized, that while these principles are plausible, there is very little experimental information to assess their causal effects, i.e., demonstrate that these principles are indeed central to the clinical change achieved by BA (Janssen *et al.*, 2021).

Several other new psychological treatments have arisen through consideration of reward and positive affect, such as Positive Affect Treatment (Craske *et al.*, 2019) and Virtual Reality Reward Training (Chen *et al.*, 2021). These approaches aim at reward anticipation and motivation for reward-driven activities, although they are still at the early stages of development and, as for BA, there is still at best only preliminary evidence for the causal involvement of reward processing in their mechanism of action. As is often the case, these treatment approaches have so far almost exclusively been tested in Western countries and their broader applicability should not be uncritically assumed.

Finally, a range of pharmacological agents have been tested in depression in relation to their actions on the reward system. These include drugs with known or likely actions on the reward system, such as pramipexole, buporopion, and amisulpiride, but also others, such as the commonly used selective serotonin reuptake inhibitors (SSRIs) and serotonin-norepinephrine reuptake inhibitors (SNRIs), and lurasidone. More recently, fast-acting antidepressants, most notably ketamine, have been tested in relation to their effects on the reward system (Stringaris & Kotoula, 2023). All these compounds show effects on the brain's reward processing, e.g., on activity in the ventral striatum during reward anticipation. Yet, none of them has strong evidence for a causal involvement of the reward system in the production or alleviation of symptoms demonstrated (Stringaris & Kotoula, 2023).

References

Adolphs, R. & Andler, D. (2018) Investigating emotions as functional states distinct from feelings. *Emotion Review* **10**, 191–201. doi:10.1177/1754073918765662.

American Psychiatric Association (2022) *Diagnostic and Statistical Manual for Mental Disorders*, 5th edn. text revision edn. American Psychiatric Association, Washington, DC. Available: https://www.psychiatry.org:443/psychiatrists/practice/dsm [19 Apr 2023].

Beesdo, K. *et al.* (2009) Anxiety and anxiety disorders in children and adolescents: developmental issues and implications for DSM-V. *The Psychiatric Clinics of North America* **32**, 483–524. doi:10.1016/j.psc.2009.06.002.

Braams, B.R. *et al.* (2015) Longitudinal changes in adolescent risk-taking: a comprehensive study of neural responses to rewards, pubertal development, and risk-taking behavior. *The Journal of Neuroscience* **35**, 7226–7238. doi:10.1523/JNEUROSCI.4764-14.2015.

Buhle, J.T. *et al.* (2014) Cognitive reappraisal of emotion: a meta-analysis of human neuroimaging studies. *Cerebral Cortex* **24**, 2981–2990. doi:10.1093/cercor/bht154.

Celeghin, A. *et al.* (2017) Basic emotions in human neuroscience: neuroimaging and beyond. *Frontiers in Psychology* **8**, 1432.

Chen, K. *et al.* (2021) Virtual reality reward training for anhedonia: a pilot study. *Frontiers in Psychology* **11**, 613617.

Cole, P.M. *et al.* (2004) Emotion regulation as a scientific construct: methodological challenges and directions for child development research. *Child Development* **75**, 317–333. doi:10.1111/j.1467-8624.2004.00673.x.

Cosmides, L. & Tooby, J. (2000) An evolutionary psychological theory of the emotions. In: *Handbook of Emotions*. (eds M. Lewis & J.M. Haviland-Jones). Guilford, New York. pp. 91–115.

Costello, E.J. *et al.* (2005) 10-year research update review: the epidemiology of child and adolescent psychiatric disorders: I. Methods and public health burden. *Journal of the American Academy of Child & Adolescent Psychiatry* **44**, 972–986. doi:10.1097/01.chi.0000172552.41596.6f.

Craske, M.G. *et al.* (2014) Maximizing exposure therapy: an inhibitory learning approach. *Behaviour Research and Therapy* **58**, 10–23. doi:10.1016/j.brat.2014.04.006.

Craske, M.G. *et al.* (2019) Positive affect treatment for depression and anxiety: a randomized clinical trial for a core feature of anhedonia. *Journal of Consulting and Clinical Psychology* **87**, 457–471. doi:10.1037/ccp0000396.

Crone, E.A. & Dahl, R.E. (2012) Understanding adolescence as a period of social–affective engagement and goal flexibility. *Nature Reviews Neuroscience* **13**, 636–650. doi:10.1038/nrn3313.

Darwin, C. (1872) *The Expression of the Emotions in Man and Animals*, 1st edn. John Murray, London. Available: http://darwin-online.org.uk/content/frameset?pageseq=1&itemID=F1142&viewtype=side [24 Apr 2023].

Davidow, J.Y. *et al.* (2016) An upside to reward sensitivity: the hippocampus supports enhanced reinforcement learning in adolescence. *Neuron* **92**, 93–99. doi:10.1016/j.neuron.2016.08.031.

deVries, M.W. (1984) Temperament and infant mortality among the Masai of East Africa. *The American Journal of Psychiatry* **141**, 1189–1194. doi:10.1176/ajp.141.10.1189.

Ekers, D. *et al.* (2014) Behavioural activation for depression; an update of meta-analysis of effectiveness and sub group analysis. *PLoS One* **9**, e100100. doi:10.1371/journal.pone.0100100.

Ekman, P. & Cordaro, D. (2011) What is meant by calling emotions basic. *Emotion Review* **3**, 364–370. doi:10.1177/1754073911410740.

Ferenczi, E.A. *et al.* (2016) Prefrontal cortical regulation of brainwide circuit dynamics and reward-related behavior. *Science* **351**, aac9698. doi:10.1126/science.aac9698.

Forbes, E.E. & Dahl, R.E. (2012) Altered reward function in adolescent depression: what, when, and how? *Journal of Child Psychology and Psychiatry* **53**, 3–15. doi:10.1111/j.1469-7610.2011.02477.x.

Foulkes, L. & Blakemore, S.-J. (2016) Is there heightened sensitivity to social reward in adolescence? *Current Opinion in Neurobiology* **40**, 81–85. doi:10.1016/j.conb.2016.06.016.

Gilmore, J.H. *et al.* (2018) Imaging structural and functional brain development in early childhood. *Nature Reviews. Neuroscience* **19**, 123–137. doi:10.1038/nrn.2018.1.

Goddings, A.-L. *et al.* (2014) The influence of puberty on subcortical brain development. *NeuroImage* **88**, 242–251. doi:10.1016/j.neuroimage.2013.09.073.

Gross, J.J. (1998) The emerging field of emotion regulation: an integrative review. *Review of General Psychology* **2**, 271–299. doi:10.1037/1089-2680.2.3.271.

Halahakoon, D.C. *et al.* (2020) Reward-processing behavior in depressed participants relative to healthy volunteers. *JAMA Psychiatry* **77**, 1286–1295. doi:10.1001/jamapsychiatry.2020.2139.

Harrewijn, A. *et al.* (2020) Associations between brain activity and endogenous and exogenous cortisol: a systematic review. *Psychoneuroendocrinology* **120**, 104775. doi:10.1016/j.psyneuen.2020.104775.

Hochschild, A.R. (1979) Emotion work, feeling rules, and social structure. *American Journal of Sociology* **85**, 551–575.

Hochschild, A.R. (2012) *The Managed Heart: Commercialization of Human Feeling*, 3rd edn. University of California Press, Berkeley, CA.

Izard, C.E. (2009) Emotion theory and research: highlights, unanswered questions, and emerging issues. *Annual Review of Psychology* **60**, 1–25. doi:10.1146/annurev.psych.60.110707.163539.

Jangraw, D.C. *et al.* (2023) A highly replicable decline in mood during rest and simple tasks. *Nat Hum Behav* **7**(4), 596–610. doi:10.1038/s41562-023-01519-7.

Janssen, N.P. *et al.* (2021) How does behavioural activation work? A systematic review of the evidence on potential mediators. *Psychotherapy and Psychosomatics* **90**, 85–93. doi:10.1159/000509820.

Jenness, J.L. *et al.* (2022) Behavioral activation as a principle-based treatment: developments from a multi-site collaboration to advance adolescent depression treatment. *Evidence-Based Practice in Child and Adolescent Mental Health* **8**, 1–18. doi:10.1080/23794925.2022.2042871.

Kaczkurkin, A.N. *et al.* (2019) Sex differences in the developing brain: insights from multimodal neuroimaging. *Neuropsychopharmacology* **44**, 71–85. doi:10.1038/s41386-018-0111-z.

Kendall, P.C. *et al.* (2014) Cognitive-behavioral therapy with children and adolescents. In: *Transdiagnostic Treatments for Children and Adolescents: Principles and Practice.* (eds J. Ehrenreich-May & B.C. Chu). Guilford Press, New York. pp. 161–182.

Keren, H. *et al.* (2018) Reward processing in depression: a conceptual and meta-analytic review across fMRI and EEG *Studies. The American Journal of Psychiatry* **175**, 1111–1120. doi:10.1176/appi.ajp.2018.17101124.

Kircanski, K. *et al.* (2018) Psychosocial treatment of irritability in youth. *Current Treatment Options in Psychiatry* **5**, 129–140. doi:10.1007/s40501-018-0141-5.

Krebs, G., Clark, B.R., Ford, T.J., Stringaris, A. *et al.* (2024) Epidemiology of body dysmorphic disorder and appearance preoccupation in youth: prevalence, comorbidity and psychosocial impairment. *J Am Acad Child Adolesc Psychiatry.* doi: 10.1016/j.jaac.2024.01.017. Online ahead of print.

Lench, H.C. *et al.* (2011) Discrete emotions predict changes in cognition, judgment, experience, behavior, and physiology: a meta-analysis of experimental emotion elicitations. *Psychological Bulletin* **137**, 834–855. doi:10.1037/a0024244.

Lewinsohn, P.M. (1974) A behavioral approach to depression. In: *The Psychology of Depression: Contemporary Theory and Research.* (eds R.J. Friedman & M.M. Katz). John Wiley & Sons, Oxford, UK. pp. xvii, 318–xvii, 318.

Lindquist, K.A. *et al.* (2012) The brain basis of emotion: a meta-analytic review. *The Behavioral and Brain Sciences* **35**, 121–143. doi:10.1017/S0140525X11000446.

Moors, A. (2022) *Demystifying Emotions: A Typology of Theories in Psychology and Philosophy.* Cambridge University Press, Cambridge, UK.

Mosing, M.A. *et al.* (2009) Genetic and environmental influences on the comorbidity between depression, panic disorder, agoraphobia and social phobia: a twin study. *Depression and Anxiety* **26**, 1004–1011. doi:10.1002/da.20611.

Nesse, R.M. (2019) *Good Reasons for Bad Feelings: Insights from the Frontier of Evolutionary Psychiatry.* Dutton, New York. Available: https://www.amazon.co.uk/Good-Reasons-Bad-Feelings-Evolutionary/dp/0241291089 [19 Apr 2023].

Nettle, D. & Bateson, M. (2012) The evolutionary origins of mood and its disorders. *Current Biology* **22**, R712–R721. doi:10.1016/j.cub.2012.06.020.

Nielson, D.M. *et al.* (2021) Great expectations: a critical review of and suggestions for the study of reward processing as a cause and predictor of depression. *Biological Psychiatry* **89**, 134–143. doi:10.1016/j.biopsych.2020.06.012.

Ohayon, M.M. & Schatzberg, A.F. (2010) Social phobia and depression: prevalence and comorbidity. *Journal of Psychosomatic Research* **68**, 235–243. doi:10.1016/j.jpsychores.2009.07.018.

Ohman, A. (2007) Fear. In: *Encyclopedia of Stress.* (ed G. Fink). Elsevier, Amsterdam.

Ortony, A. (2022) Are all "basic emotions" emotions? A problem for the (basic) emotions construct. *Perspectives on Psychological Science* **17**, 41–61. doi:10.1177/1745691620985415.

Plomin, R. *et al.* (2012) *Behavioral Genetics.* Worth Publishers, New York.

Prabhakar, J. *et al.* (2022) Origins of anhedonia in childhood and adolescence. *Current Topics in Behavioral Neurosciences* **58**, 43–60. doi:10.1007/7854_2022_356.

Rappaport, L. *et al.* (2018) Behavioral and molecular genetics of emotion dysregulation. In: *The Oxford Handbook of Emotion Dysregulation.* (eds T.P. Beauchaine & S.E. Crowell). Oxford University Press, Oxford, UK. pp. 203–220.

Rawal, A. *et al.* (2013) "The risks of playing it safe": a prospective longitudinal study of response to reward in the adolescent offspring of depressed parents. *Psychological Medicine* **43**, 27–38. doi:10.1017/S0033291712001158.

Rescorla, R.A. & Wagner, A.R. (1972) A theory of Pavlovian conditioning: variations in the effectiveness of reinforcement and nonreinforcement. In: *Classical Conditioning II: Current Research and Theory.* (eds A.H. Black & W.F. Prokasy). Appleton-Century-Crofts, New York. pp. 64–99.

Rice, F. *et al.* (2017) Antecedents of new-onset major depressive disorder in children and adolescents at high familial risk. *JAMA Psychiatry* **74**, 153–160. doi:10.1001/jamapsychiatry.2016.3140.

Rolls, E.T. (2013a) What are emotional states, and why do we have them? *Emotion Review* **5**, 241–247. doi:10.1177/1754073913477514.

Rolls, E.T. (2013b) A biased activation theory of the cognitive and attentional modulation of emotion. *Frontiers of Human Neuroscience* **7**. doi:10.3389/fnhum.2103.00074.

Rutledge, R.B. *et al.* (2014) A computational and neural model of momentary subjective well-being. *Proceedings of the National Academy of Sciences* **111**, 12252–12257. doi:10.1073/pnas.1407535111.

Saarimäki, H. *et al.* (2016) Discrete neural signatures of basic emotions. *Cerebral Cortex* **26**, 2563–2573. doi:10.1093/cercor/bhv086.

Salk, R.H. *et al.* (2017) Gender differences in depression in representative national samples: meta-analyses of diagnoses and symptoms. *Psychological Bulletin* **143**, 783–822. doi:10.1037/bul0000102.

Schultz, W. & Dickinson, A. (2000) Neuronal coding of prediction errors. *Annual Review of Neuroscience* **23**, 473–500. doi:10.1146/annurev.neuro.23.1.473.

Stringaris, A. (2011) Irritability in children and adolescents: a challenge for DSM-5. *European Child & Adolescent Psychiatry* **20**, 61–66. doi:10.1007/s00787-010-0150-4.

Stringaris, A. (2021) Sources of normativity in childhood depression. *European Child & Adolescent Psychiatry* **30**, 1663–1665. doi:10.1007/s00787-021-01891-7.

Stringaris, A. & Goodman, R. (2009) Longitudinal outcome of youth oppositionality: irritable, headstrong, and hurtful behaviors have distinctive predictions. *Journal of the American Academy of Child and Adolescent Psychiatry* **48**, 404–412. doi:10.1097/CHI.0b013e3181984f30.

Stringaris, A. & Kotoula, V. (2023) Reward processing in depression. In: *APA Handbook of Depression*. (ed D. Pizzagalli). American Psychiatric Association, Washington, DC.

Stringaris, A. *et al.* (2015) The brain's response to reward anticipation and depression in adolescence: dimensionality, specificity, and longitudinal predictions in a community-based sample. *The American Journal of Psychiatry* **172**, 1215–1223. doi:10.1176/appi.ajp.2015.14101298.

Sutton, R. & Barto, A. (2018) *Reinforcement Learning: An Introduction*, 2nd edn. The MIT Press, Cambridge, MA.

Tamir, M. (2016) Why do people regulate their emotions? A taxonomy of motives in emotion regulation. *Personality and Social Psychology Review* **20**, 199–222. doi:10.1177/1088868315586325.

Tamir, M. *et al.* (2008) Hedonic and instrumental motives in anger regulation. *Psychological Science* **19**, 324–328. doi:10.1111/j.1467-9280.2008.02088.x.

Taquet, M. *et al.* (2020) Mood homeostasis, low mood, and history of depression in 2 large population samples. *JAMA Psychiatry* **77**, 944–951. doi:10.1001/jamapsychiatry.2020.0588.

Tegegne, B.S. *et al.* (2020) Heritability and the genetic correlation of heart rate variability and blood pressure in >29 000 families. *Hypertension* **76**, 1256–1262. doi:10.1161/HYPERTENSIONAHA.120.15227.

Thapar, A. *et al.* (2022) Depression in young people. *The Lancet* **400**, 617–631. doi:10.1016/S0140-6736(22)01012-1.

Thompson, R.A. (1994) Emotion regulation: a theme in search of definition. *Monographs of the Society for Research in Child Development* **59**, 25–52. doi:10.2307/1166137.

van Duijvenvoorde, A.C.K. *et al.* (2014) A cross-sectional and longitudinal analysis of reward-related brain activation: effects of age, pubertal stage, and reward sensitivity. *Brain and Cognition* **89**, 3–14. doi:10.1016/j.bandc.2013.10.005.

Watkins, E.R. & Roberts, H. (2020) Reflecting on rumination: consequences, causes, mechanisms and treatment of rumination. *Behaviour Research and Therapy* **127**, 103573. doi:10.1016/j.brat.2020.103573.

CHAPTER 6

Attachment: normal development, individual differences, and associations with experience

Kristin Bernard[1] **and Mary Dozier**[2]

[1] Department of Psychology, Stony Brook University, Stony Brook, NY, USA

[2] Department of Psychological and Brain Sciences, University of Delaware, Newark, DE, USA

According to John Bowlby (1969/1982), the attachment system evolved to enhance reproductive fitness. Infants develop attachments to figures who are "older and wiser" than themselves and seek to maintain proximity with these attachment figures under threatening conditions. The infant's behavioral repertoire of crying, smiling, clinging, and following represents an organized system, designed to maintain or restore proximity to the caregiver. By the time the infant is capable of crawling or walking, the attachment system has developed fully such that the infant does not want to move far from the parent except when circumstances are familiar (Bretherton, 1985). Under conditions of threat, when proximity is especially important to survival, the need for proximity to the caregiver is intensified (Bowlby, 1969/1982; Rutter *et al.*, 2009). Given the basic evolutionary function of this system, attachments develop in virtually all ordinary childrearing conditions. Although the attachment system may have special significance for the infant, attachments are thought to remain important for humans throughout life.

Historical context of the development of attachment theory

Attachment theory was developed in response to psychoanalytic and social learning theories of the early to mid-20th century, and in the context of observations of the pernicious effects of privation on human and nonhuman young, and a burgeoning literature on ethology and evolution. John Bowlby articulated what has come to be known as attachment theory. Mary Ainsworth played a critical role as an astute observer of individual differences in attachment and developed a system for classifying infants' attachment quality on the basis of these observations.

Bowlby and the development of attachment theory

Bowlby was trained as a psychiatrist when psychoanalytic thinking dominated the field. Whereas many psychoanalysts of the time believed that young children's inner fantasies played a much more formative role in development than interactions with their real mothers, Bowlby insisted on the importance of a child's real caregiving experiences. Bowlby and James Robertson observed hospitalized and institutionalized children that experienced separations from their parents, documenting extreme behaviors when children experienced prolonged separations. In his 1951 World Health Organization (WHO) report, Bowlby pieced together the different conditions of neglect and deprivation, articulating the importance of the young child's relationship with the parent.

There was much criticism of this early work, with the naturalistic studies of institutional care challenged as not representative, not rigorous, and certainly not experimental. Critical to the acceptance of this work were links to Harlow's experimental findings of the effects of deprivation on infant rhesus macaques (Harlow, 1958). Finding that infant macaques became attached to the cloth diaper in their cage, even when fed by a wire mesh device, made a good case for contact comfort being separate and not simply driven by "oral needs" (as suggested by psychoanalytic theorists of the time) or reinforcement (as suggested by social learning theorists of the time).

Bowlby was struck with Lorenz's (1957) findings that goslings became imprinted on their mothers despite not depending on their mothers for food. Lorenz (1957), Tinbergen (1951), and others developed a theory of ethology, which elaborated on Darwin's theory of evolution. The behaviors described, such as imprinting, were seen as evolutionarily prepared, but dependent on the environmental conditions to elicit them. Ethology

Rutter's Child and Adolescent Psychiatry and Psychology, Seventh Edition.
Edited by Anita Thapar, Daniel S. Pine, Samuele Cortese, Cathy Creswell, Tamsin J. Ford, James F. Leckman, and Argyris Stringaris.

Companion website: www.wiley.com/go/thapar/rutterspsych7

provided a framework for thinking about how the behaviors of the young infant—crying, smiling, clinging, following—all represented evolutionarily prepared behaviors infants displayed toward the caregiver that were organized around maintaining proximity to the caregiver.

Ainsworth as methodologist

Mary Ainsworth came to work with Bowlby at the Tavistock Clinic, London, in 1950. She began a study that followed 28 Ganda babies and their 23 families over the first year of life (Ainsworth, 1967), carefully observing attachment behaviors and their precursors. Some years following her Ugandan study, Ainsworth initiated a second observational study with 26 families in Baltimore, observing each family for at least 70 hours throughout the first year of the infant's life. Close to the child's first birthday, parents brought their children in for a laboratory assessment, with this assessment among Ainsworth's key legacies. The assessment, the "Strange Situation" procedure, involves a series of separations and reunions between parent and child that provide a compelling context for observing children's behaviors toward the caregiver when distressed (Ainsworth *et al.*, 1978).

Infant attachment quality

Measurement: the Strange Situation

The Strange Situation has become the gold standard for assessing attachment quality among infants. The Strange Situation consists of eight episodes in which the child is separated from and then reunited with the parent twice. Of particular relevance for coding attachment is the child's behavior toward the parent during the reunion episodes. This behavior is thought to reflect the child's expectations of caregiver availability when distressed.

Infant attachment classifications

Whereas the *presence* of an attachment relationship is essentially universal (except under unusual conditions), there is variability in the *quality* of attachment relationships. Children's behavior during reunion episodes of the Strange Situation highlights these individual differences in attachment patterns (Table 6.1). Children who turn directly to their parents to be soothed are classified as having secure attachments. Those who turn away are classified as having avoidant attachments. Children who show a combination of proximity seeking and resistance/anger toward the parent are classified as having resistant attachments. These three types of attachment are considered organized attachments because they are thought to represent strategies that maximize caregiver availability (Main, 1990).

For the first decade after Ainsworth *et al.* (1978) published the classification system, researchers used these three categories to classify children's attachment. About a decade later, Main and Solomon (1986, 1990) introduced disorganized attachment as a distinct category. Disorganized attachment was first identified because some children (about 15% in typical samples) were difficult to classify and/or showed behaviors that fell outside of those characterized in Ainsworth *et al.*'s system. Disorganized attachment represents a breakdown in attachment strategy, with children appearing to lack a solution for dealing with their distress (Main & Solomon, 1990). Children with disorganized attachment show odd or anomalous behaviors when distressed in their parents' company, such as freezing or stilling for a period of time, contradictory attachment tendencies consecutively or simultaneously, or apprehension of the parent.

Table 6.1 Overview of Strange Situation classifications.

Strange Situation classification	Percentage[a]	Strange Situation behavior	Assumed meaning of behavior
Organized secure (B)	51.6	• Acknowledges parent's return upon reunion • Returns to play after being soothed • May or may not cry during separation	Confident in parent's availability due to history of sensitive care
Organized insecure–avoidant (A)	14.7	• Fails to acknowledge parent's return; may continue to play, or turn away • Less likely to cry during separation	Not confident in parent's availability due to history of unresponsiveness or rejecting care
Organized insecure–resistant (C)	10.2	• Mixture of seeking and resisting contact; angry quality • Highly distressed • Difficult to soothe	Not confident in parent's availability due to history of inconsistent care
Disorganized (D)	23.5	• Odd or anomalous behavior • Contradictory behaviors (e.g., crying while turning away) • Lack of organized strategy	Dysregulated in presence of caregiver due to history of frightening or atypical care (e.g., maltreatment)

[a] Percentages based on meta-analytic findings reflecting global distribution of four-way attachment classifications ($k = 285$ studies, $N = 20{,}720$ children). *Source:* Percentage data from Sheridan *et al.* (2023).

Attachment classifications versus attachment disorders

Although insecure and disorganized attachment are predictive of mental health problems, these classifications are not considered forms of pathology themselves (see Verhage *et al.* (2023) for further consideration of misconceptions about common attachment terminology). The 5th edition of the *Diagnostic and Statistical Manual of Mental Disorders* (DSM-5) recognizes two forms of attachment disorders, which are distinct from attachment classifications. Reactive attachment disorder (RAD) is characterized by inhibited and withdrawn behavior toward primary caregivers and disinhibited social engagement disorder (DSED) is characterized by reduced reticence with and overly friendly behavior toward strangers. Both disorders are thought to develop in contexts of anomalous caregiving conditions, such as severe deprivation as seen in institutional care. See Chapter 57 for more details about disorders of attachment and social engagement related to deprivation.

Cross-cultural findings

In a meta-analysis of the Strange Situation conducted in eight different countries, van IJzendoorn and Kroonenberg (1988) found that differences within cultures were typically greater than between cultures. However, some cross-cultural differences were observed. Whereas secure classifications were modal in all countries, a greater preponderance of avoidant classifications was seen in Western Europe and resistant classifications in Israel and Japan. Although cross-cultural differences in parenting norms (e.g., infants rarely being separated from mothers in Japan) may play a role in the differences in Strange Situation classification patterns (e.g., Miyake *et al.*, 1985), few studies have examined these questions empirically.

Predictors of individual differences in attachment

A number of factors contribute to individual differences in the quality of parent–child attachments. We provide an overview of these predictors, beginning with the most proximal, parental behavior, and moving to more distal factors, such as parent attachment state of mind, parent psychopathology, and environmental conditions (Figure 6.1).

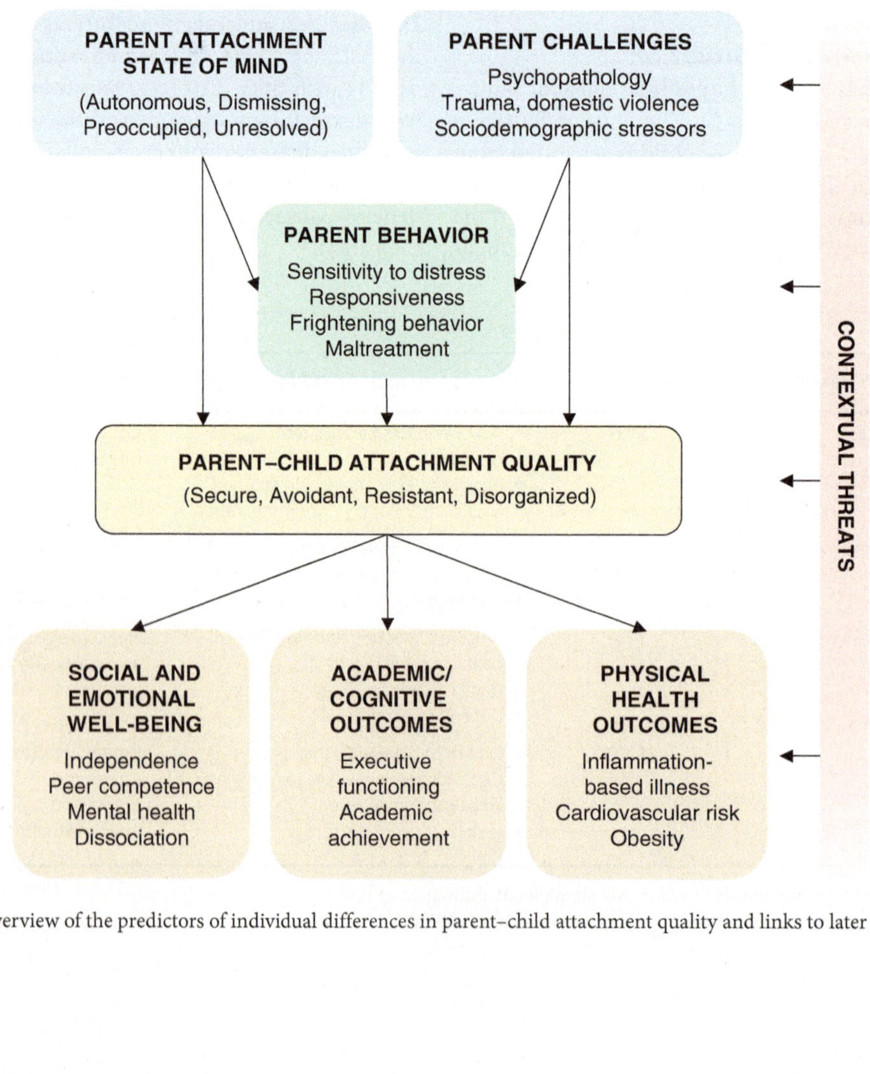

Figure 6.1 Conceptual overview of the predictors of individual differences in parent–child attachment quality and links to later outcomes.

Parental behavior

Parental behavior is seen as the critical mechanism by which individual differences in attachment develop. Attachment theory suggests that children will develop secure attachments if parents are consistently available when they are distressed, and will develop insecure attachments when parents show other patterns of behavior. In her Baltimore study, Ainsworth and colleagues found that maternal sensitivity strongly predicted infants' attachment classifications (Ainsworth *et al.*, 1978). Since Ainsworth's seminal work, parental sensitivity has been found to only moderately predict attachment security (De Wolff & van IJzendoorn, 1997).

Odd, anomalous, and/or frightening behavior appears to have associations with attachment quality that are distinct from simply insensitive behaviors. Frightening (e.g., threatening postures or aggressive movements) and frightened parental behavior (e.g., backing away from a distressed infant) have been linked specifically to the development of disorganized attachment (Lyons-Ruth *et al.*, 1999; Schuengel *et al.*, 1999; Hesse & Main, 2006; Madigan *et al.*, 2006). Other extreme and atypical parental behaviors that increase infant arousal, such as negative-intrusive behavior, role confusion, and affective withdrawal, have also been found to predict infant attachment disorganization (Lyons-Ruth *et al.*, 1999; Madigan *et al.*, 2006).

Not surprisingly, maltreatment (i.e., abuse, neglect) is associated with heightened risk for disorganized attachment (Cicchetti *et al.*, 2006). Replicating earlier findings (Cyr *et al.*, 2010), a recent meta-analysis found that rates of disorganized attachment were substantially higher in maltreated samples (64% disorganized) than nonmaltreated samples (22%; Madigan *et al.*, 2023). Children in foster care with histories of abuse and neglect show elevated rates of disorganized attachment (Vasileva & Petermann, 2018). See Chapter 25 for further consideration of child abuse and neglect.

Attachment state of mind

Attachment state of mind refers to the way in which the parent, or the adult more generally, conceptualizes their own attachment experiences. State of mind is the best-identified predictor of infant attachment (van IJzendoorn, 1995; Pederson *et al.*, 1998), although it seems to be less proximal than sensitivity. Mary Main and her colleagues deliberately developed the system of assessing attachment state of mind to match children's attachment. That is, commonalities in conceptualizations among parents of children with secure attachments were identified, as were commonalities among parents of children with avoidant, resistant, and disorganized attachment. State of mind was assessed through an interview, the adult attachment interview (AAI; George *et al.*, 1996), which asks adults to describe their parents and instantiate descriptions with particular examples, recall times from childhood when they were hurt, upset, or rejected, and consider how their adult personality is affected by the way they were raised. Finally, incidences of abuse and loss are recalled. The semistructured interview is transcribed and coded by reliable coders.

As a group, parents whose children were securely attached to them were called "autonomous" because they appeared able to evaluate attachment experiences freely. Characterizations of attachment figures matched well with specific descriptions for a rich, coherent picture, and attachment was valued. Parents whose children had avoidant attachments were called "dismissive of attachment" because they appeared to devalue attachment experiences. They typically showed a lack of memory with respect to attachment experiences and/or idealization of attachment figures. The parents of children with resistant attachments to them were termed "preoccupied with regard to attachment." These parents were caught up or enmeshed in attachment experiences, as shown by angry involvement and/or rambling discourse. Parents of children with disorganized attachments were most likely to be unresolved with regard to loss or abuse.

In a meta-analysis of the concordance between state of mind and infant attachment, Verhage *et al.* (2016) found evidence of intergenerational concordance ($r = 0.31$ for autonomous-secure concordance; $r = 0.21$ for unresolved-disorganized concordance). Parent sensitivity only partially explained this association, highlighting a "transmission gap" and a need for further research to identify mechanisms by which parental attachment state of mind influences infant attachment (Verhage *et al.*, 2016).

Parent challenges

A number of factors can interfere with parents behaving in ways that foster secure attachments. When parents face significant challenges themselves, such as psychiatric disorders, extreme poverty, and their own unresolved issues regarding attachment experiences, it often becomes more difficult to consistently parent in sensitive ways.

Psychopathology

As would be expected, parents with psychiatric disorders, such as depression, borderline personality disorder, and substance abuse, experience particular challenges in parenting. Parental depression, for example, is associated with both withdrawn and intrusive parental behaviors (Goodman & Gotlib, 1999; Bernard *et al.*, 2018). In their meta-analysis, Madigan *et al.* (2023) found that parent psychopathology was associated with lower rates of secure attachment and higher rates of disorganized attachment among infants.

Trauma exposure and domestic violence

When parents experience unresolved trauma or domestic violence, it is often difficult for them to effectively buffer children. This difficulty can be the result of children witnessing violence involving attachment figures, or the result of parents behaving in anomalous ways because of their own trauma experiences (Schuengel *et al.*, 1999). When parents are unresolved with regard to loss or trauma, they are susceptible to behaving with their children in frightening ways and children are at increased risk for disorganized attachments (Schuengel *et al.*, 1999).

Challenging environmental conditions

Living under harsh conditions can also interfere with optimal parenting and threaten the development of secure attachments. Cyr *et al.* (2010) conducted a meta-analysis of the effect of high-risk conditions on children's attachment. Children who had five or more sociodemographic risk indicators (e.g., low income, parental substance abuse, minority group, single parent, adolescent mother, and low parental education) had similar rates of disorganized attachment as maltreated children (Cyr *et al.*, 2010). Taken together, these studies suggest that adverse environmental conditions can contribute to higher rates of insecure and disorganized attachments (Madigan *et al.*, 2023).

Other factors

Child care

The National Institutes of Health in the United States invested enormous resources in assessing the effects of childcare on children's development, with a particular focus on attachment relationships (NICHD, 1997). In this study of more than 1300 children, attendance at childcare, the quality of childcare, and the amount of childcare was found to have no significant direct effects on attachment security. This was at odds with several previous studies (Belsky & Rovine, 1988; Clarke-Stewart, 1989) that had shown effects of the amount of childcare on attachment quality. These findings were sustained in assessments of children at the age of three (NICHD, 2001).

Child temperament

There has been considerable debate about whether temperament and attachment are overlapping constructs. Temperament refers to individual differences in infant reactivity or regulation across attentional, behavioral, and emotional domains. In general, studies have not found strong evidence for an association between infant temperament and security of attachment (for a review, see Vaughn *et al.*, 2008; for a meta-analysis, see Groh *et al.*, 2017). Although infant temperament does not determine the likelihood of having a secure or insecure attachment, several studies suggest that temperamental reactivity may influence the type of insecure attachment displayed. For example, infants with higher negative emotionality may be more prone to resistant patterns of insecurity (characterized by high levels of distress), whereas infants with lower negative emotionality may be more prone to avoidant patterns of insecurity (characterized by low levels of distress) (Belsky & Rovine, 1987; Marshall & Fox, 2005). Cassidy *et al.* (2011) proposed that the match between an infant's temperament and their parent's attachment state of mind may be important in predicting infant attachment quality.

Neurodevelopmental conditions

Given that autism spectrum disorder (ASD) is characterized by challenges in social communication and social–emotional reciprocity, researchers have questioned whether autistic children form attachments with primary caregivers in the same way as neurotypical children. Meta-analytic evidence has shown that autistic children do indeed demonstrate attachment behaviors (e.g., proximity seeking following separation) and develop selective preferences for their primary caregivers (Rutgers *et al.*, 2004), suggesting that autism does not preclude the formation of attachment relationships. There is some evidence to suggest that the prevalence of secure attachment is lower in autistic children relative to nonautistic children, but this may be driven in part by concurrent intellectual disability (Rutgers *et al.*, 2004). In a large meta-analysis, Madigan *et al.* (2023) found that child neurodevelopmental conditions, medical conditions, and prematurity were not associated with differences in infant attachment distributions. Similar to what is seen in neurotypical samples, maternal sensitivity is a predictor of attachment security in autistic children (Koren-Karie *et al.*, 2009; Cossette-Côté *et al.*, 2022), highlighting a similar precursor for secure attachment.

Contextual threats

Environmental conditions that threaten parents' physical and psychological safety and reduce access to resources and support pose significant threats to parent and child well-being, in ways that may undermine the development of healthy attachment relationships. War and its resulting displacement of families is one example of such a contextual threat. In a study of 1.5 to 5-year-old war-exposed Israeli children with elevated post-traumatic stress disorder (PTSD) symptoms, children showed increased avoidant attachment behaviors with their mothers (Feldman & Vengrober, 2011). Given that war often involves extreme unpredictability, loss, and threats to safety, we would expect that a parent's own ability to serve as a secure base is compromised in this context. Indeed, mothers have been found to behave in less sensitive ways in the context of ongoing armed conflict (Halevi *et al.*, 2017). See Chapter 41 for more consideration of the development of refugee, asylum-seeking, and displaced children.

Systemic and structural racism, which refers to the embedding of discriminatory or oppressive practices and policies into broader institutions or systems, has been proposed as another contextual threat that may undermine sensitive parenting and the development of secure attachments within families of color (Stern *et al.*, 2023). Few studies consider how the sociopolitical context of historical and ongoing racism may influence the development of secure attachment (Stern *et al.*, 2022). Parenting behaviors beyond sensitivity may be important in helping protect children in the context of race-related threats. For example, racial socialization (e.g., preparing children for bias) has been highlighted as an important parenting practice that supports children's socioemotional well-being in families of color (Coard, 2021; Dunbar *et al.*, 2022).

Taken together, such evidence of the impacts of major environmental threats on sensitive parenting and child attachment quality highlights the importance of considering broader ecological contexts in research and clinical practice involving parent–child relationships.

Links between infant attachment and later outcomes

Attachment quality is predictive of a number of important developmental outcomes. Although attachment theorists have primarily hypothesized about the effects of attachment on socioemotional outcomes, researchers have also found evidence of associations between attachment and other domains of functioning (e.g., academic achievement, physical health). Associations between attachment and developmental outcomes are typically stronger among children living in stable environments where conditions stay relatively constant over time than among children living in less stable environments (Weinfield *et al.*, 2000; Vondra *et al.*, 2001). Weinfield *et al.* (2000) have argued that continuity and discontinuity follow lawful patterns, with instability in care predicting discontinuity.

Social relationships in childhood

Although children remain dependent upon their attachment figures in a number of ways, secure attachment provides a secure base for exploration, theoretically allowing greater confidence in exploration (Sroufe *et al.*, 1983). Consistent with theory, empirical data suggest that secure attachments in infancy support more autonomous or independent functioning in early childhood. For example, Sroufe *et al.* (1983) found that children assessed as secure in infancy were rated by preschool teachers as more independent than avoidant and resistant children. McElwain *et al.* (2003) similarly found that infant attachment classification at 15 months predicted social behavior at age 3, controlling for concurrent attachment classifications and maternal sensitivity. In a meta-analysis based on 63 studies, there was a small effect size for the overall association between attachment security and peer relations, $r = 0.20$ (Schneider *et al.*, 2001).

Psychopathology

Two meta-analyses have found a small but significant effect for insecure attachment predicting elevated depressive and anxiety symptoms, with avoidant attachment most clearly driving the effect (Groh *et al.*, 2012; Madigan *et al.*, 2013). Based on meta-analytic effect sizes, Madigan *et al.* (2013) estimated that a child with an insecure attachment is approximately twice as likely to develop depressive/anxiety symptoms than a child with a secure attachment. Meta-analytic findings also demonstrate that insecure, and most especially disorganized, attachment is associated with behavior problems (e.g., oppositional behavior, hyperactivity) during childhood (Fearon *et al.*, 2010). Children with disorganized attachments appear most at risk for behavior problems ($d = 0.34$), with smaller effects seen among avoidant ($d = 0.12$) and resistant children ($d = 0.11$). Given that even the largest association is relatively modest in magnitude, it is important to consider that attachment is only one of many potential factors that may influence risk for psychopathology. Additionally, the relatively small magnitude of these effect sizes highlights that insecure and disorganized attachment patterns are not, themselves, reflective of pathology.

Cognitive/academic outcomes

There has been increased attention in recent years to how attachment may affect outcomes beyond those reflecting socioemotional well-being. Exposure to sensitive parenting is thought to support healthy self-regulation and brain development in ways that promote cognitive functioning. Several studies have demonstrated that attachment security is predictive of enhanced executive functioning skills, such as working memory, cognitive flexibility, and self-control (e.g., Bernier *et al.*, 2015), and school readiness (e.g., Bernier *et al.*, 2020). Furthermore, several longitudinal studies have found evidence of associations between early maternal sensitivity and academic outcomes through adolescence (Fraley *et al.*, 2013) and adulthood (Raby *et al.*, 2015).

Physical health

Emerging research suggests that attachment quality is also predictive of physical well-being (Ehrlich & Cassidy, 2021). Using data from the Minnesota Longitudinal Study, Puig *et al.* (2013) found that adults who were classified as insecurely attached during infancy were more likely to report inflammation-based illnesses as adults than those classified as securely attached. In the same sample, early maternal sensitivity was found to predict cardiometabolic risk (e.g., high blood pressure, elevated inflammation) for adults, with this association mediated by attachment-based cognitive schemas (i.e., secure base script knowledge, described more in the section on "Attachment script assessment") in early adulthood (Farrell *et al.*, 2019). Insecure attachment during infancy has been linked to increased risk of obesity for preschoolers (Anderson & Whitaker, 2011) and adolescents (Anderson *et al.*, 2012), with preliminary evidence suggesting that this association may be explained in part by increased inflammation (Bernard *et al.*, 2019).

Assessments of attachment beyond infancy

Although attachment to a caregiver has particular salience in infancy and early childhood, attachments remain important throughout life. Bowlby (1988) talked of the importance of attachment "from the cradle to the grave" (p. 62). The form that these attachments take changes across development, with children increasingly able to represent attachment figures internally over time (Main *et al.*, 2005).

Preschool

A preschool version of the Strange Situation was developed by Cassidy *et al.* (1992). Categories of attachment generally parallel infant categories. An exception is that controlling behavior is seen to a greater extent than disorganized behavior and is considered the outgrowth of disorganized attachment. That is, children become controlling of parents as a way to cope with feelings of disorganization (Main & Cassidy, 1988).

Move to the level of representation

In infancy, the organization of the child's behavioral system is the essence of attachment, with measurement of attachment based on behavioral observations. Even in infancy, though, these behaviors reflect the child's expectations of the parent's availability, and hence representations of attachment figures. With development, the "move to the level of representation" becomes more pronounced (Main *et al.*, 2005). Over time, children are thought to develop internal working models of self and caregivers based on their experiences of attachment-relevant events (Bowlby 1969/1982; Bretherton, 1992). These internal working models provide rules that guide behavior, organize attention, and permit or limit access to memory (Main *et al.*, 1985). A number of measures have been developed to assess attachment at the level of representation in childhood and adulthood.

Story stems and narratives

Semi-projective measures have been used with young children to assess their attachment representations, such as the Separation Anxiety Test (Main *et al.*, 1985) and the Attachment Story Completion Task (Bretherton *et al.*, 1990). In the Separation Anxiety Test, children are asked how they would feel and what they would do in response to a range of separation scenarios (e.g., parents leaving for two weeks); in the Attachment Story Completion Task, children are asked to describe "what happens next" in a series of story stems (e.g., a child getting hurt). Although more work is needed to validate these measures with behavioral observations of children's attachment behavior, these representational measures relate to children's behavior in separation paradigms (e.g., Slough & Greenberg, 1990) and predict children's socioemotional functioning (e.g., Easterbrooks & Abeles, 2000).

Adult attachment interview

The AAI (George *et al.*, 1996), described earlier in this chapter, is the assessment of attachment state of mind used among adolescents and adults. As predicted by theory, attachment state of mind is associated with relations with peers and parents in adolescence (Allen *et al.*, 2003), and with adult functioning in romantic relationships (Bouthillier *et al.*, 2002). Adults with psychiatric disorders are disproportionately characterized by having nonautonomous states of mind (Bakermans-Kranenburg & van IJzendoorn, 2009; Dozier *et al.*, 2008).

Attachment script assessment

The attachment script assessment (ASA; Waters & Waters, 2006) is a narrative-based task developed initially for assessing secure base script knowledge of adults. The secure base script refers to a temporal–causal sequence of cognitive expectations about interactions with an attachment figure in contexts of distress (Figure 6.2). The ASA includes prompt word outlines, from which individuals are asked to generate a story about a parent–child dyad or romantically involved couple. ASA narratives are scored for the extent to which the story demonstrates knowledge of the secure base script. Secure base script knowledge, as coded from the ASA, has been found to predict sensitive

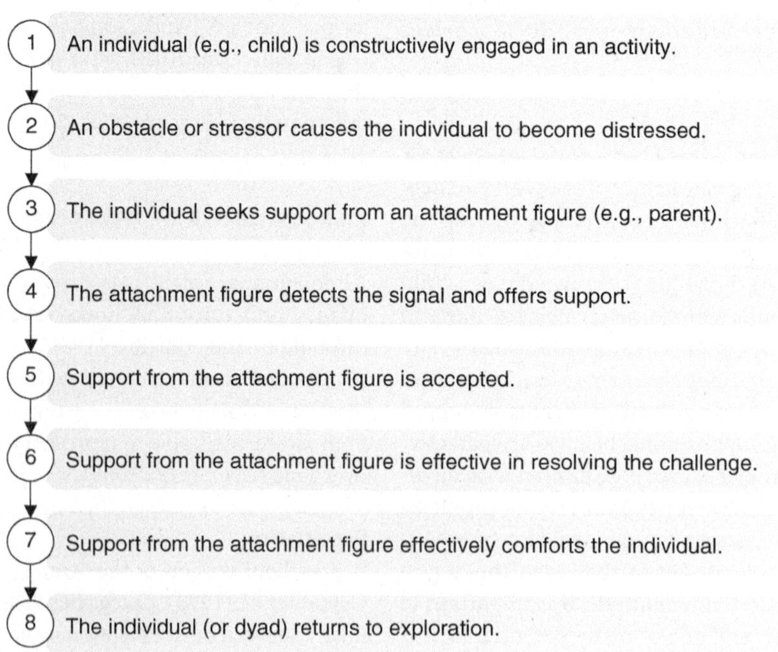

Figure 6.2 Key elements of the secure base script.

parenting (Coppola *et al.*, 2006; Hawkins *et al.*, 2015) and to be predicted by one's own history of caregiving experiences during childhood (Steele *et al.*, 2014).

Self-report assessments

Self-report assessments of attachment have been used extensively. Although self-reports are very easy to administer relative to the AAI, they relate weakly to AAI classifications (Roisman *et al.*, 2007). In a meta-analysis, Roisman *et al.* (2007) found that the AAI was very weakly related to attachment style (mean $r = 0.09$). Nonetheless, the instruments often relate to variables of interest in meaningful ways (Roisman *et al.*, 2007).

Stability and change

Evidence for the stability of attachment over time has been mixed, with effect sizes ranging from small to large (e.g., Waters, 1978; Egeland & Farber, 1984; Bar-Haim *et al.*, 2000); studies examining within-person stability from attachment quality in early childhood (assessed using the Strange Situation Procedure) through young adulthood (assessed using the AAI) suggest modest stability in normative samples (Groh *et al.*, 2014) and samples with elevated risk (Raby *et al.*, 2013). Greater instability (e.g., move from secure attachment to insecure or disorganized attachment) has been found for children who experienced more meaningful changes in the family environment, such as changes in caregiving quality or major family events or transitions (Thompson *et al.*, 1982; Vondra *et al.*, 1999).

Attachment and neurobiology

Nonhuman primate and rodent studies have provided compelling evidence for the effects of maternal care on the developing infant's neurobiology. Hofer (1994) has argued that specific maternal behaviors or processes serve as "hidden regulators" for the infant. The mother helps the infant regulate temperature, heart rate, and glucocorticoid production, for example. Hofer suggested that behavioral–sensorimotor processes, involving aspects of mother–infant attunement and synchrony, appeared particularly important to behavioral and neurobiological regulation. Not surprisingly, then, children show different physiological responses depending on caregiving quality and attachment quality.

A number of studies have examined physiological indicators of infant stress during the Strange Situation to understand the extent to which attachment quality influences children's stress system responses. The Strange Situation is designed to be stressful to all children. However, avoidant children often turn away from their parents upon reunion, appearing to distract themselves with toys, raising the question of whether these children are effectively regulating their distress. Sroufe and Waters (1977) found that children showed increased heart rate regardless of attachment classification, suggesting that avoidant children experience heightened distress despite their behavior. Cortisol is another marker of stress reactivity that has been studied during the Strange Situation. Gunnar *et al.* (2006) have argued that, in the presence of supportive caregivers, most young children do not show a cortisol response under ordinary stressful conditions. This buffering function is important in protecting the developing brain from high levels of circulating glucocorticoids. Indeed, only children with disorganized attachments to their parents have not shown significant increases in cortisol in the Strange Situation (Bernard & Dozier, 2010). These results point to the importance of attachment in helping children to regulate physiologically as well as behaviorally. See Chapter 12 for further consideration of neuroscience and attachment/affiliation.

Attachment among fathers

Increasing attention has been paid to the role that fathers play in children's development and to father–child attachment relationships (Pruett, 1998; Lamb & Lewis, 2004). As would be predicted given that attachment is considered to be relationship-specific (Sroufe, 1985), infants' attachment to fathers and to mothers is relatively orthogonal. Van IJzendoorn and De Wolff (1997) found only a modest association between infants' attachment to mothers and fathers. The association between paternal sensitivity and infant–father attachment security is weaker than the association between maternal sensitivity and infant–mother attachment security (for meta-analysis, see van IJzendoorn and De Wolff, 1997). Recent work has jointly considered the quality of children's attachment to mothers and fathers in predicting outcomes. In a recent study of 1097 children drawn from 9 studies, Dagan *et al.* (2021) found that children with an insecure attachment relationship with 1 parent (regardless of which one) or both parents had higher depressive or anxious symptoms than children who were securely attached to both parents. These results suggest that mother–child attachment quality and father–child attachment quality may both be important in predicting child mental health outcomes, although more research is needed to see whether these findings extend to other domains of development.

Attachment among children in institutional care

There are several caregiving situations that reflect deviations from species-typical parental care, such as when children experience disruptions in parental care (e.g., foster care), lack a consistent caregiver (e.g., institutional care), or experience collective caregiving, with prolonged separations from parents (e.g., kibbutz). These caregiving environments each present unique opportunities to understand how attachment relationships form under various conditions.

We focus here specifically on institutional care as it represents the most problematic of conditions for the infant and young child. Staff providing care in institutional settings typically work on shifts, with children having a number of caregivers over the day and across the week. The ratio of children to caregivers is often quite high, making it difficult for staff to provide other than perfunctory care. The adverse effects on children are striking, with children showing stunting or impaired development across physical, cognitive, and social domains (Nelson, 2007; van IJzendoorn & Juffer, 2006). The effects on attachment quality are profound. Whereas children form attachments under virtually all conditions, even when parents are abusive, many children in institutional care fail to develop consolidated attachments. Zeanah *et al.* (2005) found that 100% of never-institutionalized children formed clear, classifiable attachment behaviors, as contrasted with 3% of institutionalized children showing such behaviors. The Bucharest Early Intervention Project (BEIP; Nelson *et al.*, 2014) represents the first experimental study of the effects of institutional care. Children in institutional care in Romania were randomized to either treatment as usual (which could involve continued institutional care) or foster care. Following placement into high-quality foster care, previously institutionalized children were more likely to develop secure attachments and less likely to have disorganized attachments than children who remained in institutional care, suggesting evidence of recovery following placement into a family (Smyke *et al.*, 2010). Furthermore, timing of placement mattered. Children placed into family foster care before 24 months of age were more likely to develop secure attachments than those placed later (Smyke *et al.*, 2010). This study provides compelling evidence of the plasticity of the attachment system very early in life, and suggests that recovery from extreme deprivation may become more challenging over time.

Attachment and interventions

Infants and toddlers

There are several attachment-based interventions for parents of infants and young children with strong evidence bases. The interventions range from those that focus more on changing parents' behaviors to those that focus more on changing parents' representations of their own attachment experiences. We provide two examples below. (For more consideration of relationship-based treatments, see Chapter 36).

Attachment and Biobehavioral Catch-up

The Attachment and Biobehavioral Catch-up (ABC; Dozier & Bernard, 2019) intervention targets three issues known to affect children's attachment security and self-regulatory capabilities. First, parents are helped to behave in nurturing ways when children are distressed because nurturing behavior is associated with secure attachment (Ainsworth *et al.*, 1978). Second, parents are helped to follow children's lead, which has been demonstrated to enhance children's regulatory capabilities (Raver, 1996). Third, parents are helped to behave in ways that are not frightening because frightening behavior is associated with disorganized attachment (e.g., Schuengel *et al.*, 1999). These issues are targeted through 10 sessions implemented in families' homes with parents and children present and involves a "coaching" approach with parent coaches commenting frequently on parent–child interactions as they occur in sessions. The ABC intervention has primarily been evaluated with parents and their children with histories of early adversity (e.g., neglect, placement in foster care, poverty). The ABC intervention has been shown to be effective in randomized clinical trials in enhancing child attachment security (Bernard *et al.*, 2012). Positive outcomes for the children from the ABC intervention group have also been seen in the areas of diurnal cortisol production (Bernard *et al.*, 2015, Garnett *et al.*, 2020), emotion regulation (Lind *et al.*, 2014), and executive functioning (Lewis-Morrarty *et al.*, 2012; Lind *et al.*, 2020). In middle childhood, ABC children indicate feeling greater trust in their parents (Zajac *et al.*, 2020), and show enhanced brain development (Valadez *et al.*, 2020) relative to children in the control group. When their children were nine, the narratives of ABC mothers revealed more secure base script knowledge than mothers in the control intervention (Raby *et al.*, 2021). These effects were observed as long as eight years after the intervention, suggesting that the intervention helps parents change in fundamental, long-term ways.

Child–Parent Psychotherapy

Child–Parent Psychotherapy (CPP) focuses on traumatized parents' challenges in behaving in sensitive, nurturing ways with their young children. CPP is designed to help parents understand how their previous experiences affect parenting in a very real way. The relatively intensive, long-term intervention is intended to provide a safe, playful context. Through randomized clinical trials, CPP has been shown to reduce disorganized attachment (Cicchetti *et al.*, 2006), reduce children's negative self-representations (Toth *et al.*, 2002) among maltreated children, and reduce children's behavior problems and traumatic stress symptoms for preschoolers exposed to marital violence (Lieberman *et al.*, 2005).

Preschoolers

Several interventions for older children incorporate attachment concepts with social learning principles to greater or lesser extents. Included among these are Video-feedback Intervention to Promote Positive Parenting and Sensitive Discipline (VIPP-SD: Juffer *et al.*, 2008), Incredibly Years (Webster-Stratton *et al.*, 2001), Parent-Child Interaction Therapy (Eyberg *et al.*, 2001), and others. The most explicitly attachment-based of these interventions is the VIPP-SD, which has been tested in a wide range of samples with varying risk histories (e.g., low-income parents, foster parents, parents of autistic children, parents with depression, parents with insecure attachment). VIPP-SD has been shown to increase parents' use of more sensitive discipline strategies and children's secure attachment (see van IJzendoorn *et al.*, 2022 for a meta-analysis of 25 randomized clinical trials). Although some studies have found effects on reducing children's behavior problems (e.g., O'Farrelly *et al.*, 2021), the meta-analytic effect of VIPP-SD on behavior problems was non-significant (van IJzendoorn *et al.*, 2022).

Children and adolescents

Fewer interventions are explicitly attachment based for older children and adolescents than for younger children, although many interventions are nonetheless relevant to attachment issues. Attachment-based Family Therapy (ABFT; Diamond *et al.*, 2002) is one of the few interventions that very directly targets attachment issues for this older age group. The treatment focuses on both family and individual processes that can help build trust between the adolescent and parents, and directs attention toward enhancing a relationship in which the parent can effectively protect the child. In a randomized clinical trial, ABFT led to larger and faster reductions in suicidal ideation than enhanced usual care (Diamond *et al.*, 2010). In a subsequent study comparing ABFT to nondirective supportive therapy, ABFT and the comparison intervention both led to large and significant reductions in suicidal ideation and depressive symptoms (Diamond *et al.*, 2019). (See Chapter 35 for more information about approaches to family interventions.)

Future directions

Attachment research has been characterized by cross-cutting theoretical and methodological approaches since its earliest days. With recent developments in the fields of neurobiology, epigenetics, and translational research more generally, increasing attention has turned to understanding the role of attachment in physiological and neural development. Such interdisciplinary research that incorporates attachment into complex models of development has the potential to highlight novel opportunities for prevention and intervention. As the evidence for attachment-based interventions continues to grow, it is critical to also consider how to effectively move these interventions into the world in ways that support healthy socioemotional development across contexts. Understanding for whom and under what conditions attachment-based interventions are effective remains a critical direction for future research.

Conclusions

Attachment has emerged as a powerful construct. As Rutter pointed out (2006), much of what Bowlby proposed in the 1950s and 1960s is now accepted within psychology, social work, and even psychiatry. At the time the theory was introduced, though, it was revolutionary. A rich and growing body of empirical work has followed the seminal observational studies of Bowlby and Ainsworth, including significant longitudinal efforts and critical attention to atypical caregiving circumstances. Remarkably, these studies continue to offer strong support for key tenets of attachment theory.

References

Ainsworth, M.D.S. (1967) *Infancy in Uganda: Infant Care and the Growth of Love*. Johns Hopkins University Press, Baltimore, MD.

Ainsworth, M.D.S. *et al.* (1978) *Patterns of attachment*. Lawrence Erlbaum, Hillsdale, NJ.

Allen, J.P. *et al.* (2003) A secure base in adolescence: markers of attachment security in the mother–adolescent relationship. *Child Development* **74**, 292–307.

Anderson, S. & Whitaker, R. (2011) Attachment security and obesity in US preschool-aged children. *Archives of Pediatrics & Adolescent Medicine* **165**(3), 235–242.

Anderson, S.E. *et al.* (2012) Quality of early maternal-child relationship and risk of adolescent obesity. *Pediatrics* **129**(1), 132–140.

Bakermans-Kranenburg, M.J. & van IJzendoorn, M.H. (2009) The first 10,000 adult attachment interviews: distributions of adult attachment representations in clinical and non-clinical groups. *Attachment & Human Development* **11**(3), 223–263.

Bar-Haim, Y. *et al.* (2000) Stability and change in attachment at 14, 24, and 58 months of age: behavior, representation, and life events. *Journal of Child Psychology and Psychiatry* **41**, 381–388.

Belsky, J. & Rovine, M. (1987) Temperament and attachment security in the strange situation: an empirical rapprochement. *Child Development* **58**, 787–795.

Belsky, J. & Rovine, M. (1988) Nonmaternal care in the first year of life and the security of infant–parent attachment. *Child Development* **59**, 157–167.

Bernard, K. & Dozier, M. (2010) Examining infants' cortisol responses to laboratory tasks among children varying in attachment disorganization: stress reactivity or return to baseline? *Developmental Psychology* **46**, 1771–1778.

Bernard, K. *et al.* (2012) Enhancing attachment organization among maltreated infants: results of a randomized clinical trial. *Child Development* **83**, 623–636.

Bernard, K. *et al.* (2015) Intervention effects on diurnal cortisol rhythms of CPS-referred infants persist into early childhood: preschool follow-up results of a randomized clinical trial. *JAMA Pediatrics* **169**, 112–119.

Bernard, K. *et al.* (2018) Association between maternal depression and maternal sensitivity from birth to 12 months: a meta-analysis. *Attachment & Human Development* **20**(6), 578–599.

Bernard, K. *et al.* (2019) Longitudinal associations between attachment quality in infancy, C-reactive protein in early childhood, and BMI in middle childhood: preliminary evidence from a CPS-referred sample. *Attachment & Human Development* **21**(1), 5–22.

Bernier, A. *et al.* (2015) A secure base from which to regulate: attachment security in toddlerhood as a predictor of executive functioning at school entry. *Developmental Psychology* **51**(9), 1177–1189.

Bernier, A. *et al.* (2020) From early relationships to preacademic knowledge: a sociocognitive developmental cascade to school readiness. *Child Development* **91**(1), e134–e145.

Bouthillier, D. *et al.* (2002) Predictive validity of adult attachment measures in relation to emotion regulation behaviors in marital interactions. *Journal of Adult Development* **9**, 291–305.

Bowlby, J. (1969/1982) *Attachment and Loss: Vol. 1. Attachment*. Basic Books, New York.

Bowlby, J. (1988) *A Secure Base*. Basic Books, New York.

Bretherton, I. (1985) Attachment: retrospect and prospect. *Monographs of the Society for Research in Child Development* **50**, 3–35.

Bretherton, I. (1992) The origins of attachment theory: John Bowlby and Mary Ainsworth. *Developmental Psychology* **28**, 759–775.

Bretherton, I. *et al.* (1990) Assessing internal working models of the attachment relationship: an attachment story completion task for 3-year-olds. In: *Attachment in the Preschool Years*. (eds M.T. Greenberg, *et al.*). University of Chicago Press, Chicago. pp. 273–308.

Cassidy, J. *et al.* (1992) *Attachment Organization in Preschool Children: Coding Guidelines*, 4th edn. Unpublished manuscript, edn. University of Virginia, Charlottesville, VA.

Cassidy, J. *et al.* (2011) Enhancing infant attachment security: an examination of treatment efficacy and differential susceptibility. *Development and Psychopathology* **23**, 131–148.

Cicchetti, D. *et al.* (2006) Fostering secure attachment in infants in maltreating families through preventive interventions. *Development and Psychopathology* **18**(3), 623–649.

Clarke-Stewart, K.A. (1989) Infant day-care: maligned or malignant? *American Psychologist* **44**, 266–273.

Coard, S.I. (2021) Race, discrimination, and racism as "growing points" for consideration: attachment theory and research with African American families. *Attachment & Human Development* **24**, 373–383.

Coppola, G. *et al.* (2006) The attachment script representation procedure in an Italian sample: associations with adult attachment interview scales and with maternal sensitivity. *Attachment & Human Development* **8**(3), 209–219.

Cossette-Côté, F. *et al.* (2022) The association between maternal sensitivity/availability and attachment in children with autism spectrum disorder: a systematic review and meta-analysis. *Current Psychology: A Journal for Diverse Perspectives on Diverse Psychological Issues* **41**(11), 8236–8248.

Cyr, C. *et al.* (2010) Attachment security and disorganization in maltreating and high-risk families: a series of meta-analyses. *Development and Psychopathology* **22**, 87–108.

Dagan, O. *et al.* (2021) Configurations of mother-child and father-child attachment as predictors of internalizing and externalizing behavioral problems: an individual participant data (IPD) meta-analysis. *New Directions for Child and Adolescent Development* **2021**(180), 67–94.

De Wolff, M. & van IJzendoorn, M.H. (1997) Sensitivity and attachment: a meta-analysis on parental antecedents of infant attachment. *Child Development* **68**, 571–591.

Diamond, G.S. *et al.* (2002) Attachment-based family therapy for depressed adolescents: a treatment development study. *Journal of the Academy of Child & Adolescent Psychiatry* **41**, 1190–1196.

Diamond, G.S. *et al.* (2010) Attachment-based family therapy for adolescents with suicidal ideation: a randomized controlled trial. *Journal of the American Academy of Child & Adolescent Psychiatry* **49**, 122–131.

Diamond, S.G. *et al.* (2019) A randomized controlled trial: attachment-based family and nondirective supportive treatments for youth who are suicidal. *Journal of the American Academy of Child & Adolescent Psychiatry* **58**, 721–731.

Dozier, M. & Bernard, K. (2019) *Coaching Parents of Vulnerable Infants: The Attachment and Biobehavioral Catch-up Approach*. Guilford Press, New York.

Dozier, M. *et al.* (2008) Attachment and psychopathology in adulthood. In: *Handbook of Attachment: Theory, Research, and Clinical Implications*. (eds J. Cassidy & P.R. Shaver), 2nd edn. Guilford Press, New York. pp. 718–744.

Dunbar, A.S. *et al.* (2022) Mothers' preparation for bias and responses to children's distress predict positive adjustment among black children: an attachment perspective. *Attachment & Human Development* **24**, 287–303.

Easterbrooks, M.A. & Abeles, R. (2000) Windows to the self in 8-year-olds: bridges to attachment representation and behavioral adjustment. *Attachment & Human Development* **2**, 85–106.

Egeland, B. & Farber, E.A. (1984) Infant-mother attachment: factors related to its development and changes over time. *Child Development* **55**, 753–771.

Ehrlich, K.B. & Cassidy, J. (2021) Early attachment and later physical health. In: *Attachment: The Fundamental Questions*. (eds R.A. Thompson, *et al.*). Guilford Press, New York. pp. 204–210.

Eyberg, S.M. *et al.* (2001) Parent-child interaction therapy with behavior problems children: one and two year maintenance of treatment effects in the family. *Child and Family Behavior Therapy* **23**, 1–20.

Farrell, A.K. *et al.* (2019) Early maternal sensitivity, attachment security in young adulthood, and cardiometabolic risk at midlife. *Attachment & Human Development* **21**, 70–86.

Fearon, R.P. *et al.* (2010) The significance of insecure attachment and disorganization in the development of children's externalizing behavior: a meta-analytic study. *Child Development* **81**, 435–456.

Feldman, R. & Vengrober, A. (2011) Posttraumatic stress disorder in infants and young children exposed to war-related trauma. *Journal of the American Academy of Child and Adolescent Psychiatry* **50**, 645–658.

Fraley, R.C. *et al.* (2013) The legacy of early experiences in development: formalizing alternative models of how early experiences are carried forward over time. *Developmental Psychology* **49**, 109–125.

Garnett, M. *et al.* (2020) Parental sensitivity mediates the sustained effect of attachment and biobehavioral catch-up on cortisol in middle childhood: a randomized clinical trial. *Psychoneuroendocrinology* **121**, 1–8.

George, C. *et al.* (1996) *Adult Attachment Interview*. Unpublished manuscript,. University of California, Berkeley, CA.

Goodman, S.H. & Gotlib, I.H. (1999) Risk for psychopathology in the children of depressed mothers: a developmental model for understanding mechanisms of transmission. *Psychological Review* **106**, 458–490.

Groh, A.M. *et al.* (2012) The significance of insecure and disorganized attachment for children's internalizing symptoms: a meta-analytic study. *Child Development* **83**, 591–610.

Groh, A.M. *et al.* (2014) Stability of attachment security from infancy to late adolescence. *Monographs of the Society for Research in Child Development* **79**, 51–66.

Groh, A.M. *et al.* (2017) Attachment and temperament in the early life course: a meta-analytic review. *Child Development* **88**, 770–795.

Gunnar, M.R. *et al.* (2006) Bringing basic research on early experience and stress neurobiology to bear on preventive interventions for neglected and maltreated children. *Development and Psychopathology* **18**, 651–677.

Halevi, G. *et al.* (2017) The social transmission of risk: maternal stress physiology, synchronous parenting, and well-being mediate the effects of war exposure on child psychopathology. *Journal of Abnormal Psychology* **126**(8), 1087–1103.

Harlow, H.F. (1958) The nature of love. *American Psychologist* **13**, 673–685.

Hawkins, E. *et al.* (2015) Mediating and moderating processes underlying the association between maternal cognition and infant attachment. *Journal of Applied Developmental Psychology* **39**, 24–33.

Hesse, E. & Main, M. (2006) Frightened, threatening, and dissociative parental behavior in low-risk samples: description, discussion, and interpretations. *Development and Psychopathology* **18**, 309–343.

Hofer, M. (1994) Hidden regulators in attachment, separation, and loss. *Monographs of the Society for Research in Child Development* **59**, 192–207.

Juffer, F. *et al.* (2008) *Promoting Positive Parenting: An Attachment-based Intervention.* Lawrence Erlbaum, New York.

Koren-Karie, N. *et al.* (2009) Mothers of securely attached children with autism spectrum disorder are more sensitive than mothers of insecurely attached children. *Journal of Child Psychology and Psychiatry* **50**(5), 643–650.

Lamb, M.E. & Lewis, C. (2004) Father-child relationships. In: *Handbook of Father Involvement: Multidisciplinary Perspectives.* (eds M.E. Lamb & C. Lewis), 2nd edn. Routledge, New York. pp. 119–134.

Lewis-Morrarty, E. *et al.* (2012) Cognitive flexibility and theory of mind outcomes among foster children: preschool follow-up results of a randomized clinical trial. *Journal of Adolescent Health* **51**, 17–22.

Lieberman, A.F. *et al.* (2005) Towards evidence-based treatment: child-parent psychotherapy with preschoolers exposed to marital violence. *Journal of the American Academy of Child & Adolescent Psychiatry* **44**, 1241–1248.

Lind, T. *et al.* (2014) Intervention effects on negative affect in CPS-referred children: results of a randomized clinical trial. *Child Abuse & Neglect* **38**(9), 1459–1467.

Lind, T. *et al.* (2020) Promoting compliance in children referred to child protective services: a randomized clinical trial. *Child Development* **91**, 563–576.

Lorenz, K. (1957) *Instinctive Behavior.* International Universities Press, New York.

Lyons-Ruth, K. *et al.* (1999) Maternal frightened, frightening, or atypical behavior and disorganized infant attachment patterns. *Monographs of the Society for Research in Child Development* **64**, 67–96.

Madigan, S. *et al.* (2006) Unresolved states of mind, disorganized attachment relationships, and disrupted interactions of adolescent mothers and their infants. *Developmental Psychology* **42**, 293–304.

Madigan, S. *et al.* (2013) Attachment and internalizing behavior in early childhood: A meta-analysis. *Developmental Psychology* **49**, 672–689.

Madigan, S. *et al.* (2023) The first 20,000 strange situation procedures: a meta-analytic review. *Psychological Bulletin* **149**, 99–132. doi:10.1037/bul0000388.

Main, M. (1990) Cross-cultural studies of attachment organization: recent studies, changing methodologies, and the concept of conditional strategies. *Human Development* **33**, 48–61.

Main, M. & Cassidy, J. (1988) Categories of response to reunion with the parent at age six: predictable from infant attachment classifications and stable over a 1-month-period. *Developmental Psychology* **24**, 415–526.

Main, M. & Solomon, J. (1986) Discovery of a new, insecure-disorganized/disoriented attachment pattern. In: *Affective Development in Infancy.* (eds T.B. Brazelton & M. Yogman). Ablex, Norwood, NJ. pp. 95–124.

Main, M. & Solomon, J. (1990) Procedures for identifying infants as disorganized/disoriented during the Ainsworth Strange Situation. In: *Attachment in the Preschool Years: Theory, Research, and Intervention.* (eds M.T. Greenberg & e.a.). University of Chicago Press, Chicago. pp. 161–182.

Main, M. *et al.* (1985) Security in infancy, childhood, and adulthood: a move to the level of representation. *Monographs of the Society for Research in Child Development* **50**, 66–104.

Main, M. *et al.* (2005) Predictability of attachment behavior and representational processes at 1, 6, and 19 years of age. In: *Attachment from Infancy to Adulthood: The Major Longitudinal Studies.* (eds K.E. Grossman, *et al.*). Guilford Press, New York. pp. 245–304.

Marshall, P.J. & Fox, N.A. (2005) Relations between behavioral reactivity at 4 months and attachment classification at 14 months in a selected sample. *Infant Behavior and Development* **28**, 492–502.

McElwain, N.L. *et al.* (2003) Differentiating among insecure mother-infant attachment classifications: a focus on child-friend interaction and exploration during solitary play at 36 months. *Attachment & Human Development* **5**, 136–164.

Miyake, K. *et al.* (1985) Infant temperament, mother's mode of interaction, and attachment in Japan: an interim report. *Monographs of the Society for Research in Child Development* **50**, 276–297.

Nelson, C.A. (2007) A neurobiological perspective on early human deprivation. *Child Development Perspectives* **1**, 13–18.

Nelson, C.A. *et al.* (2014) *Romania's Abandoned Children: Deprivation, Brain Development, and the Struggle for Recovery.* Harvard University Press, Cambridge, MA.

NICHD Early Child Care Research Network (1997) The effects of infant child care on infant-mother attachment security: results of the NICHD study of early child care. *Child Development* **68**, 860–879.

NICHD Early Child Care Research Network (2001) Child-care and family predictors of preschool attachment and stability from infancy. *Developmental Psychology* **37**, 847–862.

O'Farrelly, C. *et al.* (2021) A brief home-based parenting intervention to reduce behavior problems in young children: a pragmatic randomized clinical trial. *JAMA Pediatrics* **175**, 567–576.

Pederson, D.R. *et al.* (1998) Maternal attachment representations, maternal sensitivity, and the infant-mother attachment relationship. *Developmental Psychology* **34**, 925–933.

Pruett, K.D. (1998) Role of the father. *Pediatrics* **102**(5), 1253–1261.

Puig, J. *et al.* (2013) Predicting adult physical illness from infant attachment: a prospective longitudinal study. *Health Psychology* **32**(4), 409–417.

Raby, K.L. *et al.* (2013) Genetic contributions to continuity and change in attachment security: a prospective, longitudinal investigation from infancy to young adulthood. *The Journal of Child Psychology and Psychiatry* **54**, 1223–1230.

Raby, K.L. *et al.* (2015) The enduring predictive significance of early maternal sensitivity: social and academic competence through age 32 years. *Child Development* **86**(3), 695–708.

Raby, K.L. *et al.* (2021) Increasing secure base script knowledge among parents with attachment and biobehavioral catch-up. *Development and Psychopathology* **33**, 554–564.

Raver, C. (1996) Relations between social contingency in mother-child interaction and 2-year-olds' social competence. *Developmental Psychology* **32**, 850–859.

Roisman, G.I. *et al.* (2007) The adult attachment interview and self-reports of attachment style: an empirical rapprochement. *Journal of Personality and Social Psychology* **92**, 678–697.

Rutgers, A.H. *et al.* (2004) Autism and attachment: a meta-analytic review. *Journal of Child Psychology and Psychiatry* **45**(6), 1123–1134.

Rutter, M. (2006) Review of attachment from infancy to adulthood: the major longitudinal studies. *Journal of Child Psychology and Psychiatry* **47**, 974–977.

Rutter, M. *et al.* (2009) Emanuel Miller lecture: attachment insecurity, disinhibited attachment, and attachment disorder: where do research findings leave the concepts? *Journal of Child Psychology and Psychiatry* **50**, 529–543.

Schneider, B.H. *et al.* (2001) Child-parent attachment and children's peer relations: a quantitative review. *Developmental Psychology* **37**, 86–100.

Schuengel, C. *et al.* (1999) Frightening maternal behavior linking unresolved loss and disorganized infant attachment. *Journal of Consulting and Clinical Psychology* **67**, 54–63.

Slough, N.M. & Greenberg, M.T. (1990) Five-year-olds' representations of separation from parents: responses from the perspective of self and other. *New Directions for Child Development* **48**, 67–84.

Smyke, A.T. *et al.* (2010) Placement in foster care enhances quality of attachment among young institutionalized children. *Child Development* **81**, 212–223.

Sroufe, L.A. (1985) Attachment classification from the perspective of infant-caregiver relationships and infant temperament. *Child Development* **56**, 1–14.

Sroufe, L.A. & Waters, E. (1977) Heart rate as a convergent measure in clinical and developmental research. *Merrill-Palmer Quarterly* **23**, 3–27.

Sroufe, L.A. *et al.* (1983) Attachment and dependency in developmental perspective. *Child Development* **54**, 1615–1627.

Steele, R.D. *et al.* (2014) Caregiving antecedents of secure base script knowledge: a comparative analysis of young adult attachment representations. *Developmental Psychology* **50**, 2526–2538.

Stern, J.A. *et al.* (2022) Attachment perspectives on race, prejudice, and anti-racism. *Attachment & Human Development* **24**, 253–259.

Stern, J.A. *et al.* (2023) Pathways to emotion regulation in young Black children: an attachment perspective. *Advances in Child Development and Behavior* **64**, 163–188.

Thompson, R.A. *et al.* (1982) Stability of infant-mother attachment and its relationship to changing life circumstances in an unselected middle-class sample. *Child Development* **53**, 144–148.

Tinbergen, N. (1951) *The Study of Instinct*. Clarendon Press, Oxford.

Toth, S.L. *et al.* (2002) The relative efficacy of two interventions in altering maltreated preschool children's representational models: implications for attachment theory. *Development and Psychopathology* **14**, 877–908.

Valadez, E.A. *et al.* (2020) Early parenting intervention effects on brain responses to maternal cues among high-risk children. *American Journal of Psychiatry* **177**, 818–826.

van IJzendoorn, M.H. (1995) Adult attachment representations, parental responsiveness, and infant attachment: a meta-analysis on the predictive validity of the adult attachment interview. *Psychological Bulletin* **117**, 387–403.

van IJzendoorn, M.H. & De Wolff, M.S. (1997) In search of the absent father—meta-analysis of infant-father attachment: a rejoinder to our discussants. *Child Development* **68**, 604–609.

van IJzendoorn, M.H. & Juffer, F. (2006) The Emanuel Miller memorial lecture 2006: adoption as intervention. Meta-analytic evidence for massive catch-up and plasticity in physical, socio-emotional and cognitive development. *Journal of Child Psychology & Psychiatry* **47**, 1228–1245.

van IJzendoorn, M.H. & Kroonenberg, P.M. (1988) Cross-cultural patterns of attachment: a meta-analysis of the strange situation. *Child Development* **59**, 147–156.

van IJzendoorn, M.H. *et al.* (2022) Improving parenting, child attachment, and externalizing behaviors: meta-analysis of the first 25 randomized controlled trials on the effects of video-feedback intervention to promote positive parenting and sensitive discipline. *Development and Psychopathology* **35**, 241–256.

Vasileva, M. & Petermann, F. (2018) Attachment, development, and mental health in abused and neglected preschool children in foster care: a meta-analysis. *Trauma, Violence & Abuse* **19**, 443–458.

Vaughn, B.E. *et al.* (2008) Attachment and temperament: additive and interactive influences on behavior, affect, and cognition during infancy and childhood. In: *Handbook of Attachment: Theory, Research, and Clinical Implications*. (eds J. Cassidy & P.R. Shaver), 2nd edn. Guilford Press, New York. pp. 192–216.

Verhage, M.L. *et al.* (2016) Narrowing the transmission gap: a synthesis of three decades of research on intergenerational transmission of attachment. *Psychological Bulletin* **142**(4), 337–366.

Verhage, M.L. *et al.* (2023) Editorial perspective: on the need for clarity about attachment terminology. *Journal of Child Psychology and Psychiatry* **64**, 839–843.

Vondra, J.I. *et al.* (1999) Stability and change in infant attachment style in a low-income sample. *Monographs of the Society for Research in Child Development* **64**, 119–144.

Vondra, J.I. *et al.* (2001) Attachment stability and emotional and behavioral regulation from infancy to preschool age. *Development and Psychopathology* **13**, 13–33.

Waters, E. (1978) The reliability and stability of individual differences in infant mother attachment. *Child Development* **49**, 483–494.

Waters, H.S. & Waters, E. (2006) The attachment working models concept: among other things, we build script-like representations of secure base experiences. *Attachment & Human Development* **8**(3), 185–197.

Webster-Stratton, C. *et al.* (2001) Social skills and problems-solving training for children with early-onset conduct problems: who benefits. *Journal of Child Psychology and Psychiatry* **42**, 943–952.

Weinfield, N.S. *et al.* (2000) Attachment from infancy to early adulthood in a high-risk sample: continuity, discontinuity, and their correlates. *Child Development* **71**, 695–702.

Zajac, L. *et al.* (2020) Sustained effects on attachment security in middle childhood: results from a randomized clinical trial of the attachment and biobehavioral catch-up (ABC) intervention. *Journal of Child Psychology and Psychiatry* **61**, 417–424.

Zeanah, C.H. *et al.* (2005) Attachment in institutionalized and community children in Romania. *Child Development* **76**, 1015–1028.

CHAPTER 7
Infant and early childhood mental health

Brittnie Fowler and Charles H. Zeanah
Department of Psychiatry and Behavioral Sciences, Tulane University School of Medicine, New Orleans, LA, USA

Introduction

Infant and early childhood mental health (IECMH), the clinical science of early experience, has evolved since the 1970s into an international, multidisciplinary field dedicated to supporting and enhancing the social and emotional well-being of young children (Zeanah & Zeanah, 2019). Considerable evidence has highlighted the importance of experiences in the earliest years of life as essential for healthy brain development (Fox *et al.*, 2010). Given the effects of early experiences in the developing brain, a broad-based inclusive approach aimed at reducing negative outcomes is warranted. This chapter defines IECMH and its overarching themes and explores the influences on young children's development within a variety of interrelated contexts. We consider risk and protective factors and guiding principles for the field, as well as psychopathology, assessments, and interventions developed specifically for young children.

Definitions of infant mental health

The meaning of "infant" varies across countries, cultures, and languages. Infant mental health sometimes covers the first three years of life, and sometimes the first five years of life. In this chapter, we will use the broader age range, as well as acknowledging that pregnancy is also a focus in clinical infant mental health efforts.

A widely accepted definition of infant mental health is the young child's capacity to experience, regulate, and express emotions, form close and secure relationships, and explore the environment and learn. All of these capacities will be best accomplished within the context of the caregiving environment that includes family, community, and cultural expectations for young children. Developing these capacities is synonymous with healthy social and emotional development (ZERO TO THREE, 2001). This defines infant mental health as a characteristic of the young child.

From a practice perspective, infant mental health may also be defined as "a multidisciplinary professional field of inquiry, practice and policy concerned with alleviating suffering and enhancing the social and emotional competence of young children" (Zeanah & Zeanah, 2009, p. 6). A narrower grouping of this multidisciplinary field includes mental health professionals who provide direct service to young children and families, but a broader grouping would include health care and allied health professionals who are involved in psychological and developmental problems in young children, such as pediatricians and general practitioners, nurses, speech and language therapists, occupational therapists, and others. Other nonmental health professionals, who in their roles can profoundly affect infant mental health but who approach and frame the issues very differently from the mental health frame, include child protection, legal, early care, and education professionals. Policymakers and researchers may also engage in work considered especially relevant for infant mental health.

Development and contextual issues

The rapidity of change in the earliest years of life is unprecedented in postnatal life. In 3 short years, a newborn who is completely dependent on adult caregivers becomes a young child who can move independently, express and experience complex emotions, share intentions, feelings, and ideas with others, and imagine reality different from their actual experience. Between 3 and 5 years, young children's verbal, motor, and cognitive skills advance, as does their ability to read and respond to subtle social cues. Unrelated adults (e.g., preschool teachers) and children (e.g., classmates and neighborhood peers) become increasingly important influences on the child's rapid development.

Rutter's Child and Adolescent Psychiatry and Psychology, Seventh Edition.
Edited by Anita Thapar, Daniel S. Pine, Samuele Cortese, Cathy Creswell, Tamsin J. Ford, James F. Leckman, and Argyris Stringaris.

Companion website: www.wiley.com/go/thapar/ruttерspsych7

Qualitative changes in development occur at regular intervals in the first 3 years of life in what has been called biobehavioral shifts (Stern, 1985). This means that behaviors/capabilities emerge that have not been present before across multiple domains of development. After a period of adapting to the extrauterine environment, the first biobehavioral shift occurs at 2–3 months of age when the human infant experiences a social blossoming, manifested by social smiling, responsive cooing, and more sustained eye-to-eye contact. Between 2–7 months, infants engage readily in interactions with caregivers and other adults with no strong preferences expressed for with whom these interactions occur. After the second biobehavioral shift at 7–9 months, stranger wariness and separation protest emerge, heralding the onset of focused attachment, as infants begin to turn preferentially to attachment figures who they have learned through experience will provide them with comfort, support, and protection. In addition, an important new cognitive capacity appears after 7–9 months known as intersubjectivity, which refers to the infants' new awareness that they can share thoughts feelings and intentions with others. The third major biobehavioral shift at 18–20 months involves rapid advances in symbolization, abstraction, and representational capacities, most evident in the young child's advances in expressive language. The emergence of enhanced verbal capacities changes the nature of children's social relationships, as they engage in more independent functioning. The preschool years are characterized by increasing autonomy, broadening of relationships, and social cognitive advances. These developmental processes are nested within a variety of interacting contexts, illustrated in Figure 7.1. Each context transacts with other contexts over time, influencing the young child's developmental trajectory.

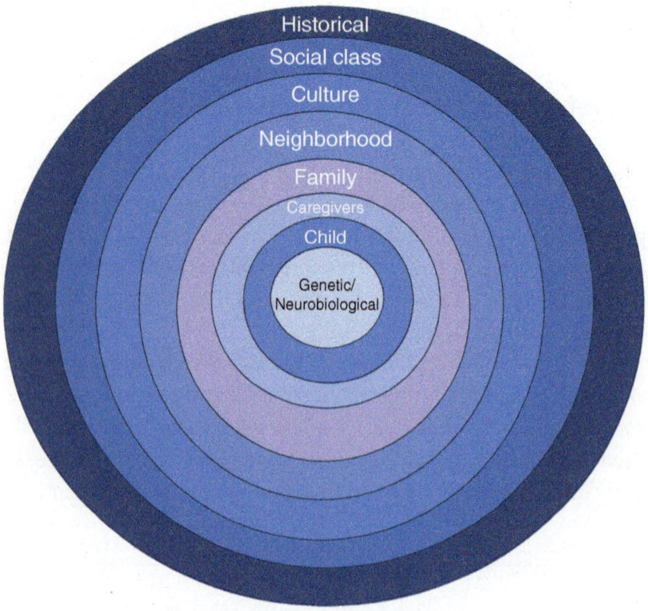

Figure 7.1 Intrinsic (black text) and extrinsic (white text) contexts for infant and early childhood development.

Genetic/neurobiological context

The intrinsic context for an individual's development derives from the expression of 20,000 genes interacting over time with various environmental characteristics. Gene–environment interactions are the most plausible explanation for how an individual's development proceeds, but the complexities of these interactions have limited our understanding about details of interactions and outcomes. Enthusiasm about studies of polymorphisms conferring risk and protection in their various configurations have waned with the realization that most published findings were spurious due to inadequate sample sizes.

Beyond genetics, the fetus is sensitive to environmental exposures that can impact the child's physiology and developmental trajectories. For example, smoking during pregnancy can increase risk for low birth weight (Nigg & Breslau, 2007) and intrauterine stress can increase susceptibility to various types of psychopathology (Glover & O'Connor, 2002; Van den Bergh, 2011). Fetal programming describes a process in which the intrauterine environment contributes to set points in physiological and metabolic responses in various organ systems that, once established, may compromise postnatal adaptation and lead to health problems later in life. The implication is that when the postnatal environment differs markedly from the prenatal environment (e.g., nutrition), the individual may be at risk for subsequent adverse health consequences.

Caregiving context

Like other altricial species, humans spend a significant amount of time dependent on a caregiver for survival. Caregiver nurturance includes care for the young child that goes beyond the child's basic needs for food, shelter, and clothing and includes emotional availability and responsiveness. Nurturing care of infants and young children facilitates skill development and competence, and buffers the young child's exposures to adversity, protecting brain structure and function which, in turn, improve health, growth, and development (Daelsman, *et al.*, 2016).

The postnatal caregiving environment also encompasses the network of individuals involved in caregiving roles with the young child, as well as siblings, "extended" relatives, and/or nonbiological caregivers. The family exerts direct and indirect impacts on child development. For example, single-parent homes are more likely to experience income inequalities, which can impact resource availability and parenting, leading to adverse child outcomes (McLanahan & Percheski, 2008). Overall, collective research suggests having a loving caregiver, stability, and economic resources seem to be key factors in better outcomes for children—socially, emotionally, cognitively, and even financially. Less is known about non-Western cultures, with different family structures and parenting strategies, with regard to key influences on infants' and young children's development (Keller, 2018).

Cultural context

The values, customs, beliefs, traditions, and ethnic or racial backgrounds and behaviors shared by a specific group influence beliefs about child caregiving practices (Rosman *et al.*, 2009). Children as young as three years-of-age may identify social norms and express discontent when these norms are changed (House, 2018). Cross-cultural studies have shown that culture influences multiple developmental domains in young children (Harkness *et al.*, 2013). Additional cross-cultural longitudinal studies are needed to better define the influence of culture on specific domains of development. Appreciating young children's cultural context may help guide clinicians and investigators to create culturally appropriate interventions, improving systems of care and changing policies to better aid young children's development.

There is increasing recognition of the importance of historical traumas as key contributors to cultural beliefs, parenting practices, and child development (Ghosh-Ippen, 2019). Historical traumas highlight the intergenerational effects of traumas inflicted on groups of people because of their race, creed, and ethnicity and may become incorporated into cultural beliefs and practices. Awareness of how the past may influence the present, as well as the strengths of diverse groups and their authentic cultural traditions, may aid understanding of approaches that can facilitate healthy development.

Social class context

Socioeconomic status (SES) is one of the most influential and best-studied constructs in child development research. Measures of SES include combinations of family income, parental education, and occupational status. Social class is associated with health, mental health, cognitive, and socioemotional outcomes in children—effects that can be demonstrated from pregnancy through adulthood (Bradley & Corwyn, 2002). A variety of mechanisms linking SES to child well-being have been proposed, with most involving differences in access to material and social resources or reactions by parents and children to stress-inducing conditions (Cano, 2022). For children, SES impacts well-being at multiple levels, including both family and neighborhood. Its effects are moderated by children's own characteristics, family structure and functioning, and cultural beliefs.

Historical context

Less well studied in the psychological sciences is the influence of the historical epoch in which young children are raised on their development, mental health, and well-being. Rapid technological advances have changed the experiences of many young children in the early 21st century compared with previous generations. The daily realities of children in Western, industrialized societies involve "screen time," phones that are also computers, geolocation systems, cameras, etc., and soon artificial intelligence (AI), all of which create vastly different experiences than the childhood experiences of their parents and other caregivers. Though it is too early to draw firm conclusions about how these different exposures and experiences relate to outcomes, this is a line of research that is actively being investigated (Przybylski & Weinstein, 2019).

Risk and protective factors

Because infant mental health is centrally concerned with young children's developmental trajectories, a focus on factors and processes that increase risk for adverse outcomes and those that bolster protection is central to clinicians (see Chapter 6 on Attachment). The best-known model of adversity is the cumulative risk model, which proposes that adverse outcomes are better predicted by the total number, rather than the specific nature of environmental risk exposures. Despite many demonstrations of its applicability (see especially Fellitti *et al.*, 1998), the cumulative risk model has been criticized primarily for its lack of specificity in delineating mechanisms and for potentially obscuring links that remain to be discovered (Zeanah & Sonuga-Barke, 2016).

Alternative models have also been proposed, attempting to clarify more specific neurobiological mechanisms that delineate pathways of risks leading to outcomes and to demonstrate how particular brain circuitry is affected by different types of environmental adversity. McLaughlin and Sheridan (2016), for example, have proposed the dimensional model of adversity and have delineated different neurobiological effects of threat and deprivation. Other dimensions, such as harshness and unpredictability also have been proposed (Ellis *et al.*, 2009). These models offer targets for prevention and intervention.

Protective factors and resilience

Protective factors buffer the young child from exposure to adversity. For example, in a study of 300 3-year-old children in the Netherlands, investigators showed increased child aggression with increasing levels of reported parenting stress, unless the children were securely attached in which case there was no increase in child aggression (Tharner *et al.*, 2012). Also, among severely deprived young children, secure attachment mediated the effects of caregiving quality on psychopathology, protecting them from the harmful effects of deprivation (McGoron *et al.*, 2012).

The United States Government's Children's Bureau endorses specific factors to support young children's well-being: (i) caregiver nurturance, (ii) effective parenting, (iii) parental resilience, (iv) social connections, (v) concrete support for caregivers, and (vi) supporting the social and emotional competence of children (Child Welfare Information Gateway, 2020). Supportive caregivers are essential to buffering the effects of adverse experiences on the developing child. Caregivers' ability to adequately manage stress, understand development, maintain healthy attachments, and access meaningful support networks all impact their ability to protect children from risk exposures.

Resilience, a related construct, includes resources and processes that help young children respond effectively to adversity by reducing harmful effects and mobilizing processes that promote recovery. Resilience has been studied as a characteristic of the child, and cognitive aptitude, personal agency, easy disposition, adaptability, and social skills have all been identified as contributors (Masten & Barnes, 2018). Beyond the individual, caregiving relationships are especially important. Following exposure to adversity, the sooner a child is placed in an adequate caregiving environment, the more likely they are to recover and the fuller their recovery is likely to be (Zeanah *et al.*, 2011). Increasingly, however, the resilience of an individual is recognized to depend not merely on intrinsic characteristics, but on interactions among many levels of systems, including caregiving and family relationships, school environments, cohesive neighborhoods, accessible health care, and other systems (Masten, 2019). These large order interconnected systems profoundly affect individual characteristics so that resilience of young children may be understood to depend on the resilience of these systems (Masten, 2019).

Guiding principles

Two important guiding principles of infant mental health are its relational focus and its emphasis on identifying strengths. It is certainly the case that these principles apply beyond the early childhood period, but these principles have been emphasized as consistently and explicitly present in infant mental health since the origins of infant mental health as a discipline of clinical science.

Relational focus

Infant mental health always has been an explicitly relational field, focusing on young children's development and psychopathology within the context of their relationships with primary caregiving adults (Zeanah & Lieberman, 2016). A relational focus is necessary for understanding young children's development and provides guidance about how to alleviate suffering and enhance well-being.

Various lines of research paved the way for a model of the parent–infant relationship introduced by Stern-Bruschweiler and Stern (1989). This model, illustrated in Figure 7.2, has broad implications for assessment and treatment. There are many formal methods of assessing interactional patterns between caregivers and young children. Caregivers' subjective experience of the infant/young child component of the relationship may also be assessed with formal coding or clinical observation. Assessing these components helps clinicians to infer the infant/young child's representation of their caregiver and relationship with their caregiver. This model highlights components of the parent–infant relationship that ought to be assessed when young children are evaluated in clinical contexts.

A broader model of relationship assessment has been advanced in the nosology of early childhood disorders *DC:0-5* (ZERO TO THREE, 2016). To emphasize the centrality context for considerations of young children's development and well-being, this nosology is multiaxial, including a relational context axis. In addition to ratings of adaptation/maladaptation of the young child's primary relationships with caregivers, the *DC:0-5* characterizes the network of family relationships in which the child develops. This includes coparenting relationships between caregivers and the broader network of close relationships that impinge on the young child's development and adaptation, including relationships with siblings.

Strengths perspective

Another important guiding principle of infant mental health is an intentional focus on strengths—in infants, in caregivers, and in infants' broader interpersonal context. Focusing solely on deficits leads not only to missing resources, it may also create and perpetuate stigma and further marginalize minoritized groups. This perspective means comprehensively assessing strengths as well as problems and their interrelations. Though it arguably applies through the life span, the strengths perspective has been a hallmark feature of infant mental health for decades. For example, reflecting the tradition of the strengths perspective, in the early 1990s the ZERO TO THREE Work Group on Developmental Assessment posited a formal shift in the assessment process of young children from a deficiency lens to a more comprehensive approach that included strengths (Greenspan & Meisels, 1994). Identifying strengths is now a focus in infant mental health training programs (Hinshaw *et al.*, 2019) and in

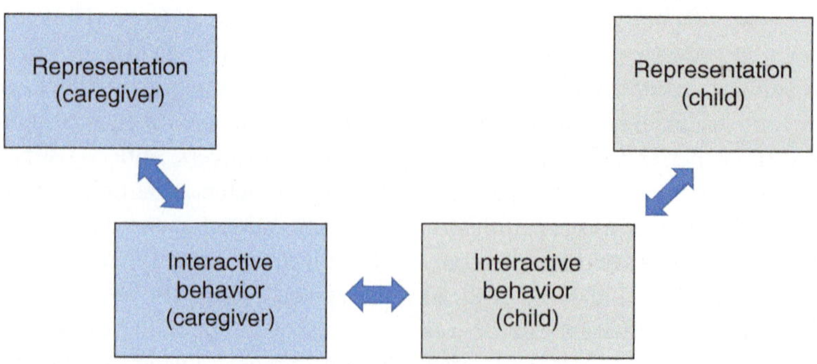

Figure 7.2 Components of the caregiver–child relationship relevant for assessment and treatment.

practice guidelines (St. John *et al.*, 2012). See Chapter 23 on resilience.

Psychopathology

There are two major lines of investigation that have contributed to conceptualizations of psychopathology in young children: research on traditional disorders and research on relational psychopathology. Each of these has faced resistance, although for different reasons. The traditional disorders approach faced an objection, suggesting that it was unreasonable to apply diagnoses to young children. Instead, young children's symptoms were asserted to be either transient responses to environmental challenges or risk factors for subsequently emerging psychopathology. Some of the common presenting problems in young children are noted in the following list:

- birth–12 months
  - excessive crying/colic
  - bedtime struggles and nightwaking
  - undereating
- 12–36 months
  - irritability
  - aggression
  - tantrums
  - food refusal/conflicts about food
  - bedtime struggles and nightwaking
  - hyperactivity/impulsivity
- 30–60 months
  - irritability
  - hyperactivity/impulsivity
  - aggression
  - oppositional/defiant behavior
  - anxiety

The relational psychopathology approach, on the other hand, has faced resistance because it runs counter to definitions of disorders as existing within, rather than between, individuals in extant nosologies.

Traditional disorders

Although infant mental health clinicians have long treated putative disorders in young children, research on early childhood psychopathology was limited until recently. Two decades ago, the American Psychiatric Association (APA) created a Task Force to review research on psychopathology in young children in order to develop criteria for early childhood disorders for which there was a sufficient empirical base. This culminated in the publication of *Research Diagnostic Criteria—Preschool Age* (Scheeringa & Task Force, 2003) and included criteria for attention deficit/hyperactivity disorder (ADHD), oppositional defiant disorder (ODD), conduct disorder (CD), major depressive disorder (MDD), post-traumatic stress disorder (PTSD), reactive attachment disorder, two types of sleep disorders, and six types of feeding disorders. This effort was necessary because many disorders require algorithm adjustments and are developmentally different manifestations of disorders identified in middle childhood or adolescence. For example, Scheeringa and colleagues (Scheeringa *et al.* 2001), showed that applying *Diagnostic and Statistical Manual of Mental Disorders IV* (DSM-IV; American Psychiatric Association, 1994) criteria to young children who had experienced trauma yielded almost no cases of PTSD, despite the fact that these traumatized young children were highly symptomatic. Adjusting the algorithm and making criteria more developmentally sensitive led to a substantial minority of these young children meeting the diagnostic threshold for PTSD. Later, these findings with clinically referred children were replicated in a population representative sample of 3202 children (Hitchcock *et al.*, 2021).

Relational pathology

Sroufe (1989) asserted that many psychiatric problems in children less than 3 years old, though poignantly expressed in child behavior, are best conceptualized as relational. A group of distinguished developmental researchers collaborated on developing a relational conceptualization of psychopathology in young children. As a foundation, they noted that several decades of research had shown that assessing the caregiving environment was essential to understanding infant development. Thus, if an individual infant was not a suitable level of analysis for infant development, therefore, "neither is the individual a suitable level of analysis for understanding infant behavioral disorders" (Sameroff & Emde, 1989, p. 222). This pioneering work was important in articulating a framework for understanding relational pathology in young children, but operationalizing relationship disorders in young children and their caregivers remained challenging until the publication of an updated nosology of early childhood disorders.

Nosology of early childhood disorders

ZERO TO THREE, an organization focused on professional training, parent support, and policy issues related to young children, created a task force to produce an updated nosology of early childhood disorders. The *Diagnostic Classification of Mental Health and Developmental Disorders of Infancy and Early Childhood* (DC:0-5; ZERO TO THREE, 2016) unites both the traditional disorders approach and the relational psychopathology approach noted in the previous section.

The nosology includes a multiaxial diagnostic characterization that emphasizes the importance of context for young children as any disorders noted are associated with a caregiving environment, physical health, stressors, and development (see Table 7.1). The disorders are clustered into sections modeled after DSM-5 (American Psychiatric Association, 2013). The criteria for disorders are informed by research, drawn from high-risk, clinical, and/or population representative samples of young children. There was an explicit effort to extend criteria to include children in the first two years of life. Several disorders that are not included in DSM-5 or *International Classification of*

Table 7.1 Multiaxial approach to diagnosis of the *Diagnostic Classification of Mental Health and Developmental Disorders of Infancy and Early Childhood (DC:0-5).*

Axis I. Clinical disorders
10 Neurodevelopmental disorders
20 Sensory processing disorders
30 Anxiety disorders
40 Mood disorders
50 Obsessive–compulsive and related disorders
60 Sleep, eating, and crying disorders
70 Trauma, stress, and deprivation disorders
80 Relationship-specific disorder
Axis II. Relational context
A. Primary caregiving relationships
B. Broader caregiving environment
Axis III. Physical health conditions and considerations
Axis IV. Psychosocial stressors
Axis V. Developmental competence

Diseases (ICD-11; World Health Organization, 2019) were introduced. For example, two new neurodevelopmental disorders (NDD) were defined that describe impairing symptoms in children less than 24 months of age but who do not meet the diagnostic threshold for their familiar counterparts in children older than 24–36 months: overactivity disorder of toddlerhood (Gleason & Humphreys, 2016), based on longitudinal evidence of continuity of signs of impairing hyperactivity/impulsivity from 18–36 months; and early atypical autism spectrum disorder (ASD; Soto *et al.*, 2016) from 9–36 months, based on impairing signs of social communication and restricted and repetitive behavior symptoms. Recognizing these disorders facilitates providing children with appropriately tailored services and improving the likelihood of optimizing their development. In addition, relationship-specific disorder of infancy and early childhood was introduced, based on research demonstrating relationship specificity, and numerous case reports of relationship-specific psychopathology (Zeanah & Lieberman, 2016).

As noted, an entire axis of this nosology describes the caregiving environment of young children in which their symptomatic behavior is embedded. First, one rates levels of adaptation in the infant or young child's primary caregiving relationships, and then, the adaptive levels of the broader caregiving environment, such as the coparenting relationship, sibling relationships, etc. Each of these aspects of the caregiving environment is rated on one of four levels of adaptation—(i) well adapted to good enough, (ii) strained to concerning, (iii) compromised to disturbed, and (iv) disordered to dangerous—with the understanding that each level includes a range of functioning. These levels can be used to determine the need for treatment, as treatment is definitely indicated for levels (iii) and (iv), and careful monitoring and perhaps treatment for level (ii).

Obviously, the health axis notes comorbid conditions, the stressors axis brings considerations of precipitants and perpetuators of symptoms, and the developmental competence axis calls attention to interrelationships between development and psychopathology. A multiaxial diagnostic profile aids clinicians in targeting their efforts.

Assessment in infant mental health

Compared to school-age children or adolescents, assessment of infants and young children includes some similar but also unique features. Though context matters at all ages, it is especially crucial in infants and young children because of the dependency of infants and young children on their caregiving environments. Individual differences in temperamental traits must be distinguished from signs of disorders (e.g., high activity versus hyperactivity; sociability versus disinhibited social behavior). Beyond determining the presence or absence of a diagnosis, assessments must also provide an understanding of the child in varying contexts (e.g., familial, cultural, etc.), identify strengths, and guide decisions related to interventions. The structure of the multiaxial frame of the DC:0-5 provides a guide for assessment.

Clinical disorders

There are structured interviews for the assessment of symptoms, disorders, and impairment that are administered to caregivers of young children. In order to reduce bias inherent in caregiver report measures, these interviews are designed to assess symptoms and impairment by specific and detailed questioning with examples to reduce inaccuracies, both by providing immediate confirmation that the question was understood and by helping the interviewer gain clarity on how the behavior compares to the standard being used by the reporter to determine the presence or absence of a disorder; probing to distinguish symptoms from typical behavioral perturbations is essential. The most commonly used diagnostic interviews for young children are interviewer-based rather than respondent-based, thus requiring interviewers to be trained clinicians.

The Preschool Age Psychiatric Assessment (PAPA) is a well-validated interviewer-based measure that assesses caregiver-reported psychiatric symptoms, disorders, and impairment in preschool children (24 months through 72 months). The PAPA requires about 1.5 hours to administer and also assesses the child's school/childcare functioning, family structure and functioning, parenting behaviors, adverse life events, and a host of demographic variables (Egger *et al.*, 2006). There is also an electronic version called the ePAPA. This interview collects detailed descriptive information from interviewees, and requires inquiring about functional impairment in each of its symptom categories and their variability across settings. Symptoms are elicited for the three months preceding the interview, in an attempt to reduce errors in recall, although there is a section for "lifetime occurrences."

The Development and Well-being Assessment (DAWBA) combines interviews, questionnaires, and rating techniques (Goodman, *et al.*, 2011). The DAWBA preschool version has been modified based on considerations of the young child's environment and considers potential variations related to development and caregiver differences. The parent/caregiver interview requires approximately 50 minutes, and explores the presence and severity of symptoms, duration of symptoms, and impact the symptoms have on the child and their environment. Teacher interviews have three sections: emotional disorders, hyperactivity–inattention, and oppositional-conduct behaviors, and requires 10–15 minutes to complete. Responses collected from the different informants are combined and then analyzed by computer which generates ICD-11 and/or DSM-5 diagnoses.

The Diagnostic Infant and Preschool Assessment (DIPA) is an interview of caregivers that provides diagnoses for young children less than six years old, requiring about 1.5 hours to administer (Scheeringa & Haslett, 2010). The DIPA is interviewer-based and semi-structured, but it does require the use of "detailed scripted probes" to inquire about specific symptoms. As with the other structured interviews, algorithms are used to determine diagnoses using DSM-5 or DC:0-5 criteria. Interviews and rating scales are discussed in Chapter 28.

Relationship context

Considering the importance of relationships with caregivers for young children, an emphasis on the relational context is unsurprising as part of the diagnostic process. Officially endorsed practice parameters for assessing young children (Thomas *et al.*, 1997), the DC:0-5 nosology (ZERO TO THREE, 2016), and texts of infant mental health (DelCarmen-Wiggins & Carter, 2019; Zeanah, 2019) place major emphasis on the relational context for the young children. Various observational and interview measures yield information about the Stern-Bruschweiler and Stern (1989) model in Figure 7.2. Each of these measures can be used for clinical and research purposes, and training is recommended for both uses.

The Parent–Child Early Relational Assessment or ERA (Clark *et al.*, 2019), assesses the relationship between caregivers and their children less than five years old and focuses on both the affective and behavioral components of parent–child interactions. It has been used for both clinical work and research. Although initially designed to identify risk and possible opportunities for early intervention for mothers with psychiatric diagnosis and their babies, later modifications incorporated additional factors such as fathers, differing functional status of parents, younger children, and elements that the child may bring to the relationship (i.e., prematurity). See Chapters 27 and 28 for further details.

The Insightfulness Assessment (IA), includes a semi-structured interview and review of a videotaped interaction between the child and caregiver (Oppenheim & Koren-Karie, 2013). The assessor selects video excerpts of a previously recorded interaction and interviews the caregiver. The questions focus on the caregiver's awareness of the child's experience and behaviors as well as the caregivers' thoughts about what they noticed. See Chapters 27 and 28 for further details.

A related method involves use a semi-structured interview and a standardized but flexible interactional assessment paradigm (Larrieu *et al.*, 2019). The Working Model of the Child Interview (WMCI) (Zeanah & Benoit 1995) is a semi-structured interview of caregivers about their child and their relationship with their child. Even without formal classifications the content and qualitative features of the interview can be useful clinically, as these provide rich information about the caregiver's subjective experience of the child. The interactional procedure with which the interview is paired involves a series of prescribed episodes: free play, clean-up the toys, bubbles, two teaching tasks, a brief separation, and a reunion (Crowell *et al.*, 1988). The dyad can be observed navigating low-demand activities (e.g., free play, bubbles) and high-demand activities (clean-up, teaching tasks), as well as how they handle transitions from one activity to another. Taken together, the interview and interactional procedure provide data that can be formally coded or made use of clinically to assess a relationship between a young child and their caregiver.

Observational procedures allow careful assessment of the young child and caregiver in standardized situations that are relevant to specific disorders and increase confidence in caregiver reports of behavior when convergent. For example, the Clinical Observation of Attachment (COA) (Boris *et al.*, 2004) involves a series of episodes that allow comparison of the child's interaction with their caregiver and interactions with the clinician, including both caregiver and clinician/stranger picking up the child and walking them around the room, reunion episodes with both caregiver and clinician/stranger, and an episode in which the child is placed between the clinician/stranger and caregiver to determine if and how the child uses the caregiver to handle response to novelty. Together with an interview such as the Disturbances of Attachment Interview (Smyke *et al.*, 2002), the COA adds a valuable component to assess attachment disorders. Similarly, the Disruptive Behavior–Diagnostic Observation Schedule (DB-DOS) is an observational procedure to assess disruptive behavior in preschool children (Wakschlag *et al.*, 2008). The procedure requires 50 minutes in which a young child interacts with both their caregiver and with an examiner in do and don't frustration tasks and social play tasks. The examiner episodes include both examiner-engaged and examiner-busy interactive sequences. In the caregiver episode, support varies by design during different tasks. Coders rate specified disruptive behaviors in two domains: problems in behavioral regulation and problems in anger modulation. These ratings may be used in combination with interview data to increase confidence in diagnosing disruptive behavior disorders.

Intervention and treatment

Both preventive interventions and treatment of clinical conditions of young children are relationship-based and typically work through changing the caregiver–young child relationship in order to change the young child's behavior. Changing the child's behavior through changing how the parent understands and responds to the young child is common to most infant mental health interventions. In order to change parenting behavior, treatment may include enhancing parenting skills, providing caregivers with need-specific resources (mental health providers; educational, housing, or financial assistance; advocacy agencies), and encouraging connections to social groups (e.g., church) and support groups to reduce isolation (Child Welfare Information Gateway, 2020). A key ingredient for healthy development is that young children receive nurturing care, and this is a central feature of interventions for young children, from promotion and prevention through treatment.

Caregiver nurturance as an intervention

The importance of nurturance was demonstrated in Harlow's famous study in which rhesus macaques preferred contact comfort over food (Harlow *et al.*, 1965). Just over a decade later, the "still face procedure" highlighted human infant's sensitivity to caregiver responsiveness (Tronick *et al.*, 1978). When caregivers are instructed to be unresponsive (by maintaining a neutral facial expression for one to two minutes), infants usually initially increase social bids to reengage with the caregiver. When the caregiver becomes unresponsive as instructed, most infants begin to display signs of emotional distress or anxiety. The past four decades have amplified these findings about the importance of caregiving nurturance in the earliest years of life (Britto *et al.*, 2017).

Because of the increasing recognition of the importance of early childhood experiences and primary caregiving relationships, early childhood is included in the World Health Organization (WHO)'s Sustainable Development Goals for 2030. In addition, *The Lancet* recently published an update of its series on early childhood development (Richter *et al.*, 2017). This series of reviews concluded that young children need nurturing care from the beginning, that multisector interventions are needed, targeting multiple risks to development, and that governments should lead efforts to take evidence-based interventions to scale. The WHO, United Nations Children's Fund (UNICEF), and World Bank Group produced a set of resources to support early childhood interventions designed to enhance nurturing care available at https://nurturing-care.org (World Health Organization, United Nations Children's Fund, World Bank Group, 2018). The emphasis on nurturing care runs from health promotion through treatment.

Introduction to promotion, prevention, and treatment

Intervention efforts begin with promotion efforts, designed to enhance development and well-being for all young children in a population, such as promoting nurturing care. Next, we focus on preventive interventions that work through and on relationships that help promote the young child's development. Finally, psychotherapeutic treatment is available for families whose children are symptomatic or have diagnosable disorders causing distress or impairment. We illustrate these different levels with evidenced-based interventions, though we note that some interventions may be used as prevention efforts in high-risk groups, as well as treatment in clinically referred children. The growth of evidenced-based work in prevention and in treatment focused on infants and young children has been considerable in the last 20 years, so that we include illustrative examples rather than a comprehensive review. A more complete discussion of universal, selected, and indicated interventions is discussed in Chapter 32.

Health promotion and universal preventive interventions

Given that there is consensus, at least in much of the developed world, about the necessary supports that enhance infant development, health promotion and universal prevention efforts are designed to promote social and emotional health and prevent onset of problems through efforts aimed at the general population. Two arenas provide access to most young children—health care settings and childcare centers. The American Academy of Pediatrics (AAP) identified 12 health promotion themes, eight of which are especially relevant to infant mental health: lifelong health for families and communities, family support, health for children and youth with special health care needs, healthy development, mental health, healthy weight, healthy nutrition, and physical activity (Hagan *et al.*, 2022). Primary care providers for young children are given directions about how to promote these goals with families of infants (defined as first year of life) and those in early childhood (defined as 1–4 years of age). In childcare settings, the AAP has published a policy statement advocating for creating multidisciplinary, evidence-based childcare practice standards, establishing state quality rating and improvement systems, improving federal and state regulations providing childcare health consultation, and initiating other innovative partnerships. The goals of these efforts are to enhance caregiving quality in early education and childcare settings.

Selected preventive interventions

Young children with identified persistent risk factors, such as poverty, are targets for selected preventive interventions. The United States government recognizes 20 different Maternal Infant and Early Childhood Home Visiting (MIECHV) programs as "evidenced-based," as determined by formal criteria. These programs aim to enhance maternal and child health, to prevent child abuse and neglect, to reduce crime and domestic violence, to increase family educational attainment and earning potential, to promote children's school readiness, and to connect families to needed community resources and supports (see Chapter 15 for additional information).

One of the best known MIECHV programs is the Nurse–Family Partnership (NFP), in which public health nurses provide in-home intervention for low-income, first-time mothers from mid-pregnancy through their child's second birthday. In addition to randomized controlled trials (RCTs) showing positive initial and long-term effects on maternal and child well-being, the NFP also reduced child maltreatment (Olds *et al.*, 1997). Though expensive to implement, the return on investment of this intervention is large (Miller, 2013). Two more recent attempts at replication, however, one in the United Kingdom (Robling *et al.*, 2016) and one in South Carolina (McConnell *et al.*, 2022), have yielded few positive results, perhaps because of a broader array of supports available in both settings.

Indicated preventive interventions

For young children who already have intrinsic (e.g., difficult temperament) or extrinsic risk (e.g., maltreatment) factors but minimally detectable symptoms that may progress to impairing psychopathology, indicated preventive interventions are offered. Many examples are well-supported by evidence. A number of video-based coaching interventions (such as those in Table 7.1) have been designed to enhance parental sensitivity and child attachment. These coaching interventions share derivation from attachment theory and research, use of video review with caregivers to enhance their reflective capacity, a central goal of enhancing caregiver sensitivity, a here-and-now focus on caregiver–child interaction, and an intentional highlighting of positive interactions. They do not require those who administer the interventions to have clinical training beyond the specific training required for each method.

Attachment and biobehavioral catch-up (ABC) (Bernard *et al.*, 2012), video-feedback intervention to promote positive parenting and sensitive discipline (VIPP-SD) (Juffer *et al.*, 2017), and attachment video-feedback intervention (AVI) (Moss *et al.*, 2018) are all attachment-derived coaching interventions generally delivered in home settings. They all include reviewing videos of interactions with caregivers to enhance their sensitive responsiveness with infants and young children. Each has a growing evidence base supporting their effectiveness with a range of indicated populations (Table 7.2).

Psychotherapeutic treatment

Psychotherapy for young children works through and on the child–caregiver relationship (see also Chapter 36 on relationship-based treatments). In some cases, this means in dyadic sessions, and in others, the caregiver watches and provides input as a therapist works with a child directly. In still other approaches, there may be parallel sessions for caregivers and for children. Even when the child's behavior is targeted directly, the caregiver's involvement is integral to the treatment. Some of the most common treatment approaches are illustrated in Table 7.3.

Child-parent psychotherapy (CPP) is an explicitly relational treatment that is one of the mostly widely used and best-studied psychotherapies for young children and their caregivers (Table 7.3). CPP focuses specifically on young children who have experienced trauma, whose caregivers have major mental illness and maladaptive parenting, and who are encumbered by ecological stressors. CPP is applicable to children from birth through 5 years of age and seeks to enhance caregivers' understanding of their child's physical and emotional needs, and to help them to create a sense of safety and security for their child.

Trauma-focused cognitive behavioral therapy (TF-CBT) for preschool children is an evidence-based intervention derived from TF-CBT for older children, used to treat trauma-related symptoms in children aged 3–6 years (see Table 7.2) (McGuire *et al.*, 2021). Treatment generally consists of 12 sessions, combining cognitive behavior techniques with family sessions, and includes using simplified language and a greater emphasis on play to help with expression of the narrative and processing of the traumatic experience(s).

Table 7.2 Selected coaching interventions for young children and caregivers.

	Age range	Format	Length of treatment	Primary target of treatment	Training required	Evidence base
Attachment and biobehavioral catch-up (ABC)	Birth–4 years	In-home sessions that include video review and in-the-moment coaching	10 one-hour weekly sessions	Caregiver behavior (following the child's lead, nurturing care, and reducing harsh and frightening behavior	Initial training is 2 days, followed by twice weekly supervision for 1 year	4 RCTs
Video-feedback Interaction to Promote Positive Parenting—Sensitive Discipline (VIPP-SD)	1–6 years	In-home sessions with video review	7 sessions of 1.5–2 hours	Sensitive caregiving	Initial training is 4 days, followed by 3 monthly individual supervision sessions	12 RCTs
Attachment video-feedback intervention (AVI)	2.5–7 years	In-home sessions with video review	9 sessions of 1.5 hours	Sensitive caregiving	Initial training is 3 days, followed by 35 hours of group supervision	2 RCTs

Table 7.3 Selected psychotherapeutic treatments for young children.

	Age range	Format	Length of treatment	Primary target of treatment	Training required	Evidence base
Child–parent psychotherapy (CPP)	Birth–5 years	Sessions of parent, child, and therapist as well as sessions of therapist and parent	1 year	Parent's representation of child	Initial training, followed by 18 months of supervision	5 RCTs
Trauma focused cognitive behavioral therapy (TF-CBT) for preschool children	3–6 years	12 sessions with therapist and child; caregiver observes	12 weeks	Child's behavior (developing skills to cope with painful memories)	1 day training followed by 3–6 months of consultation/ supervision	4 RCTs
Parent–child interaction therapy (PCIT)	2.5–7 years	Caregiver and child interact while being observed remotely by therapist. Therapist provides coaching through a remote audio.	Based on skill acquisition/ implementation, roughly 4 months	Parent verbal and behavioral responses to child (PRIDE Skills—praise, reflection, imitation, description, and enthusiasm); discipline in response to noncompliance	Initial training 40 hours, followed by twice a month supervision until 2 cases completed	Multiple RCTs

Parent–child interaction therapy (PCIT) is a well-studied psychotherapy that focuses on enhancing caregiver responsiveness and effectiveness in order to change the behavior of children aged 2–7 years (Lieneman *et al.*, 2017). Originally developed to reduce young children's disruptive behaviors, it has been applied more broadly to a variety of clinical problems, such as anxiety, depression, and selective mutism. Treatment consists of two phases: child-directed intervention focuses on strengthening the relationship by promoting positive child behaviors through coached verbal responses by caregivers, including labeled praise and behavioral descriptions, and parent-directed intervention works on bolstering the caregiver's skills to set limits on disruptive behavior and to help the child cooperate.

Additional topics

Parental mental illness

It is beyond our scope to review the vast literature on the effects of parental mental illness on young children's development, but it is not uncommon in clinical settings to encounter two generational psychiatric symptoms and disorders. For many parental disorders, the risk to children is nonspecific, children are at risk of a broad spectrum of problems and/or disorders different from their parents. On the other hand, there is more specificity for young children of parents with anxiety disorders also having anxiety disorders and young children with PTSD also having parents with PTSD (Scheeringa & Zeanah, 2001; van Santvoort *et al.*, 2015). Both may reflect genetic vulnerability, and the latter also often reflects a shared experience of traumatic events.

Equity, diversity, and inclusion

Along with increased attention to the social determinants of health (Solar & Irwin, 2010), increased efforts to address disparities within racial and ethnic minoritized groups of infants and young children have led to efforts to expand access to care, to increase diversity in the workforce, and to enhance data collection and reporting (Hill *et al.*, 2022). Because disparities are evident across income and levels of education, the effects of racism are vital to address, both within the field and beyond. Disparities in maternal and prenatal health may derive from reduced access to prenatal care for mothers, insufficient or unhealthy diets, or exposures to environmental toxins. Broader societal factors, such as structural racism, are increasingly implicated to explain racial disparities. For example, regarding maternal mortality, pregnancy-related deaths for Black women between ages 30–34 in the United States is more than four times higher than the rate for White women (48.6 versus 11.3 per 100,000). Notably, the pregnancy-related mortality rate for Black women who completed college education or higher is 5.2 times higher than the rate for White women with the same educational attainment and 1.6 times higher than the rate for White women in general (Hill *et al.*, 2022).

The field of infant mental health has recently focused more intentionally on the corrosive effects of racism internationally. For example, the flagship journal of the field, the *Infant Mental Health Journal*, has committed to ending systemic racism and promoting diversity in academic publishing (Iruka *et al.*, 2021). The Professional Development Network of the Irving Harris Foundation developed the "Diversity-informed tenets of infant mental health" (Table 7.4) (St. John *et al.*, 2012). These are aspirational principles intended to inform infant mental health practitioners to make more intentional efforts to make equity, diversity, and inclusion central in clinical work. A United States-based advocacy organization, ZERO TO THREE, has a more diverse workforce, and one committed to inclusion, that helps to ensure findings are applicable more broadly and reduce the risk of further perpetuating health disparities or creating new ones.

Table 7.4 Diversity-informed tenets of infant mental health.

Professional Development Network, Irving Harris Foundation
Self-awareness leads to better services for families
Champion children's rights globally
Work to acknowledge privilege and combat discrimination
Recognize and respect nondominant bodies of knowledge
Honor diverse family structures
Understand that language can hurt or heal
Support families in their preferred language
Allocate resources to systems change
Make space and open pathways
Advance policy that supports all families

Interventions in low- and middle-income countries

There are reasonable concerns about the application of evidence-based interventions to populations with whom they have not been studied, especially interventions developed in high-income countries applied to low- and middle-income countries. Henrich's groundbreaking review challenging universal claims in psychological science concluded that individuals from Western, educated, industrialized, rich, and democratic cultures are outliers in many key domains of psychology. Therefore, they constitute one of the most unusual subpopulations one could study for generalizing about human psychology (Henrich *et al.*, 2010). Reviewing articles published in *Psychological Science*, Rad *et al.* (2018) demonstrated that almost all research published there relied on Western samples and used these data without reflection to make inferences about humans more generally. Cultural psychologists have noted that understanding parenting strategies requires understanding the cultural beliefs and practices in which they are embedded. Therefore, interventions studied in Western settings should be applied in low- and middle-income countries only after thoroughly understanding the local context, including relying on ethnographic sources (Keller, 2018).

Conclusions and new directions

It is often said that infant mental health is in its infancy. Although IECMH lags behind the larger fields of child and adult mental health, it is not clear that the "infancy" of the field captures five decades of substantial progress in understanding risk and protective processes, developing nosologies of early childhood disorders, measurement and assessment contributions, and preventive interventions and treatment. With the substantial documentation on the profound effects of early experience, much promise awaits those who seek to understand how to favorably shape developmental trajectories. Brain development will continue to be an important and salient area of investigation, and cellular and molecular processes involved in development are promising areas of current and future research. Much remains to be learned about treatment, especially what works for whom and cultural adaptations of interventions. Promising advances in this young field are confidently anticipated.

References

American Psychiatric Association (1994) *Diagnostic and Statistical Manual of Mental Disorders*, 4th edn. American Psychiatric Association, Washington, DC.

American Psychiatric Association (2013) *Diagnostic and Statistical Manual of Mental Disorders*, 5th edn. American Psychiatric Association, Washington, DC.

Bernard, K. *et al.* (2012) Enhancing attachment organization among maltreated children: results of a randomized clinical trial. *Child Development* **83**(2), 623–636.

Boris, N.W. *et al.* (2004) Comparing criteria for attachment disorders: establishing reliability and validity in high-risk samples. *Journal of the American Academy of Child and Adolescent Psychiatry* **43**, 568–577.

Bradley, R.H. & Corwyn, R.F. (2002) Socioeconomic status and child development. *Annual Review of Psychology* **53**, 371–379.

Britto, P.R. *et al.* (2017) Nurturing care: promoting early childhood development. *The Lancet* **389**(10064), 91–102.

Cano, T. (2022) Social class, parenting, and child development: a multidimensional approach. *Research in Social Stratification and Mobility* **77**, 100648. doi:10.1016/j.rssm.2021.100648.

Child Welfare Information Gateway (2020) *Protective Factors Approaches in Child Welfare*. U.S. Department of Health and Human Services, Children's Bureau, Washington, DC.

Clark, R. *et al.* (2019) Assessment of early parent–child relationships'. In: *The Oxford Handbook of Infant, Toddler, and Preschool Mental Health Assessment*. (eds R. DelCarmen-Wiggins & A.S. Carter), 2nd edn. Oxford University Press, Oxford, UK. pp. 29–45.

Crowell, J.A. *et al.* (1988) Assessment of mother–child interaction in pre-schoolers with behavior problems. *Journal of the American Academy of Child and Adolescent Psychiatry* **27**, 303–311.

Daelsman, B. *et al.* (2016) Early childhood development: the foundation of sustainable development. *The Lancet* **389**, 9–11.

DelCarmen-Wiggins, R. & Carter, A.S. (eds) (2019) *The Oxford Handbook of Infant, Toddler, and Preschool Mental Health Assessment*, 2nd edn. Oxford University Press, Oxford, UK.

Egger, H.L. *et al.* (2006) Test-retest reliability of the preschool age psychiatric assessment (PAPA). *Journal of the American Academy of Child and Adolescent Psychiatry* **45**(5), 538–549.

Ellis, B.J. *et al.* (2009) The impact of harsh versus unpredictable environments on the evolution and development of life history strategies. *Human Nature* **20**(2), 204–268.

Felitti, V.J. *et al.* (1998) Relationship of childhood abuse and household dysfunction to many of the leading causes of death in adults. The adverse childhood experiences (ACE) study. *American Journal of Prevention Medicine* **14**(4), 245–258.

Fox, S.E. *et al.* (2010) How the timing and quality of early experiences influence the development of brain architecture. *Child Development* **81**(1), 28–40.

Ghosh-Ippen, C.M. (2019) Wounds from the past: integrating historical trauma into a multicultural infant mental health framework. In: *Handbook of Infant Mental Health.* (ed C.H. Zeanah), 4th edn. Guilford Press, New York. pp. 134–153.

Gleason, M.M. & Humphreys, K. (2016) Categorical diagnosis of extreme hyperactivity, impulsivity, and inattention in very young children. *Infant Mental Health Journal* **37**, 476–485.

Glover, V. & O'Connor, T.G. (2002) Effects of antenatal stress and anxiety: implications for development and psychiatry. *The British Journal of Psychiatry* **180**(5), 389–391.

Goodman, A. *et al.* (2011) The 'DAWBA bands' as an ordered-categorical measure of child mental health: description and validation in British and Norwegian samples. *Social Psychiatry and Psychiatric Epidemiology* **46**, 521–532.

Greenspan, S.I. & Meisels, S. (1994) Toward a new vision for the developmental assessment of infants and young children. *ZERO TO THREE* **14**(6), 1–8.

Hagan, J.F. *et al.* (eds) (2022) *Bright Futures: Guidelines for Health Supervision of Infants, Children, and Adolescents*, 4th edn. American Academy of Pediatrics, Itasca, IL.

Harkness, S. *et al.* (2013) Culture and early childhood development. In: *Handbook of Early Childhood Development Research and Its Impact on Global Policy.* (eds P.R. Britto, *et al.*). Oxford University Press, Oxford, England.

Harlow, H.F. *et al.* (1965) Total social isolation in monkeys. *Proceedings of the National Academy of Sciences of the United States of America* **54**, 90–97.

Henrich, J. *et al.* (2010) The weirdest people in the world? *Behavioral and Brain Sciences* **33**(2–3), 61–83.

Hill, L. *et al.* (2022) Racial disparities in maternal and infant health: current status and efforts to address them. KFF. Available at: https://www.kff.org/racial-equity-and-health-policy/issue-brief/racial-disparities-in-maternal-and-infant-health-current-status-and-efforts-to-address-them/ [13 August 2023]

Hinshaw, S. *et al.* (2019) Infant and early childhood mental health: updates, new directions. In: *Handbook of Infant Mental Health.* (ed C.H. Zeanah), 4th edn. Guilford Press, New York. pp. 569–584.

Hitchcock, C. *et al.* (2021) Population prevalence of the posttraumatic stress disorder subtype for young children in nationwide surveys of the British general population and of children in care. *Journal of the American Academy of Child and Adolescent Psychiatry* **60**, 1278–1287.

House, B.R. (2018) How do social norms influence prosocial development? *Current Opinion in Psychology* **20**, 87–91.

Iruka, I. *et al.* (2021) Call to action: centering Blackness and disrupting systemic racism in infant mental health research and academic publishing. *Infant Mental Health Journal* **42**(6), 745–748.

Juffer, F. *et al.* (2017) Pairing attachment theory and social learning theory in video-feedback intervention to promote positive parenting. *Current Opinion in Psychology* **15**, 189–194.

Keller, H. (2018) Universality claim of attachment theory: children's socioemotional development across cultures. *Proceedings of the National Academy of Sciences* **115**(45), 11414–11419.

Larrieu, J.A. *et al.* (2019) Assessing the relational context of infants and young children. In: *Handbook of Infant Mental Health.* (ed C.H. Zeanah), 4th edn. Guilford Press, New York. pp. 279–295.

Lieneman, C.C. *et al.* (2017) Parent–child interaction therapy: current perspectives. *Psychology Research and Behavior Management* **10**, 239–256.

Masten, A. (2019) Resilience from a developmental systems perspective. *World Psychiatry* **18**, 201–102.

Masten, A.S. & Barnes, A.J. (2018) Resilience in children: developmental perspectives. *Children* **5**(7), 98.

McConnell, M.A. *et al.* (2022) Effect of an intensive nurse home visiting program on adverse birth outcomes in a Medicaid-eligible population: a randomized clinical trial. *JAMA* **328**(1), 27–37.

McGoron, L. *et al.* (2012) Recovering from early deprivation: attachment mediates effects of caregiving on psychopathology. *Journal of the American Academy of Child and Adolescent Psychiatry* **51**(7), 683–693.

McGuire, A. *et al.* (2021) Systematic review on the application of trauma-focused cognitive behavioral therapy (TF-CBT) for preschool-aged children. *Clinical Child and Family Psychology Review* **24**, 20–37.

McLanahan, S. & Percheski, C. (2008) Family structure and the reproduction of inequalities. *Annual Review of Sociology* **34**, 257–276.

McLaughlin, K.A. & Sheridan, M.A. (2016) Beyond cumulative risk: a dimensional approach to childhood adversity. *Current Directions in Psychological Science* **25**(4), 239–245.

Miller, T. (2013) *Nurse–Family Partnership: Outcomes, Costs, and Return on Investment in New York.* Nurse–Family Partnership, Denver, CO. Available at: https://www.urmc.rochester.edu/MediaLibraries/URMCMedia/finger-lakes-regional-perinatal/documents/nfp_benefit_cost.pdf#:~:text=Estimated%20%249.56%20return%20on%20investment%20to%20society [13 August 2024].

Moss, E. *et al.* (2018) Attachment videofeedback intervention. In: *Handbook of Attachment-Based Interventions.* (eds H. Steele & M. Steele). Guilford Press, New York.

Nigg, J.T. & Breslau, N. (2007) Prenatal smoking exposure, low birth weight, and disruptive behavior disorders. *Journal of the American Academy of Child & Adolescent Psychiatry* **46**(3), 362–369. doi:10.1097/01.chi.0000246054.76167.44.

Olds, D.L. *et al.* (1997) Longterm effects of home visitation on maternal life-course and child abuse and neglect: fifteen year follow-up of a randomized controlled trial. *JAMA* **278**(8), 637–643.

Oppenheim, D. & Koren-Karie, N. (2013) The insightfulness assessment: measuring the internal processes underlying maternal sensitivity. *Attachment & Human Development* **15**(5–6), 545–561.

Przybylski, A.K. & Weinstein, N. (2019) Violent video game engagement is not associated with adolescents' aggressive behaviour: evidence from a registered report. *Royal Society Open Science* **6**, 171474. doi:10.1098/rsos.171474.

Rad, M.S. *et al.* (2018) Toward a psychology of *Homo sapiens*: making psychological science more representative of the human population. *Proceedings of the National Academy of Sciences* **115**(45), 11401–11405.

Richter, L.M. *et al.* (2017) Investing in the foundation of sustainable development: pathways to scale up for early childhood development. *The Lancet* **389**(10064), 103–118.

Robling, M. *et al.* (2016) Effectiveness of a nurse-led intensive home-visitation programme for first-time teenage mothers (Building Blocks): a pragmatic randomised controlled trial. *The Lancet* **387**, 146–155.

Rosman, A. *et al.* (2009) *The Tapestry of Culture: An Introduction to Cultural Anthropology.* Rowman Altamira, Lanham, MD.

Sameroff, A.J. & Emde, R.N. (1989) *Relationship Disturbances in Early Childhood.* Basic Books, New York.

Scheeringa, M. & Haslett, N. (2010) The reliability and criterion validity of the diagnostic infant and preschool assessment: a new diagnostic instrument for young children. *Child Psychiatry and Human Development* **41**(3), 299–312.

Scheeringa, M. & Task Force (2003) Research diagnostic criteria for infants and preschool children: the process and empirical support. *Journal of the American Academy of Child and Adolescent Psychiatry* **42**(12), 1504–1512.

Scheeringa, M. & Zeanah, C.H. (2001) A relationship perspective on PTSD in infancy. *Journal of Traumatic Stress* **14**, 799–815.

Scheeringa, M. *et al.* (2001) Towards establishing the procedural, criterion, and discriminant validity of PTSD in early childhood. *Journal of the American Academy of Child and Adolescent Psychiatry* **40**, 52–60.

Smyke, A.T. *et al.* (2002) Attachment disturbances in young children. I: the continuum of caretaking casualty. *Journal of the American Academy of Child and Adolescent Psychiatry* **41**, 972–982.

Solar, O. & Irwin, A. (2010) A Conceptual Framework for Action on the Social Determinants of Health: Social Determinants of Health Discussion Paper 2 (Policy and Practice). World Health Organization, Geneva, Switzerland. Available at: https://iris.who.int/bitstream/handle/10665/44489/9789241500852_eng.pdf?sequence=1 [13 August 2024].

Soto, T. *et al.* (2016) Symptom presentations and classification of autism spectrum disorder in early childhood: application to the diagnostic classification of mental health and developmental disorders of infancy and early childhood (DC:0-5). *Infant Mental Health Journal* **37**, 486–497.

Sroufe, L.A. (1989) Relationships and their disturbances. In: *Relationship Disturbances in Early Childhood.* (eds A.J. Sameroff & R.N. Emde). Basic Books, New York. pp. 97–124.

St. John, M. *et al.* (2012) Infant mental health professional development: together in the struggle for social justice. *ZERO TO THREE* **33**, 13–22.

Stern, D.N. (1985) *The Interpersonal World of the Infant.* Basic Books, New York.

Stern-Bruschweiler, N. & Stern, D.N. (1989) A model for conceptualizing the role of the mother's representational world in various mother-infant therapies. *Infant Mental Health Journal* **10**, 142–156.

Tharner, A. *et al.* (2012) Infant attachment, parenting stress, and child emotional and behavioral problems at age 3 years. *Parenting* ***12***(4), 261–281.

Thomas, J. *et al.* (1997) Practice parameters for the psychiatric assessment of infants and toddlers. *Journal of the American Academy of Child and Adolescent Psychiatry* **36**(10), 21s–36s.

Tronick, E.Z. *et al.* (1978) The infant's response to entrapment between contradictory messages in face-to-face interaction. *Journal of the American Academy of Child Psychiatry* **17**, 1–13.

Van den Bergh, B.R. (2011) Developmental programming of early brain and behaviour development and mental health: a conceptual framework. *Developmental Medicine and Child Neurology* **53**, 19–23.

van Santvoort, F. *et al.* (2015) The impact of various parental mental disorders on children's diagnoses: a systematic review. *Clinical Child and Family Psychology Review* **18**, 281–299.

Wakschlag, L.S. *et al.* (2008) Observational assessment of preschool disruptive behavior, part I: reliability of the disruptive behavior diagnostic observation schedule. *Journal of the American Academy of Child and Adolescent Psychiatry* **47**(6), 622–631.

World Health Organization (2019) *International Statistical Classification of Disease and Related Health Problems*, 11th edn, Geneva, Switzerland.

World Health Organization, United Nations Children's Fund, World Bank Group (2018) *Nurturing Care for Early Childhood Development: A Framework for Helping Children Survive and Thrive to Transform Health and Human Potential.* World Health Organization, Geneva, Switzerland. Licence: CC BY-NC-SA 3.0 IGO. Available at: https://nurturing-care.org [13 August 2024]

Zeanah, C.H. *et al.* (2011) Sensitive periods. In: R.B. McCall, M.H. van IJzendoorn & F. Juffer, V.K. Groza, & C.J. Groark (Eds.). *Children without permanent parental care: Research, practice, and policy. Monographs of the Society for Research in Child Development*, Serial No. 301, **76**(4), 147–162.

Zeanah, C.H. (2019) *Handbook of Infant Mental Health.* Guilford Press, New York.

Zeanah, C.H. & Benoit, D. (1995) Clinical applications of a parent perception interview. In: *Infant Psychiatry, Child Psychiatric Clinics of North America.* (ed K. Minde). W.B. Saunders, Philadelphia, PA. pp. 539–554.

Zeanah, C.H. & Lieberman, A. (2016) Defining relational pathology in early childhood: the diagnostic classification of mental health and developmental disorders of infancy and early childhood DC:0–5 approach. *Infant Mental Health Journal* **37**(5), 509–520.

Zeanah, C.H. & Sonuga-Barke, E. (2016) The effects of early trauma and deprivation on human development: from measuring cumulative risk to characterising specific mechanisms. *Journal of Child Psychology and Psychiatry* **56**(10), 1099–1102.

Zeanah, C.H. & Zeanah, P.D. (2009) The scope of infant mental health. In: *Handbook of Infant Mental Health.* (ed C.H. Zeanah), 3rd edn. Guilford Press, New York. pp. 5–21.

Zeanah, C.H. & Zeanah, P.D. (2019) Infant mental health: the clinical science of early experience. In: *Handbook of Infant Mental Health.* (ed C.H. Zeanah), 4th edn. Guilford Press, New York. pp. 5–24.

ZERO TO THREE (2001) *Definition of Infant Mental Health.* ZERO TO THREE Infant mental health steering committee, Washington, DC.

ZERO TO THREE (2016) *DC:0–5TM: Diagnostic Classification of Mental Health and Developmental Disorders of Infancy and Early Childhood (DC:0–5).* Author, Washington, DC.

CHAPTER 8

Temperament mechanisms in developmental psychopathology

Kristin A. Buss and Koraly Pérez-Edgar
Department of Psychology, The Pennsylvania State University, PA, USA

Temperament traits reflect individual differences in a child's fairly consistent strategy for, and response to, interactions with their environment, as well as their internal processing of these events. Temperamental dispositions of interest often focus on emotionality/affectivity, effortful control, activity level, and attention across time and contexts (Shiner *et al.*, 2012). Some temperamental traits, such as negative affect, are evident in the first months of life (Kagan *et al.*, 2007), while others, such as effortful control, rely on psychological processes that are later emerging (Rothbart & Posner, 2006). Often, temperament is referred to as the early appearing, biologically based component of an individual's personality (Shiner & Caspi, 2003; Anaya & Pérez-Edgar, 2019).

Temperamental variation is normative and principally reflects typical individual variation in traits across any population or community. However, there is a growing body of research suggesting that specific temperamental traits, when extreme, can increase an individual's risk for developing psychopathology, emerging in the window from early childhood through young adulthood. For example, individuals with high levels of negative affectivity (i.e., a tendency to experience negative emotions such as fear and sadness) may be at greater risk for developing anxiety or depressive disorders. Similarly, individuals with high levels of impulsivity may be more likely to develop substance-use disorders or other risky behaviors. Temperamental traits can also interact with environmental factors to increase risk for psychopathology. For instance, individuals with a genetic vulnerability for experiencing anxious feelings and thoughts may be more likely to develop an anxiety disorder if they also experience significant stress or trauma in their environment (Klein & Mumper, 2018).

Understanding an individual's temperament can help clinicians and researchers identify individuals who may be at greater risk for developing psychopathology and tailor interventions to target their specific vulnerabilities (Wakschlag *et al.*, 2018). Additionally, interventions aimed at modifying temperamental traits (e.g., through cognitive behavioral therapy [CBT] or pharmacotherapy) may be useful in reducing an individual's risk for developing psychopathology.

To constrain the chapter, we will focus on temperament throughout childhood, examining profiles with the deepest empirical support. We then briefly outline the developmental and clinical consequences of early temperament later in life. While numerous studies have documented biological, physiological, and cognitive differences associated with temperament and psychopathology (Figure 8.1), we point readers to more thorough discussions (Jarcho & Guyer, 2018). Figure 8.1 shows the types of biological systems and physiological measures that have been documented in the temperament literature.

History and major theories of temperament

While recent science has focused on outlining the neural (e.g., brain networks), physiological (e.g., cardiac functions), hormonal (e.g., cortisol reactivity), and cognitive (e.g., attention bias) markers of temperament, our basic core understanding of temperament is quite ancient.

The Greek physician Galen (Kagan, 1997) argued that four core temperaments—sanguine, melancholic, choleric, and phlegmatic—reflected stable patterns of behavior and emotion that were driven by a unique underlying balance of four bodily fluids—blood, yellow bile, black bile, and phlegm. When the fluids became imbalanced, the individual would manifest extreme distress and discomfort. Modern texts now speak of neurotransmitters rather than bodily fluids, and hormones rather than humors, but the underlying conceptualization is remarkably similar.

Rutter's Child and Adolescent Psychiatry and Psychology, Seventh Edition.
Edited by Anita Thapar, Daniel S. Pine, Samuele Cortese, Cathy Creswell, Tamsin J. Ford, James F. Leckman, and Argyris Stringaris.

Companion website: www.wiley.com/go/thapar/rutterspsych7

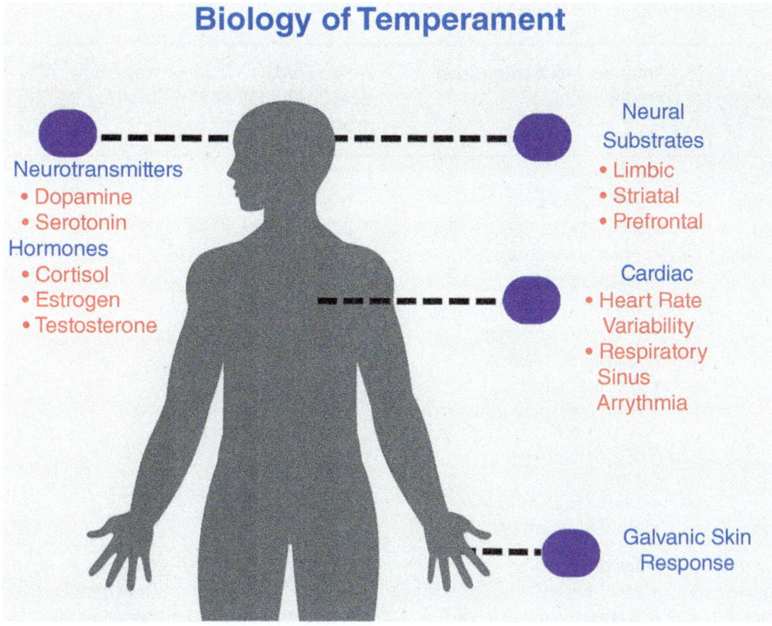

Figure 8.1 Biological components of temperament.

A core tenet of temperament theory is that a trait will show relative stability. That is, across time and contexts, temperament traits are likely to shape expectable patterns of behavior and cognitions. However, researchers have debated the extent of this stability, including whether children continue to hold their relative ranked positions over time, even with developmental changes in the expressed behavioral phenotype. For example, does the shy child in elementary school tend to remain relatively shy in comparison to peers in high school? The empirical evidence suggests that the stability is moderate at best and increases after age two, to then decline after middle childhood (Rothbart *et al.*, 2000).

That is not to say that the fingerprints of early temperament cannot be long-lasting. For example, behavioral inhibition (BI) is an early appearing temperament marked by sensitivity to novelty in the environment. Tang and colleagues (Tang *et al.*, 2020; Tang *et al.*, 2022) have found that children characterized as BI at 14 months of age displayed distinct personality and social profiles three decades later, marked by increased social withdrawal, introversion, and anxiety symptoms. That is, the phenotypic expression of a temperament trait changes over time to reflect both developmental and contextual considerations. In addition, temperamental variation is thought to reflect normative, and necessary, variability in individual traits that allow for greater heterogeneity across the population (Pérez-Edgar & Fox, 2018). It is only at the extreme, when temperament traits cause acute distress or interfere with daily functioning that temperament begins to morph into disorder (Pérez-Edgar & Guyer, 2014). For example, BI is our best characterized, and strongest, individual difference predictor of anxiety symptoms and disorder, particularly social anxiety (Chronis-Tuscano *et al.*, 2009). However, even here, the majority (50–60%) of previously inhibited children do not go on to show clinically elevated levels of anxiety (Clauss & Blackford, 2012; Sandstrom *et al.*, 2020).

Contemporary understanding of temperament

The contemporary approach to this work started to gain momentum in the 1960s. Since then, several approaches have shaped our understanding of the form, function, and impact of early appearing temperamental variation. Given the scope of this chapter, we will not delve deeply into these approaches as they have been reviewed elsewhere (Fu & Pérez-Edgar, 2015; MacNeill & Pérez-Edgar, 2020). However, we highlight some of the major schools of thought, led by Thomas and Chess, Buss and Plomin, Goldsmith, Rothbart, and Kagan (Table 8.1).

The Thomas and Chess approach

The New York Longitudinal Study stands as a landmark in temperament research. Thomas and Chess (1977) focused on behavioral styles characterized across nine dimensions: activity level, rhymicity, approach/withdrawal, adaptability, responsiveness threshold, intensity of reaction, quality of mood, attention span/persistence, and distractibility. Children are then categorized into "easy," "difficult," and "slow-to-warm-up" types based on questionnaire scores on each dimension. Chess and Thomas also introduced the concept of "goodness of fit." A good fit arises from compatibility between the child's temperament and the demands, expectations, and opportunities of the environment. A mismatch (bad fit) between temperament and environmental characteristics is more likely to result in maladaptive outcomes.

Table 8.1 Brief description of core contemporary temperament theories.

Theorists	Key ideas	Temperament categories or dimensions	Associated questionnaires or protocols	Role of biology	Criticisms
Thomas and Chess	Temperamental dimensions capture behavioral style. Dimensions are then combined to create three broad temperament categories.	Nine dimensions: • Activity level • Rhymicity • Approach/withdrawal • Adaptability • Responsiveness threshold • Intensity of reaction • Quality of mood • Distractibility • Attention span/persistence Three categories: • Easy • Difficult • Slow-to-warm-up	• Chess and Thomas' temperament survey • Carey temperament scales	Biology not central.	• Categorizing children into discrete types may hide heterogeneity. • Does not explicitly capture environmental influences on temperament.
Buss and Plomin	Temperament is heritable and influenced by genes. Shaped for evolutionary adaptation across species.	Three dimensions: • Emotionality • Activity • Sociability	• EAS temperament survey • Colorado childhood temperament inventory	Genetic underpinnings preserve traits.	• Little specificity on genetic components. • Minimizes environmental influences.
Goldsmith	Temperament is shaped by genes and environmental factors with discrete dimensions of variation.	Six dimensions: • Fear • Anger/frustration • Attentional control • Positive affect • Activity level • Pleasure seeking.	• Toddler behavior assessment questionnaire • Laboratory temperament assessment battery	Biological substrates support "pure" traits before socialization.	May have difficulty disentangling regulatory processes modulating initial temperament.
Rothbart	Temperament reflects interplay between orthogonal factors of reactivity and regulation.	Three dimensions: • Surgency • Negative affect • Effortful control	• Infant behavior questionnaire • Early childhood behavior questionnaire • Children's behavior questionnaire	Specific neural and physiological systems underlie each dimension.	Questionnaires have been translated for use cross-culturally, but may overlook culturally linked socialization.
Kagan	Temperament is early appearing and biologically based, evident in early variation in sensory reactivity.	Infant reactivity: • Negative reactivity • Positive reactivity Temperament type: • Behavioral inhibition	• Behavioral inhibition lab protocol • Behavioral inhibition questionnaire	Amygdala model suggests hypersensitive response to novelty.	Categories may minimize within group variation. Focus on relatively narrow temperament profile.

The Buss and Plomin approach

Buss and Plomin (1975) focused on temperament traits that have an early onset and are inherited, evolutionarily adaptive, present in nonhuman animals, relatively stable during development, and predictive of later behaviors, all within the framework of behavioral genetics. They identified three core dimensions based on parental report. Emotionality (E) refers to a child's general level of distress, including the ease, frequency, and intensity of their response. Activity (A) is composed of tempo and vigor, while sociability (S) is a child's preference to engage with and be around others. Their studies of twins (Buss & Plomin, 1984) suggested higher concordance in EAS traits among monozygotic (MZ) twin pairs versus dizygotic (DZ) twins, supporting genetic influences on trait variance. They also found that while children's rank orders on these traits remain stable over time, mean levels and expression changed with age.

The Goldsmith approach

Goldsmith and Campos (1982) defined temperament as individual differences in the propensity to express and experience primary emotions (e.g., joy, anger, and fear). Their definition focuses on infant temperament, obtaining a relatively "pure" conceptualization of temperament unmediated by environmental socialization influences. The emphasis on discrete emotions contrasts with other approaches that place individuals on a continuum of broad emotionality. This approach blends both questionnaire (e.g., Toddler Behavior Assessment Questionnaire (Goldsmith, 1996) and direct observation methods via the Laboratory Temperament Assessment Battery (Lab-TAB) (Goldsmith & Rothbart, 1993). This approach is unique in that: (i) motivation is a key component of emotion experience and expression, and (ii) the context of behavior needs to be considered in measuring temperament, since the eliciting situations affect the expression of temperament dimensions (Goldsmith & Gagne, 2012).

The Rothbart approach

Rothbart (Rothbart & Derryberry, 1981) provides a more inclusive conceptualization, defining temperament as biologically rooted individual differences in reactivity and regulation. Reactivity refers to levels of biological arousal triggered by changes in internal and external stimulations. Regulation refers to internal (to the child) processes that modulate reactivity. This is often termed self-regulation and is distinguished from external sources of regulation like caregiver soothing. While reactivity and regulation interact continuously over time, they are conceptualized to be orthogonal to each other (i.e., one can be high in reactivity and low in regulation, and vice versa).

Taking a dimensional approach, reactivity and regulation are operationalized in three higher-order constructs: Negative Affect, Surgency, and Effortful Control. The Rothbart model is unique in prominently placing regulation as a core component of temperament. As effortful control develops during toddlerhood, it exerts "brakes" on unregulated negative emotionality and motor activity (Derryberry & Rothbart, 2002), and enhances children's abilities to adapt to environmental demands. The continued dynamic and reciprocal interactions between temperamental reactivity and regulation contribute to the observed instability of temperament expression over time (Rothbart & Bates, 2007). The three higher-order dimensions are captured by a series of questionnaires that span from infancy through adulthood, building on the assumption of heterotypic continuity.

The Kagan approach

Distinct from dimensional approaches to temperament, Kagan and colleagues defined BI as a temperamental typology marked by a distinct profile of observed behavior in toddlerhood (Kagan, 2018). The quintessentially inhibited child, when confronted with novelty, freezes, retreats, and refuses to engage. This pattern is particularly noticeable with social stimuli. Kagan's approach emphasizes the use of behavioral observations and biological measures instead of parent-report questionnaires (Kagan, 2012), although others have created associated parent-report measures (Bishop *et al.*, 2003). BI is also linked to a distributed neural network involving limbic, striatal, and frontal regions (Blackford *et al.*, 2018).

The BI phenotype has been deeply studied, providing a broader description of its developmental trajectory relative to other temperament profiles. Retrospectively, infants who show a distinct pattern of negative reactivity to (nonsocial) sensory stimuli at four months of age are more likely to display BI later (Fox *et al.*, 2015). Prospectively, BI is the most predictive individual difference factor for the later emergence of anxiety disorders, particularly social anxiety in adolescence and early adulthood (Clauss & Blackford, 2012; Sandstrom *et al.*, 2020). The links between children's neural, physiological, and cognitive responses to novelty and avoidance behaviors may perpetuate behaviorally inhibited tendencies that can lead to social wariness, and, at the extreme, social anxiety (Pérez-Edgar & Guyer, 2014).

Temperament as a way of understanding developmental mechanisms of psychopathology

Although the various temperament approaches differ in their specific constellation of traits, and the methods used for characterizing children, they all coalesce on the conclusion that temperament traits are early appearing, have some underlying biological component, and shape how children experience dynamic, and bidirectional, interactions with their environment. Of particular interest to this discussion, temperament can be a powerful tool for understanding the emergence and developmental trajectory of early psychopathology (see also Chapter 1: Development and psychopathology: a life-course perspective; Ostlund *et al.*, 2021a).

Developmental psychopathology is an interdisciplinary field of research that seeks to understand the origins and pathways of psychological disorders across the life span. It aims to identify risk and protective mechanisms by accounting for the interactions between biological, psychological, and social factors that contribute to the development of psychopathology (Cicchetti, 1984). As a complement to child psychiatry, developmental psychopathology distinguishes itself in focusing on developmental processes that are evident prior to symptom onset and that cannot be divorced from the contexts in which they are embedded or expressed (Steinberg *et al.*, 2006). That is, a pattern of behavior that could be considered problematic or worrisome in one context may be adaptive and socially prized in another. This approach also emphasizes the importance of early identification coupled with interventions that target both the individual and the surrounding environmental context.

Conceptual boundaries between temperament, personality, and psychopathology

There are a number of temperament profiles that reappear in the literature and are most relevant to the emergence and course of psychopathology (Figure 8.2). In general, these profiles tend

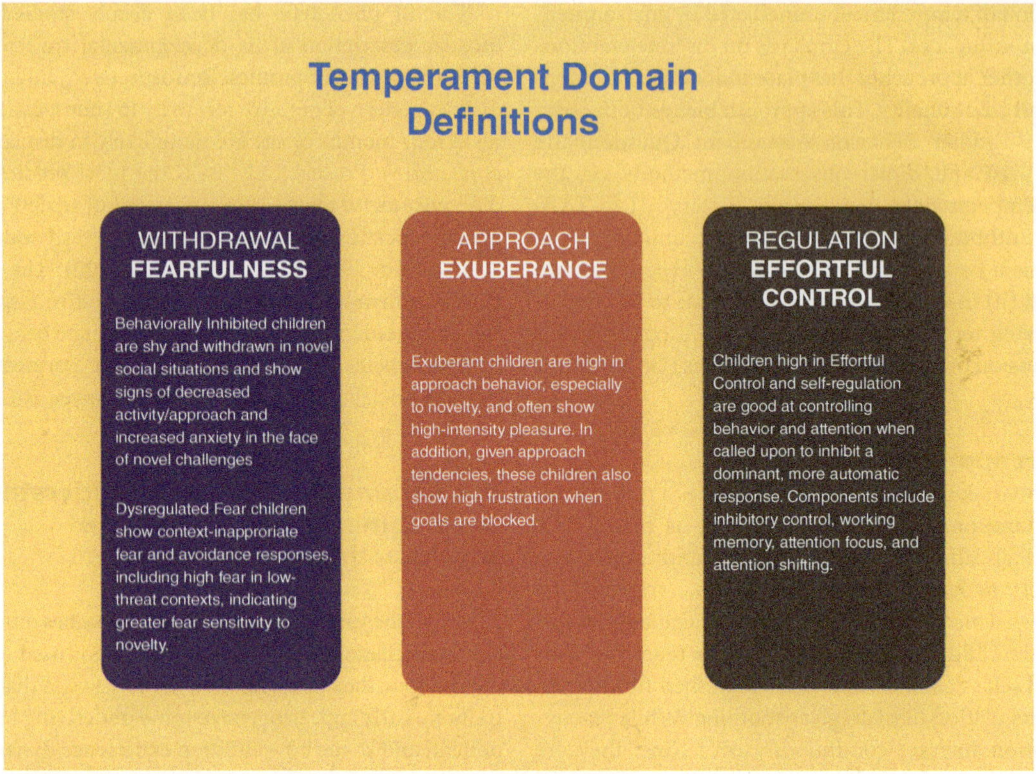

Figure 8.2 Domains of temperament that predict psychopathology.

to reflect differing combinations of reactivity and regulatory processes. A combination of high dispositional reactivity and low levels of regulation is associated with child behavior problems. The specific behavior problems would reflect the specific temperamental profiles observed in the child.

One commonly identified profile is defined by high fearfulness and low regulatory abilities (Putnam & Stifter, 2005; Beekman *et al.*, 2015) and may thus be considered an *inhibited/fearful* group of young children. A similar *negative reactive* profile also exhibits high levels of negative affect (e.g., anger, sadness) more broadly across contexts (Beekman *et al.*, 2015; Ostlund *et al.*, 2021b). A *dysregulated/irritable* profile reflects young children who display high negative affect, particularly anger, paired with high activity levels (Beekman *et al.*, 2015; Gartstein *et al.*, 2017), reminiscent of trait irritability (Wakschlag *et al.*, 2018). An *exuberant/fearless* profile is characterized by high levels of positive affect, activity, and approach-oriented behavior (Gartstein *et al.*, 2017).

While these profiles are not uncommon, they represent the consistent minority of children across studies. That is, most children tend to fall in either an *average/low reactive* profile, defined by a moderate level of emotionality, attention, and activity (Gartstein *et al.*, 2017) or a *well-regulated* profile, marked by relatively low levels of negative affect and high levels of regulation skills (Beekman *et al.*, 2015; Gartstein *et al.*, 2017).

Although there is strong agreement that specific temperamental profiles are consistently linked to fairly constrained clinical outcomes, there remains discussion concerning the potential causal relations between the two constructs. This distinction is a bit easier to make in adolescence and early adulthood—for example, the observed behaviors that go into the BI classification at 14 months are clearly different than the social anxiety symptoms reported by an adolescent at age 14 years. However, the overlap between construct and presentation can be harder to disentangle earlier in childhood. That is, temperament profiles and clinical disorders have a range of overlapping behavioral, cognitive, and neurological features in childhood (Guyer *et al.*, 2014), often due to the child's limited behavioral and cognitive repertoires.

One model suggests that temperament and psychopathology are linked by a shared common causal influence, but temperament does not cause disorder. Rather, it constrains possible socioemotional development outcomes (Kagan *et al.*, 2007). A second model emphasizes a functional continuity between temperament and psychopathology, arguing that they are simply different points within a single spectrum. Here, an individual may display a fixed clinical expression, remaining fairly static in one region of the spectrum—the socially withdrawn child becomes the introverted adult (Coplan *et al.*, 2021). Another form of the continuity model proposes that temperament is part of a single developmental sequence in which the trajectory progresses into disorder as the child "travels" across the spectrum. From this perspective, BI is a subthreshold form of social anxiety, acting as a prodromic marker for the acute disorder.

In contrast, a third set of models suggests that temperament is a separate construct, without a shared etiology, that can predispose an individual to a specific disorder (e.g., exuberance and conduct disorder [CD]) or influence the form and course of the disorder. In one formulation, temperamental fearfulness acts as a diathesis that may predispose a child to disorder when triggered by a second risk factor (Caouette & Guyer, 2014). For example, children high in both negative affect and BI may show increased social anxiety, but, in the absence of BI, would otherwise be at risk for increased depression or conduct disorder, depending on the form and context of negative affect.

Unfortunately, there has been little to no systematic study directly examining these models. Distinguishing between models is also difficult in the light of current debate regarding the best way to define, categorize, and identify discrete psychological disorders. For example, BI is rooted in observed patterns of behavior in response to novelty that are directly associated with heightened levels of limbic reactivity (Kagan, 2012). In contrast, social anxiety as defined by *Diagnostic and Statistical Manual of Mental Disorders, 5th Edition* (DSM-5; American Psychiatric Association, 2013) is identified via reported patterns of avoidance and distress in situations involving social performance and is agnostic with respect to underlying etiology or developmental course (Pine *et al.*, 2011).

Three illustrations linking temperament to psychopathology

To further outline known connections between early temperament and psychopathology, here we focus on three temperament–disorder pairs that are most common in the current literature (Figure 8.3). Some relations have already been raised to help illustrate the history and conceptualization of temperament and disorder. Here, we characterize them based on the underlying motivations typically ascribed to the pairing: Withdrawal, Approach, and Regulation.

Withdrawal: fearful temperament and anxiety

The prediction from early emerging fearful temperament, especially when extreme, to the development of anxious behaviors, clinically meaningful symptoms, and clinical disorder is

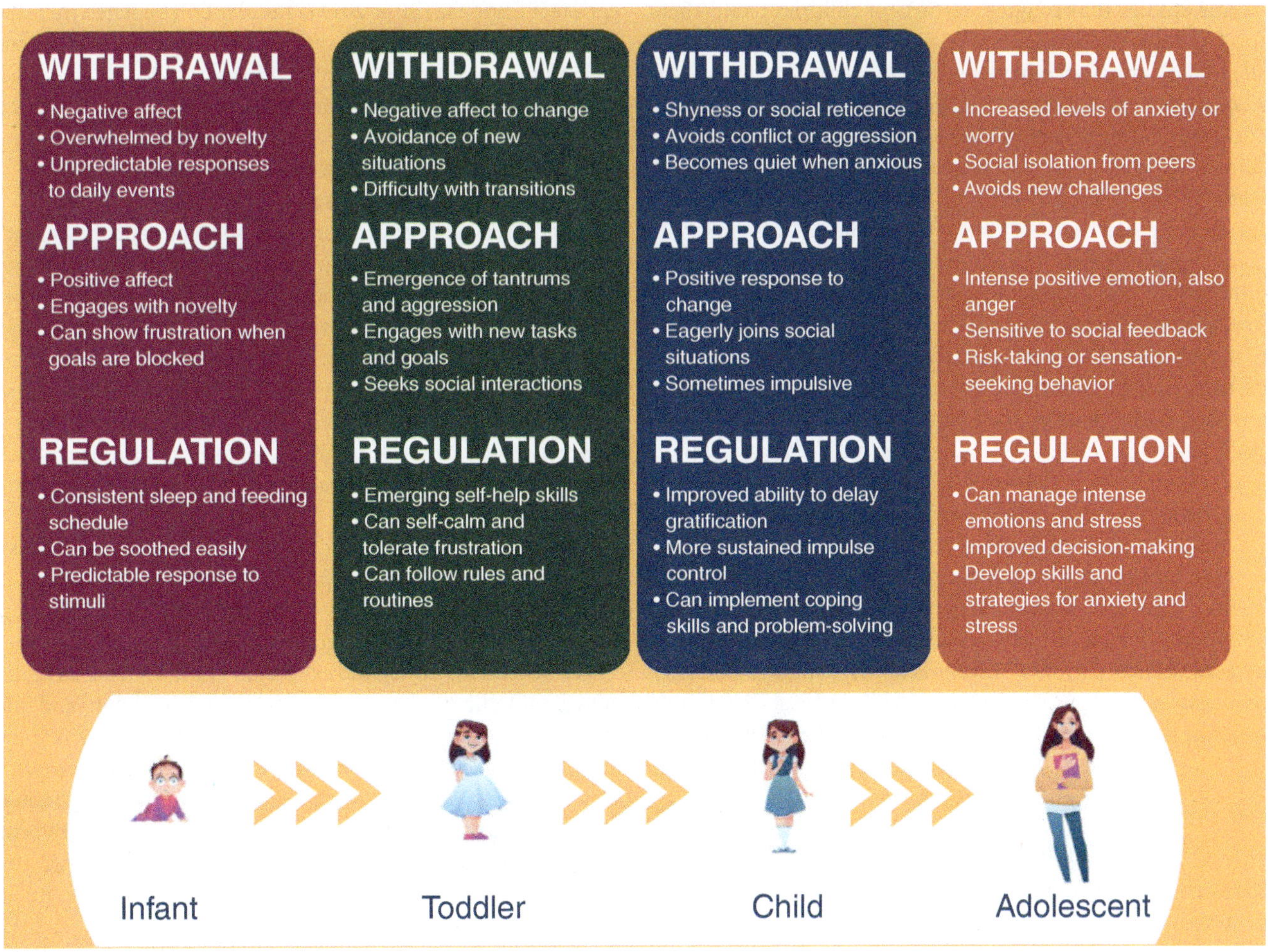

Figure 8.3 Temperament over time.

robust and very well-established (Klein & Mumper, 2018). Fearful temperament predicts anxious behaviors (i.e., social withdrawal) at early preschool age and also predicts anxiety symptoms in adolescence (Chronis-Tuscano *et al.*, 2009). Moreover, anxiety symptoms can emerge among preschoolers (Danko *et al.*, 2018) and are both: (i) associated with early and concurrent temperamental profiles (Klein & Mumper, 2018), and (ii) predict the later emergence of anxiety disorders (Clauss & Blackford, 2012; Pérez-Edgar & Guyer, 2014).

Two distinct categories or types of fearful temperament have been linked to the development of anxiety symptoms and disorder later in life: BI and dysregulated fear (DF).

Behavioral inhibition (BI)

BI children represent approximately 10–20% of infants/toddlers (between 14–24 months of age) observed in a series of situations designed to evoke individual differences in approach/withdrawal tendencies to novelty (García Coll *et al.*, 1984; Kagan *et al.*, 1984; Kagan *et al.*, 1988a). BI children are characteristically shy and withdrawn in novel social situations and show signs of decreased activity/approach and increased anxiety in the face of novel challenges.

Some studies find roughly 30–50% of children retain their inhibited status over childhood (García Coll *et al.*, 1984; Kagan *et al.*, 1988b), although other studies only reported stability for a limited subset of children (Asendorpf, 1991), and still other investigators have reported little stability (Kagan *et al.*, 1989; Rubin *et al.*, 1993). For example, in one study, inhibited group status at 3 years was unrelated to 10-year inhibited group status (Davidson & Rickman, 1999). While some of this apparent instability or change in temperament may be normative (Rothbart & Bates, 2007), it may also be related to the difficulty in measuring behavioral expression of the same construct in different developmental periods (i.e., heterotypic continuity). Even with these inconsistencies, behaviors at the extreme of the spectrum tend to be most stable (García Coll *et al.*, 1984; Kagan *et al.*, 1984; Kagan *et al.*, 1988b; Davidson and Rickman, 1999).

For example, in a follow-up of one of the Kagan cohorts (Schwartz *et al.*, 1999) 13-year-olds assessed for BI as toddlers were less likely to interact spontaneously with an experimenter and more likely to display generalized social anxiety symptoms. Stability of shy-inhibited behavior in childhood dramatically increases the likelihood of presenting with anxiety symptoms by mid-adolescence (Chronis-Tuscano *et al.*, 2009; Buss *et al.*, 2013) and recent comprehensive meta-analyses found that BI children have a three to four times increased risk for developing social anxiety disorders (SADs) by adolescence versus non-BI children (Clauss & Blackford, 2012; Sandstrom *et al.*, 2020).

Dysregulated fear (DF)

Despite consistent prediction from BI to anxiety disorder and symptoms, not all BI children develop anxiety problems. This fact led Buss and colleagues to focus on the identification of other patterns of fearful temperament (Buss, 2011). Although there are developmental and moderating influences that align with BI children "growing out" of the withdrawal behavioral pattern, Buss argued that the BI laboratory protocol may have introduced heterogeneity to the behavioral profile. This could have resulted in both "false positives" (i.e., children who sometimes appear as high fear, but are not consistently fearful) and "false negatives" (i.e., children who are extremely fearful only in particular situations).

Specifically, traditional measurement of BI is primarily based on how much *average* fear behavior is observed, or the duration or intensity of fearful and withdrawal behavior in highly novel contexts (García Coll *et al.*, 1984; Buss *et al.*, 2004). In the DF approach, behavior is measured dynamically across situations and development because children's reactions to, or interpretations of, situations (as threatening or not) will determine more precisely whether their behavior is, or will be, maladaptive. That is, does the fearful behavior match the situation? Highly threatening and novel situations should elicit fear in most children. DF is operationalized as high fear in *low-threat* situations (Buss, 2011). Importantly, you must use low-threat situations to distinguish between *well-regulated fear* and *DF* since they are indistinguishable in higher threat contexts that universally trigger a fear response (Buss, 2011). Toddler DF predicted increased social withdrawal and SAD symptoms at age 6 even while controlling for BI status (Buss, 2011; Buss *et al.*, 2013), which persisted into the transition to early adolescence (Buss *et al.*, 2021).

Approach: exuberant temperament and disruptive disorders

Approach-related temperament (e.g., surgency and exuberance) is less studied in the literature relative to withdrawal-related (fearful) and regulation (effortful control) temperament dimensions. It is the middle child in the developmental arc from temperament to psychopathology. In part, this is because exuberance is often used as a temperamental "control" for studies focused on temperamental fearfulness and its robust link to anxiety (Degnan *et al.*, 2011). It is meant to contextualize fearfulness, or act as a buffer to withdrawal, but not stand as a focus of study in and of itself.

Temperamental exuberance is characterized by high levels of positive affectivity and approach behavior, particularly in response to sensory novelty or potential social interactions. When in a room that a temperamentally fearful child may deem "risky" (Fox *et al.*, 2001), the exuberant child will instead readily engage with the novel toy, follow the unfamiliar adult, and initiate social contact with a new peer. As infants, exuberant children tend to show positive affect and fledging attempts to approach when presented with sensory stimuli, such as bubbles, blinking lights, and buzzing toys (Fox *et al.*, 2015). In the context of fearful temperament, exuberance, and its associated positive affect, is seen as a buffer or ameliorating force protecting the child from later anxiety and depression (Lahat *et al.*, 2012). Exuberance and temperamental positivity have also been linked to increased prosocial behavior, including sharing, helping, and cooperating for the purpose of benefiting someone other than the self (Eisenberg *et al.*, 2015), and has been implicated in adolescent and adult *agreeableness* (Habashi *et al.*, 2016).

However, in the context of poor regulation or less-constrained social environments, individuals with an exuberant temperament may be at increased risk for their own distinct profile of psychopathology. For example, temperamentally exuberant individuals are more likely to engage in risky behaviors in adolescence such as substance use or reckless driving (Lahat *et al.*, 2012), particularly when peers are present (Dollar *et al.*, 2017). These underling tendencies may set the stage for the development of substance-use disorders or other forms of impulsivity-related disorders, such as attention deficit/hyperactivity disorder (ADHD) or conduct disorder. In the case of conduct disorder, these children are marked by a unique combination of both positive and negative affect. However, while negative affect is central to anxiety-linked disorders, here the core negative emotion is anger, not fear or sadness. As with temperamental fear, the level of risk for psychopathology, and its ultimate form, is multiply determined by genetic vulnerability, social stressors, and societal structures.

Regulation: effortful control and emotional dysregulation

Regulation is a central, but often implicit, component of most theories of temperament (Goldsmith *et al.*, 1987; Shiner *et al.*, 2012). To illustrate, effortful control is one component of temperamental regulation connected to psychopathology (Rothbart & Rueda, 2005). Effortful control contains elements of inhibitory control, attention shifting, attention focusing, and conflict resolution (Posner & Rothbart, 2000). Most common definitions of effortful control include the ability to inhibit a dominant (sometimes inappropriate) response when an alternative, voluntary (more adaptive) response is required (Rothbart & Rueda, 2005).

Given its role in regulating behavior, effortful control plays an important role in children's socioemotional adjustment. Well-controlled behaviors that mitigate negative emotional reactions can enable cooperation and play with peers. Low effortful control in childhood is robustly associated with maladaptive outcomes, including disruptive behaviors and conduct problems (Eisenberg *et al.*, 2005). Deficits in regulation or self-control, more broadly, are predictive of several types of problematic outcomes for children and into adulthood (Moffitt *et al.*, 2011). Children high in effortful control, in contrast, are more likely to have positive socioemotional outcomes (Moffitt *et al.*, 2011).

Rothbart and Ahadi (1994) argued that changes in observed temperament occur within the context of developing systems of cognitive control. From this view, individual differences in effortful control can modulate the expression and experience of other behaviors and the expression of temperament, including both positive and negative emotionality. Thus, effortful control can shape the developmental pathways of children and may be particularly important for those who are otherwise at risk based on temperament characteristics such as shyness or exuberance. For example, one of the first studies to examine temperament-by-temperament interactions showed that greater fear reactivity from 8 to 16 months of age was linked with lower levels of effortful control in children at approximately 5 years of age (Hill-Soderlund & Braungart-Rieker, 2008). In addition, extremes in effortful control, at both ends of the spectrum, have been linked with anxiety, particularly in the context of fearful temperament (Gunther & Pérez-Edgar, 2021). For instance, low effortful control has been shown to predict poorer outcomes for highly fearful children (Muris, 2006). At the same time, high levels of inhibitory control (one component of effortful control) increase the stability of wariness and exacerbate the risk for anxiety in temperamentally fearful children—evidence that an overcontrolled pattern may be a risk factor (White *et al.*, 2011).

High levels of effortful control have also been linked with reduced psychopathology and stronger social competence, particularly in the context of exuberant temperament and lower levels of effortful control have been associated with higher risk for psychopathology. Typically, exuberant children are thought to have a propensity for positive affectivity, and often display negative emotionality, such as anger, when any reward or goal-driven behavior is blocked (Dollar & Stifter, 2012). This may indicate that exuberant children have a particularly difficult time regulating their emotions in the face of frustration and adversity. Exuberant children who have high levels of effortful control also have fewer emotional dysregulation problems (Dennis *et al.*, 2010) and effortful control moderates the relationship between exuberance, anger, and externalizing behaviors (Stifter *et al.*, 2008). Higher effortful control among exuberant children predicted less anger and externalizing behaviors. Specific to peer relationships, surgent children (who are often similar to exuberant children) with low effortful control were rated as the most aggressive by teachers, and were more likely to be rejected by peers (Gunnar *et al.*, 2003). Protective relationships also exist, such that exuberant children's increased ability to regulate predicts fewer disruptive or impulsive behaviors (Rubin *et al.*, 1995).

Individual and environmental moderators of temperament

Genetic underpinnings and the caregiving environment

The search for genetic contributions to temperament has been long and difficult. The complex nature of temperament, and the various temperaments of interest, has made it difficult to map broad behavioral constructs onto a specific genetic profile. The field lacks many of the large-scale studies needed for genome-wide association studies (GWAS), particularly those including children. The available studies are typically of adults using retrospective self-report measures (Ebstein, 2006), which can blur the line between temperament, personality, and disorder, as well as rely on the strength of individual recall.

Despite the dearth of strong GWAS data, it is clear that early temperament has a genetic component. Studies using twin samples report moderate to high heritability of BI. For example, Saudino and Cherny (2001) used longitudinal behavioral genetics models to compute covariation among twin siblings and found that continuity from 14 to 20 months and across 20, 34, and 36 months was explained, in part, by genetic influences. In addition, new genetic and nonshared environmental effects emerged at later ages, suggesting a dynamic gene–environment interaction.

In addition, there are clear relations between caregiver characteristics and child temperament profiles. Links between parent psychopathology symptoms and child temperament seem to be domain specific, mapping separately onto withdrawal and approach tendencies (Essex *et al.*, 2010), despite the two being modestly correlated in childhood (Willner *et al.*, 2016). Children of parents with higher levels of depressive and anxiety symptoms show higher rates of BI and increased inhibition in novel contexts (Rosenbaum *et al.*, 2000). In turn, children high in BI tend to have parents with higher levels of anxiety and depression (Rosenbaum *et al.*, 1992; Biederman *et al.*, 2001). Similar connections are seen between parent and child levels of approach behaviors, aggression, dysregulation, and symptom profiles, such as ADHD and conduct disorder (Chronis-Tuscano *et al.*, 2008).

Of course, it is difficult to disentangle caregiver and child factors since most studies rely on biologically related parent–child dyads. Adoption studies can provide insight into the potentially unique contributions of underlying genetic risk and environmental experiences (Reiss *et al.*, 2022), since the rearing parents do not share genetic material with their children. Brooker and colleagues (Brooker *et al.*, 2011; Brooker *et al.*, 2014) reported that higher birth mothers' social phobia was associated with higher inhibited behaviors in their 9-month-old infants in the context of higher anxiety symptoms in the adoptive parent, which was in turn directly linked to child symptom levels at 18 and 27 months. Brooker *et al.* (2014) found a direct effect of anxiety symptoms of the adoptive parent on children's anxiety symptoms and withdrawal behaviors at 18 and 27 months and. In both studies (Brooker *et al.*, 2011; Brooker *et al.*, 2014), infant effortful control modulated the relations between risk factors and the emergence of symptoms. Recent work (Anaya *et al.*, 2023) directly examining the stability of BI in early childhood found a gene–environment interaction effect, such that continued high stability of inhibited tendencies over time was specific to a higher genetic propensity for psychopathology due to birth parent psychopathology, coupled with higher anxiety levels in the adoptive family.

The emerging data suggest that a higher genetic propensity for psychopathology may condition how infants respond to, and are influenced by, their environment, an effect that may change across development. Importantly, children's temperamental profiles also influence the rearing environment (Ryan & Ollendick, 2018), as they are not passive recipients of experience. A central tenet of the developmental psychopathology perspective is that while individuals are influenced by environments, they also play an active role in shaping these same environments (Sroufe & Rutter, 1984). Children's genetically influenced characteristics can elicit distinct caregiving behaviors (Avinun & Knafo, 2013) and trigger caregiver psychopathology symptoms (Ahmadzadeh *et al.*, 2021). For example, children with a difficult temperament, characterized by negative affect, low adaptability, and high reactivity, may require more resources from caregivers and may contribute to caregiver perceptions of stress and distress.

Adaptive or "good" caregiving does not take any one form, as the specific behaviors associated with supportive caregiving will differ for children with different temperaments. As such, sensitive caregiving of a more exuberant child may look different from sensitive caregiving of a child with a fearful temperament. For example, researchers have pointed to overcontrol as a negative form of parenting for children with fearful temperaments (Kiel & Buss, 2011). Overcontrol involves demonstrations of warmth, intrusiveness, and restrictiveness in situations that do not warrant this type of behavior. In contrast, children with emotion regulation difficulties marked by parental undercontrol are likely to develop disruptive behavior problems when their mothers are more negative (Rubin *et al.*, 2003). Supportive parenting improves social competence via lower levels of child aggression, which, in turn, buffers the effects of negative peer feedback (Lahat *et al.*, 2012).

As noted, positive reactivity has been largely understudied (Degnan *et al.*, 2011). As such, we lack the needed studies to disentangle bidirectional effects and potential gene–environment correlations for children who present with the profile of extreme high approach and excitement in the face of novelty. Lengua and Kovacs (2005) did find that initial positive reactivity predicted higher levels of maternal acceptance. Valued characteristics, such as laughter and approach, may be rewarding for parents and elicit more engagement and positive reactions. Few studies have extended far enough to examine the impact of positive reactivity on later personality and psychological adjustment. Even fewer studies have considered the parenting context as a moderator of links between positive reactivity and later socioemotional adjustment, including personality development.

Sociocultural expectations

From a broad perspective, the relations between early temperament and later psychopathology are also embedded within the larger cultural context, which reflects historical trends and social expectations (Poole *et al.*, 2018). The temperament literature is dominated by research carried out in the United States and Western Europe. Within these locations, the children and families studied have been overwhelmingly white, highly educated, and solidly middle class (Chronis-Tuscano *et al.*, 2018).

This relative homogeneity may have contributed to the robust developmental trajectories seen to date, particularly with fearful temperament. However, the available data from other cultures suggest that the relations seen in the West are unlikely to be universal (García Coll, 2020) or at the very least reflect specific cultural parameters. For example, Chen and colleagues (Chen *et al.*, 1995; Chen *et al.*, 2021) reported a series of studies examining outcomes for BI children in China. Unlike in the West, children high in BI were rated as having better social relationships, stronger academic profiles, and fewer symptoms of anxiety and depression. However, follow-up work found that while these relations held true for children in rural areas, urban children with high BI profile displayed the Western profile of fewer friends, more academic difficulties, and greater risk for psychopathology. The implication is that while BI is biologically based and relatively stable, parents, caregivers, and peers socialize initial temperamental traits to fit current social ideals. The match between child and expectations, the "goodness of fit," can in turn influence socioemotional trajectories.

Implications for treatment and intervention

Modern temperament research has been informed by two core principles (Shiner *et al.*, 2012). This work (i) *focuses on the individual through development* and (ii) *cuts across multiple levels of data*. Therefore, it is quite ironic that the direct application of temperament theory and assessments in clinical settings is uncommon (Ostlund *et al.*, 2021a). To some extent, this reflects the fact that while temperament theory is focused on the individual, our methodological and analytic approaches have centered on broad averages across groups or profiles. As such, it is difficult to assess and then, if needed, intervene with any one individual child.

However, there are a number of promising approaches that could help mainstream the use of temperament in the clinic setting. As with much of the literature, the focus has been on fearful temperament and anxiety (Klein *et al.*, 2012), although more recent work is examining potential ways to ameliorate the link between temperamental irritability and disruptive disorders (Wakschlag *et al.*, 2018). Cool Little Kids is an education program developed for parents of behaviorally inhibited preschoolers (Rapee *et al.*, 2010). The focus is on educating families about BI, the link to anxiety, and the role parenting behaviors can play in diminishing risk. Facilitators also help parents address their own anxiety. The model suggests that intervention with the parent will then translate into less anxiety on the part of the child. The intervention lessens subsequent child anxiety symptoms and risk of disorder (Rapee *et al.*, 2010; Rapee, 2013) even when BI levels remain elevated. Other programs focus directly on social skills training for children (e.g., Coplan *et al.*, 2010). The Turtle Program (Chronis-Tuscano *et al.*, 2015) combines both approaches by incorporating both parent psychoeducation and group treatment for the child.

Recently, a systematic review (Ooi *et al.*, 2022) examined whether interventions for behaviorally inhibited preschool-aged children significantly reduce (i) BI, and (ii) anxiety symptoms and diagnosis. Overall, analyses of observer ratings of in-lab behavior found no significant effects of intervention on inhibited behavior. However, parents and teachers both reported significant improvement in anxiety symptoms and social behavior in daily functioning. Again, this pattern suggests a decoupling between a temperament trait and subsequent signs of psychopathology with intervention, pointing to BI and anxiety as two separate constructs.

Taking another approach, the Kaiser Permanente Child Temperament Program (Cameron *et al.*, 2013) is embedded in a broader clinical setting. Like the other programs, it is designed to help parents better understand their child's unique temperament and behavior, and to provide them with practical tools and strategies for managing challenging behaviors and promoting positive social and emotional development. Here, the focus is on activity level, adaptability, sensitivity, and mood, relying on a series of group workshops and individual coaching sessions. The unique feature of the program is that it is embedded into the typical clinical structure for the parent and child.

Not all temperament-based interventions involve early fear and anxiety risk. Wakschlag and colleagues (Wakschlag *et al.*, 2018), for example, focus on temperamental irritability. Irritability is marked by a tendency to easily become frustrated, angry, or annoyed, particularly when challenged, while normative, temperamental irritability at the extreme can be characterized by frequent and intense temper tantrums, outbursts of anger, and difficulty regulating emotions. Intervention is required when the child's irritability is persistent, intense, or interfering with their daily life. For example, Smith *et al.* (2019) employed a randomized trial to examine the potential impact of the Family Check-Up (FCU) program with children displaying elevated irritability. With intervention focused on regulation skills at age four, irritable children showed less symptomatology versus peers in the control group six years later.

Conclusion

Overall, the data suggest that while temperament is not a direct cause of psychopathology, it does play an important role in shaping the developmental trajectories that may lead to the onset of mental health disorders. By understanding the relationships between temperament and psychopathology, we can develop interventions and treatment strategies that are tailored to the specific needs of individual children. Temperament research, coupled with a developmental psychopathology approach, provides a roadmap for intervention by isolating and highlighting individual (neural, cognitive) and environmental (parenting, cultural expectations) forces that shape the ways in which a child's individual traits do, or do not, match the social world they are expected to navigate.

References

Ahmadzadeh, Y.I. *et al.* (2021) Systematic review and meta-analysis of genetically informed research: associations between parent anxiety and offspring internalizing problems. *Journal of the American Academy of Child & Adolescent Psychiatry* **60**, 823–840.

American Psychiatric Association (2013) *Diagnostic and Statistical Manual of Mental Disorders,* 5th edn. American Psychiatric Association, Washington, DC.

Anaya, B. & Pérez-Edgar, K. (2019) Personality development in the context of temperament and parenting dynamics. *New Ideas in Psychology* **53**, 37–46.

Anaya, B. *et al.* (2023) Developmental trajectories of behavioral inhibition from infancy to age seven: the role of genetic and environmental risk for psychopathology. *Child Development* **94**, e231–e245.

Asendorpf, J.B. (1991) Development of inhibited children's coping with unfamiliarity. *Child Development* **62**, 1460–1474.

Avinun, R. & Knafo, A. (2013) The longitudinal Israeli study of twins (LIST)—an integrative view of social development. *Twin Research and Human Genetics* **16**, 197–201.

Beekman, C. *et al.* (2015) The development of early profiles of temperament: characterization, continuity, and etiology. *Child Development* **86**, 1794–1811.

Biederman, J. *et al.* (2001) Further evidence of association between behavioral inhibition and social anxiety in children. *American Journal of Psychiatry* **158**, 1673–1679.

Bishop, G. *et al.* (2003) Can parents and teachers provide a reliable and valid report of behavioral inhibition? *Child Development* **74**, 1899–1917.

Blackford, J.U. *et al.* (2018) The neurobiology of behavioral inhibition as a developmental mechanism. In: *Behavioral Inhibition.* (eds K. Pérez-Edgar & N.A. Fox). Springer, Cham, Switzerland.

Brooker, R.J. *et al.* (2011) The association between infants' attention control and social inhibition is moderated by genetic and environmental risk for anxiety. *Infancy* **16**, 490–507.

Brooker, R.J. *et al.* (2014) Birth and adoptive parent anxiety symptoms moderate the link between infant attention control and internalizing problems in toddlerhood. *Development and Psychopathology* **26**, 347–359.

Buss, K.A. (2011) Which fearful toddlers should we worry about? Context, fear regulation, and anxiety risk. *Developmental Psychology* **47**, 804–819.

Buss, A.H. & Plomin, R. (1975) *A Temperament Theory of Personality Development.* Wiley, New York.

Buss, A.H. & Plomin, R. (1984) *Temperament: Early Developing Personality Traits.* Lawrence Erlbaum, Hillsdale, NJ.

Buss, K.A. *et al.* (2004) Context-specific freezing and associated physiological reactivity as a dysregulated fear response. *Developmental Psychology* **40**, 583.

Buss, K.A. *et al.* (2013) Dysregulated fear predicts social wariness and social anxiety symptoms during kindergarten. *Journal of Clinical Child and Adolescent Psychology* **42**, 603–616.

Buss, K.A. *et al.* (2021) Toddler dysregulated fear predicts continued risk for social anxiety symptoms in early adolescence. *Development and Psychopathology* **33**, 252–263. doi: 10.1017/S0954579419001743.

Cameron, J.R. *et al.* (2013) Childhood temperament-based anticipatory guidance in an HMO setting: a longitudinal study. *Journal of Community Psychology* **41**, 236–248.

Caouette, J.D. & Guyer, A.E. (2014) Gaining insight into adolescent vulnerability for social anxiety from developmental cognitive neuroscience. *Developmental Cognitive Neuroscience* **8**, 65–76.

Chen, X. *et al.* (1995) Social functioning and adjustment in Chinese children: a longitudinal study. *Developmental Psychology* **31**, 531.

Chen, X. *et al.* (2021) Behavioral inhibition in early childhood and adjustment in late adolescence in China. *Child Development* **92**, 994–1010.

Chronis-Tuscano, A. *et al.* (2008) Associations between maternal attention-deficit/hyperactivity disorder symptoms and parenting. *Journal of Abnormal Child Psychology* **36**, 1237–1250.

Chronis-Tuscano, A. *et al.* (2009) Stable behavioral inhibition during infancy and early childhood predicts the development of anxiety disorders in adolescence. *Journal of the American Academy of Child & Adolescent Psychiatry* **48**, 928–935.

Chronis-Tuscano, A. *et al.* (2015) Preliminary evaluation of a multimodal early intervention program for behaviorally inhibited preschoolers. *Journal of Consulting and Clinical Psychology* **83**, 534–540.

Chronis-Tuscano, A. *et al.* (2018) Future directions for research on early intervention for young children at risk for social anxiety. *Journal of Clinical Child and Adolescent Psychology* **47**, 655–667.

Cicchetti, D. (1984) The emergence of developmental psychopathology. *Child Development* **55**, 1–7.

Clauss, J.A. & Blackford, J.U. (2012) Behavioral inhibition and risk for developing social anxiety disorder: a meta-analytic study. *Journal of the American Academy of Child and Adolescent Psychiatry* **51**, 1066–1075.

Coplan, R.J. *et al.* (2010) 'Play skills' for shy children: development of a social skills facilitated play early intervention program for extremely inhibited preschoolers. *Infant and Child Development: An International Journal of Research and Practice* **19**, 223–237.

Coplan, R.J. *et al.* (2021) *The Handbook of Solitude: Psychological Perspectives on Social Isolation, Social Withdrawal, and Being Alone.* Wiley, Hoboken, NJ.

Danko, C.M. *et al.* (2018) The turtle program: PCIT for young children displaying behavioral inhibition. In: *Handbook of Parent-Child Interaction Therapy: Innovations and Applications for Research and Practice.* (ed L.N. Niec). Springer International Publishing, Cham, Switzerland. pp. 85–98.

Davidson, R.J. & Rickman, M. (1999) Behavioral inhibition and the emotional circuitry of the brain: stability and plasticity during the early childhood years. In: *Extreme Fear, Shyness, and Social Phobia: Origins, Biological Mechanisms, and Clinical Outcomes.* (eds L.A. Schmidt & J. Schulkin). Oxford University Press, New York. pp. 67–87.

Degnan, K.A. *et al.* (2011) Longitudinal stability of temperamental exuberance and social-emotional outcomes in early childhood. *Developmental Psychology* **47**, 765–780.

Dennis, T.A. *et al.* (2010) Do the associations between exuberance and emotion regulation depend on effortful control? *International Journal of Behavioral Development* **34**, 462–472.

Derryberry, D. & Rothbart, M.K. (2002) Temperament in children. In: *Psychology at the Turn of the Millennium, Volume 2: Social, developmental, and Clinical Perspectives.* (eds L. Blackman & C. von Hofsten). Psychology Press, Hove, UK. pp. 17–36.

Dollar, J.M. & Stifter, C.A. (2012) Temperamental surgency and emotion regulation as predictors of childhood social competence. *Journal of Experimental Child Psychology* **112**, 178–194.

Dollar, J.M., Stifter, C.A., & Buss, K.A. (2017) Exuberant and inhibited children: person-centered profiles and links to social adjustment. *Developmental Psychology* **53**, 1222.

Ebstein, R.P. (2006) The molecular genetic architecture of human personality: beyond self-report questionnaires. *Molecular Psychiatry* **11**, 427–445.

Eisenberg, N. *et al.* (2005) Relations among positive parenting, children's effortful control, and externalizing problems: a three-wave longitudinal study. *Child Development* **76**, 1055–1071.

Eisenberg, N. *et al.* (2015) The development of prosocial behavior. In: *The Oxford Handbook of Prosocial Behavior.* (eds D.A. Schroeder & W.G. Graziano). Oxford University Press, New York. pp. 114–136.

Essex, M.J. *et al.* (2010) Early risk factors and developmental pathways to chronic high inhibition and social anxiety disorder in adolescence. *American Journal of Psychiatry* **167**, 40–46.

Fox, N.A. *et al.* (2001) Continuity and discontinuity of behavioral inhibition and exuberance: psychophysiological and behavioral influences across the first four years of life. *Child Development* **72**, 1–21.

Fox, N.A. *et al.* (2015) The relations between reactivity at 4 months and behavioral inhibition in the second year: replication across three independent samples. *Infancy* **20**, 98–114.

Fu, X. & Pérez-Edgar, K. (2015) Theories of temperament development. In: *The International Encyclopedia of Social & Behavioral Sciences.* (ed J.D. Wright). Elsevier, Amsterdam. pp. 191–198.

García Coll, C. (2020) Globalization, culture, and development: are we ready for a paradigm shift? *Human Development* **64**, 245–249.

García Coll, C. *et al.* (1984) Behavioral inhibition in young children. *Child Development* **55**, 1005–1019.

Gartstein, M.A. *et al.* (2017) Latent profile and cluster analysis of infant temperament: comparisons across person-centered approaches. *Developmental Psychology* **53**, 1811–1825.

Goldsmith, H.H. (1996) Studying temperament via construction of the toddler behavior assessment questionnaire. *Child Development* **67**, 218–235.

Goldsmith, H.H. & Campos, J.J. (1982) Toward a theory of infant temperament. In: *The Development of Attachment and Affiliative Systems.* (eds R.N. Emde & R.J. Harmon). Springer, Cham, Switzerland. pp. 161–193.

Goldsmith, H.H. & Gagne, J.R. (2012) Behavioral assessment of temperament. In: *Handbook of Temperament.* (eds M. Zentner & R.L. Shiner). Guilford Press, New York. pp. 209–228.

Goldsmith, H.H. & Rothbart, M.K. (1993) *The Laboratory Temperament Assessment Battery (LAB-TAB).* University of Wisconsin Press, Madison, WI.

Goldsmith, H.H. *et al.* (1987) Roundtable: what is temperament? Four approaches. *Child Development* **58**, 505–529.

Gunnar, M.R. *et al.* (2003) Peer rejection, temperament, and cortisol activity in preschoolers. *Developmental Psychobiology* **43**, 346–358.

Gunther, K.E. & Pérez-Edgar, K. (2021) Dopaminergic associations between behavioral inhibition, executive functioning, and anxiety in development. *Developmental Review* **60**, 100966.

Guyer, A.E. *et al.* (2014) Lasting associations between early-childhood temperament and late-adolescent reward-circuitry response to peer feedback. *Development and Psychopathology* **26**, 229–243.

Habashi, M.M. *et al.* (2016) Searching for the prosocial personality: a big five approach to linking personality and prosocial behavior. *Personality and Social Psychology Bulletin* **42**, 1177–1192.

Hill-Soderlund, A.L. & Braungart-Rieker, J.M. (2008) Early individual differences in temperamental reactivity and regulation: implications for effortful control in early childhood. *Infant Behavior and Development* **31**, 386–397.

Jarcho, J.M. & Guyer, A.E. (2018) The neural mechanisms of behavioral inhibition. In: *Behavioral Inhibition.* (eds K. Pérez-Edgar & N.A. Fox). Springer, Cham, Switzerland. pp. 59–90.

Kagan, J. (1997) *Galen's Prophecy: Temperament in Human Nature.* Routledge, New York.

Kagan, J. (2012) The biography of behavioral inhibition. In: *Handbook of temperament.* (eds M. Zentner & R.L. Shiner). Guilford Press, New York. pp. 69–82.

Kagan, J. (2018) The history and theory of behavioral inhibition. In: *Behavioral Inhibition.* (eds K. Pérez-Edgar & N.A. Fox). Springer, Cham, Switzerland. pp. 1–15.

Kagan, J. *et al.* (1984) Behavioral inhibition to the unfamiliar. *Child Development* **55**, 2212–2225.

Kagan, J. *et al.* (1988a) Biological bases of childhood shyness. *Science* **240**, 167–171.

Kagan, J. *et al.* (1988b) Childhood derivatives of inhibition and lack of inhibition to the unfamiliar. *Child Development* **59**, 1580–1589.

Kagan, J. *et al.* (1989) Inhibited and uninhibited types of children. *Child Development* **60**, 838–845.

Kagan, J. *et al.* (2007) The preservation of two infant temperaments into adolescence. *Monographs of the Society for Research in Child Development* **72**, i–95.

Kiel, E.J. & Buss, K.A. (2011) Prospective relations among fearful temperament, protective parenting, and social withdrawal: the role of maternal accuracy in a moderated mediation framework. *Journal of Abnormal Child Psychology* **39**, 953–966.

Klein, D.N. & Mumper, E.E. (2018) Behavioral inhibition as a precursor to psychopathology. In: *Behavioral Inhibition.* (eds K. Pérez-Edgar & N.A. Fox). Springer, Cham, Switzerland. pp. 283–307.

Klein, D.N. *et al.* (2012) Temperament and internalizing disorders. In: *Handbook of Temperament.* (eds M. Zentner & R.L. Shiner). Guilford Press, New York. pp. 541–561.

Lahat, A. *et al.* (2012) Temperamental exuberance and executive function predict propensity for risk taking in childhood. *Development and Psychopathology* **24**, 847–856.

Lengua, L.J. & Kovacs, E.A. (2005) Bidirectional associations between temperament and parenting and the prediction of adjustment problems in middle childhood. *Journal of Applied Developmental Psychology* **26**, 21–38.

MacNeill, L. & Pérez-Edgar, K. (2020) Temperament and emotion. In: *The Encyclopedia of Child and Adolescent Development.* (eds S. Hupp & J. Jewell). Wiley, Hoboken, NJ. pp. 1–12.

Moffitt, T.E. *et al.* (2011) A gradient of childhood self-control predicts health, wealth, and public safety. *Proceedings of the National Academy of Sciences* **108**, 2693–2698.

Muris, P. (2006) The pathogenesis of childhood anxiety disorders: considerations from a developmental psychopathology perspective. *International Journal of Behavioral Development* **30**, 5–11.

Ooi, J. *et al.* (2022) The efficacy of interventions for behaviourally inhibited preschool-aged children: a meta-analysis. *Journal of Anxiety Disorders* **88**, 102559.

Ostlund, B.D. *et al.* (2021a) The centrality of temperament to the research domain criteria (RDoC): the earliest building blocks of psychopathology. *Development and Psychopathology* **33**, 1566–1583.

Ostlund, B.D. *et al.* (2021b) Prenatal substance exposure and maternal hostility from pregnancy to toddlerhood: associations with temperament profiles at 16 months of age. *Development and Psychopathology* **33**, 1566–1583.

Pérez-Edgar, K. & Fox, N.A. (2018) Next steps: behavioral inhibition as a model system. In: *Behavioral Inhibition: Integrating Theory, Research, and Clinical Perspectives.* (eds K. Pérez-Edgar & N.A. Fox). Springer, Cham, Switzerland. pp. 357–372.

Pérez-Edgar, K. & Guyer, A.E. (2014) Behavioral inhibition: temperament or prodrome? *Current Behavioral Neuroscience Reports* **1**, 182–190.

Pine, D.S. *et al.* (2011) Increasing the developmental focus in DSM-V: broad issues and specific potential applications in anxiety. In: *The Conceptual Evolution of DSM-5.* (eds D.A. Regier, *et al.*). American Psychiatric Publishing, Inc, Washington, DC. pp. 305–321.

Poole, K.L. *et al.* (2018) The temperamentally shy child as the social adult: an exemplar of multifinality. In: *Behavioral Inhibition: Integrating Theory, Research, and Clinical Perspectives.* (eds K. Pérez-Edgar & N.A. Fox). Springer, Cham, Switzerland. pp. 185–212.

Posner, M.I. & Rothbart, M.K. (2000) Developing mechanisms of self-regulation. *Development and Psychopathology* **12**, 427–441.

Putnam, S.P. & Stifter, C.A. (2005) Behavioral approach–inhibition in toddlers: prediction from infancy, positive and negative affective components, and relations with behavior problems. *Child Development* **76**, 212–226.

Rapee, R.M. (2013) The preventative effects of a brief, early intervention for preschool-aged children at risk for internalising: follow-up into middle adolescence. *Journal of Child Psychology & Psychiatry* **54**, 780–788.

Rapee, R.M. *et al.* (2010) Altering the trajectory of anxiety in at-risk young children. *American Journal of Psychiatry* **167**, 1518–1525.

Reiss, D. *et al.* (2022) Parenting in the context of the child: genetic and social processes. *Monographs of the Society for Research in Child Development* **87**, 7–188.

Rosenbaum, J.F. *et al.* (1992) Comorbidity of parental anxiety disorders as risk for childhood-onset anxiety in inhibited children. *American Journal of Psychiatry* **149**, 475–481.

Rosenbaum, J.F. *et al.* (2000) A controlled study of behavioral inhibition in children of parents with panic disorder and depression. *American Journal of Psychiatry* **157**, 2002–2010.

Rothbart, M.K. & Ahadi, S.A. (1994) Temperament and the development of personality. *Journal of Abnormal Psychology* **103**, 55–66.

Rothbart, M.K. & Bates, J.E. (2007) Temperament. In: *Handbook of Child Psychology: Vol. 3. Social, Emotional, and Personality Development.* (eds W. Damon & N. Eisenberg). Wiley, Hoboken, NJ. pp. 99–166.

Rothbart, M.K. & Derryberry, D. (1981) Development of individual differences in temperament. In: *Advances in Developmental Psychology.* (eds M.E. Lamb & A.L. Brown). Lawrence Erlbaum, Hillsdale, NJ. pp. 33–86.

Rothbart, M.K. & Posner, M.I. (2006) Temperament, attention, and developmental psychopathology. In: *Handbook of Developmental Psychopathology.* (eds D. Cicchetti & D.J. Cohen), 2nd edn. Wiley, Hoboken, NJ. pp. 465–501.

Rothbart, M.K. & Rueda, M.R. (2005) The development of effortful control. In: *Developing Individuality in the Human Brain: A Tribute to Michael I. Posner.* (eds U. Mayr, *et al.*). American Psychological Association, Washington, DC. pp. 167–188.

Rothbart, M.K. *et al.* (2000) Stability of temperament in childhood: laboratory infant assessment to parent report at seven years. In: *Temperament and Personality Development Across the Life Span.* (eds V.J. Molfese & D.L. Molfese), Vol. **85**. Lawrence Erlbaum, Hillsdale, NJ. p. 119.

Rubin, K. *et al.* (1993) Socioemotional characteristics of withdrawn and aggressive children. *Merrill-Palmer Quarterly* **39**, 518–534.

Rubin, K.H. *et al.* (1995) Emotionality, emotion regulation, and preschoolers' social adaptation. *Development and Psychopathology* **7**, 49–62.

Rubin, K.H. *et al.* (2003) Predicting preschoolers' externalizing behaviors from toddler temperament, conflict, and maternal negativity. *Developmental Psychology* **39**, 164.

Ryan, S.M. & Ollendick, T.H. (2018) The interaction between child behavioral inhibition and parenting behaviors: effects on internalizing and externalizing symptomology. *Clinical Child and Family Psychology Review* **21**, 320–339.

Sandstrom, A. *et al.* (2020) Prospective association between childhood behavioral inhibition and anxiety: a meta-analysis. *Research on Child and Adolescent Psychopathology* **48**, 57–66.

Saudino, K.J. & Cherny, S.S. (2001) Sources of continuity and change in observed temperament. In: *Infancy to Early Childhood: Genetic and Environmental Influences on Developmental Change.* (eds R.N. Emde & J.K. Hewitt). Oxford University Press, New York. pp. 89–110.

Schwartz, C.E. *et al.* (1999) Adolescent social anxiety as an outcome of inhibited temperament in childhood. *Journal of the American Academy of Child and Adolescent Psychiatry* **38**, 1008–1015.

Shiner, R. & Caspi, A. (2003) Personality differences in childhood and adolescence: measurement, development, and consequences. *Journal of Child Psychology and Psychiatry* **44**, 2–32.

Shiner, R.L. *et al.* (2012) What is temperament now? Assessing progress in temperament research on the twenty-fifth anniversary of Goldsmith et al. *Child Development Perspectives* **6**, 436–444.

Smith, J.D. *et al.* (2019) Dysregulated irritability as a window on young children's psychiatric risk: transdiagnostic effects via the family check-up. *Development and Psychopathology* **31**, 1887–1899.

Sroufe, L.A. & Rutter, M. (1984) The domain of developmental psychopathology. *Child Development* **55**, 17–29.

Steinberg, L. *et al.* (2006) The study of developmental psychopathology in adolescence: integrating affective neuroscience with the study of context. In: *Psychophysiological Methods for the Study of Developmental Psychopathology.* (eds D. Cicchetti & D.J. Cohen). Wiley, Hoboken, NJ. pp. 710–741.

Stifter, C.A. *et al.* (2008) Exuberant and inhibited toddlers: stability of temperament and risk for problem behavior. *Development and Psychopathology* **20**, 401–421.

Tang, A. *et al.* (2020) Infant behavioral inhibition predicts personality and social outcomes three decades later. *Proceedings of the National Academy of Sciences* **117**, 9800–9807.

Tang, A. *et al.* (2022) Striatal activity to reward anticipation as a moderator of the association between early behavioral inhibition and changes in anxiety and depressive symptoms from adolescence to adulthood. *JAMA Psychiatry* **79**, 1199–1208.

Thomas, A. & Chess, S. (1977) *Temperament and Development.* Brunner/Mazel, Bristol, PA.

Wakschlag, L.S. *et al.* (2018) The neurodevelopmental basis of early childhood disruptive behavior: irritable and callous phenotypes as exemplars. *American Journal of Psychiatry* **175**, 114–130.

White, L.K. *et al.* (2011) Behavioral inhibition and anxiety: the moderating roles of inhibitory control and attention shifting. *Journal of Abnormal Child Psychology* **39**, 735–747.

Willner, C.J. *et al.* (2016) The dynamics of internalizing and externalizing comorbidity across the early school years. *Development and Psychopathology* **28**, 1033–1052.

CHAPTER 9
Transdiagnostic perspectives

Giovanni Abrahão Salum[1,2] and Mauricio Scopel Hoffmann[3]
[1]Department of Psychiatry and Legal Medicine, Universidade Federal do Rio Grande do Sul, Porto Alegre, Rio Grande do Sul, Brazil
[2]Child Mind Institute, Global Programs, NY, USA
[3]Department of Neuropsychiatry, Universidade Federal de Santa Maria, Santa Maria, Rio Grande do Sul, Brazil

"All models are wrong, some are useful"

George Box

Introduction

Classifications of mental health conditions currently rely on categories based on symptoms, course duration, age of onset, and functional impairment. The two most widely used classificatory systems are the *Diagnostic and Statistical Manual of Mental Disorders* (DSM; now in a revised version of its 5th edition; American Psychiatric Association, 2022) and the *International Classification of Diseases* (ICD; now in its 11th edition; World Health Organization, 2019) (see Chapters 2 and 27 for detailed information). Despite differences in the way they are used, DSM-5-TR and ICD-11 are the cornerstones of psychiatric nosology, and both classifications played a crucial role in establishing a common language in the field of mental health and advancing the practice of mental health care to be based on scientific evidence.

Despite the historical significance and broad influence of diagnostic classifications, there is a growing belief that traditional psychiatric nosology may have reached the limits of its utility. As an alternative, transdiagnostic approaches are gaining traction. Transdiagnostic perspectives refer to approaches or practices that cut across existing categorical diagnoses and go beyond them to produce a better set of information criteria for clinical decisions. These methods offer a promising perspective that may improve our understanding of mental health conditions. The transdiagnostic approach is more than just a reclassification; it challenges traditional distinctions, leading to a deeper exploration of the fundamental theories and mechanisms behind mental disorders. In doing so, it lays the foundation for new perspectives on the emergence, persistence, treatment, and recovery of mental health conditions.

This chapter discusses how the current classifications' imperfections might be addressed by competing transdiagnostic perspectives. The first section of this chapter expands on the concept of transdiagnostic approaches and presents the main arguments for their potential to advance clinical care in child and adolescent mental health. The second section focuses on comorbidity and the pattern of covariation of symptoms and disorders, and how this literature informed the development of transdiagnostic models based on symptomatic presentations. The third section addresses evidence of shared pathophysiology, the common consequences of mental health conditions in children and adolescents, and the influence of these shared factors in generating new classification systems based on biology and prognosis. Building upon previous sections, the fourth section describes prominent transdiagnostic models (Box 9.1)—the Hierarchical Taxonomy of Psychopathology (HiTOP), the network theory of mental disorders, Research Domain Criteria (RDoC), and clinical staging. The fifth section discusses the opportunity for transdiagnostic interventions and their limitations. Finally, the last section offers some conclusions and future directions.

The ultimate question we want to address here can be summarized as follows. Is traditional psychiatric nosology still the best way to organize clinical practice? Or most importantly, what is the comparative value of the current nosology and transdiagnostic approaches?

The transdiagnostic concept

In its purest essence, the prefix "trans" carries with it the connotations of traversing, extending beyond, or encompassing various aspects. When applied to the field of mental health, the transdiagnostic approach is underpinned by three fundamental

Rutter's Child and Adolescent Psychiatry and Psychology, Seventh Edition.
Edited by Anita Thapar, Daniel S. Pine, Samuele Cortese, Cathy Creswell, Tamsin J. Ford, James F. Leckman, and Argyris Stringaris.

Companion website: www.wiley.com/go/thapar/rutterspsych7

Box 9.1 Key concepts and definitions

Term	Definition
Transdiagnostic	A characteristic that extends across (i.e., is shared by different disorders) and beyond diagnostic categories (i.e., that emerges from different disorders).
Internalizing or emotional	Mental health problems or symptoms that are experienced within the mind with typically avoidant behavior. Referred to the higher-order dimension that encompasses generalized, specific, separation and social anxiety, panic and agoraphobia, post-traumatic stress, and major depressive disorders).
Externalizing or behavioral	Mental health problems or symptoms that are typically manifested in behavior, such as impulsive and aggressive. Usually referred to the higher-order dimension that has traditionally encompassed attention deficit/hyperactivity, oppositional defiant, and conduct disorders.
HiTOP	Hierarchical Taxonomy of Psychopathology. A consortium that aims to deliver an empirical classification of mental health problems, focusing on quantitative analysis of the co-occurrence of signs and symptoms, based on dimensions of psychopathology and their hierarchy. Details at: https://www.hitop-system.org/
RDoC	Research Domain Criteria. National Institute of Mental Health (NIMH)'s research framework to investigate mental health problems as multimodal and multilevel domains of function. Details at: https://www.nimh.nih.gov/research/research-funded-by-nimh/rdoc
Network theory	Mental disorders arise from the causal interaction between symptoms in a network.
Clinical staging	Mental disorders can progress from having risk factors to a severe unremitting syndrome with functional impairment and cognitive decline unresponsive to treatment, independently of the initial phenotypic diagnosis.

principles (Fusar-Poli *et al.*, 2019), each contributing to a more comprehensive understanding of mental health.

First, there are shared characteristics across disorders. This first principle underscores the existence of commonalities that extend across various mental disorders. These commonalities encompass a wide spectrum, including behavioral patterns, cognitive functions, brain functioning, genetic factors, environment, and social determinants.

Second, there are shared characteristics beyond disorders. This principle acknowledges that beyond the characteristics that overlap across disorders, there are features that transcend specific diagnostic boundaries. These features encompass aspects such as clinical staging, where the progression of any disorder can be assessed, and the extent of functional impairment experienced by individuals.

Third, many interventions have nonspecific effects. The third principle emphasizes that mental health interventions can often produce effects that extend beyond the confines of a particular diagnosis and are effective for people with different diagnoses. This implies that treatments may impact shared aspects of mental health, offering potential benefits across a range of conditions.

While heterogeneous in their specific presentations, distinct mental disorders share characteristics and consequences. The above-mentioned principles have emerged from empirical work on transdiagnostic models (Eaton *et al.*, 2023). Before describing these model's features, the chapter discusses how research on patterns of symptom covariation moved the field to consider such alternative models that will be discussed in subsequent sections.

Comorbidity and the pattern of covariation of symptoms and disorders

Mental health conditions described in the classificatory systems frequently co-occur (McGrath *et al.*, 2020; Vasileva *et al.*, 2021). This means that having one condition substantially increases the chances of having another. The co-occurrence of more than one condition is called comorbidity, which is very high among mental disorders. Approximately 50% of individuals who meet diagnostic criteria for one disorder meet criteria for another concurrent disorder (Caspi *et al.*, 2014). Moreover, having any mental health condition early in life increases the risk of having another at a later point, either of the same type (social anxiety increasing the risk of generalized anxiety) or a distinct type (social anxiety increasing the risk of alcohol use disorder).

Comorbidity occurs in all developmental stages. By the age of seven years, studies suggest that one-third of affected children manifest at least two diagnoses (Caspi *et al.*, 2020; Vasileva *et al.*, 2021). Longitudinally, by the ages of 11–15 years, 32% of youth manifest such comorbidity, and this rate increases to 85% when participants reach the age of 45 years (Caspi *et al.*, 2020). Comorbidity cannot be attributed fully to shared symptomatology as many comorbid diagnoses share no criteria (Lahey *et al.*, 2017). Figure 9.1 presents a Venn diagram showing strong patterns of comorbidity among mental disorders in young people. Other research finds strong overlap among mental and physical disorders (Momen *et al.*, 2020).

High rates of comorbidity could arise from an underlying structure that makes clinical phenomena co-occur. Two models are frequently used to estimate patterns of symptomatic covariation, which tends to occur in clusters. These two models are grounded in two main theories: the latent and network theories (Zachar & Kendler, 2017).

The latent theory usually involves examining correlations among symptoms. Similar approaches have been applied for more than a century in psychology, reflecting the statistical framework informing the latent theory of psychopathology (van Bork, 2019). Fundamentally, the latent theory suggests that correlations among symptoms or disorders emerge from a common cause (e.g.,

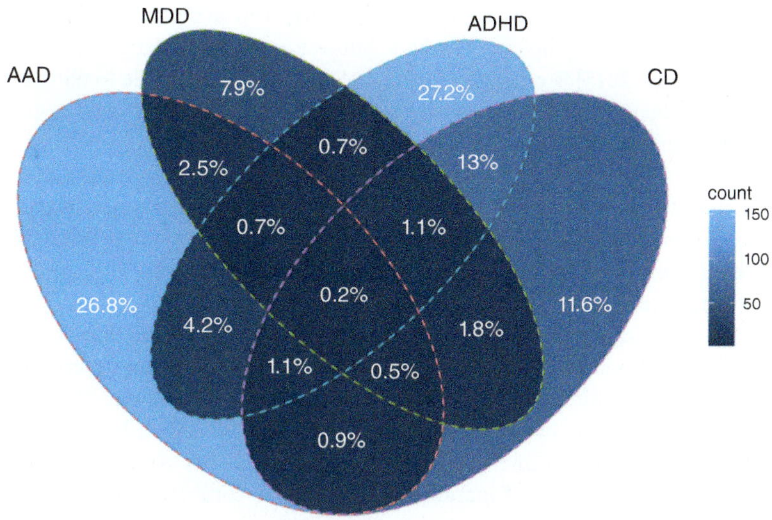

Figure 9.1 Venn diagram with mental health condition comorbidity. Data from 2511 young people aged 6-14 in Brazil (Salum *et al.*, 2015). 570 (22.7% of the total sample) presented any anxiety disorder (AAD), separation anxiety, specific or social phobia, agoraphobia, panic or generalized anxiety), major depressive disorder (MDD), attention-deficit hyperactivity disorder (ADHD) or conduct disorder (CD). 26.7% of those with any of these diagnosis have at least one comorbid condition.

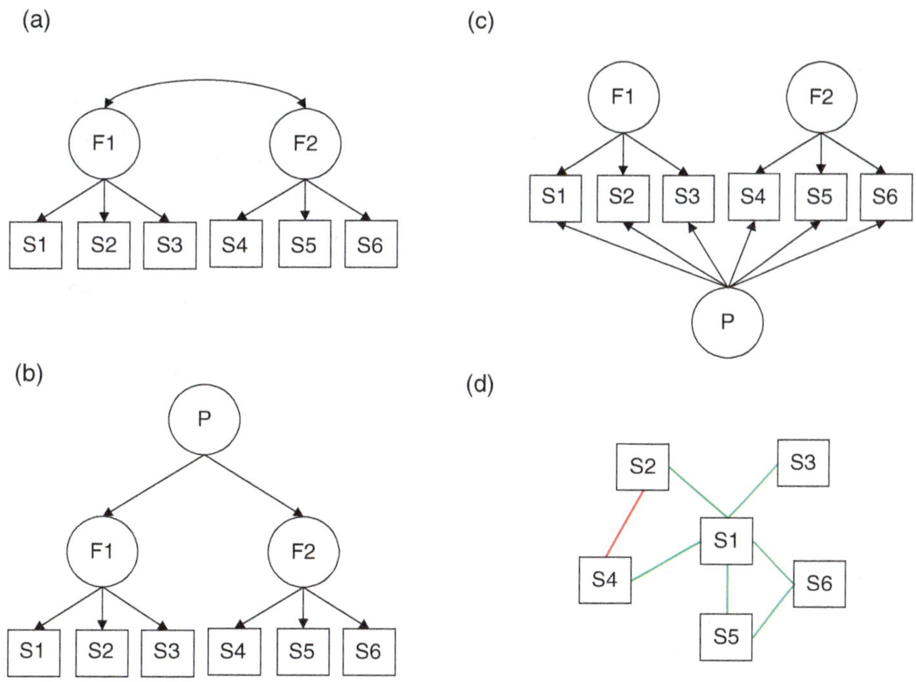

Figure 9.2 Correlated (a), second-order (b), bifactor (c) and network (d) models. Note: Assessed symptoms are represented by the letter "S" in a square. The unmeasured dimension of psychopathology is represented by the letter "F" (factor) inside a circle. The letter "P" represents the overarching p-factor, which accounts for what is common among dimensions (b) and all symptoms (c). Arrows indicate that the unmeasured dimensions are causing the symptoms to manifest. In (d), green lines represent positive correlation and red lines represent negative correlation.

unmeasured liability) (Figure 9.2). Importantly, latent factors are not directly observed but accessed through observed indicators. Many such models can be used to investigate the structure of psychopathology. One prominent model divides mental disorders into internalizing or emotional (e.g., anxiety, depression) and externalizing or behavioral (e.g., attention deficit hyperactivity disorder, conduct disorder) dimensions (e.g., Achenbach & Edelbrock 1978; Lahey *et al.*, 2008; Kessler *et al.*, 2011). Others generate a more nuanced categorization, further subdividing the internalizing dimension into two subdimensions: fear-related (e.g., phobias) and distress-related (e.g., generalized anxiety, depression) dimensions (e.g., Krueger 1999; Slade and Watson 2006; Shanmugan *et al.*, 2016;

Martel *et al.*, 2017). Finally, more recent models introduce other dimensions, focusing on thought disorders or symptoms of psychosis (Caspi *et al.*, 2014; Carragher *et al.*, 2015), a neurodevelopmental dimension encompassing inattention and hyperactivity, and a detachment dimension, which includes symptoms of social withdrawal and preference to be alone (Michelini *et al.*, 2019).

Other points arising from latent theory concern the hierarchical structure of symptom co-occurrence. The simplest, unidimensional model attributes symptom covariance to one factor. Complexity increases with the number of factors in each model (Achenbach 1966). For example, some models include two or more correlated psychopathological dimensions (Figure 9.2a). Others involve hierarchies, where dimensions manifest complex relations, either by containing overarching dimensions that encompass other dimensions as in the second-order model (Figure 9.2b), or by separating common and dissociable aspects of psychopathology as in the bifactor model (Figure 9.2c) (Lahey *et al.*, 2021). In the second-order framework, the top of the hierarchy contains overarching general dimensions (i.e., high-order factors) that explain covariance among different latent dimensions (i.e., the lower-order factors). In the bifactor models, an overarching general dimension explains the variance among all indicators (e.g., symptoms, diagnosis, etc.), and the residual variance is explained by specific dimensions uncorrelated with the general and other specific factors. The term "p-factor" has been used to describe this general factor extracted from bifactor and, to a lesser extent, second-order models (Caspi *et al.*, 2014). This naming convention resembles the convention in research on cognition. Such work dissociates cognition into specific capacities, such as verbal and visuospatial skills, in addition to an overarching competency, labeled the "g-factor." The p-factor may capture general susceptibility to psychopathology, in a way that could drive symptom covariation. Moreover, recent debate has emerged on whether psychopathology and physical diseases might reflect an underlying shared liability in children and adolescents, which has been called "d-factor" (Cortese *et al.*, 2021).

The second major model applies network theory to child and adolescent psychiatry (Borsboom, 2017; Robinaugh *et al.*, 2020). This model attributes symptom covariation to causal relations among symptoms lying within a mutualistic network (Eaton *et al.*, 2023) (Figure 9.2d). The approach resembles the approach arising from applications of percolation theory in physics, where the behavior of a symptom network changes when one symptom, considered a node in a network, joins or leaves the network (Borsboom, 2017). This implies that some symptoms might generate entire syndromes. In this case, alleviating these central symptoms might generate recovery. At times, research using this theory considers individual symptoms across diagnostic boundaries, informing understanding of symptom interplay. Such research can consider symptom interactions at a particular point in time, as part of a contemporaneous network, or across multiple time points, in a temporal network. The potential to examine how symptoms reinforce each other within the same subject is a clear transdiagnostic advantage of the network model, which is possible to obtain by measuring symptoms in a specific patient many times.

Shared pathophysiology and consequences of mental health conditions in children and adolescents

One likely explanation for comorbidity is that symptomatic presentations appearing superficially different share underlying biological, environmental (Pinto *et al.*, 2017; Lund *et al.*, 2018; Grotzinger *et al.*, 2022; Taylor *et al.*, 2023), or psychological features (Nigg, 2016). Another explanation attributes clinical presentations to combinations of overarching features, such as levels of functional impact and stages of an illness (Stringaris & Goodman 2013; Sawrikar *et al.*, 2022).

Twin studies suggest that the co-occurrence of depressive symptoms, hyperactivity, and conduct problems reflect genetic influences (Waszczuk *et al.*, 2020). Other research finds the p-factor to be highly heritable (50–73%); this heritability is stable as early as age 3 years (Allegrini *et al.*, 2020; Avinun *et al.*, 2022). From a molecular perspective, the p-factor relates to multiple polygenic risk scores, each designed to predict specific diagnoses, which can be combined for optimal prediction of this transdiagnostic dimension (Allegrini *et al.*, 2020; Neumann *et al.*, 2021). However, other research finds different patterns. Thus, while studies find frequent genetic overlap between pairs of disorders, this work fails to find a single genetic risk dimension that explains genetic overlap across disorders (Grotzinger *et al.*, 2022; Romero *et al.*, 2022).

Much like work in genetics, research on brain structure and function can be viewed from transdiagnostic perspectives (see Vanes and Dolan, 2021 for a review). Many different clinical states involve reduced gray matter volume in the dorsal anterior cingulate cortex (ACC) and insula (Goodkind *et al.*, 2015). Other research finds transdiagnostic morphometric similarities among major depressive, bipolar, schizophrenia, obsessive–compulsive, and anxiety disorders, though lower similarity exists among neurodevelopmental disorders (NDDs), such as attention deficit hyperactivity disorder (ADHD) and autism spectrum disorder (ASD) (Goodkind *et al.*, 2015; Sprooten *et al.*, 2017; Boedhoe *et al.*, 2020; Opel *et al.*, 2020). Still other findings link gray matter volume reductions associated with the p-factor to particular brain areas, such as the prefrontal cortex, which differ from reductions associated with internalizing problems, that arise in the hippocampus, amygdala, and insula (Snyder *et al.*, 2017). With development, neural networks tend to specialize (Paus *et al.*, 2008). Thus, the p-factor may express a changing pattern of relations with brain structure from adolescence (Kaczkurkin *et al.*, 2019; Durham *et al.*, 2021) to adulthood (Romer *et al.*, 2020; Romer *et al.*, 2021). A final set of findings on brain structure considers the impact of symptom persistence (Romer *et al.*, 2023) or specific facets of brain structure, such as myelination (Neumann *et al.*, 2020) or regional anatomic variation (Vanes *et al.*, 2020).

In terms of brain function, general psychopathology in youth is also associated with brain activity alterations in resting state and task activation. The p-factor relates to reduced activation in the ACC, prefrontal cortex, anterior insula, thalamus, and precuneus during executive function tasks (Shanmugan *et al.*, 2016). It may also relate to decreased functional connectivity between the dorsal ACC and caudate during resting state, as well as increased blood flow in the dorsal ACC (Kaczkurkin *et al.*, 2018). Connectivity within networks, such as in the default mode and frontoparietal network, may also manifest dysfunction across different dimensions of psychopathology, including mood, psychosis, fear, and externalizing dimensions (Xia *et al.*, 2018). Thus, alterations in brain structure or function may relate to transdiagnostic features (Vanes & Dolan 2021).

Beyond associations with brain structure or function, transdiagnostic features also correlate with altered cognitive and affective functions. The p-factor correlates with measures of negative emotionality (Tackett *et al.*, 2013; Moore *et al.*, 2020), emotion-based impulsivity (Carver *et al.*, 2017; Moore *et al.*, 2020), irritability (Hoffmann *et al.*, 2022a; Hoffmann *et al.*, 2022b), executive function (Shanmugan *et al.*, 2016; Martel *et al.*, 2017; Caspi & Moffitt 2018; Moore *et al.*, 2020), and general cognition (Caspi *et al.*, 2020). Cross-study variation in such patterns could reflect methodological features, such as aspects of assessment or sampling (Watts *et al.*, 2019; Levin-Aspenson *et al.*, 2021). Nevertheless, other findings consistently replicate. In different samples, the p-factor strongly predicts clinical impact (Hoffmann *et al.*, 2022a), reflected in multiple socioeconomic, social, and health outcomes, from childhood to mid-life, regardless of the informant or assessment tool (Caspi *et al.*, 2014; Patalay *et al.*, 2015; Sallis *et al.*, 2019; Laceulle *et al.*, 2020; Thompson *et al.*, 2021; Hoffmann *et al.*, 2022b). This might reflect common consequences of different child and adolescent psychiatric disorders (Kessler *et al.*, 1995; Kessler *et al.*, 1997; Kessler *et al.*, 1998; Erskine *et al.*, 2016; Clayborne *et al.*, 2019; Dalsgaard *et al.*, 2020; Momen *et al.*, 2020).

This overall impairment captured by the p-factor might also relate to social and environmental factors associated with multiple psychiatric disorders. Such factors increase the risk for most mental health problems (Oddy *et al.*, 2010; McLaughlin *et al.*, 2012a; McLaughlin *et al.*, 2012b; Rogers *et al.*, 2013). For example, exposure to adverse childhood experiences (ACEs) represents a nonspecific risk factor for internalizing, externalizing, and psychotic problems (McLaughlin *et al.*, 2020). Traumatic events also relate to many diagnoses, with multiple types of events linked to anxiety, mood, attentional, and conduct disorders as early as the age of 11 (Bauer *et al.*, 2022). Low socioeconomic status, perinatal exposures such as preterm birth, gestational drinking, smoking, and breastfeeding, parental psychopathology, early trauma, and peer victimization are also nonspecific risk factors for many mental health conditions (Oddy *et al.*, 2010; McLaughlin *et al.*, 2012a; McLaughlin *et al.*, 2012b; Rogers *et al.*, 2013; McLaughlin *et al.*, 2020; Leusin *et al.*, 2023).

In summary, multiple factors in many domains confer nonspecific risk to a range of mental health problems. This observation influences research in many areas, including biology, genetics, and therapeutics and informs recommendations to move from diagnosis-centric classifications to those based on prognosis or staging.

Current proposed models

Findings on symptom covariation and associated transdiagnostic relations with risk factors informed attempts to parse symptoms using approaches other than the historically defined consensus-based entities in current classificatory manuals. Such alternative approaches include four notable examples: RDoC, HiTOP, the network theory of mental disorders, and clinical staging (Cuthbert & Insel 2013; Borsboom 2017; Kotov *et al.*, 2021; Sawrikar *et al.*, 2022). Figure 9.3 depicts features of these approaches.

The National Institute of Mental Health (NIMH)'s RDoC provides a framework for research. Unlike DSM and ICD, RDoC heavily leverages neuroscientific tools. The framework includes six domains of functioning (arousal/regulatory, positive valence, negative valence, sensorimotor, cognitive, and social processes) assessed in several units of analysis (from molecular to psychological and behavioral data) (Figure 9.3a). Units of analysis are to be studied in ways that relate to developmental trajectories and associations with the environment (Cuthbert & Insel, 2013). Thus, mental health problems are viewed as alterations spanning multiple levels, and research from this perspective prioritizes a search for biomarkers as therapeutic tools. Since its launch in 2010, the RDoC has influenced research in child and adolescent psychiatry, as reflected in studies of disorders, such as ADHD, and autism, and symptoms, such as irritability (Pacheco *et al.*, 2022).

HiTOP seeks an empirical classification that leverages quantitative analysis of co-occurring signs and symptoms. The concepts and analytical strategies applied by HiTOP have been used for nearly 100 years (Achenbach 1966; Kotov *et al.*, 2022). The HiTOP framework is hierarchical (Figure 9.3b), viewing mental health problems as nested dimensions related to extremes of psychological functions. This involves an overarching domain that encompasses mid-level spectra of mental health problems, such as the above-mentioned domains of internalizing or emotional and externalizing or behavioral problems. Moreover, functional impairment is a distinct dimension from symptoms in HiTOP, similarly to the ICD system, and it recognizes that not all individuals with notable symptoms are functionally impaired (Kotov *et al.*, 2022). HiTOP dimensional operationalization has been tested against categorical classifications, and results suggest that the explained variance for several outcomes

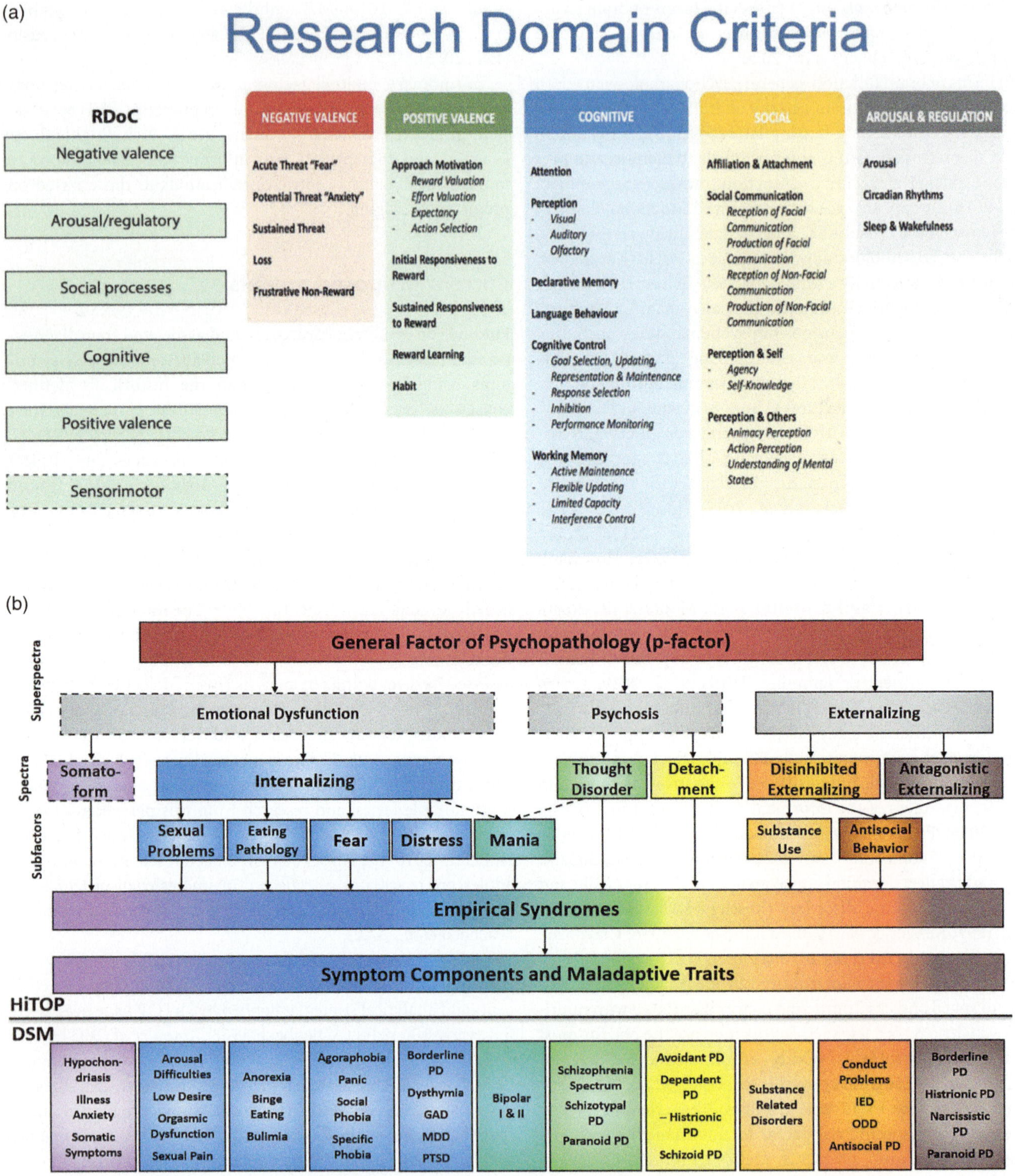

Figure 9.3 RDoC (a), HiTOP (b), Network (c) and staging (d) models.

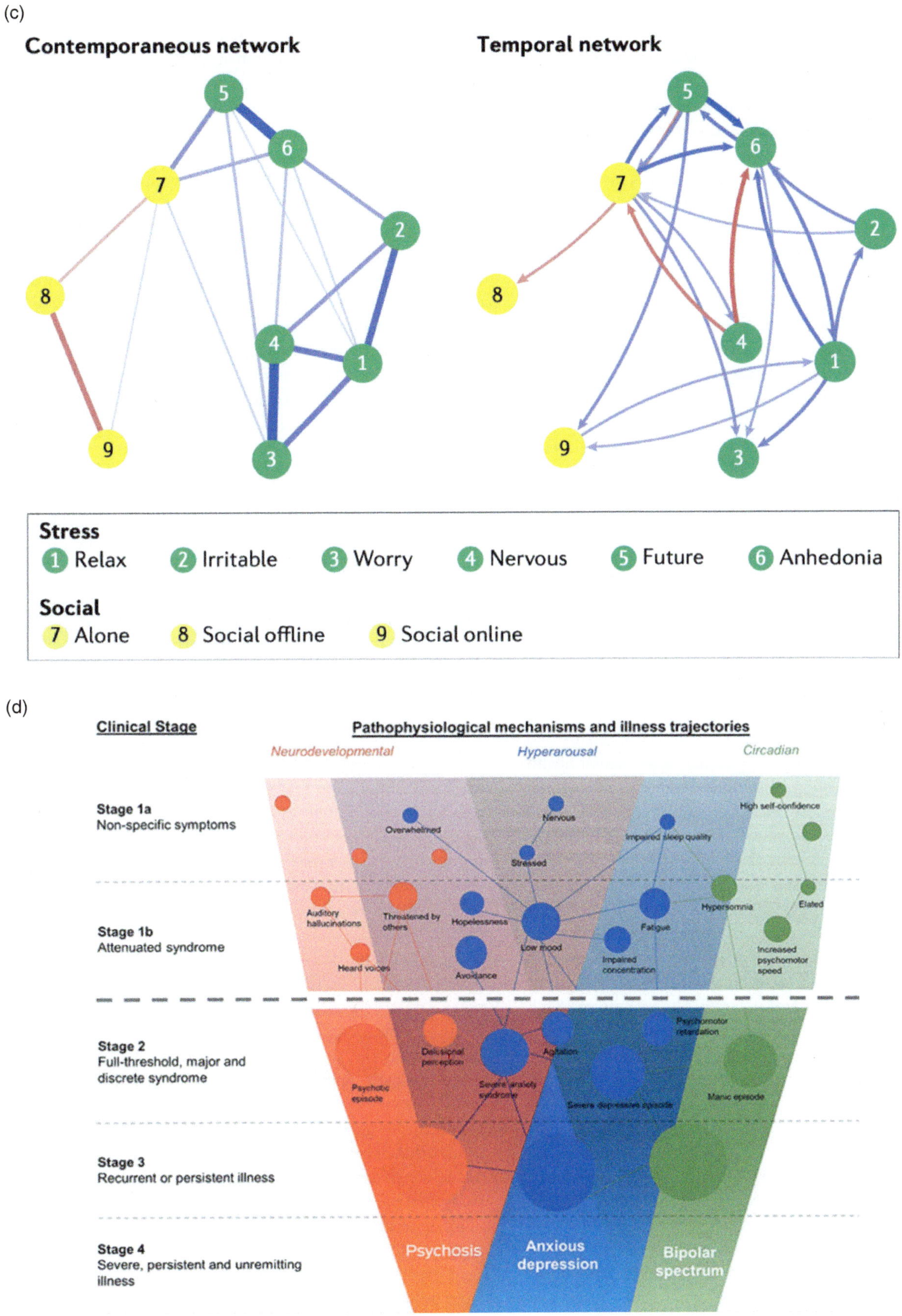

Figure 9.3 (Continued)

is superior for HiTOP when compared to their categorical counterparts (Kim *et al.*, 2021; Krueger *et al.*, 2021; Martin *et al.*, 2021; Kotov *et al.*, 2022). Thus, HiTOP may provide a clinically useful tool.

Approaches resembling HiTOP have been widely used for many years in child psychiatry. Notable examples include the Strengths and Difficulties Questionnaire (SDQ), the Child Behavior Checklist (CBCL), the Pediatric Symptom Checklist (PCS), and the Ontario Child Health Study Emotional and Behavioral Scales (OCHS-EBS). These dimensional approaches provide broadband assessments of symptoms clustered in many dimensions. Most of these symptoms lie within classical internalizing, externalizing, and attention problem domains, but other domains exist, including sleep, thought, somatic, and peer problems. The idea behind these dimensional assessments is to identify areas of functioning where a patient is struggling. Thus, the assignment of a diagnosis occurs when symptoms fall above certain severity thresholds, much like for hypertension, hypercholesterolemia, or diabetes. For instance, the CBCL uses T-scores, which convert total scores into a standardized score centered on 50 with 10-point deviations reflecting 1 standard deviation of the measure in the population. T-scores beyond 70 indicate the need for clinical attention. Figure 9.4 depicts one example while using the HiTOP system, which possesses features reflected in the CBCL.

The network model is a relatively new approach that emphasizes the dynamics of mental health problems (Borsboom, 2017; Robinaugh *et al.*, 2020). Instead of distinct categories, it treats symptoms and their correlated features, such as risk factors, as components of a mutualistic reinforcing network. The behavior of the entire network generates and maintains problems and symptoms (Figure 9.3c). Thus, the theory views mental health as entities classified through definitions of systems rather than syndromes (Fried, 2022). Dynamics arise from the features of complex systems, where one system component influences the behavior of the entire system, such that one cannot understand system function by examining isolated components. The network model has gained popularity in child and adolescent psychiatry, as it analyzes the ways that symptoms change over development by modeling temporal networks (Epskamp *et al.*, 2018). Some studies have found that some symptoms might bridge internalizing and externalizing symptoms. Such bridging symptoms could include irritability, crying, and feelings of loneliness (Rouquette *et al.*, 2018). Longitudinally, depressed mood, inattention, and worry might be symptoms that increase the likelihood of presenting other symptoms in the future (Funkhouser *et al.*, 2021). Thus, by targeting specific symptoms, the network theory generates ideas about novel therapeutics that might lead to better outcomes for young people.

Finally, clinical staging is another framework (Figure 9.3d), which emphasizes mental conditions' common underlying mechanisms (Shah *et al.*, 2020). This framework highlights the developmental course/progression of mental illness, not just the current clinical state of an individual. The clinical stage can progress from low-level risk (Stage 0) to mild/subthreshold or nonspecific symptoms (Stage 1), to recognized clinical syndrome with some functional impairment (Stage 2), moving to incomplete remission or recurrent syndromes with functional impairment and cognitive decline (Stage 3) and then to a severe unremitting syndrome with functional impairment and cognitive decline unresponsive to treatment (Stage 4). It can also extend from one dimension (e.g., anxiety symptoms) to multiple dimensions (e.g., substance use, cognitive impairment, metabolic diseases). The goal is to identify the probability of progression and extension to other dimensions of functioning based on the current stage. With that, intervention could be planned according to each stage, not to the current clinical state. This is a fundamental difference between clinical staging and current nosological systems in terms of treatment choice. In current systems, interventions, and their invasiveness (e.g., psychosocial intervention vs medication and hospitalization) are based on the current symptomatic manifestation. In clinical staging, treatment is selected based on the probability of progression, focusing on its prevention.

When assessing the value of these transdiagnostic approaches, Fusar-Poli *et al.* (2019) have proposed the TRANS Diagnostic research recommendations in psychiatry to improve research in this field encompassing six principles that are summarized here:

- Transparent definition of the gold standard: Clearly define the gold standard for diagnoses, such as ICD, DSM, or others. Specify diagnostic types, and official codes, and differentiate between primary and secondary diagnoses. Describe the diagnostic assessment interviews used.
- Reporting study details: In both the abstract and main text, provide information about the primary outcome of the study, the study design, and the precise definition of the transdiagnostic construct under investigation.
- Appraise the conceptual framework: Evaluate the conceptual framework or approach of the transdiagnostic model. Determine whether it extends across diagnoses, goes beyond diagnoses, or adopts another approach, and explain this choice.
- Numerate diagnostic categories: List the diagnostic categories, spectra, and nonclinical samples in which the transdiagnostic construct is being tested and subsequently validated.
- Show improvement: Perform specific comparative analyses to demonstrate the degree of improvement achieved by the transdiagnostic approach compared to specific diagnostic approaches.
- Demonstrate generalizability: Highlight external validation studies that demonstrate the generalizability of the transdiagnostic construct, showing its applicability beyond the initial study context.

This approach can further ensure a thorough and structured evaluation of transdiagnostic constructs within child and adolescent psychiatry, facilitating a comprehensive understanding of their utility and effectiveness.

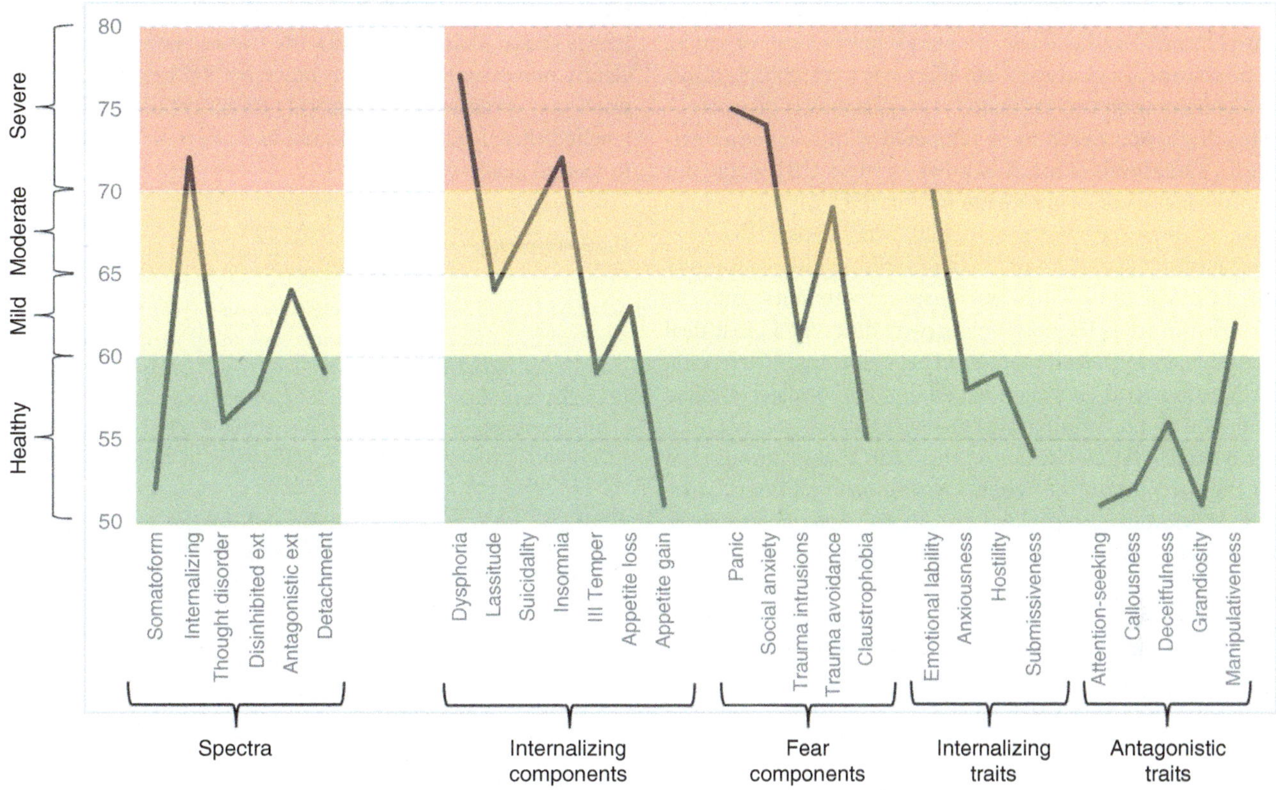

Figure 9.4 Dimensional assessment using T-score of a HiTOP. **Note:** In the present case, this hypothetical patient presents a T-score of 70 or above (meaning that this subject is beyond the 98th percentile in those symptoms) and is higher on dysphoria, insomnia, and panic symptoms, which are within the Internalizing spectra and indicate clinical attention is needed in that area (Ruggero *et al.*, 2019).

Transdiagnostic therapeutic effects of interventions in children and adolescents

When considering the value of transdiagnostic approaches, perhaps the most important issue relates to therapeutic access and discovery. Currently, some specificity does exist in the effects of some therapeutic agents, but many such agents impact multiple disorder types as described in Chapters 31–39 on therapeutics.

Perhaps the most notable psychotherapeutic example is the evidence regarding the effectiveness of a unified protocol for cognitive behavioral therapy (CBT). The unified protocol includes components such as psychoeducation, cognitive reappraisal, emotional awareness, and behavioral activation to treat emotional disorders (Ehrenreich *et al.*, 2009). Several studies have demonstrated its effectiveness in reducing the symptoms of young people with various emotional disorders, including social and generalized anxiety disorders, as well as general functioning (Carlucci *et al.*, 2021). The effect sizes of this unified approach to treat emotional disorders in children and adolescents are moderate when considering randomized trials comparing groups against passive and active controls (Carlucci *et al.*, 2021). This approach particularly enhances the evidence that the general effects of psychotherapies are probably more important than the specific effects.

This work carries many broad implications for the health sector. First, nonspecific protocols reduce barriers to dissemination contained within traditional models that require multiple treatment protocols for different disorders. Second, disorder-specific interventions rely on heterogeneous diagnostic categories and ignore the high rates of comorbidity. Finally, treatments such as those related to the unified protocol also apply to people with high levels of symptoms in the absence of a clear categorial diagnosis. Each feature could increase access to treatment for underserved populations, thereby addressing problems related to a shortage of mental health professionals and difficulties with treatment dissemination.

Medications also possess transdiagnostic effects. Selective serotonin reuptake inhibitors (SSRI) and serotonin-norepinephrine reuptake inhibitors (SNRI) are effective in multiple symptoms from many emotional and stress disorders, above and beyond specific categories (Gosmann *et al.*, 2021). Antipsychotics and stimulants have similarly broad spectrums of efficacy (Salazar de Pablo *et al.*, 2023). Quetiapine effectively reduces symptoms of bipolar depression and schizophrenia (Suttajit *et al.*, 2014; Krause *et al.*, 2018) whereas risperidone reduces symptoms of conduct and oppositional defiant disorders, with and without ADHD (Pringsheim *et al.*, 2015). Stimulants are also effective in non-ADHD conditions, such as narcolepsy, binge eating, and emotion regulation (Sinita & Coghill, 2014). Thus, many disorders can be effectively treated by therapies with unique mechanisms of action, and one pharmacological agent can effectively treat multiple disorders, highlighting constructs shared across diagnostic categories.

This discussion needs to be tempered with competing evidence for some levels of specificity. For example, CBT would not be a plausible stand-alone treatment for ASD. Lithium would not be a suitable choice for a child with anxiety disorder. Transdiagnostic effects do not mean everything works for everyone. The degree to which our current treatments could be repurposed to transdiagnostic constructs deserves a great deal of scrutiny and clinical wisdom. The main argument being made here is that there might be better ways to match clinical information to interventions that go beyond diagnostic boundaries that need to be studied and scientifically tested. It would not be in the best interest of patients to eliminate all boundaries, especially without having valid criteria for clinicians to share decision-making with their patients in the pursuit of their mental health.

Finally, people with lived experience also desire that treatments improve their lives in domains beyond their symptoms, such as quality of life, functioning, and well-being. Unfortunately, few trials in child psychiatry have been measuring them. The most common improvements that young patients desire are related to well-being, functionality, relieving distress, and coping with their symptoms (Krause *et al.*, 2021b; Krause *et al.*, 2023). Moreover, different perspectives are also important. Symptom relief has been related as an important target for young people and their parents. However, coping might be particularly important for the patients, while parents and therapists might be particularly interested in functioning (Krause *et al.*, 2021a). Nonetheless, these are transdiagnostic outcomes, in the sense of being beyond diagnosis, and are recommended measurements alongside specific symptomatic outcomes in intervention trials (Krause *et al.*, 2021b; Krause *et al.*, 2023).

Conclusions

From very early in life, symptoms of mental conditions tend to co-occur and manifest shared relations with many psychological, cognitive, emotional, biological, and environmental factors. Common factors across and beyond diagnoses might affect their incidence as well as the probability of response to interventions. Exciting research generates innovative perspectives on expressions of mental health problems as well as their risk factors and trajectories (Cuthbert & Insel 2013; Borsboom 2017; Shah *et al.*, 2020; Kotov *et al.*, 2022). However, there remains a long road ahead before transdiagnostic psychiatry can be effectively implemented in clinical practice. Consensus over transdiagnostic constructs must be achieved among clinicians, researchers, patients, and caregivers (Fusar-Poli *et al.*, 2019; Krause *et al.*, 2019). Moreover, clinical trials must reliably measure these transdiagnostic constructs that could be assessed and incorporated into health systems. Despite the enormous challenges (Fusar-Poli *et al.*, 2019), the transdiagnostic approach is clearly one prominent way to move mental health science forward as traditional categorical classifications might have reached their limits in explaining and alleviating suffering due to mental health conditions.

References

Achenbach, T.M. (1966) The classification of children's psychiatric symptoms: a factor-analytic study. *Psychological Monographs* **80**(7), 1–37. doi:10.1037/h0093906.

Achenbach, T.M. & Edelbrock, C.S. (1978) The classification of child psychopathology: a review and analysis of empirical efforts. *Psychological Bulletin* **85**(6), 1275–1301. doi:10.1037/0033-2909.85.6.1275.

Allegrini, A.G. *et al.* (2020) The p factor: genetic analyses support a general dimension of psychopathology in childhood and adolescence. *Journal of Child Psychology and Psychiatry* **61**(1), 30–39. doi:10.1111/jcpp.13113.

American Psychiatric Association (2022) *Diagnostic and Statistical Manual of Mental Disorders*, 5th edn. text revision edn. American Psychiatric Association, Washington, DC.

Avinun, R. *et al.* (2022) The general psychopathology factor from early to middle childhood: longitudinal genetic and risk analyses. *Journal of Psychopathology and Clinical Science* **131**, 705–715. doi:10.1037/abn0000780.

Bauer, A. *et al.* (2022) Associations between childhood trauma and childhood psychiatric disorders in Brazil: a population-based, prospective birth cohort study. *The Lancet Psychiatry* **9**(12), 969–977. doi:10.1016/S2215-0366(22)00337-6.

Boedhoe, P.S.W. *et al.* (2020) Subcortical brain volume, regional cortical thickness, and cortical surface area across disorders: findings from the ENIGMA ADHD, ASD, and OCD working groups. *The American Journal of Psychiatry* **177**(9), 834–843. doi:10.1176/appi.ajp.2020.19030331.

Borsboom, D. (2017) A network theory of mental disorders. *World Psychiatry* **16**(1), 5–13. doi:10.1002/wps.20375.

Carlucci, L. *et al.* (2021) On the efficacy of the unified protocol for transdiagnostic treatment of emotional disorders: a systematic review and meta-analysis. *Clinical Psychology Review* **87**, 101999. doi:10.1016/j.cpr.2021.101999.

Carragher, N. *et al.* (2015) Disorders without borders: current and future directions in the meta-structure of mental disorders. *Social Psychiatry and Psychiatric Epidemiology* **50**(3), 339–350. doi:10.1007/s00127-014-1004-z.

Carver, C.S. *et al.* (2017) Toward a functional view of the P factor in psychopathology. *Clinical Psychological Science: A Journal of the Association for Psychological Science* **5**(5), 880–889. doi:10.1177/2167702617710037.

Caspi, A. & Moffitt, T.E. (2018) All for one and one for all: mental disorders in one dimension. *American Journal of Psychiatry* **175**, p. appi.ajp.2018.17121383. doi:10.1176/appi.ajp.2018.17121383.

Caspi, A. *et al.* (2014) The p factor one general psychopathology factor in the structure of psychiatric disorders? *Clinical Psychological Science* **2**(2), 119–137. doi:10.1177/2167702613497473.

Caspi, A. *et al.* (2020) Longitudinal assessment of mental health disorders and comorbidities across 4 decades among participants in the

Dunedin birth cohort study. *JAMA Network Open* **3**(4), e203221. doi:10.1001/jamanetworkopen.2020.3221.

Clayborne, Z.M. *et al.* (2019) Systematic review and meta-analysis: adolescent depression and long-term psychosocial outcomes. *Journal of the American Academy of Child & Adolescent Psychiatry* **58**(1), 72–79. doi:10.1016/j.jaac.2018.07.896.

Cortese, S. *et al.* (2021) Beyond the p factor: is there a d factor? *JCPP Advances* **1**(4), e12051. doi:10.1002/jcv2.12051.

Cuthbert, B.N. & Insel, T.R. (2013) Toward the future of psychiatric diagnosis: the seven pillars of RDoC. *BMC Medicine* **11**(1), 126. doi:10.1186/1741-7015-11-126.

Dalsgaard, S. *et al.* (2020) Association of mental disorder in childhood and adolescence with subsequent educational achievement. *JAMA Psychiatry* **77**, 797–805. Available at: https://jamanetwork.com/journals/jamapsychiatry/fullarticle/2763443 [Accessed: 1 April 2020]

Durham, E.L. *et al.* (2021) Association of gray matter volumes with general and specific dimensions of psychopathology in children. *Neuropsychopharmacology* **46**(7), 1333–1339. doi:10.1038/s41386-020-00952-w.

Eaton, N.R. *et al.* (2023) A review of approaches and models in psychopathology conceptualization research. *Nature Reviews Psychology* **2**, 622–636. Available at: https://www.nature.com/articles/s44159-023-00218-4 [Accessed: 9 September 2023]

Ehrenreich, J.T. *et al.* (2009) Development of a unified protocol for the treatment of emotional disorders in youth. *Child & Family Behavior Therapy* **31**(1), 20–37. doi:10.1080/07317100802701228.

Epskamp, S. *et al.* (2018) Estimating psychological networks and their accuracy: a tutorial paper. *Behavior Research Methods* **50**(1), 195–212. doi:10.3758/s13428-017-0862-1.

Erskine, H.E. *et al.* (2016) Long-term outcomes of attention-deficit/hyperactivity disorder and conduct disorder: a systematic review and meta-analysis. *Journal of the American Academy of Child and Adolescent Psychiatry* **55**(10), 841–850. doi:10.1016/j.jaac.2016.06.016.

Fried, E.I. (2022) Studying mental health problems as systems, not syndromes. *Current Directions in Psychological Science* **31**(6), 500–508. doi:10.1177/09637214221114089.

Funkhouser, C.J. *et al.* (2021) Unique longitudinal relationships between symptoms of psychopathology in youth: a cross-lagged panel network analysis in the ABCD study. *Journal of Child Psychology and Psychiatry* **62**(2), 184–194. doi:10.1111/jcpp.13256.

Fusar-Poli, P. *et al.* (2019) Transdiagnostic psychiatry: a systematic review. *World Psychiatry* **18**(2), 192–207. doi:10.1002/wps.20631.

Goodkind, M. *et al.* (2015) Identification of a common neurobiological substrate for mental illness. *JAMA Psychiatry* **72**(4), 305–315. doi:10.1001/jamapsychiatry.2014.2206.

Gosmann, N.P. *et al.* (2021) Selective serotonin reuptake inhibitors, and serotonin and norepinephrine reuptake inhibitors for anxiety, obsessive-compulsive, and stress disorders: a 3-level network meta-analysis. *PLoS Medicine* **18**(6), e1003664. doi:10.1371/journal.pmed.1003664.

Grotzinger, A.D. *et al.* (2022) Genetic architecture of 11 major psychiatric disorders at biobehavioral, functional genomic and molecular genetic levels of analysis. *Nature Genetics* **54**(5), 548–559. doi:10.1038/s41588-022-01057-4.

Hoffmann, M.S. *et al.* (2022a) Reliability and validity of bifactor models of dimensional psychopathology in youth. *Journal of Psychopathology and Clinical Science* **131**(4), 407–421. doi:10.1037/abn0000749.

Hoffmann, M.S. *et al.* (2022b) Parent- and teacher-reported associations from adolescent bifactor models of psychopathology: an outcome-wide association study of 26 outcomes in mid-life. *Journal of Child Psychology and Psychiatry* **64**, 397–407. Available at: https://onlinelibrary.wiley.com/doi/abs/10.1111/jcpp.13707 [Accessed: 14 January 2023]

Kaczkurkin, A.N. *et al.* (2018) Common and dissociable regional cerebral blood flow differences associate with dimensions of psychopathology across categorical diagnoses. *Molecular Psychiatry* **23**(10), 1981–1989. doi:10.1038/mp.2017.174.

Kaczkurkin, A.N. *et al.* (2019) Dimensions of psychopathology are dissociably linked to brain structure in youth. *The American Journal of Psychiatry* **176**(12), 1000–1009. doi:10.1176/appi.ajp.2019.18070835.

Kessler, R.C. *et al.* (1995) Social consequences of psychiatric disorders, I: educational attainment. *The American Journal of Psychiatry* **152**(7), 1026–1032. doi:10.1176/ajp.152.7.1026.

Kessler, R.C. *et al.* (1997) Social consequences of psychiatric disorders, II: teenage parenthood. *The American Journal of Psychiatry* **154**(10), 1405–1411. doi:10.1176/ajp.154.10.1405.

Kessler, R.C. *et al.* (1998) The social consequences of psychiatric disorders, III: probability of marital stability. *The American Journal of Psychiatry* **155**(8), 1092–1096. doi:10.1176/ajp.155.8.1092.

Kessler, R.C. *et al.* (2011) The role of latent internalizing and externalizing predispositions in accounting for the development of comorbidity among common mental disorders. *Current Opinion in Psychiatry* **24**(4), 307–312. doi:10.1097/YCO.0b013e3283477b22.

Kim, H. *et al.* (2021) Internalizing psychopathology and all-cause mortality: a comparison of transdiagnostic vs. diagnosis-based risk prediction. *World Psychiatry* **20**(2), 276–282. doi:10.1002/wps.20859.

Kotov, R. *et al.* (2021) The hierarchical taxonomy of psychopathology (HiTOP): a quantitative nosology based on consensus of evidence. *Annual Review of Clinical Psychology* **17**(1), 83–108. Available at: https://doi.org/10.1146/annurev-clinpsy-081219-093304 [Accessed: 17 February 2021]

Kotov, R. *et al.* (2022) The hierarchical taxonomy of psychopathology (HiTOP) in psychiatric practice and research. *Psychological Medicine*, 1–13. doi:10.1017/S0033291722001301.

Krause, M. *et al.* (2018) Efficacy, acceptability, and tolerability of antipsychotics in children and adolescents with schizophrenia: a network meta-analysis. *European Neuropsychopharmacology* **28**(6), 659–674. doi:10.1016/j.euroneuro.2018.03.008.

Krause, K.R. *et al.* (2019) Review: what outcomes count? Outcomes measured for adolescent depression between 2007 and 2017. *Journal of the American Academy of Child & Adolescent Psychiatry* **58**(1), 61–71. doi:10.1016/j.jaac.2018.07.893.

Krause, K. *et al.* (2021a) A comprehensive mapping of outcomes following psychotherapy for adolescent depression: the perspectives of young people, their parents and therapists. *European Child & Adolescent Psychiatry* **30**(11), 1779–1791. doi:10.1007/s00787-020-01648-8.

Krause, K.R. *et al.* (2021b) International consensus on a standard set of outcome measures for child and youth anxiety, depression, obsessive-compulsive disorder, and post-traumatic stress disorder. *The Lancet Psychiatry* **8**(1), 76–86. doi:10.1016/S2215-0366(20)30356-4.

Krause, K.R. *et al.* (2023) What treatment outcomes matter most? A Q-study of outcome priority profiles among youth with lived experience of depression. *European Child & Adolescent Psychiatry* **32**(1), 123–137. doi:10.1007/s00787-021-01839-x.

Krueger, R.F. (1999) The structure of common mental disorders. *Archives of General Psychiatry* **56**(10), 921. doi:10.1001/archpsyc.56.10.921.

Krueger, R.F. *et al.* (2021) Validity and utility of hierarchical taxonomy of psychopathology (HiTOP): II. externalizing superspectrum. *World Psychiatry* **20**(2), 171–193. doi:10.1002/wps.20844.

Laceulle, O.M. *et al.* (2020) The wide-ranging life outcome correlates of a general psychopathology factor in adolescent psychopathology. *Personality and Mental Health* **14**(1), 9–29. doi:10.1002/pmh.1465.

Lahey, B.B. *et al.* (2008) Testing structural models of DSM-IV symptoms of common forms of child and adolescent psychopathology. *Journal of Abnormal Child Psychology* **36**(2), 187–206. doi:10.1007/s10802-007-9169-5.

Lahey, B.B. *et al.* (2017) A hierarchical causal taxonomy of psychopathology across the life span. *Psychological Bulletin* **143**(2), 142–186. doi:10.1037/bul0000069.

Lahey, B.B. *et al.* (2021) Hierarchical models of psychopathology: empirical support, implications, and remaining issues. *World Psychiatry* **20**(1), 57–63. doi:10.1002/wps.20824.

Leusin, F. *et al.* (2023) Perinatal and neonatal factors and mental disorders in children and adolescents: looking for the contributions of the early environment to common and dissociable aspects of psychopathology. *European Child & Adolescent Psychiatry*. doi:10.1007/s00787-024-02402-0.

Levin-Aspenson, H.F. *et al.* (2021) What is the general factor of psychopathology? Consistency of the p factor across samples. *Assessment* **28**(4), 1035–1049. doi:10.1177/1073191120954921.

Lund, C. *et al.* (2018) Social determinants of mental disorders and the sustainable development goals: a systematic review of reviews. *The Lancet Psychiatry* **5**(4), 357–369. doi:10.1016/S2215-0366(18)30060-9.

Martel, M.M. *et al.* (2017) A general psychopathology factor (P factor) in children: structural model analysis and external validation through familial risk and child global executive function. *Journal of Abnormal Psychology* **126**(1), 137–148. doi:10.1037/abn0000205.

Martin, E.A. *et al.* (2021) Predicting long-term outcomes in first-admission psychosis: does the hierarchical taxonomy of psychopathology aid DSM in prognostication? *Schizophrenia Bulletin* **47**, 1331–1341. (sbab043). Available at: https://doi.org/10.1093/schbul/sbab043 [Accessed: 3 June 2021]

McGrath, J.J. *et al.* (2020) Comorbidity within mental disorders: a comprehensive analysis based on 145 990 survey respondents from 27 countries. *Epidemiology and Psychiatric Sciences* **29**, e153. Available at: https://www.cambridge.org/core/journals/epidemiology-and-psychiatric-sciences/article/comorbidity-within-mental-disorders-a-comprehensive-analysis-based-on-145-990-survey-respondents-from-27-countries/7A22F65B47BDF8E52B8A1876201720E0 [Accessed: 2 June 2021].

McLaughlin, K.A. *et al.* (2012a) Parent psychopathology and offspring mental disorders: results from the WHO world mental health surveys. *The British Journal of Psychiatry* **200**, 290–299. doi:10.1192/bjp.bp.111.101253.

McLaughlin, K.A. *et al.* (2012b) Socioeconomic status and adolescent mental disorders. *American Journal of Public Health* **102**(9), 1742–1750. doi:10.2105/AJPH.2011.300477.

McLaughlin, K.A. *et al.* (2020) Mechanisms linking childhood trauma exposure and psychopathology: a transdiagnostic model of risk and resilience. *BMC Medicine* **18**(1), 96. doi:10.1186/s12916-020-01561-6.

Michelini, G. *et al.* (2019) Delineating and validating higher-order dimensions of psychopathology in the adolescent brain cognitive development (ABCD) study. *Translational Psychiatry* **9**(1), 261. doi:10.1038/s41398-019-0593-4.

Momen, N.C. *et al.* (2020) Association between mental disorders and subsequent medical conditions. *New England Journal of Medicine* **382**(18), 1721–1731. doi:10.1056/NEJMoa1915784.

Moore, T.M. *et al.* (2020) Criterion validity and relationships between alternative hierarchical dimensional models of general and specific psychopathology. *Journal of Abnormal Psychology* **129**(7), 677–688. doi:10.1037/abn0000601.

Neumann, A. *et al.* (2020) White matter microstructure and the general psychopathology factor in children. *Journal of the American Academy of Child & Adolescent Psychiatry* **59**(11), 1285–1296. doi:10.1016/j.jaac.2019.12.006.

Neumann, A. *et al.* (2021) Combined polygenic risk scores of different psychiatric traits predict general and specific psychopathology in childhood. *Journal of Child Psychology and Psychiatry, and Allied Disciplines* **63**, 636–645. doi:10.1111/jcpp.13501.

Nigg, J.T. (2016) Annual research review: on the relations among self-regulation, self-control, executive functioning, effortful control, cognitive control, impulsivity, risk-taking, and inhibition for developmental psychopathology. *Journal of Child Psychology and Psychiatry* **58**, 361–383. doi:10.1111/jcpp.12675.

Oddy, W.H. *et al.* (2010) The long-term effects of breastfeeding on child and adolescent mental health: a pregnancy cohort study followed for 14 years. *The Journal of Pediatrics* **156**(4), 568–574. doi:10.1016/j.jpeds.2009.10.020.

Opel, N. *et al.* (2020) Cross-disorder analysis of brain structural abnormalities in six major psychiatric disorders: a secondary analysis of mega- and meta-analytical findings from the ENIGMA consortium. *Biological Psychiatry* **88**(9), 678–686. doi:10.1016/j.biopsych.2020.04.027.

Pacheco, J. *et al.* (2022) Annual research review: the contributions of the RDoC research framework on understanding the neurodevelopmental origins, progression and treatment of mental illnesses. *Journal of Child Psychology and Psychiatry* **63**(4), 360–376. doi:10.1111/jcpp.13543.

Patalay, P. *et al.* (2015) A general psychopathology factor in early adolescence. *The British Journal of Psychiatry* **207**(1), 15–22. doi:10.1192/bjp.bp.114.149591.

Paus, T. *et al.* (2008) Why do many psychiatric disorders emerge during adolescence? *Nature Reviews Neuroscience* **9**(12), 947–957. doi:10.1038/nrn2513.

Pinto, J.V. *et al.* (2017) On the transdiagnostic nature of peripheral biomarkers in major psychiatric disorders: a systematic review. *Neuroscience and Biobehavioral Reviews* **83**, 97–108. doi:10.1016/j.neubiorev.2017.10.001.

Pringsheim, T. *et al.* (2015) The pharmacological management of oppositional behaviour, conduct problems, and aggression in children and adolescents with attention-deficit hyperactivity disorder, oppositional defiant disorder, and conduct disorder: a systematic review and meta-analysis. Part 2: antipsychotics and traditional mood stabilizers. *The Canadian Journal of Psychiatry* **60**(2), 52–61. doi:10.1177/070674371506000203.

Robinaugh, D.J. *et al.* (2020) The network approach to psychopathology: a review of the literature 2008–2018 and an agenda for future research. *Psychological Medicine* **50**(3), 353–366. doi:10.1017/S0033291719003404.

Rogers, C.E. *et al.* (2013) Late preterm birth, maternal depression, and risk of preschool psychiatric disorders. *Journal of the American Academy of Child and Adolescent Psychiatry* **52**(3), 309–318. doi:10.1016/j.jaac.2012.12.005.

Romer, A.L. *et al.* (2020) Pervasively thinner neocortex as a transdiagnostic feature of general psychopathology. *American Journal of Psychiatry* **178**(2), 174–182. doi:10.1176/appi.ajp.2020.19090934.

Romer, A.L. *et al.* (2021) Replicability of structural brain alterations associated with general psychopathology: evidence from a population-representative birth cohort. *Molecular Psychiatry* **26**(8), 3839–3846. doi:10.1038/s41380-019-0621-z.

Romer, A.L. *et al.* (2023) Brain structure relations with psychopathology trajectories in the adolescent brain cognitive development study. *Journal of the American Academy of Child & Adolescent Psychiatry* **62**, 895–907. Available at: https://www.jaacap.org/article/S0890-8567(23)00057-6/fulltext [Accessed: 13 February 2023]

Romero, C. *et al.* (2022) Exploring the genetic overlap between twelve psychiatric disorders. *Nature Genetics* **54**(12), 1795–1802. doi:10.1038/s41588-022-01245-2.

Rouquette, A. *et al.* (2018) Emotional and behavioral symptom network structure in elementary school girls and association with anxiety disorders and depression in adolescence and early adulthood: a network analysis. *JAMA Psychiatry* **75**(11), 1173–1181. doi:10.1001/jamapsychiatry.2018.2119.

Ruggero, C.J. *et al.* (2019) Integrating the hierarchical taxonomy of psychopathology (HiTOP) into clinical practice. *Journal of Consulting and Clinical Psychology* **87**(12), 1069–1084. doi:10.1037/ccp0000452. PMID: 31724426; PMCID: PMC6859953

Salazar de Pablo, G. *et al.* (2023) Systematic review and meta-analysis: efficacy of pharmacological interventions for irritability and emotional dysregulation in autism spectrum disorder and predictors of response. *Journal of the American Academy of Child & Adolescent Psychiatry* **62**(2), 151–168. doi:10.1016/j.jaac.2022.03.033.

Sallis, H. *et al.* (2019) General psychopathology, internalising and externalising in children and functional outcomes in late adolescence. *Journal of Child Psychology and Psychiatry* **60**(11), 1183–1190. doi:10.1111/jcpp.13067.

Salum G.A. *et al.* (2015) High risk cohort study for psychiatric disorders in childhood: rationale, design, methods and preliminary results. *Int J Methods Psychiatr Res.* **24**, 58–73.

Sawrikar, V. *et al.* (2022) Transdiagnostic clinical staging for childhood mental health: an adjunctive tool for classifying internalizing and externalizing syndromes that emerge in children aged 5-11 years. *Clinical Child and Family Psychology Review.* doi:10.1007/s10567-022-00399-z.

Shah, J.L. *et al.* (2020) Transdiagnostic clinical staging in youth mental health: a first international consensus statement. *World Psychiatry* **19**(2), 233–242. doi:10.1002/wps.20745.

Shanmugan, S. *et al.* (2016) Common and dissociable mechanisms of executive system dysfunction across psychiatric disorders in youth. *The American Journal of Psychiatry* **173**(5), 517–526. doi:10.1176/appi.ajp.2015.15060725.

Sinita, E. & Coghill, D. (2014) The use of stimulant medications for non-core aspects of ADHD and in other disorders. *Neuropharmacology* **87**, 161–172. doi:10.1016/j.neuropharm.2014.06.014.

Slade, T. & Watson, D. (2006) The structure of common DSM-IV and ICD-10 mental disorders in the Australian general population. *Psychological Medicine* **36**(11), 1593–1600. doi:10.1017/S0033291706008452.

Snyder, H.R. *et al.* (2017) Distinct patterns of reduced prefrontal and limbic gray matter volume in childhood general and internalizing psychopathology. *Clinical Psychological Science* **5**(6), 1001–1013. doi:10.1177/2167702617714563.

Sprooten, E. *et al.* (2017) Addressing reverse inference in psychiatric neuroimaging: meta-analyses of task-related brain activation in common mental disorders. *Human Brain Mapping* **38**(4), 1846–1864. doi:10.1002/hbm.23486.

Stringaris, A. & Goodman, R. (2013) The value of measuring impact alongside symptoms in children and adolescents: a longitudinal assessment in a community sample. *Journal of Abnormal Child Psychology* **41**(7), 1109–1120. doi:10.1007/s10802-013-9744-x.

Suttajit, S. *et al.* (2014) Quetiapine for acute bipolar depression: a systematic review and meta-analysis. *Drug Design, Development and Therapy* **8**, 827–838. doi:10.2147/DDDT.S63779.

Tackett, J.L. *et al.* (2013) Common genetic influences on negative emotionality and a general psychopathology factor in childhood and adolescence. *Journal of Abnormal Psychology* **122**(4), 1142–1153. doi:10.1037/a0034151.

Taylor, J.J. *et al.* (2023) A transdiagnostic network for psychiatric illness derived from atrophy and lesions. *Nature Human Behaviour*, 1–10. doi:10.1038/s41562-022-01501-9.

Thompson, E.J. *et al.* (2021) Changes in the adult consequences of adolescent mental ill-health: findings from the 1958 and 1970 British birth cohorts. *Psychological Medicine*, 1–10. doi:10.1017/S0033291721002506.

van Bork, R. (2019) *Interpreting psychometric models.* Thesis Commons. Available at: https://thesiscommons.org/x6a7s/ [Accessed: 6 February 2023].

Vanes, L.D. & Dolan, R.J. (2021) Transdiagnostic neuroimaging markers of psychiatric risk: a narrative review. *NeuroImage: Clinical* **30**, 102634. doi:10.1016/j.nicl.2021.102634.

Vanes, L.D. *et al.* (2020) White matter tract myelin maturation and its association with general psychopathology in adolescence and early adulthood. *Human Brain Mapping* **41**(3), 827–839. doi:10.1002/hbm.24842.

Vasileva, M. *et al.* (2021) Research review: a meta-analysis of the international prevalence and comorbidity of mental disorders in children between 1 and 7 years. *Journal of Child Psychology and Psychiatry* **62**(4), 372–381. doi:10.1111/jcpp.13261.

Waszczuk, M.A. *et al.* (2020) Why do depression, conduct, and hyperactivity symptoms co-occur across adolescence? The role of stable and dynamic genetic and environmental influences. *European Child & Adolescent Psychiatry.* **30**, 1013–1025. doi: 10.1007/s00787-020-01515-6.

Watts, A.L. *et al.* (2019) Riskier tests of the validity of the bifactor model of psychopathology. *Clinical Psychological Science* **7**(6), 1285–1303. doi:10.1177/2167702619855035.

World Health Organization (2019) *International Statistical Classification of Disease and Related Health Problems,* 11th edn, Geneva, Switzerland.

Xia, C.H. *et al.* (2018) Linked dimensions of psychopathology and connectivity in functional brain networks. *Nature Communications* **9**(1), 3003. doi:10.1038/s41467-018-05317-y.

Zachar, P. & Kendler, K.S. (2017) The philosophy of nosology. *Annual Review of Clinical Psychology* **13**, 49–71. doi:10.1146/annurev-clinpsy-032816-045020.

B: Neurobiology

CHAPTER 10
Neurobiological perspectives on the developing human brain

Mark H. Johnson[1,2] and Duncan E. Astle[3]
[1]Department of Psychology, University of Cambridge, Cambridge, UK
[2]Centre for Brain and Cognitive Development, School of Psychology, Birkbeck College, University of London, London, UK
[3]MRC Cognition and Brain Science Unit, Department of Psychiatry, University of Cambridge, Cambridge, UK

Introduction

Given that clinical diagnoses in child psychiatry are mainly based on parental and clinical observation of behavior, what is the relevance of understanding the underlying neurobiology? In this chapter we will see that considering the neurobiology underlying developmental brain pathways can benefit our understanding of behavior, both typical and atypical, in several different ways. First, issues and debates in developmental neurobiology often reflect those at the behavioral level and as such can be illuminating. Second, from a neurobiological perspective the natural categories of developmental diagnoses may look markedly different from those boundaries we have imposed based on behavioral traits. Third, the advent of new cellular, neuroimaging, computational, and genetic methods make a closer integration between the two fields both inevitable and desirable. Finally, neurobiological mechanisms are often posited to be causal factors in the development of behavior, and in explaining the different developmental pathways that human brain development can take.

The brain is an organ of adaptation at multiple time scales. Over evolutionary time our brain has become adapted in various ways to construct and occupy the environmental niche of our species. In ontogeny (individual development), our brain adapts both to the general features of our environment shared with others, and to the individual circumstances into which we are born. Further, on a scale of days and hours we can learn and retain information of survival relevance through the processes of learning and attention. On the scale of seconds and milliseconds our neural processes adapt to current sensory input and change state or prepare motor responses. While we can marvel at the complex and dynamic processes that underlie these adaptations, it is not surprising that there are also many different ways for them to deviate from typical.

The brain is also an organ of adaptation at multiple levels of organization. Neuroscience is one of the broadest interdisciplinary fields in biology, spanning from complex molecular interactions, through intra- and intercellular processes, to the emergent computations that result from many thousands of neurons coherently oscillating in their firing patterns. In this chapter, we review the impact on human brain and behavioral development of factors operating at the cellular and systems levels of developmental neurobiology (see also Chapter 11 for brain imaging and Chapter 21 for genetics). We will see in what follows that key issues about plasticity, timing, and constraints on development are often reflected in specific debates within the domains of genetics, cellular studies, and neural and cognitive systems.

Key issues in developmental neurobiology

Pathways from gene to behavior

The study of development necessarily requires an interdisciplinary approach in which the relevant pathways from gene to behavior are characterized. Gottlieb (1992) distinguished between two different approaches to the study of developmental biology; "deterministic epigenesis" in which it is assumed that there is a unidirectional causal path from genes to structural brain changes to psychological functions and behavior, and "probabilistic epigenesis" in which interactions among genes, structural brain changes, and psychological function are viewed as bidirectional, dynamic, and emergent. The former view still prevails in much contemporary work on child cognitive

Rutter's Child and Adolescent Psychiatry and Psychology, Seventh Edition.
Edited by Anita Thapar, Daniel S. Pine, Samuele Cortese, Cathy Creswell, Tamsin J. Ford, James F. Leckman, and Argyris Stringaris.

Companion website: www.wiley.com/go/thapar/rutterspsych7

development and psychiatry. For example, it is common to see claims about particular regions of the human brain "coming online" at specific ages, with the implication that this is a deterministic process. However, current advances are revealing how complex and context-dependent patterns of gene expression are in the brain (Cardoso-Moreira *et al.*, 2019). Thus, the development of the brain is better conceived of as an active self-organizing process involving interactions between genes, cells, and their current context, and not as simply the passive unfolding of a "genetic blueprint" on a strict maturational timetable.

The importance of interconnectivity

In many simpler organisms (such as the nematode worm *Caenorhabditis elegans*) development proceeds through cell lineages (generations) that are largely independent of each other. This process is described as a "mosaic" (Elman *et al.*, 1996) because cells will divide to yield other more specialized cells along a progression or lineage that is largely uninfluenced by the surrounding context or by other neighboring cells. In contrast, the construction of the brain in vertebrates follows a "regulatory" developmental process in which the division of cells to yield more specialized descendants is heavily dependent on their current context, including the presence or absence of other cells of similar or dissimilar types.

These two contrasting mechanisms at the cellular developmental level can also inform our thinking about the development of the human brain at a regional level. For a considerable time, functional imaging studies in human adults were dominated by the search for the specific cortical regions said to be responsible for particular perceptual, cognitive, or linguistic functions ("the region for X," where X is a cognitive function). However, over recent decades the view has emerged that the response properties of a particular brain region are largely determined by its patterns of connectivity to other regions, as well as by their current activity states, giving rise to the new study of connectomics (Vertes *et al.*, 2012; Kamps *et al.*, 2020; see Chapters 11 and 12).

Thus, in thinking about human development it is important to remember that at all postnatal stages the brain operates as an interconnected whole. While it will take years for parts of the human brain to become specialized into the microarchitecture and functions seen in adults, well before that all parts of the brain are at least partially active and can probably contribute to influencing the behaviors expressed by the child. Indeed, interactions between brain regions are critical for the development and fine-tuning of each one, and it is networks of interacting regions of the brain that give rise to emerging cognitive and emotional functions.

Changing brain structure-to-function mapping during development

One of the biggest issues in neuroscience is exactly how the cellular and connectivity patterns of the regions of the brain constrain or promote particular types of information processing; the structure-to-function mapping. The earlier assumption that different brain regions are a mosaic of isolated units with their own maturational timetable encouraged the view that the structure-to-function mapping in the brain is static and unchanging during development. In the context of typical development, this leads to the view that different regions can develop independently of other regions according to their own particular intrinsic timetable, and that childhood diagnoses could be due to "deficits" in specific regions of the brain. Contrary to this view, but consistent with the interconnected and context-dependent development of the brain, is recent evidence showing that when a new computation or skill is acquired by the child, there is a reorganization of interactions between different brain structures and regions (see Johnson, 2011 for review; Chapters 11 and 12). This reorganization process may even change how previously acquired cognitive functions are represented in the brain. Thus, different networks of brain regions can support the same overt behavior of the child at different ages during development.

Plasticity and latent possibilities

In the biological sciences, the development of structures such as the brain and its constituent parts is often considered to be a process of "restriction of fate." This notion comes from the observation of cells dividing to produce new generations of cells which are often more complex and specialized than their predecessors. In different surrounding contexts, generations of cells can specialize in different ways. Indeed, transposing the location of a group of cells within the developing embryo will often cause the cells to form a different structure from that which they would have done originally. The fact that some stem cells (regressed to an earlier developmental stage) can generate multiple different types of tissue is the basis for recent advances in medical science and psychiatry. Further, our collective ability to harness this technology to create experimental models of neurobiological systems, including primitive "mini-brain" organoids (see section on "Human structural brain development"), is allowing us to explore the complex process of self-organization in real time. These insights are then feeding back into our increasing understanding of the human brain, for instance, elucidating how gene expression and cellular plasticity are linked (see Chapter 21).

As mentioned earlier, the rapidly advancing field of human genetics has moved beyond the traditional notion of a "blueprint" that unfolds in a series of predetermined steps, to a view of the human genome as being open to a variety of factors that influence the degree of expression of different genes at different developmental points, leading to the newly emerging field of "epigenetics" (Chapter 21). At first sight, the role of epigenetic processes in the construction of a human brain seems underconstrained. Given these deep and powerful mechanisms of latent plasticity, what factors constrain the patterns of expression of the genome to give sufficient "stability" in order that the complexity and structure of the human brain results? This key question is currently the focus of much research, and a number of factors that constrain the epigenome are beginning to be described. The complexity and dynamics of gene expression derived from developing and adult postmortem human brains is now being characterized (Colantuoni *et al.*, 2011; Kang *et al.*, 2011). Ninety percent of the brain-related genes analyzed were differentially regulated across either different brain regions or points in developmental time. The majority of this differential expression occurred during prenatal development, with patterns of expression tending to become more fixed with increasing age (Kang *et al.*, 2011).

One mechanism that promotes stability within the dynamic epigenome is genomic imprinting. This is a process through which certain genes (less than 1% in mammals) are expressed according to the parent-of-origin of that variant of the gene. Effectively, genomic imprinting silences the allele from either the mother or the father, leaving the remaining one to be exclusively expressed (Keverne *et al.*, 1996). These epigenetic marks are present from the outset of an embryo and can be maintained throughout the life span. Some developmental disorders, such as Angelman syndrome and Prader-Willi syndrome are associated with deficits in this process (see Chapter 55).

Plasticity in brain development is a phenomenon that has generated much controversy, but the biological description of development as being a "restriction of fate" means we can simply view plasticity as the state of a brain region's structure or function not yet being fully specialized. That is, there is still remaining scope for developing more finely tuned neural architecture or responses. By this view the mechanisms of plasticity remain the same throughout the life span, but the expression of plasticity is more limited in adulthood because most aspects of brain structure and function have already become determined, and thus there is less scope for further change. In this way, reduced plasticity can be viewed as the flip side of advancing development. This is one reason why early life intervention, potentially prior to the onset of clinical symptoms, is favored in child psychiatry (see Chapter 32).

Box 10.1 The human brain relation to the basic vertebrate brain plan

- Human brains follow a basic vertebrate brain plan, with the major difference in higher primates being the dramatic expansion of the overlying cerebral cortex, together with associated structures such as the basal ganglia.
- The cerebral cortex of all mammals, including humans, is basically a thin (about 3–4 mm) flat sheet. Although complex, its general layered structure is relatively constant throughout its extent. The rapid expansion in the overall size of the cortex during evolution has resulted in it becoming increasingly intricately folded with various indentations (sulci) and lobes (gyri) (Figure 10.1).
- Most sensory inputs to the cortex pass through a structure known as the thalamus. Each type of sensory input has its own particular nuclei within this region. For example, the lateral geniculate nucleus (LGN) carries visual input to the cortex, while the medial geniculate nucleus (MGN) carries information from the auditory modality.
- Most areas of the neocortex are made up of six layers (Figure 10.1). The basic characteristics that define each layer appear to hold in most regions of the cortical sheet. Although this basic laminar structure holds throughout most of the neocortex, there are some regional variations that define structural areas. For example, different regions of the cortex have different input and projection patterns to other cortical and subcortical areas, are associated with a particular mix of neurotransmitters including the relative contribution of excitatory compared to inhibitory neurotransmitters, and also vary in the timing of key developmental events such as the postnatal reduction in the number of synapses.

What makes the human brain unique?

Human brains follow a basic vertebrate brain plan that is found even in species such as salamanders, frogs, and birds. Despite the evolutionary continuity in this basic plan, one of the major differences between these species and higher primates is in the dramatic expansion of the overlying cerebral cortex, together with associated structures such as the basal ganglia (Box 10.1). This raises the question of what is unique about the human brain and the developmental processes that give rise to it (and relatedly, how applicable are studies on other species to our understanding of human brain development).

As a first approximation, across different species brain size correlates with both body size and the length of developmental time it takes to reach its adult size. As large mammals, primates generally have a much more prolonged timetable for brain development than other mammals. Even between humans and other primates there is a wide difference in timing. In particular, our own species' period of postnatal cortical development is extended by roughly a factor of four compared to most other primates. What is the significance of this extended timetable of brain development?

Finlay and Darlington (1995) compared data on the size of brain structures from 131 different mammalian species, and showed that developmental landmarks are related to the relative size of parts of the adult brain in a systematic way, with disproportionately large growth occurring in the later-generated structures. From this analysis, the structure most likely to differ in size in the comparatively slowed timetable of neurogenesis in primates is the cerebral cortex (Box 10.1). Thus, the increased quantity of cortical tissue in our brains is at least, in part, a by-product of still further slowing down of the overall mammalian time course of brain development.

In addition to differences in the overall rate of brain development, however, different mammalian species are born at different stages of brain development. In this regard, while humans have the survival disadvantage of being born relatively immature and largely immobile, the resulting highly prolonged period of postnatal development allows much more scope and time for interaction with the social and physical environment of the child to contribute to the tuning and shaping of circuitry. Viewed from this perspective, the high importance of parent–infant bonding and interaction as part of the constructed niche of our species becomes evident.

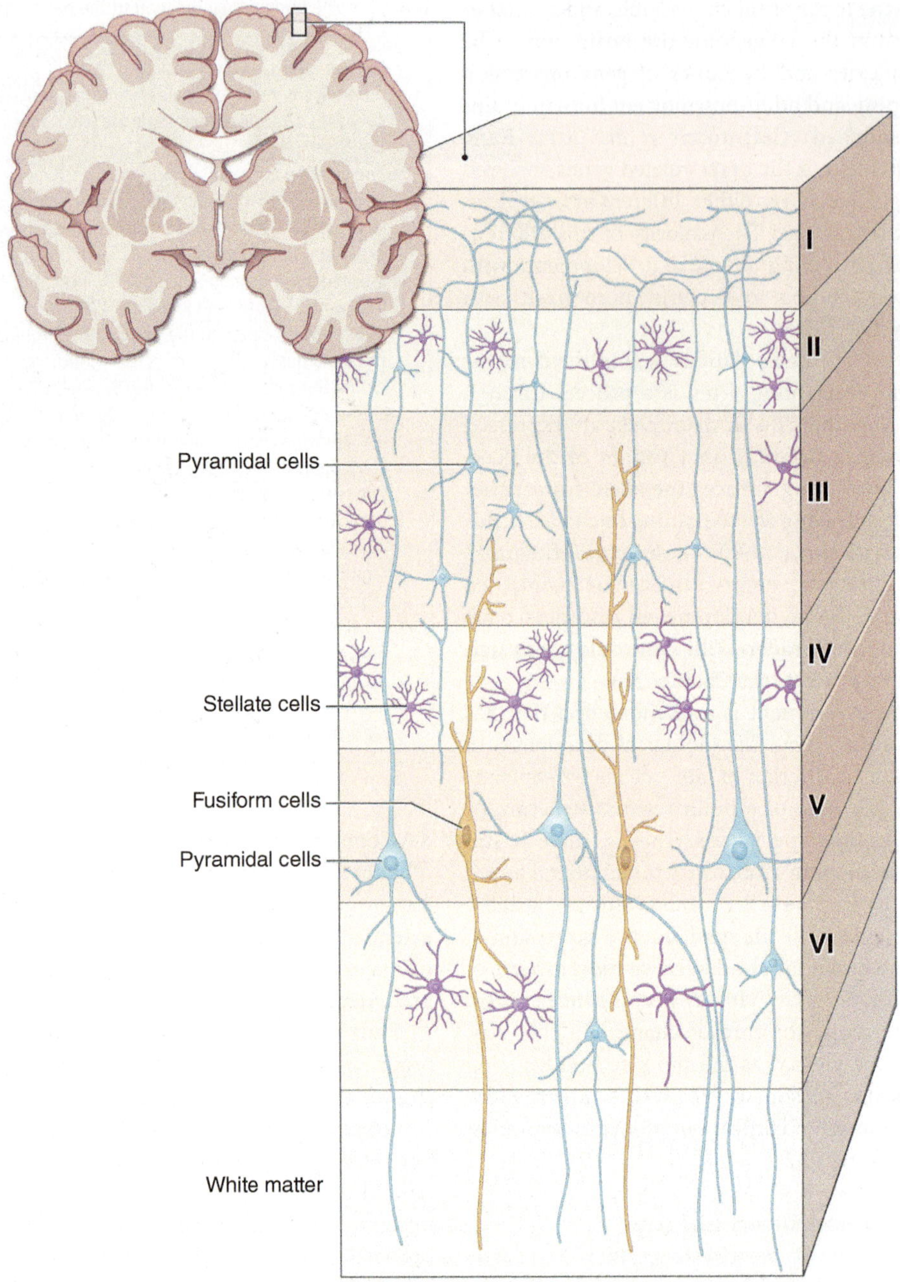

Figure 10.1 An illustration of the layered structure of the cerebral cortex. A small section of cerebral cortex is amplified in scale to illustrate how the mix of types of neurons varies between different layers. Pyramidal, stellate, and fusiform cells are common across different cortical layers.

Whether it is just the slowed timing of brain development that produces the unique human brain remains controversial. Subtle differences in the steps of brain development between primates and rodents are already known, and some reports of possibly species-specific progenitor cells or neurons in humans merit further research (Bystron *et al.*, 2008).

Human structural brain development

The sequence of events involved in the prenatal development of the human brain closely resembles that of many other vertebrates. After initial divisions of the fertilized cell, a cluster of proliferating cells (called the blastocyst) differentiates into a three-layered structure (the embryonic disk) with each of these layers further differentiating into major organ systems. The outer layer (ectoderm) gives rise to the nervous system through a process known as *neurulation*. Specifically, a portion of the ectoderm begins to fold in on itself to form a hollow cylinder called the *neural tube*, which then differentiates further to give rise to the major subdivisions of the central nervous system, with the forebrain and midbrain arising at one end and the spinal cord at the other. One end differentiates into a series of repeated units or segments to become the spinal cord, while at the other end of the neural tube a series of bulges and convolutions form. Around five weeks after conception in humans these bulges can be identified as protoforms for the cortex (telencephalon), the thalamus and hypothalamus (diencephalon), the midbrain (mesencephalon), the cerebellum (metencephalon), and the medulla (myelencephalon).

Differentiation within these different bulges gives rise to the complex layering patterns and cell types found in the adult brain (Box 10.2; Figure 10.2). Within these bulges, cells *proliferate* (are born), *migrate* (travel), and *differentiate* (change form) into particular types. The vast majority of the cells that will compose the brain are born in the so-called *proliferative zones*. These zones are close to the hollow portion of the neural tube (which subsequently become the ventricles of the brain). The first of these proliferation sites, the *ventricular zone*, may be phylogenetically older (Nowakowski,1987). The second, the *subventricular zone*, only contributes significantly to phylogenetically recent brain structures such as the neocortex (i.e., "new" cortex). These two zones yield separate glial (support and supply cells) and neuron cell lines and give rise to different forms of migration.

Neurons and glial cells are produced within these zones by the division of cells to produce clones (a clone is a group of cells which are produced by the division of a single precursor cell—such a precursor cell is said to give rise to a lineage—see earlier section on "The importance of interconnectivity"). *Glioblasts* produce a variety of different cells (subtypes of glial cells) that serve a variety of functions to support, guide, and protect neurons. In particular, recent work shows that microglia are key to development (Mehl *et al.*, 2022).

Box 10.2 The cells of the brain

- The brain has two general classes of cells—neurons and glial cells.
- Glial cells are more common than neurons, but are generally assumed to play no direct role in computation. Glial cells are, however, important for a variety of support functions including guiding young neurons to their final destinations within the cortex, and covering connecting fibers with myelin.
- The computational unit of the brain is the neuron. Neurons come in many shapes, sizes, and types, each of which reflects their particular function. There are at least 25 different neuronal types within the cerebral cortex alone, although several of these types are relatively rare, and some are restricted to particular layers. One of the most common types of neurons in the cerebral cortex is a pyramidal cell (Figure 10.2).

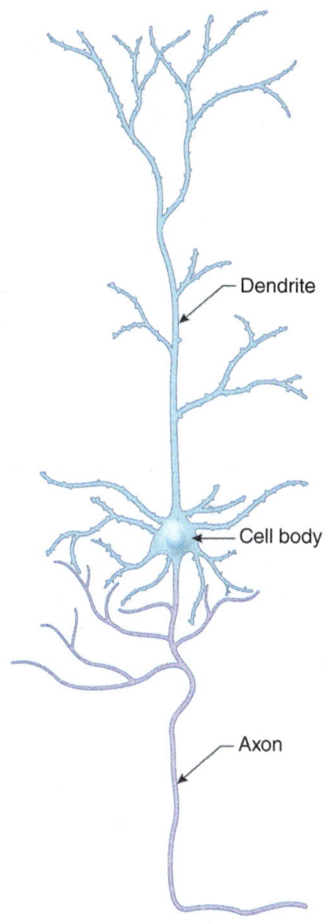

Figure 10.2 An illustration of the parts of common cortical neuron, a pyramidal cell (so-called due to its pyramid-shaped cell body). Illustrated are the dendrites (or "dendritic tree") that collects and summates signals for integration at the cell body, and the axon that transmits the discharge or firing of the neuron elsewhere in the brain.

Neuroblasts produce neurons, and in some cases particular neuroblasts also give rise to specific types of cells. For example, less than a dozen proliferating cells produce all the Purkinje cells of the cerebellar cortex, with each producing about 10,000 cells (Nowakowski, 1987). After young neurons are born, they *migrate* from the proliferative zones to the particular region where they are located in the mature brain. The first and more common type of migration is *passive cell displacement*. This occurs when cells that have been generated are then simply pushed further away from the proliferative zones by more recently born cells. This form of migration gives rise to an "outside-in" pattern with the oldest cells being pushed toward the surface of the brain, while the most recently produced cells remain closer to their place of birth. Passive migration gives rise to brain structures such as the thalamus, the dentate gyrus of the hippocampus, and parts of the brain stem.

The second form of migration is more active and involves the young cell moving past previously generated cells to create an "inside-out" pattern. This pattern is found in the cerebral cortex and in other areas that have a laminar structure (divided into parallel layers). In the case of the cerebral cortex, a "radial unit" model of neocortical differentiation gives an account of how both the layered and the regional structure of the mammalian cerebral cortex arises (Rakic, 1988). According to the model, the laminar organization of the cerebral cortex is determined by the fact that each proliferative cell (in the subventricular zone) gives rise to approximately 100 neurons. The progeny from each proliferative cell all migrate up the same route, with the latest to be born traveling past their older cousins. The route they take is determined by following a radial glial fiber—a long process that stretches from top to bottom of the cortex and originates from a specialized glial cell. These radial glial fibers act like a guidance rope to help ensure that cells produced by one proliferative unit all contribute to one radial column within the cortex.

While the "radial unit model" explains how cortical cells arrange themselves into the (approximately 100 neuron) thickness of the cortex, how does the differentiation into specific layers emerge? While we are far from being able to answer this question definitively at this point, in some cases differentiation into particular cell types occurs *before* each neuron reaches its final location. However, in other cases some of the properties that distinguish among cell types may only form later. For example, the distinctive apical dendrite of pyramidal cells, which often reaches into the upper layer of the cortex (layer 1), may be a result of the increasing distance between this layer and other layers resulting from the inside-out pattern of growth (Marin-Padilla, 1990; Figures 10.1 and 10.2).

Not all migration within the cortex follows the radial unit model (Polleux *et al.*, 2002). Interspersed between pyramidal cells are a variety of types of interneurons that help balance excitation and inhibition within the cortex. Theories of developmental conditions such as autism involve dysregulation of this balance (Le Blanc & Fagiolini, 2011), and in some cases this may be due to differences in the molecular mechanisms known to control migration processes (Polleux *et al.*, 2002).

In recent years a new approach to studying the development of the human brain has been to use cerebral organoids (Nowakowski & Salama, 2022). This entails making pluripotent stem cells (cells—sometimes derived from skin—that are regressed back to an earlier developmental stage in which they still have the potential to become a variety of other kinds of cells, including neurons and glial cells) and allowing them to grow into brain tissues within three-dimensional cultures. Advances now allow these organoids to form multiple different neuron and glial cell types, self-organize, and recapitulate the early stages of formation of the cortex including its layered structure and some regional variations. Strikingly, both spontaneous and evoked activity can be established, indicating that complex patterns of neural activity can be studied (Sharf *et al.*, 2022).

Returning to humans, by the time of birth the vast majority of neurons have been born (Box 10.3), migrated to their final locations, and have differentiated into recognizable types. The main lobes and sulci of the cortex are also developed. Nevertheless, a considerable portion of human brain development continues into postnatal years.

Box 10.3 Postnatal migration of neurons in humans

- It was thought that all neurons are already in place within the brain at birth in humans. More recent evidence, however, has revealed several instances where there is either continuing cell birth or postnatal migration of neurons.
- In the hippocampus, new neurons can be born even in adults following environmental changes (Toda *et al.*, 2019).
- During the first postnatal year streams of young migrating neurons in the temporal lobe make their way into the entorhinal cortex (that interfaces with the hippocampus) (Nascimento *et al.*, 2022) and to the prefrontal cortex where they contribute to inhibitory circuits, potentially changing plasticity and the excitation–inhibition balance (Paredes *et al.*, 2016, Kim & Paredes, 2021) (Figure 10.3).

Key features of postnatal development

As mentioned, key features of human brain development are its comparatively prolonged time schedule, and the relatively immature point on the sequence of development at which we are born. These factors combine to allow for a greatly extended period of postnatal brain development in relation to most other mammals, and a correspondingly large increase in the total volume of the brain from birth to teenage years. Since the formation of neurons and their migration to appropriate brain regions takes place almost entirely within the period of prenatal development in the human (Box 10.2), these processes do not account for the increase in volume. However, there is a dramatic postnatal increase in the size and complexity of the dendritic tree of most neurons. While the extent and reach of a cell's dendritic arbor may increase dramatically, its patterns of connectivity with other cells also become more specific. Huttenlocher and colleagues have reported a steady increase in the density of synapses in several regions of the human cerebral cortex (Huttenlocher, 1994). While an increase in synapses (synaptogenesis) begins around the time of birth in humans for all cortical areas studied to date, the most rapid bursts of increase, and the final peak density, occur at different ages in different areas. For example, in sensorimotor areas there is a rapid burst at 3–4 months, and the maximum density of around 150% of adult level is reached between 4 and 12 months. In contrast, while synaptogenesis starts at the same time in the prefrontal cortex, density increases much more slowly and does not reach its peak until well after the first year (Figure 10.4).

Similar "rise and fall" patterns of development have been observed in other measures of human brain development. For example, using positron emission tomography (PET) imaging Chugani *et al.* (2002) measured overall resting brain metabolism (the uptake of glucose from the blood is essential for cell functioning) in early postnatal development. They observed a sharp increase in glucose uptake followed by a later decline;

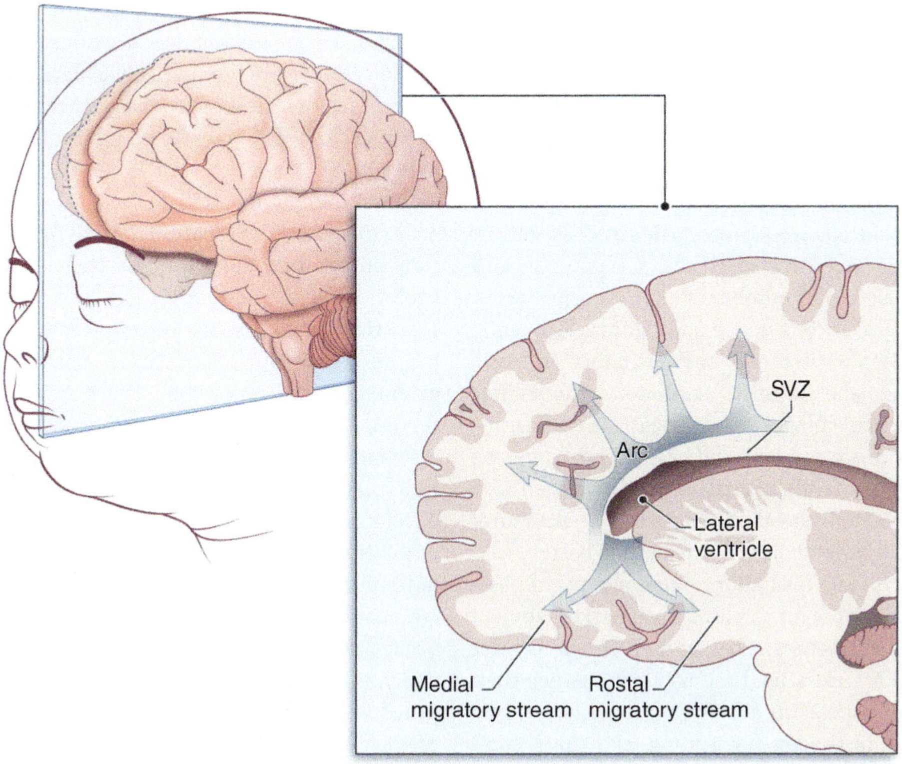

Figure 10.3 An illustration of the migratory streams of young neurons toward the temporal and frontal lobe during early postnatal human brain development. Neurons originate around the lateral ventricle (Arc, SVZ). *Source*: Paredes *et al.* (2016) with permission of American Association for the Advancement of Science (AAAS).

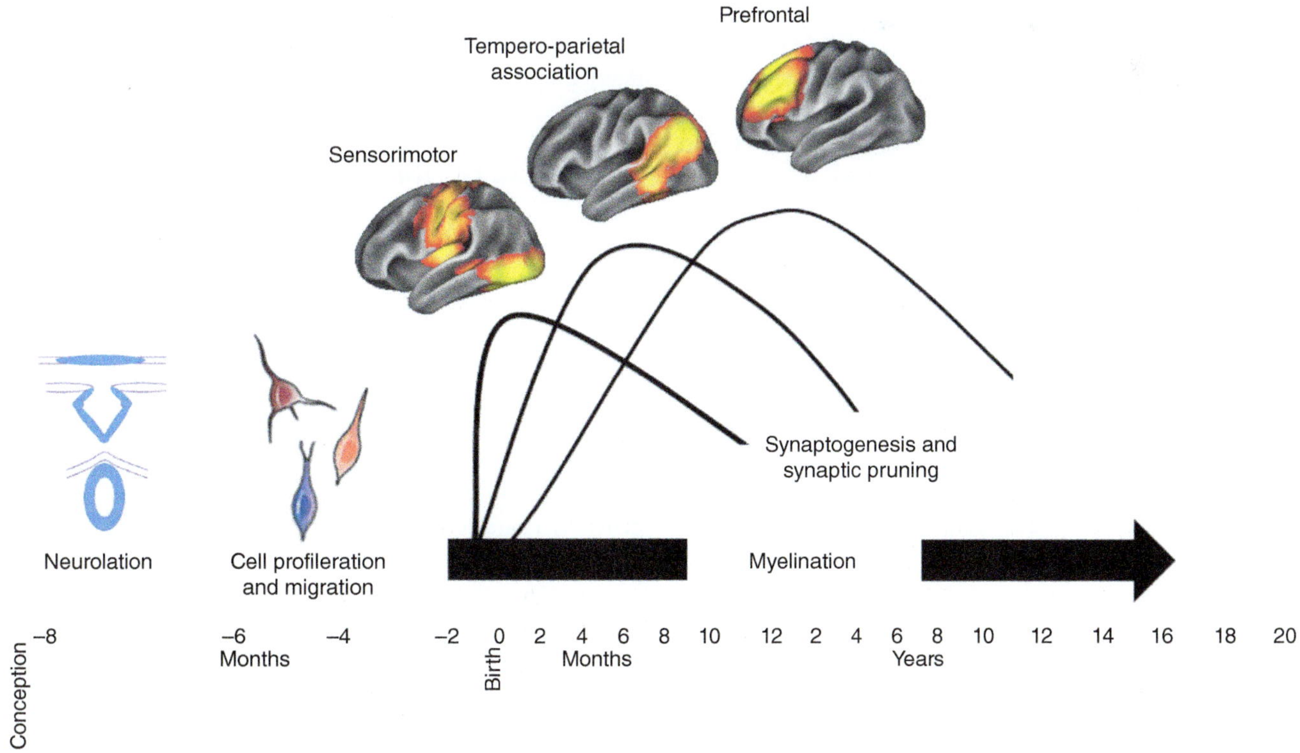

Figure 10.4 An approximate timeline for some of the most important pre- and postnatal changes during human brain development. *Source*: Adapted from Casey (2005).

with a peak approximately 150% above adult levels achieved somewhere around 4–5 years of age for some cortical areas. While this peak occurred somewhat later than that in synaptic density, an adult-like *distribution* of resting activity within and across brain regions was observed by the end of the first year.

While the developmental events discussed so far concern aspects of the structure of the brain, it is important to note that there are also significant changes in the "soft soak" aspects of neural function, molecules involved in the transmission and modulation of neural signals. A number of neurotransmitters in rodents and humans also show the rise and fall developmental pattern (Benes, 1994). For example, the excitatory intrinsic transmitter glutamate, the intrinsic inhibitory transmitter gamma-aminobutyric acid (GABA), and the extrinsic transmitter serotonin all show this same developmental trend. Thus, the distinctive "rise and fall" developmental sequence is seen in a number of microscopic and metabolic measures of structural and neurophysiological development in the human cortex.

In contrast to the rise and fall pattern, other aspects of postnatal human brain development, such as myelination, show a steady increase (Figure 10.4; see Chapter 11). In the central nervous system, sensory areas tend to myelinate earlier than motor areas. Cortical association areas are known to become myelinated last with the process continuing into the second decade of life. Because myelination is a prominent feature of postnatal development, there has been much speculation linking it to advances in behavioral and cognitive development. However, while myelination greatly increases the speed and fidelity of transmission of impulses (by as much as 100 times) it is also important to remember that undermyelinated connections in the young human brain are still capable of transmitting signals, and that some connections in the adult brain never myelinate. As we will return to later, this means that myelin does not act merely as a passive insulator, but is itself modulated by neuronal activity and experience. The end result is that it does not simply speed transmission, but rather that myelin plasticity enhances circuit functions through the increased precision of timing activity, in particular the summation and integration of information across circuits (Bonetto *et al.*, 2021).

More recently, the steady expansion of magnetic resonance imaging (MRI) methods have come to the fore in studying the structural development of the brain at a systems level, and across increasingly large sample sizes (Wood, 2022). MRI reveals brain structure at a less detailed scale than neurons and synapses, but it is sufficient to allow the measurement of gray and white matter in different cortical and subcortical regions (see Chapter 11). A rapid expansion of cortical and subcortical gray matter occurs within the first two years after birth, with the rate peaking at around six months, followed by a plateau by late childhood and a relative pruning in adolescence. By contrast there is a steadier increase in white matter, with the rate peaking at around 2–3 years from birth, and not plateauing until adulthood (Bethlehem *et al.*, 2022). There is, however, considerable variability between individuals, although larger sample sizes have revealed that the links between individual cortical regions and cognition or behavior are far subtler than previously thought with relatively crude case-control comparisons (Marek *et al.*, 2022). For some cortical regions most of the rise occurs before puberty, and most of the decline after puberty going into early adulthood (Gogtay *et al.*, 2004).

Most of the remainder of the cortex develops in a hierarchical manner, with the spatiotemporal pattern of cortical maturation proceeding along an axis that is likely to be rooted in evolution. This developmental axis appears to mirror the sensorimotor-to-association gradient (Sydnor *et al.*, 2021), and can be seen in structural, functional, metabolic, and, to some extent, gene expression data. One possibility is that this gradient serves to maximize the adaptability of the most slow-developing association cortices, although multiple theoretical perspectives now highlight that this could itself confer a vulnerability for developmental psychopathology.

Overall, a number of different measures and laboratories have found the rise and fall pattern for neurons and their local connectivity. However, it should be noted that measures such as synaptic density are but static snapshots of a dynamic process in which both additive and regressive processes are continually in progress. Thus, there are probably not distinct and separate progressive and regressive phases, but a shift in balance between these processes during development. It is also worth noting that for any given cortical region there are often multiple waves of remodeling of synaptic architecture during development. Some of these waves of change in the morphology and density of synapses correspond to sensitive periods in which sensory or environmental information can have maximum effect on the developing brain (Meredith *et al.*, 2012).

Oscillating rhythms

Even simple nervous systems show spontaneous activity that is only sometimes driven by sensory or motor events. Indeed, experiments in which stem cells were cultured *in vitro* to develop into clusters of neurons have demonstrated that simple circuits can form with primitive oscillatory firing patterns (Shi *et al.*, 2012), suggesting that oscillatory activity is a fundamental property of nervous systems. In advanced brains, oscillatory activity can occur at multiple different frequencies simultaneously. These frequencies can vary from high (40 Hz or higher, generally characteristic of local circuit activity in the cerebral cortex) to low (0.1 Hz or lower, generally characteristic of longer-range connectivity, or even glial cell activity). Oscillatory activity that is evoked by, or entrained to, sensory events can be studied noninvasively with electroencephalography (EEG), event-related potentials (ERPs), or magnetoencephalography (MEG) methods. Many evoked potentials recorded at the scalp may reflect the entrainment of ongoing oscillatory activity at specific frequencies (Palva & Palva, 2012). In development, some of these spontaneous rhythms may have particular importance in consolidating or weakening structural and functional connections between regions.

From an early stage of prenatal development, interactions between cells are critical, including the transmission of electrical signals between neurons. In one example, patterns of spontaneous firing of cells in the eyes (before they have opened and exposed themselves to light) transmit signals that appear to then help induce the layered structure of the LGN (Shatz, 2002). Thus, waves of firing neurons intrinsic to the developing organism may play an important role in specifying aspects of brain structure well before sensory inputs from the external world have any effect.

After birth, when sensory systems are bombarded with stimulation, the spontaneous oscillations of the brain can become entrained or perturbed by sensory-evoked activity in ways that are still poorly understood (see Palva & Palva, 2012). Oscillations at different frequencies are not just epiphenomena of patterns of neuron firing, but are likely to "bind" activity states across near and far regions of the brain. Indeed, some have argued that oscillation frequencies characterize distinct functional networks, and keep their information processing distinct from other concurrently active regions (Singer & Gray, 1995). In addition, high-frequency oscillations (above 30 Hz—called gamma) may play a role in sustaining interactions between regions of the cerebral cortex. Scores of studies in developmental psychopathology have focused on differences in specific ERP waveforms assumed to reflect differences in regional patterns of activation, or the time course or degree of latency jitter of these peaks of voltage change (e.g., Tye *et al.*, 2013).

Resting activity and network connectivity

It has been hypothesized that resting state activity in the brain (ongoing activity that is not task related) may provide a critical bridge between structural and functional development (Johnson, 2011). This is because this activity of the brain at rest can reflect averages of sensory- and task-driven activation patterns over an extended time period, and consolidation of experience-driven co-activation patterns between regions may require the prolonged activation that resting or default states can provide. Specifically, regions that show coherent (in phase) oscillatory activity may maintain or strengthen structural connections between them. Other regions that may oscillate at similar frequencies, but out of phase, may lose or reduce synaptic connections with the emerging coherent network.

Networks of resting state activity have been used to trace developmental changes in human brain networks and even provided the basis for a "maturational index" (Schlaggar *et al.*, 2002). Even at birth, the brain has clear characteristic patterns of network connectivity, including densely connected hub regions (Ball *et al.*, 2014). The preferential connections between these hubs over time creates a so-called "rich club" (Ball *et al.*, 2014). These hubs seem to play a role in controlling network states across the system, and, over developmental time, the strengthening versus weakening of certain modes of connectivity results in the gradual segregation of structural and functional modules, and within-module integration. The time course of this gradual modularization varies across individuals and may itself be a marker of impactful cognitive or behavioral characteristics. In turn, this conceptualization of developmental neurobiology as system-level changes in connectivity has opened the door to computational frameworks that explicitly model the formation of networks, with the aim of revealing otherwise hidden biological processes (Akarca *et al.*, 2021).

A final aspect of the transition from the child brain network to the adult one is the greater connectivity between cortical and subcortical structures seen at younger ages (Supekar *et al.*, 2009), an observation that may be fundamental for our understanding of the emergence of the social brain and memory systems, as it implies that the specialization of some cortical areas may be initially more dominated by structures such as the amygdala and hippocampus.

What determines how parts of the cortex become specialized?

A long-standing debate among those who study the developmental neurobiology of the cortex concerns the extent to which its structure and function in adults are the result of genetic, molecular, and cellular level interactions, as opposed to being the result of the pattern of activity generated by firing of neurons. In the adult primate the identity of most cortical areas can be distinguished by very detailed differences in their laminar structure, such as the precise thickness of certain layers. Often, however, the boundaries between areas are sometimes indistinct and difficult to discern. It is commonly assumed that these anatomically defined areas have particular, unique functions contained within their boundaries. While this has proved to be the case for early sensory and motor areas, there are many cases of *functional* regions that do not neatly correspond to known *neuroanatomical* divisions or borders.

Traditionally, two opposing possibilities have been put forward to account for the division of the cerebral cortex into distinct areas: *Protomap* and *Protocortex*. According to the *Protomap* (Rakic, 1988) view, differentiation into cortical regions occurs early in the formation of the cortex, and is due to intrinsic molecular factors. The alternative possibility is that different areas of cortex arise out of an undifferentiated *Protocortex*. By this view, differentiation occurs later in the development of cortex, and it depends at least partly on extrinsic factors like input from other parts of the brain or sensory systems. The activity of neurons is required for regional differentiation (O'Leary & Nakagawa, 2002). Reviews of the evidence converge on views that are midway between the protomap and protocortex hypotheses (Bystron *et al.*, 2008; Cadwell *et al.*, 2019). Most agree that graded patterns of gene expression create large-scale regions with combinations of properties that may better suit certain computations (similar to a coarse or imprecise proto-map). It is within these large-scale regions that smaller-scale functional areas arise through the activity-dependent mechanisms associated with the protocortex view. Kingsbury and Finlay (2001) refer to this as a "hyperdimensional plaid" because the patterning that emerges in a plaid is the result of small changes in many threads. Similarly, O'Leary and colleagues call this the "cooperative concentration" model since some different gradients of gene expression may act as opposing forces in shaping cortical regions (Hamasaki *et al.*, 2002).

Human functional brain development

Relating evidence on the neuroanatomical development of the brain to the remarkable changes in motor, perceptual, and cognitive abilities during the first decade or so of human life presents a considerable challenge. To briefly recap, we presented a probabilistic epigenesis view of development in which interactions between genes, structural brain changes, and psychological function are viewed as bidirectional, dynamic, and emergent, as opposed to a unidirectional causal path from genes to structural changes to psychological consequences. We also saw that mammalian neurodevelopment is best characterized as being regulatory, rather than mosaic; the response properties of a cortical area are heavily interdependent upon its connectivity to other regions and their respective activity patterns. Further, with regard to structure-to-function mappings, the same overt behavioral responses can sometimes be supported by different combinations of regional activity within the brain, thus providing potential mechanisms for adaptation. We also saw how development can be viewed as a "restriction of fate," and how plasticity becomes correspondingly reduced as potential developmental paths are reduced through the increase in specialization of cells or circuits.

Building on these foundations, the "interactive specialization" (IS) framework assumes that postnatal functional brain development, at least within the cerebral cortex, involves a process of organizing patterns of interregional interactions (Johnson, 2011), and it focuses on how the partial or immature functioning of regions transition gradually to their adult state. According to IS, the response properties of a given cortical region are partly determined by its patterns of connectivity to other regions, and their respective patterns of activity. During postnatal development, changes in the response properties of association cortex regions occur as they interact and compete with each other to acquire their role in new computational abilities. From this perspective, some cortical regions start with poorly defined, general-purpose functions, and consequently are partially activated in a wide range of different stimuli, contexts, and tasks. During development, activity-dependent interactions between regions sharpen up their functions such that their activity becomes restricted to a narrower set of circumstances (i.e., a region originally activated by a wide variety of visual objects may come to confine its response to upright human faces). The onset of new behavioral competencies will therefore be associated with changes in network activity over several regions, and not just by the onset of activity in one or more additional region(s).

Variability in neurodevelopment

Consideration of two aspects of human brain development should inform our thinking about why the process can have variable outcomes and how the differences associated with neurodevelopmental conditions emerge. On the one hand, we have seen that constructing a brain requires an exquisite and complex series of interacting events in which there are many possibilities for specific events, or their timings, to shape that construction. Indeed, some theorists argue that the stochastic nature of development, and the diverse outcomes it produces, is itself *desirable* from an evolutionary perspective (Hiesinger & Hassan, 2018). Put simply, maximizing adaptability, both as individuals and a as a species, and diverse outcomes, go hand-in-hand. From this perspective it is almost surprising that the human brain has such consistent structural and functional hallmarks. On the other hand, we have also described a number of mechanisms of stability and inherent plasticity that constrain and guide the self-organization of the brain. Viewed from this perspective, brain development is an inevitable outcome of a combination of processes, and seems to be well buffered from any minor perturbations. From the latter perspective, one might speculate that we should expect a large degree of variability stemming from multiple "minor" factors that combine to shape the way the emerging system adapts and compensates. Another possibility is that processes may be disrupted in some more fundamental way, making it difficult for the system to adapt or compensate, and resulting in more substantial divergence from the typical brain development pathway.

Many of the key points from typical human neurodevelopment discussed earlier are of direct relevance to our interpretation of developmental pathways that diverge away from the typical. We have seen that development is a process of increased differentiation of cells, neural regions, and networks. Although, for a particular environment, a specific trajectory of differentiation or specialization may characterize the majority outcome, we have also seen that apparently the same behaviors can be supported by different patterns of network activity at different ages. Even in the adult end-state, individual differences can be extensive, and research that compares groups of typical adult participants raised in different cultures has also shown a surprising degree of differences in the neural substrates of perceptual and cognitive functions (Chiao, 2009). Thus, the pathway of typical neurodevelopment should not be thought of as a single narrow track from which it is easy to deviate, but rather as a deep and broad valley whose steep sides buffer against escape.

Given that typical neurodevelopment is a broad and robust process, how are we to understand divergence from this developmental path, potentially resulting in diagnosable conditions?

Much of the neuroimaging work to date on developmental conditions such as autism and attention deficit/hyperactivity disorder (ADHD), has aimed at identifying differences in discrete brain regions, structures, or systems. These differences are then used as a basis for theory about the origins of the varied behavioral characteristics associated with these conditions (Astle & Fletcher-Watson, 2020). However, these local differences can be remarkably inconsistent across studies. Instead, the most robust differences seem to reflect broader principles of organization that subtly shape brain development (Siugzdaite *et al.*, 2020). Put simply, the conceptualization of neurodevelopmental conditions as reflecting typically developed brains with discrete and localizable "damage," has little robust support.

This conclusion also extends to many developmental disorders of known genetic etiology such as Fragile-X, Williams Syndrome, and Down Syndrome.

For example, Fragile-X involves the *FMR1* gene on the X chromosome. The changes in the gene results in a lack of the particular protein for which it codes: FMR1 protein. One of the knock-on consequences of the reduction of this protein is a disturbance in the neurotransmitter glutamate. However, despite the apparent specificity of this initial causal pathway, the effects are widespread and include several different aspects of physical and cognitive development. Thus, although Fragile-X involves only one gene, there are multiple and widespread neurodevelopmental consequences. Some of the broad phenotypic effects may be the result of compensatory processes at molecular, cellular, and system levels (Johnson *et al.*, 2021).

Factors that influence developmental pathways

Traditionally, factors that cause human brain development to deviate from the typical path (risk factors) were viewed as either intrinsic to the brain itself due to some pre- or perinatal genetic, neuroanatomical, or neurochemical atypicality, or as being environmentally caused. More recently, it has become evident that, at least for some phenotypic outcomes, intrinsic and environmental factors interact (see Chapter 23).

As mentioned, in most developmental conditions we are studying brains that have developed differently. At the point of diagnosis the relevant behavioral phenotypes are, by definition, established and embedded. It is evident from the preceding discussion of developmental neurobiology that the phenotypic end-state will include not only residual signs of the original neurobiological difference, but also compounded effects due to atypical intrinsic and environmental interactions, and the results of compensatory adaptation (Johnson *et al.*, 2021). While the vast majority of neuroscience imaging work on children and adults with developmental disorders necessarily conflate these factors, Kaiser *et al.* (2010) used functional magnetic resonance imaging (fMRI) to study patterns of brain activation in autistic children, nonautistic siblings of autistic children, and neurotypicals, while they viewed videos of biological motion. These authors found that the nonautistic siblings had some patterns of activation in common with their autistic relatives, but not neurotypicals. This "trait" activity was consistent with a "neuroendophenotype" that extends to family members, and raises the possibility that nonautistic siblings actively accommodate this neurobiological difference in some way. Encouraging this view was the existence of patterns of activation consistent with so-called "compensatory activity." These areas were not activated in either autistics or the controls, and had the hallmark of regions whose additional activity allowed children to actively accommodate a neurobiological difference elsewhere in the system, resulting in a neurotypical performance profile. Put simply, it is likely that so-called neural correlates of particular neurodevelopmental differences might reflect both some initial underlying neurobiological difference in combination with a set of adaptive mechanisms, both of which shape performance.

In considering the difficulty in interpreting neuroscience data from a brain that has undergone considerable postnatal adaptation, several groups have taken a new approach to developmental conditions based on the prospective longitudinal study of infants with an elevated familial likelihood of a particular diagnosis (most commonly infant siblings in families with an older child already diagnosed). Here the aim is to identify and study the earliest "pure" manifestations of the condition, before the establishment of confounding and compensatory factors that result from the subsequent years of adaptation and accommodation (Dawson *et al.*, 2023).

Future directions

Developmental neurobiology is an exciting and rapidly moving field, with new techniques and methods becoming available every few years. However, the allure of obtaining new kinds and quantities of empirical data should not distract us from the key questions and issues around human developmental psychopathology. It seems likely that for many developmental conditions we will need to understand how large-scale networks of neurons are influenced by alterations of their underlying molecular and cellular function. It will be important to remember that different kinds of molecular or cellular atypicalities can sometimes give rise to the same functional consequences at an overall neuronal network level. Thus, ultimately it may be at the level of whole neural systems that some developmental conditions are best understood. However, this change in focus requires us to have a better understanding of the temporal and spatial dynamics of multicellular activity in the brain, something that has been hampered by the fact that most current neuroimaging methods have either relatively poor spatial or temporal resolution.

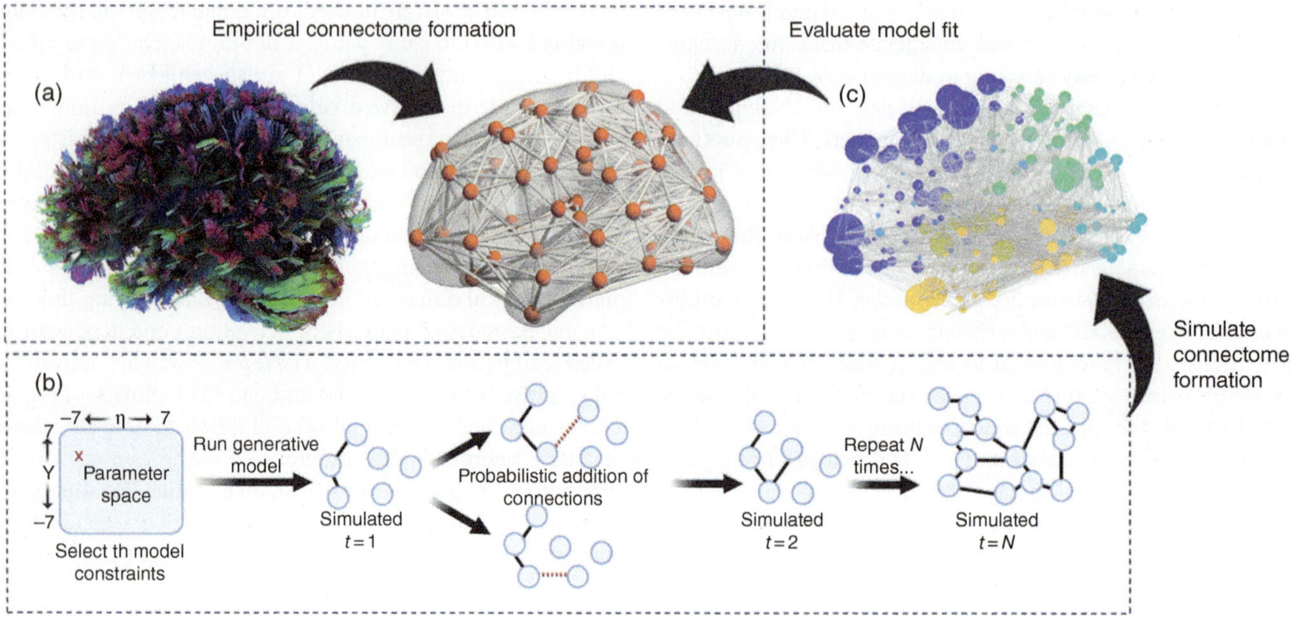

Figure 10.5 Infographic illustrating how generative artificial neural networks can be generated to simulate the growth of connectivity in real human brains: (a) illustrates how connectivity maps can be produced from structural magnetic resonance imaging (MRI) scans; (b) illustrates how generative artificial neural networks can be "grown" to produce simulated connectivity networks; and (c) represents the process of comparison between the real brain network and the simulations. The parameters of the simulation can be varied to find the best fit, allowing exploration of the developmental factors that give rise to typical and atypical brain connectivity. *Source*: Akarca *et al.* (2021)/Springer Nature/CC BY 4.0.

In recent years, one of the most exciting advances has been the application of artificial intelligence (AI)-inspired analytical tools, to build computational models of neurobiological processes. These models are themselves biophysically grounded, that is, they are artificial systems constrained within neurobiological reality. Traditionally, this type of modeling has been restricted to specific neurobiological processes like synaptogenesis, pruning, or axonal guidance. But more recently this approach is increasingly applied to whole-brain data, thereby capturing emergent organizational principles (Vertes *et al.*, 2012). These generative computational frameworks are allowing researchers to work systematically across different scales within a common empirical approach. For example, the same modeling framework can be used to identify the types of regionwise interactions that give rise to the key topological hallmarks of the human brain (Akarca *et al.*, 2021) (Figure 10.5). The same approach is being applied at a microstructural level, *in vitro*, as neuronal cell cultures self-organize over time, and in combination with experimental perturbations that allow researchers to isolate the neurochemical processes responsible for shaping this self-organization (Akarca, 2022). In other words, this revolution in the application of AI-inspired models is allowing us to fill the gap between developmental theory and neurobiological observation.

We began this chapter by stating that the brain is primarily an organ of adaptation at multiple different temporal scales and levels of organization. An exciting challenge for the future will be to understand how these processes drive variability in development, and, in cases where that development results in impactful cognitive or behavioral barriers to learning or well-being, to intervene effectively.

Definitions

Differentiation—the process through which cells take on their final (adult) morphology
EEG—electroencephalogram, the recording of brain electrical activity from sensors at the scalp
Endophenotype—an intermediate phenotype often associated with neural processes or systems
Epigenesis—the expression of genes during development
Laminar—refers to the layered structure of the cerebral cortex
MEG—magnetoencephalography, the detection of magnetic fields produced by electric currents in the brain
Migration—the traveling of cells from their location of origin
MRI—magnetic resonance imaging
Myelination—the process of depositing a fatty sheath around neural fibers
Neurogenesis—the process of generating new neurons
Progenitor cells—stem cells that give rise to neurons

Acknowledgments

MJ acknowledges financial support from the UK Medical Research Council (Programme Grant MR/T003057/1) and DA from the UK Medical Research Council (Programme Grant MC-A0606-5PQ41), and from The James S. McDonnell Foundation Opportunity Award.

References

Akarca, D. (2022) Homophilic wiring principles underpin neuronal network topology in vitro. *BioRxiv*. doi:10.1101/2022.03.09.483605.

Akarca, D. *et al.* (2021) A generative network model of neurodevelopmental diversity in structural brain organization. *Nature Communications* **12**, 4216.

Astle, D.E. & Fletcher-Watson, S. (2020) Beyond the core-deficit hypothesis in developmental disorders. *Current Directions in Psychological Science* **29**(5), 431–437.

Ball, G. *et al.* (2014) Rich-club organization of the newborn human brain. *Proceedings of the National Academy of Sciences* **111**(20), 7456–7461.

Benes, F.M. (1994) Development of the corticolimbic system. In: *Human Behavior and the Developing Brain*. (eds G. Dawson & K.W. Fischer). Guilford Press, New York. pp. 176–206.

Bethlehem, R.A.I. *et al.* (2022) Brain charts for the human lifespan. *Nature* **604**, 525–533.

Bonetto, G. *et al.* (2021) Myelin: a gatekeeper of activity-dependent circuit plasticity? *Science* **374**(6569), eaba6905. doi:10.1126/science.aba6905.

Bystron, I. *et al.* (2008) Development of the human cerebral cortex: Boulder Committee revisited. *Nature Reviews Neuroscience* **9**, 110–122.

Cadwell, C.R. *et al.* (2019) Development and arealization of the cerebral cortex. *Neuron* **103**(6), 980–1004. doi:10.1016/j.neuron.2019.07.009. PMID: 31557462; PMCID: PMC9245854

Cardoso-Moreira, M. *et al.* (2019) Gene expression across mammalian organ development. *Nature* **571**, 505–509. doi:10.1038/s41586-019-1338-5.

Casey, B.J. (2005) Imaging the developing brain: what have we learned about cognitive development? *Trends in Cognitive Science* **9**, 104–110.

Chiao, J. (ed) (2009) *Cultural Neuroscience: Cultural Influences on Brain Function. Progress in Brain Research*. Elsevier, Amsterdam.

Chugani, H.T. *et al.* (2002) Positron emission tomography study of human brain functional development. In: *Brain Development and Cognition: A Reader*. (eds M.H. Johnson, *et al.*), 2nd edn. Blackwell, Oxford, UK. pp. 101–116.

Colantuoni, C. *et al.* (2011) Temporal dynamics and genetic control of transcription in the human prefrontal cortex. *Nature* **478**, 519–523.

Dawson, G. *et al.* (2023) Prediction of autism in infants: progress and challenges. *Lancet Neurology* **22**(3), 244–254. doi:10.1016/S1474-4422(22)00407-0.

Elman, J.L. *et al.* (1996) *Rethinking Innateness: A Connectionist Perspective on Development*. MIT Press, Cambridge, MA.

Finlay, B. & Darlington, R. (1995) Linked regularities in the development and evolution of mammalian brains. *Science* **268**, 1578–1584.

Gogtay, N. *et al.* (2004) Dynamic mapping of human cortical development during childhood through early adulthood. *Proceedings of the National Academy of Sciences of the United States of America* **101**, 8174–8179.

Gottlieb, G. (1992) *Individual Development and Evolution: The Genesis of Novel Behavior*. Oxford University Press, New York.

Hamasaki, T. *et al.* (2002) EMX2 regulates sizes and positioning of the primary sensory and motor areas in neocortex by direct specification of cortical progenitors. *Neuron* **3**, 359–372.

Hiesinger, P.R. & Hassan, B.A. (2018) The evolution of variability and robustness in neural development. *Trends in Neurosciences* **41**(9), 577–586. doi:10.1016/j.tins.2018.05.007.

Huttenlocher, P.R. (1994) Synaptogenesis, synapse elimination, and neural plasticity in human cerebral cortex: threats to optimal development. In: *The Minnesota Symposia on Child Psychology*. (ed C.A. Nelson), Vol. vol. 27. Lawrence Erlbaum, Hillsdale, NJ. pp. 35–54.

Johnson, M.H. (2011) Interactive specialization: a domain-general framework for human functional brain development? *Developmental Cognitive Neuroscience* **1**, 7–21.

Johnson, M.H. *et al.* (2021) Anterior modifiers in the emergence of neurodevelopmental disorders (AMEND): a systems neuroscience approach to common developmental disorders. *Journal of Child Psychology and Psychiatry* **62**, 610–630. doi:10.1111/jcpp.13372.

Kaiser, M.D. *et al.* (2010) Neural signatures of autism. *Proceedings of the National Academy of Sciences* **107**, 21223–21228.

Kamps, F. *et al.* (2020) Connectivity at the origins of domain specificity in cortical face and place networks. *Proceedings of the National Academy of Sciences* **117**, 6163–6169.

Kang, H.J. *et al.* (2011) Spatio-temporal transcriptome of the human brain. *Nature* **478**, 483–489.

Keverne, B. *et al.* (1996) Genomic imprinting and the differential roles of parental genomes in brain development. *Developmental Brain Research* **92**(1), 91–100. doi:10.1016/0165-3806(95)00209-x. PMID: 8861727

Kim, J.-Y. & Paredes, M.F. (2021) Implications of extended inhibitory neuron development. *International Journal of Molecular Sciences* **22**, 5113. doi:10.3390/ijms22105113.

Kingsbury, M.A. & Finlay, B.L. (2001) The cortex in multidimensional space: Where do cortical areas come from? *Developmental Science* **4**, 125–142.

Le Blanc, J.J. & Fagiolini, M. (2011) Autism: a "critical period" disorder? *Neural Plasticity* **2011**, 1–17.

Marek, S. *et al.* (2022) Reproducible brain-wide association studies require thousands of individuals. *Nature* **603**(7902), 654–660.

Marin-Padilla, M. (1990) The pyramidal cell and its local-circuit interneurons: a hypothetical unit of the mammalian cerebral cortex. *Journal of Cognitive Neuroscience* **2**, 180–194.

Mehl, L.C. *et al.* (2022) Microglia in brain development and regeneration. *Development* **15**, 149.

Meredith, R.M. *et al.* (2012) Sensitive time-windows for susceptibility in neurodevelopmental disorders. *Trends in Neurosciences* **35**, 335–344.

Nascimento, M.A. *et al.* (2022) Persistent postnatal migration of interneurons into the human entorhinal cortex. *bioRxiv* [Preprint]. doi:10.1101/2022.03.19.484996.

Nowakowski, R.S. (1987) Basic concepts of CNS development. *Child Development* **58**, 568–595.

Nowakowski, T.J. & Salama, S.R. (2022) Cerebral organoids as an experimental platform for human neurogenomics. *Cells* **11**, 2803.

O'Leary, D.M. & Nakahawa, Y. (2002) Patterning centres, regulatory genes and extrinsic mechanisms controlling arealization of the neocortex. *Current Opinion in Neurobiology* **12**, 14–25.

Palva, S. & Palva, J.M. (2012) Discovering oscillatory interaction networks with M/EEG: challenges and breakthroughs. *Trends in Cognitive Science* **16**, 219–230.

Paredes, M.F. *et al.* (2016) Extensive migration of young neurons into the infant human frontal lobe. *Science* **354**(6308), aaf7073. doi:10.1126/science.aaf7073. PMID: 27846470; PMCID: PMC5436574

Polleux, F. *et al.* (2002) Control of cortical interneuron migration by neurotrophins and P13-kinase signalling. *Development* **129**, 3147–3169.

Rakic, P. (1988) Specification of cerebral cortical areas. *Science* **241**, 170–176.

Schlaggar, B.L. *et al.* (2002) Functional neuroanatomical differences between adults and school-age children in the processing of single words. *Science* **296**, 1476–1479.

Sharf, T. *et al.* (2022) Functional neuronal circuitry and oscillatory dynamics in human brain organoids. *Nature Communications* **13**, 4403.

Shatz, C.J. (2002) Emergence of order in visual system development. In: *Brain Development and Cognition: A Reader*. (eds M.H. Johnson, *et al.*), 2nd edn. Blackwell, Oxford, UK. pp. 231–244.

Shi, Y. *et al.* (2012) A human stem cell model of early Alzheimer's disease pathology in Down syndrome. *Science Translational Medicine* **4**, 24–29.

Singer, W. & Gray, C.M. (1995) Visual feature integration and the temporal correlation hypothesis. *Annual Review of Neuroscience* **18**, 555–586.

Siugzdaite, R. *et al.* (2020) Transdiagnostic brain mapping in developmental disorders. *Current Biology* **30**(7), 1245–1257.

Supekar, K. *et al.* (2009) Development of large-scale functional brain networks in children. *PLoS Biology* **7**, e1000157.

Sydnor, V.J. *et al.* (2021) Neurodevelopment of the association cortices: patterns, mechanisms, and implications for psychopathology. *Neuron* **109**(18), 2820–2846. doi:10.1016/j.neuron.2021.06.016.

Toda, T. *et al.* (2019) The role of adult hippocampal neurogenesis in brain health and disease. *Molecular Psychiatry* **24**, 67–87. doi:10.1038/s41380-018-0036-2.

Tye, C. *et al.* (2013) Neurophysiological responses to faces and gaze direction differentiate children with ASD, ADHD and ASD+ADHD. *Developmental Cognitive Neuroscience* **5**, 71–85.

Vértes, P.E. *et al.* (2012) Simple models of human brain functional networks. *Proceedings of the National Academy of Sciences of the United States of America* **109**(15), 5868–5873. doi:10.1073/pnas.1111738109.

Wood, H. (2022) Charting brain development across the human lifespan. *Nature Reviews Neurology* **18**, 317.

CHAPTER 11

Neuroimaging in child and adolescent psychiatry: the key elements

Tonya White

Section on Social and Cognitive Developmental Neuroscience, National Institutes of Mental Health, Bethesda, MD, USA

Introduction

Our understanding of the purpose and inner workings of the brain has undergone a dramatic evolution over time. The Greek philosopher Aristotle thought the brain to be a reservoir for cooling the blood (Longo, 1996). It was the heart and vascular system that carried that vital substance, blood, that controlled our thoughts and emotions. The heart, after all, alters its tempo based on experiencing emotions such as fear, contentment, and love ("I feel it in my heart"). Approximately 150 years later, around 170 BCE, the Greek physician Aelius Galenus (Galen) was one of the first to associate the brain with cognition, personality, and the control of bodily functions (Baig *et al.*, 2007). Galen's work remained authoritative until the 16th century, when his work was extended by the Belgian physician, Andreas Vesalius, who developed detailed anatomical maps of the nervous system. In the 18th century, Luigi Galvani then made a link between electrical impulses and nerve conduction, which was very important for expanding our understanding of neurophysiology (Piccolino, 1998). Our understanding of the brain has exploded over the past century, and now spans spatial and temporal resolutions from molecules to gross brain morphology, and from submilliseconds to phylogenic time scales, respectively.

Over the last half-century, neuroimaging techniques have greatly contributed to this exponential growth in knowledge. The pioneers who first began using magnetic resonance imaging (MRI) to study psychopathology believed that they would "isolate the causal lesion" for specific psychiatry disorders. However, except for tumors or other neurological disorders, bringing diagnostic, prognostic, and predictive power of neuroimaging approaches down to the individual participant has been elusive. The inherent variability within neurodevelopment, coupled with the heterogeneity of psychopathology and comorbidities of the disorders have interfered with the application of neuroimaging to precision medicine for psychiatric disorders (White, 2023), at least using current imaging methodologies. In addition, imaging approaches can have artifacts and noise that further add to the variability. These factors contribute to the mixed findings in the literature and also recent reports that thousands of participants are needed in order to show consistent brain/behavior relationships in functional neuroimaging (Marek *et al.*, 2022). Since the goal of precision medicine is toward clinical decision-making for individual patients, the need for thousands of participants to achieve reliable measures in neuroimaging studies seems to be moving us farther from the goal of precision medicine.

While there are challenges in using neuroimaging for reliable prediction and precision medicine in child and adolescent psychiatry, neuroimaging studies have taught us much about brain structure and function. These studies have provided insights into brain-based growth trajectories in both typically developing children and adolescents, and in youth with psychiatric and neurodevelopmental disorders (NDDs). When groups of participants are studied with specific disorders or traits, neuroimaging studies can identify consistent brain regions or brain connectivity patterns that are associated with specific disorders. These findings can help identify neurodevelopmental factors associated with the emergence of these disorders, or alternatively, factors related to downstream effects of the underlying psychopathology. Thus, while neuroimaging in youth with psychiatric disorders cannot yet be used for diagnosis or prediction at the level of an individual (at least in the absence of specific neurologic findings on MRI scans such as tumors, white matter lesions, etc.), neuroimaging does do well in identifying differences in groups of patients, such as the enlarged ventricular volume of cerebral spinal fluid (CSF) in youth with schizophrenia.

Rutter's Child and Adolescent Psychiatry and Psychology, Seventh Edition.
Edited by Anita Thapar, Daniel S. Pine, Samuele Cortese, Cathy Creswell, Tamsin J. Ford, James F. Leckman, and Argyris Stringaris.

Companion website: www.wiley.com/go/thapar/ruttersspsych7

The goal of this chapter is to form a basis for approaching and understanding major elements of pediatric neuroimaging. It is not the goal to go in depth regarding any one specific disorder, but rather, to build a basis to understand principles involved in neuroimaging and the types of information that these studies can provide.

Study populations and potential biases

The participants section of any study is extremely important in understanding potential biases inherent in the study. Imagine that a paper has brilliant neuroimaging methods, but the patients are drawn from two very different populations, such as recruiting youth with first-onset psychosis from a county clinic and the controls being drawn from a convenience sample of a college-prep high school near the research lab. In such a case, the neuroimaging differences could be attributed to factors other than having a psychotic disorder, such as the effects of poverty or a greater risk of exposures to toxic environmental compounds (e.g., lead). Thus, how and where the participants are recruited is key to understanding the study and potential biases that may exist due to differences in recruitment strategies.

Within the neuroimaging literature, study populations typically fall into one of four categories: clinical, population-based, high-risk, and typical developing. The advantages and disadvantages of recruitment from each of these populations are provided in Table 11.1. Each of these populations can include the recruitment of singletons, siblings, and twin populations and include cross-sectional or longitudinal studies. Differences in recruitment and attrition for individuals of certain demographics can translate to both recruitment and attrition bias, respectively. See Box 11.1 for an example of matching and potential biases in clinical studies.

Notice that there is nearly a 25-point difference in all IQ measures between the adolescent patients versus the controls. Further, the mean IQ for the controls is about 1 standard deviation above the norm. This may suggest a potential recruitment bias between patients and controls. However, the paternal and maternal education levels, which are related to parental IQ, are well matched. In fact, the paternal and maternal education levels in the patient group are slightly higher than the controls. Thus, the difference in IQ is very likely related, at least partially, to the cognitive decline associated with schizophrenia rather than a bias in recruitment. Thus, if the IQ of the child is used as a covariate, this may result in overcorrection and remove some of the true effect of schizophrenia, at least those neurobiological elements of schizophrenia that covary with IQ. Finally, the overall higher IQ and educational attainment reflect the catchment area surrounding the University of Iowa, which may also limit the generalizability.

Behavior, emotion, and cognitive measures in neuroimaging

There are a vast number of approaches used to define relationships between neuroimaging measures and behavioral, emotional, and cognitive characteristics. These approaches fall broadly into three different categories; descriptive studies (including those that describe relationships between variables), studies of prediction, and studies exploring the underlying etiology of specific disorders or traits (Ramspek *et al.*, 2021). Demonstrating etiologic relationships between brain and behavioral, emotional, or cognitive domains is challenging as associations do not imply causality. For example, finding a relationship between ADHD and decreased volume of the caudate nucleus could have several different explanations. One of the possible explanations is causal, that histological changes in the caudate are in the pathway for children to develop ADHD. However, an alternative explanation could be that problems with inattention could equate with children with ADHD having to strain to focus more, which then drives the enlarged caudate (reverse causality). Another explanation could be that children with enlarged caudate volumes and ADHD tend to have characteristics that mean they are more willing to participate in studies. Finally, children with ADHD may have greater head motion in the MRI, which results in a lower volume of the caudate, and thus the relationship could be an indirect effect of ADHD.

While there is no question that the brain is causal in generating behaviors and emotions, it is difficult to isolate causality in noninterventional neuroimaging studies. However, use of clinical data for prediction is clear for clinicians, as they use this continuously in their day-to-day process of clinical decision-making. Similar to prediction models generated by clinicians, statistical models of prediction make use of multiple variables in an attempt to predict specific outcome variables, such as diagnosis, clinical course, or other important variables. Statistical models have been applied to neuroimaging biomarkers to predict events and with the emergence of big data and machine learning algorithms, there is both much opportunity and also the potential for problems (Poldrack *et al.*, 2020). There are several key components when evaluating studies that integrate predictive models, with replication in an independent sample being the most important (Poldrack *et al.*, 2020). While approaches exist to perform replications within large datasets, if the dataset has an inherent structural bias, then performing a training and replication study in the same dataset (i.e., via *k*-fold cross validation) could propagate this bias. Testing within a completely independent dataset helps reduce the chance that there is overfitting in the predictive model. That said, some samples are so unique that testing in a completely different dataset is not possible. In these cases, creating training and test sets with independent samples is critical to prevent overfitting.

One practice to be avoided in neuroimaging studies is what is termed "double dipping" (Kriegeskorte *et al.*, 2009). Double dipping refers to approaches in which the relationship between predictors and multiple variables are first assessed, and only those that are related to the outcome are selected for further analyses. If only variables that are known to be related with the predictor are entered into the statistical model, then the relationship will be highly predictive, although this significant finding would be an artifact due to the selection of known regions. The best approach to avoid double dipping is first training a model on a dataset completely independent from the testing sample.

Table 11.1 Advantages and disadvantages of recruitment of specific populations within neuroimaging studies.

Recruitment sample[a]	Explanation	Advantages	Disadvantages	Examples
Clinical	Patients are recruited based on specific diagnoses (often based on *Diagnostic and Statistical Manual of Mental Disorders* (DSM) or *International Classification of Diseases* (ICD) diagnostic criteria) and compared to a matched control group. The control or comparison group can be typically developing or a clinical reference group, or both. The patient groups may be recruited from a single site and multisite studies can be prospective, or retrospective, such as the ENIGMA consortium (Thompson *et al.*, 2014).	Increase in power to assess youth with specific diagnoses, especially for disorders that have lower prevalence rates in the population. Well suited to integrate into clinical care.	The sample is limited by those who are help-seeking, and thus there is a potential for recruitment bias. Since recruitment occurs after the disorder has emerged, it's not possible to assess whether the differences predate or are a result of the disorder. Researchers are like "archeologists' piecing together retrospective information."	Most common approach, and thus there exist a large number of examples: pooled studies of autism spectrum disorder (ASD) via the ABIDE Network (Di Martino *et al.*, 2017) and ENIGMA for attention deficit hyperactivity disorder (ADHD) (Hoogman *et al.*, 2019), anxiety (Bas-Hoogendam *et al.*, 2022), and depression (Schmaal *et al.*, 2017).
High-risk	Participants are recruited for being either genetically at risk (offspring, siblings, genetic markers) or behaviorally at risk (nonspecific behaviors or prodromal symptoms) for the later development of psychopathology.	Can increase the sample of those who later develop psychiatric disorders, and thus can assess the brain prior to the onset of symptoms. A subgroup of those at increased risk may show subclinical symptoms or different diagnoses altogether due to genetic variations or environmental influences.	Will miss those individuals who develop the disorder due to factors other than being genetically at risk.	Brazilian High-Risk Cohort Study (Borges *et al.*, 2022), Studies of psychosis (Fusar-Poli *et al.*, 2013), bipolar affective disorder (Nery *et al.*, 2017), IBIS study of ASD (Hazlett *et al.*, 2012).
Population-based	A large number of participants are drawn from a specific population or catchment area with the goal that the children recruited reflect either the population within the catchment area or the population at-large.	Since population-based studies draw from the population at large, it is more reflective of the population. Can see the brain prior to symptoms in those who are both behaviorally and genetically at risk. Can also examine environmental factors that are associated with emerging psychopathology. It's possible to assess those with subclinical symptoms in the population, who are not help-seeking and to assess whether the relationship between symptom severity and the underlying neurobiology follow a linear versus a nonlinear trajectory (see Box 11.2).	For disorders with lower prevalence rates, the number of participants recruited from the population would need to be extremely large to have a reasonable sample size to evaluate these subgroups of participants. Due to time constraints, deep phenotyping is more challenging with large sample sizes, especially for single-site studies. Neuroimaging is expensive, and population-based studies have a large number of participants and thus funding, especially for longitudinal studies, can be challenging.	The Generation R Study (White *et al.*, 2013; White *et al.*, 2018), The GUSTO Study (Broekman *et al.*, 2014), ABCD Study[b] (Casey *et al.*, 2018).
Typically developing	Participants who show signs or symptoms of psychiatric disorders, or who are at risk due to parental or sibling psychopathology, are excluded from the sample.	Typically developing samples are often easier to recruit and tend to have less attrition over time, depending on the disorder. Often used in neuroscience to examine brain regions associated with specific tasks, emotions, or behaviors in typical development.	Rates of psychopathology are quite common in the population, and thus studies of typically developing children have an inherent bias to what is termed "super controls."	NIH Study (Raznahan *et al.*, 2011), PING[c] (Newman *et al.*, 2016).

[a] *Combinations of these approaches can also occur to enhance recruitment for specific populations.*

[b] *The ABCD Study was oversampled for youth who score higher on the Child Behavior Checklist (CBCL) and those with moderate to severe ASD were excluded, thus the ABCD Study did not employ true population-based sampling strategies.*

[c] *Did include youth with ADHD and attention problems, but all other forms of psychopathology were excluded.*

Box 11.1 Demographics: evaluating neuroimaging studies for potential biases

Consider the demographic information in a study of youth with schizophrenia in the following table (See Section on Study Populations and Potential Biases).

	Adolescent patients (n = 49)	Adolescent controls (n = 32)
Age	18.1 (1.2)	18.9 (0.3)
Sex	37/12	21/11
Educational level	11.0 (1.3)	12.6 (0.7)
Paternal educational level	13.7 (3.5)	13.6 (3.0)
Maternal educational level	13.6 (2.4)	13.0 (1.6)
Intelligence quotient (IQ)		
Full Scale IQ	91 (13)	114 (13)
Verbal IQ	93 (12)	113 (14)
Performance IQ	89 (15)	113 (11)

Source: Adapted from White *et al.* (2006).

Box 11.2 Linear versus nonlinear relationships between psychiatric symptoms and neurobiological features

There is evidence that some psychiatric symptoms extend into the population. For example, we do not all have the same levels of attention. Some individuals may be able to attend for long periods of time, whereas others have more difficulties attending, such as those with attention deficit hyperactivity disorder (ADHD). Autism spectrum disorder (ASD) embeds the word "spectrum" into the diagnostic category itself. But what is less clear is whether there is a linear or nonlinear relationship between symptoms and the underlying neurobiology.

The relationship between symptom severity and a brain imaging feature could be either linear or a nonlinear, as shown in Figure 11.1. A linear relationship between symptoms and brain measures would mean that those with subclinical symptoms also demonstrate differences in the brain, albeit fewer compared to those with clinical symptoms. Alternatively, a nonlinear relationship would infer that subclinical symptoms do not show major differences in the underlying neurobiology, whereas those with the clinical disorder do.

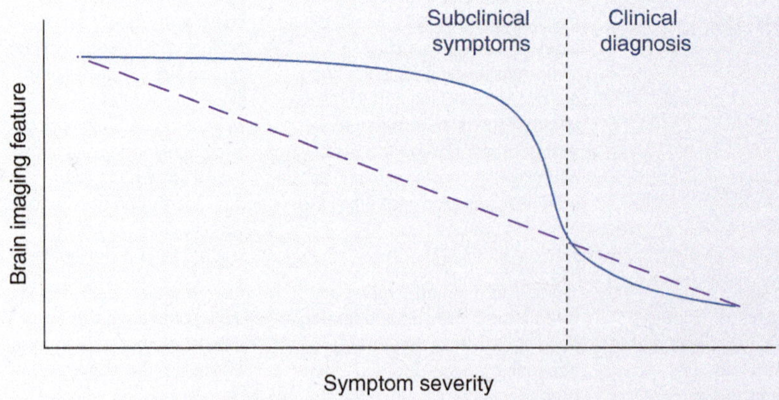

Figure 11.1 Example of linear versus nonlinear relationships between psychiatric symptoms and neurobiological features.

Covariates and confounders

Confounding variables refer to those variables that influence both the determinant and the outcome, and thus may provide an alternative pathway, or explanation, for the results. Consider a study in which researchers would like to know if the stress of growing up in an impoverished environment is associated with decreased total brain volume in a large group of children and adolescents. However, some of the neighborhoods of the participants with lower socioeconomic status (SES) also have houses with lead paint. Thus, lead paint could be a confounder, as it is related to both impoverished environments and decreased total brain volume.

Covariates are variables that can influence the outcome and are typically used to enhance precision. In the example above,

Box 11.3 Adjusting for global measures (i.e., intracranial volume) in structural neuroimaging studies

Those who have a larger total brain volume typically have larger volumes of other brain regions, such as larger total gray matter, white matter, subcortical volume, and larger individual brain structures. However, specific regions may also show regional differences, as indicated in Figure 11.2.

Even though the total brain volume (TBV) of Figure 11.2a, b (smaller), and c (larger) are different sizes, the hippocampus volume in each of these three brain images is the same volume. Both the TBV and hippocampal volume are larger for Figure 11.2d. Thus, when not covarying for intracranial volume (ICV) for Figure 11.2b and c, the relative difference in hippocampal volume in relation to TBV will not be detected. For the brain in Figure 11.2d, which has both a larger TBV and hippocampal volume, the larger hippocampal volume is a global effect, and thus will not be detected when including ICV as a covariate.

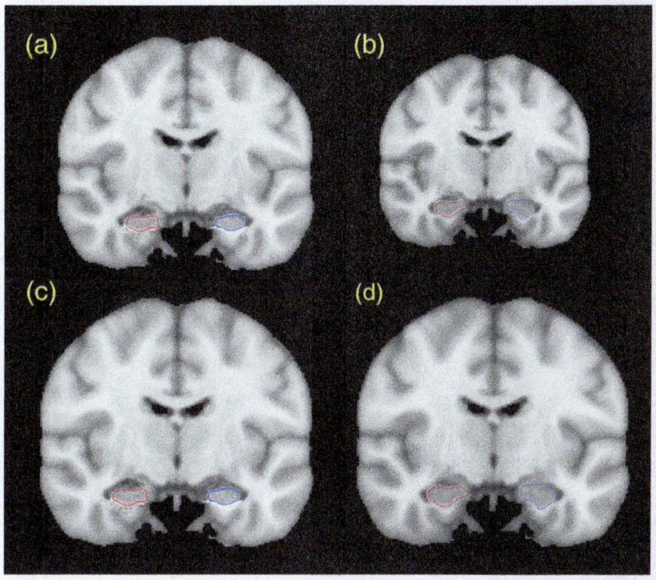

Figure 11.2 An example of controlling and not controlling for intracranial volume in structural neuroimaging studies.

age could be considered a covariate, since the brain undergoes considerable changes between childhood and adolescence, and thus adding age as a covariate will control for the variance related to age-related brain differences.

There are several covariates that are typically applied to structural and functional neuroimaging to assess localized differences in specific brain structures, regions, or connectivity patterns. The choices of the appropriate covariates and confounders is rooted in the existing literature. Brain growth that begins in prenatal life and progresses throughout childhood is driven largely by genetic mechanisms. A large element of this brain growth is global, that is individuals with larger brains will also have larger occipital, frontal, parietal, and temporal lobes. Thus, there are global processes that determine total brain size and that scale with the individual structures that make up the brain. However, certain structures could have a differential growth trajectory, for example, the link between stress exposure and decreased hippocampal volume (Carrion *et al.*, 2007). In this case, the hippocampus is smaller relative to the total brain volume and to best detect this difference, the statistical analyses should control for total brain or intracranial volume (ICV). In general, ICV would not be used as a covariate when assessing global differences or changes, but would be used when assessing regional differences that are above and beyond global differences (see Box 11.3).

ICV can be used as a covariate for regional analyses involving volume or surface area but is less useful when assessing regional differences in cortical thickness. Measures of surface area and cortical thickness are not highly correlated, and thus a global measure of cortical thickness would be best applied to assess regional differences in cortical thickness. Controlling for global effects in functional MRI (fMRI) is related and revolves around whether to adjust for the global fMRI signal, which is debated. However, one of the key reasons why the global signal is regressed out of functional connectivity analyses of the brain is due to its relationship with head motion.

Structural and diffusion tensor imaging

Structural neuroimaging includes both computer tomography (CT) and MRI. While CT acquisitions tend to be much quicker than MRI, CT has several features that make it less suitable for neuroimaging studies, especially those that involve minors. First, CT involves ionizing radiation, and so limiting exposure, especially during development, is important. Second, while CT does have excellent contrast between CSF and other brain tissues and is well-suited to measure cerebral bleeds, it does not provide optimal contrast between white and gray matter regions of the brain. Thus, it is more difficult to perform accurate segmentation of brain regions and cortical thickness with CT. However, CT was used prior to MRI and early studies in adolescents with schizophrenia showed increased ventricular volume (Schulz *et al.*, 1983), which is the most consistent neuroimaging finding in patients with schizophrenia using either CT or MRI.

Structural MRI (sMRI) provides detailed anatomic characteristics of the brain. Most sMRI sequences are tuned to quantify the concentration or properties of hydrogen molecules, and hydrogen bound to water (H_2O) is the most abundant molecule in the body. Different brain regions have different concentrations or diffusion characteristics of water, and these can be measured to highlight the differences between brain regions. Diffusion-weighted imaging, including diffusion tensor imaging (DTI), is a technique that quantifies the diffusion properties of water depending on its surrounding tissue characteristics. For example, a water molecule within the center of a cerebral ventricle could diffuse in all directions throughout the CSF. Water diffusion in gray matter also tends to be equal in all directions, but diffusion would be more restricted than in CSF due to different macromolecules within the cell impeding diffusion. Diffusion within white matter, however, is restricted in the radial direction (due to the myelinated sheaths) but diffuses more easily in the direction of the neuron. The diffusion of water that is dependent on the differences in tissue characteristics can be quantified using DTI to provide elegant maps of white matter tracts within the brain. Water within the CSF and gray matter has isotropic diffusion properties, whereas within white matter water has anisotropic diffusion properties, and thus the latter has directional diffusion properties along the white matter tracts.

Functional neuroimaging

Functional neuroimaging modalities can be subdivided into two primary categories; those that directly measure neuronal signals, and those that indirectly measure neuronal signals via secondary mechanisms. Both electroencephalography (EEG) and magnetoencephalography (MEG) directly measure diffuse neuronal activity via electromagnetic waves generated by action potentials. These electromagnetic waves can be detected at the surface of the head using sensors. Functional MRI and functional near infrared spectroscopy (fNIRS) make use of changes between the contrast of oxygenated versus deoxygenated hemoglobin in brain regions that change their activity level.

Electroencephalography (EEG)/ magnetoencephalography (MEG)

Action potentials induce electric currents that can be measured on, or close to the scalp. These electrical currents can be measured using EEG, which involves the placement of electrodes (EEG) or antennae (MEG) on the skull. If EEG is performed during a specific task, which is time-locked with the EEG, this is referred to as event-related potentials (ERP). EEG devices can have up to 512 electrodes and require a liquid or gel interface between the electrodes and the skin to increase conductance and allow for signal transduction. The advantage of EEG and MEG is that by measuring the actual neuronal signals, the temporal resolution is much higher than those that measure the response of the hemodynamic system, such as fMRI and fNIRS. However, the two primary challenges related to EEG are that the signal is blurred by the skull and thus has limited spatial resolution; and second, it is difficult to measure structures deep within the brain.

Whenever an electric field is generated, there is a corresponding magnetic field that is orthogonal to the electric field. This magnetic field can be detected using MEG, which while typically requiring a superconducting environment using liquid helium, has greater precision as the magnetic signal is not blurred by the skull. However, MEG also has limitations, being similar to EEG, in that it is difficult to measure signals from deep in the brain. Second, the requirement of a superconducting environment is very susceptible to noise, and must be well-isolated from environmental electromagnetic noise. New MEG devices, however, are being developed that do not require a superconducting environment.

Both fMRI and fNIRS do not directly measure neuronal activity, but rather measure the hemodynamic response that is associated with changes in neuronal activity. The hemodynamics are measured via differences between oxygenated and deoxygenated hemoglobin. When a region of the brain becomes "active," there are feedback mechanisms in the circulatory system that result in an excess of blood flow to the activated region of the brain, resulting in a difference in the ratio of oxy- to deoxyhemoglobin. This ratio can be measured because deoxygenated hemoglobin is paramagnetic, whereas oxygenated hemoglobin is not.

Similarly, fNIRS is measured using the changes in the absorption differences between oxygenated and deoxygenated hemoglobin. Thus, similar to fMRI, the color properties between oxygenated and deoxygenated hemoglobin can be measured by shining light through the skull and measuring the reflected signal. Functional MRI has the advantage, however, of being able to measure functional changes deep within the brain, whereas fNIRS can only measure signals on the surface of the skull and with much less precision.

Magnetic resonance spectroscopy

Magnetic resonance spectroscopy (MRS) is an MR method that, rather than providing anatomical information, is able to measure the neurochemical properties within regions of the brain. The output of MRS is a frequency spectrum, of which different peaks within that spectrum can be measured and used to calculate the concentration of specific neurochemicals within the measurement area. For MRS, the higher the field strength, the better the ability to more accurately measure the neurochemicals, especially allowing for the differentiation between neurochemicals that fall within similar frequencies. For example, concentrations of glutamine versus glutamate are much easier to differentiate at 7 Tesla compared to 3 Tesla MR field strength.

Image processing

Once imaging data is collected, it can undergo what is considered pre- and postprocessing. Preprocessing refers to the steps applied to the data to curate and clean the data, removing artifacts and processing the data so that different postprocessing analysis strategies can be applied. However, these two steps may be merged. Irrespective of which imaging modality is applied, an initial step includes visual and automated inspection of the data with the correction or removal of artifacts or poor-quality data. Different neuroimaging modalities have different approaches to curate the data prior to processing.

Movement artifacts are extremely common in younger children and become less of a problem during late childhood and into adolescence, although in some populations, such as some children with developmental delays, movement continues to be a major issue. While experts in pediatric brain MRI agree that movement artifacts can influence results, there is no clear consensus regarding how much movement is too much movement. The typical approach to movement in MRI scans is to first remove those above a set threshold of motion; and second, to either residualize or control for movement using automatically derived measures of movement. It is not possible to completely remove all movement artifacts from MR and it's important that studies provide metrics for movement and data quality.

Analysis strategies for a structural magnetic resonance image

Postprocessing of sMRI can be performed using several different techniques (Figure 11. 3). A very common approach is to parse the images based on anatomic features of the brain and extract metrics from the segmented images. Metrics may be global variables (i.e., total brain volume, total gray or white matter, total CSF) or regional variables (i.e., prefrontal cortex, hippocampus, amygdala volumes). The extracted variables can include a number of different metrics, such as volume, surface area, thickness, or gyrification of cortical regions. These variables can then be entered into statistical models to assess relationships between the brain measures and other variables.

The images in Figure 11.3 providing the following analyses: (a) In voxel-based analysis, all the subjects are registered to a common template in order to establish voxel-to-voxel correspondence among all participants. Then the values at each voxel (for example, diffusion derived properties, or gray matter concentrations) can be compared using voxel-by-voxel statistical

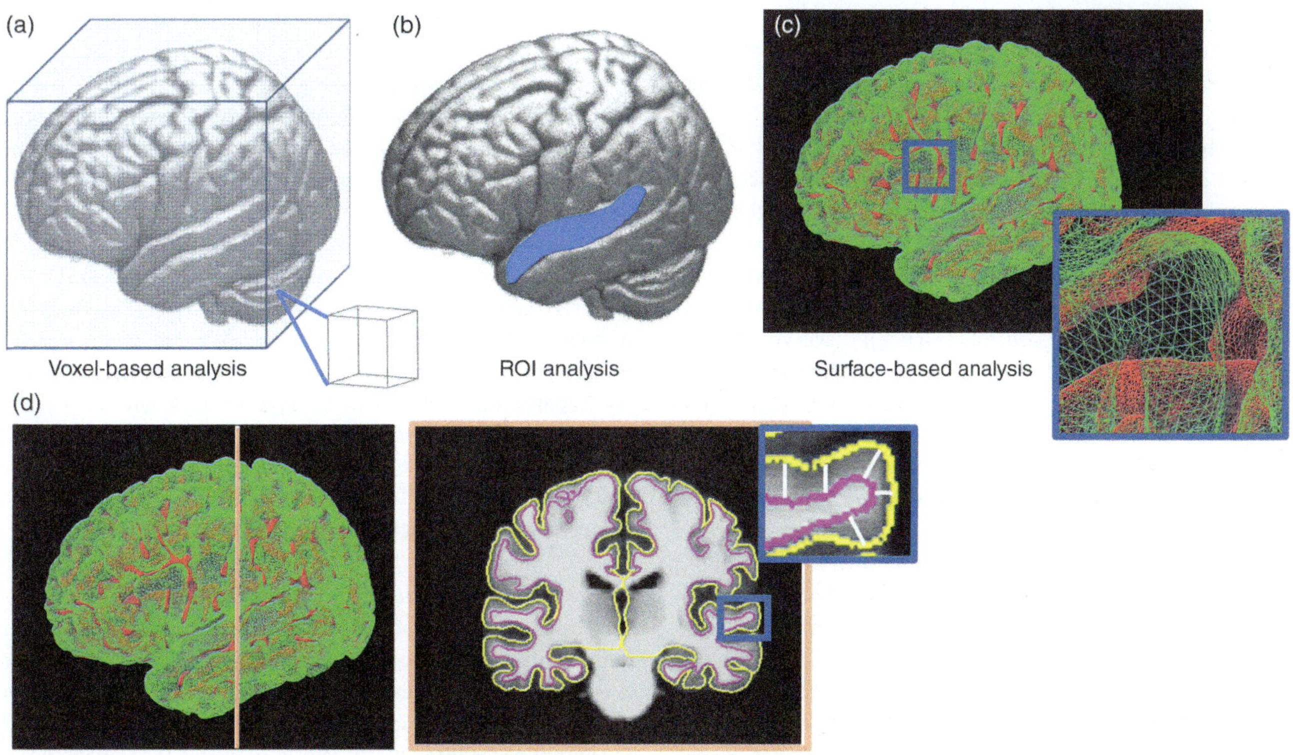

Figure 11.3 Analysis strategies for a structural magnetic resonance image (sMRI). See text for explanation of the different methods. *Source*: Photo by Neda Sadeghi and Siobhan Lawler.

analyses, controlling for multiple testing. (b) In region of interest (ROI) analysis, metrics (i.e., volumes, intensity, etc.) of brain regions are extracted from each individual and compared among participants or groups. (c) In surface-based analyses, pial and white matter surfaces are modeled as tessellated triangles and different metrics are extracted based on the properties of these triangles. For example, cortical thickness at each triangular isosurface can be measured as the distance between the white/gray matter interface on the inner cortex and pial surface, as shown in (d), or surface area would be calculated as the sum of areas of triangles within a region. The area of each triangle can be added for a specific brain region to provide the surface area for that region.

An alternative or complementary approach to the region-of-interest (ROI) approach is that statistical analyses can be applied to 2- or 3-dimensional models of the brain, using either surface-based or voxel-based analyses, respectively. Surface-based analyses are applied to the cortical surface of the brain and make use of a surface map that is applied to both the external (pial) brain surface and the gray/white matter interface on the cortex. Image processing software, such as FreeSurfer or CIVET, creates a tessellated isosurface along each of these layers, made up of thousands of small equilateral triangles. The distance between these two isosurfaces, the pial surface and the gray/white matter interface, can be used to measure cortical thickness at any small point along the brain (Figure 11.3b and c). The area of each triangle can be added for a specific brain region to provide the surface area for that region. Finally, since the brain is a curved surface, the angle between the different triangles can be measured to quantify whether the region is a sulci or a gyri, and also to calculate the amount of gyrification between different regions.

Voxel-based analyses utilize nonlinear algorithms that warp the sMRI images into a defined standard space and then iteratively apply statistics to the same voxel within the participants, or within masked regions of the brain. The statistical analyses of all participants are then performed in 3-D, yielding results also within a 3-D space of regional differences or changes between, for example, patients and controls (Figure 11.3a). Voxel-based analyses can also be applied to DTI images, where the statistical analyses are typically restricted to only white matter regions and the results show voxel-based differences in white matter microstructure.

Region-of-interest analyses can also be performed on DTI data after measures of specific white matter fiber tracts have been quantified. Alternatively, a method known as tractography can be applied to DTI images, which uses directional diffusion-weighted information to generate white matter tracts. Tractography uses DTI-derived directional information combined with atlases to segment different regions of interest, from which the specific metrics can then be extracted and used in subsequent analyses.

Analysis approaches to EEG, MEG, fMRI, and fNIRS have both overlaps and differences in postprocessing algorithms. Each of these approaches can be time-locked to specific tasks that are performed during the imaging sessions. For EEG/MEG, this is termed event-related potentials, in which the waveform in different regions of the brain is extracted and averaged over trials, to define a waveform associated with the task. The temporal resolution for EEG/MEG is high, in the order of milliseconds, thus analyses assessing the power spectrum within different frequency ranges associated with a task can also be assessed. Task-fMRI is used to describe when specific tasks are performed in the scanner and can demonstrate which regions of the brain are associated with task performance or where brain regions are different between patients and controls when performing specific tasks.

Even when not performing a task, the brain is always active. In fact, the term "rest" in reference to the brain has been termed "random episodic spontaneous thought." Thus, for all imaging modalities, data can be collected during the "resting-state," meaning that the individuals participate in the imaging session without performing any specific task. Connectivity analyses can be performed to assess the distributed brain networks at rest and differences in connectivity patterns between patients and controls.

Neuroanatomy in child and adolescent psychiatric disorders

Whereas each of the individual chapters will describe brain regions and functional patterns that are associated with specific disorders, this chapter provides a general overview of imaging neuroanatomy and approaches to understanding the literature. There is considerable variability in the results of neuroimaging studies, and different brain regions or networks tend to come more to the forefront in different studies. These systems include the limbic system, especially in mood and anxiety disorders, the striatum, notably in ADHD and externalizing disorders, the cerebellum and regions of the temporal lobe in ASD, and the prefrontal cortex in nearly all disorders, especially the dorsolateral prefrontal cortex in those with associated cognitive deficits. A brief overview of brain regions associated with psychopathology are shown in Figures 11.4 and 11.5 and a description is presented in Table 11.2.

Stochasticity and the brain

Nature and nurture are often considered the only two factors that influence brain development. Nature involves genetic factors, nurture involves environmental factors, and epigenetics results from the interaction between nature and nurture. However, stochastic factors also have an effect on brain development (White, 2019). While identical twins have nearly identical DNA and experience much of the same environment, they are not completely identical (Machin, 1996). While some of

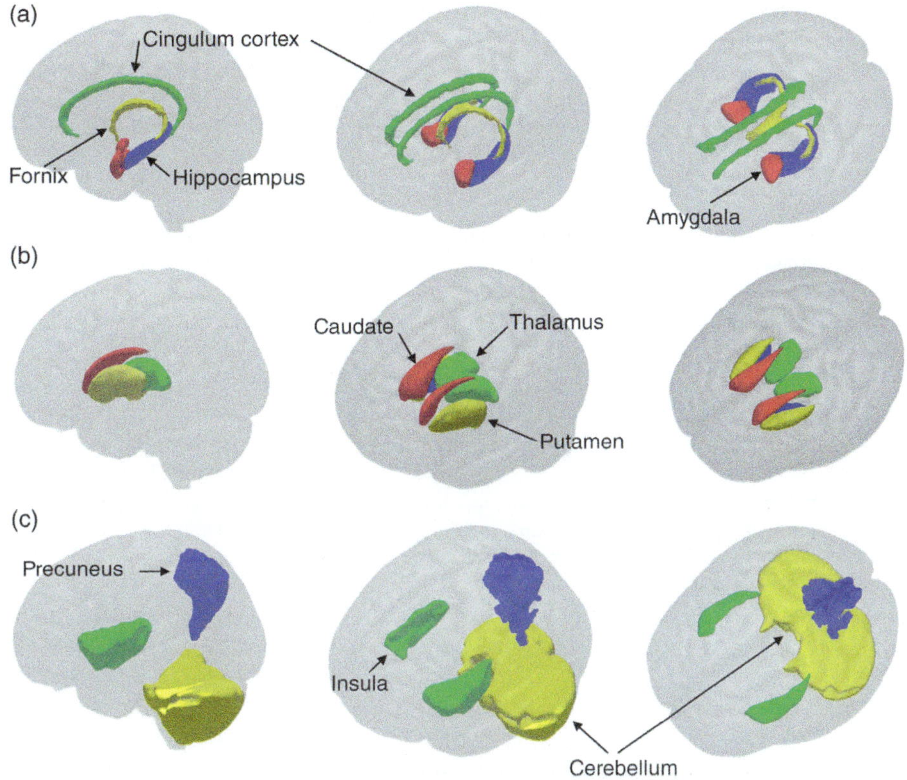

Figure 11.4 Brain regions often implicated in pediatric neuropsychiatric disorders. (a) cingulum (green), fornix (yellow), hippocampus (blue), amygdala (red); (b) head of caudate (red), thalamus (green), putamen (yellow), pallidum (blue); (c) insula (green), precuneus (blue), cerebellum (yellow). Additional info: Each 3-D brain image above was generated using FSLeyes version 1.5.0 using MNI152 T1 average brain and MNI atlas for the cerebellum, Juelich atlas for the cingulum and fornix, and the Harvard-Oxford atlas for the rest of the brain. *Source*: Generated for this chapter by Neda Sadeghi and Siobhan Lawler.

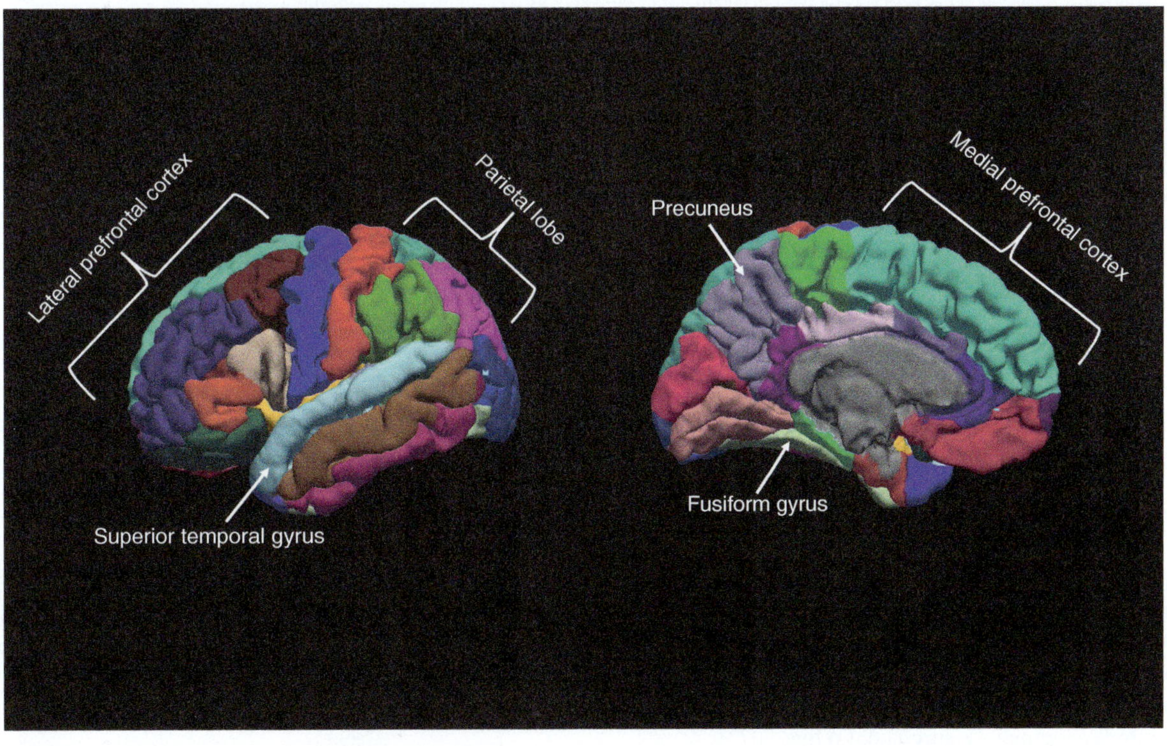

Figure 11.5 Surface map of brain regions often implicated in pediatric neuropsychiatric disorders. *Source*: Adapted from Fischl, 2012.

Table 11.2 A selection of brain regions commonly associated with psychiatric disorders in children and adolescents.

Brain region	Function	Examples of implicated psychiatric disorders (not exhaustive)
Prefrontal cortex	Higher-order cognitive functions, working memory, inhibition, problem-solving, attention, emotion regulation, decision-making.	Depression (Halari *et al.*, 2009), schizophrenia (Seidman *et al.*, 2006), ASD (Goldberg *et al.*, 2011), ADHD (Shaw & Rabin, 2009; Davenport *et al.*, 2010).
Cingulate cortex	Involved in cognition, selective attention, inhibition, award- and aversion-related decisions.	Obsessive–compulsive disorder (OCD) (Gilbert *et al.*, 2018), ADHD (Shaw & Rabin, 2009), major depressive disorder (MDD) (Halari *et al.*, 2009).
Hippocampus	Integration of multimodal sensory information, memory, regulation of stress response.	Schizophrenia (White *et al.*, 2008; White *et al.*, 2007), ADHD (Shaw & Rabin, 2009), post-traumatic stress disorder (PTSD) (Carrion *et al.*, 2007).
Amygdala	Processing of emotions, especially anxiety- and fear-related emotions.	Anxiety disorders (Bas-Hoogendam *et al.*, 2022; Monk *et al.*, 2008), depression (Musgrove *et al.*, 2015), ASD (Schumann *et al.*, 2004; Nordahl *et al.*, 2012).
Basal ganglia	The basal ganglia include the striatum (caudate, putamen, and nucleus accumbens), the globus pallidus, the ventral pallidum, and the substantia nigra. The striatum is involved in motivation, reward processing, and motor function.	Schizophrenia (Lang *et al.*, 2004; Walther *et al.*, 2011), ADHD (Shaw & Rabin, 2009).
Cerebellum	Involved in motor and cognitive functions, timing of events.	ASD (Piven *et al.*, 1992; Alemany *et al.*, 2021; Durkut *et al.*, 2022), ADHD (Shaw & Rabin, 2009; Shaw *et al.*, 2018), schizophrenia (PMID: 25309350)
Superior temporal lobe	Involved in auditory processing, language, social cognition, visual memories.	Schizophrenia (Crossley *et al.*, 2009; Davenport *et al.*, 2010), ASD (Poustka *et al.*, 2012; Alemany *et al.*, 2021; Durkut *et al.*, 2022).
Parietal lobe/ precuneus/ fusiform gyrus	Processing of sensory information. The precuneus is involved in perception, mental imagery, and episodic memory. The fusiform gyrus is involved in the processing of faces and highly familiar objects.	Schizophrenia (Cavanna, 2007), ASD (Schultz, 2005; Trontel *et al.*, 2013).
Insula	Important for interoception (awareness of the body state). Has abundant connections with the limbic system and cerebral cortex and integrates visceral sensory and motor information, as well as pain, attention, and emotion.	Schizophrenia (Aryutova *et al.*, 2021; Steenkamp *et al.*, 2022), ADHD (Vetter *et al.*, 2018), ASD (Odriozola *et al.*, 2016), OCD (Shuren *et al.*, 1995).

Note: This is not an exhaustive list, as nearly every brain region has been associated with nearly all psychiatric disorders in children and adolescents.

these differences can stem from genetic factors (Jonsson *et al.*, 2021), differences in twins can also be a result of variations in the nonshared environment, such as has been reported in children with ASD (Castelbaum *et al.*, 2020). Random factors in genetics are common, however, random (or random-equivalent) events also take place during the course of neurodevelopment.

Consider the construction of the human brain as an engineering problem. The human genome is made up of approximately 21,000 protein-coding genes (Willyard, 2018). Of these genes, approximately one-third to one-half are expressed in the brain (Naumova *et al.*, 2013). Thus, between 7,000–10,000 genes are used to create and locate the approximately 80 billion neurons, their supporting cells, and the trillions of synapses that make up the human brain. The only way that this engineering problem can be solved is via considerable redundancy; by setting up boundary conditions so that specific neurodevelopmental features have freedom to develop, but are confined within the boundaries of typical neurodevelopment (Figure 11.6) (White, 2023).

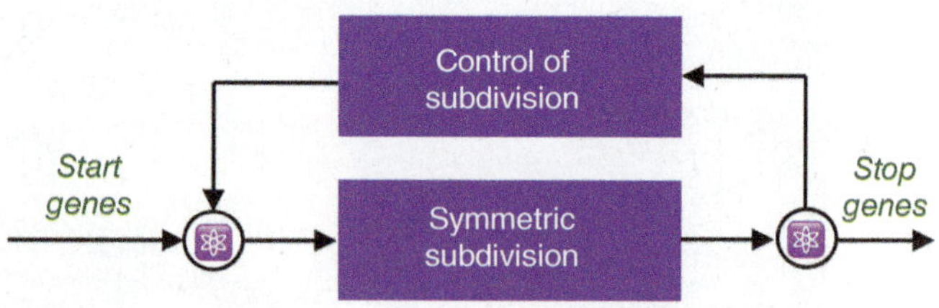

Figure 11.6 Consider an early step in neurodevelopment to highlight the role of stochasticity in brain development. Neuronal precursors divide symmetrically along the ventricular zone starting at approximately two weeks and ending at approximately six weeks, following conception. Since, with each successive division of cells, the number of neurons essentially doubles, there must be very tight regulation of this developmental process. However, small variations in the location of the dividing cells or the speed of the subdivisions could contribute to minor differences in the total number of neurons and their eventual location in cortical regions, which can in turn contribute to minor variations in neurodevelopment even when the genetic code is identical.

Conclusions

Despite the challenges in using neuroimaging for precision medicine in child and adolescent psychiatry, neuroimaging methods have dramatically shaped our understanding of neurodevelopment and characteristic features associated with psychopathology. Many psychiatric disorders that occur during childhood and adolescence are considered NDDs, meaning that the emergence of the disorder itself arises from abnormalities, or deviations, in typical development (Reiss, 2009). Thus, in order to have an in-depth understanding of the neurobiology of NDDs, such as ASD, ADHD, and schizophrenia, it's crucial to also have an understanding of typical brain development. The relationship between neurodevelopment and psychopathology can deviate from typical development in many ways (Box 11.4). Studies of childhood- and adolescent-onset schizophrenia tend to show decreased growth trajectories (Gogtay *et al.*, 2008), whereas ADHD has shown a delay in growth trajectories (Shaw & Rabin, 2009). Finally, longitudinal studies that collect the same measure at multiple time points can assess the interplay

Box 11.4 Overview of possible aberrations in typical brain development in youth with psychopathology

Not all children develop at the same rate, and certain differences in children may actually reflect slower or more rapid aspects of neurodevelopment compared to children at the same age. In addition, for children with psychiatric disorders, neuroimaging trajectories can help define when the brain changes first occurred and how psychopathology interacts with brain development (Figure 11.7).

Longitudinal studies in which the same brain and behavioral measures are collected during the different waves allow for the opportunity to study how specific brain regions are related to later behavior, or alternatively, how earlier behavioral issues can alter later brain structure and function.

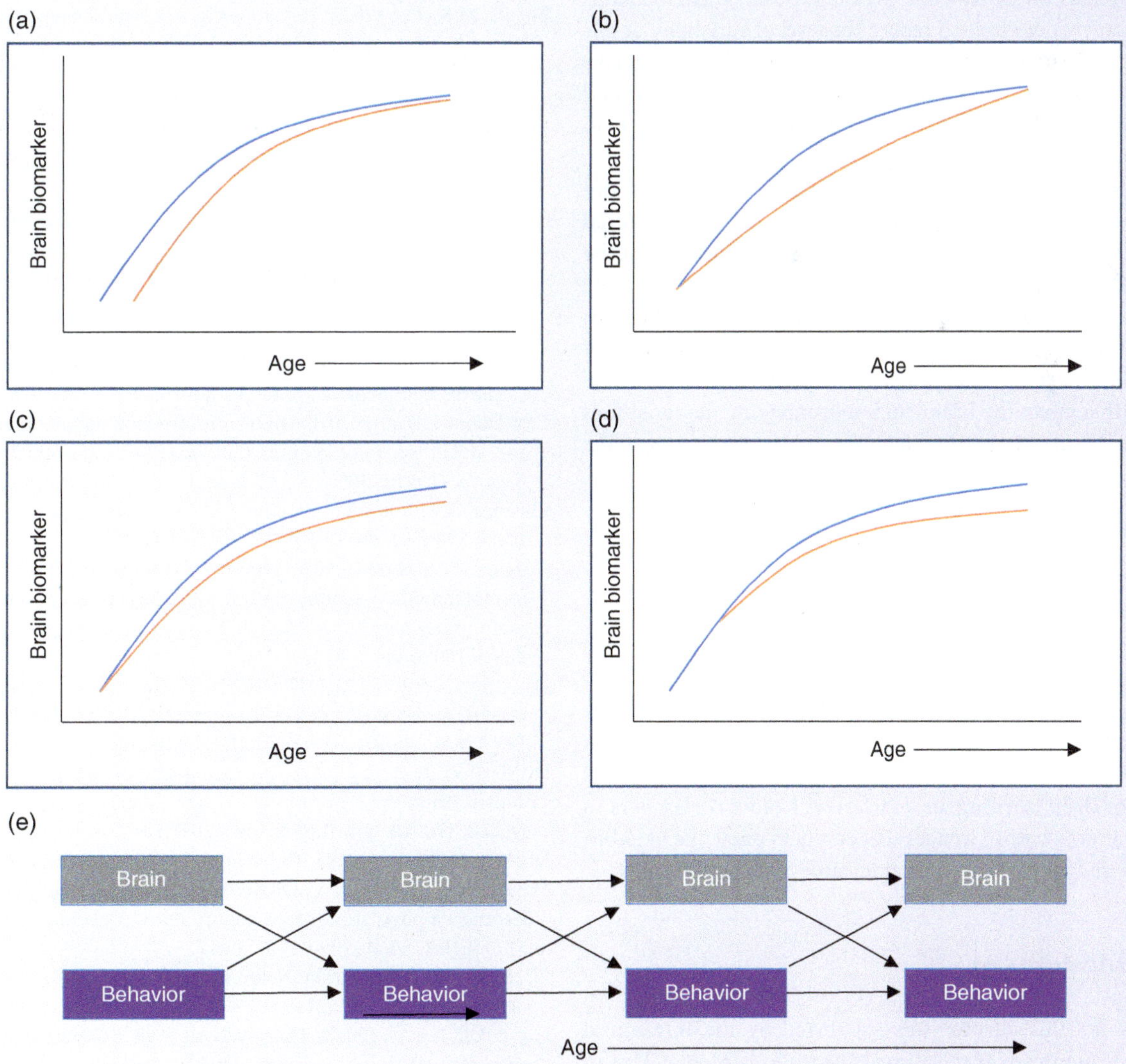

Figure 11.7 Overview of possible aberrations in typical brain development in youth with psychopathology: (a) Delayed neurodevelopment with catch-up growth. (b) Slowing in the rate of neurodevelopment, but the end effect of growth is the same. (c) Slowing in the rate of neurodevelopment and a lower value of the variable at maturity. (d) Similar developmental trajectory to a point in time, at which point a deviation takes place. (e) Brain or behavior characteristics from earlier timepoints can effect measures at later timepoints.

between brain and behavior. While there are a number of studies that demonstrate that brain differences can predict later symptoms (Jarvers *et al.*, 2022; Steenkamp *et al.*, 2022), studies have also shown the opposite, with behavioral symptoms predicting later brain changes (Blok *et al.*, 2022; Muetzel *et al.*, 2018). Timing of the measurements can also play a role, as findings of no brain/behavior interplay in ASD between late childhood and early adolescence, may indicate that the events occurred earlier in development and remain stable over time (Durkut *et al.*, 2022).

While neuroimaging has many strengths and has made many significant contributions to our understanding of neurodevelopment, neuroscience, and psychopathology, it is also not without its challenges. The tremendous variability of the human brain, driven by genetic, environmental, and stochastic factors, is extraordinarily important on an evolutionary scale, but brings challenges for infusing precision medicine approaches using neuroimaging techniques. Studies that attempted to standardize laboratory animals by using animals with identical DNA and exposing them to identical environments did little to reduce the level of variability of different organ systems between animals (Gartner, 2012). This heterogeneity is one of the reasons why many epidemiologic and neuroimaging studies require a larger number of participants to demonstrate statistically significant effects.

Even though neuroimaging of psychopathology has not entered precision medicine in clinical settings, it has entered clinical care and public health settings. The ability to demonstrate that there are brain differences or changes based on the emergence of different disorders provides helpful information for parents and children and has helped reduce the stigma of psychiatric disorders. Psychiatric disorders are medical disorders that affect the brain, and neuroimaging demonstrates the regions and networks that are implicated in specific disorders, although not yet down to the individual.

Future directions

The future is already upon us in some areas of medicine, and this future is moving into the field of neuroimaging. The use of big data and machine learning approaches will also move into the field of radiology, augmenting the radiologist's ability to detect differences. It's also possible that the use of big data and machine or deep learning approaches will allow researchers to identify patterns within images that can help parse the variability so that imaging can become applicable in clinical settings.

Acknowledgment

The work for this chapter was supported by the Intramural Research Program of the National Institute of Mental Health project number ZIA-MH002986.

References

Alemany, S. *et al.* (2021) Brain morphology, autistic traits, and polygenic risk for autism: a population-based neuroimaging study. *Autism Research* **14**(10), 2085–2099. doi:10.1002/aur.2576.

Aryutova, K. *et al.* (2021) Differential aberrant connectivity of precuneus and anterior insula may underpin the diagnosis of schizophrenia and mood disorders. *World Journal of Psychiatry* **11**(12), 1274–1287. doi:10.5498/wjp.v11.i12.1274.

Baig, M.N. *et al.* (2007) The Eastern heart and Galen's ventricle: a historical review of the purpose of the brain. *Neurosurgical Focus* **23**(1), E3. Available at: https://pubmed.ncbi.nlm.nih.gov/17961055/.

Bas-Hoogendam, J.M. *et al.* (2022) Structural brain correlates of childhood inhibited temperament: an ENIGMA-anxiety mega-analysis. *Journal of the American Academy of Child and Adolescent Psychiatry* **61**(9), 1182–1188. doi:10.1016/j.jaac.2022.04.023.

Blok, E. *et al.* (2022) The bidirectional relationship between brain features and the dysregulation profile: a longitudinal, multimodal approach. *Journal of the American Academy of Child and Adolescent Psychiatry* **61**(6), 830–831. doi:10.1016/j.jaac.2022.03.008.

Borges, M.S. *et al.* (2022) Deviations from a typical development of the cerebellum in youth are associated with psychopathology, executive functions and educational outcomes. *Psychological Medicine*, 1–11. doi:10.1017/S0033291722002926.

Broekman, B.F. *et al.* (2014) Gestational age and neonatal brain microstructure in term born infants: a birth cohort study. *PLoS One* **9**(12), e115229. doi:10.1371/journal.pone.0115229.

Carrion, V.G. *et al.* (2007) Stress predicts brain changes in children: a pilot longitudinal study on youth stress, posttraumatic stress disorder, and the hippocampus. *Pediatrics* **119**(3), 509–516. doi:10.1542/peds.2006-2028.

Casey, B.J. *et al.* (2018) The adolescent brain cognitive development (ABCD) study: imaging acquisition across 21 sites. *Developmental Cognitive Neuroscience* **32**, 43–54. doi:10.1016/j.dcn.2018.03.001.

Castelbaum, L. *et al.* (2020) On the nature of monozygotic twin concordance and discordance for autistic trait severity: a quantitative analysis. *Behavior Genetics* **50**(4), 263–272. doi:10.1007/s10519-019-09987-2.

Cavanna, A.E. (2007) The precuneus and consciousness. *CNS Spectrums* **12**(7), 545–552. doi:10.1017/s1092852900021295.

Crossley, N.A. *et al.* (2009) Superior temporal lobe dysfunction and frontotemporal dysconnectivity in subjects at risk of psychosis and in first-episode psychosis. *Human Brain Mapping* **30**(12), 4129–4137. doi:10.1002/hbm.20834.

Davenport, N.D. *et al.* (2010) Differential fractional anisotropy abnormalities in adolescents with ADHD or schizophrenia. *Psychiatry Research* **181**(3), 193–198. doi:10.1016/j.pscychresns.2009.10.012.

Di Martino, A. *et al.* (2017) Enhancing studies of the connectome in autism using the autism brain imaging data exchange II. *Scientific Data* **4**, 170010. doi:10.1038/sdata.2017.10.

Durkut, M. *et al.* (2022) The longitudinal bidirectional relationship between autistic traits and brain morphology from childhood to adolescence: a population-based cohort study. *Molecular Autism* **13**(1), 31. doi:10.1186/s13229-022-00504-7.

Fischl, B. (2012) FreeSurfer. *NeuroImage* **62**(2), 774–781. doi:10.1016/j.neuroimage.2012.01.021.

Fusar-Poli, P. *et al.* (2013) The psychosis high-risk state: a comprehensive state-of-the-art review. *JAMA Psychiatry* **70**(1), 107–120. doi:10.1001/jamapsychiatry.2013.269.

Gartner, K. (2012) A third component causing random variability beside environment and genotype. A reason for the limited success of a 30 year long effort to standardize laboratory animals? *International Journal of Epidemiology* **41**(2), 335–341. doi:10.1093/ije/dyr219.

Gilbert, K.E. *et al.* (2018) Associations of observed performance monitoring during preschool with obsessive-compulsive disorder and anterior cingulate cortex volume over 12 years. *JAMA Psychiatry* **75**(9), 940–948. doi:10.1001/jamapsychiatry.2018.1805.

Gogtay, N. *et al.* (2008) Three-dimensional brain growth abnormalities in childhood-onset schizophrenia visualized by using tensor-based morphometry. *Proceedings of the National Academy of Sciences of the United States of America* **105**(41), 15979–15984. doi:10.1073/pnas.0806485105.

Goldberg, M.C. *et al.* (2011) Children with high functioning autism show increased prefrontal and temporal cortex activity during error monitoring. *Developmental Cognitive Neuroscience* **1**(1), 47–56. doi:10.1016/j.dcn.2010.07.002.

Halari, R. *et al.* (2009) Reduced activation in lateral prefrontal cortex and anterior cingulate during attention and cognitive control functions in medication-naive adolescents with depression compared to controls. *Journal of Child Psychology and Psychiatry* **50**(3), 307–316. doi:10.1111/j.1469-7610.2008.01972.x.

Hazlett, H.C. *et al.* (2012) Brain volume findings in 6-month-old infants at high familial risk for autism. *The American Journal of Psychiatry* **169**(6), 601–608. doi:10.1176/appi.ajp.2012.11091425.

Hoogman, M. *et al.* (2019) Brain imaging of the cortex in ADHD: a coordinated analysis of large-scale clinical and population-based samples. *The American Journal of Psychiatry* **176**(7), 531–542. doi:10.1176/appi.ajp.2019.18091033.

Jarvers, I. *et al.* (2022) The relationship between adolescents' externalizing and internalizing symptoms and brain development over a period of three years. *NeuroImage. Clinical* **36**, 103195. doi:10.1016/j.nicl.2022.103195.

Jonsson, H. *et al.* (2021) Differences between germline genomes of monozygotic twins. *Nature Genetics* **53**(1), 27–34. doi:10.1038/s41588-020-00755-1.

Kriegeskorte, N. *et al.* (2009) Circular analysis in systems neuroscience: the dangers of double dipping. *Nature Neuroscience* **12**(5), 535–540. doi:10.1038/nn.2303.

Lang, D.J. *et al.* (2004) Reduced basal ganglia volumes after switching to olanzapine in chronically treated patients with schizophrenia. *The American Journal of Psychiatry* **161**(10), 1829–1836. doi:10.1176/ajp.161.10.1829.

Longo, O. (1996) Hot heads and cold brains. Aristotle, Galen and the "radiator theory". *Physis; Rivista Internazionale di Storia della Scienza* **33**(1–3), 259–266. https://www.ncbi.nlm.nih.gov/pubmed/11619385

Machin, G.A. (1996) Some causes of genotypic and phenotypic discordance in monozygotic twin pairs. *American Journal of Medical Genetics* **61**(3), 216–228. doi:10.1002/(SICI)1096-8628(19960122)61:3<216::AID-AJMG5>3.0.CO;2-S.

Marek, S. *et al.* (2022) Reproducible brain-wide association studies require thousands of individuals. *Nature* **603**(7902), 654–660. doi:10.1038/s41586-022-04492-9.

Monk, C.S. *et al.* (2008) Amygdala and ventrolateral prefrontal cortex activation to masked angry faces in children and adolescents with generalized anxiety disorder. *Archives of General Psychiatry* **65**(5), 568–576. doi:10.1001/archpsyc.65.5.568.

Muetzel, R.L. *et al.* (2018) Tracking brain development and dimensional psychiatric symptoms in children: a longitudinal population-based neuroimaging study. *The American Journal of Psychiatry* **175**(1), 54–62. doi:10.1176/appi.ajp.2017.16070813.

Musgrove, D.R. *et al.* (2015) Impaired bottom-up effective connectivity between amygdala and subgenual anterior cingulate cortex in unmedicated adolescents with major depression: results from a dynamic causal modeling analysis. *Brain Connectivity* **5**(10), 608--619. doi:10.1089/brain.2014.0312.

Naumova, O.Y. *et al.* (2013) Gene expression in the human brain: the current state of the study of specificity and spatiotemporal dynamics. *Child Development* **84**(1), 76–88. doi:10.1111/cdev.12014.

Nery, F.G. *et al.* (2017) White matter volumes in youth offspring of bipolar parents. *Journal of Affective Disorders* **209**, 246–253. doi:10.1016/j.jad.2016.11.023.

Newman, E. *et al.* (2016) Anxiety is related to indices of cortical maturation in typically developing children and adolescents. *Brain Structure & Function* **221**(6), 3013–3025. doi:10.1007/s00429-015-1085-9.

Nordahl, C.W. *et al.* (2012) Increased rate of amygdala growth in children aged 2 to 4 years with autism spectrum disorders: a longitudinal study. *Archives of General Psychiatry* **69**(1), 53–61. doi:10.1001/archgenpsychiatry.2011.145.

Odriozola, P. *et al.* (2016) Insula response and connectivity during social and non-social attention in children with autism. *Social Cognitive and Affective Neuroscience* **11**(3), 433–444. doi:10.1093/scan/nsv126.

Piccolino, M. (1998) Animal electricity and the birth of electrophysiology: the legacy of Luigi Galvani. *Brain Research Bulletin* **46**(5), 381–407. doi:10.1016/s0361-9230(98)00026-4.

Piven, J. *et al.* (1992) Magnetic resonance imaging in autism: measurement of the cerebellum, pons, and fourth ventricle. *Biological Psychiatry* **31**(5), 491–504. doi:10.1016/0006-3223(92)90260-7.

Poldrack, R.A. *et al.* (2020) Establishment of best practices for evidence for prediction: a review. *JAMA Psychiatry* **77**(5), 534–540. doi:10.1001/jamapsychiatry.2019.3671.

Poustka, L. *et al.* (2012) Fronto-temporal disconnectivity and symptom severity in children with autism spectrum disorder. *The World Journal of Biological Psychiatry* **13**(4), 269–280. doi:10.3109/15622975.2011.591824.

Ramspek, C.L. *et al.* (2021) Prediction or causality? A scoping review of their conflation within current observational research. *European Journal of Epidemiology* **36**(9), 889–898. doi:10.1007/s10654-021-00794-w.

Raznahan, A. *et al.* (2011) Patterns of coordinated anatomical change in human cortical development: a longitudinal neuroimaging study of maturational coupling. *Neuron* **72**(5), 873–884. doi:10.1016/j.neuron.2011.09.028.

Reiss, A.L. (2009) Childhood developmental disorders: an academic and clinical convergence point for psychiatry, neurology, psychology and pediatrics. *Journal of Child Psychology and Psychiatry* **50**(1–2), 87–98. doi:10.1111/j.1469-7610.2008.02046.x.

Schmaal, L. *et al.* (2017) Cortical abnormalities in adults and adolescents with major depression based on brain scans from 20 cohorts worldwide in the ENIGMA major depressive disorder working group. *Molecular Psychiatry* **22**(6), 900–909. doi:10.1038/mp.2016.60.

Schultz, R.T. (2005) Developmental deficits in social perception in autism: the role of the amygdala and fusiform face area. *International Journal of Developmental Neuroscience* **23**(2–3), 125–141. doi:10.1016/j.ijdevneu.2004.12.012.

Schulz, S.C. *et al.* (1983) Ventricular enlargement in teenage patients with schizophrenia spectrum disorder. *The American Journal of Psychiatry* **140**(12), 1592–1595. doi:10.1176/ajp.140.12.1592.

Schumann, C.M. *et al.* (2004) The amygdala is enlarged in children but not adolescents with autism; the hippocampus is enlarged at all ages. *The Journal of Neuroscience* **24**(28), 6392–6401. doi:10.1523/JNEUROSCI.1297-04.2004.

Seidman, L.J. *et al.* (2006) Altered brain activation in dorsolateral prefrontal cortex in adolescents and young adults at genetic risk for schizophrenia: an fMRI study of working memory. *Schizophrenia Research* **85**(1–3), 58–72. doi:10.1016/j.schres.2006.03.019.

Shaw, P. & Rabin, C. (2009) New insights into attention-deficit/hyperactivity disorder using structural neuroimaging. *Current Psychiatry Reports* **11**(5), 393–398. doi:10.1007/s11920-009-0059-0.

Shaw, P. *et al.* (2018) A multicohort, longitudinal study of cerebellar development in attention deficit hyperactivity disorder. *Journal of Child Psychology and Psychiatry* **59**(10), 1114–1123. doi:10.1111/jcpp.12920.

Shuren, J.E. *et al.* (1995) Insula and obsessive-compulsive disorder. *Canadian Journal of Psychiatry* **40**(2), 112. doi:10.1177/070674379504000215.

Steenkamp, L.R. *et al.* (2022) Hallucinations and brain morphology across early adolescence: a longitudinal neuroimaging study. *Biological Psychiatry* **92**(10), 781–790. doi:10.1016/j.biopsych.2022.05.013.

Thompson, P.M. *et al.* (2014) The ENIGMA consortium: large-scale collaborative analyses of neuroimaging and genetic data. *Brain Imaging and Behavior* **8**(2), 153–182. doi:10.1007/s11682-013-9269-5.

Trontel, H.G. *et al.* (2013) Fusiform correlates of facial memory in autism. *Behavioral Sciences* **3**(3), 348–371. doi:10.3390/bs3030348.

Vetter, N.C. *et al.* (2018) Anterior insula hyperactivation in ADHD when faced with distracting negative stimuli. *Human Brain Mapping* **39**(7), 2972–2986. doi:10.1002/hbm.24053.

Walther, S. *et al.* (2011) Resting state cerebral blood flow and objective motor activity reveal basal ganglia dysfunction in schizophrenia. *Psychiatry Research* **192**(2), 117–124. doi:10.1016/j.pscychresns.2010.12.002.

White, T. (2023) Behavioral phenotypes, stochastic processes, entropy, evolution, and individual variability: toward a unified field theory for neurodevelopment and psychopathology. *Aperture Neuro* **2**, 1–3. doi:10.52294/c900ce20-3ffd-4545-8c15-3ec532b2ee3b.

White, T. *et al.* (2006) Neuropsychological performance in first-episode adolescents with schizophrenia: a comparison with first-episode adults and adolescent control subjects. *Biological Psychiatry* **60**, 463–471.

White, T. *et al.* (2007) Disruption of hippocampal connectivity in children and adolescents with schizophrenia: a voxel-based diffusion tensor imaging study. *Schizophrenia Research* **90**(1–3), 302–307. doi:10.1016/j.schres.2006.09.032.

White, T. *et al.* (2008) Limbic structures and networks in children and adolescents with schizophrenia. *Schizophrenia Bulletin* **34**(1), 18–29. doi:10.1093/schbul/sbm110.

White, T. *et al.* (2013) Pediatric population-based neuroimaging and the generation R study: the intersection of developmental neuroscience and epidemiology. *European Journal of Epidemiology* **28**(1), 99–111. doi:10.1007/s10654-013-9768-0.

White, T. *et al.* (2018) Paediatric population neuroimaging and the generation R study: the second wave. *European Journal of Epidemiology* **33**(1), 99–125. doi:10.1007/s10654-017-0319-y.

White, T.J.H. (2019) Brain development and stochastic processes during prenatal and early life: you can't lose it if you've never had it; but it's better to have it and lose it, than never to have had it at all. *Journal of the American Academy of Child and Adolescent Psychiatry* **58**(11), 1042–1050. doi:10.1016/j.jaac.2019.02.010.

Willyard, C. (2018) New human gene tally reignites debate. *Nature* **558**(7710), 354–355. doi:10.1038/d41586-018-05462-w.

CHAPTER 12

Systems neuroscience

Daniel S. Pine
Section on Development and Affective Neuroscience, National Institute of Mental Health (NIMH) Intramural Research Program, Bethesda, MD, USA

Introduction

The current chapter includes seven sections. The first section defines key terms, highlights clinical relevance, and delineates levels of inquiry targeted in systems neuroscience. The chapter next reviews important contexts by describing relevant material in other chapters and summarizing information on the brain that informs research in systems neuroscience. The final five sections describe examples connecting systems neuroscience to clinical research in key areas: (i) cognitive control, (ii) reward anticipation, (iii) defensive behavior, (iv) attachment and affiliation, and (v) brain development. The chapter leverages these examples to make broader points on the clinical relevance of neuroscience. Examples are selected both for the diverse clinical areas they highlight and for the novel neuroscience techniques they employ.

Key terms and clinical relevance

The term "systems neuroscience" refers to research on neural circuits, which are collections of neurons that can either be localized in one brain area or be broadly scattered across many areas. Neurons form circuits to function as a unit and perform computations that alter how animals behave. The term "computation" refers to calculations performed by circuits expressed through neurons' action potentials, which allow events in the world to influence an animal's behavior. For example, a group of neurons connected to the retina may respond to light by generating action potentials. Mathematical functions describe how patterns of photons striking the retina generate patterns of action potentials in these neurons and how this first pattern of firing alters action-potential firing rates in a second group of neurons. When this second group of neurons is connected to muscles, computations describe the calculations performed by neurons that translate sensory input into behavior. By describing this process, system neuroscience studies how computations performed by neural circuits relate to behavior. Such work is clinically relevant when it targets meaningful behaviors associated with neural circuits and the computations they perform.

Research in systems neuroscience closely relates to the field of computational psychiatry, which seeks to show how the brain represents information in ways that relate to clinical endpoints. From this perspective, computational psychiatry seeks to define the precise rules used by the brain when it performs calculations. Such calculations explain how certain patterns of sensory input leads to particular patterns of motor output and associated changes in behavior. Both systems neuroscience and computational psychiatry examine the functions of neural circuits. However, computational psychiatry focuses relatively narrowly on applications of mathematical tools, whereas systems neuroscience includes these tools and other techniques to study how brain circuits generate behavior. Computational psychiatry typically involves two sets of research approaches (Huys *et al.*, 2016a, Huys *et al.*, 2016b). One approach, often using relatively large datasets, applies mathematical tools to parsimoniously define relations among collections of neural circuits and clinically meaningful behaviors. This first approach often assesses large numbers of neural circuits and many associated behaviors that are only loosely connected by a theory. The second approach uses equations to test predictions from an explicit theory relating functioning of selected neural circuits to clinically meaningful behaviors. With this second approach, preexisting research has often identified relevant neural circuits and has made initial observations that support a theory precisely linking circuitry function to behavior. Both approaches help scholars use computational tools from mathematics and engineering to quantify information processing functions that mediate links between the brain and behavior.

Systems neuroscience helps clinicians in at least three ways. First, considerable efforts seek to improve diagnosis and treatment by applying systems neuroscience. These efforts inform pathophysiological theories of many conditions described in this textbook. When clinicians understand these efforts, they

Rutter's Child and Adolescent Psychiatry and Psychology, Seventh Edition.
Edited by Anita Thapar, Daniel S. Pine, Samuele Cortese, Cathy Creswell, Tamsin J. Ford, James F. Leckman, and Argyris Stringaris.

Companion website: www.wiley.com/go/thapar/rutterspsych7

are better poised to anticipate possible forthcoming theory-driven influences on the classification, outcome-prediction, and treatment of mental illnesses. Second, communications to the public can mislead families about the current capabilities of neuroscience to improve diagnosis and treatment. When clinicians understand systems neuroscience, they are better placed to evaluate such claims and frame realistic expectations with families. Finally, people often struggle to understand factors influencing behavior, particularly behaviors related to mental illness. Besides measures of brain function, many factors, including the availability of resources and exposure to stress, relate powerfully to children's behavior. Nevertheless, brain function strongly shapes behaviors related to clinical outcomes in ways that systems neuroscience can parsimoniously describe. When clinicians can explain these influences, patients and families can feel supported and appreciate the pace of research progress.

Like these guides, other clinical benefits are likely to remain relatively abstract for years. While some readers might expect more immediate effects on practice, multiple complications limit clinical translation. For example, great excitement followed the discovery of optogenetics, which allows scientists to alter activity in neurons with much greater precision than older techniques (Deisseroth, 2012). While the technique continues to evolve, its invasive nature makes it unlikely to be applicable to large groups of children in the coming decades. Other concerns limit applications of less invasive tools. For example, imaging provides impactful ways to chart the connections between behavior and brain function. However, recent work also suggests that brain imaging is unlikely to yield broadly applicable clinical tools in the coming decade. This work tempers enthusiasm by suggesting that earlier studies overestimated the sensitivity of imaging to clinically meaningful features (Marek *et al.*, 2022).

Systems neuroscience research involves experts in many areas. This includes scholars in psychology, psychiatry, information technology, genetics, and engineering, to name just a few areas. It is difficult to delineate boundaries separating systems neuroscience from allied fields, given the rapid pace of research in these many areas. Arguably, brain imaging is uniquely relevant, but many areas discussed in this textbook inform a search for clinical relevance.

Levels of inquiry

The phenomena connected in Figure 12.1 encompass multiple spatial layers of inquiry, extending from microscopic targets to phenomena involving multiple people. Together, these areas operate to support brain–behavior relations through mechanisms, a term that refers to chains of events that interact in ways that cause changes in the behavior of an organism (Bechtel, 2016). At the microscopic level, the top left corner of Figure 12.1 displays a section of the genome, which affects behavior by altering functions within individual neurons that coalesce to function as a circuit. Circuits can be viewed at a microscopic level, as studied using invasive techniques, or at a macroscopic level, as studied noninvasively through brain imaging, as illustrated by the two pictures at the top right and center of Figure 12.1. Finally, when people interact, systems neuroscience research can track the ways in which the brain of one individual alters their behavior in ways that induce changes in the brain and behaviors of the other person. In this way, Figure 12.1 extends research that examines processes operating within cells to processes operating in societies.

Studies in multiple species are needed to identify the connections appearing in Figure 12.1. This is because work in nonhuman animals can utilize invasive techniques not appropriate for use in most people. An evolutionary perspective frames conclusions in cross-species research at multiple levels (Pine *et al.*, 2021). At the microscopic level, humans' differences from other primates and primates' differences from rodents involve distinct genetic regulatory elements supporting brain development. Accordingly, similarities and differences in the ways that genes influence behavior in people and other mammals reflect the shared and unique evolutionary history in each species. Similarly, at the macroscopic level, while humans share some brain regions with many mammalian species, other regions in humans have no such homologs (Murray *et al.*, 2017). Accordingly, research in other species provides clearer insights about human brain–behavior relations when the work targets regions shared across species. Thus, studies of the amygdala can compare function in mammals, nonhuman primates, and people, but studies of the prefrontal cortex (PFC) can only compare function among primates.

Context for systems neuroscience

Research contexts

Systems neuroscience provides a unique perspective by integrating insights arising from other areas of research. Like systems neuroscience, these other areas also concern relations that brain function shows with behavior. However, whereas systems neuroscience connects levels in Figure 12.1, other areas focus more narrowly on isolated components. Systems neuroscience is well placed to impact clinical thinking by addressing questions relevant to a whole person. Nevertheless, the success of this integrative approach rests on other work; integration succeeds when it binds established observations concerning individual components.

Multiple textbook chapters review specific findings and the techniques employed to generate them, reflecting Figure 12.1 components. Readers can more fully appreciate this integration when they read the current chapter alongside these other chapters. Thus, Chapter 21 describes how researchers discover genes that are linked to behavior, and it delineates how techniques identify the different types of genes that influence risk for different groups of mental disorders. While genetic concepts vitally shape the field, equally impactful are the described

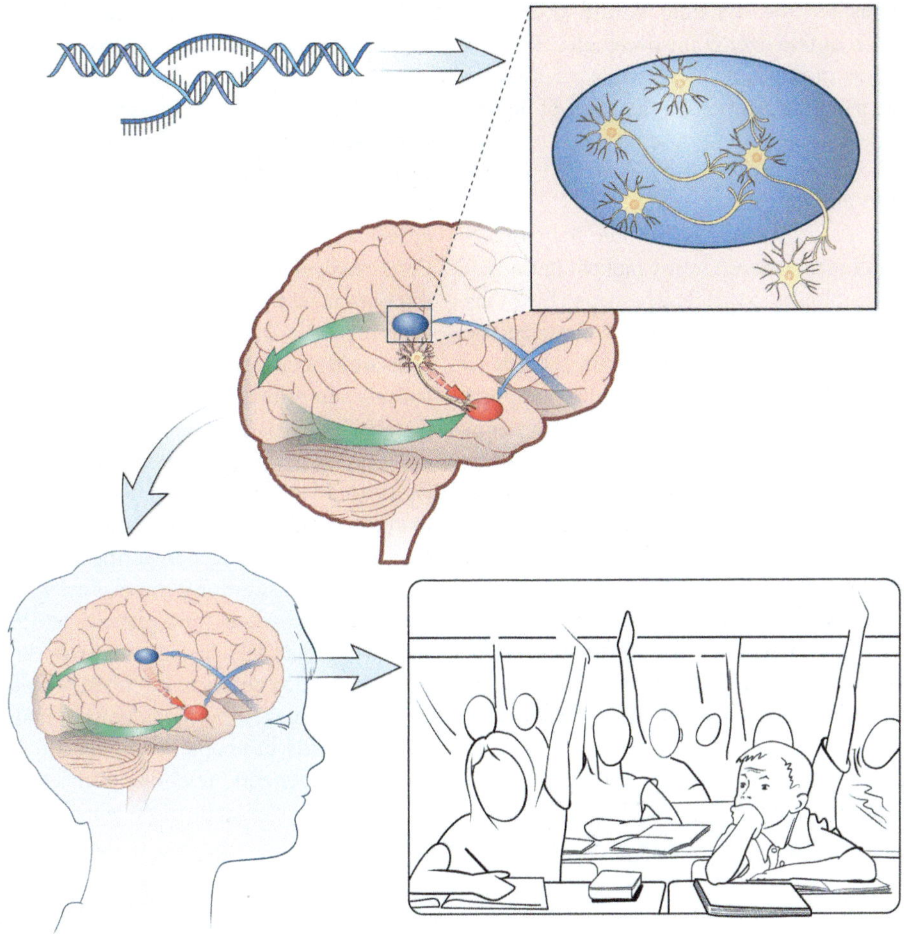

Figure 12.1 Depicts the relationships among constructs targeted in systems neuroscience. The upper-left-hand corner depicts molecular-genetic targets in DNA, as they relate to neuron function, depicted toward the right. Individual neuron function relates to the functions of neural circuits, composed of collections of neurons, as also depicted in this figure. Finally, functioning within these neural circuits represented by the blue, green, and red arrows can be studied through imaging, in structures that can be assessed in children using brain imaging. With this technique, the functions of the circuit in the child can be related to the functions that the child displays in their world, as depicted by a child with his hand on his chin attending school. Finally, the environment interacts with each level of this multitiered system, extending from the classroom through molecular-genetic targets.

technological advances. Similarly, Chapters 20 and 22 describe research on environmental factors related to psychopathology. These factors can act either independently or in concert with genes through gene–environment correlations and interactions. Influence from genes or environments on brain function are better understood when examined in comprehensive fashions.

Research on brain function in humans uniquely positions systems neuroscience as a clinically relevant area. Chapters 10, 11, and 26 describe details about brain functions. As one aspect of the material, Chapters 10 and 26 explain how the effects of genes and the environment are mediated through their influences on brain development and function. As another aspect, Chapter 11 discusses brain-imaging research that applies principles from systems neuroscience to study patients using multiple noninvasive techniques. Briefly summarized, this includes electroencephalography (EEG) and magnetoencephalography (MEG), tools with millisecond-level temporal resolution. This allows researchers to quantify the many important features of brain function that unfold very rapidly. Chapter 11 also describes many magnetic resonance imaging (MRI)-based techniques, which assess aspects of brain structure, function, and chemistry. Perhaps more than any other suite of imaging techniques, MRI-based tools provide great clinical promise, due to exquisite spatial resolution.

Finally, the computational approach employed in systems neuroscience research benefits from research on psychological processes (Ferrante *et al.*, 2019). Such research defines the functions performed by these processes and provides a basis for generating equations leveraged in computational psychiatry and systems neuroscience. Most of the textbook's first 10 chapters describe psychological processes in typical and atypical development. This focus on development reminds readers about the complexity of applying systems neuroscience to children.

Applications must consider the dynamic nature of brain–behavior relations, which unfold over many timescales. Readers are encouraged to review multiple chapters, while referring to Figure 12.1 and considering mechanistic explanation of behaviors arising from neural circuits.

Fundamental brain functions

Readers can appreciate systems neuroscience when they understand principles of brain organization. The top half of Figure 12.2 schematically depicts homologies in vertebrates shaped by events spanning hundreds of millions of years. Circuitry connects the cerebral cortex, or its homologs in nonmammalian species, to subcortical structures (Murray *et al.*, 2017), which supports interactions among structures, enabling seamless coordination of perception and action. This "perception–action" coordination proved advantageous for our ancestors by facilitating access to resources, assisting in predator avoidance, and enabling procreation (Cisek, 2019). Behavior can be understood by localizing information processing functions to each of the circuitry components schematized in the top half of Figure 12.2. Species similarities and differences reflect evolution's impact on the individual components in the figure. Circuits having similar components in many mammals support broad ideas about perception–action coordination. However, more narrow ideas reflect cross-species differences and the complex cortical circuitry of primates (Giarrocco & Averbeck, 2022). Vertebrate brain structures are linked by one set of neurons, shown as green arrows in Figure 12.2, which activate targets, as well as another set of neurons, shown as red lines, which inhibit targets.

Among mammals, cross-species similarities and differences manifest in parts of the cerebral cortex labeled in the bottom half of Figure 12.2. Areas appearing in yellow, such as motor cortex, somatosensory cortex, auditory cortex, and visual cortex, show strong cross-species similarities. These regions perform concrete functions closely related to interactions with the environment: perceiving objects or performing simple acts. Figure 12.2 depicts other areas in purple. These include the cingulate and orbito-frontal cortices, which show greater similarities among primates than between rodents and primates, as well as the dorsolateral prefrontal cortex (DLPFC), and parietal and temporal association cortices, which differ even among primates. These and other purple-shaded regions tend to perform more abstract functions less closely related to interactions with the environment. These include the representation of complex plans for acquiring resources.

Parallels exist among the evolution of brain structures, the age in people when they mature, and the relation structures show with disorders. Some structures, such as subcortical components of the canonical circuit schematized in the top half of Figure 12.2, have homologs among many vertebrates, mature relatively early in people, and may show similarities across age in the components' relations with clinical conditions. Other structures, such as some of the purple darkly shaded association

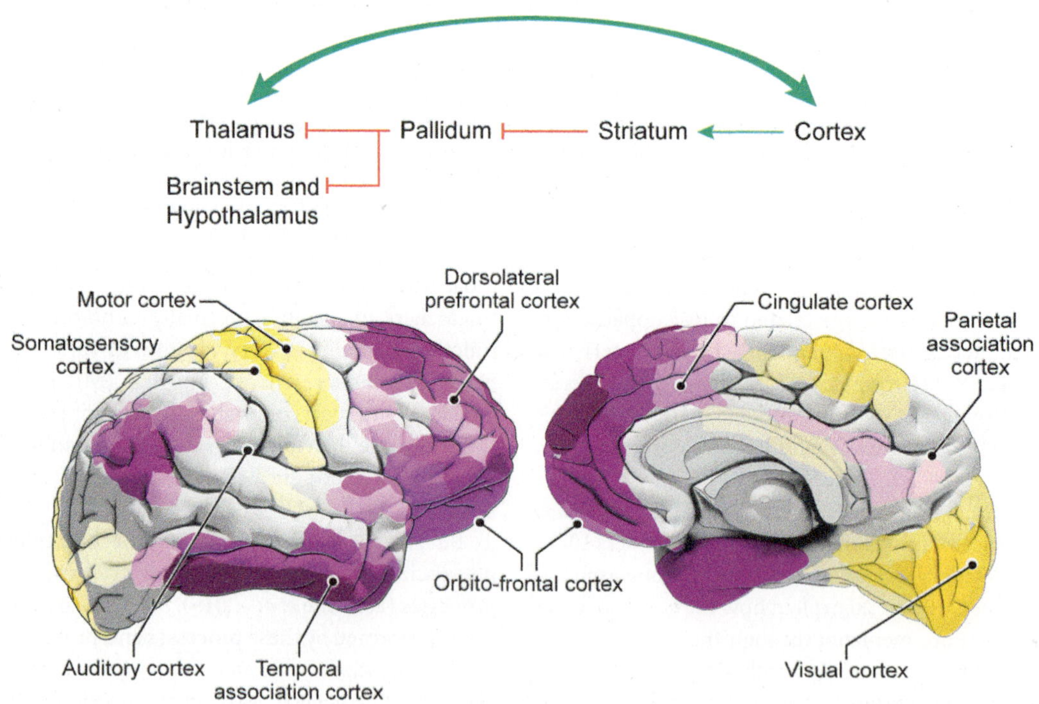

Figure 12.2 The top half of this figure depicts a schematic display of vertebrate brain circuitry, with red lines indicating inhibitory connections and green lines indicating excitatory connections. The bottom half of this figure depicts cortical regions in ways that reflect cross-species similarities. Areas with yellow shading show relatively strong cross-mammalian similarities, with purple shading identifying areas unique to primates or hominins when the shading is dark.

areas in Figure 12.2, only exist in primates, mature relatively late in people, and may show strong age differences in their relations with clinical conditions.

Cognitive control

Defining behaviors, psychological processes, and clinical endpoints

Cognitive control is a psychological process that facilitates adaptation by suppressing neural activity inappropriate to the context. Clinical studies of cognitive control typically ask children to perform routine motor tasks while the researcher assesses task performance (Cohen *et al.*, 2004; Carter, 2005; Carter, 2006; van Veen *et al.*, 2008). Work in this area provides clues about the tools that systems neuroscience research may yield for the prediction of outcomes, particularly among children with complex clinical pictures involving comorbid disorders.

Figure 12.3a depicts a trial from one typical cognitive control task (Nigg, 2007; Geburek *et al.*, 2012). In this task, subjects choose a response signaled by rightward- or leftward-pointing arrows. This can be difficult for a child to do when the task proceeds rapidly, when stimuli are difficult to see, or when a rightward-pointing central target arrow appears amidst many, darker leftward-pointing distractor arrows. Hence, these and other aspects of difficult trials signal the need to engage

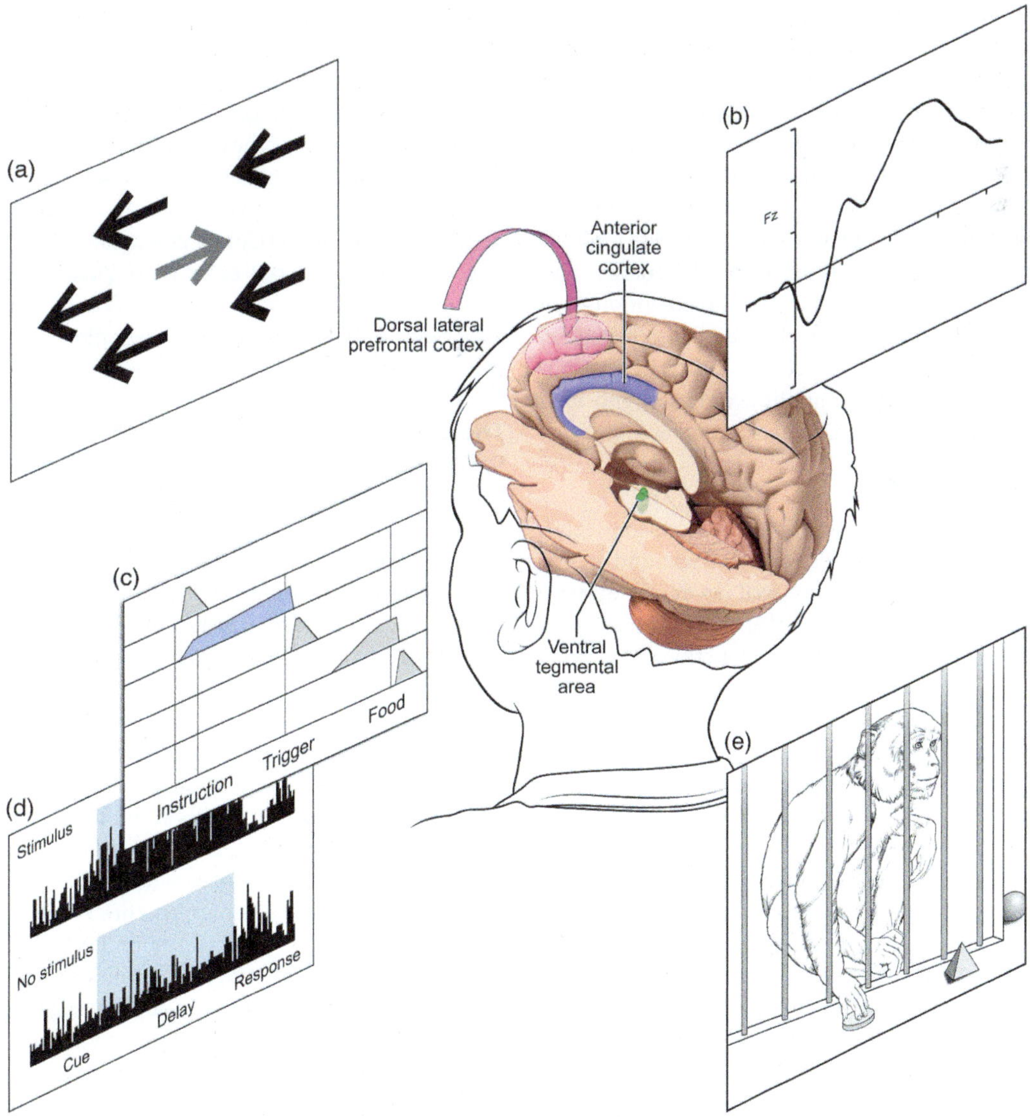

Figure 12.3 Depicts research on cognitive control, with panels indicated by letters appearing around a view of a boy's brain displaying regions that support cognitive control. (a) Displays the flanker task on a screen that can be used in brain imaging or electrophysiology studies. (b) Depicts the error-related negativity (ERN) response, which is recorded from a child's scalp using electroencephalography. (c) Summarizes data collected from the individual neuron plots that appear in figure (d) recorded from a monkey performing a task shown in the figure (e). Blue shading in (c) highlights the way activity in dopamine neurons reflects reward anticipation. Other plots in (c) illustrate characteristic responses in different parts of the cognitive control circuit to instructions, triggers, and food cues.

cognitive control to maintain performance. Multiple psychological processes and computations manifest on such tasks, dissociable by their unique neural correlates. For example, one process involves the maintenance of task rules (e.g., push right-hand button to a faint central-appearing, rightward-pointing arrow). Another involves the monitoring of errors (e.g., mistaken commission of a left-hand button response to a faint, central-appearing, rightward-pointing arrow).

Clinical applications link the processes associated with behaviors observed in the laboratory to behaviors that occur in children's daily lives. For example, children with attention deficit hyperactivity disorder (ADHD) and obsessive–compulsive disorder (OCD) perform poorly on cognitive control tasks, though the nature of these deficits varies in the two disorders (Nigg, 2007; Geburek *et al.*, 2012; Bellato *et al.*, 2021). In children with ADHD, clinical reflections of deficient cognitive control could be seen as a failure to suppress boisterous behavior appropriate when the child's class is playing an outside game but inappropriate when the class transitions to the schoolroom to begin reading time. In children with OCD, clinical reflections could be seen as a failure to suppress the urge to wash one's hands, after one has already washed one's hands multiple times. As such, difficulties quantified in the laboratory may reflect unique features of symptoms in the two conditions that manifest as in these examples where children fail to engage in their daily lives cognitive control processes studied in the laboratory. More information concerning these disorders and their pathophysiology can be found in Chapters 54 and 60.

Neural circuitry and behavior

Systems neuroscience research links brain functions to psychological processes by deploying electrophysiologic and brain-imaging techniques with people as well as more invasive techniques in nonhuman primates or patients who require invasive clinical monitoring. The structure and function of the nervous system share features across vertebrates, reflecting a pattern labeled as the "canonical vertebrate brain." Figure 12.2 shows how this pattern is arranged into a loop in mammals that connects the neocortex to structures lying beneath it, comprising the so-called "subcortical structures." Referring to this pattern when imaging functions of the brain allows clinicians to place neural perturbations in a broader context of systems neuroscience research. Cognitive control studies detect perturbations in four structures: (i) the anterior cingulate gyrus, which is shaded in blue in Figure 12.3, and associated medial prefrontal cortex (mPFC), structures with homologs in rodents and nonhuman primates, (ii) the DLPFC, a structure shaded pink in Figure 12.3 with homologs only in primates, as well as the (iii) basal ganglia, and (iv) dopaminergic neurons of the ventral tegmental area (VTA), two subcortical structures with homologs in most vertebrates (Schultz, 2001; Cohen *et al.*, 2004; Corbetta *et al.*, 2008). Figure 12.3 illustrates the architecture of this circuit, where functioning has been mapped with invasive studies in nonhuman primates.

This circuit enables behavior by supporting a range of psychological processes that work together to shape behavior. For example, research suggests that the DLPFC represents stimulus–action rules (Miller & Cohen, 2001), whereas the VTA generates a prediction error signal when events violate expectations (Schultz, 2001). Research in computational psychiatry illustrates how circuitry understandings connect behavior to brain functions and thereby generate ideas about the pathophysiology of mental disorders (Geana *et al.*, 2022). Extensions of this work use electrophysiology techniques to contrast cognitive control perturbations in ADHD and OCD. In ADHD, findings suggest a degraded representation of error signals, whereas in OCD, findings suggest somewhat opposing patterns, an enhanced representation of error signals (Bellato *et al.*, 2021). This is exemplified by research on the error-related negativity (ERN), an electrophysiological signal that is illustrated in Figure 12.3b. The ERN reflects the rapid propagation of a brain signal that occurs in the earliest stages of error commission before an individual has awareness of the error. This signal can be recorded on the surface of the head using EEG, and this scalp-detected signal is thought to arise from reflections of VTA-to-mPFC signaling deep within the brain (Cohen *et al.*, 2004). From this perspective, in ADHD, reduced error representation manifests as an attenuation of the ERN, whereas in OCD, the opposite manifests, with enhanced error representation manifesting as an enhancement of the ERN.

The search for clinical applications

Differentiating ADHD and OCD with electrophysiology represents a reasonable first step in clinical applications. However, to be useful, systems neuroscience should address questions not answered with clinical knowledge. This must go beyond a mere differentiation between ADHD and OCD, as these two conditions can be readily distinguished on clinical grounds. For example, ADHD and OCD commonly co-occur, and it is difficult to anticipate how symptoms in children with both problems will manifest over time, either with or without treatment. As techniques improve, neural measures could quantify cognitive control functions in children with increasing reliability and sensitivity. These next-generation measures could longitudinally differentiate clinical outcomes in children with ADHD and OCD in ways that go beyond predictions generated from only clinical data.

Such research resembles approaches in other areas of medicine, where prognosis reflects data on both clinical and pathophysiological factors. Current electrophysiology measures remain insufficiently sensitive to support such applications, and even if future measures prove more sensitive, efforts need to adapt these future measures for large-scale clinical use. Findings suggest the potential fruition of continued pursuit of this research: the ERN predicts risks for adult psychopathology related to early-life temperaments (Tang *et al.*, 2020). Future efforts might attempt to predict outcomes in patients presenting for treatment who manifest signs of both ADHD and OCD. Nevertheless, clinicians should appreciate the time it will require for these possibilities to be realized. Research in this section summarizes some of the best supported work using electrophysiology to predict outcomes in common pediatric mental illnesses. Despite providing important clues, wide-scale clinical application remains many years away.

Reward anticipation

Defining behaviors, psychological processes, and brain circuitry

Tasks employed in research on cognitive control among nonhuman primates can also be used to study features of reward anticipation, a psychological process distinct from cognitive control. The term "reward" refers to stimuli that animals will extend effort to obtain, and nonhuman primates extend effort on cognitive-control tasks so that they will obtain rewards, such as a squirt of fruit juice. Studies of reward processing examine psychological processes and associated neural events that manifest around the times of reward anticipation and receipt.

Beyond research on cognitive control in nonhuman primates, studies in diverse species examine other facets of reward processing. In the 1950s, rats were shown to extend effort to receive stimulation in certain brain regions, including the VTA that appears in Figure 12.3. With this work, Olds and Milner initiated a thematic series of studies (Olds & Milner, 1954). While the broad role of dopamine was recognized early in this series, almost 40 years later, Robinson and Berridge emphasized the particular role for dopamine in representing incentive features of rewards (Robinson & Berridge, 1993). Phasic responses in dopamine neurons occur when animals anticipate forthcoming rewards, as is depicted in Figure 12.3c and d. Brain-imaging studies extended such research to patients by differentiating regions in humans that responded to the anticipation as opposed to receipt of a reward (Keren *et al.*, 2018).

The search for clinical applications

Research on reward anticipation illustrates the many ways that systems neuroscience could impact clinicians' daily lives. Studies in this area are notable both for similarities with research on cognitive control and for informing clinicians about other issues, such as safety and possible utility of medications. This illustrates diversity in the promise of systems neuroscience.

Across the life span, brain-imaging studies in patients generate findings on reward anticipation that resemble results in studies on relations among the ERN, ADHD, and OCD. However, unlike work on the ERN, studies of reward anticipation find the most consistent relations with major depressive disorder (MDD), with some evidence of particularly strong associations in adolescence (Keren *et al.*, 2018). This includes cross-sectional functional MRI (fMRI) studies that show adolescents with MDD to manifest lower levels of engagement in the striatum than healthy adolescents when anticipating receipt of a reward.

Research on reward anticipation demonstrates how systems neuroscience combines tools to understand brain function in patients. The spatial resolution of fMRI inspires confidence in scientists attempting to localize brain regions expressing reduced engagement to reward anticipation; precise localization is needed when comparing findings in people and other species. However, low temporal resolution leaves some uncertainty about timing; findings on fMRI scans possibly could reflect MDD-related differences in either reward anticipation or receipt. This uncertainty is addressed by studies using EEG, which, compared to fMRI, possesses converse strengths and weaknesses: stronger temporal but weaker spatial resolution. EEG studies implicate altered reward anticipation in MDD. Moreover, longitudinal studies using both MRI and EEG suggest that patterns observed in cross-sectional data might also predict future risk for depressive symptoms (Burani *et al.*, 2021; Tang *et al.*, 2022). Nevertheless, similar problems limiting applications of the ERN restrict clinical application, where findings for the ERN even may appear closer to clinical application.

Beyond understandings of outcome prediction, research on reward anticipation may inform ideas about therapeutics. This is because systems neuroscience studies of psychostimulant effects in rodents and nonhuman primates delineate mechanisms that causally connect the medications to clinically relevant behaviors (Robinson & Berridge, 1993; Berridge & Arnsten, 2013). One set of studies outlines mechanisms that could underlie the medications' abuse liability. These studies could inform the creation of novel medications with reduced risk for abuse or the safer use of available stimulants in the treatment of ADHD. Clearly, clinical studies inform such treatment practices by examining relations among ADHD, stimulant use, and risk for substance abuse (Lee *et al.*, 2011). However, ethical restrictions preclude implementation of experiments that would more definitively reveal a stimulant's potential causal role in generating substance abuse problems. Studies in rodents and nonhuman primates use experimental designs to fill this causality-related gap.

Other studies in rodents and nonhuman primates might inform development of novel antidepressants. Many such new treatments for MDD in adults affect brain dopamine pathways, which relate intimately to reward anticipation, as shown in Figure 12.3c for the blue-shaded area (Marwaha *et al.*, 2022). The abuse liability of these new treatments could derive from such effects on the brain. While these neural effects provide a target for continued development of new treatments, the effects also raise questions about abuse liability. These questions appear particularly heightened among youth, where systems neuroscience research delineates important facets of development (Spear, 2018). The immature state of the adolescent brain could affect the use of new antidepressants for MDD in this age group. Systems neuroscience can generate important information in this arena to help guide clinicians.

Defensive behavior

Defining behaviors, psychological processes, and brain circuitry

The term "defensive behaviors" refers to actions that animals perform when confronted by threats, stimuli capable of harming the animal. Like studies of cognitive control and reward anticipation, research on defensive behavior maps the neural architecture that responds to events in the environment in ways that generate particular actions. One set of clinically relevant defensive behaviors manifest similarly in many organisms. These behaviors relate to functions in neural circuits that operate similarly among rodents, nonhuman primates, and people.

Mammalian brains possess limited resources, and the term "attention" refers to psychological processes that efficiently allocate these resources based on goal relevance and stimulus salience (Corbetta *et al.*, 2008). In contexts involving the potential for harm, threats receive priority for processing, even when they are irrelevant to current goals (LeDoux, 2000; Bar-Haim *et al.*, 2007; Pagliaccio *et al.*, 2019). Computations supporting attention allocation in these situations can be quantified with cognitive tasks (Naim *et al.*, 2022), thereby linking brain functions to behavior. Such tasks rely on a panoply of measures, including relatively indirect measures of computational outputs, such as reaction time or eye-gaze patterns, and more direct measures of computations acquired through brain imaging. Across these various measures, studies consistently find that children with anxiety disorders allocate more attention to threats than children without anxiety disorders (Bar-Haim *et al.*, 2007; Pine *et al.*, 2009; White *et al.*, 2017; Abend *et al.*, 2021). In fact, relations with perturbed attention may be the most consistent finding in all available research on the pathophysiology of anxiety. Such findings can manifest even when threats are presented so briefly that children remain unaware of their presence (Monk *et al.*, 2008).

The search for clinical applications

Research on attention is unique from a systems neuroscience standpoint. This work more directly informs novel therapeutics than work in many other areas, including cognitive control and reward anticipation. Attention problems in anxiety may involve brain circuits dissociable from circuits supporting language that are engaged in psychotherapy (LeDoux & Pine, 2016). Problems with attention show features that resemble habits, which can be altered by repetitive motor training (Murray *et al.*, 2017). Habits differ from processes that are learned primarily through language in that they are more powerfully shaped by practice and training than by cognitive understanding. These observations inform the creation of novel therapies that use repetitive motor training to alleviate attention problems in pediatric anxiety disorders. One set of studies suggests that active forms of these therapies produce stronger clinical effects than control therapies (Price *et al.*, 2016). Another set of studies suggests that these therapies affect brain systems and associated computations that are distinct from the systems engaged in cognitive behavioral therapy (CBT). When considering clinical trial data, adding active attention-training therapies to CBT might target multiple brain systems and thereby produce more robust clinical effects than adding control therapies to CBT (Shechner *et al.*, 2014; White *et al.*, 2017).

Behavior studies generate progress in research on attention, based on promising findings from clinical trials. However, when attempting to quantify pathophysiology, assessments of behavior remain incomplete; more complete insights can follow by assessing both behavior and brain function. This is because many structures in the brain can perform the same functions, which suggests that a behavioral correlate of anxiety could arise from one of many potential problems in the brain. Hence, when attempting to study processes that generate behavior, combined assessments of brain and behavior more precisely differentiate phenomena than assessments of behavior on their own (Edelman & Gally, 2001). This linking of many structures to one underlying function has been termed degeneracy, and it is ubiquitous in the control of defensive behaviors (LeDoux & Daw, 2018). As a result, many possible neural problems could produce the signatures of anxiety expressed through perturbations in attention.

Research on defensive behavior is relevant to treatment. While premature to support widespread use, some scholars are already beginning to consider clinical applications of neuroscience studies of defensive behavior in contexts where potential treatment-related risks can be justified (Wald *et al.*, 2016). Additional problems must be solved for this trend to continue. For example, few brain-imaging studies on novel treatments examine attention, which leaves questions open on relations between treatment and brain function. Moreover, the psychometric properties of measures used to assess attention correlates of anxiety are poor, and treatments exert relatively small effects (Price *et al.*, 2015). Next-generation measures may address these limitations (Linetzky *et al.*, 2020), but large-scale randomized controlled trials are needed. Despite promise, years of work are needed before this research can affect routine care of children.

Attachment and affiliation

Defining specific behaviors

The fourth example considers the neural underpinnings of attachment and affiliation. These areas differ from defensive behavior, where attachment and affiliation show stark differences among rodents, nonhuman primates, and humans. This illuminates a puzzle in cross-species research: questions must be addressed in each species at an appropriate level of abstraction, so that species-typical behaviors can be studied in a form that still applies to other species. Research on attachment and affiliation probes the complex array of behaviors that bond people (Carter, 1998). This includes studies on infants and their mothers' interactions that ground social development (Paukner *et al.*, 2011).

Important work examines rodents, particularly two species of vole that differ markedly in their social behavior (Insel *et al.*, 1993; Carter, 1998). One highly social species, the prairie vole, expresses rich social behavior at virtually all life stages. In contrast, the other species, the isolated-living montane vole, only expresses such behaviors when infant voles are raised by their mothers. These differences relate to neuropeptide signaling. Figure 12.4a contrasts the solitary-appearing montane vole and the social prairie vole, whose differences in behavior relate to differing neural distributions of receptors for neuropeptides, including oxytocin. This work also highlights the role of another neuropeptide, vasopressin, which compliments oxytocin in its effects.

Studies in this area illustrate the integrative capacity of systems neuroscience by connecting components in Figure 12.1 (Boender & Young, 2020). This links genetic variation at the microscopic level to social behavior at the macroscopic level, in research that successfully traverses the many complex paths connecting genes to behavior. As described in Chapter 21, isolated genes typically exert small influences on behavior that are transduced through complex arrays of neurons and the circuits they form. Benefiting patients by applying genetic knowledge requires scientists to find causal links connecting genes to neurons and neurons to behavior of complicated organisms, much in the way that has been done for oxytocin. Studies of neuropeptides in voles map mechanistic, localized, and precisely timed influences that genes initiate. Whereas species differences reflect brain distributions, changes in the montane vole may reflect precisely timed changes in gene expression. Finally, while relatively consistent findings exist over 30 years relating oxytocin to vole behavior, new technologies raise questions about such findings. In particular, clustered regularly interspaced short palindromic repeats (CRISPR) refers to a technique for altering genes in many species. This technique provides more precise genetic tools than available during years when many findings accrued, and recent findings using this technology raise questions on the precise role of oxytocin in vole behavior (Berendzen *et al.*, 2023).

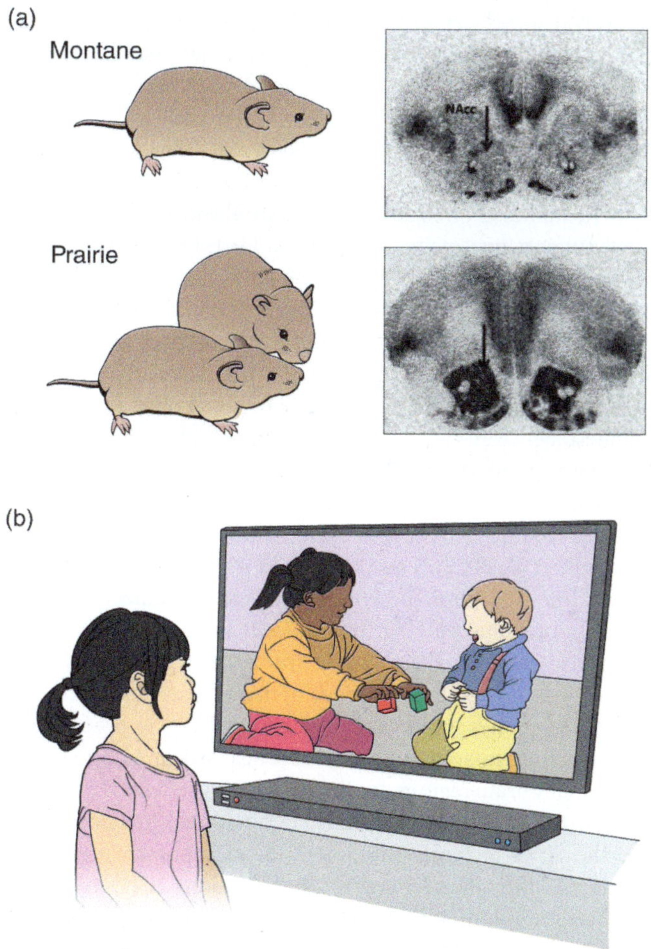

Figure 12.4 Depicts work on aspects of attachment. (a) Shows two species of voles and associated brain slices depicting differences in the brain chemistry. (b) Depicts a task that might be used to study brain systems in children related to attachment.

Linking the behavior to clinical questions and neural circuitry

Brain circuitry that supports attachment in voles relates to an array of developmental psychopathologies. Research on autism spectrum disorders (ASDs) provides one example. Of note, readers should recognize the harmful effect of outdated theories incorrectly relating attachment in infants to ASD. Research finds no relation in humans between attachment during infancy and ASD. Additional relevant discussion appears in Chapter 50, focused specifically on ASDs, as well as in Chapters 1 and 3, which describe ASDs as one example of neurodevelopmental disorders (NDDs). The current section focuses on relations in people between social behavior and brain circuitry, where circuitry has been shown to relate to attachment in voles as opposed to people.

Precise quantification of infants' social behavior with caregivers is difficult, particularly as it relates to brain function. This reflects the complex interactions that unfold over time between infants and caregivers. Success in research follows from studies that attempt to model isolated features of these behaviors, either in infants or children. This has been achieved in studies that present infants and children with pictures of faces or movies showing social behaviors, such as when two children share, as shown in Figure 12.4b. In these studies, children view such material while scientists monitor their viewing patterns or brain function, which some studies successfully link to clinical features of ASD (Constantino *et al.*, 2017; Klin & Jones, 2018). Nevertheless, inconsistent findings remain (Webb *et al.*, 2022).

The search for clinical applications

Attempts to clinically apply insights gained from basic research on oxytocin demonstrate potential promise and pitfalls in research on novel therapeutics. Most new therapies arise from serendipitous clinical observations. Even some of the newest treatments, such as antidepressants discussed in the section on reward anticipation, arose from this path. Studies on defensive behavior describe an alternative route that arises from basic science. This informed the development of a therapy that indirectly targets neural circuitry through repetitive training of particular behaviors. Novel treatments for ASDs more directly target brain function by using pharmacology to extend insights on attachment and affiliation in rodents. Such treatments use medications that may carry greater risks than the type of repetitive cognitive training used to treat pediatric anxiety disorders. Risk for adverse effects of such medications can be justified among patients who suffer from particularly severe forms of ASDs.

Systems neuroscience research relating neuropeptides to attachment and affiliation illustrates the obstacles on the path toward clinical translation. Research in voles first stimulated work examining the effects of oxytocin in healthy humans (Meyer-Lindenberg & Tost, 2012), which found relations with social behavior. Next, studies followed that utilized oxytocin as a novel treatment for ASD. These and other initial findings were suggestive of a possible role in treatment. Nevertheless, as with many treatments identified through pathophysiological research, the most definitive evaluation of the therapy found no benefit (Sikich *et al.*, 2021). While disappointing, these findings show the tortuous nature of the path connecting pathophysiology to treatment, reflecting the early stage of systems neuroscience applications. Caution is needed when evaluating new treatments arising through this path.

Brain development

Defining behaviors

This final example considers different behaviors than other areas in the chapter. Other examples leverage invasive studies of neural architecture in rodents or nonhuman primates. This final example primarily follows from brain-imaging research with children. Moreover, unlike earlier examples on precise behaviors, the final example considers broader behaviors and depicts the dual directions in which systems neuroscience can flow, where insights, initially in children with ADHD, inform studies in other species. Chapter 54 describes ADHD, which involves behaviors considered to be pathological, based as much on the age during which the child expresses these behaviors as the form of these behaviors. For example, hyperactivity manifests in age-specific manners; the same level of hyperactivity considered pathological for a 10-year-old might appear normal in a six-year-old child. Development alters the absolute threshold for defining hyperactivity, reflecting changes in children's mean level of activity.

Appropriate developmental contextualization of behavior underlies assessment of NDDs. As described in Chapter 3, many features of ADHD besides hyperactivity involve behaviors that would be appropriate at younger ages but are viewed as pathological in a relatively old child. Longitudinal research suggests that this might reflect a generalized slowing of typical developmental processes, but this research primarily examines behavior in the absence of relations with brain function. As described for defensive behaviors, degeneracy in brain–behavior relations necessitates incorporation of neural data for precise classification of behavior. This view raises questions for systems neuroscience. Does pathophysiology in ADHD involve atypical brain development, or does pathophysiology involve a mere slowing of otherwise normal processes, commensurate with the form of the behaviors being expressed? If the latter, can we learn to accelerate development in some children, or should we recommend activities for children, based on levels of neural development as opposed to chronological age? Finally, if ADHD results from different as opposed to slowed development, how do we view changing behavior with maturity? Does this reflect some form of atypical compensatory response? Thus, systems neuroscience seeks to ground a view of ADHD in data on brain structure and function.

The search for clinical applications

As noted above, MRI provides impactful tools for applications of systems neuroscience in children. This technique allows safe, highly reliable assessments of brain structure, which supports an ever-growing series of longitudinal MRI investigations relevant to core questions about neurodevelopment and its relation to ADHD. This work continues to accelerate and support MRI studies in thousands of children, assessed with tens-of-thousands of scans, across most phases of development. This research generates rich insights on ADHD.

MRI studies of brain structure in typical and atypical development support two major conclusions. First, brain development involves amazingly complex, slow processes, findings unsurprising based on basic research (Bethlehem *et al.*, 2022). These processes involve multiple patterns of increases and decreases in structural components of various brain regions and types of brain tissue, visible into the 20s. Second, cross-sectional associations manifest between various clinical factors and brain structure. However, recent studies utilizing relatively large samples find associations that are smaller than in older studies that were based on smaller samples (Hoogman *et al.*, 2019; Boedhoe *et al.*, 2020; Bernanke *et al.*, 2022). Thus, for a child with ADHD who is otherwise free of neurological illness, the measurement of brain structure provides limited if any clinically useful information.

Two interacting sets of future studies may generate clinical applications related to neurodevelopmental features of ADHD. One set of studies might extend ongoing efforts in brain imaging. Structural imaging suggests that correlates of ADHD manifest in many brain regions, each showing small effects (Hoogman *et al.*, 2019; Bernanke *et al.*, 2022). Functional imaging might use the types of large-scale longitudinal approach previously employed in structural imaging (Shaw & Sudre, 2021). Available data suggest that functional studies often detect larger associations with cognition and behavior than structural studies (Marek *et al.*, 2022). As a result, functional studies generating larger effect sizes might differentiate features of ADHD that result from distinct types of development. The other set of studies might extend ongoing efforts in basic science. Strong findings on the genetics of ADHD could inform such basic research, as it seeks to define the ways in which genetic influences shape risk through effects on various neural processes. The availability of invasive tools allows basic research to identify such processes more quickly than clinical research. Such interacting clinical and basic avenues differentiates systems neuroscience approaches in this final example. While the first four examples emphasized the flow of ideas from basic to clinical avenues, this final example involves a flow of ideas in the other direction. Nevertheless, as with the other four examples, this final one also highlights the complexity of systems neuroscience, which makes it unlikely that research in this area will broadly impact clinical practice for many years.

Conclusion

The current chapter conveys three fundamental themes. First, the chapter introduces the reader to systems neuroscience and computational psychiatry research, emphasizing the multidisciplinary nature of these rapidly changing fields. Second, clinicians are given reasons to consider systems neuroscience as relevant to their practice, and findings in other chapters are highlighted to show how systems neuroscience integrates many themes appearing in chapters across the textbook. Finally, five specific examples illustrate the range of questions targeted using various techniques. These examples suggest that systems neuroscience primarily impacts clinical thinking by abstractly shaping views of mental illness. Concrete tools useful for diagnosis or treatment in the care of most patients are unlikely to appear before publication of the next edition of this textbook.

Acknowledgment

The work for this chapter was supported by projects ZIA-MH002781 and ZIA-MH002782 in the Intramural Research Program of the National Institute of Mental Health.

References

Abend, R. *et al.* (2021) Converging multi-modal evidence for implicit threat-related bias in pediatric anxiety disorders. *Research on Child and Adolescent Psychopathology* **49**, 227–240.

Bar-Haim, Y. *et al.* (2007) Threat-related attentional bias in anxious and nonanxious individuals: a meta-analytic study. *Psychological Bulletin* **133**, 1–24.

Bechtel, W. (2016) Mechanists must be holists too! Perspectives from circadian biology. *Journal of the History of Biology* **49**, 705–731.

Bellato, A. *et al.* (2021) A systematic review and meta-analysis of altered electrophysiological markers of performance monitoring in Obsessive-compulsive disorder (OCD), Gilles de la Tourette Syndrome (GTS), Attention-deficit/hyperactivity disorder (ADHD) and autism. *Neuroscience and Biobehavioral Reviews* **131**, 964–987.

Berendzen, K.M. *et al.* (2023) Oxytocin receptor is not required for social attachment in prairie voles. *Neuron* **111**, 787–796.e4.

Bernanke, J. *et al.* (2022) Structural brain measures among children with and without ADHD in the adolescent brain and cognitive development study cohort: a cross-sectional US population-based study. *Lancet Psychiatry* **9**, 222–231.

Berridge, C.W. & Arnsten, A.F. (2013) Psychostimulants and motivated behavior: arousal and cognition. *Neuroscience and Biobehavioral Reviews* **37**, 1976–1984.

Bethlehem, R.A.I. *et al.* (2022) Brain charts for the human lifespan. *Nature* **604**, 525–533.

Boedhoe, P.S.W. *et al.* (2020) Subcortical brain volume, regional cortical thickness, and cortical surface area across disorders: findings from the ENIGMA ADHD, ASD, and OCD working groups. *The American Journal of Psychiatry* **177**, 834–843.

Boender, A.J. & Young, L.J. (2020) Oxytocin, vasopressin and social behavior in the age of genome editing: a comparative perspective. *Hormones and Behavior* **124**, 104780.

Burani, K. *et al.* (2021) Neural response to rewards, stress and sleep interact to prospectively predict depressive symptoms in adolescent girls. *Journal of Clinical Child and Adolescent Psychology* **50**, 131–140.

Carter, C.S. (1998) Neuroendocrine perspectives on social attachment and love. *Psychoneuroendocrinology* **23**, 779–818.

Carter, C.S. (2005) Applying new approaches from cognitive neuroscience to enhance drug development for the treatment of impaired cognition in schizophrenia. *Schizophrenia Bulletin* **31**, 810–815.

Carter, C.S. (2006) Re-conceptualizing schizophrenia as a disorder of cognitive and emotional processing: a shot in the arm for translational research. *Biological Psychiatry* **60**, 1169–1170.

Cisek, P. (2019) Resynthesizing behavior through phylogenetic refinement. *Attention, Perception, & Psychophysics* **81**, 2265–2287.

Cohen, J.D. *et al.* (2004) A systems-level perspective on attention and cognitive control: guided activation, adaptive gating, conflict monitoring, and exploitation versus exploration. In: *Cognitive Neuroscience of Attention.* (ed M.I. Posner). Guilford Press, New York. pp. 71–90.

Constantino, J.N. *et al.* (2017) Infant viewing of social scenes is under genetic control and is atypical in autism. *Nature* **547**, 340–344.

Corbetta, M. *et al.* (2008) The reorienting system of the human brain: from environment to theory of mind. *Neuron* **58**, 306–324.

Deisseroth, K. (2012) Optogenetics and psychiatry: applications, challenges, and opportunities. *Biological Psychiatry* **71**, 1030–1032.

Edelman, G.M. & Gally, J.A. (2001) Degeneracy and complexity in biological systems. *Proceedings of the National Academy of Sciences of the United States of America* **98**, 13763–13768.

Ferrante, M. *et al.* (2019) Computational psychiatry: a report from the 2017 NIMH workshop on opportunities and challenges. *Molecular Psychiatry* **24**, 479–483.

Geana, A. *et al.* (2022) Using computational modeling to capture schizophrenia-specific reinforcement learning differences and their implications on patient classification. *Biological Psychiatry: Cognitive Neuroscience and Neuroimaging* **7**, 1035–1046.

Geburek, A.J. *et al.* (2012) Electrophysiological indices of error monitoring in juvenile and adult attention deficit hyperactivity disorder (ADHD): a meta-analytic appraisal. *International Journal of Psychophysiology* **87**, 349–362.

Giarrocco, F. & Averbeck, B.B. (2022) Anatomical organization of forebrain circuits in the primate. *Brain Structure & Function* **228**, 393–411.

Hoogman, M. *et al.* (2019) Brain imaging of the cortex in ADHD: a coordinated analysis of large-scale clinical and population-based samples. *The American Journal of Psychiatry* **176**, 531–542.

Huys, Q.J. *et al.* (2016a) Computational psychiatry as a bridge from neuroscience to clinical applications. *Nature Neuroscience* **19**, 404–413.

Huys, Q.J.M. *et al.* (2016b) Computational psychiatry: from mechanistic insights to the development of new treatments. *Biological Psychiatry: Cognitive Neuroscience and Neuroimaging* **1**, 382–385.

Insel, T.R. *et al.* (1993) The role of neurohypophyseal peptides in the central mediation of complex social processes: evidence from comparative studies. *Regulatory Peptides* **45**, 127–131.

Keren, H. *et al.* (2018) Reward processing in depression: a conceptual and meta-analytic review across fMRI and EEG studies. *The American Journal of Psychiatry* **175**, 1111–1120.

Klin, A. & Jones, W. (2018) An agenda for 21st century neurodevelopmental medicine: lessons from autism. *Revista de Neurologia* **66**, S3–S15.

LeDoux, J.E. (2000) Emotion circuits in the brain. *Annual Review of Neuroscience* **23**, 155–184.

LeDoux, J. & Daw, N.D. (2018) Surviving threats: neural circuit and computational implications of a new taxonomy of defensive behaviour. *Nature Reviews. Neuroscience* **19**, 269–282.

LeDoux, J.E. & Pine, D.S. (2016) Using neuroscience to help understand fear and anxiety: a two-system framework. *The American Journal of Psychiatry* **173**, 1083–1093.

Lee, S.S. *et al.* (2011) Prospective association of childhood attention-deficit/hyperactivity disorder (ADHD) and substance use and abuse/dependence: a meta-analytic review. *Clinical Psychology Review* **31**, 328–341.

Linetzky, M. *et al.* (2020) Gaze-contingent music reward therapy for clinically anxious 7- to 10-year-olds: an open multiple baseline feasibility study. *Journal of Clinical Child and Adolescent Psychology* **49**, 618–625.

Marek, S. *et al.* (2022) Reproducible brain-wide association studies require thousands of individuals. *Nature* **603**, 654–660.

Marwaha, S. *et al.* (2022) Novel and emerging treatments for major depression. *The Lancet* **401**, 141–153.

Meyer-Lindenberg, A. & Tost, H. (2012) Neural mechanisms of social risk for psychiatric disorders. *Nature Neuroscience* **15**, 663–668.

Miller, E.K. & Cohen, J.D. (2001) An integrative theory of prefrontal cortex function. *Annual Review of Neuroscience* **24**, 167–202.

Monk, C.S. *et al.* (2008) Amygdala and ventrolateral prefrontal cortex activation to masked angry faces in children and adolescents with generalized anxiety disorder. *Archives of General Psychiatry* **65**, 568–576.

Murray, E.A. *et al.* (2017) *The Evolution of Memory Systems: Ancestors, Anatomy, and Adaptations*. Oxford University, Oxford, UK.

Naim, R. *et al.* (2022) Context-dependent amygdala-prefrontal connectivity during the dot-probe task varies by irritability and attention bias to angry faces. *Neuropsychopharmacology* **47**, 2283–2291.

Nigg, J. (2007) *What Causes ADHD?* Guilford Press, New York.

Olds, J. & Milner, P. (1954) Positive reinforcement produced by electrical stimulation of septal area and other regions of rat brain. *Journal of Comparative and Physiological Psychology* **47**, 419–427.

Pagliaccio, D. *et al.* (2019) Cross-species convergence in pupillary response: understanding human anxiety via non-human primate amygdala lesion. *Social Cognitive and Affective Neuroscience* **14**, 591–599.

Paukner, A. *et al.* (2011) Delayed imitation of lipsmacking gestures by infant rhesus macaques (*Macaca mulatta*). *PLoS One* **6**, e28848.

Pine, D.S. *et al.* (2009) Challenges in developing novel treatments for childhood disorders: lessons from research on anxiety. *Neuropsychopharmacology* **34**, 213–228.

Pine, D.S. *et al.* (2021) Evolution, emotion, and episodic engagement. *The American Journal of Psychiatry* **178**, 701–714.

Price, R.B. *et al.* (2015) Empirical recommendations for improving the stability of the dot-probe task in clinical research. *Psychological Assessment* **27**, 365–376.

Price, R.B. *et al.* (2016) Pooled patient-level meta-analysis of children and adults completing a computer-based anxiety intervention targeting attentional bias. *Clinical Psychology Review* **50**, 37–49.

Robinson, T.E. & Berridge, K.C. (1993) The neural basis of drug craving: an incentive-sensitization theory of addiction. *Brain Research Reviews* **18**, 247–291.

Schultz, W. (2001) Reward signaling by dopamine neurons. *The Neuroscientist* **7**, 293–302.

Shaw, P. & Sudre, G. (2021) Adolescent attention-deficit/hyperactivity disorder: understanding teenage symptom trajectories. *Biological Psychiatry* **89**, 152–161.

Shechner, T. *et al.* (2014) Attention bias modification treatment augmenting effects on cognitive behavioral therapy in children with anxiety: randomized controlled trial. *Journal of the American Academy of Child and Adolescent Psychiatry* **53**, 61–71.

Sikich, L. *et al.* (2021) Intranasal oxytocin in children and adolescents with autism spectrum disorder. *The New England Journal of Medicine* **385**, 1462–1473.

Spear, L.P. (2018) Effects of adolescent alcohol consumption on the brain and behaviour. *Nature Reviews Neuroscience* **19**, 197–214.

Tang, A. *et al.* (2020) Infant behavioral inhibition predicts personality and social outcomes three decades later. *Proceedings of the National Academy of Sciences of the United States of America* **117**, 9800–9807.

Tang, A. *et al.* (2022) Striatal activity to reward anticipation as a moderator of the association between early behavioral inhibition and changes in anxiety and depressive symptoms from adolescence to adulthood. *JAMA Psychiatry* **79**, 1199–1208.

van Veen, V. *et al.* (2008) The neural and computational basis of controlled speed-accuracy tradeoff during task performance. *Journal of Cognitive Neuroscience* **20**, 1952–1965.

Wald, I. *et al.* (2016) Selective prevention of combat-related post-traumatic stress disorder using attention bias modification training: a randomized controlled trial. *Psychological Medicine* **46**, 2627–2636.

Webb, S.J. *et al.* (2022) The autism biomarkers consortium for clinical trials: initial evaluation of a battery of candidate EEG biomarkers. *The American Journal of Psychiatry* **180**, 41–49.

White, L.K. *et al.* (2017) Complementary features of attention bias modification therapy and cognitive-behavioral therapy in pediatric anxiety disorders. *The American Journal of Psychiatry* **174**, 775–784.

C: Research approaches and service planning

CHAPTER 13
Identifying causal effects using natural experiments and other designs

Anita Thapar[1,2,3] and Kate Tilling[4]

[1] Child and Adolescent Psychiatry Section, Division of Psychological Medicine and Clinical Neurosciences, Cardiff University School of Medicine, Cardiff, UK
[2] Centre for Neuropsychiatric Genetics and Genomics, Division of Psychological Medicine and Clinical Neurosciences, Cardiff University School of Medicine, Cardiff, UK
[3] Wolfson Centre for Young People's Mental Health, Division of Psychological Medicine and Clinical Neurosciences, Cardiff University School of Medicine, Cardiff, UK
[4] Bristol Medical School, University of Bristol, Bristol, UK

Introduction

What is a causal effect?

There have been many philosophical discussions about what it means to say that "X causes Y." One definition is that binary exposure (X) causes an outcome (Y) if a person is exposed and their outcome is different to their outcome if not exposed (Hernán, 2004). We can then define the causal effect for a person as the difference between these two outcomes (outcome if exposed and outcome if not exposed), and this leads on to a definition of the average causal effect for a population. The outcomes for a person if exposed/not exposed are sometimes referred to as "potential" or "counterfactual" outcomes—because they are not both observed (since the same person cannot be both exposed and not exposed at the same moment). This framework can be expanded to continuous/categorical exposures, for example, estimating the causal effect of a blood pressure of 120 mmHg compared to 122 mmHg (at age 50 years) on 10-year risk of stroke.

Why is identifying causal effects important?

Estimating the causal effects of an exposure on health outcomes is a key goal in epidemiology. The motivation for such research is to inform disease/ill-health prevention strategies, by reducing or eliminating causes, and to identify effective interventions (Box 13.1 shows key definitions; see Chapter 14). Good examples include legislation to reduce rates of cigarette smoking and treating high blood pressure because of its causal effects on stroke and ischemic heart disease. Identifying and targeting genuinely causal effects is important if prevention or treatment is to be effective.

Given the high global prevalence of mental health problems in young people and limited resources for intervention, there are strong economic as well as ethical pressures to identify genuine causal effects so that prevention and public health strategies, as well as treatment interventions, are likely to be effective and succeed. Another important motivation is to provide accurate information for families and young people who wish to understand why someone has developed a mental disorder. This is especially important given the history of erroneous assumptions about causation; for example, epidemiological findings that Vitamin E protects against heart disease which were later refuted by randomized controlled trials (RCTs) and Mendelian randomization (MR) (see section on "Using genetic instruments: Mendelian randomization"; Davey Smith & Ebrahim, 2005).

Challenges to identifying causal effects from observational data

A first step to identifying potentially causal effects is observing association or correlation between an exposure and outcome; an approach employed in case control and cohort studies. Association or correlation, however, are not causation. Bradford Hill (1965) proposed nine criteria (Table 13.1) to infer causality from association data although thinking on causality has developed considerably since then as we will discuss in this chapter. As shown in Figure 13.1, observed associations can also arise from: an unmeasured third variable that causes both the exposure and the outcome, known as confounding; reverse causation; or conditioning on a variable that is caused by both exposure and outcome (collider bias).

For example, an association between parent mental disorder (exposure) and adolescent depression (outcome) could arise from the confounding effects of poverty or shared genetic liability. An association could also arise because of the impact of the young person's mental disorder on parental mental health (reverse causation). If exposure (parent mental disorder) and outcome

Rutter's Child and Adolescent Psychiatry and Psychology, Seventh Edition.
Edited by Anita Thapar, Daniel S. Pine, Samuele Cortese, Cathy Creswell, Tamsin J. Ford, James F. Leckman, and Argyris Stringaris.

Companion website: www.wiley.com/go/thapar/rutterspsych7

Box 13.1 Key terms and what they mean

Causal risk factor	A risk factor that changes the probability of an outcome when altered.
Causal prognostic factor	A variable in people with a given disorder that changes the outcome of that disorder when altered.
Selection bias	Difference between the causal effect in the study sample and target population—can occur due to nonrandom participation in the study or dropouts/missing data.
Confounding	A variable that lies on a back-door path from exposure to outcome (see directed acyclic graphs (DAGs)). This can be a variable that causes both the exposure and outcome. Conditioning on the variable blocks the back-door path.
Reverse causation	The outcome causes the exposure.
Instrumental variable (IV)	A variable that is associated with the exposure but has no direct effect on the outcome and is not associated with confounders of the exposure and outcome.
Negative control (could be exposure or outcome)	A negative exposure is an exposure that is subject to similar bias as the exposure of interest but that cannot plausibly cause the outcome. A negative outcome is one that is thought to be subject to similar bias as the outcome of interest, but is not caused by the exposure.

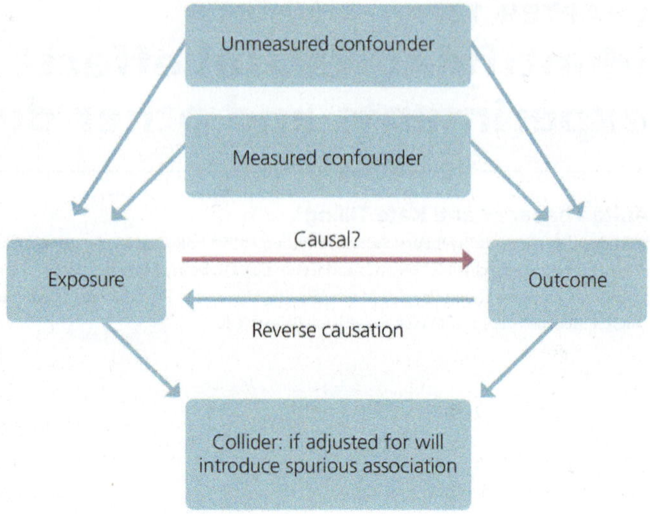

Figure 13.1 Threats to causal inference.

Table 13.1 A historical perspective: Bradford Hill criteria for evaluating association—first steps toward inferring causation[a].

Criterion	Meaning
Strength of association	Strong association between exposure and outcome
Consistency of association	Across samples and methods
Specificity	Ideally, specific outcome arising from exposure
Temporality	Exposure precedes outcome
Dose–response relationship	Higher levels of exposure increase outcome level
Biological plausibility	Plausible biological mechanism explaining how exposure could lead to outcome
Coherence	Across study designs; e.g., between epidemiological and laboratory findings
Experimental evidence	Experimental approaches show consistent findings
Analogy	Similar associations observed for analogous exposure and outcome or exposure and analogous outcome

[a] None provide an alternative to RCTs, some are considered outdated now.

(adolescent depression) both influence a third variable (e.g., educational attainment of the adolescent), then including this collider as a covariate in the analysis would induce a spurious association between the exposure and the outcome. Collider bias refers to the situation where two variables both influence a third variable, termed a "collider." If the collider is included in analyses, it induces a spurious association between the two causes of the collider. This is especially relevant for mental health research, where covariates are often included to try to control for confounders (e.g., including educational attainment to attempt to control for socioeconomic position). Collider bias can also arise via selection into or voluntary participation in a study. If participants who have both a parent with a mental disorder and depression themselves are less likely to join the study, this could cause an erroneous observed association between exposure and outcome in the study sample. This is known as selection bias, which is often a type of collider bias.

A further challenge is definition of the exposure itself, and identifying the people to whom the conclusions of the study will apply. This has been well-explained in the framework of "trial emulation" (Hernán et al., 2022). This involves careful thought about how an ideal randomized trial would be conducted and ensuring that the observational analysis replicates this as closely as possible. This includes consideration of the sample to be included (e.g., newly exposed versus those who have already been exposed), and identification of the start of the "trial."

A final point is that the causal effect may be different across subgroups of the population, known as "effect modification" or "moderation"; for example, young children may respond differently than adults to an exposure such as parent depression. The effect modifiers may be known and measured, or not known/measured. However, the estimated causal effect will only generalize to a population with the same distribution of effect modifiers. For example, if age is an effect modifier, the causal effect estimated by a study of children would not generalize to a population of young adults.

How can we identify causal effects?

Causal effects are most robustly identified in rigorously controlled experimental situations where confounding and reverse causation cannot occur, and where care is taken to avoid collider bias. Examples include laboratory settings using animal or cellular models. For human research, an RCT provides the gold standard for testing the causal effects of any intervention (see Chapter 15). In particular, a within-person (cross-over) RCT comes close to observing the "potential" or "counterfactual" outcome for each person, if we can assume that the person does not change between treatments. A between-person (parallel group) RCT relies on the assumption that randomization ensures balance of individual characteristics across arms of the trial. However, an RCT is not ethical or feasible for many exposures (e.g., randomizing children to a potentially toxic exposure). Thus, causal evidence tends to rely on observational data—where confounding is always an issue. A multitude of different statistical methods (see Chapter 16) and research designs (see Chapter 14) are used as an alternative to the RCT gold standard. Each approach attempts to overcome confounding and other biases, essentially attempting to mimic an RCT. Every method makes specific assumptions that are often not verifiable given the observed data, so ultimately, we are limited to inferring rather than determining causation. A first step is to recognize potential biases and for this, DAGs are invaluable (Shrier & Platt, 2008; Digitale *et al.*, 2022; see section on "Directed acyclic graphs"). Also, for research evidence to be robust, valid, and to obtain more reliable answers to the questions we ask, we require many different lines of evidence to converge across diverse research designs. This is known as triangulation (Lawlor *et al.*, 2016; see section on "Triangulation").

In this chapter we consider a range of research designs that can be used to infer causation. We will describe the methods, explain what they can be used for, and highlight examples relevant to mental health. We also consider their limitations and strengths (Table 13.2). For additional statistical methods, we direct the reader to Chapter 16 on statistics. A useful first step is to begin with a DAG.

Directed acyclic graphs

This type of graph (Figure 13.2) is a way of showing associations between variables that are included as "nodes" on the graph; lines or arrows connect them to show the assumed relationships (Digitale *et al.*, 2022). A "directed" graph can only include arrows between these variables—thus the direction of causation must be specified for every pair of related variables. A "path" from variable X (e.g., parent depression) to variable Y (e.g., adolescent depression) is a way to get from X to Y along lines or arrows; a "directed path" is one which follows the direction of arrows. An "acyclic" graph is one where there can be no cycles, i.e., there are no paths from X that come back to X. An absence of an arrow between X and Y makes a very strong statement—i.e., that X does not cause Y, and Y does not cause X.

A DAG has three main uses. The first is to show the assumptions being made about how variables relate to each other. Figure 13.2 is hypothetical and shows that we are assuming that parental depression has direct causal effects on adolescent depression and, via anxiety, that provides another path to adolescent depression (mediator).

The second use is to identify which variables should be conditioned on to minimize confounding. Although a confounder has traditionally been thought of as a variable that causes both X and Y, a DAG allows this definition to be widened to include any variable that could block a confounding path. A confounding, or "back-door" path is a noncausal path from X to Y. In figure 13.2, there is only one such path—from the exposure (parental depression) backwards (hence the "back door") to neighborhood violence, and then forwards from neighborhood violence to the outcome (offspring depression). Conditioning on (i.e., adjusting for or stratifying on) any variable along a back-door path blocks that path, and therefore removes that confounding. For example, Figure 13.2 shows that we should condition on neighborhood violence to minimize confounding of the relationship between parent and adolescent depression. However, in reality, the DAG will be more complex; for example, if parental education has causal effects on both parental depression and parental income, and parental income affects adolescent depression. In this case, we have a choice of "confounding variables"—conditioning on either of parental education or parental income, and would block this back-door path. There are a set of guidelines to identify when there is confounding of a relationship between exposure and outcome, and to ascertain which variable(s) can be conditioned on to minimize the confounding (Greenland *et al.*, 1999).

The third use of a DAG is to identify potential sources of bias; e.g., whether some variables conditioned on might be colliders, or whether a complete-case analysis might be biased. For example, Figure 13.2 shows that we assume that both parent and adolescent depression influence school nonattendance, and therefore we should not condition on this variable (e.g., by stratifying or by adjusting for it in analyses). Underlying all these uses is the requirement that the DAG must be correct and include all relevant variables (whether or not they are measured in a given dataset). A DAG is a useful tool for describing assumed causal relationships, and is best drawn before conducting any analyses or research to visualize potential confounders, colliders, and selection biases.

Statistical approaches for dealing with measured confounding

Multivariable regression

The most common way to minimize confounding when estimating an association between exposure and outcome is to include all known, measured confounders in a multivariable regression model. For example, from Figure 13.2, we could use linear regression to relate an outcome (adolescent depression, measured using a

Table 13.2 Different genetic/family-based designs, what they are used for and their main strengths and limitations/biases.

Study design	Prenatal exposures	Postnatal exposures	Cross-generational environmental transmission	Main strengths and limitations
Bivariate twin design: decomposing covariance between exposure and outcome	–	+	–	Tests whether an environmental exposure is associated with outcome after controlling for twin genetic similarity (active, evocative gene–environment correlation) Does not include parent genetic contributions (passive gene–environment correlation) Equal environments assumption (EEA) Assumes random mating Unmeasured nongenetic factors may contribute to "environmental mediation" i.e., unmeasured confounding
Monozygotic (MZ) twin differences and discordance	–	+	–	MZ co-twin is a negative control; controls for offspring but not parent genetic confounders EEA Assumes random mating The measured risk exposure may be a proxy for the true risk exposure that impacts on one twin and not the other i.e., unmeasured confounding Discordant MZ twin pairs are atypical for highly heritable traits MZ twins are not necessarily 100% genetically identical
Children-of-twins (CoT) design	+	+	+	Main strength is in testing intergenerational environmental similarity/transmission of psychopathology EEA for twins Further assumes offspring of MZ twins have as much environmental sharing with their aunt/uncle as dizygotic (DZ) twins Assumes random mating Association between parent and offspring phenotype could be explained by another confounding variable (e.g., different parent psychopathology; other unmeasured confounding) Limited power compared to other designs e.g., adoption Does not allow for contributions of active and evocative gene-environment correlation Can be difficult to resolve direction of effects i.e., parent to child versus child to parent Cousins are not the same age which may affect phenotype manifestation and its etiology at that age
Adoption design	–	+	+	Atypical family situation Low prevalence of risk exposures Does not allow for prenatal environmental contributions Removes passive gene-environment correlation

Assisted reproductive technology (ART) design	+	+	+	Main strength is for examining prenatal exposures as removes parental genetic contribution to exposure (passive gene–environment correlation) Atypical family/parental situation Low prevalence of risk exposures Cross-generational links can be bidirectional i.e., parent to child versus child to parent Association between parent and offspring phenotype could be explained by another confounding variable (e.g., different parent psychopathology; other unmeasured confounding)
Discordant sibling pair design (see section on "Negative controls")	+	+	–	Main strength is for examining prenatal exposures where unexposed sibling provides the negative control Unknown why mother behaves differently in different pregnancies-selection of siblings who are differentially exposed can lead to confounding by a nonshared environment factor (e.g., traumatic event leading to mother smoking in one pregnancy and not the other) Siblings are born at different times and risk exposures can change over time for family or at population level Random measurement error can attenuate association Exposure or outcome in first sibling could influence exposure or outcome in second sibling and result in reversal of association Weak design for postnatal exposures as siblings share 50% of their genome and differ in age, so preferable to use twin pairs
Maternal versus paternal exposure (see section on "Negative controls")	+	–	–	Main strength is for examining prenatal exposures as father provides the negative control Limited range of exposures that can be tested Assumes random mating when parents may show similarities in behavior Maternal risky behaviors in pregnancy, e.g., smoking, are subject to different selection biases to paternal behavior in pregnancy

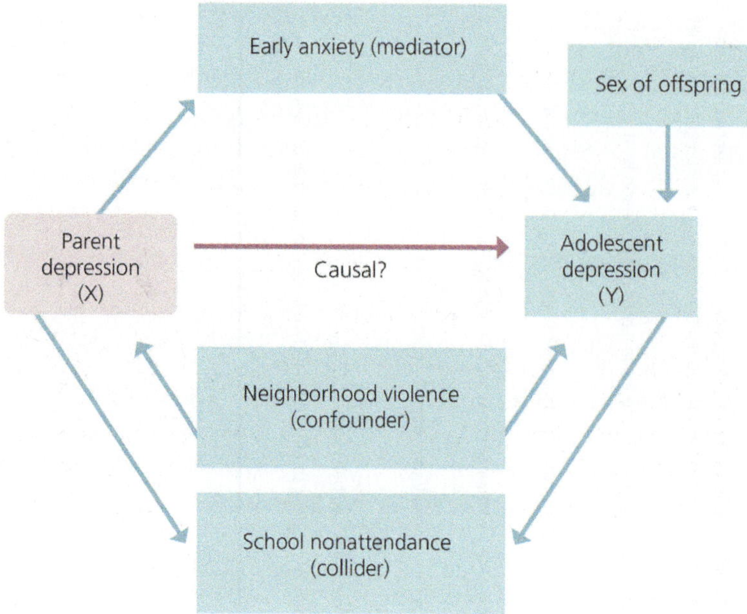

Figure 13.2 Hypothetical example of a simple directed acyclic graph (DAG).

validated scale) to an exposure (parental depression), also measured using a validated scale. This approach will estimate the causal effect of exposure on outcome given two main assumptions: the model is correctly specified, and there is no unmeasured confounding. It is worth noting that it is very unlikely that these assumptions are met for this and all other approaches. The first assumption means that in our example, parental depression should have a linear effect on adolescent depression (e.g., increasing the parental depression score from 0 to 1 has the same effect as increasing it from 29 to 30). Also, that the effect of parental depression on adolescent depression is the same for everyone, and that we correctly specify the error structure of the model. These assumptions can, to an extent, be tested using the observed data. The second assumption is there are no further confounders that have not been included in the model. This can be examined partially using measured confounders, but the assumption that there are no unmeasured confounders cannot be assessed using the observed data.

Propensity scores

A related way to adjust for measured confounding is using a "propensity score." This predicts the chance of each individual receiving a binary intervention or exposure, given their values of the confounding variables (Rosenbaum & Rubin, 1983; Harder *et al.*, 2010). For example, propensity scores were used in a UK observational cohort study to examine the reduction of depression in 14-year-olds who had contact with mental health services in the last year compared to those who had not had contact (Neufeld *et al.*, 2017). Those with contact showed a greater decrease in depression symptom scores and also lower odds of reporting clinical depression at age 17 compared to those who had been similarly depressed at baseline.

The propensity score can be used in several different ways. First, to match individuals, either by matching each individual who received the intervention to another individual with the same *a priori* chance of having the intervention, but who did not receive it, or by categorizing the propensity score and conducting the analysis within each propensity score category (Senn *et al.*, 2007). The analysis would then be carried out only using the sample of matched individuals. Second, propensity scores also can be used to weight individuals (inverse probability weighting) by the inverse of their chance of the exposure or treatment received. Third, the scores can be included as a covariate in the regression model (Fu *et al.*, 2019). When using propensity scores, it is important to assess the extent to which they balance observed confounders in the exposed and unexposed groups (Kainz *et al.*, 2017; Fu *et al.*, 2019).

A key assumption again is that there is no unmeasured confounding. An advantage of propensity scores is that it is easier to include a large number of covariates (especially if intervention or exposure is common but outcome is rare).

Prognostic scores

A prognostic score relates the outcome (e.g., chronicity of psychosis) to observed covariates excluding the exposure (e.g., substance misuse) (Hansen, 2008). A prognostic score may be derived from historic data and can then be used to match individuals for analysis or included as a covariate in the regression model. As with propensity scores, it is important to assess covariate balance, and prognostic score overlap between those experiencing and not experiencing the exposure. This method also assumes no unmeasured confounding.

Marginal structural models

The marginal structural model (Robins *et al.*, 2000) was developed to deal with time-varying confounding and is also suitable when exposure is time varying (e.g., childhood risk factors for alcohol-related problems in adolescence; (Kendler *et al.*, 2018a)). Analyses are conducted using weights for the chance of exposure at each given time point. The intention is to eliminate confounding. This is achieved by creating a "pseudopopulation" in which each subject has the same probability of receiving the exposure and back-door paths from exposure to outcome via confounders are removed.

These multiple analyses are then pooled, with robust standard errors used to account for the fact that each individual is now included in the analyses several times. They assume no unmeasured confounding. For example, Kendler *et al.* (2018a) found that associations between parent and offspring alcohol problems were not attenuated after using marginal structural models, whereas the association between low parental monitoring and offspring alcohol problems declined substantially, suggesting that a proportion of the association here was due to confounding.

Designs that take familial or genetic confounding into account

Many risk exposures relevant to mental health (e.g., maternal depression, prenatal exposures) are correlated with parental genetic liability; known as passive gene–environment correlation. For example, offspring depression could be explained by parent nontransmitted genes that influence stressful environments which the offspring is exposed to, as well as by transmitted parental genes. Other exposures are associated with offspring genetic liability (e.g., stressful life events), referred to as active and evocative gene–environment correlation (see Chapter 21, Genetics). This means that observed associations between an exposure and mental health outcome could arise because of shared family and/or genetic risks, that is, confounding, rather than because of causal effects of the exposure. There are a range of different genetically informative designs that separate out the effects of genetic confounding, thereby enabling inference about causality. However, each has its own set of assumptions, as well as limitations and strengths. Also, different designs are required to investigate environmental exposures before and after birth (Rice *et al.*, 2018) (Table 13.2). For exposures after birth, some designs consider contributions of offspring genetic liability only, while others include parental genetic contributions only. Although genetically informative designs are considered separately, they represent a type of natural experiment (see section on "Natural experiments") because they pull apart genetic and environmental contributions by serendipity and use an IV approach (e.g., twin birth is the instrument; see section on "Methods robust to unmeasured confounding: instrumental variables").

Twin design

Monozygotic (MZ) twins, in principle, share 100% of their genotypes (see Chapter 21 for assumptions), whereas dizygotic (DZ) twins, like siblings, share on average 50% of their genome. By examining the similarity of MZ and DZ twin pairs, it becomes possible to separate offspring (twin) genetic influences from environmental influences on the outcome or exposure of interest. One key assumption is that MZ and DZ twins share environments to the same extent as each other: the equal environments assumption (EEA). Causal inference in relation to environmental risk exposures involves using a multivariate twin design. Here, association between an exposure and an outcome (e.g., stressful life events and depression) is decomposed into genetic (confounding) and environmental (covariance) factors. Such studies allow us to test whether the association between exposure and outcome remains after including "genetic confounding." This is sometimes called environmental mediation. Twin designs enable us to test environmental exposures after birth, but not prenatal exposures as they include twin genetic contributions to the environmental exposure but not parental genotype (i.e., passive gene–environment correlation). For example, stressful life events are robustly associated with depression. However, such stressors can arise as a result of depression itself or its early features (reverse causation). Association could also be explained by shared genetic liability (confounding) because stressful life events are to some extent heritable and also share genetic liability with depression. Nevertheless, twin and longitudinal studies consistently observe that stressful life events show an environmental link with depression; however, associations are more modest once genetic contributions are included (Kendler *et al.*, 1999). Some twin studies also involve full and half-siblings.

Co-twin control or discordant twin pair designs

These studies focus on MZ twins where one has developed the psychopathology outcome of interest and the other has not. An alternative involves examining twins where one twin has been exposed to an environmental exposure and the co-twin has not. As MZ twin pairs share 100% of their genome, discordance in psychopathology is attributable to environmental exposures that are not shared by the twins. Essentially, the co-twin serves as a negative control (see section on "Negative controls"). Some studies also include DZ twin pairs where co-twin inclusion controls for family-/sibling-level confounding but not all genetic factors. For example, a co-twin design has shown that even after genetic confounding is considered, exposure to stressful life events remains associated with depression (Bjørndal *et al.*, 2023).

Children-of-twins design

The children-of-twins (CoT) design take advantage of the fact that offspring of MZ and DZ twins are socially cousins but that offspring of MZ twins are genetically half siblings whereas DZ twin offspring share on average one-eighth of their genes (like all first cousins). Thus, MZ twins will share 50% of their genome with their biological aunt. This design has been used to examine cross-generational transmission of psychopathology as well as to a lesser extent investigate the impact of prenatal exposures. The CoT design has suggested that the cross-generational transmission of depression is explained by environmental or rearing factors with no evidence of shared genetic liability, although the latter is difficult to rule out (Ahmadzadeh *et al.*, 2021). There are limitations of the CoT design (see McAdams *et al.* (2014)). Although it enables controlling for genetic confounds, assortative mating (mating with a partner who is phenotypically and/or genetically similar to oneself) and other unmeasured confounders (e.g., social contact) could still contribute and cross-generational associations can be bidirectional (child psychopathology effects on parent). Also, offspring will not have passed through the period of risk in many instances (adolescence or adulthood for disorders such as psychosis and depression). Where possible, it is preferable to include spouse information.

Adoption design

As parents transmit DNA to their offspring, association between parenting or other types of rearing and offspring psychopathology could arise from shared genetic contribution to the exposure and outcome (i.e., genetic confounding). Adoption studies involve children who have been adopted away and reared by parents who are biologically unrelated to them, or other variations of this differential genetic relatedness (see Chapter 21, Genetics). This provides a powerful design for testing the impacts of family-related environments (e.g., parental depression, parenting) on offspring outcomes. That is because any genetic contributions to rearing are independent of genes shared by rearing parent and offspring. The adoption design removes passive environment gene–environment correlation effects but only after birth (i.e., the rearing but not the pregnancy environment), so cannot be used to test prenatal exposures because those are correlated with biological maternal genetic liability.

Multiple adoption studies have shown that maternal or parental depression is associated with offspring depression mainly due to rearing/environmental factors with some but not all observing inherited contributions (McAdams *et al.*, 2015; Kendler *et al.*, 2018b, 2020). These findings mainly converge with those from CoT studies. Adoption studies have also observed that genetically influenced behaviors in offspring impact on adoptive parent rearing (evocative gene–environment correlation). The best example here is in relation to coercive parenting and antisocial behavior where the link with child antisocial behavior remained even once child genetic contributions were included (Ge *et al.*, 1996). Adoption studies also provide a powerful and robust means of testing whether environmental exposures can moderate the manifestations of genetic liability—so called gene–environment interaction. For example, this type of design has shown that being reared in more socioeconomically advantaged homes increases cognitive ability in adopted-away children relative to their nonadopted siblings (Kendler *et al.*, 2015).

Assisted reproduction technologies (ART)/*in vitro* fertilization (IVF) design

An alternative design is based on offspring who differ in genetic relatedness to their mother because they were conceived via ART (Rice *et al.*, 2009). This approach is essentially an *in utero* adoption study. However, unlike twin and adoption studies, this design is especially useful for testing prenatal exposures. The ART approach also can be used to examine cross-generational transmission. ART provides a unique opportunity because if a prenatal exposure has genuinely causal intrauterine environmental effects on the offspring, then it will not matter if the child is genetically related (homologous *in vitro* fertilization, sperm donation) or unrelated (egg donation and in some cases embryo donation) to the mother. This novel design showed that maternal cigarette smoking in pregnancy was associated with lower offspring birth weight regardless of mother–offspring relatedness. In contrast, cigarette smoking in pregnancy was only associated with attention deficit hyperactivity disorder (ADHD) in genetically related dyads (Thapar *et al.*, 2009). These findings triangulate with observations from CoT and negative control designs.

Methods robust to unmeasured confounding: instrumental variables (IV)

An instrument is a variable that predicts exposure but, crucially, is unrelated to the outcome except via the exposure. The key assumptions are that the IV affects the outcome only via the exposure (Figure 13.3), that the IV causes exposure, and that IV is unrelated to any confounders of the exposure and outcome (Greenland, 2000). If these assumptions hold, then an association between the IV and outcome can only occur if the exposure causes the outcome. The only assumptions that can be tested using observed data are whether the IV is associated with exposure, and whether the IV is associated with any measured confounders of exposure and outcome. If all the assumptions hold, then we can examine whether exposure causes outcome by testing whether the IV (as an indicator of exposure) is associated with the outcome; this test is unaffected by unmeasured confounding. Further assumptions are needed to use the IV to estimate the causal effect. Potential IVs include natural experiments, physician preference, thresholds for exposure (regression discontinuity), and genetic instruments.

Natural experiments

Natural experiments take advantage of situations where the exposure or intervention has not been provided by the researcher and it is assumed that exposure is "as-if random" (de Vocht *et al.*, 2021). Historically, natural experiments have utilized external shocks such as famines, or changes in legislation or policy, to investigate the causal effects of an exposure. However, the use of natural experiments to infer causality depends on the plausibility of the "as-if random" assumption.

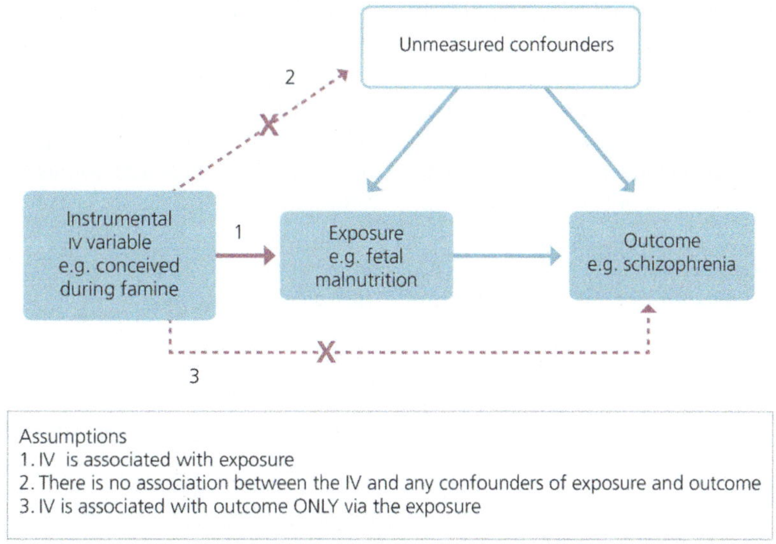

Figure 13.3 Instrumental variable (IV) assumptions.

Universal introduction of risk

The most well-known example relevant to psychopathology is time-limited starvation/famine. Exposure to the Dutch Hunger Winter (Susser *et al.*, 1996) and the Chinese famine studies (St Clair *et al.*, 2005) both examined the cognitive and psychiatric impacts of exposure to famine that serves as an IV for prenatal nutritional deficiencies. In both these situations, exposure was universal and there is nothing to suggest that there was selection bias in terms of exposure. In 1944–1945, during World War II, 4.5 million Dutch people experienced famine owing to a food blockade of the Netherlands. Those conceived during the height of the famine showed an increased risk of congenital nervous system anomalies including neural tube defects and schizophrenia.

The famine in China occurred between 1959 and 1961 and the impacts were studied by examining rates of schizophrenia in one of the most affected areas before, during, and after the famine years. The risks of schizophrenia rose from 0.84% in 1959 to 2.15% in 1960. The mortality-adjusted relative risks in the famine years ranged between 2.30 (95% confidence interval, 1.99–2.65) and 1.93 (95% confidence interval, 1.68–2.23) (St Clair *et al.*, 2005). The Dutch and Chinese famine studies took place in different countries, at different times and included populations of diverse ancestry yet findings were replicated. However, exposure to such extreme fetal malnutrition is rare and thus unlikely to represent a key causal exposure for schizophrenia in higher income countries.

The "as-if randomized" assumption here is that being born/conceived just before, during, or after the famine is essentially random—i.e., there are no systematic differences between these groups before birth/conception. The main IV assumption is that the famine is only acting on the outcome via the exposure (fetal malnutrition, in this case)—whereas there could be other effects of the famine, for example, via stress of the mother while pregnant.

Universal removal of risk

This design takes advantage of situations where risk is removed universally such that there is no evidence of selection or allocation bias. One renowned example comes from the Great Smoky Mountains study, a US longitudinal epidemiological study of children. During this study, a casino was opened on a Native American reserve. This led to a substantial increase in income of US$4000 a year per person for around a quarter of the 1000 participating families. The researchers took advantage of this situation to examine the causal effects of poverty on child and adolescent mental health by examining rates of disorder before and after the casino opened. Here, the opening of the casino serves as the IV for poverty. The researchers showed reductions in oppositional defiant disorder (ODD) and conduct disorder (CD) in those who were lifted out of poverty but no changes in anxiety or depression (Costello *et al.*, 2003). The effects appeared to be explained by higher levels of parental supervision and the rise in income had no mental health benefits to the never-poor families. Exposure to family income supplements in childhood remained associated with better mental health and functioning in adult life (Copeland *et al.* 2022). The "as-if randomized" assumption here is that there were no systematic differences between the population before and after the casino opened. The main IV assumption is that opening the casino is only related to outcomes via its effect on poverty.

Changes in legislation and policies

Where these are introduced to an entire population it becomes possible to assess the impact of an exposure altered by the IV of legislation or policies. One Swedish study examined the effects of prenatal alcohol exposure on offspring by taking advantage of changes in a policy addressing alcohol sales in two different regions (Nilsson, 2017). The original intention of this policy was to shift the population toward consuming drinks with lower levels of alcohol and away from high alcohol percentage spirits by changing the pricing of alcoholic beverages. However, the policy had to be terminated abruptly in 1968 once it transpired that, inadvertently, consumption of strong beer had risen, especially among teenagers. Using registry data, the researchers were able to examine the offspring of women who were pregnant during the time that the legislation was in place in two regions of Sweden. One region was exposed and the other unexposed to this legislation; they also examined adjacent time-unexposed cohorts. At age 30 years, the exposed group showed reduced cognitive ability, lower educational achievement, lower earnings, and higher rates of welfare dependence than those born in unexposed cohorts. These outcomes were most marked in males, those born to younger mothers, and those exposed to the policy for the longest period *in utero*. These results suggested that prenatal alcohol exposure may have an impact on cognitive ability and educational attainment. However, there are weaknesses to this type of policy-based design, including the limitation in this instance that the results apply to the whole population and not necessarily at an individual level.

Physician preference

Preference-based instruments are based on the assumptions that individual health care providers may systematically allocate individuals to certain interventions, but that individual selection/allocation to physicians is independent of their outcome (or factors affecting the outcome) (Brookhart & Schneeweiss, 2007). For example, one clinician may prescribe cognitive behavioral therapy (CBT) for mild depression when another may not suggest CBT until the depression has become more severe. Comparison of outcomes in those allocated to CBT in the care of either/both of these clinicians would be biased due to confounding. However, we could use preference of the clinician for prescribing CBT as an instrument—assuming that clinician preference only affects patient outcome via the treatment they actually receive, and that there are no systematic differences between patients of clinicians with different prescribing preferences. If outcomes are better in those under the care of clinicians with a higher preference for prescribing CBT, then that would provide evidence for a causal effect of CBT on depression outcome.

Regression discontinuity

Many clinical and policy decisions, such as eligibility for early years intervention, involve exposure or intervention only when a continuous variable (e.g., poverty level) meets a specific and known threshold. Regression discontinuity is a statistical approach that capitalizes on this threshold to infer causal effects of an intervention or policy decision by examining those just below and above the threshold (Venkataramani *et al.*, 2016). For example, in many countries, including the UK, the school entry threshold is the 1st September; this means that the youngest in any school year, born in August, will be almost a year younger than the oldest child, born in September. Several studies have suggested worse mental health in children who are youngest in their school (e.g., Kuntsi *et al.*, 2022; Broughton *et al.*, 2023). Large sample sizes are needed for this design, with assumptions that there are no confounders of exposure (e.g., age at starting school) or outcome (e.g., mental health) that also are associated with the threshold for exposure/intervention. Another assumption is that the outcome ordinarily would not show a discontinuity at the threshold (e.g., worse mental health if born in August versus September) if there was no exposure (i.e., school entry).

Using genetic instruments: Mendelian randomization (MR)

MR is a type of natural experiment that uses variation in DNA (see Chapter 21) as the IV to infer potentially causal effects of an exposure (e.g., depression) on the outcome (e.g., educational attainment) (Davies *et al.*, 2018).

The genetic instruments are gene variants that have been found to be indicators of the exposure (e.g., depression), usually because they show association in very large genome-wide association discovery studies (GWAS; see Chapter 21). As genetic instruments (DNA variation) are fixed at conception, with few exceptions (see Chapter 21), they are not subject to reverse causation effects. Also, as alleles are randomly allocated from parent to offspring, there is no confounding of instrument and outcome/exposure. As MR uses genetic instruments, these capture lifelong liability to an exposure, rather than exposure at one time point for a discrete time period, as would happen in an RCT.

MR is a valuable tool for causal inference for many physical health problems, as long as biases are carefully considered. It can involve the genetic instrument for exposure and outcome being assessed in the same sample, or each in a separate sample (two-sample MR (Choi *et al.*, 2020)). Here, genetic instruments for an exposure (e.g., ADHD) are taken from one GWAS and instruments for an outcome (e.g., a physical health outcome) taken from an independent GWAS. For example, ADHD genetic liability appears to have a causal effect on obesity and coronary artery disease (Leppert *et al.*, 2021). Similarly, MR suggests that ADHD and autism spectrum disorder (ASD) genetic liability affect educational attainment (Dardani *et al.*, 2021). When this approach is used, it is recommended that associations with the genetic instruments are tested in both directions; that is, from exposure to outcome and from outcome to exposure. Large databases of GWAS data to identify suitable genetic instruments, such as MR-base and GWAS catalog, are available to interested researchers (Davies *et al.*, 2018).

The genetic instruments need to meet all the criteria that are needed for any IV (Figure 13.4). However, it can be difficult to meet all the assumptions of MR, especially when investigating psychopathology. One key assumption is that the genetic instrument only influences the outcome (e.g., educational attainment) via the exposure (e.g., child ADHD) (Figure 13.4a). However, as Figure 13.4b shows, if the genetic variant is associated with the outcome (e.g., educational attainment) through another

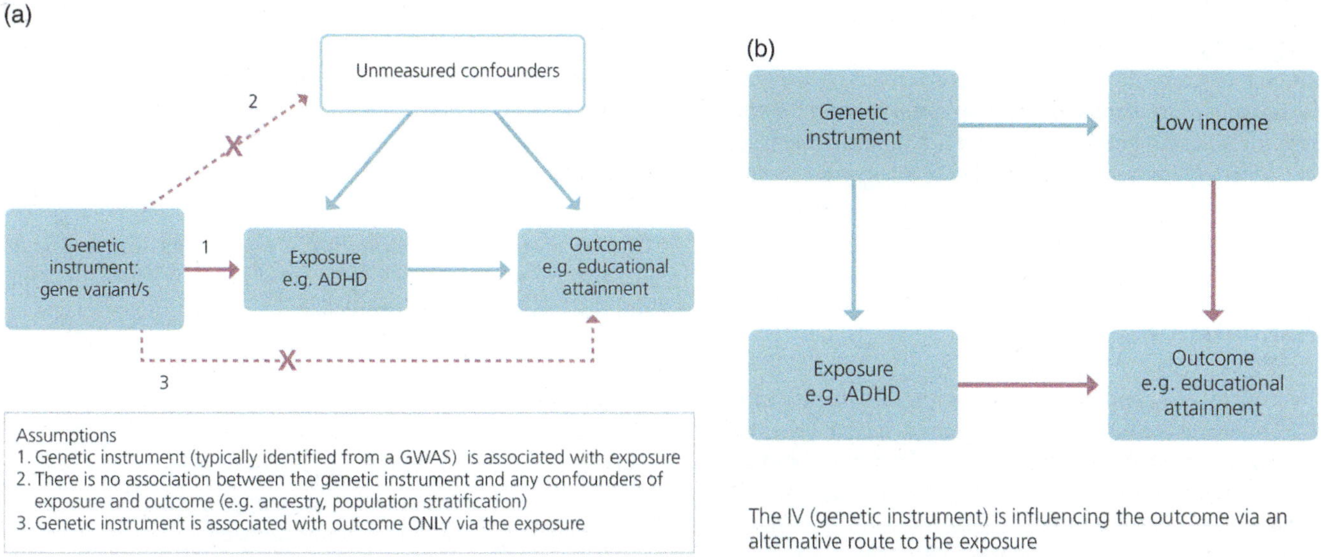

Figure 13.4 (a) Mendelian randomization (MR) and its assumptions. (b) Horizontal pleiotropy: one violation of Mendelian randomization and an instrumental variable (IV) approach.

pathway to the one under investigation (e.g., via low income), this is known as horizontal pleiotropy and represents a violation of an IV assumption. If the genetic instrument is associated with the outcome through another trait that is downstream to the exposure (e.g., cognitive differences resulting from ADHD adversely affecting educational attainment), that is known as vertical pleiotropy and is not a violation of the IV assumptions.

Another problem is that the genetic instruments observed in GWAS of psychopathology are weak and only predict a small proportion of the variance in exposure. However, it is possible to use multiple genetic instruments in MR including composite measures of nominally associated risk alleles (polygenic risk scores; see Chapter 21). A weak instrument is a concern because it results in greater horizontal pleiotropic effects of the gene variant. Also, weak instruments show bias toward observing association with the outcome for single-sample MR and toward null findings when two-sample MR is used (Davies *et al.*, 2018). It is useful to consider how the MR estimate (i.e., association of genetic instruments with outcome) compares with the observational estimate (e.g., ADHD with educational attainment). Finally, if there are ancestral differences in the genetic risk variants and the outcome of interest, that too violates the assumption that there is no confounding. Any researcher using MR should include further examination of pleiotropy and other potential biases using a variety of different statistical methods, including MR Egger, inverse variance weighted (IVW) regression approaches, and median and mode estimators (Yang *et al.*, 2022). Other threats include the potential for parental genotypes to influence offspring outcomes (e.g., educational attainment), known as dynastic effects, and assortative mating where parental genotypes are more similar than expected for some traits (e.g., height, educational attainment). Within-family MR, which uses parent as well as offspring DNA variation, can help address some biases.

Negative controls

A negative control can help identify if there is confounding, selection, or measurement bias (Lipsitch *et al.*, 2010; Sanderson *et al.*, 2018). The negative control can refer to an exposure or outcome and works especially well for pregnancy or intrauterine exposures (Davey Smith, 2012) where maternal versus paternal exposures are used and their associations with offspring outcomes compared. Other situations that provide plausible negative controls are MZ co-twin studies where both twins share inherited DNA but are discordant for environment exposure (or psychopathology), and also pre- versus postnatal exposures where it is thought that exposure during pregnancy only is the harmful exposure.

Maternal versus paternal exposure in pregnancy

In this situation, paternal behaviors in pregnancy serve as the negative control for a maternal exposure in pregnancy that is thought to have an intrauterine effect on offspring outcomes. For example, cigarette smoking in pregnancy, when exposure is maternal, is associated with lower offspring birth weight but paternal exposure is not. Different findings have been observed in relation to ADHD (Rice *et al.*, 2018) where both maternal and paternal exposure are associated with the offspring outcome of ADHD. However, there are limitations to this design such that they do not provide definitive evidence of bias being absent. One assumption is that the negative exposure and outcome are subject to the same bias (e.g., confounding, selection) as the exposure and outcome, which is not necessarily the case. For example, pregnant mothers may change their behaviors in pregnancy and the factors that influence this maybe different to fathers.

Sibling pairs discordant to exposure in pregnancy

Another negative control design involves sibling pairs where one is exposed *in utero* and the other not, for example, where a mother smoked in one pregnancy but not the other. Such studies have generally suggested that the sibling unexposed to cigarette smoking *in utero* does not show elevated ADHD levels compared to the exposed siblings (Rice *et al.*, 2018).

Triangulation

The designs and approaches described in this chapter can only infer not prove causality. Each method has its own set of limitations, so what does the researcher and clinician believe? Triangulation brings together different approaches, ideally where each has different biases. Causal inference is strengthened where findings from different approaches all converge on the same conclusion. It is helpful, if the types of biases of every study design or method are explicitly considered or stated, to then seek evidence from alternative approaches with biases in different directions. We have provided several different examples in this chapter where findings have been similar across different designs. Lawlor *et al.* (2016) proposed a framework for triangulation. At least two, but preferably more, different approaches that address the same causal question are needed. The scientist needs to consider explicitly what the biases of each approach are and preferably use approaches that would be thought to have biases in opposite directions *a priori*. Finally, there needs to be consideration of the exposure duration and its timing. Typically, triangulation is achieved by using different study approaches in different samples, although it can be achieved using a single dataset when known as triangulation within a study (TWIST) (Bowden *et al.*, 2021).

The ideal situation is where different study designs are employed, for example, MR, standard regression analyses, and twin approaches across populations with different confounding structures, such as across culture and time. For example, a systematic review of cigarette smoking in pregnancy and offspring ADHD found this causal question was addressed in one IVF study, eight discordant sibling studies, and two maternal versus paternal comparisons (Rice *et al.*, 2018). Most suggested it unlikely that there is a substantial intrauterine effect of cigarette smoking on ADHD but that it does appear to have a causal effect on offspring birth weight. Another study used cross-time cohorts to examine links between maternal smoking in pregnancy and offspring outcomes; this was achieved by comparing two national UK cohorts born in 1958 and 2000–2001 (Sellers *et al.*, 2021). These cohorts had different confounding structures because smoking in pregnancy was actively discouraged in later years. As might be expected, maternal smoking in pregnancy was less common and more strongly associated with social disadvantage in 2000–2001 compared with 1958. Although maternal smoking in pregnancy was strongly and equally associated with offspring low birth weight in both cohorts, associations with offspring ADHD symptoms in the 2000–2001 cohort were much stronger than in the 1958 cohort.

Conclusions

To conclude, a variety of different methods and research designs are available to infer causation. However, clinicians and researchers need to appreciate the many different biases in any single approach and how easy it is to jump to erroneous conclusions about causality. This can lead to ineffective prevention and intervention strategies, wasting time and resources in providing interventions that later transpire to be ineffective, and also creates unnecessary distress to families, for example, by incorrectly assigning blame. Thus, it is important for all to have some knowledge of the different biases and strengths of different approaches and to be wary of making causal conclusions without considering how findings triangulate.

References

Ahmadzadeh, Y.I. *et al.* (2021) Systematic review and meta-analysis of genetically informed research: associations between parent anxiety and offspring internalizing problems. *Journal of the American Academy of Child and Adolescent Psychiatry* **60**, 823–840.

Bjørndal, L.D. *et al.* (2023) Stressful life events increase the risk of major depressive episodes: a population-based twin study. *Psychological Medicine* **53**(11), 5194–5202.

Bowden, J. *et al.* (2021) The triangulation within a STudy (TWIST) framework for causal inference within pharmacogenetic research. *PLoS Genetics* **17**, e1009783.

Bradford Hill, A. (1965) The environment and disease: association or causation? *Proceedings of the Royal Society of Medicine* **58**(5), 295–300.

Brookhart, M.A. & Schneeweiss, S. (2007) Preference-based instrumental variable methods for the estimation of treatment effects: assessing validity and interpreting results. *International Journal of Biostatistics* **3**, 14.

Broughton, T. *et al.* (2023) Relative age in the school year and risk of mental health problems in childhood, adolescence and young adulthood. *The Journal of Child Psychology and Psychiatry and Allied Disciplines* **64**, 185–196.

Choi, K.W. *et al.* (2020) An exposure-wide and Mendelian randomization approach to identifying modifiable factors for the prevention of depression. *The American Journal of Psychiatry* **177**, 944–954.

Copeland, W.E. *et al.* (2022) Long-term outcomes of childhood family income supplements on adult functioning. *JAMA Pediatrics* **176**(10), 1020–1026.

Costello, E.J. *et al.* (2003) Relationships between poverty and psychopathology: a natural experiment. *JAMA* **290**, 2023–2029.

Dardani, C. *et al.* (2021) Is genetic liability to ADHD and ASD causally linked to educational attainment? *International Journal of Epidemiology* **50**, 2011–2023.

Davey Smith, G. (2012) Negative control exposures in epidemiologic studies. *Epidemiology* **23**, 350–351.

Davey Smith, G. & Ebrahim, S. (2005) What can Mendelian randomisation tell us about modifiable behavioural and environmental exposures? *BMJ* **330**(7499), 1076–1079.

Davies, N.M. *et al.* (2018) Reading Mendelian randomisation studies: a guide, glossary, and checklist for clinicians. *BMJ* **362**, 601.

de Vocht, F. *et al.* (2021) Conceptualising natural and quasi experiments in public health. *BMC Medical Research Methodology* **21**, 1–8.

Digitale, J.C. *et al.* (2022) Tutorial on directed acyclic graphs. *Journal of Clinical Epidemiology* **142**, 264–267.

Fu, E.L. *et al.* (2019) Merits and caveats of propensity scores to adjust for confounding. *Nephrology, Dialysis, Transplantation* **34**, 1629–1635.

Ge, X. *et al.* (1996) The developmental interface between nature and nurture: a mutual influence model of child antisocial behavior and parent behaviors. *Developmental Psychology* **32**, 574–589.

Greenland, S. (2000) An introduction to instrumental variables for epidemiologists. *International Journal of Epidemiology* **29**, 722–729.

Greenland, S. *et al.* (1999) Causal diagrams for epidemiologic research. *Epidemiology* **10**, 37–48.

Hansen, B.B. (2008) The prognostic analogue of the propensity score. *Biometrika* **95**, 481–488.

Harder, V.S. *et al.* (2010) Propensity score techniques and the assessment of measured covariate balance to test causal associations in psychological research. *Psychological Methods* **15**, 234–249.

Hernán, M.A. (2004) A definition of causal effect for epidemiological research. *Journal of Epidemiology & Community Health* **258**, 265–271.

Hernán, M.A. *et al.* (2022) Target trial emulation: a framework for causal inference from observational data. *Journal of the American Medical Association* **328**(24), 2446–2447.

Kainz, K. *et al.* (2017) Improving causal inference: recommendations for covariate selection and balance in propensity score methods. *Journal of the Society for Social Work and Research* **8**, 279–303.

Kendler, K.S. *et al.* (1999) Causal relationship between stressful life events and the onset of major depression. *The American Journal of Psychiatry* **156**, 837–841.

Kendler, K.S. *et al.* (2015) Family environment and the malleability of cognitive ability a Swedish national home-reared and adopted-away cosibling control study. *Proceedings of the National Academy of Sciences of the United States of America* **112**, 4612–4617.

Kendler, K.S. *et al.* (2018a) Childhood risk factors for heavy episodic alcohol use and alcohol problems in late adolescence: a marginal structural model analysis. *Journal of Studies on Alcohol and Drugs* **79**, 370–379.

Kendler, K.S. *et al.* (2018b) Sources of parent-offspring resemblance for major depression in a national Swedish extended adoption study. *JAMA Psychiatry* **75**, 194–200.

Kendler, K.S. *et al.* (2020) The sources of parent-child transmission of risk for suicide attempt and deaths by suicide in Swedish national samples. *The American Journal of Psychiatry* **177**, 928–935.

Kuntsi, J. *et al.* (2022) The combined effects of young relative age and attention-deficit/hyperactivity disorder on negative long-term outcomes. *Journal of the American Academy of Child and Adolescent Psychiatry* **61**, 291–297.

Lawlor, D.A. *et al.* (2016) Triangulation in aetiological epidemiology. *International Journal of Epidemiology* **45**, 1866–1886.

Leppert, B. *et al.* (2021) The effect of attention deficit/hyperactivity disorder on physical health outcomes: a 2-sample Mendelian randomization study. *American Journal of Epidemiology* **190**, 1047–1055.

Lipsitch, M. *et al.* (2010) Negative controls: a tool for detecting confounding and bias in observational studies. *Epidemiology* **21**, 383–388.

McAdams, T.A. *et al.* (2014) Accounting for genetic and environmental confounds in associations between parent and child characteristics: a systematic review of children-of-twins studies. *Psychological Bulletin* **140**, 1138–1173.

McAdams, T.A. *et al.* (2015) The relationship between parental depressive symptoms and offspring psychopathology: evidence from a children-of-twins study and an adoption study. *Psychological Medicine* **45**, 2583–2594.

Neufeld, S.A.S. *et al.* (2017) Reduction in adolescent depression after contact with mental health services: a longitudinal cohort study in the UK. *The Lancet Psychiatry* **4**, 120–127.

Nilsson, J.P. (2017) Alcohol availability, prenatal conditions, and long-term economic outcomes. *Journal of Political Economy* **125**, 1149–1207.

Rice, F. *et al.* (2009) Disentangling prenatal and inherited influences in humans with an experimental design. *Proceedings of the National Academy of Sciences of the United States of America* **106**, 2464–2467.

Rice, F. *et al.* (2018) Identifying the contribution of prenatal risk factors to offspring development and psychopathology: what designs to use and a critique of literature on maternal smoking and stress in pregnancy. *Development and Psychopathology* **30**, 1107–1128.

Robins, J.M. *et al.* (2000) Marginal structural models and causal inference in epidemiology. *Epidemiology* **11**, 550–560.

Rosenbaum, P.R. & Rubin, D.B. (1983) The central role of the propensity score in observational studies for causal effects. *Biometrika* **70**, 41–55.

Sanderson, E. *et al.* (2018) Negative control exposure studies in the presence of measurement error: implications for attempted effect estimate calibration. *International Journal of Epidemiology* **47**, 587–596.

Sellers, R. *et al.* (2021) Using a cross-cohort comparison design to test the role of maternal smoking in pregnancy in child mental health and learning: evidence from two UK cohorts born four decades apart. *International Journal of Epidemiology* **49**, 390–399.

Senn, S. *et al.* (2007) Stratification for the propensity score compared with linear regression techniques to assess the effect of treatment or exposure. *Statistics in Medicine* **26**, 5529–5544.

Shrier, I. & Platt, R.W. (2008) Reducing bias through directed acyclic graphs. *BMC Medical Research Methodology* **8**, 1–15.

St Clair, D. *et al.* (2005) Rates of adult schizophrenia following prenatal exposure to the Chinese famine of 1959–1961. *JAMA* **294**, 557–562.

Susser, E. *et al.* (1996) Schizophrenia after prenatal famine. Further evidence. *Archives of General Psychiatry* **53**, 25–31.

Thapar, A. *et al.* (2009) Prenatal smoking might not cause attention-deficit/hyperactivity disorder: evidence from a novel design. *Biological Psychiatry* **66**, 722–727.

Venkataramani, A.S. *et al.* (2016) Regression discontinuity designs in healthcare research. *BMJ* **352**, i1216–i1216.

Yang, Q. *et al.* (2022) Exploring and mitigating potential bias when genetic instrumental variables are associated with multiple non-exposure traits in Mendelian randomization. *European Journal of Epidemiology* **37**(7), 683–700.

CHAPTER 14
The role of epidemiology and youth voice in planning, organizing, and improving mental health services

Tamsin J. Ford[1] and Tamsin Newlove-Delgado[2]
[1]Department of Psychiatry, University of Cambridge, Cambridge, UK
[2]Medical School, University of Exeter, Exeter, UK

Epidemiology is the basic science that underpins public health and comprises the study of who gets what (disorder, risk/protective factor, recovery), as well as when, where, how, and why (Nature Communications, 2018). The COVID-19 pandemic not only emphasized the scientific importance of epidemiology, but also demonstrated its social and political elements. COVID-19 was arguably a *syndemic,* as social and biological factors interacted to amplify the impact of the virus on certain parts of the population (Mendenhall, 2020). In this chapter, we explain how epidemiological findings and data can be used to plan, organize, and improve mental health services, working with experts by experience (Sunkel & Sartor 2022). Our focus throughout is on practical advice for those involved in the "swampy lowlands" (Schön, 1987) of real-world practice. These services may provide *universal* (prevention and mental health promotion, and provided to all children in the population), *targeted* (groups identified as vulnerable), or *indicated* (children with identified needs) interventions. Overviews of child psychiatric epidemiological findings are covered in the relevant disorder chapters, while universal or primary preventions are described in Chapter 17.

Why bother?

The use of epidemiological findings is fundamental to evidence-based policy and service provision but involves a nuanced assessment of the available data and the context from which it was obtained and is being applied (Gray, 2004). Without reference to epidemiological prevalence studies and the predictors of access to support, *service planning* is subject to historical accidents, fluctuating political priorities, and responses to moral panics. For example, surveillance surveys of pediatric and mental health service practice in relation to attention deficit/hyperactivity disorder (ADHD) revealed some pediatric services where access after the age of 16 was related to continued full-time education, but adult services for ADHD only served those aged 18 plus (Eke *et al.*, 2020).

Equally, decisions about service provision should not solely rely on current access because only a small and atypical group of children currently access services and are not necessarily those most in need. Many factors influence presentation to services, including the (perceived) availability of support (Anderson *et al.*, 2021), willingness to seek help, which has increased over the last two decades (Pitchforth *et al.*, 2018), and recognition by practitioners. The 78% increase in clinical diagnoses of autism recorded in primary care in the United Kingdom (UK), likely reflects broadening diagnostic criteria and improved recognition rather than a true increase in the prevalence (Russell *et al.*, 2022).

Epidemiological data can aid decisions about where to target resources in relation to service *organization*. Ongoing reference to locality-based epidemiological data is essential for services to meet the needs of groups prioritized for intervention and underserved communities (Islam *et al.*, 2021). The current interest and activity in the use of administrative and epidemiological data to predict those most at risk of adverse outcomes (Skarda *et al.*, 2021; Soneson *et al.*, 2023) is insufficiently developed for practical application but offers great potential. Epidemiological analyses may also inform decisions in relation to individual cases attending services. For example, Lambert and Shimokawa (2011) demonstrated that giving feedback to therapists on patient symptoms against anticipated progress can improve patient outcomes.

Rutter's Child and Adolescent Psychiatry and Psychology, Seventh Edition.
Edited by Anita Thapar, Daniel S. Pine, Samuele Cortese, Cathy Creswell, Tamsin J. Ford, James F. Leckman, and Argyris Stringaris.

Companion website: www.wiley.com/go/thapar/rutterspsych7

Epidemiological data and tools are important to service *evaluation and quality improvement*. Routine collection of outcome data is now mandated in England's Children's and Young People's Mental Health Programme and not only provide powerful evidence of service impact at a national level but also identify subgroups who might need alternative approaches (Clark, 2018). Randomized controlled trials (RCTs) are the gold standard for measuring the impact of a change, with other approaches more prone to bias. As Clark and colleagues (2008) note "in the absence of randomization, one has to work very hard to demonstrate that unbalanced patient characteristics or referral practices could not have substantially influenced the treatment outcome comparison." Mental health service attenders inevitably score highly on symptom scales as referral is often sought when difficulties peak. Their scores will tend to reduce over time because of regression to the mean, attenuation, and the fluctuating nature of childhood psychopathology, regardless of intervention (Wolff *et al.*, 2018). Regression to the mean occurs because of random measurement error; low or high scorers on any scale will tend to be closer to the mean when remeasured (Porta, 2014). In epidemiological studies, people tend to report more problems in the first than subsequent responses (attenuation), perhaps because of respondent fatigue (Jensen *et al.*, 1995).

Epidemiological data provide useful comparison data. For example, by propensity score matching children who attended school-based counseling to children from the British Child and Adolescent Mental Health Survey (BCAMHS), Finning demonstrated sustained reduction in psychopathology scores among children attending counseling which were not seen in the national survey reference sample (Finning *et al.*, 2020). Similarly, the "added-value" score is an algorithm based on parental report on the Strengths and Difficulties Questionnaire (SDQ; Ford *et al.*, 2009) from BCAMHS data that clinicians can apply to their patients' follow-up parental SDQ total difficulties score to estimate the impact of treatment. This approach is only appropriate for clinical interventions and should only be used to assess change at team, regional, or national levels, as the estimates are insufficiently precise to accurately measure individual progress. Funnel plots, which are graphs that plot average clinic/service outcome against the precision of the estimate or 95% confidence interval (Fugard *et al.*, 2015) can assess whether services are functioning within expected levels of clinical outcome scores to assess clinic/service effectiveness. Ranking, a frequent alternative provides no information about quality; all services may be excellent or poor, while those ranked low are likely to be demoralized.

Other approaches to assess clinically significant change in outcomes over time include *reliable change indices*, *difference scores*, and whether scores cross a validated *clinical threshold* after treatment (Wolpert *et al.*, 2015). *Reliable change indices* attempt to factor out changes that occur randomly due to measurement error and, like clinical thresholds, can be used to assess universal as well as targeted or indicated interventions, in addition to individual progress. *Difference scores* measure the average difference in outcome measure scores before and after treatment across groups. This value is often divided by the standard deviation of the scale (how much scores vary), to estimate how much the patients have changed as a group to provide an *effect size*. Context is important when interpreting effect sizes, as even small changes in an average score can translate into a large increase in those scoring above the clinical threshold on a population level (Carey *et al.*, 2023).

Epidemiological data alone should never drive service planning, organization, evaluation, or funding. Nuanced consideration of methodological limitations and complexities are essential. Wolpert and Ford (2015) emphasize the need to consider the effectiveness of interventions, accessibility, and acceptability of services for families, and the skills and abilities of potential service providers. Indeed, working with the populations served by services is essential. We explore engagement and involvement in the next section before outlining the main methodological issues that affect epidemiological data. Despite the limitations and complexities of the application of epidemiological data to service planning, evaluation, and improvement, empirical data provides a firmer foundation for services than historical levels of provision or politically determined policy priorities (Jenkins, 2001).

"Nothing about us without us"

Initially adopted by disability activists arguing for self-determination, this phrase is used by many groups arguing for increased participation, including experts by their experience of mental health services. The involvement of patients and carers in research, policy, and service development ensures meaningful benefit and avoids wasting resources (Burn *et al.*, 2022). Limited empirical evidence from the James Lind Alliance (https://www.jla.nihr.ac.uk/) indicates that involving the youth can lead to more efficient research processes and improved research outcomes. Liabo *et al.* (2020) and our accompanying video (Video Clip 1) provide practical advice on how to successfully involve young people and parents/carers in your work. Young people and parents should contribute at every stage of the research or quality improvement process, from codeveloping the research agenda, to choosing the most important constructs to measure and the most acceptable tools to measure them with, as well as advising on protocol development to maximize recruitment and retention (Liabo *et al.*, 2020). Figure 14.1 provides examples of some of the ways in which young people and parents can be involved at different stages of research.

Young people and parents' involvement in dissemination can broaden the impact of research. For example, the James Lind Alliance completed a research prioritization exercise in relation to mental health in children and young people, with 25 ranked questions (see https://www.jla.nihr.ac.uk/priority-setting-partnerships/Mental-health-in-children-and-young-people/top-10-priorities.htm). Other stakeholders are also important, such as practitioners working in services or referring to them,

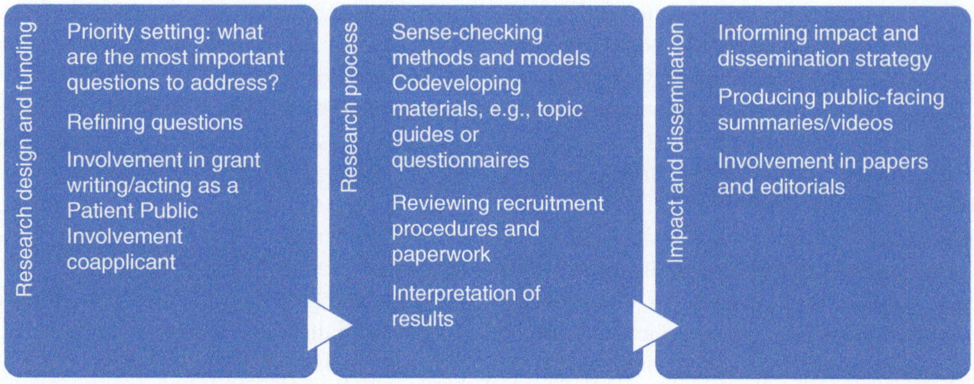

Figure 14.1 Examples of ways that young people and parents can be involved in different stages of research or quality improvement.

school staff, and mental health practitioners. Researchers must engage those from underserved groups to ensure adequate representation, which may require outreach to community leaders to encourage participation (Moreton *et al.*, 2022).

Key questions to consider when using epidemiological data

The starting point of any project is to define the question to be addressed, from which other important considerations cascade, particularly the *study design*, measures, or *data* required. All approaches have advantages and limitations (Table 14.1).

Study design

Epidemiological studies can be experimental, such as RCTs, or observational, where the researcher does not influence events but draws conclusions through observation of people defined by their exposure (risk or protective factor) or outcome (usually a disorder). Sampling and measurement error are generally random and reduce the precision of a study's estimate; they can be reduced by larger samples and more accurate measures. In contrast, nonrandom error introduced by bias (systematic errors) or confounding (a nonexplanatory characteristic that is associated with both outcome and exposure) reduces the validity of findings. Study design and measurement selection are key factors to minimize nonrandom error.

Randomized controlled trials (RCTs)

RCTs (see Chapter 7) provide the most robust evidence because random allocation of the intervention (exposure) should ensure treatment groups are similar in respect to *all confounders, both known and unknown*. Perceptions about the interventions may influence self-reported or researcher-ascertained outcomes, so researchers and participants should be unaware of which intervention they receive (*double-blind*) to prevent *information bias*.

Quasi-experimental studies

Quasi-experimental studies (see Chapter 15) aim to establish causality without randomization or active intervention by leveraging other factors such as unplanned events or genetic variants. For instance, Rutter *et al.* (2007) studied extreme adversity in infancy by following the developmental trajectory of Romanian orphans.

Cross-sectional surveys

Cross-sectional surveys estimate prevalence for service planning or to identify potential risk factors. Surveys are a poor choice of design for rare disorders; for example, the 2017 Mental Health of Children and Young People survey, which included more than 9000 participants aged between 2 and 19 years, detected only 23 participants meeting diagnostic criteria for eating disorders (O'Logbon *et al.*, 2022).

Surveys collect data from a sample selected from a *defined population*, for example, children aged 5–16 years living in private households (Ford *et al.*, 2020) using a sample frame. As disorder and exposures are measured simultaneously, surveys cannot provide direct evidence of causality. The *sampling frame* must be representative of the base population to avoid *selection bias* or systematic over-or-underestimation of prevalence. For example, the first two UK national prevalence surveys of children and young people's mental health used the child benefit register as the sample frame, because it was then a universal benefit (Ford *et al.*, 2020). The most recent UK survey could not use the child benefit register because it now excludes more affluent eligible families and the resulting sample would underestimate the prevalence of psychiatric disorder. Nonresponders often differ from responders in any study, so comparison with responders is important. For example, Wolke *et al.* (2009) demonstrated dropouts from the Avon Longitudinal Study of Parents and Childhood (ALSPAC) were more likely to have teacher-reported behavioral difficulties than responders, so ALSPAC would underestimate prevalence. In contrast, the associations of background characteristics with these behavioral difficulties were no different between those who stayed in and dropouts, supporting the exploration of predictors and mechanisms in ALSPAC.

Case-control studies

Case-control studies recruit cases and noncases (controls) from the *same defined population* to explore past exposures, which are

Table 14.1 Strengths and limitations of different types of study design.

	Cross-sectional survey	Case-control	Cohort	Ecological	Clinical trial	Clinical evaluation	Qualitative
Who is studied?	Defined population—more generalizable if known sample frame versus convenience sample	Caseness/outcome—controls should only differ by outcome (common source of bias)	Exposure and followed forward to study outcome(s)	Data on outcome or exposure is collected at group level (e.g., national alcohol consumption)	Caseness/outcome	Caseness—quasi-experimental, including a nonrandomized control group, but may just be pre- and posttreatment	Defined groups with interest in topic—often patients, carers, or practitioners
What is measured?	Prevalence	Odds ratio	Relative risk	Correlation/regression coefficient	Mean difference, relative risk, odds ratio	Mean difference, relative risk, odds ratio	Experiences and beliefs about conditions, services, and interventions
Applications	Planning services Mapping secular and geographical trends Identifying correlates	Multiple exposures Rare and single outcomes which are difficult to study in surveys	Rare and single exposure exposures but can study multiple outcomes	Rare outcomes Rare exposures Multiple exposures Population exposures such as air pollution	Efficacy /effectiveness of new interventions Hypothesis testing mechanisms	Monitoring clinical outcomes or initial evaluation of innovations	Understanding of barriers, facilitators, outcomes, and experience Hypothesis generating
Probability of confounding	Medium	Medium	Low	High	Very low, if randomization successful	High	Not applicable
Resources	Quick and cheap	Relatively quick and cheap	Lengthy and expensive	Relatively quick and cheap	Relatively expensive	Quick and cheap Should be routine	Relatively quick and cheap
Source of bias	Selection nonresponse information (recall and observer)	Selection information (recall and observer)	Information (observer only) Loss to follow up (selection)	Selection of population ecological fallacy	Selection information (reduced by blinding)	Selection nonresponse information (recall and observer)	Not generalizable beyond sample
Recent examples	Mental Health of Children and Young People in England Series (https://digital.nhs.uk/data-and-information/publications/statistical/mental-health-of-children-and-young-people-in-england/2022-follow-up-to-the-2017-survey)	Preexisting mental health disorders and risk of opioid use disorder in young people: a case-control study (Marshall *et al.*, 2023)	Physical and mental health three months after Sar-Cov-2 infection (long COVID) among adolescents in England (CLoCk): a national matched cohort study (Stephenson *et al.*, 2022)	Rising suicide rates among adolescents in England and Wales (Bould *et al.*, 2019)	Mental Health Intervention for Children with Epilepsy (MICE) (Bennett *et al.*, 2024)	Mindfulness-based cognitive therapy for young people and their carers: a mixed-methods feasibility study (Racey *et al.*, 2018)	Communication in youth mental health encounters: introducing the agential stance (Bergen *et al.*, 2022)

most useful for the initial investigation of rare disorders or events. Parker *et al.* (2016) explored the relationship between psychopathology, academic attainment, and developmental level with exclusion from school using this method. Case-control studies are highly vulnerable to *selection bias*; cases and controls should ONLY vary in relation to outcome status, requiring careful definition of the reference population. Information is often biased by health status. *Observer bias* occurs if researchers push harder for evidence of exposure in cases than controls. *Recall bias* occurs if participants with the disorder think more deeply about the potential causes—that differs from controls ("search after meaning"). Both can be mitigated using objective measures such as blood tests and medical records, by blinding researchers to participants' outcome status, and concealing the study hypothesis.

Participants in *cohort studies* are defined by their exposure status and followed forwards in time. *Information bias* is limited by prospective follow-up so cohort studies can suggest the direction of causality, at least by temporal relationship. *Population cohort studies* permit the study of multiple exposures as well as multiple outcomes. For example, the UK's Millennium Cohort Study has followed children born at the turn of this century at regular intervals, providing rich data about disparate issues affecting health and development (www.cls.ioe.ac.uk/page.aspx?&sitesectionid=851).

Ecological studies

Ecological studies assess correlations between the average level of one or more exposures and the prevalence of an outcome in different populations. Both exposure and outcome are aggregated across individuals. For example, child well-being is negatively correlated with income inequality in developed countries (Pickett & Wilkinson, 2007). Both child well-being and income inequality were reported at *group level* across the population, yet will vary within each country. Application of results obtained from aggregated population-level data to individuals is known as the "*ecological fallacy*." Information on potential confounding factors is often lacking and as data on the exposure and the outcome are frequently gathered simultaneously, we cannot draw inference about the direction of causality.

Qualitative studies

Qualitative studies gather data about experiences, beliefs, and attitudes, and aim to document the breadth of experience or opinion, rather than to generate generalizable findings. Data collection involves in-depth interviews or focus groups, and samples sizes are necessarily smaller. For instance, process evaluations accompanying RCTs explore barriers and facilitators that might influence implementation and are particularly important for complex psychosocial interventions. Shafran and colleagues drew on focus groups, Plan-Do-Study-Act (PDSA) service improvement methods, and semi-structured patient interviews to optimize an existing modular psychological intervention for children with epilepsy (Shafran *et al.*, 2020). The PDSA framework ensures clarity in what service improvement aims to accomplish, what indicates success, and what change is required, with cycles of planning, doing, studying, and acting to ensure incremental change. An RCT of this optimized intervention included further qualitative research of patient and practitioner experiences (Bennett *et al.*, 2021). Qualitative or mixed method (combining and triangulating quantitative and qualitative methods) studies can also provide insights into mechanisms by which moderators and mediators may act.

Measures

After study design, the next important step is measure selection (see Chapter 28). Measurement development constitutes a highly specialized and time-consuming endeavor, which inexperienced researchers often underestimate and undermine their work by applying rapidly developed, untested, bespoke measures. Even small changes in the wording of validated questionnaires can generate large differences in how a questionnaire functions, so this should be avoided (Goodman *et al.*, 2007). Translation from one language to another requires iterative translation and back-translation by bilingual experts to get to an approved version which then needs discussions with local community leaders in terms of cultural issues prior to testing for validity and reliability. Most measures are developed for use in high-income countries and the concepts measured do not necessarily translate to lower- or middle-income countries, (Kusi-Mensah *et al.*, 2022).

For service planning, organization, and evaluation, traditional symptom-based measures are most relevant, despite recent criticisms for their focus on phenomenology, course, and outcome rather than biomarkers of pathophysiological dysfunction (for a recent summary see Morris *et al.*, 2022). *Validity* refers to how well a measure captures the concept that it is supposed to be measuring and comprises several components (Box 14.1). *Reliability* refers to a measure's stability and repeatability; do you get the same answer when it is used more than once (*test–retest reliability*) or by two or more people (*inter-rater*

Box 14.1 Types of validity

- **Construct validity:** the extent to which the construct is a real and coherent entity, and the salience of the measure to that construct.
- **Concurrent validity:** the extent to which the new measure relates, as hypothesized, to other measures taken at the same time.
- **Convergent and divergent validity:** a measure will be more closely related to an alternative measure of the same construct than it will be to measures of different constructs.
- **Predictive validity:** assesses the extent to which a new measure can predict future occurrences.
- **Factorial/structural validity:** a test of theoretical meaning in our measurements. Using exploratory factor analysis (EFA), factorial validation starts with exploring the pattern of correlations between responses; stronger correlations among certain items suggest that these items belong to a specific topic and we can deduce meaning from this structure to help generate a theory about what is it that we are measuring.

or inter-observer reliability)? Validity requires reliability, but a reliable test may not be valid. For example, a thermometer giving widely different readings is clearly unreliable, but even similar (reliable) recordings could still be consistently over-or-underestimating the temperature (lack validity).

Most self-report scales and some diagnostic interviews (for example, the Diagnostic Interview Schedule for Children) are *structured* using closed questions with constrained responses. These tend to be highly reliable but cannot detect or respond to misunderstandings so may lack validity. Perhaps as a result, they tend to provide higher prevalence estimates (Angold *et al.*, 2012) than *semi-structured measures*, such as the Schedule for Affective Disorders and Schizophrenia for Children (K-SADS; Ambrosini, 2000). The latter often requires training or clinical qualification to administer and allows flexibility for the interviewer to ask supplementary questions, and to exercise their judgment as to the clinical significance of the symptoms and signs elicited. Validity is improved but these measures are inherently less reliable, given the variation in questions and judgments involved. The Development and Well-being Assessment (DAWBA), used in the UK national survey series as well as in many clinical services, combines both approaches, with highly structured questions about each type of disorder expanding into qualitative questions about any problem areas (Goodman *et al.*, 2000; www.dawba.info).

Research with children and young children requires multiple informants, usually parents, teachers, and the young person themselves, to increase diagnostic accuracy (Garb, 2005). Correlations between informants reporting about the same child are surprisingly low ($r \sim 0.2$–0.4; Collishaw *et al.*, 2009), not only relating to measurement error but also because each informant brings their own frame of reference. Young people are best placed to report on emotional symptoms, which may not be evident to parents or to teachers in busy classrooms, but the latter have a broader frame of reference in relation to behavior and peer relationships while parents are likely to be more familiar with their own child than teachers. Early epidemiological studies set rules about how many informants were required to report a difficulty for it to be accepted as present, with all or only one at the extremes and obvious impacts on prevalence estimates. The DAWBA allow trained clinical raters to combine reports applying the same judgments as they would in clinical practice (Goodman *et al.*, 2000).

Development influences the reliable completion of measures, so we cannot assume that a measure functions similarly across all ages. Schlechter and colleagues studied *measurement invariance* of the short Moods and Feelings Questionnaire in the ALSPAC cohort, which was completed 10 times between the ages of 11 and 26 (Schlechter *et al.*, 2023). They reported measurement invariance between 14 and 26 years but recommended caution when comparing depressive symptoms reported by children under 13 and over 17 years of age, when measurement models were not fully invariant.

The sheer volume of measures of similar constructs limits comparability between studies. Computerized adaptive testing (CAT) offers a potential solution. CAT uses individual questions in "item banks" which include information about patterns of responses to component items (their "calibration") from samples of the target population (Stochl *et al.*, 2021). An algorithm selects questions for each informant on psychometric models and mathematical formulae that maximize the information until a prespecified level of confidence in the individual's score is reached. CAT reduces participant burden via shorter and more varied question completion.

Data

Organizations working with children and families collect a huge amount of data, which is a potential gold mine for service organization, planning, and quality improvement (Soneson *et al.*, 2023). In some countries, national patient registry data provide full population capture of service contacts and diagnoses. While administrative datasets will contain more variations in recording practice and missing information than those completed by small research teams working to a protocol, they offer opportunities that would be difficult to achieve through individually funded research studies, particularly sample size and generalizability. The accuracy and standardization of records are inevitably compromised by the large numbers of staff with limited training. Intrinsic biases can arise from recording practices, so it is essential to understand the source data. For example, if clinician-reported scales, such as the Health of the Nation Scales for Children and Adolescents (HoNOSCA), are used in funding decisions, there is a clear incentive for staff to maximize severity at initial assessment but minimize it at discharge. Clinical services only record episodes of care, providing "windows" of time when information is available on individuals, interspersed with data-free periods, which are contingent on clinical improvement or disengagement and must be accounted for in the analyses.

Increasing the structure of records may increase the volume of immediately accessible data points, provided that practitioners complete them, but structured data are *not* intrinsically more accurate. *Machine learning* and *natural language processing* of text fields could extract additional detail from unstructured data (Downs *et al.*, 2018). The development of portals for patients to provide their own information, as well as linkage of administrative health data to data from wearables and other devices may also greatly enhance the use of routine data in the future.

What is a need?

Using epidemiological data to inform service planning and organization requires careful consideration of what is defined as a "need."

Need for health care in general can be conceptualized in different ways. Acheson (1978) describes need, first, as any "disturbance of health and wellbeing" or, second, as requiring some

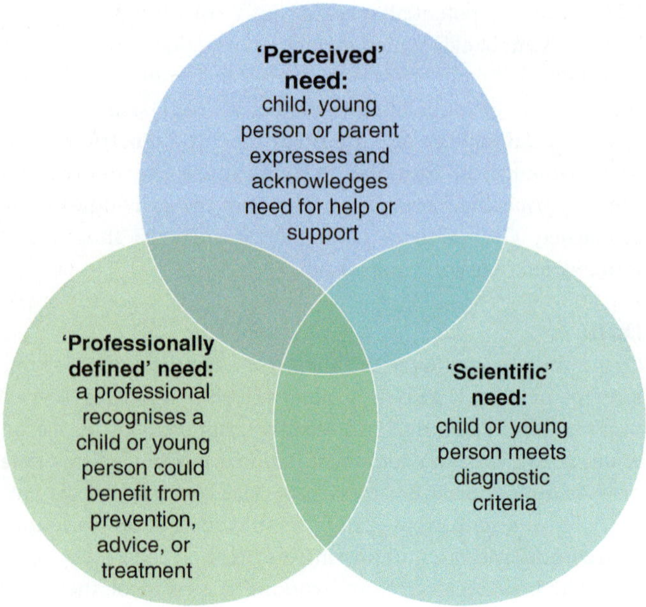

Figure 14.2 World Health Organization definitions of need for health care for children and young people.

capacity to benefit from medical intervention "at reasonable cost," i.e., subject to the context of resources and prioritization. The World Health Organization (https://www.who.int/docs/default-source/documents/health-systems-strengthening-glossary.pdf) uses three further definitions, shown in Figure 14.2. Children and young people may meet all three of these definitions, or only one or two.

Defining mental health needs in children and young people is complex. A modified version of the groups of children with needs proposed in the previous edition of this textbook (Wolpert & Ford, 2015) included: (i) those at risk of developing diagnosable mental health problems, or where children and families are adjusting to mild or temporary difficulties, (ii) those with diagnosable mental health conditions, and (iii) those with levels of impairment resulting from symptoms that make it difficult for them to function in their community or culture. A "need" may be recognized by a parent, teacher, or the child or young person themselves. Differences in perception of need may affect the likelihood of seeking help and of pathways to care, discussed later in this chapter. There is also an important question of "a need for what?" Many children in the groups mentioned may not require specialist child mental health services or meet thresholds for access. However, targeted early intervention from education or social care may not only benefit these children but also prevent their needs from increasing.

Individual clinical assessments (see Chapter 27) can take a holistic view of the needs of the child and family but needs assessment can also form part of a more structured process of triage, by using standardized measures completed by informants as part of the referral process. This can streamline and standardize processes, and potentially increase accuracy in identifying children who can benefit from services. For example, a study in Denmark (Hansen *et al.*, 2023) suggested that use of the DAWBA (Goodman *et al.*, 2000) led to a higher number of "correct" referral decisions, in terms of children with disorders and impact being accepted into services. In many countries, high demand and low availability of child and adolescent mental health services lead to strict criteria-based referral processes as a tool to manage demand, which is concerning if the measures being used are less valid for some types of difficulties.

Determining need at a population level using epidemiological data raises different issues. Planning universal and targeted services aimed at prevention and early intervention requires an understanding of the level and distribution of risk and protective factors in the population. This will include as a minimum the use of routine data on the structure of the population in terms of age, gender, and ethnicity, as well as data on factors such as deprivation. Other important sources of data include education, social care, and health services, which may be able to inform on factors such as adverse family circumstances, school readiness, or numbers of children with special educational needs and disabilities.

Planning services also requires an understanding of the prevalence of symptoms, impairment, and diagnoses in the population. The most common way of collecting these data is through cross-sectional surveys, such as England's Mental Health of Children and Young People survey series (Ford *et al.*, 2020), or the Australian Child and Adolescent Survey of Mental Health and Wellbeing (Hafekost *et al.*, 2016). Surveys may use measures designed to identify difficulties on a dimensional scale, such as the SDQ (Goodman, 1997), and/or standardized diagnostic assessments, such as the DAWBA. Population surveys must be regular and timely, or those planning services risk "working in the dark" with old data that no longer represents the needs of the population.

Data also need to be available for the appropriate geography or population groups, but surveys may include insufficient numbers of some children to produce accurate estimates, for example, for children in certain minority ethnic groups or with other less common characteristics (Ford, 2008). In such cases, "booster" samples or targeted surveys may be required (Berthoud *et al.*, 2009). For more localized data, school, county, or state surveys of child mental health may provide regional breakdowns, or modeled estimates can be produced based on knowledge of local risk factors.

Service access

Using epidemiology to understand access to services can help describe "met" and "unmet" needs. While service activity data is essential to examine variation, and in understanding the demands on services, it is limited by exclusion of children who are not referred for help. Commonly, in population surveys, parents or young people are asked to report contact with services in a given time frame. There are limitations to the accuracy of these data where respondents have limited recall or may misclassify contacts with services (e.g., reporting having seen a psychiatrist when they saw a school counselor). Children and young people may also approach services unknown to their parents, or interventions at school level may take place with considerable discussion and resource allocation but no direct interaction with parents or young people so will not be reported using this method. However, validation of the Children's Service Interview demonstrated moderate or better concordance with medical records about appointments and interventions, although agreement was poorer about the type of professional seen (Ford *et al.*, 2007a). Other study designs include the use of linked routine or administrative data to examine metrics such as referrals or clinic attendances (Edwards *et al.*, 2022).

Comparisons of rates of service contact across countries are complex due to variations in the definition, finance, and organization of services. Nonetheless, research consistently suggests that only a minority of children with a psychiatric disorder reach mental health services, and that many are supported by other services, such as education, while a large proportion receive no input at all (Newlove-Delgado *et al.*, 2015; Kovess-Masfety *et al.*, 2017). A recent meta-analysis of studies from high-income countries found that on average, only 44.2% of children with a disorder received any services (Barican *et al.*, 2022). No similar reviews are available from low- and middle-income countries, but evidence points toward an even more marked gap between need and service provision in these settings, with challenges in data collection, plus a lack of clear policy drive and appropriate investment (Kumar *et al.*, 2021).

It is equally important to bear in mind that "contact" alone with services does not necessarily equal "effective" treatment. The limited but growing literature on the effectiveness of routine services provides inconsistent evidence of positive outcomes (Neufeld *et al.*, 2017). Receipt of "adequate" or "evidence-based" treatment (as opposed to access alone) is considerably more difficult to measure. Definitions vary and will naturally be relatively crude owing to the impossibility of determining whether treatment reported is adequate. However, some studies do suggest that a high proportion of children who are in contact with services only have a few contacts with professionals or do not receive what the study defines as "minimally adequate treatment." For example, data from the Australian Child and Adolescent Survey of Mental Health and Wellbeing reported that only 11.6% of children with disorders had a minimum of four contacts or sessions plus medication, or eight without medication (Sawyer *et al.*, 2019). These findings underline the importance of collecting more nuanced data on type, duration, and nature of service contacts to fully understand the "treatment gap." This may be most feasibly achieved using linked routine data.

Underserved populations

The most significant factor predicting access to services remains the presence of disorder or categorical measures of difficulty and impact (Merikangas *et al.*, 2011; Kovess-Masfety *et al.*, 2017). Unfortunately, it is also clear from the evidence that need and access to services are often not evenly matched. Contact with key gatekeepers strongly predicts specialist service contact (Ford *et al.*, 2007b). In many health systems, primary care professionals are central gatekeepers, but schools also have an important role in identification and onward referral of mental health difficulties. Research shows that various factors may impact the likelihood of teachers recognizing and referring mental health problems, including teacher gender, child's ethnicity, and the teacher–student relationship (Halladay *et al.* 2020). Symptoms such as hyperactivity and impulsivity are more strongly associated with contact with a range of services, including education and specialist mental health services, than symptoms of anxiety and depression (Ford *et al.*, 2007b; Costello *et al.*, 2014; Kovess-Masfety *et al.*, 2017).

Poor physical health, poor academic performance, nontraditional family structure, parental psychopathology, and adverse life events are all frequently associated with service contact, although they are also strongly associated with the presence of a psychiatric disorder (e.g., Ford *et al.*, 2008). There remains mixed evidence on the relationship between service contact and socioeconomic status. Some investigators report that children from lower-income groups may be less likely to be in contact relative to markers of need, which is known as Tudor-Hart's *inverse care law* (Newacheck *et al.*, 2003). Other studies have reported no statistical association, or more contact by disadvantaged groups (e.g., Staghezza-Jaramillo *et al.*, 1995). These findings may be partly explained by differences in mental health systems and funding structures, or by families of different socioeconomic status accessing different settings, such as middle-class families opting for education-based services instead of mental health services. Studies examining ethnicity in high-income countries are equally complex to interpret, and in general report both underrepresentation and overrepresentation of children from ethnic minorities, although more recent studies from the United States and Canada have reported such children were less likely to have contact with services after adjusting for symptoms (Merikangas *et al.*, 2011; Edwards *et al.*, 2022).

Contextual determinants are also important. A recent systematic review identified a positive association between use of children and young people's mental health services and various determinants including access to a school-based health center, region of residence, living in an urban area, and living in an area with high socioeconomic status (Verhoog *et al.*, 2022).

Olsson *et al.* (2021) propose an extended definition of unmet mental health needs, in which unmet needs can occur at three stages of the pathway to adequate care: (i) not perceiving a need, (ii) not seeking care, and (iii) not receiving (sufficient or adequate) care. While epidemiology can tell us who does not receive care, qualitative research which draws on the voices of children, young people, parents, and practitioners, is likely to be best placed to provide insights into pathways and barriers to care, and how they can be addressed. Qualitative research with parents and young people has highlighted a range of influences, including knowledge and awareness of mental health, social stigma and embarrassment, perceptions of the therapeutic relationship with professionals and of confidentiality and trust, and more systemic and structural barriers which include financial and other costs, availability, and accessibility of services (Radez *et al.*, 2021; Coelho *et al.*, 2022). Understanding the perspectives of underserved communities is particularly important. For example, studies of young people from ethnic minorities in high-income countries emphasize the need for cultural understanding of mental health professionals (Coelho *et al.*, 2022; Ilozumba *et al.*, 2022). Improving the diversity and representativeness of the mental health workforce could therefore support help-seeking and facilitate pathways to care.

Much of the literature discussed above relates to the prepandemic context. With an immediate focus on acute care for COVID-19, in many settings the availability and delivery of usual health care, including mental health, was severely disrupted (World Health Organization, 2020). Studies from various countries reported initial falls in referrals to services, as well as a decline in primary care consultations and psychotropic prescribing in the early part of the pandemic (Carr *et al.* 2021; McNicholas *et al.* 2021; Evensen *et al.* 2022).

Changes in mode of access may also have affected both access to, and experience of, services. Studies highlighted concerns over a large-scale switch to online delivery, with parents reporting difficulties in online engagement and rapport, and professionals perceiving that remote delivery was often not accessible or suitable for more vulnerable groups, or for those where the therapeutic relationship was more difficult to establish (Johnson *et al.*, 2021; Werling *et al.*, 2022). However, prepandemic, access to digital and online mental health services was often proposed as a means of widening access and improving young people's engagement (Hollis *et al.*, 2015). Despite the expansion of online provision, there remains uncertainty over whether digital services can effectively reach underserved populations of children and young people and address the treatment gap (Hollis *et al.*, 2017).

Striving for excellence: active epidemiology

One of the central aims of epidemiology is to understand the distribution of risk and resilience factors, as well as their prevalence. This will identify areas of need and support the case for service improvement. For example, epidemiological incidence data pinpoints late adolescence as a key period of transition and difficulty for many young people, informing a gradual shift toward the introduction of enhanced support for the transition from child to adult services (Anderson *et al.*, 2021). New service models are designed specifically for adolescents and young adults, removing the "cliff edge" at 18 years of age, and include the Headspace model in Australia (Rickwood *et al.*, 2019), which was designed to provide holistic and integrated health care for those aged 12–25 years. Models using epidemiological data can also be used to forecast need for health care for specific conditions at a local level, using a combination of empirical incidence data and small-area data. These models will only be as good as the data inputted. The use of outdated, inaccurate, incomplete, or unrepresentative epidemiological data will result in estimates or predictions that risk significantly under- or over-representing need. The assumptions made in modeling also need to be explicit, to enable use by others, and to increase trust by model users (Stiglic *et al.*, 2020). Caution should also be used when applying estimates to other settings or areas where the original assumptions may not hold.

Another example of the use of epidemiology to improve access to services is screening. The World Health Organization (2018) defines screening as "the presumptive identification of unrecognized disease in an apparently healthy, asymptomatic population by means of tests, examinations or other procedures that can be applied rapidly and easily to the target population" (https://www.who.int/cancer/prevention/diagnosis-screening/screening/en/).

The intention of screening should be to improve outcomes rather than just "detect" disease, and the benefits of screening must outweigh the risks. Screening in child mental health should therefore aim to identify children who may (i) have risk factors for the development of a disorder, and/or (ii) have raised levels of psychopathology or experience psychiatric symptoms, and who therefore could potentially benefit from early intervention. Children who "screen positive" can be referred for more comprehensive assessments, and then for appropriate intervention, if required. A full discussion of screening approaches and methods is outside the scope of this chapter, however, there are some key criteria that all screening programs should meet, originally proposed by Wilson *et al.*, (1968). Some essential questions to ask when planning screening in child mental health are briefly outlined in Box 14.2.

Screening may be offered to the whole age group (universal screening), or to a population who are selected due to having an "at risk" characteristic or that are being subjected to a risk factor (targeted screening). Examples of where targeted screening may be appropriate include children who are cared for by the state, those who have been displaced by war or other events, or young people in the criminal justice system (Ford *et al.*, 2007c; Chitsabesan *et al.*, 2014; Gadeberg *et al.*, 2017; Clemente *et al.*, 2022).

Schools offer the opportunity for universal mental health screening, as they are likely to be the most inclusive setting for this age group, with the widest reach, but there remains a challenge in demonstrating benefits which outweigh potential costs. Anderson, Ford, and colleagues reported a lack of strong evidence regarding the accuracy of different identification models, and most crucially on their effectiveness in increasing access to

Box 14.2 Eight essential questions to ask when planning a screening program in child mental health

1. Is the clinical course well-understood and is there a window for early detection and intervention?
2. Is the proposed screening procedure safe, simple, and acceptable?
3. How accurate is the proposed screening tool? For example:
   - How good is the tool at identifying children with the target disorder (i.e., identifying true positives)?
   - How good is the tool at identifying most children without the target disorder (i.e., identifying true negatives)?
   - How good is a positive test result at indicating whether a disorder is present (i.e., the positive predictive value)?
   - How good is a negative test result at indicating whether a disorder is not present (i.e., the negative predictive value)?
   - Has the tool been validated in a similar population?
4. What could a false negative result mean for the child and their family, and how can any impact be mitigated?
5. What could a false positive result mean for the child and their family, and how can any impact be mitigated?
6. Is there a clear pathway for what happens once a child has "screened positive"? And is it sufficiently resourced?
7. What is the evidence that the screening is leading to better outcomes?
8. Are the right data being collected to monitor the safety, success, and cost-effectiveness of the program, and any unintended consequences?

appropriate specialist support (Anderson *et al.*, 2018). The latter is a particularly salient point in relation to this chapter's earlier discussion of access to services, as it can only be ethical to screen if the child or young person being screened has the potential to benefit, and this applies to all forms of screening.

Conclusion

Epidemiological data should play an active and central part in planning, organizing, evaluating, and commissioning services. Population data are especially vital in capturing information on children who are not referred for help, and when linked with service activity data can be a powerful tool in understanding pathways to care and the nuances of any "treatment gap." Epidemiological data and tools also increasingly play a role in service evaluation and quality improvement, for example, using routine outcome measurement. Developing areas which may enhance the use of such data in future include patient portals for patients to provide their own data, linkages to wearables, and the use of machine learning and natural language processing to "mine" routine textual data. These may all add to the efficiency, flexibility, timeliness, and relevance of epidemiological data.

However, if such data are to meaningfully contribute to any of these aspects it is crucial that all involved remain mindful of the methodological limitations and complexities involved, as well as the need to draw on other relevant information covered in other chapters in this volume, including information as to the effectiveness of interventions, acceptability of services to potential service users and their parents, and the skills and abilities of potential service providers. Finally, as discussed under "Nothing about us without us," excellent epidemiology should strongly reflect the voices and perspectives of children, young people, and families. Epidemiology is a live science, and must be responsive to changing contexts and the needs of those who contribute and use data.

References

Acheson, R.M. (1978) The definition and identification of need for health care. *Journal of Epidemiology and Community Health* **32**(1), 10–15.

Ambrosini, P.J. (2000) Historical development and present status of the schedule for affective disorders and schizophrenia for school-age children (K-SADS). *Journal of the American Academy of Child & Adolescent Psychiatry* **39**(1), 49–58. ISSN 0890-8567

Anderson, J.K. *et al.* (2018) A systematic review of effectiveness and cost-effectiveness of school-based identification of children and young people at risk of, or currently experiencing mental health difficulties. *Psychological Medicine* **49**(1), 9–19. doi:10.1017/S0033291718002490.

Anderson, J.K. *et al.* (2021) Annual research review: a systematic review of mental health services for emerging adults—moulding a precipice into a smooth passage. *Journal of Child Psychology and Psychiatry.* doi:10.1111/jcpp.13561.

Angold, A. *et al.* (2012) Psychiatric diagnostic interviews for children and adolescents: a comparative study. *Journal of the American Academy of Child and Adolescent Psychiatry* **51**(5), 506–517.

Barican, J.L. *et al.* (2022) Prevalence of childhood mental disorders in high-income countries: a systematic review and meta-analysis to inform policymaking. *Evidence-Based Mental Health.* doi:10.1136/ebmental-2021-300277.

Bennett, S. *et al.* (2021) M.I.C.E.—Mental health intervention for children with epilepsy: a randomised controlled, multi-centre clinical trial evaluating the clinical and cost-effectiveness of MATCH-ADTC in addition to usual care compared to usual care alone for children and young people with common mental health disorders and epilepsy—study protocol. *Trials* **22**, 132. doi:10.1186/s13063-020-05003-9.

Bennett, S.D. *et al.* (2024) Clinical effectiveness of the psychological therapy Mental Health Intervention for Children with Epilepsy in addition to usual care compared with assessment-enhanced usual care alone: a multicentre, randomised controlled clinical trial in the UK. *The Lancet* **403**(10433), 1254–1266. doi:10.1016/S0140-6736(23)02791-5.

Bergen, C. *et al.* (2022) Communication in youth mental health clinical encounters: introducing the agential stance. *Theory & Psychology* **32**(5), 667–690.

Berthoud, R. *et al.* (2009) *Design of the Understanding Society Ethnic Minority Boost Sample.* Understanding Society Working Paper Series No. 2009-02, Institute for Social and Economic Research University of Essex.

Bould, H. *et al.* (2019) Rising suicide rates among adolescents in England and Wales. *The Lancet* **393**(10193), 116–119.

Burn, A. *et al.* (2022) Developing a web-based app to assess mental health difficulties in secondary school pupils: qualitative user-centered design study. *JMIR Formative Research* **6**(1), e30565.

Carey, E. *et al.* (2023) When Is A "Small Effect" Actually Large And Impactful? [Online]. Available: Psyarxiv.Com/V3fjk.

Carr, M.J. *et al.* (2021) Effects of the COVID-19 pandemic on primary care-recorded mental illness and self-harm episodes in the UK: a population-based cohort study. *The Lancet Public Health*. doi:10.1016/S2468-2667(20)30288-7.

Chitsabesan, P. *et al.* (2014) The development of the comprehensive health assessment tool for young offenders within the secure estate. *The Journal of Forensic Psychiatry & Psychology* **25**(1), 1–25.

Clark, D.M. (2018) Realizing the mass public benefit of evidence-based psychological therapies: the IAPT program. *Annual Review of Clinical Psychology* **14**, 159–183. doi:10.1146/annurev-clinpsy-050817-084833.

Clemente, N.S. *et al.* (2022) A whole-child, whole-family approach to health assessments for asylum-seeking children. *BMJ Paediatrics Open* **6**(1), e001575. doi:10.1136/bmjpo-2022-001575. PMID: 36645766; PMCID: PMC9693674

Coelho, H. *et al.* (2022) Experiences of children and young people from ethnic minorities in accessing mental health care and support: rapid scoping review. *Health and Social Care Delivery Research* **10**(22).

Collishaw, S. *et al.* (2009) How far are associations between child, family and community factors and child psychopathology informant-specific and informant-general? *Journal of Child Psychology and Psychiatry* **50**, 571–580. doi:10.1111/j.1469-7610.2008.02026.x.

Costello, E.J. *et al.* (2014) Services for adolescents with psychiatric disorders: 12-month data from the national comorbidity survey. *Psychiatric Services* **65**(3), 359–366.

Downs, J. *et al.* (2018) Detection of suicidality in adolescents with autism spectrum disorders: developing a natural language processing approach for use in electronic health records. *American Medical Informatics Association Annual Symposium Proceedings* **2017**, 641–649. PMID: 29854129; PMCID: PMC5977628

Edwards, J. *et al.* (2022) Characterizing mental health related service contacts in children and youth: a linkage study of health survey and administrative data. *Child and Adolescent Psychiatry and Mental Health* **16**, 48. doi:10.1186/s13034-022-00483-w.

Eke, H. *et al.* (2020) Transition between child and adult services for young people with attention-deficit hyperactivity disorder (ADHD): findings from a British national surveillance study. *The British Journal of Psychiatry* **217**(5), 616–622. doi:10.1192/bjp.2019.131.

Evensen, M. *et al.* (2022) Impact of the COVID-19 pandemic on mental healthcare consultations among children and adolescents in Norway: a nationwide registry study. *European Child & Adolescent Psychiatry*. doi:10.1007/s00787-022-02046-y.

Finning, K. *et al.* (2020) Emotional disorder and absence from school: findings from the 2004 British child and adolescent mental health survey. *European Child & Adolescent Psychiatry* **29**(2), 187–198. doi:10.1007/s00787-019-01342-4.

Ford, T. (2008) Practitioner review: how can epidemiology help us plan and deliver effective child and adolescent mental health services? *Journal of Child Psychology and Psychiatry*. doi:10.1111/j.1469-7610.2008.01927.x.

Ford, T. *et al.* (2007a) The children's services interview: validity and reliability. *Social Psychiatry and Psychiatric Epidemiology* **42**, 36–49. doi:10.1007/s00127-006-0092-9.

Ford, T. *et al.* (2007b) Child mental health is everybody's business: the prevalence of contact with public sector services by type of disorder among British school children in a three-year period. *Child and Adolescent Mental Health* **12**(1), 13–20.

Ford, T. *et al.* (2007c) Psychiatric disorder among British children looked after by local authorities: comparison with children living in private households. *British Journal of Psychiatry* **190**(4), 319–325.

Ford, T. *et al.* (2008) Five years on: public sector service use related to mental health in young people with ADHD or hyperkinetic disorder five years after diagnosis. *Child and Adolescent Mental Health* **13**, 122–129.

Ford, T. *et al.* (2009) Strengths and Difficulties Questionnaire Added Value Scores: evaluating effectiveness in child mental health interventions. *The British Journal of Psychiatry* **194**(6), 552–558. doi:10.1192/bjp.bp.108.052373.

Ford, T. *et al.* (2020) Data resource profile: Mental Health of Children and Young People (MHCYP) surveys. *International Journal of Epidemiology* **49**(2), 363–364g. doi:10.1093/ije/dyz259. PMID: 31953946

Fugard, A.J.B. *et al.* (2015) Analysing and reporting UK CAMHS outcomes: an application of funnel plots. *Child and Adolescent Mental Health* **20**, 155–162. doi:10.1111/camh.12086.

Gadeberg, A.K. *et al.* (2017) Assessing trauma and mental health in refugee children and youth: a systematic review of validated screening and measurement tools. *European Journal of Public Health* **27**(3), 439–446.

Garb, H.N. (2005) Clinical judgement and decision making. *Clinical Psychology* **1**, 67.

Goodman, R. (1997) The Strengths and Difficulties Questionnaire: a research note. *Journal of Child Psychology and Psychiatry* **38**(5), 581–586.

Goodman, R. *et al.* (2000) The development and well-being assessment: description and initial validation of an integrated assessment of child and adolescent psychopathology. *Journal of Child Psychology and Psychiatry* **41**(5), 645–655. doi:10.1111/j.1469-7610.2000.tb02345.x.

Goodman, R. *et al.* (2007) Seemingly minor changes to a questionnaire can make a big difference to mean scores: a cautionary tale. *Social Psychiatry and Psychiatric Epidemiology* **42**(4), 322–327. doi:10.1007/s00127-007-0169-0.

Gray, D.E. (2004) *Doing Research in the Real World*. SAGE Publications, London.

Hafekost, J. *et al.* (2016) Methodology of young minds matter: the second Australian Child and Adolescent Survey of Mental Health and Wellbeing. *The Australian and New Zealand Journal of Psychiatry*. doi:10.1177/0004867415622270.

Halladay, J. *et al.* (2020) Teacher-student relationships and mental health help seeking behaviors among elementary and secondary students in Ontario Canada. *Journal of School Psychology*. doi:10.1016/j.jsp.2020.05.003.

Hansen, A.S. *et al.* (2023) The effect of the development and well-being assessment as an adjunct to standard referral letters on referral decisions by child and adolescent mental health services: a randomized feasibility trial. *Clinical Child Psychology and Psychiatry* **28**(2), 434–449. doi:10.1177/13591045221081384.

Hollis, C. *et al.* (2015) Technological innovations in mental healthcare: harnessing the digital revolution. *The British Journal of Psychiatry* **206**, 263–265.

Hollis, C. *et al.* (2017) Annual research review: digital health interventions for children and young people with mental health problems—a systematic and meta-review. *Journal of Child Psychology and Psychiatry* **58**, 474–503. doi:10.1111/jcpp.12663.

Ilozumba, O. *et al.* (2022) Ethnic minority experiences of mental health services in the Netherlands: an exploratory study. *BMC Research Notes* **15**, 266. doi:10.1186/s13104-022-06159-0.

Islam, S. *et al.* (2021) "We are not hard to reach, but we may find it hard to trust" .... Involving and engaging 'seldom listened to' community voices in clinical translational health research: a social innovation approach. *Research Involvement and Engagement* **7**, 46. doi:10.1186/s40900-021-00292-z.

Jenkins, R. (2001) Making psychiatric epidemiology useful: the contribution of epidemiology to government policy. *Acta Psychiatrica Scandinavica* **103**, 2–14. doi:10.1111/j.1600-0447.2001.00004.x.

Jensen, P.S. *et al.* (1995) Test–retest reliability of the diagnostic interview schedule for children (DISC 2.1). *Archives of General Psychiatry* **52**, 61–71.

Johnson, S. *et al.* (2021) Impact on mental health care and on mental health service users of the COVID-19 pandemic: a mixed methods survey of UK mental health care staff. *Social Psychiatry and Psychiatric Epidemiology* **56**, 25–37. doi:10.1007/s00127-020-01927-4.

Kovess-Masfety, V. *et al.* (2017) Unmet need for specialty mental health services among children across Europe. *Psychiatric Services* **68**(8), 789–795. doi:10.1176/appi.ps.201600409.

Kumar, M. *et al.* (2021) Editorial: strengthening child and adolescent mental health (CAMH) services and systems in lower-and-middle-income countries (LMICs). *Frontiers in Psychiatry* **12**. doi:10.3389/fpsyt.2021.645073.

Kusi-Mensah, K. *et al.* (2022) A systematic review of the validity and reliability of assessment tools for executive function and adaptive function following brain pathology among children and adolescents in low- and middle-income countries. *Neuropsychology Review* **32**, 974–1016. doi:10.1007/s11065-022-09538-3.

Lambert, M.J. & Shimokawa, K. (2011) Collecting client feedback. *Psychotherapy* **48**(1), 72–79. doi:10.1037/a0022238.

Liabo, K. *et al.* (2020) Public involvement in health research: what does 'good' look like in practice? *Research Involvement and Engagement* **6**, 11. doi:10.1186/s40900-020-0183-x.

Marshall, T. *et al.* (2023) Preexisting mental health orders and risk of opioid use disorder in young people: a case-control study. *Early Intervention in Psychiatry* **17**(10), 963–973. doi:10.1111/eip.13385.

McNicholas, F. *et al.* (2021) Referral patterns for specialist child and adolescent mental health services in the Republic of Ireland during the COVID-19 pandemic compared with 2019 and 2018. *British Journal of Psychiatry Open* **7**(3), E91. doi:10.1192/bjo.2021.48.

Mendenhall, E. (2020) The COVID-19 syndemic is not global: context matters. *The Lancet* **396**(10264), P1731. doi:10.1016/S0140-6736(20)32218-2.

Merikangas, K.R. *et al.* (2011) Service utilization for lifetime mental disorders in U.S. adolescents: results of the national comorbidity survey-adolescent supplement (NCS-A). *Journal of the American Academy of Child and Adolescent Psychiatry* **50**, 32–45.

Moreton, R. *et al.* (2022) Creating systems change: evaluating the contribution of the Fulfilling Lives programme. CFE Research. Community Fund. Available: https://www.tnlcommunityfund.org.uk/media/insights/documents/Creating-Systems-Change-Evaluating-the-contribution-of-the-Fulfilling-Lives-programme-2022.pdf?mtime=20220926141204&focal=none [24 September 2024].

Morris, S.E. *et al.* (2022) Revisiting the seven pillars of RDoC. *BMC Medicine* **20**, 220. doi:10.1186/s12916-022-02414-0.

Nature Communications (2018) Epidemiology is a science of high importance. *Nature Communications* **9**, 1703. doi:10.1038/s41467-018-04243-3.

Neufeld, S.A.S. *et al.* (2017) Reduction in adolescent depression after contact with mental health services: a longitudinal cohort study in the UK. *The Lancet Psychiatry*. doi:10.1016/S2215-0366(17)30002-0.

Newacheck, P.W. *et al.* (2003) Disparities in adolescent health and health care: does socioeconomic status matter? *Health Services Research* **38**(5), 1235–1252.

Newlove-Delgado, T. *et al.* (2015) Mental health related contact with education professionals in the British child and adolescent mental health survey 2004. *The Journal of Mental Health Training, Education and Practice* **10**(3), 159–169.

O'Logbon, J. *et al.* (2022) How does the increase in eating difficulties according to the development and well-being assessment screening items relate to the population prevalence of eating disorders? An analysis of the 2017 mental health in children and young people survey. *International Journal of Eating Disorders* **55**(12), 1777–1787. doi:10.1002/eat.23833.

Olsson, S. *et al.* (2021) Unmet need for mental healthcare in a population sample in Sweden: a cross-sectional study of inequalities based on gender, education, and country of birth. *Community Mental Health Journal*. doi:10.1007/s10597-020-00668-7.

Parker, C. *et al.* (2016) The "supporting kids, avoiding problems" (SKIP) study: relationships between school exclusion, psychopathology, development and attainment—case control study. *Journal of Children's Services* **11**(2), 91–110. doi:10.1108/JCS-03-2015-0014.

Pickett, K. & Wilkinson, R.G. (2007) Child well-being and income inequality in rich societies; an ecological cross-sectional survey. *BMJ* **335**, 1080–1087.

Pitchforth, J. *et al.* (2018) Mental health and well-being trends among children and young people in the UK, 1995-2014: analysis of repeated cross-sectional national health surveys. *Psychological Medicine*. doi:10.1017/S0033291718001757.

Porta, M. (2014) *A Dictionary of Epidemiology*, 6th edn. Oxford University Press, New York.

Racey, D.N. *et al.* (2018) Mindfulness-based cognitive therapy for young people and their carers: a mixed-method feasibility study. *Mindfulness* **9**(4), 1063–1075.

Radez, J. *et al.* (2021) Why do children and adolescents (not) seek and access professional help for their mental health problems? A systematic review of quantitative and qualitative studies. *European Child & Adolescent Psychiatry* **30**(2), 183–211. doi:10.1007/s00787-019-01469-4.

Rickwood, D. *et al.* (2019) Australia's innovation in youth mental health care: the headspace centre model. *Early Intervention in Psychiatry* **13**(1), 159–166. doi:10.1111/eip.12740.

Russell, G. *et al.* (2022) Time trends in autism diagnosis over 20 years: a UK population-based cohort study. *Journal of Child Psychology and Psychiatry* **63**, 674–682. doi:10.1111/jcpp.13505.

Rutter, M. *et al.* (2007) Effects of profound early institutional deprivation: an overview of findings from a UK longitudinal study of Romanian adoptees. *European Journal of Developmental Psychology* **4**(3), 332–350. doi:10.1080/17405620701401846.

Sawyer, M.G. *et al.* (2019) Adequacy of treatment for child and adolescent mental disorders in Australia: a national study. *The Australian and New Zealand Journal of Psychiatry* **53**(4), 326–335. doi:10.1177/0004867418808895.

Schlechter, P. *et al.* (2023) The short mood and feelings questionnaire from adolescence to emerging adulthood: measurement invariance across time and sex. *Psychological Assessment* **35**(5), 405–418. doi:10.1037/pas0001222.

Schön, D.A. (1987) *Educating the Reflective Practitioner: Toward a New Design for Teaching and Learning in the Professions.* Jossy-Bass Publishers, San Francisco, CA.

Shafran, R. *et al.* (2020) Optimising evidence-based psychological treatment for the mental health needs of children with epilepsy: principles and methods. *Clinical Child and Family Psychology Review* **23**, 284–295. doi:10.1007/s10567-019-00310-3.

Skarda, I. *et al.* (2021) LifeSim: a lifecourse dynamic microsimulation model of the Millennium birth cohort in England. *International Journal of Microsimulation* **14**(1), 2–42. doi:10.34196/IJM.00228.

Soneson, E. *et al.* (2023) Leveraging administrative data to better understand and address child maltreatment: a scoping review of data linkage studies. *Child Maltreatment* **28**(1), 176–195. doi:10.1177/10775595221079308.

Staghezza-Jaramillo, B. *et al.* (1995) Mental health service utilisation among Puerto Rican children. *Journal of Child and Family Studies* **4**, 399–418.

Stephenson, T. *et al.* (2022) Physical and mental health 3 months after SARS-CoV-2 infection (long COVID) among adolescents in England (CLoCk): a national matched cohort study. *The Lancet. Child & Adolescent Health* **6**(4), 230–239.

Stiglic, G. *et al.* (2020) Interpretability of machine learning-based prediction models in healthcare. *Data Mining and Knowledge Discovery* **10**, 1–13.

Stochl, J. *et al.* (2021) Modernising measurement in psychiatry: item banks and computerised adaptive testing. *The Lancet. Psychiatry* **8**(5), 354–356. ISSN 2215-0366

Sunkel, C. & Sartor, C. (2022) Perspectives: involving persons with lived experience of mental health conditions in service delivery, development and leadership. *BJPsych Bulletin* **46**(3), 160–164. doi:10.1192/bjb.2021.51.

Verhoog, S. *et al.* (2022) Contextual determinants associated with children's and adolescents' mental health care utilization: a systematic review. *European Child & Adolescent Psychiatry* **33**, 2051–2064. doi:10.1007/s00787-022-02077-5.

Werling, A.M. *et al.* (2022) The impact of the COVID-19 pandemic on mental health care of children and adolescents in Switzerland: results of a survey among mental health care professionals after one year of COVID-19. *International Journal of Environmental Research and Public Health* **19**(6), 3252. doi:10.3390/ijerph19063252. PMID: 35328941; PMCID: PMC8953578

Wilson, J.M.G. *et al.* (1968) *Principles and Practice of Screening for Disease.* World Health Organization, Geneva, Switzerland. https://apps.who.int/iris/handle/10665/37650

Wolff, J.C. *et al.* (2018) Trajectories of suicidal ideation among adolescents following psychiatric hospitalization. *Journal of Abnormal Child Psychology* **46**(2), 355–363.

Wolke, D. *et al.* (2009) Selective drop-out in longitudinal studies and non-biased prediction of behaviour disorders. *The British Journal of Psychiatry* **195**(3), 249–256. doi:10.1192/bjp.bp.108.053751.

Wolport, M. & Ford, T. (2015) Using epidemiology to plan, organize, and evaluate services for children and adolescents with mental health problems. In: *Rutter's Child and Adolescent Psychiatry.* (eds A. Thapar, *et al.*), 6th edn. John Wiley & Sons, Ltd, Chichester, UK. pp. 163–176.

Wolpert, M. *et al.* (2015) Comparison of indices of clinically meaningful change in child and adolescent mental health services: difference scores, reliable change, crossing clinical thresholds and 'added value'—an exploration using parent rated scores on the SDQ. *Child and Adolescent Mental Health* **20**(2), 94–101. doi:10.1111/camh.12080.

World Health Organization (2018) Cancer. Available: https://www.who.int/cancer/prevention/diagnosis-screening/screening/en/ [24 September 2024].

World Health Organization (2020) The impact of covid-19 on mental, neurological and substance use services. Available: https://www.who.int/publications/i/item/978924012455 [27 April 2023].

CHAPTER 15

Establishing the clinical effectiveness of interventions and implementations

Helena Chmura Kraemer
Department of Psychiatry and Behavioral Sciences, Stanford University, Stanford, CA, USA

Scores of books and papers exist advising researchers on how to do studies to evaluate treatment efficacy or effectiveness or reporting their results, but few guiding clinical consumers to process such research for their decision-making. Clinical consumers include clinicians making decisions concerning their patients' care, policymakers for their communities' care, or patients seeking information for their own care, who need to know what results in published research papers they might well ignore, what is suggestive but not conclusive, and what should be seriously considered in making decisions.

A major source of problems is that of words used capriciously, inaccurately, or inconsistently. For example, "quasi-experimental" means nonexperimental and "modified intent-to-treat" means not by intent-to-treat, both terms encouraging readers to treat the results as if experimental or done by intent-to-treat. Moreover, many researchers report and interpret "p-values" and "statistical significance" inconsistently with their precise definitions. Consequently, definition of terms is a focus here.

To start, an "intervention" is any strategy, injection, ingestion, incision, or instruction, to be prescribed by a clinician in hopes of improving the well-being of a patient. An intervention may be delivered to prevent future onset of a disorder or to treat an existing disorder. Moreover, one intervention can often be delivered in multiple ways: "implementations." For example, cognitive behavior therapy (CBT) is an intervention that can be delivered by a clinician face-to-face with a patient, or with a group of patients, and either might be delivered online instead of face-to-face. Is CBT equally effective in all four implementations, or more effective in some and perhaps useless in others? For convenience here, an intervention plus its implementation is called a "treatment."

The "efficacy" of a treatment refers to how successfully it achieves its goal under ideal conditions, when given only to carefully selected patients, by those expert in its delivery or under controlled conditions. "Effectiveness" refers to how successful a treatment is under the conditions treatment would usually be delivered to patients (Hoagwood *et al.*, 1995). In an effectiveness study all patients with the disorder of interest who might benefit from treatment are eligible for inclusion, excluding only those who will be harmed by participation and those unwilling to participate. The treatment is delivered under ordinary conditions by clinicians like those who would usually deliver the treatment.

To whom is the treatment to be delivered, the "target" of the treatment? In most cases, treatment is delivered to individual patients who have no interaction with each other. However, in evaluation of group therapy, the target is a group of patients, who communicate with each other during therapy and may influence each other's response. In such cases, the effect of treatment may be augmented by the insights and support patients within the group provide each other or may be diminished by the decrease in personal attention to individuals by the therapist. In other studies, the target of intervention may be a clinician to be given special training, with the effect of that training assessed on that clinician's patients. The target of intervention may be a class of students, with the effect assessed on the individual students within each class. In all such cases, the evaluation principles here apply to the "cluster," the group, not to the individuals within a cluster, and the analysis must account for any nonindependence of patients within each cluster. In what follows the term "cluster" might be substituted for "patient," but the principles remain the same.

The very earliest clinical trials of a new treatment are likely to be efficacy trials, because if a treatment does not work under ideal conditions, it is hardly likely to work under usual conditions, and efficacy trials are less difficult and costly. Efficacy studies are crucial in the early stages of research, necessary to

Rutter's Child and Adolescent Psychiatry and Psychology, Seventh Edition.
Edited by Anita Thapar, Daniel S. Pine, Samuele Cortese, Cathy Creswell, Tamsin J. Ford, James F. Leckman, and Argyris Stringaris.

Companion website: www.wiley.com/go/thapar/rutterspsych7

developing safe treatments and to designing subsequent clinical trials, but questionable as a basis of clinical decision-making. For that reason, consumers should be reluctant to base clinical decisions only on efficacy studies. The focus of this discussion is on effectiveness studies.

Effectiveness is a comparative judgment: the treatment "works" if the patients will have a better outcome with the treatment than without. Studies relevant to clinical decision-making must always compare two (or more) different treatments, at least a treatment of interest (T) and a control/comparison treatment (C) that assesses the outcome "without T." Often T is a new treatment and C an established one, with T the one the researchers would bet on. In some cases, C is an established treatment whose effectiveness or safety has come under question, with T an alternative treatment choice, one researchers would bet on. Whatever the motivation for the comparison, the goal is to decide which of T or C is to be preferred. Which of the two treatments being compared is labeled T and which C is arbitrary, for both must be fairly evaluated against each other. In a study comparing more than two treatments, the principles apply to each pair of treatments.

What of pre-post studies, studies in which a sample of patients with a disorder are assessed pretreatment, all patients given *one* treatment, then assessed over the course of the intervention? Surely, if improvement in the clinical course is shown, isn't that proof that the treatment is effective?

No, the patients in any treatment study are included because they satisfy the inclusion/exclusion criteria. Diagnoses, symptoms, risk-level assessments, and other such criteria are never perfectly reliable: there are false positive and false negative identifications. All negatives, true or false, are excluded from the trial, but false positives are included along with true positives. If a treatment has no effect (e.g., a placebo), there will be an appearance of improvement, as the false positives migrate back to their true values and the true positives maintain theirs—a statistical artifact called "statistical regression to the mean" (James, 1973; Blomqvist, 1986; Campbell & Kenny, 1999). Moreover, there are expectation effects. Patients beginning a new treatment, and the evaluators of treatment response, expect and hope for improvement. What outcomes they report may be biased by those expectations and hopes. Finally, there are natural trends. Patients already improving at the time of entry to the study might simply continue that course, which may also produce a false appearance of a treatment effect.

Such artifacts produce the appearance of improvement with any treatment, including an inert placebo: the "placebo effect." When two treatments are compared in a well-designed trial, the placebo effect equally affects outcomes for both treatments. In contrasting the outcomes between treatments, the artifacts cancel out, and the difference between the two groups correctly reflects the differential effect of the two treatments. That is effectiveness. For that reason, pre-post studies provide useful information, particularly related to patient compliance or to adverse events, but are misleading in providing evidence of effectiveness.

Expectation bias also exists when the patient and those evaluating response to treatment know which of two treatments that patient is receiving. Knowing that this patient is being given an active drug expected to have benefit, while that patient is being given an inert placebo or a less favored treatment, can influence how patients' responses are evaluated. Consequently, effectiveness trials should "blind" outcome assessments as much as possible, i.e., use procedures that prevent those evaluating treatment outcomes (patients or evaluators) from being biased by knowledge of which treatment is being given to whom.

Most importantly, the results of any study apply to the population of patients represented by those included in the study. Generalization beyond those limits is risky. This is particularly problematic for evaluation of treatments for children and adolescents, for such studies are challenging to design and to execute. Generalizing the results of studies done on adults to children and adolescents, can be misleading. Moreover, if a treatment is shown to be effective in reducing illicit drug use for adolescents in a trial excluding smokers, those with any mental health diagnosis, those who also use alcohol, or those who have a history of other risky behaviors, that treatment may not be effective for the general population of adolescent drug users that would include all of these groups. Researchers reporting the results of trials state their inclusion/exclusion criteria, and what percentage of those excluded and why, information important to clinical consumers. To evaluate the effectiveness of any treatment (T) against any control/comparison (C), both must be delivered to samples from the *same* population.

What of observational studies? There, a sample of patients given T is compared with a sample of patients given C, where the decision to give T or C was that of the patients or clinicians. In such cases, the two samples of patients may be from two different populations, differentiated by whatever factors patients or clinicians used to make those decisions, factors not consistently used and unknown to researchers. If the populations sampled for T and C differ, then the T outcome in the T-population may be better than the C outcome in the C-population, but it may be that C is more effective than T in both those different populations. In observational studies, it is impossible to separate the effects determining treatment choice from the outcomes of such choices on patients.

But surely mathematical models can be used to "control for" or "adjust for" such selection factors used to choose T versus C? No, since the factors that determine which patients get T and which get C are unknown to the researchers, the factors that need to be adjusted for are guesswork. Moreover, the mathematical models used for adjustment are based on various assumptions: linearity, equal variances, normal distributions, noncollinearity, absence of interactions, etc., that the researchers make. If any of those assumptions are wrong, the answers that result from such analyses are also wrong.

Moreover, if there is to be adjusting in hypothesis testing, what factors are to be adjusted for and how must be justified and stated, and assumptions checked, before the study is started (*a priori*). The sample size must then be increased for adequate power. However, in many cases, it is only after the study is completed that researchers decide to adjust, perhaps because of observed baseline imbalances between the T and C groups: *post hoc* testing. Then the p-values are miscomputed and any claims of statistical significance are unsupported. To do such *post hoc* analysis is useful, even crucial, for elucidating the results or generating hypotheses for future work but is not the basis of clinical decision-making.

Researchers will recognize that these considerations lead inexorably to a recommendation that the evaluation of treatment effectiveness, while informed by pre-post studies, observational studies, efficacy studies, and *post hoc* studies, should focus on randomized controlled clinical trials (RCTs). In what follows, we consider first what is needed to lead up to an RCT (hypothesis-generating exploratory studies), then what clinical consumers should look for in RCT-reported results, and finally what should follow a valid RCT (*post hoc exploratory* analyses) that might lead to development of even more effective treatments for some or all the population, hypotheses to be tested in future RCTs.

What leads up to a valid randomized controlled clinical trial (RCT)?

Explorations/hypothesis generation

All clinical research starts in the lab and in the clinic. In the lab, there are experiments done *in vitro*, and studies done on animal models *in vivo*, but what happens in a Petri dish or in a lab rat cannot be immediately generalized to patients. In the clinic, observations of patterns in patients are informative but can mislead. Beyond this are many hypothesis-generating or exploratory studies, not definitive in guiding clinical decision-making, but necessary both to develop viable hypotheses to be tested in RCTs, to guide the delivery of treatments safely to patients, and to generate the information necessary to design valid and adequately powered RCTs to guide clinical decision-making. Such hypothesis-generating studies include not only pre-post studies and observational studies, as already noted, but also re-analyses of existing datasets obtained for a variety of reasons: clinical, government, or industrial databases, data collected in epidemiological studies, and data collected in completed hypothesis-testing studies, including completed RCTs. Such studies are the foundation on which the evidence necessary for evidence-based clinical decision-making is based, the first steps, not the last (see Hypothesis-generating/Exploration level in Figure 15.1).

Ethically, to conduct an RCT, there must be rationale and justification from previous studies for hypothesizing that T and C will have different effects on patient outcomes for patients in the population sampled, and that these different effects may potentially be of clinical importance. The researchers proposing a study should be in "clinical equipoise" (Freedman, 1987). Based on what is known, they should see it as likely that there is some outcome difference between T and C, but nowhere near certain that there is a difference, or if the difference is large

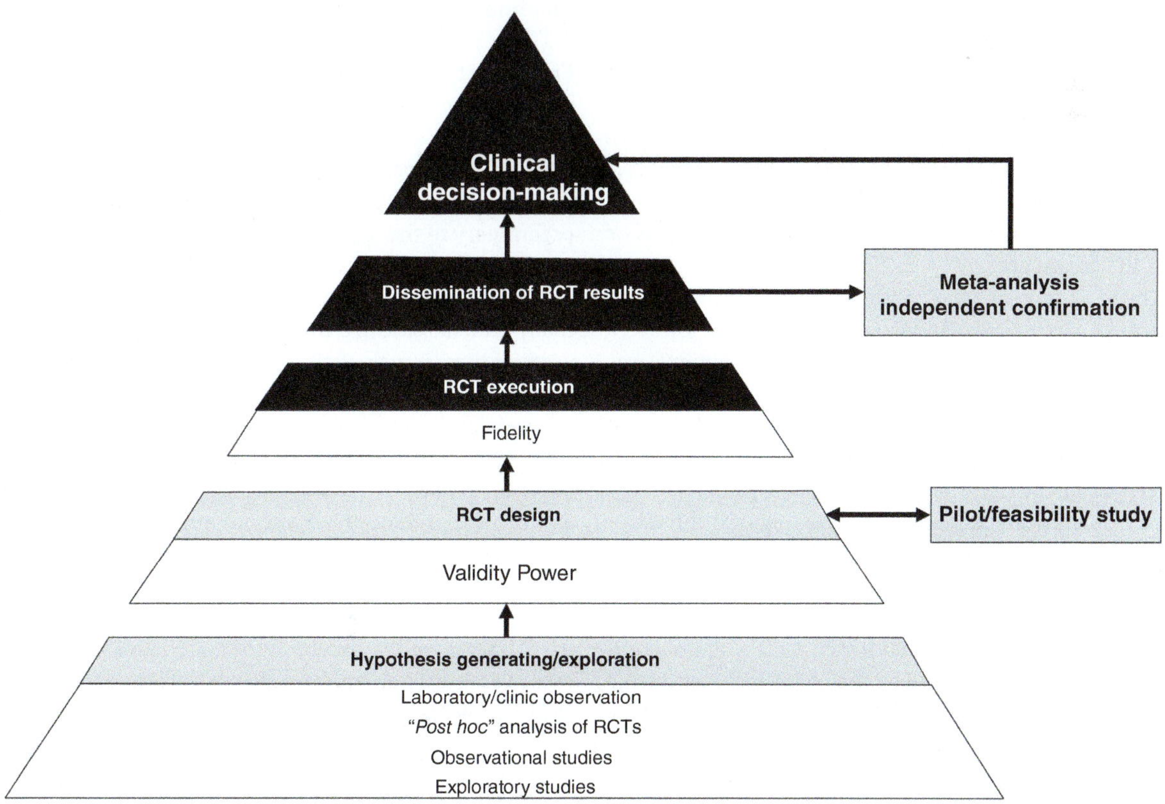

Figure 15.1 A depiction of the overall structure of research leading to randomized clinical trials (RCTs), ultimately to clinical decision-making.

enough to be of "clinical significance," i.e., large enough to impact patient care. Clinical equipoise is necessary both to avoid placing a burden of participation in an RCT on patients that can result in no progress, and to ensure that the research is done as free as possible from any bias of the researchers.

Research design

From information in those exploratory studies, the researchers specify the population to whom the results are meant to apply (sampling plan, inclusion/exclusion criteria, whether the target is the individual patient or a cluster), and the protocols for T and C, necessary both to allow other independent researchers to replicate or confirm any conclusion the RCT reaches and for clinicians to use in treating their patients. Also necessary is specification of the clinical outcome the treatment is meant to improve and of how that outcome is to be measured, as well as the design and analysis plans. There are many decisions to be made in designing an RCT, based on what is learned in the Exploratory phase (Figure 15.1) and unbiased by any researchers "knowing" what the "correct" answer is.

If the target of the intervention is an individual patient, patients recruited to the RCT are then *randomly* assigned to T and to C, so that the patients given each treatment are *random* samples from the *same* patient population. If the target is a cluster of patients, the clusters are randomly assigned to T and to C, so that the clusters are *random* samples from the *same* population of clusters. It must be noted that random samples from the same population will be similar in their baseline characteristics, but they are not matched samples. Two samples that are very different, as well as two samples that are too well matched, would both raise questions about how randomization was done. The more effort researchers invest in trying to match samples on certain characteristics, the more likely there will be very serious imbalances on other characteristics.

All patients randomized must be included in the analysis or results in the treatment group to which they were assigned: analysis "by intention to treat." Patients often do not comply with treatment recommendations or drop out of an RCT because of a negative reaction to whichever treatment was assigned, dropping out when they feel that treatment is not benefitting them, or when they find compliance with the treatment protocol impossible. Such patients exist in the population sampled as well as in the sample. Excluding such patients in the analysis of results means excluding evidence against the effectiveness of the treatment, resulting in samples from two different populations in the two different treatment groups converting what was planned as an RCT to an observational study. Part of the proposed analytic plan for a valid RCT deals with how randomized patients with missing data are to be included in the analysis by intention to treat, and again decisions guided by the exploratory phase.

The most crucial part of the research plan is the proposed "statistical test" of the hypothesis, a declaration before the study is begun (*a priori*), of the condition under which the researchers will conclude that T is recommended over C (T > C) or that C is recommended over T (C > T) for patients in the population sampled. This declaration is usually in the form of a proposal to compute a statistic, the p-value. If the p-value correctly computed is found to be less than 0.05, the result is labeled "statistically significant at the 5% level," indicating support for a treatment difference. The goal is an RCT that is both valid and adequately powered.

For validity, there should be very little chance of claiming an advantage of T over C or of C over T when there is none, usually less than 5% chance—the "significance level." To be adequately powered, there should be quite a good chance, perhaps greater than 80%—the "statistical power"—that if there is an advantage of one treatment over the other large enough to be of clinical significance, that will be found statistically significant. Like the odds set on a horse prior to a horse race, the significance level and power are probabilities calculated *before* an RCT is begun: *a priori*. If computed after the race/trial is underway or completed, the calculations would be very different. Once again: clinical significance means an advantage of one treatment over another large enough to have a meaningful impact on patient outcomes. The figure of 5% is set by tradition, reflecting what was deemed a tolerable limit of false positive research results in the research literature. Some recommend that it be made more stringent, say 1% or 0.5%. The value of 80% for power is negotiable but it should be kept reasonably high to prevent useless burdening of patient participants in the RCT, and wasting of time and resources for the researchers.

Feasibility/pilot studies

Once a study design is proposed, researchers should be reasonably sure that what they propose they should and could do (with "fidelity" to the research plan).

This motivates a study of some kind (Eldridge *et al.*, 2016) preliminary to the RCT. If there is any doubt that enough available patients will be eligible and willing to participate, that might be checked by reviewing clinic records to find out how many patients satisfied inclusion/exclusion criteria in previous years. If there is lack of clarity on exactly how to deliver T or C, a small study might be done to finalize the manuals for treatment delivery, and to train participating clinicians to deliver those treatments. If there is doubt as to which measure of outcome is best to use, a methodological study comparing the reliabilities and validities on various proposed measures of that outcome might be done. If there is any doubt that patients will agree to randomization or can comply with the demands of the RCT, or that the treatment can be delivered and outcomes measured as proposed, a small number of eligible patients might be recruited into a miniature version of the proposed RCT, a "mini-RCT," to check. What is crucial is that this is a preliminary study, not one that provides information on the effectiveness of treatments.

One particular use of the mini-RCT pilot/feasibility study is discouraged: that of using the study to estimate the relative effectiveness of the treatments as a basis of power computations and sample size for the proposed RCT to follow (Kraemer *et al.*, 2006). Because the sample size in such a pilot study is small, the estimate of effectiveness can be very inaccurate. It may be seriously underestimated, which would discourage funding, or seriously overestimated, which would result in an underpowered RCT and a failed RCT.

In short, the researchers do a small study to assure themselves (and proposal reviewers) that what they propose for the RCT they can and should do. The results of such pilot/feasibility studies are used to "tweak" the research design. While there are exceptions (e.g., a finalized treatment manual or a comparison of measures), pilot/feasibility studies are usually not publishable because they typically deal with local conditions.

The term "pilot" in pilot studies corresponds to the same term in pilot boat. A pilot boat is a small simple boat that leads a large ship, a luxury liner, or an aircraft carrier, safely into port. A pilot study is a small simple study that leads an RCT to correct conclusions. One cannot expect that a pilot boat performs the functions of a large ship (house or feed hundreds of tourists or land aircraft), no more than one can expect to draw conclusions about effectiveness of any T versus C from a pilot study. Moreover, it is as pointless to send a pilot boat out in the absence of any ship to guide into port, as it is to do a pilot study when there is no intent to do a full-scale RCT. However, some researchers have appropriated the term "pilot study" to label a small, poorly designed, or underpowered study to encourage publication. A published study labeled "pilot/feasibility," correctly so labeled or not, may be crucial to further research, often of interest to researchers, but is not the basis of clinical decision-making (see Pilot/Feasibility study level in Figure 15.1). It is important as the basis of a proposal for an RCT.

The review process

Once the research proposal is finalized, its ethical basis is usually evaluated by an institutional review board (IRB). RCTs generally require funding, and after ethical approval, are usually evaluated on behalf of the funder by an independent review committee comprising a wide range of expertise. Once approved and funded, the RCT plan is registered (in the United States, at clinicaltrials.gov), open to anyone to review, and the RCT can get under way. It is crucial that researchers execute their RCT with fidelity to their research plan, for deviations can undermine both the validity and the power of any RCT. Sometimes there is an independent review committee that monitors the ongoing conduct of an RCT (Data Safety and Monitoring Board: DSMB). Once the RCT is completed, any report of its research results for publication in a professional journal is evaluated by editors and reviewers to assure that the RCT reports conclusions accurately and completely, with conclusions supported by the evidence (see RCT execution and dissemination of RCT results levels in Figure 15.1).

In short, by the time clinical consumers read a published RCT report (the peak in Figure 15.1), if the system works as it should, they should be assured that the RCT has undergone multiple levels of reviews by multiple experts, before, during, and after its completion. Reviewers, as well as researchers, bear responsibility for preventing execution and publication of studies that might mislead clinical decision-making. If all this is so, what is left for clinical consumers to do in evaluating RCT results for decision-making? Why not just read the conclusion section of the abstract of the published paper of an RCT and act on that? The problem is that the conclusion section represents how the researchers interpret their findings, which may or may not correspond to how individual consumers should interpret those findings for their own use.

The clinical consumer evaluating an RCT

Is this an RCT?

It is usually obvious from the title of a paper, but if, for example, the analysis is not done by intention to treat, or if the outcome measures are biased in an "unblinded" RCT, it may not be a valid RCT.

Is the research question of clinical relevance to this clinical consumer?

The rationale and justification for the study is reported in the introductory section of the paper. If, for example, the disorder or the population is not one of interest to the consumer, the report is obviously irrelevant to their decision-making.

Is the population sampled the one of concern to this consumer?

For example, if a patient has the disorder of interest, but with comorbidities that are excluded in the RCT, the conclusions are not likely to apply to that patient. The inclusion/exclusion criteria should always be clearly stated in the paper. Statistics describing the population sampled are usually presented in the first table of a paper, and a CONSORT diagram (Schulz *et al.*, 2010) typically also reports on patient flow. If the population sampled does not correspond to that of interest, the results of the RCT are irrelevant to that clinical consumer.

Is the comparison between T and C relevant for this consumer?

If, for example, the RCT compares a new treatment (T) against a placebo control group (C), but a clinician generally uses another treatment already known to be more effective than placebo (C), and possibly more effective than T as well, that RCT may be irrelevant to that clinician's decision-making. Many researchers choose to use placebo controls even when treatments known to be more effective than the placebo are readily available.

A more informative choice of a control group, from a medical consumer's viewpoint, might be "treatment as usual" (TAU). Then patients in the study would be randomized either to the new treatment (T) or to be treated as they would have been had they not been RCT participants (C is TAU). Both treatment groups should be evaluated with the same blinded procedures. The research question then would be whether T is a better choice than whatever clinicians are generally using. In exploratory *post hoc* analysis, which treatments are being used, and how, in TAU might be reported. Some exploration of how each such treatments fared relative to T might also guide design of future RCTs.

A TAU control group has a distinct advantage over a placebo. Informed consent for patients recruited into any RCT requires that patients know what T and C are. If they know that C is a placebo, well-informed patients, highly motivated to get well, who know there are effective treatments available from community clinicians (TAU), may well refuse to participate. This is often seen in the CONSORT diagram as a high percentage of eligible patients refusing randomization, and in a nonblinded RCT, dropping out without accepting the assigned treatment. The resulting samples in the RCT may be biased relative to the population of interest to clinical consumers. On the other hand, with TAU as C, patients are assured that they will either get what they would have if they had refused participation in the RCT, or perhaps something better (T), and are more likely to participate and comply.

Researchers, on the other hand, may distrust a TAU control group, for community clinicians may differ from each other not only in what treatments they deliver, but also in the quality of their delivery. For example, in an RCT comparing a drug treatment for attention deficit hyperactivity disorder (ADHD) against TAU (The MTA Cooperative Group, 1999), clinicians in the TAU group often prescribed the same drug as that used in the drug treatment group. However, the outcomes for patients given that drug in the TAU group were inferior to those for patients randomized to the same drug. In this case, the assessments were not blinded. Part of that effect may have been due to expectation bias. However, it was also true that the dosage schedules, monitoring, and control specified in the protocol for the drug treatment group (the implementation) was not followed by TAU clinicians prescribing that drug. That also might account for the differences.

In general, a TAU control group is heterogeneous in treatments and in treatment outcomes. The sample size necessary for adequate power is usually much larger than that needed for a placebo-controlled RCT. A valid, adequately powered such RCT will take longer and cost more than a valid, adequately powered placebo-controlled RCT.

Another possible C is treatment thought to be the best available for the patients, but, the sample size, duration, and cost of the RCT would then be much greater.

Does the primary outcome define the consumer's primary goal of treatment?

Is the selected outcome measure the "right" one (one that clearly signals the impact on the patient, often hard to measure well), or is it merely a "good" one (an interesting measure that is easy to obtain and reliable but not the right one) (Tukey, 1979)? For example, in evaluating the effect of an intervention for low birthweight, premature infants on child health, a mother's report might be used, only to find that the primary influence on such reports is not the child's health, but the mother's educational level (Gross *et al.*, 1997). This is a problem often encountered with research with children, where parents' reports are often the most accessible source of information about the child (good), but often reflect parents' characteristics and expectations as much as or more than the child's (right) outcome.

It may also be that the outcome is one in which consumers are most interested, but is poorly measured in the RCT, for example, an arbitrary dichotomization of an important outcome measure, such as 6-month survival time. Outcome measures insensitive to individual differences important to a clinician may be good measures but not necessarily the right measures. In this case, for example, it would be far preferable to compare the T and C survival curves, showing the comparison between T and C at every time point (not merely at 6 months) up to the end of follow-up. It is better for consumers, and since power is increased, better for the researchers as well.

Finally, the outcome measure may be the result of a technically complex procedure done on patients, laboratory tests, scans, easily "blinded," highly reliable, and of scientific importance. However, if what is important to the medical consumer is whether symptoms have decreased and functioning increased, reporting differences in brain structure and function, or changes in biochemical measures, may be irrelevant outcomes for clinical decision-making—again good measures, not the right ones. Such measures may well be included as secondary outcome measures to further scientific knowledge, but are not the basis of clinical decision-making.

How much better is T than C in this population?

If the RCT passes muster with the clinician's interest and goals, then the final crucial question is: "How much better is T than C (or vice versa)?" To be specific: "What is the probability that a patient in this population given T will have a better outcome than one given C, less the probability that the reverse is true?" This is an effect size, "success rate difference" (SRD), that can be estimated from any RCT comparing T versus C, no matter the outcome measure (Kraemer & Kupfer, 2006; Kraemer *et al.*, 2020).

If, in an RCT, there are m patients randomly assigned to T and n to C, there are mn possible T-C pairs of patients. The proportion of pairs in which the T patient has a better outcome than the paired C patient (a "T-success") less the proportion of pairs in which C patient has a better outcome than the paired T patient (a "C-success") estimates SRD. Researchers can obtain a 95% confidence interval for the true SRD using bootstrap methods: 95% of such confidence intervals would cover the true population value of SRD.

The true SRD reflects the relative effectiveness of T to C in the population sampled, ranging from −1 to +1. The null value of SRD is when the T and C are equally effective and SRD is zero (which should never happen with strong rationale and justification for the RCT), although SRD = 0 does not necessarily mean T and C are equally effective. Switching the T and C labels reverses the sign of SRD. The primary determinant of estimation precision, the length of the confidence interval, is sample size, and it is also the primary determinant of the p-value or statistical significance. In turn, factors affecting the necessary sample size are related to the quality of research decision-making: the reliability of outcome measures and their sensitivity to individual differences in outcome, balance in group size, fidelity to the research plan, choice of test, etc.

SRD equal to +1 means that every patient will respond better to T than to C; SRD equal to −1 means that every patient will respond better to C than to T. A large magnitude SRD indicates that most patients in the population sampled will respond better to the preferred treatment. On the other hand, SRD near, or even equal to, zero is ambiguous. SRD = 0 does not necessarily mean that T and C are equally effective in the population sampled, a common misinterpretation of nonstatistically significant RCT results (p-value ≥ 0.05) or a small effect size. It may mean that there are unknown patient factors (moderators of treatment outcome) that divide the sampled population into two subpopulations, those for whom T is better than C (T > C), and those for whom C is equally better than T (C > T) (e.g., Wallace *et al.*, 2013). Alternatively, a small effect size or a nonstatistically significant result may simply mean a poorly designed or executed RCT.

Closely related to SRD is number needed to treat (NNT = 1/SRD) (Bogarty & Brophy, 2005; Shearer-Underhill & Marker, 2010), difficult to use in calculations, but perhaps more interpretable to clinicians. Roughly, NNT calculates how many patients need to be treated with T to have one more success than if they had all been treated with C (NNT)? Or to express this differently: how many patients would have to be treated with T unnecessarily (since they would have much the same results as with C) (NNT-1)? If SRD = +0.001, NNT = 1000. If SRD = 0.5, NNT = 2.

SRDs are not commonly reported. Instead, sometimes other effect sizes are reported, some valid only in special circumstances, but used, valid or not, and with widely different scales (Table 15.1). If the outcome were a time to an event, e.g., "How long to remission?", and certain assumptions apply, hazard ratio (HR) might be used and SRD = (HR −1)/(HR+1) or (1 −HR)/(1+HR), depending on whether the outcome is a welcome (remission) or unwelcome (death) one. If the outcome measure were a continuous measure, e.g., the answer to "What is the decrease in symptoms over 6 months?", under certain assumptions, Cohen's d (standardized mean difference) is used, and SRD is a mathematical rescaling of d (Table 15.1). If the outcome measure were ordinal, SRD = 2U/(mn) −1, where U/mn is the area under a receiver operating characteristic (ROC) curve, and U is the Mann-Whitney U-statistic with m and n the two sample sizes. Finally, if the outcome was binary, e.g., "Is the patient cured?" (yes/no), SRD is simply the difference between the two success rates. In short, there are many valid effect sizes, most valid only under certain conditions, and/or measured on different scales, but clinically interpretable ones can be rescaled to SRD, and SRD can always be used (Table 15.1).

Table 15.1 Conversions from the number needed to treat (NNT), Cohen's d (standardized mean difference), and Hazard ratio to the corresponding success rate difference (SRD) for SRD ≥ 0.

			Hazard ratio	
SRD	NNT	Cohen's d	Positive	Negative
0.00	∞	0.0	1.0	1.00
0.05	20.0	0.1	1.1	0.90
0.10	10.0	0.2	1.2	0.82
0.15	6.7	0.3	1.4	0.74
0.20	5.0	0.4	1.5	0.67
0.25	4.0	0.5	1.7	0.60
0.30	3.3	0.5	1.9	0.54
0.35	2.9	0.6	2.1	0.48
0.40	2.5	0.7	2.3	0.43
0.45	2.2	0.8	2.6	0.38
0.50	2.0	1.0	3.0	0.33
0.55	1.8	1.1	3.4	0.29
0.60	1.7	1.2	4.0	0.25
0.65	1.5	1.3	4.7	0.21
0.70	1.4	1.5	5.7	0.18
0.75	1.3	1.6	7.0	0.14
0.80	1.3	1.8	9.0	0.11
0.85	1.2	2.0	12.3	0.08
0.90	1.1	2.3	19.0	0.05
0.95	1.1	2.8	39.0	0.03
1.00	1.0	∞	∞	0.00

The major exception is the odds ratio (OR), which is not an interpretable effect size, but is often reported as such, comparing two binary outcomes (Sackett *et al.*, 1996). OR = 1 if and only if SRD = 0, but otherwise SRD lies anywhere between zero and $Y = (OR^{1/2}-1)/(OR^{1/2}+1)$. For example, if OR = 4, then Y = 1/3, and the SRD lies somewhere between 0 and 1/3, with NNT greater than 3. That means that SRD may be 0.001 and NNT = 1000, or that SRD may be 0.3 and NNT = 3, a huge difference to those making clinical decisions. OR indicates which of T and C is preferable, but merely puts a "cap" on the magnitude of SRD. No matter how large or small a non-null OR is (OR unequal to 1), the corresponding SRD may be very near zero and NNT very large, useless for clinical decision-making.

Now for a critical and challenging question for clinical consumers: "How large an effect size is large enough to be considered of clinical significance, to make the choice of T over C non-negotiable for you?" That value of SRD we denote as SRD*, of NNT as NNT*, is the threshold of clinical significance. For an RCT to be "adequately powered," the researchers set their required significance level (usually 5%) and power (80%?) and *their* critical effect size (SRD*). That determines the sample size necessary for an adequately powered trial. Whether that is reasonably done is assessed in the proposal review process.

While the true SRD or NNT comparing T versus C is based on comparison of the primary outcomes objectively achieved, their critical values are determined subjectively by researchers and clinical consumers and may differ from one to another

For example, Cohen (Cohen, 1988) proposed that for a treatment RCT, under certain circumstances d = 0.2, 0.5, or 0.8 would be considered a small, medium, or large effect size. That translates into SRD = 0.11, 0.28, 0.43 or NNT = 9, 4, 2. If the condition to be treated is potentially fatal, even the smallest increase in the chance of survival might be of importance, and one might set SRD* = 0.1 and NNT* = 9. However, if the condition were not that serious (common cold?) and the treatment onerous, costly, or associated with side effects, much greater assurance of benefit might be required, e.g., SRD* = 0.43, NNT* = 2. The question for each clinical consumer is how small an effect size is too small to warrant clear preference of one treatment over the other? How much risk of failure are you willing to take? 1 in 9? 1 in 2?

For any situation, clinical consumers may (appropriately) have very different standards for that critical value, SRD*, than do the researchers. Individual patients might have different SRD* from their clinicians, and clinicians making decisions for patients might have SRD* different from medical policymakers making decisions for communities of patients. Moreover, any individual may set SRD* very differently depending on what the disorder is (common cold versus cancer), on what the costs and risks of treatment are (surgery versus medication versus psychotherapy), on what C is (placebo versus TAU), and on what the primary outcome impact would be.

Consumers' interpretation of RCT results should be based on their own critical effect size, not necessarily on that of the researchers, although the researchers' choice is often a good start. What medical consumers need to see is not the p-value reported by the researchers, but the 95% confidence interval for SRD to allow them to make their decisions relative to their own SRD*. Figure 15.2 shows all possible configurations of the 95% confidence interval for SRD from an RCT, using the SRD* set by an individual medical consumer.

Before proposing an RCT, the researchers should be in clinical equipoise. Essentially, that means that if the researchers were asked, in proposing the RCT, based on all exploratory/hypothesis-generating work, to present a *subjective* 95% confidence interval for SRD, they should report confidence intervals like A or B (Figure 15.2), each including SRD = 0 and some SRDs with magnitude greater than SRD*, their "critical value." If at the end of an RCT, the now *objective* 95% confidence interval for SRD, based on the RCT results, is still like A or B, that study is a "failed RCT," for it fails to disturb clinical equipoise.

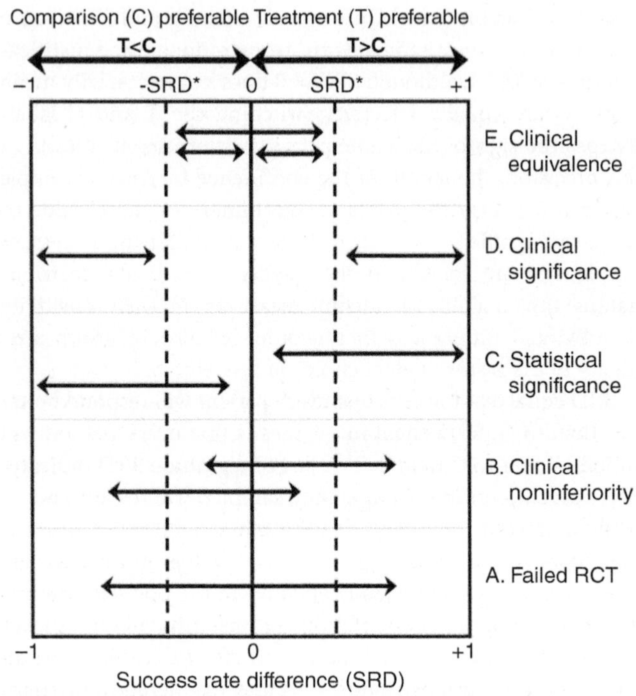

Figure 15.2 All possible configurations of the 95% confidence interval for an effect size (ES; here ES = SRD) using the consumer's critical value ES*, the threshold of clinical significance, which is the lower limit of effect sizes likely to have clinical impact on patient welfare.

Noninferiority RCTs (B) are considered by some to be unethical, but defended by others (Garattini & Bertele, 2008; Kaji & Lewis, 2015; Rehal *et al.*, 2016; Graber *et al.*, 2018). An RCT result showing noninferiority of T over C means that T may be inferior to C, just not inferior enough to be clinically significantly inferior by the researchers' standard, effect size* (ES*). Such RCTs are attractive to researchers, because the necessary sample size is smaller than an RCT designed to show superiority—the larger their SRD*, the smaller the necessary sample size. However, to consumers with a smaller SRD* than that of the researchers', such an RCT will simply be a failed RCT.

If researchers report a result with "$p < 0.05$", the 95% confidence interval would be like that in C, D, or the bottom two lines in E (Figure 15.2), a statistically significant result. Statistical significance at the 5% level ($p < 0.05$) means that the 95% confidence interval does not include SRD = 0, but it may come very close to SRD = 0 (like the bottom two lines in E). In short, a statistically significant difference between T and C may be trivial, or it may be clinically significant—an ambiguous result.

Clinical significance means that the 95% confidence interval lies totally beyond the critical value SRD* (D in Figure 15.2), in which case clinical superiority of the preferred treatment is indicated. A clinically significant result is always statistically significant, but not vice versa. This is the type of assurance that clinical consumers need for unambiguous treatment preference.

Finally, clinical equivalence means that the 95% confidence interval contains no clinically significant effect size (E in Figure 15.2).

This is the situation in which the choice between T and C in that population might be totally based on subjective assessments of availability, cost, and preference. It should be noted that T and C may be clinically equivalent but one treatment may be statistically significant and therefore better than the other or not. Again, statistical significance is an ambiguous result for clinical decision-making.

As suggested by the lengths of confidence intervals, the largest sample sizes are generally needed to establish clinical equivalence, next largest for clinical significance, next largest for statistical significance, less for noninferiority, and least for a failed RCT.

Can the conclusion be independently verified?

Clinical decision-making requires either clinical significance or clinical equivalence. However, most RCT researchers are satisfied with aiming for statistical significance in proposing an RCT, perhaps the best choice. To establish either clinical significance or clinical equivalence generally requires sample sizes far larger than usually possible in one RCT, and there are advantages to requiring *independent* replication and confirmation of any scientific conclusion.

Multiple independent RCTs addressing the same research question (same T versus same C in the same clinical population, the same outcome) provide the opportunity to compare the effect sizes not only across sites tapping populations with different sociodemographic characteristics (but the same inclusion/exclusion criteria), different medical policies, different staff, etc., but also possibly different measures of the same outcome. This checks whether the RCT results are generalizable. Then the effect sizes can be pooled using cumulative meta-analysis (Lau *et al.*, 1992).

If there were multiple *valid* RCTs for the *same* research question, one could present the confidence interval for SRD from the first RCT, then pool the results from the first two studies, then from the first three studies, etc. What one should see, if these confidence intervals were stacked one above the other, is that each successive confidence interval would overlap the last but be smaller, forming an "arrow" pointing to an unequivocal result for clinical decision-making (Lau *et al.*, 1992) (each clinical consumer using their own ES*). If each study included were valid for the same research question and adequately powered, it might take no more than 2–5 RCTs for an unequivocal result. If all studies were valid but many not adequately powered, it would take more. However, if invalid studies (different clinical populations, different outcomes, poorly designed studies) are included, a correct unequivocal result might never be reached. In short, inadequately powered but valid RCTs for a research question slow the process to a clinical resolution, but invalid studies, RCTs or not, may derail it entirely.

After an RCT, what then?

Any well-done research study, including RCTs, should first address the research questions for which the study was designed. In an RCT, that would be the effectiveness of T versus C in the population sampled, but thereafter the study would be a source of further information about the population, about the disorder, about the outcomes, and about treatments. This is particularly true of RCTs, especially in identifying possible moderators or mediators of treatment outcome, to gain a better understanding of patient impact.

Moderators of treatment outcome

In a valid RCT, a large SRD indicates a relatively homogeneous population, most or all responding better to the preferred treatment. However, large SRDs are rare. A small SRD, even SRD = 0, does not necessarily mean clinical equivalence of T and C. It may indicate a heterogeneous population, some responding much better to T than to C, and an equal number responding equally much better to C than to T.

What might well follow such an RCT is a *post hoc*, exploratory analysis (no statistical tests, no p-values) seeking to identify those baseline factors (potential moderators) that distinguish patients with T > C from those with C > T. If such factors can be found, subsequent RCTs might evaluate T versus C separately in the subpopulations so defined. It may be that in the original RCT population ES = 0, but in the two such subpopulations one of the two treatments is much more effective, just not the same one. This is the basis of "personalized" or "precision" medicine. It would be unwise to discard treatments, not because they are generally ineffective, but because the wrong population was sampled in the RCT to detect that effectiveness.

Likely candidates for moderators of treatment outcome are sociodemographic factors (age, sex, race/ethnicity), clinical factors (duration of illness, baseline severity of symptoms), and biomarkers (genotype, results of brain scans, biochemical responses).

Mediators of treatment outcome

To push the boundary even further, following moderator analyses, one might ask *why* one treatment is better than the other in each subpopulation: mediators of treatment outcome (Baron & Kenny, 1986, Kraemer *et al.*, 2008, MacKinnon, 2008). While moderators of treatment outcome are baseline, pretreatment factors, that stratify the population into subpopulations that respond differently to T versus C, mediators of treatment outcome are events or changes that occur during treatment that may explain all or part of why T is preferred to C in that population (Kraemer *et al.*, 2008). If such mediators can be identified in exploratory analyses after a valid RCT and after any moderators are used to subdivide the population, these may be clues as to how the preferred treatment might be further improved.

The most common candidate for a mediator is patient compliance with treatment. If all or part of the effect of T over C is explained by differential patient compliance, one might consider modifying the protocol for T to facilitate compliance, to further increase the effect size, which can be tested in subsequent RCTs. Other important mediators to be considered might be changes in psychological measures such as depression, anxiety, self-esteem, or self-confidence, and in biological measures such rate of drug absorption or change in biomarkers.

Secondary outcomes

The decision to recommend one treatment over another in an RCT is based on the primary outcome measure, but often there are other outcomes measured as "secondary outcomes," selected to help interpret the primary outcome results and inform future RCTs. Secondary outcomes should be distinct from the primary outcome and from each other, not multiple measures of the same outcome. Secondary outcomes do not change the RCT conclusion but may be useful in guiding treatment development in future RCTs.

In short, just as an RCT is not the first study done in evaluating T versus C in a population, no RCT should be the last study done. There is always more to be learned from any well-done RCT that would inform future research. However, it is important for clinical consumers to understand that the preliminary studies (hypothesis-generating) and the *post-hoc* exploratory studies are meant to inform the conduct and design of future RCTs, not to inform clinical decision-making (Figure 15.1).

What are the areas of particular difficulty for consumers?

It is simple enough for consumers to ascertain that the report concerns an RCT, to decide whether the disorder is of interest to them or not, to consider whether the population corresponds to that of the patient(s) under their consideration, to decide whether the chosen T and C matter to them or not, and whether the analysis was done blinded and by intention to treat or not. Whether the statistical analyses were done and reported correctly should have been checked by expert reviewers both at the proposal stage and the journal submission. However, there are areas that particularly challenge clinical interpretation in the way research results are reported.

The problems of multiple outcomes

First is the choice of outcome measure. Discussion here has focused on "the primary outcome" as if there were only one, but many researchers test multiple primary outcomes. This is problematic for several reasons. With a 5% significance level and a valid test, the probability of a false positive with one outcome measure is 5%. However, with each additional outcome measure tested at the 5% level, the probability of one or more false positives increases. With 14 independent outcome measures, that probability is greater than 50%. There is no way to distinguish the true positives from the false positives.

The statistical solution is to reduce the significance level from 5% sufficiently to keep the overall probability of one or more false positives below the required 5%, which would then require an increase in sample size for adequate power to avoid proliferation of false negatives. For consumers, this statistical solution only worsens the situation.

Does that mean that multiple outcomes should not be examined? No, it means that the primary outcome in an RCT, the one on which the decision between T and C is to be based, should be the one that most clearly reflects the overall impact of treatment on patients, whether that is one measure or a combination of several. If, for example, the primary outcome was a decrease of symptoms over the 12 months of treatment, the results should not be tested separately at 3, 6, 9, 12 months; the primary outcome should be the overall change over the entire time period combining the 5 timed results per patient. If the primary outcome were change, for example, in a symptom assessment scale, only the total score should be tested, not each of the subscale scores as well. In general, multiple measures reflecting the same outcome should not be used; a composite should be used. If several distinct outcomes are clinically relevant, say benefit and harm, a decision should be made *a priori* as to how to balance one against the other in assessing the impact on the patients. All measures might separately be used in *post hoc* exploration to develop a more substantial depiction of treatment outcome that might influence what the primary outcome measure might be in future RCTs.

Many RCTs do not report valid interpretable effect sizes

Many RCTs report invalid Odds Ratios. When valid effect sizes, other than SRD, are reported, they can usually be converted to SRD (Table 15.1). As seen in Table 15.1, the scales on which valid effect sizes are measured are vastly different from each other, some ranging from minus to plus infinity (Cohen's d or NNT), some ranging from 0 to infinity (Hazard Ratio), and some ranging from −1 to +1 (SRD), making it difficult to set standards for the critical values or to compare results with different measures of the same outcome. Converting all to SRD (or another effect size that could be used whatever the outcome measure) would alleviate that problem.

How does one set that critical value?

In setting a critical value for their power computations, researchers often fall back on the suggestions made by Cohen (Cohen, 1988), who posited that for Cohen's d, for treatment (not prevention), d = 0.2, 0.5, and 0.8 are "small," "medium," and "large," effect sizes. This would correspond (Table 15.1) to SRD = 0.11, 0.28, and 0.43. Cohen's standards were based on his long experience in psychological/psychiatric research and correspond well with the results of treatment studies in many fields of medical research. Cohen himself warned against reifying those standards, but they provide a starting point. One might set d = 0.8 if C were a placebo, d = 0.5 if C were TAU, and d = 0.2 if C were the optimal existing treatment. Or one might set d = 0.2 for a relatively inexpensive, safe, and easy to manage treatment, d = 0.5 for a more expensive or more difficult one, and d = 0.8 for a very expensive and difficult treatment. With enough experience in seeing and judging effect sizes and their subsequent impact on patient care, exposure few now have, consumers would gain the experience to set their own standards, as Cohen did his. But this would require that every RCT report a valid effect size and measured on one scale, with its 95% confidence interval, to provide that experience.

Conclusion

It is unreasonable to expect any clinical consumer to process all the vast and constantly growing research literature, and in the case of clinicians, all the research literature for all the disorders they deal with. Thus, we conclude with a flight of fancy: a patient is diagnosed with a disorder requiring treatment. The clinician opens a computer application, specifying the diagnosis and giving access to that patient's medical history: current age, height, weight, blood pressure, and any results of tests done etc., from the patient's clinic records. Then the database in the application (which is constantly updated) has access to all *valid* RCTs done to date. From that database, all valid RCTs for that diagnosis are compiled, selecting those done on populations most closely matching the patient's characteristics, and with outcomes reflecting the patient's priority, comparing various treatments. Any valid RCTs that address the same research question (same population, same T and C, same outcome) are pooled using cumulative meta-analysis to end with the most precise estimate of effect size for that particular comparison. Shortly thereafter, patient and clinician have a listing of available treatment options (intervention plus implementation) in order of likely impact (effect sizes) on that patient. Any patient preferences would be applied with both clinician and patient knowing what the benefits and costs of choosing one treatment over another are likely to be for that patient, based on all science can currently bring to bear on the question. References to the relevant RCTs are provided as well, should clinician or patient want to check out the evidence.

Is that possible now? Certainly, technology is up to the task, given the necessary information. Most clinics today have computerized clinical records. Evaluation of emerging RCTs for validity and compiling the pertinent information for each valid RCT (inclusion/exclusion criteria, labeling of T and C, outcome, outcome measure, effect size and its 95% confidence interval) could be done using expert panels. If a valid RCT reports no valid effect size and its confidence interval in submission for publication, the reviewers and editors might demand that information.

To do this would require an effect size (like SRD) that could be used for any outcome measure. However, except in special cases, neither SRD nor any other of the known interpretable effect sizes would currently allow the rank ordering of treatments unless every pair of treatments were compared in one or more valid RCTs. What could now be done is to present the choices pairwise, the pairs compared in one or more valid RCTs in the population—not an ideal solution, but that would help.

Researchers, many themselves clinicians and all potential patients, structure research to address scientific concerns and interests, not specifically to improve patient care, and argue that addressing scientific concerns and interests will eventually serve the needs and wants of patients. They are right, of course, but improvement may be very slow in the process, and misinterpretation of research reports may, in the meantime, harm patients. Understanding which research should be the focus, and how to process that research, is, in the meantime, of value to clinicians, to patients, and to clinical consumers.

References

Baron, R.M. & Kenny, D.A. (1986) The moderator-mediator variable distinction in social psychological research: conceptual, strategic, and statistical considerations. *Journal of Personality and Social Psychology* **51**, 1173–1182.

Blomqvist, N. (1986) On the bias caused by regression toward the mean in studying the relation between change and the initial value. *Journal of Clinical Periodontology* **13**, 34–37.

Bogarty, P. & Brophy, J. (2005) Numbers needed to treat (needlessly?). *The Lancet* **365**, 1307–1308.

Campbell, D.T. & Kenny, D.A. (1999) *A Primer on Regression Artifacts.* Guilford Press, New York.

Cohen, J. (1988) *Statistical Power Analysis for the Behavioral Sciences.* Lawrence Erlbaum, Hillsdale, NJ.

Eldridge, S.M. *et al.* (2016). *Defining feasibility and pilot studies in preparation for randomised controlled trials: development of a conceptual framework. PLoS One* **11**, 1–22.

Freedman, B. (1987) Equipoise and the ethics of clinical research. *The New England Journal of Medicine* **317**, 141–145.

Garattini, S. & Bertele, V. (2008) The ethics of non-inferiority trials. *The Lancet* **895**.

Graber, M.A. *et al.* (2018) Are noninferiority studies ethically inferior? *American Journal of Health-System Pharmacy* **75**, 911–914.

Gross, R.T. *et al.* (1997) *Helping Low Birth Weight, Premature Babies.* Stanford University Press, Stanford, CA.

Hoagwood, K. *et al.* (1995) Introduction to the special section: efficacy and effectiveness in studies of child and adolescent psychotherapy. *Journal of Consulting and Clinical Psychology* **63**, 683–687.

James, K.E. (1973) Regression toward the mean in uncontrolled clinical studies. *Biometrics* **29**, 121–130.

Kaji, A.H. & Lewis, R.J. (2015) Noninferiority trials: is a new treatment almost as effective as another? *JAMA* **313**, 2371–2372.

Kraemer, H.C. & Kupfer, D.J. (2006) Size of treatment effects and their importance to clinical research and practice. *Biological Psychiatry* **59**, 990–996.

Kraemer, H.C. *et al.* (2006) Caution regarding the use of pilot studies to guide power calculations for study proposals. *Archives of General Psychiatry* **63**, 484–489.

Kraemer, H.C. *et al.* (2008) How and why criteria defining moderators and mediators differ between the Baron & Kenny and Macarthur approaches. *Health Psychology* **27**, S101–S108.

Kraemer, H.C. *et al.* (2020) Wrangling with p-values versus effect sizes to improve clinical decision making: a tutorial. *The International Journal of Eating Disorders* **53**, 302–308.

Lau, J. *et al.* (1992) Cumulative meta-analysis of therapeutic trials for myocardial infarction. *New England Journal of Medicine* **327**, 248–254.

MacKinnon, D.P. (2008) *Introduction to Statistical Mediation Analysis.* Lawrence Erlbaum, New York.

MTA Cooperative Group, The (1999) Treatment strategies for attention-deficit/hyperactivity disorder. *Archives of General Psychiatry* **56**, 1073–1086.

Rehal, S. *et al.* (2016) Non-inferiority trials: are they inferior? A systematic review of reporting in major medical journals. *BMJ Open* **6**, e012594.

Sackett, D.L. *et al.* (1996) Down with odds ratios! *Evidence-Based Medicine* **1**, 164–166.

Schulz, K.F. *et al.* (2010) CONSORT 2010 statement: updated guidelines for reporting parallel group randomised trials. *British Medical Journal* **340**, 698–702.

Shearer-Underhill, C. & Marker, C. (2010) The use of number needed to treat (NNT) in randomized clinical trials in psychological treatment. *Clinical Psychology: Science and Practice* **17**, 41–48.

Tukey, J.W. (1979) Methodology, and the statistician's responsibility for BOTH accuracy AND relevance. *Journal of the American Statistical Association* **74**, 786–793.

Wallace, M.L. *et al.* (2013) A novel approach for developing and interpreting treatment moderator profiles in randomized clinical trials. *JAMA Psychiatry* **70**, 1241–1247.

CHAPTER 16
What clinicians need to know about statistical methods

Rachael Bedford[1] and Daniel Stahl[2]

[1]Centre for Brain Behaviour, Department of Psychology, Queen Mary University of London, London, UK
[2]Department of Biostatistics and Health Informatics, Institute of Psychiatry, Psychology and Neuroscience, King's College London, London, UK

Overview

In recent years, it has become evident that psychology and psychiatry face a replication crisis; findings from many studies cannot be replicated, including well-known and established phenomena. Members of the scientific community have called for increased scrutiny of research practices in conducting scientific studies. Statistical methodology plays a critical role in the progression of our scientific understanding by providing a framework which enables hypotheses to be operationalized and tested. Key concepts, such as effect sizes, sample size calculations, bias, confounding, measurement error, and latent variables will be introduced. We explain how easily false positive or negative results can come about, and how to reduce the likelihood of this. Finally, we discuss recent advances in personalized approaches, such as precision medicine. Robust statistical approaches alone, however, are not sufficient. Tackling the replication crisis requires a multifaceted approach, which encompasses rigorous consideration of modern statistical methodology together with open science practices, including preregistration of study design, hypotheses and planned analyses, reporting guidelines, uploading of code, syntax, and data, and publishing in open-source journals.

Understanding and tackling the reproducibility crisis

There is a common natural history for many "findings" in psychology and psychiatry (Stahl & Pickles, 2018). First, a small study finds a significant association and the authors of the study persuade an editor of its value. Many small studies fail to replicate the finding, but since everyone knows that small studies have "low power" this comes as no surprise; few if any such findings are published. Any small replication studies that do find a significant association are published, apparently confirming the interesting finding. Eventually, a large study fails to replicate the finding, and because of the study's size and the fact this failure is now seen as overturning a received wisdom, the results are published in a prominent journal. Complicating the issue further is the fact that nonreplicable findings remain highly cited even after a failure to replicate (Serra-Garcia & Gneezy, 2021).

Statistics plays a pivotal part in addressing the replication crisis. By implementing appropriate statistical practices throughout the research process, we can significantly improve the reproducibility of scientific findings. This starts with study design, through to data collection and analyses, including estimation of uncertainty and interpretation of results. Reproducibility can be further improved by open science research practices which promote transparency by sharing data, methods, protocols, and analysis code, allowing others to evaluate and reproduce findings.

There are several factors which increase the problem of non-reproducible findings. These include so-called "researcher degrees of freedom"—the flexibility of the researcher to make decisions about study design and analysis, which can lead to "chasing significance" (Simmons *et al.*, 2011), conducting studies with small sample sizes that can result in biased estimates, and the publication bias toward "significant" findings, commonly referred to as the "file drawer" effect. A key issue is the fact that readers and editors of papers are drawn to reports of significant associations of novel findings and undervalue negative, non-significant results. As a consequence, the p-value remains the statistic upon which the success or failure of a study is seen to rest.

Rutter's Child and Adolescent Psychiatry and Psychology, Seventh Edition.
Edited by Anita Thapar, Daniel S. Pine, Samuele Cortese, Cathy Creswell, Tamsin J. Ford, James F. Leckman, and Argyris Stringaris.

Companion website: www.wiley.com/go/thapar/rutterspsych7

Multiple testing

Every study, regardless of size, has a fixed chance of identifying a significant effect in the sample drawn when there is no such effect in the population. Known as the type I error, we usually set this risk, rather arbitrarily, as one in twenty, or 0.05. If we test for the presence of two effects or study the same effect in two samples, then the risk that at least one of these shows a significant finding is now slightly less than one in ten. Test for the presence of enough effects or conduct enough studies (and just how many student projects do you have?) and the so-called family-wise error rate is increased, i.e., the chance of a false positive when running multiple comparisons. The Bonferroni correction—dividing the alpha error by the number of tests conducted—can be used to set a meaningful significance criterion. More efficient alternative methods can also be applied, such as Holm or permutation procedures, that account for the correlation of tests. Research areas like genetics, which test for associations between a particular disorder and hundreds of thousands of single nucleotide polymorphisms, often use the less stringent False Discovery Rate control. This approach allows for a certain proportion of false positive results among the significant associations (Benjamini & Hochberg, 1995). However, the problem becomes inflated by the many choices that researchers have when designing studies, collecting data, preprocessing and analyzing results, and interpreting findings. These practices typically go unnoticed in multiple testing considerations and can inadvertently inflate the likelihood of finding a statistically significant result even when no true effect exists. Preregistration of the study and transparent reporting of any deviation from the preregistered plan is an effective strategy to reduce the potential issues caused by these researcher degrees of freedom (Simmons *et al.*, 2011).

Effect size and confidence intervals

Instead of focusing solely on significance, statisticians advise that the size of the effect, together with some measure of precision, preferably a confidence interval (CI) should be reported in addition to the p-value. Effect sizes are the best estimate of the strength of the true effect. Standardized effect sizes, such as Cohen's d, correlation coefficients, or standardized betas, allow for comparison across scales and studies. In contrast, CIs indicate the likely range of the true effect in the underlying population, reflecting our confidence in our estimate. The CI gives the opportunity to reflect upon the range of possible values of the true effect that are potentially consistent with the data and to assess whether effects of this magnitude would be, say, of clinical importance.

Consideration of clinically relevant outcomes (Cepeda *et al.*, 2020)

Statistical significance does not necessarily equate to clinical significance. For example, imagine an intervention testing the efficacy of an antidepressant in improving depression symptoms, where the primary outcome is Beck's Depression Inventory II (BDI-II), which ranges from 0 to 62; with a large enough sample size, a difference of just 1 point may be significant, but that does not reflect a *clinically meaningful* change in depression symptoms. Defining a clinically meaningful effect size is context-dependent—it takes into consideration broader factors, such as initial severity, side effects, costs, and stakeholder interests (NCCMH, 2004; Button *et al.*, 2015).

Type I and type II errors

In inferential statistics, we can encounter two types of errors when performing a statistical hypothesis test. A false positive error involves rejecting the null hypothesis (which states no effect) when there is no genuine effect in the population. We represent this type error I as α, and by setting the conventional α level to 0.05, we accept a 5% chance of a false-positive result per test. A false negative, or type II error, occurs if we do not reject the null hypothesis when there is a true effect in the population. The probability of a type II error is represented by β and is related to the power of a test ($1-\beta$). The power is the probability of detecting an effect size in the population if it exists.

Power calculations

For *a priori* sample size calculations, it is necessary to specify a two-tailed or a one-tailed test. Typically, statistical tests are two-tailed, which allows the possibility of both positive and negative differences. A one-tailed test needs to be prespecified and is only appropriate if we are interested in a difference in one direction but not interested if the opposite outcome could be true. This is the case in non-inferiority trials, where the aim is to show that a new treatment is not worse than the standard treatment by a specific margin. Here, the null hypotheses is that the new treatment is worse and the alternative hypothesis that the new treatment is not worse than a specific margin. The main advantage of one-sided tests is the greater statistical power compared to the two-tailed test. The main disadvantage of one-tailed test is the difficulty in interpreting the non-rejection of the null hypothesis. In the next step, we need to choose an effect size, such as the difference in depression score between two treatment arms, to calculate power.

Researchers often rely on previous pilot studies to choose an effect size or even just opt for a Cohen's medium effect size (Cohen's d = 0.5), with little consideration of how and whether this applies to their specific study. Cohen's d is defined as the difference between two groups, divided by the standard deviation. Using standard definitions of small, medium, and large effect sizes to select an effect size can be problematic. The choice is usually somewhat arbitrary and the oft-picked medium effect size is, in many cases, a rather optimistic choice. It is important to note that even a small effect can have a significant impact at the population level (Carey *et al.*, 2023). The choice of effect size should also not be based on observed effect sizes from previous small or pilot studies because these are inherently unreliable. Practices like publication bias, data dredging to achieve statistical significance, and unchecked researcher degrees of freedom can inflate effect sizes. This in turn can systematically result in underpowered studies (Albers & Lakens, 2018). Pilot studies have other uses, such as determining the feasibility of performing the designed study in practice (Leon *et al.*, 2011).

The effect size should instead be based on recommendations in the literature, meta-analyses, or discussions with clinical experts and other stakeholders. For example, NICE recommends a difference of at least three points in BDI-II as a meaningful treatment effect for people with depression (NCCMH, 2004; Button *et al.*, 2015). Previous studies suggest that the standard deviation on BDI-II scores for this population is about 13 (Beck *et al.*, 1996). Our standardized minimum meaningful effect size is therefore d = 3/13 = 0.23, corresponding to a small effect size. The required sample size to detect an effect of 0.23 (or larger) with 90% power at an alpha level of 0.05 is 325 per arm. This is considerably higher than the estimated sample size using a medium effect size of d = 0.5, where only 70 participants per arm would be required. Recruiting 70 participants per arm would result in a power of only 39% with our assumed population effect size of 0.23! This drastically reduces the probability of finding a true positive effect, assuming such an effect does exist in the population.

Although the power analysis procedure described above is the most popular in health research, there are other, often more appropriate approaches to sample size calculations. In many instances, a researcher may focus on the precision with which the effect can be estimated, which is represented by the width of the standard error for estimating a treatment effect. Sample size calculation for precision is often desired when estimating prevalence. For example, we need a sample size of 256 people to estimate an expected proportion of 20% with a precision of plus or minus 5% at a 95% confidence level, which would be equivalent to an estimate of the prevalence with a CI of plus or minus 10% (Sergeant, 2018).

Software for sample size calculations is available for many standard tests but not for more complex studies, for which power formulae do not exist. An alternative approach to sample size, power, or precision calculations is Monte Carlo simulation. This computer-intensive simulation method mimics the data-generating process in order to evaluate the properties of a test statistic or CI (Landau & Stahl, 2013). Unlike standard sample size tools, we can simulate violations of assumptions, such as normally distributed data, when data are skewed, or the effects of loss of follow-up on power patterns. Modern software has built-in simulation tools to estimate sample sizes for a variety of settings, including multilevel models and structural equation models. Additionally, researchers can develop their own simulation tools within these software packages to tailor the simulation to their research needs.

In the absence of adequate power analyses, sample size needs to be considered when assessing the likely importance of significant effects. It is a common misconception that finding a significant large effect in a small study must mean that the effect is substantial. In small studies, the magnitude of the estimate must be large for it to appear as significant—in a small study all small effect estimates are non-significant—and just because the estimate is large, does not mean that the true effect is necessarily so. The large CIs around the estimate underscore the limitations of small sample sizes in accurately estimating the true effect size. Large CIs around a non-significant effect can indicate that the study was not informative, as the wide range of values that are consistent with the data precludes drawing any definitive conclusions from the study. In psychology and psychiatry, true effect sizes are often relatively small, yet many published studies have small sample sizes and are underpowered to detect effects. It was estimated that the median power for neuroscience and psychiatric disorder studies is only 20–30% (Dumas-Mallet *et al.*, 2017). The consequence is a low probability of finding true effects, low positive predictive value (PPV), and an exaggerated estimate of the magnitude of the effect when a true effect is discovered. This is further amplified by publication bias, selective data analysis, and selective reporting of outcomes, which are more likely to affect low-powered studies (Button *et al.*, 2013). Studies with small sample sizes, that do not have appropriate power analyses, undermine scientific research and are a major contributor to the replication crisis.

This concern was highlighted by Ioannidis (2005) who posited that over half of published "significant" research findings in natural sciences might be false (Figure 16.1). The reliability of a positive "significant" result, represented by the PPV, relies on prior probability, study power, and the alpha error. We therefore need to make assumptions about the prior probability of a test. For instance, imagine assessing 1000 risk factors for anxiety, where 10% (i.e., 100) are genuinely related to anxiety but we do not know which ones. Given a statistical test with 80% power at an alpha-error level of 0.05 or 5%, we would expect to detect 80% of the 100 risk factors (i.e., 80 true positive results) but 20 risk factors would not be detected (false negative results). The remaining 900 factors are not risk factors, but we would expect that 5% or 45 would be falsely declared as such (false positives). We would therefore obtain 80 + 45 = 125 positive results, but only 80 (64%) are true positives, making nearly one-third of the positive results false—much higher than the alpha error of 5% suggests.

Bayesian statistics may offer a solution to this dilemma by incorporating prior knowledge and beliefs about the phenomenon under investigation. This approach can potentially yield a clearer and more accurate representation of the true associations (Beard & West, 2017). However, defining prior knowledge often involves subjectivity and typically requires both specialist knowledge and advanced statistical software.

Meta-analysis

Meta-analysis attempts to overcome the problem of small sample sizes, by establishing a consensus across multiple studies (Cooper *et al.*, 2009). It is the statistical method used to combine studies included in a systematic review, and consists of four steps: (i) assembling an exhaustive list of the potentially relevant

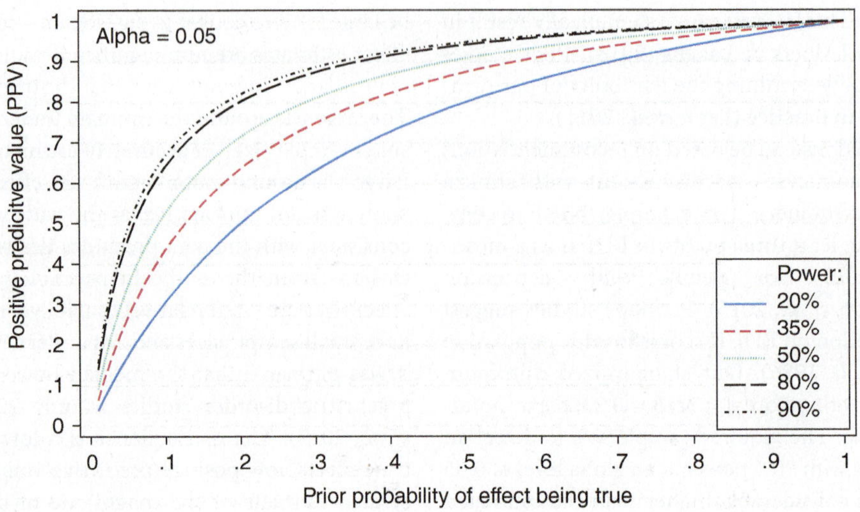

Figure 16.1 Plot showing the positive predictive value (PPV) (Y-axis) against the probability that a hypothesis is true for different powered studies (20%, 30%, 40%, 50%, 80%, and 90%) at an alpha error of 0.05. Even without publication bias toward positive results, the PPV of positive statistical results is far less than we may have expected. This underlines the importance of conducting and presenting a power analysis where feasible (Stahl & Pickles, 2018/ Cambridge University Press.).

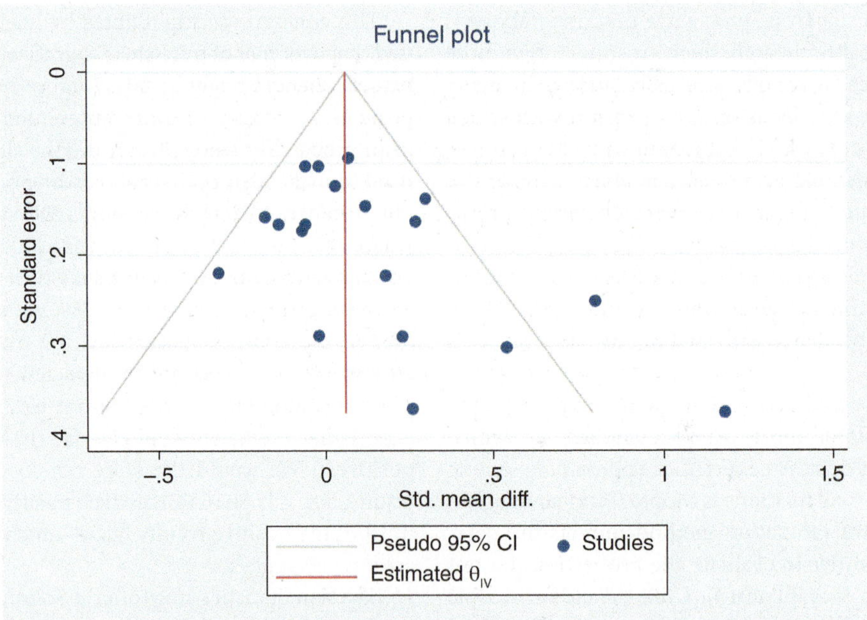

Figure 16.2 A funnel plot is used to assess publication bias or, more generally, small-study effects in meta-analysis. On the x-axis, we have the standardized mean difference or the effect size. The y-axis shows the standard error of each study's effect size, with individual studies represented as blue dots. The red line in this plot represents the weighted effect size, denoted as estimated theta θ. The pseudo 95% confidence intervals (CI) delineate the range within which we would expect 95% of the studies' results to fall. Asymmetry may indicate publication bias. This funnel plot suggests an asymmetry caused by the absence of small studies in the region where studies did not show positive effect sizes.

published studies; (ii) selecting against a predefined list of criteria a subset whose design, implementation, and clarity of reporting suggest that they are appropriate and of good quality (ideally blind to authorship and the actual findings of the study); (iii) displaying the findings in a funnel plot (Light & Pillemer, 1984). Figure 16.2 shows data from several acupuncture studies illustrating the diminution of effect size reported as the sample sizes increase, to the point where the study with the largest sample size shows no effect. If the true effect is zero, then Figure 16.2 also shows evidence of publication bias, since, if all studies with smaller sample sizes were published, one would expect their estimates to be scattered symmetrically around those of the studies with larger sample sizes. Such evidence of publication bias should prompt significant concern and a search for unpublished studies; (iv) pooling the information to derive a single weighted overall estimate of the average effect and a 95% CI. Typically, a weighted mean of the effect sizes using the inverse variance of the individual studies as weights is used. Despite the advantages of meta-analyses, it is important to note that biases in primary studies still affect the meta-analytic syntheses and effect sizes are often inflated and should be interpreted with caution (Sotola, 2022).

Testing associations in psychopathology

Key Readings:

- Hernán, M.A. & Robins, J.M. (2020) *Causal Inference: What If.* Chapman & Hall/CRC. NB: Available online only: https://www.hsph.harvard.edu/miguel-hernan/causal-inference-book/.
- MacKinnon, D. (2012) *Introduction to Statistical Mediation Analysis*. Routledge.
- MacKinnon, D.P. *et al.* (2007) Mediation analysis. *Annual Review of Psychology* **58**, 593–614.

Bias and confounding

Rarely is an outcome of psychiatric interest related to a single causal factor. It is important to consider whether an observed effect can be attributed solely to the association between the exposure and the outcome, or whether alternative explanations are possible. Perhaps the two biggest problems in observational studies are bias and confounding (see Chapter 13 for further detail) and they also contribute to the non-reproducibility of findings. Bias refers to any systematic error in the design, conduct, or analysis of a study that leads to an incorrect estimate of the association between exposure and outcome. Examples include selection bias, which occurs when the selection of participants is not random, leading to a non-representative sample, or due to differential dropout in follow-up assessments. If the source of the sampling bias and its effects are known, they can be adjusted for using methods such as regression adjustment or inverse probability weighting regression adjustment. Regression adjustment involves including variables in the analysis that relate to both the outcome variable and the sampling bias. Inverse probability weighting involves assigning weights to the observations in the sample based on the probability of being selected. This approach effectively upweights observations that are less likely to be selected and downweights those more likely to be selected. If sample size is sufficient, these methods can help to control for the impact of bias in the analysis, yielding more accurate results.

Unlike bias, which refers to a systematic error in the exposure–outcome association, confounding, refers to a real but noncausal association between the exposure and the outcome, which makes it difficult to determine the true effect of the exposure on the outcome. For example, predictors of poorer mental health outcomes often co-occur. Low-income families are more likely to live in less affluent neighborhoods, with a lower quality of educational opportunities, and an increased exposure to psychosocial risk factors and stressful life events, which are associated with poor mental health outcomes. A child who is high in any one of these potential risk factors is also likely to be high in other factors. There are two important aspects of this problem. The first, "independent effects of confounders," relates to the fact that these other factors may have effects on both exposure and outcome, which should be accounted for. The second, "selection effects," refers to the variation among subjects in their exposure to the factor of interest being correlated with variation in these other factors. In other words, those who are selected to be exposed to one risk factor have commonly experienced and are experiencing these other risks as well. The effect of our factor of interest will be confounded with the effects of these other risks. Broadly speaking, we can attempt to solve our problem if we can deal with either of the two aspects of the problem. While it is best to control for confounding in the design of the study itself, there are several ways to tackle confounding in the analytic phase, including standardization, multiple regression analyses, and stratification.

We present an example of regression adjustment based on data from a prospective study of autism when children are 2 and 9 years of age (Lord *et al.*, 2006). Initial verbal IQ (VIQ) is lower in the autism diagnosis group than both pervasive developmental disorder not-otherwise-specified (PDD-NOS) and non-autistic spectrum (NS) groups (Figure 16.3). To assess if diagnosis group at 2 years is associated with later social communication symptoms at 9 years (measured by the Autism Diagnostic Observation Schedule (ADOS); Lord *et al.*, 2000), it is necessary to control for the potential confounding effect of VIQ. This could be done by including both the 2-year diagnosis and VIQ as main effects in a regression model. Taking this approach, the results indicate that the PDD-NOS and NS groups score lower

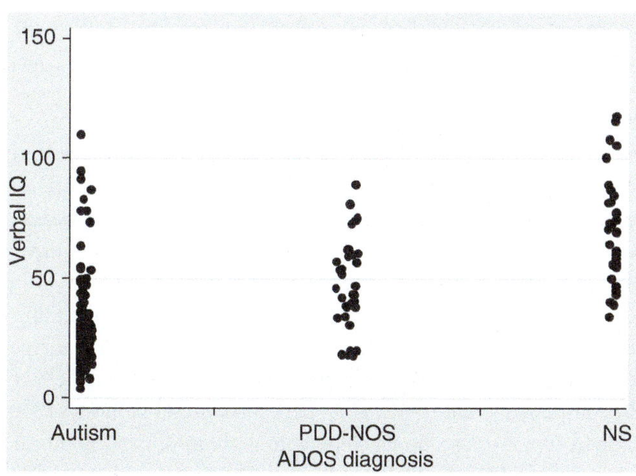

Figure 16.3 Distribution of baseline verbal IQ and ADOS diagnostic groups (PDD-NOS = autistic spectrum but not autism).

on the ADOS at 9 years compared to those initially diagnosed with autism, with VIQ associated with a lower ADOS score. Important in adjusting for confounders is understanding the underlying assumptions of the chosen method, particularly linearity across diagnostic groups. The model assumes a consistent linear relationship between VIQ and outcome across all three groups. However, examining the data, most children (71%) diagnosed with autism at 2 years have a VIQ below the lowest in the NS group. This means within the autistic group we may wrongly extrapolate for higher VIQ values. If we instead control for VIQ by matching, a nonparametric approach that does not assume linearity, there would be no match in the NS group for the autistic children with low VIQ and they would be dropped from the analysis. Alternatively, we could restrict the regression adjustment to the VIQ range shared by all three diagnostic groups. This narrowed analysis of 78 children (instead of 167 in the full sample) presents outcome differences that are smaller and less precise than previous estimates. Adjusting across the whole sample can provide greater statistical power and may control for confounding, but this comes at the cost of assuming that VIQ adjustment is correct for all three groups; this cannot be assessed in areas of the scale where the adjustment is based solely on children from a single diagnostic group.

When deciding whether adjustment is appropriate, it is important to understand the directionality and mechanism of the effects. VIQ can only be considered a confounder if it influences the predictor and outcome (Figure 16.4). Often, it remains uncertain whether one variable influences another, and in such cases, we can only make assumptions. Establishing causality requires careful consideration of factors such as temporality, strength of association, dose–response relationship, biologic plausibility, and recognizing the potential for bias and confounding in the study design and analysis. In 1965, Bradford Hill proposed a framework to determine whether an observed association can be justifiably considered a causal relationship, which remains relevant today. Modern statistics have also provided new methods for establishing causality (Hernán & Robins, 2020), see Chapter 13 for more detailed information on identifying causal effects.

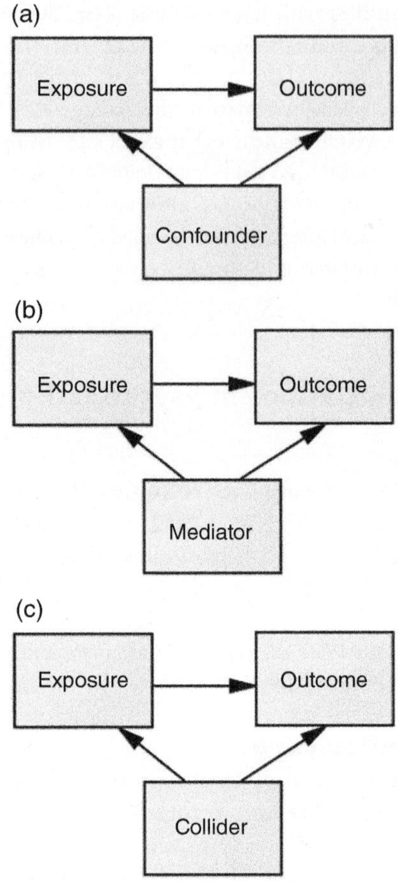

Figure 16.4 Third variable effect. Visualizing the concepts of confounder, mediator, and collider: (a) A confounder effects both exposure and outcome and needs to be controlled for to avoid biased exposure–outcome estimates; (b) A mediator lies between exposure and outcome. Controlling for a mediator will change the exposure–outcome relationship as it contributes to the overall effect; (c) A collider is influenced by both exposure and outcome and should not be included in the model as conditioning on it can imply a correlation ("collider bias") between uncorrelated variables.

Mediation and moderation

The problem of controlling for confounding effects can become more complex when distinguishing between confounders, mediators, and moderators. This is because each of these variables operates differently in relation to the outcome and requires distinct strategies to effectively address their effects.

A mediator is a variable that represents an explanatory linking mechanism between an exposure and outcome. A mediation analysis attempts to decompose an assumed or hypothesized causal effect into components that occur along particular causal pathways. For example, in a cross-sectional study with a group of participants at high risk for psychosis, McDonnell *et al.* (2018) found that heightened interpersonal sensitivity (the excessive awareness of both the behavior and feelings of others) mediated the association between childhood history of bullying victimization and later paranoid ideation (the feeling of being threatened, persecuted, or conspired against). In a cross-sectional study, it is not possible to differentiate between mediating and confounding effects in a statistical model, because the underlying correlation matrix on which the statistical model is based does not specify a direction of causality as is shown in Figure 16.4. These effects can only be distinguished conceptually, based on theory or previous research. It is important to differentiate between a mediator and a confounder because, although their effects on the exposure are identical, the interpretation of the results can differ. Controlling for a confounding variable reduces the effect size of the exposure on the outcome, while controlling for a mediator represents overadjustment and can lead to underestimation of the true effect. Therefore, careful consideration and proper identification of mediating and confounding variables is critical for accurate interpretation of study results.

Mediation analysis models can be expanded to include multiple mediators or multiple outcomes using path analysis. Path analysis is a statistical technique that allows researchers to examine the assumed causal relationships between multiple variables simultaneously. In path analysis, researchers specify a theoretical model that includes the direct and indirect effects of the independent variable (i.e., the predictor measure) on the dependent variable (i.e., the outcome measure), as well as the direct and indirect effects of the independent variable on the mediators. The model can also include the effects of confounding variables, which can be controlled for by including them as additional variables in the model. It can be further expanded to include repeated measurements over time, the latter allowing possible temporal relationships between variables to be identified (Goldsmith *et al.*, 2018). Finally, recent work in statistics has attempted to place the more informal early work (Judd & Kenny, 1981; Baron & Kenny, 1986) into a more rigorous and formal framework of causal inference with an emphasis on the assumptions required for identification (Pearl, 2014).

Moderation refers to the influence of a third variable, the 'moderator', which affects the relationship between an independent variable and an outcome. In statistical terms, moderation is an interaction. Consider the role of risk and resilience in psychopathology. For example, we cannot say that divorce is a universal risk factor for childhood antisocial behavior, since divorce may be beneficial if the absenting father is themselves antisocial (Jaffee *et al.*, 2003). Indeed, many behavioral responses may be adaptive or maladaptive depending upon the context.

Where the outcome variable is continuous, analysis and interpretation of interaction terms is relatively straightforward. Next, we return to our example from above on VIQ and autism. Figure 16.4 shows the estimated association for each group, obtained from fitting a model that allowed an interaction term between diagnostic group and VIQ. This is an example of moderation. Although the interaction term was non-significant, Figure 16.5 clearly shows nonparallel lines. These imply that the difference in ADOS outcome score may depend upon the child's VIQ, and that adjusting for VIQ could hide important variations. For example, there may be larger differences in ADOS score between the autism and PDD-NOS diagnosis groups if VIQ is low, but less difference when VIQ is high. Unless designed in advance, for example, by selecting subjects matched on VIQ, most studies do not have the power to test effectively for such variation. Unfortunately, designing a study to be powerful in this regard would make it clumsier to analyze for all but the designed comparison. Moreover, the design would have increased power only with respect to the matched variables, and may exclude important subgroups of children, in this case the many autistic children with low VIQs.

When the outcome is binary, logistic regression models are commonly applied. Logistic regression assumes a multiplicative association with outcome (Pickles & De Stavola, 2007), due to the nature to the logistic function that has an S-shaped curve that approaches the limits of 0 and 1. This means that the effect

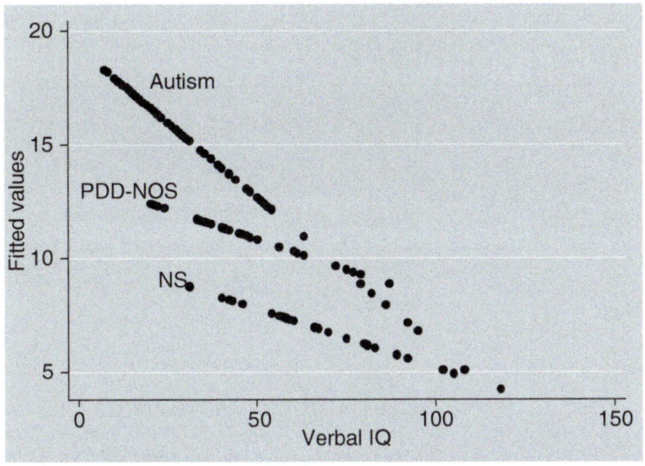

Figure 16.5 Relationship between baseline verbal IQ and follow-up fitted ADOS score by initial diagnosis (NS = nonautism spectrum; PDD-NOS = autistic spectrum but not autism).

of an independent variable on the probability of the outcome is not constant but varies depending on the value of the independent variable. Figure 16.6 shows a hypothetical example of the association between drug-dose and the probability of recovery for boys and girls separately. The estimated odds ratio (OR) is 2.41 (95% CI 2.31–2.51): a single unit increase in drug-dose from −2 to −1 for females results in an 25% chance improvement in recovering while an increase by one unit from 1 to 2 is less than 5%. The effect of dose on the probability to recover is not parallel between males and females although no interaction was modeled.

In summary, given the complexity of confounders, interactions and mediators, health psychology studies require a strong theoretical framework. Furthermore, while linear relationships are often assumed in models, this is not always sufficient and nonlinear models using polynomials, splines, or general additive models are necessary to ensure accurate representation of relationships and mechanisms in statistical models. By addressing these complexities, researchers can gain deeper insights, leading to more effective interventions and evidence-based health practices.

Missing data

Missing data are a common problem and can arise for a variety of reasons ranging from missing questionnaire items to attrition from the study. There are three categories of missing data (Little & Rubin, 1987, 1989): missing completely at random (MCAR), missing at random (MAR), and nonignorable missing or not missing at random (NMAR). MCAR suggests that missingness is not related to any observed (variables you measured) or unobserved variables (variables which were not measured in the study, or have not directly been observed, so-called "latent" variables, discussed later in this chapter). An example is some data are missing in an online survey due to technical issues with the survey platform. In this case, an analysis of complete data

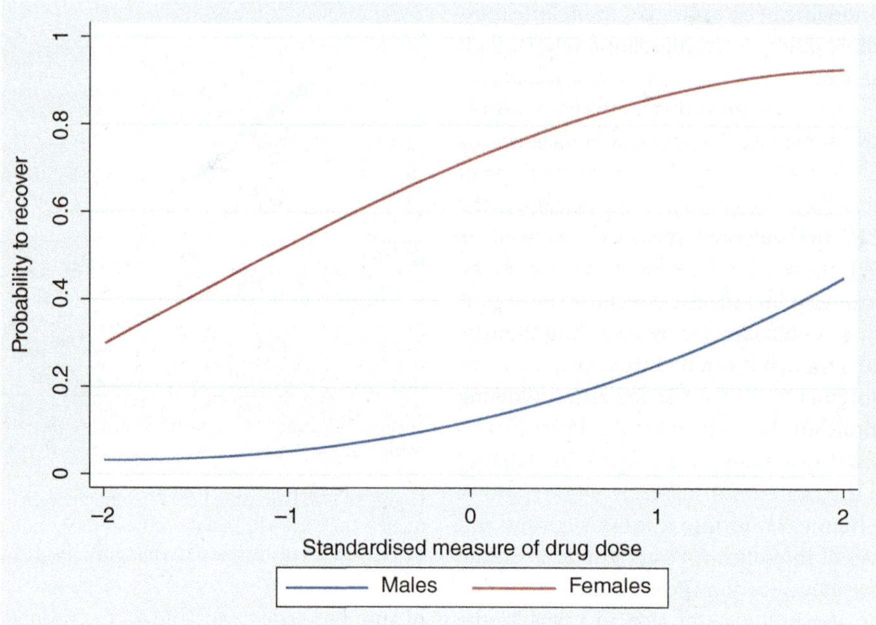

Figure 16.6 Hypothetical example of a (standardized) drug dose and its effect on the probability to recover from a disease for males and females.

cases does not lead to bias but does reduce statistical power and precision because of the reduced sample size. In reality, missing data are rarely unrelated to observed or unobserved variables and a complete case analysis approach is typically biased. MAR assumes that the reason data are missing is related to one or more observed variables but is not related to unobserved factors or the actual values that are missing. For instance, suppose boys are more likely to be late and miss a language test, causing their test data to be missing. If actual language ability of boys does not drive the test's missing data, then accounting for gender would classify the data as MAR. If gender is not included in the model, the data are not considered MAR, and results would be biased if there is a gender difference in language ability.

Data which are MAR can be analyzed with standard full information maximum likelihood (FIML) approaches but this is only available for complex models in specialist software. An alternative approach for tackling missing data is multiple imputation (MI; Schafer, 1999) that has been widely adopted due to its flexibility and ease of implementation but should be used with caution and not be seen as a panacea (Sullivan *et al.*, 2018). MI is a statistical technique that involves fitting a model to the observed data and using it to estimate values for each missing observation. Several datasets are created that have the same observed data but missing data are filled in with values that differ between datasets, the variability depending upon the uncertainty of the missing values. Chained equations, also known as fully conditional specification, are a commonly used method for implementing MI in complex datasets. Each dataset is analyzed and the results pooled using simple formulae (Rubin, 1987), which uses the variability in results from dataset to dataset as the source of the information on how the missing data contributes to uncertainty. Although MI methods are increasingly common and easy to undertake, mistakes are easy to make and often hard to detect. MI can also be less efficient than standard maximum likelihood approaches, particularly when data are only missing for the outcome variable.

When missingness is dependent on both observed and unobserved values, missing data are nonignorable, e.g., those with higher depression have more missing data because they were less likely to complete a depression assessment. Such missingness requires more specialist and speculative methods and is probably better thought of as part of a sensitivity analysis testing the robustness of findings (White *et al.*, 2011). For instance, in a clinical trial with missing data, a sensitivity analysis may assume that the individuals who are lost to follow-up experience systematically worse outcomes, by adding a clinically plausible amount to the imputed outcomes from MI analyses. As well as testing the robustness of the conclusions, this method can be used to determine the degree of change in the imputed outcomes required to change the clinical interpretation of the trial.

Researchers in psychology and psychiatry must not sideline the evaluation of missing data patterns. It is critical to understand that in many cases proceeding with full cases only, under the assumption data are missing completely at random, will lead to biased effect estimates and unreliable conclusions.

Measurement error

Linear regression assumes that both the predictors and outcome are free of measurement error. Many researchers are familiar with the idea that if a risk factor is measured with error, then in any bivariate regression model where the measure is used to predict an outcome, the estimated coefficient will be "attenuated," i.e., the coefficient magnitude will be lower than if the risk factor had been perfectly measured. In fact, where there are several potentially correlated exposures, with one or more measured with error, such error can have far more pernicious effects, where the partial regression coefficient can be overestimated. In addition, measurement error in the outcome can result in inflated standard error estimates for the coefficient. Measurement error is a common challenge in psychology and psychiatry, where the focus is often on studying unobservable constructs such as emotions and cognitions. Because these constructs cannot be directly measured, researchers rely on indirect measures or proxies to assess them, such as self-report questionnaires or observer ratings. The use of multiple items to measure a construct (as seen in many psychological scales) can help in offsetting individual item errors and provide more accurate measures.

Latent variables and structural equation modeling

Latent variables can address the problem of measurement error by representing unobserved constructs (e.g., depression) through observed indicators (e.g., questionnaire items about observable symptoms like loss of interest in play or sleep problems), see Figure 16.7. These indicators, potentially measured with error, are analyzed using factor analysis to fit a model that links the latent variable "depression" to the observed symptoms. The link between each observed indicator and the latent variable has a factor loading, which represents the strength of the association. The latent construct, in this case depression, represents the shared variance (i.e., variability in scores for each indicator which overlaps across all the indicators). This removes any item-specific measurement error from the latent variable (i.e., if a parent misinterpreted one item).

The model's adequacy is then assessed using fit indices like the root mean squared error of approximation (RMSEA), comparative fit index, and standardized root mean square residual (SRMR). However, while these indices evaluate the model's fit to the observed data, they do not confirm the validity and reliability of the construct measurement. For example, it would also be important to test whether responses are the same if you ask the questions again a few days later (test–retest reliability), and whether the depression construct relates to other existing measures of depression (construct validity). The reliability of the questionnaire measure across different populations is also important. While the latent variable approach removes any item-specific measurement error, any shared bias in responding across items, for example, if depressed mothers generally rate their children as more depressed, would be included in the latent factor. Finally, it is often necessary to validate the applicability of scales across genders or cultural contexts by conducting measurement invariance analyses, which assess whether the latent variable model remains consistent across different groups. Both validation and reliability are central concepts to latent variable modeling and psychometric scale development.

Latent variables in the form of factor models can be expanded into structural equation modeling (SEM). SEM allows for the examination of complex relationships between observed and latent variables, as well as the interrelationships among the latent variables themselves. SEM comprises two parts: a measurement model, which encompasses the latent variables and their indicators, and a structural model which describes the relationships among the latent variables—see Figure 16.8 for SEM notation.

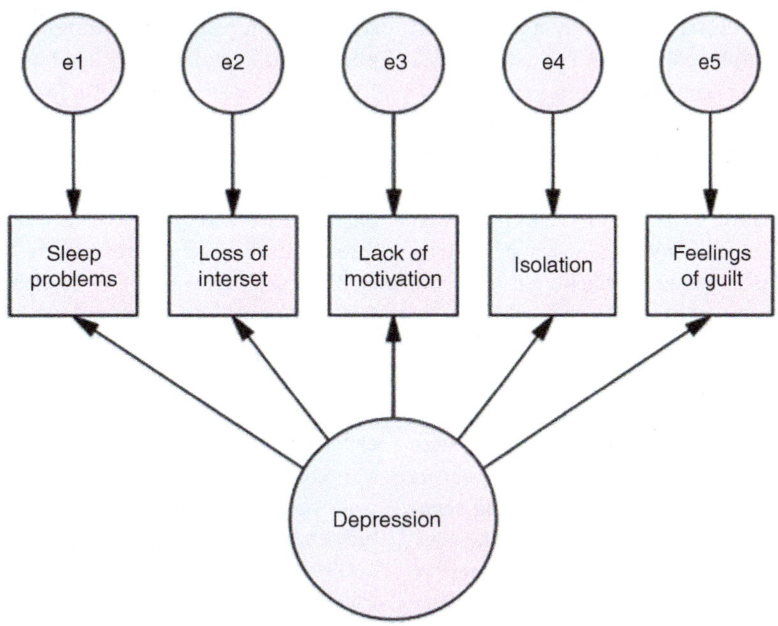

Figure 16.7 A latent variable model for depression.

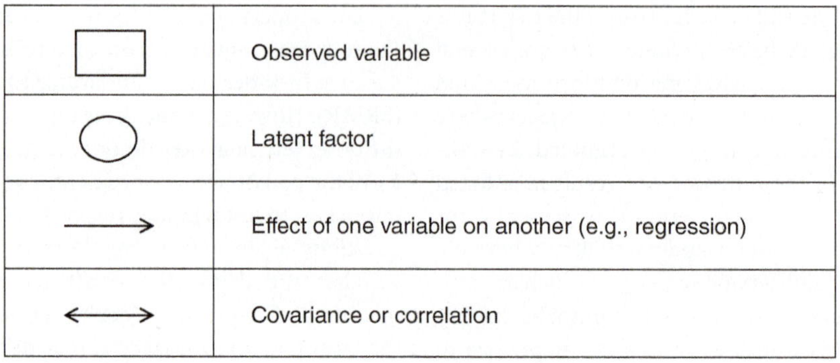

Figure 16.8 Notation for structural equation models.

Longitudinal data analysis

Key Reading:

- Diggle, P. *et al.* (2013) *Analysis of Longitudinal Data*. 2nd edn. Oxford University Press.

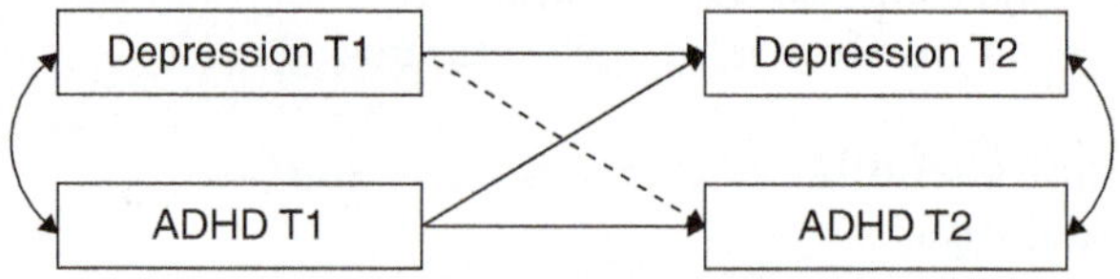

Figure 16.9 Cross-lag model showing an association between attention deficit/hyperactivity disorder (ADHD) at T1 and depression at T2, but not vice versa.

Longitudinal data arise from repeated observations on one or more variables over time. This repeated-measures nature of the data makes it expensive to collect both in terms of the number of measurements (at least two for each participant) and the cost of tracking participants over time. However, for addressing questions in development, longitudinal data provide the only real way to examine change over time. Unlike cross-sectional data, which allow only within-time correlations to be examined, longitudinal data enable the ordering of correlations over time to be assessed and thus come closer to addressing questions of causality. There are several modeling approaches which are well-suited to the analysis of longitudinal data.

Autoregressive cross-lag models are commonly applied to test bidirectional associations between constructs. For example, we may want to test evidence for homotypic and heterotypic continuity in mental health diagnoses over time. Homotypic continuity refers to the fact that having a particular disorder, such as depression, predicts an increased likelihood of having the same disorder later on, whereas heterotypic continuity relates to cross-disorder prediction—e.g., having attention deficit/hyperactivity disorder (ADHD) at time one increases the likelihood of having a different disorder, such as depression at a later time point (Figure 16.9). More recently, an extension to cross-lag models, so-called random intercept cross-lag panel models have increased in popularity. These models include a random intercept to account for time-invariant, between-subjects differences (Hamaker *et al.*, 2015). This method enables between- versus within-subjects change to be partitioned, by accounting separately for the "trait-like" stability in a particular construct.

An alternative for longitudinal data is a growth curve model in which each child is considered as having a trajectory defined by an initial ability (represented by a latent intercept factor or random effect) and a rate of improvement (represented by a latent slope factor, or random coefficient). When both autoregressive and growth curve models fit well, model choice is likely to rest upon theoretical considerations. The growth curve model has fewer parameters as well as the advantage of partitioning initial cross-sectional variation from subsequent change.

Much theory in developmental psychopathology relates to groups or a categorical typology of individuals. A classic example is Moffitt's (1993) three antisocial behavior groups defined in terms of their longitudinal trajectory; life-course persistent, adolescent limited, and never antisocial. Empirically defining cutoffs for these groups may be somewhat arbitrary, so a data-driven method that can identify subgroups directly from the data is desirable. Such a model can be considered as a form of latent class model or a model-based cluster analysis (Everitt *et al.*, 2011). Models with different numbers of classes can be estimated, and the relative fit of these different models compared. Latent class and latent trajectory models, however, should not be considered as a tool to identify how many classes exist. First, the number of classes which yields the best fit according to some standard information criterion, e.g., Bayesian or Akaike information criterion, varies depending on the extent of the data available. Second, even when the data are truly continuous, a latent class model with only a small number of classes often provides a better fit than a model assuming the continuous variability of the "true" model. Nonetheless, these models allow for an effective summary of the data, which can be helpful for theory building and constructing tests of clinical interest.

Beyond observational studies: randomized clinical trials

Key Reading:

- Shih, W. J. & Aisner, J. (2021) *Statistical Design, Monitoring, and Analysis of Clinical Trials: Principles and Methods*. 2nd edn. Chapman & Hall.

The field of epidemiology focuses on understanding the distribution and determinants of health and disease in populations. The field applies this knowledge to prevent and control health problems through various observational study designs. However, to establish the efficacy and effectiveness of treatments, more rigorous methods need to be employed.

Randomized control trials (RCTs) have long been seen in medicine as the gold standard for establishing a causal effect (see Chapter 15 for detailed coverage of this topic). RCTs are typically used to test the effectiveness of an intervention or drug treatment. In a standard RCT design, participants are recruited and complete a baseline assessment, before being randomly allocated to one of two groups or "arms"—treatment or control. Participants in the treatment arm receive the target treatment or intervention, while participants in the control arm typically receive no treatment, or, depending on the trial design, they may receive a placebo or an alternative treatment. At treatment endpoint all participants are assessed again and change from baseline to outcome is compared across the groups. The process of random assignment is key to testing causality, as it means that any unmeasured confounders should be balanced across the two groups.

The standard analytic approach in RCTs is "intention to treat," which compares change across all participants in the treatment arm, with all participants in the control arm, not taking into account whether the participants actually complied with the intervention (e.g., did they take the drug/adhere to the intervention). While compliance can be measured in the treatment arm, and therefore could be taken into account, modeling noncompliance within the control arm is more challenging—how do we know who the "compliers" are in the control arm? Which control participants would have complied/not complied if hypothetically allocated to the intervention arm? Instrumental variable approaches can be used to deal with this complexity (Emsley *et al.*, 2010).

RCTs and observational studies differ in their design and purpose, and discrepancies may be resolved if the formal attention to detail in specifying eligibility, treatment, and outcome that characterizes an RCT is applied to the epidemiological data (Hernán *et al.*, 2008). Such a proposal, for greater care, clarity, and objectivity in the analysis of epidemiological data, in an attempt to emulate the rigor employed by randomized trials, is important and of wide relevance, especially with the availability of electronic health records and other big databases (Hernán & Robbins, 2016).

Precision/personalized medicine

Key Readings:

- James, G. *et al.* (2021) *An Introduction to Statistical Learning with Applications in R*. 2nd edn. Springer.
- Steyerberg, E. (2019) *Clinical Prediction Models: A Practical Approach to Development, Validation, and Updating*. 2nd edn. Springer.

In recent years, there has been a shift from classical, evidence-based medicine toward precision medicine. It recognizes that focusing on the average treatment response, as typically studied in traditional RCTs, may not be the most appropriate approach to evaluating the best treatment for an individual (Figure 16.10). Precision medicine instead focuses on identifying which treatment or health-related approaches will be effective for an individual based on their genetic, environmental, and lifestyle factors.

Modern precision medicine is made possible by the provision of "new" data such as electronic health records, imaging, omics, sensors in smartphones and wearables, and internet and smartphone usage, along with high-performance computing technology that effectively collects, processes, stores, and analyses "big data" from a variety of modalities (Figure 16.11). Prediction modeling is a key component of precision medicine, using statistical models and machine learning (ML) techniques to identify patterns in patient data and predict the likelihood of a particular outcome, such as the risk of developing a disease, to make a prognosis about the likely course of a clinical condition or the response to a specific treatment. These models can guide clinical decision-making, suggesting preventive programs or tailoring treatment to the specific needs of individual patients. For example, Fusar-Poli *et al.* (2017) developed and validated a clinical web-based risk calculator for the transdiagnostic prediction of psychoses in secondary mental health care using electronic health records. Using this calculator can potentially aid in the individualized provision of preventive interventions and improve outcomes of first-episode psychosis.

Prediction modeling in health research differs from statistical or explanatory modeling by primarily focusing on reliably forecasting the outcome of individuals rather than explaining the specific nature of the underlying relationships between variables. The primary objective is to identify a model with a suitable subset of predictor variables that shows good generalizability across different settings. Prediction models, therefore, are optimized for the purpose of predicting new or future observations, while in explanatory research the average response of a population is of interest and minimizing the bias (difference between estimated and true population parameter) is the key criterion for selecting the best model. Consequently, there is tension between explanatory and predictive modeling because the best explanatory model may differ from the best predictive model (Shmueli, 2010).

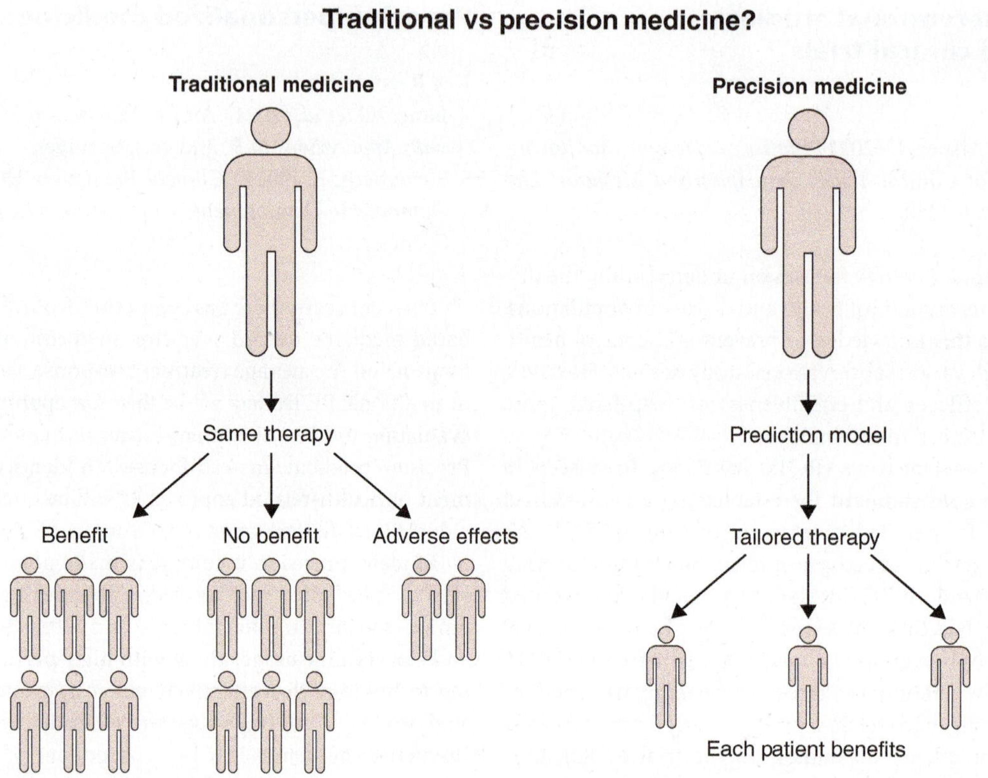

Figure 16.10 In traditional medicine, all patients are treated but only some benefit (others do not or even experience adverse effects). In precision medicine, treatments are tailored to individual patients based on specific characteristics (e.g., biomarkers like gene variants) to maximize patient benefit.

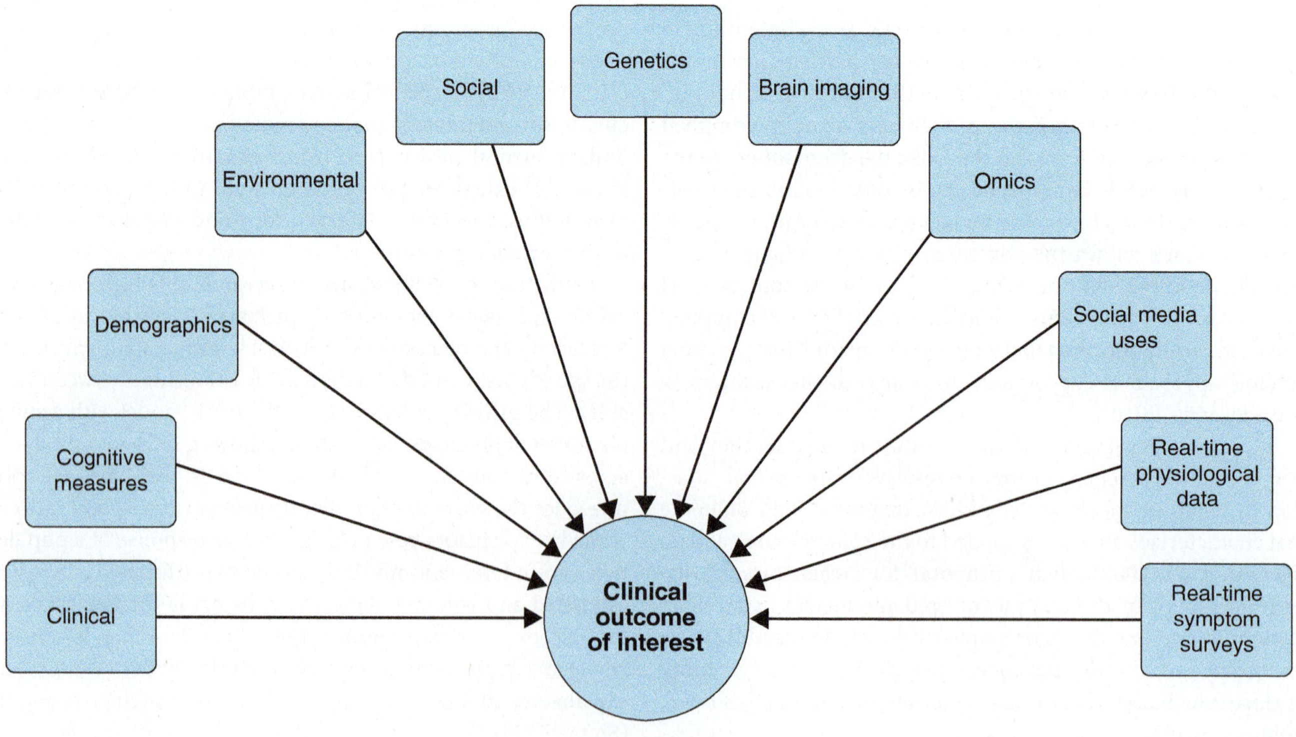

Figure 16.11 Example of 'big data' from a variety of modalities.

In prediction modeling, assessing the prediction accuracy of unseen cases is a key measure of evidence to validate a model. In internal validation, we assess the performance of a model to predict the outcome of unseen cases of the same population. Here, we often use cross-validation or bootstrapping to assess the prediction accuracy. In n-fold cross-validation, the single available dataset is randomly divided into n-folds (equal subsets). In turn, each fold is used as the unseen data (test set) with the remaining n-1 folds pooled together as the training set (Figure 16.12). Prediction performance is the average over the n-folds. Typically, 5–10-fold cross-validation is used. If a prediction model shows good performance, it needs to be externally validated in completely different settings to evaluate the generalizability of the model and its ability to predict outcomes in real-world scenarios. Prediction performance metrics commonly focus on discrimination and calibration. Discrimination, often measured by metrics like mean squared error (MSE) or area under the curve (AUC), evaluates a model's ability to distinguish between different outcomes. Calibration, on the other hand, assesses how closely the predicted probabilities align with the actual outcomes. Both are crucial for determining the accuracy and reliability of predictive models.

In medical research, large, complex datasets with a high number of variables relative to sample size, known as "big data" have arisen in recent years. ML is used to analyze such datasets. ML models, such as random forests, support vector machines, or neural networks, are algorithms that can learn from and make predictions on data. When using ML methods for model building, which permits the exploration of numerous different models, it is essential to implement proper model selection or hyperparameter tuning. Here, even more computer-intensive methods, such as nested cross-validation or double bootstrap, are required for internal model validation.

In prediction models, the theoretical model itself is not of primary interest ("black box"). However, classical statistical methods such as logistic or Cox regression often perform equally or even better than ML methods if datasets with moderate numbers of variables and predictive power are analyzed. Unlike ML, these models are easy to interpret and provide clarity on how predictions are being made. This is important for building trust and ensuring that these systems are used in a fair and ethical manner and for advancing scientific knowledge and understanding. Biases in ML models can arise if the training data are biased, and the model produces systematically prejudiced outcomes due to erroneous assumptions in the learning process. It is difficult to identify such bias. For example, in health care, an algorithm used to identify patients with health care needs generated differential risk scores for Black and White patients, meaning that sicker Black patients were assigned risk scores equivalent to healthier White patients, which could lead to disparities in health care access (Obermeyer *et al.*, 2019). In recent years, explainable artificial intelligence (AI) tries to decipher the "black box" to better understand how an ML model works and identify any potential biases or errors that may arise. Finally, it is a myth that ML models can be applied to small datasets. ML models generally require large amounts of data to accurately identify patterns and relationships between variables, are prone to overfitting, and often fail to generalize to new settings. Classical statistical methods may be more appropriate for analyzing limited data, and it is important to carefully consider the strengths and limitations of different approaches before applying them to a given problem. Additionally, ensuring proper assessment of model validity is essential.

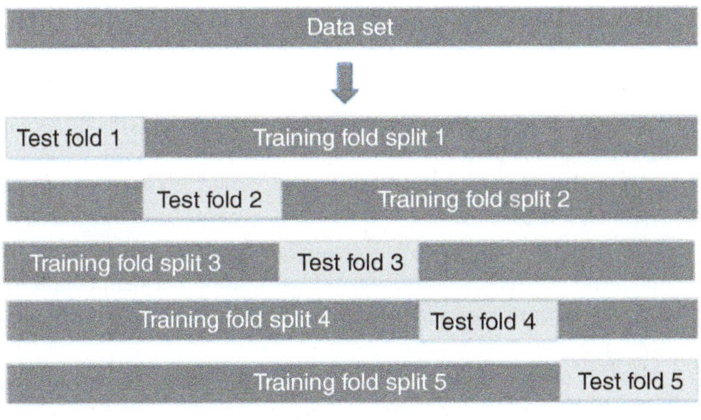

Figure 16.12 For internal assessment, we often employ n-fold cross-validation. Fivefold cross-validation sets aside one-fifth of the data as an independent test set, while the rest is used for training. This process is carried out across five different data splits, ensuring each data point is used once for validation. The outcomes from these five test folds are then averaged, and the final model is developed using the entire dataset.

Going beyond statistics: open science

The replication crisis in psychology and psychiatry has highlighted the need for a comprehensive approach that incorporates modern statistical methodology and open science practices, including adherence to ethical guidelines for research with human subjects and animals. This involves pre-registering study designs, hypotheses, and planned analyses to reduce the chance of false positives. It is also essential to follow reporting guidelines. For instance, for the reporting of results from trials, guidelines exist (e.g., www.consort-statement.org), while for epidemiologic studies, guidelines are still developing (e.g., www.strobe-statement.org). Sharing code, syntax, and data for replication and verification of results is also crucial. Additionally, it is important to publish both positive and negative findings in open-source journals to avoid the file-drawer effect. To promote an open science "mindset," researchers should commit to these practices and embrace transparency and accountability in their work (Hagger, 2022). By doing so, they can contribute to the advancement of knowledge in psychology and psychiatry and promote the credibility of the field.

Acknowledgments

We acknowledge Professor Andrew Pickles for an earlier version of this chapter. DS received financial support by the National Institute for Health Research (NIHR) Biomedical Research Centre at South London and Maudsley NHS Foundation Trust and King's College London. The views expressed are those of the author(s) and not necessarily those of the NHS, the NIHR, or the Department of Health.

References

Albers, C. & Lakens, D. (2018) When power analyses based on pilot data are biased: inaccurate effect size estimators and follow-up bias. *Journal of Experimental Social Psychology* **74**, 187–195. doi:10.1016/j.jesp.2017.09.004.

Baron, R.M. & Kenny, D.A. (1986) The moderator-mediator variable distinction in social psychological research: conceptual, strategic, and statistical considerations. *Journal of Personality and Social Psychology* **51**, 1173–1182.

Beard, E. & West, R. (2017) Using Bayesian statistics in health psychology: a comment on Depaoli *et al.* (2017). *Health Psychology Review* **11**(3), 298–301.

Beck, A. *et al.* (1996) *Beck Depression Inventory*, 2nd edn. Psychological Corporation, San Antonio, TX.

Benjamini, Y. & Hochberg, Y. (1995) Controlling the false discovery rate: a practical and powerful approach to multiple testing. *Journal of the Royal Statistical Society: Series B (Methodological)* **57**, 289–300.

Button, K. *et al.* (2013) Power failure: why small sample size undermines the reliability of neuroscience. *Nature Reviews. Neuroscience* **14**, 365–376. doi:10.1038/nrn3475.

Button, K.S. *et al.* (2015) Minimal clinically important difference on the Beck Depression Inventory II according to the patient's perspective. *Psychological Medicine* **45**(15), 3269–3279. doi:10.1017/S0033291715001270.

Carey, E.G. *et al.* (2023) Editorial perspective: when is a 'small effect' actually large and impactful? *Journal of Child Psychology and Psychiatry*. doi:10.1111/jcpp.13817.

Cepeda, N.A. *et al.* (2020) A primer on clinically important outcome values: going beyond relying on P values alone. *The Journal of Bone & Joint Surgery* **102**(3), 262–268. doi:10.2106/JBJS.19.00817.

Cooper, H. *et al.* (2009) *The Handbook of Research Synthesis and Meta-Analysis*, 2nd edn. Russell Sage Foundation, New York.

Diggle, P. *et al.* (2013) *Analysis of Longitudinal Data*, 2nd edn. Oxford University Press, Oxford, UK.

Dumas-Mallet, E. *et al.* (2017) Low statistical power in biomedical science: a review of three human research domains. *Royal Society Open Science* **4**(2), 160254.

Emsley, R. *et al.* (2010) Mediation and moderation of treatment effects in randomised controlled trials of complex interventions. *Statistical Methods in Medical Research* **19**(3), 237–270.

Everitt, B.S. *et al.* (2011) *Cluster Analysis*, Wiley Series in Probability and Statistics, 5th edn. doi:10.1002/9780470977811.

Fusar-Poli, P. *et al.* (2017) Development and validation of a clinically based risk calculator for the transdiagnostic prediction of psychosis. *JAMA Psychiatry* **74**(5), 493–500. doi:10.1001/jamapsychiatry.2017.0284. Erratum in: JAMA Psychiatry

Goldsmith, K.A. *et al.* (2018) Measurement error, time lag, unmeasured confounding: considerations for longitudinal estimation of the effect of a mediator in randomised clinical trials. *Statistical Methods in Medical Research* **27**(6), 1615–1633.

Hagger, M.S. (2022) Developing an open science 'mindset'. *Health Psychology and Behavioral Medicine* **10**(1), 1–21.

Hamaker, E.L. *et al.* (2015) A critique of the cross-lagged panel model. *Psychological Methods* **20**(1), 102.

Hernán, M.A. & Robins, J.M. (2016) Using big data to emulate a target trial when a randomized trial is not available. *American Journal of Epidemiology* **183**(8), 758–764.

Hernán, M.A. & Robins, J. (2020) *Causal Inference: What If*. Chapman & Hill/CRC, Boca Raton, FL. Available: https://www.hsph.harvard.edu/miguel-hernan/causal-inference-book/

Hernán, M.A. *et al.* (2008) Observational studies analyzed like randomized experiments: an application to postmenopausal hormone therapy and coronary heart disease. *Epidemiology* **19**, 766–779.

Ioannidis, J.P. (2005) Why most published research findings are false. *PLoS Medicine* **2**(8), e124.

Jaffee, S.R. *et al.* (2003) Life with (or without) father: the benefits of living with two biological parents depend on the father's antisocial behavior. *Child Development* **74**, 109–126.

James, G. *et al.* (2021) *An Introduction to Statistical Learning with Applications in R*, 2nd edn. Springer, Cham, Switzerland.

Judd, C.M. & Kenny, D.A. (1981) Process analysis: estimating mediation in treatment evaluations. *Evaluation Review* **5**, 602–619.

Landau, S. & Stahl, D. (2013) Sample size and power calculations for medical studies by simulation when closed form expressions are not available. *Statistical Methods in Medical Research* **22**(3), 324–345.

Leon, A.C. *et al.* (2011) The role and interpretation of pilot studies in clinical research. *Journal of Psychiatric Research* **45**(5), 626–629.

Light, R.J. & Pillemer, D.B. (1984) *Summing Up. The Science of Reviewing Research*. Harvard University Press, Cambridge, MA.

Little, R.J.A. & Rubin, D.B. (1987) *Statistical Analysis with Missing Data*. Wiley, New York.

Little, R.J.A. & Rubin, D.B. (1989) The analysis of social science data with missing values. *Sociological Methods & Research* **18**, 292–326.

Lord, C. *et al.* (2000) The autism diagnostic observation schedule-generic: a standard measure of social and communication deficits associated with the spectrum of autism. *Journal of Autism and Developmental Disorders* **30**, 205–223.

Lord, C. *et al.* (2006) Autism from two to nine. *Archives of General Psychiatry* **63**, 694–701.

MacKinnon, D. (2012) *Introduction to Statistical Mediation Analysis*. Routledge, New York.

MacKinnon, D.P. *et al.* (2007) Mediation analysis. *Annual Review of Psychology* **58**, 593–614.

McDonnell, J. *et al.* (2018) Interpersonal sensitivity in those at clinical high risk for psychosis mediates the association between childhood bullying victimisation and paranoid ideation: a virtual reality study. *Schizophrenia Research* **192**, 89–95.

Moffitt, T.E. (1993) Adolescence-limited and life-course persistent antisocial behavior: a developmental taxonomy. *Psychological Review* **100**, 674–701.

NCCMH (2004) *Depression: Management of Depression in Primary and Secondary Care*. British Psychological Society and Royal College of Psychiatrists, Leicester and London.

Obermeyer, Z. *et al.* (2019) Dissecting racial bias in an algorithm used to manage the health of populations. *Science* **366**(6464), 447–453.

Pearl, J. (2014) Interpretation and identification of causal mediation. *Psychological Methods* **19**(4), 459.

Pickles, A. & De Stavola, B. (2007) An overview of models and methods for life course analysis. In: *Methods in Life Course Epidemiology*. (eds A. Pickles, *et al.*). Oxford University Press, Oxford, UK. pp. 181–120.

Rubin, D.B. (1987) *Multiple Imputation for Nonresponse in Surveys*. J. Wiley & Sons, New York.

Schafer, J.L. (1999) Multiple imputation: a primer. *Statistical Methods in Medical Research* **8**, 3–16.

Sergeant, E.S.G. (2018) Epitools – Epidemiological Calculators. Ausvet. Available: http://epitools.ausvet.com.au [4 September 2024].

Serra-Garcia, M. & Gneezy, U. (2021) Nonreplicable publications are cited more than replicable ones. *Science Advances* **7**(21), eabd1705.

Shih, W.J. & Aisner, J. (2021) *Statistical Design, Monitoring, and Analysis of Clinical Trials: Principles and Methods*, 2nd edn. Chapman & Hall/CRC, Boca Raton, FL.

Shmueli, G. (2010) To explain or to predict? *Statistical Science* **25**(3), 289–310.

Simmons, J.P. *et al.* (2011) False-positive psychology: undisclosed flexibility in data collection and analysis allows presenting anything as significant. *Psychological Science* **22**(11), 1359–1366. doi:10.1177/0956797611417632.

Sotola, L.K. (2022) Garbage in, garbage out? Evaluating the evidentiary value of published meta-analyses using z-curve analysis. *Collabra: Psychology* **8**(1), 32571.

Stahl, D. & Pickles, A. (2018) Fact or fiction: reducing the proportion and impact of false positives. *Psychological Medicine* **48**(7), 1084–1091. doi:10.1017/S003329171700294X.

Steyerberg, E. (2019) *Clinical Prediction Models: A Practical Approach to Development, Validation, and Updating*, 2nd edn. Springer, Cham, Switzerland.

Sullivan, T.R. *et al.* (2018) Should multiple imputation be the method of choice for handling missing data in randomized trials? *Statistical Methods in Medical Research* **27**(9), 2610–2626.

White, I.R. *et al.* (2011) Strategy for intention to treat analyses in randomised trials with missing outcome data. *British Medical Journal* **342**, 1–4.

CHAPTER 17

How can economics help decision-makers to improve child and adolescent mental health equitably and efficiently?

Martin Knapp and Sara Evans-Lacko
Care Policy and Evaluation Centre, London School of Economics and Political Science, London, UK

Introduction

For better or for worse, money is a key consideration in policy and practice discussions, even if it sometimes lurks below the surface. Although the professional delivering one-to-one therapy, prescribing medication, or arranging group activities might not have to be concerned about the associated costs, further along the management chain someone will be monitoring expenditure and trying to balance the books. And while the budget holder may be focused on avoiding a deficit at year end, someone higher up in the health, education, or social care system will be considering wider strategic options and looking to achieve best value for money in the use of available resources. If a new treatment (such as a new medication, mode of family therapy, or care arrangement) is introduced—and known to be effective—budget holders will want to know whether it is affordable and whether it is worth what it costs. If needs and their consequences are enduring, governments will want to know the associated long-term expenditure implications and how to contain them.

The underlying challenge common to all these wants or concerns is scarcity: there are never enough resources to meet all needs. This is the most fundamental, pervasive, durable, and important justification for understanding the economics of child and adolescent mental health. Scarcity is a permanent feature of all health and related systems and is the reason why choices must be made between alternative uses of resources. As we shall see, those choices between alternative uses give meaning to costs. Economics, and particularly economic evaluation, provides evidence to inform both professional practice and strategic decisions about allocating available resources to get more out of them—e.g., better outcomes for children and families, fairer distributions of access to services—and about the incentives needed to achieve those allocations.

Although the primary aim of any mental health system is to alleviate symptoms to improve functioning and quality of life, it is increasingly recognized that pursuit of such a laudable, fundamental objective cannot proceed without regard for the economic consequences. Awareness of this need to improve not only effectiveness but also cost-effectiveness produces various demands for economic evidence. There are requests for measures of overall resource or cost impact of a particular health problem. There are demands for *cost-effectiveness* and similar analyses of particular treatments or policies: these are evaluations that compare the outcomes of two or more interventions and the relative costs of achieving them and any economic payoffs. There are searches for new system and service reconfigurations that improve efficiency of resource use, and for improved incentive structures that alter how resources are deployed.

Economic methods provide helpful answers to decision-making questions faced by health professionals, budget holders, and governments. Considerations around health care decisions are always relevant, given the perennially high demand for mental health support but—as the global economic context changes—decisions, preferences, and social conditions may also change. For instance, economic methods are especially relevant to countries which are experiencing or recovering from financial or other types of shocks, such as those affected by natural disasters, conflicts, political instability, economic recession, or a pandemic. Methods such as cost, cost-offset analyses (comparing amounts expended with amounts saved), and the various forms of economic evaluation (comparing costs and the outcomes achieved)—often *cost-effectiveness analysis* (CEA) for short—can support better, more informed decisions about efficient ways of

Rutter's Child and Adolescent Psychiatry and Psychology, Seventh Edition.
Edited by Anita Thapar, Daniel S. Pine, Samuele Cortese, Cathy Creswell, Tamsin J. Ford, James F. Leckman, and Argyris Stringaris.

Companion website: www.wiley.com/go/thapar/rutterspsych7

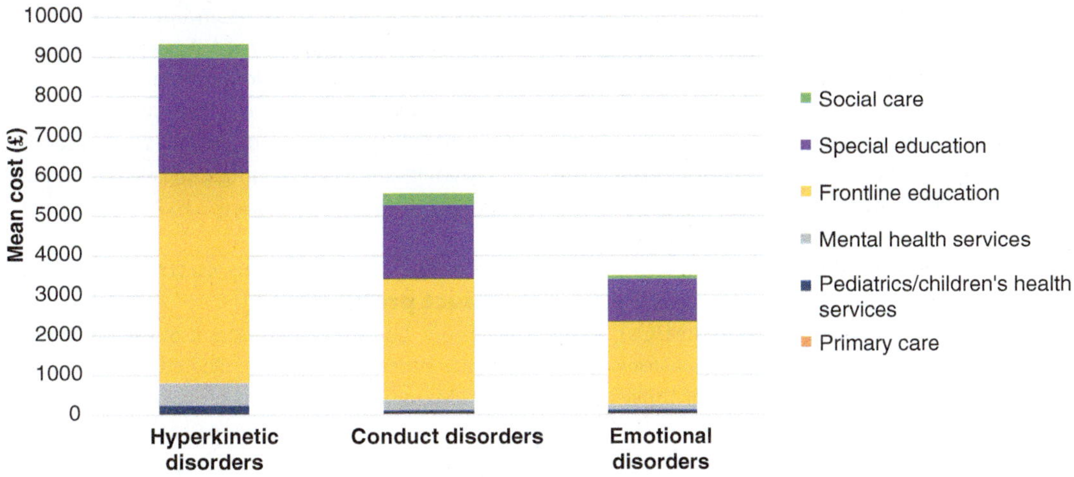

Figure 17.1 Health, social service, and education resource use: mean cost over three-year follow-up for all children/young people with a disorder (adapted from Snell *et al.*, 2013). Note: Costs can be converted from £ sterling to US$ by dividing the £ figures by 0.681.

allocating resources during times of economic transition. We explain the main types of economic evaluation in more detail later in the section, Exploring cost-effectiveness. It may be that increasing investment in interventions or services to alleviate the consequences of an economic recession could be associated with long-term savings. During times of economic growth, economic methods can help identify efficient ways to scale up services. Growing evidence demonstrates the case for further government investment in child and adolescent mental health care to support delivery of these evidence-based interventions across countries worldwide (McDaid & Evans-Lacko, 2021).

Costs in childhood

Mental health problems have cost implications. The most obvious effect is on health service utilization, but there may be contacts with special education, social work, public housing, criminal justice, and other service-delivering agencies. Indeed, this multiplicity of contacts and services is a marked and welcome characteristic of well-developed mental health systems (Knapp & Wong, 2020). If needs are not appropriately addressed, there could be adverse effects on functioning, with implications for educational engagement and attainment, employment, income, and wealth, and effects on families.

Studies have described these costs during childhood and adolescence. Snell *et al.* (2013) demonstrate the substantial additional health care, social care, and education costs[1] associated with childhood psychiatric disorders (Figure 17.1). They show the large costs and the wide range of sectors affected by childhood psychiatric disorders. The cost of frontline education services was more than twelve times that of specialty mental health services; special education services were also costly. Cost differed by type of problem: higher costs were associated with children with hyperkinetic and conduct disorders, compared to children with emotional disorders. Severity and impact of mental illness are often important cost drivers, while socioeconomic characteristics and parental stigma may also influence service utilization and associated costs (Ribeiro *et al.*, 2022; Ziebold *et al.*, 2022).

Romeo *et al.* (2006) examined impacts across sectors and estimated broad implications for families and the wider economy for children referred for severe antisocial behavior. There were considerable nonservice costs: almost half the total costs were borne by families. The mean annual cost of care was £5960, equivalent to US$8752, using the OECD purchasing power parity exchange rate (Organisation for Economic Cooperation and Development, 2013): the same conversion rate is used throughout the chapter. Costs varied by a factor of more than 400, emphasizing the inherent heterogeneity in children with mental health needs.

A further example points to the high and enduring costs of autism in the United States and United Kingdom. Combining data from multiple studies on accommodation, medical services, nonmedical services, out-of-pocket payments by families, and prevalence, Buescher *et al.* (2014) found similar lifetime costs of someone with autism and intellectual disability across the two countries. The study also found—similarly to Snell and colleagues discussed above—high costs carried by the education sector, with parental productivity losses also high. A later review of evidence found similar patterns internationally (Rogge & Janssen, 2019).

These studies show the breadth of economic impact across service sectors and on families, although they can only measure what is provided (in terms of service-related costs) or what impacts are recognized (in terms of indirect costs). We shall see in the next section that, if mental health problems in childhood

[1] Mean costs based on data from 2007–2008.

or adolescence are inadequately addressed, there can be substantial costs stretching long into adulthood.

The extent to which the resource (cost) consequences of childhood or adolescent mental health problems fall outside the health sector depends on how different sectors, such as health, social services, education, and housing are organized. But regardless of system boundaries, many young people with mental health problems have needs in multiple life domains, each potentially with economic ramifications.

Few studies explore how costs may be distributed across sectors in low- and middle-income countries (LMICs). One study using data from the Brazilian high-risk cohort found the costs to be greatest in the health sector. Overall, for those using services, average annual cost of service use was US$527.14 per user, although costs varied by severity and type of condition. Other research has looked at differences according to type of mental health condition. Global figures from the UNICEF report, *The State of the World's Children 2021*, suggest that anxiety disorders, behavioral disorders, and depression accounted for the greatest economic impacts among children and adolescents. Detailed Danish registry data found that all types of mental health conditions were associated with income loss, excess health care costs, and excess public transfer payments (Christensen *et al.*, 2022).

These multiple impacts are obviously hard to measure, and harder still to factor into decision-making. Not only does the decision-maker in, for example, the health sector need to find out the implications of their actions for other sectors, they must also establish the mechanisms to do something about them. A common problem is "silo budgeting": resources located in specific agencies or budgets cannot easily be shifted, indeed might be rigorously protected (Knapp & Wong, 2020). Professional rivalry, myopic budget protection, performance assessment regimes, or slowly churning bureaucratic processes could leave one agency unwilling or unable to devote more of its own resources so that another agency can achieve savings, or for the broader system of treatment and support to achieve greater effectiveness or cost-effectiveness.

Costs continuing into adulthood

Mental health problems experienced in childhood or adolescence can have many and often serious adverse effects on psychosocial outcomes such as crime, relationships, substance misuse, and quality of life (see Chapter 1). Mental health needs in childhood could also be associated with later physical health needs. Physical and mental comorbidities tend to co-occur and can increase costs in childhood due particularly to increased service use (Guevara *et al.* 2001; Nelson *et al.* 2013). These comorbidities may worsen in adulthood, leading to higher service costs, lower workforce participation, and higher absenteeism (Simon *et al.*, 2023). Surprisingly, there is little research on how these comorbidities interact, their economic consequences, or how best to evaluate costs and outcomes of complex combinations of interventions aimed at addressing them.

A few studies have explored connections between childhood disorders and adulthood *economic* consequences: they demonstrate higher utilization of health and other services, lower employment, reduced earnings, and increased poverty. We offer examples from three areas.

Evidence for long-term costs associated with conduct problems

The Inner London Longitudinal Study collected data on 2281 ten-year olds in 1970 and selected 228 of them for intensive study (Maughan, 1989). This group was interviewed again at age 28. Service-related costs were derived from the information gathered (Scott *et al.*, 2001). This is an early study of the long-term economic impacts of childhood problems. Costs were incomplete because data collection did not cover relevant impacts such as social work, voluntary sector service use, primary health care contacts, lost employment, divorce, undetected crime, effects of crime on victims, emotional impacts on others, and transmitted effects to family members or children. Despite these omissions, conduct disorder (CD) in childhood (found for the most antisocial 3% of the sample studied) and conduct problems (found for the next 9%) led to greatly elevated costs in adulthood in many sectors, especially the criminal justice system (Figure 17.2).

Links between conduct problems and CD in childhood and service-related costs in early adulthood were further explored statistically, adjusting for gender, parental social class, reading age, and number of primary schools attended. The estimated coefficient on the CD variable—the additional cost between the ages of 10 and 28 (aggregating across all 18 years) of having CD at age 10 compared to not having any antisocial behavior problems—was £40,784 (2004–2005 prices; equivalent to US$59,888). The additional cost of having conduct problems (the next 9% of the group) compared to having no such problems was £17,017 (US$24,988). Given the underdeveloped, underresourced nature of child and adolescent mental health services in the United Kingdom in the early 1970s, these cost differences might indicate the economic consequences of not (or only rather poorly) addressing antisocial behavior in 10-year-olds.

More recent research has compared the economic impacts of conduct problems with other types of mental health conditions (Knapp *et al.*, 2011; Gronholm *et al.*, 2022; King *et al.*, 2023). Rivenbark *et al.* (2018) linked data from the Dunedin cohort of 1037 individuals born in New Zealand in 1972–1973 with administrative records including: health service use, prescription drug fills, social welfare benefits, and crime convictions. Those with persistent problems had greater economic impacts across all outcomes. King *et al.* also found that child and adolescent conduct problems were associated with greater costs of general practitioner health care utilization up to age 50, especially when co-occurring with emotional problems.

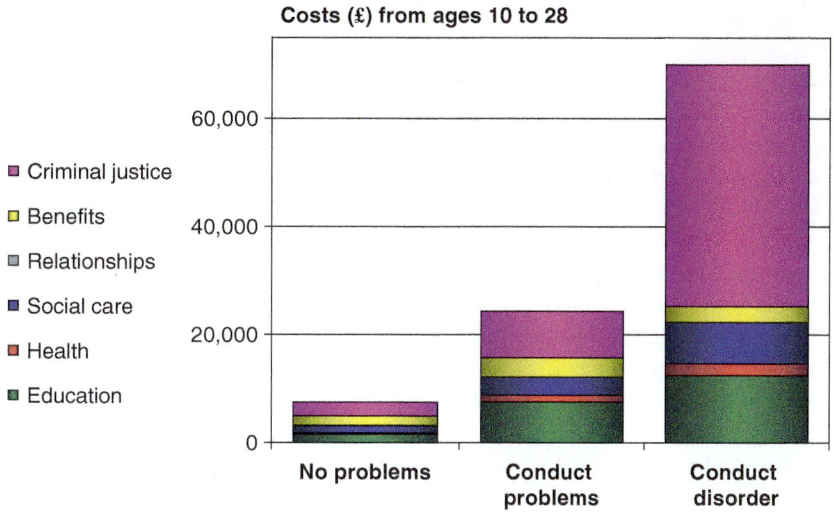

Figure 17.2 Costs in early adulthood from childhood conduct disorder (adapted from Scott *et al.*, 2001).

Evidence of early prevention and intervention programs for young people

Aos and colleagues (Aos *et al.*, 2004) were commissioned by Washington state legislature to investigate the long-term costs and benefits of early prevention and intervention programs for young people, and to recommend (i) whether prevention and early intervention programs were good investments, and (ii) which programs provide the best investment. They modeled costs and benefits across six areas: education, crime, substance abuse, child abuse and neglect, teen pregnancy, and public assistance. Programs which performed a rigorous evaluation of at least one key outcome were identified from the literature.

The report concluded that some prevention and early intervention programs provide good return on investment to taxpayers. However, findings were mixed, with some interventions resulting in clear benefits while for others the benefits did not outweigh the costs. Their findings emphasized the importance of rigorous evaluation and quality control when implementing programs. Some of the most effective public policies which demonstrated positive long-term impacts for youth with mental health conditions include: Functional Family Therapy for youth post-release, following confinement in residential or correctional facilities (benefit-cost ratio of US$18.75 and 100% chance of positive net benefits); Dialectical Behavior Therapy for youth in state institutions (benefit-cost ratio of US$32.59 and 93% chance of positive net benefits); and Nurse Family Partnership for low-income families (benefit-cost ratio of US$3.02 and 99% chance of positive net benefits). However, these results may not generalize to other contexts, as studies of the Nurse Family Partnership and Functional Family Therapy in the United Kingdom did not suggest similar effectiveness, indicating local conditions and program implementation are also important factors (Skivington *et al.*, 2021).

Evaluation of the long-term impact of risk factors such as child maltreatment and bullying

Child maltreatment can have long-term economic impacts, such as mental health care utilization and productivity losses. Analysis of the Netherlands Mental Health Survey and Incidence Study (NEMESIS), which included 5618 individuals in a large, population-based cohort, found excess costs of child maltreatment at one-year follow-up were between US$2610–3666. At population-level, child maltreatment was associated with excess costs of between US$203–655 million per million people per year. Importantly, the study also found that certain protective factors, such as high internal locus of control, ameliorated onset of mental disorder and subsequently reduced associated economic consequences (Thielen *et al.* 2016).

More recent UK research using longitudinal cohort data estimated lifetime costs of various outcomes associated with child maltreatment, including physical and mental health problems, social care use, and labor market outcomes. Average lifetime incidence costs were £89,390 per nonfatal case (with significant proportions attributed to mental health problems: short-term mental health problems £18,553, anxiety £954; depression £5,145; alcohol abuse £537) and £940,759 for cases of child maltreatment resulting in death (Conti *et al.*, 2021).

Research on the long-term impacts of childhood bullying using the 1958 British Birth Cohort found economic impacts across many domains, including reductions in employment, earnings (among females), and wealth. These impacts are likely to be partly mediated by poorer mental health among victims of bullying, as demonstrated through greater health service costs associated with mental illness among those who were bullied versus those who were not (Brimblecombe *et al.*, 2018).

Cost-offset considerations

A question that governments and other macrolevel decision-makers often want answering is whether investment in preventive measures or better treatments during (say) a child's early years will reduce economic impacts in adolescence and in adulthood. This is the *cost-offset* question: what is the balance between expenditure and savings? Evaluation of the Early Start Denver Model (ESDM), a comprehensive behavioral intervention for autistic children in the United States, found that children who received ESDM had significantly higher annual health-related intervention costs compared to children receiving community-based treatment (Cidav *et al.*, 2017). However, within a few years, these high intervention costs were fully offset by reductions in other types of service use and costs. Children who received ESDM used less applied behavior analysis (ABA), early intensive behavioral intervention (EIBI), occupational therapy, physical therapy, and speech therapy compared with children who received community-based treatment, amounting to savings of c.US$19,000 per child per year.

Bonin *et al.* studied the effect of group parenting interventions for young people with CD using simulation modeling (Bonin *et al.*, 2011) (see Box 17.1 for a summary of simulation modeling and other health economics designs; Chapter 13 on causal inference, and Chapter 14 on study designs.) Petrou and Gray (2011) provide an excellent introduction to modeling designs in health economics. Bonin suggested the parenting intervention resulted in long-term benefits to the public sector and to society as a whole by reducing the chance that CD persisted into adulthood. Long-term benefits were greatest in the health and criminal justice sectors.

Bonin's study was based on hypothetical (simulated) valuations, whereas a second example—the High/Scope Perry Preschool Study—was based on direct observations. Although not focused on children with mental health problems, this well-known intervention has been influential because of its finding of substantial savings in relation to crime, education, and welfare payments, as well as higher taxes paid by individuals who went through the preschool program (e.g., see summary by Heckman *et al.*, 2010). However, these findings relate to a very small sample of individuals, and generalizability is far from straightforward.

The importance of taking a long-term view is further illustrated by studies of a school-based anti-bullying intervention, KiVa, developed in Finland (Kärnä *et al.*, 2011). KiVa can be delivered by teachers, focusing on enhancing empathy, self-efficacy, and antibullying attitudes. Simulation modeling in the English context showed that the total costs of KiVa are more than offset by immediate savings, suggesting a short-term return on investment of £1.58 for every £1 invested (McDaid *et al.*, 2017a). There were considerably larger cost-offsets when the effects of averting longer-term adverse consequences were measured, including reduced impacts on specialist mental health services, primary care, hospital costs, and productivity (McDaid *et al.*, 2017b).

Exploring cost-effectiveness

Knowing the costs in childhood associated with mental health problems helps decision-makers gauge the component and overall societal impact of these conditions. Knowing what economic consequences these problems lead to in adulthood helps decision-makers focus on the need for better preventive or treatment interventions. But neither of these bodies of evidence can tell a decision-maker how to make better use of available resources. It is necessary to examine not just costs but also outcomes of different uses of those resources.

Consider what happens following the introduction of a new treatment (say a new medication for treating childhood depression). Decision-makers face two central questions when considering whether to use or recommend this medication. The clinical question is whether the medication is effective in alleviating depressive symptoms and generally improving child health. Or, when considering two or more different drugs, which has better outcomes? If the answer to the clinical question is that the new medication is no better than existing treatments, there is usually no need to consider its use any further, nor probably to look at relative costs. But if the new medication looks clinically effective, the decision-maker will then want to know if

Box 17.1 Examples of health economics study designs

Randomized controlled trial (RCT)

An RCT is an experimental study design where study participants are randomly assigned to two or more groups. The design has high internal validity, but may not produce widely generalizable results (see Cunningham *et al.*, 1995; Byford *et al.*, 2007a, 2007b; Domino *et al.* 2009; Byford *et al.*, 2015;Cidav *et al.*, 2017; Shearer *et al.*, 2018; Chatterton *et al.*, 2019; Ford *et al.*, 2019.)

Quasi-experimental study design

Quasi-experimental studies cover a range of designs and investigate the effect of an intervention without using randomization. They tend to have lower internal validity compared to RCTs. When performing economic evaluation, it is important to consider causality and account for confounding factors.

Simulation modeling

Simulation modeling uses existing data to estimate the impacts of an intervention for different hypothetical scenarios. For example, what are the costs and outcomes if an intervention studied in an RCT for one year was extended for a further two years? It may incorporate epidemiological or cost data from other sources to model costs and outcomes (see Bonin *et al.*, 2011; McDaid *et al.*, 2017a, 2017b; Tinelli *et al.*, 2023.)

it is cost-effective: does treatment achieve the improved child outcomes at a cost that is worth paying?

These two questions (Is the treatment effective? Is it worth it?) are at the heart of CEA. It is important to emphasize CEA does what it says on the label: it looks at *both* costs and effectiveness (outcomes). Comparing costs of one intervention with costs of another, without evidence on outcomes, might be interesting but does not provide enough evidence for decision-makers to make informed choices between alternative uses of scarce resources. Similarly, calculating and in some way comparing costs and outcomes of a single intervention could be revealing, but is not especially helpful unless comparison is made with equivalent data for another service (or with the "do nothing" option), for otherwise decision-makers will have no benchmark against which to judge whether observed costs and outcomes are attractive enough to justify action.

Note that the second question in a CEA asks whether improved outcomes are "worth" the extra cost. Deciding what is or is not "worth" the cost is not straightforward and not without controversy, as discussed below.

There are different variants of cost-effectiveness that can be applied to decision-making (Box 17.2). They share a common approach to conceptualization, definition, and measurement of costs, but adopt different approaches to outcome measurement, reflecting what decision-making questions need answering. There is, however, some potential for terminological confusion. "Cost-effectiveness" can refer to a specific variant of economic evaluation or to the group of *all* such evaluations. In this chapter, we use the term in its generic sense, unless otherwise stated. These types of evaluation are described in detail in health economics textbooks, the classic text being Drummond *et al.* (2015). There are also shorter, introductory guides such as the one from the Office for Health Improvement and Disparities (2021).

Question and perspective

The evaluative approach depends on the question. If the question is clinical—what is the most appropriate treatment for a child with particular needs and circumstances, and whether to opt for one therapeutic package or another—information is needed on the comparative costs of the different therapies and the comparative outcomes measured as symptom alleviation, improved functioning, and so on. In these circumstances, CEA (in the narrow sense) would be appropriate and sufficient (see section on "Effectiveness measurement" below).

If, to take a broader stance, the question is whether to invest available health system resources to treat either childhood depression or asthma, then decision-makers need to know the relative costs of the alternatives, and the relative effectiveness of the two options measured using a common metric. The most commonly used measure is "utility," generated from health-related quality-of-life scales (see section on "Utility measurement" below). In these circumstances, a cost-utility analysis (CUA) is needed.

To widen the perspective further, if the question is whether to invest more money in health care or more money in improving transport, launching a new environmental policy, or bolstering a country's defense forces, then the research question becomes one of asking what are the comparative costs and merits of these different investment options, where "merit" will now need to be measured in some common unit across all these areas of public policy. The usual choice of broad measure is monetary, leading to cost-benefit analysis (CBA) (see section on "Benefit measurement" below).

The choice of question influences the type of evaluation needed, but a single study could support more than one type of analysis and address more than one policy or practice-related question. A body of evidence well-located within the clinical

Box 17.2 Types of economic evaluation

Cost-consequences analysis

Cost-consequence analysis (CCA) looks at a wide range of costs and outcomes from the interventions being compared, and reports them separately. It can include a range of different outcomes. It gives decision-makers a comprehensive summary of the economic, health, and quality-of-life consequences. Because it reports the various costs and outcomes separately, each decision-maker can focus on those costs and outcomes most relevant to their context.

Cost-effectiveness analysis

Cost-effectiveness analysis (CEA) is similar to CCA but concentrates on just one outcome measure, usually a clinical measure (e.g., symptoms). Outcomes are measured in what might be the most "natural" indicator for clinical purposes. The advantage over CCA is that the differences in costs and outcome between interventions can be expressed as a simple ratio, making it easier to compare between studies. The disadvantage is lack of breadth.

Cost utility analysis

Cost utility analysis (CUA) differs from other types of evaluation in measuring outcome ("utility") in terms of quantity and (health-related) quality of life. The most common measure of utility in high-income countries is quality-adjusted life years (QALYs). CUAs are most helpful when looking across different illnesses/conditions because the utility measure is intended to have generic validity. In England, CUAs are favored by the National Institute for Health and Care Excellence (NICE) for health technology assessments, intended to help the National Health Service make strategic resource allocation decisions across specialties.

Cost–benefit analysis

Cost-benefit analysis (CBA) differs from other evaluations in putting a monetary value on health outcomes. CBAs also usually include nonhealth impacts of interventions, including cost savings and productivity gains (if patients return to work). Because costs and outcomes are measured in the same units (money), decision-making is arguably clearer and simpler. An intervention whose benefits exceed its costs would be recommended. If two interventions are compared, the one with the bigger excess of benefits over costs would be recommended as offering better value for money. CBAs can support high-level strategic decisions. The main disadvantage is the considerable difficulty of attaching monetary values to outcomes.

domain will be exactly what health care professionals need but may not be appropriate for higher-level decision-making, such as by a health ministry. The broader the question, the harder it is to measure outcomes satisfactorily.

Linked to the specification of the question is the *perspective* to be adopted. Is the evaluation needed to help resource allocation within a particular agency (e.g., a mental health service), a particular system (e.g., health care or education), a particular sector (e.g., government), or for the whole society? Breadth of perspective determines breadth of cost measurement and choice of measures of outcomes.

Cost measurement

There are various ways to categorize costs. There are costs directly associated with treatment and associated supports, some delivered by nonhealth agencies. There are wider costs which fall to families or are seen in terms of lost productivity because of future disruptions to employment patterns for children once they reach adulthood, or current disruptions to parents' employment. There are unmeasured costs, perhaps reflecting family impacts, or societal concerns about antisocial behavior. Evaluations usually measure these elements as long-run marginal opportunity costs (Knapp, 1997). This helps ensure a long-term perspective on resource implications is employed, that only those effects on resources attributable to the program or service user are counted, and that costs are reckoned as opportunities forgone, not just money expended. How broadly costs are measured depends on the perspective taken for the evaluation and purpose of the study.

In carrying out evaluations in practice, economists would look for data on service use patterns. These data might come from organizational "billing" systems, recording amounts transferred between payers and service providers. This is a common approach in US research, for example (although usually only spanning one system—such as health care—at a time). In care systems without such payment mechanisms, there might nevertheless be routine information systems that record service contacts and referrals, potentially providing data for an evaluation. However, in many countries, billing data and information systems are unavailable or unreliable for cost calculation. In these circumstances, patterns of service use can be collected through interviews with individuals, family members, or service professionals using tools like the Client Service Receipt Inventory (Beecham & Knapp, 1999).

Researchers would then attach unit cost estimates to these data on service utilization. It is not always necessary to calculate these unit costs anew. In England, for example, there is an excellent annual compendium of unit costs, widely used in applied research (Jones *et al.*, 2023). Nonservice costs are harder to measure, partly because of the difficulty of identifying impacts (e.g., on parental employment patterns, or on a child's own future earning capacity) and partly because of the difficulty of then attaching a monetary value (see Johnston *et al.*, 1999; Brouwer *et al.*, 2001).

Effectiveness measurement

Probably the most intuitive mode of economic evaluation is CEA: it measures costs as set out above, and measures outcomes using instruments and scales familiar from clinical studies, because its focus is symptoms, behavior, functioning, peer-group integration, and so on. A CEA can help decision-makers choose between alternative interventions available to or aimed at specific patient groups. An analysis would study a single outcome dimension (e.g., change in a behavioral measure, or symptom-free days) and then compute and compare the ratio of difference in costs between two treatments to difference in (primary) outcome (the so-called incremental cost-effectiveness ratio). Certain areas of child mental health lack robust studies, such as programs for learning disorders (see Box 17.3).

An example of cost-effectiveness based on an RCT comes from Domino *et al.* (2009). The study compared the cost-effectiveness of three treatments for major depression among adolescents: (i) fluoxetine; (ii) cognitive behavioral therapy (CBT); and (iii) fluoxetine plus CBT. Costs of service use of study participants were evaluated at 36 weeks follow-up in relation to the number of depression-free days and QALYs. Although combination treatment was most costly, it was found to be most cost-effective overall.

Ford *et al.* were more tentative in their conclusions from an RCT comparing the Incredible Years® Teacher Classroom Management (TCM) program with Teaching as Usual (Ford *et al.*, 2019). The outcome measure for the CEA was the Strengths and Difficulties Questionnaire (SDQ). Uncertainty in

Box 17.3 Cost and benefits of programs for learning disorders

Learning disorders represent one area for which there is little published evidence on cost-effectiveness of programs. Some encouraging evidence using intervention data combined with various cohort data is available, but more robust study designs are needed.

Challen *et al.* examined the association between learning difficulties and various social and economic outcomes later on (Challen *et al.*, 2008). Combining these data with intervention data from a phonological awareness intervention for kindergartners (Schneider *et al.* 1997) allowed cost-effectiveness to be explored. The substantial effect size found in the evaluation (spelling improved by 0.57 and reading by 0.26 standard deviations) suggested that the intervention was potentially very cost-effective. This finding appears promising, but there are several caveats in that the evaluation of the intervention was too small to look specifically at the effects for individuals with learning disorders and did not include a long-term follow up.

Machin and McNally investigated the cost-effectiveness of the "literacy hour" (Machin & McNally, 2008), a reading intervention for 5–11-year-olds in English primary schools. The program improved literacy and school achievement through a teaching framework incorporating focused literacy instruction and effective classroom management. Birth cohort data were combined with intervention data to estimate the impact of the intervention (in terms of reading score improvement) on future earnings. As the cost of the intervention was low (£26 (US$38) per pupil per year), even with very conservative estimates of the impact, the economic benefits were between £1375–3581 (US$2019–5258).

the economic analyses was explored by constructing cost-effectiveness acceptability curves (CEACs) that indicate the likelihood that an intervention would be seen as cost-effective when compared with a range of willingness-to-pay thresholds. This approach is helpful when an intervention is both more effective and more costly than its comparator. The TCM approach may be both effective and cost-effective, particularly when used to support primary school children identified by teachers as "struggling." The study was relatively long-term, with data collected for 30 months, but positive outcome findings for the whole population of primary school pupils were only observed up to 9 months, though they persisted throughout for those with poor teacher-reported mental health at baseline.

An obvious weakness with the strict cost-effectiveness methodology is its focus on a single outcome when children and adolescents with mental health problems often have multiple needs for support and when most clinicians would expect to achieve improvements in more than one area. Therefore, cost-effectiveness ratios are sometimes computed in turn for two or more outcome measures. This is sometimes called CCA (see Box 17.2). It has more breadth but poses a challenge if two or more cost-effectiveness ratios point to different interventions as being more cost-effective. If that happens, the decision-maker must weigh up the strength of evidence.

An example is provided by the evaluation of an intervention to support parents of preschool autistic children (Byford *et al.*, 2015). In the Pre-School Autism Communication Trial (PACT), 152 preschool children received either treatment as usual or an add-on, parent-mediated, communication-focused therapy. The new approach was effective in improving parent and child dyadic behaviors, such as parental synchrony and child initiations, when interacting with each other, but not effective in symptom reduction at immediate follow-up (Green *et al.*, 2010). The CCA adopted two perspectives. From a service perspective (health, social care, and education services), PACT was less cost-effective than treatment as usual, mainly because of the cost of the intervention itself. In contrast, from a societal perspective (including wider societal costs associated with schooling and childcare, parental out-of-pocket expenditure, productivity losses, and unpaid care time), the cost difference between the interventions was no longer significant. Byford *et al.* concluded that it was difficult to recommend PACT on cost-effectiveness grounds (Byford *et al.*, 2015).

These are the short-term findings (up to the 13-month follow-up point). However, a 6-year follow-up to mid-childhood found that more children in the intervention group had a reduction in severe symptoms compared to controls (Pickles *et al.*, 2016). There were also comparative improvements in children's communication with their parents, and parents in the intervention group reported improvements in peer relationships, social communication, and repetitive behaviors. A subsequent modeling study calculated that PACT is likely to become cost-saving by the 6-year follow-up point, particularly because it reduces the costs associated with parental support (Tinelli *et al.*, 2023).

Making trade-offs

Many evaluations of new interventions find them both more effective (the outcome profiles are better than for old/current interventions) but simultaneously more expensive. For example, one study found that a group-parenting program had better outcomes but slightly higher costs than an individual program (Cunningham *et al.*, 1995). How is the trade-off to be made between better outcomes and the higher expenditure necessary to achieve them?

The net benefit approach seeks to explicate the nature of the trade-off, and is most commonly seen in the construction of CEACs. These curves show the probability that a new intervention will be cost-effective for each of multiple prespecified or implicit valuations of an outcome improvement by the decision-maker. CEACs makes the trade-offs faced by decision-makers more transparent.

Two studies by Byford and colleagues illustrate this approach. The first example examines the cost-effectiveness of treating adolescents with major depression using selective serotonin reuptake inhibitors (SSRI) and routine specialist care alone, or in conjunction with CBT (Byford *et al.*, 2007a). The latter intervention was both more costly and less effective: adding CBT to SSRI and the usual treatment did not look economically attractive. The researchers plotted a CEAC to address uncertainty in the data—reproduced as Figure 17.3. This CEAC shows that, even at a value of £50,000 per one-point improvement in mental health (measured by the Health of the Nation Outcome Scales for Children and Adolescents (HoNOSCA)), the probability that adding CBT to SSRI treatment would be seen as cost-effective was low (only 25%). When QALYs were used to measure outcomes, the probability of adding CBT to SSRI being cost-effective was even lower, no higher than 4%.

The second study by Byford and colleagues compared three treatment options for adolescents with anorexia: inpatient psychiatric services, specialist outpatient psychiatric services, and general outpatient services (Byford *et al.*, 2007b). Specialist outpatient treatment tended to cost less and be more effective. The plotted CEAC showed that, at two-year follow-up, if a decision-maker's willingness to pay for a unit increase in Morgan–Russell Average Outcome Scale score was zero, there was a 78% probability that the specialty outpatient services would be cost-effective. At higher willingness-to-pay levels, the probability actually decreased, but specialist outpatient services remained the most cost-effective of the options.

Utility measurement

CUA measures and then values the impact of an intervention in terms of improvements in preference-weighted, health-related quality of life. The value of the quality-of-life improvement is gauged in units of "utility," usually expressed by a combined

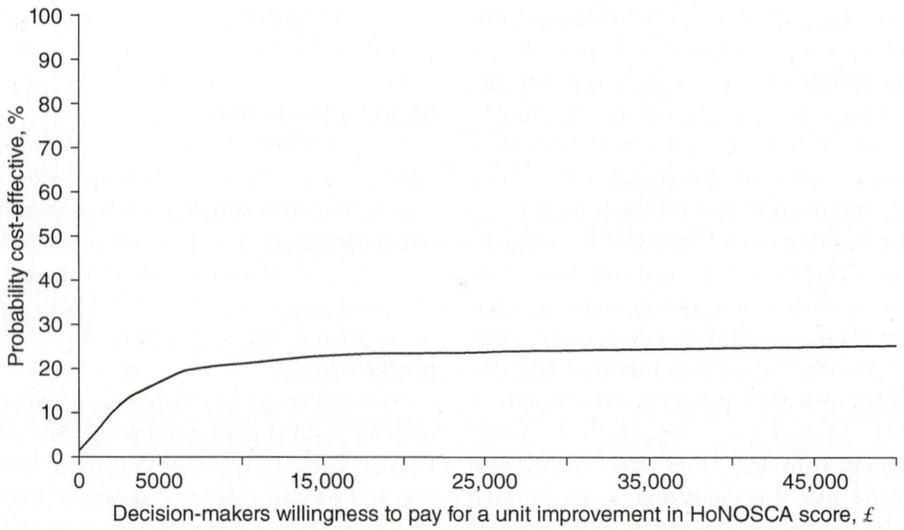

Figure 17.3 Cost-effectiveness acceptability curve for Health of the Nation Outcome Scales for Children and Adolescents (HoNOSCA) showing the probability that selective serotonin reuptake inhibitors (SSRIs) plus cognitive-behavioral therapy (CBT) is more cost-effective than SSRIs alone.

index of the mortality and quality-of-life effects of an intervention. The best known and most robust such index is the QALY.

Another generic measure sometimes used is the disability-adjusted life year (DALY) which combines reduction in life expectancy and diminished quality of life ("disability"). The aim of a health care intervention is then to avert DALYs (i.e., reduce the so-called "burden of disease") or increase QALYs (i.e., increase health-related quality of life). Although there are differences in orientation and measurement, the two approaches have the same overall aim—to provide a generic measure that can be applied across different health conditions to support strategic resource allocation decisions. QALYs are recommended by most health technology assessment agencies in high-income countries (such as NICE in England) because they use preference weights and are more sensitive to changes in health state. DALYs are more commonly used in studies conducted in LMICs, use standardized disability weights (making them easier to compute), but may not pick up small changes in health (or associated quality of life) so well (Feng *et al.*, 2020). We focus on QALYs in this chapter.

Cost-utility analyses are increasingly being used in health economics evaluations. They have some advantages, including using a unidimensional measure of impact, a generic measure which allows comparisons to be made across diagnostic or clinical groups (e.g., comparing psychiatry with oncology or cardiology) and an explicit methodology for weighting preferences and valuing health states. But these same features have sometimes been seen as disadvantages: the utility measure may be seen as too reductionist; the generic quality-of-life indicator may be insufficiently sensitive to the kinds of change expected in some mental health areas, such as schizophrenia treatment; and a transparent approach to scale construction paradoxically opens the approach to criticism from those who question the values thereby obtained. There are worries that the generic utility-generating instruments, such the EQ-5D (EuroQol Group, 1990), which is recommended by NICE, and the SF-6D (Brazier *et al.*, 2002) and HUI3 (Petrou *et al.*, 2010), are insufficiently sensitive to the symptom and functioning changes observed for people with mental health problems (Mulhern *et al.*, 2014). There are now QALY-generating tools specifically designed for mental health, such as ReQoL (Keetharuth *et al.*, 2018), and for children and youth, such as CHU9D (Stevens, 2010). Condition-specific QALY-generating tools should be more sensitive to context, but complicate strategic resource allocation decisions because different measures are being used for different conditions.

The advantage of cost-utility analyses is that they avoid potential ambiguities with multidimensional outcomes in cost-consequences studies. The transparency of the approach should generally also be welcomed. Such an approach produces an estimate of cost per QALY-gain from one intervention over another. NICE, which has responsibility in England and Wales for providing national guidance on promoting good health and preventing and treating ill health, has a well-developed process for assessing economic evidence (NICE, 2008) and cost-utility values certainly influence guideline development (NICE, 2008; Cerri *et al.* 2013).

Cost-utility analyses are becoming more common in the child and adolescent mental health area. The study by Byford *et al.* summarized above was one of the first (Byford *et al.*, 2007a). An Australian cost-utility study illustrates the importance of study perspective—something emphasized earlier in the chapter. Chatterton *et al.* investigated a stepped care approach for managing childhood anxiety (Chatterton *et al.*, 2019). Their RCT found that outcomes (QALYs) were the same between stepped care compared to a validated manualized treatment approach. Health sector costs were also the same between the two groups, but there were lower costs for the stepped care model when account was taken of lost productivity resulting from disruption to parental employment.

A final example comes from a study of cost-effectiveness of cognitive therapy as an early treatment for post-traumatic stress disorder (PTSD) for children and adolescents (Shearer *et al.*, 2018). The authors analyzed data from an RCT comparing cognitive therapy for PTSD with usual care in children and adolescents who experienced a traumatic event in the previous 2–6 months. Benefits were measured in terms of QALYs, and data on costs and QALYs were collected during the 11-week RCT and then projected over a 3-year time horizon using decision analytic modeling. Although there was uncertainty in the model when estimating over a longer time horizon, findings suggested a 60–90% probability of being cost-effective and, over 3 years, the cost of achieving an additional QALY was £2205, which is significantly below the NICE threshold of £20,000–30,000 per QALY conventionally used to decide whether to recommend an intervention for use within England's National Health Service.

There is a quandary facing researchers and decision-makers in the United Kingdom today, and in some other countries that have chosen a strategic evidence-based approach to health technology appraisal. A generic outcome measure, such as the QALY, when combined with cost estimates, can point to ways of achieving improved value for money when decisions need to be taken across a broad area (such as across a number of diagnostic areas), but if that QALY measure is not sensitive enough to reflect all relevant differences in effectiveness, then it might not be a sound enough basis for such an important task.

Benefit measurement

CBA asks whether the benefits of a treatment or policy exceed the costs, supporting cross-sector strategic decision-making. All costs and outcomes (benefits) are valued in the same (monetary) units. If benefits exceed costs, the evaluation would provide support for the treatment, and vice versa. With two or more alternatives, the treatment with the greatest net benefit would be deemed the most efficient. CBAs are intrinsically attractive but conducting them is especially problematic because of the difficulty of valuing outcomes in monetary terms.

Comparing costs incurred (e.g., on treatments) with costs saved (e.g., on future health services no longer needed) is not a CBA but a *cost-offset* comparison. This confusion is unfortunately still quite common. A CBA must measure outcomes (in terms of improved health or improved quality of life) and then convert them to monetary values. Consequently, studies such as that by Jacobson *et al.* of an early intensive behavioral program for children with pervasive development disorder (PDD) or autism, which compared the costs of the intervention with cost savings into adulthood, are certainly interesting but not as helpful as studies that compare the costs *and* the outcomes of interventions (Jacobson *et al.*, 1998). Attaching values to the outcomes of child and adolescent mental health interventions is inherently

Box 17.4 Good reporting guidelines

The CHEERS tool (Husereau *et al.*, 2022) summarizes issues to be considered when conducting an economic evaluation:

- title
- abstract
- background and objectives
- target population and subgroups
- setting and location
- study perspective
- comparators
- time horizon
- discount rate
- choice of health outcomes
- measurement of effectiveness
- measurement and valuation of preference-based outcomes
- estimating resources and costs
- currency, price date, and conversion
- choice of model
- assumptions
- analytical methods
- study parameters
- incremental costs and outcomes
- characterizing uncertainty
- characterizing heterogeneity
- study findings, limitations, generalizability, and current knowledge
- source of funding
- conflicts of interest

complicated. Health economists have suggested ways to obtain direct valuations of health outcomes by patients, relatives, or others. These techniques ask individuals to state the amount they would be prepared to pay (hypothetically) to achieve a given health state or health gain, or they observe actual behavior and impute the implicit values (Olsen & Smith, 2001). These methods may be difficult to apply in mental health contexts. Conjoint analysis is an alternative method that asks individuals to rank different "real-world" scenarios, with multiple dimensions (e.g., health outcomes, quality of life, time, discomfort, and stigma), including cost as one of these dimensions. Conjoint analysis is more complex but may be easier to administer than willingness-to-pay studies. It has the advantage of not specifically asking individuals to put a monetary value on health states or health gain, which can make the technique easier to administer than traditional willingness-to-pay studies (Ryan, 1999).

Bodies, such as NICE, provide recommendations for conducting economic evaluations. The CHEERS tool (Husereau *et al.*, 2022) summarizes considerations for conducting a good-quality economic evaluation (Box 17.4).

Conclusion

Interest in the economics of child and adolescent mental health is driven by scarcity: there are not, and there never will be, enough resources available to meet all mental health (or other) needs of all children and families. It would be irrationally utopian to imagine that incremental growth in budgets will gradually remove all need. We cannot and *must* not avoid facing up to the choices that have to be made in the face of scarcity. In making those choices we would want our decision-makers to be transparent about the criteria they are employing. For instance, are they looking to maximize effectiveness in symptom alleviation or quality of life, or to redistribute resources to poorer communities, or to equalize access to skilled resources for every family?

Within this set of criteria, cost-effectiveness obviously has a role to play. As noted earlier, it should probably be seen as secondary. If, for example, a therapeutic intervention improves the well-being of children and families and appears to be more effective than currently available therapies, then it would be natural to ask about the relative costs of the two options and compare those costs with the outcome gains. Balancing outcome improvements with higher costs is, however, quite a challenge.

Many economic evaluations across the health spectrum find that new therapies (whether pharmacological, psychological, or organizational) offer better outcome profiles than current ones, but at higher costs. The decision-maker, whether this is the individual care professional, or their line manager and budget holder, or someone near the top of the health ministry, then faces a difficult trade-off: are the better outcomes from the new intervention worth the higher cost? Indeed, there are many potential challenges in translating the findings from economic evaluations to better policy or practice. The evidence may be incomplete, may only look at short-term effects and costs, may point to interventions that are cost-effective but not deliverable (e.g., because of skilled staff), or ignore hidden impacts on families, and may be prone to disincentives linked to silo-budgeting when multiple sectors are involved (Knapp & Wong, 2020).

Heckman argues that we need a better understanding of life-course dynamics to identify optimal time points for intervention (Heckman, 2012). A developmental approach which models early, intermediate, and longer-term outcomes, and examines how interventions and consequences vary over time, would help those allocating resources to consider the relative benefits of various approaches to prevention and treatment. In addition to considering life course and timing, context is also important. Some cost-effective interventions could be prenatal, which could be important for global mental health: investing in sustainable prenatal interventions could make good economic and clinical sense (Bauer *et al.*, 2015) in LIMCs (Bauer *et al.*, 2022).

Requests for economic insights in the child and adolescent mental health field are of many kinds. We have illustrated some of them, including requests to measure the overall cost impact of a particular disorder or diagnosis. Second, there are cost-offset studies that compare the amounts expended on interventions with the longer-term savings from introducing those interventions. Third, and most powerfully, cost-effectiveness studies (using the term generically to also include the rarely feasible cost–benefit and the increasingly common cost-utility studies) weigh up and compare costs *and* outcomes, and therefore give a more complete and rounded view as to the consequences of introducing different interventions.

Most economic studies found in the international literature today are from North America, Western Europe, and Australia. Results from these studies may not transfer well to other countries because of differences in health system structure, financing arrangements, incentive structures, and relative price levels. There might also be differences in the appropriate choice of comparator: a new therapeutic approach might look attractive compared to current arrangements in one country but not in comparison to the norm elsewhere. It is infeasible and certainly unnecessary to do an evaluation for every policy decision, but evidence-based decisions are generally thought to be better than evidence-free decisions. This could mean using the results from another country, updating a previous study, or carrying out a modest adaptation to adjust for context.

The available economics evidence base in the child and adolescent mental health field is growing, but only slowly. It is disappointingly underdeveloped at present in high-income countries and mostly absent in LMICs, but more is now being invested in the area, including some new studies that will—in time—offer valuable new insights into the resource consequences and cost-effectiveness of different interventions for children and families. Further developments are also needed in response to the changing global context. For example, there has been growth in developing and implementing digital mental health care for children and adolescents, some of which was accelerated in response to restrictions in availability of face-to-face mental health care during the COVID-19 pandemic.

These solutions have the potential to improve the accessibility, affordability, and acceptability of mental health care for children and adolescents, especially for those who face barriers to more traditional services or who prefer online modes of delivery. However, the evidence base for their cost-effectiveness is particularly limited (Goldberg *et al.*, 2022), which makes this another important gap for future consideration.

There is a need to continue rigorous and comprehensive economic evaluations of child and adolescent mental health interventions so that the evidence base is relevant for broader and more diverse target groups, contexts, and types of interventions and delivery modalities. These evaluations should take account of not only their direct costs and benefits, but also their broader impacts on the quality of life, well-being, and productivity of children and adolescents and their families. Economists need to address these new challenges and opportunities from the changing global context and in collaboration with a variety of stakeholders including health professionals, individuals and families with lived experience, and other types of decision-makers.

References

Aos, S. *et al.* (2004) *Benefits and Costs of Prevention and Early Intervention Programs for Youth*. [Online]. Washington State Institute for Public Policy, Olympia, WA. Available: https://www.scirp.org/reference/ReferencesPapers.aspx?ReferenceID=2179824 [a12 May 2023].

Bauer, A. *et al.* (2015) Perinatal depression and child development: exploring the economic consequences from a South London cohort. *Psychological Medicine* **45**(1), 51–61.

Bauer, A. *et al.* (2022) Costs of common perinatal mental health problems in South Africa. *Global Mental Health* **9**, 429–438.

Beecham, J. & Knapp, M. (1999) Costing psychiatric interventions. In: *Measuring Mental Health Needs.* (eds G. Thornicroft, *et al.*). Gaskell, London. pp. 200–224.

Bonin, E.M. *et al.* (2011) Costs and longer-term savings of parenting programmes for the prevention of persistent conduct disorder: a modelling study. *BMC Public Health* **11**(1), 1–10.

Brazier, J. *et al.* (2002) The estimation of a preference-based measure of health from the SF-36. *Journal of Health Economics* **21**(2), 271–292.

Brimblecombe, N. *et al.* (2018) Long term economic impact associated with childhood bullying victimisation. *Social Science & Medicine* **208**, 134–141.

Brouwer, W. *et al.* (2001) Costing in economic evaluations. In: *Economic Evaluation in Healthcare: Merging Theory with Practice.* Oxford University Press, New York. pp. 68–93.

Buescher, A.V. *et al.* (2014) Costs of autism spectrum disorders in the United Kingdom and the United States. *JAMA Pediatrics* **168**(8), 721–728. doi:10.1001/jamapediatrics.2014.210.

Byford, S. *et al.* (2007a) Cost-effectiveness of selective serotonin reuptake inhibitors and routine specialist care with and without cognitive–behavioural therapy in adolescents with major depression. *The British Journal of Psychiatry* **191**(6), 521–527.

Byford, S. *et al.* (2007b) Economic evaluation of a randomised controlled trial for anorexia nervosa in adolescents. *The British Journal of Psychiatry* **191**, 436–440.

Byford, S. *et al.* (2015) Cost-effectiveness analysis of a communication-focused therapy for pre-school children with autism: results from a randomised controlled trial. *BMC Psychiatry* **15**(1), 316.

Cerri, K.H. *et al.* (2013) Decision making by NICE: examining the influences of evidence, process and context. *Health Economics, Policy & Law*, 1–23.

Challen, A. *et al.* (2008) *Economic Modeling for Foresight Project: Mental Capital and Wellbeing, Working paper, Centre for Economic Policy.* London School of Economics, London.

Chatterton, M.L. *et al.* (2019) Economic evaluation of stepped care for the management of childhood anxiety disorders: results from a randomised trial. *The Australian and New Zealand Journal of Psychiatry* **53**(7), 673–682.

Christensen, M.K. *et al.* (2022) The cost of mental disorders in Denmark: a register-based study. *NPJ Mental Health Research* **1**(1), 1–7.

Cidav, Z. *et al.* (2017) Cost offset associated with early start Denver model for children with autism. *Journal of the American Academy of Child and Adolescent Psychiatry* **56**(9), 777–783.

Conti, G. *et al.* (2021) The economic costs of child maltreatment in UK. *Health Economics* **30**(12), 3087–3105.

Cunningham, C.E. *et al.* (1995) Large group community-based parenting programs for families of preschoolers at risk for disruptive behaviour disorders: utilization, cost effectiveness, and outcome. *Journal of Child Psychology and Psychiatry* **36**(7), 1141–1159.

Domino, M.E. *et al.* (2009) Relative cost-effectiveness of treatments for adolescent depression: 36-week results from the TADS randomized trial. *Journal of the American Academy of Child and Adolescent Psychiatry* **48**(7), 711–720.

Drummond, M.F. *et al.* (2015) *Methods for the Economic Evaluation of Health Care Programmes*, 4th edn. Oxford University Press, Oxford, UK.

EuroQol Group (1990) EuroQol—a new facility for the measurement of health-related quality of life. *Health Policy* **16**, 199–208.

Feng, X. *et al.* (2020) Using QALYs versus DALYs to measure cost-effectiveness: how much does it matter? *International Journal of Technology Assessment in Health Care* **36**(2), 96–103.

Ford, T. *et al.* (2019) The effectiveness and cost-effectiveness of the Incredible Years® Teacher Classroom Management programme in primary school children: results of the STARS cluster randomised controlled trial. *Psychological Medicine* **49**(5), 828–842.

Goldberg, S.B. *et al.* (2022) Mobile phone-based interventions for mental health: a systematic meta-review of 14 meta-analyses of randomized controlled trials. *PLOS Digital Health* **1**(1), e0000002. [Online]

Green, J. *et al.* (2010) Parent-mediated communication-focused treatment in children with autism (PACT): a randomised controlled trial. *Lancet* **375**(9732), 2152–2160.

Gronholm, P.C. *et al.* (2022) Health service costs in adulthood associated with adolescent mental health problems in three British cohorts. *Journal of Mental Health Policy and Economics* **25**, 39–52.

Guevara, J. *et al.* (2001) Utilization and cost of health care services for children with attention-deficit/hyperactivity disorder. *Pediatrics* **108**(1), 71–78.

Heckman, J.J. (2012) The developmental origins of health. *Health Economics* **21**(1), 24–29.

Heckman, J.J. *et al.* (2010) The rate of return to the High/Scope Perry Preschool Program. *Journal of Public Economics* **94**(1–2), 114–128.

Husereau, D. *et al.* (2022) Consolidated health economic evaluation reporting standards 2022 (CHEERS 2022) statement: updated reporting guidance for health economic evaluations. *BMC Medicine* **20**, 23. doi:10.1186/s12916-021-02204-0.

Jacobson, J.W. *et al.* (1998) Cost benefit estimates for early behavioral intervention for young children with autism: general model and single state case study. *Behavioral Interventions* **13**, 201–226.

Johnston, K. *et al.* (1999) Assessing the costs of healthcare technologies in clinical trials. *Health Technology Assessment* **3**(6), 1–76.

Jones K *et al.* (2023) *Unit Costs of Health and Social Care programme (2022 - 2027).* Personal Social Services Research Unit (PSSRU), University of Kent, Canterbury, UK. Available: https://www.pssru.ac.uk/unitcostsreport/ [12 May 2023].

Kärnä, A. *et al.* (2011) Going to scale: a nonrandomized nationwide trial of the KiVa antibullying program for grades 1-9. *Journal of Consulting and Clinical Psychology* **79**(6), 796–805.

Keetharuth, A.D. *et al.* (2018) Recovering quality of life (ReQoL): a new generic self-reported outcome measure for use with people experiencing mental health difficulties. *British Journal of Psychiatry* **212**(1), 42–49.

King, D. *et al.* (2023) Effects of mental health status during adolescence on primary care costs in adulthood across three British cohorts. *Social Psychiatry and Psychiatric Epidemiology* **59**(6), 917–928.

Knapp, M. (1997) Economic evaluations and interventions for children and adolescents with mental health problems. *Journal of Child Psychology and Psychiatry* **38**(1), 3–25.

Knapp, M. & Wong, G. (2020) Economics and mental health: the current scenario. *World Psychiatry* **19**(1), 3.

Knapp, M. *et al.* (2011) Economic outcomes in adulthood and their associations with antisocial conduct, attention deficit and anxiety problems in childhood. *The Journal of Mental Health Policy and Economics* **14**(3), 137–147.

Machin, S. & McNally, S. (2008) The literacy hour. *Journal of Public Economics* **92**, 1441–1462.

Maughan, B. (1989) Growing up in the inner city: findings from the inner London longitudinal study. *Paediatric and Perinatal Epidemiology* **3**(2), 195–215.

McDaid, D. & Evans-Lacko, S. (2021) *The Case for Investing in the Mental Health and Well-being of Children, Background Paper for The State of the World's Children 2021.* UNICEF, New York.

McDaid, D. *et al.* (2017a) *Commissioning Cost-Effective Services for Promotion of Mental Health and Wellbeing and Prevention of Mental Ill-Health.* Public Health England, London. Available: https://www.gov.uk/government/publications/mental-health-services-cost-effective-commissioning [13 October 2024].

McDaid, D. *et al.* (2017b) *The Economic Case for Prevention in Young People's Mental Health: Bullying.* MQ, London.

Mulhern, B. *et al.* (2014) Using generic preference-based measures in mental health: psychometric validity of the EQ-5D and SF-6D. *The British Journal of Psychiatry* **205**(3), 236–243.

Nelson, T.D. *et al.* (2013) Psychopathology as a predictor of medical service utilization for youth in residential treatment. *The Journal of Behavioral Health Services & Research* **40**(1), 36–45.

National Institute for Health and Clinical Excellence (NICE) (2008) *Guide to the Methods of Technology Appraisal.* National Institute for Health and Clinical Excellence (NICE), London.

Office for Health Improvement and Disparities (2021) Economic evaluation: health economic studies. Office for Health Improvement and Disparities, London. Available: https://www.gov.uk/guidance/economic-evaluation-health-economic-studies.

Olsen, J.A. & Smith, R.D. (2001) Theory versus practice: a review of 'willingness-to-pay' in health and health care. *Health Economics* **10**(1), 39–52.

Organisation for Economic Cooperation and Development (2013) *PPPs and Exchange Rates* OECD, Paris. Available: https://stats.oecd.org/Index.aspx?DataSetCode=SNA_TABLE4 [11 May 2023].

Petrou, S. & Gray, A. (2011) Economic evaluation using decision analytical modelling: design, conduct, analysis, and reporting. *BMJ* **342**, d1766.

Petrou, S. *et al.* (2010) Economic costs and preference-based health-related quality of life outcomes associated with childhood psychiatric disorders. *The British Journal of Psychiatry* **197**(5), 395–404.

Pickles, A. *et al.* (2016) Parent-mediated social communication therapy for young children with autism (PACT): long-term follow-up of a randomised controlled trial. *The Lancet* **388**(10059), 2501–2509.

Ribeiro, W.S. *et al.* (2022) Influence of stigma, sociodemographic and clinical characteristics on mental health-related service use and associated costs among young people in the United Kingdom. *European Child & Adolescent Psychiatry* **32**(8), 1363–1373.

Rivenbark, J.G. *et al.* (2018) The high societal costs of childhood conduct problems: evidence from administrative records up to age 38 in a longitudinal birth cohort. *Journal of Child Psychology and Psychiatry* **59**(6), 703–710.

Rogge, N. & Janssen, J. (2019) The economic costs of autism spectrum disorder: a literature review. *Journal of Autism and Developmental Disorders* **49**(7), 2873–2900.

Romeo, R. *et al.* (2006) Economic cost of severe antisocial behaviour in children—and who pays it. *British Journal of Psychiatry* **188**, 547–553.

Ryan, M. (1999) Using conjoint analysis to take account of patient preferences and go beyond health outcomes: an application to in vitro fertilization. *Social Science & Medicine* **48**(4), 535–546.

Schneider, W. *et al.* (1997) Short- and long-term effects of training phonological awareness in kindergarten: evidence from two German studies. *Journal of Experimental Child Psychology* **66**(3), 311–340.

Scott, S. *et al.* (2001) Financial cost of social exclusion: follow up study of antisocial children into adulthood. *BMJ* **323**(7306), 191–194.

Shearer, J. *et al.* (2018) Cost-effectiveness of cognitive therapy as an early intervention for post-traumatic stress disorder in children and adolescents: a trial based evaluation and model. *Journal of Child Psychology and Psychiatry* **59**(7), 773–780.

Simon, J. *et al.* (2023) Excess resource use and costs of physical comorbidities in individuals with mental health disorders: a systematic literature review and meta-analysis. *European Neuropsychopharmacology* **66**, 14–27.

Skivington, K. *et al.* (2021) A new framework for developing and evaluating complex interventions: update of medical research council guidance. *BMJ* **374**, n206.

Snell, T. *et al.* (2013) Economic impact of childhood psychiatric disorder on public sector services in Britain: estimates from national survey data. *Journal of Child Psychology and Psychiatry* **54**(9), 977–985.

Stevens, K.J. (2010) Working with children to develop dimensions for a preference-based, generic, pediatric, health-related quality-of-life measure. *Qualitative Health Research* **20**(3), 340–351.

Thielen, F.W. *et al.* (2016) Long-term economic consequences of child maltreatment: a population-based study. *European Child & Adolescent Psychiatry* **25**, 1297–1305. doi:10.1007/s00787-016-0850-5.

Tinelli, M. *et al.* (2023) Cost-consequence analysis of early intervention for autistic children: findings from four case studies in England, Ireland, Italy and Spain. *European Psychiatry* **66**(1), e76.

Ziebold, C. *et al.* (2022) Utilisation and costs of mental health-related service use among adolescents. *PLoS One* **17**(9), e0273628.

CHAPTER 18
Public health challenges in child and adolescent mental health: dealing with global and local threats

Lucie Cluver[1,2], Isang Awah[1] and Andrea Danese[3,4,5]
[1] Department of Social Policy and Intervention, University of Oxford, Oxford, UK
[2] Department of Psychiatry and Mental Health, University of Cape Town, Cape Town, South Africa
[3] Social, Genetic and Developmental Psychiatry Centre, Institute of Psychiatry, Psychology and Neuroscience, King's College London, London, UK
[4] Department of Child and Adolescent Psychiatry, Institute of Psychiatry, Psychology and Neuroscience, King's College London, London, UK
[5] National and Specialist CAMHS Clinic for Trauma, Anxiety, and Depression, South London and Maudsley NHS Foundation Trust, London, UK

Background

Child and adolescent mental health problems are prevalent. In the United Kingdom, recent estimates suggest that one in five young people have a diagnosable mental health disorder (NHS Digital, 2022). Globally, the pooled prevalence of mental disorders in children and adolescents is 13.4% (Polanczyk *et al.*, 2015). The burden of child and adolescent mental health problems is greatest in low- and middle-income countries (LMICs) (Jorns-Presentati *et al.*, 2021), where around 90% of all children and young people live (Kieling *et al.*, 2011). LMICs are also disproportionally affected by emergencies and disasters, such as war and political violence, as well as climate- and contagion-related emergencies.

The study of trauma-related psychopathology offers a lens to understand the impact of emergencies and disasters on psychopathology. In a recent UK cohort study, 1 in 4 young people who reported exposure to traumatic events developed post-traumatic stress disorder (PTSD) by the age of 18 (Lewis *et al.*, 2019), with the highest rates among young people who reported exposure to direct, interpersonal trauma. However, PTSD was not the most common form of psychopathology in this group, as common mental health problems were also the most prevalent disorders in young people exposed to trauma: while the 12-month prevalence of PTSD in trauma-exposed children was 14%, the prevalence of depression was nearly 30%, conduct disorder (CD) 23%, and alcohol dependence 16%. Overall, these rates reflect a two to threefold increase in the prevalence of mental health problems in young people who reported exposure to traumatic events compared to peers without such experiences. Beyond psychopathology, 1 in 4 young people who reported exposure to traumatic events engaged in self-harm (two-fold increase), 1 in 12 attempted suicide (>four-fold increase), and 1 in 6 was not in education, employment, or training (NEET; two-fold increase). However, only 10% of young people who reported exposure to traumatic events sought support from a mental health professional.

In emergencies and disasters, the balance of risk and resilience is further affected (Danese *et al.*, 2020b); further discussion is presented in Chapter 41 on refugee, asylum-seeking and displaced children. On the one hand, the risk of psychopathology linked with trauma exposure is often compounded by additional risks, such as the interpersonal nature of the trauma, the accumulation of multiple traumatic experiences and daily stressors over time, and the loss or separation from loved ones (Miller & Rasmussen, 2010). On the other hand, family support may be limited by parental psychopathology and stress, and normal daily routines and activities may be disrupted by damage to infrastructure and forcible displacement.

The World Health Organization (WHO) prevalence estimates of mental disorders in conflict settings suggest that the age-specific mean prevalence of PTSD was about 15%, anxiety disorders 20%, and depression 10% in young people (Charlson *et al.*, 2019). Furthermore, a meta-analysis of mental health problems in young refugees and asylum seekers found that the prevalence of PTSD was 22.71%, anxiety disorders 15.77%, and depression 13.81% (Blackmore *et al.*, 2020). A recent study comparing affected and nonaffected areas during the early stages of the Russian invasion of Ukraine found a fourfold increase in the prevalence of PTSD and a threefold increase in the prevalence of depression and anxiety linked to the invasion (Osokina *et al.*, 2023).

Rutter's Child and Adolescent Psychiatry and Psychology, Seventh Edition.
Edited by Anita Thapar, Daniel S. Pine, Samuele Cortese, Cathy Creswell, Tamsin J. Ford, James F. Leckman, and Argyris Stringaris.

Companion website: www.wiley.com/go/thapar/rutterspsych7

Climate-related emergencies have increased, and also appear related to higher rates of psychopathology. For example, half of a small group of children exposed to Hurricane Katrina, described as one of the worst natural disasters in U.S. history, met criteria for PTSD (Scheeringa & Zeanah, 2008), and exposure was also associated with a threefold increase in the rates of emotional disorders in children and young people (McLaughlin *et al.*, 2009). In tsunami-affected areas in southern Thailand, displaced children living in camps had a twofold increase in the rate of PTSD and depression compared to peers in unaffected villages (Thienkrua *et al.*, 2006).

The COVID-19 pandemic is a recent example of a global contagion-related emergency. Looking at time trends in England, rates of probable mental disorders have increased between 2017 and 2022 from 1 in 9 (12.1%) to 1 in 6 (16.7%) in 7–16-year-olds, and from 1 in 10 (10.1%) to 1 in 4 (25.7%) in 17–19-year-olds, with the greatest increase in emotional disorders (NHS Digital, 2022). These examples highlight the significant mental health needs of young people affected by emergencies and disasters. They also demonstrate that the threats to child and adolescent mental health are both global—that is, at a worldwide scale—and local, that is, specific to a community, country, or region.

In this chapter, we will first introduce key principles for work in emergencies and disasters such as equity, scalability, and long-term support. Building on these principles, we will describe a framework for emergency preparedness and response, also considering critical issues around implementation. We will also reflect on the need for supporting responders' mental health. Finally, we will discuss future research challenges and directions.

Key principles and considerations

As climate, health, and conflict-related emergencies proliferate and become more severe (UNDP, 2022), there is a clear need for effective, scaled-up mental health support for children and adolescents (El-Khani *et al.*, 2023). But this raises an immediate set of considerations around core principles of provision. First, equity. Mental health care is insufficient everywhere, but is most scarce in LMICs (Lund *et al.*, 2010; Patel *et al.*, 2018) and in emergency contexts (Belkin *et al.*, 2017). If we are committed to mental health as a public health priority, we must consider a set of interventions that can be delivered across the Global South and North, in contexts with minimal or no mental health professionals, and weak health systems (Sherr *et al.*, 2021). Achieving equity may also require striving to develop new health services to enable the delivery of the most effective, evidence-based clinical interventions through innovative approaches.

Second, there is growing critique of short-term responses in emergency contexts for their lack of comprehensive and sustainable solutions for long-term recovery (Harris, 2021). Both immediate support and stable, long-term provision is needed. Third, we need to consider whether mental health support is targeted or universal. Ideally, mental health support is tailored to different needs, but there are substantial added challenges of delivering differentiated interventions in crisis contexts. There is increasing evidence that universally delivered light-touch interventions can be feasible and effective in low-resource settings (Lund, 2018), and may support a "pyramid" approach with targeted, more intensive support for the most vulnerable (Cluver *et al.*, 2022b).

Especially vulnerable groups may include children with pre-existing mental health problems, children with disabilities, those exposed directly to violence, refugee and migrant children, and children living on the streets (Watters & O'Callaghan, 2016; Fellmeth *et al.*, 2018; Buckley *et al.*, 2020). These children are often harder to find and reach than general populations, and mental health care for these groups may be ideally delivered through more specialist services. However, the scalability and durability of intensive and targeted interventions remains a major challenge, especially in contexts of low resources, rural areas, and where there are few or no mental health workers.

Emergency preparedness

Emergencies and disasters may occur suddenly and require resources to be mobilized rapidly. It is important to invest in advance planning to enable adequate delivery of care. Emergency preparedness includes the actions that can be taken to ensure that "emergency planning enables the effective and efficient prevention, reduction, control, mitigation of, and response to emergencies" (NHS England, n.d.). While the details of the advance plans may vary based on the assets available in different countries, there are some essential elements that can be used to develop local frameworks: building resources, reducing barriers, coordinating actions, and evaluating outcomes.

To begin with, it is essential to build sufficient child and adolescent mental health resources. The resilience of mental health systems amidst emergencies and disasters is a function of their strength during "peacetime." Specialist child and adolescent mental health services are vastly underdeveloped and underresourced around the world, and local investment in training and capacity building is necessary to develop local expertise and leadership. Because trauma-related psychopathology is both prevalent (Lewis *et al.*, 2019) and poorly diagnosed and treated (Danese *et al.*, 2020a), even in high-income countries, and likely to account for a significant burden of mental health problems during emergencies and disasters (Charlson *et al.*, 2019; Blackmore *et al.*, 2020), training needs to include assessment of the psychological responses to trauma, and the ability to deliver evidence-based treatments. It is very unlikely that specialist services will ever be able to provide sufficient levels of care to address the needs in the population, and stepped-care models can expand capacity to nonspecialist care workers. As such, it is similarly important to identify and train lay workers to provide nonspecialist mental health care (Tol *et al.*, 2011), for example, considering the materials provided by the Inter-Agency Standing Committee (IASC) Reference Group on Mental Health and Psychosocial Support (MHPSS) in Emergency Settings (MHPSS, n.d.). Finally, it is helpful to prepare in advance accessible materials based on evidence that can be rapidly disseminated in the population through written leaflets, traditional media, and social media directly to young people and their families (see "Implementation principles" section below).

To ensure that these resources can reach children, young people, and families, it is important to map and address barriers in health-care utilization (Gulliver *et al.*, 2010; Danese *et al.*, 2020a). Some of the barriers may be psychological, related to common reactions to psychological trauma (e.g., avoidance, distrust). Others may be cultural, including limited access to mental health knowledge or stigma around mental illness. And yet others may be structural, for example, limited availability of local-language resources or lack of transportation. The involvement of the local communities and stakeholders is necessary to develop acceptable and feasible plans to address barriers.

The implementation of emergency plans requires significant coordination of resources and agencies, which needs to be considered in advance. It is important to identify local and national experts in child and adolescent mental health who can provide leadership and guidance. Furthermore, it is important to test and resolve issues of jurisdiction, data sharing, and quality assurance for collaborative work across health services, police, and the third sector, including international aid organizations. Finally, because the evidence base in this area is limited, it is important to plan continued evaluation in order to identify helpful and unhelpful practices and consequently adapt delivery.

Scalable mental health interventions

The IASC guidelines on *Mental Health and Psychosocial Support in Emergency Settings* were developed to plan and coordinate minimum responses in crisis contexts (Inter-agency Standing Committee, 2007). The guidelines outline a pyramid of responses at different levels to meet not only the needs of different groups, but also the needs of a range of disorders, prevalence, and severity (Figure 18.1). Each layer represents a smaller proportion of the affected population. The first—universal—layer highlights basic services such as food, water, and safety. The second layer focuses on identifying and supporting family-based and community-based support for mental health. This includes services such as family reunification, parenting programs, and youth groups. The third layer includes focused support, delivered primarily by nonspecialists such as community workers, and mental health first aid delivered through the primary health care system. The top layer of the pyramid focuses on specialized services for those experiencing very severe mental health distress or those with preexisting severe mental disorders. It recommends referral to specialized mental health services if those exist, or long-term training and supervision of primary health care workers.

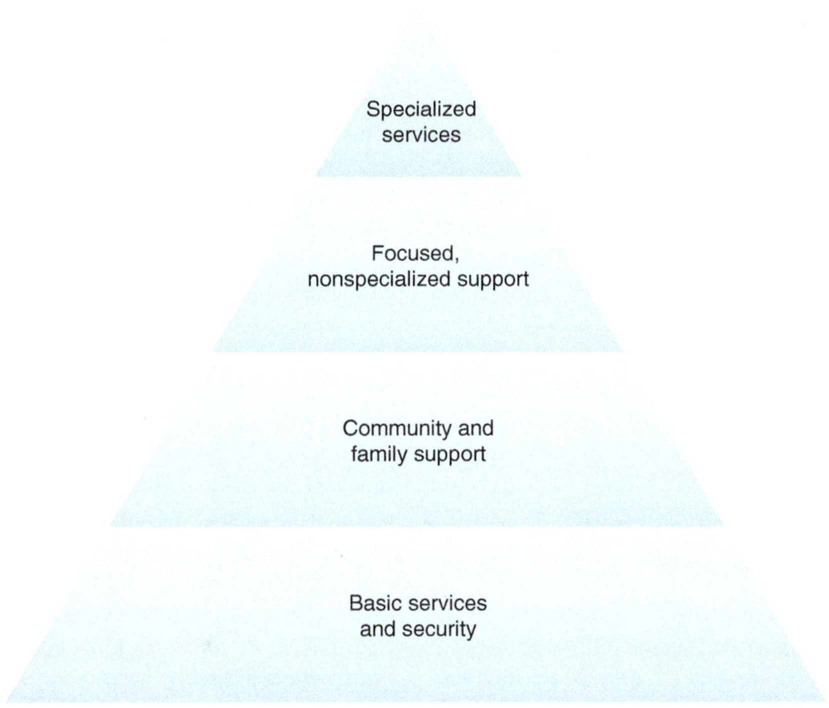

Figure 18.1 Intervention pyramid for mental health and psychosocial support in emergencies.

This pyramid reflects a global necessity to deliver evidence-based mental health care through differentiated approaches. There remains a stark gap in child and adolescent mental health services across most settings (Patel *et al.*, 2007; Jörns-Presentati *et al.*, 2021), and scarcity of psychiatric professionals in the Global South: for example, ratios are 1 mental health worker per 140,000 people in the African WHO region (Lund, 2018). There is increasing evidence for broadened approaches to provision, for example, the Programme for Improving Mental Health Care (Lund *et al.*, 2012), which worked with ministries of health and partners in five Global South countries to integrate evidence-based psychosocial and pharmacological interventions into existing primary health care systems using WHO's Mental Health Gap Action Programme (mhGAP) guidelines (Lund *et al.*, 2016). Recently, the WHO established a population-level action plan to integrate mental health service provision for children and adolescents in the Global South (WHO, 2018).

There is increasing evidence for self-help and psychoeducation services, for example, self-help problem-solving booklets (guided by trained community workers, or self-guided) were found to reduce mental health problems among vulnerable adolescents in a low-resource setting in India (Michelson *et al.*, 2020). However, none of these approaches alone will be sufficient to reach across the population of children and adolescents who require mental health support in the context of threats, and innovative system-level combinations may be the way forward.

Where there are no services

During humanitarian crises, access to essential health care services can be hampered by displacement, remoteness, insecurity, or access constraints (Bamforth, 2022). Nonetheless, parents and caregivers can provide mental health and psychosocial support for children and adolescents through positive parenting (Reed *et al.*, 2012). Although caregivers' own exposure to trauma could be a source of risk (Tol *et al.*, 2013) and are associated with a higher risk of harsh parenting resulting in increased child mental health problems (Bryant *et al.*, 2018, Sim *et al.*, 2018), parenting interventions can provide psychosocial support for parents and caregivers, improve parenting, and consequently improve the well-being of parents and children in emergency contexts including natural disasters (Cobham *et al.*, 2018), conflict (El-Khani *et al.*, 2020), and health emergencies (Sherr *et al.*, 2022). Mental health and psychosocial support for parents and caregivers could be channeled through innovative mechanisms of delivery such as social media (Cluver *et al.*, 2020; Sherr *et al.*, 2022) and routine food delivery (El-Khani *et al.*, 2016), and through collaborations with the faith sector and private sector (Sherr *et al.*, 2022).

The mental health of children and adolescents affected by humanitarian crises could also be improved through psychological first aid (Simonds *et al.*, 2022), family-based interventions (Frounfelker *et al.*, 2019), child-friendly spaces (Borja Jr. *et al.*, 2019; Metzler *et al.*, 2019), and school-based interventions (Sim *et al.*, 2018) including emergency education programs that integrate psychosocial support (Thienou, 2022). However, the evidence is still emerging. For instance, OperationSAFE, designed to reduce PTSD symptoms in children exposed to community trauma, was found to improve child mental health in five Asian countries (Simonds *et al.*, 2022). However, the intervention is yet to be tested in controlled studies.

Task-sharing may be a key tool (Frounfelker *et al.*, 2019; Sherr *et al.*, 2022; Simonds *et al.*, 2022). A parenting intervention that was effective in preventing child maltreatment and improving parental and child mental health among Syrian refugees in Lebanon was delivered by local International Rescue Committee staff and refugee volunteers who were given short but relevant trainings (Sim *et al.*, 2021). Similarly, the COVID-19 parenting resources (Box 18.1) were successfully delivered by nonhealth specialists (Sherr *et al.*, 2022). Effective interventions could be scaled within programs by humanitarian organizations. However, sustaining lay workers is challenging and there is need to explore ways to better support their commitment and retention (Padmanathan & De Silva, 2013).

Another innovative strategy is the provision of shorter interventions. For example, single session interventions, which focus on delivering key elements of evidence-based treatments in a single installment, were effectively implemented during the COVID-19 pandemic (Schleider *et al.*, 2022) and used in LMICs (Osborn *et al.*, 2020).

Stepping up mental health care delivery

To achieve equity, it is also important to consider how effective, evidence-based interventions can be scaled up through innovative approaches, in order to support young people with key risk factors or more severe clinical presentations. It is valuable to consider how this more vulnerable group can be identified through systematic screening of trauma-exposed young people, using brief history-taking and short, validated questionnaires (e.g., the Children's Revised Impact of Event Scale, and the Strengths and Difficulties Questionnaire) (see Box 18.2 for an implementation example).

As detailed in the PTSD chapter in this book, Chapter 58, the strongest evidence for efficacy in the treatment of young people with trauma-related psychopathology is for individual delivery of trauma-focused cognitive-behavioral therapy (TF-CBT) (NICE, 2018), which is not only effective in treating PTSD but also in reducing comorbid anxiety and depressive symptoms. Individual eye movement desensitization and reprocessing (EMDR) has also shown some evidence of efficacy (de Roos *et al.*, 2017). However, individual treatment is unlikely to be feasible in large-scale emergencies and disasters, even in high-income countries. Initial evidence suggests that these interventions can be provided within groups to improve scalability (Davis *et al.*, 2023). Only some of these group interventions were delivered by lay providers, and there are concerns of reduced effectiveness than those delivered by professionals (Venturo-Conerly *et al.*, 2022). It is important to establish the

Box 18.1 Emergency mental health responses during COVID-19

As the world went into lockdown in March 2020, 1.8 billion children were out of school and restricted to their homes, in the context of a health and economic emergency. This presented a major risk for mental health and household-level violence. Good parenting and positive family functioning can act as a buffer for mental health risks (Prime *et al.*, 2020; Kreniske *et al.*, 2019), and there was an urgent need for evidence-based mental health and violence prevention support for families that could be delivered remotely and rapidly (Pedersen *et al.*, 2019).

Globally, Parenting for Lifelong Health brought together a coalition of UN agencies, including the United Nations Children's Fund (UNICEF) and WHO, to adapt parenting programs that had been tested in 15 randomized trials in LMICs (Ward *et al.*, 2019; Lachman *et al.*, 2021) into open-source brief resources (Cluver *et al.*, 2020). These included mindfulness techniques for adults to reduce parenting stress and boost mental health (Williams and Kuyken, 2012), daily strategies to improve caregiver–child relationships, such as five minutes of one-to-one time, and simple breathing techniques to de-escalate conflict.

From 2020–2022, these were shared in multiple formats—from WHO's global Viber account, to loudspeakers in 27,000 villages in Laos, to radio programs in Malawi—to 210 million people in 198 countries (Perks & Cluver, 2020). Over 250 nongovernmental organizations distributed the resources, and 34 governments used them in their national COVID responses. Pre-post and retrospective studies, as well as qualitative evaluation in 10 countries showed positive impacts on parental mental health and reduced violence against children (Sherr *et al.*, 2022). These resources have subsequently been adapted for the Ukraine war, floods in Pakistan, and earthquake survivors in Syria and Turkey, reaching over 15 million people (Cluver *et al.*, 2022a). However, further evidence-building is essential to refine and improve effectiveness and delivery mechanisms for light-touch, family-based mental health support in crisis contexts.

In the United Kingdom, basic aspects of behavioral activation (BA) for depression were presented in a BBC Bitesize blog: *How to boost positivity for your family at home* (www.bbc.co.uk/bitesize/articles/zykkvwx). Furthermore, key elements from evidence-based parenting interventions for emotional and behavioral problems were adapted for media dissemination using animations and voiceovers from well-known parents in the *Families Under Pressure* series (https://maudsleycharity.org/familiesunderpressure-emotions), which was then adapted and translated in Australia and Germany.

The delivery of mental health support for adolescents needs to account for special considerations: adolescents cannot be treated as passive recipients of expert advice as they strive to separate from their parents and gain agency; they can be withdrawn and difficult to reach through conventional services, and highly sensitive to the cultural norms of the society they live in, including stigma. Projects targeting adolescents need to account for these factors. For example, the *KeepCool* project (www.kcl.ac.uk/research/keepcool), which was built around codevelopment and coproduction, was delivered through popular social media platforms, and focused on universal emotional experiences of anxiety, anger, and sadness, reaching almost 1 million adolescents.

Box 18.2 Response to terrorism and war in Europe

Digital delivery provides a possible approach to population-level mental health support in contexts of global and local threats, with emerging evidence suggesting potential effectiveness, but almost no evidence from LMICs (Lehtimaki *et al.*, 2021). WHO systematic reviews find that digitally-delivered parenting programs have similar effectiveness to in-person versions (Gardner *et al.*, 2021). There is also initial evidence that self-guided digital mental health interventions targeting symptoms of PTSD and depression may be effective (Merry *et al.*, 2012; Ruggiero *et al.*, 2015; Kassam-Adams *et al.*, 2016). However, a key concern remains on the digital divide, and often the most vulnerable children and families are the ones who lack access to digital capacity, internet access, and literacy. If we are to deliver mental health care at scale through remote platforms, it must be offline-first, open-source, and locally adaptable.

It is important to plan routine screening of young people involved in terrorist attacks and provide treatment when necessary (Whalley & Brewin, 2007). One such screen-and-treat program was commissioned by the UK Government and undertaken by the South London and Maudsley (SLaM) NHS Foundation Trust after the terrorist attacks in Tunisia, Paris, and Brussels in 2015–2016 (Gobin *et al.*, 2018).

Stage 1 included completion of a brief questionnaire returned to the screening team at Public Health England (PHE), using the parent-completed Children's Revised Impact of Event Scale (Perrin *et al.*, 2005) and Diagnostic Infant and Preschool Assessment (Scheeringa & Haslett, 2010). In Stage 2, children and young people who screened positive on the questionnaire underwent a more detailed clinical assessment led by SLaM. Treatment was arranged through the local NHS-run Child and Adolescent Mental Health Services, with regular clinical supervision provided by SLaM personnel by phone, if requested.

Based on this work, in order to improve detection of mental illness in children and young people affected by terrorist attacks, future programs should implement a more comprehensive and proactive screening of all young people in the identified families with self-completed measures and provide brief psychoeducation materials about the impact of trauma on children.

right balance between efficacy and scalability in different emergency scenarios (Lewis & Danese, 2023). Further discussion is presented in the low resources setting chapter in this book, Chapter 46.

Implementation principles

Global threats may bring new opportunities for nonproprietary and collaborative responses. Increasingly, mental health and family strengthening services for LMIC contexts and in humanitarian situations are using open-source approaches. For example, evidence-based resources are freely available from the International Rescue Committee, UNICEF, and WHO (International Rescue Committee, 2016; WHO, 2019; UNICEF and WHO, 2022), and the IASC's Reference Group on Mental Health and Psychosocial Support in Emergency Settings shares local language resources across agencies in contexts such as natural disasters and conflict.

A key principle of mental health support in contexts of global and local threats is to ensure availability of services and resources in all local languages and dialects, and this can require rapid coordination of translation, and supporting local organizations with rapid mental health training and supervision (Box 18.3).

Box 18.3 Examples of mental health care delivered during contexts of armed conflict

In South Sudan, a locally-led USAID/PEPFAR-supported program provides psychosocial counseling and parenting programs to adolescents and their families living with HIV (Janowski *et al.*, 2021). In northern Nigeria, nongovernmental organizations (NGOs) like the International Organization of Migration (IOM) and *Médecins du Monde* (MDM) have been instrumental in responding to the mental health needs of adolescents affected by the Boko Haram insurgency. These organizations have trained frontline health workers in internally displaced persons camps and host communities using the WHO mhGAP *Humanitarian Intervention Guide* (WHO & UNHCR, 2015).

Also important is local contextual adaptation—which needs to be balanced with maintaining core components of evidence-based mental health content (Castro *et al.*, 2004). The extent and type of adaptation can vary by context, but examples include adjustments for relevant customs, such as traditions around children's involvement in burial and grieving rituals. In many contexts across the Global South and North, inclusion of religious or spiritual content is considered valuable or essential in supporting mental health, and this can require careful engagement and collaboration to ensure that services are not only effective, but also inclusive and nondiscriminatory. "Surface level" adaptations are also often considered important, such as visual resources reflecting local clothing. There can be challenges in recruiting and retaining families into programs that lack cultural sensitivity (Kumpfer *et al.*, 2002).

More broadly, collaboration and coproduction with implementing organizations and practitioners is important to increase relevance, uptake, and scalability of mental health and psychosocial support. The IASC guidelines emphasize key principles of building local capacity, supporting self-help, and strengthening resources already present, even in the early stages of an emergency (Inter-agency Standing Committee, 2007). They also emphasize the goal of building capacity in government and civil society. Such partnership has resulted in increased innovation and integration of mental health resources and training into other systems and services, for example, the United Nations Office on Drugs and Crime (UNODC)'s provision of evidence-based parenting resources wrapped around daily bread provisions in Syria (El-Khani *et al.*, 2016). Recently, there has been progress in combining evidence-based services for associated challenges to mental health—for example, the International Rescue Committee's program effectively combined prevention of violence against children and intimate partner violence (Falb et al., 2023).

Public and population health responses

Mental health distress may also be reduced through services that reduce stressors on children, adolescents, and their families. For example, social protection services such as cash transfers for poverty reduction and for crisis responses have been shown to improve child and adolescent mental health outcomes (Zimmerman *et al.*, 2021) across low-, middle-, and high-income countries (Zaneva *et al.*, 2022). Access to education or remote education may be essential for children to maintain hope for their futures, especially in protracted emergencies (Aber *et al.*, 2021). Access to sexual and reproductive health care is crucial for adolescent girls. In particular, those with long-term negative mental health impacts of unwanted pregnancy and HIV-infection (Toska *et al.*, 2020; Steventon Roberts *et al.*, 2022). These examples suggest an approach to mental health care that not only goes beyond a practitioner–patient model, but also suggests opportunities to provide combined services that may maximize effectiveness. For example, emergency social protection services are increasingly provided through mobile technology, as are innovative mental health services. These could be bundled to give "cash plus care" protection to the most vulnerable.

Supporting responders' mental health

The critical work of emergency responders can have a heavy mental health toll through compounded effects of exposure to high levels of distress and loss of important resilience factors. While supporting others during emergencies and disasters, responders can be directly affected by traumatic events, such as loss. They can witness war atrocities or the life-changing consequences of natural disasters. They can be indirectly exposed to aversive details of the trauma through their work. They can also face situations that deeply violate their conscience or threaten their core values, for example, grappling with avoidable limitations in resources or staffing during the pandemic response, leading to moral injuries. At the same time, because of the restriction in activities and the difficult living circumstances, responders may be unable to engage in heathy behaviors, such as adequate diet, sufficient sleep, social interaction, or other regular positive activities. All these conditions have been linked to increased risk of mental health problems ranging from PTSD, anxiety, depression, substance misuse, and others (Benedek *et al.*, 2007; Williamson *et al.*, 2018; Kisely *et al.*, 2020).

Warning signs for mental health problems often include: distress, loss of interest in previously enjoyable activities, irritability/anger outbursts, intrusive thoughts, distressing thoughts about work or the future, poor attention, insomnia, fatigue, poor appetite, poor diet, social isolation, and alcohol consumption. It is important to support mental health screening of emergency responders (Brackbill *et al.*, 2009), and provide access to specialist services (Danese *et al.*, 2020b). It is also important to map and minimize the barriers that emergency responders often face in seeking help. These may include difficulties in scheduling an appointment, not knowing where to get help, concerns about confidentiality, and fear that seeking psychological services would have a negative impact on one's career, or perceived stigma, for example, through feelings of negative judgment from co-workers and leadership (Haugen *et al.*, 2017).

To build emotional resilience and cope with distress, it is essential to look after physical health, for example, balanced diet, sufficient sleep, and regular physical activity. It is also important to maintain social connections with family and friends, even if only phone/video calls may be possible. Similarly, it is important to continue meaningful positive activities, and other coping strategies through psychological first aid training (WHO, 2011). For example, it can be helpful to use relaxation techniques (e.g., breathing exercises, muscle relaxation) and grounding techniques to cope with acute distress, and have a regular practice of journaling and mindfulness, self-compassion, and kindness. Any of these activities take time, but their mental health benefits will also likely be reflected in increased productivity and capacity to support long-term responses.

Research challenges and directions

The importance of mental health and psychosocial support in contexts of local and global threats is now widely recognized (Mohan *et al.*, 2022). The evidence-base is slowly increasing for psychological and psychosocial interventions for children affected by humanitarian emergencies (Purgato *et al.*, 2018; Barbui *et al.*, 2020) but still lags behind the number of randomized trials in noncrisis contexts, and behind the evidence for adults. Much of the evidence is from randomized controlled trials (RCTs) conducted in noncrisis situations (Cluver *et al.*, 2018; Skar *et al.*, 2021), and evidence from humanitarian settings is limited both in quantity and quality (Blanchet *et al.*, 2017). For example, although war has affected several Middle Eastern countries for decades, a recent systematic review of PTSD interventions for children and adolescents affected by war in LMICs in the Middle East highlights few available RCTs and scant evidence for effective treatment options (Alzaghoul *et al.*, 2022).

Research in humanitarian contexts is challenging for several reasons. First, there are concerns about conducting randomized trials in humanitarian settings with huge need and urgency for relief aid. Second, traditional research designs may not be feasible in humanitarian settings, and study designs may require changes with little notice (Kohrt *et al.*, 2019). Additionally, challenges faced by potential participants make them particularly vulnerable to harm, burden, or undue influence in research (Seagle *et al.*, 2020), further creating a tension between the need to develop evidence-based emergency health measures and the need to protect vulnerable populations (Leaning, 2001). The possibility that talking about traumatic experiences could reactivate in participants' distressing accounts of trauma has also been raised (Ford *et al.*, 2009; El-Khani *et al.*, 2013), with recommendations to do so in the context of safe therapeutic settings.

Third, while longitudinal evidence could help in understanding, measuring, and addressing the long-term impact of humanitarian crises (Metzler *et al.*, 2023), high levels of movement and migration make long-term follow-up challenging. There may be opportunities to utilize recent advances in quasi-experimental designs that boost causal inference while reducing some of the complexities associated with randomization. Support for evaluation of existing mental health services in crisis contexts would be valuable.

Other challenges with research in humanitarian settings include limited capacity to provide scientific and technical guidance and monitor research ethics, lack of infrastructure and human resources which could limit both access to populations over time and the ability to conduct research, and political pressure and barriers to research, especially in cases where study findings might be sensitive (Ford *et al.*, 2009). Having to coordinate with many local and international actors and stakeholders who are rapidly changing also presents challenges, as does the very limited funding opportunities for humanitarian research.

However, humanitarian health is integral to global health, and humanitarian research is needed to determine which mental health interventions are most effective for children and adolescents, when new or adapted interventions are needed, and how best to deliver care in crisis settings (Kohrt *et al.*, 2019). Researchers should use flexible and adaptive methodologies, including RCTs when feasible, while maintaining rigor and quality as much as possible (Kohrt *et al.*, 2019). Other research actors, including ethical review boards, funders, and journal publishers, should be advised on the need for flexible and adaptive methodologies in these settings (El-Khani *et al.*, 2013; Kohrt *et al.*, 2019).

There are some clear directions for future research. First, to build a robust evidence base for mental health and psychosocial interventions that are delivered at scale in the contexts of global threats. The COVID-19 crisis has demonstrated that there is a need to move beyond a reliance on specialist mental health practitioners when large-scale emergencies occur. Second, there is a need for evidence that has long-term follow-up of the impacts of interventions delivered in crisis contexts and allows understanding of effects (or lack of effects) on children and adolescents as they develop and become adults. Third, the development and use of digital mental health interventions in recent years (Wright *et al.*, 2023) also calls for research into how digital tools can be used to promote child and adolescent mental health in the context of emergencies and disasters (Danese *et al.*, 2024).

Other important recommendations for humanitarian research include engaging with affected communities, local leadership, early stakeholder engagement, leveraging existing tools and networks, building local and global humanitarian research capacity, validating survey tools, establishing clear protocols, respecting cultural norms, avoiding retraumatization, collaborating across disciplines, and building collaborative partnerships between academic institutions and humanitarian organizations (Ford *et al.*, 2009; Kohrt *et al.*, 2019; Seagle *et al.*, 2020). Research collaborations could also occur among health care systems, community, and faith-based organizations, state and local public health departments, and relevant federal and international agencies. These collaborations could increase information sharing and influence policy makers (Payton *et al.*, 2022). There could be substantial value in centers of excellence for mental health support for children and adolescents in crisis contexts: to conduct research, and train practitioners and academics. Addressing mental health during global threats may be the next, essential frontier challenge for child and adolescent mental health services.

Acknowledgments

With thanks to Dr. Bothaina Eltigani for literature reviews and support in the writing of this manuscript, and to Jenny Chen-Charles for editing and reviewing.

References

Aber, J.L. *et al.* (2021) Children's learning and development in conflict- and crisis-affected countries: building a science for action. *Development and Psychopathology* **33**, 506–521.

Alzaghoul, A.F. *et al.* (2022) Post-traumatic stress disorder interventions for children and adolescents affected by war in low- and middle-income countries in the Middle East: systematic review. *British Journal of Psychiatry Open* **8**, e153.

Bamforth, L. (2022) *Providing Emergency Health in Humanitarian Emergencies* [Online]. Available: https://www.medair.org/stories/providing-emergency-health-in-humanitarian-emergencies [1 March 2023].

Barbui, C. *et al.* (2020) Efficacy of psychosocial interventions for mental health outcomes in low-income and middle-income countries: an umbrella review. *The Lancet Psychiatry* **7**, 162–172.

Belkin, G. *et al.* (2017) Converging on child mental health: toward shared global action for child development. *Global Mental Health* **4**, e20.

Benedek, D.M. *et al.* (2007) First responders: mental health consequences of natural and human-made disasters for public health and public safety workers. *Annual Review of Public Health* **28**, 55–68.

Blackmore, R. *et al.* (2020) Systematic review and meta-analysis: the prevalence of mental illness in child and adolescent refugees and asylum seekers. *Journal of the American Academy of Child and Adolescent Psychiatry* **59**, 705–714.

Blanchet, K. *et al.* (2017) Evidence on public health interventions in humanitarian crises. *The Lancet* **390**, 2287–2296.

Borja, A., Jr. *et al.* (2019) Child-centred, cross-sectoral mental health and psychosocial support interventions in the Rohingya response: a field report by save the children. *Intervention* **17**, 231–237.

Brackbill, R.M. *et al.* (2009) Asthma and posttraumatic stress symptoms 5 to 6 years following exposure to the World Trade Center terrorist attack. *JAMA* **302**, 502–516.

Bryant, R.A. *et al.* (2018) The effect of post-traumatic stress disorder on refugees' parenting and their children's mental health: a cohort study. *The Lancet Public Health* **3**, e249–e258.

Buckley, N. *et al.* (2020) Prevalence estimates of mental health problems in children and adolescents with intellectual disability: a systematic review and meta-analysis. *The Australian and New Zealand Journal of Psychiatry* **54**, 970–984.

Castro, F. *et al.* (2004) The cultural adaptation of prevention interventions: resolving tensions between fidelity and fit. *Prevention Science* **5**, 41–45.

Charlson, F. *et al.* (2019) New WHO prevalence estimates of mental disorders in conflict settings: a systematic review and meta-analysis. *The Lancet* **394**, 240–248.

Cluver, L.D. *et al.* (2018) Parenting for lifelong health: a pragmatic cluster randomised controlled trial of a non-commercialised parenting programme for adolescents and their families in South Africa. *BMJ Global Health* **3**, e000539.

Cluver, L. *et al.* (2020) Parenting in a time of COVID-19. *The Lancet* **395**, e64.

Cluver, L. *et al.* (2022a) Ukraine's children: use evidence to support child protection in emergencies. *BMJ* **376**, o781.

Cluver, L.D. *et al.* (2022b) From surviving to thriving: integrating mental health care into HIV, community, and family services for adolescents living with HIV. *The Lancet Child & Adolescent Health* **6**, 582–592.

Cobham, V.E. *et al.* (2018) Parenting support in the context of natural disaster. In: *The Power of Positive Parenting: Transforming the Lives of Children, Parents, and Communities Using the Triple P System.* (eds M.R. Sanders & T.G. Mazzucchelli). Oxford University Press, New York. pp. 272–283.

Danese, A. *et al.* (2020a) Psychopathology in children exposed to trauma: detection and intervention needed to reduce downstream burden. *BMJ* **371**, m3073.

Danese, A. *et al.* (2020b) Child and adolescent mental health amidst emergencies and disasters. *The British Journal of Psychiatry* **216**, 159–162.

Danese, A. *et al.* (2024) Scoping review: Digital mental health interventions for children and adolescents affected by war. *Journal of the American Academy of Child & Adolescent Psychiatry.* doi:10.1016/j.jaac.2024.02.017.

Davis, R.S. *et al.* (2023) Meta-analytic review: group-based interventions for treating posttraumatic stress symptoms in children and adolescents. *Journal of the American Academy of Child and Adolescent Psychiatry* **62**, 1217–1232.

de Roos, C. *et al.* (2017) Comparison of eye movement desensitization and reprocessing therapy, cognitive behavioral writing therapy, and wait-list in pediatric posttraumatic stress disorder following single-incident trauma: a multicenter randomized clinical trial. *Journal of Child Psychology and Psychiatry* **58**, 1219–1228.

El-Khani, A. *et al.* (2023) Urgent help needed for children affected by the earthquake in Syria and Turkiye. *The Lancet Psychiatry* **10**, 246–247.

El-Khani, A. *et al.* (2013) Ethical issues in research into conflict and displacement. *The Lancet* **382**, 764–765.

El-Khani, A. *et al.* (2016) Daily bread: a novel vehicle for dissemination and evaluation of psychological first aid for families exposed to armed conflict in Syria. *Global Mental Health* **3**, e15.

El-Khani, A. *et al.* (2020) Caregiving for children through conflict and displacement: a pilot study testing the feasibility of delivering and evaluating a light touch parenting intervention for caregivers in the West Bank. *International Journal of Psychology* **55**(Suppl 1), 26–39.

Falb, K.L. *et al.* (2023) Improving family functioning and reducing violence in the home in north Kivu, Democratic Republic of Congo: a pilot cluster-randomised controlled trial of safe at home. *BMJ Open* **13**, e065759.

Fellmeth, G. *et al.* (2018) Health impacts of parental migration on left-behind children and adolescents: a systematic review and meta-analysis. *The Lancet* **392**, 2567–2582.

Ford, N. *et al.* (2009) Ethics of conducting research in conflict settings. *Conflict and Health* **3**, 7.

Frounfelker, R.L. *et al.* (2019) Living through war: mental health of children and youth in conflict-affected areas. *International Review of the Red Cross* **101**, 481–506.

Gardner, F. *et al.* (2021) *Global Review of Evidence for the WHO Parenting Program Guidelines Process*. WHO, Geneva, Switzerland.

Gobin, M. *et al.* (2018) Outcomes of mental health screening for United Kingdom nationals affected by the 2015-2016 terrorist attacks in Tunisia, Paris, and Brussels. *Journal of Traumatic Stress* **31**, 471–479.

Gulliver, A. *et al.* (2010) Perceived barriers and facilitators to mental health help-seeking in young people: a systematic review. *BMC Psychiatry* **10**, 113.

Harris, D. (2021) *Rapid emergency and humanitarian responses: how fast is fast enough?* Oxford Policy Management. [Online]. Available: www.opml.co.uk/blog/rapid-emergency-humanitarian-responses-how-fast-enough [22 September 2023].

Haugen, P.T. *et al.* (2017) Mental health stigma and barriers to mental health care for first responders: a systematic review and meta-analysis. *Journal of Psychiatric Research* **94**, 218–229.

Inter-Agency Standing Committee (2007) *Guidelines on Mental Health and Psychosocial Sup-port in Emergency Settings*. UNGA, New York.

International Rescue Committee (2016) Parenting Skills Trainers Manuals. Available: https://inee.org/sites/default/files/resources/IRCJ4060_PAR_Training_Manual_220616_clean.pdf [25 September 2024].

Janowski, R. *et al.* (2021) Transferability of evidence-based parenting programs to routine implementation in postconflict South Sudan. *Research on Social Work Practice* **30**, 858–869.

Jörns-Presentati, A. *et al.* (2021) The prevalence of mental health problems in sub-Saharan adolescents: a systematic review. *PLoS One* **16**, e0251689.

Kassam-Adams, N. *et al.* (2016) Pilot randomized controlled trial of a novel web-based intervention to prevent posttraumatic stress in children following medical events. *Journal of Pediatric Psychology* **41**, 138–148.

Kieling, C. *et al.* (2011) Child and adolescent mental health worldwide: evidence for action. *The Lancet* **378**, 1515–1525.

Kisely, S. *et al.* (2020) Occurrence, prevention, and management of the psychological effects of emerging virus outbreaks on healthcare workers: rapid review and meta-analysis. *BMJ* **369**, m1642.

Kohrt, B.A. *et al.* (2019) Health research in humanitarian crises: an urgent global imperative. *BMJ Global Health* **4**, e001870.

Kreniske, P. *et al.* (2019) Sounding the alarm: perinatally HIV-infected youth more likely to attempt suicide than their uninfected cohort peers. *The Journal of Adolescent Health* **65**, 702–705.

Kumpfer, K.L. *et al.* (2002) Cultural sensitivity and adaptation in family-based prevention interventions. *Prevention Science* **3**, 241–246.

Lachman, J.M. *et al.* (2021) Effectiveness of a parenting programme to reduce violence in a cash transfer system in the Philippines: RCT with follow-up. *The Lancet Regional Health. Western Pacific* **17**, 100279.

Leaning, J. (2001) Ethics of research in refugee populations. *The Lancet* **357**, 1432–1433.

Lehtimaki, S. *et al.* (2021) Evidence on digital mental health interventions for adolescents and young people: systematic overview. *JMIR Mental Health* **8**, e25847.

Lewis, S.J. & Danese, A. (2023) Editorial: are group-based interventions effective for treating trauma-related psychopathology in children and young people? *Journal of the American Academy of Child and Adolescent Psychiatry* **62**, 1188–1190.

Lewis, S.J. *et al.* (2019) The epidemiology of trauma and post-traumatic stress disorder in a representative cohort of young people in England and Wales. *The Lancet Psychiatry* **6**, 247–256.

Lund, C. (2018) Improving quality of mental health care in low-resource settings: lessons from PRIME. *World Psychiatry* **17**, 47–48.

Lund, C. *et al.* (2010) Poverty and common mental disorders in low and middle income countries: a systematic review. *Social Science & Medicine* **71**, 517–528.

Lund, C. *et al.* (2012) PRIME: a programme to reduce the treatment gap for mental disorders in five low- and middle-income countries. *PLoS Medicine* **9**, e1001359.

Lund, C. *et al.* (2016) Integration of mental health into primary care in low- and middle-income countries: the PRIME mental healthcare plans. *The British Journal of Psychiatry* **208**(Suppl 56), s1–s3.

McLaughlin, K.A. *et al.* (2009) Serious emotional disturbance among youths exposed to Hurricane Katrina 2 years postdisaster. *Journal of the American Academy of Child and Adolescent Psychiatry* **48**, 1069–1078.

Merry, S.N. *et al.* (2012) The effectiveness of SPARX, a computerised self help intervention for adolescents seeking help for depression: randomised controlled non-inferiority trial. *British Medical Journal* **344**, e2598.

Metzler, J. *et al.* (2019) Short- and longer-term impacts of child friendly space interventions in Rwamwanja refugee settlement, Uganda. *Journal of Child Psychology and Psychiatry* **60**, 1152–1163.

Metzler, J. *et al.* (2023) Improving adolescent mental health and protection in humanitarian settings: longitudinal findings from a multi-arm randomized controlled trial of child-friendly spaces among south Sudanese refugees in Uganda. *Journal of Child Psychology and Psychiatry* **64**, 907–917.

MHPSS (n.d.) *The Mental Health & Psychosocial Support Network* [Online]. Available: www.mhpss.net [6 September 2024].

Michelson, D. *et al.* (2020) Effectiveness of a brief lay counsellor-delivered, problem-solving intervention for adolescent mental health problems in urban, low-income schools in India: a randomised controlled trial. *The Lancet. Child & Adolescent Health* **4**, 571–582.

Miller, K.E. & Rasmussen, A. (2010) War exposure, daily stressors, and mental health in conflict and post-conflict settings: bridging the divide between trauma-focused and psychosocial frameworks. *Social Science & Medicine* **70**, 7–16.

Mohan, A. *et al.* (2022) Improving adolescent wellbeing is an urgent global priority. *BMJ* **379**, o2551.

NHS Digital (2022) *Mental Health of Children and Young People in England 2022: Wave 3 Follow Up to the 2017 Survey* [Online]. Available: https://digital.nhs.uk/data-and-information/publications/statistical/mental-health-of-children-and-young-people-in-england/2022-follow-up-to-the-2017-survey [6 September 2024].

NHS England (n.d.) *Emergency Preparedness, Resilience and Response (EPRR)* [Online]. Available: https://www.england.nhs.uk/ourwork/eprr [6 September 2024].

NICE (2018) *Post-traumatic Stress Disorder* [Online]. Available: www.nice.org.uk/guidance/ng116 [6 September 2024].

Osborn, T.L. *et al.* (2020) Single-session digital intervention for adolescent depression, anxiety, and well-being: outcomes of a randomized controlled trial with Kenyan adolescents. *Journal of Consulting and Clinical Psychology* **88**, 657–668.

Osokina, O. *et al.* (2023) Impact of the Russian invasion on mental health of adolescents in Ukraine. *Journal of the American Academy of Child and Adolescent Psychiatry* **62**, 335–343.

Padmanathan, P. & De Silva, M.J. (2013) The acceptability and feasibility of task-sharing for mental healthcare in low and middle income countries: a systematic review. *Social Science & Medicine* **97**, 82–86.

Patel, V. *et al.* (2007) Mental health of young people: a global public-health challenge. *The Lancet* **369**, 1302–1313.

Patel, V. *et al.* (2018) The lancet commission on global mental health and sustainable development. *The Lancet* **392**, 1553–1598.

Payton, C. *et al.* (2022) A logic model framework for planning an international refugee health research, evaluation, and ethics committee. *Health Promotion Practice* **23**, 852–860.

Pedersen, G.A. *et al.* (2019) A systematic review of the evidence for family and parenting interventions in low- and middle-income countries: child and youth mental health outcomes. *Journal of Child and Family Studies* **28**, 2036–2055.

Perks, B. & Cluver, L. (2020) The parenting vaccine. *Nature Human Behaviour* **4**, 985.

Perrin, S. *et al.* (2005) The children's revised impact of event scale (CRIES): validity as a screening instrument for PTSD. *Behavioural and Cognitive Psychotherapy* **33**, 487–498.

Polanczyk, G.V. *et al.* (2015) Annual research review: a meta-analysis of the worldwide prevalence of mental disorders in children and adolescents. *Journal of Child Psychology and Psychiatry* **56**, 345–365.

Prime, H. *et al.* (2020) Risk and resilience in family well-being during the COVID-19 pandemic. *The American Psychologist* **75**, 631–643.

Purgato, M. *et al.* (2018) Psychological therapies for the treatment of mental disorders in low- and middle-income countries affected by humanitarian crises. *The Cochrane Database of Systematic Reviews* **7**, Cd011849.

Reed, R.V. *et al.* (2012) Mental health of displaced and refugee children resettled in low-income and middle-income countries: risk and protective factors. *The Lancet* **379**, 250–265.

Ruggiero, K.J. *et al.* (2015) Web intervention for adolescents affected by disaster: population-based randomized controlled trial. *Journal of the American Academy of Child & Adolescent Psychiatry* **54**, 709–717.

Scheeringa, M.S. & Haslett, N. (2010) The reliability and criterion validity of the diagnostic infant and preschool assessment: a new diagnostic instrument for young children. *Child Psychiatry and Human Development* **41**, 299–312.

Scheeringa, M.S. & Zeanah, C.H. (2008) Reconsideration of harm's way: onsets and comorbidity patterns of disorders in preschool children and their caregivers following hurricane Katrina. *Journal of Clinical Child and Adolescent Psychology* **37**, 508–518.

Schleider, J.L. *et al.* (2022) A randomized trial of online single-session interventions for adolescent depression during COVID-19. *Nature Human Behaviour* **6**, 258–268.

Seagle, E.E. *et al.* (2020) Research ethics and refugee health: a review of reported considerations and applications in published refugee health literature, 2015–2018. *Conflict and Health* **14**, 39.

Sherr, L. *et al.* (2021) Mind Matters: Lessons from Past Crises for Child and Adolescent Mental Health during COVID-19. Innocenti Research Report, UNICEF Office of Research - Innocenti, Florence, Italy.

Sherr, L. *et al.* (2022) 'Tipping the balance': an evaluation of COVID-19 parenting resources developed and adapted for child protection during global emergency responses. *Health Psychology and Behavioral Medicine* **10**, 676–694.

Sim, A. *et al.* (2018) Modeling the effects of war exposure and daily stressors on maternal mental health, parenting, and child psychosocial adjustment: a cross-sectional study with Syrian refugees in Lebanon. *Global Mental Health* **5**, e40.

Sim, A.L. *et al.* (2021) Acceptability and preliminary outcomes of a parenting intervention for Syrian refugees. *Research on Social Work Practice* **31**, 14–25.

Simonds, E.A. *et al.* (2022) Trauma functioning and well-being in children who receive mental health aid after natural disaster or war. *Children* **9**, 951.

Skar, A.S. *et al.* (2021) Evaluation of parenting interventions to prevent violence against children in Colombia: a randomized controlled trial. *Journal of Interpersonal Violence* **36**, NP1098–NP1126.

Steventon Roberts, K. *et al.* (2022) Risk factors for poor mental health among adolescent mothers in South Africa. *Psychology, Health & Medicine*, 1–18.

Thienkrua, W. *et al.* (2006) Symptoms of posttraumatic stress disorder and depression among children in tsunami-affected areas in southern Thailand. *JAMA* **296**, 549–559.

Thienou, A. (2022) *Sahel: The Importance of Mental Health for Children in Conflict*. European Commission, Brussels. [Online]. Available: https://civil-protection-humanitarian-aid.ec.europa.eu/news-stories/stories/sahel-importance-mental-health-children-conflict_en [12 March 2023].

Tol, W.A. *et al.* (2011) Mental health and psychosocial support in humanitarian settings: linking practice and research. *The Lancet* **378**, 1581–1591.

Tol, W.A. *et al.* (2013) Annual research review: resilience and mental health in children and adolescents living in areas of armed conflict—a systematic review of findings in low- and middle-income countries. *Journal of Child Psychology and Psychiatry* **54**, 445–460.

Toska, E. *et al.* (2020) Adolescent mothers affected by HIV and their children: a scoping review of evidence and experiences from sub-Saharan Africa. *Global Public Health*, 1–19.

UNDP (2022) *Human Development Report 2022: Uncertain Times, Unsettled Lives: Shaping Our Future in a Transforming World*. UNDP, New York.

UNICEF & WHO (2022) *Helping Adolescents Thrive Toolkit*. UNICEF, New York.

Venturo-Conerly, K.E. *et al.* (2022) Meta-analysis: the effectiveness of youth psychotherapy interventions in low- and middle-income countries. *Journal of the American Academy of Child and Adolescent Psychiatry* **62**, 859–873.

Ward, C.L. *et al.* (2019) Parenting for lifelong health for young children: a randomized controlled trial of a parenting program in South Africa to prevent harsh parenting and child conduct problems. *Journal of Child Psychology and Psychiatry* **61**, 503–512.

Watters, C. & O'Callaghan, P. (2016) Mental health and psychosocial interventions for children and adolescents in street situations in low- and middle-income countries: a systematic review. *Child Abuse & Neglect* **60**, 18–26.

Whalley, M.G. & Brewin, C.R. (2007) Mental health following terrorist attacks. *The British Journal of Psychiatry* **190**, 94–96.

WHO (2011) *Psychological First Aid: Guide for Field Workers* [Online]. Available: https://apps.who.int/iris/bitstream/handle/10665/44615/9789241548205_eng.pdf [6 September 2024].

WHO (2018) *WHO Mental Health Gap Action Programme (mhGAP)*. World Health Organization, Geneva, Switzerland.

WHO (2019) *mhGAP Intervention Guide Version 2.0 for Mental, Neurological and Substance Use Disorders in Non-specialised Health Settings*. World Health Organization, Geneva, Switzerland. [Online]. Available: https://www.who.int/publications/i/item/9789241549790 [6 September 2024].

WHO & UNHCR (2015) *mhGAP Humanitarian Intervention Guide (mhGAP-HIG): Clinical Management of Mental, Neurological and Substance Use Conditions in Humanitarian Emergencies*. World Health Organization, Geneva, Switzerland.

Williams, J.M. & Kuyken, W. (2012) Mindfulness-based cognitive therapy: a promising new approach to preventing depressive relapse. *The British Journal of Psychiatry* **200**, 359–360.

Williamson, V. *et al.* (2018) Occupational moral injury and mental health: systematic review and meta-analysis. *The British Journal of Psychiatry* **212**, 339–346.

Wright, M. *et al.* (2023) Interventions with digital tools for mental health promotion among 11-18 year olds: a systematic review and meta-analysis. *Journal of Youth and Adolescence* **52**, 754–779.

Zaneva, M. *et al.* (2022) The impact of monetary poverty alleviation programs on children's and adolescents' mental health: a systematic review and meta-analysis across low-, middle-, and high-income countries. *The Journal of Adolescent Health* **71**, 147–156.

Zimmerman, A. *et al.* (2021) The impact of cash transfers on mental health in children and young people in low-income and middle-income countries: a systematic review and meta-analysis. *BMJ Global Health* **6**, e004661.

CHAPTER 19
Legal issues in the care and treatment of children with mental health problems

Brenda Hale[1] and Jonathan Herring[2,3]
[1]Formerly President, Supreme Court of the United Kingdom, London, UK
[2]Faculty of Law, University of Oxford, Oxford, UK
[3]Exeter College, University of Oxford, Oxford, UK

The universality of human rights

The issues are universal: how are mental health professionals to navigate their way between the responsibilities of the parents, the autonomy of the child, and their professional duties toward their patient or client? In this chapter we shall illustrate the relevant concepts by reference to the law of England.[1] But it is likely that the legal principles will be very similar in those Western countries whose legal systems are derived from the common law of England and Wales, including Canada, Australia, New Zealand, and most of the United States of America. This chapter covers human rights, and legal aspects in relation to the protection of children and providing treatment.

The issues engage with the human rights of both parents and child. These include the right to liberty and security of person, the right not to be subjected to torture or inhuman or degrading treatment or punishment, the right to physical and psychological integrity, the right to respect for family life, and the right to a fair trial. Such rights have been recognized since the United Nations Universal Declaration of Human Rights in 1948, later translated into the binding International Covenants on Civil and Political Rights and Economic, Social and Cultural Rights in 1966, and supplemented by UN Conventions catering for specific groups, of which the Convention on the Rights of the Child (CRC) 1989 and the Convention on the Rights of Persons with Disabilities (CRPD) 2006 are the most relevant. In addition, members of the Council of Europe must become parties to the European Convention on Human Rights (ECHR) 1950.

In common law countries,[2] such international treaties are binding in international law once ratified, but do not generally become part of the ordinary law of the land unless the national Parliament so provides. Under the United Kingdom's Human Rights Act 1998 (HRA), the rights guaranteed by the ECHR became rights recognized in UK law. The UK has not legislated to incorporate the whole of the CRC or the CRPD into its domestic law; but the European Court of Human Rights in Strasbourg interprets the ECHR rights in the light of other international human rights instruments; so the CRC is increasingly finding its way into both the Strasbourg and the UK courts' judgments on children's rights issues (Gilmore, 2017).[3] Under the influence of the ECHR there is "further support for the general movement towards now giving young people greater rights concerning their own future while reducing the supervisory rights of their parents."[4]

Most Western-style democracies have written constitutions which also protect fundamental rights. The oldest is the Constitution of the United States of America, with its Bill of Rights of 1791 and later Amendments. The modern Constitutions of the independent Commonwealth countries protect enumerated fundamental rights which are largely based upon those in the ECHR. In between are the "old" Commonwealth countries, which (apart from Australia) have their own Bill or Charter of Rights, such as the Canadian Charter of Rights and Freedoms 1982. National laws dealing with mental health issues

[1] Scotland and Northern Ireland are separate jurisdictions with their own laws. Much of the law in Wales is the same as in England but statute law can differ.

[2] In short, a common law jurisdiction is one whose legal system originated from the English common law, and would include Australia, New Zealand, Canada, and most of the United States.

[3] E.g., *Neulinger and Shuruk v Switzerland* (2012) 54 EHRR 31; *R (Williamson and Others) v Secretary of State for Education* [2005] UKHL 15 [80].

[4] *R (Axon) v Secretary of State for Health and another* [2006] EWHC 37 (Admin), [115].

Rutter's Child and Adolescent Psychiatry and Psychology, Seventh Edition.
Edited by Anita Thapar, Daniel S. Pine, Samuele Cortese, Cathy Creswell, Tamsin J. Ford, James F. Leckman, and Argyris Stringaris.

Companion website: www.wiley.com/go/thapar/rutterspsych7

have therefore to be judged against these constitutional standards.

Legal rights have become a core aspect of citizenship, as well as a powerful tool for recognizing the value of each person (Freeman, 2020). Where people are denied rights, this reflects a clear statement about their place in the legal and political community. This is why children's rights advocates insist on the importance of recognizing that children have rights (Todres & King, 2020).

The different roles of the mental health professional

Most commonly, of course, a mental health professional will encounter a child or young person as a patient. In the UK, health care is a universal service, free to all (apart from some "persons from abroad") at the point of need, regardless of ability to pay. Unlike both the education and social care services, however, the National Health Service (NHS) can rarely be obliged to offer treatment or care which it does not wish or is unable to offer. In recent years in United Kingdom, there have been grave concerns over long waiting lists for young people with mental health difficulties (Young Minds, 2022).[5] There are long waiting lists for mental health services across Europe (Bencharif, 2022). However, mental health professionals, like all other professionals, owe a duty of care to their own patients. If they negligently fail to diagnose or to treat, and the patient suffers harm as a result, they may be held liable in damages: for example, a child psychologist who fails to diagnose dyslexia[6]. The duty is owed only to their child patient and not to the child's parents. The courts here and elsewhere recognize that if professionals also owed a duty to the parents, they might hesitate to diagnose abuse and the child would go unprotected (Box 19.1).[7]

Box 19.1 Three ways for health professionals to treat children without parental consent (UK)

> If health professionals wish to provide treatment for a child with mental health problems and either the child or their family resist this, they have a range of options available. These include
> - persuading an approved mental health professional (AMHP) to invoke the compulsory procedures under the Mental Health Act 1983,
> - persuading the local children's services authority (social services) to bring care proceedings under the Children Act 1989 (CA) (meaning the children can be looked after by social services), or
> - themselves applying to the family court for an order authorizing the treatment.

The choice between these options will depend upon whether it is the parents or the child who are seen as the principal obstacle and what it is ultimately sought to achieve—treatment for the child or a different family environment or both. These are discussed in the next two sections. Any court proceedings are likely to require expert evidence from mental health professionals, discussed in the concluding section.

Mental health professionals may also be involved in providing advice to other statutory agencies. Thus, for example, in England psychological reports are part of the formal process of assessing and providing an Education, Health and Care Plan for the child who has special educational needs[8] or a disability. The education authorities are then under a legal duty to meet the duties set out in the Plan.[9] Unlike the health and social care services, the education services can be ordered by a tribunal to provide an individual child with the education which the tribunal decides that he needs. Occasionally, psychiatric reports are required in the criminal justice system, on those rare occasions where a child or young person needs a specialist mental health disposal and there is one available (see Chapter 47 on Forensic Psychiatry).

Intervening against the parents

If health or social care professionals encounter opposition to what they believe to be in the best interests of an individual child, the first question is whether it is appropriate to take action against the parents or against the child. With older children, the obstacle may well be the child. With younger children, the obstacle is generally the authority of the parents, known in English law as "parental responsibility." In England and Wales, the mother automatically has parental responsibility, sharing it with the father if they are married to one another, or if an unmarried father has acquired it by agreement, court order, or by registration on the child's birth certificate (CA, ss 2(1), (2) and (4)). The great majority of unmarried fathers are registered on the birth certificate and so will have parental responsibility in that way.

General principles

In Western democratic legal systems, it is parents and families, rather than the State, who have the primary right and the primary responsibility to bring up their children: to meet their claims for nurture, care, and upbringing and to decide for themselves how this will be done. It is the hallmark of a dictatorship to gain control of the children and distance them from the varied and "subversive" influences of their families (Hale, 2005: 5). Hence article 8 of the ECHR, drafted in 1950 in the twin shadows of the Nazi totalitarianism of the recent past and the Stalinist totalitarianism of the then present, guarantees to everyone,

[5] Sometimes the courts have expressed serious concerns about the lack of provision for vulnerable young people with mental health issues: *Re X (A Child) (No. 4)* [2017] EWHC 2084 (Fam).

[6] *Phelps v Hillingdon London Borough Council* [2001] 2 AC 619 (none has succeeded).

[7] *D v East Berkshire Community Health NHS Trust and Others* [2005] UKHL 23.

[8] Known as additional learning needs in Wales.

[9] Children and Families Act 2014, Part 3.

parents and children alike, the right to respect for their private and family life, their home, and their correspondence. The CRC also requires States Parties to recognize that "parents or, as the case may be, legal guardians, have the primary responsibility for the upbringing and development of the child. The best interests of the child will be *their* basic concern" (article 18.1, emphasis added). States Parties must also recognize "the right of the child to the enjoyment of the highest attainable standard of health and to facilities for the treatment of illness and rehabilitation of health" (article 24.1) and "that a mentally or physically disabled child should enjoy a full and decent life, in conditions which ensure dignity, promote self-reliance and facilitate the child's active participation in the community" (article 23.1).

The rights of parents are not absolute, and there are various ways of overcoming their neglect of or opposition to treatment. The CA provides in section 3(5) that a person who does not have parental responsibility for a child but has care of the child may "do what is reasonable in all the circumstances of the case for the purpose of safeguarding or promoting the child's welfare." This provision would clearly authorize emergency treatment to save a child's life or prevent serious deterioration in the child's health whatever the parents said. It would also authorize routine measures where the parents' views were not known and could not be obtained within a reasonable time. But it would not be reasonable to proceed with major nonurgent interventions without consulting the parents, and if necessary, obtaining court authorization.

Securing parental compliance

Historically, the only means of putting pressure upon the parents to agree to treatment was the threat of prosecution for child neglect or abuse.[10] Some legal systems are still reluctant to go beyond this threat to secure parental compliance, but this will not help the child unless it is effective. And it is least likely to be effective against struggling parents who simply do not appreciate the risks.[11]

Dealing with single issues

For one-off situations, where the child is being properly looked after in other respects but there are concerns about a particular issue, a hospital or health care professional can apply to a court for permission to override the parent's objections. In English law this can be done either by invoking the ancient "inherent" (that is, nonstatutory) jurisdiction of the High Court to safeguard children or by a "specific issue" order (CA 1989, s 8) authorizing the treatment: for example, a blood transfusion for the child of Jehovah's Witnesses. The Court will determine what order will best promote the welfare of the child. The views of the parents will be taken into account in that assessment, but ultimately the focus will be on the best interests of the child.[12]

Where two or more people have parental responsibility, each of them may act alone and without the other in meeting it (CA, s 2(7)), so the consent of one parent will usually suffice. But where they disagree, in the UK, the other parent can take steps to prohibit the treatment until the matter is resolved by the court, so in practice such disputes may have to be taken to court. The same procedures can also be invoked by a professional who wants to *prevent* treatment to which a parent has agreed: for example, the sterilization of an 11-year-old girl with Sotos' syndrome.[13]

Long-term responses

Many children with mental health problems or learning difficulties are likely to present more long-term and complex problems. The family environment and dynamics may be an important part of the child's difficulties. If so, it may be necessary to bring proceedings to remove the child from the harmful environment. Indeed, in some cases, it may be thought necessary to remove the child at or soon after birth, in order to prevent their suffering harm to their mental or psychological health in the future. In England and Wales, responsibility for undertaking care proceedings lies, not with the health authorities, but with the local children's services authorities (social services), which have the statutory responsibility to protect children from harm (CA, s 47 and Sched 2). This is because the eventual outcome of most care proceedings is that the authority will have to take parental responsibility for the child. Care by a local authority may not be ideal, but at least the authority should have, or have access to, the full range of facilities needed to take care of the child, including the health and education services. Neither the health nor the education services are equipped to cater for everything which parents should provide for their children, nor can they find alternative homes for children who need them.

The legal need for "actual" or "likely" harm

It is not enough that such intervention is in the child's best interests. While some legal systems have a list of specific grounds for taking children into care, section 31(2) of the CA focuses on actual or likely harm to the child. First, it must be shown that the child is suffering or likely to suffer significant harm. "Harm" means ill-treatment or the impairment of health or development. "Health" means physical or mental health. "Development" means physical, intellectual, emotional, social, or behavioral development. "Ill-treatment" includes sexual abuse and forms of ill-treatment which are not physical. Hence, it is very likely that a child with mental health problems whose health or educational needs are not being met will be suffering or likely to suffer significant harm. But it is not the object of the Act to supply children with ideal parents to replace the less-than-ideal parents which we all are. It is not enough that the children might do better with different

[10] Children and Young Persons Act 1933, s 1(1).

[11] *R v Sheppard* [1981] AC 394.

[12] *Fixsler v Manchester University Foundation NHS Trust* [2021] EWCA Civ 1018.

[13] *Re D (A Minor) (Wardship: Sterilization)*[1976] Fam 185.

parents. As Hedley J said in *Re L (Care: Threshold Criteria)*,[14] which was a case about the children of parents with quite serious learning difficulties, "... society must be able to tolerate very diverse standards of parenting, including the eccentric, the barely adequate and the inconsistent. It follows too that children will inevitably have both very different experiences of parenting and very unequal consequences flowing from it." So, one problem is to distinguish "significant harm" from the ordinary consequences of growing up with parents who have learning disabilities, mental ill health, addictions, or whatever.

"Likely" does not mean "probable," but simply "a real possibility, a possibility which cannot sensibly be ignored having regard to the nature and gravity of the feared harm in the particular case".[15] So, quite a low risk of really serious harm might justify preventive action, whereas if the feared harm is less serious, a greater risk may be required. Section 31(2) also requires that the harm, or likelihood of harm, is attributable to a lack of reasonable parental care, because the child's carers have not provided or will not provide it, and not because the services themselves are failing to deliver what the child needs. This is important because a child may be found to be suffering harm owing to mental health difficulties, but these may not result from a lack of parental care. By contrast, a parent's failure to take reasonable steps to get mental health interventions for a child could form the basis of an application for a care order.

Removal of child from the parents and other interventions

Once the harm threshold is crossed, the court can decide what order will be best for the child. It may be better for the child to make no order at all; but unless there is someone else (such as another family member) who is willing and able to take parental responsibility for the child, the only other choices are a supervision order and a care order. A supervision order places the child under the local authority's supervision, but without affecting the parents' own parental responsibility. Conditions for medical or psychiatric examination and treatment of the child can be imposed, if there is medical evidence to support it (CA, s 35 and Sched 3, paras 4 and 5). But supervision is rarely thought sufficient to protect the child from significant harm. A care order gives the designated local authority (social services) parental responsibility for the child, and the power to limit the parents' exercise of their responsibility. In England and Wales, the court has no power to impose conditions or to insist that the local authority discharge their parental responsibilities in a particular way. This puts the court in a quandary. How can it know whether the order will be in the best interests of the child unless it knows how the authority plan to look after the child and has some confidence that the plan will be carried out? This can be a source of frustration both for courts and for health care professionals whose recommendations for treatment are not always adopted by the local authority (social services), but courts have neither the resources nor the expertise to act as substitute parents for children.

In most cases, the real choice is between planning to reunite the child with the family and planning to place the child with a permanent alternative family. This raises an even greater dilemma. If the authorities intervene early, before a child suffers permanent harm, the more likely it is that the child can be successfully placed for adoption or special guardianship with new carers. The later things are left, the more harm is done, and the more difficult it will be to successfully repair the damage. The dilemma is particularly acute with emotional neglect or abuse, which may take many years to result in significant harm to the child, if indeed they ever do. But can such early intervention be justified in human rights terms?

Article 8(2) of the ECHR permits interference by a public authority with the right to respect for family life only if three conditions are fulfilled. First, the intervention must be "in accordance with the law"; this means that it must comply with a national law which is sufficiently clear and certain for people to be able to conduct themselves accordingly. Second, the interference must be for one of the legitimate aims laid down; in this case, for the protection of the "health or morals" or the "rights and freedoms" of the child. Third, and most important, the interference must be "necessary in a democratic society"; this means that the steps taken must be proportionate to the legitimate aim pursued and the reasons given must be relevant and sufficient. The Strasbourg court generally allows a wide "margin of appreciation" to the national authorities in deciding whether to take a child into public care.[16] But the aim when doing so must generally be to reunite the family; so, steps which cut children off from their families of birth will be scrutinized with much more care. Permanent removal, through adoption, for example, requires exceptional justification in the interests of the child.

Separate court authorization is needed under the Adoption and Children Act 2002 if the child is to be placed for adoption without the parents' consent. This can be done at the same time as a care order is made or later. Parental consent can only be dispensed with if the court is satisfied that the welfare of the child *requires* this (s 52). This is a test of necessity, not desirability.[17] Compulsory adoption is clearly the most drastic possible interference in the family life of a child, the parents, and the wider family and UK law is unusual in allowing this. But in *R and H v United Kingdom*,[18] the Strasbourg court held that it was justifiable to free a child for adoption without parental consent when it was clear that the child could not go back to parents who had a long history of alcohol abuse. This was despite the expert evidence that the child needed to retain contact with her parents, so that every effort should be made to find adopters who would support that contact, and the proceedings should be adjourned

[14] [2007] 1 FLR 2050, 2063.

[15] *Re H (Minors) (Sexual Abuse: Standard of Proof)* [1996] AC 563, 585F.

[16] E.g., *KA v Finland* (2001) 2 FLR 696.

[17] *S v L* [2012] UKSC 30.

[18] [2011] 2 FLR 1236.

to enable that to be done. But the Strasbourg court reiterated that "measures which deprive biological parents of the parental responsibilities and authorise adoption should only be applied in exceptional circumstances and can only be justified if they are motivated by overriding requirements pertaining to the child's welfare" (para 81).

Two vignettes follow which give a flavor of how courts deal with cases where there is a dispute between parents and medical professionals.

Vignette 1 (a UK example): assessing harm and proportionality

The particular dilemmas arising where it is feared that a parent's mental health problems may cause psychological harm to a child in the future are well illustrated in the Supreme Court case of *Re B*.[19] The mother had a history of sexual abuse in childhood and had begun a long and abusive relationship with her controlling and violent stepfather when she was still under 16. She also had a history of presenting herself to many different hospitals and doctors with a variety of symptoms, some of which had a physical explanation, but the history satisfied the diagnostic criteria for somatization disorder. There were also indications of factitious illness disorder, though not of the so-called Munchausen syndrome by proxy. Eventually, she succeeded in extricating herself from the relationship with her stepfather (leaving behind their daughter, then aged 10) and formed a relationship with the father of her new baby. When the baby was born, there was such a confusion of accusation and counteraccusation from the mother and her stepfather, in which the dreaded word "Munchausen's" featured, that the child was removed on an interim care order shortly after birth. But the parents showed during regular contact that they were devoted to her and well able to cater for her immediate needs and she became strongly attached to them. The trial judge found that there was a risk that she would suffer psychological harm from her mother's somatization disorder, and quite extraordinary propensity for lying and deceptive behavior, and some risk of her being exposed to unnecessary medical examinations and treatment. The judge also found that the parents would not be able to cooperate with social services in a program of monitoring and support to avoid these risks, so there was no alternative but to agree to the local authority's plan for adoption.

Was this "significant harm" or was it just the ordinary risk that a child might pick up bad behaviors from her parents? Was the unquantified risk of the child doing so a sufficiently "real possibility" to justify compulsory preventive action? Above all, was an unquantified risk of this sort of psychological or emotional harm at some time in the distant future sufficient to justify the most drastic step of all, the separation of the child from her parents at birth and placement in a closed adoption? The Supreme Court upheld the judge's decision, but Lady Hale dissented on the ground that this was not a proportionate response to the risk presented.

[19] [2013] UKSC 33.

Vignette 2: parents wanting treatment which doctors opposed

There has been extensive litigation in England over Charlie Gard.[20] The case made headlines around the world. Charlie was born with a rare genetic condition that caused multiple disabilities including severe brain damage. The medical team at the London hospital caring for him decided it would be best to withdraw ventilation and enable him to die peacefully. His parents wanted him to be taken to the United States and receive "nucleoside bypass therapy." During the court proceedings it became clear this therapy had not been used before on humans and there was little evidence to suggest it would succeed. The consistent medical opinion was that it was not appropriate to attempt it. Nevertheless, there was an American doctor willing to offer it.

The legal principle at the heart of the case was relatively straightforward: the case must be decided on what was in Charlie's best interests. All the judges who heard the case agreed on that. Francis J determined that the therapy had no realistic chance of success. The trip to America carried clear risks of harm. The medical interventions necessary to keep Charlie alive were not providing him with a benefit (and it was not known whether they caused him pain). It was therefore in his best interests to remain in England and to withdraw the treatment. This was upheld by the Court of Appeal and leave to appeal to the Supreme Court was refused. Lady Hale stated that "parents are not entitled to insist upon treatment by anyone which is not in their child's best interests." The case went to the European Court of Human Rights where the parents' case was again rejected. It finally returned to Francis J who again approved the withdrawal.

The argument the parents made was that the state should only interfere in their decision about Charlie if it could be shown it would cause him significant harm.[21] This argument was rejected by the courts. The views of parents should be taken into account and given weight. However, at the end of the day the court had the authority to decide what was best for Charlie, and could not authorize a course of action which was against his best interests.

Intervening against the child to authorize treatment

When health or social care professionals encounter opposition to what they believe to be in the best interests of an individual child, the source of the problem may be the child's own resistance.

[20] E.g., *Yates and Another v Great Ormond Street Hospital for Children NHS Foundation Trust and Another* [2017] EWCA Civ 410. See Goold *et al.* (2020).

[21] For academic arguments in favor and against this approach see Goold *et al.* (2020).

Traditionally, the assumption was that the right to decide the medical treatment of a child rested with the parents. Today, this approach is being reassessed, particularly in relation to adolescents, many of whom have an intellectual development on a par with many adults. Although most countries have a relatively high age of legal majority (18 is the most common in EU countries), there has been a growing realization worldwide that long before this, many adolescents acquire a strong personal interest in taking responsibility for decisions affecting their future.

The child's right to consent to treatment

In England and Wales, where the age of majority is 18, legislation enables 16- and 17-year-olds to consent to surgical, medical, or dental treatment themselves with no need to seek parental consent.[22] But what of those under the age of 16?

In the late 1980s, the groundbreaking decision of the House of Lords in *Gillick v West Norfolk and Wisbech Area Health Authority* (*Gillick*)[23] established that even a child under 16 who had sufficient understanding was able to give a valid consent to medical treatment and advice. It was a question of fact, to be decided on a case-by-case basis, whether the child had "sufficient understanding of what is involved to give a valid consent in law."[24] If the child was competent to consent, the parents need not be involved. The notion of "*Gillick* competence" (or the "mature minor" doctrine) became widely used in common law countries by doctors dealing with young patients (Box 19.2).[25]

Box 19.2 Gillick capacity (England and Wales)

> Gillick Capacity is the phrase used in English and Welsh law to describe a child who has sufficient understanding to be able to consent to medical treatment. A child will be Gillick-competent if they have sufficient maturity and understanding of the issues relating to the decision. That said, a doctor is required to take reasonable steps to provide the child with the information he or she needs to gain the understanding to have capacity.[26]

Box 19.3 Assessing mental capacity (England and Wales)

> Some guidance may be sought from the test of capacity laid down in section 3 of the English and Welsh Mental Capacity Act 2005 (MCA), which applies to those over 16. Adults are presumed to have capacity and are only unable to make a decision for themselves if they are unable
> - to understand the information relevant to the decision;
> - to retain that information; and
> - to use or weigh that information as part of the process of making the decision; or
> - to communicate his decision (whether by talking, using sign language or by any other means).
>
> Although the Act only applies to adults, doctors may find that the same concepts are helpful when deciding whether a child is *Gillick*-competent.[27] However, there is case law to support the view that there may be issues in addition to those listed in the MCA when considering children, such as issues around maturity and life experience. It might also be important to bear in mind that a child can be more readily subject to external pressures and influences than many adults. So, while the MCA test can be useful to assist in determining capacity for children, it does not provide a definitive test.[28]
>
> *Source:* Adapted from Bencharif, 2022.

Assessing child competence

The "*Gillick*-competence" test has been criticized for its ambiguities. In particular, it contains no guidance as to the extent to which an adjustment should be made for factors affecting adolescents' understanding, such as peer pressure, drug and substance abuse, family stress, emotional disturbance, risk taking, and physical and mental illness—all matters which might radically influence their ability to attain *Gillick* competence (Fortin, 2012: 94) (Box 19.3).

Easy cases will be where the child does not understand the key facts about the illness or the proposed treatment. Clearly the child will then not be *Gillick*-competent.

Are there treatments no child could have capacity to consent to?

In *Bell v The Tavistock and Portman NHS Foundation Trust*[29] the Court of Appeal had to address the question of whether a trans child under the age of 16 could consent to take puberty blockers as a response to the child's gender identity. The Court of Appeal emphasized that this was a matter to be determined by the individual doctor and child patient. It would not be right for the court to state as a matter of principle that no child would have the capacity to consent to puberty blockers. This emphasizes the point that a medical professional must assess each child as an individual and determine his or her level of capacity, rather than relying on assumptions about what children generally do or do not understand (Jowett 2022; Chua, 2023).

---

22 Family Law Reform Act 1969, section 8 (2). See also Age of Legal Capacity (Scotland) Act 1991, section 2(4).

23 [1986] AC 112.

24 Lord Fraser in *Gillick* stated that the doctor should be satisfied: (i) that the girl (although under 16) will understand his advice; (ii) that he cannot persuade her to inform her parents or allow him to inform the parents that she is seeking contraceptive advice; (iii) that she is very likely to begin or to continue having sexual intercourse with or without contraceptive treatment; (iv) that unless she receives contraceptive advice or treatment her physical or mental health or both are likely to suffer; and (v) that her best interests require him to give her contraceptive advice, treatment or both without the parental consent.

25 E.g., *Secretary, Department of Health and Community Services v JWB (Marion's case)* (1992) 175 CLR 218 (Australia).

26 *Bell v The Tavistock and Portman NHS Foundation Trust* [2022] 1 FLR 30.

27 *Re S (Child as parent: Adoption: Consent)* [2017] EWHC 2729 (Fam).

28 *Re X (A Child) (No 2)* [2021] EWHC 65 (Fam).

29 [2022] 1 FLR 30.

Fluctuating capacity

One point that may be particularly relevant in cases of mental illness is that if the child is fluctuating between competence and incompetence, a court might regard the child as not competent. This was the approach taken in a case in the 1990s.[30] The decision might be justified on the basis that, otherwise, the hospital would be in a very difficult position in having to decide each time the child was touched whether she was competent or not.

Children's capacity and human rights

It is not entirely clear how the concept of *Gillick* competence fits with the principles of human rights law. The CRC and the CRPD deliver a rather different message from the one sent out by *Gillick*. Article 12(1) of the CRC requires States to give all children, who are capable of forming their own views, the right to express these freely in all matters affecting them and the right to have their views given "due weight in accordance with the age and maturity of the child." Article 7(3) of the CRPD requires children with disabilities to be given that right on an equal basis with other children, and to be provided with disability- and age-appropriate assistance to realize that right. This gives every child, not merely a *Gillick*-competent child, the right to *participate* in decision-making about themselves, and (in the CRPD) to be helped to be able to do so. But, unlike *Gillick*, this right to be consulted is not about autonomy: it does not give children the right to decide matters for themselves.

Turning to the ECHR, one might assume that article 8 of the ECHR reinforces the concept of *Gillick* competence and autonomy. In case law concerning adults, the Strasbourg court has emphasized that it protects the right to respect for physical and psychological integrity, and includes the right to self-determination or the "notion of autonomy";[31] it protects against compulsory medical intervention even if that intervention is of minor importance.[32] In theory, these rights are available to everyone, irrespective of age and certainly irrespective of opposition from third parties, such as parents. But in a rare (and controversial) early decision about the psychiatric care of a child, the European court adopted a conservative approach to the notion of children having rights against their parents.[33] Nevertheless, the High Court has since held that the concept of *Gillick* competence is unaffected by a mother's article 8 right to bring up her daughters free from state interference—that her rights are not so extensive that they override her daughters' own article 8 right to medical privacy.[34] Indeed, where a child is *Gillick*-competent she has the same rights to confidentiality as any other patient, meaning a medical professional should not disclose private information about a competent child to a parent without the child's consent.

Overriding the child's refusal to consent to treatment

But where does this leave the "*Gillick*-competent" child who wishes to refuse consent to what is proposed? Controversially, the courts have suggested (*obiter*) that the *Gillick* decision still allows a parent with parental responsibility to give effective consent, even where a child is refusing treatment. In two English cases decided in the 1990s, doctors faced with adolescents refusing lifesaving treatment made their patients wards of court in order to sidestep that refusal. Both applications involved adolescents with serious psychological problems.[35] The Court of Appeal held that under its inherent jurisdiction it could override a young patient's wishes and authorize lifesaving treatment in his or her best interests. As it was put in one case a doctor only needs one "flak jacket" providing legal authorization for treatment.[36] That can be given by a *Gillick*-competent child or a parent with parental responsibility. In practice, medical professionals would be wise to seek court authorization in cases where a *Gillick*-competent child is objecting to treatment, rather than rely on the authorization of a parent.

This approach in the 1990s cases is objected to by those who argue that if a child has sufficient capacity to make the decision it should be respected whether they are consenting to medical treatment or refusing it. There is a danger that the law is recognizing children's autonomy only where the child is giving the "right" answer, by agreeing with doctors. And, of course, only supporting autonomy when the "right" answer is given is not supporting autonomy at all. Most of all, it is one thing to allow a *court* to override the child's decision after a fair hearing in which all sides of the argument have been properly ventilated. It is another thing to allow a parent—or worse still a local authority (social services) with parental responsibility—the right to force unwanted treatment upon a competent child. This may explain why many medical professionals faced with a teenager objecting to treatment will prefer to seek a court authorization for the intervention. This is wise, given that the Supreme Court has decided that the parents of a child aged 16 or 17 who lacks the capacity to decide on their living arrangements cannot consent to depriving the child of their liberty in residential accommodation providing for their special needs.[37]

[30] *Re R (A Minor) (Wardship: Consent to Medical Treatment)* [1992] 1 FLR 190.

[31] *Pretty v United Kingdom* [2002] 2 FLR 45, [61].

[32] *YF v Turkey* (2004) 39 EHRR 34, para [33]: "A person's body concerns the most intimate aspect of one's private life."

[33] *Nielsen v Denmark* (1988) 11 EHRR 175.

[34] *R (Axon) v Secretary of State for Health and the Family Planning Association* [2006] EWCA 37 (Admin).

[35] *Re R (A Minor) (Wardship: Consent to Treatment)* [1992] Fam 11, authorizing the compulsory use of antipsychotic drugs to treat a 15-year-old suffering from increasingly paranoid and disturbed behavior; *Re W (A Minor) (Medical Treatment: Court's Jurisdiction)* [1993] Fam 64, authorizing the compulsory treatment of a 16-year-old in a dangerously anorexic state.

[36] *Re W (A Minor) (Medical Treatment: Court's Jurisdiction)* [1993] Fam 64, 78.

[37] *In re D (A Child)* [2019] UKSC 42. See also the guidance in the Mental Health Act Code of Practice, discussed in the section "Using mental health law for intervention and treatment."

If a case involving a child objecting to treatment comes to court, the focus will be on the welfare of the child. While it is clear that the courts may well determine that it is in a child's best interests to receive treatment recommended by doctors, they will need to take into account the impact on the child of being forced to receive treatment (Daly, 2018). Forcing a child to receive treatment to which they object can be seen as degrading and can only be done in cases where the child will face death or a very serious harm without it.

Vignettes

In *Re E and F (Minors: Blood Transfusion)*[38] two young people aged 16 and 17 refused potentially lifesaving blood transfusions because of their religious beliefs. The Court of Appeal confirmed that the court could authorize the treatment of a *Gillick*-competent or 16- or 17-year-old child even where they had capacity and refused to consent. However, that was only appropriate where the treatment was in the welfare of the child and that the competent child's views should be "upheld where possible." This case was one of the "rare circumstances" where the "imperative to preserve life" required the court to intervene.[39] This suggests in other cases, including most psychiatric cases, where there is no threat to life a court is unlikely to override the opposition of a 16- or 17-year-old.

That case should be contrasted with *A Teaching Hospital NHS Trust v DV (A Child)*[40] where a 17-year-old had been diagnosed with bone cancer. His religious views led him to object to a blood transfusion, although he consented to other interventions. It was held, given his age and the strength of his religious convictions, that forcing treatment on him would be deeply traumatic and could not be said to be in his best interests. Interestingly the doctors in that case had agreed that it would not be appropriate to use force to provide the blood transfusion.

As these vignettes indicate, the issues become particularly complex when religious beliefs are involved. Generally, the courts here and abroad have shown little appetite for allowing the wishes of adolescents with strong religious views to dictate a fatal outcome.[41] As it was put in *Re E (A Minor) (Wardship: Medical Treatment)*:[42] a court "should be very slow to allow an infant to martyr himself."

This particular issue has not so far reached the UK Supreme Court. But in *AC v Manitoba (Director of Child and Family Services)*,[43] the Supreme Court of Canada dealt with a challenge from AC, a 14-year-old Jehovah's Witness, forced to undergo blood transfusion treatment for a life-threatening condition. Its survey of international approaches to this problem showed that other jurisdictions were finding it equally difficult to allow adolescents to reject lifesaving treatment: ". . . courts . . . have generally not seen the 'mature minor' doctrine as dictating guaranteed outcomes, particularly where the consequences for the young person are catastrophic" (para 69). The majority[44] considered that the provincial legislation giving the courts a discretionary power to authorize medical treatment for adolescents under the age of 16, even against their wishes, did not unduly infringe AC's constitutional right to freedom from forced medical treatment. The State had a legitimate concern to protect younger adolescents, as a vulnerable group, from making decisions before attaining capacity for truly mature and independent thought.

Does human rights law hold the key to this problem? It provides child patients, like adults, with a right to freedom from arbitrary deprivation of liberty,[45] an absolute right to protection from inhuman and degrading treatment, and a qualified right to respect for their physical and psychological integrity.[46] On the other hand, like adults, they also have a right to life, which in certain circumstances includes the right of a vulnerable patient or prisoner to be prevented from harming themselves.[47] Perhaps Strasbourg would regard an adolescent refusing lifesaving treatment in the same light. Furthermore, it takes the view that, in principle, treatment which is a "medical necessity" infringes neither article 3 nor article 8.[48] But that is in the context of detained psychiatric patients. It remains to be seen what view the Strasbourg court would take of a human rights challenge to the power of either the parents or the courts to impose treatment upon a competent child who refuses it. In *Storck v Germany*,[49] the Strasbourg court held that an 18-year-old's right to liberty was infringed when she was detained in a psychiatric hospital on her father's authority. It has been suggested that *Storck* sent out "a clear message indicating a different approach to the personal autonomy of young people."[50] The UK Supreme Court has held that parents cannot consent to depriving a 16- or 17-year-old of liberty,[51] but it has not yet decided whether a court can impose treatment against the will of a competent child who refuses it.

Using mental health law for intervention and treatment

Sometimes children, more commonly adolescents, require specialized treatment for mental health problems and, rarely, their doctors need compulsory powers to ensure that this occurs. The Mental Health Act 1983 in England and Wales (MHA) applies to all patients requiring treatment for mental disorder,

[38] [2021] EWCA Civ 188.
[39] Para 63.
[40] [2021] EWHC 1037 (Fam).
[41] E.g., *Minister for Health v AS* [2004] WASC 286.
[42] [1993] 1 FLR 386, 394.
[43] [2009] 2 SCR 181.

[44] Binnie J gave a strong dissenting judgment.
[45] ECHR, article 5; also CRC, article 37(b).
[46] ECHR, articles 3 and 8; also CRC article 19(a).
[47] *Rabone v Pennine Care NHS Trust* [2012] UKSC 2.
[48] *Herczegfalvy v Austria* (1993) 15 EHRR 437.
[49] (2006) 43 EHRR 96.
[50] *Austin v Metropolitan Police Commissioner* [2009] UKHL 5, [45], Lord Walker.
[51] *In re D (A Child)* [2019] UKSC 42.

irrespective of their age (for a full account, see Hale *et al.*, 2017). Where hospital treatment for mental disorder is needed, most patients are admitted informally[52] under section 131(1), thereby avoiding the compulsory procedures.

The Mental Health Amendment Act (England and Wales) 2007 introduced important new legal safeguards for older adolescents regarding their informal admission. This responded to critics arguing that children, whether competent or not, had liberty interests which should be protected against the well-meaning but possibly arbitrary decisions of their parents. Now, where a patient aged 16 or 17 has capacity (i.e., has sufficient understanding and maturity) to consent to informal admission to hospital for treatment for mental disorder, and does consent, the arrangements may be made on the child's authority, even though there are one or more persons who have parental responsibility for the child (MHA, section (s) 131 (2), (3)); and where such a patient does *not* consent, the arrangements may *not* be made, even though a person with parental responsibility does consent (MHA, s 131(2), (4)). So, doctors can no longer bypass the refusal of a patient aged 16 or 17 who has capacity, by obtaining parental consent. They will have to choose between using compulsion under the MHA and going to court. The young patient's capacity to consent should be judged, not by the broad test of *Gillick* competence, but by the more explicit criteria of the MCA (s 3; see Box 19.3).

The MHA does not deal with the position where a child under the age of 16 also has that capacity. Presumably, therefore, the *Gillick* principle will apply where a competent child does consent to admission. Where a competent child refuses to agree to admission, the Code of Practice (Department of Health, 2015) states that "it is not advisable" to rely on the consent of a parent with parental responsibility (para 19.39). This is reinforced if the admission will amount to a deprivation of liberty: whether it does so depends upon the age of the child and the conditions in the hospital. The test is whether the restrictions are stricter than those which are normal for a child of that age.[53] If so, as with the older age group, the professionals will have to choose between the compulsory procedures in the MHA or asking the court to authorize admission and treatment.

Where a child of any age is not competent, or expresses no view about the admission, it will generally be possible to rely upon parental consent to an informal admission. The Code points out that the child may have the intellectual capacity to make a decision but in fact be so overwhelmed by the situation as to be unable to do so (para 19.31). But parents cannot consent to the admission of a 16- or 17-year-old who lacks capacity if this will amount to a deprivation of liberty.[54] The view has been expressed that this may also be true in relation to a younger child who lacks competence.[55]

Admission and treatment are different matters legally. Informal patients may not be treated without valid consent or some other lawful justification, so the same legal principles as those discussed earlier will apply. In other words, for those aged between 16 and 17, their competence to consent to treatment will be assessed by the criteria set out by the MCA; competence to consent for those under 16 is assessed by the *Gillick*-competence criterion.

Where informal admission or treatment is not possible, the same compulsory powers to admit for up to 28 days assessment (under MHA section 2,), or for up to 72 hours in an emergency (under MHA section 4), or longer term for treatment (under MHA section 3) are available for patients of any age. Although, as noted below, these procedures have features designed to protect the human rights of mental patients, they must obviously be effective to overcome the objections of the patient and, when relevant, the objections of a parent. A patient's nearest relative (usually a parent, if the patient is a minor) has no right to prevent an AMHP making an application for short-term admission under MHA section 2 or section 4, although "before or within a reasonable time," the AMHP must "take such steps as are practicable" to inform the nearest relative that the application is to be or has been made (MHA, s 11(3)). An AMHP cannot make an application for long-term admission for treatment under section 3 without first consulting the nearest relative, unless this is not reasonably practicable or would involve unreasonable delay (MHA, s 11(4)(b)); active consent of the nearest relative is not required, but the application cannot be made if that person objects (MHA, s 11(4)(a)). But there is a process for applying to a court to replace a nearest relative who unreasonably objects to the admission or is otherwise unsuitable (MHA, s 29).

The Act recognizes that removing a person's liberty in order to compel the patient to accept treatment is a drastic step and so the criteria, the procedures, and the consequences are clearly defined. Most forms of treatment for mental disorder may be given without the patient's consent when the MHA is used (MHA, s 63); this includes force-feeding for anorexia nervosa.[56] There are special safeguards for neurosurgery, long-term medication, and electroconvulsive therapy (ECT) (MHA, ss 57, 58, 58A). Neurosurgery cannot be performed on any patient, whether informal or detained, unless the patient is capable of consenting to it, does so consent, and an independent multidisciplinary team certify that it should be given (MHA, s 57). Patients under 18, whether informal or detained, cannot be given ECT without the benefit of an independent second opinion (MHA, ss 56(5) and 58A). Detained patients also have the right to apply to a tribunal for their discharge.[57]

It appears that attitudes to the use of the MHA for minors are gradually changing and that, particularly when treating eating disorders in older adolescents, doctors are now more prepared

[52] By informal patients we mean patients who are not compulsorily detained under legislation, but who voluntarily receive treatment.

[53] *Cheshire West and Chester Council v P; Surrey County Council v P and Q* [2014] UKSC 19.

[54] *Re D (A Child)* [2019] UKSC 42.

[55] Lady Black in *Re D* above.

[56] *Riverside Mental Health NHS Trust v Fox* [1994] 1 FLR 614.

[57] Now the Health, Education and Social Care (HESC) Chamber within the First-tier Tribunal.

to envisage its use. As discussed above, the law now acknowledges the autonomy rights of mentally ill or behaviorally disturbed 16- and 17-year-olds so far as informal admission is concerned. But in other respects, because of the law's complexity and uncertainty, young patients' rights can be overlooked. There is a difficult balance to be struck between the protection given by legal formalities and the stigma they are sometimes thought to bring.

Expert witnesses in court proceedings

Experts and the Mental Health Act and court proceedings

Compulsory procedures under the MHA require the prescribed medical recommendations explaining that the statutory criteria for detention and/or treatment are established (MHA, s 12). The patient's responsible clinician will usually be called upon to give evidence if the detention is challenged in a mental health tribunal (a panel that reviews cases where a patient detained under the MHA/their representative requests this) and the patient may have the benefit of an independent psychiatric report. Mental health professionals are also frequently called upon to give expert evidence in court proceedings about a child's future, assessing either the parents' mental health or parenting capacities, or the child's mental health, development, and well-being, or both. Experts differ from other witnesses in that they are permitted to give evidence, not only as to the facts, but also as to their opinions. In children proceedings they are allowed to base those opinions upon hearsay.[58] But they should be willing to acknowledge that medical records are not always perfectly accurate or complete and may from time to time repeat or rely upon unverified hearsay.

Categories of expert witnesses

Expert witnesses fall into two broad categories, although the distinction between them is not always clear cut. Professionals who are already working with the child or the family may be asked to report on the history, diagnosis, and treatment to date, together with their assessment and recommendations for the future. Independent experts may be commissioned to investigate, sometimes only on paper and sometimes also by seeing the parties, and to make a report and recommendations to the court.[59] This might be to assess the severity of a harm a patient has suffered or to assess capacity. Such reports may be commissioned by any of the parties to the case, but the court is in charge of whether and how many experts may be instructed and in which disciplines.[60] One aim is to prevent the child being subjected to multiple examinations and assessments (Butler-Sloss, 1988). Another is to prevent the proceedings becoming unnecessarily prolonged and expensive.

[58] Children Act 1989, s 96(3) to (7) and Children (Admissibility of Hearsay Evidence) Order 1993.

[59] *Re B (Sexual Abuse: Expert's Report)* [2000] 1 FLR 871.

[60] Family Proceedings Rules 2010, rule 25.1; Civil Procedure Rules 1998, rule 35.4.

Experts and assessment of children

The court has power to require an assessment of the child but not the treatment of the parents.[61] This does not always reflect the realities of psychiatric practice. In some of the most complex and difficult cases, it is not possible to separate the assessment of the child from the assessment of the parents.[62] What requires assessment is the relationship between them all and the capacities of the parents to meet the needs of the child. What begins as assessment may move into assessment with therapy and move again into therapy with continuing assessment. Our nice legal distinctions mean nothing to health care professionals who are assessing their patients all the time. This would not matter were it not for the problems of funding the very specialist resources which some of these deeply damaged families require. The court can only require the parties to pay for an assessment which is necessary to enable the court to perform its own function of deciding what order to make.

Single and jointly instructed experts

The court may require the parties to agree upon a single, jointly instructed expert. Even then, some cases require expertise in more than one discipline.[63] And while the battle between separately instructed experts can be unedifying, especially if one or other is seen as a "hired gun" for the instructing party, a single joint expert brings problems for a party who wishes to challenge their conclusions. Parents or children's guardians, who have serious concerns about the accuracy or rigor of an expert's report, face formidable difficulties if they try to challenge it without expert evidence of their own. It is not easy to reconcile the need of the child to be spared multiple and intrusive investigations, and to have the issues about their future resolved without delay, with the right (guaranteed by article 6 of the ECHR as well as the common law) of both the child and their family to a fair trial of the issues.

The use of expert evidence

Expert evidence can now only be commissioned where it is *necessary* to resolve the case and the information is not already available from other sources.[64] The court, rather than the parties, should decide what questions the expert should address. The expert's overriding duty is to the court and takes precedence over any duty to the party who instructs them. Although it is important for professionals to recall their obligations to protect client confidentiality and ensure they have the consent of patients or other legal authorization before disclosing private information. Expert witnesses enjoy immunity from suit in respect of their evidence but not the investigations leading up to

[61] Children Act 1989, s 38(6); *Re G (A Child) (Interim Care Order: Residential Assessment)* [2005] UKHL 68.

[62] *Re C (A Minor) (Interim Care Order: Residential Assessment)* [1997] AC 489.

[63] E.g., *Re B*, above.

[64] *Children and Families Act 2014, s 13*; Family Procedure Rules 2010, Part 25, also PD25B and PD25C.

it;[65] but this does not protect them from professional discipline if, for example, they go beyond the limits of their expertise;[66] and they may be held liable in negligence to the party who instructs them.[67] In family proceedings, a lack of contradiction or opposition will place a heightened duty of independent professionalism upon the expert witness and of vigilance upon the court. In Re C (Parental Alienation: instruction of expert)[68] grave concerns were raised at the use of unregulated psychologists in family cases. The President of the Family Division emphasized that expert evidence could only be given by a person who was qualified as an expert to give such evidence.

Conclusion

Children with mental health problems present more legal issues than do adults: there is the parents' responsibility for and authority over the child, as well as the more problematic question of the child's own autonomy. Mental health professionals are now much more aware of such questions than once they were. Fortunately, most of the time they are able to treat their patients without disputes or challenge. It is always better to try and reach agreement rather than to resort to the blunt instrument of legal proceedings which may polarize positions and make future cooperation for the sake of the patient more difficult.

[65] *D v East Berkshire Community NHS Trust* [2003] EWCA Civ 1151.
[66] *Meadow v General Medical Council* [2006] EWCA Civ 1390.
[67] *Jones v Kaney* [2011] UKSC 13.
[68] [2023] EWHC 345 (Fam).

References

Bencharif, S.-T. (2022) Europe's growing mental health care gap. *Politico.*

Butler-Sloss, L.J., (Chairman) (1988) *Report of the Inquiry into Child Abuse in Cleveland 1987* Cm 412. HMSO, London.

Chua, H. (2023) Consent to treatment for transgender youth: the next chapter—*Bell & Anor* v *the Tavistock and Portman NHS Foundation Trust & Ors. Modern Law Review* **86**, 214–225.

Daly, A. (2018) No weight for "due weight"? A children's autonomy principle in best interest proceedings. *International Journal of Children's Rights* **26**, 61–82.

Department of Health (2015) *Code of Practice: Mental Health Act 1983.* TSO, London.

Fortin, J. (2012) *Children's Rights and the Developing Law*, 3rd edn. Cambridge University Press, Cambridge, UK.

Freeman, M. (2020) *A Magna Carta for Children? Rethinking Children's Rights.* Cambridge University Press, Cambridge, UK.

Gilmore, S. (2017) Use of the UNCRC in family law cases in England and Wales. *International Journal of Children's Rights* **25**, 500–524.

Goold, I. *et al.* (eds) (2020) *Parental Rights, Best Interests, and Significant Harm.* Hart, Oxford, UK.

Hale, B. (2005) Understanding children's rights: theory and practice. *Childright* **216**, 3–8.

Hale, B. *et al.* (2017) *Mental Health Law*, 6th edn. Sweet and Maxwell, London.

Jowett, S. (2022) *Consent for Medical Treatment of Trans Youth.* Cambridge University Press, Cambridge, UK.

Todres, J. & King, S. (eds) (2020) *The Oxford Handbook of Children's Rights Law.* Oxford University Press, Oxford, UK.

Young Minds (2022) *Mental Health Waiting Times Harming Young People* Young Minds. Available: https://www.youngminds.org.uk/about-us/media-centre/press-releases/mental-health-waiting-times-harming-young-people/ [9 September 2024].

PART II

Influences on psychopathology

CHAPTER 20

Biological mechanisms linking childhood adversity to mental health problems

Andrea Danese[1,2,3] and Eamon McCrory[4,5]

[1] Social, Genetic and Developmental Psychiatry Centre, Institute of Psychiatry, Psychology and Neuroscience, King's College London, London, UK
[2] Department of Child and Adolescent Psychiatry, Institute of Psychiatry, Psychology and Neuroscience, King's College London, London, UK
[3] National and Specialist CAMHS Clinic for Trauma, Anxiety, and Depression, South London and Maudsley NHS Foundation Trust, London, UK
[4] Division of Psychology and Language Sciences, University College London, London, UK
[5] Anna Freud, London, UK

Introduction

Childhood adversities are experiences that challenge basic safety and support, requiring significant adaptation by the developing child. Although systemic, neurobiological, psychological, and sociocultural adaptations occur, these mechanisms may in some cases lead to maladaptive outcomes including mental health problems. These experiences are common in the population and became even more prevalent during the COVID-19 pandemic. In the chapter, we will present an overview of the intertwined set of mechanisms that are thought to explain the association between childhood adversity and mental health problems. We will also discuss key methodological and conceptual challenges to provide a balanced interpretation of the research findings in this area. Finally, we will reflect on how knowledge about mechanisms linking childhood adversity and mental health problems can inform the development of new interventions.

Conceptualizing childhood adversity

Childhood adversity encompasses several types of experiences: interpersonal adversities in childhood, such as maltreatment and bullying, that often have a chronic course (Box 20.1); absolute or relative poverty; discrimination (for example, based on race, sexual orientation, or gender); other psychosocial adversities with acute course, such as emergencies and disasters (see Chapter 18); and environmental adversities, such as pollution, traumatic brain injury, and infections. The term therefore captures a broad construct that is often difficult to measure or define comprehensively or with precision. Awareness of the ongoing measurement issues within the field (Box 20.2) is important to provide a balanced interpretation of clinical and biological findings discussed later in this chapter.

Childhood adversities are not randomly distributed in the population. They often occur together—both within and across types—in the same children (Felitti *et al.*, 1998; Finkelhor *et al.*, 2007). They also have cumulative effects on health outcomes (Felitti *et al.*, 1998; Finkelhor *et al.*, 2007; Danese *et al.*, 2009). As such, it is often difficult to study individual types of childhood adversity in humans in the same way that they can be studied in animal models, where experimental manipulation creates specific and unique exposures. The epidemiological evidence mirrors the findings from biological research. There is likely some specificity in the biological mechanisms linking individual types of childhood adversity to mental health problems—particularly with regard to environmental adversities. However, the mechanisms currently hypothesized to mediate the impact of childhood adversity on mental health typically converge on a common set of stress-sensitive pathways (Danese & McEwen, 2012), which are discussed in the following sections. Chronic interpersonal adversities in childhood often display the most detrimental clinical outcomes and have been most frequently studied (Lewis *et al.*, 2021). As such, they will be the primary focus of our discussion of biological mechanisms.

Rutter's Child and Adolescent Psychiatry and Psychology, Seventh Edition.
Edited by Anita Thapar, Daniel S. Pine, Samuele Cortese, Cathy Creswell, Tamsin J. Ford, James F. Leckman, and Argyris Stringaris.

Companion website: www.wiley.com/go/thapar/ruttterspsych7

Box 20.1 Definitions of childhood adversity

Childhood adversity. Experiences that challenge basic safety and support, requiring significant adaptation by the developing child.
Adverse childhood experiences (ACEs). The definition of ACEs can be ambiguous. The origin of the term goes back to the Adverse Childhood Experiences Study, which selected 10 experiences for a survey in adults accessing an American health maintenance organization: physical abuse, emotional abuse, sexual abuse, physical neglect, emotional neglect, parental mental illness, parental substance abuse, parental divorce, domestic violence, and incarcerated relative. However, the term is often used as a larger umbrella category that includes several other (nonspecified) adverse experiences in children.
Childhood physical abuse. Intentional use of physical force or implements against a child that results in, or has the potential to result in, physical injury.
Childhood sexual abuse. Any completed or attempted sexual act, sexual contact, or noncontact sexual interaction with a child by a caregiver.
Childhood emotional (psychological) abuse. Behavior that conveys to a child that he/she is worthless, flawed, unloved, unwanted, endangered, or valued only in meeting another's needs.
Childhood neglect. Failure to meet a child's basic physical, emotional, medical/dental, or educational needs; failure to provide adequate nutrition, hygiene, or shelter; or failure to ensure a child's safety.
Childhood maltreatment. Any act of commission or omission by a parent or other caregiver that results in harm, potential for harm, or threat of harm to a child. Harm does not need to be intended. Maltreatment includes physical, sexual, and emotional abuse and neglect.
Bullying (peer) victimization. Repeated hurtful actions between peers where an imbalance of power exists.
Childhood victimization. This umbrella term is used to indicate the combination of maltreatment by adults and bullying by peers.
Childhood trauma. The definition of childhood trauma can be ambiguous. A narrow definition is based on classification systems for mental illness (American Psychiatric Association, 2013; World Health Organization, 2018), where trauma exposure is defined in order to identify individuals with post-traumatic stress disorder (PTSD). For example, in the most recent DSM-5-TR (American Psychiatric Association, 2022), criteria for trauma exposure are met when a person was exposed to death, threatened death, actual or threatened serious injury, or actual or threatened sexual violence through direct exposure, witnessing the trauma, learning that a relative or close friend was exposed to a trauma, or indirect exposure to aversive details of the trauma. However, the term is often used as a larger umbrella category that includes several other (nonspecified) adverse experiences in children.

Source: Adapted from Danese, 2020.

Box 20.2 Measurement issues

Dimensional versus cumulative approaches

In recent years, there has been a focus on the potential explanatory value of dimensional versus cumulative approaches to the investigation of brain mechanisms. A long-standing framework is the cumulative risk perspective (Felitti *et al.*, 1998) within which accruing a greater number of risk experiences is associated with more compromised developmental outcomes. The emphasis is on cumulative risk rather than the role of any particular form of adversity.

By contrast, dimensional models focus on the putative impact of specific forms of adversity. One prominent model has sought to contrast the impact of *deprivation* (experiences characterized by a paucity of social and cognitive inputs, such as neglect and deprivation) with the impact of *threat* (experiences characterized by actual harm, like physical abuse). The model derives from the premise that different environmental experiences have differential impacts on neurodevelopmental mechanisms and these in turn have different implications for mental health and cognitive outcomes. There is evidence that threat-related experiences are associated with altered structure and function of several brain regions implicated in emotion processing, including the amygdala and hippocampus (McLaughlin *et al.*, 2019). In contrast, evidence of the impact of deprivation points to a more distributed set of alterations in brain regions associated with executive functioning (Sheridan *et al.*, 2017; Puetz *et al.*, 2019).

The dimensional approach has been critiqued (Smith & Pollak, 2021) because adversity types are highly overlapping, both conceptually and in their distribution in community samples (Debowska *et al.*, 2017), undermining the explanatory value of focusing on any individual adversity types. There also remains a paucity of experimental data supporting unique or specific effects for different types of childhood adversity. Finally, it has been highlighted that the impact of any form of adversity is mediated by appraisal—a child's perception of the experience (Danese & Widom, 2020). That is, how an individual constructs their experience of an event is instrumental in determining the impact that experience then has—psychologically as well as biologically—and in this way the specific category of the event itself is arguably of secondary importance (Smith & Pollak, 2021).

Prospective versus retrospective measures

A cross-cutting measurement issue relates to the data source used to capture the experience of adversity. Childhood adversity is rarely measured based on the account of children in childhood. Prospective measures of adversity collected in childhood typically rely on observer reports (e.g., parents, teachers, child protection services), which capture—with variable degrees of objectivity—the third-person perspective on the events. Most studies on adversity are based on retrospective measures, namely self-reports typically collected in adult life, which capture the subjective, first-person perspective on the events. Because of the assumption that prospective and retrospective measures identify the same groups of individuals, the two measures have long been used interchangeably (Danese, 2020). However, this assumption is not supported by the available data. In a meta-analysis of the agreement between prospective and retrospective measures of childhood maltreatment, the overlap between groups was very limited ($k = 0.19$) (Baldwin *et al.*, 2019). This indicated that prospective and retrospective measures of childhood maltreatment capture different constructs and should not be used interchangeably. For example, it is inappropriate to conflate the findings (e.g., brain-imaging differences, associations with health outcomes) based on retrospective measures of childhood maltreatment with explanatory models based on prospective measures (Danese, 2020).

Different levels of explanation

The following section provides an overview of the intertwined mechanisms that are thought to explain the association between childhood adversity and mental health problems. Our description of these mechanisms centers around a multilevel model of biological mediation that attempts to integrate relevant systemic, neurobiological, psychological, and sociocultural factors (Figure 20.1). This developmental model explicitly challenges biological reductionism by highlighting how mental health problems may emerge over time as a result of the interaction between these levels. The model also challenges all-encompassing but poorly specified theories by providing examples grounded in empirical research.

At a systemic level, the mechanisms described capture evolutionarily well-conserved responses to (originally physical) threats in the environment. At the neurobiological level, the mechanisms reflect functional brain adaptations that drive defensive behaviors. At the psychological level, the mechanisms ensure that aversive emotions are minimized, that new experiences are appraised by individuals based on their existing knowledge, and that new knowledge guides future behaviors by shaping perception and the formation of memories, identity, and schemas. At the sociocultural level, the mechanisms enable individuals to engage or disengage with others to maximize survival and fitness. Mechanisms at different levels of explanation influence each other and interact with other social, genetic, and developmental factors to create highly individualized patterns of response to childhood adversity. Mapping these complex processes and interactions can help explain resilience and vulnerability to psychopathology after childhood adversity.

Systemic mechanisms

Childhood adversities can trigger systemic biological responses aimed at maintaining the stability of human physiology (or homeostasis) in the face of external stressors (Danese & McEwen, 2012). The process of maintaining homeostasis through adaptive changes in the organism, or allostasis, involves hormonal and immune pathways that, in the short term, protect the body from damage and promote survival. Childhood adversities occur early in life when the allostatic systems, like the hormonal and immune systems, are still developing and are more sensitive to environmental stimuli. As such, they may lead to long-term activation of the allostatic systems, meaning that they persist well after childhood adversities have ended. The resulting allostatic load, or chronic overactivation of once-adaptive stress-responsive hormonal and immune systems, has been associated with later mental health and physical health problems (Danese & McEwen, 2012).

The main hormonal system promoting adaptation to stress is the hypothalamic–pituitary–adrenal (HPA) axis. There is now a comprehensive body of work indicating that altered activity of the HPA axis is associated with exposure to childhood adversity. Acute psychosocial stressors are known to trigger the HPA axis, leading to the secretion of cortisol in humans. Cortisol first supports the increased metabolic demands for fight-or-flight responses by mobilizing stored energy and then inhibiting physiological arousal (Danese & McEwen, 2012). This adaptive role of cortisol is diminished during chronic stress, either because hormonal production abates (hypocortisolism) or because the biological efficacy of cortisol is reduced in the context of chronic hyperproduction, which over time leads to reduced sensitivity of the cortisol receptor (glucocorticoid receptor resistance) (Danese & McEwen, 2012). These types of alterations of the HPA axis have been reported in several mental health problems, pointing to the HPA axis as a biologically plausible mediator between childhood adversity and psychopathology (Koss & Gunnar, 2017). Several studies have tested multiple indices of HPA axis abnormalities in individuals with histories of childhood adversity. Meta-analytical studies have found that childhood maltreatment may be associated with small elevations in hair cortisol, suggesting chronic cortisol overproduction (Khoury *et al.*, 2019), and with small reductions in wake-up cortisol levels (particularly in agency-referred samples), suggesting possible hypocortisolism (Bernard *et al.*, 2017). Findings have been inconsistent with regard to the cortisol awakening response (CAR), which reflects the degree of change in cortisol levels from wake to peak 30 minutes later (Bernard *et al.*, 2017; Fogelman & Canli, 2018), and to cortisol reactivity to acute psychosocial stressors (Bunea *et al.*, 2017; Fogelman & Canli, 2018). No association has been found between childhood maltreatment and diurnal slope, or unstimulated daytime cortisol levels (Bernard *et al.*, 2017; Bunea *et al.*, 2017). This complex pattern of findings likely reflects significant methodological heterogeneity across studies.

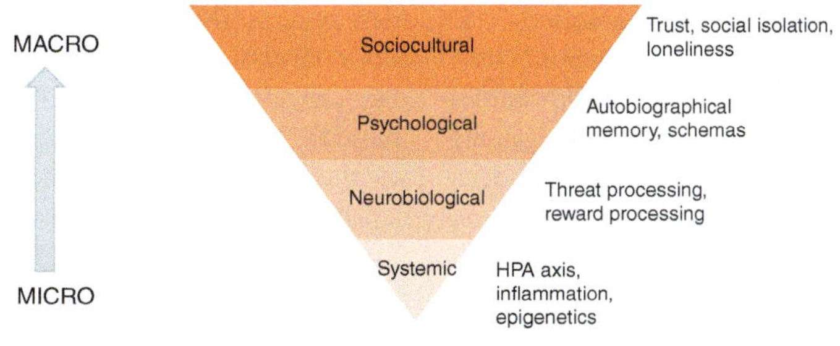

Figure 20.1 The different levels of explanation.

Childhood adversity has also been associated with overactivation of the immune system, and particularly the component of the immune system that is already active during early development—the innate inflammatory response. An inflammatory response can be adaptive in the short term, for example, if adversities are accompanied by physical injury. However, chronic activation of the inflammatory response can be detrimental, negatively affecting brain development, key behavioral domains (e.g., cognition, positive valence systems, negative valence systems), reactivity to subsequent stressors, and, ultimately, risk for psychopathology (Danese & Baldwin, 2017; Danese & Lewis, 2017). Childhood adversity may influence the inflammatory response owing to the HPA axis abnormalities described above, leading to impaired anti-inflammatory effects of cortisol (Danese & Baldwin, 2017; Danese & Lewis, 2017). Childhood adversity may also be related to inflammation directly or indirectly because of behavioral mechanisms linked to obesity, substance misuse, or poor sleep (Danese & Baldwin, 2017; Danese & Lewis, 2017). Initial evidence for the association between childhood maltreatment and chronic inflammation in humans was reported in a long-term cohort study (Danese *et al.*, 2007), replicated in dozens of studies in adults (Baumeister *et al.*, 2015), but less clearly in young people (Kuhlman *et al.*, 2020), and back-translated in multiple animal models (Dutcher *et al.*, 2020; Lumertz *et al.*, 2022). Despite the causal evidence from experimental animal models (Lumertz *et al.*, 2022), the origins of the association between childhood adversity and inflammation in humans remain unclear and require further investigation. For example, a Mendelian randomization analysis indicated noncausal links between childhood maltreatment and inflammation (Warrier *et al.*, 2021).

In the turn of the century, research has also begun to investigate the molecular mechanisms underpinning the biological responses to childhood adversity. For example, experiments in animal models have shown that early life stress can exert long-term influence on HPA axis functioning through neuronal DNA methylation (Weaver *et al.*, 2004), a molecular process that prevents the binding of transcriptional factors to DNA and, thus, inhibits gene transcription. This seminal preclinical work sparked several human studies testing epigenetic changes in peripheral cells, examining both candidate genes as well as epigenome-wide differences between individuals with or without a history of childhood maltreatment (Cecil *et al.*, 2020; Parade *et al.*, 2021). Systematic reviews found that childhood maltreatment was associated with heterogeneous patterns of epigenome-wide differences (Cecil *et al.*, 2020; Parade *et al.*, 2021), although studies in large population-representative samples found no epigenetic differences particularly when accounting for basic confounders, including smoking (Marzi *et al.*, 2018). Epigenetic modification offers an intriguing molecular mechanism to map the effects of environmental adversity in childhood on stress biology. However, further research is needed to address several methodological challenges in human epigenetic studies (Gladish *et al.*, 2022) including adequate control for known confounders, better understanding of tissue specificity, sufficient statistical power, direction of effects, and more direct mapping of links between childhood adversity-related epigenetic differences, and biological and clinical outcomes.

Although the examples considered above have focused on chronic interpersonal adversities in childhood, such as maltreatment, other types of childhood adversity have shown some associations with the same stress-sensitive pathways. For example, in one study examining the links with poverty, a sample of adults with low early-life socioeconomic status (SES; as defined by parental occupation during the first five years of life) showed greater cortisol secretion during the day and downregulation of genes responding to the glucocorticoid receptor, as well as upregulation of genes responding to proinflammatory stimuli and greater production of cytokines (inflammatory biomarkers) compared to adults who had higher SES in childhood (Miller *et al.*, 2009). A small correlation between lower childhood socioeconomic status and higher inflammation has also been identified in a meta-analysis (Milaniak & Jaffee, 2019). Similarly, racial discrimination in young people is associated with stronger acute cortisol reactivity, higher overall cortisol output, and a flatter diurnal cortisol slope (Adam *et al.*, 2020), as well as high inflammation levels (Brody *et al.*, 2015). Furthermore, in studies that have examined the impact of war, hair cortisol concentration was found to be positively, but weakly, associated with the number of war-related events experienced in a cohort of Syrian refugee young people and decreased with time since leaving Syria (Smeeth *et al.*, 2023). These findings await replication and clarification in future studies.

Neurobiological mechanisms

Studies employing functional magnetic resonance imaging (MRI) have investigated a range of potential neurocognitive mechanisms contributing to elevated psychiatric risk in children who have experienced maltreatment (McCrory *et al.*, 2017a; McCrory *et al.*, 2017b). Although inconsistencies remain in the literature, these studies have described altered functioning in several neurocognitive domains that have also been shown to characterize individuals presenting with psychiatric disorder, including threat processing and emotion regulation, reward processing, and autobiographical memory (ABM) functioning (McCrory *et al.*, 2011, 2017a, 2017b). The biological embedding of adverse experience may be associated with recalibration of these systems (Danese & McEwen, 2012; McCrory & Viding, 2015; McCrory *et al.* 2017a) representing (at least partly) adaptations that provide proximal benefits for a child in dangerous or unpredictable environments. There is a lively debate as to whether experiencing specific kinds of adversity (for example, deprivation versus threat) have specific effects on the brain—see Box 20.2 for a consideration of this issue. According to the theory of latent vulnerability, brain adaptations following adversity may be poorly optimized for normative environments, contributing to an increased risk of psychopathology (McCrory &

Viding, 2015; McCrory *et al.*, 2017a). Such risk may arise directly (e.g., as a result of maladaptive emotional processing). However, as we discuss in more detail later, latent factors may increase the risk of psychiatric disorder indirectly by influencing how an individual interacts with their social world. Here we focus on the evidence for altered functioning of three neurocognitive domains: threat processing and emotion regulation, reward processing, and ABM.

Threat processing and emotion regulation

Studies have shown that adverse experiences, including maltreatment, are associated with disrupted threat processing, with evidence for both hypervigilance toward and avoidance of threat cues, depending on the experimental context (see Hein and Monk (2017) for a meta-analytic review; see also the "defensive behavior" section of Chapter 12). A variety of specific processes may be implicated, including preattentive threat evaluation, cognitive, affective, and physiological resource allocation (including selective attention), and metacognitive voluntary response (including effortful control or avoidance). For example, studies of incidental processing and preattentive threat processing have reported heightened reactivity in response to angry faces in the amygdala, a key threat processing region, in both adults and children with a history of maltreatment (McCrory *et al.*, 2011, 2013). Amygdala hyperactivity has also been reported in children exposed to community disadvantage (Suarez *et al.*, 2022). Conversely, other studies show that maltreated children, as well as children exposed to community violence, present with amygdala hypoactivation in response to threat-related cues (Puetz *et al.*, 2016; Huggins *et al.*, 2022) and patterns of behavioral avoidance to social threat cues (Kelly *et al.*, 2015). A bias toward or away from threat is likely to be adaptive when a child is in a dangerous environment—it might be useful for a child to be highly alert to threat, or protective to disengage from it (McCrory & Viding, 2015). However, over time, these strategies may increase risk—especially as heightened reactivity is typically associated with reduced emotion regulation and cognitive control (Jenness *et al.*, 2021). Hypervigilance, poorer emotion regulation, and neural hyperreactivity to threat have been implicated in conduct disorder and anxiety disorders (Cisler & Koster, 2010), and similar patterns of neural response have been found in individuals with depression and post-traumatic stress disorder (PTSD) (Etkin & Wager, 2007), showing the role that altered threat processing and poor emotion regulation plays in a broad range of psychiatric disorders. Prior differences in neural reactivity to threat may help account for the impact of adverse experiences, including the impact of natural disasters on subsequent mental health problems (e.g., Kujawa *et al.*, 2016).

Reward processing

Children and adolescents who have experienced adversity have also shown attenuated response in the neural circuitry underpinning reward processing (see Oltean *et al.*, (2023) for a recent meta-analysis; see also Chapter 12 for a general overview of reward anticipation circuitry and clinical applications). This includes altered reward processing associated with maltreatment experience (McCrory *et al.*, 2017a), social deprivation (Hein *et al.*, 2020), lower family income (Palacios-Barrios *et al.*, 2021), and general family adversity (Holz *et al.*, 2017). Reward processing relates to a set of neurocognitive mechanisms that respond to desirable stimuli, largely underpinned by a mesocorticolimbic dopaminergic circuit (Delgado, 2007). Such alterations may arise in abusive and particularly neglectful environments characterized by scarce and unpredictable rewards, which may also act to constrain reward learning (Glynn & Baram, 2019; Blair *et al.*, 2022). Blunted responses to reward might be appropriate and adaptive in such contexts, potentially reducing disappointment and effort expenditure where there is a low likelihood of rewarding outcomes. However, attenuated response to rewarding stimuli has been implicated in the development of depression (Mackin *et al.*, 2019) and with several other disorders, including attention deficit hyperactivity disorder (ADHD), eating disorders, and schizophrenia (Aldridge-Waddon *et al.*, 2020).

Autobiographical memory

Detailed memories of personally experienced events—known as ABM—are central to our sense of self and guide how we perceive and respond to our present experience. The neural basis of ABM has been assessed experimentally using paradigms in which participants recall well-specified emotionally valenced memories in the scanner (e.g., Young *et al.*, 2014; McCrory *et al.*, 2017b). Such ABM retrieval engages a distributed network of prefrontal, parietal, and temporal regions that are differentially weighted in individuals with depression and PTSD (St Jacques *et al.*, 2013; Young *et al.*, 2013). Children and adolescents have been found to engage a similar neural network during ABM retrieval as adults (McCrory *et al.*, 2017b). Those who have experienced maltreatment show a distinct pattern of neural activity in this network, similar to that seen in adults with depression, including reduced activation in the hippocampus (when recalling positive memories), and increased activation in the amygdala (when recalling negative memories) (McCrory *et al.*, 2017b). Such a pattern may reflect greater salience accorded to negative versus positive memories and increase the likelihood of a negative inferential style, negative self-schemata, and a ruminative response style—all cognitive vulnerabilities associated with maltreatment experience and psychiatric vulnerability (McCrory *et al.*, 2017b).

Psychological mechanisms

Formation and retrieval of autobiographical memories are also understood to operate mechanistically at the psychological level in influencing long-term mental health outcomes following adversity exposure. ABM is a uniquely human form of memory that moves beyond recall of experienced events to integrate perspective, interpretation, and evaluation across self, other, and time to create a personal history. Childhood adversity can affect the formation of negative autobiographical memories in childhood and, thus, exert profound and detrimental influences on the developing mental representations (models or schemas) of self and the world (Conway *et al.*, 2005; Goodman *et al.*, 2010). In turn, retrieval of memories about childhood adversity and related maladaptive schemas play a central role in transdiagnostic cognitive models psychopathology (Danese, 2020; Dalgleish & Hitchcock, 2023). Furthermore, it has long been known that ABM is not an accurate representation but rather an "imaginative reconstruction" of experience (Schacter, 1999). Regardless of their veracity, autobiographical memories of childhood adversity may, therefore, influence risk of psychopathology (Danese, 2020). Selected examples provide empirical evidence for these mechanisms.

A cohort of 1196 children that was followed up to the age of 30 years has investigated the role of ABM of childhood maltreatment in psychopathology (Danese & Widom, 2020). Roughly half of the study members had a documented history of childhood maltreatment based on court records (or "objective" experience of maltreatment), whereas the remaining study members did not have such history and were demographically matched. The retrospective recall of childhood maltreatment memories (or "subjective" experience of maltreatment) was measured at age 30 years. Even for the severe cases of childhood maltreatment identified through court records, the risk of lifetime psychopathology at 30 years was not associated with objective measures in the absence of subjective reports. In contrast, the risk of lifetime psychopathology was associated with subjective reports of childhood maltreatment, whether or not the reports were consistent with objective measures.

Beyond recollection of memories of childhood adversity, distortion of ABM more generally (Dalgleish & Hitchcock, 2023) may contribute to later mental health problems. In particular, meta-analytical evidence suggests that inability to deliberately recollect details of personal events, or overgeneral memory, is a transdiagnostic risk factor for psychopathology (Barry *et al.*, 2021). In the context of childhood adversity, overgeneral memory may be adaptive in the short term, by promoting recall of less vivid or detailed memories of negative experiences. However, it may prove maladaptive in the longer term, by reducing access to previously successful strategies to cope with distress. Consistent with this hypothesis, children (Valentino *et al.*, 2009; McCrory *et al.*, 2017b) and adults (Kuyken & Brewin, 1995) with histories of childhood maltreatment show a pattern of overgeneral memory. Furthermore, in adolescents with a documented history of childhood maltreatment, overgeneral memory has been associated with subsequent reduced prosocial behavior and showed a trend-level association with elevated depressive symptoms (Puetz *et al.*, 2020).

Sociocultural mechanisms

Significant childhood adversity, including experiences of maltreatment, is robustly associated with an increased risk of difficulties in social relationships in adulthood, including social isolation, loneliness, increased peer victimization, violence in romantic relationships, and reduced levels of social support (McCrory *et al.*, 2022). Individuals with a history of maltreatment, for example, typically have smaller social networks (defined as fewer social relationships and less frequent social contacts) than those who did not experience maltreatment (Hanlon *et al.*, 2020). These social difficulties are thought, in turn, to contribute to an increased risk of mental health problems because they compromise the construction of an adaptive "social architecture" which includes: (i) social status, which is one's position within a hierarchy, indexing access to resources; (ii) social integration, which is one's ability to maintain affiliative or supportive relationships; and (iii) social stress, which is one's experience of interpersonal stressful or adverse events (McCrory *et al.*, 2022). Human and animal studies have demonstrated that these aspects of social architecture are impacted by adverse early experience (Snyder-Mackler *et al.*, 2020). How does this happen? What role do biological mechanisms play in this risk pathway?

The patterns of neurocognitive and psychological adaptation following significant adversity reviewed above may contribute to poorly optimized social functioning in more normative environments. This may arise in at least two main ways. First, if social functioning is poorly optimized there is a greater risk of conflict or stress in our interpersonal interactions. This phenomenon, known as stress generation, was originally identified in individuals with depression (Hammen, 2006) and acknowledges that the individual is not just a passive recipient of their environment but an active agent in its construction. Multiple studies have found that stress generation is associated with childhood maltreatment (Hernandez *et al.*, 2016; McCrory *et al.*, 2022) including, for example, increased interpersonal stress (including in romantic relationships) and rejection compared to typically developing individuals. Further empirical studies are required to establish how precisely altered neurocognitive functioning (for example, heightened threat reactivity or attenuated reward processing) may influence affective and behavioral functioning in ways that increase the risk of generating interpersonal stress.

A second way that neurocognitive adaptation to early adverse early environments may lead to poorly optimized social functioning is via "social thinning." This refers to the attenuation of a child's network of affiliative or supportive relationships over time or their potential to develop such relationships in the first place (McCrory, 2020; McCrory *et al.* 2022). Individuals with a history of maltreatment, for example, present with social thinning during childhood and adolescence and impoverished social networks even many years later. Adults who reported adverse childhood events, including maltreatment, experience less social support from both family and friends than adults who reported few or no adverse events (Duncan *et al.*, 2015). Another study of more than 150,000 adults found that adults who self-reported one type of childhood maltreatment (either physical, sexual, or emotional abuse, or neglect) were more likely to experience loneliness and social isolation than were individuals who experienced no maltreatment (Hanlon *et al.*, 2020). It is widely accepted that reduced levels of social support contribute to psychiatric risk; several studies have found that social support moderates or partly mediates the association between childhood maltreatment and later psychiatric disorder (Cicchetti & Doyle, 2016).

How do alterations in neurocognitive systems following significant adversity (including maltreatment) impact social functioning in ways that increase the risk of stress generation and social thinning? Such research is in its infancy. It is plausible that heightened threat reactivity, poorer emotion regulation, attenuated response to reward and altered memory processing each—in different ways—lead to poorly optimized social functioning. In addition, alterations in trust processing—that are commonly experienced in clinical practice—have now been established experimentally in children and young people with history of maltreatment (Neil *et al.*, 2022). This group found unfamiliar faces significantly less trustworthy than their non-maltreated peers. Over time, alterations in one or more of these domains may contribute to the construction of a maladaptive social architecture that, in turn, will influence future brain development. This is illustrated in Figures 20.2.

In Figure 20.2a, a relatively high number of risk factors and a paucity of protective influences lead to stress generation and social thinning. These processes influence ongoing canalization within neurocognitive systems, such that, over time, the systems have reduced ability to optimally support individuals when they negotiate new social challenges. This in turn leads to a social architecture characterized by more stressful interpersonal interactions and fewer protective social relationships. By

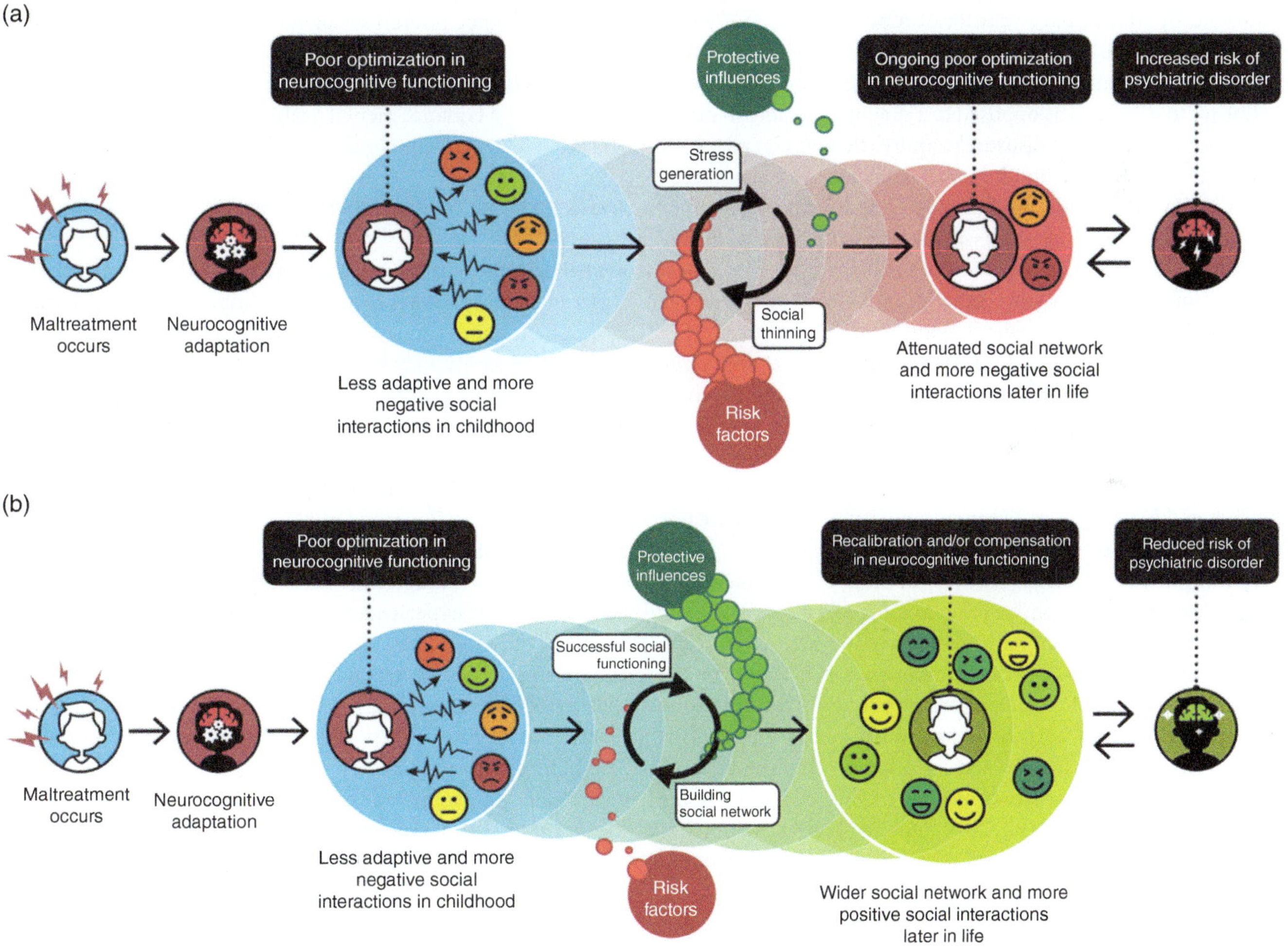

Figure 20.2 Mechanisms in action. Part (a): The neurocognitive social transactional model: a risk trajectory. This scenario depicts a child who has experienced maltreatment (repeated exposure to abuse or neglect, or both) and subsequently experiences further risk factors and a paucity of protective influences. In this context, increased stress generation and social thinning lead to an impoverished social architecture, contributing ultimately to an increased risk of psychiatric disorder. Part (b): The neurocognitive social transactional model: a resilient trajectory. This scenario depicts a child who has experienced maltreatment (repeated exposure to abuse or neglect, or both) and subsequently experiences a range of protective influences that help build and maintain their social relationships, and relatively few risk factors. In this context, less stress generation and social thinning lead to a richer, more adaptive social architecture, contributing ultimately to a decreased risk of psychiatric disorder. *Source:* McCrory *et al.*, 2022/with permission of Elsevier.

contrast, in Figure 20.2b, the same initial neurocognitive adaptations after maltreatment arise within a context of more protective influences and fewer risk factors. In this pathway, a child is able gradually to build a more positive, supportive social architecture, which in turn contributes to recalibration or compensation of neurocognitive functioning. Over time, the risk of psychiatric disorder is lowered as a function of both more adaptive neurocognitive functioning and a more protective social architecture.

Interplay among different levels

When we think about the relationship between adversity and psychiatric risk it is necessary to embed our understanding of biology within a multilevel framework that encompasses cognitive, emotional, and social systems. The interplay between each of these levels of explanation is essential for any comprehensive understanding of illness, a position originally informed by Engel's biopsychosocial model (Engel, 1977) (see Savalescu *et al.* (2020) for a contemporary perspective). In other words, a mechanistic understanding (that sheds light on pathways to disorder) as opposed to a diagnostic understanding (that simply categorizes disorder) requires that we consider how one level is shaped by another. Such interactions are complex and not fully predictable, but rather act in a probabilistic manner across development. A very simple example relates to the importance of cognitive appraisal in influencing the biological impact of a stressor—in general, stressors *perceived* as uncontrollable have a greater impact on HPA reactivity (Liu *et al.*, 2021). With regard to abuse and neglect, the same experience may elicit different cognitive appraisals that, in turn, elicit different biological reactions across individuals, with long-term implications for mental health vulnerability (Danese & Widom, 2020). The lesson here is simple: cognition impacts biology and biology impacts cognition. It is neither possible nor sensible to see one level as privileged.

ABM provides a helpful exemplar of multilevel interaction in the context of adversity and psychopathology. At a systemic level, adaptive response to traumatic events requires activation of the HPA axis, and low basal cortisol levels are a risk factor for the development of PTSD, while administration of hydrocortisone (a synthetic form of cortisol) may reduce memory intrusions (Hennessy *et al.*, 2022). As such, HPA axis abnormalities or linked inflammatory abnormalities described in some maltreated children may contribute to the formation of intrusive autobiographical memories of childhood maltreatment (Danese & Baldwin, 2017; Danese & Lewis, 2017). At the neurobiological level, maltreatment experience is associated with reduced activation in the hippocampus and increased activation in the parahippocampal gyrus (when recalling positive memories), and increased activation in the amygdala (when recalling negative memories). At the cognitive level, these changes may increase the propensity for rumination, contributing to increased risk of depression (McCrory *et al.*, 2017b). As previously noted, a pattern of overgeneral memory following adversity can also emerge, potentially serving to minimize negative affect (Dalgleish & Werner-Seidler, 2014). This memory style is associated with poor problem-solving abilities and negative self-representations (Valentino *et al.*, 2009) such that affected individuals may be less able to generate effective solutions to interpersonal problems. For example, people with overgeneral memory may find it harder than those without this memory style to remember what behavior exacerbated previous similar challenges, and what led to a successful resolution. In other words, a pattern of overgeneral ABM may lead to poorly optimized social functioning. The presence of memory biases, such as intrusive recollection or overgeneral memory, can affect risk for psychopathology directly or indirectly modifying the social environment of maltreated children (Danese & Widom, 2020, 2021). In line with this, children and adolescents who have experienced adversity show a pattern of overgeneral memory that has been found to predict poorer social functioning with peers (Puetz *et al.*, 2020). Such difficulties may contribute to stress generation and social thinning over time, act cumulatively to compromise resilience, and enhance mental health risk (McCrory *et al.*, 2022).

Addressing misconceptions

The importance of a developmental perspective

It is important to always consider the impact of adversity within a developmental framework. Brain changes associated with early life adversity may be evident in children and adolescents but not in adults (Pollok *et al.*, 2022). Moreover, the timing of exposure *during* childhood and adolescence matters, with evidence of earlier exposure having a greater impact on brain, cognitive, and HPA function (McCrory *et al.*, 2013; Sonuga-Barke *et al.*, 2017; Raymond *et al.*, 2021) and possibly the same form of adversity having different regional impacts on the brain at different ages (Andersen *et al.*, 2008). For example, Romanian adoptees who experienced institutionalization beyond six months of age were found to present with particularly compromised emotional and cognitive outcomes, indicating that extended early deprivation is associated with long-term deleterious effects on well-being (Sonuga-Barke *et al.*, 2017). Initial findings suggest that adults who experienced famine, specifically during gestation, show altered white matter across the entire cerebrum (Hulshoff Pol *et al.*, 2000), while adolescents (but not infants) who experience sexual abuse show reductions in gray matter volume in the frontal cortex (Andersen *et al.*, 2008).

It has been argued that such findings indicate the presence of critical periods of development during which adversity can exert particularly deleterious effects. These effects are thought to emerge when there are violations in the expectable environment (both in relation to biological and psychosocial hazards) at critical periods of brain maturation and plasticity (Nelson & Gabard-Durnam, 2020). Such changes can contribute to cumulative risk by impacting brain development at key periods of maturation, as well as impacting cognition and behavior. In other words, adversity influences transactional and iterative neurocognitive, behavioral, and social processes that can interact in important ways with a child's developmental stage and stage of brain maturation. These interactions will play out over development in ways that are always important to consider in the context of psychiatric risk (McCrory *et al.*, 2022).

The importance of the longitudinal design

In building explanatory models for the association between childhood adversity and psychopathology, it is important to recognize that many of the studies in humans discussed above rely on cross-sectional design with single measures of biological pathways that cannot disentangle longitudinal changes from stable preexisting vulnerabilities (Danese, 2020). For example, several studies in humans have identified cognitive deficits in individuals with a history of childhood maltreatment compared to nonmaltreatment individuals—interpreting such differences as changes in cognitive abilities linked to maltreatment. However, longitudinal analyses with repeated cognitive measures and twin analyses found that group differences in cognitive abilities between maltreated and nonmaltreatment individuals were largely explained by cognitive deficits already observed *prior* to exposure to maltreatment (Danese *et al.*, 2017). In contrast to prior interpretations, these findings suggest that cognitive deficits are stable, preexisting vulnerabilities rather than consequences of maltreatment, and risk factors for exposure to maltreatment. Animal models can provide initial, suggestive evidence of causal mechanisms, but their relevance to humans is unclear. In addition to indirect evidence from animal models, human studies with longitudinal and genetically sensitive designs are needed to strengthen causal inference in the associations between childhood adversity and putative biological pathways for psychopathology (Danese, 2020), as further discussed in Chapter 13.

Deterministic explanations for the effects of childhood adversity versus individual differences

Explanatory models for the association between childhood adversity and psychopathology commonly describe average differences in biomarkers between groups with or without histories of childhood adversity. Such models can be misinterpreted to provide deterministic explanations—suggesting that all individuals within a group show similar abnormalities. However, probabilistic effects have consistently been found across clinical and biological studies. For example, ACEs have been repeatedly associated with negative health outcomes in the population (Felitti *et al.*, 1998), but many individuals reporting a high ACE score do not develop negative health outcomes, and many individuals with negative health outcomes do not have a high ACE score (Baldwin *et al.*, 2021; Meehan *et al.*, 2022). As such, ACEs are not helpful to develop individual risk prediction models from population screening (Danese, 2020). Similar observations are also common in biological research. For example, although childhood maltreatment is associated with heightened inflammation in the population, not all individuals with a history of childhood maltreatment have high inflammation, and many individuals with high inflammation do not have a history of childhood maltreatment (Danese *et al.*, 2007). Of note, the probabilistic nature of these associations underscores the significant individual differences found in the face of childhood adversities. Better understanding of the differences in biological responses among individuals exposed to childhood adversity will help identify resilience mechanisms and new treatment targets.

Interpreting brain differences

Interpreting the meaning of differences in brain structure or function in individuals who have experienced adversity, and their relevance to psychopathology, is not as straightforward as it might first appear. First, it is often assumed that brain differences associated with adversity are fixed. This is not necessarily the case. Changes in activation in regions associated with PTSD in children exposed to adversity have been reported following trauma-focused cognitive behavioral therapy (CBT) (Garrett *et al.*, 2019). This points to malleability in brain response. Moreover, preliminary evidence has shown that, over time, functional brain differences can attenuate, even in the absence of specific intervention (Puetz *et al.*, 2021). A second common assumption is that the meaning of alterations in brain structure or function following adverse experience is self-evident. In practice, the opposite is often true. For example, there is a thin empirical basis to infer what greater or smaller gray matter in a given region actually means in functional terms. For example, decreased amygdala *volumes* have frequently been observed in PTSD but (rather counterintuitively) individuals with PTSD typically present with increased amygdala functional *activation* (Ganzel *et al.*, 2008). In other words, altered structure is not readily interpretable in functional terms. Functional studies are more interpretable when triangulated with experimental task and group performance. But here again we are often reliant on assumptions about the cognitive processes thought to be associated with a given brain region or task and the putative mechanistic role they play in mental health disorder or etiology. As a general rule, therefore, the significance and meaning of brain findings should always be judged with caution (especially those that have not been replicated) and interpreted alongside what we know from clinical and psychological studies.

Translational implications

The mechanisms described have important implications for clinical advancement. For example, ABM offers an excellent example of how we might advance mechanistically informed approaches for clinical interventions. Evidence-based treatments for trauma-related psychopathology, including trauma-focused CBT, already target some aspects of the ABM for childhood adversity, for example, by updating them or challenging maladaptive cognitions. Novel memory therapeutics have the potential to target distortion in memory recollection, for example: by reducing affective biases through selective emphasis on recollecting and savoring positive memories; by reducing the frequency of memory intrusions through imagery rescripting or visuospatial cognitive interference; and by reducing overgeneral recollections through repeated practice in retrieving specific memories in response to word or picture cues (Dalgleish & Hitchcock, 2023). Other, more experimental memory therapeutics aim to directly modify memory consolidation or reconsolidation (Monfils & Holmes, 2018; Phelps & Hofmann, 2019).

Emerging neurobiological research is also helping to shed light on the complex transactional and longitudinal pathways that influence psychiatric risk following adversity. While there is a need to better understand the mechanisms that shape these pathways to improve our prevention and intervention approaches, it is clear that trusted, stable, and supportive relationships play a central role in resilience and recovery following adversity. To reduce rates of psychiatric disorder and their associated economic costs, a radical shift toward prevention is needed. This requires a social transactional approach informed by neuroscience research that moves away from an exclusively proximal, individual-specific, and symptom-based approach: risk and vulnerability mechanisms are not simply located within the child. Social care and educational systems should develop approaches that foster trusted, stable, and supportive relationships.

Acknowledgments

We are grateful to Harriet Phillips who kindly assisted with the referencing of this chapter.

References

Adam, E.K. *et al.* (2020) Racial discrimination and ethnic racial identity in adolescence as modulators of HPA axis activity. *Development and Psychopathology* **32**(5), 1669–1684. doi:10.1017/S095457942000111X.

Aldridge-Waddon, L. *et al.* (2020) Atypical social reward anticipation as a transdiagnostic characteristic of psychopathology: a meta-analytic review and critical evaluation of current evidence. *Clinical Psychology Review* **82**, 101942. doi:10.1016/j.cpr.2020.101942.

American Psychiatric Association (2013) *Diagnostic and Statistical Manual of Mental Disorders*, 5th edn. American Psychiatric Association, Washington, DC.

American Psychiatric Association (2022) *Diagnostic and Statistical Manual of Mental Disorders*, 5th edn. text revision edn. American Psychiatric Association, Washington, DC.

Andersen, S.L. *et al.* (2008) Preliminary evidence for sensitive periods in the effect of childhood sexual abuse on regional brain development. *Journal of Neuropsychiatry and Clinical Neurosciences* **20**(3), 292–301. doi:10.1176/jnp.2008.20.3.292.

Baldwin, J.R. *et al.* (2019) Agreement between prospective and retrospective measures of childhood maltreatment: a systematic review and meta-analysis. *JAMA Psychiatry* **76**(6), 584–593. doi:10.1001/jamapsychiatry.2019.0097.

Baldwin, J.R. *et al.* (2021) Population vs individual prediction of poor health from results of adverse childhood experiences screening. *JAMA Pediatrics* **175**(4), 385–393. doi:10.1001/jamapediatrics.2020.5602.

Barry, T.J. *et al.* (2021) Autobiographical memory impairments as a transdiagnostic feature of mental illness: a meta-analytic review of investigations into autobiographical memory specificity and overgenerality among people with psychiatric diagnoses. *Psychological Bulletin* **147**(10), 1054–1074. doi:10.1037/bul0000345.

Baumeister, D. *et al.* (2015) Childhood trauma and adulthood inflammation: a meta-analysis of peripheral C-reactive protein, interleukin-6 and tumour necrosis factor-α. *Molecular Psychiatry* **21**, 642–649. doi:10.1038/mp.2015.67.

Bernard, K. *et al.* (2017) Maltreatment and diurnal cortisol regulation: a meta-analysis. *Psychoneuroendocrinology* **78**, 57–67. doi:10.1016/j.psyneuen.2017.01.005.

Blair, K.S. *et al.* (2022) Different forms of childhood maltreatment have different impacts on the neural systems involved in the representation of reinforcement value. *Developmental Cognitive Neuroscience* **53**, 101051. doi:10.1016/j.dcn.2021.101051.

Brody, G.H. *et al.* (2015) Discrimination, racial identity, and cytokine levels among African-American adolescents. *Journal of Adolescent Health* **56**(5), 496–501. doi:10.1016/j.jadohealth.2015.01.017.

Bunea, I.M. *et al.* (2017) Early-life adversity and cortisol response to social stress: a meta-analysis. *Translational Psychiatry* **7**(12), 1–8. doi:10.1038/s41398-017-0032-3.

Cecil, C.A.M. *et al.* (2020) Childhood maltreatment and DNA methylation: a systematic review. *Neuroscience & Biobehavioral Reviews* **112**, 392–409. doi:10.1016/j.neubiorev.2020.02.019.

Cicchetti, D. & Doyle, C. (2016) Child maltreatment, attachment and psychopathology: mediating relations. *World Psychiatry* **15**(2), 89–90. doi:10.1002/wps.20337.

Cisler, J.M. & Koster, E.H.W. (2010) Mechanisms of attentional biases towards threat in anxiety disorders: an integrative review. *Clinical Psychology Review* **30**(2), 203–216. doi:10.1016/j.cpr.2009.11.003.

Conway, M.A. *et al.* (2005) The self and autobiographical memory: correspondence and coherence. *Social Cognition* **22**(5), 491–529. doi:10.1521/soco.22.5.491.50768.

Dalgleish, T. & Hitchcock, C. (2023) Transdiagnostic distortions in autobiographical memory recollection. *Nature Reviews Psychology* **2**(3), 166–182. doi:10.1038/s44159-023-00148-1.

Dalgleish, T. & Werner-Seidler, A. (2014) Disruptions in autobiographical memory processing in depression and the emergence of memory therapeutics. *Trends in Cognitive Sciences* **18**(11), 596–604. doi:10.1016/j.tics.2014.06.010.

Danese, A. (2020) Annual research review: rethinking childhood trauma-new research directions for measurement, study design and analytical strategies. *Journal of Child Psychology and Psychiatry* **61**(3), 236–250. doi:10.1111/jcpp.13160.

Danese, A. & Baldwin, J.R. (2017) Hidden wounds? Inflammatory links between childhood trauma and psychopathology. *Annual Review of Psychology* **68**, 517–544. doi:10.1146/annurev-psych-010416-044208.

Danese, A. & Lewis, S.J. (2017) Psychoneuroimmunology of early-life stress: the hidden wounds of childhood trauma? *Neuropsychopharmacology* **42**, 99–114. doi:10.1038/npp.2016.198.

Danese, A. & McEwen, B.S. (2012) Adverse childhood experiences, allostasis, allostatic load, and age-related disease. *Physiology & Behavior* **106**(1), 29–39. doi:10.1016/j.physbeh.2011.08.019.

Danese, A. & Widom, C.S. (2020) Objective and subjective experiences of child maltreatment and their relationships with psychopathology. *Nature Human Behaviour* **4**(8), 811–818. doi:10.1038/s41562-020-0880-3.

Danese, A. & Widom, C.S. (2021) The subjective experience of childhood maltreatment in psychopathology. *JAMA Psychiatry* **78**(12), 1307–1308. doi:10.1001/jamapsychiatry.2021.2874.

Danese, A. *et al.* (2007) Childhood maltreatment predicts adult inflammation in a life-course study. *Proceedings of the National Academy of Sciences of the United States of America* **104**(4), 1319–1324. doi:10.1073/pnas.0610362104.

Danese, A. *et al.* (2009) Adverse childhood experiences and adult risk factors for age-related disease: depression, inflammation, and clustering of metabolic risk markers. *Archives of Pediatrics & Adolescent Medicine* **163**(12), 1135–1143. doi:10.1001/archpediatrics.2009.214.

Danese, A. *et al.* (2017) The origins of cognitive deficits in victimized children: implications for neuroscientists and clinicians. *The American Journal of Psychiatry* **174**(4), 349–361. doi:10.1176/appi.ajp.2016.16030333.

Debowska, A. *et al.* (2017) What do we know about child abuse and neglect patterns of co-occurrence? A systematic review of profiling studies and recommendations for future research. *Child Abuse & Neglect* **70**, 100–111. doi:10.1016/j.chiabu.2017.06.014.

Delgado, M.R. (2007) Reward-related responses in the human striatum. *Annals of the New York Academy of Sciences* **1104**, 70–88. doi:10.1196/annals.1390.002.

Duncan, A.E. *et al.* (2015) Associations between body mass index, post-traumatic stress disorder, and child maltreatment in young women. *Child Abuse & Neglect* **45**, 154–162. doi:10.1016/j.chiabu.2015.02.007.

Dutcher, E.G. *et al.* (2020) Early-life stress and inflammation: a systematic review of a key experimental approach in rodents. *Brain and Neuroscience Advances* **4**, 2398212820978049.

Engel, G.L. (1977) The need for a new medical model: a challenge for biomedicine. *Science* **196**(4286), 129–136. doi:10.1126/science.847460.

Etkin, A. & Wager, T.D. (2007) Functional neuroimaging of anxiety: a meta-analysis of emotional processing in PTSD, social anxiety disorder, and specific phobia. *American Journal of Psychiatry* **164**(10), 1476–1488. doi:10.1176/appi.ajp.2007.07030504.

Felitti, V.J. *et al.* (1998) Relationship of childhood abuse and household dysfunction to many of the leading causes of death in adults:the adverse childhood experiences (ACE) study. *American Journal of Preventive Medicine* **14**(4), 245–258. doi:10.1016/s0749-3797(98)00017-8.

Finkelhor, D. *et al.* (2007) Poly-victimization: a neglected component in child victimization. *Child Abuse & Neglect* **31**(1), 7–26. doi:10.1016/j.chiabu.2006.06.008.

Fogelman, N. & Canli, T. (2018) Early life stress and cortisol: a meta-analysis. *Hormones and Behavior* **98**, 63–76. doi:10.1016/j.yhbeh.2017.12.014.

Ganzel, B.L. *et al.* (2008) Resilience after 9/11: multimodal neuroimaging evidence for stress-related change in the healthy adult brain. *NeuroImage* **40**(2), 788–795. doi:10.1016/j.neuroimage.2007.12.010.

Garrett, A. *et al.* (2019) Longitudinal changes in brain function associated with symptom improvement in youth with PTSD. *Journal of Psychiatric Research* **114**, 161–169. doi:10.1016/j.jpsychires.2019.04.021.

Gladish, N. *et al.* (2022) Childhood trauma and epigenetics: state of the science and future. *Current Environmental Health Reports* **9**(4), 661–672. doi:10.1007/s40572-022-00381-5.

Glynn, L.M. & Baram, T.Z. (2019) The influence of unpredictable, fragmented parental signals on the developing brain. *Frontiers in Neuroendocrinology* **53**, 100736. doi:10.1016/j.yfrne.2019.01.002.

Goodman, G.S. *et al.* (2010) Child maltreatment and memory. *Annual Review of Psychology* **61**(1), 325–351. doi:10.1146/annurev.psych.093008.100403.

Hammen, C. (2006) Stress generation in depression: reflections on origins, research, and future directions. *Journal of Clinical Psychology* **62**(9), 1065–1082. doi:10.1002/jclp.20293.

Hanlon, P. *et al.* (2020) Association between childhood maltreatment and the prevalence and complexity of multimorbidity: a cross-sectional analysis of 157, 357 UK biobank participants. *Journal of Comorbidity* **10**, 2235042X10944344. doi:10.1177/2235042X10944344.

Hein, T.C. & Monk, C.S. (2017) Research review: neural response to threat in children, adolescents, and adults after child maltreatment—a quantitative meta-analysis. *Journal of Child Psychology and Psychiatry* **58**(3), 222–230. doi:10.1111/jcpp.12651.

Hein, T.C. *et al.* (2020) Childhood violence exposure and social deprivation are linked to adolescent threat and reward neural function. *Social Cognitive and Affective Neuroscience* **15**(11), 1252–1259. doi:10.1093/scan/nsaa144.

Hennessy, V.E. *et al.* (2022) Accelerated forgetting of a trauma-like event in healthy men and women after a single dose of hydrocortisone. *Translational Psychiatry* **12**(354), 1–9. doi:10.1038/s41398-022-02126-2.

Hernandez, E.M. *et al.* (2016) Vulnerability-specific stress generation: childhood emotional abuse and the mediating role of depressogenic interpersonal processes. *Child Abuse & Neglect* **62**, 132–141. doi:10.1016/j.chiabu.2016.10.019.

Holz, N.E. *et al.* (2017) Ventral striatum and amygdala activity as convergence sites for early adversity and conduct disorder. *Social Cognitive and Affective Neuroscience* **12**(2), 261–272. doi:10.1093/scan/nsw120.

Huggins, A.A. *et al.* (2022) Neighborhood disadvantage associated with blunted amygdala reactivity to predictable and unpredictable threat in a community sample of youth. *Biological Psychiatry Global Open Science* **2**(3), 242–252. doi:10.1016/j.bpsgos.2022.03.006.

Hulshoff Pol, H.E. *et al.* (2000) Prenatal exposure to famine and brain morphology in schizophrenia. *American Journal of Psychiatry* **157**(7), 1170–1172. doi:10.1176/appi.ajp.157.7.1170.

Jenness, J.L. *et al.* (2021) Alterations in neural circuits underlying emotion regulation following child maltreatment: a mechanism underlying trauma-related psychopathology. *Psychological Medicine* **51**(11), 1880–1889. doi:10.1017/S0033291720000641.

Kelly, P.A. *et al.* (2015) Sex differences in socioemotional functioning, attentional bias, and gray matter volume in maltreated children: a multilevel investigation. *Development and Psychopathology* **27**(4), 1591–1609. doi:10.1017/S0954579415000966.

Khoury, J.E. *et al.* (2019) The association between adversity and hair cortisol levels in humans: a meta-analysis. *Psychoneuroendocrinology* **103**, 104–117. doi:10.1016/j.psyneuen.2019.01.009.

Koss, K.J. & Gunnar, M.R. (2017) Annual research review: early adversity, the hypothalamic-pituitary-adrenocortical axis, and child psychopathology. *Journal of Child Psychology and Psychiatry* **59**(4), 327–346. doi:10.1111/jcpp.12784.

Kuhlman, K.R. *et al.* (2020) Early life adversity exposure and circulating markers of inflammation in children and adolescents: a systematic review and meta-analysis. *Brain, Behavior, and Immunity* **86**, 30–42. doi:10.1016/j.bbi.2019.04.028.

Kujawa, A. *et al.* (2016) Neural reactivity to emotional stimuli prospectively predicts the impact of a natural disaster on psychiatric symptoms in children. *Biological Psychiatry* **80**(5), 381–389. doi:10.1016/j.biopsych.2015.09.008.

Kuyken, W. & Brewin, C.R. (1995) Autobiographical memory functioning in depression and reports of early abuse. *Journal of Abnormal Psychology* **104**(4), 585–591. doi:10.1037/0021-843X.104.4.585.

Lewis, S.J. *et al.* (2021) Unravelling the contribution of complex trauma to psychopathology and cognitive deficits: a cohort study. *The British Journal of Psychiatry: The Journal of Mental Science* **219**(2), 448–455. doi:10.1192/bjp.2021.57.

Liu, Q. *et al.* (2021) The relationship between perceived control and hypothalamic-pituitary-adrenal axis reactivity to the trier social stress test in healthy young adults. *Frontiers in Psychology* **12**, 683914. doi:10.3389/fpsyg.2021.683914.

Lumertz, F.S. *et al.* (2022) Effects of early life stress on brain cytokines: a systematic review and meta-analysis of rodent studies. *Neuroscience & Biobehavioral Reviews* **139**, 104746. doi:10.1016/j.neubiorev.2022.104746.

Mackin, D.M. *et al.* (2019) Reward processing and future life stress: stress generation pathway to depression. *Journal of Abnormal Psychology* **128**(4), 305–314. doi:10.1037/abn0000427.

Marzi, S.J. *et al.* (2018) Analysis of DNA methylation in young people: limited evidence for an association between victimization stress and epigenetic variation in blood. *American Journal of Psychiatry* **175**(6), 517–529. doi:10.1176/appi.ajp.2017.17060693.

McCrory, E. (2020) The case for a preventative approach to mental health: childhood maltreatment, neuroimaging, and the theory of latent vulnerability. In: *Psychiatry Reborn: Biopsychosocial Psychiatry in Modern Medicine*. (eds J. Savulescu, *et al.*). Oxford University Press, Oxford, UK. pp. 175–189.

McCrory, E.J. & Viding, E. (2015) The theory of latent vulnerability: reconceptualizing the link between childhood maltreatment and psychiatric disorder. *Development and Psychopathology* **27**(2), 493–505. doi:10.1017/S0954579415000115.

McCrory, E.J. *et al.* (2011) Heightened neural reactivity to threat in child victims of family violence. *Current Biology* **21**(23), 947–948. doi:10.1016/j.cub.2011.10.015.

McCrory, E.J. *et al.* (2013) Amygdala activation in maltreated children during pre-attentive emotional processing. *British Journal of Psychiatry* **202**(4), 269–276. doi:10.1192/bjp.bp.112.116624.

McCrory, E.J. *et al.* (2017a) Annual research review: childhood maltreatment, latent vulnerability and the shift to preventative psychiatry—the contribution of functional brain imaging. *Journal of Child Psychology and Psychiatry* **58**(4), 338–357. doi:10.1111/jcpp.12713.

McCrory, E.J. *et al.* (2017b) Autobiographical memory: a candidate latent vulnerability mechanism for psychiatric disorder following childhood maltreatment. *British Journal of Psychiatry* **211**(4), 216–222. doi:10.1192/bjp.bp.117.201798.

McCrory, E. *et al.* (2022) Social thinning and stress generation after childhood maltreatment: a neurocognitive social transactional model of psychiatric vulnerability. *The Lancet Psychiatry* **9**(10), 828–837. doi:10.1016/S2215-0366(22)00202-4.

McLaughlin, K.A. *et al.* (2019) Childhood adversity and neural development: a systematic review. *Annual Review of Developmental Psychology* **1**, 277–312. doi:10.1146/annurev-devpsych-121318-084950.

Meehan, A.J. *et al.* (2022) Poor individual risk classification from adverse childhood experiences screening. *American Journal of Preventive Medicine* **62**(3), 427–432. doi:10.1016/j.amepre.2021.08.008.

Milaniak, I. & Jaffee, S.R. (2019) Childhood socioeconomic status and inflammation: a systematic review and meta-analysis. *Brain, Behavior, and Immunity* **78**, 161–176. doi:10.1016/j.bbi.2019.01.018.

Miller, G.E. *et al.* (2009) Low early-life social class leaves a biological residue manifested by decreased glucocorticoid and increased proinflammatory signaling. *Proceedings of the National Academy of Sciences* **106**(34), 14716–14721. doi:10.1073/pnas.0902971106.

Monfils, M.H. & Holmes, E.A. (2018) Memory boundaries: opening a window inspired by reconsolidation to treat anxiety, trauma-related, and addiction disorders. *The Lancet Psychiatry* **5**(12), 1032–1042. doi:10.1016/S2215-0366(18)30270-0.

Neil, L. *et al.* (2022) Trust and childhood maltreatment: evidence of bias in appraisal of unfamiliar faces. *Journal of Child Psychology and Psychiatry* **63**(6), 655–662. doi:10.1111/jcpp.13503.

Nelson, C.A. & Gabard-Durnam, L. (2020) Early adversity and critical periods: neurodevelopmental consequences of violating the expectable environment. *Trends in Neurosciences* **43**(3), 133–143. doi:10.1016/j.tins.2020.01.002.

Oltean, L.E. *et al.* (2023) Childhood adversity and impaired reward processing: a meta-analysis. *Child Abuse & Neglect* **142**, 105596. doi:10.1016/j.chiabu.2022.105596.

Palacios-Barrios, E.E. *et al.* (2021) Lower neural value signaling in the prefrontal cortex is related to childhood family income and depressive symptomatology during adolescence. *Developmental Cognitive Neuroscience* **48**, 100920. doi:10.1016/j.dcn.2021.100920.

Parade, S.H. *et al.* (2021) A systematic review of childhood maltreatment and DNA methylation: candidate gene and epigenome-wide approaches. *Translational Psychiatry* **11**(134), 1–33. doi:10.1038/s41398-021-01207-y.

Phelps, E.A. & Hofmann, S.G. (2019) Memory editing from science fiction to clinical practice. *Nature* **572**, 43–50. doi:10.1038/s41586-019-1433-7.

Pollok, T.M. *et al.* (2022) Neurostructural traces of early life adversities: a meta-analysis exploring age- and adversity-specific effects. *Neuroscience & Biobehavioral Reviews* **135**, 104589. doi:10.1016/j.neubiorev.2022.104589.

Puetz, V.B. *et al.* (2016) Altered neural response to rejection-related words in children exposed to maltreatment. *Journal of Child Psychology and Psychiatry* **57**(10), 1165–1173. doi:10.1111/jcpp.12595.

Puetz, V.B. *et al.* (2019) Investigating patterns of neural response associated with childhood abuse v. childhood neglect. *Psychological Medicine* **50**(8), 1398–1407. doi:10.1017/S003329171900134X.

Puetz, V.B. *et al.* (2020) Autobiographical memory as a latent vulnerability mechanism following childhood maltreatment: association with future depression symptoms and prosocial behavior. *Development and Psychopathology* **33**(4), 1300–1307. doi:10.1017/S0954579420000504.

Puetz, V.B. *et al.* (2021) Functional brain plasticity following childhood maltreatment: a longitudinal fMRI investigation of autobiographical memory processing. *Development and Psychopathology*, 1–8. doi:10.1017/S0954579421001292.

Raymond, C. *et al.* (2021) Early childhood adversity and HPA axis activity in adulthood: the importance of considering minimal age at exposure. *Psychoneuroendocrinology* **124**, 105042. doi:10.1016/j.psyneuen.2020.105042.

Savalescu, P.J. *et al.* (2020) *Psychiatry Reborn: Biopsychosocial Psychiatry in Modern Medicine.* Oxford University Press, Oxford, UK.

Schacter, D.L. (1999) The seven sins of memory: insights from psychology and cognitive neuroscience. *American Psychologist* **54**(3), 182–203. doi:10.1037/0003-066X.54.3.182.

Sheridan, M.A. *et al.* (2017) Dimensions of childhood adversity have distinct associations with neural systems underlying executive functioning. *Development and Psychopathology* **29**(5), 1777–1794. doi:10.1017/S0954579417001390.

Smeeth, D. *et al.* (2023) War exposure, post-traumatic stress symptoms and hair cortisol concentrations in Syrian refugee children. *Molecular Psychiatry* **28**(2), 647–656. doi:10.1038/s41380-022-01859-2.

Smith, K.E. & Pollak, S.D. (2021) Rethinking concepts and categories for understanding the neurodevelopmental effects of childhood adversity. *Perspectives on Psychological Science* **16**(1), 67–93. doi:10.1177/1745691620920725.

Snyder-Mackler, N. *et al.* (2020) Social determinants of health and survival in humans and other animals. *Science* **368**(6493), eaax9553. doi:10.1126/science.aax9553.

Sonuga-Barke, E.J.S. *et al.* (2017) Child-to-adult neurodevelopmental and mental health trajectories after early life deprivation: the young adult follow-up of the longitudinal English and Romanian adoptees study. *The Lancet* **389**(10078), 1539–1548. doi:10.1016/S0140-6736(17)30045-4.

St Jacques, P.L. *et al.* (2013) Neural networks supporting autobiographical memory retrieval in posttraumatic stress disorder. *Cognitive, Affective, & Behavioral Neuroscience* **13**(3), 554–566. doi:10.3758/s13415-013-0157-7.

Suarez, G.L. *et al.* (2022) The impact of neighborhood disadvantage on amygdala reactivity: pathways through neighborhood social processes. *Developmental Cognitive Neuroscience* **54**, 101061. doi:10.1016/j.dcn.2022.101061.

Valentino, K. *et al.* (2009) Autobiographical memory functioning among abused, neglected, and nonmaltreated children: the overgeneral memory effect. *Journal of Child Psychology and Psychiatry* **50**(8), 1029–1038. doi:10.1111/j.1469-7610.2009.02072.x.

Warrier, V. *et al.* (2021) Gene–environment correlations and causal effects of childhood maltreatment on physical and mental health: a genetically informed approach. *The Lancet Psychiatry* **8**(5), 373–386. doi:10.1016/S2215-0366(20)30569-1.

Weaver, I.C.G. *et al.* (2004) Epigenetic programming by maternal behavior. *Nature Neuroscience* **7**(8), 847–854. doi:10.1038/nn1276.

World Health Organization (2018) *International Classification of Diseases.* 11th revision, Geneva, Switzerland. Available: https://icd.who.int/en [11 September 2024].

Young, K.D. *et al.* (2013) Behavioral and neurophysiological correlates of autobiographical memory deficits in patients with depression and individuals at high risk for depression. *JAMA Psychiatry* **70**(7), 698–708. doi:10.1001/jamapsychiatry.2013.1189.

Young, K.D. *et al.* (2014) Neurophysiological correlates of autobiographical memory deficits in currently and formerly depressed subjects. *Psychological Medicine* **44**(14), 2951–2963. doi:10.1017/S0033291714000464.

CHAPTER 21
Genetics

Anita Thapar[1,2,3] and Matthew W. State[4]

[1] Child and Adolescent Psychiatry Section, Division of Psychological Medicine and Clinical Neurosciences, Cardiff University School of Medicine, Cardiff, UK
[2] Centre for Neuropsychiatric Genetics and Genomics, Division of Psychological Medicine and Clinical Neurosciences, Cardiff University School of Medicine, Cardiff, UK
[3] Wolfson Centre for Young People's Mental Health, Division of Psychological Medicine and Clinical Neurosciences, Cardiff University School of Medicine, Cardiff, UK
[4] Department of Psychiatry and Behavioral Sciences, Langley Porter Psychiatric Institute, Weill Institute for Neurosciences, University of California San Francisco, San Francisco, CA, USA

Introduction

The 21st century has witnessed astonishing advances in genomic technologies and in the reliability of genetics research methods, leading to a remarkable array of scientific discoveries. How these findings have influenced the understanding of child psychiatric syndromes and neurodevelopmental disorders (NDDs), and their relevance to those working in clinical services, is the focus of this chapter.

The motivation for investment in genetics is that an increased understanding of the nature of these risks and an associated illumination of molecular, cellular, and circuit mechanisms underlying psychiatric disorders can potentially lead to improved diagnosis, novel therapeutics development, and effective prevention strategies. This promise has been enticing for mental health disorders, particularly given the poor understanding of pathophysiology and paucity of new treatments. However, while the pace of progress in psychiatric genomics has, in some cases, led all of medicine, the path from genes to mental health clinics has remained frustratingly slow.

This chapter will address the recent successes that have emerged since the turn of the millennium, consider the impact of these findings on child and adolescent psychiatry, and explore the opportunities and obstacles to harnessing this understanding to improve human health.

What is a gene and how does it work?

DNA

The human genome is composed of DNA, deoxyribonucleic acid, a large molecule that contains all the genetic instructions for the development, growth, functioning, and reproduction of living organisms. DNA is made up of subunits called *nucleotides*, which include: a phosphate group, a sugar molecule (deoxyribose), and a nitrogenous base: adenine (A), guanine (G), cytosine (C), and thymine (T). DNA exists as a double helix structure where two strands of DNA molecules twist around each other in a spiral shape, held together by hydrogen bonds between the base pairs in which adenine always pairs with thymine (A-T), and guanine always pairs with cytosine (G-C). In human cells, genomic DNA, which represents the majority of genetic material, is carried in the nucleus. The mitochondrial genome is much smaller and is inherited through the maternal line.

Genes

At the most fundamental level, a gene is a distinct sequence of nucleotides; the specific content and sequence of nucleotides defines the structure and function of that gene.

As described later, genes have tangible biological impact through the processes of *transcription*, in which a DNA segment serves as a template for the production of RNA molecules, and *translation*, in which the corresponding RNA molecules lead to the creation of proteins made up of amino acids (AAs) (Figure 21.1). At present, genes can best be thought of as specific DNA sequences contained within a circumscribed region of the genome which encodes a biologically functional product.

Genes include a promoter, "exons," "introns," and untranslated regions (UTRs) (Figure 21.1). The human genome contains approximately 20,000–25,000 genes, corresponding to about 1.5% of the genomic DNA in every cell (~30,000,000 of the 3 billion bases in the human genome). The remaining ~99% of the nuclear genome is noncoding. Collectively, these noncoding sequences were long referred to as "junk" DNA but are now recognized to have enormous impact on the coordinated expression of genes. Noncoding DNA sequences that modify

Rutter's Child and Adolescent Psychiatry and Psychology, Seventh Edition.
Edited by Anita Thapar, Daniel S. Pine, Samuele Cortese, Cathy Creswell, Tamsin J. Ford, James F. Leckman, and Argyris Stringaris.

Companion website: www.wiley.com/go/thapar/rutterspsych7

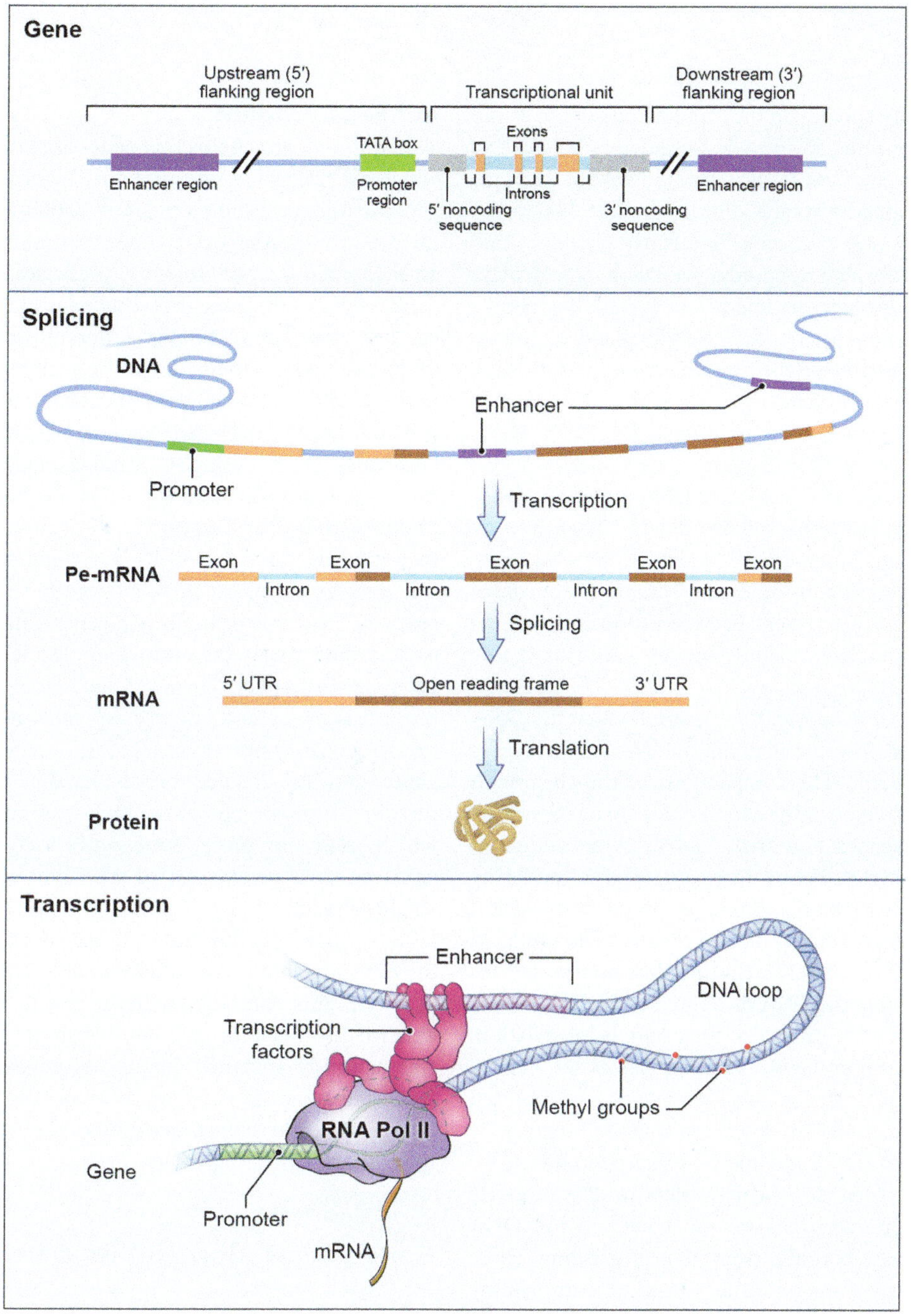

Figure 21.1 Genes, splicing, and transcription: The top panel, "Gene," is a highly simplified representation of a human gene, including surrounding regions of the genome that contain DNA sequences contributing to the regulation of gene expression. The promoter is a sequence motif typically in the upstream (or 5′) region of the gene which defines where the RNA polymerase II molecule, an enzyme that transcribes the gene, binds to the DNA and initiates transcription. Untranslated regions, both upstream (5′) and downstream (3′) of a gene, flank the "transcriptional unit" and play crucial roles in regulating gene expression including in controlling the timing and efficiency of transcription. Selected examples of commonly identified sequence motifs in humans are shown in the diagram including the "TATA box," a promoter sequence that helps define the direction of transcription and which strand of DNA is "read" during this process. The transcriptional unit, which will be transcribed into mRNA (see top and central panels), includes both "coding" and "noncoding" sequences, including introns and exons. During the process of translation, mRNA derived from DNA is "read" in sequential units of three nucleotides, called *triplets* or *codons*. 61 of the 64 possible triplets derived from the 4 DNA bases correspond to 1 of 20 specific amino acids (AAs) which are the building blocks of proteins. Three triplets are "stop" signals. If a section of DNA downstream of the transcription start site provides the instructions for a biologically meaningful series of amino acids and contains certain canonical sequences, it is referred to as an "exon." "Introns" are the intervening DNA sequences between exons that may contain regulatory motifs and are removed during splicing. The central panel, "Splicing," provides a conceptual overview of mRNA splicing. The transcriptional machinery is directed to a gene via regulatory sequences and produces a "pre-messenger RNA (pre-mRNA) molecule." In the human genome most genes include both introns and exons. Pre-mRNA is spliced into mRNA via a highly regulated process that can yield a variety of transcripts from a single pre-mRNA molecule through "alternative splicing" in which different exons may be skipped or included, often regulated spatiotemporally (that is different protein isoforms may be produced in specific cell types at specific time points during development). Consequently, a single pre-mRNA molecule can produce multiple different mRNA molecules and, ultimately, multiple different protein isoforms which may have divergent biological functions. The bottom panel, "Transcription," provides a view of the human transcriptional machinery that includes RNA polymerase II, a complex multiunit enzyme, along with multiple additional proteins, including transcription factors, that are required to initiate and maintain transcription. The diagram reflects the importance of the three-dimensional nature of transcription. While simplified diagrams typically show DNA and mRNA in two dimensions, in reality, transcription is carried out and regulated in three dimensions, where "distant" regulatory elements may be brought into contact with each other through looping of the DNA molecule and are often mediated by DNA-binding regulatory proteins.

transcriptional activity and are on the same chromosome as the impacted gene(s) are referred to as "cis-regulatory" elements. These include *enhancers*, *silencers*, that may increase or decrease gene expression respectively, and *insulators* that block the activity of enhancers and silencers. Regulatory elements that impact gene activity through the production of an intermediate molecule (typically a protein) are referred to as trans-regulatory elements. Typically, these act on multiple genes and at greater distances than cis-regulatory elements, which tend to influence a smaller number of nearby genes.

Chromosomes

Each human chromosome is a long, linear DNA molecule within the cell nucleus. It is tightly packed around and organized by proteins called histones. Humans have 23 pairs of chromosomes, numbered 1–22, known as autosomes and 1pair of sex chromosomes (XX in females, XY in males). Each chromosome contains hundreds to thousands of genes, along with intra- and intergenic DNA.

Histone proteins serve as a scaffold around which the DNA is wound or packaged. The combination of DNA and protein is referred to as chromatin. The compactness of the chromatin varies from region to region of the genome and changes through the cell cycle. Chromosomes are particularly tightly condensed at the point of the cycle referred to as metaphase, rendering them visible under the light microscope, as is seen in the typical karyotype. The degree of condensation of chromatin is regulated through a number of processes, including (but not limited to) chemical modification of the DNA through methylation, as well as histone protein modification, via, for example, acetylation, methylation, and phosphorylation. These processes act, in part, by defining the three-dimensional architecture of the DNA and by regulating the "access" of the transcriptional and regulatory machinery to the DNA. DNA and histone protein modifications play a key role in epigenetics—which refers to alterations in gene activity or expression that are not coded in the DNA sequence and which are heritable through cell divisions. These epigenetic mechanisms also contribute to genomic imprinting whereby the expression of specific alleles is silenced depending on the sex of the parent from whom the chromosome was inherited; defects in this process can result in important disorders such as Prader-Willi syndrome. Environmental exposures can also lead to epigenetic changes (see Chapter 20).

Finally, telomeres, are repetitive DNA sequences located at the ends of chromosomes. They act as protective caps, preventing the degradation of essential genetic information during DNA replication. These may serve as a marker of cellular aging as they shorten each time a cell divides and eventually reach a critical length that triggers cell death. Telomere length is influenced by genetics. In addition, multiple nongenetic factors, ranging from diet to stress, exposure to trauma, and environmental toxins, have also been associated with telomere length. The impact of both genes and environment on cellular aging is an active area of investigation.

Genes to proteins

The central dogma holds that genes are transcribed into mRNA which are translated into proteins (Figure 21.1). In the human genome, the total complement of 20,000–25,000 genes leads to the production of about 5 times that many proteins underling an enormous array of biological processes.

20,000–25,000 protein-coding genes in the human genome can give rise to up to 100,000 different proteins because the set of instructions contained within a single gene may lead to multiple mRNA molecules through regulatory elements and splicing events that can yield multiple different isoforms (versions). The resulting RNA molecule(s), in turn, may have a direct biological function or lead to the production of multiple proteins from a single gene. Each of these RNAs and proteins may subserve the same or different functions in a given cell and this may be regulated in a temporally (developmentally) and spatially (cell-type or brain region) specific manner. Moreover, as described earlier, the multiple molecules encoded by a single gene may be impacted by DNA sequences thousands, hundreds of thousands, or millions of base pairs away through cis- and trans-regulatory processes. In addition, the biological impact of genes may be dictated by chemical alterations of encoded proteins through so-called post-translational modifications which occur after proteins are synthesized by the ribosome and can lead to a diverse set of physiological outcomes from a single protein.

In sum, tracing the path from genetics to biology to behavior for even a single gene represents a "many to many to many" problem. This, combined with the genetic heterogeneity of psychiatric disorders, the cellular diversity of the human brain, the tremendously dynamic nature of development, and highly restricted access to pathological tissue in psychiatric disorders, has conspired to make translation of the success in genetics into the clinic a frustratingly slow process.

Genetic variation and its detection

Genetic variation

Any two randomly selected humans share ~98–99% of their genetic material; it is the small remaining portion of the genome that varies among individuals which carries the answers to questions about genetic risks for disease. At any genomic location, if the sequence or structure of the DNA carries any variation, either within an individual or within a population, it is referred to as an *allele*. An individual inherits DNA on one chromosome from one parent, and the other chromosome from the other parent. If someone carries the same allele on both chromosomes, the person is referred to as a homozygote at that genomic location. If they carry different alleles, they are referred to as heterozygotes. The interaction between alleles at a genomic site can vary. If the effect of one allele on a trait supersedes the other, this is known as dominance. For recessive traits, an individual must carry both alleles to manifest the trait.

It had long been known that the DNA sequence varies between any two individuals, except for monozygotic (MZ) twins. Similarly, any two individuals also vary with respect to the microstructure of their chromosomes (Figure 21.2). When these changes are small enough that they cannot readily be detected by a light microscope, they are often referred to as copy number variations (CNVs) or *structural variants*.

Another important dimension of DNA variation is its frequency in the population: variation is considered common when it exceeds an arbitrary threshold (typically 1% of individuals) and rare when it does not. For genes that influence disease traits, especially for phenotypes that emerge before the end of reproductive age, there tends to be an inverse relationship between the population frequency of an allele and the magnitude of its risk. For all common psychiatric conditions studied to date, common variants (also called single nucleotide polymorphisms (SNPs)) have been found to confer very small individual effects, whereas rare variants (also referred to as rare mutations) tend to carry larger effects (Figure 21.3).

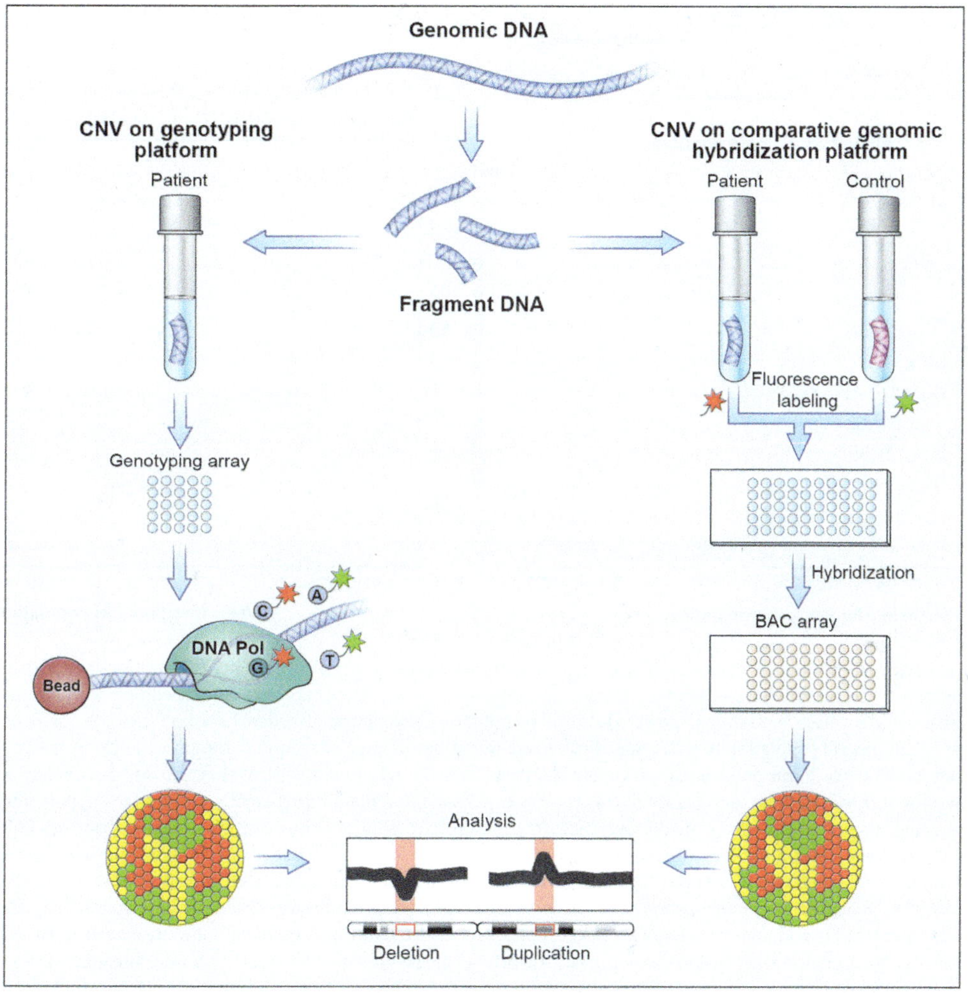

Figure 21.2 Chromosomal microarrays (CMA): Two of the most commonly used current methods for the detection of copy number variation (CNV) are diagrammed. On the left, the use of a genotyping approach is shown. In this method, DNA only from a patient is used. Sheared DNA is prepared and hybridized to synthetic oligonucleotides maintained on a solid substrate (a microarray of beads in this figure). These synthetic nucleotides are specific sequences that bind to cognate sequences in the patient DNA. A single base reaction then takes place in the presence of fluorescently labeled nucleotides. The incorporation of a given nucleotide base leads to the incorporation of a distinct color probe depending on the sequence of the patient DNA at that position. Consequently, this platform provides genotyping data. In addition, there are many copies of each synthetic oligonucleotide on the array. Consequently, the amount of input DNA from the patient can be inferred by the strength of the fluorescence signal that results. The signal is compared to a large group of controls that have been genotyped on the array. This signal strength for the subject is displayed relative to that from the group control (shown at the very bottom of the diagram). The right side of the figure shows a comparative genomic hybridization array. Sheared patient and control DNA (either an individual or a group of controls) is prepared and hybridized together on an array containing segments of the human genome. Patient and control are tagged with different fluorescence probes. The relative amounts of the patient signal and the control signal are then determined. An increase in patient signal is predicted to be a duplication or further amplification of the DNA copy number, and a relative paucity of patient DNA is inferred to be a deletion. For both types of assays, the inferences from the relative fluorescence signal are typically subject to some confirmatory process using an alternative assay.

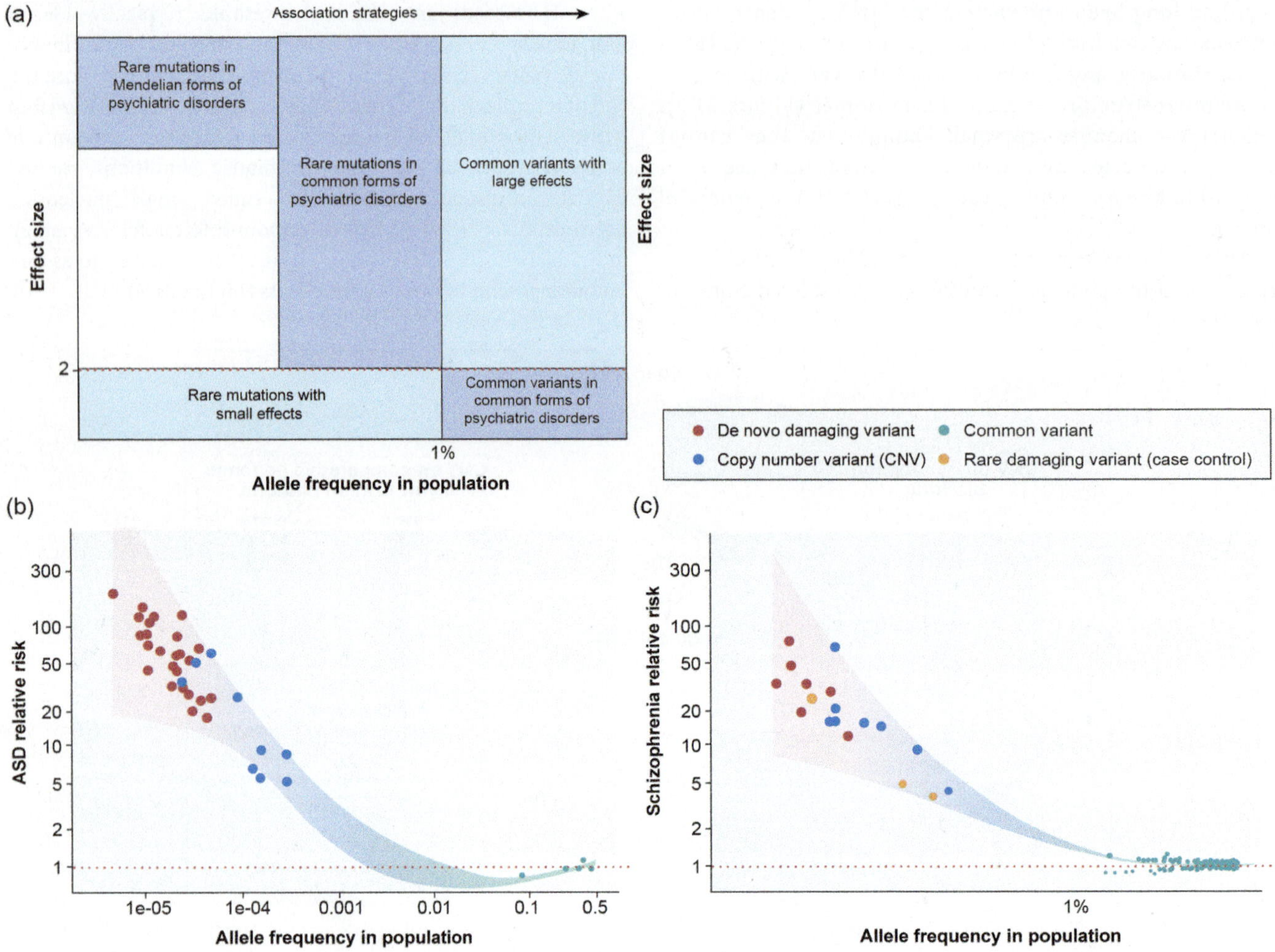

Figure 21.3 Genetic architecture of psychiatric disorders: The genetic or allelic architecture of a disorder refers to the types and distributions of variants that contribute to a condition. Panel (a) shows a plot of predictions from the prior version of this chapter, in the 6th edition of this book (p. 307), regarding the types of variations that could be discovered in well-powered studies of childhood psychiatric disorders based on their effect size (y-axis) and the frequency of the variant in the general population (x-axis). Specifically, rare mutations of large effect and common variants of small effect were anticipated to be discoverable (darker blue), while common variants carrying large effects were thought to not exist, as they should have already been identified via prior genetic studies. Studies of rare mutations carrying small effects were anticipated to remain insufficiently powered to support replicable findings. Panels (b) and (c) show a summary of results from gene discovery efforts through 2021 in "idiopathic" autism spectrum disorders (ASDs) and schizophrenia, respectively. (b) Both rare large-effect mutations and common small-effect risk alleles have been identified as contributing to common forms of ASD. The scale of the effects of rare, spontaneous heterozygous sequence variants has been larger than anticipated and rival those of so-called simple or Mendelian genetic syndromes. Gene discovery efforts for other childhood onset disorders, including attention deficit hyperactivity disorder (ADHD), obsessive–compulsive disorder (OCD). and Tourette's Disorder have similarly identified contributions from both rare and de novo mutations of large effect and common alleles carrying modest risks (not shown). (c) The majority of alleles confirmed to carry risk for schizophrenia so far identified are common alleles of small effect. This pattern of relative enrichment of common risk alleles is also reflected in findings from studies of later onset mood, anxiety, and substance use disorders (not shown). *Source:* Adapted from Willsey, H.R. *et al.* (2022).

A third important distinction is that a variation passed from one generation to the next is termed "transmitted" or "inherited." In contrast, in the generation in which a mutation first occurs, it is referred to as "*de novo*." De novo mutations can occur in any cell; those that arise in germ cells, i.e., sperm or egg, occur regularly in every generation at a low rate. If this spontaneous mutation occurs prior to a germ cell being fertilized, the mutation will be present in all the genomic DNA of the offspring but not in either parent.

Genomic assays

Currently three broad types of DNA assays are in common use: these include genotyping, sequencing, and CNV detection. Genotyping evaluates for the presence or absence of a known genetic (typically common) sequence variation. The development of microarray technology currently allows for the simultaneous testing of millions of SNPs in a single individual at low cost.

DNA sequencing, in contrast to genotyping, identifies individual nucleotides without the requirement of knowing, in advance, the position or population frequency of a potential variation. Whole exome sequencing (WES), capturing the sequence comprising ~21,000 genes, is now widely available. Increasingly, whole genome sequencing (WGS), encompassing nearly all 3 billion bases in the human genome, is also available at a price that is becoming feasible for large-scale studies and clinical testing. Currently, CNVs are most often detected via chromosomal microarrays (CMA) using either comparative genomic hybridization (CGH) or genotyping arrays (Figure 21.2). More recently, CNVs may also be detected using WES or WGS.

Genetic approaches relevant to child and adolescent psychiatry

Classic methods

Prior to the advent of large-scale molecular studies, genetics research was based on groups of individuals who differ in their degree of genetic relatedness. Genetic and environmental risk contributions to a disorder or trait (phenotype) are inferred statistically by examining similarities and differences between relatives. With a few emerging exceptions, these designs are more powerful than current molecular genetic studies in capturing genetic liability at the population-level but do not tell us about the individual. We will focus on classic family, twin, and adoption studies. The use of these and other genetic designs in epidemiology is explained in Chapter 13.

Family studies

These involve investigating the rate of disorder in the biological relatives of an affected individual (proband) compared with relatives of unaffected controls. One limitation is that some published studies have biased ascertainment; for example, if probands were selected from hospitals. Another challenge is determining whether someone is affected or unaffected as they may not have passed through the relevant age of risk (e.g., schizophrenia) or show subthreshold disorder. Finally, asking the index family to report on relatives is unreliable and it is preferable to directly interview relatives to ascertain whether or not they are affected.

Family studies show that all psychiatric disorders and NDDs run in families, although this clustering could be explained by shared environment as well as genetic liability. These familial risks are known as recurrence risks and are potentially relevant to genetic counseling (Table 21.1). For some psychiatric disorders, such as depression, bipolar disorder, and schizophrenia, familial risk may be higher when there is an early age-at-onset, where multiple relatives are affected, especially if both parents are affected, and for more narrow, severe definitions of disorder that involve recurrence and hospitalization (Kendall *et al.*, 2021). Newer family studies are taking advantage of large health record/registry data and utilizing data on distantly related family members as well as first degree relatives. Risks can be weighted to account for the degree of genetic sharing and the effects of relatives cohabiting (Kendler *et al.*, 2021). There are two major drawbacks to using familial recurrence risks to estimate individual risk. First, assumed genetic sharing between relatives (e.g., 50% between siblings) is only an average estimate, it is not precise, and does not allow for gene–gene interaction. Also, we now know that noninherited rare, large effect mutations contribute to risk and these would not necessarily be captured by familial risk estimates. In addition, familial risks are probabilistic and nonspecific; they cross diagnostic boundaries. That means, for example, a parent could have bipolar disorder, but the familial liability could manifest as attention deficit hyperactivity disorder (ADHD), anxiety, or conduct disorder (CD) rather than bipolar disorder in offspring (Birmaher *et al.*, 2021).

Table 21.1 Familial risk in first degree relatives and twin heritability for selected psychiatric and neurodevelopmental disorders.

	Relative risk (RR)	Twin heritability (h^2)
Schizophrenia	7	81%
Bipolar disorder	7	75%
Major depressive disorder	1.5	37%
ADHD	3.5	75%
ASD	8.7	80%
Anorexia nervosa	5.1	56%

Note: Psychiatric disorders are based on adult data so relative risks will likely be higher in children and adolescents.
Source: Baselmans *et al.* (2021).

Twin designs

These are based on the premise that MZ twins are genetically identical, whereas dizygotic (DZ) twins share on average 50% of their genome. Differences in MZ versus DZ twin correlations are used to infer genetic and environmental influences on a given phenotype. Phenotypic variation within the study population that is explained by all the genetic risks added up together is known as heritability (h^2). A heritability estimate has no meaning for an individual and applies to the population studied. Thus, such estimates might differ by country, age, or sex. Other limitations of twin heritability are that it encompasses additive genetic variation, genetic dominance, gene–gene interaction, and gene–environment interplay (see section on "Gene–environment interplay"). Where nonadditive dominant genetic effects are included in the heritability estimate, it is known as broad-sense rather than narrow heritability.

Initially, twin studies were utilized to estimate the heritability of different traits and disorders. A meta-analysis of 17,804 traits showed that all are heritable to some extent (Polderman *et al.*, 2015) with additive genetic variation being the major contributor. One important exception is CD, where shared environment contributes (Polderman *et al.*, 2015). For common psychiatric disorders, estimated heritabilities are highest for autism spectrum disorder (ASD), schizophrenia, ADHD, and bipolar disorder (Table 21.1).

Twin studies have also been used to examine the relationship between different phenotypes and have shown that the same genetic liability contributes to multiple different psychiatric syndromes and NDDs. They can also be used to examine the genetic relationship between diagnoses (or those with high trait scores) and variation in the rest of the population, for example, showing that ADHD diagnoses lie at the extreme of a population continuum. Finally, the twin design provides a valuable approach for examining the environment (see Chapter 13 and gene–environment interplay). Despite many strengths, twin studies have limitations including assumptions that are not necessarily valid. MZ twins are not necessarily genetically identical because of postzygotic mutations. Also, it is assumed that MZ and DZ twins share environment to the same extent, but this is not always correct. For example, greater intrauterine sharing for MZ twins and spending more time together could inflate MZ twin concordance.

Adoption studies

These involve investigating biological and unrelated adoptive relatives' similarities. Such studies have highlighted the genetic contribution to schizophrenia, bipolar disorder, depression, and ADHD among others. They have also highlighted the cross-generational environmental (as well as genetic) contribution to depression and suicide (Kendler *et al.*, 2020). However, adoption studies have a range of limitations including the fact that adoptive families typically come from more advantaged homes thereby restricting variation in environmental exposures. Also, even if offspring are adopted at birth, they will have been exposed to genetically influenced prenatal environments which would inflate similarity of the adoptive child with their biological mother.

Gene–environment interplay

Classic twin and adoption studies can be used to examine the relationship between genetic liability and environment (see Chapter 13). Such studies have shown that many environmental risks (e.g., life events, maltreatment, parenting, some prenatal exposures) are correlated with genetic liability and this is known as gene–environment correlation. Where environmental exposures are associated with parental genetic liability, this is known as "passive" gene–environment correlation (e.g., parent reading to child). When related to offspring genetic liability, gene–environment correlation is known as "active" where environments are selected (e.g., peer group) or "evocative" where genetic propensities are associated with other's responses (e.g., hostility from others). Gene–environment interaction refers to the situation where the manifestation of genetic liability varies depending on the environment. For example, a cross-fostering design showed that genetic liability contributes to petty criminality but the risk effects are much greater when those individuals are placed in homes with low social status (Cloninger *et al.*, 1982).

Identifying specific genetic risks

Common variants

Genome-wide association studies

Genome-wide association studies (GWAS) use a hypothesis-free approach, simultaneously testing common genetic variation across the genome. This approach has been used for more than 5700 traits and has proved extremely successful as it has led to the discovery of hundreds of loci associated with common health conditions and traits (Uffelmann *et al.*, 2021).

GWAS now have almost completely supplanted hypothesis-driven or "candidate gene" approaches to identifying common risk alleles, which previously dominated the field. Both GWAS and candidate gene studies most commonly test for differences in allele frequencies between cases and controls, however the latter focuses on a small number of alleles corresponding to one or a small number of nearby genes. With the benefit of hindsight, it is clear that the probability of guessing correctly which gene or allele to study was low, that a statistical threshold that only accounted for experiment-wide error, as was often used, was insufficient to prevent false positive findings, and that candidate studies tended to overestimate plausible effect sizes. Moreover, the limited genotyping done in candidate studies made accurate assessments of ancestry problematic. In practice this led to the identification of differences in allele frequencies between cases and controls due to "population stratification"—that is variation in frequencies related to the ancestral origins of case versus controls. While candidate gene studies of common alleles have not completely disappeared from the literature, they are now widely considered to be a wholly unreliable approach.

The emergence of genome-wide genotyping, a dramatic expansion of patient cohorts, and the development of methods to control for differences in ancestry between cases and controls, has led to highly reproducible common variant findings. While GWAS for common psychiatric disorders have turned out to require very large sample sizes, often reaching hundreds of thousands to millions of cases, these have been enabled by highly effective data sharing through international consortia such as the Psychiatric Genomics Consortium (PGC). At the time of writing, 287 genetic loci had been identified via GWAS for schizophrenia (Trubetskoy *et al.*, 2022), 636 for depression (Adams *et al.*, 2024), 64 for bipolar disorder (Mullins *et al.*, 2021), and 27 for ADHD (Demontis *et al.*, 2023). Although deep phenotyping may be important to address specific clinical questions (e.g., clinical subtypes), for gene discovery it remains preferable to maximize the sample size. So far, genetic correlations between deeply and minimally phenotyped samples have been shown to be very high.

Despite the success of GWAS, there are still important limitations and considerations. GWAS are not designed to detect the contribution of rare or de novo variations. Moreover, as is the case in any observational association study (see Chapter 13), biases and spurious associations can arise. Challenges include relatedness within samples and assortative mating (mate choice associated with phenotypic similarity, e.g., height). Importantly, genome-wide significant alleles are markers of increased (or decreased) risk but may not mediate that risk. For example, the associated SNPs may only be physically close to other alleles that impact gene expression. Importantly, GWAS test alleles, not genes, and a bona fide risk allele may be found ultimately to alter expression in nearby genes or those at a considerable distance. Therefore, to establish both that a GWAS variant is causal and which gene is implicated, other research is needed. This includes fine mapping the genomic region around the associated loci, conducting meta-analysis across different ancestry groups that will break up linkage disequilibrium (co-inheritance of one genetic locus with a nearby variant), and examining the biological impact of the genetic variation(s) (see section on "Understanding biology and pathophysiology").

Nevertheless, GWAS have revealed a number of key findings (Andreassen *et al.*, 2023). First, psychiatric disorders and NDDs show extreme polygenicity with most population risk explained by thousands of common genetic loci, each of small effect (typical odds ratios: 1.1–1.2). Second, SNP heritability estimates are substantially lower than twin heritabilities. This missing heritability is thought to be explained, at least in part, by variation that is not captured by GWAS, including rare variants and gene–environment correlation and interaction. Third, GWAS have been based predominantly on people of European ancestry which may or may not accurately reflect risk in non-Europeans (see polygenic scores (PGS)). Fourth, GWAS have been used to examine genetic correlations between different disorders and have found substantial genetic correlations between different psychiatric disorders and NDDs, known as pleiotropy. Genetic correlations have also been observed with physical health and lifestyle parameters, as well as environmental exposures.

Using GWAS data to infer causality

Mendelian randomization (MR) (Davies *et al.*, 2018), which is described extensively in Chapter 13, uses GWAS data to select loci that are associated with the phenotype or exposure of interest (e.g., cholesterol) as a genetic indicator (instrumental variable). The researcher then tests whether the genetic instrument(s) is associated with the outcome of interest (e.g., coronary artery disease). MR mimics randomized controlled trials (RCTs) because alleles are allocated randomly in meiosis and can be used to infer causality. While widely used in epidemiology, MR has also been used to test whether GWAS-identified risk alleles have a likely causal effect on molecular phenotypes such as gene expression profiles. Although MR is used widely, there are many assumptions and limitations (see Chapter 13).

Indirect genetic effects ("genetic nurture")

This approach requires genotyped data on both biological parents and their offspring (trios). Offspring will inherit 50% of their alleles from each parent. Where these inherited alleles contribute to a phenotype in the offspring, this is known as a direct genetic effect. If noninherited/transmitted alleles of the parent are associated with offspring phenotype, this is an indirect genetic effect and could be explained by nontransmitted alleles influencing the environments provided for offspring (passive gene–environment correlation) (Kong *et al.*, 2018). This contribution has been referred to as "genetic nurture" and has been shown to be important for educational attainment (Wang *et al.*, 2021). However, genetic nurture does not appear to contribute to the cross-generational transmission of ADHD (Martin *et al.*, 2023).

Polygenic scores (PGS)

These are a measure of the cumulative common variant risk for a given disorder or trait. Typically, they are captured through a composite of nominally associated SNPs—in contrast to the process of identifying individual risk alleles for a trait or disorder, which requires much more stringent statistical thresholds (Murray *et al.*, 2021). PGS are generated using data from a large GWAS, known as the discovery sample. Where an allele is more common in cases than controls, these are coded as "risk alleles." The researcher then defines these risk alleles in a second, independent target sample and weights each by effect size using estimates from the discovery data. The sum of these risk alleles multiplied by effect size is known as the PGS for that phenotype in that individual. In recent years, there has been an explosion of research utilizing PGS. A key advantage is that if a large discovery cohort includes measures of multiple traits/disorders (e.g., height, blood pressure, depression), then one sample can be used to generate PGS for multiple phenotypes with only one genotyping array. They are also easy to generate in any target genotyped dataset and provide an indicator of genetic liability for each person. Unlike indirect measures of genetic liability (e.g., family history), a PGS applies to the individual; that is, it provides a personalized indicator of risk.

PGS findings

PGS for psychiatric syndromes and NDDs show extensive pleiotropy. For example, schizophrenia PGS not only predict other psychiatric disorders, such as depression and bipolar disorder, they also predict worse cognitive, communication, social, behavioral, and emotional symptom scores in childhood and adolescence. Psychiatric disorder and NDD PGS also predict multiple other phenotypes including measures of brain structure and function (Thompson *et al.*, 2020), personality (e.g., neuroticism), lifestyle, and physical health (Leppert *et al.*, 2020). These associations could arise because of pleiotropy between different phenotypes or because of a causal relationship; for example, if higher psychiatric genetic liability leads to obesity (see Chapter 13). Another observation is that PGS associated with certain psychiatric disorders and NDDs predict trait levels for similar phenotypes in the population (e.g., ADHD, psychotic experiences, tic disorders, and adolescent depression), lending support to the idea that some, but not all clinical diagnoses lie at the extreme of a continuously distributed population trait or set of traits (e.g., Taylor *et al.*, 2019). A further observation is that, psychiatric disorder and NDD PGS show gene–environment correlation for many environmental exposures including lower socioeconomic status (SES), maltreatment, and bullying (Machlitt-Northen *et al.*, 2022; Thapar *et al.*, 2022) among others.

Limitations of PGS

Despite enormous interest, it is important that clinicians and scientists recognize the multiple weaknesses of PGS. As they capture characteristics of a discovery population, the target population must be similar. This is especially important when it comes to matching ancestries. Nearly all discovery GWAS have been based on individuals of European ancestry and PGS derived from these cohorts do not work so well in individuals with a different ancestry. Given the potential for future clinical benefits in using PGS, this is a serious concern as it will further exacerbate global health inequalities. There are now growing efforts to conduct GWAS across different ethnicities, but the disparities remain large. Another limitation is that predictive power is very reliant on the discovery sample size and these samples are smaller for psychiatric disorders and NDD in comparison to many physical health conditions. Thus, psychiatric syndrome and NDD PGS explain only a small amount of variance; that is, they have very weak predictive ability. Another limitation is that PGS are the sum of multiply associated risk alleles anywhere across the genome. Thus, they have no biological meaning. Finally, PGS only include common gene variants without consideration of rare variant contributions to risk. (See section on "Incorporating polygenic scores into clinics—when will this happen?" for a further discussion of the potential applications to PGS in the clinical setting.)

Gene–environment interaction

Psychiatric disorders and NDDs are multifactorial, and environmental factors also contribute. Rigorously controlled laboratory studies of rodents and fruit flies have demonstrated that the manifestation of genotype varies depending on environmental exposure. However, currently identifying gene–environment interaction at a molecular level in humans is fraught with challenges despite publications that assert otherwise. That is because, for example, investigating gene–environment interactions involving common alleles demands even larger sample sizes than those required for GWAS to adequately power for the increased burden of multiple comparisons. As we cannot know, *a priori*, what gene variants are likely to be modified by specific environmental exposures, and candidate gene approaches have been widely discredited, these types of studies must rely on genome-wide methods. Moreover, it can be challenging to measure the degree or timing of a given environmental exposure with precision. Thus, at present, we urge readers to remain cautious about observational gene–environment findings in our field using human molecular genetic data. The same issues in relation to adequate sample size also applies to gene–gene interaction and identifying common alleles involved in treatment response, where environmental exposure is the treatment provided (e.g., cognitive behavioral therapy (CBT), antidepressant medication), although in this instance, the exposure can be measured and controlled.

Rare risk variants of larger effect

Parametric linkage analysis

This approach has been extremely successful for discovering hundreds of genes involved Mendelian conditions—in which the relationship between a single gene or mutation and clinical outcomes is highly predictable (sometimes referred to as a single gene disorder). Linkage analysis involves investigating the transmission of genetic variants in a given family or set of families. If the marker is close to the disorder-causing gene, it will be inherited together with the disease despite homologous recombination; that is, they are linked. Although this approach has proved exceptionally fruitful for Mendelian disorders, it has not shown success for common, multifactorial disorders that include most NDDs and psychiatric disorders.

Cytogenetics

Historically, the study of chromosome structure, or cytogenetics, relied on the light microscope and was able to identify an individual as having too many (aneuploidy, e.g., 47XX +21 Down syndrome; 49XXY) or too few (e.g., Turner syndrome 46XO) chromosomes or the loss, gain, or rearrangement of (only) large amounts of chromosomal material measured ultimately in millions of DNA base pairs. By the 1990s, techniques had developed to use fluorescent probes to increase the resolution of chromosomal studies leading to the characterization of various recurrent abnormalities such as the 22q11 microdeletion (causing velocardiofacial syndrome) and deletions on the proximal long arm of chromosome 15 (causing Prader-Willi and Angelman syndromes).

Copy number variation (CNV) analysis

The development of microarray technology increased the resolution of routine chromosomal analyses further (Figure 21.2), allowing for the detection of submicroscopic losses and gains of DNA ranging as low as hundreds to thousands of DNA bases. Initially, the most striking finding from this technology was that, like sequence variation, chromosomal or structural variation was a normal characteristic of the human genome. However, it also soon became apparent that some CNVs, particularly those that were rare and corresponded to the coding portion of the genome, could also carry risks for common neurodevelopmental and psychiatric disorders. These CNVs can vary in their size, and, therefore, how many genes they span, and are located at different sites across the genome. Some genomic locations are especially prone to harboring CNVs. Rare recurrent (at the same location) CNVs, in some cases arising de novo, are now known to contribute risk for an extremely broad range of phenotypes, including, but not limited to, intellectual disability (ID) and developmental disorders (DD), ASD, ADHD, Tourette's syndrome, and schizophrenia (Mollon *et al.*, 2023).

Importantly, in many cases, specific recurrent CNVs impacting multiple genes have been found to carry risks for a wide range of different phenotypes, raising challenges for linking individual genes to specific psychiatric and developmental phenotypes. However, some CNVs have been found, on average, to have a more reliable link between genotype and psychiatric phenotype. For example, 22q11 microdeletions are associated with schizophrenia, while duplications appear to be protective. 7q11.23 deletions are associated with Williams syndrome, characterized by hypersocial behavior, while 7q11.23 duplications tend to be associated with ASD.

Next-generation sequencing

Next-generation sequencing refers to a variety of methods that allow for the high-throughput assessment of DNA sequence without relying on the prior identification of variants of interest. These new approaches enabled the routine identification of rare mutations at single base resolution across essentially the entire coding portion of the genome (also known as WES), and, more recently, the whole genome (WGS).

Just as with common alleles, rare variants may or may not have any functional significance. Consequently, similar to GWAS methods, statistical approaches have been developed to reliably identify rare risk mutations. In part, because of relatively large effect sizes when mutations are associated with a phenotype, and, in part, because of increased statistical power associated with the study of rare de novo mutations, studies have not uniformly required the extremely large samples required for GWAS. For example, the initial discovery of rare, de novo mutations associated with idiopathic ASD involved only several hundred families.

In some cases, the process of identifying rare alleles associated with neurodevelopmental phenotypes can be aided by leveraging a broad understanding of the functional significance of specific types of coding mutations. For example, for some early onset NDDs, particularly large effects have been observed for mutations in the exome that are predicted to lead to the premature termination of a protein. Focusing gene discovery on these so-called "likely gene disrupting" (LGD) mutations has proven to be highly productive, particularly in early onset disorders such as ASD, epilepsy, and ID. Moreover, now that sequencing databases include hundreds of thousands of unaffected individuals, it is also possible to calculate how likely any gene is to carry damaging mutations in the general population, and conversely to specify how resistant a gene is to specific types of variation. Germline LGD de novo mutations in highly resistant genes have been found to carry particularly large effects on associated phenotypes. This is consistent with our understanding of natural selection: A de novo mutation may carry very large risks for serious developmental abnormalities. As long as the mutation is not lethal prenatally, it may be detected in the developing individual in which it arose, as natural selection has not had even a single generation to act on that damaging variant.

Exome sequencing has so far been most successful in the study of early onset disorders such as ID (Wright *et al.*, 2023) and ASD (Satterstrom *et al.*, 2020; Fu *et al.*, 2022). In addition, as cohort sizes grow, studies have been increasingly successful in identifying mutations across a wider range of psychiatric and neurodevelopmental phenotypes including schizophrenia (Singh *et al.*, 2022), Tourette's disorder, ADHD, and obsessive–compulsive disorder (OCD) (Satterstrom *et al.*, 2018; Andreassen *et al.*, 2023).

The emergence of low-cost, rapid WGS, which provides a nearly complete picture of genomic variation in a single assay, promises to make significant contributions to the detection and understanding of genetic risks. Already, WGS has improved the detection of damaging mutations in the coding portion of the genome compared to WES. However, not surprisingly, the interpretation of the many rare variants seen in the noncoding genome is proving comparatively difficult and, given evidence that these types of variants carry more modest biological risks versus rare coding mutations, it is likely successful gene discovery efforts will require patient cohorts that begin to approach the size required for successful GWAS.

What we have learned and where next in molecular genetics?

Both common and rare variants contribute to risk

There have been hundreds of genetic discoveries which have helped clarify, broadly, the nature of the genetic architecture of common psychiatric disorders and NDDs. For example, we have learned that the population risk for essentially all psychiatric disorders and NDDs is explained mainly by the contribution of thousands of common gene variants, each with very small effect, and most often mapping to the noncoding portions of the genome.

We have also found that rare variations in the coding portion of the genome may contribute marked clinical risks for some common psychiatric disorders and NDDs (Figures 21.3 and 21.4). For example, current estimates are that rare variants account for less than 5% of the genetic variance for ASD in the general population. However, among clinical samples, rare coding mutations are found at higher rates; from 10% to more than 50% of individuals being evaluated in the clinic, depending on the ascertainment criteria.

To date, rare risk variants have been found to be especially enriched in those with NDDs and schizophrenia. As noted, in these cases, in contrast to the polygenic inheritance of common variants, the cumulative evidence points to single mutations in

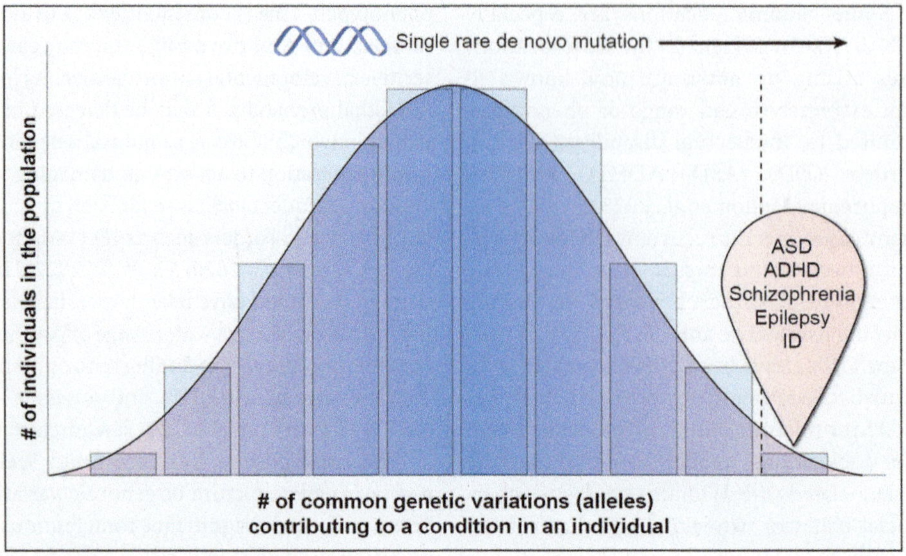

Figure 21.4 Common and rare alleles contribute to childhood onset disorders: The figure is a conceptual illustration of the contribution of common and rare alleles to common psychiatric disorders first diagnosed in childhood. To date, large-scale studies across multiple diagnoses confirm that common alleles carry the vast majority of population risk through variants of individually small effect. Moreover, to date, these alleles show evidence of additive effect and normal distribution. This is represented by the curve which is divided into deciles (vertical bars) to represent cumulative genetic risks (which may be calculated as polygenic risk scores). Of note, the vast majority of individuals carrying common risk alleles will not show symptoms or meet diagnostic thresholds. While, on average, individuals with higher levels of genetic risk are more likely to be symptomatic and to meet categorical diagnostic thresholds (as shown by the vertical dotted line and red bubble), individuals across the spectrum of genetic risks may be affected (which is not represented in this diagram). The DNA image at the top of the figure represents the potential contribution of a rare (in this case de novo) mutation carrying large risks. To date, available data most strongly supports a model where these types of rare mutations combine with common variant risk and have the potential to "move" a proband from a "baseline" predisposition derived from transmitted common variants inherited from parents toward a higher level of risk and greater likelihood of affected status. This contrasts with Mendelian, or single gene, inheritance in which there is a highly reliable relationship between a mutation or single gene and a clinical outcome, for example in Huntington's disease. The model illustrated in this figure of the contribution of rare mutations to common neurodevelopmental disorders (NDDs) helps explain why not all rare de novo mutations, even in very large effect genes, lead to a diagnosis. The diagram also illustrates the repeated empirical observation that the same or similar rare mutation/copy number variant (CNV) may lead to a wide range of distinct diagnostic outcomes. This has led to the working hypothesis, based on an increasing volume of empirical data from polygenic scores (PGS) and other studies, that the nature of the cumulative common variant "background"—almost certainly along with environmental inputs and stochastic events—helps determine which disorders—either alone or in combination—may emerge in the presence of a single very large effect rare mutation.

individuals carrying very large effects (Figure 21.4). For example, on average, a single damaging mutation in an ASD risk gene is estimated to carry risks to an individual that rival or exceed individuals falling in the top decile of polygenic risk for schizophrenia.

However, there is an important difference between the risks conferred by these rare large effect mutations in common psychiatric syndromes and NDDs versus so-called Mendelian or single gene inheritance. There is already considerable evidence that in common psychiatric conditions, rare large effect variants interact with common polygenic risk in the individual in determining outcomes (Figure 21.4). For example, in those with a 22q11 microdeletion, a higher burden of schizophrenia common genetic risk variants increases the likelihood of developing that disorder. It is also anticipated that for some disorders environmental factors will be found to influence the trajectory of large effect rare mutations, contributing to the high degree of phenotypic variability seen for identical mutations in a given large effect gene or CNV.

Understanding biology and pathophysiology

The discovery of both rare and common risk variants has contributed to our understanding of the biology of psychiatric disorders and NDDs. It is also the case that different classes or types of variants offer distinct challenges and opportunities in moving from gene discovery to the illumination of pathological mechanisms. For example, when rare, damaging variants are found to carry large effects, the path from gene identification to examining biology is relatively direct, for instance, the creation of "construct valid" animal models or, increasingly, recapitulating the precise mutation in human stem cell-derived assays (Dixon & Muotri, 2023).

With regard to GWAS findings and common risk alleles, the path to investigating biology is more complex. As noted, the finding of an associated common allele in the noncoding region of the genome requires several additional steps to confirm that the observed variant is functional, as well as to identify which gene is being impacted. Given the small individual effects of common alleles in all psychiatric disorders, the conceptual ideal would then be to study the biological impact of many alleles simultaneously, but this is not currently technically feasible. So, while it is not uncommon to see, for example, manipulation of a single risk gene implicated by a common allele in a mouse model, the interpretation of these studies and their relevance to human pathophysiology poses some additional challenges.

Despite these differences, studies of the biology of common alleles and rare risk mutations share the "many to many to many" problem noted at the outset of this chapter. In the case of common alleles, the first "many" typically refers to the multiple risk alleles that must act together to measurably increase risk. For rare variants, the "many" may refer to the multiple different mutations or genes that all carry large individual risks for a given phenotype. Moreover, while in any individual a rare large effect mutation in a single gene may be carrying the majority of risk, most genes produce multiple protein versions (or isoforms) that may have different functions at different times in different cell types, which themselves may contribute to different brain circuits in a developmentally regulated fashion. So, despite the tantalizing simplicity of coding mutations of large effect, in practice, efforts to elaborate pathophysiological mechanisms from single genes in psychiatric disorders has been far more complex than initially hoped or anticipated.

To address the challenges of illuminating pathophysiology from either common or rare variant risks, researchers have increasingly sought to look for points of convergence among disparate genetic risks. For example, in ASD, success in rare variant gene discovery led quickly to the observation that many of the different genes involved could readily be grouped by their established function either at the synapse or in regulating gene expression. Soon thereafter, studies were able to pinpoint a convergence of activity among many different ASD risk genes in cortical excitatory neurons, particularly during mid-fetal development. As the discovery of rare mutations and the search for convergence in gene expression and gene function has continued, these findings have been widely replicated and the contribution of striatal interneurons and of neurogenesis have emerged as additional important biological themes. In addition, investigators have searched for convergence among varying animal or induced pluripotent stem cell (IPSC) derived models of specific mutations that have supported and extended these findings. In short, the pursuit of rare mutations has provided reproducible insights into molecular and cellular mechanisms. How and whether these findings may lead to rational therapeutics remains to be seen.

Similarly, in the pursuit of common variants, the search for convergence has become a key strategy in elaborating biology, with a particularly heavy reliance on bioinformatic approaches—given the challenges of directly modeling multiple risk alleles simultaneously *in vivo*. For example, once the many risk alleles identified can be translated into a reliable list of impacted genes, these can be investigated with respect to bioinformatic data characterizing RNA expression, protein expression, and other molecular phenotypes (e.g., indicators of gene modifiers such as methylation). These data can be derived from model systems or from human samples, including from human brain or induced stem cells, and from both cases and controls.

To date, such approaches have suggested that for schizophrenia, bipolar disorder, depression, and ADHD, expression is greatest in neurons. Integrating gene variant data with other data on function and biological networks has suggested that schizophrenia, bipolar disorder, and ADHD common variants are also enriched in excitatory and inhibitory neurons and that schizophrenia variants are enriched for glutamatergic neurotransmission.

Potential clinical implications

Genetic testing and counseling

Genetics research has now advanced to a stage where it is crucial for all practitioners to regularly review testing guidelines as this is a rapidly evolving field. Current reports and guidance include those published by the UK Royal College of Psychiatrists (in press), the International Society for Psychiatric Genetics (ISPG, 2019) and the American Academy of Child & Adolescent Psychiatry (American Academy of Child & Adolescent Psychiatry, 2020).

Diagnostic testing for rare gene variants

First, there is the consideration of when to do a diagnostic test. An important guide to decision-making is whether clinical benefit is likely to result from testing; for example, if there are actionable physical health implications. We recommend that all clinicians familiarize themselves with national and local guidelines on genetic testing, as well as finding out what sorts of families their local clinical genetics service would be interested in assessing. Testing is not currently useful for the purpose of making a psychiatric or NDD diagnosis.

In the UK, genetic testing within the NHS is starting to move toward WGS. However, in many countries there is limited availability of genetic testing or challenges in obtaining reimbursement for such investigations. So far, guidelines, at least in the UK, have not recommended routine genetic testing for any psychiatric disorder or NDD (ADHD, ASD), except for ID. In contrast, in the US, CMA testing in individuals being evaluated for ASD is recommended by several professional societies, irrespective of the presence or absence of ID or other comorbid features.

More broadly, across countries there are some situations where genetic testing is already clearly relevant for the child and adolescent mental health practitioner. For example, in schizophrenia, the yield of CNVs, such as 22q11 microdeletion, is sufficiently high with potentially clinically actionable results, that in the UK, testing is now recommended in new guidance from the Royal College of Psychiatrists (2023). In early onset NDDs, there is an emerging consensus that if the presenting child/young person has comorbid ID/DD, shows unusual physical health presentations (e.g., epilepsy, congenital heart defect), minor congenital anomalies, or dysmorphic features, genetic testing is warranted.

Our view is that mental health clinicians should speak to their local clinical geneticist about the appropriate approach locally as genetic counseling, as well as full assessment, is an important part of the process of testing. That is because there are many complex ethical considerations involved around genetic testing for families that include advice on family planning (e.g., where there are multiple children with severe ASD with ID), implications for relatives of the index child who are not involved with the service, and the issue of child consent.

Pharmacogenetic testing

All clinicians will be familiar with individuals responding differently to the same medication and dose, not only in terms of clinical response but also in experiencing adverse side effects. Some of this variation is attributable to genetic factors that influence the way that medication affects the brain and other biological systems (pharmacodynamics). Other variation is explained by differences in the way that the body metabolizes the medication (pharmacokinetics). Currently, there is no clear agreement on whether pharmacogenetic testing is cost-effective or has clinical utility. Thus, most current guidelines in Europe (Royal College of Psychiatrists, 2023; van Schaik *et al.*, 2020) and the US (American Academy of Child & Adolescent Psychiatry, 2020) do not recommend routine pharmacogenetic testing in mental health clinics.

Nonetheless, commercial and direct-to-consumer pharmacogenetic arrays are currently available in some countries (e.g., US). Given the lack of evidence for clinical utility as well the very weak scientific foundation for many of the alleles being tested, often including many derived from fundamentally flawed candidate gene studies, we caution clinicians to avoid using such tests.

What may become relevant in the future is genetic testing of variants influencing enzymes involved in drug metabolism, especially in those who are treatment resistant. A major caveat here is that there are many nongenetic influences on treatment response and side effects (e.g., noncompliance, drug–drug interactions). Many medications are metabolized in the liver by cytochrome 450 enzymes (CYP) with CYP2D6 and CYP2C19 being especially important for psychotropic drugs. Genetic variation influences how active these enzymes are in breaking down medications. For example, a proportion of the population have little or no CYP2D6 enzyme activity with marked ethnic variations in the frequency of the low- and high-activity enzyme variants.

Genomic testing is not of benefit for clozapine or lithium where blood testing is required. While some have suggested genotyping could be considered for other psychotropic medications in certain situations (Swen *et al.*, 2023), we reiterate, the American Academy of Child & Adolescent Psychiatry in 2020 (American Academy of Child & Adolescent Psychiatry, 2020) and the UK Royal College of Psychiatrists in 2023 do not currently recommend pharmacogenetic testing. However, one relevant genetic difference relates to agranulocytosis, a serious adverse reaction to clozapine. Full blood count monitoring, not pharmacogenetic testing, is required to identify this. Importantly, in those of African and Middle Eastern ancestries, the Duffy-null genotype (AKCKR1 gene) is robustly associated with a benign form of neutropenia (Legge *et al.*, 2019). Clinicians need to be aware of this so that clozapine is not unnecessarily withheld or terminated as a treatment choice for these individuals. Our view is that if in doubt about pharmacogenetic issues, clinicians should consult with their local pharmacology team.

Incorporating polygenic scores into clinics—when will this happen?

There is growing interest in the potential for using PGS to predict disorder onset, clinical course, and prognosis, as well as for predicting likely treatment benefits and side effects. More broadly there is also the possibility that PGS could aid the process of clinical diagnosis and decision-making (Murray *et al.*, 2021). It is generally accepted that PGS on their own have limited utility but could be helpful when combined with clinical variables. If we take the example of coronary artery disease, risk prediction tools include risk factors, such as family history and elevated blood pressure, and are already part of routine clinical practice. A number of studies, although not all, suggest that combining PGS with these conventional risk factors substantially improves the accuracy of coronary artery disease risk score prediction (King *et al.*, 2022). As a result, several countries are evaluating the use of PGS for certain physical health disorders.

In psychiatry, predicting onset is challenging, as PGS are currently only weakly predictive, risk scoring is not part of routine clinical practice, and unlike coronary artery disease, where risks can be easily modified (e.g., antihypertensive medication), that is not the case for psychiatric disorders. One possible exception is using PGS in recognized high-risk groups who are already under clinical attention (e.g., 22q11 microdeletion carriers). It also seems unlikely that PGS will aid the diagnostic process because of their nonspecificity. However, what is conceivable is that PGS add to the weighting process undertaken routinely by all clinicians to aid decision-making. For example, could PGS help identify adolescents who are more likely to switch from depression to bipolar disorder? Before PGS are implemented, much more research is needed to evaluate the clinical utility and potential risks of using PGS in clinic settings. There needs to be increased genetic literacy and counseling skills among practitioners and consideration of potentially adverse impacts of genetic information on people (e.g., unhealthy change), as well as careful review of ethical issues and the potential for discrimination. A new, emerging concern is the use of commercially available polygenic embryo screening for psychiatric and cognitive traits. The International Society of Psychiatric Genetics has highlighted the social and ethical implications of such practice, and the need for caution and proper oversight (Lencz *et al.*, 2022).

Emerging treatments for rare mutations

For both rare Mendelian forms of DDs, for example Fragile X or Rett syndrome, as well as for rare large effect mutations leading to common forms of NDDs, there is growing interest in directly targeting the genome for treatment. Current proven strategies include gene replacement as well as targeting RNA with antisense oligonucleotides (ASOs), which are single-stranded nucleic acid molecules able to bind RNA and alter the expression of nearby genes. For example, Angelman syndrome affects the maternally inherited ubiquitin protein ligase E3A (*UBE3A*) gene. The paternal gene is normally silenced—an example of imprinting—leading to no UBE3A expression in affected individuals. Trials using ASOs that "release" the expression of the paternal allele are currently in progress. Moreover, clinical trials of genetic therapies are emerging for some individuals carrying large effect de novo "ASD" mutations. These trials are currently targeting severe phenotypes, including epilepsy, that may be comorbid with ASD. Efforts to target social development in individuals with large effect ASD mutations are likely on the horizon, but will confront a host of practical and ethical challenges.

Conclusion

To conclude, genetics has progressed to the point where it is no longer possible for any child and adolescent mental health clinician to ignore findings, if only to be able to understand enough to explain what is scientifically robust to families (Box 21.1). Genetics already has implications for the clinician because all the disorders we see run in families and if unrecognized may jeopardize the success of intervention (e.g., treatment compliance) and clinic engagement. Genetics has also highlighted that familial and genetic risks disrupt our diagnostic boundaries. This means that biological relatives of the index child with one disorder may show a different clinical disorder. The genetic findings also warn against excessive reification of current diagnostic categories.

Genetic discoveries have implications in terms of knowing when to consider genetic testing. This will evolve rapidly as WGS is introduced into routine health care, at least in higher income countries. Commercial direct-to-consumer genotyping is already available, so clinicians need to be poised as to what to say when such tests are brought to the clinic. In our view, it is now important to conduct clinical research alongside gene discovery efforts and biological investigations. For example, evaluating the potential clinical utility of different types of genetic testing in different contexts. The growing number of gene discoveries is leading to increased biological insight which may soon be able to inform the identification of subgroups that improve our diagnostic categories and offer clues to new treatments. It is equally important to conduct research examining ethical issues and potential risks or unforeseen adverse consequences, as well as the benefits of genetic testing in clinical settings. Finally, the global and ethnic inequalities in genetics are a concern that both scientists and clinicians will need to address more strongly going forward.

Box 21.1 Key questions for clinicians

Question	Author recommendations
Can we use genetic tests to diagnose psychiatric disorders and NDDs now?	No
Should we be aware of when to consider genetic testing for rare, large effect variants?	Yes
Can we use genetic testing to inform our treatment choice?	Not currently
Are their implications for family members when a child has a specific diagnosis (e.g., ASD, ADHD)?	Yes Is a parent or sibling similarly affected? Recognize this as it could impact on clinical management
Does the same diagnosis always run in families?	No Multiple genes and environment contribute risk Genetic and familial liabilities cross diagnostic boundaries
If a disorder is genetic, then does environment matter?	Yes Genes and environment work together Even for single gene disorders, environments can influence outcomes and functioning

Acknowledgments

We thank Professor Michael O'Donovan, Cardiff University, for advice and expert review of this chapter.

References

Adams, M.J. et al. (2024) Genome-wide study of major depression in 685,808 diverse individuals identifies 697 independent associations, infers causal neuronal subtypes and biological targets for novel pharmacotherapies. medRxiv 2024.04.29.24306535. doi: https://doi.org/10.1101/2024.04.29.24306535.

American Academy of Child & Adolescent Psychiatry (2020) *Clinical Use of Pharmacogenetic Tests in Prescribing Psychotropic Medications for Children and Adolescents* [Online]. Available: https://www.aacap.org/aacap/Policy_Statements/2020/Clinical-Use-Pharmacogenetic-Tests-Prescribing-Psychotropic-Medications-for-Children-Adolescents.aspx [2 October 2023].

Andreassen, O.A. *et al.* (2023) New insights from the last decade of research in psychiatric genetics: discoveries, challenges and clinical implications. *World Psychiatry* **22**, 4–24.

Baselmans, B.M.L. *et al.* (2021) Risk in relatives, heritability, SNP-based heritability, and genetic correlations in psychiatric disorders: a review. *Biological Psychiatry* **89**(1), 11–19.

Birmaher, B. *et al.* (2021) A longitudinal study of psychiatric disorders in offspring of parents with bipolar disorder from preschool to adolescence. *Journal of the American Academy of Child and Adolescent Psychiatry* **60**, 1419–1429.

Cloninger, C.R. *et al.* (1982) Predisposition to petty criminality in Swedish adoptees: II. Cross-fostering analysis of gene–environment interaction. *Archives of General Psychiatry* **39**, 1242–1247.

Davies, N.M. *et al.* (2018) Reading Mendelian randomisation studies: a guide, glossary, and checklist for clinicians. *BMJ* **362**, 601.

Demontis, D. *et al.* (2023) Genome-wide analyses of ADHD identify 27 risk loci, refine the genetic architecture and implicate several cognitive domains. *Nature Genetics* **55**, 198–208.

Dixon, T.A. & Muotri, A.R. (2023) Advancing preclinical models of psychiatric disorders with human brain organoid cultures. *Molecular Psychiatry* **28**(1), 83–95.

Fu, J.M. *et al.* (2022) Rare coding variation provides insight into the genetic architecture and phenotypic context of autism. *Nature Genetics* **54**(9), 1320–1331.

ISPG (2019) Genetic Testing and Psychiatric Disorders: A Statement from the International Society of Psychiatric Genetics International Society of Psychiatric Genetics [Online]. Available: https://ispg.net/genetic-testing-statement [2 October 2023].

Kendall, K.M. *et al.* (2021) The genetic basis of major depression. *Psychological Medicine* **51**, 2217–2230.

Kendler, K.S. *et al.* (2020) The sources of parent-child transmission of risk for suicide attempt and deaths by suicide in Swedish national samples. *The American Journal of Psychiatry* **177**, 928–935.

Kendler, K.S. *et al.* (2021) The patterns of family genetic risk scores for eleven major psychiatric and substance use disorders in a Swedish national sample. *Translational Psychiatry* **11**(1), 326.

King, A. *et al.* (2022) Polygenic risk score improves the accuracy of a clinical risk score for coronary artery disease. *BMC Medicine* **20**, 1–14.

Kong, A. *et al.* (2018) The nature of nurture: effects of parental genotypes. *Science* **359**(6374), 424–428.

Legge, S.E. *et al.* (2019) Association of genetic liability to psychotic experiences with neuropsychotic disorders and traits. *JAMA Psychiatry* **76**, 1256–1265.

Lencz, T. *et al.* (2022) Concerns about the use of polygenic embryo screening for psychiatric and cognitive traits. *The Lancet Psychiatry* **9**(10), 838–844.

Leppert, B. *et al.* (2020) A cross-disorder PRS-pheWAS of 5 major psychiatric disorders in UK biobank. *PLoS Genetics* **16**(5), e1008185.

Machlitt-Northen, S. *et al.* (2022) Polygenic scores for schizophrenia and major depression are associated with psychosocial risk factors in children: evidence of gene–environment correlation. *The Journal of Child Psychology and Psychiatry and Allied Disciplines* **63**, 1140–1152.

Martin, J. *et al.* (2023) Investigating direct and indirect genetic effects in attention-deficit/hyperactivity disorder using parent-offspring trios. *Biological Psychiatry* **93**, 37–44.

Mollon, J. *et al.* (2023) The contribution of copy number variants to psychiatric symptoms and cognitive ability. *Molecular Psychiatry*. doi:10.1038/s41380-023-01978-4.

Mullins, N. *et al.* (2021) Genome-wide association study of more than 40,000 bipolar disorder cases provides new insights into the underlying biology. *Nature Genetics* **53**, 817–829.

Murray, G.K. *et al.* (2021) Could polygenic risk scores be useful in psychiatry?: a review. *JAMA Psychiatry* **78**(2), 210–219.

Polderman, T.J.C. *et al.* (2015) Meta-analysis of the heritability of human traits based on fifty years of twin studies. *Nature Genetics* **47**(7), 702–709.

Royal College of Psychiatrists (2023) *The Role of Genetic Testing in Mental Health Settings. CR237.* Royal College of Psychiatrists, London, UK. Available: https://www.rcpsych.ac.uk/improving-care/campaigning-for-better-mental-health-policy/college-reports/2023-college-reports/the-role-of-genetic-testing-in-mental-health-settings-(cr237) [25 September 2024].

Satterstrom, F.K. *et al.* (2018) ASD and ADHD have a similar burden of rare protein-truncating variants. *Nature Neuroscience* **22**(12), 1961–1965.

Satterstrom, F.K. *et al.* (2020) Large-scale exome sequencing study implicates both developmental and functional changes in the neurobiology of autism. *Cell* **180**, 568–584.e23.

Singh, T. *et al.* (2022) Rare coding variants in ten genes confer substantial risk for schizophrenia. *Nature* **604**, 509–516.

Swen, J.J. *et al.* (2023) A 12-gene pharmacogenetic panel to prevent adverse drug reactions: an open-label, multicentre, controlled, cluster-randomised crossover implementation study. *The Lancet* **401**, 347–356.

Taylor, M.J. *et al.* (2019) Association of genetic risk factors for psychiatric disorders and traits of these disorders in a Swedish population twin sample. *JAMA Psychiatry* **76**(3), 280–289.

Thapar, A. *et al.* (2022) Practitioner review: attention-deficit hyperactivity disorder and autism spectrum disorder—the importance of depression. *Journal of Child Psychology and Psychiatry* **64**(1), 4–15.

Thompson, P.M. *et al.* (2020) ENIGMA and global neuroscience: a decade of large-scale studies of the brain in health and disease across more than 40 countries. *Translational Psychiatry* **10**(1), 100.

Trubetskoy, V. *et al.* (2022) Mapping genomic loci implicates genes and synaptic biology in schizophrenia. *Nature* **604**, 502–508.

Uffelmann, E. *et al.* (2021) Genome-wide association studies. *Nature Reviews Methods Primers* **1**, 59.

van Schaik, R.H.N. *et al.* (2020) Pharmacogenetics in psychiatry: an update on clinical usability. *Frontiers in Pharmacology* **11**, 575540.

Wang, B. *et al.* (2021) Robust genetic nurture effects on education: a systematic review and meta-analysis based on 38,654 families across 8 cohorts. *American Journal of Human Genetics* **108**, 1780–1791.

Willsey, H.R. *et al.* (2022) Genomics, convergent neuroscience and progress in understanding autism spectrum disorder. *Nature Reviews Neuroscience* **23**(6), 323–341.

Wright, C.F. *et al.* (2023) Genomic diagnosis of rare pediatric disease in the United Kingdom and Ireland. *The New England Journal of Medicine* **388**(17), 1559–1571.

CHAPTER 22
Psychosocial adversity

Jennifer Jenkins[1], Sheri Madigan[2] and Louise Arseneault[3]

[1] Applied Psychology and Human Development, University of Toronto, Toronto, Ontario, Canada

[2] Department of Psychology, University of Calgary, Calgary, Alberta, Canada

[3] Institute of Psychiatry, Psychology and Neuroscience, King's College London, London, UK

Introduction

Human development is the process of individual adaptation to a complex and ever-changing environment. At times the adaptation is smooth; the environment provides support to the individual and the individual can use their own skills in a successful adaptation. At other times, however, the adaptation of the individual fails. This may be because the challenges in the environment are too great, the individual's abilities in adapting are insufficient, or a combination of the two (Rutter, 2012). Until recently, most of our knowledge about psychosocial adversities and their effect on children's mental health came from cross-sectional correlational studies that could not determine the direction of effect. Some environmental adversities such as poverty and war exposure are so distal to children, that children cannot affect their occurrence. Proximal adversities, however, are all about children's relationships (with caregivers, siblings, peers, and teachers). These are co-constructed, with a component of that relationship attributable to what the child brings to the interaction. To accurately attribute the ways in which psychosocial adversity affects children we must use research designs that allow us to distinguish between effects of the individual and effects of social partners on the individual.

Methodological designs to disambiguate causal effects between children and their relational environment

Several novel designs have emerged since 2000 that help to establish causality rather than merely correlated processes. Because of the high level of heritability in mental health problems, one of the emphases in psychosocial adversity research has been to show that there are effects of adversity over and above genetic ones, by using genetically sensitive designs. These are fully discussed in Chapter 21. More recently, the emphasis has shifted to novel designs that use stability and change during person interactions, to differentiate a person's "individual effect" from the effect of other people on their behavior (i.e., what individuals bring to interactions/relationships and how they are changed by these relationships). For further details see Figure 22.1.

The role of the individual in the relationship

Many findings in psychosocial adversity show that negative parent–child or peer relationships relate to an individual's mental health, but perhaps a lot of that relationship is attributable to just one person in the dyad. The social relations model (Kenny *et al.*, 2006) is a data collection and statistical technique in which each member of a family interacts with all other members. The analysis isolates two types of person effect: what a person *expresses to,* and *evokes from,* multiple other family members. This design captures the "individual effects" by identifying the consistency of a person's behavior as they interact with different people. If people are highly consistent across *different* partners, then relationships are more about the challenges of the individual, than the relationship per se. Adolescents and adults have been found to show consistency of behavior across family members of between 30% and 60% (Ackerman *et al.*, 2011; Rasbash *et al.*, 2011). Thus, person effects on the relationship are strong.

The use of cross-lag panel models

Bidirectional effects are most often measured using cross-lagged designs (Hamaker *et al.*, 2018). In these designs, two processes that covary (e.g., parental and child depression) are examined over time, and the goal is to determine which of the two processes predicts change in the other more strongly. These designs

Rutter's Child and Adolescent Psychiatry and Psychology, Seventh Edition.
Edited by Anita Thapar, Daniel S. Pine, Samuele Cortese, Cathy Creswell, Tamsin J. Ford, James F. Leckman, and Argyris Stringaris.

Companion website: www.wiley.com/go/thapar/rutterspsych7

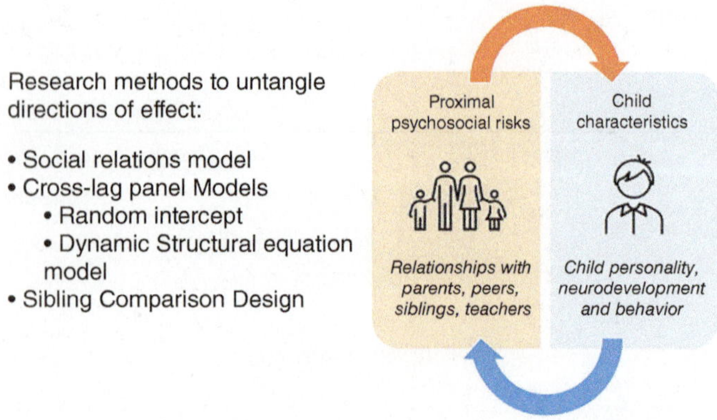

Figure 22.1 Research methods to disentangle directions of effect from children to their environments and vice-versa. *Note*: Drawn by Hazel Ngo with thanks.

are considered to closely approximate causality in observational studies, particularly when there are many waves of data. There are two types of structural equation models that are proving to be very useful in this regard. The random intercept cross-lag panel model (RI-CLPM) differentiates stabilities in the behaviors of individuals, from time-varying behaviors of each person (Racine *et al.*, 2019). The dynamic structural equation model (DSEM) does something similar, but it can accommodate many more time points which results in a better estimate of the stabilities (Hamaker *et al.*, 2018).

The sibling comparison design

Within-family heterogeneity in response to family psychosocial stressors can be utilized to understand causal mechanisms in children's mental health. Most psychosocial adversity research has utilized single unit designs (i.e., one child per family is sampled). The drawback of this design is that because family- and child-level variances are not separated, the effects of family- and child-level predictors are confounded. Lahey and D'Onofrio (2010) have shown that the sibling comparison design allows for a greater degree of causal inference and better differentiation of family- and child-specific risks than a single unit design. For instance, Browne *et al.*, (2018) found that socioeconomic status (SES) was associated with greater sibling differences on birthweight and that siblings with higher birthweights elicited higher maternal sensitivity than their siblings.

Mediation: from distal to proximal risks

Bronfenbrenner (1977) proposed a model for understanding context effects on child behavior (now also extended to brain development (Hyde *et al.*, 2020)). Ecological models hold that development occurs within embedded "layers" of context, from distal systems (country and community influences) to proximal systems (effectively, children's experiences in close relationships, across contexts such as families and schools). These terms are generally utilized within mediation models. A mediation model requires a significant pathway from the distal process to the child outcome, through the proximal process, e.g., cumulative environmental risk leads to greater problems in parenting which in turn explains child behavior. Mediation models are "causal" models: the mediator is conceptualized as the active agent that is causally responsible for the relationship between a distal and an outcome variable. Studies compare multiple potential mediators to determine pathways of influence. Generally, a mediator only explains some of the relationship between the distal predictor and the outcome and this is referred to as partial mediation. Theories of causation are very discipline-based and influenced by our scientific knowledge. For example, although "parenting" offers a causal mechanism for behavioral scientists, for neuroscientists mediation is about brain mechanism. A novel development in mediation studies is the use of a meta-analysis to test for mediation processes (Cheung, 2015).

Developmental timing

Psychosocial adversity has its effect on mental health through the embedding of stress in biological and cognitive systems (see Chapter 20). Are children more vulnerable to the ill effects of adversity at certain points of development? Because the brain is developing so rapidly in early childhood some have argued that effects of stress may be worse in this period than at other points in development (Dunn *et al.*, 2019). Evidence of developmental timing effects is very mixed, however. Some single studies find that the magnitude of the childhood adversity/adult outcome association does vary as a function of age of adversity exposure (e.g., Riem & Kerreman, 2019) and meta-analyses confirm this (Brindle *et al.*, 2022). Most studies examining this issue are correlational, rely on retrospective reports for the timing of childhood adversities, and have small samples. The strongest evidence for an early sensitive period comes from the Bucharest Adoption Study. Children within orphanages were randomly assigned to family foster care early in life or care as usual (i.e., longer exposure to the orphanage). Early placement in families was associated with better neural and behavioral outcomes (Sheridan *et al.*, 2012). As Rutter (2012) pointed out, however, adversity may leave its marks on some biological systems more profoundly at some life stages compared to others. Although the body is constantly adapting to the environment, no developmental period is immune to the effect of stress and its reversibility.

Cumulative, additive, and multiplicative risks versus the effect of single risk factors

Risk factors rarely operate in isolation. Although researchers may only study one risk, more may go underinvestigated in a child's life. For example, living in poverty is associated with parental psychiatric disorders, exposure to intimate partner violence, and increased likelihood of child victimization. This means that by looking at the impact of single risks we may fail to capture the degree of risk exposure that children experience. Cumulative risk indices are simply a count of the number of risks to which children are exposed and this has been found to explain more variance in child and adult outcomes than single risks (Evans *et al.*, 2013). For instance, 48% of adults reporting 4 or more adverse childhood experiences (ACEs), which include abuse, neglect, and household dysfunction, have mental health problems, whereas in adults with 0 ACEs it is only 15% (Madigan *et al.*, 2023a).

Some researchers have cautioned against the use of simple cumulative risk scores as they may oversimplify how risk factors combine in unique ways to predict child mental health (e.g., Putnam *et al.*, 2020). The occurrence of two risks may combine additively (each factor carries its own level of risk and the combination of the two risks is simply an addition of the risk attached to each factor). In multiplicative models, two risks may multiply the effects of one another. The interaction of exposure to marital conflict *and* receiving harsh parenting amplifies child conduct problems compared to either of these risks in isolation. These models are often tested against each other, and results can vary depending on the factors combining, the outcome or the populations being examined. Putnam *et al.* (2020) have shown that certain pairs of ACEs (e.g., emotional abuse and neglect) can account for a large proportion (61%) of the variance in conduct problems, in males specifically. In other studies, it has been shown that the combined effects of experiencing sexual assault, physical assault, and family violence in childhood had the greatest impact on adult male mental disorders and suicidality (Wiens *et al.*, 2020).

Empirical findings on distal risk factors

Socioeconomic status (SES)

Societies are hierarchically organized along an economic dimension. Both absolute levels of income and the extent of the difference between rich and poor members of the society have been found to be consistent correlates of mental and physical health (Peverill *et al.* 2021). Low SES, through lack of parental resources and high stress (Evans *et al.*, 2013), results in a cascade of proximal risks: to the developing fetus (poor nutrition, drug and alcohol exposure) and postnatally (e.g., negative parenting, interpersonal violence). SES effects on children's developing brains have been noted to be strongest for brain areas related to language, executive function, and attention in children (Hackman & Farah, 2009; Raver & Blair, 2020), and to be more strongly associated with externalizing than internalizing psychopathology (Peverill *et al.*, 2021). Randomized studies of cash transfers have shown mixed results. While some show beneficial effects (Zimmerman *et al.* 2021; Troller-Renfree *et al.*, 2022), others show little or no impact (Morris *et al.*, 2017; Zaneva *et al.*, 2022) depending on factors such as context and outcome. A recent meta-analysis shows a large amount of heterogeneity across studies (Zimmerman *et al.*, 2021). Some studies have shown that combining cash transfers with parenting interventions may be advantageous and some suggest that cash transfers during pregnancy may be effective. Relative income also plays a role in health outcomes. Wilkinson and Pickett (2009) developed an inequality metric by examining the ratio of incomes for the top and bottom 20% of a society across countries, which explained variation across countries in health and learning outcomes for children.

Neighborhood influences

Deprived neighborhoods are characterized by high unemployment rates, predominately minority populations, dense public housing, crime, and violence, as well as social isolation. Research on the influence of neighborhoods on children's mental health has the challenge of differentiating between the impact of families' SES and the neighborhood in which they live, given that SES constrains families' choice of neighborhood (Peverill *et al.*, 2021). One review estimated that effects of deprived neighborhoods accounted for between 5% and 10% of variance observed in children's developmental outcomes (Leventhal & Brooks-Gunn, 2000); however, because of the design of these studies it remains possible that uncontrolled effects at the individual and family levels are misattributed to neighborhoods.

Results from an experimental study, the Moving to Opportunity (MTO) program, provide more compelling causal data. Families recruited from high-poverty neighborhoods in the US were randomly assigned to the experimental or control condition. Members of the experimental group were given vouchers to move to a low-poverty area. Approximately 40% of families in the experimental condition took up the option of moving and effects were calculated for all families. Although beneficial effects on school achievement were initially reported for both girls and boys, later follow-ups suggested that only girls benefited from the intervention (Ludwig *et al.*, 2013), and lasting effects were only seen for some outcomes. One study reported that the intervention may even have been harmful for adolescent boy's mental health (Kessler *et al.*, 2014). Positive effects have been described, however, on college attendance and earnings, when children moved neighborhoods prior to age 13 (Chetty *et al.*, 2016).

Immigration

Immigration across the world is common. Studies have investigated adjustment among immigrant children, using first- (those not born in the host country) and second-generation status as an indicator of acculturation. Studies have reported better psychiatric and school achievement among first-generation children than second-generation immigrants and also better than host country peers (Gadermann *et al.*, 2022), a phenomenon referred to as "the immigrant paradox." This might be explained by educational and family characteristics associated with immigration, both because of the challenging criteria for immigration that governments demand (education, finances) and the characteristics of families that lead them to seek opportunities in other countries. Other studies, including a recent meta-analysis, are showing the opposite pattern, however, with second-generation children doing better than first-generation children

(Sirin & Sin, 2023). Critical multilevel factors at child, family, and host country levels, as well as their unique combination of benefits and harm, are thought to explain this variation. Factors include children's experience of loneliness, discrimination, bullying, and not feeling that they belong (Alegria *et al.*, 2019). Children's sense of belonging has been found to be higher when their own ethnicity is well represented in the school (Georgiades *et al.*, 2013). It is important for schools to attend to the sense of belonging because it predicts whether children remain in education.

The COVID-19 pandemic

The COVID-19 pandemic was a global event experienced by all, with 1.5 billion children experiencing school closures (UNICEF, 2021) and >11 million children losing a caregiver (Hillis *et al.*, 2022). Moreover, to mitigate the spread of the COVID-19 virus, measures were taken to limit social interactions (e.g., canceling extracurricular activities, gym closures), which may have unintentionally led to increased risks for mental distress and increases in screen time (Madigan *et al.*, 2022). A meta-analysis of over 50 longitudinal cohort studies with data before and during the pandemic shows that depression (and anxiety to a lesser extent) increased in children and adolescents (Madigan *et al.*, 2023c). Moreover, a comparison of >11 million pediatric emergency department visits before and during the pandemic showed that visits for suicide attempts increased by 22% (Madigan *et al.*, 2023b).

Empirical findings on proximal risk factors: development in the context of close relationships

Child effects: child anger, inattention/hyperactivity, shyness

During interactions we affect one another and co-construct the relationship that evolves. Children who are more temperamentally difficult (i.e., negative mood or a readiness to anger at low levels of provocation) are hard for their parents to manage. Mood-related problems in children are influenced by a range of factors but biological influences in operation before birth (e.g., heritability, low birthweight, prematurity, and adverse exposures) have been documented to increase emotional dysregulation in child- and adulthood (Wolke *et al.*, 2019). Although most of the evidence for child effects having an impact on relationships comes from child negativity and externalizing behavior (Plamondon *et al.*, 2018), other aspects of child behavior, such as shyness and positivity, also elicit characteristic responses from interaction partners (Liu *et al.*, 2018). Furthermore, sibling studies that differentiate between from within-family processes, show that relatively minor differences in the birthweights of siblings do result in differences in the caregiving that siblings receive (Browne *et al.*, 2018). Differential child effects on parenting have been shown to be stronger when families are under stress. In a longitudinal study during the COVID-19 pandemic, sibling differences in externalizing behavior increased over the period of study, when economic and relational family stress was high (Browne *et al.*, 2021). As designs get better at differentiating the stable effects of children, from the stable effects of parents (e.g., DSEM, RI-CLPM), we are seeing children play a strong role in how interactions proceed (Sokolovic *et al.*, 2021; Yirmiya *et al.*, 2021).

Gender identity

In the last decade, growing empirical attention is being paid to the role of children's gender identity or expression on their mental health (see Chapter 40). Children who identify as transgender and gender nonconforming often experience stigmatization and discrimination, which are precipitants to mental distress. In addition to higher rates of mental health problems, gender diverse children experience barriers to accessing health care (e.g., care refusal, doctor avoidance), which can exacerbate mental distress. A meta-analysis of 23 studies by Lucassen *et al.* (2017) shows that gender diverse youth reported higher rates of both depressive symptoms and depressive disorders, compared to cisgendered youth. However, consistent with models of resilience, research also suggests that the presence of gender-affirming parents (i.e., buffering supports) can mitigate a gender diverse child's risk for mental health problems (Olson *et al.*, 2016).

Parental responsivity for young children

Bowlby (1971) proposed that the infant's attachment system is a biobehavioral system developed for protection. Infants elicit caregiving through signals such as crying and clinging, which are designed to maintain close proximity to a parent. This biobehavioral system motivates the child to use the parent as a secure base from which to explore the world, and as a haven of safety in times of perceived threat or distress. The central mechanism was originally thought to be sensitive responding to child distress, but it may be more related to reading the thoughts and feelings of the infant and responding appropriately (Prime *et al.*, 2015; Giovanelli *et al.*, 2020). Sensitive responding by both mothers and fathers is associated with attachment relationships, mental health, and multiple aspects of cognitive development (Madigan *et al.*, 2019; Rodrigues *et al.*, 2021). See Figure 22.2 for effect sizes of the relationship between father sensitivity and children's outcomes. Effects are enduring (e.g., Raby *et al.*, 2015). Intervention research has demonstrated that enhancing parental responsiveness can significantly impact the child's language and cognitive development, supporting its causal influence on child outcomes (Landry *et al.*, 2008). Recent research has focused on the development of efficient measurement in families and childcare settings (Sokolovic *et al.*, 2022), interventions (Alvarenga *et al.*, 2020; Sokolovic *et al.*, 2021), and the application of the concept in a global health context.

Other behaviors that are correlated with parental sensitivity are speech directed to children, cognitive stimulation, and turn-taking, all of which have been consistently implicated in child

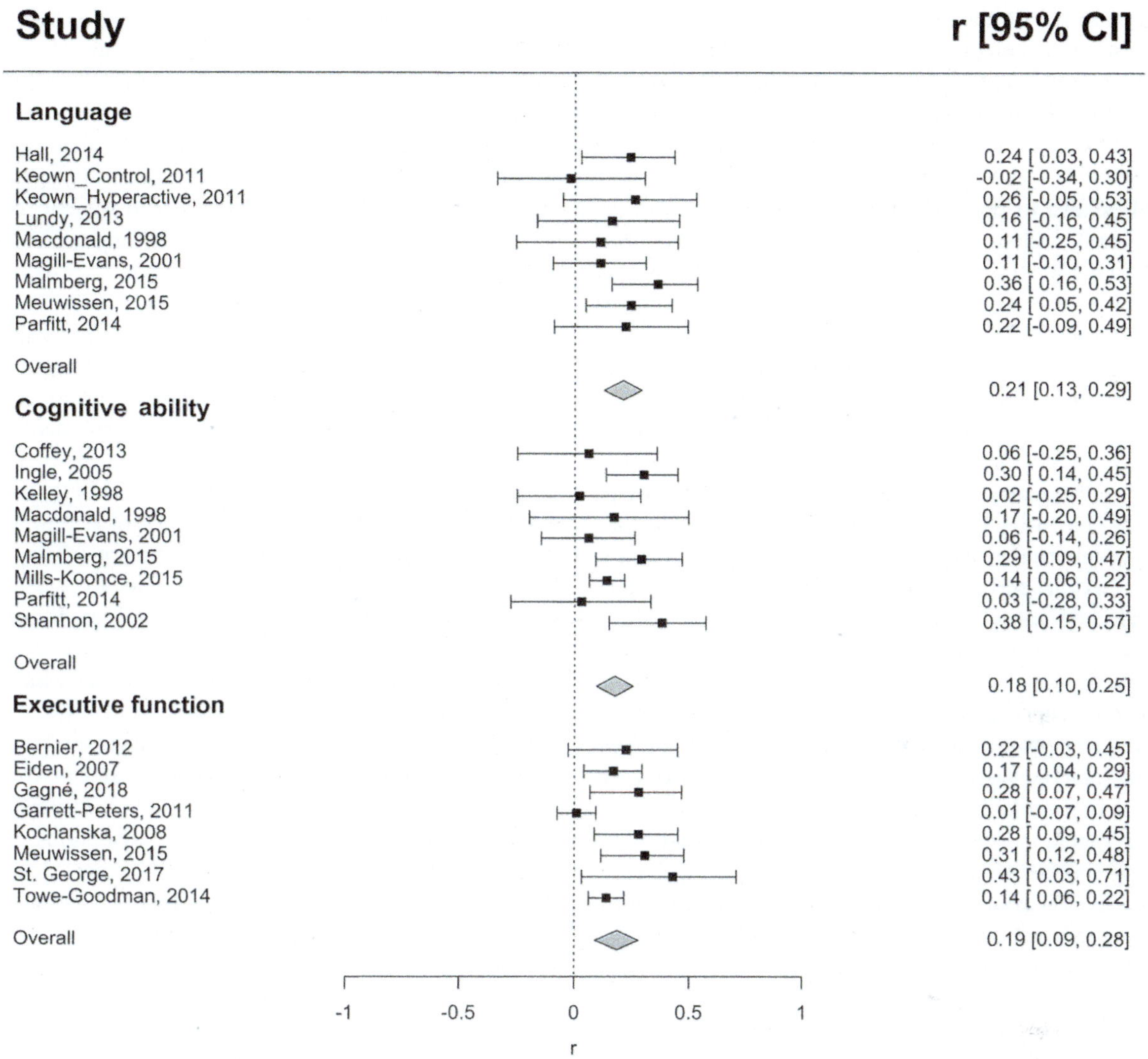

Figure 22.2 Magnitude of association between father's sensitivity and children's skills using meta-analysis. Observed effect sizes and 95% confidence intervals (CIs) are indicated for each sample. *Source*: Rodrigues *et al.*, 2021, with permission of John Wiley & Sons.

language and cognition (Romeo *et al.*, 2018; Madigan *et al.*, 2019; Anderson *et al.*, 2021). One of the explanations for the slower language development of children in low socioeconomic homes is less parental speech matched to the child's focus of attention and actions (Golinkoff *et al.*, 2019). In a meta-analysis of 17 studies, Borairi *et al.* (2021) showed that the association between SES and children's language development was mediated by maternal sensitivity.

Parenting harshness, monitoring

The domain of parenting most consistently linked to psychopathology is parental harshness (see Chapter 65), which has the most consistent links to children's externalizing behavior (Pinquart, 2017a, 2017b). Harsh parenting involves verbal aggression, hostility, and criticism toward children. Even from an early age, children who are recipients of harsh and controlling interchanges with parents are more likely to show non-compliance, aggressive behavior with peers, and externalizing problems (Smith *et al.*, 2004). Harsh parenting to one sibling more than another has been shown to predict *change* in sibling externalizing, suggesting a causal effect (Plamondon *et al.*, 2018). Effects of harshness on adult antisocial behavior (ASB) have been found to be mediated by amygdala reactivity to facial expressions in toddlerhood (Gard *et al.*, 2017).

Another dimension of parenting that is associated with adolescent psychopathology is lack of parental monitoring. Common indicators of parental monitoring include parental knowledge about where children are, who they are with and what they are doing, parental control of the child's activities and associations, and, finally, the child's voluntary disclosure of information. Meta-analytic evidence suggests that all indicators of parental monitoring are more strongly related to externalizing than internalizing (Pinquart, 2017a, 2017b). Research into parenting factors that predict a child's willingness to self-disclose suggest that a warm and responsive family climate is likely to influence the child's proclivity to disclose information (Soenens *et al.*, 2006).

Cultural issues in parenting research

Parenting goals, values, and specific practices (e.g., cognitive stimulation, discipline) show both similarities and differences across cultures (Bornstein *et al.*, 2015; Lansford, 2022). Although initially it was thought that certain aspects of parenting, like harshness, were associated with child behavior (e.g., externalizing behavior) in one culture but not another, as more studies across more cultures have been done, results have become more mixed (Davidov, 2021). Factors such as the emphasis a culture places on individuality and collectivism, the normativity of parental and child behaviors, and the macro and micro processes operating in countries explain some of this variation in findings. For both clinicians and researchers, analyzing the meaning of parent and child behaviors within culture will be critical for understanding the relationship between parenting and culture.

The childhoods of parents

Parents who experienced harsh or warm parenting in their own childhoods are more likely to engage in the same with their own children (Belsky *et al.*, 2005). The same is true for attachment styles intergenerationally (Fraley & Roisman, 2019). These intergenerational continuities are also affected by an individual's partner choice. Conger *et al.* (2012) initially assessed the parenting that children received when they were young and then followed them up after they became parents themselves. Children who had been parented harshly were more likely, once they became adults, to choose partners who were harsh. Adults who had experienced harsh parenting in their childhoods were also more likely to parent harshly if their partner used harsh parenting methods.

Siblings

Clustering in sibling behavior is well documented for behaviors such as delinquency and aggression, sexual risk, and early pregnancy (East, 1998; McHale *et al.*, 2009), with both genetic and environmental influences operating. Using time-varying designs to examine causal influences on sibling behavior, both younger to older and older to younger influences are evident (Borairi *et al.*, 2023). Siblings shape one another by matching one another's affect: positivity elicits subsequent positivity, while negativity elicits subsequent negativity. Sibling relationship quality influences mental health over time (Pike & Oliver, 2017) and operates to buffer children who experience adversity (Gass *et al.*, 2007).

Bullying victimization

Bullying is a common form of peer abuse involving repeated hurtful actions between peers where an imbalance of power exists. Evidence demonstrates that being bullied is harmful to children's well-being and increases the risk of psychopathology: victims are more at risk for anxiety, depression, self-harm, violent behavior, and psychotic symptoms than nonvictims and these problems can last until adulthood (for a review, see Arseneault, 2018; McDougall & Vaillancourt, 2015). The effects of victimization on mental health have been shown to be over and above other forms of hardship and genetic confound (Arseneault *et al.*, 2008; Silberg *et al.*, 2016; Singham *et al.*, 2017).

The risk of being bullied is related to internalizing and externalizing problems (Bowes *et al.*, 2009). The family environment also plays a role in placing children at risk of being bullied via factors like physical maltreatment (Bowes *et al.*, 2009), parental depression (Beran & Violato, 2004), and low SES (Wolke *et al.* 2001). Genetic and environmental factors, such as physical maltreatment, contribute to the continuity of bullying victimization over time (Bowes *et al.*, 2013). Children who are victims of abuse often enter a cycle of victimization that perpetuates itself over time and across situations. Being a victim of violence places the child at increased risk of various forms of further violence (revictimization) including emotional abuse, physical abuse, sexual abuse, and Internet harassment (polyvictimization). Child victims of physical assaults were twice as likely to experience another assault a year later, and victims of sexual abuse were seven times more likely to experience the same form of abuse in that same period of time (Finkelhor *et al.*, 2007). Furthermore, children who experienced polyvictimization suffer from increased symptoms of mental health problems, irrespective of more recent victimization experiences. Factors, such as having older siblings and friends, were associated with desistence of victimization from one year to another while moving to a bad neighborhood was associated with persistence. Altogether, this body of evidence suggests that efforts aimed at reducing bullying victimization in childhood and adolescence should be strongly supported.

School-based prevention and intervention programs aimed at reducing bullying behavior are common and some countries have mandatory antibullying policies in all schools. Examples of antibullying programs include the Olweus Bullying Prevention Program (Olweus, 1994) and the KiVa Antibullying Program (Salmivalli *et al.*, 2005). A meta-analysis showed that these interventions have a small effect on reducing symptoms, such as anxiety and depression, in young victims suggesting we need to find new avenues to reduce the harmful effect of being bullied in childhood (Guzman-Holst *et al.*, 2022).

Social isolation

Young people are constantly learning from each other and limited opportunities for peer-to-peer interactions can be detrimental to health (Holt-Lunstad *et al.*, 2015). Social isolation occurs when children experience a lack of positive peer-based social connections that typically provide support (Cacioppo *et al.*, 2011). Childhood and adolescence are periods of substantial psychological and social transformations (Blakemore & Mills, 2014). Thus, peer connections are increasingly important for young people as cognitive processes rapidly develop and mental health problems become apparent and persistent. Research has shown concurrent and longitudinal associations between social isolation and symptoms of psychiatric conditions such as depression, anxiety, and attention-deficit hyperactivity disorder (ADHD) (Loades *et al.*, 2020; Thompson *et al.*, 2022a and 2022b, 2023). Thompson *et al.* (2022a; 2023) have highlighted the complex associations between social isolation and poor mental health (Figure 22.3). They emphasize the importance of not only thinking of social isolation as a risk factor for psychiatric disorders, but also recognizing social isolation in children and adolescents as a key component of mental health difficulties. Social functioning around peers has even been shown to have a shared genetic basis with ADHD, major depression, and autistic spectrum disorder (ASD) (Schlag *et al.*, 2022). Interventions based on social support and inclusion show potential for valuable individual-based prevention of psychiatric conditions (Ma *et al.*, 2020).

Marital conflict, separation, divorce

Based on a large meta-analysis, marital conflict has been found to be associated with a wide range of mental health, emotion dysregulation, and attributional processes. All types of conflict (e.g., frequency, hostility, disengaged, child-related) predict child outcomes (van Eldik *et al.*, 2020). Difficult children generate increases in conflict between parents (Jenkins *et al.*, 2005). Short and accessible interventions improve marital functioning (Doss *et al.*, 2020).

The rates of both divorce and childbearing outside of marriage have been steadily climbing in many countries, and accordingly, the proportion of children living apart from a biological parent is on the rise. Meta-analyses have confirmed long-term negative effects on child, adolescent, and adult mental health problems, relationships, and achievement. Although such effects are now very consistently demonstrated across outcomes, they are small in magnitude (Auersperg *et al.*, 2019). Family stressors such as continued parental conflict, economic hardship, coparenting challenges, and diminution of non-custodial parent–child contact are possible mediators (Barnhart *et al.*, 2022).

Childcare influences

Childcare is a core element of many industrial societies as most children attend childcare or nursery prior to school entry. A meta-analysis of 20 independent samples revealed that across all ages, children in higher quality childcare had better academic,

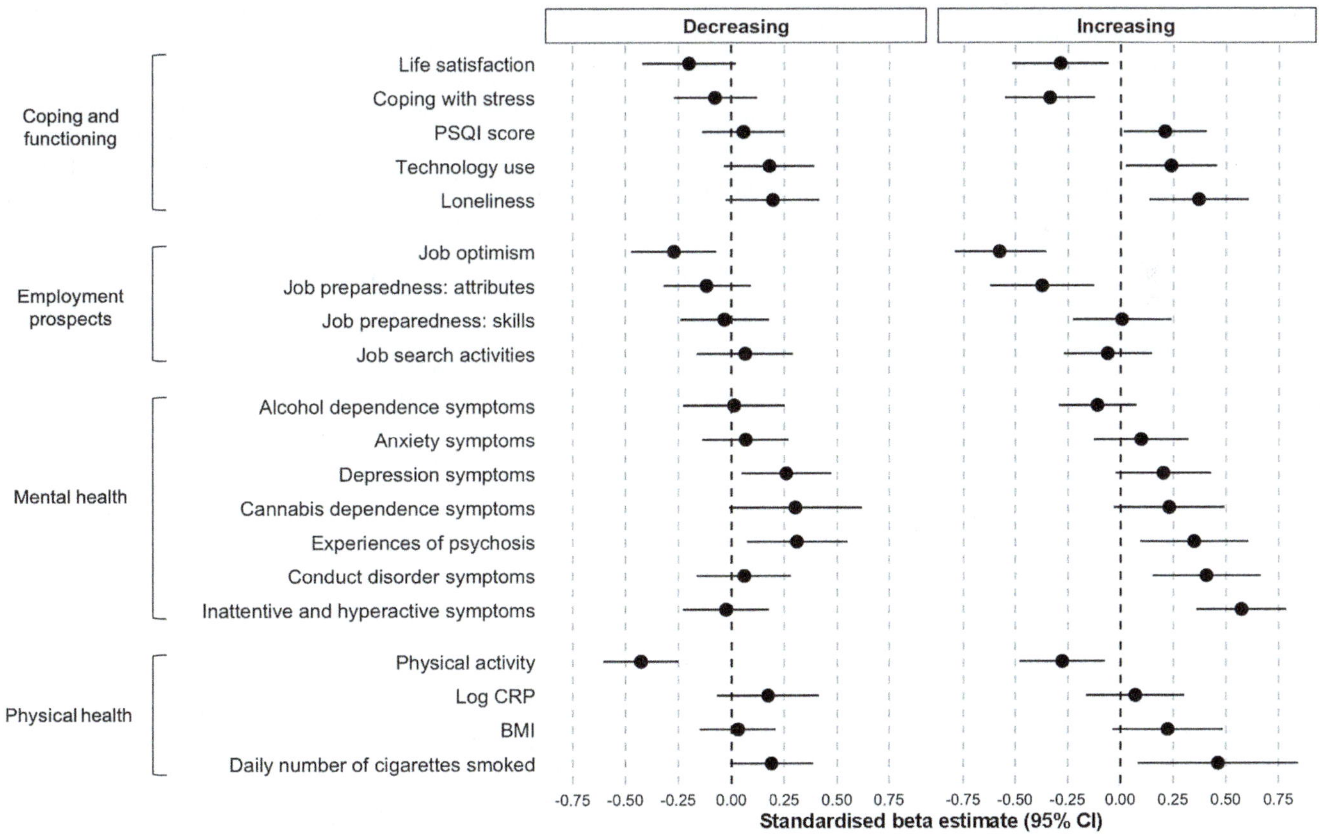

Figure 22.3 Decreasing and increasing trajectories of childhood social isolation are associated with poor outcomes in emerging adulthood. *Source:* Thompson *et al.* 2022a/John Wiley & Sons/CC-BY-4.0. *Note:* N total = 2232, N increasing = 106, N decreasing = 117. Beta (β) estimates and 95% confidence intervals (CI) for all associations.

language, and social skills outcomes (Burchinal *et al.*, 2011). Quality refers to the interaction between educators and children, as well as structural features such as adult/child ratios. Peisner-Feinberg *et al.* (2001) demonstrated that, after adjusting for child and family characteristics, children's cognitive, language, and social skill gains were evident into early elementary school and the NICHD follow-up to 15 years has shown the same (Vandell *et al.*, 2010). A meta-analysis of ratios and class size found that cognitive outcomes benefited from better teacher to child ratios (Bowne *et al.*, 2017). A meta-analysis of interventions has shown that it is possible to improve the quality of educator–child interactions (Werner *et al.*, 2016). Age of entry into childcare does not seem to influence the development of children's social skills (Zhu *et al.*, 2023). It is important to note that parenting quality appears to be a far stronger and more consistent predictor of child developmental outcomes than childcare experience (Belsky *et al.*, 2007).

Summary of findings related to psychosocial adversity causing child psychopathology

Evidence suggests that exposure to a range of environmental adversities and their combinations increases the risk of children's psychopathology. Environmental influences are best conceptualized as embedded layers of context with distal risks influencing proximal risks which, in turn, have effects on children's development. Poverty and social position in society, the pandemic and problematic neighbourhoods have all been shown to have influences on the development of child psychopathology. Some of this influence operates indirectly through the proximal environment while some of the effect has a direct impact. Children influence their exposure to proximal risk, as characteristics of children influence the quality of relationships that they co-construct with parents, siblings, teachers, and peers. It is very important to recognize that children's vulnerability to the effects of distal and proximal risk varies enormously, an issue discussed in Chapter 16.

Directions for future research

One of the most significant issues in this area is the extent to which proximal adversities such as parenting, peer, and sibling influences are non-independent of the individual and designs that allow for this distinction are critical. Second, issues related to timing and sequence of risk exposure, as well as the vulnerability of individuals to timing and sequence, will become increasingly important as we gain a better understanding of developmental timing in risk exposure. Third, there have been successful randomized controlled trial related to reducing children's exposure to environmental adversities and thus improving behavioral outcomes. It would be valuable to combine these with measurement of brain structures, and neuroendocrine and immune function, to examine the extent to which these biological processes mediate the relationship between exposure to adversity and child behavior (see Chapters 10–12). Fourth, the utilization of neural networks will be central to understanding how the constitutional vulnerabilities of children combine with psychosocial adversities in the environment to result in mental health problems for children. Artificial intelligence (AI) models (unsupervised learning algorithms) have been found to achieve higher levels of outcome prediction than more traditional statistical models. One of the reasons for their superiority is that unlimited (i.e., multiway) and previously unknown interactions become part of the "black box" that enables the higher levels of prediction (LeCun *et al.*, 2015). Tools are being rapidly developed to increase the "interpretability" of the "black-box" networks (Linardatos *et al.*, 2020).

References

Ackerman, R.A. *et al.* (2011) Positive-engagement behaviors in observed family interactions: a social relations perspective. *Journal of Family Psychology* **25**(5), 719–730. doi:10.1037/a0025288.

Alegria, M. *et al.* (2019) The effect of minority status and social context on the development of depression and anxiety: a longitudinal study of Puerto Rican descent youth. *World Psychiatry* **18**(3), 298–307.

Alvarenga, P. *et al.* (2020) Effects of a short video feedback intervention on enhancing maternal sensitivity and infant development in low-income families. *Attachment & Human Development* **22**(5), 534–554. doi:10.1080/14616734.2019.1602660.

Anderson, N.J. *et al.* (2021) Linking quality and quantity of parental linguistic input to child language skills: a meta-analysis. *Child Development* **92**(2), 484–501. doi:10.1111/cdev.13508.

Arseneault, L. (2018) Annual research review: the persistent and pervasive impact of being bullied in childhood and adolescence: implications for policy and practice. *Journal of Child Psychology and Psychiatry* **59**(4), 405–421. doi:10.1111/jcpp.12841.

Arseneault, L. *et al.* (2008) Being bullied as an environmentally mediated contributing factor to children's internalizing problems: a study of twins discordant for victimization. *Archives of Pediatrics & Adolescent Medicine* **162**(2), 145–150. doi:10.1001/archpediatrics.2007.53.

Auersperg, F. *et al.* (2019) Long-term effects of parental divorce on mental health—a meta-analysis. *Journal of Psychiatric Research* **119**, 107–115. doi:10.1016/j.jpsychires.2019.09.011.

Barnhart, S. *et al.* (2022) Adolescent mental health and family economic hardships: the roles of adverse childhood experiences and family conflict. *Journal of Youth and Adolescence* **51**(12), 2294–2311.

Belsky, J. *et al.* (2005) Intergenerational transmission of warm-sensitive-stimulating parenting: a prospective study of mothers and fathers of 3-year-olds. *Child Development* **76**(2), 384–396. doi:10.1111/j.1467-8624.2005.00852.x.

Belsky, J. *et al.* (2007) Are there long-term effects of early child care? *Child Development* **78**(2), 681–701. doi:10.1111/j.1467-8624.2007.01021.x.

Beran, T.N. & Violato, C. (2004) A model of childhood perceived peer harassment: analyses of the Canadian national longitudinal survey of children and youth data. *The Journal of Psychology* **138**(2), 129–148. doi:10.3200/JRLP.138.2.129-148.

Blakemore, S.J. & Mills, K.L. (2014) Is adolescence a sensitive period for sociocultural processing? *Annual Review of Psychology* **65**, 187–207. doi:10.1146/annurev-psych-010213-115202.

Borairi, S. *et al.* (2021) A mediation meta-analysis of the role of maternal responsivity in the association between socioeconomic risk and children's language. *Child Development* **92**(6), 2177–2193. doi:10.1111/cdev.13800.

Borairi, S. *et al.* (2023) Do siblings influence one another? Unpacking processes that occur during sibling conflict. *Child Development* **94**(1), 110–125. doi:10.1111/cdev.13842.

Bornstein, M.H. *et al.* (2015) A developmental analysis of caregiving modalities across infancy in 38 low- and middle-income countries. *Child Development* **86**(5), 1571–1587. doi:10.1111/cdev.12402.

Bowes, L. *et al.* (2009) School, neighborhood, and family factors are associated with Children's bullying involvement: a nationally representative longitudinal study. *Journal of the American Academy of Child and Adolescent Psychiatry* **48**(5), 545–553. doi:10.1097/CHI.0b013e31819cb017.

Bowes, L. *et al.* (2013) Chronic bullying victimization across school transitions: the role of genetic and environmental influences. *Development and Psychopathology* **25**(2), 333–346. doi:10.1017/S0954579412001095.

Bowlby, J. (1971) *Attachment and Loss, Volume 1. Attachment.* Hogarth Press, London.

Bowne, J.B. *et al.* (2017) A meta-analysis of class sizes and ratios in early childhood education programs: are thresholds of quality associated with greater impacts on cognitive, achievement, and socioemotional outcomes? *Educational Evaluation and Policy Analysis* **39**(3), 407–428. doi:10.3102/0162373716689489.

Brindle, R.C. *et al.* (2022) Adverse childhood experiences (ACEs) relate to blunted cardiovascular and cortisol reactivity to acute laboratory stress: a systematic review and meta-analysis. *Neuroscience and Biobehavioral Reviews* **134**, 104530–104530. doi:10.1016/j.neubiorev.2022.104530.

Bronfenbrenner, U. (1977) Toward an experimental ecology of human development. *The American Psychologist* **32**(7), 513–531. doi:10.1037/0003-066X.32.7.513.

Browne, D.T. *et al.* (2018) Child and contextual effects in the emergence of differential maternal sensitivity across siblings. *Developmental Psychology* **54**(7), 1265–1276. doi:10.1037/dev0000506.

Browne, D.T. *et al.* (2021) COVID-19 disruption gets inside the family: a two-month multilevel study of family stress during the pandemic. *Developmental Psychology* **57**(10), 1681–1692. doi:10.1037/dev0001237.

Burchinal, M. *et al.* (2011) How well do our measures of quality predict child outcomes? A meta-analysis and coordinated analysis of data from large-scale studies of early childhood settings. In: *Quality Measurement in Early Childhood Settings.* (eds M. Zaslow, *et al.*). Paul H. Brookes Publishing Co, Baltimore. pp. 11–31.

Cacioppo, J.T. *et al.* (2011) Social isolation. *Annals of the New York Academy of Sciences* **1231**(1), 17–22. doi:10.1111/j.1749-6632.2011.06028.x.

Chetty, R. *et al.* (2016) The effects of exposure to better neighborhoods on children: new evidence from the moving to opportunity experiment. *The American Economic Review* **106**(4), 855–902. doi:10.1257/aer.20150572.

Cheung, M.W.L. (2015) metaSEM: an R package for meta-analysis using structural equation modeling. *Frontiers in Psychology* **5**, 1521.

Conger, R.D. *et al.* (2012) Intergenerational continuity and discontinuity in harsh parenting. *Parenting, Science and Practice* **12**(2–3), 222–231. doi:10.1080/15295192.2012.683360.

Davidov, M. (2021) Cultural moderation of the effects of parenting: answered and unanswered questions. *Child Development Perspectives* **15**(3), 189–195. doi:10.1111/cdep.12422.

Doss, B.D. *et al.* (2020) Online programs improve relationship functioning for distressed low-income couples: results from a nationwide randomized controlled trial. *Journal of Consulting and Clinical Psychology* **88**(4), 283–294. doi:10.1037/ccp0000479.

Dunn, E.C. *et al.* (2019) Sensitive periods for the effect of childhood adversity on DNA methylation: results from a prospective, longitudinal study. *Biological Psychiatry* **85**(10), 838–849. doi:10.1016/j.biopsych.2018.12.023.

East, P.L. (1998) Impact of adolescent childbearing on families and younger sibling: effects that increase younger siblings' risk for early pregnancy. *Applied Developmental Science* **2**(2), 62–74. doi:10.1207/s1532480xads0202_1.

Evans, G.W. *et al.* (2013) Cumulative risk and child development. *Psychological Bulletin* **139**(6), 1342–1396. doi:10.1037/a0031808.

Finkelhor, D. *et al.* (2007) Poly-victimization: a neglected component in child victimization. *Child Abuse & Neglect* **31**(1), 7–26. doi:10.1016/j.chiabu.2006.06.008.

Fraley, R.C. & Roisman, G.I. (2019) The development of adult attachment styles: four lessons. *Current Opinion in Psychology* **25**, 26–30. doi:10.1016/j.copsyc.2018.02.008.

Gadermann, A.M. *et al.* (2022) Prevalence of mental health disorders among immigrant, refugee, and nonimmigrant children and youth in British Columbia, Canada. *JAMA Network Open* **5**(2), e2144934. doi:10.1001/jamanetworkopen.2021.44934.

Gard, A.M. *et al.* (2017) The long reach of early adversity: parenting, stress, and neural pathways to antisocial behavior in adulthood. *Biological Psychiatry: Cognitive Neuroscience and Neuroimaging* **2**(7), 582–590. doi:10.1016/j.bpsc.2017.06.005.

Gass, K. *et al.* (2007) Are sibling relationships protective? A longitudinal study. *Journal of Child Psychology and Psychiatry* **48**(2), 167–175. doi:10.1111/j.1469-7610.2006.01699.x.

Georgiades, K. *et al.* (2013) Emotional and behavioral problems among adolescent students: the role of immigrant, racial/ethnic congruence and belongingness in schools. *Journal of Youth and Adolescence* **42**, 1473–1492.

Giovanelli, C. *et al.* (2020) Exploring the relation between maternal mind-mindedness and children's symbolic play: a longitudinal study from 6 to 18 months. *Infancy* **25**(1), 67–83. doi:10.1111/infa.12317.

Golinkoff, R.M. *et al.* (2019) Language matters: denying the existence of the 30-million-word gap has serious consequences. *Child Development* **90**(3), 985–992. doi:10.1111/cdev.13128.

Guzman-Holst, C. *et al.* (2022) Research review: do antibullying interventions reduce internalizing symptoms? A systematic review, meta-analysis, and meta-regression exploring intervention components, moderators, and mechanisms. *Journal of Child Psychology and Psychiatry* **63**(12), 1454–1465. doi:10.1111/jcpp.13620.

Hackman, D.A. & Farah, M.J. (2009) Socioeconomic status and the developing brain. *Trends in Cognitive Science* **13**(2), 65–73.

Hamaker, E.L. *et al.* (2018) At the frontiers of modeling intensive longitudinal data: dynamic structural equation models for the affective measurements from the COGITO study. *Multivariate Behavioral Research* **53**(6), 820–841. doi:10.1080/00273171.2018.1446819.

Hillis, S. *et al.* (2022) Orphanhood and caregiver loss among children based on new global excess COVID-19 death estimates. *JAMA Pediatrics* **176**(11), 1145–1148. doi:10.1001/jamapediatrics.2022.3157.

Holt-Lunstad, J. *et al.* (2015) Loneliness and social isolation as risk factors for mortality: a meta-analytic review. *Perspectives on Psychological Science* **10**(2), 227–237. doi:10.1177/1745691614568352.

Hyde, L.W. *et al.* (2020) An ecological approach to understanding the developing brain: examples linking poverty, parenting, neighborhoods, and the brain. *The American Psychologist* **75**(9), 1245–1259. doi:10.1037/amp0000741.

Jenkins, J. *et al.* (2005) Mutual influence of marital conflict and children's behavior problems: shared and nonshared family risks. *Child Development* **76**(1), 24–39. doi:10.1111/j.1467-8624.2005.00827.x.

Kenny, D.A. *et al.* (2006) *Dyadic Data Analysis.* Guilford Press, New York.

Kessler, R.C. *et al.* (2014) Associations of housing mobility interventions for children in high-poverty neighborhoods with subsequent mental disorders during adolescence. *JAMA* **311**(9), 937–947.

Lahey, B.B. & D'Onofrio, B.M. (2010) All in the family: comparing siblings to test causal hypotheses regarding environmental influences on behavior. *Current Directions in Psychological Science* **19**(5), 319–323. doi:10.1177/0963721410383977.

Landry, S.H. *et al.* (2008) A responsive parenting intervention: the optimal timing across early childhood for impacting maternal behaviors and child outcomes. *Developmental Psychology* **44**(5), 1335–1353. doi:10.1037/a0013030.

Lansford, J.E. (2022) Annual research review: cross-cultural similarities and differences in parenting. *Journal of Child Psychology and Psychiatry* **63**(4), 466–479. doi:10.1111/jcpp.13539.

LeCun, Y. *et al.* (2015) Deep learning. *Nature* **521**(7553), 436–444.

Leventhal, T. & Brooks-Gunn, J. (2000) The neighborhoods they live in: the effects of neighborhood residence on child and adolescent outcomes. *Psychological Bulletin* **126**(2), 309–337. doi:10.1037/0033-2909.126.2.309.

Linardatos, P. *et al.* (2020) Explainable AI: a review of machine learning interpretability methods. *Entropy* **23**(1), 18.

Liu, J. *et al.* (2018) Cross-lagged panel analyses of child shyness, maternal and paternal authoritarian parenting, and teacher-child relationships in mainland China. *Journal of Child and Family Studies* **27**(12), 4116–4125. doi:10.1007/s10826-018-1229-7.

Loades, M.E. *et al.* (2020) Rapid systematic review: the impact of social isolation and loneliness on the mental health of children and adolescents in the context of COVID-19. *Journal of the American Academy of Child and Adolescent Psychiatry* **59**(11), 1218–1239.e3. doi:10.1016/j.jaac.2020.05.009.

Lucassen, M.F. *et al.* (2017) Sexual minority youth and depressive symptoms or depressive disorder: a systematic review and meta-analysis of population-based studies. *The Australian and New Zealand Journal of Psychiatry* **51**(8), 774–787. doi:10.1177/0004867417713664.

Ludwig, J. *et al.* (2013) Long-term neighborhood effects on low-income families: evidence from Moving to Opportunity. *The American Economic Review* **103**(3), 226–231. doi:10.1257/aer.103.3.226.

Ma, R. *et al.* (2020) The effectiveness of interventions for reducing subjective and objective social isolation among people with mental health problems: a systematic review. *Social Psychiatry and Psychiatric Epidemiology* **55**, 839–876.

Madigan, S. *et al.* (2019) Parenting behavior and child language: a meta-analysis. *Pediatrics* **144**(4). doi:10.1542/peds.2018-3556.

Madigan, S. *et al.* (2022) Assessment of changes in child and adolescent screen time during the COVID-19 pandemic: a systematic review and meta-analysis. *JAMA Pediatrics* **176**(12), 1188–1198. doi:10.1001/jamapediatrics.2022.4116.

Madigan, S. *et al.* (2023a) Adverse childhood experiences: a meta-analysis of prevalence and moderators among half a million adults in 206 studies. *World Psychiatry* **22**, 463–471.

Madigan, S. *et al.* (2023b) Comparison of paediatric emergency department visits for attempted suicide, self-harm, and suicidal ideation before and during the COVID-19 pandemic: a systematic review and meta-analysis. *The Lancet Psychiatry* **10**(5), 342–351. doi:10.1016/S2215-0366(23)00036-6.

Madigan, S. *et al.* (2023c) Changes in depression and anxiety among children and adolescents from before to during the COVID-19 pandemic: a systematic review and meta-analysis. *JAMA Pediatrics* **177**(6), 567–581. doi:10.1001/jamapediatrics.2023.0846.

McDougall, P. & Vaillancourt, T. (2015) Long-term adult outcomes of peer victimization in childhood and adolescence: pathways to adjustment and maladjustment. *The American Psychologist* **70**(4), 300–310. doi:10.1037/a0039174.

McHale, S.M. *et al.* (2009) Sibling relationship, family, and genetic factors in sibling similarity in sexual risk. *Journal of Family Psychology* **23**(4), 562–572. doi:10.1037/a0014982.

Morris, P.A. *et al.* (2017) Impacts of family rewards on adolescents' mental health and problem behavior: understanding the full range of effects of a conditional cash transfer program. *Prevention Science* **18**, 326–336.

Olson, K.R. *et al.* (2016) Mental health of transgender children who are supported in their identities. *Pediatrics* **137**(3), e20153223. doi:10.1542/peds.2015-3223.

Olweus, D. (1994) Bullying at school: basic facts and effects of a school-based intervention program. *Journal of Child Psychology and Psychiatry* **35**(7), 1171–1190.

Peisner-Feinberg, E.S. *et al.* (2001) The relation of preschool child-care quality to children's cognitive and social developmental trajectories through second grade. *Child Development* **72**(5), 1534–1553. doi:10.1111/1467-8624.00364.

Peverill, M. *et al.* (2021) Socioeconomic status and child psychopathology in the United States: a meta-analysis of population-based studies. *Clinical Psychology Review* **83**, 101933. doi:10.1016/j.cpr.2020.101933.

Pike, A. & Oliver, B.R. (2017) Child behavior and sibling relationship quality: a cross-lagged analysis. *Journal of Family Psychology* **31**(2), 250–255. doi:10.1037/fam0000248.

Pinquart, M. (2017a) Associations of parenting dimensions and styles with externalizing problems of children and adolescents: an updated meta-analysis. *Developmental Psychology* **53**(5), 873–932. doi:10.1037/dev0000295.

Pinquart, M. (2017b) Associations of parenting dimensions and styles with internalizing symptoms in children and adolescents: a meta-analysis. *Marriage & Family Review* **53**(7), 613–640. doi:10.1080/01494929.2016.1247761.

Plamondon, A. *et al.* (2018) Disentangling child-specific and family-wide processes underlying negative mother-child transactions. *Journal of Abnormal Child Psychology* **46**(3), 437–447. doi:10.1007/s10802-017-0309-2.

Prime, H. *et al.* (2015) The development of a measure of maternal cognitive sensitivity appropriate for use in primary care health settings.

Journal of Child Psychology and Psychiatry **56**(4), 488–495. doi:10.1111/jcpp.12322.

Putnam, F.W. *et al.* (2020) Synergistic adversities and behavioral problems in traumatized children and adolescents. *Child Abuse & Neglect* **106**, 104492–104410. doi:10.1016/j.chiabu.2020.104492.

Raby, K.L. *et al.* (2015) The enduring predictive significance of early maternal sensitivity: social and academic competence through age 32 years. *Child Development* **86**(3), 695–708. doi:10.1111/cdev.12325.

Racine, N. *et al.* (2019) Dynamic and bidirectional associations between maternal stress, anxiety, and social support: the critical role of partner and family support. *Journal of Affective Disorders* **252**, 19–24. doi:10.1016/j.jad.2019.03.083.

Rasbash, J. *et al.* (2011) A social relations model of observed family negativity and positivity using a genetically informative sample. *Journal of Personality and Social Psychology* **100**(3), 474.

Raver, C.C. & Blair, C. (2020) Developmental science aimed at reducing inequality: maximizing the social impact of research on executive function in context. *Infant and Child Development* **29**(1), e2175. doi:10.1002/icd.2175.

Riem, M.M. & Karreman, A. (2019) Childhood adversity and adult health: the role of developmental timing and associations with accelerated aging. *Child Maltreatment* **24**(1), 17–25. doi:10.1177/1077559518795058.

Rodrigues, M. *et al.* (2021) Paternal sensitivity and children's cognitive and socioemotional outcomes: a meta-analytic review. *Child Development* **92**(2), 554–577. doi:10.1111/cdev.13545.

Romeo, R.R. *et al.* (2018) Beyond the 30-million-word gap: children's conversational exposure is associated with language-related brain function. *Psychological Science* **29**(5), 700–710. doi:10.1177/0956797617742725.

Rutter, M. (2012) Resilience as a dynamic concept. *Development and Psychopathology* **24**(2), 335–344. doi:10.1017/s0954579412000028.

Salmivalli, C. *et al.* (2005) Anti-bullying intervention: implementation and outcome. *British Journal of Educational Psychology* **75**(3), 465–487. doi:10.1348/000709905X26011.

Schlag, F. *et al.* (2022) Polygenic risk for mental disorder reveals distinct association profiles across social behaviour in the general population. *Molecular Psychiatry* **27**(3), 1588–1598. doi:10.1038/s41380-021-01419-0.

Sheridan, M.A. *et al.* (2012) Variation in neural development as a result of exposure to institutionalization early in childhood. *Proceedings of the National Academy of Sciences of the United States of America* **109**(32), 12927–12932. doi:10.1073/pnas.1200041109.

Silberg, J.L. *et al.* (2016) Psychiatric outcomes of bullying victimization: a study of discordant monozygotic twins. *Psychological Medicine* **46**(9), 1875–1883. doi:10.1017/S0033291716000362.

Singham, T. *et al.* (2017) Concurrent and longitudinal contribution of exposure to bullying in childhood to mental health: the role of vulnerability and resilience. *JAMA Psychiatry* **74**(11), 1112–1119. doi:10.1001/jamapsychiatry.2017.2678.

Sirin, S.R. & Sin, E.J. (2023) Meta-analysis on the relation between acculturation and academic performance: testing the immigrant paradox. *Educational Research Review* **252**, 100526. doi:10.1016/j.edurev.2023.100526.

Smith, C.L. *et al.* (2004) Predicting stability and change in toddler behavior problems: contributions of maternal behavior and child gender. *Developmental Psychology* **40**(1), 29. doi:10.1037/0012-1649.40.1.29.

Soenens, B. *et al.* (2006) Parenting and adolescent problem behavior: an integrated model with adolescent self-disclosure and perceived parental knowledge as intervening variables. *Developmental Psychology* **42**(2), 305–318. doi:10.1037/0012-1649.42.2.305.

Sokolovic, N. *et al.* (2021) Do mothers or children lead the dance? Disentangling individual and influence effects during conflict. *Child Development* **92**(2), e143–e157. doi:10.1111/cdev.13447.

Sokolovic, N. *et al.* (2022) Assessing quality quickly: validation of the responsive interactions for learning—educator (RIFL-Ed.) measure. *Early Education and Development* **33**(6), 1061–1076. doi:10.1080/10409289.2021.1922851.

Thompson, K.N. *et al.* (2022a) Do children with attention-deficit/hyperactivity disorder symptoms become socially isolated? Longitudinal within-person associations in a nationally representative cohort. *JAACAP Open* **1**(1), 12–13. doi:10.1016/j.jaacop.2023.02.001.

Thompson, K.N. *et al.* (2022b) Trajectories of childhood social isolation in a nationally representative cohort: associations with antecedents and early adulthood outcomes. *JCPP Advances* **2**(2), e12073. 1–10. doi:10.1002/jcv2.12073.

Thompson, K.N. *et al.* (2023) Do children with deficit/hyperactivity disorder symptoms become socially isolated? Longitudinal within-person associations in a nationally representative cohort. *JAACAP Open* **1**, 12–23.

Troller-Renfree, S.V. *et al.* (2022) The impact of a poverty reduction intervention on infant brain activity. *Proceedings of the National Academy of Sciences* **119**(5), e2115649119.

UNICEF (2021) *Framework for re-opening schools supplement: from re-opening to recovery—key resources*. Available: https://www.unicef.org/media/94871/file/Framework%20for%20Reopening%20Schools%20Supplement-From%20Reopening%20to%20Recovery-Key%20Resources.pdf [13 September 2024].

van Eldik, W.M. *et al.* (2020) The interparental relationship: meta-analytic associations with children's maladjustment and responses to interparental conflict. *Psychological Bulletin* **146**(7), 553–594. doi:10.1037/bul0000233.

Vandell, D.L. *et al.* (2010) Do effects of early child care extend to age 15 years? Results from the NICHD study of early child care and youth development. *Child Development* **81**(3), 737–756. doi:10.1111/j.1467-8624.2010.01431.x.

Werner, C.D. *et al.* (2016) Do intervention programs in child care promote the quality of caregiver-child interactions? A meta-analysis of randomized controlled trials. *Prevention Science* **17**(2), 259–273. doi:10.1007/s11121-015-0602-7.

Wiens, K. *et al.* (2020) Capturing risk associated with childhood adversity: independent, cumulative, and multiplicative effects of physical abuse, sexual abuse, and family violence on mental disorders and suicidality. *The Permanente Journal* **24**(2). doi:10.7812/TPP/19.079.

Wilkinson, R. & Pickett, K. (2009) *The Spirit Level: Why More Equal Societies Almost Always Do Better*. Allen Lane, London.

Wolke, D. *et al.* (2001) Bullying and victimization of primary school children in England and Germany: prevalence and school factors. *The British Journal of Psychology* **92**(4), 673–696. doi:10.1348/000712601162419.

Wolke, D. *et al.* (2019) The life course consequences of very preterm birth. *Annual Review of Developmental Psychology* **1**(1), 69–92. doi:10.1146/annurev-devpsych-121318-084804.

Yirmiya, K. *et al.* (2021) From mothers to children and back: bidirectional processes in the cross-generational transmission of anxiety from early childhood to early adolescence. *Depression and Anxiety* **38**(12), 1298–1312. doi:10.1002/da.23196.

Zaneva, M. *et al.* (2022) The impact of monetary poverty alleviation programs on children's and adolescents' mental health: a systematic review and meta-analysis across low-, middle-, and high-income countries. *Journal of Adolescent Health* **71**(2), 147–156.

Zhu, Y. *et al.* (2023) Bidirectional relations between self-control and cooperation among Japanese preschoolers: a random-intercept cross-lagged panel analysis. *Early Childhood Research Quarterly* **64**, 139–147. doi:10.1016/j.ecresq.2023.02.010.

Zimmerman, A. *et al.* (2021) The impact of cash transfers on mental health in children and young people in low-income and middle-income countries: a systematic review and meta-analysis. *BMJ Global Health* **6**(4), e004661.

CHAPTER 23

Resilience: a multilevel developmental psychopathology perspective

Dante Cicchetti

Institute of Child Development, University of Minnesota, Minneapolis, MN, USA

Developmental psychopathologists stress that there is multifinality in developmental processes such that the manner in which persons respond to and interact with vulnerability and protective factors at each level of the ecology (i.e., culture, community, family, and their transactions) allows for heterogeneity in developmental outcomes (Cicchetti & Lynch, 1993; Cicchetti & Rogosch, 1996; Causadias, 2013). Individuals may begin on the same major developmental trajectory yet exhibit very different patterns of adaptation or maladaptation. The pathway to either psychopathology or resilience is influenced by a complex matrix of the individual's level of biological and psychological organization, current experiences, active choices, the social context, the timing of positive and adverse events and experiences, and the developmental history of the individual (Egeland *et al.*, 1993; Luthar *et al.*, 2000; Narayan *et al.*, 2023).

Just as deviations from the average expectable environment potentiate some individuals toward the development of maladaptation, others demonstrate adaptation in the face of the same challenges (Rutter, 1987; Masten *et al.*, 1990; Cicchetti & Lynch, 1995; Ellis *et al.*, 2017). Accordingly, it is equally important to comprehend the mechanisms that promote adaptation among individuals experiencing adversity as it is to investigate the developmental trajectories toward maladaptation. Research on biological, as well as psychological, protective factors is critically important for discovering mechanisms and processes that contribute to the development of either the recovery of function or resilient adaptation in the face of significant adversity (Masten, 2001; Curtis & Cicchetti, 2003; Charney, 2004).

Resilience refers to a dynamic developmental process encompassing positive adaptation within the context of significant adversity. Implicit within this conceptualization are two essential conditions: (i) exposure to or experiencing significant adversity; and (ii) the achievement of positive adaptation despite major assaults on developmental processes (Masten *et al.*, 1990; Rutter, 1990).

Historical context

Since the 1970s, researchers interested in children who develop well in the context of significant adversity have endeavored to enhance understanding of the diverse pathways to psychopathology, to elucidate the processes that eventuate in normal development, and to inform preventive interventions and social policies that could improve the lives of vulnerable children and families (Garmezy, 1971; Cicchetti & Garmezy, 1993; Luthar & Cicchetti, 2000). Investigations of risk and resilience have led scientists to rethink their prior assumptions about the causes and course of psychopathology and have resulted in a reformulation of the deficit etiological models that characterized earlier viewpoints about the development of children who have experienced disadvantage and great adversity (Garmezy & Streitman, 1974; Rutter, 1985).

Studies conducted on individuals at high risk for psychopathology and on persons with mental disorders, frequently portrayed the developmental course as deterministic, inevitably resulting in maladaptive and pathological outcomes. Investigations focusing on genetic and biological predispositions to psychopathology, assaults on development associated with inadequate caregiving, and traumatic occurrences within the home—such as child maltreatment and domestic violence, exposure to community violence, chronic illness, and catastrophic life events—graphically convey the multiplicity of risks that can eventuate in disordered outcomes. Epidemiological investigations of families exhibiting disharmony and disruption with no parental disorder (Rutter & Quinton, 1984) and studies

Rutter's Child and Adolescent Psychiatry and Psychology, Seventh Edition.
Edited by Anita Thapar, Daniel S. Pine, Samuele Cortese, Cathy Creswell, Tamsin J. Ford, James F. Leckman, and Argyris Stringaris.

Companion website: www.wiley.com/go/thapar/rutterspsych7

of links between cumulative risk factors and developmental outcome were also instrumental in the field's emergence (Rutter, 1979; Sameroff *et al.*, 1987). As researchers discovered that not all high-risk children manifested the dire consequences that extant theories of psychopathology predicted, comprehending the processes through which children at risk did not develop psychopathology became viewed as important for informing theories of maladaptation and pathology.

The investigation of factors that result in adaptive outcomes in the presence of adversity has a long and illustrious history with the empirical literature on schizophrenia constituting a salient founding base (Garmezy & Streitman, 1974; Masten *et al.*, 1990). Early investigations of severely disordered patients were focused primarily on understanding maladaptive behavior, and the patients who showed relatively adaptive patterns were considered atypical and afforded little attention. By the 1970s, researchers had discovered that people with schizophrenia with the least severe course of illness were characterized by a premorbid history of relative competence at work, social relations, marriage, and capacity to fulfill responsibility (Garmezy, 1970; Zigler & Glick, 1986). Although resilience was not part of the descriptive picture of these atypical individuals with schizophrenia, these aspects of premorbid social competence might be viewed today as prognostic of relative resilient trajectories. In parallel fashion, studies of children of mothers with schizophrenia played a crucial role in the emergence of childhood resilience as a major theoretical and empirical topic (Garmezy, 1974; Garmezy & Streitman, 1974). Evidence that many of these children thrived despite their high-risk status led to increasing empirical efforts to understand individual variation in response to adversity.

Following Emmy Werner's groundbreaking studies on children in Hawaii (Werner & Smith, 1977), research on resilience expanded to include multiple adverse conditions such as socioeconomic disadvantage and associated risks (Rutter *et al.*, 1997; Werner & Smith, 1982, 1992), parental mental illness (Masten & Coatsworth, 1998), maltreatment (Cicchetti & Rogosch, 1997), urban poverty and community violence (Richters & Martinez, 1993; Luthar, 1999), chronic illness (Wells & Schwebel, 1987), and catastrophic life events (O'Dougherty-Wright *et al.*, 1997). The thrust of this research was a systematic search for protective forces, that is, those which differentiated children with healthy adaptation profiles from those who were comparatively less well adjusted.

Early efforts were primarily focused on the personal qualities of "resilient children," such as autonomy or high self-esteem (see Masten & Garmezy, 1985). Subsequent research led to the delineation of three sets of factors implicated in the development of resilience: (i) attributes of the children themselves; (ii) aspects of their families; and (iii) characteristics of their wider social environments (Werner & Smith, 1982, 1992; Masten & Garmezy, 1985).

During the last several decades, the focus of empirical work has shifted away from identifying protective factors to understanding underlying protective processes. Rather than simply studying which child, family, and environmental factors are involved in resilience, researchers are increasingly striving to understand how such factors may contribute to positive outcomes (Cowen *et al.*, 1997; Luthar, 1999). Such attention to underlying mechanisms is viewed as essential for advancing theory and research in the field, as well as for designing appropriate prevention and intervention strategies for individuals facing adversity (Cicchetti & Hinshaw, 2002). Randomized controlled trials (RCTs) and epidemiologically based preventive interventions may be conceptualized as true experiments in altering the course of development (Kellam & Rebok, 1992; Costello, 2008; Rutter & Stevenson, 2008), thereby presenting opportunities to test existing developmental theories as well as to provide insights into the etiology and course of positive adaptational outcomes in individuals experiencing significant adversity.

Finally, conceptions of resilience as absolute or global, as opposed to relative or circumscribed, have also changed over the years (Luthar *et al.*, 2000). In some early writings, those who did well despite multiple risks were labeled "invulnerable" (Anthony, 1974). This term was misleading because it implied that risk evasion was absolute and unchanging. As research evolved, it became clear that positive adaptation despite exposure to adversity involves a developmental progression, such that new vulnerabilities and/or strengths often emerge with changing life circumstances (Werner & Smith, 1982; Masten & Garmezy, 1985). Thus, the term "resilient," which more accurately describes the relative as opposed to fixed nature of the concept, came to encompass those once referred to as "invulnerable."

The investigators and clinicians who would become pioneers in resilience science recognized that it was vitally important to know why some children do well under very high-risk circumstances, while others do poorly in the tasks of life or develop serious mental health problems. They realized, further, that this knowledge could have profound implications for promoting positive development when conditions were not optimal and also for intervention to prevent, ameliorate, or treat symptoms and psychopathological disorders.

Research on resilience in development has a number of roots. Many of these roots are intertwined with the history of developmental psychopathology and the study of competence in human development (White, 1959; Cicchetti, 1990; Cicchetti & Garmezy, 1993; Masten & Coatsworth, 1998). These roots include psychoanalytic theory about the protective roles of the ego and mechanisms of defense, the concepts of adaptation and competence in developmental theory, and studies of coping and adaptation to stress in clinical psychology and psychiatry. The systematic study of variation dates to the nineteenth century, shaped particularly by Darwinian and Freudian theory (Masten, *et al.*, 2006).

The study of resilience has matured and changed over the past half-century of work, in part reflecting the normal progression in any maturing area of inquiry and in part reflecting the dramatic advances in developmental theory and the technologies and methods for research in related fields (Luthar, 2006;

Cicchetti, 2010; Masten *et al.*, 2021). Resilience science advanced from basic descriptive goals to studies of processes and experiments to test resilience theory by trying to promote positive adaptation in contexts of risk or adversity. Definitions of resilience became more dynamic and multilevel as developmental systems theory became the prevailing perspective in developmental theory and science more broadly considered (Cicchetti, 2010, 2013; Masten, 2011). Advances in techniques for modeling complex data, observing the human brain in action, and studying how genes work and other biological processes provided traction for more sophisticated research on processes proposed in resilience theories or models. There was also a growing interest in and efforts to study resilience in more diverse contexts (Ungar, 2012; Ungar *et al.*, 2013).

Resilience is not something that an individual "has"; it is a multiply determined developmental process that is not fixed or immutable (Egeland *et al.*, 1993). Moreover, since resilient adaptation may be achieved at any point in the life cycle, there is a need for research on the achievement of positive outcomes at different points in development, including in adulthood and in later life (Luthar *et al.*, 2000).

Defining resilience

Resilience has been defined in various ways in extant theoretical writings. For example, Rutter (1987, 1990) has conceptualized resilience as the positive end of the distribution of developmental outcomes among individuals at high risk. Masten *et al.* (1990) have distinguished among three groups of resilient phenomena: (i) at-risk individuals who show better than expected outcomes; (ii) individuals whose positive adaptation is maintained despite the occurrence of stressful experiences; and (iii) individuals who exhibit a good recovery from trauma (van der Kolk, 2014).

Discrepancies also exist in conceptualizations of resilience as a personal trait versus a dynamic process. Researchers often use these terms interchangeably. A major source of the confusion regarding the issue of trait versus process derives from the influential literature on ego-resiliency, a construct developed in longitudinal research conducted by Block and Block (1980) that refers to a personal characteristic of the individual. Ego-resiliency encompasses a set of traits reflecting general resourcefulness and sturdiness of character, and flexibility of functioning in response to varying environmental circumstances.

Although adversity of some kind may actually have been experienced by a child labeled as ego-resilient, by definition, one cannot necessarily assume that this is true. In contrast, when the term resilience is used to refer to a process, the experience of significant adversity is a given. Thus, the terms ego-resiliency and resilience differ on two major dimensions (Luthar, 1996). First, ego-resiliency is a personality characteristic of the individual, whereas resilience is a dynamic developmental process. Second, ego-resiliency does not presuppose exposure to substantial adversity, whereas resilience, by definition, does.

Despite the various ways that resilience has been defined, there is broad agreement that resilience refers to a subset of adaptive processes or outcomes when there is a significant threat. In situations where there are few or no adversity experiences, children should be described in terms of how they are developing rather than their resilience.

Definitions of resilience have shifted to be reflective of the growing influence of developmental systems theory and the expanding need to integrate knowledge about resilience processes across multiple systems, levels of analysis, and disciplines in order to address multisystem threats (Cicchetti & Dawson, 2002; Masten *et al.*, 2021). Resilient functioning is not irreversible. Transitional "turning points" (Rutter, 2012) provide opportunities and challenges for individuals either to remain on a positive trajectory despite ongoing adversity, to "bounce back" from a decline in functioning, to persist on a maladaptive trajectory, or to exhibit a decline in functioning from positive functioning (Cicchetti & Rogosch, 1997). Resilience should be conceptualized as a multidomain, multidimensional construct. Changes in one domain of competent functioning can cascade to affect other developmental domains over time (Cicchetti & Tucker, 1994; Masten & Cicchetti, 2010).

Resilience in developing systems

Recently, Masten *et al.* (2021) defined resilience "as the capacity of a dynamic system to adapt successfully through multisystem processes to challenges that threaten the function, survival, or development of the system" (p. 524). This broad definition integrates ideas from ecological theory (Bronfenbrenner & Morris 1998), general systems theory (von Bertalanffy, 1968), systems thinking in biology (Gottlieb, 2007; Likliter, 2013), and developmental psychopathology (Gottesman, 1974; Sroufe & Rutter, 1984; Cicchetti, 2006; Sroufe *et al.*, 2009).

Multiple systems are involved in the processes leading to successful adaptation in a child, family, or community. Moreover, systems that are interconnected across levels will influence the resilience of each other. Thus, the resilience of an individual child that is manifested at the level of behavior depends on many other systems, both within the child (e.g., immune system; stress response system), in relationships or family resilience, or in the larger sociocultural and ecological systems in which that child's life and development are embedded.

Since its emergence, developmental psychopathology has been an interdisciplinary science (Cicchetti, 1984). It advocates multidisciplinary approaches that examine the biological, psychological, and social-contextual aspects of development. Risk and protective factors cut across multiple levels of analysis, from the molecular and cellular through the psychological and social systems levels. Moreover, risk factors tend to co-occur rather than exist in isolation (Sameroff & Chandler, 1975; Rutter, 1987).

For research to progress toward a process-level understanding of resilience will require incorporating research designs and strategies that call for the simultaneous assessment of multiple domains of variables both within and outside the developing person. Resilience cannot be understood fully unless all levels are examined and integrated. Moreover, the influence of levels on one another is almost always bidirectional.

Because different levels of analysis constrain other levels, as scientists learn more about multiple levels of analyses, researchers conducting their work at each level will need to develop theories that are consistent across all levels. Just as is the case in systems neuroscience (Chapter 12), it is critical that there be an integrative framework that incorporates all levels of analysis about complex systems in the development of resilience. The sophisticated and comprehensive portrayal of resilience that will ensue will serve not only to advance scientific understanding but also to inform efforts to promote resilience.

In summary, a developmental systems perspective on resilience includes the following principles derived from Masten *et al.*, 2021:

- Human adaptation and development—in both low- and high-risk environments—arise from continuous interactions across levels of function within individuals and between individuals and their environments.
- Many interacting systems shape the course of development and the processes involved in resilience.
- The capacity for adaptation can be conceptualized at multiple levels.
- The capacity for adaptation in challenging circumstances (resilience) depends on many interacting systems.
- Manifested resilience emerges from many interacting systems and always reflects the current context as well as the history of the child (or system).
- Living systems are self-organizing with emergent properties that can be surprising or unpredictable from lower levels of analysis.
- Resilience is dynamic—always changing—because the systems involved in the capacity for adaptation are developing or changing.
- Resilience—potential or manifested—should not be construed as a trait, although many traits could influence resilience.

Developmental cascades

Theoretical and empirical work in developmental science has been interested in the processes by which one domain or level of system influences another system or level of function over time to shape the course of development. These effects reflect the processes by which interactions and transactions influence development in complex living systems that have cumulative effects on the course of a system's development (Gottlieb, 1998, 2007; Thelen & Smith, 1998; Sameroff, 2000; Masten & Cicchetti, 2010). Developmental cascades refer to the cumulative consequences for development of the many interactions and transactions occurring in developmental systems that result in spreading effects across levels, among domains at the same level, and across different systems or generations. These effects may be direct and unidirectional, direct and bidirectional, or indirect through various pathways; however, the consequences are not transient: developmental cascades alter the course of development (Masten & Cicchetti, 2010).

Cascade effects could explain why some problems in childhood predict widespread effects in adulthood, whereas others do not. Cascade effects encompass a broad array of phenomena investigated in developmental science within and across multiple levels of function, from the molecular level to the macro level. They may account for the pathways by which gene–environment interplay unfolds over time in epigenesis to shape development, linking genes to neural levels of function to behavior to social experience, through processes of multilevel dynamics (Gottlieb, 1998, 2007; Cicchetti, 2002). The processes by which genetic disorders result in the development of behavioral anomalies have been described as cascades (Jarvinen-Pasley *et al.* 2008). Developmental cascades may be positive or negative in their consequences with respect to adaptive behavior. Research on resilience has highlighted the cascade effects pertinent to positive adaptation (Masten & Cicchetti, 2010).

Pathways of resilience and maladaptation

Resilience theory also highlights positive pathways of adaptation through time. Pathway models of adaptive function have a long history, dating back to the work of early embryologists describing development, including the epigenetic landscape of Waddington (1957) and pathways delineated by Gottesman (1974) and his collaborations with Shields (Gottesman & Shields, 1972, 1982) portraying the combined effects of epigenetic processes in shaping the life course toward and away from schizophrenia. In resilience science, pathway models represented efforts to capture the course of adaptive function over time, in the relation to changes in adversity and other circumstances. Even prior to the emergence of a mental disorder, certain pathways signify adaptational failure and probabilistically forebode subsequent psychopathology.

Developmental psychopathologists have articulated the expectations that there are multiple contributors to adaptive or maladaptive outcomes in any individual, that these factors and their relative contributions vary among individuals, and that there are myriad pathways to any particular manifestation of adaptive or disordered behavior (Sroufe & Jacobvitz, 1989; Robins & Rutter, 1990). In accord with this view, the principles of equifinality and multifinality derived from general systems theory (von Bertalanffy, 1968) are germane.

Equifinality refers to the observation that in any open system, a diversity of pathways may lead to the same outcome. Equifinality possesses significant implications for biological and psychological regulatory systems and for behavioral and biological plasticity (Cicchetti & Tucker, 1994). Initial descriptions of equifinality emanated from work in embryology. For example, the development of a normal organism was shown to occur from a whole ovum, a divided ovum, or two fused ova. Further, it was demonstrated that different initial sizes and different courses of growth can eventuate in the same ultimate size of an organism (Waddington, 1957; von Bertalanffy, 1968). Within the discipline of developmental psychopathology, equifinality has been invoked to explain why a variety of developmental pathways may eventuate in a given outcome, rather than expecting a singular primary pathway to the adaptive or maladaptive outcome (Cicchetti & Rogosch, 1996).

The principle of multifinality states that a particular adverse event should not necessarily be seen as leading to the same psychopathological or nonpsychopathological outcome. Individuals may begin on the same major pathway and, as a function of their subsequent choices, exhibit very different patterns of adaptation or maladaptation (Sroufe *et al.*, 1990; Cicchetti & Rogosch, 1996).

Steeling effects and post-traumatic growth

One of the most intriguing pathways is post-traumatic growth, whereby adaptive function appears to improve following exposure to adversity. The idea that some exposure to adverse experiences and challenges is better than none or too much exposure for longer-term adaptive function is a concept with a long history in resilience science. In 1987, Rutter described the steeling effects of exposure (see also Rutter, 2012). The possibility that adapting to adversity can alter an individual (child, adolescent, or adult) in positive ways for future adaptation is fundamental to preventive interventions. However, an overprotected child may not end up with the adaptive capacity for responding successfully to the vicissitudes of life that will inevitably occur.

A multilevel perspective on resilience

Because self-righting, one of the basic mechanisms underlying resilience, has historical roots in the fields of embryology and genetics, it is unfortunate that researchers investigating the pathways to resilient adaptation have largely eschewed the inclusion of genetic and biological measures (Curtis & Cicchetti, 2003). Until the past several decades, the empirical study of resilience predominantly focused on behavioral and psychosocial correlates of, and contributors to, the resilience and did not examine biological correlates or contributors (Luthar *et al.*, 2000; Curtis & Cicchetti, 2003; Charney, 2004; Feder *et al.*, 2009). These studies were undertaken prior to the inception of modern techniques for examining the molecular genetic, neurobiological, and biological correlates of human behavior and development.

Evidence from earlier variable-oriented and person-oriented investigations of resilience converge on a short list of attributes and environment that have been demonstrated to be well-established correlates of competent adaptation and psychopathology. Contemporary investigations continue to corroborate the following factors associated with resilient functioning: (i) close relationships with competent and caring adults in the family and community; (ii) self-regulation abilities; (iii) positive views of self; (iv) motivation to be effective in the environment (self-efficacy and self-determination); and (v) friendships and romantic attachments with prosocial and well-regulated peers (Masten, 2007, 2014). Furthermore, good executive functions, active coping strategies, and the capacity to confront fears directly, minimizing denial, disengagement, and avoidant coping have all been associated with resilient functioning (Masten, 2001; Luthar, 2006; Cicchetti & Bendezú, 2023). Moreover, optimism, positive emotionality, perceiving stressful occurrences in less threatening ways, the ability to reframe adverse experiences in a positive vein, spirituality, and being able to find meaning amidst trauma have each been linked to resilience (Feder *et al.*, 2009).

Undoubtedly, the relative neglect of biology as relevant to developmental theorizing on the unfolding of adaptive behavioral outcomes in the face of adversity was primarily due to the paucity of information that existed about the structural and functional organization of the brain (see Chapter 11), and the immature state of chemical neuroscience There simply was not enough knowledge about brain development and function to articulate their role in the genesis and epigenesis of normal mental processes let alone in their contribution to the development of resilient adaptation (Segalowitz, 1994; Johnson, 1998).

In recent decades, scientists have urged researchers to incorporate molecular genetic, neurobiological, and biological assessments into their investigations of the developmental pathways to resilient functioning (Curtis & Cicchetti, 2003; Charney, 2004; Cicchetti & Blender, 2006; Feder *et al.*, 2009). Technological advances in molecular genetics, neuroimaging, magnetoencephalography (MEG), electroencephalography (EEG) recording, and hormonal assay techniques have made it more feasible to conduct research on the development of resilience from a multilevel perspective. The role of biological factors in resilience is also suggested by evidence on neural, neuroendocrine, and immune system functions in relation to stress sensitivity (McEwen & Stellar, 1993), and in behavior–genetic research on nonshared environment effects (Plomin *et al.*, 1991).

Additionally, the advent of modern neuroscience, along with its many associated subdisciplines, represented an unprecedented opportunity to augment extant conceptual and methodological approaches to the investigation of resilience (see Chapter 10). Regardless, it is critically important to keep in mind that biological domains do not function independently; rather, more commonly the functioning of one system influences the functional properties of one or more other systems, through a developmental cascade of bidirectionally influenced processes (Masten & Cicchetti, 2010). Given this increasing recognition of the importance of considering many levels of interdependent processes simultaneously, in order to advance the understanding of a multifaceted phenomenon such as resilience, it is incumbent upon resilience researchers to meet the challenge of simultaneously incorporating multiple levels of analysis both across and within systems (Cicchetti, 2008). Biological and psychological domains are both essential to include in basic research on resilience and in resilience-promoting interventions (Cicchetti & Gunnar, 2008). Each level both informs and constrains all other levels of analysis. Moreover, the influences of levels on one another are almost always bidirectional.

When disciplines function in isolation, they run the risk of creating theories that will ultimately be incorrect, because vital information from other disciplines has either been ignored or is unknown. Just as is the case in systems neuroscience (Albright *et al.*, 2000; Frodl, 2016), it is critical that there be an integrative framework that incorporates all levels of analysis about complex systems in the development of resilience.

Neural plasticity and resilience

Experience-expectant and experience-dependent mechanisms of neural plasticity are integral to the very structure of cortical tissue and cause the formation of the brain to be an extended malleable process (Cicchetti & Tucker, 1994). Developmental psychopathologists and neuroscientists can utilize this knowledge as an avenue for understanding the vulnerability and protective processes of brain development as contributors to the genesis and epigenesis of psychopathology and resilience. Moreover, because the mechanisms of plasticity cause the brain's anatomical differentiation to be dependent on stimulation from the environment, it is clear that the cytoarchitecture of the cerebral cortex is shaped by input from the social environment (Eisenberg, 1995). Because the human cortex is only diffusely structured by the genetic plan, and because its eventual differentiation is highly reactive to the active coping strategies of the individual in a particular environment, it is highly likely that normal, atypical, and resilient outcomes of this process would encompass a diverse range of cortical network anatomies and individual personalities.

The neurobiology of some children who have experienced significant adversity does not appear to be structurally or functionally aberrant and may be reflective of an enhanced neural plasticity in resilient individuals (Cicchetti & Curtis, 2006; Demers *et al.*, 2019). Studies must be conducted that examine whether some neural systems may be more plastic than other neural systems or whether particular neural systems may be more refractory to change, or have a more time-limited window when neural plasticity can occur. In addition, investigations strive to ascertain whether there are differences in connectivity, assessed through diffusion tensor imaging, between regions of the cerebral cortex, possibly providing evidence of neural plasticity as one of the underlying mechanisms of resilient outcomes.

In self-organizing brain development, some regions of the brain serve to stabilize and organize information for other areas, whereas other regions utilize experience to fine-tune their anatomy for optimal function (Singer, 1995). In this manner, individuals can benefit from the interaction of genetic constraints and environmental information to self-organize their highly complex neural systems. Accordingly, children manifesting resilience, who develop in positive and adaptive ways even though they have experienced adversity, may be likely to function adaptively in a wide array of environments. Through experience-dependent processes, children who function adaptively are likely to seek out experiences that serve to modify and/or protect their brain development in ways that foster future adaptive developmental outcomes and generate resilience. Because experience-dependent plasticity is a central feature of the mammalian brain, neither early brain anomalies nor aberrant experiences should be viewed as determining the ultimate fate of the individual (Cicchetti & Tucker, 1994). That is, early experience and prior levels of adaptation neither doom the individual to continued maladaptive functioning nor inoculate them from future problems in functioning (McLaughlin *et al.*, 2022). Change takes place in a system as new needs and environmental challenges destabilize the existing organizations, necessitating the emergence of new organizations that may prove to be more adaptive than the preexisting ones in their current context.

The organization that takes place is often dramatic, with observable changes in the neural substrate that are translated into changes observable at the behavioral level (Curtis & Nelson, 2003). Such central nervous system changes that are the hallmarks of plasticity can take place at one or more levels of analysis, including molecular, cellular, neurochemical, and anatomical and at the level of brain systems (Nelson, 1999; van Praag *et al.*, 2000). Plasticity also plays a prominent role in neurodevelopmental processes (Cicchetti & Cannon, 1999; Cicchetti & Walker, 2003; see Chapter 3).

Neurobiological promotive and protective processes and resilience

Experience-dependent processes involve the adaptation of the brain to information that is unique to the individual. An important central mechanism for experience-dependent development is the formation of new neural connections. Because all persons encounter distinctive environments, each brain is modified in a singular fashion. This heterogeneity in experience-dependent plasticity is likely to emanate from existing differences between neural subsystems in rates of maturation, the extent and timing of reductant connectivity, and the presence of the neuromodulators and receptors that are critical for neural modifiability. Unlike the case with experience-expectant processes, experience-dependent processes do not take place within a stringent temporal interval because the timing or nature of experience that the person engages or chooses cannot be entirely and dependably envisioned (Greenough *et al.*, 1987).

Biological factors influence psychological processes; in addition, social and psychological experiences also exert actions on the brain by feeding back upon it to modify gene expression and brain structure, function, and organization (Cicchetti & Tucker, 1994; Eisenberg, 1995; Kandel, 1998; see Chapter 11). Because the brain is only diffusely structured by gene-driven processes and the eventual differentiation of the brain is very reactive to the individual's active coping in a particular environment, the normal, atypical, and resilient outcomes of this developmental process should encompass a diverse range of neural, synaptic, and associative networks that are the physiological determinants of many possible individual psychological organizations, including resilience (Kandel, 1999).

Gene–environment interaction (GxE)

Advances in molecular biology have helped to usher in a renascence of interest in the contribution that studies in GxE can make to unravel the complex pathways of adaptive and maladaptive development, including resilience processes (Rutter, 2006).

In GxE, environmental experiences moderate genetic effects (or vice versa) on adaptive function and development, including normal, pathological, or optimal outcomes (see Chapter 21). Risk-exposed individuals who carry the "protective" version (or allele) of a gene with respect to that risk condition develop significantly lower levels of maladaptation or psychopathology compared to comparably risk-exposed individuals with the "vulnerable" allele.

Much of the GxE research that is relevant to resilience has focused on how genes may serve as protective factors against developing psychopathology or maladaptive development. GxE studies are instructive and relevant for resilience research because they provide an illustration of how genetic variation may confer protection against mental disorder. Moreover, the presence of mental disorder does not preclude the attainment of resilient functioning. Many persons with mental disorder not only experience periods of remission, but also an appreciable number manage to function in an adaptive fashion for prolonged periods of their lives (Hinshaw & Cicchetti, 2000). Stated differently, in some individuals, deviations from the "average expectable" environment increase the likelihood of developing maladaptive functioning, whereas other individuals demonstrate positive adaptation in the face of the same challenges. Resilience is not a magical phenomenon (Masten, 2001, 2014). The same developmental cascades that can amplify maladaptive outcomes over time can perpetuate or amplify positive outcomes when the individual benefits from some combination of experiences and/or biological propensities that tip the initial balance toward adaptive outcomes (Cicchetti, 2013).

Although there has been an abundance of research conducted on GxE interactions and evidence for GxE interactions in the etiological pathways of psychopathology, as well as a small number of GxE studies on manifest resilience, it is important to note that several criticisms have been levied against GxE research (e.g., Duncan & Keller, 2011). These include small sample sizes that can yield low statistical power, failure to control for all potential confounders in all models, failure to compute all relevant interaction terms in the same model, and a paucity of replication studies.

Epigenetics

Although it is in its early stages, epigenetics broadly refers to the way the environment results in the modification of genes, which change the way genes are expressed. Epigenetics involves functionally relevant changes to the genome that do not result in changes in the nucleotide sequence, but rather operates like a light switch and can turn genes "on" or "off" or act as a dimmer to increase the way the gene is expressed. Chronic severe stressors, such as child maltreatment, can initiate epigenetic changes, representing one potential process by which chronic stress leads to adverse physical and mental health outcomes (Cicchetti *et al.*, 2016a). Research on epigenetic processes holds high promise, both for basic research investigations and translational intervention research on the determinants of resilience, providing a potential mechanism by which environmental experiences (natural or in the form of intervention) may exert their impact on gene expression that can last throughout the life span or even across generations (Lenroot & Giedd, 2008).

The dynamic nature of epigenetic processes demonstrates that genetic influences on behavior are responsive to experience and the environmental surround. Protective factors in the environment may bring about alterations in gene expression and thereby set in motion a cascade of positive adaptation to stress that is promotive of resilience (Masten & Cicchetti, 2010; Bowes & Jaffee, 2013).

Resilience-promoting interventions: a multilevel perspective

Research on the processes underlying resilience has substantial potential to guide the development and implementation of interventions for facilitating the promotion of resilient functioning in diverse high-risk populations who have experienced significant adversity (Luthar & Cicchetti, 2000). Such interventions should target protective and vulnerability forces at multiple levels of influence-culture, community, family, and the individual (Causadias, 2013; Masten, 2014).

Although several of the resilience-promoting interventions that have been implemented have employed a multifaceted approach in order to ensure sensitivity to the diverse transactions between children and their environmental contexts, there have been relatively few interventions that have incorporated biological measures as part of their pre-post evaluation battery (Curtis & Cicchetti, 2003; Cicchetti & Gunnar, 2008). However, there is growing evidence that successful intervention modifies not only maladaptive behavior, but also the cellular and physiological correlates of behavior (Eisenberg, 1995; Kandel, 1998; Fisher *et al.*, 2007; Dozier *et al.*, 2008; Cicchetti *et al.*, 2011). Because one of the primary objectives of the field of prevention science is to intervene in the course of development to foster the recovery of function and to promote resilient adaptation in individuals at high risk for maladaptation and/or psychopathology (Ialongo *et al.*, 2006), it is now critical to utilize multiple levels of analysis perspective ranging from DNA sequences to culture in research evaluations aimed at assessing the efficacy of RCT interventions whose goal is to foster the development of resilient adaptation. Thus, it is important for prevention scientists to investigate the means by which changes in experience and psychological functioning resulting from preventive interventions may modify biological processes.

Determining the multiple levels at which change is engendered through RCT prevention trials will provide more insights into the mechanisms of change, the extent to which neural plasticity may be promoted, and the interrelations between biological and psychological processes in maladaptation, psychopathology, and resilience (Cicchetti & Curtis, 2006). Moreover, preventive interventions with the most in-depth empirical support, based on integrative multilevel theories of normality, psychopathology, and resilience, can be implemented in effectiveness trials in community or real-world settings to reach the broadest number of people and prevent, alleviate, and ultimately cure, suffering from mental disorders (Insel & Scolnick 2006; Cicchetti *et al.*, 2016b). Furthermore, the inclusion of biological assessments in evaluations of interventions designed to foster resilience will enable scientists to discover whether the various components of multifaceted interventions each exert a differential impact on separate brain systems. If RCTs alter neurobiological systems associated with disorders and it can be shown that they mediate changes in psychosocial and behavioral functioning, then this fosters a better understanding of the neurobiological underpinnings of the disorder. If biological systems recover in response to the intervention, then this provides support for arguments that the systems under study are sensitive to environmental input during development. It is thus possible to conceptualize successful resilience-promoting interventions as examples of experience-dependent neural plasticity.

It also is extremely important to ascertain whether resilience-promoting interventions are more effective when implemented in the early years of life. Are such interventions more likely to achieve their goal of promoting resilience if they are conducted as closely as possible to the identification of the adverse event(s) or experience? The incorporation of a multiple levels of analysis perspective will enable scientists to learn whether, for example, resilience-promoting interventions implemented in the early years of life are better for brain development and functioning, even if improvement occurs in individuals who receive resilience-promoting interventions further removed in time from their adverse event(s) or traumatic experiences.

The incorporation of a multilevel perspective into research on resilience would still require adherence to a dynamic developmental viewpoint that respects the importance of context. Omitting biology and genetics from research and interventions on resilience is tantamount to omitting psychology. Biological, genetic, and psychological domains are each essential to include in basic research on resilience and in resilience-promoting interventions.

Future directions

Recommendations for continuing to improve future research on multisystem integration of resilience are listed below.

- The brain is a dynamic, self-organizing system that is mutable. Accordingly, future neuroimaging research should strive to ascertain whether the brain structure and functioning of resilient individuals differ from those of nonresilient individuals. Before we can be completely confident of the results, psychometric properties for brain-imaging measures must be thoroughly evaluated.
- Although research on cultural processes has grown, additional investigations are needed in order to identify unique processes and practices that promote resilience in particular sociocultural contexts (Masten *et al.*, 2021).
- It is important to conduct multisystem research on biological wear and tear (allostatic overload) or premature aging on youth who have successfully adapted to living in dangerous environments or in situations with large amounts of discrimination and oppression in order to ascertain whether there are skin-deep costs that may occur in resilient youth who strive to overcome structural inequality (Brody *et al.*, 2020; Masten *et al.*, 2021).
- The effects of genes and experience at a particular period may be influenced by the effects of prior development. Additionally, there are experience effects on the epigenome, and these may also operate differently across the course of development. Thus, GxE interaction and epigenetic research should begin to incorporate a developmental perspective.
- Prevention and intervention strive to alter the environment in order to bring about positive outcomes. Research on epigenetics suggests that prevention and intervention may also change the epigenome and that this could improve outcomes. If researchers are to understand the processes through which early adverse experiences impact maladaptation, psychopathology, or resilience, then it is crucial that genetic variation and epigenetic modifications be examined.
- Fetal programming posits that *in utero* exposures have a lifelong influence on physical and mental health (O'Donnell & Meaney, 2017). Programming refers to the effects of an environmental period to influence the construction of organ systems (Rutter, 2016). Because the fetal brain and other organ

systems are rapidly developing, they are particularly vulnerable to the programming effects of environmental signals of stress. Pregnancy is also a sensitive window of development for the mother during which the maternal brain is also susceptible to the programming effects of stressors (Howland & Cicchetti, 2021). Research on fetal development may provide an early insight into the effects of gestational stress on future outcomes of adolescence and young adulthood.

- Gestational resilience research can also focus on uncovering protective factors that might explain better-than-expected outcomes in the face of risk. Such investigation can be informed by existing resilience research into factors which support positive functioning during gestation. Given that both the fetal and the maternal brain exhibit heightened plasticity, it is possible that gestation is a sensitive period during which the achievement of resilience is more probable (Howland & Cicchetti, 2021). Gestational resilience research can inform prevention and intervention efforts, and, given heightened fetal and maternal developmental plasticity, it is possible that interventions to enhance resilience may be particularly efficacious during this period.

Conclusion

Resilience is a dynamic developmental concept. It changes with experience and from the interactions of many systems, both within and outside the individual. Resilience varies by context, domain, and level of analysis. Adversity and stress processes can have positive effects on the development of resilience. Efficacious interventions can generate positive cascade effects over time, domains, and generations (Szyf & Bick, 2013). In order to comprehend fully how individuals achieve resilient functioning in the face of adversity, it is incumbent to investigate it with a commensurate level of complexity.

References

Albright, T.D. *et al.* (2000) Neural science: a century of progress and the mysteries that remain. *Cell* **100**, S1–S55.

Anthony, E.J. (1974) The syndrome of the psychologically invulnerable child. In: *The Child in his Family: Children at Psychiatric Risk.* (eds E.J. Anthony & C. Koupernik). John Wiley & Sons, New York. pp. 201–230.

Block, J. & Block, J.H. (1980) The role of ego-control and ego-resiliency in the organization of behavior. In: *The Minnesota Symposia on Child Psychology: Development of Cognition, Affect, and Social Relations.* (ed W.A. Collins). Lawrence Erlbaum, Hillsdale, NJ. pp. 39–101.

Bowes, L. & Jaffee, S.R. (2013) Biology, genes, and resilience: toward a multidisciplinary approach. *Trauma Violence Abuse* **14**, 195–208.

Brody, G.H. *et al.* (2020) Persistence of skin-deep resilience in African American adults. *Health Psychology* **39**, 921–926.

Bronfenbrenner, U. & Morris, P.A. (1998) The ecology of developmental processes. In: *Handbook of Child Psychology: Theoretical Models of Human Development.* (eds W. Damon & R.M. Lerner). John Wiley & Sons, New York. pp. 993–1028.

Causadias, J.M. (2013) A roadmap for the integration of culture into developmental psychopathology. *Development and Psychopathology* **25**, 1375–1398.

Charney, D. (2004) Psychobiological mechanisms of resilience and vulnerability: implications for successful adaptation to extreme stress. *American Journal of Psychiatry* **161**, 195–216.

Cicchetti, D. (1984) The emergence of developmental psychopathology. *Child Development* **55**, 1–7.

Cicchetti, D. (1990) A historical perspective on the discipline of developmental psychopathology. In: *Risk and Protective Factors in the Development of Psychopathology.* (eds J. Rolf, *et al.*). Cambridge University Press, New York. pp. 2–28.

Cicchetti, D. (2002) The impact of social experience on neurobiological systems: illustration from a constructivist view of child maltreatment. *Cognitive Development* **17**, 1407–1428.

Cicchetti, D. (2006) Development and psychopathology. In: *Developmental Psychopathology.* (eds D. Cicchetti & D.J. Cohen), 2nd edn, Vol. *1*. John Wiley & Sons, New York. pp. 1–23.

Cicchetti, D. (2008) A multiple-levels-of-analysis perspective on research in development and psychopathology. In: *Child and Adolescent Psychopathology.* (eds T.P. Beauchaine & S.P. Hinshaw). John Wiley & Sons, New York. pp. 27–57.

Cicchetti, D. (2010) Resilience under conditions of extreme stress: a multilevel perspective. *World Psychiatry* **9**(3), 145–154. doi:10.1002/j.2051-5545.2010.tb00297.x.

Cicchetti, D. (2013) Annual research review: resilient functioning in maltreated children—past, present, and future perspectives. *Journal of Child Psychology and Psychiatry* **54**, 402–422.

Cicchetti, D. & Bendezú, J.J. (2023) Childhood adversity and the development of coping. In: *The Cambridge Handbook of the Development of Coping.* (eds E. Skinner & M. Zimmer-Gembeck). Cambridge University Press, Cambridge, UK. pp. 246–275.

Cicchetti, D. & Blender, J.A. (2006) A multiple-levels-of-analysis perspective on resilience: implications for the developing brain, neural plasticity, and preventive interventions. *Annals of the New York Academy of Sciences* **1094**, 248–258. doi:10.1196/annals.1376.029.

Cicchetti, D. & Cannon, T.D. (1999) Neurodevelopmental processes in the ontogenesis and epigenesis of psychopathology. *Development and Psychopathology* **11**, 375–393.

Cicchetti, D. & Curtis, W.J. (2006) The developing brain and neural plasticity: implications for normality, psychopathology, and resilience. In: *Developmental Psychopathology (2nd ed.), Vol. 2: Developmental Neuroscience.* (eds D. Cicchetti & D.J. Cohen). John Wiley & Sons, New York. pp. 1–64.

Cicchetti, D. & Dawson, G. (2002) Multiple levels of analysis. *Development and Psychopathology* **14**, 417–420.

Cicchetti, D. & Garmezy, N. (1993) Prospects and promises in the study of resilience. *Development and Psychopathology* **5**, 497–502.

Cicchetti, D. & Gunnar, M.R. (2008) Integrating biological measures into the design and evaluation of preventive interventions. *Development and Psychopathology* **20**, 737–743.

Cicchetti, D. & Hinshaw, S.P. (2002) Prevention and intervention science: contributions to developmental theory [Special Issue]. *Development and Psychopathology* **14**(4), 667–981.

Cicchetti, D. & Lynch, M. (1993) Toward an ecological/transactional model of community violence and child maltreatment: consequences for children's development. *Psychiatry* **56**, 96–118.

Cicchetti, D. & Lynch, M. (1995) Failures in the expectable environment and their impact on individual development: the case of child maltreatment. In: *Developmental Psychopathology: Risk, Disorder, and Adaptation.* (eds D. Cicchetti & D.J. Cohen), Vol. *2*. John Wiley & Sons, New York. pp. 32–71.

Cicchetti, D. & Rogosch, F.A. (1996) Equifinality and multifinality in developmental psychopathology. *Development and Psychopathology* **8**, 597–600.

Cicchetti, D. & Rogosch, F.A. (1997) The role of self-organization in the promotion of resilience in maltreated children. *Development and Psychopathology* **9**, 797–815.

Cicchetti, D. & Tucker, D. (1994) Development and self-regulatory structures of the mind. *Development and Psychopathology* **6**, 533–549.

Cicchetti, D. & Walker, E.F. (eds) (2003) *Neurodevelopmental Mechanisms in Psychopathology.* Cambridge University Press, New York.

Cicchetti, D. *et al.* (2011) Normalizing the development of cortisol regulation in maltreated infants through preventive interventions. *Development and Psychopathology* **23**, 789–800.

Cicchetti, D. *et al.* (2016a) An investigation of child maltreatment and epigenetic mechanisms of mental and physical health risk. *Development and Psychopathology* **28**, 1305–1317.

Cicchetti, D. *et al.* (2016b) What do we know and why does it matter? The dissemination of evidence-based interventions for child maltreatment. In: *The Wiley Handbook of Developmental Psychology in Practice: Implementation and Impact.* (eds K. Durkin & H.R. Schaffer). Blackwell, Oxford, UK. pp. 369–406.

Costello, E.J. (2008) Using epidemiological and longitudinal approaches to study causal hypotheses. In: *Rutter's Child and Adolescent Psychiatry.* (eds M. Rutter, *et al.*), 5th edn. Blackwell, Oxford, UK. pp. 58–70.

Cowen, E. *et al.* (1997) Rochester child resilience project (RSRP): facts found, lessons learned, future directions divined. In: *Developmental Psychopathology: Perspectives on Adjustment, Risk, and Disorder.* (eds S. Luthar, *et al.*). Cambridge University Press, New York. pp. 527–547.

Curtis, W.J. & Cicchetti, D. (2003) Moving research on resilience into the 21st century: theoretical and methodological considerations in examining the biological contributors to resilience. *Development and Psychopathology* **15**, 773–810.

Curtis, W.J. & Nelson, C.A. (2003) Toward building a better brain: neurobehavioral outcomes, mechanisms, and processes of environmental enrichment. In: *Resilience and Vulnerability: Adaptation in the Context of Childhood Adversities.* (ed Luthar). Cambridge University Press, New York. pp. 463–488.

Demers, L.A. *et al.* (2019) Childhood maltreatment disrupts brain-mediated pathways between adolescent maternal relationship quality and positive adult outcomes. *Child Maltreatment* **24**, 424–434.

Dozier, M. *et al.* (2008) Effects of an attachment-based intervention on the cortisol production of infants and toddlers in foster care. *Development and Psychopathology* **20**(3), 845–859. doi:10.1017/S0954579408000400.

Duncan, L.E. & Keller, M.C. (2011) A critical review of the first 10 years of candidate gene-by-environment interaction research in psychiatry. *American Journal of Psychiatry* **168**, 1041–1049.

Egeland, B. *et al.* (1993) Resilience as process. *Development and Psychopathology* **5**, 517–528.

Eisenberg, L. (1995) The social construction of the human brain. *American Journal of Psychiatry* **152**, 1563–1575.

Ellis, B.J. *et al.* (2017) Beyond risk and protective factors: an adaptation-based approach to resilience. *Perspectives on Psychological Science* **12**, 561–587.

Feder, A. *et al.* (2009) Psychobiology and molecular genetics of resilience. *Nature Reviews Neuroscience* **10**, 446–457.

Fisher, P.A. *et al.* (2007) Effects of a therapeutic intervention for foster preschoolers on diurnal cortisol activity. *Psychoneuroendocrinology* **32**, 892–905.

Frodl, T. (ed) (2016) *Systems Neuroscience in Depression.* Elsevier, Amsterdam.

Garmezy, N. (1970) Process and reactive schizophrenia: some conceptions and issues. *Schizophrenia Bulletin* **2**, 30–74.

Garmezy, N. (1971) Vulnerability research and the issue of primary prevention. *American Journal of Orthopsychiatry* **41**, 101–116.

Garmezy, N. (1974) The study of competence in children at risk for severe psychopathology. In: *The Child in his Family. Vol. 3 Children at Psychiatric Risk.* (eds E.J. Anthony & C. Koupernick). John Wiley & Sons, New York. pp. 77–97.

Garmezy, N. & Streitman, S. (1974) Children at risk: conceptual models and research methods. *Schizophrenia Bulletin* **9**, 55–125.

Gottesman, I.I. (1974) Developmental genetics and ontogenetic psychology: overdue detente and propositions from a matchmaker. In: *Minnesota Symposium on Child Psychology.* (ed A. Pick). University of Minnesota Press, Minneapolis, MN.

Gottesman, I.I. & Shields, J. (1972) *Schizophrenia and Genetics: A Twin Study Vantage Point.* Academic Press, New York.

Gottesman, I.I. & Shields, J. (1982) *Schizophrenia: The Epigenetic Puzzle.* Cambridge University Press, New York.

Gottlieb, G. (1998) The significance of biology for human development: a developmental psychobiological systems view. In: *Handbook of Child Psychology.* (eds W. Damon & R.M. Lerner), 5th edn, Vol. *1*. John Wiley & Sons, New York. pp. 233–273.

Gottlieb, G. (2007) Probabilistic epigenesis. *Developmental Science* **10**, 1–11.

Greenough, W.T. *et al.* (1987) Experience and brain development. *Child Development* **58**(3), 539–559.

Hinshaw, S.P. & Cicchetti, D. (2000) Stigma and mental disorder: conceptions of illness, public attitudes, personal disclosure, and social policy. *Development and Psychopathology* **12**, 555–598.

Howland, M.A. & Cicchetti, D. (2021) Gestational stress and resilience: perspectives to guide interdisciplinary research. In: *Prenatal Stress and Child Development.* (eds A. Wazana, *et al.*). Springer, Cham, Switzerland. pp. 387–431.

Ialongo, N. *et al.* (2006) The importance of utilizing and translating basic research knowledge on normal and abnormal development into preventive interventions. In: *Developmental Psychopathology (2nd ed.): Theory and Method.* (eds D. Cicchetti & D.J. Cohen). John Wiley & Sons, New York. pp. 968–1018.

Insel, T.R. & Scolnick, E.M. (2006) Cure therapeutics and strategic prevention: raising the bar for mental health research. *Molecular Psychiatry* **11**, 11–17.

Jarvinen-Pasley, A. *et al.* (2008) Defining the social phenotype in Williams syndrome: a model for linking gene, the brain, and behavior. *Development and Psychopathology* **20**, 1–35.

Johnson, M.H. (1998) The neural basis of cognitive development. In: *Handbook of Child Psychology: Cognition, Perception, and Language.* (eds D. Kuhn & R. Siegler). John Wiley & Sons, New York. pp. 1–49.

Kandel, E.R. (1998) A new intellectual framework for psychiatry. *American Journal of Psychiatry* **155**, 475–469.

Kandel, E.R. (1999) Biology and the future of psychoanalysis: a new intellectual framework for psychiatry revisited. *American Journal of Psychiatry* **156**, 505–524.

Kellam, S.G. & Rebok, G.W. (1992) Building developmental and etiological theory through epidemiologically based preventive intervention trials. In: *Preventing Antisocial Behavior: Interventions from Birth Through Adolescence.* (eds J. McCord & R.E. Tremblay). Guilford Press, New York. pp. 162–195.

Lenroot, R.K. & Giedd, J.N. (2008) The changing impact of genes and environment on brain development during childhood and adolescence: initial findings from a neuroimaging study of pediatric twins. *Development and Psychopathology* **20**, 1161–1175.

Likliter, R. (2013) Modeling psychobiological development in the postgenomic era. *International Journal of Developmental Science* **77**, 79–82.

Luthar, S. (1999) *Poverty and Children's Adjustment.* Sage Publications Thousand Oaks, CA.

Luthar, S.S. (1996) Resilience: A Construct of Value? Paper Presented at the 104th Annual Convention of the American Psychological Association, Toronto.

Luthar, S.S. (2006) Resilience in development: a synthesis of research across five decades. In: *Developmental Psychopathology: Risk, Disorder, and Adaptation.* (eds D. Cicchetti & D.J. Cohen). John Wiley & Sons, New York. pp. 739–795.

Luthar, S.S. & Cicchetti, D. (2000) The construct of resilience: implications for interventions and social policies. *Development and Psychopathology* **12**, 857–885.

Luthar, S.S. *et al.* (2000) The construct of resilience: a critical evaluation and guidelines for future work. *Child Development* **71**, 543–562.

Masten, A.S. (2001) Ordinary magic: resilience processes in development. *American Psychologist* **56**(3), 227.

Masten, A.S. (2007) Resilience in developing systems: progress and promise as the fourth wave rises. *Development and Psychopathology* **19**(3), 921–930.

Masten, A.S. (2011) Resilience in children threatened by extreme adversity: frameworks for research, practice, and translational synergy. *Development and Psychopathology* **23**(2), 493–506.

Masten, A.S. (2014) *Ordinary Magic.* Guilford Press, New York.

Masten, A.S. & Cicchetti, D. (2010) Developmental cascades. *Development and Psychopathology* **22**(3), 491–495.

Masten, A.S. & Coatsworth, J.D. (1998) The development of competence in favorable and unfavorable environments: lessons from research on successful children. *American Psychologist* **53**(2), 205.

Masten, A.S. & Garmezy, N. (1985) Risk, vulnerability, and protective factors in developmental psychopathology. *Advances in Clinical Child Psychology* **8**, 1–52.

Masten, A.S. *et al.* (1990) Resilience and development: contributions from the study of children who overcome adversity. *Development and Psychopathology* **2**(4), 425–444.

Masten, A.S. *et al.* (1995) The structure and coherence of competence from childhood through adolescence. *Child Development* **66**(6), 1635–1659. https://www.ncbi.nlm.nih.gov/pubmed/8556890

Masten, A.S. *et al.* (2006) Competence and psychopathology in development. In: *Developmental Psychopathology (2nd ed.), Vol. 3: Risk, Disorder, and Adaptation.* (eds D. Cicchetti & D.J. Cohen). John Wiley & Sons, New York. pp. 696–738.

Masten, A.S. *et al.* (2021) Resilience in development and psychopathology: multisystem perspectives. *Annual Review of Clinical Psychology* **17**, 521–549.

McEwen, B.S. & Stellar, E. (1993) Stress and the individual mechanisms leading to disease. *Archives of Internal Medicine* **153**, 2093–2101.

McLaughlin, K.A. *et al.* (eds) (2022) Dimensions of early experience and adaptive and maladaptive development. [Special Issue]. *Development and Psychopathology* **34**(2), 447–754.

Narayan, A. *et al.* (2023) A multisystem, dimensional interplay of assets versus adversities: revised benevolent childhood experiences (BCEs) in the context of childhood maltreatment, threat, and deprivation. *Development and Psychopathology* **35**(5), 2444–2463.

Nelson, C.A. (1999) Neural plasticity and human development. *Current Directions in Psychological Science* **8**, 42–45.

O'Donnell, K.J. & Meaney, M.J. (2017) Fetal origins of mental health: the developmental origins of health and disease hypothesis. *American Journal of Psychiatry* **174**, 319–328.

O'Dougherty-Wright, M. *et al.* (1997) Long-term effects of massive trauma: developmental and psychobiological perspectives. In: *Rochester Symposium on Developmental Psychopathology, Vol. 8, The Effects of Trauma on the Developmental Process.* (eds D. Cicchetti & S.L. Toth). University of Rochester Press, Rochester. pp. 181–225.

Plomin, R. *et al.* (1991) Quantitative genetics and developmental psychopathology. In: *Rochester Symposium on Developmental Psychopathology: Internalizing and Externalizing Expressions of Dysfunction.* (eds D. Cicchetti & S.L. Toth). Lawrence Erlbaum, Hillsdale, NJ. pp. 155–202.

Richters, J.E. & Martinez, P. (1993) Violent communities, family choices, and children's chances: an algorithm for improving the odds. *Development and Psychopathology* **60**, 1068–1075.

Robins, L.N. & Rutter, M. (eds) (1990) *Straight and Devious Pathways from Childhood to Adulthood.* Cambridge University Press, Cambridge, UK.

Rutter, M. (1979) Protective factors in children's responses to stress and disadvantage. *Annual Academy of Medicine, Singapore* **8**, 324–338.

Rutter, M. (1985) Resilience in the face of adversity: protective factors and resistance to psychiatric disorder. *British Journal of Psychiatry* **128**, 493–509.

Rutter, M. (1987) Psychosocial resilience and protective mechanisms. *American Journal of Orthopsychiatry* **57**, 316–331.

Rutter, M. (1990) Psychosocial resilience and protective mechanisms. In: *Risk and Protective Factors in the Development of Psychopathology.* (eds J. Rolf, *et al.*). Cambridge University Press, New York. pp. 181–214.

Rutter, M. (2006) *Genes and Behavior: Nature—Nurture Interplay Explained.* Blackwell, Malden, MA; Oxford, UK.

Rutter, M. (2012) Resilience as a dynamic concept. *Development and Psychopathology* **24**, 335–344.

Rutter, M. (2016) Why is the topic of the biological embedding of experiences important for translation? *Development and Psychopathology* **28**, 1245–1258.

Rutter, M. & Quinton, D. (1984) Parental psychiatric disorder: effects on children. *Psychological Medicine* **14**, 853–880.

Rutter, M. & Stevenson, J. (2008) Developments in child and adolescent psychiatry over the last 50 years. In: *Rutter's Child and Adolescent Psychiatry.* (eds M. Rutter, *et al.*). Wiley Blackwell, Oxford, UK. pp. 3–17.

Rutter, M. *et al.* (1997) Integrating nature and nurture: implications of person-environment correlations and interactions for developmental psychopathology. *Development and Psychopathology* **9**, 335–364.

Sameroff, A.J. (2000) Developmental systems and psychopathology. *Development and Psychopathology* **12**, 297–312.

Sameroff, A.J. & Chandler, M.J. (1975) Reproductive risk and the continuum of caretaking casualty. *Review of Child Development Research* **4**, 187–244.

Sameroff, A.J. *et al.* (1987) Intelligence quotient scores of 4-year-old children: social-environmental risk factors. *Pediatrics* **79**, 343–350.

Segalowitz, S.J. (1994) Developmental psychology and brain development: a historical perspective. In: *Human Behavior and the Developing Brain*. (eds G. Dawson & K.W. Fischer). Guilford Press, New York. pp. 67–92.

Singer, W. (1995) Development and plasticity of cortical processing architectures. *Science* **270**(5237), 758–764.

Sroufe, L.A. & Jacobvitz, D. (1989) Diverging pathways, developmental transformations, multiple etiologies, and the problem of continuity in development. *Human Development* **32**, 196–203.

Sroufe, L.A. & Rutter, M. (1984) The domain of developmental psychopathology. *Child Development* **55**, 17–29.

Sroufe, L.A. *et al.* (1990) The fate of early experience following developmental change: longitudinal approaches to individual adaptation in childhood. *Child Development* **61**, 1363–1373.

Sroufe, L.A. *et al.* (2009) *The Development of the Person: The Minnesota Study of Risk and Adaptation from Birth to Adulthood*. Guilford Press, New York.

Szyf, M. & Bick, J. (2013) DNA methylation: a mechanism for embedding early life experiences in the genome. *Child Development* **84**, 49–57.

Thelen, E. & Smith, L.B. (1998) Dynamic systems theories. In: *Handbook of Child Psychology: Theoretical Models of Human Development*. (eds W. Damon & R.M. Lerner), 5th edn. John Wiley & Sons, New York. pp. 563–634.

Ungar, M. (2012) Researching and theorizing resilience across cultures and contexts. *Preventive Medicine* **55**, 387–389.

Ungar, M. *et al.* (2013) Annual research review: what is resilience within the social ecology of human development? *Journal of Child Psychology and Psychiatry* **54**, 348–366.

Van Der Kolk, B. (2014) *The Body Keeps the Score*. Penguin Books, London.

Van Praag, H. *et al.* (2000) Neural consequences of environmental enrichment. *Nature Reviews Neuroscience* **1**(3), 191–198.

von Bertalanffy, L. (1968) *General System Theory: Foundations, Development*. George Braziller, New York.

Waddington, C.H. (1957) *The Strategy of Genes*. Allen & Unwin, London.

Wells, R.D. & Schwebel, A.I. (1987) Chronically ill children and their mothers: predictors of resilience and vulnerability to hospitalization and surgical stress. *Journal of Development and Behavioral Pediatrics* **8**, 83–89.

Werner, E.E. & Smith, R.S. (1977) *Kauai's Children Come of Age*. University Press of Hawaii, Honolulu, HW.

Werner, E.E. & Smith, R.S. (1982) *Vulnerable but Invincible: A Study of Resilient Children*. McGraw-Hill, New York.

Werner, E.E. & Smith, R.S. (1992) *Overcoming the Odds: High Risk Children from Birth to Adulthood*. Cornell University, Ithaca, NY.

White, R.W. (1959) Motivation reconsidered: the concept of competence. *Psychological Review* **66**, 297–333.

Zigler, E. & Glick, M. (1986) *A Developmental Approach to Adult Psychopathology*. John Wiley & Sons, New York.

CHAPTER 24

Impact of parental psychiatric disorder on children's psychological outcomes

Alan Stein[1], Rebecca M. Pearson[2] and Gordon Harold[3,4]
[1]Blavatnik School of Government, University of Oxford, Oxford, UK
[2]School of Psychology and Institute of Children's Futures, Manchester Metropolitan University, Manchester, UK
[3]Faculty of Education, University of Cambridge, Cambridge, UK
[4]Child and Adolsecent Psychiatry Unit, School of Medicine, University College Dublin, Dublin, Ireland

A substantial body of evidence links psychiatric disorders in parents to increased risk of psychological difficulties in their children across development. However, it should be emphasized that negative associations are not inevitable, and that many children of parents with psychiatric disorders develop without psychological difficulties. It should also be noted that considerable evidence points to a two-way process with children's difficulties affecting parental mental health. Given the frequency of parental and child mental health disorders, there is a need for further understanding of the processes involved in the intergenerational transmission of mental health problems. To understand the conditions that make a parental disorder more likely to lead to adverse psychological outcomes in children, research has moved away from the inevitability of simple cause–effect notions toward appreciating the individual differences that exist in the outcomes of children. As a result, a range of studies aiming to understand potential mechanisms of transmission, have shown the role of mediating variables, explaining links between parent and offspring psychiatric symptoms, as well as moderating variables that alter the strength of these links (Stein *et al.*, 2014). This then allows mechanisms to be clinically targeted, with an understanding of mediators enabling the remediation of risk as well as drawing upon family strengths; and moderators to guide which groups or populations to focus on. Clinically, it also provides critical information to guide clinicians, communities, and policy-makers in helping families.

Intergenerational transmission of psychiatric disorder: conceptual and theoretical overview

One of the strongest predictors of transdiagnostic psychiatric challenges in children is having a parent with a current, or history of, psychiatric disorder (Newlove-Delgado *et al.*, 2022). Intergenerational transmission of mental illness describes manifestations of symptoms or disorders across generations. Homotypic and heterotypic continuity refer to the transmission of the same (e.g., anxiety) or different traits (e.g., parent substance misuse to child conduct problems) being passed from one generation to the next, respectively (Branje *et al.*, 2020; Costantini, 2023). The intergenerational transmission of psychiatric disorders is a complex and multifaceted process (Serbin & Karp, 2004), with several reviews already available (Branje *et al.*, 2020; Goodman, 2020).

We consider four processes involved in intergenerational transmission: genetic transmission; fetal exposure to mental health and associated physiological stress *in utero*; the parent–child relationship and modeling of cognitions and behaviors; and finally, family and socioenvironmental stress and resources (Goodman, 2020).

We propose an integrated theoretical model that conveys the complex and multifaceted processes through which parental psychiatric disorder may confer developmental risk to children (Figure 24.1). In this figure, we draw on the causal diagram framework described in Chapter 13 and elucidate a number of

Rutter's Child and Adolescent Psychiatry and Psychology, Seventh Edition.
Edited by Anita Thapar, Daniel S. Pine, Samuele Cortese, Cathy Creswell, Tamsin J. Ford, James F. Leckman, and Argyris Stringaris.

Companion website: www.wiley.com/go/thapar/rutterspsych7

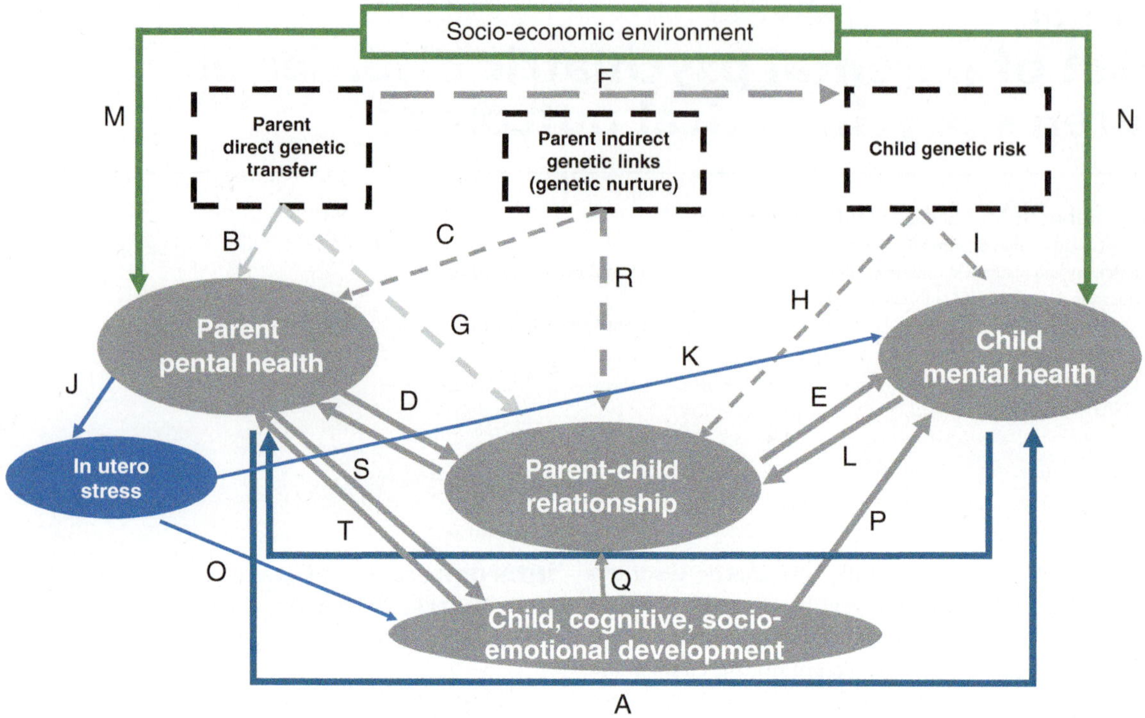

Figure 24.1 Pathways from parent psychiatric disorder to child psychological risk.

pathways. The simple link between parental and child disorder (Path A) is also underpinned by a complex interplay of multiple pathways and processes (Paths B–Q).

Specifically, factors that mediate (i.e., *are on the causal pathway*) and moderate (*change the causal pathway qualitatively or quantitatively*) paths are examined (see also Chapter 16). They can offer opportunities through which intervention targets may be directed to prevent or reduce the intergenerational transmission. For example, parental psychiatric disorder has been linked to disruptions in children's neurobiological functioning (e.g., hypothalamic–pituitary–adrenal (HPA) axis dysregulation), cognitive–emotional–social processing (e.g., negative attributions, emotional regulation, social skills), and disrupted patterns of family functioning (e.g., interparental conflict, struggles with parenting, and the parent–child relationship). As noted in Figure 24.1, each sequence of paths offers a unique mediating process (e.g., *in utero* pathways—Path J) which is in turn linked to child mental health (Path K). Any intervening domain (e.g., support with family relationships—Path D) may present further mediation. In other words, a potential break in the causal chain or cascade. Several other possibilities exist (e.g., all combinations of pathways), capturing unidirectional, bidirectional, and transactional patterns (e.g., changing the direction of the arrows).

Importantly, confounding pathways, including shared genetic and environmental risk factors, also influence both specific mediating and direct pathways (see Chapter 13).

We briefly outline theories and evidence for the four above-mentioned processes of transmission with reference to the multiple pathways in Figure 24.1. These processes are explained further in Video 24.1 on the book's companion website, brought to life by real-life experiences.

Processes

Process 1: genetic transmission

Direct genetic (Path F)

Children born to parents with psychiatric problems inherit DNA placing them at elevated risk (see also Chapter 21). Twin heritability estimates suggest contribution of genetic factors to all mental health phenotypes but with some variation (see Chapter 21). Jami *et al.* (2021) review multiple genetically-informed studies of cross-generational transmission and provide evidence of both genetic and environmental transmission for many psychiatric phenotypes. It should be emphasized that any genetic transmission occurs not through a single genetic variant, but rather through a substantial number of genetic variants, each with relatively small effects (although less common, inherited rare genetic variants of large effect size also contribute to some phenotypes (see Chapter 21)).

Indirect genetic (Paths C–D, C–A, R–E)

Indirect genetic pathways describe pathways from parental genetic risk that are *not* passed to children (i.e., untransmitted parental DNA) but still influence offspring via parent phenotypes (e.g., mental health or parenting behavior). This environmental mediation of genetic propensity has been referred to as passive gene–environment correlation or genetic nurture (see Chapter 21). More recently, so-called "genetic nurture" has also been investigated at a molecular level by using genetic data from parent–offspring trios to examine the contribution of parental untransmitted alleles on offspring phenotypes. The most consistent evidence of genetic nurture has been observed for educational attainment (Wang *et al.*, 2021), with mixed results for mental health.

Evocative/bidirectional

Recent studies have highlighted how a child's own genetic liability to psychopathology manifests early in life (Riglin *et al.*, 2022; Costantini *et al.*, 2023b). Therefore, another type of gene–environment correlation (child evocative effects) may occur, and it refers to the influence of genetic liabilities in the child on parental behavior and/or mental health (Reiss *et al.*, 2022). Previous work has provided evidence for evocative genetic effects: where genetic liability for behavioral problems (as inferred from biological family history), for example, are associated with harsher parenting in adoptive parents (Reiss *et al.*, 2022).

Interaction with environment

Environments may modify genetic transmission of risk as shown in cross-fostering adoption studies of criminality and cognitive ability (see Chapters 13 and 21). Molecular genetic studies however are inadequately powered to examine interactions across the genome. Further highlighting our process-orientated approach to understanding the intergenerational transmission of psychopathology via environmental mechanisms, each of the proposed mediators presented in Figure 24.1 may also represent moderation. For example, socioeconomic status (SES), access to resources, or conflictual family interactions may accentuate associations between parental psychiatric disorder and children's psychopathology (Paths M and N).

Process 2: fetal exposure to mental health and associated physiological stress *in utero* (Paths J–K, J–O–P)

The fetal programming hypothesis of development posits that adverse intrauterine exposures can result in biological changes to the fetus (Path J). This in turn can have long-term consequences on offspring Development (Path O), including mental health (Path K) (Talge *et al.*, 2007). Indeed, there is some evidence that antenatal exposure to depression is linked to child depression (Pearson *et al.*, 2013a). Overall, it should be emphasized that it is hard to separate fetal exposure from genetic and postnatal paths, with a number of studies also showing that the postnatal environment modifies the impact of prenatal exposure (Clayborne *et al.*, 2022) (see Chapter 13).

Process 3: the parent–child relationship and modeling of cognitions and behaviors (Path D, Path E)

Evidence suggests that various aspects of parenting can be both mediators and moderators of the association between parent psychiatric disorder and child outcomes (Leve *et al.*, 2009). There are several related processes involved, most prominently mediation. In particular, there is substantial evidence that depression is linked with challenges in the parent–child relationship (Stein *et al.*, 2014) which, in turn, can increase the risk of child emotional and behavioral problems. However, it is important to note that even if there is evidence that parenting is part of the causal pathway, this does not mean parents are somehow to blame. Rather, through no fault of their own, as described in the later section on "Psychiatric disorders and parenting," the symptoms of mental health problems are likely to interfere with thought and behavior processes key to parenting. Strengths-based approaches within intervention models may be especially helpful (Box 24.1). For example, focusing on examples where parents show regulation and management of emotional distress and reinforcing positive moments rather than focusing on moments of conflict highlight the potential strengths in parenting in buffering risk.

Box 24.1 Harnessing parenting power and reducing stigma and blame

Whether or not parenting has a causal role in intergenerational transmission is complicated to disentangle, even for researchers and clinicians. It can be even more confusing for parents, especially if they are referred to parenting interventions. It is important to be aware how parents or children may interpret the suggestion that parenting support can be helpful. In working with parents with lived experience of mental health who have been referred to parenting support, focusing on the strengths of parenting to minimize risk rather than parenting as the "problem" that needs to be fixed, has been well received.

To illustrate this point, let us consider examples in completely different areas of life (from medicine to football).

Scenario 1: An individual feels fatigued. Their blood tests show they have low thyroxine levels. They are prescribed thyroxine, which brings their thyroxine levels to normal, and they no longer feel tired. Here the intervention is directly linked to the cause (low levels of thyroxine); "fix" the thyroid levels and the problematic symptom (fatigue) is prevented.

Scenario 2: In another example, a footballer is unable to run following an injury after being fouled by a defender on the pitch. The intervention given to restore functioning is physiotherapy. Physiotherapists cannot prevent future injury on the football pitch by a foul from other players; however, physiotherapy can minimize the damage and rebuild strength.

Parenting will never be as simple as either of these examples, however, it is possible to build parents' existing skills to flexibly adapt and support child behavior when needed; much like training a football coach in physiotherapy on the sidelines, so that they are ready to act quickly to manage injuries to prevent harm. Indeed, no one would blame a physiotherapist for a foul-related injury, but they would be considered the solution. Strengths-based approaches to parenting may increase uptake and engagement with parenting interventions and reduce stigma.

Psychiatric disorders and parenting (Path D)

Symptoms of a psychiatric disorder can affect a person's ability to respond to their environment, and thereby their parenting. For example, rumination (the core cognitive process in depression) can make it difficult for a parent to provide sensitive parenting.

Rumination comprises a state of narrowed, or self-focused, attention in which one's mind is dominated by recurrent intrusive thoughts that are difficult to control and dismiss. Rumination has been shown to interfere with both attention and responsiveness to the environment. There are three capacities that may be affected by caregivers who are ruminating or preoccupied.

First, maternal focus of attention to child signals, and associated contingent responsiveness which, if impaired, compromises the development of the child's attentional capacities and cognitive ability. This has been confirmed specifically in studies with depressed mothers. Experimental evidence indicates that maternal cognitions associated with depression and anxiety make it difficult for the parent to attend to the child's signals. This, in turn, impacts negatively on mother–child interactions (Stein *et al.*, 2012a) and the infant's ability to sustain attention, and thus process information effectively. Second, maternal emotional scaffolding, principally through warmth, consistent support, and low levels of intrusiveness and coercion, during stressful situations, which, if impaired, adversely affects child emotional regulation and behavior. One of the most important tasks for a parent is to support young children, when distressed, to maintain or recover their emotional equilibrium. Central to this process is the parent's promotion of child emotional regulation; this concerns the monitoring, evaluating, and modifying of emotional reactions to both internal and external stimuli so as to achieve a well-regulated state. The development of the capacity for emotional regulation begins very early (Jahromi *et al.*, 2004) and plays an important role in subsequent child adjustment (Kochanska *et al.*, 1998). Third, parental availability and responsiveness to a child's attachment needs and the ability to treat the child as a psychological agent, which, if impaired, increases the risk for insecure attachment.

We give rumination as an example, but other features of depression and anxiety can also be important. For example, hopelessness can link to low motivation and withdrawal; irritability and emotional dysregulation can link to inconsistent parenting.

Evidence for parenting differences and child outcomes (Path E) and mediation via parenting (Paths D and E)

We have discussed how parenting may be challenged in the context of parent mental health and its impacts on children are considered in Chapters 6, 7, 22 and 33.

As well as ample evidence provided for the two paths D (parent mental health to parent–child relationship) and E (parent–child relationship to child mental health) separately, there is good evidence that parenting mediates part of the relationship between some types of parental mental health and offspring psychopathology (e.g., Stein *et al.*, 2014; Culpin *et al.*, 2021). Triangulating this with randomized controlled trial (RCT) evidence suggests that parenting interventions could be a potential target for clinicians working with families (Costantini *et al.*, 2023a) (see Chapter 33).

Modeling of parent symptoms (Path S)

As well as the parenting relationship itself, another related process is the modeling of parenting behavior. According to Bandura's social learning theory (Bandura, 1977), humans learn from one another via modeling, observation, and imitation. Thus, a child may, for example, learn from a socially anxious parent to fear social situations and interactions. Similarly, a child may also acquire different cognitive biases that may sustain or provoke a negative mood from a depressed or anxious parent (Spence & Rapee, 2016). Such behaviors may not be linked to parenting directly but rather involve the child observing the depressed and anxious behaviors of their parent in other situations (e.g., interaction with the partner or other family components, or outside the familial environment).

Disorder specific behaviors, such as speech and affect, manifested by a parent may also be modeled by or otherwise transmitted to the child leading to outcomes in the child that resemble the parent's disorder. For example, in experimental studies, if non-anxious mothers "mimic" socially anxious behaviors, their infant is more likely to show fearful and avoidance behaviors in subsequent interactions in the short term (Murray *et al.*, 2009). There is some evidence that mother and offspring depressogenic cognitive styles, measured 18 years apart, are correlated and partially mediate the association between perinatal maternal depression and offspring depression at age 18 (Pearson *et al.*, 2013b). Furthermore, when parents have negative thoughts, e.g., of the future such as hopelessness, or see potential threats persistently in the environment, this can translate into the nature of the language they use when speaking to their children (Murray *et al.*, 2009). Children then begin to internalize these kinds of negative views of their family and the outside world.

Bidirectional effects and the transactional model (Paths L, Q, and T)

As mentioned earlier, it should not be assumed that the direction of effects is only from parent to child (Figure 24.1, Path L). Some children are more difficult to rear because, for example, they cry a great deal, sleep poorly, and are very emotionally reactive. Indeed, high irritability in young infants is associated with the onset of maternal depression by eight weeks postpartum and a recent study has shown that genetic liability for neuroticism manifests in different temperaments as early as infancy (Costantini, I. *et al.*, 2023b).

Process 4: family and socioenvironmental stress and resources (Paths M and N)

The context of the family, their social network, education level, and access to resources is also important. Such factors provide the ecosystem and generally act as moderators, i.e., factors that modify the strength of the association, but are not part of the causal pathway. Important moderators relate to emotional support, education, and material support (socioeconomic factors). For example, there is a wide range of literature concerning depression that suggests that material and emotional support can moderate the impact of depression on parenting. Thus, parents with adequate emotional and material support are less likely to have their parenting affected in the face of depression, and those without emotional and, especially, material support are more likely to have their parenting affected (Lovejoy *et al.*, 2000; Stein *et al.*, 2008). In addition, the role of the parents' relationship, marital breakdown, and father absence are all linked to mental health outcomes in both parents and child and moderate associations between parent and child mental health (Culpin *et al.*, 2022).

Psychiatric disorders in fathers

The issue of the potential impact of parental disorder on children applies both to mothers and fathers, with the majority of research having been conducted with mothers (Ramchandani & Psychogiou, 2009). Where relevant the effects of paternal disorders have been mentioned. Overall, most psychiatric disorders that affect fathers are associated with an increased risk of behavioral and emotional difficulties in their children, similar in magnitude to that of maternal psychiatric disorders. A systematic review (Sweeney & MacBeth, 2016) suggested that paternal depression can play a role on infant, child, and adolescent development. The pattern of associations between paternal depression and increased risk of internalizing and externalizing behaviors was demonstrated in offspring from 2 months to 21 years, however, fewer studies investigated outcomes after 13 years (Sweeney & MacBeth, 2016). Early childhood was suggested to represent a particularly sensitive period of development with associations being stronger and more common during these years. The authors note that the associations were small to moderate and subject to multiple mediators: for example, paternal negative expressiveness, involvement, and marital conflict. When considering adolescent outcomes, evidence was found in a systematic review for associations between paternal depression and adolescent depression and anxiety (Wickersham *et al.*, 2020). Similar patterns of depressed mood in offspring up to age 24 were seen following exposure to paternal depression as they had been following exposure to maternal depression, albeit to a smaller degree (Rajyaguru *et al.*, 2021). The fathers' role can also buffer the potential impact of maternal depression (Martin *et al.*, 2022) and both parents' depression and the parent relationship can act as moderators, especially regarding the bidirectional parenting pathway (Paths D, E, and D–E–L).

Specific disorders

We now discuss the major specific disorders in order to understand the needs of people with these disorders as well as opportunities for more personalized approaches. As discussed in Chapter 21, offspring are at elevated risk of the same and different psychiatric disorders to their parent.

Depression

Depression and anxiety disorders are among the most common mental health problems worldwide, with 1 in 10 women in high-income countries and 1 in 5 women in low- and middle-income countries (LMICs) experiencing high levels of these disorders in the perinatal period (Gelaye *et al.*, 2016; Woody *et al.*, 2017). Antenatal depression has increased in comparable populations of pregnant women from the 1990s to the 2010s (Pearson *et al.*, 2018). There is evidence that both depression and anxiety have risen in parents during and since the COVID-19 pandemic (Kwong *et al.*, 2021). Several studies link maternal depression to multiple outcomes (Goodman *et al.*, 2011) up to adulthood (Weissman *et al.*, 2006b; Netsi *et al.*, 2018). More severe and chronic parental depression is associated with a higher risk for offspring disorder (Goodman *et al.*, 2011; Netsi *et al.*, 2018), more specifically, an increased risk of behavioral problems, such as conduct disorder (CD) in school-aged children, and an increased risk of some psychiatric disorders in adolescents, particularly depression and anxiety disorders.

Anxiety

The number of studies reporting prevalence estimates specifically for perinatal anxiety disorders has grown. Although there is wide variation in the estimates provided, it is reported that up to 39% of women experience "any anxiety disorder." Depression and anxiety (especially generalized anxiety disorder; GAD) are often comorbid, and a specific rise in anxiety symptom items, such as feeling overwhelmed, has been shown to explain the rise in emotional disorders across generations and since the COVID-19 pandemic (Pearson *et al.*, 2018; Kwong *et al.*, 2021). There is also evidence that comorbidity between depression and anxiety is linked to greater risks for child psychopathology, with a cross-cohort study finding that a combined depression/anxiety factor was the stronger predictor of child outcomes (Szekely *et al.*, 2021). A meta-analyses including 25 studies assessed risk for anxiety and depressive disorders among children of parents with anxiety disorders (Lawrence *et al.*, 2019). Children were found to be at increased risk for both anxiety and depressive disorders but the risk for offspring anxiety disorders was higher than the risk for depression. Furthermore, the risk was significant regarding some anxiety disorders (GAD, separation anxiety disorder, and specific phobia), but not others (panic disorder or social anxiety disorder) in the offspring. Maternal anxiety and depression have also been linked to specific and differential mediating pathways via different aspects of child executive function (Pearson *et al.*, 2016).

Eating disorders

Eating disorders (EDs) are common among women of childbearing age, with 1 in 20 women meeting diagnostic criteria for EDs during pregnancy (Martínez-Olcina *et al.*, 2020). Rates of EDs are rising among males and in low/middle-income settings (Hoek, 2016; Ayala *et al.*, 2022). The majority of women with EDs suffer from bulimia nervosa or eating disorder not otherwise specified (EDNOS). Beyond the independent risk factors that may contribute to the onset and maintenance of EDs throughout development, there is evidence that parental disorders increase the risk of EDs in children, especially from mothers to their female children (Bould *et al.*, 2015a). This intergenerational risk for EDs is transmitted both homotypically (e.g., mothers' EDs to children's EDs) and heterotypically (e.g., mothers' depression or anxiety to children's EDs) (Bould *et al.*, 2015b). Data from one UK cohort study showed that children whose mothers had a history of anorexia nervosa or bulimia nervosa were at increased risk in the preschool period of a range of difficulties, such as emotional, conduct, and hyperactivity disorders for girls, and emotional problems for boys, for children of women with anorexia nervosa. Girls of mothers with bulimia nervosa were more likely to show hyperactivity while boys showed an increase of emotional and CDs (Martini *et al.*, 2020).

Alcohol and substance misuse

The worldwide prevalence of alcohol use during pregnancy is around 9.8% (95% CI: 8.9–11.1), with an estimated prevalence of fetal alcohol syndrome (FAS) at 14.6% (95% CI: 9.4–23.3) per 10,000 people in the general population (Popova *et al.*, 2017). Alcoholism and substance misuse are not uncommon disorders among adults of childbearing age and are associated with higher risks among the children. Heavy alcohol consumption during pregnancy has been recognized as potentially harmful to the fetus. In particular, it may result in FAS which is characterized by minor facial anomalies, impaired growth, and developmental delay.

Alcohol and drug problems can exist alone, but often coexist with depressive disorder. With regard to problems in older children, a large longitudinal study found that adult children of alcoholics had an increased lifetime prevalence of mood, anxiety, and abuse/dependence disorders and possibly also schizophrenia when compared to offspring of nonalcoholic parents. Rates were especially high for the children of fathers with drinking problems (Thor *et al.*, 2022). However, the evidence of longitudinal associations with child outcomes is inconsistent (Westman *et al.*, 2022). Intergenerational transmission of substance abuse and alcohol use disorder has recently been investigated. A genetically informed study provided evidence for both the role of genetic factors and the rearing environment, as well as the combination of the two, as sources of parent–offspring transmission of substance abuse and alcohol use disorder (Kendler *et al.*, 2019).

Severe mental health disorders, schizophrenia, and other psychoses

Schizophrenia affects 1% of the world population, and its incidence is rising (He *et al.*, 2020). Schizophrenia, together with some other psychotic conditions, has been historically associated with reduced fertility (MacBeth *et al.*, 2023), although there is increasing evidence that, throughout their life span, individuals with schizophrenia are likely to have children and should be supported in starting a family (Howard & Khalifeh, 2020). There are similar considerations for those with bipolar disorder. The early postnatal period is high risk for new and recurrent episodes of severe mental illness (SMI), with around 1–2 women in 1000 requiring admissions in the first few months after birth. Women were around 22 times more likely to have a psychiatric admission in the month following birth than in the prepregnancy period (Howard & Khalifeh, 2020). Episodes are usually affective in type and the most notable risk factor is a past or family history of affective psychosis. These disorders can have a major impact on the family. The infant may be affected in terms of a mother's ability to care for herself and her infant (poorer quality practical caregiving and responsiveness), and by the infant becoming the focus of a mother's delusional beliefs. Compared with the general population, children of parents with SMI, including schizophrenia, bipolar disorder, and major depressive disorder, have approximately twice the risk of developing any psychiatric disorder (Rasic *et al.*, 2014).

Personality disorders

A recent systematic review and meta-analysis of observational studies reported rates of borderline personality disorders (BPDs) during the perinatal period in both a clinical and a nonclinical population. Among the nonclinical sample, the pooled prevalence rate of BPD during the perinatal period ranged between 0.7–1.7%, while in the clinical sample it was 14% (Prasad *et al.*, 2022). There is also research showing a high level of possible BPD in women admitted to mother and baby units (Gressier *et al.*, 2022). Maternal personality disorders are also associated with specific disruptions to attachment security and early infant emotional response (Conroy *et al.*, 2012; Eyden *et al.*, 2016).

Clinical implications

It is important to be aware, when seeing parents with psychiatric problems, that this may have present and future implications for the whole family, including the child, if they are not supported. A helpful overall framework for assessing the potential risks to children, where a parent has a psychiatric disorder, was originally provided by Rutter (1989). Careful assessment should include the areas which are most likely to be affected by the parental disorder. These are outlined above but include specific difficulties in the interaction between parents and children, the quality and type of care the parent can provide, the presence of extended family, and the quality of the interparental relationship. Review of these factors in the history, as well as at the present time, can give useful insight into any potential areas of difficulty that may exist, as well as resilience and strengths in the parent–child relationship (both with the affected parent and the partner/spouse) that can be drawn upon. An individualized assessment of this kind will be the best guide to the areas where intervention (if required) is most likely to be of benefit with growing evidence for person-centered approaches. Clinicians can also play a practical, positive role in providing support, information, and treatment to parents affected by psychiatric disorder. There is considerable evidence to suggest that treating parental psychiatric difficulties will, in many cases, lead to better outcomes for the child and family (Weissman *et al.*, 2006b).

One critical issue is how to sensitively approach parents about the possible effects on their children while avoiding blame, especially as it is likely that the parents are already worried about the effect on the children. Nonetheless, it will be important to enquire about the parental relationship as well as the children's well-being, what children appear to understand of their parent's difficulties, and what they have been told. It will be helpful to emphasize that the difficulties the family are facing are common and that the parents can be supported in talking to their children and assisted in reducing the possibility of problems. From a very young age, children perceive changes in the parents' mood and facial expressions and their understanding increases with developmental maturity (see Stein *et al.* (2018) for a description of developmental changes). By five years old they begin to develop a conscience and are able to experience guilt. When children see their parents become irritable, frequently upset, or angry without explanation, they can blame themselves. In the context of separations (e.g., if a parent needs admission to a psychiatric facility), it is especially important that children understand what is happening and that it is not their fault; and that they receive support.

Understandably, parents want to protect their children from any distress or worry yet research shows that when children are not told about what is happening within their families, they reach their own, often mistaken, conclusions. Children generally want and need age-appropriate and honest information about changes they notice such as in their parent's behavior. Telling children about parental illness allows them to make sense of what they are seeing and be emotionally supported by their family network. Furthermore, effective communication with children has benefits both for children's mental health, and also trust and relationships within the family. However, it is difficult for parents to do this by themselves, especially if they are struggling. Therefore, families need their clinicians to help them navigate these sensitive conversations. Accurate and nonstigmatizing information about parental mental illness, treatment, and recovery can help young people understand their parent's symptoms and behavior and reduce the stigma and burden of worrying about their parent (Pihkala *et al.*, 2012; Riebschleger *et al.*, 2017).

A number of parent- and family-based interventions have been developed with the aim of improving outcomes for children of parents with depression (Beardslee *et al.*, 2007). There has also been a meta-analysis of preventative interventions (mainly focused on depression), which has shown substantial benefits for the child (Siegenthaler *et al.*, 2012) (see later section 'Interventions'). However, no effective interventions have yet been developed for use in routine practice and this should be a research priority.

Parents of children with mental health problems

Similarly, when children are referred for psychiatric problems, clinicians should again be aware that their parents may have a disorder and that assessing the parent's mental health, and treating any disorders found, may be an important part of the overall treatment package. This is now being recognized in treatment guidelines; for example, the UK National Institute for Health and Care Excellence (NICE) guidelines for the treatment of depression in children and young people specifically recommend the assessment of possible parental psychiatric problems (especially depression) as part of the clinical assessment and wider formulation. It can be helpful to involve adult mental health services, although this is not always possible. Clearly assessments need to be conducted cautiously and sensitively as parents can easily feel blamed. When children are referred for problems and the family is being seen, it may not be immediately evident that parents have underlying difficulties. It may be necessary, with parental consent, to obtain information from people outside the immediate family about the situation at home. For example, parents may be reluctant to acknowledge that they spend long periods of time in bed and are unable to provide necessary support for their children. The establishment of close collaborative links with adult psychiatric services is likely to lead to the most positive outcomes for families where a parent has chronic, severe psychiatric difficulties. However, this is not always possible, either because such services are not readily available, or because of differences in thresholds for accepting referrals. The decision about treatment can sometimes be a difficult clinical judgment. When the ideal circumstance of close joint management with adult services is not available, a clinician might be able to liaise with the parent's general practitioner or other primary health care services, but in some circumstances provision of treatment directly to the parent within the child and adolescent mental health setting may be appropriate, i.e., family therapy.

Family interventions are recommended in the treatment of adolescent mental health disorders including CD, EDs, and depression (Bülow *et al.*, 2022; NICE, 2023a, 2023b; Van Ijzendoorn *et al.*, 2023) and, in the UK, relational approaches are a priority for children with mental health needs and complex developmental circumstances (NICE, 2023a, 2023b). This may be more challenging if a parent has not received appropriate treatment for their own illness.

Occasionally, in very serious cases, there may be a concern about neglect and maltreatment, in which case social services may need to be involved (see Chapter 29).

Interventions

There is substantial research literature on the treatment of children who are diagnosed with a psychiatric disorder. However, there is less research on interventions to help families where a parent has such a disorder (Loechner *et al.*, 2018); to either prevent or manage problems in the children (Costantini *et al.*, 2020; Costantini *et al.*, 2023a). Studies that have addressed this question have mainly concerned parental depression, and it has become clear that it is essential to treat parental disorders to improve child outcomes. One large treatment trial of 7–17-year-old children whose mothers were treated with antidepressant medication found that maternal remission within 3 months (occurring in approximately one-third of women) was associated with a significant decrease in child and adolescent disorder and symptoms, particularly of the internalizing kind (Weissman *et al.*, 2006a). In a small experimental study, it was found that adults given 7 days of antidepressants rated infant faces more positively than those receiving a placebo (Stein *et al.*, 2012b). A meta-analysis of 13 preventative interventions (treatment trials mainly focused on depression) found these substantially reduced the risk of children and adolescents developing the same condition as their parents (Siegenthaler *et al.*, 2012). The risk of developing the same illness as the parent was decreased by 40% and internalizing symptoms specifically were decreased. Some trials found benefits for externalizing symptoms but, overall, this was not significant. The trials comprised interventions directed at the parent, the couple, and the family but there were no differences across these groups. The authors suggest that the positive effects may have been due to more nonspecific factors, such as attention and empathy, which are common to most treatments. However, it should be noted that all treatments in their meta-analysis were structured with a clear focus and therefore may not generalize to treatments with less structure and a more general focus. An RCT for children with anxiety disorders, whose mothers also had a current anxiety disorder, evaluated whether cognitive behavioral therapy (CBT) for child anxiety would be improved by adjunct treatments focusing on the mother's anxiety disorders or mother–child interactions (Creswell *et al.*, 2020). The study demonstrated that good clinical outcomes can be achieved through the provision of individual child CBT alongside parental support, while adding CBT for maternal anxiety or treatment focused on the mother–child relationship to individual child-focused CBT were not found to be significantly beneficial to the children. A number of studies have specifically aimed at preventing depression among adolescents of depressed parents. One trial of a group CBT intervention for adolescents of depressed parents found that the treatment reduced the risk of depression for up to 15 months post-treatment. At the two-year follow-up, a significant preventative effect persisted but at a diminished level (Clarke *et al.*, 2001). A large trial using a group cognitive behavior prevention program targeting a similar group, added six-monthly continuation sessions with the aim of prolonging the effects. This trial showed significant sustained benefits in terms of preventing onset of depressive disorders at the three-year follow-up (Beardslee *et al.*, 2013). See Chapter 32 for more information on prevention.

Parenting interventions

Parenting interventions are often defined as those that have a central focus on parenting behaviors and beliefs (Costantini *et al.*, 2020). Parenting interventions are covered in detail in Chapters 7 and 33, but are relevant here in relation to when a parent has mental illness with a need for interventions to be personalized where possible. A recent network-based meta-analysis of 59 RCTs (n = 18,349) found early parenting intervention, with a specific focus on dyadic relationships, may be more effective in preventing internalizing and externalizing problems in children, at least in the short term as compared to treatment as usual (Costantini *et al.*, 2023a).

In daily clinical practice, it is important to remember that disturbed parental cognitions are key mediators of the effects on children (see the earlier section on "Psychiatric disorders and parenting"). As mentioned in the parenting section (Box 24.2), these core cognitive disturbances comprise a narrowed state of attention, where the parent is overwhelmed by recurrent intrusive thoughts (Watkins, 2008). This narrowed focus of attention can have profound adverse effects on an individual's capacity to attend and respond to the outside world. This is likely to affect appropriate responsiveness and attention to a child. It is critical to help a parent to attend to a child's communication, especially facial cues, speech, and mood, and to respond appropriately in order to move the parent's focus of attention from their own internal thoughts to those of their children's communication (Stein *et al.*, 2009, 2014). An example of how to help parents notice and respond to infant cues is provided for the case of postnatal EDs (Box 24.2). Video feedback or other in-person parent coaching is adaptable to more person-centered

Box 24.2 Responding to infant cues, an example of maternal eating disorders

> In the postnatal year, mothers who have a history of eating disorders (EDs) often experience a re-emergence of symptoms as a result of the changes in their body shape and weight. Mealtimes can become challenging as the infant attempts to self-feed (one of the first experiences of autonomy), often making a mess and eating at a pace that means any attempts from the parent to hasten feeding can result in food refusal. Given that mealtimes are already stressful for people with EDs, this can lead to conflict. Guiding the parent to focus on infant cues by watching the infant and carefully responding to the infant's experiences of pleasure around food and to wait while the baby's mouth is closed can be particularly helpful. It can be useful to explain that this is a time for children to learn about their own hunger, satiety, and tastes, as well as exploring different textures in food and communicating with those around them with vocal and facial gestures about food and nonfood experiences.

approaches across different presentations of parental mental health. The micromoments that the film segments can highlight can be carefully selected depending on need. It has shown to be effective in the context of EDs in parents (Stein *et al.*, 2009, 2014) and in a range of other contexts. It is yet to be systematically evaluated in older children, however, see Video 24.1 for potential applications.

Interventions in severe psychiatric disorders

Children of parents with psychotic disorders often experience substantial unpredictability and lack of consistency in the household, as well as occasional absences due to hospital admissions. Parents often display major fluctuations in mood and behavior. Children need support not only to cope with these fluctuations, but also to realize that such behavior is part of their parent's illness. They may need time and care from other adults, as well as opportunities to have positive experiences with their ill parent. Children often want to know whether they are also likely to develop the disorder and thus supportive and open discussions at age-appropriate times are necessary. Mothers with puerperal psychosis will often require in-patient care, ideally in a specialist mother and baby unit, where the baby can remain with her mother in all but the most extreme of presentations, and where experienced, skilled staff can provide the level of care and supervision necessary. It is in these circumstances that clinicians have to be particularly aware of the potential danger to the child's well-being, either through direct risk from a mother with delusional beliefs and/or hallucinations, or through neglect of the child. The need to balance the risk (to mother and child) with the desire to keep families together to promote the development of a positive relationship and facilitate the mother's recovery requires experienced clinical judgment. Health care professionals should always enquire about whether patients have children, their well-being, and the extent to which they are involved in the care of the parent. Hospitals and other clinical facilities should provide space and facilities to allow children to visit and spend time with their parents. Emotional support for such children is critical. Advice on how and where they can obtain help, and liaison with social services to provide practical support in the home, is invaluable. Where "young carer" groups exist, these can provide emotional support and respite.

Low- and middle-income countries

In LMICs, where trained health-care professionals may not be available, local community health workers can play an invaluable role in supporting families and can be trained to provide interventions for parents and young children. In particular, a small number of randomized trials in LMICs have demonstrated that psychological interventions delivered by local health workers may be helpful in reducing maternal depression and may have a positive impact on some aspects of child development. For example, in Pakistan, a perinatal intervention program using cognitive behavioral principles delivered by primary care health workers, compared with enhanced usual care, reduced rates of maternal depression, although infant growth was not affected (the principal outcome). Parents reported that they played more with their children, although the quality of parent–child interaction was not measured. In addition, a reduction in maternal reports of diarrhea and higher rates of completed courses of immunization were found (Rahman *et al.*, 2008). A second study was conducted in a socioeconomically disadvantaged South African community, although not specifically in the context of depression. The home-based intervention focused specifically on helping mothers to attend to the details of the infant's communication and to respond sensitively. It led to improvements in the quality of mother–child interaction and increased rates of secure attachment (Cooper *et al.*, 2009). Interventions that focus on the wider family and partner support may also be especially relevant given the strong influence of challenges with the partner in the African context (Redinger *et al.*, 2018). See Chapter 46 for more information on low-resource settings.

Summary

In summary, there is evidence that parental psychiatric disorders are associated with a range of psychological sequelae in children. However, it is crucial to be aware that children are not invariably adversely affected, and the relationship is complex with evidence of multiple bidirectional processes. It is also very important to support families and see their strengths, countering out-of-date ideas on blame, help them understand that these kinds of problems are common, and avoid stigmatizing them. Recent research has also moved from assuming traditional causal models to process-orientated models, whereby the aim is to understand why an association exists between parent risk and child outcome (mediation), and under what conditions the risk may be accentuated or ameliorated (moderation) and to separate this from confounding and genetic pathways. A number of high-quality intervention studies have informed both clinical practice and policy. However, much remains to be done to improve child outcomes and support families, especially as the child gets older. Furthermore, much can be learnt from children who thrive despite adversity, and a focus on resilience is critical for the future (see Chapter 23 on resilience).

Finally, it is important to note that much of the burden of the impact of parental psychiatric disorder occurs in LMICs. However, most of the research on parental psychiatric disorders has been conducted in high-income settings, with uncertainty about the applicability of these findings across different LMIC settings. While there have been a number of recent studies, much less research, especially treatment trials, has been conducted in LMICs, and this omission needs to be addressed.

Acknowledgments

We are very grateful to Ilaria Costantini and Gaby Illingworth for their enormous help in putting together this chapter.

References

Ayala, C.O. *et al.* (2022) Assessing eating disorder symptoms in low and middle-income countries: a systematic review of psychometric studies of commonly used instruments. *Journal of Eating Disorders* **10**(1), 124.

Bandura, A. (1977) *Social Learning Theory*. Prentice-Hall, Oxford, UK.

Beardslee, W.R. *et al.* (2007) Long-term effects from a randomized trial of two public health preventive interventions for parental depression. *Journal of Family Psychology* **21**(4), 703.

Beardslee, W.R. *et al.* (2013) Prevention of depression in at-risk adolescents: longer-term effects. *JAMA Psychiatry* **70**(11), 1161–1170.

Bould, H. *et al.* (2015a) Do eating disorders in parents predict eating disorders in children? Evidence from a Swedish cohort. *Acta Psychiatrica Scandinavica* **132**(1), 51–59. doi:10.1111/acps.12389.

Bould, H. *et al.* (2015b) Parental mental illness and eating disorders in offspring. *International Journal of Eating Disorders* **48**(4), 383–391.

Branje, S. *et al.* (2020) Intergenerational transmission: theoretical and methodological issues and an introduction to four Dutch cohorts. *Developmental Cognitive Neuroscience* **45**, 100835.

Bülow, A. *et al.* (2022) Parent–adolescent interaction quality and adolescent affect—an experience sampling study on effect heterogeneity. *Child Development* **93**(3), e315–e331.

Clarke, G.N. *et al.* (2001) A randomized trial of a group cognitive intervention for preventing depression in adolescent offspring of depressed parents. *Archives of General Psychiatry* **58**(12), 1127–1134.

Clayborne, Z.M. *et al.* (2022) Positive maternal mental health attenuates the associations between prenatal stress and children's internalizing and externalizing symptoms. *European Child & Adolescent Psychiatry*, 1–14.

Conroy, S. *et al.* (2012) Maternal psychopathology and infant development at 18 months: the impact of maternal personality disorder and depression. *Journal of the American Academy of Child & Adolescent Psychiatry* **51**(1), 51–61.

Cooper, P.J. *et al.* (2009) Improving quality of mother-infant relationship and infant attachment in socioeconomically deprived community in South Africa: randomised controlled trial. *BMJ* **338**, b974.

Costantini, I. (2023) *Childhood internalising problems: a multi-method approach to explore intergenerational pathways*. Thesis, University College London.

Costantini, I. *et al.* (2020) Protocol for a systematic review and network meta-analysis of randomised controlled trials examining the effectiveness of early parenting interventions in preventing internalising problems in children and adolescents. *Systematic Reviews* **9**(1), 244. doi:10.1186/s13643-020-01500-9.

Costantini, I. *et al.* (2023a) Early parenting interventions to prevent internalising problems in children and adolescents: a global systematic review and network meta-analysis. *BMJ Mental Health* **26**(1), e300811. doi:10.1136/bmjment-2023-300811.

Costantini, I. *et al.* (2023b) Childhood trajectories of internalising and externalising problems associated with a polygenic risk score for neuroticism in a UK birth cohort study. *JCPP Advances* **3**, e12141. doi:10.1002/jcv2.12141.

Creswell, C. *et al.* (2020) A randomised controlled trial of treatments of childhood anxiety disorder in the context of maternal anxiety disorder: clinical and cost-effectiveness outcomes. *Journal of Child Psychology and Psychiatry* **61**(1), 62–76.

Culpin, I. *et al.* (2021) Maternal postnatal depression and offspring depression at age 24 years in a UK-birth cohort: the mediating role of maternal nurturing behaviours concerning feeding, crying and sleeping. *Wellcome Open Research* **6**, 187.

Culpin, I. *et al.* (2022) Father absence and trajectories of offspring mental health across adolescence and young adulthood: findings from a UK-birth cohort. *Journal of Affective Disorders* **314**, 150–159.

Eyden, J. *et al.* (2016) A systematic review of the parenting and outcomes experienced by offspring of mothers with borderline personality pathology: potential mechanisms and clinical implications. *Clinical Psychology Review* **47**, 85–105.

Gelaye, B. *et al.* (2016) Epidemiology of maternal depression, risk factors, and child outcomes in low-income and middle-income countries. *The Lancet Psychiatry* **3**(10), 973–982. doi:10.1016/S2215-0366(16)30284-X.

Goodman, S.H. (2020) Intergenerational transmission of depression. *Annual Review of Clinical Psychology* **16**(1), 213–238. doi:10.1146/annurev-clinpsy-071519-113915.

Goodman, S.H. *et al.* (2011) Maternal depression and child psychopathology: a meta-analytic review. *Clinical Child and Family Psychology Review* **14**(1), 1–27.

Gressier, F. *et al.* (2022) Comorbid borderline personality disorders in women with post-partum depression admitted to mother-baby units. *Journal of Psychiatric Research* **146**, 149–155.

He, H. *et al.* (2020) Trends in the incidence and DALYs of schizophrenia at the global, regional and national levels: results from the global burden of disease study 2017. *Epidemiology and Psychiatric Sciences* **29**, e91.

Hoek, H.W. (2016) Review of the worldwide epidemiology of eating disorders. *Current Opinion in Psychiatry* **29**(6), 336–339.

Howard, L.M. & Khalifeh, H. (2020) Perinatal mental health: a review of progress and challenges. *World Psychiatry* **19**(3), 313–327.

Jahromi, L.B. *et al.* (2004) Maternal regulation of infant reactivity from 2 to 6 months. *Developmental Psychology* **40**(4), 477.

Jami, E.S. *et al.* (2021) Parental characteristics and offspring mental health and related outcomes: a systematic review of genetically informative literature. *Translational Psychiatry* **11**(1), 197. doi:10.1038/s41398-021-01300-2.

Kendler, K.S. *et al.* (2019) Parent-offspring transmission of drug abuse and alcohol use disorder: application of the multiple parenting relationships design. *American Journal of Medical Genetics Part B: Neuropsychiatric Genetics* **180**(4), 249–257.

Kochanska, G. *et al.* (1998) Children's emerging regulation of conduct: restraint, compliance, and internalization from infancy to the second year. *Child Development* **69**(5), 1378–1389.

Kwong, A.S.F. *et al.* (2021) Mental health before and during the COVID-19 pandemic in two longitudinal UK population cohorts. *The British Journal of Psychiatry* **218**(6), 334–343.

Lawrence, P.J. *et al.* (2019) Systematic review and meta-analysis: anxiety and depressive disorders in offspring of parents with anxiety disorders. *Journal of the American Academy of Child & Adolescent Psychiatry* **58**(1), 46–60.

Leve, L.D. *et al.* (2009) Structured parenting of toddlers at high versus low genetic risk: two pathways to child problems. *Journal of the*

American Academy of Child & Adolescent Psychiatry **48**(11), 1102–1109.

Loechner, J. *et al.* (2018) Preventing depression in the offspring of parents with depression: a systematic review and meta-analysis of randomized controlled trials. *Clinical Psychology Review* **60**, 1–14. doi:10.1016/j.cpr.2017.11.009.

Lovejoy, M.C. *et al.* (2000) Maternal depression and parenting behavior: a meta-analytic review. *Clinical Psychology Review* **20**(5), 561–592.

MacBeth, A. *et al.* (2023) General and age-specific fertility rates in non-affective psychosis: population-based analysis of Scottish women. *Social Psychiatry and Psychiatric Epidemiology* **58**(1), 105–112. doi:10.1007/s00127-022-02313-y.

Martin, A.F. *et al.* (2022) The protective role of father behaviour in the relationship between maternal postnatal depression and child mental health. *JCPP Advances* **2**(2), e12075.

Martínez-Olcina, M. *et al.* (2020) Eating disorders in pregnant and breastfeeding women: a systematic review. *Medicina* **56**(7), 352.

Martini, M.G. *et al.* (2020) Eating disorders mothers and their children: a systematic review of the literature. *Archives of Women's Mental Health* **23**(4), 449–467. doi:10.1007/s00737-020-01019-x.

Murray, L. *et al.* (2009) The development of anxiety disorders in childhood: an integrative review. *Psychological Medicine* **39**(9), 1413–1423.

National Institute for Health and Care Excellence (NICE) (2023a) *Depression in children and young people: identification and management: NICE guideline [NG134]*. Available: www.nice.org.uk/guidance/ng134 [26 July 2023].

National Institute for Health and Care Excellence (NICE) (2023b) *Eating disorders: recognition and treatment: NICE guideline [NG69]*. Available: www.nice.org.uk/guidance/ng69 [26 July 2023].

Netsi, E. *et al.* (2018) Association of persistent and severe postnatal depression with child outcomes. *JAMA Psychiatry* **75**(3), 247–253.

Newlove-Delgado, T. *et al.* (2022) *Mental Health of Children and Young People in England*. NHS Digital, Leeds, UK.

Pearson, R.M. *et al.* (2013a) Association between maternal depressogenic cognitive style during pregnancy and offspring cognitive style 18 years later. *American Journal of Psychiatry* **170**(4), 434–441.

Pearson, R.M. *et al.* (2013b) Maternal depression during pregnancy and the postnatal period: risks and possible mechanisms for offspring depression at age 18 years. *JAMA Psychiatry* **70**(12), 1312–1319. doi:10.1001/jamapsychiatry.2013.2163.

Pearson, R.M. *et al.* (2016) Maternal perinatal mental health and offspring academic achievement at age 16: the mediating role of childhood executive function. *Journal of Child Psychology and Psychiatry* **57**(4), 491–501.

Pearson, R.M. *et al.* (2018) Prevalence of prenatal depression symptoms among 2 generations of pregnant mothers: the Avon longitudinal study of parents and children. *JAMA Network Open* **1**(3), e180725.

Pihkala, H. *et al.* (2012) Children in Beardslee's family intervention: relieved by understanding of parental mental illness. *International Journal of Social Psychiatry* **58**(6), 623–628.

Popova, S. *et al.* (2017) Estimation of national, regional, and global prevalence of alcohol use during pregnancy and fetal alcohol syndrome: a systematic review and meta-analysis. *The Lancet Global Health* **5**(3), e290–e299. doi:10.1016/S2214-109X(17)30021-9.

Prasad, D. *et al.* (2022) The prevalence of borderline personality features and borderline personality disorder during the perinatal period: a systematic review and meta-analysis. *Archives of Women's Mental Health* **25**(2), 277–289.

Rahman, A. *et al.* (2008) Cognitive behaviour therapy-based intervention by community health workers for mothers with depression and their infants in rural Pakistan: a cluster-randomised controlled trial. *The Lancet* **372**(9642), 902–909.

Rajyaguru, P. *et al.* (2021) Maternal and paternal depression and child mental health trajectories: evidence from the Avon longitudinal study of parents and children. *BJPsych Open* **7**(5), e166.

Ramchandani, P. & Psychogiou, L. (2009) Paternal psychiatric disorders and children's psychosocial development. *The Lancet* **374**(9690), 646–653. doi:10.1016/S0140-6736(09)60238-5.

Rasic, D. *et al.* (2014) Risk of mental illness in offspring of parents with schizophrenia, bipolar disorder, and major depressive disorder: a meta-analysis of family high-risk studies. *Schizophrenia Bulletin* **40**(1), 28–38. doi:10.1093/schbul/sbt114.

Redinger, S. *et al.* (2018) First trimester antenatal depression and anxiety: prevalence and associated factors in an urban population in Soweto, South Africa. *Journal of Developmental Origins of Health and Disease* **9**(1), 30–40.

Reiss, D. *et al.* (2022) Parenting in the context of the child: genetic and social processes. *Monographs of the Society for Research in Child Development* **87**(1–3), 7–188. doi:10.1111/mono.12460.

Riebschleger, J. *et al.* (2017) Mental health literacy content for children of parents with a mental illness: thematic analysis of a literature review. *Brain Sciences* **7**(11), 141.

Riglin, L. *et al.* (2022) Early manifestations of genetic liability for ADHD, autism and schizophrenia at ages 18 and 24 months. *JCPP Advances* **2**(3), e12093. doi:10.1002/jcv2.12093.

Rutter, M. (1989) Pathways from childhood to adult life. *Archives of General Psychiatry* **30**, 23–51.

Serbin, L.A. & Karp, J. (2004) The intergenerational transfer of psychosocial risk: mediators of vulnerability and resilience. *Annual Review of Psychology* **55**(1), 333–363. doi:10.1146/annurev.psych.54.101601.145228.

Siegenthaler, E. *et al.* (2012) Effect of preventive interventions in mentally ill parents on the mental health of the offspring: systematic review and meta-analysis. *Journal of the American Academy of Child & Adolescent Psychiatry* **51**(1), 8–17.

Spence, S.H. & Rapee, R.M. (2016) The etiology of social anxiety disorder: an evidence-based model. *Behaviour Research and Therapy* **86**, 50–67.

Stein, A. *et al.* (2008) The influence of maternal depression, caregiving, and socioeconomic status in the post-natal year on children's language development. *Child: Care, Health and Development* **34**(5), 603–612.

Stein, A. *et al.* (2009) The influence of postnatal psychiatric disorder on child development: is maternal preoccupation one of the key underlying processes? *Psychopathology* **42**(1), 11–21.

Stein, A. *et al.* (2012a) Maternal cognitions and mother–infant interaction in postnatal depression and generalized anxiety disorder. *Journal of Abnormal Psychology* **121**(4), 795.

Stein, A. *et al.* (2012b) Effects of reboxetine and citalopram on appraisal of infant facial expressions and attentional biases. *Journal of Psychopharmacology* **26**(5), 670–676.

Stein, A. *et al.* (2014) Effects of perinatal mental disorders on the fetus and child. *The Lancet* **384**(9956), 1800–1819. doi:10.1016/S0140-6736(14)61277-0.

Stein, A. *et al.* (2018) Mitigating the effect of persistent postnatal depression on child outcomes through an intervention to treat depression and improve parenting: a randomised controlled trial. *The Lancet Psychiatry* **5**(2), 134–144.

Sweeney, S. & MacBeth, A. (2016) The effects of paternal depression on child and adolescent outcomes: a systematic review. *Journal of Affective Disorders* **205**, 44–59. doi:10.1016/j.jad.2016.05.073.

Szekely, E. *et al.* (2021) Maternal prenatal mood, pregnancy-specific worries, and early child psychopathology: findings from the DREAM BIG consortium. *Journal of the American Academy of Child & Adolescent Psychiatry* **60**(1), 186–197.

Talge, N.M. *et al.* (2007) Antenatal maternal stress and long-term effects on child neurodevelopment: how and why? *Journal of Child Psychology and Psychiatry* **48**(3–4), 245–261.

Thor, S. *et al.* (2022) Fathers' alcohol consumption and risk of substance-related disorders in offspring. *Drug and Alcohol Dependence* **233**, 109354.

Van Ijzendoorn, M.H. *et al.* (2023) Improving parenting, child attachment, and externalizing behaviors: meta-analysis of the first 25 randomized controlled trials on the effects of video-feedback intervention to promote positive parenting and sensitive discipline. *Development and Psychopathology* **35**(1), 241–256.

Wang, B. *et al.* (2021) Robust genetic nurture effects on education: a systematic review and meta-analysis based on 38,654 families across 8 cohorts. *American Journal of Human Genetics* **108**(9), 1780–1791. doi:10.1016/j.ajhg.2021.07.010.

Watkins, E.R. (2008) Constructive and unconstructive repetitive thought. *Psychological Bulletin* **134**(2), 163.

Weissman, M.M. *et al.* (2006a) Remissions in maternal depression and child psychopathology: a STAR* D-child report. *JAMA* **295**(12), 1389–1398.

Weissman, M.M. *et al.* (2006b) Offspring of depressed parents: 20 years later. *American Journal of Psychiatry* **163**(6), 1001–1008.

Westman, J. *et al.* (2022) Mortality in adult children of parents with alcohol use disorder: a nationwide register study. *European Journal of Epidemiology* **37**(8), 815–826.

Wickersham, A. *et al.* (2020) The association between paternal psychopathology and adolescent depression and anxiety: a systematic review. *Journal of Adolescence* **79**, 232–246.

Woody, C.A. *et al.* (2017) A systematic review and meta-regression of the prevalence and incidence of perinatal depression. *Journal of Affective Disorders* **219**, 86–92. doi:10.1016/j.jad.2017.05.003.

CHAPTER 25

Child abuse and neglect

Danya Glaser
Formerly at Great Ormond Street Hospital for Children NHS Foundation Trust, London, UK

Introduction

Child abuse and neglect or child maltreatment (terms used interchangeably) are a universal phenomenon (Hillis *et al.*, 2016) affecting girls and boys equally (Pinheiro, 2006). Child maltreatment violates children's rights to safety and protection (UN, 1989). It is common, harmful, and being caused by human behavior, is potentially preventable. Most of the manifest harm is psychological and behavioral, and has particular relevance to both child and adult mental health services. Much of the harm is enduring, with an intergenerational pattern. While child maltreatment may occur within different relationships such as from teachers or caregiving staff, the commonest setting is intrafamilial (Pinheiro, 2006). It is also a public health issue (Shonkoff *et al.*, 2012) and impacts on professionals involved. Child abuse and neglect carries a high cost to society. It includes the labor-intensive cost of multiagency child protection, resources for interventions both in childhood and adulthood, the costs of some subsequent antisocial behavior and crime, poor parenting, and the wasted potential and unemployment which often follow childhood maltreatment.

What constitutes child abuse and neglect or maltreatment?

Child maltreatment constitutes both omission, such as in physical and emotional neglect, and commission, as in psychological, physical, and sexual abuse. It can be grouped into persistent and episodic patterns. The persistent forms are intrinsic to the caregiver—child relationship. As a result, the child may regard it as a "normal" attribute of this relationship and may not be able to recall specific incidents, while others may dismiss its significance, regarding it as merely an aspect of this family. Physical neglect, emotional abuse, and emotional neglect are usually persistent, although occasionally may occur as a single incident which may be salient to the child. The episodic forms are often repeated and usually have a beginning and an end, which may facilitate the child's recall. The child may experience periods free of maltreatment. While the child may be able to anticipate abuse, uncertainty and the fear of recurrence is ever present. Physical and sexual abuse can be regarded as episodic.

Definitions

There are several definitions for the forms of maltreatment. Some overall definitions use the, arguably unhelpful, term "violence" against children, where violence incudes not only abuse but also neglect and negligent treatment. Definitions vary according to context, which may be local or national. Definitions also depend on their purpose, for instance, when decisions need to be made about the threshold for recognition, or for legal criminal or child protective proceedings (Laajasalo *et al.*, 2023).

The term trauma has been used interchangeably both for child abuse and neglect and for its effects. Trauma is not synonymous with either and is most usefully applied when the nature of the experience leads to a clinical picture of post-traumatic stress.

Neglect

Neglect includes lack of provision of food, clothing, shelter and safe living conditions, health care, and education. Lack of supervision or negligent care is responsible for many so-called accidental injuries, which are often predictable and preventable. It also includes use of inadequate caregivers. Some definitions include psychological/emotional (nonphysical) neglect, while others include this aspect under psychological maltreatment. While all definitions include persistent neglect, some allow for isolated incidents. The World Health Organization (WHO) and the International Society for the Prevention of Child Abuse and Neglect (ISPCAN) (WHO, 2006) confine neglect to a "parent (who) is in a position to" provide for the child's need. The WHO

Rutter's Child and Adolescent Psychiatry and Psychology, Seventh Edition.
Edited by Anita Thapar, Daniel S. Pine, Samuele Cortese, Cathy Creswell, Tamsin J. Ford, James F. Leckman, and Argyris Stringaris.

Companion website: www.wiley.com/go/thapar/rutterspsych7

also helpfully states that "the parents of neglected children are not necessarily poor." Definitions assume neglect to be harmful. The United Kingdom (UK) definition (HM Government, 2023) includes prebirth neglect such as maternal substance misuse.

Emotional abuse and neglect/psychological maltreatment

While the UK usage of the term "emotional abuse" on its own does not include neglect, the US term "psychological maltreatment" does. The most recent proposed overarching definition refers to "caregiver behaviors toward or involving a child (excluding physical/sexual abuse and physical neglect) which cause or have a strong potential to cause serious harm to a child's emotional, cognitive, social, interpersonal, or physical wellbeing or development. Psychological maltreatment could occasionally reflect a single caregiver act or omission or more usually repeated caregiver behaviors" (Slep *et al.*, 2022). Most research tools and many professionals consider emotional abuse to comprise only verbal hostility and denigration. There are several other forms which belong under the overarching term (Table 25.1).

Physical abuse

One definition (World Health Organization, 2006) captures elements in most other definitions: "Intentional use of physical force against the child that is likely to or results in harm to the child's health, survival, development or dignity." This includes hitting, beating, kicking, shaking, biting, strangling, scalding, burning, poisoning, and suffocating. Much physical violence against children in the home is inflicted with the object of punishing. There has been debate about the inclusion of corporal punishment or physical discipline under physical abuse. If punishment or discipline

Table 25.1 Forms of psychological maltreatment.

Forms of psychological maltreatment	Examples of caregiver behavior toward child
Psychological neglect	Ignoring; unavailable; unresponsive; lack of affection
Spurning	Hostile; denigrating; blaming; scapegoating; rejecting
Developmentally inappropriate interactions	Developmentally inappropriate expectations including infantilization and parentification
Inappropriate discipline	Confining; unreasonable limitations on child's social interactions; depriving of necessities
Terrorizing	Exposing a child to traumatizing experiences (including domestic violence); threatening
Exploiting/using the child to fulfill caregiver needs	Involving child in interparental disputes; Munchausen by proxy/fabricated or induced illness (FII): parent using child's reported, rarely induced, ill-health for own gain (Glaser, 2020)
Failure to promote socialization/corruption	Social isolation; encouraging antisocial behavior

include using an implement, forced ingestion, or leaving a physical mark, it would generally be regarded as physical abuse. In some jurisdictions, for instance in the UK, fabricated or induced illness (FII) (Munchausen by proxy) is currently included under physical abuse. This inclusion might be revised since: (i) it includes psychological as well as physical harm; (ii) in many cases the harm results from erroneous reporting by the caregiver rather than the rarer physical acts; and (iii) some of the harm is caused inadvertently by doctors' responses (RCPCH, 2021).

Sexual abuse and child sexual exploitation

The WHO defines sexual abuse as "the involvement of a child in sexual activity that she/he does not fully comprehend, is unable to give informed consent to, for which the child is not developmentally prepared, or that violates the laws or social taboos of society. Children can be sexually abused by both adults and other children who are, by virtue of their age or stage of development, in a position of responsibility, trust, or power over the victim" (World Health Organization, 2006). Recent UK government guidance expands this: "Sexual abuse may also include non-contact activities, such as involving children in looking at, or in the production of, sexual images, watching sexual activities, encouraging children to behave in sexually inappropriate ways or grooming a child in preparation for abuse. Sexual abuse can take place online, and technology can be used to facilitate offline abuse." "Child sexual exploitation is a form of child sexual abuse (CSA). It occurs where an individual or group takes advantage of an imbalance of power to coerce, manipulate or deceive a child or young person under the age of 18 into sexual activity (i) in exchange for something the victim needs or wants, and/or (ii) for the financial advantage or increased status of the perpetrator or facilitator. The victim may have been sexually exploited even if the sexual activity appears consensual. Child sexual exploitation does not always involve physical contact; it can also occur through the use of technology" (HM Government, 2023).

Overall experience

Regardless of the individual forms of child maltreatment, the overall experience of being maltreated is stressful, unpredictable, confers a sense of unsafety, and often includes deprivation, lack of empathy by caregivers, exposure to conflict resolution by violence, and the absence of external affect regulation.

Cultural aspects

There are culturally different parenting and child-rearing practices, e.g., the question of acceptability of physical discipline. While international organizations, such as the WHO, provide universal definitions for child maltreatment, each jurisdiction adapts these. A particular concern arises for children from families with individual cultural practices and norms, living in multicultural societies. The question is to what extent seemingly cultural behaviors toward children are to be acceptable, when they are considered as abusive or neglectful by the "host" country's legislation and social norms. It might therefore be difficult to establish whether maltreatment has occurred. Ultimately, if the practices are regarded as harmful to the child, an "explanation based on cultural practice is unsuitable because this should not justify hurting or harming a child or young person" (NICE, 2009).

Adverse childhood experience (ACEs)

Considerable attention has been accorded to adverse childhood experiences (ACEs) which were compiled by US adult physicians (see Chapter 20). They noted poor health outcomes in their adult patients who had ACEs, with a direct relationship between the number of ACEs, and illness severity and mortality. However, not all ACEs are synonymous with child maltreatment. Nor do they include thresholds for severity, frequency, and qualifiers in the definitions, and therefore are not collectively predictive of future ill-health (Baldwin & Danese, 2021). They are, nevertheless, important to note.

Epidemiology

Data on prevalence vary (Gilbert *et al.*, 2009). There are several reasons for variation in rates (Jud *et al.*, 2016; Prevoo *et al.*, 2017).

First, the source of data determines the rates. The highest rates are consistently found in clinical samples and self- and parent reports, both retrospective and concurrent. For instance, Radford *et al.* (2013) in England, using a modified version of the Juvenile Victimization Questionnaire (JVQ) (Hamby *et al.*, 2004) found that, based on parent reports, 8.9% of under 11s, and on self-reports, 21.9% of 11–17s, had maltreatment by a parent or guardian during their childhood. These rates were far higher than the 0.35% of the child population with substantiated cases of child maltreatment at the time of the study. Self-reports have been shown to be reliable (Pinto Pereira *et al.*, 2021). However, not all verified child maltreatment is perceived or reported by adult survivors (Danese & Widom, 2023). Prospective and administrative data from child protective services and legal records show lower rates, for instance, for sexual abuse (Karsna & Bromley, 2023). Prospective and retrospective reports yield different results and should not be used interchangeably (Danese & Widom, 2020).

Second, rates vary between different countries, partly due to the quality of data collection and particularly because of variations in definitions and the acceptability of various forms of maltreatment (Wadji *et al.*, 2023).

Third, rates will vary according to the form(s) of maltreatment being studied. Forms may be found in isolation, although commonly co-occur (Smith & Pollak, 2021) with polyvictimization (Turner 2010). The common co-occurrence makes the precise prevalence of each form difficult to determine. Physical neglect and psychological maltreatment are the commonest, followed by physical and sexual abuse (Prevoo *et al.*, 2017). Sexual abuse within the family is uncommonly found in isolation.

Fourth, social circumstances vary, and social deprivation is associated with greater risk (Bywaters & Skinner, 2022), particularly physical and psychological abuse and neglect (Lee *et al.*, 2017). Other social stressors such as migration, wars, and natural disasters confer greater vulnerability.

Even in comparable settings, it is unclear whether variation in rates over time reflect true prevalence or are due to more active recognition and recording. Rates of CSA have reduced (Jud *et al.*, 2016). Particular circumstances temporarily elevate rates of child maltreatment. The most recent has been the COVID-19 pandemic.

The COVID-19 pandemic

Variation in prevalence of different forms of child maltreatment has been found during the COVID-19 pandemic. Factors contributing include the nature of studies—cross-sectional, retrospective, or longitudinal, and sources of information. A decline in allegations, and data from surveillance and official reports suggest reduction. This is partly explained by school closures whereby children were not observed by teachers and others, and signs of maltreatment were not recognized. By contrast, individual surveys and clinical settings have found increases. Enforced social isolation, decreased income, reduced access to supportive services, and increased intrafamily proximity all increased risk. Neglect, and emotional and physical abuse increased as stressed parents struggled to combine work and childcare and cope with decreased income (Lee & Kim 2022; Park & Walsh 2022; Blumenthal, 2023).

Who maltreats?

Physical neglect, psychological neglect, and emotional abuse are mostly brought about by primary caregivers. Sexual abusers include fathers, stepfathers, adolescent siblings (often underrecognized), family members, and nonfamily members already known to the child or who may have groomed the child. Much sexual abuse occurs in educational, religious, sporting, and other settings. About 10% of sexual abusers are female.

Risk factors for child abuse and neglect

There are risk factors relating to individual parents or children, the quality of the partner relationship, and parent–child interaction, and risks in the wider environment surrounding the family. Contextual risk factors can be both distal and proximal to the child (Figure 25.1). Distal risk factors include especially low socioeconomic status associated with poverty, poor housing, social isolation, and migration. These indirect influences on the child are largely mediated by their effects on the parents, affecting the parents' capacity to interact with their children safely. Some distal factors impinge directly on the

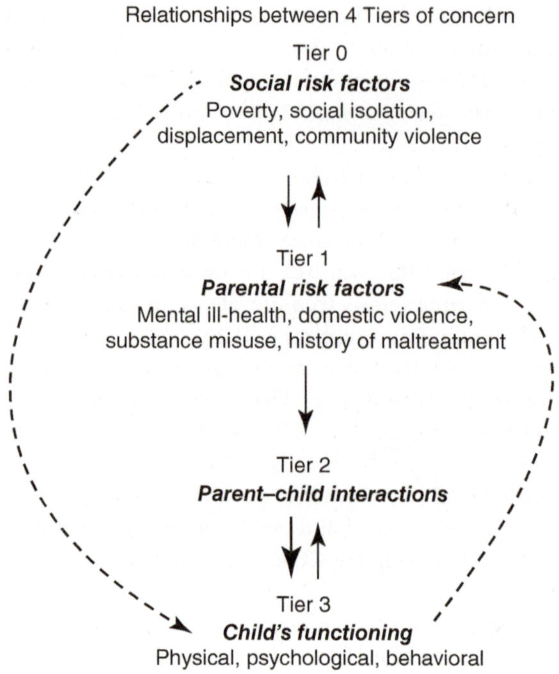

Figure 25.1 Relationships between 4 Tiers of concern.

child's well-being. Exposure to community violence has been shown to mediate the effects of physical abuse on the child's behavioral and trauma symptoms (Cecil *et al.*, 2017). Parental risk factors are well recognized and include interparental violence, parental dependent personality, insecure attachment patterns (Van IJzendoorn *et al.*, 2020), mental ill-health, drug misuse, and criminality. Adults who maltreat children are more likely to have suffered maltreatment in their own childhood. An example is sexual abuse, both off- and online (Chopin *et al.*, 2022). There are several mechanisms to explain this intergenerational transmission of child maltreatment (Alink *et al.*, 2019). Last, without assigning blame, the behavior of maltreated children may, in turn, affect the quality of the parent–child interactions, as well as affecting the parents' own well-being. Arguably, some behaviors associated with disorders with a strong genetic basis, such as attention deficit hyperactivity disorder (ADHD) (see Chapter 54) and difficulties at the severe end of the autism spectrum, can manifest regardless of parents' behaviors. They may pose challenges to parents, particularly those with their own difficulties. These interactions are illustrated in Figure 25.1.

There are also risk factors in children themselves. Children with disabilities are particularly vulnerable to all forms of maltreatment (Sullivan & Knutson, 2000). They may experience neglect of their needs when highly dependent on personal care, with attendant vulnerability to sexual abuse. Difficulties in communication make it harder for children with disabilities to report maltreatment. Challenging behavior may inadvertently elicit aggressive responses.

The impact of maltreatment

Child maltreatment can adversely affect all aspects of a child's and adolescent's health and functioning (Gilbert *et al.*, 2009), extending into adulthood (Anda *et al.*, 2006), with particularly serious psychological and behavioral consequences (Magalhães & Camilo, 2023).

Determinants of harm

Several factors contribute to the nature, severity, and timing of the harm from maltreatment, beyond the specific form(s) of maltreatment (Smith & Pollak, 2021).

Child factors

The effects of maltreatment depend, in part, on the stage of the child's brain development (Malave *et al.*, 2022). Differential susceptibility, also described as "orchids and dandelions" (Boyce, 2019), refers to a postulated continuum (Zhang *et al.*, 2023) of sensitivity to proximal environmental factors, both positive and negative. At one end, children termed "orchids" are genetically, stress-reactively, and temperamentally extremely sensitive to their environment, and will be particularly adversely affected by, for instance, maltreatment. (They will, however, thrive with good care.) "Dandelion" children will be more resilient to moderate forms of maltreatment. (See also Chapter 21.)

Timing of manifestations of harm

Children may not show symptoms of harm at the time of abuse. Some neurobiological changes found in childhood following maltreatment are not associated with functional impairment at the time but may show later psychopathology, indicating latent vulnerability (McCrory *et al.*, 2017) (see Chapter 20). Drug and alcohol misuse and self-harm may first manifest in adolescence, following earlier abuse or neglect. Some effects manifest in adulthood.

Subjective experience of childhood maltreatment has been associated with subsequent greater chronicity of emotional disorders, regardless of agreement between subjective recall and objective measures of past maltreatment (Danese & Widom, 2023).

Maltreatment factors

In light of the frequent coexistence of different forms of maltreatment, aspects of their context, and the many risk and protective factors, it is not possible to predict outcome in individual cases. There is evidence of the cumulative effect of maltreatment on mental health (Cecil *et al.*, 2017). Duration, intensity, and developmental timing are more predictive. Hostility and negativity, which exist on their own and also underpin other forms of maltreatment, may be predictors of internalizing disorders and post-traumatic stress disorder (PTSD) (see Chapter 58) (Cecil *et al.*, 2017).

Protective factors

Not all maltreated children will be adversely affected. Some children develop coping and adaptive responses, with enhanced skills (Ellis *et al.*, 2022) (see Chapter 23). Resilience (Masten, 2019) and a variety of protective factors, especially early secure attachment, family and school support, and peer relationships (Meng *et al.*, 2018) can mitigate the harm.

Neurobiological mechanisms underlying harm

The physical effects of adverse psychosocial experiences have been termed biological embedding (Hertzman, 1999). Neurobiological effects are manifest in various brain structures, sites, and functions, hormones, and neurotransmitters (Teicher *et al.* 2016) (see Chapters 10, 11, 20).

Developmental effects (see also Chapter 10)

Brain development proceeds in a predetermined, stepwise sequence of sensitive periods during which overproduction of axons, dendrites, and synapses is followed by necessary pruning. The social environment—the young child's experiences—may influence what will be pruned. In many areas of the associated cortex, including the prefrontal cortex, this process continues to maturation in late adolescence, allowing not only for prolonged neural plasticity and recalibration, but also rendering that part of the brain vulnerable to continued adverse effects.

Many effects can be regarded as adaptive responses to the (maltreating) environment at that time, in anticipation that these environmental factors will endure, even when the child's circumstances and care actually improve (Teicher *et al.*, 2003). This is regarded as experience-adaptive programming (Rutter, 2002), which is neither deterministic nor fully amenable to plasticity. One possible example of experience-adaptive programming is a study in which children, previously exposed to physical abuse and anger, showed enhanced recognition of anger within a series of morphed facial expressions ranging from neutral to angry (Pollak *et al.*, 2009). This enhanced recognition of anger is adaptive only in a threatening environment. It could lead a child to preemptive or reactive aggression. Privileging aggressive cues occurs at the cost of attending to other social cues. There may be effects on the amygdalae which undergo rapid development early in life. Children, adopted at a mean age of 19 months out of orphanages were found, using functional magnetic resonance imaging (fMRI), to have heightened amygdala activity in response to fearful faces and distractor stimuli, but not to neutral facial expressions (Tottenham *et al.*, 2011). They also showed reduced eye-contact, postulated to be the child's attempt to regulate overarousal caused by face-to-face interactions. However, the cost is impaired social interaction (see also Chapter 20).

In experience-expectant development, lack of exposure to experiences that are developmentally expected during their sensitive periods, will lead to largely irreversible pruning of related neural connections with attendant loss of function. This is particularly relevant to neglect with deprivation of experience at key developmental stages (McLaughlin & Gabard-Durnam, 2022). An example relevant to child and adolescent mental health (CAMH) is disinhibited social engagement disorder (DSED) in which stranger wariness is not developed (see Chapter 57). A further example is the smaller total brain volume found in adults adopted in childhood from extremely depriving institutions. These findings mediate the relationship between the early deprivation and lower general intelligence and ADHD symptoms in adulthood (Mackes *et al.*, 2020).

Harm related to the stress response

While much stress is tolerable, in toxic stress the stressors are intense and prolonged "in the absence of the buffering protection of adult support" (Shonkoff *et al.*, 2009). Both abuse and neglect are stressful (Smith & Pollak, 2021), often amounting to toxic stress, due to feelings of terror, fear, pain, shame, powerlessness, helplessness, an unpredictable future, and abandonment. The stress response is necessary for survival. It has several aspects, immediately involving the sympathetic nervous system and, particularly, the hypothalamic-pituitary-adrenal (HPA) axis, including increased cortisol secretion (see Chapter 20). Cortisol reduces glial cell division, affecting myelination (Lauder, 1983), thus reducing speed of conduction. In one study, the volume of various tracts of the corpus callosum, which consists entirely of white matter, has been found to be reduced in children with PTSD who had been sexually and physically abused and exposed to domestic violence (De Bellis *et al.*, 1999) (but note Chapter 11) with reduced right–left hemispheric integration (Yazgan *et al.*, 1995) The right hemisphere is associated with negative emotions and social avoidance. Following maltreatment, right hemispheric lateralization is increased.

Infancy is a potentially stressful period with exposure to myriad unfamiliar and incomprehensible experiences (see Chapter 7). After early infancy, both rodents and human infants undergo a stress-hyporesponsive period, presumably to protect the developing brain from the elevated cortisol stress response. The precise duration of this period until preschool age is not yet clear. The stress response of infants and young children with secure attachments (see Chapter 6) is buffered, despite evident distress, even in infants who are temperamentally very stress-reactive (Koss & Gunnar, 2018). Conversely, insecurely attached infants and young children whose caregivers are neglectful and unresponsive to their distress, mount the usual stress response with elevated cortisol (Gunnar & Donzella, 2002).

Oxytocin, associated with affiliative love, social bonding, maternal caregiving, and attachment, is involved in reducing HPA axis activity. In the presence of stressors, the reciprocal, mutual regulation between the HPA and oxytocin systems may become dysregulated (Li *et al.*, 2019). There is an indication of a sensitive period for the development of the oxytocin system (Fries *et al.*, 2005)

The harm: symptoms and disorders

Insecure and disorganized attachment patterns (see Chapter 6) and attachment disorders (see Chapter 57) are related, in part, to child maltreatment. Internalizing difficulties which include depression, anxiety, poor emotion regulation, and PTSD often follow earlier child maltreatment. The recent diagnosis of complex PTSD in *International Classification of Diseases 11th Revision* (ICD-11) incorporates both core PTSD symptoms, which not all maltreated children show, and affect dysregulation, negative self-concept, and difficulties in relationships (DeJong & Wilkinson, 2019).

Some maltreated children present with features similar to autism spectrum disorder (ASD) (see Chapter 50). Some may have confirmed ASD and, of those, some may have been maltreated due to the difficulties which they posed to their caregivers. Due to their experiences, some maltreated children have difficulties in recognizing facial emotions, a lack of social and emotional responsiveness, vulnerability to changes in routine, and sensitivity to sensory indicators of threat (Wilkinson *et al.*, 2023). Furthermore, reactive attachment disorder (RAD) (see Chapter 57) includes social withdrawal and emotional inhibition. However, there are some differences between ASD and post-maltreatment. The latter may show less limited social reciprocity and social use of language, and no repetitive and stereotyped behavior (Wolstencroft *et al.*, 2023). RAD is primarily characterized by minimal seeking and accepting of comfort. Distinguishing between ASD and post-maltreatment may be difficult in a one-off assessment. ASD features are enduring while difficulties due to maltreatment may abate with a change in caregiving.

Behavioral difficulties are common. Aggression sometimes extends to violence and may be expressed as antisocial behavior and criminality. Self-injurious behavior is used, more often by adolescent girls, as a way of distraction from post-traumatic intruding reminders. Suicidality may follow maltreatment. Many children have low self-esteem and a sense of shame. Adolescent drug and alcohol misuse may be a delayed sequel of earlier maltreatment. Sexually inappropriate behavior in young children (Davies *et al.*, 2000) is a common sequel of sexual abuse. Sexual disinhibition in adolescence may follow both sexual and physical abuse. Children and adolescents who have been maltreated often experience difficulties in their interpersonal, especially peer, relationships (McCrory *et al.*, 2019), which may be exacerbated by their lack of trust in others (Neil *et al.*, 2022).

Abuse and, particularly, neglect are subsequently associated with educational underachievement, with delayed language development, impaired cognition, poor executive function, and difficulties in visuospatial processing (Romano *et al.*, 2015). Interestingly, Lewis *et al.*, (2021) report that maltreated children with cognitive deficits in adolescence and adulthood had low cognitive ability which predated the maltreatment (only measured from age five) and correlated with maternal IQ.

The variability of post-maltreatment mental health difficulties, with complex attachment- and trauma-related symptomatology, are not captured by the two main classifications of disorders—Diagnostic and Statistical Manual of Mental Disorders 5th edition (DSM-5) and International Classification of Diseases 11th Revision (ICD-11) (DeJong, 2010; Tarren-Sweeney, 2021). It is important to seek for clinically significant problems as well as items on the Child Behavior Checklist (CBCL) and Strengths and Difficulties Questionnaire (SDQ). In childhood (C) and adolescence (A), the Assessment Checklist for Children (ACC) (Tarren-Sweeney, 2007) and adolescent version (ACA) (Tarren-Sweeney, 2013), parent report rating instruments capture a broader set of symptoms in several scales. The scales, each with constituent items are: sexual behavior (C&A), pseudomature (C), nonreciprocal (C&A), indiscriminate(C) and insecure (C), interpersonal behavior (C), anxious–distrustful (C), abnormal pain response (C), food maintenance (C&A), self-injury (C), suicide discourse (C&A), negative self-image (C&A), low confidence (C&A), social instability/behavioral dysregulation (A), emotional dysregulation/distorted social cognition (A), and dissociation/trauma symptoms (A).

Core features of borderline personality disorder (BPD) may well apply to some adolescents who have experienced severe maltreatment (Lawless & Tarren-Sweeney, 2022).

Sequelae in adulthood

Using adult self-reports in a large, controlled study, Struck *et al.*, (2020) found an overrepresentation of different forms of child maltreatment associated with adult mental illness. In a prospective, record-linkage study, Kisely *et al.* (2018) found that neglect, and particularly emotional abuse, were followed by serious mental ill-health in early adulthood. Dutra *et al.* (2009) found that in young adulthood, dissociation was significantly predicted by both lack of parental responsiveness in infancy and verbal abuse in childhood.

Indicators and recognition

The process of recognizing maltreatment is not straightforward and may be troubling for professionals. There is a fine line between missing or ignoring indicators of, or actual, maltreatment and overcautious, unjustified concern and hasty action. The former is often based on a wish to maintain a therapeutic relationship with the child and family and concern about child protective and/or possible criminal proceedings against the parents. The latter is motivated by concern for children and also, in some jurisdictions, mandatory reporting laws which place a duty on professionals to report, even suspicions, to child protective services.

There are some general principles:

- A child's disclosure or description of abuse, especially if unsolicited, is of particular concern.
- A troubled child with mental health difficulties for which there is no obvious explanation, may be or have been maltreated, and explanations need to be sought.

- An understanding of parents' difficulties which lead to maltreatment, even when there is no intention to harm the child, does not negate the fact of maltreatment. An example would be postnatal depression leading to psychological neglect.
- Maltreatment in children with disabilities may be difficult to recognize.
- Considering or suspecting child maltreatment can be stressful and calls for consultation with a suitably qualified colleague, and will involve several agencies. In the UK, all health services have assigned safeguarding or "named" professionals, whose role is to advise and consult to staff who have concerns about possible maltreatment. In the US, child abuse pediatricians are helpful (Raz *et al.*, 2023). In some countries, suspicion of maltreatment requires reporting to child protective services or law enforcement.

Indicators

Within the sphere of CAMH, there are several, observed or reported, emotional and behavioral presentations. Marked change in behavior or emotional state without a clear precipitant, or uncharacteristically intense emotional responses and out of proportion to the situation, are indicators of possible abuse. They include: fearfulness; indiscriminate contact with affection-seeking from, and over-friendliness to, strangers; excessive clinginess and persistent attention-seeking; dissociation; self-injurious behavior (Liu *et al.*, 2018); running away from home; and age-inappropriate sexualized behavior (NICE, 2009). Presentation of children by parents who report symptoms not observed by others and who insist on medically unwarranted investigations and treatments indicate possible FII (Glaser, 2020).

Disclosure and description

In the course of assessment or therapeutic consultations, some children and young persons disclose or describe actual abuse.

Observation

During consultations it is possible to observe actual emotional abuse or neglect within parent–child interactions. A child may present as physically neglected or behave in a sexually inappropriate way.

Child and adolescent mental health services (CAMHS) response to concerns

Possible sexual abuse

CSA is suspected when there is an unexplained change in the child's behavior or emotional state, a disclosure or description of sexual abuse, self-harm, or observed or reported age-inappropriate sexualized behavior (Davies *et al.*, 2000). While repeated questioning of a child is undesirable, and a formal interview should be set up (see later section on "Child sexual abuse (CSA)"), research has found that unless a young child has already described some aspect of abuse, she/he is unlikely to talk about abuse at a formal interview (Keary & Fitzpatrick, 1994). There is considerable delay in children's reports of sexual abuse. Victims of sexual abuse have often described that, despite indicators, no one had ever asked them for the reasons. Therefore, it is possible to talk on their own with a child who is suspected of being sexually abused, using nonleading open questions, seeking their explanations for the concerns (CSA Centre, 2022). With a self-harming adolescent, following open questions it is not inappropriate to enquire about sexual abuse. Careful notes need to be made about the child's descriptions and the course of these conversations. Any indication by the child of sexual abuse needs to be reported immediately to child protective services, with an explanation to the child. The child's reservations about reporting should be explored and reassurance given as far as possible. This needs to be followed by a formal, forensic interview. In some jurisdictions, parents are immediately informed of suspicions, while this may not be in the child's best interests. The reason is that in sexual abuse, the child's description is usually the single most important piece of evidence. A potentially unsupportive, denying, or disbelieving parent could silence the child.

Other concerns

Openness in communication with the family enhances therapeutic work. With nonsexual abuse concerns, open discussion is important about reported concerns and especially those observed in the parent–child interactions and in the child. In some cases of psychological maltreatment, therapeutic work may bring about sufficient change to reduce the concerns (Glaser, 2011). However, reporting laws, the severity of the abuse, or insufficient change require reporting to child protective services, with full explanation to the family.

Evidence of child maltreatment

There are several aspects to evidence of child abuse and neglect, which rely heavily on information-sharing. Psychiatrists and other CAMH professionals play an important role in compiling and constructing evidence.

Uses of evidence

At its most basic, evidence is required to justify expenditure of human resources for social work and therapeutic services. More importantly, evidence is needed to establish whether child maltreatment has occurred or is occurring, in order to decide whether the child needs protecting and how to achieve this. Unless parents are fully engaged in and able to work toward change, evidence is needed to justify stepped, mandated intervention. Administrative child protective procedures enable protective, supportive, and therapeutic work to proceed. In more severe cases, where the need to separate the child from their caregivers is contemplated, the decision is determined in the (civil) family court. In the UK, the family court requires evidence of "significant harm," an interesting concept, allowing for one or two forms of evidence. One is *ill-treatment* causing actual or likely harm, allowing for protection of a child before harm has occurred. This applies to psychological and sexual abuse, and neglect. The other is *impairment* to all aspects of the child's health and development, attributable to the treatment the child has/has not received. This mainly applies to physical abuse and neglect, and less so to psychological maltreatment.

Evidence may also be required for criminal court proceedings, which determine the guilt or innocence of the alleged abuser or neglectful parent, but are scarcely concerned with the child's welfare. While the evidential threshold for civil family proceedings is "on balance of probabilities," evidence in criminal prosecutions of abusers requires the higher threshold of "beyond reasonable doubt"; in the latter case the evidence is stringently tested in a wholly adversarial process.

The nature of evidence required and the role of CAMH professionals

The different forms of child maltreatment require evidence in answer to different questions (Box 25.1).

Child sexual abuse (CSA)

In the case of CSA, the question is first whether it has happened and, if so, who the abuser was. CSA is essentially a secret activity, without witnesses unless several children are involved, and is mostly denied by the alleged abuser. Conclusive physical signs are only found in a minority of sexually abused children and DNA evidence is rare. There may be supporting circumstantial evidence. The primary evidence is, therefore, the child's account, its veracity being tested. The child may mention abuse to their caregiver, teacher, or friend. These early words may be spontaneous as an unintentional disclosure, a wish for the abuse to stop, concern to protect a sibling, or in response to questions. Thereafter, the account will inevitably change due to repetition, altered recall, and further conversations and interviews. Also, importantly, by the time of disclosure, sexual abuse will usually have occurred repeatedly. Descriptions and their circumstances—time, place, and nature of the abuse—will therefore inevitably vary, without the child's account being inaccurate or untruthful.

Much importance is accorded to a forensic, video-recorded interview of the child, usually carried out by police together with a social worker. There are protocols, applicable in different jurisdictions, for the process of the interview in which open, rather than leading questions should be used, followed by questions clarifying details (Lamb *et al.*, 2007). Usually, only one interview is carried out. Children with communication difficulties may be interviewed by a specially trained psychologist. For validating accounts of abuse, the context and the child's first mention of abuse are particularly important. Other important factors for validation are any findings from medical examination, family circumstances, and the nature of the child's relationship with the alleged abuser. Spontaneous false allegations by children are possible but rare. False descriptions most commonly occur in the context of interparental disputes (Faller, 2005). The results of the formal interview are a central aspect of court evidence, although in criminal cases the child will also be cross-examined, increasingly via a video link.

Child psychologists and psychiatrists may be witnesses of fact, describing the child's account given to them. More often, they are called to provide their opinion as expert witnesses regarding the child's veracity.

Box 25.1 Different evidential questions and their sources

Child sexual abuse (CSA)
(secret, not witnessed, denied)
Question: *Has it happened?*
Source: *Child's testimony*
Challenges: *Veracity*

Physical abuse
(not observed)
Question: *Was injury inflicted or accidental?*
Source: *Medical findings*
Challenge: *Medical interpretation*

Psychological maltreatment and neglect
(observable, likely effects)
Question: *Is it harmful?*
Source: *Observations/descriptions*
Challenges: *How harmful?*
Is harm attributable to maltreatment?

Psychological maltreatment, neglect, and physical abuse

In the case of psychological maltreatment (and neglect), the evidence is observable and describable, being the nature or absence of parent–child interactions. The question here is whether the interactions of concern conform to the overall definition and the several subtypes of psychological maltreatment, but mainly whether they are actually harmful, and the nature and extent of harm to the child. This constitutes the expert opinion and evidence of CAMH professionals. However, the state of a child's mental health cannot be adduced as conclusive evidence of maltreatment. (In the case of physical harm or abuse, the question for pediatricians is whether the physical harm or injury is inflicted or "accidental," although many accidental injuries are predictable and preventable and are aspects of neglect.)

Intervention in cases of likely or actual maltreatment

Prevention

There are 3 levels of prevention:

- Universal prevention targets whole populations to prevent harm, such as minimizing poverty (Bullinger & Boy, 2023) and programs in schools to raise awareness of sexual abuse.

- Selective prevention in the case of child maltreatment is targeted toward identified high-risk groups and factors. Attachment-based programs aim at enhancing sensitive parenting of young children by vulnerable and young parents and dealing with behavior problems (NICE, 2017; Tobon *et al.*, 2022).
- Indicated prevention includes both protection from further harm and treating the effects of harm (Figure 25.2).

Indicated prevention: protection

There are two aspects to protecting a child from further harm: immediate protection and working toward protection.

Immediate protection

Forms of CSA which require immediate protection are a risk of further abuse after a child has been abused, or a child in close contact with a known sexual abuser. Immediate protection may also be required in some aspects of physical abuse, severe neglect, and risk of immediate serious harm to a child's health or life from FII when the caregiver induces illness in the child in order to convince doctors about her contention that the child is ill (RCPCH, 2021). Immediate protection requires separation of the maltreating person from the child, which often necessitates moving the child. In cases of sexual abuse, the safety of the child is, in part, determined by the closeness of the relationship between the nonabusing caregiver(s) and the alleged abuser. The closer that relationship, the less is the child protected. The initial focus is to support nonabusing caregiver(s). In the immediate aftermath of removal, a child may well be distressed and traumatized and feel guilt for the separation. They require age-appropriate explanations, and their caregivers need support to respond sensitively to these very troubled children. Children who are moved from home need safe continuity of relationships with the birth family. Minimizing further moves is essential. These steps will mitigate some of the subsequent emotional and behavioral difficulties.

Working toward protection

While a sexual abuser is often not an attachment figure, in emotional abuse and neglect the maltreating parent(s) is also an attachment figure. In these many cases, the intervention is working *toward* protection by maintaining attachment relationships. In assessing hierarchy of need and planning interventions, the 4-tier explanatory model is useful (Figure 25.1). Having identified the focus of work, working toward protection is a time-limited trial of the parents' capacity to change and sustain change, with support. Child protective services will determine when failure of a sustained change indicates the need to provide the children with alternative permanent care (Cyr *et al.*, 2022). Age at alternative permanent placement is related

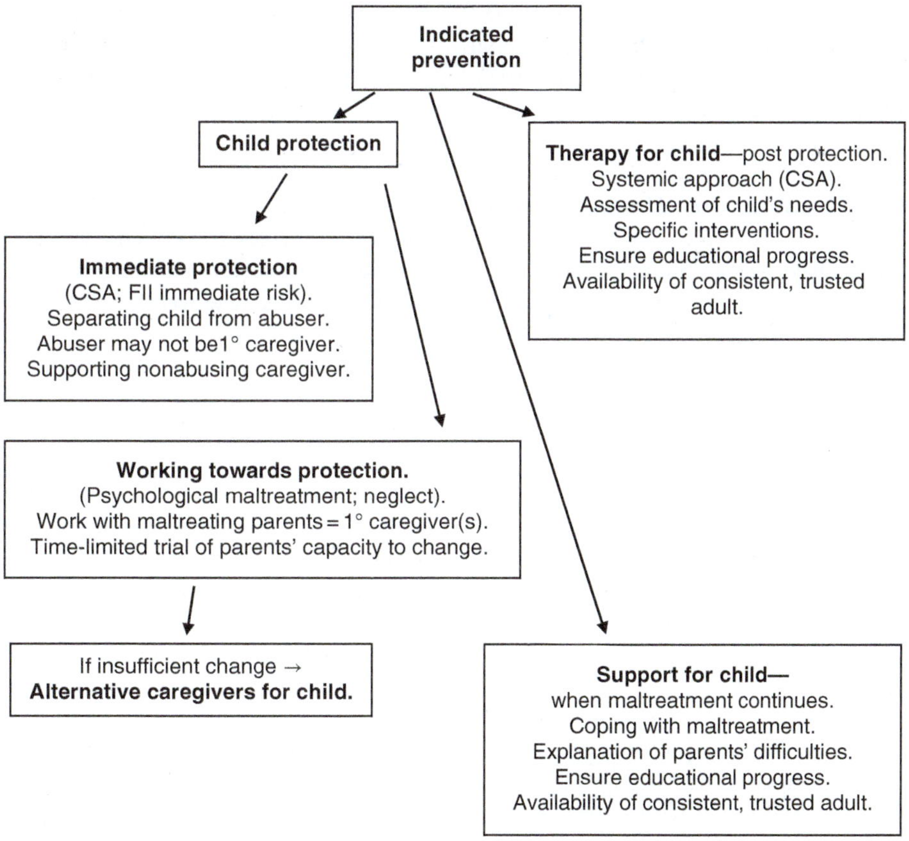

Figure 25.2 Indicated prevention.

to severity of emotional and behavioral difficulties (Burge, 2007).

Therapeutic work with caregivers and family (see also Chapter 36) depends on the form(s) of maltreatment. Arguably, it will be most effective with parents who are more differentially susceptible/sensitive (see orchids and dandelions in earlier "Child factors" section) (Van IJzendoorn *et al.*, 2020). With infants and young children, the maltreatment is often psychological or physical abuse and neglect, with associated disorganized attachment. Interventions for caregivers of young children are aimed at changing the maltreating caregiving with attendant improvement in the attachments (Toth *et al.*, 2013). The work focuses on parent and young child together, such as child–parent psychotherapy (CPP) (Alto *et al.*, 2021), attachment and biobehavioral catch-up (ABC) (Bernard *et al.*, 2012), or a brief attachment-based intervention using video feedback (Moss *et al.*, 2011), which enables parents to reflect on their own past as well as improving their sensitive responsiveness to their child. There is a good evidence base for these interventions, while evidence for some widely used therapies is lacking (Wright *et al.*, 2023). For parents of children up to secondary school age, parenting interventions and parent–child interaction therapy (Thomas & Zimmer-Gembeck, 2011) are recommended (NICE, 2017), the latter based on both attachment and social learning theories and also addressing physical abuse. Multisystemic therapy for child abuse and neglect (MST-CAN) (Buderer *et al.*, 2020) has been found to reduce neglect. Some of the categories of emotional abuse require more specific work with the parents (Glaser, 2011). The child's school attendance and educational progress also need to be ensured.

Indicated prevention: treating the effects of harm

Sexual abuse

Fulfilling the child's immediate needs requires a relationship with caregivers who are not blaming the child and believe her/his account. The caregiver(s) often feels guilt for not protecting the child, having divided loyalties between the child and the abuser (who may be an adolescent brother), sometimes losing of the relationship with the abuser, and possible reawakening of their own previous abuse. They therefore require early therapeutic support. Direct work with the child should be based on symptoms included in the ACC and ACA (Tarren-Sweeney, 2007, 2013). Trauma-focused CBT has a strong evidence base (Wang *et al.*, 2023). Both individual and group work for children and caregivers is useful.

Child maltreatment

As there is no consistently recognizable post-maltreatment syndrome, work with children and adolescents who have been maltreated is based on their particular symptoms and difficulties, which may be additional to effects of maltreatment, such as ASD. Difficulties require a thorough, systemic, and often extended, assessment (see earlier section on "The harm: symptoms and disorders") which needs to take into account the effects of the child's current, possibly unstable, placement with lack of consistent attachment persons. Some children require immediate help with acute distress or post-traumatic stress.

Broadly, as well as addressing depression and anxiety, children may require specific help with PTSD and therapy to process the meaning of the maltreatment in terms of their self-view as well as the fact of having been maltreated by one's parents. Part of this work is constructing a coherent narrative of their experiences. Many of the children need help with affect regulation, emotion recognition, and peer relationships. All of these aspects will enhance educational progress. Much work will involve the child's family.

Some older children may remain living with the maltreating parents whose capacity to change is limited, for instance, due to substance misuse or fluctuating mental illness. These children require particular support to cope with their situation. This includes explanations about the nature of their parents' difficulties, dealing with a sense of shame or guilt, opportunities to talk about their predicament, ensuring continued education, and, most importantly, having a sustained relationship with a trusted adult.

The discreet aspects of protective and therapeutic work involve several professionals and agencies including health, social services, education, and the law. Close coordination of work among the professionals, as well as with the caregivers and the child, is required of this multiagency work.

Conclusions

Child maltreatment is universal and common. It is both a children's rights matter and a public health issue. Its harm extends to the long term and is largely psychological and behavioral, variously affecting all aspects of the child's functioning. Beyond prevention by reducing risk factors, there is a need for early recognition and intervention, to protect the child, mitigate the harm, and prevent further maltreatment. Some children will necessarily be moved from their birth families, which adds a further layer of difficulty, particularly if the children are repeatedly moved. Much of the intervention is rightly focused on supporting caregivers to enable sensitive caregiving. Interventions are complex, costly, and require interprofessional cooperation and multiagency coordination.

CAMHS play an important role in the management of child maltreatment in various situations. Emotional abuse and neglect may be observable during consultations. They may be requested for an opinion regarding the provenance of a child's emotional or behavioral difficulties or to assess the nature and extent of harm to the child. CAMHS may be involved in work with parents to change maltreating behavior. Treating the child for effects of maltreatment is a central task for CAMHS. Lastly, CAMHS professionals may provide expert evidence about all these aspects.

References

Alink, L.R. *et al.* (2019) The effect of maltreatment experiences on maltreating and dysfunctional parenting: a search for mechanisms. *Development and Psychopathology* **31**(1), 1–7.

Alto, M.E. *et al.* (2021) Longitudinal outcomes of child parent psychotherapy: response to commentaries. *Research on Child and Adolescent Psychopathology* **49**, 595–601.

Anda, R.F. *et al.* (2006) The enduring effects of abuse and related adverse experiences in childhood: a convergence of evidence from neurobiology and epidemiology. *European Archives of Psychiatry and Clinical Neuroscience* **256**, 174–186.

Baldwin, J.R. & Danese, A. (2021) Research, practice, and policy implications of adverse childhood events—reply. *JAMA Pediatrics* **175**(8), 867–868. doi:10.1001/jamapediatrics.2021.0813.

Bernard, K. *et al.* (2012) Enhancing attachment organization among maltreated children: results of a randomized clinical trial. *Child Development* **83**, 623–636.

Blumenthal, A. (2023) A bad time for kids in lockdown: the relationship between negative pandemic events, parenting stress, and maltreatment related parenting behaviors. *Child Abuse & Neglect* **138**, 106060.

Boyce, W.T. (2019) *The Orchid and the Dandelion: Why Sensitive People Struggle and How All Can Thrive*. Pan MacMillan, London.

Buderer, C. *et al.* (2020) Effects of multisystemic therapy for child abuse and neglect on severity of neglect, behavioral and emotional problems, and attachment disorder symptoms in children. *Children and Youth Services Review* **119**, 105626.

Bullinger, L.R. & Boy, A. (2023) Association of expanded child tax credit payments with child abuse and neglect emergency department visits. *JAMA Network Open* **6**(2), e2255639–e2255639.

Burge, P. (2007) Prevalence of mental disorders and associated service variables among Ontario children who are permanent wards. *The Canadian Journal of Psychiatry* **52**(5), 305–314.

Bywaters, P. & Skinner, G. (2022) *The Relationship Between Poverty and Child Abuse and Neglect: New Evidence*. Nuffield Foundation, London.

Cecil, C. *et al.* (2017) Disentangling the mental health impact of childhood abuse and neglect. *Child Abuse & Neglect* **63**, 106–119.

Chopin, J. *et al.* (2022) Childhood victimization and poly-victimization of online sexual offenders: a developmental psychopathology perspective. *Child Abuse & Neglect* **129**, 105659.

CSA Centre (2022) Communicating with children: a guide for those working with children who have or may have been sexually abused. Available: www.csacentre.org.uk [20 September 2024].

Cyr, C. *et al.* (2022) An attachment-based parental capacity assessment to orient decision-making in child protection cases: a randomized control trial. *Child Maltreatment* **27**(1), 66–77.

Danese, A. & Widom, C.S. (2020) Objective and subjective experiences of child maltreatment and their relationships with psychopathology. *Nature Human Behaviour* **4**, 811–818.

Danese, A. & Widom, C.S. (2023) *Associations between objective and subjective experiences of childhood maltreatment and the course of emotional disorders in adulthood. JAMA Psychiatry*, Vol. 80. pp. 1009–1016.

Davies, S.L. *et al.* (2000) Children's sexual play and behavior in preschool settings: staff's perceptions, reports, and responses. *Child Abuse & Neglect* **24**(10), 1329–1343.

De Bellis, M. *et al.* (1999) Developmental traumatology part II: brain development. *Biological Psychiatry* **45**(10), 1271–1284.

DeJong, M. (2010) Some reflections on the use of psychiatric diagnosis in the looked after or 'in care' child population. *Clinical Child Psychology and Psychiatry* **15**(4), 589–599.

DeJong, M. & Wilkinson, S. (2019) Assessment of mental health problems in children following early maltreatment: what will the new diagnosis of complex PTSD add? *Developmental Child Welfare* **1**(4), 360–373.

Dutra, L. *et al.* (2009) Quality of early care and childhood trauma: a prospective study of developmental pathways to dissociation. *The Journal of Nervous and Mental Disease* **197**, 383.

Ellis, B.J. *et al.* (2022) Hidden talents in harsh environments. *Development and Psychopathology* **34**(1), 95–113.

Faller, K.C. (2005) False accusations of child maltreatment: a contested issue. *Child Abuse & Neglect* **29**(12), 1327–1331.

Fries, A.B. *et al.* (2005) Early experience in humans is associated with changes in neuropeptides critical for regulating social behavior. *Proceedings of the National Academy of Sciences of the United States of America* **102**(47), 17237–17240.

Gilbert, R. *et al.* (2009) Burden and consequences of child maltreatment in high-income countries. *The Lancet* **373**(9657), 68–81.

Glaser, D. (2011) How to deal with emotional abuse and neglect: further development of a conceptual framework (FRAMEA). *Child Abuse & Neglect* **35**(10), 866–875.

Glaser, D. (2020) Fabricated or induced illness: from "Munchausen by proxy" to child and family-oriented action. *Child Abuse & Neglect* **108**, 104649.

Gunnar, M.R. & Donzella, B. (2002) Social regulation of the cortisol levels in early human development. *Psychoneuroendocrinology* **27**(1–2), 199–220.

Hamby, S. *et al.* (2004) *The Comprehensive JVQ Administration and Scoring Manual*. University of New Hampshire, Crimes Against Children Research Centre, Durham, NH.

Hertzman, C. (1999) The biological embedding of early experience and its effects on health in adulthood. *Annals of the New York Academy of Sciences* **896**(1), 85–95.

Hillis, S. *et al.* (2016) Global prevalence of past-year violence against children: a systematic review and minimum estimates. *Pediatrics* **137**(3), e20154079.

HM Government (2023) *Working Together to Safeguard Children 2023*. HM Government, London, UK.

Jud, A. *et al.* (2016) On the incidence and prevalence of child maltreatment: a research agenda. *Child and Adolescent Psychiatry and Mental Health* **10**(1), 1–5.

Karsna, K. & Bromley, P. (2023) *Child Sexual Abuse in 2021/22: Trends in Official Data*. Centre of Expertise on Child Sexual Abuse, Barkingside, UK.

Keary, K. & Fitzpatrick, C. (1994) Children's disclosure of sexual abuse during formal investigation. *Child Abuse & Neglect* **18**(7), 543–548.

Kisely, S. *et al.* (2018) Child maltreatment and mental health problems in adulthood: birth cohort study. *The British Journal of Psychiatry* **213**(6), 698–703.

Koss, K.J. & Gunnar, M.R. (2018) Annual research review: early adversity, the hypothalamic–pituitary–adrenocortical axis, and child psychopathology. *Journal of Child Psychology and Psychiatry* **59**(4), 327–346.

Laajasalo, T. *et al.* (2023) Current issues and challenges in the definition and operationalization of child maltreatment: a scoping review. *Child Abuse & Neglect* **140**, 106187.

Lamb, M.E. *et al.* (2007) A structured forensic interview protocol improves the quality and informativeness of investigative interviews with children: a review of research using the NICHD investigative interview protocol. *Child Abuse & Neglect* **31**(11), 1201–1231.

Lauder, J.M. (1983) Hormonal and humoral influences on brain development. *Psychoneuroendocrinology* **8**(2), 121–155.

Lawless, J. & Tarren-Sweeney, M. (2022) Alignment of borderline personality disorder and complex post-traumatic stress disorder with complex developmental symptomatology. *Journal of Child & Adolescent Trauma* **16**, 1–14.

Lee, H. & Kim, E. (2022) Global prevalence of physical and psychological child abuse during COVID-19: a systematic review and meta-analysis. *Child Abuse & Neglect* **135**, 105984.

Lee, C. *et al.* (2017) Social disadvantage, severe child abuse, and biological profiles in adulthood. *Journal of Health and Social Behavior* **58**(3), 371–386.

Lewis, S.J. *et al.* (2021) Unravelling the contribution of complex trauma to psychopathology and cognitive deficits: a cohort study. *The British Journal of Psychiatry* **219**(2), 448–455.

Li, Y. *et al.* (2019) Exploring the mutual regulation between oxytocin and cortisol as a marker of resilience. *Archives of Psychiatric Nursing* **33**(2), 164–173.

Liu, R.T. *et al.* (2018) Childhood maltreatment and non-suicidal self-injury: a systematic review and meta-analysis. *The Lancet Psychiatry* **5**(1), 51–64.

Mackes, N.K. *et al.* (2020) Early childhood deprivation is associated with alterations in adult brain structure despite subsequent environmental enrichment. *Proceedings of the National Academy of Sciences of the United States of America* **117**, 641–649.

Magalhães, E. & Camilo, C. (2023) Maltreatment history and internalizing and externalizing symptoms in out-of-home care: a three-level Meta-analysis. *The European Journal of Psychology Applied to Legal Context* **15**(2), 89–103.

Malave, L. *et al.* (2022) Early life adversity shapes neural circuit function during sensitive postnatal developmental periods. *Translational Psychiatry* **12**, 306.

Masten, A.S. (2019) Resilience from a developmental systems perspective. *World Psychiatry* **18**(1), 101.

McCrory, E.J. *et al.* (2017) Annual research review: childhood maltreatment, latent vulnerability and the shift to preventative psychiatry–the contribution of functional brain imaging. *Journal of Child Psychology and Psychiatry* **58**(4), 338–357.

McCrory, E. *et al.* (2019) Neurocognitive adaptation and mental health vulnerability following maltreatment: the role of social functioning. *Child Maltreatment* **24**(4), 435–451.

McLaughlin, K.A. & Gabard-Durnam, L. (2022) Experience-driven plasticity and the emergence of psychopathology: a mechanistic framework integrating development and the environment into the Research Domain Criteria (RDoC) model. *Journal of Psychopathology and Clinical Science* **131**(6), 575.

Meng, X. *et al.* (2018) Resilience and protective factors among people with a history of child maltreatment: a systematic review. *Social Psychiatry and Psychiatric Epidemiology* **53**, 453–475.

Moss, E. *et al.* (2011) Efficacy of a home visiting intervention aimed at improving maternal sensitivity, child attachment, and behavioral outcomes for maltreated children: a randomized control trial. *Development and Psychopathology* **23**, 195–210.

Neil, L. *et al.* (2022) Trust and childhood maltreatment: evidence of bias in appraisal of unfamiliar faces. *Journal of Child Psychology and Psychiatry* **63**(6), 655–662.

NICE (2009) Child maltreatment: when to suspect maltreatment in under 18s. National Institute for Health and Care Excellence, London. Available: https://www.nice.org.uk/guidance/CG89/ [20 September 2024].

NICE (2017) Child abuse and neglect. National Institute for Health and Care Excellence, London. Available: https://www.nice.org.uk/guidance/ng76 [20 September 2024].

Park, W.J. & Walsh, K.A. (2022) COVID-19 and the unseen pandemic of child abuse. *BMJ Paediatrics Open* **6**(1), e001553.

Pinheiro, P.S. (2006) *World Report on Violence Against Children*. United Nations, Geneva, Switzerland.

Pinto Pereira, S.M. *et al.* (2021) Adult retrospective report of child abuse and prospective indicators of childhood harm: a population birth cohort study. *BMC Medicine* **19**(1), 1–11.

Pollak, S.D. *et al.* (2009) Development of perceptual expertise in emotion recognition. *Cognition* **110**(2), 242–247.

Prevoo, M.J. *et al.* (2017) Methodological moderators in prevalence studies on child maltreatment: review of a series of meta-analyses. *Child Abuse Review* **26**, 141–157.

Radford, L. *et al.* (2013) The prevalence and impact of child maltreatment and other types of victimization in the UK: findings from a population survey of caregivers, children and young people and young adults. *Child Abuse & Neglect* **37**(10), 801–813.

Raz, M. *et al.* (2023) Using child abuse specialists to reduce unnecessary child protective services reports and investigations. *JAMA Pediatrics* **177**(12), 1249–1250. doi:10.1001/jamapediatrics.2023.3676.

RCPCH (2021) *Perplexing Presentations (PP)/Fabricated or Induced Illness (FII) in Children*. Royal College of Paediatrics and Child Health, London.

Romano, E. *et al.* (2015) Childhood maltreatment and educational outcomes. *Trauma, Violence, & Abuse* **16**(4), 418–437.

Rutter, M. (2002) Nature, nurture, and development: from evangelism through science toward policy and practice. *Child Development* **73**(1), 1–21.

Shonkoff, J.P. *et al.* (2009) Neuroscience, molecular biology, and the childhood roots of health disparities: building a new framework for health promotion and disease prevention. *JAMA* **301**(21), 2252–2259.

Shonkoff, J.P. *et al.* (2012) The lifelong effects of early childhood adversity and toxic stress. *Pediatrics* **129**(1), e232–e246.

Slep, A.M.S. *et al.* (2022) Psychological maltreatment: an operationalized definition and path toward application. *Child Abuse and Neglect* **134**, 105882.

Smith, K.E. & Pollak, S.D. (2021) Rethinking concepts and categories for understanding the neurodevelopmental effects of childhood adversity. *Perspectives on Psychological Science* **16**(1), 67–93.

Struck, N. *et al.* (2020) Childhood maltreatment and adult mental disorders: the prevalence of different types of maltreatment and associations with age of onset and severity of symptoms. *Psychiatry Research* **293**, 113398.

Sullivan, P.M. & Knutson, J.F. (2000) Maltreatment and disabilities: a population-based epidemiological study. *Child Abuse & Neglect* **24**(10), 1257–1273.

Tarren-Sweeney, M. (2007) The assessment checklist for children—ACC: a behavioral rating scale for children in foster, kinship and residential care. *Children and Youth Services Review* **29**, 672–691.

Tarren-Sweeney, M. (2013) The assessment checklist for adolescents—ACA: a scale for measuring the mental health of young people in foster kinship residential and adoptive care. *Children and Youth Services Review* **35**(3), 384–393.

Tarren-Sweeney, M. (2021) Mental health symptom profiles of adolescents in foster care. *Journal of Child & Adolescent Trauma*, 1–13.

Teicher, M.H. *et al.* (2016) Annual research review. Enduring neurobiological effects of childhood abuse and neglect. *Journal of Child Psychology and Psychiatry* **57**(3), 241–266.

Teicher, M. *et al.* (2003) The neurobiological consequences of early stress and childhood maltreatment. *Neuroscience and Biobehavioral Reviews* **27**(1–2), 33–44.

Thomas, R. & Zimmer-Gembeck, M.J. (2011) Accumulating evidence for parent–child interaction therapy in the prevention of child maltreatment. *Child Development* **82**, 177–192.

Tobon, A.L. *et al.* (2022) School age effects of minding the baby—an attachment-based home-visiting intervention—on parenting and child behaviors. *Development and Psychopathology* **34**(1), 55–67.

Toth, S.L. *et al.* (2013) Relational interventions for child maltreatment: past, present, and future perspectives. *Development and Psychopathology* **25**(4pt2), 1601–1617.

Tottenham, N. *et al.* (2011) Elevated amygdala response to faces following early deprivation. *Developmental Science* **14**(2), 190–204.

Turner, H.A. (2010) Poly-victimization in a national sample of children and youth. *American Journal of Preventive Medicine* **38**(3), 323–330.

UN (1989) *Convention on the Rights of the Child.* United Nations, New York.

Van IJzendoorn, M.H. *et al.* (2020) Umbrella synthesis of meta-analyses on child maltreatment antecedents and interventions: differential susceptibility perspective on risk and resilience. *Journal of Child Psychology and Psychiatry* **61**(3), 272–290.

Wadji, D.L. *et al.* (2023) Associations between experiences of childhood maltreatment and perceived acceptability of child maltreatment: a cross-cultural and exploratory study. *Child Abuse & Neglect* **143**, 106270.

Wang, W. *et al.* (2023) Effectiveness of trauma-focused cognitive behavioral therapy among maltreated children: a meta-analysis. *Research on Social Work Practice* **33**(8), 913–928.

Wilkinson, S. *et al.* (2023) Assessing autism spectrum disorder in children with a background of maltreatment: challenges and guidance. *Archives of Disease in Childhood* **108**(8), 597–600.

Wolstencroft, J. *et al.* (2023) Can we distinguish the consequences of early maltreatment on child behaviour from idiopathic autism? *Archives of Disease in Childhood* **108**, 392–397.

World Health Organization (WHO) (2006) The prevention of child maltreatment. In: *Preventing Child Maltreatment: A Guide to Taking Action and Generating Evidence.* World Health Organization (WHO) and International Society for Prevention of Child Abuse and Neglect (ISPCAN), Geneva, Switzerland. pp. 32–49.

Wright, B. *et al.* (2023) Routinely used interventions to improve attachment in infants and young children: a national survey and two systematic reviews. *Health Technology Assessment* **27**(2).

Yazgan, M. *et al.* (1995) Functional significance of individual variations in callosal area. *Neuropsychologia* **33**(6), 769–779.

Zhang, X. *et al.* (2023) Beyond orchids and dandelions: susceptibility to environmental influences is not bimodal. *Development and Psychopathology* **35**(1), 191–203.

CHAPTER 26

Neurological disorders and psychopathology

Isobel Heyman[1], David Skuse[1] and Ashley Liew[2,3]

[1] Great Ormond Street Institute of Child Health, University College London, London, UK

[2] South London and Maudsley NHS Foundation Trust, London, UK

[3] University of Warwick, Warwick, UK

The concepts and conditions discussed in this chapter, as well as throughout this textbook, should dispel any notion that a dichotomy exists between "brain" and "mind," or between "neurology" and "psychiatry," fallacies that have been perpetuated since the concept of mind–body dualism was argued by Descartes in the 17th century. Nevertheless, most health care services persist in treating neurological disorders and mental/psychiatric disorders as though they are conceptually distinct conditions and this is reflected in both training, staffing, and facilities. Fortunately, a paradigm shift is beginning, toward integration. The emergence of integrated care services for brain-based disorders, like epilepsy and brain injuries, has already provided evidence for better outcomes, efficiencies, economics, and safety, as well as an improved experience for children and their families. At its most basic level, integration is reflected in better interprofessional communication and co-location of services, but, in due course, should lead to a situation in which child and adolescent psychiatrists and others from a multidisciplinary mental health service work closely with pediatricians or pediatric neurologists and their clinical teams (Fazel *et al.*, 2021). Building the foundations of such integrated services is critical, and a successful model is provided by Triple Board certification in Pediatrics, Psychiatry, and Child Psychiatry in the United States of America (USA). Reflecting on the benefits of joint training and service provision, we aim, within this chapter, to provide supportive evidence for both clinicians and researchers in child and adolescent psychiatry to consider when managing pediatric neurological disorders. A main goal is to ensure that children with neurological conditions get timely, accessible, and effective mental health treatment when it is needed (Box 26.1)

Epidemiology

Rutter's landmark epidemiological studies on the Isle of Wight were some of the first research studies to demonstrate that psychiatric disorders were more prevalent in children with physical disorders, and that these rates were much higher in those who had brain-based disorders like epilepsy and cerebral palsy (Rutter *et al.*, 1976). More contemporary population studies have not only demonstrated rates of 80% for mental health disorders in children with active epilepsy, but also that two-thirds of the children had not received relevant diagnoses (Reilly *et al.*, 2014), suggesting possible diagnostic overshadowing, which may occur across children with epilepsy and other neurological disorders. The most common comorbid mental disorders in epilepsy are neurodevelopmental conditions like intellectual disability (ID), attention deficit hyperactivity disorder (ADHD), and autism spectrum disorder (ASD), which occur in 20–40% of children with epilepsy. The rate of psychiatric symptoms is even higher in neuroinflammatory conditions, like autoimmune encephalitis, where during acute presentations, almost 90% of cases will display mental health symptoms. Symptoms include emotional lability, repetitive behaviors, and visual hallucinations; and more than one-third of children have psychiatric symptoms in the long term (Nguyen *et al.*, 2022). Depression and anxiety are common mental health disorders in childhood which have been identified as global public health issues due to their contribution to the risk of mental disorders in adulthood. Despite children with neurological disorders making up less than 5% of the child population, they may represent 15–18% of those in population samples with depression and anxiety

Rutter's Child and Adolescent Psychiatry and Psychology, Seventh Edition.
Edited by Anita Thapar, Daniel S. Pine, Samuele Cortese, Cathy Creswell, Tamsin J. Ford, James F. Leckman, and Argyris Stringaris.

Companion website: www.wiley.com/go/thapar/rutterspsych7

Box 26.1 Key points to an integrated approach

- Children with neurological conditions have increased rates of mental and neurodevelopmental disorders (NDDs).
- Always consider detection and diagnosis of these coexisting mental disorders when seeing a child with a neurological disorder.
- These children should receive the standard evidence-based mental health treatments—taking into account any medical interaction with their neurological condition and tailoring psychological treatments to their developmental needs.

(Whitney *et al.*, 2019c), suggesting both clinical and financial value in diagnosing and treating mental disorders in this group of children. It has therefore been suggested that children with a neurological disorder receive routine screening for mental ill health (Downs *et al.*, 2018).

Mechanisms

Genetic factors

The evidence that brain disorders arising from genetic risk lead directly to specific childhood psychopathology is largely circumstantial. Recent research with animal models for genetic risk are beginning to illuminate causal mechanisms (Teal *et al.*, 2023; see Chapter 21). Neurological disorders in childhood can be caused by a variety of genetic risk factors, some of which are due to spontaneous mutations in parental autosomes or sex chromosomes, or to anomalies that are transmitted by both parents. For instance, familial forms of epilepsy can be inherited in different ways depending on the specific genetic mutation involved. Forms of familial epilepsy resulting from autosomal dominant inheritance include benign familial neonatal epilepsy and other familial focal epilepsies (Gooley *et al.*, 2022). Rarely, epilepsies have autosomal recessive inheritance. Other conditions result from X-linked inheritance (mutations on the X chromosome), hence the disorder is usually more common in males than females. A few epilepsy syndromes are caused by mutations in mitochondrial DNA. Affected mothers can pass the disorder to both sons and daughters, but affected fathers cannot pass it to their children. Examples of epilepsy syndromes with mitochondrial inheritance include myoclonic epilepsy with ragged-red fibers (MERRF) and mitochondrial encephalomyopathy, lactic acidosis, and stroke-like episodes (MELAS). It is important to note that while familial forms of epilepsy can be inherited, many cases of epilepsy are not due to a single genetic mutation, but instead involve complex interactions between multiple genes (polygenic risk) and environmental factors. In a relatively common group of patients with a familial focal epilepsy due to mutations in genes related to GAATOR1 and the mTOR pathway, there are implications for management, prognosis, and genetic counseling (Gooley *et al.*, 2022). Testing for specific epilepsy or other neurological disorder-related genes is not currently available in all clinical centers. The child psychiatrist needs to be aware of rapid genetic advances being made in neurological fields such as epilepsy, and to collaborate with colleagues where appropriate to consider these aspects.

Perinatal factors

The perinatal period refers to pregnancy, childbirth, and the first year of the child's postnatal development. During this time, several factors can increase the likelihood of a child developing a neurological disorder. Preterm birth (<37 completed weeks) is associated with increased incidence of neurological disorders, such as cerebral palsy and developmental delays, as well as neurodevelopmental conditions including autism. Preterm birthrates are rising and are currently up to 10% of live births worldwide. The earlier a child is born, the greater the risk of neurological impairment, and this escalates substantially for infants born before 28 weeks' gestation. Although the incidence of more severe conditions, such as cerebral palsy, blindness, and deafness, in this particularly vulnerable group has fallen in recent years (due to innovations in neonatal care), poor cognitive outcomes (especially in terms of executive functions) remain unchanged (Cheong *et al.*, 2020). Being born with a low birth weight is another significant risk factor for developmental delays and learning disabilities (Silva *et al.*, 2021), as is birth asphyxia.

Other perinatal factors that put infants at risk of neurological complications include specific infections during pregnancy, such as rubella, cytomegalovirus, and toxoplasmosis (Bălălău *et al.*, 2020). These are especially likely to impact mothers in low- and middle-income countries (LMICs), as is maternal substance abuse, including alcohol, tobacco, and illicit drugs (Faruk *et al.*, 2020). Chronic maternal health conditions, such as diabetes and hypertension, increase the risk of neurological disorders in the developing fetus, as can some medications taken during pregnancy such as sodium valproate (Wartman & VandenBerg, 2022).

Medication for neurological conditions

Pharmacological treatments for child neurological disorders can have both desired therapeutic effects and potential side effects. The specific side effects depend on the medication used and the individual child's response to it. For instance, while drugs such as antiseizure medications (ASMs) can be effective in controlling seizures, they can also have side effects such as drowsiness, concentration difficulties, and memory problems. We discuss this further in the section on epilepsy. Cognitive difficulties in childhood epilepsy are often attributed in part to the effects of ASMs but the connection is not straightforward, and may be related to the underlying etiology, age of onset of the seizures, their frequency and location, and potentially the nature of associated epileptiform abnormalities (Nickels *et al.*, 2016).

How do neurological and nonneurological factors interact?

Vulnerability to environmental factors

Environmental factors can play a significant role in the risk of neurological disorders in children. These can be considered in the context of early development. First, there is the potential risk of prenatal exposure to maternal use of alcohol, tobacco, and medications, and substance misuse. In addition, in some circumstances, mothers will be inadvertently exposed to environmental toxins, such as lead. There is evidence of a weak placental–fetal barrier to lead, suggesting that maternal lead exposure potentially affects the fetus (Bui *et al.*, 2022). Many potential environmental sources of lead persist, even though petrol has been deleaded for nearly 50 years in the USA and United Kingdom (UK). Lead plumbing and lead paint dust still exist in older housing stock, for instance. There is substantial lifelong risk to cognitive development after childhood lead exposure, and in some countries lead exposure continues to be relatively common (Obeng-Gyasi, 2019). Organophosphate pesticides are another source of toxicity, especially in some LMICs, exposure in early pregnancy being associated with impaired infant cognitive development in the first postnatal year (Suwannakul *et al.*, 2021).

As discussed, certain infections during pregnancy, such as rubella, cytomegalovirus, and toxoplasmosis, have been linked to an increased risk of neurodevelopmental disorders (NDD) (Bergdolt & Dunaevsky, 2019). There is evidence that infection with the original SARS-CoV-2 Delta variant was associated with an increased risk of maternal mortality and morbidity, as well as neonatal morbidity, but not stillbirth or intrauterine growth retardation (Smith *et al.*, 2023). Zika virus exposure has been associated with microcephaly and a pattern of abnormalities described as Congenital Zika Syndrome (da Silva *et al.*, 2020). Maternal health and nutrition during pregnancy can have a significant impact on fetal brain development. Poor maternal nutrition, maternal obesity, and gestational diabetes have all been linked to an increased risk of NDDs.

There is increasing interest in the prospect that maternal immune activation during pregnancy can have an adverse impact on fetal neurodevelopment, and acts as a final common pathway for a wide variety of environmental adversities (Han *et al.*, 2021). Potentially, environmental factors including diet, exercise, sleep, socioeconomic status, stress, exposure to environmental pollutants, and the gut microbiome, have the capacity to alter the transcription of susceptibility genes by inducing pathological imprinting of the immune system (Gumusoglu & Stevens, 2019).

Sex differences

There is no one definitive answer to what mechanisms make males more vulnerable to neurological and NDDs in childhood, as the causes of these disorders can be complex and multifactorial (see Chapter 3). Furthermore, the magnitude of those sex differences in prevalence may be diminishing due to improved, less biased ascertainment. For instance, the male–female sex ratio in autism has fallen from 4:1 to less than 3:1 in recent years (Santos *et al.*, 2022). Several hypotheses and theories have been proposed. First, there are genetic differences where males may be more vulnerable to genetic mutations that affect the X chromosome, which can play a role in certain neurological or NDDs, especially those that are X-linked (Brand *et al.*, 2021). Second, a role could be played by prenatal exposure to testosterone, because the brains of male fetuses are exposed to higher levels of testosterone than female fetuses. While the hypothesis was strongly advocated in the past, current evidence that this mechanism could affect brain development and increase the risk of certain NDDs, such as autism, has little empirical support (Carlsson *et al.*, 2021). Males may be more susceptible to environmental factors that can affect brain development, such as exposure to toxins such as lead, mercury, and certain pesticides, especially during the prenatal period, which can affect brain development and increase the risk of neurological and NDDs (DiPietro & Voegtline, 2017).

Differences in patterns of brain development between males and females may contribute to the differential risk. Certain brain regions develop differently in males and females, and these differences may play a role in the susceptibility to certain neurological disorders. For example, there are replicable differences in the corpus callosum which tends to be larger in females than in males, the amygdala which may be larger in males than in females, and the cerebellum which may develop more rapidly in males than in females. Some studies have shown that the prefrontal cortex may develop more slowly in males than in females, and that there are sex differences in brain functional connectivity in both the prefrontal and limbic regions (Bölte *et al.*, 2023).

While there is no doubt that males in general are more vulnerable to some neurodevelopmental conditions, there is also increasing evidence that males are more likely to be diagnosed with certain disorders simply because they exhibit more visible or disruptive symptoms, while females may exhibit more subtle or internalized symptoms that are less likely to be recognized as a disorder (Hollingdale *et al.*, 2022).

Impact of mental disorders in children with neurological disorders

It is not unusual in the clinic to hear families describe how they are used to coping with their child's neurological disorder—seizures, mobility difficulties, and other issues; but the new onset of low mood, anxiety, refusal to attend school, or other emotional and behavioral difficulties have created a new and disruptive set of problems. The impact on the child's social, educational, emotional, and behavioral well-being can be more impairing than the physical condition itself (Baca *et al.*, 2011). Studies have shown that children who have both physical and mental health needs remain in hospital for much longer, have repeated admissions, and their care is more costly than for children with physical health problems only (Zima *et al.*, 2016).

In our clinical practice, we often encounter children with severe, but unrecognized specific learning difficulties (see Chapter 52)—these are more common in children with neurological disorders. Because the nature of the cognitive deficits is not obvious (and may be uncovered only by specialist testing) they may go unrecognized. The child cannot keep up with his or her lessons, and that engenders marked frustration with schooling, leading on to defiant and disruptive behavior in class. Specific learning problems and below-average intelligence are common psychoeducational correlates of neurological abnormalities (e.g., Rutter *et al.*, 1970; Sorg *et al.*, 2022). There is often a direct link between the impact of the underlying neurological disorder on neural functioning and impaired cognitive processing. On the other hand, risk is sometimes aggravated by restricted educational opportunities, lower expectations, and lengthy absences from school for therapy or operations. For children with epilepsy, their cognitive and scholastic skills can be disrupted not only by clinical and subclinical seizures, but also by the effects of antiepileptic medication.

The presence of a neurological disorder might also lead to mental health difficulties as a consequence of parental overprotectiveness, or from inconsistent discipline provided by a parent who is suffering guilt because they blame themselves for their child's neurological disorder. The capacity of parents to inflict blame on themselves (or on their child's medical care), based on the most tenuous of presumed causal events, is remarkable and must be addressed by clinicians. Parents of children with long-term health conditions, and especially epilepsy, are known to have high rates of stress and mental health needs (Reilly *et al.*, 2018), and also experience stigma (Song *et al.*, 2018). The beliefs and attitudes of the family and the wider social world also have a major impact on emotions and behavior in the child. Parents, teachers, and peers respond to a child with a neurological disorder in the light of their beliefs and prejudices. These beliefs influence the likelihood of overprotection, peer rejection, and unrealistic expectations. Unhelpful attitudes about the nature of their child's condition can interfere with parents' abilities to set limits to unacceptable behaviors. Some parents assume that all bad behavior is driven by the neurological abnormality and that it is therefore beyond the child's control. Others fear that any reproof will trigger off an epileptic seizure and further damage the child's brain. Family relationships can be disrupted for other reasons as well. Sibling rivalry, for example, can be fueled by the resentment of disabled children who see themselves being overtaken by younger siblings, or by the resentment of nondisabled siblings who feel they are missing out on parental attention. These are only a few of the many possible psychosocial pathways from neurological disorders to child psychiatric difficulties. In a recent study of children with epilepsy, factors that most compromised quality of life included impaired cognitive ability and disrupted family functioning (Puka *et al.*, 2020).

In summary, neurological disorders can have a multitude of psychosocial consequences. Physical disabilities can result in teasing, poor self-image, and reduced opportunities for peer interaction. Repeated hospitalizations may disrupt friendships and predispose to behavioral disorders, perhaps as a result of repeated separations from family. Many neurological disorders also have behavioral consequences, especially poor attention, hyperactivity, and an impaired ability to decipher social and emotional cues. While these consequences are relatively nonspecific, they may, in turn, have adverse effects on family relationships, as well as the ability to make and sustain friendships at school and elsewhere outside the home.

Psychiatric consequences of specific neurological disorders

Epilepsy

Epilepsy is the most common neurological disorder in childhood, affecting up to 1% of children. The cornerstone of diagnosis remains a careful clinical history, although this is increasingly supplemented by videos recorded by parents/carers. An electroencephalogram (EEG) may also be helpful and even diagnostic in certain epilepsy syndromes (e.g., childhood absence epilepsy) but it is important to bear in mind that up to 8% of healthy children may display nonspecific changes on the EEG. A contemporary clinical approach also aims to identify possible underlying causes, as this may lead to more precise individualized treatments like epilepsy surgery, or the use or avoidance of certain ASMs. Increasingly, magnetic resonance imaging (MRI) and other imaging modalities (e.g., magnetoencephalography (MEG)) may be used (e.g., to identify focal cortical dysplasia, which can be resected surgically), or genetic testing including specific epilepsy gene panels (e.g., to identify Dravet Syndrome, a rare genetic epileptic encephalopathy), which may open up access to specific treatments. Consequently, the current international classification of seizures attempts to classify more defined epilepsy syndromes on the basis of etiology, clinical, and EEG features, as well as prognosis (Specchio *et al.*, 2022b). Importantly for child and adolescent psychiatrists, it also aims to describe significant intellectual, psychiatric, and other comorbidities associated with each syndrome.

Psychiatrists may also become involved in the diagnostic process to distinguish possible nonepileptic seizures (also known as functional seizures—see Chapter 69). This may prove a challenging task since many children with functional seizures will also have epileptic seizures, and certain epilepsy types (e.g., frontal lobe epilepsy) can present with unusual features which mimic behaviors associated with functional seizures. A collaborative multidisciplinary approach with the neurologist/pediatrician and family is essential so that a positive diagnosis of functional seizures is made on the basis of features that support the diagnosis, rather than a process which may include multiple investigations to result in a diagnosis of exclusion (Vassilopoulos *et al.*, 2022).

Comorbid neurodevelopmental disorders

ADHD occurs in about one-third of children with active epilepsy (Reilly *et al.*, 2014) and does show some differences compared to ADHD in the general population. For example, studies suggest a more equal gender ratio and that the predominantly inattentive subtype occurs more frequently compared to the hyperactive/impulsive subtype. Consequently, ADHD is less likely to be identified in children with epilepsy compared to the general population, and also less likely to be treated with stimulant medication. Children with ADHD and epilepsy are also typically younger when seizures commence and are more likely to progress to have more frequent seizures (Dunn *et al.*, 2016). These may be some of the factors, along with the fallacy that stimulants greatly worsen seizures, that lead to reduced rates of treatment.

ASD occurs in about 21% of children with active epilepsy (Reilly *et al.*, 2014) and there is a bidirectional relationship where children with ASD also have higher rates of epilepsy (Kwon *et al.*, 2022). This significant association between ASD and epilepsy is probably due to a number of shared causes including perinatal factors (e.g., congenital rubella), genetic variants (e.g., sodium channelopathies like SCN1A), and metabolic conditions (e.g., Sanfilippo syndrome and other lysosomal storage disorders), which lead to neuronal dysfunction (e.g., excessive synaptic growth or anomalous synaptic plasticity) (Specchio *et al.*, 2022a). One particular example is tuberous sclerosis where rates of epilepsy and ASD are much higher than the general population and where the underlying mechanism of dysfunction in the mammalian target of rapamycin (mTOR) pathway appears to be a shared risk factor. There is emerging evidence that the degree of ASD symptoms may correlate with the severity of mTOR overactivation and that treatment using an mTOR inhibitor may result in improvements in both the epilepsy and ASD profiles of affected children (Mizuguchi *et al.*, 2019).

Comorbid anxiety, depression, and psychosis

The risk of anxiety and depression in children with epilepsy is increased in association with a lower IQ and language delays. Age of seizure onset and seizure type have not been observed consistently to be risk factors for anxiety and depression, but persistence of seizures compared to more stable seizure control has been noted to be a risk factor. The latter observation may be related to shared neurobiological mechanisms but may also be related to increased social anxiety about having a seizure in public, or separation anxiety from being apart from parents or carers. There may also be a systemic impact from parental anxiety about the child with epilepsy engaging in risky activities or being alone (Dagar & Falcone, 2020). A higher seizure frequency in juvenile myoclonic epilepsy appears to correlate with the severity of anxiety symptoms, as well as impacts on psychosocial functioning (Paiva *et al.*, 2020). Depression symptoms may also be a side effect of some ASMs like phenobarbital, levetiracetam, and topiramate. Psychosis has been reported in adolescents during both the postictal and interictal phases, whereas ictal psychosis (as seen in adults) has not been well described in children. The concepts of alternative/reciprocal psychosis (where clinically, psychosis worsens when seizures improve) or forced normalization (where psychosis worsens when the EEG appearance has improved or resolved) remain controversial, typically when confounded by the presence of ASM which may have adverse effects resembling psychotic symptoms. Both topiramate and vigabatrin, among other ASMs, have been noted to induce psychosis in adolescents (Besag *et al.*, 2016). Possible effects of different ASMs which may result in mental health difficulties are summarized in Table 26.1.

Table 26.1 Possible effects of different antiseizure medicines (ASMs) which may result in mental health difficulties.

	Possibly negative impacts	Possibly positive impacts
Cognition	Phenobarbitone Zonisamide Topiramate	Lamotrigine Rufinamide Lacosamide
Mood	Levetiracetam Vigabatrin Perampanel	Carbamazepine Lamotrigine Valproate
Behavior	Phenytoin Topiramate	Lamotrigine

Psychiatric features in specific epilepsy syndromes or types

The 2022 International League Against Epilepsy (ILAE) classification of seizures has further emphasized the delineation of epilepsy syndromes which include phenotypes comprised of unique psychiatric features (Specchio *et al.*, 2022b). For example, self-limited epilepsy with centrotemporal spikes (previously referred to as Benign Rolandic epilepsy) is associated with a positive prognosis from an epilepsy perspective since it generally does not require treatment with ASM and may resolve by late adolescence, but one-third of affected children may have behavioral difficulties, and an EEG with increased spikes may be associated with raised symptoms of depression, anxiety, and aggression (Dagar & Falcone, 2020). Furthermore, the rate of psychiatric features for all types of epilepsy may vary depending on seizure type. For example, children with temporal lobe epilepsy appear to have higher rates of depression compared to those with frontal lobe epilepsy (Schraegle & Titus, 2017).

Bringing together an integrated approach to mental health features/disorders in childhood epilepsy

We advocate a care coordinated or integrated care approach (Fazel *et al.*, 2021) when assessing and treating mental health features or disorders in children with epilepsy. Aspects to consider within such an approach are suggested below:

- Consider any possible shared underlying causes (e.g., specific genetic mutation or structural pathology like tuberous sclerosis) for both epileptic seizures and psychopathology.

- Consider any possible *direct* impacts from the epilepsy seizures or epilepsy syndrome on mental health features (e.g., dysphoria or depression in children with temporal lobe epilepsy, or ADHD features in children with developmental and/or epileptic encephalopathy with spike-wave activation in sleep).
- Consider any possible *indirect* impacts from the child or young person living with epilepsy (e.g., anxiety when engaging in sports or watching a film with strobe effects) or from sociocultural stigma.
- Consider the *systemic* impact of parents'/carers' mental states (e.g., parental anxiety limiting opportunities for peer interactions) and increased carer burden.
- Consider the impact of any interventions to treat epilepsy (e.g., adverse effects of medication like agitation or hallucinations with sodium valproate, enzyme inhibitor effects associated with carbamazepine, or the dietary restrictions posed by being on the ketogenic diet).
- Proceed with the established evidence-based treatments including psychological therapies and/or medications for the identified mental health presentation.

The above approach serves as an exemplar when approaching mental health presentations in other neurological disorders as in the following sections and is summarized in Figure 26.1.

Readers are advised to read a more detailed and contemporary account of pediatric epilepsy by Gogou and Cross (2022) and further understand the mental health presentations in children with epilepsy by accessing the report of the Child Neuropsychiatry Taskforce of ILAE by Besag *et al.* (2016) and the paper by Nickels *et al.* (2016) reviewing the cognitive and neurodevelopmental comorbidities.

Neuroinflammatory conditions

Young people are particularly susceptible to bacterial meningitis and in low-income countries, two-thirds of meningitis deaths are in children under age 15 (World Health Organization, 2004). Mental disorders like depression and anxiety are likely to be underdetected in meningitis survivors and may further worsen quality of life in addition to typical sequelae like cognitive impairments and hearing loss (Kostenniemi *et al.*, 2020). Tuberculous meningitis, in particular, can commonly cause infarctions in the basal ganglia, leading to increased risks for executive dysfunction, autism, and ADHD (Riva *et al.*, 2019).

Autoimmune conditions, like systemic lupus erythematosus (SLE), have long been observed to have mental health features, secondary to systemic inflammation and consequent tissue damage. So, it is unsurprising that immune-mediated inflammatory conditions of the central nervous system (CNS), like multiple sclerosis and acute disseminated encephalomyelitis (ADEM), are also associated with a high prevalence of mental health presentations like depression and psychosis. In the 21st century, the discovery of anti-NMDA (n-methyl-D-aspartate) receptor encephalitis and the subsequent detection of other CNS autoantibodies causing encephalitis, has led to an appreciation of how neuropsychiatric features may predominate or even be exclusively how autoimmune encephalitis presents acutely (e.g., mania, psychotic features like hallucinations, agitation, catatonia, and mood lability) (Hauptman & Ferrafiat, 2023). Further longitudinal research also suggests that over one-third of children with anti-NMDA receptor encephalitis may have persistent mental health features (Nguyen *et al.*, 2022). Child and adolescent psychiatrists should therefore be aware of relevant investigations, particularly serology and lumbar puncture for autoantibodies

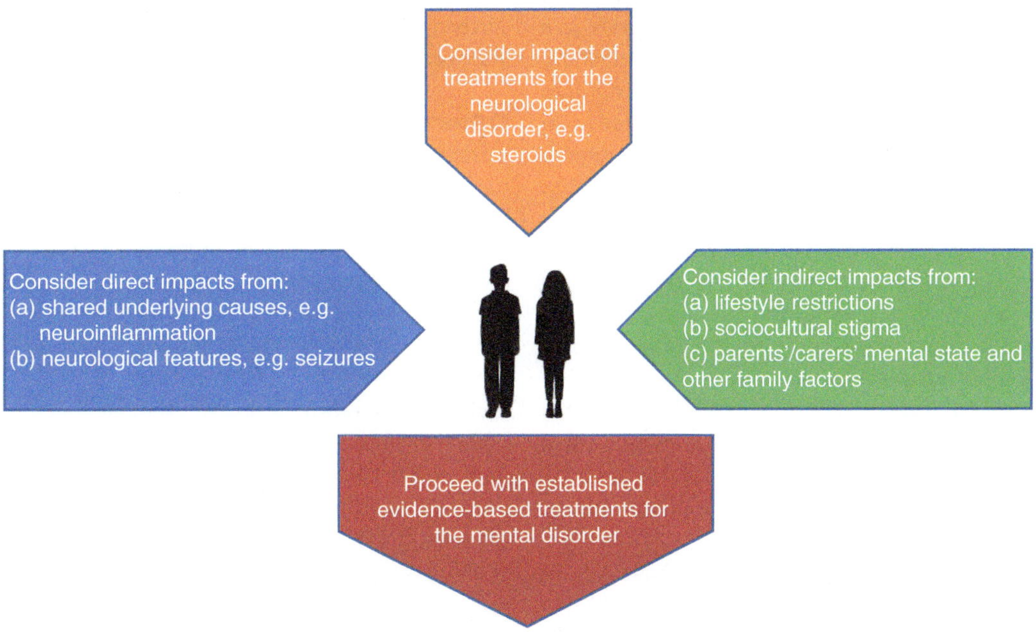

Figure 26.1 A suggested clinical approach when assessing children with mental disorder comorbid with neurological disorder.

and inflammatory markers, and also EEG and neuroimaging. Neuropsychiatric features alongside other investigation findings (e.g., neuroimaging features), in the absence of autoantibody identification, may also aid the diagnosis of seronegative autoimmune encephalitis (Cellucci *et al.*, 2020). There is little international consensus at present regarding psychiatric treatments in pediatric autoimmune encephalitis, but what is clear is that multidisciplinary care in collaboration with other treating medical specialties is essential (Mooneyham *et al.*, 2021)

The evidence base surrounding the concepts of pediatric acute-onset neuropsychiatric syndrome (PANS) and pediatric autoimmune neuropsychiatric disorder associated with streptococcal infection (PANDAS) remains an area for further research. The description of acute-onset mental health symptoms, like obsessive compulsive behaviors, food restriction, and tics, following exposure to streptococcus or other infections, makes identification challenging due to complexities related to laboratory testing and the clinical assessment of acute-onset features in a child. The treatment evidence base in PANS is limited and a systematic review concluded a low certainty of evidence for beneficial effects from anti-inflammatory, antibacterial, and immunomodulatory interventions; and a moderate certainty of evidence for adverse effects (Johnson *et al.*, 2021).

Interested readers are directed to a review of pediatric neuroinflammatory syndromes by Hauptman and Ferrafiat (2023) and practical guidance to assessing and diagnosing autoimmune encephalitis (Cellucci *et al.*, 2020).

Traumatic and acquired brain injuries

Pediatric traumatic and acquired brain injuries are a major cause of mortality and morbidity in children and adolescents, with a prevalence of about 280 per 100,000 globally. There can be longer-term complications because such injuries are associated with the development of emotional dysregulation, including mood swings and irritability, that persists into adulthood (Arif *et al.*, 2021). These difficulties contribute to an increased incidence of anxiety and depression and require additional support and interventions (Schorr *et al.*, 2020). Executive functions seem to be particularly vulnerable to early brain trauma, leading to impairments in attention, memory, and problem-solving skills. These deficits can themselves lead to impairments in academic and social functioning; one of the most frequent outcomes being secondary ADHD, a term implying the condition arose as a consequence of the trauma but did not precede it (Narad *et al.*, 2020).

Children who are already disinhibited and impulsive are at greater risk of traumatic and acquired brain lesions, and boys are twice as likely as girls to sustain a traumatic brain injury, especially in the first four years of life, largely from falls. In older children, the impact of medical treatment for ADHD is to reduce the risk of injuries (Ghirardi *et al.*, 2020). Overall, traumatic and acquired brain lesions can have a significant impact on mental health in childhood and beyond. It is important for health care providers to carefully monitor and manage the mental health needs of children with these conditions and provide appropriate interventions and support for emotional regulation, cognitive deficits, and behavioral and social difficulties (Jones *et al.*, 2020).

Neurometabolic and neurodegenerative disorders

Neurodegenerative disorders are associated with a progressive loss of cognitive, language, and motor skills resulting in significant impairments to all aspects of functioning and eventually death, often during childhood. Conditions associated with neurodegeneration include several inherited metabolic disorders like Hunter Syndrome (mucopolysaccharidosis type II) and Batten Disease (neuronal ceroid lipofuscinosis), as well as other rare neurological disorders like Wilson Disease and Cockayne Syndrome. Behaviors of concern, including hyperactivity, aggression, self-injury, and repetitive behaviors, occur frequently across the spectrum of neurometabolic and neurodegenerative disorders and may fluctuate or progressively worsen as per the clinical course of the disease. The significant carer burden posed by caring for a child with profound disabilities and a life-limiting condition also has significant impacts to the mental health of both the child and the parent/carer. Child and adolescent psychiatrists should be especially alert to any atypical pattern of regression in developmental skills (as opposed to regression or plateauing of language skills observed at age 18–24 months, often seen in autism). This can be challenging as depending on the age of the child, reverting to more childish behaviors and speech may be associated with an emotional reaction to being physically ill or under stress. Likewise, depression, or an evolving psychosis in a child, may also sometimes present with an apparent loss of cognitive and language skills. Readers can access a topical review by Djafar (2023) to understand neurodegenerative disorders further, as well as a practical approach to developmental regression by Smith and Ram (2019).

Other neurological disorders

Cerebral palsy is the most common cause of pervasive physical disability originating from childhood and represents a group of conditions that used to be considered to impact mainly the development of movement and posture, but are now known to have wide-ranging intellectual and neuropsychiatric effects. Cerebral palsy is due to a nonprogressive brain-based cause occurring during the fetal or infant periods. The increased survival rates of very premature babies have led to an increased incidence, currently estimated at about 1 in every 500 births. Children with cerebral palsy are at risk of impaired academic and social functioning, with bullying victimization and difficulties with friendships contributing to anxiety and depression (Whitney *et al.*, 2019a,2019b). In general terms, cerebral palsy is associated with an increased risk of ADHD and ASD, but these remain underrecognized and can contribute to social and academic difficulties requiring additional interventions (Påhlman *et al.*, 2020).

Functional neurological disorder (FND) has been described as involving "the biological embedding of lived experience in the body and brain, culminating in stress-system activation or dysregulation and in aberrant changes in neural network function." (Kozlowska *et al.*, 2023). This group of children can have neurological symptoms often indistinguishable from neurological disorders such as epilepsy or movement disorders, and can represent up to 20% of referrals to pediatric neurology (Doss & Plioplys, 2018). We have discussed functional seizures already and further elaboration of a clinical approach to somatoform disorders can be found in Chapter 69. While pediatric FND services remain scarce internationally, probably reinforced in part by the dualistic manner of health services organization and training, it is important to note that good outcomes have been demonstrated following a prompt positive diagnosis and utilizing a stepped-care multidisciplinary treatment model (Kozlowska *et al.*, 2023).

Assessment and treatment considerations

The mental health problems of children with brain disorders can be treated in just the same ways as those of neurologically intact children, and psychological and biological treatments are neither more nor less useful. There is no empirical basis, for example, for expecting greater success in treating a child's disruptive behavior disorder with risperidone rather than with parent training simply because the child also has a neurological disorder. Individual, family, and school-based treatment approaches can all be helpful. Children with neurological disorders, such as epilepsy, have traditionally been excluded from randomized controlled trials (RCTs) of therapeutic interventions so there is little systematic information on response to psychological, or psychotropic drug, treatment. However, clinical experience suggests that children with epilepsy and an additional mental health problem, such as oppositional defiant disorder (ODD), respond just as well, if not better, to the current best evidence-based interventions like parent training programs (see Chapter 33 or Shafran *et al.*, 2020). For example, a recent RCT of evidence-based psychological interventions for children with mental health needs and epilepsy has demonstrated that these treatments can be used successfully in this population (MICE Study Team *et al.*, 2021). Similarly, although there are very few studies in adults or children, children with depression and epilepsy respond well to antidepressants (Maguire *et al.*, 2021), and children with anxiety and epilepsy to cognitive behavior therapy (CBT) (MICE Study Team *et al.*, 2021). In each of these examples, the treatment is an evidence-based intervention for these conditions in children *without* epilepsy, so should be the treatment of choice for children with epilepsy, until there is evidence to the contrary.

Some of the most common and impairing disorders of childhood, such as anxiety, can be treated successfully with methods that achieve 80% good outcomes. Such success is associated with some of the largest effect-sizes in medicine (Dickson *et al.*, 2022). Parents and children, if asked, often rate the psychiatric disorder as having a larger negative impact on quality of life than the physical condition, yet the mental health problem may be quicker and easier to treat. For example, one study which looked at a 5-year follow-up of children with epilepsy and their quality of life, showed that presence or absence of seizures did not affect quality-of-life ratings. Yet, the presence of a psychiatric disorder was associated with significantly reduced quality of life, as rated by both parents and children (Baca *et al.*, 2011). Pediatricians may lack the time or skills to diagnose an associated psychiatric disorder, the physical illness may "overshadow" the mental illness (Hendriksen *et al.*, 2015), and even if they did detect such a disorder, they are often unaware of its significant functional impact.

As far as drug treatment is concerned, four points are worth emphasizing. First, the indications for, and choice of, psychotropic medication differs little from standard practice (see Chapter 39). Second, epilepsy is not a strong contraindication to using antipsychotics or antidepressants even though these drugs may increase seizure frequency. In practice, an increase in seizure frequency is rarely a major problem, and can often be countered by adjusting the dose of ASM. Most of the second-generation antipsychotic drugs, such as risperidone, are probably less likely than older drugs to exacerbate seizures, while olanzapine and clozapine are better avoided, if possible, because they are associated with a particularly high risk of seizures. Third, stimulant medication can be very helpful for children with ADHD who also have a neurological disorder such as epilepsy. Trials have confirmed that methylphenidate appears to be safe and effective for children with epilepsy (Santos *et al.*, 2013). Stimulant treatment does not overall increase seizures and may even be associated with reduced seizure frequency (Liu *et al.*, 2018). Finally, when children with epilepsy develop behavioral problems, changing the type or dosage of anti-epileptic medication can sometimes help, although there are few systematic or consistent findings. Changes in ASM should obviously be discussed with the child's pediatrician or neurologist.

Mental health professionals are often alarmed by a clinical encounter with a child who has active epilepsy, or severe cerebral palsy. Their discomfiture distracts them from recognizing and treating coexisting mental health problems, because their initial response is to think the child's problems lie outside their area of expertise. Yet the most effective and acceptable services for children with brain illnesses are likely to have physical and mental health professionals working closely together. New service models are developing around the world where physical and mental health care will be fully integrated. Joint clinical discussions, in which each expert's professional skills are recognized and valued, should ensure that these children do not suffer the double disadvantage of having both a neurological illness and an untreated, yet usually treatable, mental illness too (Box 26.2).

Box 26.2 Benefits to delivering neurological and psychiatric care in an integrated model

- Closer communication between clinicians resulting in improved clinician learning and satisfaction
- More integrated clinical formulations and treatments—this may be critical for certain situations like a child with epilepsy who also presents with comorbid functional seizures
- Increased child/young person and parent/carer satisfaction
- Reduced health utilization with probable cost savings

Policy and research

International policies

International policies for the management of children with neurological and NDDs aim to promote early detection, accurate diagnosis, and timely interventions to optimize the health and well-being of affected children and their families. Broadly, these include the Convention on the Rights of the Child and the Convention on the Rights of Persons with Disabilities. In an effort to standardize the description of health, functional abilities, and disabilities of individuals in the context of a chronic health condition, the World Health Organization (WHO) created the International Classification of Functioning, Disability and Health (ICF). To encourage the application of the ICF in day-to-day practice, ICF Core Sets, have been developed (http://icf-core-sets.org). There are currently Core Sets for cerebral palsy, ASD, and ADHD. These aim to provide service providers and stakeholders with an age-appropriate framework to record an individual's level of functioning and disability to guide assessment, treatment, and evaluation, and for policy purposes. Conceptually, the value of Core Sets is in measuring functioning that represents what a person *can do or is able to do every day*. In practical terms, this represents a more concrete and practical notion of "health" than can be inferred from a "diagnosis" alone. The WHO framework emphasizes the need for comprehensive and integrated approaches to care, including early detection and diagnosis, access to affordable and effective treatments, and support for families and caregivers (Schiariti *et al.*, 2021).

Additionally, some countries have developed national policies and guidelines for the management of children with neurological disorders. For example, the five Nordic countries have enacted social safety nets for the families of children with disabilities (Alriksson-Schmidt *et al.*, 2021). The National Institute for Health and Care Excellence (NICE) in the UK has published guidelines for the management of various neurological conditions in children, including epilepsy and cerebral palsy—many of these guidelines also cover the associated mental health and well-being for these conditions. Overall, international policies for the management of children with neurological disorders recognize the need for a coordinated and multidisciplinary approach to care, which involves collaboration between health care providers, educators, social services, and families. These policies also highlight the importance of addressing the social and environmental factors that can impact the health and well-being of affected children and their families. However, in many less developed countries, policies aimed at supporting children with disabilities have often not been fully implemented (Loucaides *et al.*, 2022).

Low- and middle-income countries (LMICs)

In rural areas of less developed countries, children are important for the economic productivity of the family and children with severe disability may be perceived as a misfortune by parents because they cannot contribute to the family's welfare (Kamiya, 2021). This perception may affect the quality of caregiving, the value attributed to the child, and the psychological stress associated with caregiving (Nyante & Carpenter, 2019). Traditional beliefs in society can contribute to feelings of stigma and shame experienced by families of children with disability. Community beliefs and superstitions may regard a child born with disability as a form of punishment from God and superstition about bewitchment and demonic possession (Mkabile *et al.*, 2021). Consequently, parents may believe their child is vulnerable to "spiritual sickness" and in need of spiritual protection, leading them to simultaneously access multiple interventions from ethnomedicine and local faith healers (Fonzi *et al.*, 2021). Even in countries such as those in East Asia where the practices and values of Confucianism are influential, valuing family interdependence, hierarchy of human relationships, a sense of duty and honor to the family, individual self-help, and filial piety as social virtues, there can be negative public attitudes to children with neurological and neurodevelopmental disabilities (Lee *et al.*, 2023).

Future directions

Children with disabilities (including neurological and mental disorders as a significant proportion) comprise about 150 million of the 1 billion people with disabilities in the world (World Health Organization, 2011). Yet despite declaring that support for such children is a human rights issue, some parts of the world lack disability awareness, services, or research into this subject. For instance, in many sub-Saharan African countries, access to health care services and rehabilitation services for children with disabilities is limited to urban areas, if it exists at all (Adugna *et al.*, 2020). A paucity of services for children with NDDs is far more widespread (Divan *et al.*, 2021) and, as these authors point out, the health care priorities of many LMICs are to manage communicable diseases, immunizations, and acute illnesses. Consequently, both the awareness of and services for children with chronic neurodevelopmental disabilities are lacking. A call for more research into how to provide universal health coverage is inevitable and Divan *et al.* (2021) provide a comprehensive Theory of Change framework for that purpose. On the other hand, for many families living in impoverished communities, national policies alone will not produce the evolution of societal attitudes to disability that are needed to

Gene	Recommended treatments	ASMs to avoid
SCN1A	Stiripentol, valproate, clobazam, cannabidiol, fenfluramine	Carbamazepine, lamotrigine
TSC1/TSC2	Vigabatrin for infantile spasms, everolimus	
SLC2A1	Ketogenic diet	Phenobarbitone
ALDH7A1	Pryridoxine (vitamin B6)	

Figure 26.2 A precision medicine approach in the field of pediatric genetic epilepsies have led to clinicians having more specific guidance for recommended treatments, as well as antiseizure medicines (ASMs) to avoid.

deliver change. Potential collaborative links between conventional health and educational services and the traditional healers who play such an important role in rural communities, both in Africa and Asia, would be useful, as well as initiatives to reduce the prevalence of stigma (Sanchez *et al.*, 2021).

One advance in the clinical care of pediatric genetic epilepsies has been the translation of multimodal research to inform a precision medicine approach (Knowles *et al.*, 2022)—see Figure 26.2 for a summary of how identified genes can guide epilepsy treatments to use and also to avoid. As the specific mental health presentations associated with these genetic epilepsies are understood further, an exciting future direction is a similar precision medicine approach to mental disorders.

We hope that our synthesis in this chapter of the current landscape of evidence-based approaches to mental disorders presenting as a result and as part of neurological disorders, as well as these future directions, will further break down the dualistic dichotomy of "brain" versus "mind" and lead to more integrated clinical approaches, service developments, and academic research in the future.

References

Adugna, M.B. *et al.* (2020) Barriers and facilitators to healthcare access for children with disabilities in low and middle income sub-Saharan African countries: a scoping review. *BMC Health Services Research* **20**, 1–11.

Alriksson-Schmidt, A.I. *et al.* (2021) Living life with cerebral palsy? A description of the social safety nets for individuals with cerebral palsy in the Nordic countries. *Scandinavian Journal of Public Health* **49**(6), 653–665.

Arif, H. *et al.* (2021) Long-term psychiatric outcomes in adults with history of pediatric traumatic brain injury. *Journal of Neurotrauma* **38**(11), 1515–1525.

Baca, C.B. *et al.* (2011) Psychiatric and medical comorbidity and quality of life outcomes in childhood-onset epilepsy. *Pediatrics* **128**(6), 532–1543.

Bălălău, O.D. *et al.* (2020) Maternal infections with an increased risk of transmission to the foetus; a literature review. *Journal of Clinical and Investigative Surgery* **5**(2), 66–72.

Bergdolt, L. & Dunaevsky, A. (2019) Brain changes in a maternal immune activation model of neurodevelopmental brain disorders. *Progress in Neurobiology* **175**, 1–19.

Besag, F. *et al.* (2016) Psychiatric and behavioural disorders in children with epilepsy (ILAE Task Force Report): epilepsy and psychosis in children and teenagers. *Epileptic Disorders* **18**, 1–86.

Bölte, S. *et al.* (2023) Sex and gender in neurodevelopmental conditions. *Nature Reviews Neurology* **19**(3), 135–159.

Brand, B.A. *et al.* (2021) The impact of X-chromosome inactivation on phenotypic expression of X-linked neurodevelopmental disorders. *Brain Sciences* **11**(7), 904.

Bui, L.T. *et al.* (2022) Does short-term, airborne lead exposure during pregnancy affect birth outcomes? Quasi-experimental evidence from NASCAR's deleading policy. *Environment International* **166**, 107354.

Carlsson, T. *et al.* (2021) Early environmental risk factors for neurodevelopmental disorders: a systematic review of twin and sibling studies. *Development and Psychopathology* **33**(4), 1448–1495.

Cellucci, T. *et al.* (2020) Clinical approach to the diagnosis of autoimmune encephalitis in the pediatric patient. *Neurology Neuroimmunology & Neuroinflammation* **7**, e663.

Cheong, J.L. *et al.* (2020) Have outcomes following extremely preterm birth improved over time? *Seminars in Fetal and Neonatal Medicine* **25**(3), 101114.

da Silva, P.F.S. *et al.* (2020) Pediatric neurodevelopment by prenatal Zika virus exposure: a cross-sectional study of the microcephaly epidemic research group cohort. *BMC Pediatrics* **20**, 472.

Dagar, A. & Falcone, T. (2020) Psychiatric comorbidities in pediatric epilepsy. *Current Psychiatry Reports* **22**, 77.

Dickson, S.J. *et al.* (2022) Impact of psychotherapy for children and adolescents with anxiety disorders on global and domain-specific functioning: a systematic review and meta-analysis. *Clinical Child and Family Psychology Review* **25**(4), 720–736.

DiPietro, J.A. & Voegtline, K.M. (2017) The gestational foundation of sex differences in development and vulnerability. *Neuroscience* **342**, 4–20.

Divan, G. *et al.* (2021) Annual research review: achieving universal health coverage for young children with autism spectrum disorder in low-and middle-income countries: a review of reviews. *Journal of Child Psychology and Psychiatry* **62**(5), 514–535.

Djafar, J.V. (2023) Childhood dementia: a collective clinical approach to advance therapeutic development and care. *Pediatric Neurology* **139**, 76–85.

Doss, J.L. & Plioplys, S. (2018) Pediatric psychogenic nonepileptic seizures. *Child and Adolescent Psychiatric Clinics of North America* **27**, 53–61.

Downs, J. *et al.* (2018) The prevalence of mental health disorders and symptoms in children and adolescents with cerebral palsy: a systematic review and meta-analysis. *Developmental Medicine and Child Neurology* **60**, 30–38.

Dunn, D. *et al.* (2016) Epilepsy and attention-deficit hyperactivity disorder: links, risks, and challenges. *Neuropsychiatric Disease and Treatment* **12**, 287–296.

Faruk, T. *et al.* (2020) Screening tools for early identification of children with developmental delay in low-and middle-income countries: a systematic review. *BMJ Open* **10**(11), e038182.

Fazel, M. *et al.* (2021) Integrated care to address child and adolescent health in the 21st century: a clinical review. *JCPP Advances* **1**, e12045.

Fonzi, V. *et al.* (2021) The multifaceted care-seeking practices among caregivers of children with cerebral palsy: perspectives from mothers and providers in Ghana. *PLoS One* **16**(10), e0258650.

Ghirardi, L. *et al.* (2020) Attention-deficit/hyperactivity disorder medication and unintentional injuries in children and adolescents. *Journal of the American Academy of Child & Adolescent Psychiatry* **59**(8), 944–951.

Gogou, M. & Cross, J.H. (2022) Seizures and epilepsy in childhood. *CONTINUUM: Lifelong Learning in Neurology* **28**, 428–456.

Gooley, S. *et al.* (2022) ILAE Genetic Literacy series: familial focal epilepsy syndromes. *Epileptic Disorders* **24**(2), 221–228.

Gumusoglu, S.B. & Stevens, H.E. (2019) Maternal inflammation and neurodevelopmental programming: a review of preclinical outcomes and implications for translational psychiatry. *Biological Psychiatry* **85**(2), 107–121.

Han, V.X. *et al.* (2021) Maternal immune activation and neuroinflammation in human neurodevelopmental disorders. *Nature Reviews Neurology* **17**(9), 564–579.

Hauptman, A.J. & Ferrafiat, V. (2023) Neuroinflammatory syndromes in children. *Current Opinion in Psychiatry* **36**, 87–95.

Hendriksen, J.G.M. *et al.* (2015) Diagnostic overshadowing in a population of children with neurological disabilities: a cross sectional descriptive study on acquired ADHD. *European Journal of Paediatric Neurology* **19**, 521–524.

Hollingdale, J. *et al.* (2022) Sex differences in conduct and emotional outcomes for young people with hyperactive/inattentive traits and social communication difficulties between 9 and 16 years of age: a growth curve analysis. *Psychological Medicine* **53**(10), 4539–4549.

Johnson, M. *et al.* (2021) Anti-inflammatory, antibacterial and immunomodulatory treatment in children with symptoms corresponding to the research condition PANS (pediatric acute-onset neuropsychiatric syndrome): a systematic review. *PLoS One* **16**, e0253844.

Jones, S. *et al.* (2020) Qualitative study of the needs of injured children and their families after a child's traumatic injury. *BMJ Open* **10**(11), e036682.

Kamiya, Y. (2021) Current situation of children with disabilities in low- and middle-income countries. *Pediatrics International* **63**(11), 1277–1281.

Knowles, J.K. *et al.* (2022) Precision medicine for genetic epilepsy on the horizon: recent advances, present challenges, and suggestions for continued progress. *Epilepsia* **63**, 2461–2475.

Kostenniemi, U.J. *et al.* (2020) Psychiatric disabilities and other long-term consequences of childhood bacterial meningitis. *The Pediatric Infectious Disease Journal* **40**, 26–31.

Kozlowska, K. *et al.* (2023) Evidence-based mind-body interventions for children and adolescents with functional neurological disorder. *Harvard Review of Psychiatry* **31**, 60–82.

Kwon, C.-S. *et al.* (2022) Autism spectrum disorder and epilepsy. *Neurologic Clinics* **40**, 831–847.

Lee, C.E. *et al.* (2023) Caregiving and future planning perspectives of siblings of individuals with intellectual and developmental disabilities: insights from South Korea, Japan and Taiwan. *Journal of Applied Research in Intellectual Disabilities* **36**, 50–57.

Liu, X. *et al.* (2018) Stimulants do not increase the risk of seizure-related hospitalizations in children with epilepsy. *Journal of Child and Adolescent Psychopharmacology* **28**(2), 111–116.

Loucaides, E.M. *et al.* (2022) Livelihood support for caregivers of children with developmental disabilities: findings from a scoping review and stakeholder survey. *Disability and Rehabilitation* **46**(2), 293–308.

Maguire, M.J. *et al.* (2021) Antidepressants for people with epilepsy and depression. *Cochrane Database of Systematic Reviews* **4**(4), CD010682.

MICE Study Team *et al.* (2021) M.I.C.E—Mental Health Intervention for Children with Epilepsy: a randomised controlled, multi-centre clinical trial evaluating the clinical and cost-effectiveness of MATCH-ADTC in addition to usual care compared to usual care alone for children and young people with common mental health disorders and epilepsy—study protocol. *Trials* **22**, 132.

Mizuguchi, M. *et al.* (2019) Everolimus for epilepsy and autism spectrum disorder in tuberous sclerosis complex: EXIST-3 substudy in Japan. *Brain and Development* **41**, 1–10.

Mkabile, S. *et al.* (2021) African families' and caregivers' experiences of raising a child with intellectual disability: a narrative synthesis of qualitative studies. *African Journal of Disability* **10**, 1–10.

Mooneyham, G.C. *et al.* (2021) Developing consensus in the assessment and treatment pathways for autoimmune encephalitis in child and adolescent psychiatry. *Frontiers in Psychiatry* **12**, 638901.

Narad, M.E. *et al.* (2020) Impact of secondary ADHD on long-term outcomes after early childhood traumatic brain injury. *The Journal of Head Trauma Rehabilitation* **35**(3), E271.

Nguyen, L. *et al.* (2022) A systematic review and quantitative synthesis of the long-term psychiatric sequelae of pediatric autoimmune encephalitis. *Journal of Affective Disorders* **308**, 449–457.

Nickels, K.C. *et al.* (2016) Cognitive and neurodevelopmental comorbidities in paediatric epilepsy. *Nature Reviews Neurology* **12**, 465–476.

Nyante, G.G. & Carpenter, C. (2019) The experience of carers of children with cerebral palsy living in rural areas of Ghana who have received no rehabilitation services: a qualitative study. *Child: Care, Health and Development* **45**(6), 815–822.

Obeng-Gyasi, E. (2019) Sources of lead exposure in various countries. *Reviews on Environmental Health* **34**(1), 25–34.

Påhlman, M. *et al.* (2020) Autism spectrum disorder and attention-deficit/hyperactivity disorder in children with cerebral palsy: results from screening in a population-based group. *European Child & Adolescent Psychiatry* **29**, 1569–1579.

Paiva, M.L. *et al.* (2020) Seizure control and anxiety: which factor plays a major role in social adjustment in patients with juvenile myoclonic epilepsy? *Seizure* **80**, 234–239.

Puka, K. *et al.* (2020) Trajectories of quality of life 10 years following a diagnosis of epilepsy in childhood. *Epilepsia* **61**(7), 1453–1463.

Reilly, C. *et al.* (2014) Neurobehavioral comorbidities in children with active epilepsy: a population-based study. *Pediatrics* **133**, e1586–e1593.

Reilly, C. *et al.* (2018) Symptoms of depression, anxiety, and stress in parents of young children with epilepsy: a case controlled population-based study. *Epilepsy & Behavior* **80**, 177–183.

Riva, D. *et al.* (2019) Language cerebro-cerebellar reorganization in children after surgery of right cerebellar astrocytoma: a fMRI study. *Cerebellum* **18**(4), 791–806.

Rutter, M. *et al.* (1970) *A Neuropsychiatric Study in Childhood. Clinics in Developmental Medicine Nos. 35/36*. S.I.M.P./Heinemann, London.

Rutter, M. *et al.* (1976) Isle of Wight studies, 1964–1974. *Psychological Medicine* **6**, 313–332.

Sanchez, N. *et al.* (2021) Stakeholder views of the practical and cultural barriers to epilepsy care in Uganda. *Epilepsy & Behavior* **114**, 107314.

Santos, K. *et al.* (2013) The impact of methylphenidate on seizure frequency and severity in children with attention-deficit-hyperactivity disorder and difficult-to-treat epilepsies. *Developmental Medicine and Child Neurology* **55**, 654–660.

Santos, S. *et al.* (2022) Male sex bias in early and late onset neurodevelopmental disorders: shared aspects and differences in autism spectrum disorder, attention deficit/hyperactivity disorder, and schizophrenia. *Neuroscience and Biobehavioral Reviews* **135**, 104577.

Schiariti, V. *et al.* (2021) Promoting developmental potential in early childhood: a global framework for health and education. *International Journal of Environmental Research and Public Health* **18**(4), 2007.

Schorr, E. *et al.* (2020) Parenting styles as a predictor of long-term psychosocial outcomes after traumatic brain injury (TBI) in early childhood. *Disability and Rehabilitation* **42**(17), 2437–2443.

Schraegle, W.A. & Titus, J.B. (2017) The relationship of seizure focus with depression, anxiety, and health-related quality of life in children and adolescents with epilepsy. *Epilepsy & Behavior* **68**, 115–122.

Shafran, R. *et al.* (2020) Optimising evidence-based psychological treatment for the mental health needs of children with epilepsy: principles and methods. *Clinical Child and Family Psychology Review* **23**, 284–295.

Silva, C.C. *et al.* (2021) Patterns of fetal and infant growth and brain morphology at age 10 years. *JAMA Network Open* **4**(12), e2138214.

Smith, T. & Ram, D. (2019) Fifteen-minute consultation: a practical approach to developmental regression in children. *Archives of Disease in Childhood—Education & Practice Edition* **104**, 173–177.

Smith, E.R. *et al.* (2023) Adverse maternal, fetal, and newborn outcomes among pregnant women with SARS-CoV-2 infection: an individual participant data meta-analysis. *BMJ Global Health* **8**(1), e009495.

Song, J. *et al.* (2018) Health of parents of individuals with developmental disorders or mental health problems: impacts of stigma. *Social Science & Medicine* **217**, 152–158.

Sorg, A.L. *et al.* (2022) Cognitive disorders in childhood epilepsy: a comparative longitudinal study using administrative healthcare data. *Journal of Neurology* **269**(7), 3789–3799.

Specchio, N. *et al.* (2022a) The epilepsy–autism spectrum disorder phenotype in the era of molecular genetics and precision therapy. *Epilepsia* **63**, 6–21.

Specchio, N. *et al.* (2022b) International League Against Epilepsy classification and definition of epilepsy syndromes with onset in childhood: position paper by the ILAE Task Force on Nosology and Definitions. *Epilepsia* **63**, 1398–1442.

Suwannakul, B. *et al.* (2021) Organophosphate pesticide exposures in early and late pregnancy influence different aspects of infant developmental performance. *Toxics* **9**(5), 99.

Teal, L.B. *et al.* (2023) The evolving role of animal models in the discovery and development of novel treatments for psychiatric disorders. *Advances in Neurobiology* **30**, 37–99.

Vassilopoulos, A. *et al.* (2022) Treatment approaches for functional neurological disorders in children. *Current Treatment Options in Neurology* **24**, 77–97.

Wartman, C. & VandenBerg, A. (2022) Valproate: not all boxed warnings are created equal. *Annals of Pharmacotherapy* **56**(12), 1349–1355.

Whitney, D.G. *et al.* (2019a) Mental health disorders, participation, and bullying in children with cerebral palsy. *Developmental Medicine and Child Neurology* **61**, 937–942.

Whitney, D.G. *et al.* (2019b) Factors associated with depression and anxiety in children with intellectual disabilities. *Journal of Intellectual Disability Research* **63**, 408–417.

Whitney, D.G. *et al.* (2019c) The contribution of neurologic disorders to the national prevalence of depression and anxiety problems among children and adolescents. *Annals of Epidemiology* **29**, 81–84.

World Health Organization (2004) *The Global Burden of Disease 2004 Update*. World Health Organization, Geneva, Switzerland.

World Health Organization (2011) *World Report on Disability 2011*. World Health Organization, Geneva, Switzerland.

Zima, B.T. *et al.* (2016) Psychiatric disorders and trends in resource use in pediatric hospitals. *Pediatrics* **138**, e20160909.

PART III

Approaching the clinical encounter

A: The clinical assessment

CHAPTER 27

Clinical assessment and formulation

James F. Leckman
Child Study Center, Yale University, New Haven, CT, USA

Introduction

The goal of clinical assessments is to identify the presence of psychopathology as well as risk and protective factors. If indicated, clinicians also need to develop a plan to initiate treatment in partnership with the parents and/or other providers. This is a multistep process that involves complex and conscientious decision-making based upon the available evidence from multiple sources. The nature and progression of the child's symptoms (past and present) within and across multiple contexts (family, peers, school, and cultural background) is crucial. It is important to consider the child's developmental and medical histories, their family's psychiatric history, and exposure to adversity (acute or chronic), as well as the child's strengths and interests. Indeed, the presence of protective and resilience factors can certainly impact the child's prognosis and treatment outcome. Another important goal is the formation of a therapeutic alliance with the family. The formulation and prioritization of treatment goals with the family should involve a collaborative, problem-solving, hypothesis-generating, and hypothesis-testing approach that is based both on the available scientific evidence concerning potential risks and benefits of specific interventions, and on the child's and the family's knowledge-base and their attitudes concerning various treatment options and opportunities (Chapter 2). Consequently, clinical assessments often need to include a psychoeducational component. Less frequently, clinical assessments of children and adolescents are conducted in a more focused and circumscribed fashion to address immediate safety, forensic, and/or research issues. Regardless of the scope, clinical assessments of children and adolescents are complex in nature and vary a good deal across the globe. This is particularly true in our digital age and in the aftermath of the COVID-19 pandemic when so many clinical assessments continue to be "online" (Chapters 18 and 49). This chapter addresses each of these assessment components (Table 27.1) before moving on to consider how best to "formulate" the child's difficulties and develop an initial treatment plan. We begin by addressing the reasons for the referral and the need to understand the intentions of the person or agency requesting the clinical assessment.

Initial questions regarding referral

Children are usually referred to practitioners by someone with a focused question. Clarity about why the referral was initiated (and by whom) is an essential ingredient for the evaluation to be a success. Typically, the child's presenting symptoms are a greater source of concern for the parents or others in their environment than they are for the child. Many clinicians, based on their training and a traditional medical model of care, may choose to focus on whether or not the child meets criteria for a particular disorder; but this question may not be foremost in the mind of the person making the referral. For example, parents are often worried that the child's current symptoms may portend the emergence of a more serious mental disorder that is thought to run in the family. The child's behavior at school may be much more problematic than it is judged to be at home. Not infrequently, the parties involved may not see the situation in the same way. Parents may be seeking an evaluation for the child to return to school. In other instances, the referral source may be asking for an opinion concerning the legal status of the child—whether the child should be removed from the family or what the custody arrangements should be (Chapter 47). Because of this broad range of possibilities, procedures need to be in place to clarify questions about the referral. What are the key questions to be addressed? Who made the referral? What prompted the referral? Are there differing points of view concerning the need for a clinical assessment? Based on the answers to these questions, one should also consider whether the clinical team that has been approached is the one best suited to undertake the assessment. For example, depending on the clarity of the issues

Rutter's Child and Adolescent Psychiatry and Psychology, Seventh Edition.
Edited by Anita Thapar, Daniel S. Pine, Samuele Cortese, Cathy Creswell, Tamsin J. Ford, James F. Leckman, and Argyris Stringaris.

Companion website: www.wiley.com/go/thapar/rutterspsych7

Table 27.1 Basic elements in child and adolescent psychiatric assessments.

Content	Informants	Resources	Goals
Why this child? Why now?			
Reason(s) for referral	Parent, guardian, school personnel, and health care provider(s)	Referral letters and conversations from school personnel and other health care providers	Clarity concerning reasons for the assessment; potentially different perspectives; opportunity to build therapeutic alliance; initial opinions concerning potential treatment options
Child's strengths, talents and interests, and environmental supports How the family members interact with one another	Parents, child, other family members, peers, teachers, coaches	Parent- and self-reports about areas of interest and excellence Nature of the observed interactions between and among family members	Clarity concerning how the child is viewed within the family Opportunity to build trust and establish a therapeutic alliance and promote resiliency
Who is this child?			
History of present illness Comorbid conditions Past psychiatric history and treatment response Treatment response by other family members Current neighborhood	Parents, child, other family members Past psychiatric evaluations and mental health records Medical records, treating clinicians Parents, teachers, new media	Review of parent-, teacher-, and self-reports; questionnaires; diagnostic interviews; videotapes Previous evaluations, therapies, treatments, medications (including dietary supplements); hospitalizations Identify interventions that were helpful for other family members Frequency of criminal acts that could impact the child's and the family's well-being	Clarity concerning the course and function of the symptoms, accommodation, intervening stressors, or associated changes in life circumstances Success of prior interventions Initial impressions concerning treatment priorities Success of prior interventions for family members Clarity concerning the safety of the child's current home environment
What is the nature of the problem?			
Developmental, educational, and medical history	Parents, guardian, school personnel, and health care provider(s)	Review of birth and pediatric records; education evaluations (Chapters 36 and 43)	Presence of developmental or medical disorders, as well as traumatic events that may have impacted the child
Family history	Parent, guardian, school personnel, and health care provider(s)	Review of structured and unstructured questionnaires; Genogram (Chapters 25 and 29)	Presence of familial vulnerabilities relevant to prognosis Treatment response of family members
Home, school, and community environment	Parents, child, other family members	Parental self-esteem and psychopathology, parental strain, partial discord, sibling conflicts, level of hubbub, computer/video games, access to the internet; family resources including pets and neighbors (Chapters 27 and 29); How safe is the family's neighborhood?	To inform intervention strategies and identify challenges that will be faced by the treatment team; potential targets for adjunctive interventions
Mental status examination	Child	Structured assessments of appearance, mood, orientation, adaptive functioning, attention, memory, fund of knowledge, judgment, insight, thought (coherence, speed, and content). Presence of hallucinations or delusions.	Assess the child's interaction with the clinician; screen for overt psychiatric symptoms that impact the child's behavior, adjustment, and cognitive functioning
Neuropsychological evaluation	Child	Optional standardized assessments of intelligence, memory, receptive and expressive language, reading, executive function, visuospatial skills, and motor coordination (Chapter 35)	Clarify nature of the child's interaction with the psychologist; characterize the child's pattern of cognitive and linguistic strengths and weaknesses, relative to same-aged peers
Physical and neurological examination, laboratory testing, electrophysiological assessment, and brain imaging	Child	Optional examinations to identify body dysmorphic features and evaluate the child's somatic, metabolic, and neurological status, as well as brain structure and function (Chapters 11, 25 and 36)	Identify any genetic, medical, metabolic, endocrine, or neurological disorders that may impact the child's course of illness and treatment

and the health care system, it may make sense to refer the family to another provider who is better positioned to intervene with the appropriate services. However, parents may become upset with the idea that they need to be seen and evaluated by another practitioner. This decision needs to be made as early as possible.

Many of these questions can be clarified by direct contact with the referral source and by review of any relevant documents. If privacy and confidentiality can be assured, direct contact by telephone or via the internet may be of great benefit and lead to requests for additional information. Many clinicians and health care systems have found the use of structured and semistructured questionnaires and well-validated parent, teacher, and self-reports to be invaluable in preparing for clinical assessments. However, rating scales are no substitute for an in-person assessment.

Some of the widely used parent-report instruments, with excellent psychometric properties, provide a preliminary assessment of the child's mood and anxiety level, attentional and disruptive behavioral problems (e.g., difficulties with their peers at school), and the child's perceived level of psychosocial stress, as well as the parents' well-being (e.g., the child's mother had recently been diagnosed with cancer), the home environment, and the level of caregiver strain (Chapter 28). At times, this information may point to other important problems that had not been previously identified and that need to be considered during the course of the evaluation. In many health care systems, it is required to ask families for prior authorization to contact other relevant parties including medical and school personnel.

At the beginning of the assessment, practitioners often use open-ended questions such as, "Because we want to be sure to address your primary concerns, please briefly tell us how we can best be of service to you." Typically, the parents are asked with and without the child present, and the child is asked as well. This will help the clinician gain greater clarity concerning the motivation to seek an assessment, and can also be very useful in setting the stage for the development of a positive therapeutic alliance. A positive therapeutic alliance is associated with improved outcomes for children and their families. This has been clearly documented in children and families dealing with severe anxiety and those with disruptive behaviors (Chapters 59 and 65).

Observations of the family

Attitudes to referral, disorder, and treatment

From the initial contact with the family, it is important to be attentive to the nature of the parents' attitudes to their child and to each other, as well as to the professionals involved in the case. How did they describe their child and were there any hints as to the nature of the communication between the parents? What are their fears and expectations? How important is the family's cultural background as they consider their child's difficulties? What is their explanation, if any, for the problem? Often, these attitudes shift to some degree as the assessment process takes place, and as the family recognizes the inherently collaborative nature of the process. When clinicians show respect and a positive attitude during the assessment, it can make a difference.

Patterns of interaction

Among the sources of information that the clinician has available during the assessment, one of the most important is the nature of the interactions within the family. Patterns of dyadic reciprocity, sensitivity, and intrusiveness are often remarkably stable over the course of development. Opportunities to observe these interactions abound, beginning with how the family members position themselves during the assessment, be it online or in-person.

Regardless of how the later stages of the assessment are organized, it is often beneficial to have a brief meeting with the family all together to explain what will be taking place and to sort out who will be seeing whom for what purpose. This provides another opportunity to monitor closely the nature of the verbal and the nonverbal communication among family members. After welcoming the family, making any further introductions, and thanking them for coming in and filling out the questionnaires and parent reports, many clinicians have found that asking the parents to reflect on their child's positive features is a useful starting point. "What strengths and talents and favorite activities does your child have?" This can set the stage for a successful encounter, as well as providing clues as to how one might foster resilience in the child and the family. Each of the family members should be asked to share their perspective. The clinician may ask, "What questions do you have for us? We will do our best to answer each of them before you leave today." Other open-ended questions such as, "I wonder how much you have talked together about why you are here to see us?" or "Have you had a family discussion about your reasons for coming in today?" or "How did you feel about the referral?" are often more informative than making more specific inquiries. This approach also provides opportunities for the clinician to observe interactions among family members, as well as to identify any conflicting viewpoints that will need to be reconciled if the recommended interventions will be adhered to and successfully implemented. Depending on the age of the child, some of these questions should be repeated when the child is no longer present.

Naturally, during this initial portion of the interview when the family is together, care needs to be taken to make the child feel as comfortable as possible. In the case of some adolescents, it is important to consider changing the order of the interviews in the assessment as they may feel "disrespected" if parents are interviewed at length before they are interviewed alone. For younger children, the availability of toys, paper and crayons, other play materials, or even websites make good sense. Whatever the circumstance, seeing what the child decides to do and how they interact with their parents and the clinician throughout the assessment is informative. Likewise, if the child becomes distressed or starts to display disruptive behavior, this provides another opportunity to monitor the parent's response, as well as to intervene in a sensitive fashion by encouraging the parents to respond in a way that they find the most appropriate.

Basic elements in the clinical assessment

Other key elements in the assessment include interviewing the child and interviewing the parents separately. The sequence and organization of these interviews depend on the child's age and developmental level, as well as the clinician's best judgment about how best to proceed.

Interview with the child

When possible, it is important to see the child without either of their parents present. The cardinal aim of the interview is to help the child relax with the interviewer and to lay a foundation of trust. Without trust little can be achieved. If a modicum of trust does develop, the clinician will be able to ascertain how the child perceives problems in his or her life, evaluate the child's affect and capacity to relate to the interviewer, and catch a glimpse of their family life. The age, developmental level, personality, and expectations of the child matter and will shape the course and content of the interview.

The clinical assessment of young children differs fundamentally from that of adults and adolescents. While it is useful to monitor the child's behavior and social interactions in various contexts, including when the parents are present, it is also crucial to interview and interconnect with the child separately. Care needs to be taken to minimize the child's distress when being separated from their parents. This can be done by reassuring the child that they can be reunited with their parents as needed. The child also needs to know exactly where their parents will be located during their interview with the clinician. If the assessment is being completed by a team, often the parental interview will occur simultaneously with the child's interview. Under such circumstances, having the parents accompany the child to the room set aside for his/her assessment makes sense and can be a source of comfort for the child.

For younger children, the opportunity to play and interact in a less structured fashion with the clinician can help put the child at ease. For example, asking the child to talk about what they enjoy doing is a good place to start. Having an ongoing activity, e.g., drawing a picture or using building blocks, permits the child to respond more spontaneously and openly to the clinician's queries. Intermittently praising the child's work and positioning oneself at the child's eye-level, i.e., sitting on the floor, can facilitate a positive dyadic interaction between child and clinician. Some clinicians find it helpful to ask the child questions such as, "If I were a magician and could give you three wishes, what would those be?"

Eventually the clinician will need to address the behaviors and emotional issues that prompted the referral. People of all ages are open to the influence of suggestions, but none more so than young children. Open-ended questions will work the best and be the least prone to distortion and suggestion: "What did your parents say about why you were coming in to see us today?" "What is most upsetting to you?" "What do you wish might be different?" "Is there anything you worry about every day?" Also, when assessing any symptom, it can be helpful to ask the child to give it a rating out of 10, where zero is "not a problem" and 10 is "awful, it couldn't be worse." Once the child provides some insight into their difficulties, it will be important for the clinician to contextualize the problem in terms of where and when and in relation to whom these problems occur. "How do each of your parents respond when that happens?" The issues for older children and adolescents vary and may reflect their reluctance to be open with an "adult." Even though it is almost always possible to establish rapport and collect information from adolescents, it can be a challenge. Being respectful and curious about the adolescent's perspective is very important. While it is important for the assessments of children of all ages to have an appropriate degree of structure and standardization, the clinician also needs to be open to the unexpected. Otherwise, important information and insights may be missed. Variations in the style and content of the interview may differ considerably depending on the child's symptoms, and on their cognitive and sensory impairments, if any (Chapters 48, 52–70). The interview with the child should also include many elements of the mental status examination (MSE) (Box 27.1). At the end of the interview, the clinician should review with the child what they have both learned about the child's strengths and interests, as well as the reasons for why they were being seen.

Parental interview

The parental interview is focused on the child's presenting problems, medical and family history, early development, school progress, and peer relations, as well as on gathering information concerning the home and family environment including the parents' child-rearing techniques and the methods of discipline used (Table 27.1). The best place to start is to address the *reason for referral* and determine what it is about the child's day-to-day feelings, behaviors, and social interactions that are of greatest concern to the parents and that prompted the assessment. What impact do these problems have on the day-to-day life of the child and their family? Do they interfere with the child's ability to socialize with friends and/or family members? Does the child engage in any violent behavior directed toward themselves or others family members? It is also important to mention that the results of the assessment will be confidential.

How do the parents understand their child's problems?

Context is critically important. How predictable are the child's symptoms in a given set of circumstances? How much do they vary depending upon which parent is there? Are there other contextual features that make the situation better or worse?

Box 27.1 Mental status examination (MSE)[a]

- **Appearance:** Patient's age, sex, body mass index, and ethnicity. How is the patient dressed? Does the patient have any distinguishing features—for example, tattoos or scars? How is the patient's personal hygiene?
- **Behavior:** Is the patient talkative, timid, or aggressive? What is their facial expression? Do they maintain eye contact? Do they have any abnormal movements, such as facial or body tic?
- **Speech:** What is the rate, volume, tone, and flow of their speech?
- **Mood and affect:** A patient's mood is their own perception of how they feel. Their affect is the clinician's objective assessment of their mood. Does the patient appear elated, depressed, anxious, irritable, or withdrawn?
- **Thought content:** What are the patients' beliefs and ideas?
  - Does the patient have any ***Obsessions***—repetitive thoughts about something that he or she is anxious about? Does the patient have any ***Compulsions***—such that they feel compelled to repeat actions—for example, hand washing or counting?
  - Do they have any ***Delusions*** (fixed, false beliefs not consistent with the person's background)? The most common types of delusions include delusions of persecution, grandiose delusions, delusions of reference, delusions of control, and delusions of guilt.
  - Does the patient currently have or have they had any ***Thoughts of Harming*** themselves or others? If present, were these planned or spur-of-the-moment decisions? Was there a trigger? What has stopped the patient from acting on them?
- **Thought process:** Write down how the patient is expressing his or her thoughts. Do the patient's sentences link together, or is the patient hopping from one topic to another with no apparent association?
- **Perception:** How does this patient perceive the world? Is the patient experiencing external stimuli differently than the objective reality? For example, is he or she misinterpreting a cat for a hat?
  - ***Hallucinations:*** Does the patient see (visual), hear (auditory), smell (olfactory), taste (gustatory), and feel (tactile) external stimuli that cannot be experienced by others?
  - ***Dissociative symptoms:*** Does the patient feel detached from him- or herself or think that any part of his or her body is unreal (depersonalization)?
- **Cognition:** The clinician needs to assess the patient's alertness, orientation, attention, concentration, and memory.
  - ***Consciousness:*** Is the patient alert, intoxicated, drowsy, or in a coma? Has the patient been able to give coherent answers?
  - ***Orientation:*** Can the patient recall the date, where they are, and can they recognize three people who they know?
  - ***Attention and concentration:*** Ask the patient to recite the days of the week backwards.
  - ***Memory:*** Test short-term memory by giving patients three objects to remember, then asking them to repeat the series until they can repeat all of them correctly. Test them again later in the conversation to test long-term memory.
- **Insight:** A patients' insight into their mental state is usually on a spectrum. It is not simply present or absent. It is important to determine whether or not the patient recognizes when they experience an unusual mental event. Are they aware that they have a mental illness? Ask questions such as: "Do you think there is anything wrong with you at the moment?" "Do you think your friends would say that there is something unusual going on?" "What do you think might be causing you to feel this way?" and "Do you think you might benefit from receiving some form of treatment?"

[a] Adapted from Soltan and Girguis (2017).

Identifying specific antecedents and precipitants can provide valuable clues to what *function* the symptoms have. What has been the parents' response? Anxiety in children will often trigger behaviors in their parents. At times, the parent's efforts to comfort and reassure the child can have unforeseen negative consequences by providing a form of re-enforcement that may lead the symptoms to persist and intensify. Although accommodation of this sort has been studied extensively in obsessive–compulsive disorder (OCD), it is commonplace among other childhood anxiety disorders (Kitt *et al.*, 2022). How have others in the family or at school responded? What has worked in the past and what has not? Is there any hint of secondary gain? Here it is important to move beyond general answers (such as mentioning efforts to comfort, admonish, or punish the child) and to obtain a more detailed sequential account of how this has been done and how the child responded. Often asking the parents to recall specific recent episodes can be useful. This can provide some clarity about how things have progressed from the onset and if there were any precipitating events or predisposing factors. It is important to ask for detailed examples of the child's symptoms from the previous week and then determine if these were typical of the past month as well. There is always a dynamic interplay between the child's presenting symptoms and their home and school environments.

Do these symptoms reflect an underlying disorder, or do they reveal problems within the child's social–emotional environment? It is also important to be vigilant about the parents' state of mind and their possible embarrassment, ambivalence, or shame in seeking professional advice. "What did we do wrong?" and "Is it my fault?" are common unspoken questions. Echoes of the parents' memories of their own experiences while growing up are often part of the unspoken dialogue.

Beyond the immediate reason for referral, the assessment team also needs to consider the presence of any *co-occurring symptoms*, as well as any significant *past psychiatric* and *neurodevelopmental problems*. Many services now ask parents to complete questionnaires to screen for possible co-occurring conditions (see Chapter 28). However, clinicians still need to be alert to the presence of co-occurring and past symptoms. "In addition to these symptoms and concerns, have there been any other emotional or behavioral difficulties that your child currently has or has had in the past?"

Next, asking the parents to review their child's *developmental history* will allow the clinician to gain a clear perspective on the child's somatic, psychomotor, neurocognitive, linguistic, social, temperamental, and emotional development. Parents can vary a great deal in terms of their ability to recall specific developmental milestones. Often, it is useful to ask the parents to complete a structured questionnaire and for the clinician to review this information prior to the time of the in-person assessment. This will allow the clinician to be knowledgeable and relatively expeditious. Understanding the child's gender identity is another element in the child's developmental history (Chapter 40).

It is also important to review the child's *educational history*, starting with nursery school and kindergarten. Then in later schooling "What did the parents hear from the teachers?" "What were their peer interactions like?" "How easy was it for them to make good friends?" "What pastimes did they enjoy most and excel at?"

Another important component of the parental interview concerns the child's medical history (Chapter 30). Major influences on neural development can occur during embryonic and fetal development (Chapter 9). Consequently, this history needs to proceed from conception onward and include any difficulties the mother had in becoming pregnant and the use of any interventions (such as *in vitro* fertilization), as well as any pregnancy and birth complications, including the mother's emotional state and level of psychosocial stress during the pregnancy. Any allergies should be carefully documented. Likewise, the use of any medications over the course of development should also be noted (Chapter 36).

Family history has been well-researched as a factor that can increase risk for developing a mental disorder. As a result, the child's family history of mental and medical disorders needs to be carefully documented.

The *MSE* is another essential part of the initial clinical assessment (Soltan & Girguis, 2017, Box 27.1). An MSE gives the clinician a snapshot of a patient's emotions, thoughts, and behavior at the time of their evaluation. It can help identify the presence and severity of mental disorders and the risk the patient poses to him- or herself, or to others. It includes a description of the child's appearance and behavior; the fluency of their speech and their ability to communicate effectively; their affect and mood; their patterns of interaction with parents, siblings, and clinicians; their orientation to person, place, and time; their attention and apparent intellectual ability; their thought form and content; the speed, content, and coherence of their cognitive processing; their current affect and reactivity; the appropriateness of their affect and perception, e.g., hallucinations; and their insight regarding the possibility that they are experiencing a mental disorder.

The MSE also serves as a useful opportunity to screen for organic conditions and serves as a prelude to recommending further psychological, medical, and/or neurological examinations (Chapters 35 and 36). Although the MSE is conceptualized as being distinct from other portions of the assessment, it serves to summarize the clinician's impressions from the interviews with the family and with the child. Some components, however, do require specific inquiries (such as the child's orientation to person, place, and time, and their fund of knowledge and memory).

Finally, while some clinicians prefer to conduct the entire diagnostic assessment in a conjoint family setting, this approach has some inherent disadvantages. Context matters and individuals do not behave the same when everyone in the family is present. Indeed, there are circumstances when spending time with each parent individually can be important, as in the case of parental divorce and joint custody arrangements. Some time spent with each parent may be useful even if there is no obvious discord between them. However, being open to the parents' preferences in this matter also makes good sense, especially as the team needs to continue to build therapeutic alliances collaboratively with the parents and child. Also, when the parents are divorced and both have involvement and/or "supervisory rights" over the child, it is important to have permission from both parents, even before scheduling the evaluation.

School reports and direct contact with teachers

Children may behave differently in the school setting than they do at home. Therefore, it is often useful for the clinician to access and review school reports, as well as to speak directly with the teachers and other school personnel. This is particularly true of reports related to academic performance and any special education services that the child may currently be receiving or have received in the past. Educational difficulties are frequently associated with psychopathology, and parents and teachers may only partially agree on the presence of particular symptoms such as inattentiveness, hyperactivity-impulsivity, and oppositionality (Chapter 54). While there are advantages to using standardized teacher-report questionnaires (Chapter 34), it also is useful to have teachers express their own concerns and report on the child's behavior and response to directives. If special services have been provided, it is important to review their impact on the child's behavior and academic performance over the course of time. Being attentive to cultural differences in the educational context is also important, especially if the child has recently relocated from their home country. Even with the teacher and school reports in hand, it is often the case that specific queries will arise that will prompt a member of the assessment team to contact the school personnel directly. In some instances, if there are persistent differences of opinion concerning the child's behavior at home and at school, visits to observe the child in both settings may be useful. Efforts to build a collaborative alliance with the teachers and other professionals at the school will bode well for the child's long-term outcome. In many instances treatment components focus on the school environment in terms of advocacy, services, accommodations, and opportunities for resilience (Chapter 23).

Medical assessment

The initial assessment needs to be informed by knowledge of previous assessments and screening (e.g., for hearing) (Chapter 30); a specific referral may be needed.

Standardization of clinical assessment

Standardized approaches and the use of structured interviews, rating scales, and observational methods constitute an important part of a clinical assessment (Chapter 29), but there is also a clear need to look beyond the diagnosis to consider factors that might be important in the causation of the disorder and its course and prognosis, and that will inform therapeutic planning.

Standardized interviews are particularly relevant in clinical settings where child and adolescent mental health professionals, and other clinicians, are forced to make decisions about treatment in imperfect situations within a limited time period and with incomplete information. For example, the Development and Well-being Assessment (DAWBA) is a package of interviews, questionnaires, and rating techniques designed to generate psychiatric diagnoses, reflecting *International Classification of Diseases* (ICD)/*Diagnostic and Statistical Manual of Mental Disorders* (DSM) criteria, on 5–17-year-olds based on information provided from multiple informants (parents, youth over 11 years old, and teachers) and is now available, free and with computer algorithms, in more than 20 languages (http://www.dawba.info/a0.html). However, the accuracy of the results of the DAWBA should be carefully considered. Another reason for caution is the high frequency of idiosyncratic but clinically significant information that may be missed. Despite recent efforts to revise and validate the DSM and ICD diagnostic categories, they remain imperfect (Chapter 2). Additionally, the much debated and carefully chosen wording of these criteria rarely matches the complex presentations of the children referred for assessment.

Moving beyond diagnosis, as the assessment team formulates a narrative concerning the nature of the child's problems, they need to consider how a given child's symptoms resemble those seen in other children, as well as what aspects of the presentation are unique to this child and this family. These considerations will allow them to frame an initial set of hypotheses concerning what factors will influence response to treatment, while building a strong therapeutic alliance. This is a key step in the problem-solving, hypothesis-generating, and hypothesis-testing approach needed to formulate and prioritize treatment goals with the child and the family.

Presence/absence of clinically significant psychopathology

Care needs to be taken not to "pathologize the normal." One basic question underlying the assessment process is whether or not the child's problems are *clinically significant*. This raises the important issue of how to establish thresholds that distinguish normal developmental traits and emotional states from those that are indicative of pathology. Relevant questions include: "Does their intensity go beyond the range of normal variation given the child's age and temperamental predisposition?" "Do these symptoms reflect a clear, substantial change from the child's usual emotional state?" "Are they pervasive across interpersonal and social contexts?" "How much time do they consume in a typical day?" "To what extent can the child control these symptoms by means of distraction or engagement in pleasurable activities?" Many of these questions are embedded in symptom-specific rating scales (Krause *et al.*, 2021) (Chapter 28), which can track the child's progress. Despite the potential benefits associated with the use of these scales, they are no substitute for the practitioner's judgment concerning whether or not the child's presenting symptoms are clinically significant following the in-person assessment described in this chapter. In addition, the usefulness of these scales may be limited depending on the child's age, the need for specific informants (parent, teacher, self, expert clinician), the variable time periods that are assessed (current, past week, etc.), idiosyncratic scoring paradigms, their potential cost, and, in some cases, the need for formal training to establish the rater's reliability. Then there is the reality that these scales are available only in a limited number of languages.

In other instances, clinical interventions may not be indicated even if the level of distress is high. For example, a serious grief reaction following the death of a loved one is quite common and a source of distress. In many cases, the emotional distress of the parents and family members contributes to the intensity of the child's reaction. The passage of time and supportive counseling may be sufficient (Chapter 35).

Assessment of psychosocial impairment and safety

Efforts to determine the degree of impairment in psychosocial functioning is another key consideration in establishing the clinical significance of a child's presenting symptoms. The assessment of impairment is a standard part of the assessment of children and adolescents. Progress in incorporating the level of *psychosocial impairment* associated with various forms of psychopathology was given further impetus by subsequent epidemiological surveys that reported remarkably high prevalence rates of psychiatric disorders. Current classification systems for mental disorders, including the ICD-11 and the DSM-5-TR, require an assessment of the degree of psychosocial impairment. For example, are the features of the disorder(s) distressing the child? Is their schoolwork suffering? Are they held back from social activities, or victimized, or unable to make friends?

The assessment of the child's *safety* is another important topic. In the case of younger children this may focus on the child's risk of injury, because of abuse or neglect (Chapter 25). For older children and adolescents, the assessment concerns the risk of violence to self or others (Chapters 64 and 65). In some instances, the referral itself may have been prompted by these concerns. If so, the person making the referral will often be directed immediately to seek emergency services, which in turn may lead to psychiatric hospitalization or legal actions to protect the safety of the child and to specialized forensic assessment services. In any case, the clinical assessment team, in nonemergency settings, needs to be alert to issues of safety. The clinician may also need to determine whether the child or others are in immediate danger. Relevant information includes the presence of current or past ideation or acts that indicate a significant risk to self or others, as well as a range of risk factors (explicit plans, cognitive distortions, mood state, impulsivity, personality, and a range of environmental stress factors involving family psychopathology and conflict) (Chapter 64). In addition to self-harm with clear suicidal intent, acts of intentional self-harm (cutting, burning, etc.) to provide temporary relief from intense dysphoria have become more common over the past two decades among adolescents and young adults (Clements *et al.*, 2023). Acts of nonsuicidal self-injury need to be carefully documented and understood and, if present, need to be considered in the formulation of the initial treatment plan.

Violent behavior in children and adolescents can include a wide range of behaviors: explosive temper tantrums, physical aggression, cruelty toward animals, and intentional destruction of property and vandalism. Other serious risks during adolescence include unplanned pregnancies due to reckless and hypersexual behaviors associated with bipolar disorder (Chapter 62).

Duration and timing of disorder

The timing and duration of psychopathological states are two other features that contribute to an understanding of their clinical significance. Many classification systems specify a duration criterion—the minimum time period the symptoms need to be present in order for a diagnosis to be made. In the case of DSM-5-TR, panels of experts came up with a very broad range of required periods, currently: 2 weeks for major depressive disorder; 3 months for bulimia nervosa; 6 months for generalized anxiety disorder, 12 months for conduct disorder; and 2 years for persistent depressive disorder (American Psychiatric Association, 2022). While these time periods are based on the consensus of experts, they remain opinions and are somewhat arbitrary. For other diagnoses, such as attention deficit hyperactivity disorder (ADHD), the DSM criteria specify that the symptoms being considered must have been present prior to a certain age. In many instances, establishing a clear onset or estimating the duration can be problematic given the retrospective nature of the information provided by multiple informants and concerning multiple potentially interrelated psychiatric symptoms. Apart from possible reporting biases, it may well be that many psychiatric disorders do not, in fact, have a clear-cut onset. Frequently, symptomatology gradually builds up over time when new symptoms become evident or when psychosocial impairment is manifest (Sandberg *et al.*, 2001). In contrast, other disorders are defined in part by their sudden, overnight onset. While clinicians need to take the necessary time to clarify as much as possible the onset, course, and timing of the presenting symptoms, as well as the points of remission and exacerbation, this is usually an imperfect science. Therefore, a slavish adherence to diagnostic criteria that specify symptom duration makes little sense.

Formulation: integration and synthesis

As noted above, formulation in child and adolescent psychiatry is a complex and iterative process that distills information from multiple sources into a meaningful narrative and establishes a set of hypotheses about the child and his or her presentation that then shape the initial treatment priorities (Chapter 2; Table 27.2). There are several approaches to presenting the formulation of the child's difficulties ranging from a simply biological perspective to a more systemic model, or to psychodynamic formulation. "What symptoms are causing the greatest degree of difficulty for the child and for others in his or her immediate environments?" "When and why did these problems arise and how long have they been present?" "What can be done to ameliorate them?" "Are there any proximal risk mechanisms that, if addressed, might have a positive impact?" "What else is going on in the environment (acute or chronic stressors, etc.) that is having an impact on these symptoms?" "What new knowledge could we provide that would be useful for the family and others directly involved in the case (peers, teachers, etc.) to know, e.g., evidence-based knowledge concerning the natural history, treatment, and prognosis?" "Can everyone agree regarding the nature of these difficulties and what the best course of action would be to address them?"

Diagnoses are one element in this formulation, and they provide a succinct summary of some aspects of what has been learned over the course of the evaluation. Ultimately, the clinician's judgment in integrating all the available information into a "best estimate" diagnosis is key. However, care needs to be taken not to "reify" the diagnosis. When a specific disorder is reified by the clinicians there is a risk that the child is no longer viewed as a unique human entity but is instead viewed as "a case of X disorder." We need to focus on "the whole child" including his/her strengths, interests, and abilities, not just his/her "diagnosis." Indeed, we need to work with the child and her or his family to "formulate" what the nature of the of the child's problems is that led to the referral (Hoyos & Cortese, 2023).

Table 27.2 Formulation matrix.

Factors	Biological	Psychological	Social
Predisposing	Genetic Birth trauma Brain injury Illness—psychiatric/ physical Medication Drug use/alcohol Pain	Personality Modeling Defenses (unconscious) Coping strategies Self-esteem Body image Cognition	Socioeconomic status Trauma
Precipitating	Medication Trauma Drug use/alcohol Acute illness Pain		Work Finances Connections Relationships
Protective	Physical health	Engagement Insight Adherence Coping strategies Intelligence	

Source: Adapted from Selzer and Ellen (2010).

Formulations and diagnoses allow for "informed" communication between professionals and researchers, e.g., what interventions have the strongest evidence base for a specific disorder, or as record keeping, e.g., health care systems that need to monitor the prevalence of disorders as well as track service delivery (Chapter 2). In putting the clinical information together to establish a set of hypotheses about the child, the clinician needs to consider the source of the information and the context within which it was obtained. In cases of divorce and parental discord, the parents may not agree with regard to the presence of specific symptoms or their importance. Parents, teachers, and other informants may also disagree on the importance of specific symptoms. It is also important to consider the knowledge base of the informants. "Are there other family members with a similar condition and how did this condition impact that individual over the course of his/her life?" "How much information has the family gleaned from various sources, including the internet, and how accurate is their understanding of the condition and its course and treatment?" Given the iterative nature of assessments and treatment planning, the clinician always needs to ask—"What information am I lacking and what would be the best source(s) to gain a more complete view of the child and a deeper understanding of their psychopathology?"

Psychoeducation

The basics

Psychoeducation can be a key ingredient leading to a successful intervention. Given the incremental advances in our understanding of the etiology, course, and treatment of childhood-onset neurodevelopmental disorders and/or psychiatric disorders, providing families with accessible, user-friendly sources of information can be enormously helpful. Most involved family members of children and adolescents with mental illnesses need information and support to best assist their ill family member. Ideally, this information will include content about the nature of the disorder (etiology, course, and outcome), as well as expanding social support networks. Advocacy organizations are often an excellent source of such information. Indeed, providing the parents with the web links to such organizations can be very helpful and may initiate an interconnection that will be useful to everyone involved in the United Kingdom (UK) and beyond (https://www.pohwer.net/childrens-and-young-peoples-advocacy).

Another dimension of psychoeducation, for both the clinician and the family, is the need to be acquainted with the available evidence base concerning the efficacy of various therapeutic interventions. Major organizations, including The Centre for Evidence-Based Medicine (http://www.cebm.net) and Cochrane (http://www.cochrane.org), provide rigorous synthesis of the evidence informing clinical practice. In addition, clinical practice guidelines are also available from professional organizations including the National Institute for Health and Clinical Excellence (NICE) in the UK, the American Academy of Child and Adolescent Psychiatry, and the European Society for Child and Adolescent Psychiatry, among others. The decision on which course of action to follow remains subject to input from personal, political, philosophical, ethical, economic, and esthetic values as well as the imperative to minimize the potential for doing harm to the child.

Alert the family to the potential for *stigma*

In order to improve access to care and treatment, and optimize the well-being of children and adolescents affected by a mental disorder, it is crucial that the potential for *stigma* needs to be addressed during the course of the evaluation and subsequent care. This is particularly important for families without much prior exposure to mental health encounters.

Treatment planning

Once the assessment nears completion and a meaningful narrative has been formulated that summarizes the information from multiple sources, the next step is to build a consensus to embark on treatment planning. Although setting forth a "diagnosis" is important, relying solely on the "diagnosis" to guide a treatment plan can be problematic. Seldom does our current state of knowledge allow for "the diagnosis" by itself to dictate the intervention (Hoyos & Cortese, 2023). For example, Johnny's (an 8-year-old boy) increasing separation anxiety at home and his increasing social isolation and, at times, his disruptive behavior at school is based, in part, on his parents' hostile estrangement from one another and on his need to transition back and forth between two residences. In such a case, it may make sense to engage the family in a therapeutic intervention that seeks to help the parents recognize the negative consequences of their hostile interactions on their child and to provide a neutral therapist to explore with the child his or her understanding of the situation (Chapters 28, 35, and 36). This in turn may help the estranged parents refocus on their child and find ways to support and celebrate jointly the child's interests and abilities. In contrast, if the child's anxiety is long-standing and a reflection of a shy or inhibited temperament manifested by being socially awkward, withdrawn, and avoidant, a course of an increasing number of psychological interventions using cognitive behavioral therapy (CBT), or pharmacotherapy, or both may be indicated depending on the family's willingness to pursue one of these interventions (Chapter 59). Other principles that are key to treatment planning include: safety (to do no harm); building on the child's strengths (as a way to foster resilience and keep the child's development "on track") (Chapter 28); and working as a collaborative team with the patients, the family, the school, and other providers to ensure coordination and continuity of culturally appropriate care.

Safety

Just as safety is a key issue to consider during the course of an assessment, it has no less a role in the initial phase of treatment planning. This is always a balance. In situations with the potential for child abuse or neglect, care needs to be taken to ensure the protection of the child, as well as the rights of the child's caregivers in accordance with the legal and ethical guidelines that are in place (Chapters 25, 57, and 64). The initiation of pharmacological treatment also requires that the family and the patient have a clear grasp of the risks and benefits. Often it is useful to delay the initiation of medications. The experience of going through an evaluation, learning about the disorder through psychoeducation, and giving voice to the child's and family's concerns can have a positive impact on the clinical picture. Simply having someone who understands the situation and is committed to working with the family and other practitioners can make a real difference. Likewise, given the increasing number of psychological interventions, including CBT interventions with proven efficacy, pharmacotherapy may not be the first agreed upon intervention. Often the major problem is finding a clinician with the necessary skills and experience to provide the CBT with fidelity. However, once the joint decision is made to initiate medication, it is important for the child and family to "commit" to completing an adequate trial unless untoward side effects are clinically significant, even after making any necessary adjustments in dosage or the timing of drug administration.

Build on strengths, foster resilience, and keep development "on track"

Supporting the positive elements of the child's life is always an important part of the initial treatment planning (Chapter 23). This is especially true if there are opportunities to build on the child's talents and interests (music, sports activities, etc.). The child's continued engagement in such activities provides something for him/her to be "proud of" and is a source of positive re-enforcement. Physical exercise can also have a positive impact on the brain and there is some evidence to support its use across a range of conditions from ADHD to depressive mood (Purgato *et al.*, 2023; Svedell *et al.*, 2023). Likewise, healthy sleep habits are important to ensure the well-being of the child (Schlier & Han, 2021). It is also very important to emphasize with the patient and the parents the need to keep the child's development "on track." Almost invariably this means finding ways to continue the child's life with others outside the home. Withdrawal and isolation are a prescription for ongoing self-doubt and low self-esteem, as well as problematic interactions in the home. For example, children with ADHD often have major difficulties with social acceptance and this can create a vicious cycle that involves a degree of social isolation, peer rejection, and an increased risk of being bullied. Depending on the child's developmental level, efforts to keep development on track may involve identifying opportunities for the child in question to interact with younger or older children rather than with their same aged peers, e.g., in religious groups or scouting or outdoor activities. In these contexts, the child with impaired social skills can interact with younger (as a mentor) or older peers (as a mentee). These new settings provide an opportunity for the child to be resilient in the face of continuing adversity (peer rejection, bullying, etc.) (Chapter 23).

Team building with the child and the parents

Optional treatment planning and the willingness of the family to engage in treatment interventions depend on consensus building within the therapeutic alliance. This step can be problematic if the parents are in conflict and can easily provoke each other. In such instances, separate interactions with each parent may be of value in re-enforcing the merits of a specific intervention, as viewed from that parent's unique perspective. Encouraging acceptance of the realities of their lives and circumstances may lessen the anger and distress that distract them from their child's needs.

Interface with school personnel, pediatricians, and other practitioners

Often, the therapeutic team needs to involve other practitioners and professionals. Multiple examples come to mind. For example, autism spectrum disorders, and speech and language and other learning disorders, including ADHD, will often involve working with school personnel and other professionals and medical disciplines (Chapters 50–54). In these complex situations, someone, besides a parent, needs to serve as the coordinator and convener as the child matures.

Cultural appropriateness

It is also important that clinicians not lose sight of the unique cultural and religious background of the family during the treatment planning process. Attrition is a long-standing problem in mental health centers serving youth (Gibbons *et al.*, 2021). Ethnicity is a consistent predictor of attrition, particularly when the treatment provider is not from the same ethnic or religious background. Likewise, a family's ethnic and cultural background may influence their choice of various treatment alternatives. For example, Naydeline Mejia and Isabeth Mendoza pointed out on National Public Radio, "If you were raised in a Latinx household, you'll know that when it comes to mental health, we don't grow up talking about it." (Mejia *et al.*, 2022). Although enduring therapeutic alliances are possible across ethnic and cultural backgrounds, a careful appraisal of the match between the mental health service providers and the family in question is encouraged.

Standards for practice

Clinical practice must be performed under a variety of administrative, financial, and legal constraints. This chapter outlines what is needed to complete a psychiatric assessment. However, health services may not provide adequate time or resources and may require burdensome administrative tasks, all of which compromise one's ability to complete a meaningful psychiatric assessment. In some instances, a short period of time may be sufficient, if the presenting problems are straightforward and not particularly worrisome, e.g., uncomplicated bedwetting or parental "overconcern" about a preschool child's age-appropriate behavior toward siblings. However, when the presenting problems are substantial and context dependent, it is critical for the clinician to address each of the areas mentioned above in order to formulate a coherent narrative concerning the child's condition. Almost invariably this will require multiple sources of information and a degree of professional judgment (Hoyos & Cortese, 2023). Clinicians must also act in accordance with the legal and ethical guidelines that are in place to ensure the safety of the child (Chapter 19).

Approaches to assessment and treatment planning across the globe

Health care systems vary widely across the world. Even in some low- and middle-income countries, such as Brazil, health care is seen as a right not a privilege. On the other hand, in some of the wealthier countries, e.g., the United States, marked disparities are still in place. In addition to access, the question of the quality of the services that are available is significant, especially given the stigma associated with mental disorders and the shortage of well-trained practitioners (Chapters 18 and 41). Often, the issues of access to, and the availability of, well-trained professionals mean that the task of assessment falls to primary care clinicians, pediatricians, and professionals in settings outside of medical centers, e.g., school-based programs (Chapter 43). In these contexts, the availability of expert consultants and the existence of sustainable programs to train professionals in school settings are an important focus for health care planning. Innovative approaches are needed to address these barriers and to improve access to care. Options to consider include the use of screening measures for the detection of children at high risk coupled with a more complete second-stage diagnostic assessment and the use of nonspecialist workers in community and school settings for the delivery of psychosocial interventions (Aggarwal *et al.*, 2020). One of the most promising emerging strategies is through the empowerment of existing human resources, e.g., parents and other members of the extended families, through innovative technologies, such as mobile health, with the necessary skills for the detection and treatment of child mental disorders. The increasing use of electronic medical records, e-mail and social media is also transforming aspects of referral and clinical assessments, as well as treatment planning. For example, some interventions are now available online for a range of neuropsychiatric and developmental disorders (Chapter 49), including autism (McLay *et al.*, 2023); ADHD (Lee *et al.*, 2023), anxiety and depression (Casella *et al.*, 2022); and OCD (Aspyall *et al.*, 2021; Lauri *et al.*, 2023)). The internet is also an expanding source of information and misinformation, increasingly used by parents as a guide to decision-making. Additionally, telemedicine is being increasingly used to provide mental health assessments and services at a distance (Döpfner *et al.*, 2024).

Conclusions

This chapter has sought to stress the importance of forming an alliance with the child and family, keeping in mind their cultural background and family milieu, their developmental status, and their perspective (as well as that of those around them) on their child's symptoms. The approach outlined requires multiple sources of information and clinical judgment, and sharing of the information with the child and the family along with an honest appraisal of the child's prognosis. Treatment planning can then build on the child's strengths in order to foster resilience and keep the child's development "on track." The child's response to treatment will indicate whether or not the formulation and therapeutic hypotheses were correct and what modifications are needed to ensure a path to recovery.

References

Aggarwal, S. *et al.* (2020) Explanatory style in youth self-harm: an Indian qualitative study to inform intervention design. *Evidence-Based Mental Health* **23**(3), 100–106. doi:10.1136/ebmental-2020-300159.

American Psychiatric Association (2022) *Diagnostic and Statistical Manual of Mental Disorders*, 5th edn, text Revision edn. American Psychiatric Association, Washington, DC.

Aspyall, K. *et al.* (2021) Effect of an internet-delivered stepped-care program vs in-person cognitive behavioral therapy on obsessive-compulsive disorder symptoms in children and adolescents. *Journal of the American Medical Association* **325**(18), 1863–1873. doi:10.1001/jama.2021.3839.

Casella, C.B. *et al.* (2022) Brief internet-delivered cognitive-behavioural intervention for children and adolescents with symptoms of anxiety and depression during the COVID-19 pandemic: a randomised controlled trial protocol. *Trials* **23**(1), 899. doi:10.1186/s13063-022-06836-2.

Clements, C. *et al.* (2023) Self-harm in university students: a comparative analysis of data from the multicentre study of self-harm in England. *Journal of Affective Disorders* **335**, 67–74. doi:10.1016/j.jad.2023.04.112.

Döpfner, M. *et al.* (2024) Feasibility, satisfaction, and goal attainment in routine telemedicine consultation in child and adolescent psychiatry and psychotherapy. *European Child & Adolescent Psychiatry*. doi:10.1007/s00787-024-02477-9. Online ahead of print

Gibbons, N. *et al.* (2021) Making sense of child and adolescent mental health services. *Clinical Child Psychology and Psychiatry* **26**(3), 760–769. doi:10.1177/1359104521999709.

Hoyos, C. & Cortese, S. (2023) Beyond diagnosis: formulation-storytelling and maps. *Journal of the American Academy of Child and Adolescent Psychiatry* **62**(2), 120–122. doi:10.1016/j.jaac.2022.06.008.

Kitt, E.R. *et al.* (2022) Family accommodation in pediatric anxiety: relations with avoidance and self-efficacy. *Behaviour Research and*

Therapy **154**, 104107. doi:10.1016/j.brat.2022.104107. PMID: 35613517

Krause, K.R. *et al.* (2021) International consensus on a standard set of outcome measures for child and youth anxiety, depression, obsessive-compulsive disorder, and post-traumatic stress disorder. *The Lancet Psychiatry* **8**(1), 76–86. doi:10.1016/S2215-0366(20)30356-4.

Lauri, K.O. *et al.* (2023) Long-term effect of stepped-care vs in-person cognitive behavioral therapy for pediatric obsessive-compulsive disorder. *Internet Interventions* **32**, 100613. doi:10.1016/j.invent.2023.100613.

Lee, K.-Y. *et al.* (2023) Exploring mediational roles for self-stigma in associations between types of problematic use of internet and psychological distress in youth with ADHD. *Research in Developmental Disabilities* **133**, 104410. doi:10.1016/j.ridd.2022.104410.

McLay, L. *et al.* (2023) Telehealth-delivered naturalistic developmental behavioural intervention with and without caregiver acceptance and commitment therapy for autistic children and their caregivers. *BMJ* **13**(5), e071235. doi:10.1136/bmjopen-2022-071235.

Mejia, N. et al. (2022) 4 tips for talking to your Latinx parents about mental health. *NPR.* Available: https://www.npr.org/2022/01/13/1072763217/talking-to-latinx-parents-about-mental-health-and-stigma [27 September 2024].

Purgato, M. *et al.* (2023) Umbrella systematic review and meta-analysis: physical activity as an effective therapeutic strategy for improving psychosocial outcomes in children and adolescents. *Journal of the American Academy of Child and Adolescent Psychiatry* 63(2), 172–183. doi:10.1016/j.jaac.2023.04.017.

Sandberg, S. *et al.* (2001) Do high-threat life events really provoke the onset of psychiatric disorder in children? *Journal of Child Psychology and Psychiatry* **42**(4), 523–532.

Schlier, M. & Han, J. (2021) The role of sleep in young children's development: a review. *The Journal of Genetic Psychology* **182**(4), 205–217.

Selzer, R. & Ellen, S. (2010) Twelve tools for teaching medical students. *Australasian Psychiatry* **18**(2), 170–173. doi:10.3109/10398560903471425.

Soltan, S. & Girguis, J. (2017) How to approach the mental state examination. *BMJ* **357**. doi:10.1136/sbmj.j1821.

Svedell, L.A. *et al.* (2023) Feasibility and tolerability of moderate intensity regular physical exercise as treatment for core symptoms of attention deficit hyperactivity disorder. *Frontiers in Sports and Active Living* **5**, 1133256. doi:10.3389/fspor.2023.1133256.

CHAPTER 28

Use of structured interviews, rating scales, and observational methods in clinical settings

Argyris Stringaris

[1] Faculty of Brain Sciences, University College London, London, UK

[2] First Department of Psychiatry, Aiginiteio Hospital, National and Kapodistrian University of Athens, Athens, Greece

Overview

The use of structured interviews, rating scales, and observational methods is now standard in child and adolescent psychiatry research and becoming more common in clinical practice. Here, I provide a conceptual overview of these assessments, including their central assumptions and their challenges. I then discuss some major instruments used in the field. I will use the term *assessment instruments* to refer collectively to structured interviews, rating scales, and observational methods where necessary.

Background to assessment instruments

Importance of using assessment instruments

There are several reasons why using assessment instruments is important in clinical practice. First, using outcome measures can enhance quality of care for young people. In this context, the term measurement-based outcomes or measurement-based care refers to employing standardized measures to regularly monitor a patient's symptoms, functioning, and treatment progress over time. Indeed, feeding back to clinicians on measurement appears to be useful. For example, Bickman and colleagues (Bickman *et al.*, 2011) conducted a randomized cluster trial that evaluated the effects of routine feedback to clinicians on mental health outcomes in youths receiving mental health services. They found that patients treated at sites where clinicians could receive weekly feedback improved faster than youths treated at sites where clinicians did not receive weekly feedback. Recent meta-analyses further support the use of measurement feedback, though the effect sizes may be relatively modest (Cohen's $d \sim 0.15$) (Rognstad *et al.*, 2023). There are some similar findings specific to using standardized diagnostic instruments, and there is evidence from a randomized controlled trial (RCT) that disclosing a standardized diagnosis to clinicians prior to clinical decision-making improved agreement between clinicians for emotional disorders and led to the consideration of a broader range of diagnoses (Aebi *et al.*, 2012). However, other trials found the effect to be modest and specific to only some anxiety disorders (Ford *et al.*, 2013). An ongoing trial in a large sample examines the impact that standardized diagnostic assessments have on the rate of diagnosis (Day *et al.*, 2022).

The second reason is the imperative of integrating patients' views into clinical decision-making. It is important to think of the patient as an individual with unique needs, preferences, and values and reflect this in the assessment. Indeed, the importance of patient-reported outcome measures (PROMS) has recently been emphasized and is now government policy (NHS England, 2015), and is reflected in funders expectations in relation to child and adolescent mental health (CAMH). Standardized measures are one way of incorporating patients' views into clinical decision-making.

The third reason concerns the utility of standardized instruments in freeing up clinician time. For example, asking patients to complete standardized measures before seeing them can reduce the time that a clinician spends on screening for problems and thus free up time to focus on discussing with the patient what is most important to them. However, there is, to my knowledge, no empirical demonstration of this yet.

The fourth reason concerns the ability to translate clinical constructs to quantities which can be statistically evaluated and compared with each other. This is a prerequisite for being able to offer patients evidence-based medicine.

All these are compelling reasons for using assessment instruments in clinical practice. Yet, there are several reasons to be

Rutter's Child and Adolescent Psychiatry and Psychology, Seventh Edition.
Edited by Anita Thapar, Daniel S. Pine, Samuele Cortese, Cathy Creswell, Tamsin J. Ford, James F. Leckman, and Argyris Stringaris.

Companion website: www.wiley.com/go/thapar/rutterspsych7

cautious with their use and knowledgeable about their limitations. I expand on their conceptual, statistical, and pragmatic challenges at the end of this chapter.

Assessment instruments as standardized measures of feelings and behavior

Structured interviews, rating scales, and observational methods are increasingly used in clinical practice. Their use is meant to allow clinicians to obtain "an objective and standardized measure of samples of behavior," as neatly summarized by two of the pioneers of psychometric assessment (Anastasi & Urbina, 1997). These *samples of behavior* can come in any format, including responses to a rating scale or observations made by the clinician during parent–child interactions, and they can include behaviors in the broad sense, e.g., feelings and displays of emotion. The word *objective* can be confusing—here it should be taken to refer to the fact that the process and outcome of a test is empirically demonstrable and therefore subject to scrutiny. They are *standardized* in two senses: first, that they are meant to be administered and scored in a uniform and systematic way to everybody (with exceptions in cases where linguistic, cultural, or other adjustments are required); second, that their interpretation is based on some standard (e.g., performance of a population) and uses some criterion (e.g., total score on a scale).

The information derived by such instruments is then used for various clinical purposes, including: to arrive at a diagnosis, to formulate a person's problems, to develop a treatment plan, and to monitor the child's progress over time.

Assumptions of assessment instruments and main methodological approaches

The assumption underlying assessment instruments is that there exists a true score, e.g., a true score of depression severity. The word *true* here does not need to imply that depression is a naturally occurring entity, it is fine to consider this as a construct.

This assumption underlies both main approaches to assessment instruments, their design and interpretation, namely *standard test theory (STT)* and *item response theory (IRT)*.

STT (Lord *et al.*, 1968) posits that a test score is composed of a true score and an error score. The true score is the hypothetical construct that represents an individual's actual level of ability or trait, e.g., depression severity. The error score reflects sources of fallibility, such as factors associated with taking the test (e.g., being particularly tired on the day, or completing a questionnaire in a noisy environment), as well as problems with the test itself (e.g., poor wording or ambiguity of questions in depression). In STT the aim is to minimize the impact of measurement error and obtain accurate estimates of the true score.

In contrast, IRT models (Embretson & Reise, 2000) the probability of an individual responding correctly to an item as a function of their ability level and the characteristics of the item, such as how difficult a question is to answer (e.g., the difficulty of a question is too vaguely or too precisely specified) and discrimination (how well an item differentiates between people with depression—questions about suicidality provide high discrimination). IRT assumes that an individual's level of ability is a continuous latent variable that is normally distributed across the population and models the measurement error as a function of the individual's level of ability. IRT has become increasingly popular in educational and psychological testing.

Basic psychometric parameters of assessment instruments

Assessment instruments are measures and this means that numbers are allocated to concepts (be it symptoms or syndromes) according to some rules that follow statistical principles. Here, I discuss three key aspects of measures, namely reliability, validity, and accuracy.

Reliability

When we measure an outcome, such as depression severity, in a group of people there is variability—outcomes vary between individuals. Reliability is central to psychometric theory and reflects the ratio of the true variability between people in the construct measured (e.g., depression severity) over the total variability of the measure (that includes the sources of error mentioned above) (Nunnally & Bernstein, 1994). True variability cannot be measured directly and is therefore estimated in two main ways.

Cronbach's alpha

This measures how strongly related the items of a measurement are to each other e.g., different symptoms of depression. When we measure an outcome, such as depression severity, in a group of people, each item on that scale will have a correlation with the other items. Cronbach's alpha is proportional to the average of those correlations as well as the total number of items in the scale and is inversely related to the total variability of the items. Values with a Cronbach's alpha of 0.8 and above are considered reliable, or internally consistent, though cut-offs should be applied with care.

There are two important things to know about Cronbach's alpha. First, a very high alpha can be obtained simply by creating very long scales (as intuited by the fact that alpha is proportional to the number of items). This is not only meaningless to strive for, but also a waste of precious patient time. Second, a high alpha can be obtained by asking the same question in various ways, creating scales with high redundancy.

Test–retest reliability

This most commonly assesses the consistency of scores obtained from the same individuals on the same instrument at two or more different points in time, such as when the same patients are assessed on depression severity several days apart. It is easiest to intuit as the correlation between the same measure at the two different time points, although the use of different types of

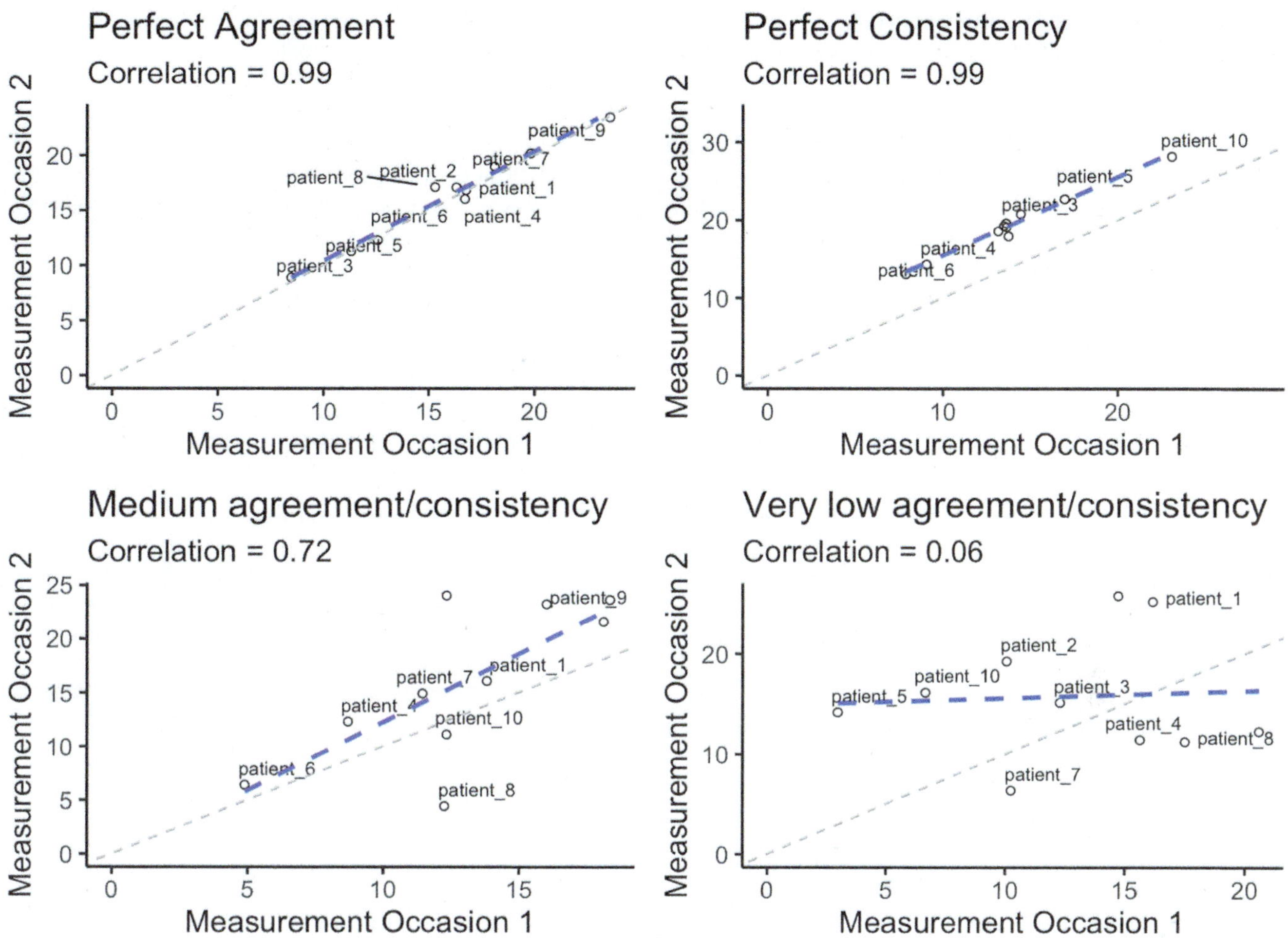

Figure 28.1 Illustrating patterns of reliability for two measurement occasions. In the top left-hand corner, is an occasion of perfect agreement. In this fictitious (and highly unlikely) situation, patients score exactly the same on average on the measure, on both occasions. In the top right, measurements of perfect consistency are displayed—every patient has shifted by 5 points between the two occasions (note that the correlation coefficient is the same as for the perfect agreement). In the bottom left, the more usual situation is depicted of medium agreement/consistency between the two measurement occasions. In the bottom right is an instance of random ratings on the scale on each occasion. Data come from simulations by the author.

intraclass correlation coefficient is more appropriate depending on purpose. The higher the absolute test-reliability coefficient, the better, with values above 0.2 indicating at least fair reliability.

Figure 28.1 illustrates reliability using 10 clinic patients in four prototypical cases.

Validity

Validity in psychometrics refers to the extent to which an instrument measures what it is intended to measure. There are several types of validity that can be assessed to determine the extent to which an instrument is valid:

Content validity assesses the extent to which the items of a measure cover the aspects of interest to be measured. For example, does a depression questionnaire adequately represent the breadth of the experience of depression?

Face validity assesses whether the items of a measure are appropriate and relevant to the people who use them. For example, how well do the items of a questionnaire ask about, say, low mood or anhedonia.

Criterion-related validity assesses how correlated a measure is with a criterion, or benchmark instrument, of the construct being measured. In psychiatry, a standard interview, or a previously used scale, are used as criteria against which a new scale will be measured. For example, one would expect any new measure of depression severity to demonstrate that it is strongly correlated with ones that are already in use.

Construct validity refers to the extent to which an instrument measures the construct it is intended to measure, rather than other constructs that may be related but distinct. For example, a questionnaire that purports to measure depression severity should correlate better with other scales that measure depression severity, rather than with scales that measure, say, attention deficit/hyperactivity disorder (ADHD).

Sensitivity, specificity, and accuracy

In clinical practice, scales are often used to make predictions, such as assess membership of a group, e.g., does the score on this questionnaire indicate that the patient is suffering from depression or not. Below, I discuss the parameters that are important in this regard based on a scenario.

Let there be a population of 2000 young people, half of whom have depression and the other half are healthy. You, the clinician, are using two different scales in order to screen this population with regards to depression. Obviously, your goal is to detect as many as possible of those who have depression and to avoid classifying healthy people as having depression. Figure 28.2a and b shows the results received from using each rating scale in this population and of applying different thresholds for each scale.

Figure 28.2a shows a good depression rating scale, one that differentiates well between people with depression (depicted as red dots) and those without (depicted as green dots). This is evident as those with depression generally score substantially higher than those without. By contrast, Figure 28.2b shows a

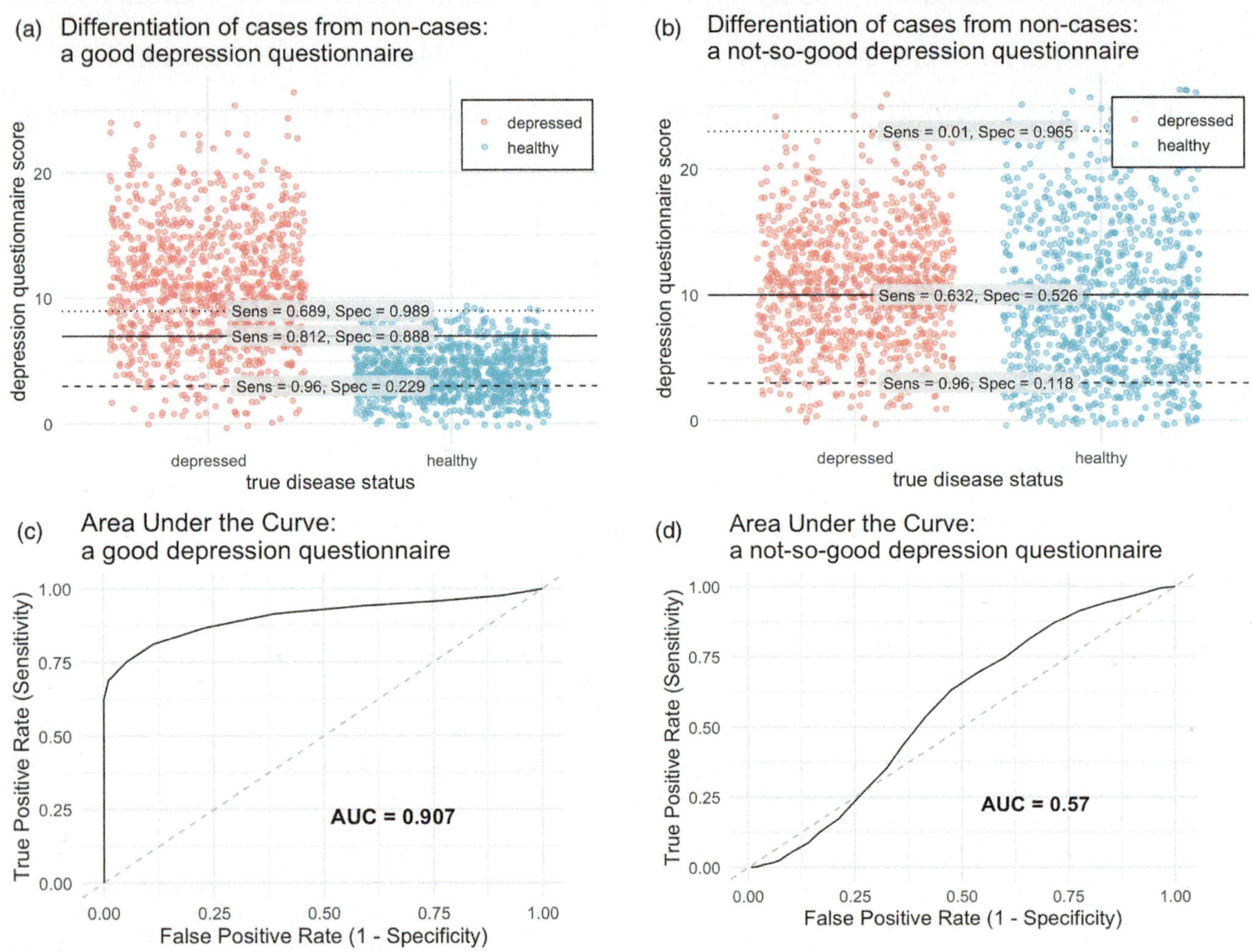

Figure 28.2 In this figure I illustrate some basic psychometric properties using a good (28.2a and 28.2c) and a not so good depression questionnaire (28.2b, and 28.2d). The good and not-so-good depression rating scale differ in terms of their ability to differentiate between people with depression from those without, as shown in Figures 28.2a and 28.2b. These two figures also depict sensitivities and specificities at different thresholds (questionnaire cut-offs). The red dots are the values in a depression questionnaire of patients with depression and the green dots are the scores of healthy people. The horizontal solid black line is the value of the questionnaire (threshold or cut-off score) which maximizes both sensitivity and specificity. As one moves upwards (e.g., dotted line) the specificity increases but the sensitivity decreases (many false negatives, missed cases of depression), and as one moves downwards (e.g., dashed line) the sensitivity increases at the cost of specificity (many false positives, mislabelled healthy people). Figures 28.2c and 28.2d depict the difference in the area under the curve (AUC, the integral of the curve) for the good and not-so-good rating scale, respectively. All data come from simulations done by the author. Code available upon request.

not-so-good depression rating scales, one where the differentiation between those who are depressed and those who are not is generally poor. There are many possible reasons for the difference in performance between the two scales, for example the not-so-good performing scale may be using questions that are irrelevant to people, or the questions may be phrased in a way that is not clear to people, compared to the good scale.

Also, on each Figure 28.2a and 28.2b, there are three lines that represent thresholds, cut-off scores, for each questionnaire: these are points at which a clinician may declare that patients scoring above it are "a case" (and those scoring below it are "not a case"). Where the threshold is set determines how *sensitive* and how *specific* the test will be for detecting caseness. I explain the terms below.

Sensitivity (also called true positive rate) refers to the ability of a test to correctly identify individuals who have the condition of interest. It is calculated as the proportion of people who are identified as having depression among all those who actually have depression (as measured against the gold standard of depression, e.g., an interview assessing depression). A high sensitivity (the bottom dashed black line shows an extreme version) may be desired of screening instruments to make sure that cases are not missed. The horizontal solid line in Figure 28.2a (good questionnaire) shows a sensitivity of 0.81, or expressed in absolute numbers, the questionnaire correctly identified 812 out of 1000 people with depression as having the disease (but also missed 188 of them). This is the point where the accuracy (explained below), is maximal.

Specificity (also called true negative rate), refers to the ability of a test or model to correctly identify individuals who do not have the condition of interest. A high specificity is desirable post-screening, particularly when making important treatment decisions (an extreme of this is depicted by the top dotted black line). The horizontal solid line in Figure 28.2a (good questionnaire) shows a specificity of 0.89, or expressed in absolute numbers, the questionnaire correctly identified 888 out of 1000 people *without* depression as *not* having the disease (but also misclassified 112 of them as having it when they didn't). This is the point where the accuracy (explained below), is maximal.

Accuracy refers to the overall performance of a test or model at a specified threshold, by finding the best balance between sensitivity and specificity, but also the prevalence (in this case, how common depression is in the sample). In the depression case it would be the sum of true positives and true negatives divided over the whole population (true positives and negatives as well as false positives and negatives). The accuracy is much higher for the good (accuracy_good = 0.85) than for the not-so-good questionnaire (accuracy_not-so_good = 0.58).

Area under the curve (AUC) refers to an evaluation of how good a binary is (e.g., depression versus no depression, that is, how clear the separation between the two groups would be). Figure 28.2c (corresponding to the good questionnaire) and 28.2d (corresponding to the not-so-good questionnaire), depict this relationship in a plot where the true positive rate (sensitivity) is plotted on the y-axis and the false positive rate (specificity reversely plotted) on the x-axis. This is, for historical reasons, called a receiver operating characteristic (ROC) curve. The test with the biggest AUC, is the best. An optimal test would be at (x, y) coordinates of 0, 1 and it would have the maximal area; by contrast a test that performs as well as a coin flip, would be at 0.5, 0.5, that is on the diagonal, the line that cuts the ROC curve into two equal triangles. It is evident that the AUC is much higher for the good than for the not-so-good questionnaire.

It is worth noting here that clinicians are often faced with the reverse scenario, namely: if a test for depression is positive (or negative), what is the probability that their patient has (or, respectively, does not have) depression? The positive predictive value (PPV) is the ratio of true positives over all positive tests (true+false positives). This (and the equivalently calculated negative predictive value, NPV) are of practical relevance. The PPV in our example of the good questionnaire is pretty good (PPV = 0.88) not least because the prevalence of depression is high (50%). But the same questionnaire would have a PPV = 0.6, i.e. much lower, if the prevalence had been at 10% (e.g. at a depression prevalence common in the adolescent general population). This is an important public health insight and the relative excess of false positives one of the challenges of broad screening.

Types of assessment instruments

Interviews

Semistructured interviews are instruments that are typically conducted by clinicians (or researchers supervised by clinicians). They typically involve a set of standardized questions that the interviewer can use as a guide, and also allow for flexibility to explore areas of particular relevance to the individual being assessed. This type of interview is useful for gathering detailed information about specific symptoms or areas of concern, while still allowing for individual differences in presentation.

Structured interviews, on the other hand, are highly standardized and typically include a set of predetermined questions and response options. This type of interview is useful for ensuring consistency in the assessment process across different patients and assessors and can be particularly helpful for research purposes.

Most semistructured and structured interviews follow either DSM-IV or DSM-5 criteria, some also ICD-10, to assess a wide range of mental health symptoms and disorders in children and

Table 28.1 Common interviews for general psychopathology in child and adolescent psychiatry.

Child and Adolescent Psychiatric Assessment (CAPA)	Structured diagnostic interview used to assess a wide range of psychiatric disorders and substance abuse in children and adolescents	Angold *et al.* (1995)
Development and Well-being Assessment (DAWBA)	Structured diagnostic interview used to assess a wide range of mental disorders in children and adolescents	Goodman *et al.* (2000)
Diagnostic Interview Schedule for Children (DISC)	Structured diagnostic interview used to assess a wide range of mental disorders in children and adolescents	Shaffer *et al.* (1996)
Kiddie Schedule for Affective Disorders and Schizophrenia (K-SADS)	Semi-structured diagnostic interview used to assess current and past episodes of psychopathology in children and adolescents	Kaufman *et al.* (1997)

adolescents, including anxiety, depression, and autism spectrum disorder (ASD). Please refer to Table 28.1, for some of the most widely used of such instruments.

Rating scales

Rating scales provide a standardized way of measuring a range of mental health issues, such as anxiety, depression, ADHD, and ASD, among others. Rating scales can be completed by various sources, including parents, teachers, the child or adolescent themselves, and clinicians. Please refer to Table 28.2, for some of the most widely used rating scales for depression, anxiety, and behavior problems. Rating scales typically enquire about symptoms or signs of problems—their intensity and/or frequency, as well as resulting impairments. Some scales explicitly enquire about the strengths of the person. Some rating scales also assess situational factors (e.g., when a problem arises), though, in practice, these are used less frequently.

There are broadband scales that enquire about psychopathology overall, with the Strengths and Difficulties Questionnaire (SDQ) and the Child Behavior Checklist (CBCL) being prime examples. These are used at assessment and sometimes at follow up.

There are specific scales used at assessment, such as the Mood and Feelings Questionnaire (MFQ) or the Screen for Child Anxiety Related Emotional Disorders (SCARED) for depression and anxiety, respectively.

Some scales are designed for assessing treatment progress, such as the Children's Depression Rating Scale-Revised (CDRS-R).

Observational measures

These measures involve the systematic observation and recording of a child's behavior, either through real-time observation or video recordings. Such measures can be used for diagnostic purposes, typically in ASD, or for the purposes of treatment planning and monitoring. Observations offer insights into the processes that may underlie the genesis or maintenance of psychopathology, such as parent–child conflict and understanding behavioral problems in children (such as oppositionality) and their treatment. They are particularly useful for very young children (e.g., mother–infant observations) and children who are limited in their verbal expression, and their use in core autism reflects such issues. Observational methods are limited in their utility by the effort and time they require to be set up, conducted, and coded

Perhaps the most widely used observational measure is the Autism Diagnostic Observation Schedule (ADOS). The ADOS contains both structured and semistructured elements that assess the symptoms of ASD in children and adolescents. It contains tasks and activities that assess social interaction, communication, and repetitive behaviors, and is considered the gold standard for diagnosing ASD (Lord *et al.*, 2000).

Other widely used instruments include the Disruptive Behavior–Diagnostic Observation Schedule (DB-DOS), a structured clinic-based assessment designed to elicit clinically salient behaviors relevant to the diagnosis of disruptive behavior in preschoolers (Wakschlag *et al.*, 2008).

The Student Observation System (SOS) is another observation tool used to assess the behavior of children and adolescents in the classroom setting. The SOS includes a set of standardized codes that capture behaviors such as academic engagement, disruptive behavior, and social interactions (Reynolds *et al.*, 2015).

Coding Interactive Behavior (CIB) is an observational measure used to assess the quality of parent–child interactions. The CIB includes a set of standardized codes that capture behaviors such as sensitivity, intrusiveness, and positive affect (Feldman, 2012).

Ecological momentary assessment (EMA)

EMA typically involves the use of electronic devices, such as smartphones or wearable sensors, to prompt participants to provide data multiple times a day, for several days or weeks. Young people are usually asked to respond to brief questionnaires or surveys, report their mood, activities, or events, or provide other types of information, such as physiological or geolocation data.

The main advantage of EMA is that it provides a more detailed and accurate picture of people's behaviors and experiences in their everyday lives, compared to traditional methods that rely on retrospective self-reports (which are liable to several memory biases, particularly over longer time frames) or laboratory settings. The promise of EMA is that it assesses the dynamic nature of mental health symptoms and behaviors in children and adolescents (Myin-Germeys *et al.*, 2018). Here, dynamic refers to how symptoms change over different time scales (e.g., how suicidal ideation fluctuates in real time) and how they may depend on environmental factors (e.g., how going to school or interacting with peers may affect depression severity) (Kleiman *et al.*, 2017). Challenges to using EMA

Table 28.2 Common rating scales in child and adolescent psychiatry.

Assessment instrument	Description	Reporter(s)	No. of items	Reference
Affective Reactivity Index (ARI)	Irritability: preschool to age 18 years	Parent, self	7	Stringaris *et al.* (2012)
Beck Depression Inventory (BDI-II)	Measures severity of depressive symptoms	Self	21	Beck *et al.* (1996)
Center for Epidemiological Studies Depression Scale (CES-D)	Measures depressive symptoms in the general population	Self	20	Garrison *et al.* (1991)
Child Behavior Checklist (CBCL)	Broadband psychopathology	Parent or self-report	113	Achenbach & Rescorla (2004)
Children's Depression Inventory (CDI)	Measures depressive symptoms in children and adolescents	Self, parent	27	Kovacs (1985)
Children's Depression Rating Scale - Revised (CDRS-R)	Measures severity of depressive symptoms in children and adolescents	Clinician, parent	17	Poznanski *et al.* (1984)
Clinician Affective Reactivity Index (CL-ARI)	Irritability: 6–18 years of age	Clinician	12	Haller *et al.* (2020)
Conners' Rating Scales - Revised (CRS-R)	Measures symptoms of attention deficit/hyperactivity disorder (ADHD)	Parent, teacher	27	Conners *et al.* (1998)
Emotion Dysregulation Inventory (EDI)	Emotion dysregulation with subscales for reactivity and dysphoria	Parent	30	Mazefsky *et al.* (2018)
Mood and Feelings Questionnaire (MFQ)	Measures depressive symptoms in children and adolescents	Self, parent	33	Angold *et al.* (1995)
Multidimensional Anxiety Scale for Children (MASC)	Measures anxiety symptoms in children and adolescents	Self, parent	39	March *et al.* (1997)
Revised Children's Anxiety and Depression Scale (RCADS)	Measures anxiety and depressive symptoms in children and adolescents	Self, parent	47	Chorpita *et al.* (2000)
Reynolds Adolescent Depression Scale (RADS-2)	Measures depressive symptoms in adolescents	Self, clinician	30	Reynolds (2004)
Screen for Child Anxiety Related Emotional Disorders (SCARED)	Measures anxiety symptoms in children and adolescents	Self, parent	41	Birmaher *et al.* (1997)
Spence Children's Anxiety Scale (SCAS)	Measures anxiety symptoms in children and adolescents	Self, parent	44	Spence *et al.* (2003)
SNAP-IV ADHD	Measures symptoms of ADHD	Parent, teacher	26	Swanson *et al.* (2001)
Social Communications Questionnaire (SCQ)	Assessing social communication skills in autism spectrum disorder (ASD)	Parent	40	Rutter *et al.* (2003)
Social Responsiveness Scale (SRS)	Assessing social responsiveness in ASD	Parent, teacher	65	Constantino & Gruber (2005)
Strengths and Difficulties Questionnaire (SDQ)	Broadband psychopathology	Self, parent, teacher	25	Goodman (1997)

include: (i) compliance and engagement as young people, particularly those at school or in other activities, may forget or be unable to respond to questions; (ii) technical issues, which include variations in young people's ability to use devices; and (iii) ethical issues around not only data sharing, but also potential overexposure to electronic devices.

Chatbots

Chatbots are computer programs that have been designed to simulate conversation with human users. Chatbots have been used for a variety of purposes, for both assessment and treatment delivery, and may, overall, be acceptable to young people (Dosovitsky & Bunge, 2023), and also in trials (Nicol *et al.*, 2022), though further research is required into their use.

The basic ingredients of scale development and interpretation

In this section, I discuss the importance of how standardized assessment instruments should take account of the perspectives of young people, describe briefly how scales developed (most recently in co-research with young people), and discuss two key components of their interpretation, namely the derivation of norms and standards, and the integration of different informant sources.

Lived experience, and youth goals and preferences

Here, I discuss the value of the perspective of people with lived experience in the design and application of assessment instruments and provide two examples of such instruments.

Involving young people and families with lived experience in the design and development of assessment instruments is currently considered best practice for two main reasons (Scrutton, 2017). First, for reasons of epistemic justice, because it is unethical to ignore the perspective of the person with lived experiences themselves and devalue their knowledge about their own self. Second, for practical reasons, as it is expected to lead to more relevant, understandable, and acceptable assessment tools (i.e., improve both content and face validity, see earlier section on "Validity"), that also empower young people in their mental health care. It will also be interesting to have empirical demonstration of how involving young people can lead to measurable improvements in health care.

It is relevant to discuss two types of instruments here that reflect the importance allocated to the views of health care users themselves. The first is *preference-based measurement*: this is in keeping with the idea of the importance of patients' perspectives on their own health and is a method used to measure the health-related quality of life (HRQoL) of children and adolescents. It is primarily used by economists to assesses individuals' preferences for different health states and allows for the calculation of quality-adjusted life years (QALYs), a measure of the value of a particular health state. A typical example of this is the Child Health Utility 9D (CHU9D) (Stevens & Ratcliffe, 2012). The second is *goal-based measurement* which focuses on the achievement of specific goals that are collaboratively set between the patient and the provider. This approach is particularly important in child and adolescent psychiatry, where treatment goals may involve not only symptom reduction but also improvements in social, academic, and family functioning. Goals are defined as working on the existing gap between current and desired states and the relevant changes in how one feels and acts that they want to achieve through therapy. It involves questions such as: "What do you want to be different?," and "Where do you want to go from here?"

Overall, people with lived experience can be involved as members of the research team, as advisors (e.g., youth advisory board) and as part of the team that disseminates outputs.

How are scales developed?

In order to understand the advantages and challenges of assessment instruments, it may help the clinical reader to have an overview of how scales are developed (Streiner *et al.*, 2014). Here, I provide a simplified set of steps that are typically involved. I use the development of a depression measurement scale as an example.

Step 1: Conceptualization and item generation

The first step in developing a psychometric scale is to identify the construct that the scale will measure. In this case, the DSM-5 criteria for depression will be reviewed along with the literature of existing scales. Involving people with lived experience as researchers at this stage can be quite helpful in considering aspects of depression experience that academic researchers may not be aware of. It may also facilitate engagement with other young people with lived experience as research participants, and encourage them to offer views about the moods, feelings, and cognitive and bodily experiences that are typically left out of scales. A recent historical review indicates how our current concept of depression may be unduly narrow (Kendler, 2016a). The development team can use the results of such reviews and develop them further in order to generate a pool of items that represent the various symptoms and features of depression, i.e., have face and content validity (see earlier section on "Validity").

Step 2: Item selection

The next step is to select the most appropriate items from the pool generated in Step 1. This process involves a thorough review of each depression item, and items that are poorly worded, redundant (e.g., asking about sadness in various different ways), or not relevant to the construct being measured are removed. The remaining items are then reviewed to ensure that they have good face validity and coverage of pertinent themes (e.g., anhedonia in depression). Again, involving young people at this stage can be very helpful and methodologies, such as cognitive interviewing, exist that provide a framework to scrutinize items for how understandable, acceptable, and relevant they are.

Step 3: Scale administration

Once the items have been selected, they are administered to a sample of individuals who have experience with the construct being measured—in this case, depression. The sample should be representative of the population of interest, and its size should be sufficient to provide adequate statistical power. Typically, respondents are asked to rate the extent to which they agree or disagree with each item using a Likert scale or another appropriate response format, such as a visual analog scale.

Step 4: Analysis of acceptability and basic psychometric properties

The primary question is whether the scale is acceptable to people. One can ask young people directly about it, but rates of response can also be quite helpful in this. It is worth giving young people the opportunity to comment on individual items, as well as on the scale as a whole.

The data collected from the scale administration are analyzed to evaluate the psychometric properties of the scale. This involves steps such as the following:

Factor analysis is used to identify the underlying structure of the scale items. In the case of a depression scale, this would involve identifying whether the questions all measure one dimension (e.g., depression) or whether subscales can be identified (e.g., representing sadness versus loss of interest or somatic problems).

Reliability analysis involves estimating Cronbach's alpha and test–retest reliability as described in the earlier section on "Reliability".

Validity analysis where the various forms of validity described above are estimated. Existing depression scales are used as outcomes (bearing in mind that very high coefficients of correlation may not be desired as this would indicate that a new scale might not be needed).

Step 5: Scale revision and new data collection

Based on the results of the first-round data analysis, the scale may need to be revised. This involves removing or modifying items or delivery format and collecting new data. Again, involving young people at each stage of the above process can help make scale development relevant to those who are meant to benefit from it.

Another important question about rating scales and, more generally, assessment instruments is whether they measure the same thing across time and across cultures. The frequency of behavior/symptoms changes over time (e.g., think about temper outbursts) but their significance will also change over time (e.g., stealing at the age of 5, which may refer to taking out more chocolate than told to out of a bowl, versus stealing at the age of 16, which may refer to theft). Statistical approaches from the factor analysis tradition, chiefly *measurement invariance* evaluation, are primarily deployed to examine how much a test evaluates the same construct across time and place.

How are standards, norms, and thresholds derived?

Using measured outcome to inform clinical decision-making entails making normative judgments; that is, deciding what is bad or worse than before, and what is good or may have gotten better. This is true both for outcomes measured in a binary way (diagnosis or not) and those measured as a spectrum; this is because clinical decision-making is categorical, e.g., treat or not, refer further or not, discharge or not, improved or not, etc.

Normative judgments are often implicit as they rely on societal expectations about age, gender, and social position. They matter not only in terms of how questions are asked and measures are designed, but also in how feedback is conveyed (Stringaris, 2021).

One way of developing norms is based on what position a person occupies in a distribution of test scores. It involves collecting data from a representative sample of individuals who are similar to those for whom the test is intended, e.g., depressed adolescents. Once data are collected from the sample, the scores are analyzed to determine the distribution of scores and the average score, in this case of depression. This then allows the placing of the individual in their position on the distribution of depression scores, e.g., finding out that their score corresponds to the ninety-fifth percentile of the population.

Another way of developing norms is based on a criterion. For example, when validating an instrument for depression, one could use the diagnosis of depression as a criterion and establish the score that predicts depression with high enough accuracy. This is then used as a threshold for depression diagnosis and people can be above or below that criterion.

It should be obvious that in both of these examples, the choice of the norm (the percentile or the diagnostic threshold) is an arbitrary one; it is not inherent in the quantitative measurement but rather a judgment that is influenced by values that prevail in society.

Dealing with informant sources

CAMH classically involves collecting information from various informants, including the young person, their parents, and teachers. Research has consistently shown that there is often at best moderate agreement between informants about youth psychopathology. For example, a meta-analysis (Achenbach *et al.*, 1987) found correlations between informants of around $r = 0.28$, a fairly modest agreement. Other studies have found similarly modest levels of agreement between informants on measures of depression, anxiety, and other mental health outcomes (De Los Reyes & Kazdin, 2005). There are several hypotheses about such disagreements and they include measurement problems (e.g., the inability of young people to report reliably on their problems), limited knowledge (e.g., of parents and particularly teachers about a child's emotional problems, to which the only the child has privileged access), and the different settings at which children are observed (e.g., a child may behave differently at home than at school).

Another factor that may contribute to informant disagreement is the degree to which informants are aware of each other's reports. For example, a recent study of informant sources of irritability showed substantial disagreement between parent and child reports of irritability despite good psychometric properties (Cronbach's alpha and test–retest reliability) for each informant report (Mallidi *et al.*, 2023). This has led the authors to propose that children and parents interpret items differently and that this may be an indication of heterogeneity of the irritability construct.

In any case, clinicians should try to avoid simply averaging informant sources, as information may be lost. Similarly, they should also be cautious about simply applying an "or" rule to decide whether a diagnosis is present or not: again, prevalence estimates can vary substantially depending on how informant reports are handled (Schwab-Stone *et al.*, 1996). There is no recipe on what to do with informant disagreement, except perhaps to be open-minded about the possibility that either or both informants may be right in their rating (each from their own perspective, perhaps). A clinician ought to document such differences and, where appropriate, try to resolve them in follow-up interviews enquiring further with each informant or even by interviewing them together—differences in perspective are revealing for assessment and treatment

Practical aspects of assessment

Ethics and conditions for assessment

Ensuring confidentiality and being upfront about what conditions may necessitate breaching it (in the case of certain risks to self or others) is expected of every clinician conducting an assessment. Ensuring confidentiality can be tricky when conducting assessments remotely and when storing assessments online or electronically. Following best practices in the clinician's country and organization is important and identifying information should be used sparingly—de-identification should be used whenever possible.

In general, the informant (patient or carer) should have easy access to the outcomes of the assessment and the assumption should be that the data belong to them.

The conditions should be conducive to assessment. This starts with "electronic convenience,"—the ease with which electronic assessments can be accessed and completed. There is some evidence that providing electronic platforms for completion of PROMS leads to higher completion rates compared to in-clinic completion (Morris *et al.*, 2023). When in a clinic, patients and carers should be given enough time and a quiet space to complete their measures.

Clinicians should also be understanding if patients and carers have not had time to complete questionnaires—families with children with mental health difficulties will very often be disadvantaged in multiple other ways and short of time and resources (e.g., childcare). Making time to complete the questionnaires in a clinic can be helpful.

How to choose assessment instruments

Different assessment instruments will be used for different purposes. In general, the best screening instruments will have a high sensitivity at the expense of specificity, whereas more specificity will be required when treatment decisions become necessary. Also, in the initial phases of assessment, broadband instruments (e.g., the SDQ (Goodman, 1997)) will be more useful in getting a general sense of the breadth of problems, allowing the clinician to then hone in more at later stages using specific instruments, e.g., for depression or ADHD.

Efficiency is important at every stage. Asking too many questions (having assessment batteries that are too long) risks attrition and dysphoria.

It is probably best for a service to have a standard battery of tests that everyone receives initially (e.g., a broadband scale), which can then be refined, though this will also depend on the profile of the service—those that specialize in a certain condition, e.g., mood disorders, will want to screen for that condition in sufficient depth in advance.

Considerations when collecting and interpreting data from assessment instruments

What is the issue?

The first question is "What is the problem?" The leading problem may be different for children than for parents and carers. It can be elicited by simple open questions of the type: "I would like to hear from you about the reasons that we are meeting here," or "From your point of view, why are we meeting here today?" Instruments for assessing leading problems include the Top Problems tool, developed by Weisz and colleagues (Weisz *et al.*, 2011), particularly at the outset and monitoring of treatment.

Establishing a common language

Parents and children often refer to the same problem in different ways. Neither patients nor their parents/carers will necessarily use DSM-based terminology to communicate their problems. Words such as "bored" may be used to denote depressive feelings, while "I am naughty" may be the only thing that a child can say initially to describe their behavior problems. It is important to pick up on such cues and encourage the person interviewed to tell you more about them during an interview. Both null findings as well as overestimation of pathology in questionnaires can arise because the wording is outdated or inappropriate. Going through individual questions with the patient or carer can help, particularly when aspects of the assessment are known to be ambiguous.

Who reports the problem?

This will vary by the age of the children referred to the clinic, or the area of the problems (e.g., obsessive–compulsive disorder (OCD) versus autism or ADHD) that the clinic specializes in. Both parents and teachers will be good at noticing the behaviors, and will therefore be good informants about behavioral equivalents of say irritability, i.e., the temper outbursts. However, teachers, in particular, may not be as good at describing accompanying feelings of anxiety or low mood, or the more persistent and often not externalized irritable mood. Typically developing children as young as seven years may provide meaningful accounts of their own feelings and of accompanying circumstances.

Placing the problem in a time frame

In a semistructured interview, it is generally a good idea to elicit accounts of symptoms related to specific events. Commonly, this is achieved by asking the parents or young people to refer to "the most recent," the "most severe," or the "one you can best remember." If the problem is a daily occurrence, asking the person interviewed to take you through a "typical day" can be very helpful too. Using a whiteboard or a sheet of paper to achieve this can help identify patterns. Trying to do this with both informant sources can be useful—disparate views on concrete events are revealing, as is the coincidence of opinion.

Establishing a comparator

The first comparator, used in many questionnaires and interviews, asks the parent to rate children compared to other children of that age. This is particularly useful when asking about problems that occur repeatedly over time or are chronic.

The second comparator is the child themselves over time. This is the basis of assessing change over the last week or month. It is particularly useful when assessing episodic problems (e.g., depression) or those that have potentially sharply demarcated onsets (e.g., behavioral changes following abuse).

Intensity of the problem

When assessing intensity, it is important not to simply rely on the labels that the informant provides. Descriptions such as: "he is depressed" or "she had a tantrum" should be explored further and the clinician should look for individual signs or symptoms through their interview. Questionnaires serve the same purpose by asking about several possible symptoms.

The clinician will look at the report of the parent, carer, or teacher for signs of distress. For example, the following information is useful in judging a child's tantrum: the extent of angry facial expressions, being red in the face, yelling, screaming, and stamping of feet. Breaking things and attacking others are obvious signs of escalation and higher intensity.

Looking at the total score of questionnaires is important but can also be misleading. Certain conditions, such as OCD or body dysmorphic disorder (BDD), may be very impairing even when monosymptomatic—one single symptom, such as hand washing, can be so frequent or of such long duration as to be devastating.

Chronicity

The time of onset of a problem is not always clear and research instruments may avoid such questions to avoid recall biases. However, hearing about onset can be quite helpful for understanding perceptions of the problem. Characteristically in the case of irritability, one may receive answers from the parent of the type: "forever, ever since he was born." Similarly, in depression the time of onset may be blurry. By contrast, there may be very clear and sharply demarcated onsets, and these can give clues about important life events, such as trauma.

Clinicians will want to know whether depression, anxiety, or irritability occur as discrete episodes (e.g., a period of one week of very intense low mood or irritability) or as something chronic, that is, a set of feelings and behaviors that have been typical of the young person for a considerable period of time. Drawing a timeline—perhaps on a board or a large sheet of paper—can be quite helpful.

Context and antecedents

Some symptoms will manifest in certain circumstances only, such as when reminded of traumatic events or when confronted with particular challenges, e.g., when a child with autism is faced with an unannounced change. Other symptoms are pervasive, i.e., they can occur at home as much as at school, or during leisure activities. Pervasiveness is generally regarded as an indicator of severity. However, symptoms that occur only in particular contexts can also be debilitating—characteristically, oppositionality that is restricted to the parents. Conventional questionnaires and interviews are often not designed to assess this and thus deprive the clinician of important information. Diary keeping and recording by tablets or smartphones can be particularly helpful.

Impact and consequences

It is worth thinking about these problems along two axes. The first axis concerns the domains or environment in which problems manifest. Often these are divided into family life, school environment (to include academic performance and behavior), leisure time, and peer relationships. This division of domains is reflected in several instruments, including in the impact supplement of the SDQ.

The second axis concerns the time scale of impact and consequences, and is typically divided into immediate (or short-term), medium-, and long-term consequences.

There are several scales one can use for assessing functioning and impact, including the clinician-rated Children's Global Assessment Scale (CGAS) (Shaffer *et al.*, 1983) and the parent-, teacher-, or youth-reported SDQ impact supplement.

Limitations and criticisms concerning assessment instruments

As mentioned at the beginning of this chapter, the use of assessment instruments offers several advantages and is becoming more common in clinical practice. However, there are several reasons to be cautious in the interpretation of results from assessment instruments. I enumerate these below.

Undue reification

It is common to view psychiatric diagnoses or dimensions as real entities, as if our classification had carved nature at its joints. This is very unlikely to be the case for most psychiatric and psychological disorders, and alternative explanations have been proposed (Kendler, 2016b). In any case, it is important to display sufficient epistemic humility when referring to diagnoses and dimensions arrived at through assessment instruments: it is very unlikely that, at least for the moment, our measurement in psychiatry resembles that of, say, temperature measurement using mercury.

Narrow representation

It is striking that most assessment instruments have been developed in a subset of Western industrialized countries. Many of these instruments have been translated and applied to populations outside those countries, but the fact that they are inspired and driven primarily by concerns in one part of the world may constrain our knowledge about variation in psychological phenomena. It may lead to either over- or underrecognition of problems in people. Perhaps inevitably, most instruments are developed within the bounds of the normativities (Stringaris, 2021) of a certain historical epoch and of a dominant class of people within a society. Such normativities shape how instruments are developed and what is measured. As a result, experiences of those less represented, including those of different sexual orientation or gender minorities, may be absent. This is a particular problem given the disproportionately higher rates of psychopathology in certain underrepresented groups (Reisner *et al.*, 2016). Similar issues arise when applying criteria developed for boys (as in ADHD research) onto girls, or vice versa, and when symptom thresholds are applied uncritically across age ranges.

Psychometric criticism

Criticisms that apply to the DSM or ICD classification systems also apply to assessment instruments. For example, based on current criteria, one can arrive at thousands of different depression syndromes, simply based on combinatorics, and this heterogeneity is also demonstrable empirically (Fried & Nesse, 2015). Similarly, instruments are developed in ways that are not always transparent; some items are simply used ad hoc, decisions about the inclusion or exclusion of items and the statistics are often not clear, and several instruments may be developed that purport to measure the same thing but measure something different, or purport to measure different things but actually show great overlap.

Access

Many instruments are behind paywalls, even though public funds have been used (sometimes exclusively) for their development and despite the fact that the income from such instruments is reasonably thought to far exceed maintenance and related costs. This is particularly frustrating when it concerns instruments that have become "gold standard" as it means that cash-strapped clinics and health care systems will not have access to them and that patients will not benefit from their use.

References

Achenbach, T.M. & Rescorla, L.A. (2004) The Achenbach System of Empirically Based Assessment (ASEBA) for ages 1.5 to 18 years. In: *The Use of Psychological Testing for Treatment Planning and Outcomes Assessment: Instruments for Children and Adolescents.* (ed M.E. Maruish), 3rd edn, Vol. 2. Lawrence Erlbaum, Mahwah, NJ. pp. 179–213.

Achenbach, T.M. *et al.* (1987) Child/adolescent behavioral and emotional problems: implications of cross-informant correlations for situational specificity. *Psychological Bulletin* **101**, 213–232. doi:10.1037/0033-2909.101.2.213.

Aebi, M. *et al.* (2012) The use of the Development and Well-being Assessment (DAWBA) in clinical practice: a randomized trial. *European Child & Adolescent Psychiatry* **21**, 559–567. doi:10.1007/s00787-012-0293-6.

Anastasi, A. & Urbina, S. (1997) *Psychological Testing*, 7th edn. Prentice Hall/Pearson Education, Upper Saddle River, NJ.

Angold, A. *et al.* (1995) Development of a short questionnaire for use in epidemiological studies of depression in children and adolescents. *International Journal of Methods in Psychiatric Research* **5**, 237–249.

Beck, A.T. *et al.* (1996) Comparison of Beck Depression Inventories-IA and -II in psychiatric outpatients. *Journal of Personality Assessment* **67**, 588–597. doi:10.1207/s15327752jpa6703_13.

Bickman, L. *et al.* (2011) Effects of routine feedback to clinicians on mental health outcomes of youths: results of a randomized trial. *Psychiatric Services* **62**, 1423–1429. doi:10.1176/appi.ps.002052011.

Birmaher, B. *et al.* (1997) The Screen for Child Anxiety Related Emotional Disorders (SCARED): scale construction and psychometric characteristics. *Journal of the American Academy of Child and Adolescent Psychiatry* **36**, 545–553. doi:10.1097/00004583-199704000-00018.

Chorpita, B.F. *et al.* (2000) Assessment of symptoms of DSM-IV anxiety and depression in children: a revised child anxiety and depression scale. *Behaviour Research and Therapy* **38**, 835–855. doi:10.1016/s0005-7967(99)00130-8.

Conners, C. *et al.* (1998) The revised Conners' Parent Rating Scale (CPRS-R): factor structure, reliability, and criterion validity. *Journal of Abnormal Child Psychology* **26**, 257–268. doi:10.1023/A:1022602400621.

Constantino, J. & Gruber, C. (2005) *The Social Responsiveness Scale.* Western Psychological Sciences, Los Angeles, CA.

Day, F. *et al.* (2022) STAndardised DIagnostic Assessment for children and young people with emotional difficulties (STADIA): protocol for a multicentre randomised controlled trial. *BMJ Open* **12**, e053043. doi:10.1136/bmjopen-2021-053043.

De Los Reyes, A. & Kazdin, A.E. (2005) Informant discrepancies in the assessment of childhood psychopathology: a critical review, theoretical framework, and recommendations for further study. *Psychological Bulletin* **131**, 483–509. doi:10.1037/0033-2909.131.4.483.

Dosovitsky, G. & Bunge, E. (2023) Development of a chatbot for depression: adolescent perceptions and recommendations. *Child and Adolescent Mental Health* **28**, 124–127. doi:10.1111/camh.12627.

Embretson, S.E. & Reise, S.P. (2000) *Item Response Theory for Psychologists.* Psychology Press, New York. doi:10.4324/9781410605269.

Feldman, R. (2012) Parenting behavior as the environment where children grow. In: *The Cambridge Handbook of Environment in Human Development, Cambridge Handbooks in Psychology.* (eds L.C. Mayes & M. Lewis). Cambridge University Press, New York, NY. pp. 535–567. doi:10.1017/CBO9781139016827.031.

Ford, T. *et al.* (2013) Can standardized diagnostic assessment be a useful adjunct to clinical assessment in child mental health services? A randomized controlled trial of disclosure of the Development and Well-being Assessment to practitioners. *Social Psychiatry and Psychiatric Epidemiology* **48**, 583–593. doi:10.1007/s00127-012-0564-z.

Fried, E.I. & Nesse, R.M. (2015) Depression is not a consistent syndrome: an investigation of unique symptom patterns in the STAR*D study. *Journal of Affective Disorders* **172**, 96–102. doi:10.1016/j.jad.2014.10.010.

Garrison, C.Z. *et al.* (1991) The CES-D as a screen for depression and other psychiatric disorders in adolescents. *Journal of the American Academy of Child & Adolescent Psychiatry* **30**, 636–641. doi:10.1097/00004583-199107000-00017.

Goodman, R. (1997) The Strengths and Difficulties Questionnaire: a research note. *Journal of Child Psychology and Psychiatry* **38**, 581–586. doi:10.1111/j.1469-7610.1997.tb01545.x.

Goodman, R. *et al.* (2000) The Development and Well-being Assessment: description and initial validation of an integrated assessment of child and adolescent psychopathology. *Journal of Child Psychology and Psychiatry* **41**, 645–655.

Haller, S.P. *et al.* (2020) The Clinician Affective Reactivity Index: validity and reliability of a clinician-rated assessment of irritability. *Behavior Therapy* **51**, 283–293. doi:10.1016/j.beth.2019.10.005.

Kaufman, J. *et al.* (1997) Schedule for Affective Disorders and Schizophrenia for school-age children-Present and Lifetime version (K-SADS-PL): initial reliability and validity data. *Journal of the American Academy of Child and Adolescent Psychiatry* **36**, 980–988. doi:10.1097/00004583-199707000-00021.

Kendler, K.S. (2016a) The phenomenology of major depression and the representativeness and nature of DSM criteria. *The American Journal of Psychiatry* **173**, 771–780. doi:10.1176/appi.ajp.2016.15121509.

Kendler, K.S. (2016b) The nature of psychiatric disorders. *World Psychiatry* **15**, 5–12. doi:10.1002/wps.20292.

Kleiman, E.M. *et al.* (2017) Examination of real-time fluctuations in suicidal ideation and its risk factors: results from two ecological momentary assessment studies. *Journal of Abnormal Psychology* **126**, 726–738. doi:10.1037/abn0000273.

Kovacs, M. (1985) The Children's Depression, Inventory (CDI). *Psychopharmacology Bulletin* **21**, 995–998.

Lord, F.M. *et al.* (1968) *Statistical Theories of Mental Test Scores.* Addison-Wesley, Oxford, UK.

Lord, C. *et al.* (2000) The Autism Diagnostic Observation Schedule—generic: a standard measure of social and communication deficits associated with the spectrum of autism. *Journal of Autism and Developmental Disorders* **30**, 205–223. doi:10.1023/A:1005592401947.

Mallidi, A. *et al.* (2023) Robust caregiver-youth discrepancies in irritability ratings on the affective reactivity index: an investigation of its origins. *Journal of Affective Disorders* S0165-0327(23)00451–2. doi:10.1016/j.jad.2023.03.091.

March, J.S. *et al.* (1997) The Multidimensional Anxiety Scale for Children (MASC): factor structure, reliability, and validity. *Journal of the American Academy of Child & Adolescent Psychiatry* **36**, 554–565. doi:10.1097/00004583-199704000-00019.

Mazefsky, C.A. *et al.* (2018) Development of the emotion dysregulation inventory: a PROMIS®ing method for creating sensitive and unbiased questionnaires for autism spectrum disorder. *Journal of Autism and Developmental Disorders* **48**, 3736–3746. doi:10.1007/s10803-016-2907-1.

Morris, A.C. *et al.* (2023) Assessing the feasibility of a web-based outcome measurement system in child and adolescent mental health services—myHealthE a randomised controlled feasibility pilot study. *Child and Adolescent Mental Health* **28**, 128–147. doi:10.1111/camh.12571.

Myin-Germeys, I. *et al.* (2018) Experience sampling methodology in mental health research: new insights and technical developments. *World Psychiatry* **17**, 123–132. doi:10.1002/wps.20513.

NHS England 2015) Future in Mind: Children and Young People's Mental Wellbeing [online]. Available: https://www.england.nhs.uk/blog/martin-mcshane-14 [4 September 2023].

Nicol, G. *et al.* (2022) Chatbot-delivered cognitive behavioral therapy in adolescents with depression and anxiety during the COVID-19 pandemic: feasibility and acceptability study. *JMIR Formative Research* **6**, e40242. doi:10.2196/40242.

Nunnally, J. & Bernstein, I. (1994) *Psychometric Theory*, 3rd edn. McGraw-Hill, New York.

Poznanski, E.O. *et al.* (1984) Preliminary studies of the reliability and validity of the children's depression rating scale. *Journal of the American Academy of Child Psychiatry* **23**, 191–197. doi:10.1097/00004583-198403000-00011.

Reisner, S.L. *et al.* (2016) Social epidemiology of depression and anxiety by gender identity. *The Journal of Adolescent Health* **59**, 203–208. doi:10.1016/j.jadohealth.2016.04.006.

Reynolds, W.M. (2004) The Reynolds Adolescent Depression Scale-second edition (RADS-2). In: *Comprehensive Handbook of Psychological Assessment, Vol. 2: Personality Assessment.* (eds M.J. Hilsenroth & D.L. Segal). John Wiley & Sons, Inc, Hoboken, NJ. pp. 224–236.

Reynolds, C. et al. 2015 BASC-3 | The Behavior Assessment System for Children [online]. Available: https://www.pearsonassessments.com/store/usassessments/en/Store/Professional-Assessments/Behavior/BASC-3-Family-of-Assessments/p/P100010000.html?gclid=CjwKCAjw586hBhBrEiwAQYEnHYy-voOJRDXZFG5YPxGKvvRIpEqievQmm9OzcKmV3mhmqzCOmKt8bxoCmMQQAvD_BwE [4 October 2023].

Rognstad, K. *et al.* (2023) A systematic review and meta-analysis of measurement feedback systems in treatment for common mental health disorders. *Administration and Policy in Mental Health* **50**, 269–282. doi:10.1007/s10488-022-01236-9.

Rutter, M. *et al.* (2003) *The Social Communication Questionnaire.* Western Psychological Sciences, Los Angeles, CA.

Schwab-Stone, M.E. *et al.* (1996) Criterion validity of the NIMH Diagnostic Interview Schedule for Children version 2.3 (DISC-2.3). *Journal of the American Academy of Child and Adolescent Psychiatry* **35**, 878–888. doi:10.1097/00004583-199607000-00013.

Scrutton, A.P. (2017) Epistemic injustice and mental illness. In: *The Routledge Handbook of Epistemic Injustice.* (eds I.J. Kidd, *et al.*). Routledge, New York.

Shaffer, D. *et al.* (1983) A Children's Global Assessment Scale (CGAS). *Archives of General Psychiatry* **40**, 1228–1231. doi:10.1001/archpsyc.1983.01790100074010.

Shaffer, D. *et al.* (1996) The NIMH Diagnostic Interview Schedule for Children version 2.3 (DISC-2.3): description, acceptability, prevalence rates, and performance in the MECA study. Methods for the epidemiology of child and adolescent mental disorders study. *Journal of the American Academy of Child and Adolescent Psychiatry* **35**, 865–877. doi:10.1097/00004583-199607000-00012.

Spence, S.H. *et al.* (2003) Psychometric properties of the Spence Children's Anxiety Scale with young adolescents. *Journal of Anxiety Disorders* **17**, 605–625. doi:10.1016/S0887-6185(02)00236-0.

Stevens, K. & Ratcliffe, J. (2012) Measuring and valuing health benefits for economic evaluation in adolescence: an assessment of the practicality and validity of the Child Health Utility 9D in the Australian adolescent population. *Value in Health* **15**, 1092–1099. doi:10.1016/j.jval.2012.07.011.

Streiner, D.L. *et al.* (2014) *Health Measurement Scales: A Practical Guide to Their Development and Use.* Oxford University Press, Oxford, UK.

Stringaris, A. (2021) Sources of normativity in childhood depression. *European Child & Adolescent Psychiatry* **30**, 1663–1665. doi:10.1007/s00787-021-01891-7.

Stringaris, A. *et al.* (2012) The Affective Reactivity Index: a concise irritability scale for clinical and research settings. *Journal of Child Psychology and Psychiatry* **53**, 1109–1117. doi:10.1111/j.1469-7610.2012.02561.x.

Swanson, J. *et al.* (2001) Genes and attention-deficit hyperactivity disorder. *Clinical Neuroscience Research* **1**, 207–216. doi:10.1016/S1566-2772(01)00007-X.

Wakschlag, L.S. *et al.* (2008) Observational assessment of preschool disruptive behavior, part I: reliability of the Disruptive Behavior Diagnostic Observation Schedule (DB-DOS). *Journal of the American Academy of Child and Adolescent Psychiatry* **47**, 622–631. doi:10.1097/CHI.0b013e31816c5bdb.

Weisz, J.R. *et al.* (2011) Youth top problems: using idiographic, consumer-guided assessment to identify treatment needs and to track change during psychotherapy. *Journal of Consulting and Clinical Psychology* **79**, 369–380. doi:10.1037/a0023307.

CHAPTER 29

Psychological assessment in the clinical context

William Mandy[1], Jennifer L. Hudson[2] and Tara Murphy[3]

[1] Department of Clinical, Educational and Health Psychology, University College London, London, UK

[2] Black Dog Institute, Faculty of Medicine and Health, University of New South Wales, Sydney, NSW, Australia

[3] Great Ormond Street Hospital for Children, London, UK

The distinctive characteristics of psychological assessment in the clinical context

Psychologists bring a diverse set of skills and approaches to the clinical assessment of children and young people[1] with mental health difficulties, but their work in this area has one core, common characteristic: it involves applying psychological theory to illuminate the clinical presentations of their clients. A related principle that is common to clinical psychological work is that it should be "evidence-based," meaning that it should be guided by the latest relevant scientific findings. For psychologists, such evidence-based assessment should engender a collaborative and flexible way of working that integrates the latest scientific evidence, clinical expertise, and individual client preferences (e.g., Spring, 2007; Tolin *et al.*, 2015). This approach was summarized by the American Psychological Association's Presidential Task Force on Evidence Based Practice as "the integration of the best available research with clinical expertise in the context of patient characteristics, culture, and preferences" (American Psychological Association, Presidential Task Force on Evidence-Based Practice, 2006).

While the application of psychological theory and knowledge is at the heart of all psychology practice, the activities of psychologists in clinical assessment are diverse. In this chapter, we aim to acknowledge the variety of such psychological work, while also drawing out its commonalities and, thereby, its fundamental characteristics.

[1] In this chapter "child" refers to someone aged 9 years or younger and "young person" refers to adolescents, aged 10 to 19 years.

Different applied psychology roles in child and adolescent mental health (CAMH) work

One indicator of the variety of applied psychological work is that there are several different practitioner disciplines, each with its own culture, identity, training, and focus. The distinctions between these can be bemusing to clients, colleagues, and even to psychologists themselves. Here, we briefly outline four key professional roles of practitioner psychologists working in child and adolescent mental health (CAMH). We stress that the routes to qualification and precise definition of each practitioner discipline vary globally, and the below account undeniably reflects the authors' experiences working as psychologists in health services of anglophone, high-income countries.

Clinical psychology

Clinical psychologists usually have a bachelor's degree in psychology, followed by a postgraduate qualification at masters or doctoral level. They work with clients across the life span in both mental and physical health settings, with the aim of promoting well-being and functioning. Since its beginnings at the end of the 19th century, the scope of the profession has expanded to include assessment, intervention, development of the evidence base, and clinical leadership (Marzillier & Hall, 1998). In the early years of clinical psychology, activity was largely limited to assessment, with practitioners deploying their expertise in measurement, based on such theoretical disciplines as psychometrics, intelligence research, and neuropsychology (Marzillier & Hall, 1998). Subsequently, in the second half of the 20th century, the clinical application of learning theory opened the door to clinical psychologists delivering interventions, initially mostly for common problems of childhood, such as enuresis and sleep disturbances (Buchanan, 2010; Hall *et al.*, 2015). The close association between clinical psychology and the

Rutter's Child and Adolescent Psychiatry and Psychology, Seventh Edition.
Edited by Anita Thapar, Daniel S. Pine, Samuele Cortese, Cathy Creswell, Tamsin J. Ford, James F. Leckman, and Argyris Stringaris.

Companion website: www.wiley.com/go/thapar/rutterspsych7

burgeoning field of cognitive behavioral therapy (CBT) from the late 1970s onwards further allowed clinical psychologists to increase their reach, as they delivered interventions for a growing range of problems across the life span (Hall *et al.*, 2015) and played a significant role in extending the evidence base for mental health interventions (Layard & Clark, 2014) (see Chapter 34). In addition to CBT and behavioral work, clinical psychologists as a group can be informed by various psychological models, for example, drawing on ideas from psychoanalysis and systemic theory (see Chapter 31). Another development in the professional role has been a growing emphasis on clinical leadership, that involves activities such as teaching, service development, and management.

Educational psychology

Educational psychologists typically have an undergraduate psychology degree and have completed a specific postgraduate educational psychology qualification, commonly a doctorate. They draw on psychological science to promote their clients' ability to learn, retain, and use new knowledge and capacities. The majority of their activity is with children and adolescents, in educational settings. The role includes assessment, intervention, and consultancy. Areas of activity of particular relevance to CAMH assessment include: supporting neurodiverse young people in their learning, including those with dyslexia, autism, and attention deficit hyperactivity disorder (ADHD); assessment of intellectual and cognitive development; work with emotional and behavioral difficulties in educational settings; and consulting to educational systems to promote inclusive education, including for those with mental health difficulties and/or neurodevelopmental conditions.

Counseling psychology

Counseling psychologists usually have a psychology degree, followed by further specialist postgraduate training that emphasizes supervised practice. Traditionally, compared to clinical psychology, counseling psychology has had a greater emphasis on intervention for mental health problems, with less focus on assessment and treating severe and enduring mental illness. In some settings, counseling and clinical psychologists have overlapping functions, making it hard to always draw clear boundaries between the two professions. While, increasingly, counseling psychologists deliver CBT interventions, traditionally their work is guided by different psychological models (e.g., psychodynamic and Rogerian theory) that focus on the relationship between the client and the therapist, both as a source of information about the client's difficulties and as an instrument by which to intervene on these difficulties (see Chapter 36 on relationship-based treatments).

Clinical neuropsychology

Clinical neuropsychologists are qualified practitioner psychologists (e.g., clinical or educational psychologists) who have completed formal training in knowledge of brain–behavior relations, that involves research, teaching, and supervised clinical practice (Collins *et al.*, 2015). They are concerned with how disease or atypical development within the brain can be associated with impairment and, in some cases, this can be carefully monitored through neurocognitive assessment and neuroradiological measures (see Chapters 10, 11, and 12). However, for neuropsychological assessment within child and adolescent mental health services (CAMHS), the focus will likely be on characterizing the client's cognitive profile with a goal of improving well-being and functioning.

In CAMHS assessment, a major role for clinical neuropsychologists is standardized assessment of cognitive functioning and development, for example, for those with neurodevelopmental conditions, traumatic brain injuries, or epilepsy. This can include a monitoring function, benchmarking, and tracking change in situations where there is a risk of cognitive decline, for example, for children and young people with Rasmussen encephalitis, pediatric dementia, or epilepsy. A key part of neuropsychological assessment is formulating how brain-based strengths and difficulties influence adaptive functioning; and what strategies can be employed to promote better functioning and quality of life.

This list of subtypes of practitioner psychologists is not exhaustive. Rather, it is designed to cover the disciplines most likely to be involved in CAMH assessments. In several health care systems, including those of the United Kingdom (UK) and Australia, psychologists working in paraprofessional roles are making a growing contribution (Ludlow *et al.*, 2020). This is an initiative to expand the psychological workforce, to reduce waiting times, and generally improve access to services. These practitioner psychologists tend to have a psychology degree, plus some additional specialist training, and work under the supervision of more extensively trained professionals, often clinical psychologists.

Below, we describe a set of key characteristics of the contribution by psychologists to clinical assessment of CAMH.

Theory-based formulation

All psychological assessments should aim to inform theory-based case formulation, which involves developing a conceptual understanding of the child or young person's presenting concerns (Persons, 2022). This formulation includes the psychologist's understanding of the factors that have contributed to the development of symptoms and, importantly, it also includes the modifiable factors that maintain symptoms, which are crucial for intervention. A good clinical formulation considers the child or young person's cultural context instead of viewing them in isolation. The formulation is typically a dynamic model (or "working hypothesis") that can be adapted and expanded upon during the intervention as more information becomes available or as changes occur. The psychologist uses this formulation to determine treatment options.

There are a wide variety of theoretical models that psychologists might use to build a case formulation. The main schools of thought include behavioral, cognitive, cognitive-behavioral, interpersonal, systemic, and psychodynamic approaches. Each of these theoretical frameworks emphasize different causal and maintaining factors. For instance, a behavioral case formulation primarily focuses on the patterns of behavior the child or young person has learned from their environment. It may include consideration of operant conditioning, for example, how carers have shaped the child or young person's behaviors through positive and/or negative reinforcement; and of classical conditioning, for example, by identifying in the environment antecedents (i.e., triggers or prompts) that evoke behaviors of interest (please see Chapter 34 for more on behavioral approaches). By contrast, a psychodynamic model focuses on the relationship between client and therapist, to understand unconscious processes and internal conflicts thought to explain the child or young person's behavior. Such therapeutic approaches commonly emphasize the role of early experience, particularly in the context of relationships with caregivers.

The psychologist's preferred model will vary depending on the evidence base, as well as the context in which they are working, their own culture, identity, personality, training, and experience. There is an ambition within the mental health field to increase the adoption of evidence-based approaches in therapeutic practice. Currently, in CAMH, the best-evidenced assessment and intervention models are behavioral or cognitive-behavioral (e.g., Hudson *et al.*, 2023) (see Chapter 34). There is also evidence supporting other approaches such as Maudsley family-focused therapy for anorexia nervosa (NICE, 2020) or group interpersonal therapy for depression (NICE, 2022). Other approaches (e.g., systemic and psychodynamic) may have value but are currently underresearched in CAMH (e.g., Palmer *et al.*, 2013). Please see Chapters 31 and 36 for deeper consideration of the evidence base for interventions that draw on psychological theories other than CBT or behaviorism.

Cognitive and neuropsychological assessment

What is a cognitive assessment?

Cognitive assessment can be included as part of a psychological assessment as a means of establishing the child or young person's relative strengths and weaknesses with thinking processes. If the assessment is used to describe the behavioral level, without reference to brain mechanisms, then this is typically referred to as a cognitive or psychoeducational assessment. When the client has an acquired brain injury or specific neuropathology, a neuropsychological assessment may be warranted, which is guided by information about the brain. Typically, neuropsychological assessments are more focused, and may be informed by findings from neuroradiological investigations such as magnetic resonance imaging (MRI) and/or electroencephalography (EEG). Psychologists who carry out neuropsychological assessment typically have further training in brain–behavior relationships (see above section on "Clinical neuropsychologists") whereas cognitive assessment, which seeks to describe cognitive data alone, is more broadly applied to everyday clinical work with children and young people. The information gained from a cognitive assessment can inform psychological formulation and help explain patterns of behavior.

Why include cognitive testing?

Cognitive or neuropsychological assessment can guide the tailoring of clinical assessment and intervention to specifically meet the needs of the client; and to estimate future needs for adolescent or adult life. It also has an important role in understanding educational performance and support needs. It is a time-consuming element of the evaluation but can contribute a unique perspective to assessment and formulation. This is particularly important as many children and young people seen for assessment of neurodevelopmental and mental health concerns are likely to have varied cognitive profiles, a formal specific learning disorder, and educational vulnerability. Cognitive assessments vary in their depth and scope. However, there are several key principles that should be considered. The focus of the assessment should be hypothesis-driven and guided by referral information, collateral information from carers and teachers, and, if he or she is at sufficient age to give their opinion, the client themselves. The hypothesis testing approach to neuropsychological assessment is flexible, as compared with a fixed-battery approach. The former enables the psychologist to create tentative explanations for the client's challenge to be tested and subsequently supported or unsupported (Lezak *et al.*, 2004), whereas the latter follows a predetermined protocol to include or exclude a particular profile, such as a specific learning disorder, for example, dyslexia. Evidence shows that the detection of specific learning disorders, such as dyslexia or dyscalculia, is important as children and young people with these conditions may be predisposed to low self-esteem, attentional, and emotional difficulties (Snowling *et al.*, 2007; Pennington & Bishop, 2009).

Intelligence and adaptive behavior

The most commonly assessed domain of cognition evaluated in children and young people is intellectual function. There are several reasons for this. While the concept of intelligence is a hotly debated area in psychology, a measure of intelligence may provide a global description of the individual's abilities or capacity to comprehend abstract ideas, recognize patterns, learn from experience, and engage in various forms of reasoning in order to achieve goals in a broad range of environments (Neisser, 2014). It is increasingly acknowledged that the greatest clinical utility comes from mapping a client's pattern of intellectual strengths and difficulties. This is done via interpretation of the analyses of the index scores, which describe different areas of cognitive function encompassed by contemporary models of intelligence (Weiss *et al.*, 2016).

Intimately related to intellectual function, and a key element to diagnosing intellectual disability (ID), is adaptive function, which refers to a collection of conceptual skills (e.g., language, problem-solving), social skills (e.g., interpersonal communication), and practical skills (e.g., self-care, money management, recreation, academic progress) that are learned and performed by individuals in their day-to-day lives to achieve personal independence and social responsibility (American Psychiatric Association, 2013). Assessment of intellectual functional and adaptive behavior offers a basic understanding of how a child is functioning across most cognitive domains.

Intellectual disability

Adaptive behavior and intellectual function are strongly related (Harrison & Oakland, 2015). In addition to characterizing the child or young person's cognitive profile, measures of intellectual function and adaptive behavior enable the psychologist to assess for ID along a spectrum of severity (see Chapter 53 for consideration of ID). Guidelines from the *International Statistical Classification of Diseases and Related Health Problems* (ICD-11; World Health Organization, 2022), and the *Diagnostic and Statistical Manual of Mental Disorders, Fifth Edition* (DSM-5; American Psychiatric Association, 2013) require deficits in both intellectual and adaptive functioning presenting before 18 years of age to diagnose ID. This shift from focusing merely on intelligence quotient (IQ) scores means that psychologists now need to understand how the individual is functioning in daily life, which naturally has significant culturally specific characteristics and demands, especially given that our standardized measures of adaptive function have all been developed in the United States and may not apply across cultures and contexts. Commonly used assessments of intellectual and developmental functioning are given in Table 29.1.

Table 29.1 Commonly used measures to assess intellectual and developmental functioning.

Name of test	Age range	Rationale for inclusion in assessment
Wechsler Preschool and Primary Scale of Intelligence, Fourth Edition (WPPSI-IV)	2 years, 6 months–7 years, 7 months	A broad test encompassing verbal comprehension, motor skills, fluid reasoning, and working memory for young children
Wechsler Intelligence Scale for Children, Fifth Edition (WISC-V)	6–16 years, 11 months	A widely used measure assessing verbal comprehension, visual-spatial skills, fluid reasoning, working memory, and processing speed. It provides a broad overview of ability within a short time period and potentially indicates additional assessment needed
British Ability Scales, Third Edition (BAS-3)	3–17 years	A measure of verbal ability, nonverbal reasoning ability, and spatial ability
Leiter International Performance Scale, Third Edition (Leiter-3)	3–75+ years	A measure of nonverbal intelligence quotient (IQ), nonverbal attention, and nonverbal memory, particularly useful in the assessment of nonverbal children and young people
Bayley Scales of Infant Development, Third Edition	1–42 months	Broad range assessment of cognitive, language, motor, social-emotional, and adaptive behavior in preschool children. Helpfully, co-normed with the ABAS-III (see below)
Adaptive Behavior Assessment System, Third Edition (ABAS-III)	Available for completion by self, parent/carer, and teacher. Spans birth to 89 years	A broad measure which assesses everyday skills relating to conceptual, social, and practical skills
Vineland Adaptive Behavior Scale, Second Edition (Vineland-II)	Completion by parent and teacher. Spans birth to 90 years Parent interview also available	A broad-ranging informant-report measure which assesses communication, daily living skills, socialization, and motor skills (in younger children)

Beyond IQ—further cognitive assessment

When the formulation and hypotheses require it, expertise is available, and time allows, a more detailed cognitive assessment which explores certain cognitive domains will be conducted. In these cases, assessment of a child or young person's function in one or more specific areas may be beneficial, including: visual-spatial skills; expressive and receptive language (see Chapter 51); executive functions, attention, and memory; and motor skills (see Chapter 52). Some of these areas may be assessed by members of the multidisciplinary team who are not psychologists, for example, occupational therapists or speech and language therapists. There is likely to be overlap between two or more cognitive domains (e.g., memory and attention) and this should always be considered in any assessment: the measures used to test performance are not thought to assess for a single domain alone. Although it is beyond the remit of this chapter to offer a detailed account of assessments for every cognitive domain, including motor skills, visual-spatial skills, and auditory processing, there are compendia available for this (Baron 2018; Booth *et al.*, 2022).

Executive functioning, attention, and memory

Cognitive assessments of attention and executive functioning can be useful, especially alongside self-report measures, particularly in clients struggling to accomplish everyday, age-appropriate tasks or educational targets. Beyond their formal scores on such measures, how a child or young person responds to the tests' demands can be informative, providing insights into their most effective approach to different types of effortful cognitive task. Cognitive tests of executive function and attention are highly structured in design, so that the scores they yield can be consistent and standardized. It should be acknowledged that this tends to involve providing a high level of scaffolding, which can result in children "overperforming" during formal testing, compared to how they manage real-life, less structured situations. A further challenge is that most tests of executive function have been adapted from adult measures which can impact their validity when used with children and young people, in particular their ecological validity (Souissi *et al.*, 2022). For this reason, inclusion of informant-report measures from carers and teachers, such as the Behavior Rating Inventory of Executive Functioning, Second Edition (BRIEF—II; Gioia *et al.*, 2015), can provide a more well-rounded description of overall abilities in daily life, at home, and at school. There is often a weak relationship between informant reports and the child or young person's performance on structured, individually administered standardized tests of executive function. While sometimes hard for clinicians to explain, such discrepancies can be informative. It is often helpful to consider factors such as who the respondent is, what the assessment context is, and how much the structured testing situation may differ from the situations in which the informant-report ratings were given. For further discussion, please see Chapter 28 on measurement. The most commonly used cognitive tests of executive function include: the Delis-Kaplan Executive Functions System (Delis *et al.*, 2001) and the Behavioral Assessment of the Dysexecutive Syndrome in Children (BADS-C; Emslie *et al.*, 2003). The BADS-C is a battery of executive tasks that seeks to prioritize ecological validity and generally applies well to everyday tasks that the child might be involved in such as homework preparation.

For attention, the Test of Everyday Attention for Children, Second Edition (TEA-Ch-2; Manly *et al.*, 2016) and the Conners' Continuous Performance Test, Third Edition (Conners, 2014) are well validated and widely used. They can be partially or fully administered via a laptop, which can facilitate engagement. The measures include assessment of many different aspects of attention, including sustained attention, divided attention, selective attention, and inhibitory control. The referral question and hypothesis that is guiding the clinician may be used to clarify which aspects of attention are evaluated. Once again, these performance measures are likely to give the most informative data if administered alongside measures that take informant reports (e.g., Conners 4th Edition; Conners, 2022) and, if developmentally appropriate, self-report.

Finally, there are several batteries which include assessment of attention, memory, and executive function such as the NIH Toolbox Cognition Battery (Gershon *et al.*, 2013), the Developmental NEuroPSYchological Assessment, Second Edition (NEPSY-II; Korkman *et al.*, 1998) and the Repeatable Battery for the Assessment of Neuropsychological Status (Randolph *et al.*, 1998). These allow for assessment of a broader range of cognitive domains, using the same normative sample, rather than across different tests. Each test has its own merits in terms of depth of assessment and modality of delivery. The psychologist should have a clear rationale for selecting the measure and how the data can be used to answer the diagnostic or formulation question.

Assessment of memory should be led by the presenting concerns and information about potential brain injury, neurodevelopmental condition, or psychiatric disorder. There are several different aspects of memory including working memory, semantic memory, episodic memory, and autobiographical memory (see Booth *et al.*, 2022 for an introduction to this complex topic). There are batteries of tests which include both visual and verbal memory, immediate and delayed recall alongside recognition, such as the Child and Adolescent Memory Profile (Sherman & Brooks, 2015), Children's Memory Scale (Cohen, 1997), the Test of Memory and Learning, Second Edition (Reynolds & Voress, 2007), and the Wide Range Assessment of Memory and Learning, Third Edition (Sheslow & Adams, 2021). Everyday memory, referred to as episodic memory, may be relevant, and for this the Rivermead Behavioral Memory Test for Children (Wilson *et al.*, 1991) can be useful. In addition, assessment of verbal learning can also be useful to assess verbal recall, and recall and recognition, and can be assessed using the California Verbal Learning Test—Children's Version (Delis *et al.*, 1994) and Children's Auditory Verbal Learning Test, Second Edition (Talley, 1993). As with other cognitive domains, self-report questionnaires from important people within the child or young person's system will help to triangulate findings and give important information on the impact of any cognitive impairments. For the memory domain, the Everyday Memory Questionnaire (Drysdale *et al.*, 2004) may be helpful.

Achievement tests

Assessments of school-based attainments, including reading, writing, and math are important because these skills are essential in school and give insight into how the child or young person is accessing and responding to education. It is useful to employ batteries that are co-normed with measures of intellectual ability so that clinical discrepancies between, on the one hand, intelligence, and on the other hand, academic attainment can be measured, although the discrepancies are no longer used to inform diagnosis of specific learning disorders, which was previously the case. Batteries such as the Wechsler Individual Achievement Test, Fourth Edition (Wechsler, 2020) and the Woodcock-Johnson, Third Edition Tests of Achievement (Woodcock *et al.*, 2001) are designed to be used alongside the Wechsler IQ tests. Assessments that measure literacy usually focus on various capacities that contribute to reading performance, namely, word reading accuracy, passage reading fluency, phonological decoding, reading comprehension, and spelling. Math skills are important to assess and are often neglected, even in comprehensive psychological evaluations. Several groups presenting for assessment in child and adolescent services are at elevated risk of mathematical difficulties, such as those born prematurely (Hellgren *et al.*, 2013) and those with fetal alcohol syndrome (Rasmussen & Bisanz, 2009) or Turner syndrome (Bruandet *et al.*, 2004). Finally, writing skills are an aspect of educational attainment which encompass both spelling and handwriting and may also be important to consider when children or young people experience slow performance and legibility concerns. There are assessments of handwriting in many of the larger batteries and also stand-alone assessments, such as the Detailed Assessment of Speed of Handwriting (Barnett *et al.*, 2007), and attention, motor, and scanning skills should be considered alongside in assessment. For more detailed information on specific learning disorders, see Chapter 52.

Interpretation of cognitive test results

Psychologists must have mastery over the interpretation of their cognitive assessments and results. Most cognitive tests use a bell curve model, outputting age-standardized scores with a mean of 100 and a standard deviation of 15 (Figure 29.1). Such standardized scales allow for comparison of performance across different measures and can (i) show how someone performs compared to others their age, and (ii) their distinctive pattern of strengths and difficulties across the cognitive domains tested. Other standardized scores may be used such as T-scores. There are also tests which use a more flexible and qualitative approach to interpreting scores and performance. One of these approaches is the Boston process approach, which was developed by Kaplan and colleagues (Hebben & Milberg, 2009) and focuses on observing the process and solutions that enable the child to conclude a task.

Interpretation of cognitive data

Cognitive data are best included in the formulation with other information gathered at the assessment and should always be considered in context. Several factors influence how a child or young person performs during cognitive assessment. Their mental state, including their level of anxiety and mood, may be influential. Assessors should always aim to follow the standardized instructions in any test manual, to ensure the resultant test scores are valid. Nevertheless, sometimes modifications are required, such as simplification of instruction for a child with language difficulties or use of an interpreter for a young person who is being assessed in English when it is their second language. In addition, minor adaptations may be needed to increase a client's engagement with the tasks, but again these should be explicitly recorded and used to interpret results. Having a parent or carer in the room should be avoided, unless testing a very young child and, if required in an older client, their need for this, as well as its potential effect on test performance, should be considered. Finally, lengthy testing sessions and potential practice effects from recent assessments may influence how a child performs in the assessment and should be considered. Importantly, the clinician carrying out the assessment can learn much from carefully observing how the child or young person approaches testing. For example, this can provide first-hand information on how the client approaches problems, responds to frustration, and their level of persistence and confidence. As such, observations during testing are a crucial part of the assessment process, often yielding insights and clinical recommendations to be applied in everyday life.

When to carry out a cognitive assessment

If reports do not indicate difficulty with day-to-day function, then there may be no need to offer a cognitive assessment. Once concerns have been identified then behavioral difficulties can be formulated, usually through interview, use of questionnaires, and standardized assessment in a range of domains. The role of any cognitive assessment is to identify the underlying cognitive

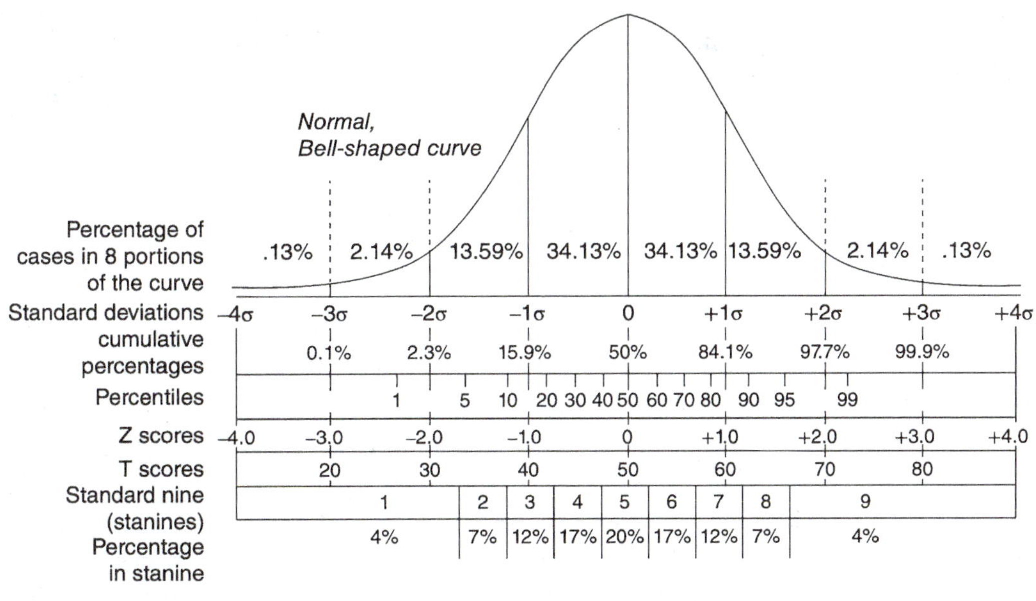

Figure 29.1 The bell curve—marked with different types of standardized scores.

difficulties that need to be addressed to support the child or young person. From here, interventions can be identified and made available to them to support their cognitive strengths and weakness. Ellen Braaten describes, the "3 As of intervention": accepting a child or young person's unique learning style, helping him or her to accommodate any learning challenges, and advocating for their need (Braaten & Willoughby, 2014).

The framework for formulation is important. Once the general cognitive level Is established for the individual then educational attainments and specific cognitive impairments can be identified. From this information, the impact of these impairments on the individual's functioning at school or in other settings can be monitored. It is important that relative cognitive strengths and other protective factors (e.g., well-developed social skills, supportive teachers/colleagues) are used as compensatory strategies to aid the individual with their difficulties.

Telepsychology for cognitive assessment

Prior to, and even more since, the COVID-19 pandemic, there has been an increase in the use of telepsychology, which is the use of video-teleconferencing techniques to administer psychological services without face-to-face contact (Cullum *et al.*, 2014). This is advantageous to those living long distances from services or in geographically remote communities. Use of telepsychology involves a high level of technology, use of screens, a reliable internet connection, and well-honed clinical skills. There are several models available to facilitate administration which can be explored further in Roberts *et al.* (2022). Many commonly used standardized measures, such as the WISC-V and Clinical Evaluation of Language Fundamentals, Fourth Edition, Australian Adaptation (Semel *et al.*, 2006), have been shown to be valid for remote administration (e.g., Hodge *et al.*, 2019; Harder *et al.* 2020). This is an area that requires further research but has currently been adopted in everyday clinical practice and is predicted to be a practice that may develop and become more common in coming years.

Assessment in context

Emotional and behavioral difficulties of children and young people occur within a context that influences their onset, maintenance, impact, and outcomes. Even for conditions that are largely the result of genetic variation, such as autism, context matters in terms of influencing the well-being and functioning of a young person and those around them (Mandy & Lai, 2016). Psychologists working from systemic perspectives (including family therapy models) and/or trained in developmental psychopathology, will place great emphasis on context. But so do psychologists guided by more individualist approaches, as when a behavioralist looks for environmental triggers and reinforcers of a problematic behavior or a CBT therapist considers feedback loops whereby a child with social anxiety is encouraged to avoid frightening social settings, thereby further entrenching their fears of being negatively evaluated.

There is a long tradition within academic psychology of seeking to understand the ways in which a person's environment influences their development, and this body of knowledge is valuable for shaping the work of practitioner psychologists. It is beyond the scope of this chapter to summarize all clinically relevant psychological science on environmental influences on development. So, here we have selected the work of two psychologists, whose work is both influential and directly relevant to the practical task of clinical assessment in CAMHS.

The work of the Soviet psychologist, Lev Vygotsky (1896–1934), has been enormously influential on psychological and educational practice. At the heart of Vygotsky's work is the idea that the social environment profoundly shapes the development of children's cognitions, emotions, and behavior (Vygotsky & Cole, 1978). A key mechanism in this process is the "zone of proximal development" (ZPD)—which is the space between what a child can do on their own and what they can accomplish when scaffolded by an adult or more capable peer. In Vygotskian thought, the ZPD is the optimal state in which intellectual development takes place; and it represents a useful heuristic in clinical assessment for formulating the nurturing experiences a child or young person is receiving, and how these might need to be adapted to enhance development (Vygotsky & Cole, 1978).

Another Russian-born psychologist, Urie Bronfenbrenner (1917–2005), elaborated an "ecological systems theory" to provide a detailed and concrete account of how the environment influences human development, including mental health. Bronfenbrenner articulated a principle that is key to clinical assessment of children and young people: that human development arises from a dynamic interaction between the individual and their environment (Bronfenbrenner, 1979, 2005). For example, conduct problems can develop and persist because: (i) a child's tendency to behavioral dysregulation can evoke harsh and inconsistent parenting; and (ii) such parenting further promotes behavioral and emotional dysregulation (e.g., Rutter, 2006). When a child or young person presents with mental health difficulties, their context, including how it shapes them and is shaped by them over time, needs to be formulated; and this is a common focus of psychological assessment.

Another intellectual contribution of Bronfenbrenner's, which is relevant to psychological assessment, was his broad conceptualization of the environment that not only incorporated proximal features (the family, the classroom) but also wider, more distal structures such as the community in which a family lives, and the economic and political conditions under which that community exists. Thus, Bronfenbrenner's ideas direct the clinician to consider that "interpersonal relationships, including even microprocesses in the parent–child relationship, do not exist in a social vacuum but are embedded in the larger social structures of community, society, economics, and politics" (Ceci, 2006). Furthermore, Bronfenbrenner pointed out that the ways in which different elements of the environment interact with each other is influential on development, thus providing another valuable principle to shape psychological assessment. For example, it is commonly valuable in clinical assessment to understand the relationship between a child's parents and their school, and to consider how this may enhance or diminish the child's chances of well-being and adaptive functioning.

In practitioner psychology, as well as in other clinical disciplines, there is a regrettable history of underplaying the impact of societal factors, such as poverty, sexism, homophobia, and racism, as a contextual influence on children and young people's well-being. However, in the face of shifting social attitudes and a growing evidence base that social injustice impinges on well-being and functioning in multiple ways, this is starting to change (e.g., Lugo-Candelas *et al.*, 2021). For example, clinical psychology training courses increasingly focus on the need to address social inequality and prejudice as key contextual risk factors; and increasingly practitioner psychologists should seek to incorporate them in their assessments and formulations.

Selecting culturally sensitive and developmentally appropriate assessment tools

Before selecting the assessment tool, or formulating conclusions about the assessment results, it is essential that the psychologist considers the child or young person's cultural background. Most measures were developed from white, middle- to high-income samples that lack diversity in terms of ethnicity, race, sexuality, and gender. This means it cannot be assumed that the items will be culturally sensitive or appropriate for all children and young people. Furthermore, the normative data used to determine assessment results and care decisions may also not be relevant to the client's distinctive cultural context and may lead to over- or underdetection of the construct.

For First Nations peoples in Australia, their experience of what current psychiatric nosology might term "mental health symptoms" may not be relevant or appropriate, and may not acknowledge First Nations ways of being or knowing. For instance, in First Nations cultures, a young person may experience deep longing and sadness when they are not "on country," that is when they have traveled away from the land on which they were born (Westerman, 2004; Gee *et al.*, 2014). These symptoms may mimic major depression but would be considered normative within the young person's cultural context; and likely require a different intervention compared to depression.

Moreover, many assessment tools rely on decisions that are based on sex-aggregated normative data that use a binary classification of gender and may not be appropriate for children with diverse gender identities. Using data that has not included gender minorities or that is not aligned with the child or young person's gender identity may lead to over- or underdetection of the assessment construct and impact on access to care (Weber *et al.*, 2019).

Since interpretation of many psychometric tools is based on normative data that may not apply to the client, making treatment decisions based on this could be unhelpful, or even harmful. These issues will become increasingly important as treatment decision-making becomes more reliant on artificial intelligence (AI) methods (see Bertie & Hudson, 2021) that depend on datasets that lack cultural diversity. Until the field develops and establishes culturally sensitive assessment tools, the responsibility is on the psychologist and the professional care team to ensure that they consider the child or young person's cultural context when conducting the assessment and interpreting the findings.

In addition to cultural context, the child or young person's developmental context must also be considered when selecting and interpreting assessments, particularly self-report measures. Many measures have often been developed and tested as downward extensions of adult measures, rather than designed to reflect the developmental characteristics of children and young people. As a result, they typically rely on written tests and often require an understanding of Likert scales. First and foremost, the psychologist needs to ensure that the selected measures have appropriate normative data that matches the client's age. As age is only ever a rough indication of development, the psychologist must also consider cognitive level when selecting measures. Many psychological measures have been developed for typically developing children and young people with average-range reading and cognitive abilities, and, as a result, may not be well understood by those with reading delays. This is particularly relevant if the client's age is on the cusp of the recommended suitability for the assessment tool. For example, the RCADS (Ebesutani *et al.*, 2012) includes a self-report measure suitable for those aged 8–18 years. However, for an 8-year-old child who is struggling at school to read, some items may be difficult to understand, such as "I have problems with my appetite" or "I have to do some things over and over again (like washing my hands, cleaning, or putting things in a certain order)." As a result, the psychologist must consider their client's developmental needs, including cognitive capacity and reading ability, when selecting self-report or direct assessment measures and, where appropriate, consider observational measures or parent-report measures as an alternative. Further, psychologists need to be aware that on many measures, there will be markedly different average raw scores seen at different ages, reflecting development, so clinicians should be cautious when interpreting within-person differences in raw scores that occur over time.

Additional cultural factors are important to consider when planning, carrying out cognitive assessment, and interpreting data. Few tests were developed with cultural factors in mind and have their development and background in less diverse populations than we currently have in modern society. Although many cognitive skills are recognized as universal across nationalities, their development may differ. It is important to consider the use of cognitive assessments in a language which differs from the child's family language. There are helpful guidelines for psychologists working with interpreters. More broadly, the clinician should also be aware of construct bias, instrument or item bias, and administration bias

(Fernández & Abe, 2018) when selecting and using assessment materials. See Stark (2022) for a more detailed account of culture in cognitive and neuropsychological settings.

The psychologist's role in communicating findings

Psychologists play a critical role in communicating the findings of a CAMH assessment to relevant stakeholders. Despite its importance, this aspect of assessment is often given the least attention and planning. The data collection process demands significant time investment, not only from the psychologist, but also from the child or young person and their family. To fully leverage the benefits of this investment, it is best to conduct a carefully planned and executed feedback session, following a carefully written report.

A well-executed feedback session has the potential to help children or young people and their families make informed decisions about intervention and increase the likelihood of receiving appropriate care at the right time. Further, it can strengthen the therapeutic alliance between the psychologist, the client, and/or the family by building trust and establishing a shared understanding of the issues. When sensitive and effective communication is achieved, the feedback session can instill hope for a better future. On the other hand, when assessment feedback is not provided accurately, sensitively, and effectively, families may lose confidence in the ability of health care professionals to listen, understand their experiences, and respect their privacy.

Effective assessment can also contribute to positive change and symptom improvement by increasing understanding of the issues and shifting core beliefs that may be maintaining the child or young person's symptoms. This new understanding can help shape their identity and personal narrative. For instance, a child who has struggled with reading may have consequently developed anxiety and low mood due to beliefs like "I am dumb" and "people will think I am dumb." Upon receiving a diagnosis of dyslexia, they might experience great relief, as their negative beliefs are challenged with the new information provided by the assessment. A well-delivered feedback session has a capacity to develop insights not only to weakness and vulnerability but also to highlight strengths, and advise on how these challenges can be compensated for, or ameliorated by, relative strengths.

When planning the feedback session, psychologists need to make several decisions, including who to involve, what to share, when to share it, and how to do so in a developmentally appropriate, safe, and sensitive manner. Given the complexity of this task, and the potential benefits and risks involved, it is crucial that psychologists and the broader mental health care team allocate sufficient time for planning and delivering the findings effectively, both in terms of verbal and written feedback. A detailed account drawing on expert data on how to understand and optimize feedback following cognitive or neuropsychological assessment is available in Postal and Armstrong (2013).

What to share with whom in the feedback session

CAMH assessments typically involve more stakeholders than adult assessments. In addition to the child or young person and their health care team, the psychologist may also need to involve parents, carers, and/or teachers in the feedback. The psychologist needs to be extremely careful when sharing information across stakeholders, and only share information when appropriate consent has been obtained.

Information sharing among stakeholders is impacted by law. The psychologist must be clear on the child or young person's and parent's legal rights when it comes to sharing medical information, as this can differ from country to country and even within a country (e.g., state to state). As a result, the clinician needs to be acutely aware of legal constraints on privacy, not only to prevent harm to the child or young person, but also for recording and sharing confidential information that others could access by law.

Sharing information among different stakeholders can create various dilemmas for psychologists, which require careful consideration (see also Chapter 19 for consideration of legal issues in clinical work with children and young people). For instance, during the data collection phase of an assessment, a child may disclose information that is unknown to others in their life. Similarly, parents or caregivers may disclose private information that they do not wish to share with the child, school, or other health care providers. Another common dilemma arises when parents or caregivers request access to information that they have a legal right to obtain, but the child or young person has asked to be kept private. These situations can become even more complex if the child or young person's caregivers are in conflict, going through a separation or divorce, or involved in legal proceedings. Countries under the Convention on the Rights of the Child are obligated to prioritize the child or young person's rights and well-being in their decisions. Therefore, the psychologist is responsible for making decisions that are in the best interests of the child or young person. Regardless of the decision made, it is recommended that the psychologist work with the child or young person to plan how the sharing of information should occur or if it should be kept private.

When sharing assessment information with stakeholders, psychologists must decide which components of the assessment are essential for their client's best care. Although psychologists are familiar with diagnostic labels, symptoms, formulations, standard bell curves, and cut-off scores, these terms can be foreign and potentially damaging to children or young people and families new to mental health care. Improper use or poor understanding of such terms could alienate families, increase stigma, and negatively affect willingness to continue with care. Additionally, cultural factors such as race, ethnicity, religion, and family context must be considered when choosing what information to share to which parties.

The use of diagnostic labels and classifications is important in treatment decision-making and can aid in communication between health practitioners. Sometimes, a diagnostic label is necessary for a child or young person to access much-needed care. It can also be helpful for the client to understand their experience and for the family to understand the need for treatment. However, in some cases, diagnostic terminology may be unnecessary and potentially harmful. There is no universal rule to follow, as assessment contexts vary greatly. Therefore, the psychologist must take time to understand the child or young person's context and best interests, and use this to guide decisions about what information to communicate with whom.

The developmental stage and level of the child or young person is an important factor to consider when deciding what assessment information to share and with whom. However, since age is only a proxy for development, it may not always be the best guide for making these decisions. Instead, psychologists should consider cognitive, emotional, and physical development when determining which aspects of the assessment results should be shared with the child or young person and other stakeholders.

How to provide feedback

Once the decision has been made about what information should be shared with specific stakeholders, the psychologist must determine the best way to deliver this information to achieve the best outcomes. If the psychologist decides that the parent and child or young person need to receive specific scores from an assessment, it is important to provide context and background information to the scores. A score of 25 on the DASS-21 Depression Scale and the corresponding "severe depression" category may be well understood by a psychologist, but a 17-year-old may be far less likely to know what this label means. Providing this feedback without context is likely to be distressing for the young person and their family. An example of sensitive delivery of assessment results is given in Box 29.1.

When starting an assessment feedback session, it is valuable for the psychologist to first determine and clarify how those present understand the purpose of the feedback session. The psychologist should provide clear information about the decision points regarding the options and next steps. During the feedback process, it is important to be mindful of the family's reactions to the information provided as this will vary from situation to situation and may result in varied reactions including, but not limited to, relief, shock, anger, guilt, or confusion. The psychologist should provide the child or young person and their family with an opportunity to share their reaction to the information provided and normalize their reactions when appropriate. This discussion can also be helpful to identify any misunderstandings and add to a shared understanding of the presenting issues.

Some children and young people will interpret feedback in a way that is consistent with their mental disorder. For example, a child with major depressive disorder, hearing information about their diagnosis might confirm their feelings of worthlessness or being "problematic." It is important for psychologists to approach feedback in a sensitive and compassionate manner, considering these potential interpretation biases, to avoid exacerbating any negative beliefs or self-perceptions. This is also true for parent's beliefs as well. Given that mental health difficulties run in families, interpretation biases may also be present in parents. This may be particularly relevant for parents experiencing anxiety and depression, who on hearing the information about their child's assessment, may experience guilt and sadness.

Box 29.1 Example feedback to a child about elevated questionnaire scores

> "The answers you and your parents gave to the questions, show me that you are really feeling down at the moment and this is having a big impact on you. Your answers also show me that it could be really useful to get some help so that you do not feel this way all the time. Other young people I see who gave similar answers have found this really helpful."

Conclusion

In this chapter we have sought to show how the science of psychology, when applied in the clinical setting, can contribute to assessing and formulating the mental health challenges of children and young people. In clinical assessment, applied psychologists with varied roles and professional identities seek to practice in a way that is both evidence-based and responsive to the unique circumstances of each client. This involves the application of a range of theories and methods, including those pertaining to measurement, cognition, learning, cross-cultural difference, and the psychological and social mechanisms that contribute to mental health.

References

American Psychiatric Association (2013) *Diagnostic and Statistical Manual of Mental Disorders*, 5th edn. American Psychiatric Association, Washington, DC.

American Psychological Association, Presidential Task Force on Evidence-Based Practice (2006) Evidence-based practice in psychology. *American psychologist* **61**, 271–285.

Barnett, A. *et al.* (2007) Development and standardization of a new handwriting speed test: The Detailed Assessment of Speed of Handwriting. In: *BJEP Monograph Series II: Part 6 Teaching and Learning Writing*. (eds V. Connelly, *et al.*). British Psychological Society, Leicester, UK. https://explore.bps.org.uk/content/monograph/bpsmono.2005.cat538

Baron, I.S. (2018) *Neuropsychological Evaluation of the Child: Domains, Methods, & Case Studies*. Oxford University Press, New York.

Bertie, L.A. & Hudson, J.L. (2021) CBT for childhood anxiety: reviewing the state of personalised intervention research. *Frontiers in Psychology* **12**, 722546.

Booth, R. *et al.* (2022) *Paediatric Neuropsychology Within the Multidisciplinary Context*. Mac Keith Press, London.

Braaten, E. & Willoughby, B. (2014) *Bright Kids Who Can't Keep Up: Help your Child Overcome Slow Processing Speed and Succeed in a Fast-paced World*. Guilford Press, New York.

Bronfenbrenner, U. (1979) *The Ecology of Human Development: Experiments by Nature and Design.* Harvard University Press, Cambridge, MA.

Bronfenbrenner, U. (2005) *Making Human Beings Human: Bioecological Perspectives on Human Development.* Sage Publishing, Thousand Oaks, CA.

Bruandet, M. *et al.* (2004) A cognitive characterization of dyscalculia in Turner syndrome. *Neuropsychologia* **42**(3), 288–298.

Buchanan, R.D. (2010) *Playing with Fire: The Controversial Career of Hans J. Eysenck.* Oxford University Press, Oxford, UK.

Ceci, S.J. (2006) Urie Bronfenbrenner (1917-2005). *American Psychologist* **61**(2), 173–174.

Ebesutani, C. *et al.* (2012) The Revised Children's Anxiety and Depression Scale – Short Version: scale reduction via exploratory bifactor modeling of the broad anxiety factor. *Psychological Assessment* **24**, 833–845.

Cohen, M.J. (1997) *Children's Memory Scale: Administration Manual.* The Psychological Corporation, San Antonio, TX.

Collins, A. *et al.* (2015) History of neuropsychology. In: *Clinical Psychology in Britain: Historical Perspectives.* (eds J. Hall, *et al.*). British Psychological Society, Leicester, UK. pp. 270–282.

Conners, C.K. (2014) *Conners' Continuous Performance Test*, 3rd edn. Pearson, London.

Conners, C.K. (2022) *Conners*, 4th edn. Pearson, London.

Cullum, C.M. *et al.* (2014) Teleneuropsychology: evidence for video teleconference-based neuropsychological assessment. *Journal of the International Neuropsychological Society* **20**(10), 1028–1033.

Delis, D.C. *et al.* (1994) *California Verbal Learning Test-Children's Version (CVLT-C).* The Psychological Corporation, San Antonio, TX.

Delis, D.C. *et al.* (2001) *Delis-Kaplan Executive Function System.* The Psychological Corporation, San Antonio, TX.

Drysdale, K. *et al.* (2004) Use of the Everyday Memory Questionnaire with children. *Child Neuropsychology* **10**(2), 67–75.

Emslie, H. *et al.* (2003) *Behavioural Assessment of the Dysexecutive Syndrome for Children (BADS-C).* APA PsycTests. Harcourt Assessment/The Psychological Corporation, London. doi: 10.1037/t89186-000.

Fernández, A.L. & Abe, J. (2018) Bias in cross-cultural neuropsychological testing: problems and possible solutions. *Culture and Brain* **6**(1), 1–35.

Gee, G. *et al.* (2014) Aboriginal and Torres Strait Islander social and emotional wellbeing. *Working Together: Aboriginal and Torres Strait Islander Mental Health and Wellbeing Principles and Practice* **2**, 55–68.

Gershon, R.C. *et al.* (2013) NIH toolbox for assessment of neurological and behavioral function. *Neurology* **80**(11 Supplement 3), S2–S6.

Gioia, G.A. *et al.* (2015) *BRIEF-2: Behavior Rating Inventory of Executive Function.* Psychological Assessment Resources, Lutz, FL.

Hall, J. *et al.* (2015) *Clinical Psychology in Britain: Historical Perspectives.* British Psychological Society, Leicester, UK.

Harder, L. *et al.* (2020) Home-based pediatric teleneuropsychology: a validation study. *Archives of Clinical Neuropsychology* **35**(8), 1266–1275.

Harrison, P.L. & Oakland, T. (2015) *ABAS-3.* Western Psychological Services, Torrance, CA.

Hebben, N. & Milberg, W. (2009) *Essentials of Neuropsychological Assessment.* John Wiley & Sons, Hoboken, NJ.

Hellgren, K. *et al.* (2013) Compromised approximate number system acuity in extremely preterm school-aged children. *Developmental Medicine & Child Neurology* **55**(12), 1109–1114.

Hodge, M.A. *et al.* (2019) Agreement between telehealth and face-to-face assessment of intellectual ability in children with specific learning disorder. *Journal of Telemedicine and Telecare* **25**(7), 431–437.

Hudson, J.L. *et al.* (2023) Interventions for young children's mental health: a review of reviews. *Clinical Child and Family Psychology Review* **26**, 593–641. doi:10.1007/s10567-023-00443-6.

Korkman, M. *et al.* (1998) *NESPY: A Developmental Neuropsychological Assessment.* The Psychological Corporation, San Antonio, TX.

Layard, R. & Clark, D.M. (2014) *Thrive: The Power of Psychological Therapy.* Penguin, London.

Lezak, M.D. *et al.* (2004) *Neuropsychological Assessment.* Oxford University Press, New York.

Ludlow, C. *et al.* (2020) A current review of the children and young people's improving access to psychological therapies (CYP IAPT) program: perspectives on developing an accessible workforce. *Adolescent Health, Medicine and Therapeutics* **11**, 21–28.

Lugo-Candelas, C. *et al.* (2021) Intergenerational effects of racism: can psychiatry and psychology make a difference for future generations? *JAMA Psychiatry* **78**(10), 1065–1066.

Mandy, W. & Lai, M.C. (2016) Annual research review: the role of the environment in the developmental psychopathology of autism spectrum condition. *Journal of Child Psychology and Psychiatry* **57**(3), 271–292.

Manly, T. *et al.* (2016) *The Test of Everyday Attention for Children, Second Edition (TEA-Ch-2).* Pearson, London.

Marzillier, J. & Hall, J. (1998) *What is Clinical Psychology?* 2nd edn. Oxford University Press, Oxford, UK.

National Institute for Health and Care Excellence (2020) Eating Disorders: Recognition and Treatment [NICE Guideline No. 69]. [Online]. Available: www.nice.org.uk/guidance/ng69 [2October 2024].

National Institute for Health and Care Excellence (2022) Depression in Adults: Treatment and Management. [NICE Guideline No. 222]. [Online]. Available: www.nice.org.uk/Guidance/ng222 [26 October 2024].

Neisser, U. (2014) *Cognitive Psychology: Classic Edition.* Psychology Press, Abingdon, UK.

Palmer, R. *et al.* (2013) The state of the evidence base for psychodynamic psychotherapy for children and adolescents. *Child and Adolescent Psychiatric Clinics* **22**(2), 149–214.

Pennington, B.F. & Bishop, D.V. (2009) Relations among speech, language, and reading disorders. *Annual Review of Psychology* **60**, 283–306.

Persons, J.B. (2022) Case formulation. *Cognitive and Behavioral Practice* **29**(3), 537–540.

Postal, K. & Armstrong, K. (2013) *Feedback That Sticks: The Art of Effectively Communicating Neuropsychological Assessment Results.* Oxford University Press, New York.

Randolph, C. *et al.* (1998) The Repeatable Battery for the Assessment of Neuropsychological Status (RBANS): preliminary clinical validity. *Journal of Clinical and Experimental Neuropsychology* **20**(3), 310–319.

Rasmussen, C. & Bisanz, J. (2009) Executive functioning in children with fetal alcohol spectrum disorders: profiles and age-related differences. *Child Neuropsychology* **15**(3), 201–215.

Reynolds, C. & Voress, J.K. (2007) *Test of Memory and Learning,* 2nd edn) edn. PRO-ED, Austin, TX.

Roberts, E. *et al.* (2022) Paediatric teleneuropsychology. In: *Paediatric Neuropsychology Within the Multidisciplinary Context.* (eds R. Booth, *et al.*). MacKeith Press Practical Guides, MacKeith Press, London.

Rutter, M. (2006) *Genes and Behaviour*. Blackwell, Oxford, UK.

Semel, E.M. *et al.* (2006) *Clinical Evaluation of Language Fundamentals, (4th Australian standardised edn)*. Harcourt Assessment, Marrickville, NSW, Australia.

Sherman, E.M.S. & Brooks, B.L. (2015) *Child and Adolescent Memory Profile (ChAMP)*. Psychological Assessment Resources, Lutz, FL.

Sheslow, D. & Adams, W. (2021) *Wide Range Assessment of Memory and Learning, Third Edition: Administration Manual*. Jastak Associates Inc, Wilmington, DE.

Snowling, M.J. *et al.* (2007) Children at family risk of dyslexia: a follow-up in early adolescence. *Journal of Child Psychology and Psychiatry* **48**(6), 609–618.

Souissi, S. *et al.* (2022) Assessment of executive functions in school-aged children: a narrative review. *Frontiers in Psychology* **13**, 991699.

Spring, B. (2007) Evidence-based practice in clinical psychology: what it is, why it matters; what you need to know. *Journal of Clinical Psychology* **63**(7), 611–631.

Stark, D. (2022) Culture. In: *Paediatric Neuropsychology Within the Multidisciplinary Context*. (eds R. Booth, *et al.*). MacKeith Press Practical Guides, MacKeith Press, London.

Talley, J.T. (1993) *Children's Auditory Verbal Learning Test*, 2nd edn. Psychological Assessment Resources, Lutz, FL.

Tolin, D.F. *et al.* (2015) Empirically supported treatment: recommendations for a new model. *Clinical Psychology: Science and Practice* **22**(4), 317–338. doi:10.1037/h0101729.

Vygotsky, L.S. & Cole, M. (1978) *Mind in Society: Development of Higher Psychological Processes*. Harvard University Press, Cambridge, MA.

Weber, A.M. *et al.* (2019) Gender norms and health: insights from global survey data. *The Lancet* **393**(10189), 2455–2468.

Wechsler, D. (2020) *Wechsler Individual Achievement Test*. APA PsycTests.

Weiss, L.C. *et al.* (2016) *Theoretical and Clinical Foundations of the WISC-V Index Scores*. Elsevier Academic Press, Amsterdam.

Westerman, T. (2004) Guest editorial: engagement of indigenous clients in mental health services: what role do cultural differences play? *Australian e-journal for the Advancement of Mental Health* **3**(3), 88–93.

Wilson, B. *et al.* (1991) *The Rivermead Behavioural Memory Test for Children aged 5 to 10 Years*. Thames Valley Test Company, Bury St. Edmunds, UK.

Woodcock, R.W. *et al.* (2001) *Woodcock-Johnson III Tests of Cognitive Abilities*. Riverside Publishing Company, Itasca, IL.

World Health Organization (2022) *International Statistical Classification of Disease and Related Health Problems*, 11th edn, World Health Organization, Geneva, Switzerland.

CHAPTER 30

Physical examination and medical investigation

Kenneth E. Towbin

[1] Emotion and Development Branch, National Institute of Mental Health, Intramural Research Program, Bethesda, MD, USA

[2] Department of Psychiatry and Behavioral Health, The George Washington University School of Medicine, Washington, DC, USA

Introduction

Child psychiatry is a medical subspecialty in a nexus with child neurology and general pediatrics. While the primary focus of child psychiatry is mental disorders, practitioners must be ever mindful of the close relationship among "mental," "neurological," and other "medical" symptoms. The boundaries among these may not be sharp (as discussed in Chapters 2 and 26). A fundamental principle of psychiatry is that mental disorders are also brain disorders that affect perception, thinking, learning, behavior, social interaction, and mood. Thus, when considering diagnoses and treatment, child mental health professionals must be alert to medical and neurological disorders that produce psychiatric symptoms, influence treatment interventions, and affect outcome.

The purpose of this chapter is to provide guidelines for clinicians to follow for a standard medical assessment of the child. The need for medical assessment arises from a fundamental principle: it is essential to discover, through observations and measures, biological contributions to mental disorders. These may be signs of medical illness, somatic consequences of ongoing psychiatric disorders, or features indicating risks (constitutional or acquired) for mental disorders. However, the astute clinician knows that physical and laboratory investigations are only one part of a comprehensive grasp of the patient's condition.

Modern child psychiatry sees conditions as rooted in both biology and the mind, and it acknowledges the continuous interplay between them. Child mental health professionals recognize that a child's body is affected by the child's environment and by the way that child thinks and acts. Clearly, psychiatric disorders (e.g., eating disorders, depression, psychosis, psychosomatic fatigue, conversion symptoms), and the somatic therapies that are often prescribed to treat them, can affect pediatric growth and general medical health. Reciprocally, as child mental health professionals know, medical problems can influence a child's development and mental well-being. For these reasons, the physical examination and evaluation of the patient—drawing information from what is reported and an examination of the patient's body—are fundamental to a comprehensive understanding of that individual.

There are other influences to be considered along with biomedical processes. It is equally fundamental to our field to appreciate the power of experiences, relationships, and the context of a child's life. These have a formidable effect on how that child develops and thinks; one must account for them in formulating the child's condition and treatment. The sophisticated, modern view is that the course of development and disorders (e.g., onset, severity) are a function of biological *and* environmental forces acting through a complex interaction of risk and protective factors (Rutter *et al.*, 2006; Kendler & Baker 2007; Rutter, 2013; Dick *et al.* 2015; O'Donnell & Meaney 2020).

The physical examination in child psychiatry takes place within the doctor's relationships with the patient, the patient's family, and in many cases, other health care providers in the patient's life. Physicians are mindful of this as they approach their patients and their patients' families. The manner with which the examination is conducted communicates a great deal, much of it nonverbally, to the patient; the psychiatrist's way of conducting the examination plainly conveys how the patient's identity, thoughts, emotions, and physical feelings are regarded. Similarly, most parents are keenly aware that physical contact with their child has profound significance; it arouses concern and invites protective instincts. This is one reason why a parent or chaperone must always be present for the physical examination, as discussed below.

The medical examination reflects a scientific approach. Physicians begin with gathering data, such as the primary complaint and the history of its onset and course. As data are being gathered, practitioners consider hypotheses about the differential diagnosis, potential contributions to the expression of those

Rutter's Child and Adolescent Psychiatry and Psychology, Seventh Edition.
Edited by Anita Thapar, Daniel S. Pine, Samuele Cortese, Cathy Creswell, Tamsin J. Ford, James F. Leckman, and Argyris Stringaris.

Companion website: www.wiley.com/go/thapar/rutterspsych7

symptoms, and prognosis. Medical and laboratory assessments are not "fishing expeditions"; they test specific hypotheses that arise from listening carefully to the chief complaint(s) and history. Laboratory and medical evaluations are tools that facilitate the process of narrowing the differential diagnosis and hypotheses into a workable treatment plan and approach to the child's care. The process is a "two-way street" in which laboratory and medical data can raise new hypotheses, support existing ones, and refute others (see Chapter 2 for further discussion of this approach).

All child mental health professionals consider the context of their patients' health care to guide their examination. Thus, the medical evaluation entails more than the basic history and course of illness. Child mental health professionals consider the scope of their involvement and their role in the team of those providing overall medical health care to their patients. Child mental health professionals should be mindful of what is feasible under the current condition where care is being delivered, what part of their patients' care falls to them alone, who has the most expertise to pursue a more extensive workup, and what should be performed by (or in collaboration) with others. It is common sense that a child without basic health care or any access to care will face insurmountable barriers to fulfilling recommendations for various forms of ancillary medical tests, such as magnetic resonance imaging (MRI) scans or extensive metabolic assessments. Conversely, when a child has ready access to routine pediatric care, the approach should take this into account when planning the workup and ordering tests. Child mental health professionals consider the context of care, and their patients' general health, history of prior assessments, and current health care relationships. It follows that mental health professionals routinely communicate their findings and plans and coordinate their assessments with those providing primary care to their patients be they pediatricians, nurse practitioners, or family medical doctors. When a child's care includes other health care providers, child mental health professionals think about the basic data others will need to pursue more focused, additional studies. Child mental health professionals consider these collaborations carefully and frame specific questions or hypotheses for their collaborators. For example, if a psychiatrist believes a child might have anemia, it is logical to confirm this by obtaining a complete blood count, serum hemoglobin, and hematocrit prior to referring the child for a more comprehensive hematological workup.

The medical history

The medical history is a cornerstone of the medical evaluation. It encompasses the child's current general health, health history, developmental health history, socioeconomic circumstances, and family medical history.

The current health history is generally understood to include all current illnesses, recurrent conditions, allergies, and current and past medications, particularly psychoactive medications, and medications that might affect mood and behavior. In the context of psychiatric care, it should also include the child's living conditions, socioeconomic conditions, and access to health care. In high-income countries clinicians may make a tacit assumption that children have primary care providers, satisfactory nutrition, and everything they need for basic hygiene. However, one should refrain from such assumptions. Children may lack basic health care because they reside in low- and middle-income countries (LMICs), or in poverty (whether in high-income countries or LMICs), or in homes or communities where they face deprivation and/or neglect. A routine medical history ought to include queries about the child's diet, activity/exercise level, and whether either parent or child has concerns about how the child is growing or feeling physically. These questions become particularly salient when assessing the possibility of an eating disorder, contamination fears, or depression.

The developmental history informs the clinician about a broad range of risks. When exploring the prenatal history, one listens for significant risks prior to the child's birth, such as family medical/psychiatric history, sources of stress for the family, how the family coped with those stressors, and the barriers to health care. The course of the pregnancy conveys information about constitutional and environmental influences and perinatal events. These deserve further exploration because prenatal and perinatal environments continue to affect that child's development and risk for psychopathology (Monk *et al.*, 2019; Lautarescu *et al.*, 2020). As in general pediatrics, the developmental history includes a review of developmental milestones, the feeding history, development of gross and fine motor skills, coordination, language, social abilities (including peer relationships), school/academic functioning, and overall adaptive functioning in communication, daily living skills, socialization, and motor domains (Gerber *et al.*, 2010; Wilks *et al.*, 2010; Gerber *et al.*, 2011). There are established norms for many of these milestones and screening instruments (Frankenburg *et al.*, 1992; Drotar *et al.*, 2008; CDC, 2022; Sparrow *et al.*, 2016) that are helpful when acquiring information about past or ongoing delays or deficits. A history of developmental delays and deviances should alert the clinician to the possibility of a neurodevelopmental disorder (see Chapter 3). For older children, it is important to gather a history of work activities. Also, standard practice is to inquire about past or recent exposure to traumatic events (interpersonal or natural), abuse, being victimized or bullied (in person or "online" via social media), and exposure to violence at home, in the community, or at school.

The past medical history typically includes the patient's past and current medical illnesses, surgical history, any hospitalizations, and a review of complications arising from common childhood illnesses or medications. As suggested above, the history may raise questions that go beyond medical interventions. The past medical history may reveal features of the context of the child's past and present. Medical illness can impair a child's psychological health and a family's relationship with the child. Juvenile onset conditions (e.g., diabetes, cancer, epilepsy, rheumatoid arthritis, or inflammatory bowel disease) or congenital disorders (e.g., heart, blood, or immune diseases) will have profound effects on psychological, social, and physical development. Even seemingly ordinary childhood events might cue the child mental health professional to relevant psychiatric concerns. For example, a history of repeated accidents, fractures, or injuries (particularly concussions) could lead to questions about safety, supervision of the patient, impulsivity, thrill-seeking, mood disorder, or risk-taking. Some psychiatric conditions, such as attention deficit hyperactivity disorder (ADHD), post-traumatic stress disorder (PTSD), or a depressive disorder might drive such behavior. Similarly, relatively common chronic or recurrent childhood maladies can shape the child's perspective on the world. Asking about asthma, bowel, and bladder function, headaches, ear infections, and tics (and other repetitive movements) is important because these conditions may associate with psychiatric symptoms, influence psychological development, have profound effects on a child's day-to-day life, and/or involve treatments that affect mood and behavior. This is also a time to review past use of prescription medications and "complementary/alternative" agents or "supplements" for medical or psychiatric conditions. A child psychiatrist will need to know whether psychotropic medications will interact with drugs that are already being taken for other conditions. There are online resources that can assist prescribers in this effort such as, Drugbank online (https://go.drugbank.com/drug-interaction-checker), Drugs.com (https://www.drugs.com/drug_interactions.html), or Medscape (https://reference.medscape.com/drug-interactionchecker) (WebMD operates both http://RxList.com and Medscape). Learning about unusual reactions to any drugs alerts those who prescribe psychiatric medications to the risks of adverse effects that might arise.

The family medical history is a major part of the patient's medical history. The family's medical history informs the child mental health professional about the risks for developing medical and psychiatric disorders and suggests possible medical disorders that produce psychiatric symptoms. A parent, grandparent, guardian, or sibling with a serious medical or psychiatric disorder is likely to affect the family's life and the child. Learning the family medical history can inform the mental health professional about troubling events and circumstances in the patient's life and influence the patient's psychological development. Although, it is well beyond the scope of this chapter to catalog all the ways a medical disorder might influence a child or family, here are some examples of conditions that are relatively more heritable, particularly likely to produce psychiatric symptoms, or convey an elevated risk of adverse reactions to somatic treatments.

A family history of cardiac illness is an exemplar. A family history of cardiac disease in elderly relatives is common. Yet, family history of cardiac disease assumes compelling relevance for the child's medical and psychiatric care when there is a childhood onset (e.g., malformations, arrhythmias) or sudden death in young family members. A family history for myocardial infarction or sudden death in young family members indicates risk for cardiac conduction or myocardial diseases in the patient (Tan & Judge, 2012). Moreover, some psychiatric medications can increase a risk for a cardiac event in vulnerable patients (Jensen *et al.* 2015; Beach *et al.*, 2018). Compared to those with no concerning family history of heart conditions, children with such a family history, particularly sudden death before age 40 or arrhythmias, may have a greater risk of adverse cardiovascular effects of psychostimulant medications or atypical antipsychotic medications. This would prompt a more thorough characterization of the patient's current cardiac function (e.g., a baseline electrocardiogram (ECG), exercise stress testing) and monitoring for ECG changes during initiation and following dose increments with some medications (Cortese *et al.*, 2013; Jensen *et al.* 2015). Consultations with the child's usual pediatric care provider would certainly be indicated.

A family history of endocrine disorders is another example. A family history of diabetes or hypothyroidism can increase the likelihood that the patient will have a similar disorder contributing psychiatric symptoms. A family history of Type 2 Diabetes (T2D) is a risk factor for developing T2D (Shah *et al.*, 2022a). An overweight child who presents with depression and a strong family history for T2D warrants consideration of hyperglycemia contributing to depression (Copeland *et al.*, 2013; Hannon *et al.*, 2013) and monitoring for development of T2D (Schmitz *et al.*, 2016). A family history of diabetes also increases the risk for additional weight gain, developing diabetes while on psychotropic medication, and developing arrythmias on some medications (de Hert *et al.* 2011; Jensen *et al.* 2015; Jensen *et al.*, 2019).

Similarly, there are major genetic contributions to hyperthyroidism and to Hashimoto's thyroiditis (which can lead to hypothyroidism) (Lane *et al.* 2023; McLachlan & Rapoport 2023). Compared to patients with no family history of thyroid disease, those with depression plus a family history of thyroid disease have greater risk of possible thyroid dysfunction.

A family history of neurological disorders is relevant. While the most common severe inherited neurological disorders arise in infancy (e.g., gangliosidoses), or in adulthood (e.g., Huntington's disease, dementia), a few begin in childhood or adolescence (e.g., Wilson's disease). Family and personal history is often the first clue to their presence. Some less severe, more commonly inherited neurological conditions, that produce psychiatric symptoms (e.g., chronic tic disorders), have their peak incidence during childhood.

Family history may be important for treatment. For example, a family history of glaucoma increases the patient's risk of developing it with pharmacological treatments such as selective serotonin reuptake inhibitors (SSRIs) and atypical antipsychotic drugs (Jain *et al.*, 2021). Box 30.1 summarizes the key points of the medical history.

Box 30.1 Summary of the key points of "The medical history"

- It is essential to be aware of medical disorders that produce or result from psychiatric disorders.
- Being mindful of the context of psychiatric care within the patient's overall health care means recognizing one's role, communicating with other care providers, and discussing who will do what parts of the examination.
- The medical history is a cornerstone of the medical evaluation.
- The medical examination reflects a deductive scientific approach. The history raises possible disorders that might explain the symptoms and course of illness (see Chapter 27).
- The history includes the child's current general health, medical health history, developmental history, and family medical history.
- Inquiring about a family history of cardiac, endocrine, autoimmune, psychiatric, or neurological illness can be instrumental.

The physical examination

How patients construe their physical examination varies by individual, development, and over time. Thus, one must be attuned to how pediatric patients might perceive their examination and explain the reasons for it. This also includes talking about the timing of the examination within the overall evaluation. Typically, a physical examination is conducted within the first few meetings with the child and repeated whenever new symptoms surface, additional history suggesting of a medical contribution is revealed, or there is a marked deterioration in the patient's functioning. Most children and adolescents view psychiatric care, focusing on mood, "feelings," and behavior, as fundamentally different from pediatric health care that focuses on general heath (well-child care), ordinary infections (e.g., colds, flu, otitis), or injury. Thus, patients may be surprised that the psychiatrist will examine them. In addition, for many children, the mind and the body are such separate entities that those who do not feel physically ill will not see the logic of performing the examination. It may not be obvious that a problem affecting thinking, mood, or behavior would have a connection to their body.

The physician also must be aware of, and protect, the patient's modesty and anxiety. Being mindful about modesty makes it imperative that a parent (or guardian) chaperone, and/or another health care provider be with the physician at all times during the physical examination (Committee on Practice and Ambulatory Medicine, 2011). Physicians should refrain from physical contact whenever they are alone with their patients. The rationale for keeping this boundary embraces therapeutic, psychological, ethical, and legal principles.

This awareness should also lead the physician to help the patient understand what will be done and why. One cannot assume that all children will understand and interpret the physician's intentions correctly. Explaining what will be done before doing it allows anxious or confused children to anticipate the procedures of the examination and to see the point to the doctor's requests. Furthermore, compared to healthy children, children with severe psychiatric disorders have a greater risk of misunderstanding physical interactions. There may also be cultural beliefs about physical contact to consider and these should be raised and discussed with the parent(s) in advance.

When examining children, physicians also must be attuned to developmental considerations. Creating an environment in which a child can ask questions and exercise some choice over the examination is important. The space used for the examination should be well lit, large enough to move around comfortably, and protect privacy. The art of examining developmentally younger children is gathering neurological information from observations of a child who is engaged in ordinary actions or playing simple games. For a child with a psychiatric disorder, the examination will be less invasive and distressing when one uses techniques that include toys, observations, and games, rather than mechanical requests to perform movements or actions.

As generally described above, the decision about who should examine the child will depend on the circumstances and the context of that child's general health care. When a child has an established pediatric care provider, the onus falls to the doctors to reach a mutual decision about who will perform the examination. In some cases, it is desirable for each doctor to perform some segments of the examination. For children who are being seen for psychiatric care, the mental status/neurological examination is the principal focus (see also Chapter 27). Attention should be given to other elements of the physical examination as dictated by the details of the history, observed signs, and the symptoms (e.g., signs of encephalopathy, intellectual disability) or "dysmorphic features" (such as misshapen or unusual position of eyes, ears, or other face parts, or disproportion of the head, face, or other body parts). In other circumstances, such as when a child is admitted to an inpatient or intensive psychiatric care facility, or there are no other medical care providers available, a psychiatrist may do the entire physical examination.

Repeating the relevant portions of the physical examination (e.g., mental status and neurological system, perhaps blood tests) is an appropriate consideration whenever new symptoms arise that point to onset of another condition, when there is a possibility that the patient is experiencing an adverse reaction to a new drug or dose, or when a patient's functioning deteriorates.

Recommendations to limit in-person contact in response to the COVID-19 virus pandemic, pushed practitioners to expand remote telehealth technology for mental health care. When those recommendations were loosened, many practitioners continued with solely remote, or adopted "hybrid" (some visits in-person, others remote), care. Arguing over whether "in-person" or remote telehealth care is superior is an oversimplified false equivalence; everything depends on the environmental conditions, population, features of the disorder being treated, physical condition of the patient, family resources for remote technology access, and availability of care. Within limitations, psychiatric assessments of youth and older children can be performed via telehealth, but some information will be lost (e.g., reliable weight/vital signs, highly confidential disclosures). Even so, remote assessment may be superior to no care. Being mindful of telehealth limitations, practitioners can gather key features of the mental status examination and observable physical signs. However, knowledge of and proficiency in conducting telehealth assessments (or care) cannot be presumed. Just as with conventional care, they require training and practice. In addition, the quality of the evidence comparing in-person assessment to telehealth assessment for children and youth is poor, and as of this writing, most reports are anecdotal.

There are excellent texts available for methods and techniques of the physical examination (e.g., Bickley *et al.*, 2020; Suneja *et al.* 2020). A complete review of techniques and methods exceeds the scope of a single chapter of guidelines. Generally, practitioners have a standard, systematic, practiced routine for performing the examination. Some findings have greater relevance for child psychiatric assessment. Few symptoms are pathognomonic of any disorder; most diagnoses emerge from an iterative process drawing on history and physical signs to raise hypotheses, which are then confirmed or refuted by evidence from additional findings (e.g., laboratory investigation).

By convention, the examination begins with obtaining vital signs—the patient's height, weight, blood pressure, pulse, and respiratory rate. Plotting height, weight, and head circumference on a growth chart allows one to track them over time. Vital signs assume greater salience when one is considering pharmacological treatments that may affect weight or cardiovascular function. Vital signs that fall significantly above or below the normal range may signal the presence of a medical and/or psychiatric condition.

For example, acquired low weight might result from protein-calorie malnutrition, an eating disorder, depression with loss of appetite, hyperthyroidism, celiac disease, anemia, cancer, infection, autoimmune disorder, or another primary medical condition. As part of obtaining weight data, careful attention should be paid to the child's growth. Evidence of deviation in the typical course of height or weight can provide clues to various changes in the child's medical well-being. In addition, some medications, such as SSRIs or psychostimulants, can alter the child's growth. Thus, it is important to track the child's growth trajectory when initiating these treatments. It is also crucial to recognize and monitor excessive weight or obesity. Obesity elevates risks to psychological and physiological health that should be reflected when gathering the history, performing the physical examination, and selecting any laboratory/medical tests. Obesity may generate sleep apnea, which, in turn, may produce or exacerbate psychiatric symptoms (Sateia, 2009) and may be associated with ADHD (Cortese & Tessari, 2017).

The examination of the skin, which includes lesions, skin texture, and color variations, can reveal systemic illness or signal noteworthy behaviors. Abnormalities in skin and hair texture point to thyroid disease as a contribution to depression or cognitive changes. Common skin lesions, such as scars, may also be informative and reflect intentional self-injury, repeated accidents, or past physical trauma (e.g., abuse). Some clinicians may be reluctant to ask patients about or examine sites of self-injury. As with so many delicate but necessary parts of psychiatric assessment, (e.g., suicidal ideation, embarrassing obsessions or compulsive behaviors, bodily concerns, gender identification, and sexual attraction/activity) skilled clinicians can foster a trusting rapport that allows patients to talk about the sources of their stress and adaptations. Most patients will not volunteer information about such sensitive topics, and thus, it is incumbent on the practitioner to ask, and be prepared to respond, in constructive, therapeutic ways. The clinician's discomfort with asking and apprehension about how best to respond are understandable and appropriate foci for training, repetition, and proficiency.

Acne, while very common, may cause distress, particularly among those who have social anxiety or body dysmorphic disorder. Skin hygiene can point to loss of self-care or parental neglect, particularly when accompanied by parasitic infections such as lice and scabies. The skin also may show active lesions from picking (dermatotillomania), pinching (tics), abrasions (from compulsive behaviors), petechia (especially around the eyes, suggestive of self-induced choking), abuse (welts, bruising, petechia in specific patterns such as grip marks or ligatures, burns, wounds), or sexual preferences. Assessing hair distribution and texture may reveal systemic illness or trichotillomania. The skin examination may also show dramatic hair color or styles, skin piercings, and tattoos that, while not pathological, certainly open avenues to learn about the patient's self-image, interests, and social world.

Neurocutaneous disorders that link to central nervous system disease and neuropsychiatric disorders may display areas of hyperpigmentation (neurofibromatosis), or pink or red bumps (angiofibromas) on the face (tuberous sclerosis). Though rare, tuberous sclerosis carries a high risk for neuropsychiatric disorders (de Vries *et al.*, 2018).

The head, eyes, ears, nose, and throat examination bundles a few signs that can be psychiatrically important. Head shape can reflect environmental risks from neglect or genetic risks from craniosynostosis (Knight *et al.*, 2014), particularly in intellectually disabled children. Head circumference, like other physical measures, may be excessively large or small and suggest genetic and neurological disorders with behavioral features. Similarly, highly characteristic dysmorphic facial features may suggest specific genetic disorders such as trisomy 21, Fragile X, Prader-Willi, Angelman, Klinefelter, velo-cardio-facial (VCF), Williams, or Turner syndrome. There is a wide range of facial abnormalities in VCF but cleft palate, particularly involving the soft palate, and elongated face, wide nose, and small ears are frequently seen with this disorder. Characteristic facial features also are seen with repeated fetal exposure to alcohol. Deprivation or neglect may lead to poor dental hygiene and severely damaged teeth and gums that are observed on examination of the mouth and throat. Inspection of the mouth can also reveal signs of self-induced vomiting, such as erosion of teeth and lesions in the mouth. Lesions from sexually transmitted diseases may be visible. Examination of the appearance of the eyes may uncover disorders affecting genetic/metabolic (e.g., Wilson's disease, neurofibromatosis) or endocrine (thyroid) function. Systemic and infectious diseases can influence eye function such as pupillary responses to light and accommodation. A quick examination of vision may be conducted by having the patient view a hand-held pocket vision screener (or an E-chart) card at 14 in (36 cm) or copy drawings of familiar geometric shapes. Disorders that produce dysmorphic facial features, like those mentioned above, could affect the shape, size, and placement of the ears. Limited or loss of hearing affects language acquisition in young children. Any concerns about hearing should be assessed by an audiologist, but a screening assessment can be performed in a quiet room by asking if the child can hear the clinician rubbing a forefinger and thumb together at 13–14 in (35–36 cm) from the ear.

Pediatric psychiatric disorders have many fewer specific associations with examination of the neck, heart, lungs, and abdomen. Major exceptions include the size of the thyroid gland, and in asthmatic children, the presence of wheezing. Genetic disorders like the ones noted above may affect cardiac hemodynamics and auscultation.

The circumstances that require a psychiatrist to perform a genital examination are rare. It is generally recognized that psychiatric care providers should refrain from genital examinations. When other features of the physical examination suggest a pattern that requires inspection of the genitals in order to winnow the differential diagnosis (such as Fragile X, Klinefelter, or Prader-Willi syndrome, or disorders of sexual development), arrangements for another provider to perform a genital examination should be made. If it is necessary, such an examination demands the utmost of attention to the patient's comfort and modesty. Unless there are extraordinary circumstances, one should never examine a patient's genitals unless a parent/guardian is present. If a genital examination is essential, the psychiatrist must explain and give a clear rationale for it in advance.

The examination of the extremities may reveal picking, bruising, scarring, or recent evidence of self-injury. Much less commonly, one may see signs of abnormal shape or growth that suggest genetic disorders with psychiatric symptoms such as Smith-Magenis (Gropman *et al.*, 2006) or Prader-Willi syndrome (Angulo *et al.*, 2015).

The neurological examination is highly relevant to child psychiatric care and to resolving hypotheses about the diagnosis (see Chapter 33). Many pediatric neurological conditions produce psychiatric symptoms; discussing each of them exceeds the scope of this chapter. However, physicians should be mindful of behavioral and emotional changes that may be the first sign of a progressive neurological condition. The neurological examination should assess the cranial nerves, motor system (strength and tone), sensory system, balance and coordination, reflexes, and mental status.

A great deal can be learned by carefully observing the patient during an ordinary interview or, with younger children, while playing age-appropriate games such as throwing or kicking a ball. Fine motor coordination skills can be observed from playing a game of copying geometric figures or simply asking the child to make a drawing. How the child walks, gets up from the floor, or moves during conversation can provide leads for a more focused examination. Motor coordination difficulties are also relevant though much remains to be understood about them. While common in children, motor coordination disorders may have prognostic implications when concurrent with ADHD or executive function disorders (Meachon *et al.*, 2022). Observing repetitive movements, mannerisms, voice quality, articulation, gait, gaze, and coordination can be accomplished during a typical interview.

The mental status examination is central to the child psychiatric examination (see also Chapter 27). The basic elements of the mental status examination focus on the patient's capacities and current function in the context of their developmental level. As with the examination of adults, the mental status examination begins with the patient's appearance, mood, and affect. The clinician notes the variations and range of mood and affect during the interview. Inquiring about current or past suicidal ideation or thoughts/plans to harm others should be a routine part of the examination. Observations are made of the patient's speech and language. Behaviors are noted including stereotyped motor movements, capacity to sit calmly, and use of nonverbal communication such as gestures, facial expressions, and eye gaze. Changes in behavior during the interview are important, too. Cognitive capacity can be estimated from the patient's vocabulary, the coherence of the patient's ideas, and complexity of the patient's language construction. The child's narrative provides information on major themes and contents of the patient's thoughts. Spontaneous comments convey information about the flow of the child's thoughts and whether there is perseveration, developmentally immature thinking, frankly odd or bizarre ideas, or reason to have concerns about delusional beliefs, hallucinations, or perceptual distortions. When considering the presence of hallucinations, it is important to inquire whether they arise exclusively in a pattern of falling off to sleep (hypnagogic) or upon awakening from sleep (hypnopompic). It is also useful to learn whether they are vivid, frightening to the child, can be summoned or dismissed easily, and whether the child is convinced they are caused by an outside source rather than his or her mind (Sikich, 2013). A great deal about the patient's mental status can be learned from ordinary conversation. Features of orientation, mood, affect, intelligence, fund of knowledge, judgment, memory, attention, and abstracting abilities can be readily noted. When a child performs well academically without accommodations at school, this usually reflects at least average general intelligence. The mental status examination traditionally includes comments on the manner of the

Box 30.2 Summary of the key points of "The physical examination"

- Physical examination is basic to a comprehensive understanding of the patient and the neurological and mental status examinations are pivotal for a child psychiatry assessment.
- Sensitivity to the patient's past experiences, current state, culture, and developmental and cognitive levels should be foremost.
- The physical examination should be done only when a parent (or chaperone) is present.
- Protecting the patient's modesty and providing reassurance by explaining what will be done before doing it are key.
- The physical examination includes vital signs and follows with a systematic approach for each segment of the body.
- It is generally recognized that psychiatric care providers should refrain from genital examinations.

child's relating to the examiner over the course of the interview(s) and on any changes in that manner of relating with time and topics. Box 30.2 summarizes the key points of the physical examination.

Laboratory investigation

The laboratory investigation flows from the same rubric as the physical examination. The physical examination is guided by thoughtfully listening to the chief complaint, being mindful of patterns that emerge as one hears about symptoms, narrowing the range of possible conditions to a differential diagnosis, using observation and examination to further narrow the possibilities, and, ultimately, gauging the likelihood that a condition is contributing to the child's impairment. The laboratory investigation provides additional data to support or refute the diagnostic possibilities that are raised by the history and physical examination. Like the physical examination, laboratory testing is part of an iterative process that refines the differential diagnosis. The decision about which additional studies to pursue should consider the context of the child's usual health care, the hypotheses about the most likely conditions, and clinical judgment about risk (such as whether there could be an acute illness posing immediate danger). Figure 30.1 offers a conceptual overview of this kind of deductive, iterative process. There are risks, costs, delays, and waste that arise from obtaining laboratory data using a scattershot approach that ignores the fundamentals of a considered differential diagnosis.

The laboratory investigation also occurs in a treatment context. Under the optimal circumstances a child will have regular health care and will have been followed by a pediatric or family medical doctor. If so, the physicians should confer, discuss possible medical contributions to the patient's symptoms, and come to a consensus about the need and direction for any laboratory workup. Typically, the laboratory evaluation will be the purview of the care provider who oversees the child's general medical health. As with the physical examination, the decision about who should order and follow the laboratory investigation and tests will depend on the circumstances and the context of that child's general health care. Thus, the psychiatric practitioner should be alert to the patient's treatment team; ordering highly specific laboratory tests and interpreting those results should go to the provider who has the greatest competence and knowledge of them. This is particularly important when parents seek specific laboratory tests for autoimmune conditions, hair mineral analyses, or vitamin D levels. However, there may be suboptimal circumstances or extenuating situations that

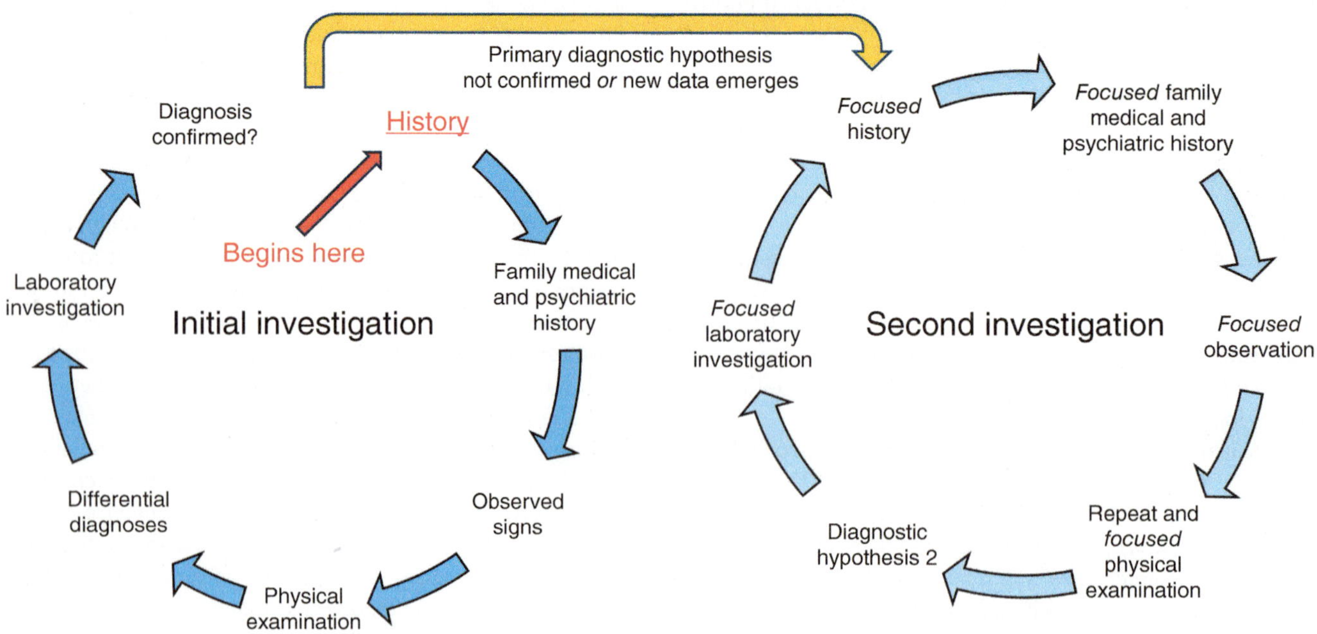

Figure 30.1 The iterative process of physical examination and laboratory investigation.

shift the responsibility to the psychiatrist. If so, then one should consider a stepwise medical evaluation, beginning with what a subspecialist might need prior to a more focused and specific evaluation that might follow. For example, if following considerable weight gain, a patient describes fatigue, polyuria, persistent thirst, and increased appetite, then the psychiatrist ought to confer with the child's general medical provider (de Hert *et al.*, 2011) and discuss who will obtain a fasting blood sugar, glycosylated hemoglobin level (HbA_{1c}), and, if possible, an oral glucose tolerance test before referring the child to a diabetic subspecialist (Shah *et al.*, 2022b).

The attuned clinician will also consider the impact that laboratory procedures have on the patient. On casual consideration, phlebotomy, an ECG, or an electroencephalogram (EEG) might seem minor, but these procedures can make children highly anxious. Therefore, it is important to explain, in developmentally compatible terms, what will happen and why.

Laboratory investigations often proceed in sequential steps; initial findings may raise questions that require additional studies to resolve. Thus, the laboratory evaluation unfolds over time and the psychiatric provider should be mindful of how requesting additional studies affects parents. In some situations, laboratory results may be needed urgently, but others may be deferred. Thought should be given to who will need the results and one should avoid any unnecessary repetition of studies. For example, for a child who has ready access to a general health care provider and complains of abdominal pain that could be due to gastro-esophageal reflux or anxiety, one might pass the medical workup to the pediatric care provider who follows that patient.

There is no "standard battery" of laboratory tests for psychiatric disorders, and laboratory studies should never be ordered simply to assess "general health." However, when one suspects the presence of a specific condition, a focused laboratory assessment should be performed. For example, if there are concerns about anemia or bleeding problems then obtaining a complete blood count with differential count, hemoglobin, hematocrit, and coagulation indices, such as a prothrombin time and partial thromboplastin time, are warranted. If one is starting medications that might worsen anemia or bleeding, it would be important to obtain premedication, baseline measures. For one example, SSRIs may cause changes in coagulation and, rarely, anemia, and therefore obtaining a baseline complete blood count with differential count would be reasonable. For another, where the history suggests recurrent infections, symptoms of neurological problems with weakness and/or coordination, and weight loss, the physician might pursue assessment for human immunodeficiency virus (HIV).

Similarly, there is no "standard battery" of laboratory tests to obtain prior to starting any psychotropic medication (see Chapter 39). The selection of the tests and recommendations for ongoing monitoring will depend on the patients' individual risk factors and the agent(s) being prescribed. Generally, the laboratory tests and monitoring follow from the "Warnings" or "Warnings and Precautions" sections of the package insert or drug information for each specific medication. These sections typically recommend screening procedures, including what baseline studies should be obtained, risks of concurrent medications, and clinical signs and symptoms that should be monitored (see Chapter 39).

Fortunately, most children have healthy kidney function. But when there are concerns about kidney impairment, or if one is starting a drug that is primarily excreted through the kidneys, such as lithium, then obtaining baseline kidney function tests are important. Also, basic urine analysis would follow from concerns about infection, or the presence of metabolic conditions.

Primary liver disease is rare in children. However, since some medications can affect liver function, obtaining liver function tests becomes salient prior to starting them (see Chapter 39). When high rates of hepatitis are to be found among children in some locales, results of these indices might lead one to obtain measures of serum hepatitis antibodies.

A further example would be concerns about cognitive function presenting along with attentional problems and disruptive behaviors in a child who resides where environmental conditions carry a high risk of exposure to lead. Obtaining a serum lead level would be even more compelling if the child was young and had not had a lead level measured previously, or while residing at the child's current address.

The decision to obtain thyroid function studies should be based on the examination (e.g., thin hair, puffy face, dry skin, bradycardia, muscle weakness) and symptom profile (depression, constipation, fatigue, cold sensitivity, impaired memory). However, even if there are few of such symptoms, a child who resides in a region where iodine deficiency is endemic (such as mountainous regions, areas of the northern Ganges River (India), or in North Africa) would spur one to obtain serum thyroid stimulating hormone (TSH) and thyroxine (T4) (Zimmerman, 2009).

Additional medical studies, such as an ECG, EEG, or neuropsychological testing should be ordered when the indications are clear. For example, when prescribing medications, such as atypical antipsychotic medications or noradrenergic antagonists that may change cardiac conduction, it is prudent to obtain a baseline ECG. Ongoing monitoring for any changes as the dose is increased may be appropriate (see Chapter 39). This is particularly important in children who have a family history of sudden death in young relatives, have a family history of cardiac anomalies or conduction disorders such as Wolff-Parkinson-White syndrome, or have a personal history of symptoms such as syncope, severe shortness of breath during exercise, prolonged or very significant fatigue, or, on routine ECG, borderline cardiac indices. As discussed in Chapter 39, evidence of cardiac risk of stimulant medication appears to be lower than previously suspected (Zhang *et al.*, 2022), even among those with cardiac illness (Topriceanu *et al.*, 2022).

The decision to obtain an EEG should follow from the history and symptoms that are reported or observed. The yield of clinically meaningful information from routine EEGs in children with generic psychiatric disorders is low (Camfield & Camfield, 2000; Raybould *et al.*, 2012) and does not offset the cost, inconvenience, and discomfort to the patient. Conversely, when there is a history of paroxysmal events, with motor and/or psychomotor events, a prior history of serious head injury, acute onset psychosis or catatonia, or the presence of disorders with a high likelihood of comorbid epilepsy, such as intellectual disability, specific genetic disorders, or autism spectrum disorders (ASDs), then a compelling case can be made for an EEG. In the case of possible epilepsy, obtaining a detailed history for stereotyped symptoms that precede the psychomotor events or any "post-ictal" symptoms such as fatigue, cognitive dulling, or confusion that typically follow them is warranted. Similarly, any rapid onset psychosis or catatonia that presents along with a decline in previously acquired skills, language, or intellect, and is accompanied by a history of antecedent viral infection or unusual responses to antipsychotic medications, raises the possibility of an autoimmune encephalitis (Abboud *et al.*, 2021; Adams *et al.*, 2021; Hageboutros *et al.*, 2023). Such a presentation warrants evaluation that includes an EEG. Such a history accompanied by seizures or family history of autoimmune disorders raises even greater concern for such conditions.

Since the likelihood of finding clinically useful information from routine neuroimaging of child psychiatric patients is so low, it has a limited role in general child and adolescent assessments (see Chapter 11). MRI is indicated when focal neurological findings suggest a tumor or diffuse focal findings of autoimmune neuroinflammatory conditions are suspected (Hardy, 2022).

Obtaining chromosomal and/or genetic studies assessments follows from the physical examination or likelihood of intellectual disabilities (as discussed in Chapter 53 and Chapter 21). In addition, in the future, there may be a role for obtaining genetic studies when the patient gives a personal or family history of adverse drug reactions that raise a possibility of hyper- or hypometabolism of specific agents (e.g., codeine, tramadol) (Crews *et al.*, 2021). Currently, studies cast doubt on its benefit and evidence does not support obtaining genetic assessments as a routine part of evaluation and treatment (Namerow *et al.* 2020; Vande Voort *et al.*, 2022) (see Chapter 39).

Assessment of cognitive functions should also flow from the history and physical examination. When the history points to consistent problems with learning and/or reaching social and cognitive milestones this prompts the clinician to consider obtaining a standard assessment of intellectual function (as discussed in Chapter 53). Similarly, specific patterns of impairment may emerge from the history, or arise from interviewing the child. A review of the child's academic history will provide essential data when considering the need for subsequent specific evaluations. For example, impairments in receptive language (e.g., problems with understanding instructions or explanations that use simple vocabulary), word finding, expressive language (e.g., problems in expressing thoughts, using appropriate length of utterances, using age- and culturally appropriate vocabulary), or organization of language would prompt one to obtain a focused evaluation of language function from a speech pathologist (see Chapter 51).

Two examples (Examples 30.1 and 30.2), that follow the iterative processes in Figures 30.2 and 30.3, show the flow information and what the physician might consider during the examination.

Example 30.1

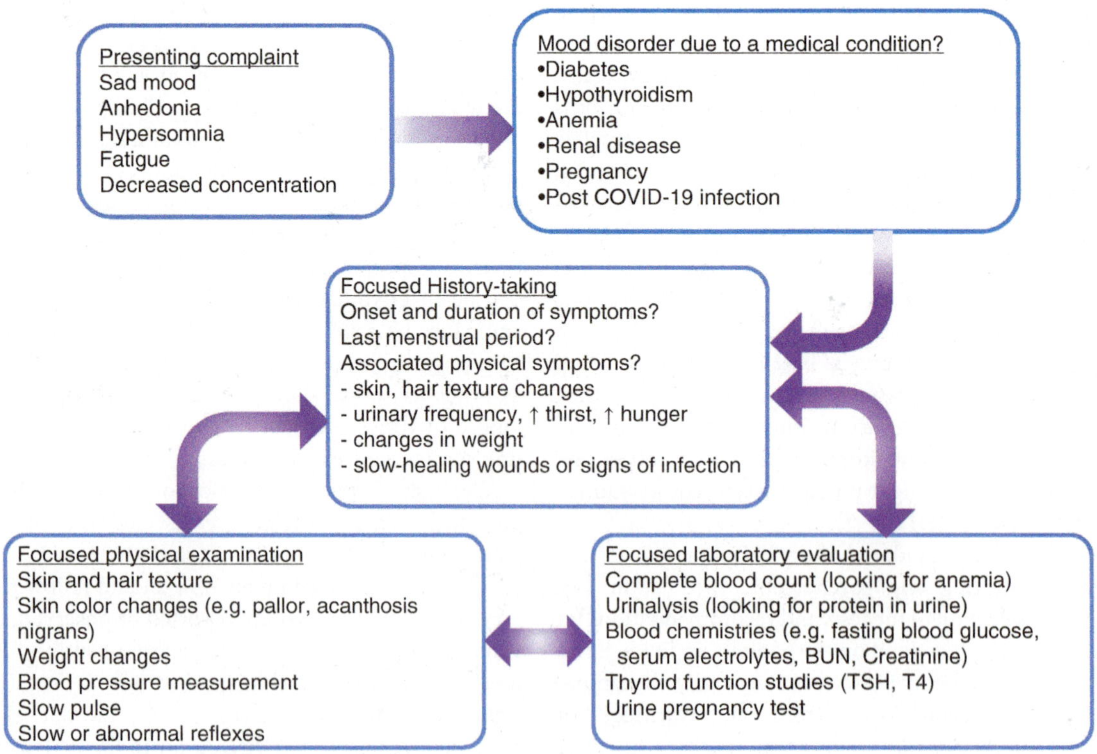

Figure 30.2 Flow chart of the assessment for a hypothetical 16-year-old female who presents with symptoms of a depressive disorder.

Example 30.2

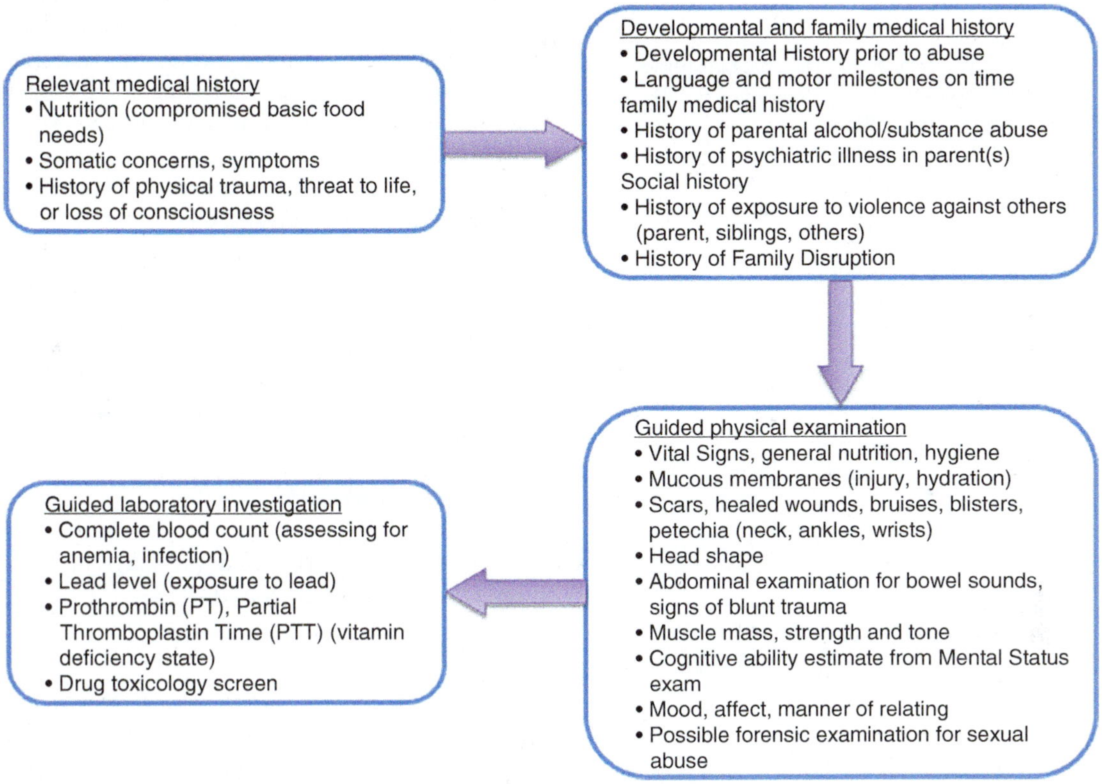

Figure 30.3 Flow chart of the assessment for a hypothetical 8-year-old female who, after physical abuse and neglect, was removed from her home by Protective Services and is reported to be listless and fearful, and complaining of stomach aches and headaches. PT = Prothrombin Time; PTT = Partial Thromboplastin Time.

A complex example: the evaluation of new onset psychosis

As a further example, consider the patient with new onset psychosis. The differential diagnosis of psychotic conditions in children and adolescents is extensive (Sikich, 2013; Staal *et al.*, 2019) (see Chapter 56). The general grouping of etiologies parallels the many causes of delirium and mental status changes in adults (Table 30.1). Despite this long list of disorders, the probability that a child will have any one of these conditions is 1–2/10,000. When the presentation includes focal neurological signs, changes in cognition, loss of skills, co-occurring movement disorder, seizures, or mutism, then the likelihood of a somatic etiology rises (Staal *et al.*, 2019).

As shown in Figure 30.1, the assessment, including the laboratory examination, flows systematically from the history, family history, signs, and symptoms. Particular attention should be paid to sudden co-occurring changes in cognitive functions and emotions since this may signal progressive and acute conditions (Staal *et al.*, 2019; Hardy, 2022). Resisting a haphazard approach, laboratory assessments should consider the most common etiologies first. For acute onset psychoses, it is reasonable to begin with a drug screen, complete blood count with differential (to consider infectious etiologies), serum electrolytes, urine analysis (for specific gravity, glucose, drugs of abuse, porphobilinogen, infection), thyroid function studies, and, if neurological symptoms or history suggesting seizures, an EEG. Though rare, an assessment for autoimmune encephalitis would be indicated for those who develop a rapid decline following a viral illness leading to seizures, psychotic symptoms, movement disorder, memory disturbance, and changes in consciousness/catatonia (Hardy, 2022). Box 30.3 summarizes the key points of the laboratory investigation.

Summary

The physical examination of the child is a deductive process of gathering information and arriving at a best estimate of the diagnoses. Physical examination of child psychiatric patients routinely includes all the basic elements of medical inquiry: the chief complaint, history of current illness, past medical and psychiatric history, family medical and psychiatric history, and a physical examination. Following the leads from these data, the psychiatrist may confer with a medical provider to plan for

Table 30.1 Differential diagnosis of delirium/psychosis.

- I Toxic conditions (such as):
  - (a) Substance abuse (amphetamines, bath salts, cocaine, 3,4-methylenedioxy-N-methylamphetamine (MDMA), hallucinogens)
  - (b) Acute lead encephalopathy
  - (c) Neuroleptic malignant syndrome
  - (d) Drug-induced delirium
- II Metabolic disorders (such as):
  - (a) Adrenoleukodystrophy
  - (b) GM2 gangliosidoses
  - (c) Neimann pick disease
  - (d) Acute intermittent porphyria
  - (e) Homocystinuria
- III Endocrinological disorders (such as):
  - (a) Thyrotoxicosis
  - (b) Hypothyroidism
  - (c) Addison's disease
  - (d) Cushing syndrome
  - (e) Hyperparathyroidism
- IV Infectious diseases (such as):
  - (a) Viral encephalitis
  - (b) Bacterial encephalitis
  - (c) Post-infectious encephalitis
  - (d) Fungal encephalitis (e.g., Cryptococcus)
  - (e) Spirochetal infections
- V Structural neurological lesions (such as):
  - (a) Temporal lobe glioma
- VI Autoimmune disorders (such as):
  - (a) Systemic lupus erythematosus
  - (b) Sarcoidosis
  - (c) Autoimmune encephalitis (e.g., s N-methyl-D-aspartate receptor (NMDAR)-antibody and leucine-rich glioma inactivated (LGI1)-antibody)
- VII Paroxysmal disorders (such as):
  - (a) Temporal lobe epilepsy
  - (b) Partial complex status epilepticus
  - (c) Post-ictal psychosis
- VIII Specific genetic disorders (such as):
  - (a) Huntington's disease
  - (b) Wilson's disease
  - (c) Parkinson's disease
  - (d) Fahr's disease

Box 30.3 Summary of the key points of "Laboratory investigation"

- The laboratory investigation provides additional data to narrow diagnostic possibilities raised by the history and physical examination.
- The decision about which additional studies to pursue considers the context of the child's usual health care (e.g., who is best to interpret the results), the hypotheses about the most likely conditions, and clinical judgment about whether there may be an acute problem that poses immediate risk.
- There is no standard battery of laboratory tests for psychiatric disorders and laboratory studies should not simply assess "general health."
- When one suspects the presence of a specific condition, a focused laboratory assessment should be performed.
- Acquiring additional medical assessments, such as ECG, EEG, genetics, cognitive testing, and language/communication evaluations, follows from the history and physical examination.
- Currently, routine use of neuroimaging in child psychiatry has a low yield of clinically useful information and is not recommended.

focused laboratory and other clinical evaluations that will reduce the differential diagnosis in a logical manner. Generally, that child's medical provider conducts the direct physical examination of the child, but there are occasions and situations when psychiatrists may be required to examine their patients. If so, the sensitivity of the physician to the patient's past experiences, current state, culture, and developmental and cognitive levels should be foremost. The components of the examination that require touching the patient should occur in the presence of a parent or guardian or a chaperone. Perhaps one of the most vital skills in obtaining data from the history and physical examination is the mental health professional's capacity for observation. A great deal can be learned about cognitive and neurological functions from close observation of the patient during interviews, simple requests, and ordinary interactions.

Acknowledgment

This research was supported (in part) by the Intramural Research Program of the NIMH.

References

Abboud, H. *et al.* (2021) Autoimmune encephalitis: proposed best practice recommendations for diagnosis and acute management. *Journal of Neurology, Neurosurgery, and Psychiatry* **92**(7), 757–768.

Adams, A.V. *et al.* (2021) Psychiatric phenotypes of pediatric patients with seropositive autoimmune encephalitis. *Hospital Pediatrics* **11**(7), 743–750.

Angulo, M.A. *et al.* (2015) Prader-Willi syndrome: a review of clinical, genetic, and endocrine findings. *Journal of Endocrinological Investigation* **38**(12), 1249–1263.

Beach, S.R. *et al.* (2018) QT prolongation, Torsades de pointes, and psychotropic medications: a 5-year update. *Psychosomatics* **59**(2), 105–122.

Bickley, L.S. *et al.* (2020) *Bates' Guide to Physical Examination and History Taking.* Lippincott Williams & Wilkins, Philadelphia, PA.

Camfield, P. & Camfield, C. (2000) How often does routine pediatric EEG have an important unexpected result? *The Canadian Journal of Neurological Sciences* **27**(4), 321–324.

CDC (Centers for Disease Control and Prevention) (2022) *CDC's Developmental Milestones.* Available: https://www.cdc.gov/ncbddd/actearly/milestones/index.html [18 April 2023].

Committee on Practice and Ambulatory Medicine (2011) Use of chaperones during the physical examination of the pediatric patient. *Pediatrics* **127**(5), 991–993.

Copeland, K.C. *et al.* (2013) American Academy of Pediatrics. Management of newly diagnosed type 2 diabetes mellitus (T2DM) in children and adolescents. *Pediatrics* **131**(2), 364–382.

Cortese, S. & Tessari, L. (2017) Attention-deficit/hyperactivity disorder (ADHD) and obesity: update 2016. *Current Psychiatry Reports* **19**(1), 4.

Cortese, S. *et al.* (2013) European ADHD Guidelines Group. Practitioner review: current best practice in the management of adverse events during treatment with ADHD medications in children and adolescents. *Journal of Child Psychology and Psychiatry* **54**(3), 227–246.

Crews, K.R. *et al.* (2021) Clinical pharmacogenetics implementation consortium guideline for CYP2D6, OPRM1, and COMT genotypes and select opioid therapy. *Clinical Pharmacology and Therapeutics* **110**(4), 888–896.

de Hert, M. *et al.* (2011) Metabolic and endocrine adverse effects of second-generation antipsychotics in children and adolescents: a systematic review of randomized, placebo controlled trials and guidelines for clinical practice. *European Psychiatry* **26**(3), 144–158.

de Vries, P.J. *et al.* (2018) A clinical update on tuberous sclerosis complex-associated neuropsychiatric disorders (TAND). *American Journal of Medical Genetics. Part C, Seminars in Medical Genetics* **178**(3), 309–320.

Dick, D.M. *et al.* (2015) Candidate gene–environment interaction research: reflections and recommendations. *Perspectives on Psychological Science* **10**(1), 37–59.

Drotar, D. *et al.* (2008) Selecting developmental surveillance and screening tools. *Pediatrics in Review* **29**(10), e52–e58.

Frankenburg, W.K. *et al.* (1992) The DENVER II: a major revision and restandardization of the Denver Developmental Screening Test. *Pediatrics* **89**, 91–97.

Gerber, R.J. *et al.* (2010) Developmental milestones: motor development. *Pediatrics in Review* **31**(7), 267–276.

Gerber, R.J. *et al.* (2011) Developmental milestones 3: social-emotional development. *Pediatrics in Review* **32**(12), 533–536.

Gropman, A.L. *et al.* (2006) Neurologic and developmental features of the Smith-Magenis syndrome (del 17p11.2). *Pediatric Neurology* **34**(5), 337–350.

Hageboutros, K. *et al.* (2023) Neuropsychological functioning in children and adolescents with anti-NMDA receptor encephalitis (anti-NMDARE). *Journal of Neurology* **270**(1), 402–412.

Hannon, T.S. *et al.* (2013) Depressive symptoms and metabolic markers of risk for type 2 diabetes in obese adolescents. *Pediatric Diabetes* **14**(7), 497–503.

Hardy, D. (2022) Autoimmune encephalitis in children. *Pediatric Neurology* **132**, 56–66.

Jain, N.S. *et al.* (2021) Psychotropic drug-induced glaucoma: a practical guide to diagnosis and management. *CNS Drugs* **35**, 283–289.

Jensen, K.G. *et al.* (2015) Corrected QT changes during antipsychotic treatment of children and adolescents: a systematic review and meta-analysis of clinical trials. *Journal of the American Academy of Child and Adolescent Psychiatry* **54**(1), 25–36.

Jensen, K.G. *et al.* (2019) Cardiometabolic adverse effects and its predictors in children and adolescents with first-episode psychosis during treatment with quetiapine-extended release versus aripiprazole: 12-week results from the tolerance and effect of antipsychotics in children and adolescents with psychosis (tea) trial. *Journal of the American Academy of Child and Adolescent Psychiatry* **58**(11), 1062–1078.

Kendler, K.S. & Baker, J. (2007) Genetic influences on measures of the environment: a systematic review. *Psychological Medicine* **37**, 615–626.

Knight, S.J. *et al.* (2014) Neurodevelopmental outcomes in infants and children with single-suture craniosynostosis: a systematic review. *Developmental Neuropsychology* **39**(3), 159–186.

Lane, L.C. *et al.* (2023) Graves' disease: moving forwards. *Archives of Disease in Childhood* **108**(4), 276–281.

Lautarescu, A. *et al.* (2020) Prenatal stress: effects on fetal and child brain development. *International Review of Neurobiology* **150**, 17–40.

McLachlan, S.M. & Rapoport, B. (2023) Discoveries in thyroid autoimmunity in the past century. *Thyroid* **33**(3), 278–286.

Meachon, E.J. *et al.* (2022) Developmental coordination disorder (DCD): relevance for clinical psychologists in Europe. *Clinical Psychology in Europe* **4**(2), e4165.

Monk, C. *et al.* (2019) Prenatal developmental origins of future psychopathology: mechanisms and pathways. *Annual Review of Clinical Psychology* **15**, 317–344.

Namerow, L.B. *et al.* (2020) Pharmacogenomics: an update for child and adolescent psychiatry. *Current Psychiatry Reports* **22**(5), 26.

O'Donnell, K.J. & Meaney, M.J. (2020) Epigenetics, development, and psychopathology. *Annual Review of Clinical Psychology* **16**, 327–350.

Raybould, J.E. *et al.* (2012) EEG screening for temporal lobe epilepsy in patients with acute psychosis. *The Journal of Neuropsychiatry and Clinical Neurosciences* **24**(4), 452–457.

Rutter, M. (2013) Annual research review: resilience—clinical implications. *Journal of Child Psychology and Psychiatry* **54**(4), 474–487.

Rutter, M. *et al.* (2006) Gene-environment interplay and psychopathology: multiple varieties but real effects. *Journal of Child Psychology and Psychiatry* **47**(3–4), 226–261.

Sateia, M.J. (2009) Update on sleep and psychiatric disorders. *Chest* **135**(5), 1370–1379.

Schmitz, N. *et al.* (2016) Depression and risk of type 2 diabetes: the potential role of metabolic factors. *Molecular Psychiatry* **21**(12), 1726–1732.

Shah, A.S. *et al.* (2022a) Spectrum of phenotypes and causes of type 2 diabetes in children. *Annual Review of Medicine* **73**, 501–515.

Shah, A.S. *et al.* (2022b) ISPAD Clinical Practice Consensus Guidelines 2022: type 2 diabetes in children and adolescents. *Pediatric Diabetes* **23**(7), 872–902.

Sikich, L. (2013) Diagnosis and evaluation of hallucinations and other psychotic symptoms in children and adolescents. *Child and Adolescent Psychiatric Clinics of North America* **22**(4), 655–673.

Sparrow, S.S. *et al.* (2016) *Vineland-3: Vineland Adaptive Behavior Scales. Manual*, 3rd edn. Pearson Assessments, Minneapolis, MN.

Staal, M. *et al.* (2019) Early warning signs in misrecognized secondary pediatric psychotic disorders: a systematic review. *European Child & Adolescent Psychiatry* **28**(9), 1159–1167.

Suneja, M. *et al.* (2020) *DeGowin's Diagnostic Examination*, 11th edn. McGraw Hill, New York.

Tan, B.Y. & Judge, D.P. (2012) A clinical approach to a family history of sudden death. *Circulation. Cardiovascular Genetics* **5**(6), 697–705.

Topriceanu, C.C. *et al.* (2022) The use of attention-deficit hyperactivity disorder medications in cardiac disease. *Frontiers in Neuroscience* **16**, 1020961.

Vande Voort, J.L. *et al.* (2022) A randomized controlled trial of combinatorial pharmacogenetics testing in adolescent depression. *Journal of the American Academy of Child and Adolescent Psychiatry* **61**(1), 46–55.

Wilks, T. *et al.* (2010) Developmental milestones: cognitive development. *Pediatrics in Review* **31**(9), 364–367.

Zhang, L. *et al.* (2022) Risk of cardiovascular diseases associated with medications used in attention-deficit/hyperactivity disorder: a systematic review and meta-analysis. *JAMA Network Open* **5**(11), e2243597.

Zimmerman, M.B. (2009) Iodine deficiency. *Endocrine Reviews* **30**, 376–408.

B: Interventions

CHAPTER 31

Psychological interventions: overview and critical issues for the field

V. Robin Weersing[1] and Michelle Rozenman[2]

[1] Joint Doctoral Program in Clinical Psychology, San Diego State University, San Diego, CA, USA
[2] College of Arts, Humanities, and Social Sciences, University of Denver, Denver, CO, USA

The study of psychological interventions for youth mental health problems began over 60 years ago (Weisz *et al.*, 2017), and, for the first four decades of this history, the main focus of research was to determine if psychotherapy "worked." To answer this question, clinical trial methodologies were adapted to map onto challenges of operationalizing and measuring psychosocial interventions and outcomes, with innovations including the development of therapy manuals, standardized diagnostic and clinical assessments, and "control" conditions for psychotherapy. A large body of rigorous clinical trials accumulated, indicating that therapy for youth is almost always better than nothing (no treatment control; Weisz *et al.*, 2017), often better than something (nonspecific therapies and placebo/attention controls; Weisz *et al.*, 2017), and, that some specific treatments might be better than others (e.g., exposure-based therapies for anxiety versus treatments that do not include exposure; Whiteside *et al.*, 2020).

As the field matured, attention has turned from this question of efficacy (does psychotherapy work?) to two important and related concerns. First, rather than demonstrating that psychosocial treatments can work in carefully controlled clinical trials, work has pivoted to testing whether interventions are or can be *effective in practice*, with more diverse populations of youth, delivered by frontline clinicians, embedded in organizational structures with economic constraints. Second, there has been a greater emphasis on studying the mechanisms of psychosocial interventions, and understanding *how* treatments work. Intervention research provides a unique context to experimentally manipulate and test theories of psychopathology to advance our scientific understanding of mental health problems. Understanding the mechanisms of treatment should allow for intervention refinement, improved potency of treatment programs, and enhanced outcomes. The questions of effectiveness and mechanism are complementary; for treatments to be effective under the demands of practice they will need to be quite potent, and as brief and efficient as possible.

In this chapter, we provide our understanding of the state of the field and suggest useful future directions for research and practice. As background, we begin with a review of what evidence-based psychotherapy (EBT) is and current research support for disorder-specific interventions, including for whom and how interventions likely work. We then turn to youth intervention innovations in the last decade, including efforts to utilize evidence-based treatment strategies in efficient and accessible packages that might be suited to clinical practice in real-world settings. Finally, we discuss challenges in the field, with steps that will need to be addressed to improve the potency and reach of mental health services for children and adolescents.

What is evidence-based psychotherapy?

"Evidence-based psychotherapies" refer to interventions that (i) have been tested in randomized controlled clinical trials (RCTs), in which (ii) the intervention components, participants, and outcomes have been clearly specified, (iii) the intervention outperforms a meaningful control condition, and, for the highest levels of support, (iv) where results have been replicated by independent research teams (Southam-Gerow & Prinstein, 2014). Criteria for exactly what "counts" as an EBT have varied across organizations and over time. Current definitions employed by the Society for Clinical Child and Adolescent Psychology (American Psychological Association Division 53) emphasize a two tier-system for EBTs: (i) a well-established EBT has two (or more) RCTs by at least two independent research teams in different settings that show the intervention to be "superior to pill, psychological placebo, or another treatment"

Rutter's Child and Adolescent Psychiatry and Psychology, Seventh Edition.
Edited by Anita Thapar, Daniel S. Pine, Samuele Cortese, Cathy Creswell, Tamsin J. Ford, James F. Leckman, and Argyris Stringaris.

Companion website: www.wiley.com/go/thapar/rutterspsych7

or "not significantly different from an already well-established treatment in experiments,"; in contrast, (ii) a probably efficacious EBT requires that "at least two good experiments show the treatment is superior. . .to wait-list control" but without the requirement for independent replication of intervention effects (Southam-Gerow & Prinstein, 2014). Definitions for lower levels of empirical support (e.g., "possibly efficacious" treatments) are also provided, although interventions meeting these less rigorous outcome criteria are not considered EBTs.

The bulk of evidence for these well-established interventions have been obtained from studies with the goal of demonstrating efficacy. An efficacy RCT is one in which a treatment is tested in the context of well-controlled experimental procedures, such as random assignment to treatment or control conditions, manualized protocols, and supervision of clinicians. While these design features allow for strong causal inferences about intervention effects, they are limited in their generalization outside of the laboratory or specialty clinic. In contrast, an effectiveness study tests the treatment in settings and under circumstances in which the treatment would be delivered in the real world (e.g., community mental health clinic; Silverman & Hinshaw, 2008). The distinction between efficacy and effectiveness highlights the "research–practice gap" (Kazdin, 2017), whereby, even today, well-established interventions that we know have potential to improve youth mental health have not been sufficiently tested in or extended to clinical practice settings.

Table 31.1 provides the types of interventions that are currently considered well-established and their proposed active treatment components. Across interventions for this wide variety of mental health concerns, five empirically supported principles of change that reflect specific intervention strategies taught to youth have been identified. These include: calming

Table 31.1 Evidence-based outpatient youth psychotherapies for specific mental health problems and proposed mechanisms of action[a].

Psychotherapy	Most common core components	Proposed mechanisms of action
Anxiety		
Behavior therapy (BT)/ Cognitive behavior therapy (CBT)	• Psychoeducation • Relaxation strategies • Cognitive restructuring/coping (may not be in BT) • Graded exposure	• Cognitive skills for threat-focused thinking • Exposure/increased approach for avoidance
Depression		
Behavior therapy (BT)/ Cognitive behavior therapy (CBT)	• Psychoeducation • Problem-solving • Cognitive restructuring/coping (not a focus in BT) • Behavioral activation	• Cognitive skills for negative thinking • Behavioral activation for withdrawal • Problem-solving for effective communication/ decision-making
Interpersonal psychotherapy (IPT)	• Psychoeducation and linking interpersonal events/conflicts to mood • Identifying sources of social support • Problem-solving • Communication skills	• Identifying sources of support for loneliness, low mood • Problem-solving interpersonal challenges and practicing communication skills to improve social interactions/ functioning • Parent involvement for younger children to increase skill implementation
Obsessive–compulsive disorder (OCD)		
Behavior therapy (or Exposure and response prevention [ERP])/ Cognitive behavioral therapy (CBT)	• Psychoeducation • Relaxation strategies • Cognitive restructuring/coping (not a focus in BT/ERP) • Exposure and response prevention (ERP)	• Cognitive skills for responding to obsessions • ERP for distress tolerance and reducing compulsions • Parent involvement may facilitate between-session exposure practice and reduce accommodation
Trauma exposure and post-traumatic stress disorder (PTSD)		
Trauma-focused CBT (TF-CBT)	• Psychoeducation and normalization of symptoms • Relaxation strategies and affect modulation • Cognitive coping (can also involve cognitive processing) • Trauma narrative and prolonged exposure to narrative • Skills to enhance safety • Can involve parallel sessions for youth and parent	• Relaxation and affect modulation strategies for responding to physiological reactivity • Cognitive coping for unhelpful thoughts causing distress • Exposure to reducing distress from memories and reducing avoidance • Parent involvement may facilitate communication about youth's trauma and skills to support youth regulation and managing responses to trauma cues
Attention deficit hyperactivity disorder (ADHD)		
Behavioral classroom management	• Teacher involved in or primary interventionist • Reward system for positive behaviors • Consequences/no rewards for negative behaviors	• Reinforcement/planned ignoring for adaptive behavior • Rewards/consequences for motivation

Table 31.1 (Continued)

Psychotherapy	Most common core components	Proposed mechanisms of action
Organizational skills training	• Behavioral techniques taught to parents: prompting, rehearsal, contingency management • Time-management skills • Rewards to reinforce use of behavioral techniques • Some may include parent–child relationships or homework strategies	• Organization, time management, and planning for improving academic outcome • Parent involvement might improve at-home behavior
Behavioral parent training	• Creating house rules and structural/organizational routines • Clear instructions/directives for behavior: rule-setting, time-out, and planned ignoring of mild, unwanted behavior • Rewards, praise, and positive attention for desirable behavior • Improving parent–child interactions • Can include parent–child positive time	• Reinforcement/planned ignoring for adaptive behavior • Rewards/consequences for motivation • Parent–child strategies for reducing conflict and improving interactions
Disruptive behavior		
Functional family therapy	• Engagement: psychoeducation and therapeutic alliance • Increasing motivation to change with cognitive strategies to disrupt dysfunctional thoughts about self and family • Relational assessment to identify family interaction patterns and individual behaviors • Communication and conflict management skills toward behavior change • May also include specific parenting strategies	• Treatment motivation or motivation to change over time for engagement in behavior change • Improvement in family interaction/parenting strategies for youth behavior
Multidimensional family therapy	• Cognitive and behavioral coping • Problem-solving • Decision-making skills • Family/caregiver enhancement of family functioning	• Coping and problem-solving strategies to reduce family conflict • Skills to improve parenting behaviors for youth behavior change
Multisystemic therapy (MST)	• Integration of evidence-based psychotherapy (EBT) strategies to address risk factors in family, peer, school, and community • Promotion of behavioral change in youth environment • Behavioral parent training to increase supervision, appropriate discipline, manage familial relationships, and help youth cope with family, peer, school, and neighborhood problems	• Improving family functioning for reducing risk with peers, school, and community • Reduction in risk to reduce problem behavior/improve functioning
Autism spectrum disorder (ASD)		
Applied behavior analysis (in young children, called early/intensive behavioral intervention)	• Communication and language skills • Social skills training • Behavioral self-management • Pre-academic skills (e.g., imitation, letter, number concepts)	• Social skills training to improve social interaction • Behavioral strategies to improve activities of daily living/ functioning
Behavior therapy (BT)/ Cognitive behavior therapy (CBT)	• Psychoeducation • Relaxation strategies • Cognitive restructuring/coping (may not be in BT) • Graded exposure toward functional behaviors (e.g., social approach) • Can also include social skills and/or communication skills training	• Cognitive skills for threat-focused thinking • Exposure/increased approach for avoidance • Social skills training for more effective social interactions
Eating disorders		
Family therapy including CBT for refeeding/eating	• Restoration of physical health, often including CBT or exposures for refeeding/eating and/or dietary/nutritional programs, with parents taking responsibility for what, when, and how much youth eats. Over time, responsibility transferred to youth • Family mealtimes with behavioral coaching • Parent modeling of behavior • Can include rewards and consequences for food-related behavior	• Behavior change/exposures for refeeding and increasing health • Behavior change for modifying family interactions/ conflict around food
Adolescent substance/alcohol abuse		
Cognitive behavioral therapy (CBT)	• Psychoeducation and functional analysis of use/abuse • Cognitive and motivational strategies for change • Can involve contingency management following abstinence • Coping skills • Behavioral and problem-solving strategies to avoid triggers	• Coping skills for responding to urges • Behavioral and problem solving for behavioral change and reduction in use

(*Continued*)

Table 31.1 (Continued)

Psychotherapy	Most common core components	Proposed mechanisms of action
Multisystemic therapy (MST)	• Integration of EBT strategies to address risk factors in family, peer, school, and community • Promotion of behavioral change in youth environment • Behavioral parent training to increase supervision, appropriate discipline, manage familial relationships, and help youth cope with family, peer, school, and neighborhood problems	• Improving family functioning to reduce risk related to peers, school, and community • Reduction in risk to reduce problem behavior/improve functioning • Behavioral modifications to environment to reduce risk
Functional family therapy	• Engagement: psychoeducation and therapeutic alliance • Increasing motivation to change with cognitive strategies to disrupt dysfunctional thoughts about self and family • Relational assessment to identify family interaction patterns and individual behaviors • Communication and conflict management skills toward behavior change • May also include specific parenting strategies	• Treatment motivation or motivation to change over time for engagement in behavior change • Problem-solving coping may reduce substance/alcohol use
Motivational interviewing/ Enhancement treatment (typically used in combination with CBT)	• Engaging: establishing a therapeutic relationship • Focusing: developing and maintaining specific conversations about change • Evoking: eliciting client's motivations about change • Planning: developing a commitment to change and formulating a concrete plan of action	• Behavioral change may occur following client change language and/or client experience of discrepancy • Decisional balance, or thinking through pros/cons of making versus not making change may also lead to behavioral change
Additional transdiagnostic treatment across emotional and behavioral regulation challenges		
Dialectical behavior therapy (DBT)	• Mindfulness skills • Distress tolerance skills • Emotion regulation skills • Interpersonal effectiveness/communication • Dialectical balancing between acceptance versus change, or "walking the middle path"	• Mindfulness, distress tolerance, and emotion regulation skills to improve regulation and related behavior • Interpersonal effectiveness skills to reduce conflict/ improve interpersonal functioning

[a] Society for Clinical Child and Adolescent Psychology (SCCAP) (https://effectivechildtherapy.org). Last accessed on April 5, 2024.

skills such as progressive muscle relaxation, deep breathing, and guided imagery; increasing motivation with tangible rewards, differential attention, and praise; changing unhelpful thoughts with cognitive restructuring, cognitive defusion (noticing thoughts without responding to them, and letting thoughts come and go), and cognitive coping; problem-solving in a sequential way (e.g., identifying a problem, brainstorming solutions, examining pros/cons, selecting a solution, and trying it); and practicing the positive opposite with graded exposure, behavioral activation, and emotion regulation strategies (Fitzpatrick *et al.*, 2022).

How strong is the intervention evidence base for youth mental health problems?

Identifying specific *well-established* treatments (Table 31.1) is one way to characterize the strength of research support behind psychosocial interventions. Another important technique is meta-analysis. A meta-analysis is a statistical approach that pools and synthesizes data across RCTs or from pre-to-post-treatment in studies without a comparison condition to examine average effect sizes for all available studies targeting a common domain. Psychotherapy meta-analyses have been conducted across youth mental health problems and intervention packages (e.g., Weisz *et al.*, 2013b; Venturo-Conerly *et al.*, 2023a). These tend to focus on relatively common problem domains such as anxiety, depression, attention deficit hyperactivity disorder (ADHD), and disruptive behavior (e.g., oppositional defiant disorder (ODD), conduct disorder (CD)), and often collapse findings across age groups and intervention type. Overall, mean effect sizes that reflect pre-to-post-treatment changes for psychosocial interventions across youth mental health problems (compared to control conditions, typically comprised of wait list, supportive talk therapy, or other approaches that are not well-established or probably efficacious) are within the medium (i.e., 0.5) to large (0.8) effect size range (Cohen, 1988) at post-treatment, with effects well-maintained over the course of 12-month follow-up (Rith-Najarian *et al.*, 2019; Pilling *et al.*, 2020). These data indicate that, on average, evidence-based interventions for youth lead to significant symptom/diagnostic improvement, with treated participants being at the 60–80% percentile compared to youth in the control conditions.

Meta-analyses that examine interventions for specific disorder groupings (e.g., youth anxiety, youth depression) indicate comparable effect sizes to those examining psychotherapy across psychopathology. Figure 31.1 compares effects from the

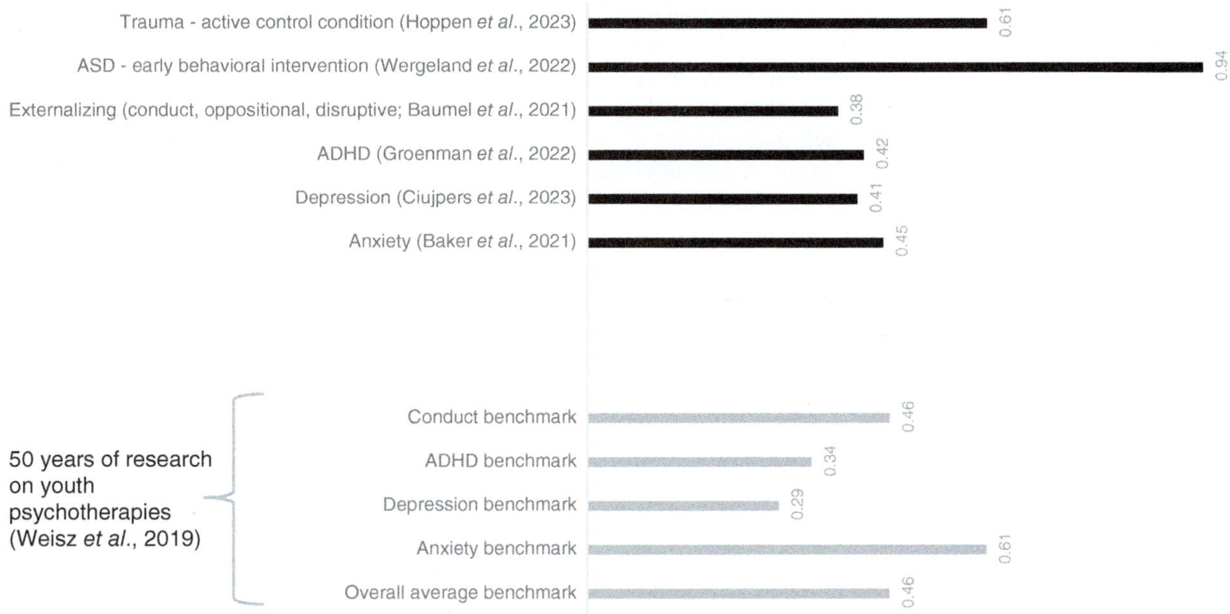

Figure 31.1 Selected disorder-specific meta-analyses benchmarked against comprehensive effect sizes from 50 years of youth psychotherapy research. *Note:* Autism spectrum disorder (ASD); attention deficit hyperactivity disorder (ADHD); some meta-analyses include studies without an active comparison group or independent outcome ratings by evaluators masked to treatment condition, which may inflate effects.

most recent large meta-analysis inclusive of interventions across youth mental health problems (Weisz *et al.*, 2017) to disorder-specific meta-analyses published during 2021–2023. Evidence-based interventions tested in efficacy trials have support for the treatment of youth anxiety (see Chapter 59). While effects from these meta-analyses appear comparably robust for other disorders, data should be interpreted with caution. For these other disorders, some of the included studies focus on pre-to-post-treatment effects and do not include a randomly assigned comparison condition and/or outcome ratings by independent evaluators who are unaware of treatment condition, which may inflate effect sizes. (See Chapter 50 for ASD, Chapter 54 for ADHD, Chapter 58 for PTSD, Chapter 60 for OCD, Chapter 62 for bipolar disorder, and Chapter 63 for depressive disorders.) Collectively, these data suggest that evidence-based interventions have at least some support in improving a variety of mental health and neurodevelopmental symptoms in youth, although effects for specific disorders may vary.

Mediators of treatment: how do psychosocial treatments work?

The last decade has seen secondary analysis of RCT data to determine how and for whom treatments work. *How* a treatment works requires identifying mechanisms, or the processes through which the treatment exerts its effects on treatment outcome (i.e., symptoms/diagnoses). Knowing what an intervention's core mechanisms are (and are not) would allow for increasing the amount of active treatment ingredient(s) and decreasing or even removing treatment components that do not contribute to symptom improvement. This approach could ultimately improve intervention potency so that youth might experience greater symptom improvement more quickly. This would also be time- and cost-saving for providers and settings/systems. A critical step in identifying intervention mechanisms is testing whether a particular component of, or process in, treatment is a *mediator*, or variable, that precedes and predicts changes in treatment outcome (e.g., symptoms of a disorder being treated). As we describe mediators in youth psychotherapy below, we note that most studies have not tested the temporal precedence of change necessary to truly establish mediation (i.e., that changes in the proposed mediator *precede* and predict improvements in treatment outcome/symptoms).

Here we focus on domain-specific processes implicated in individual disorders and their relevant treatments. For example, avoidance is a core symptom of anxiety and behavioral withdrawal is a core symptom of depression. In cognitive behavioral therapy (CBT), avoidance in youth anxiety is targeted with graded behavioral exposure, and withdrawal/inactivity in youth depression is targeted with behavioral activation. Meta-analytic data provide strong evidence that these behavioral approach strategies are critical components associated with symptom improvement in CBT for youth anxiety and depression (Martin & Oliver, 2019; Schopf *et al.*, 2020; Whiteside *et al.*, 2020). Similarly, negative thinking and avoidance of, or withdrawal from, daily life activities have been tested as candidate change processes in cognitive-behavioral and behavioral treatments for youth anxiety and depression. This reflects the cognitive-behavioral theory that individuals with anxiety and depression tend to think more negative and threatening thoughts than unaffected peers, and teaching youth cognitive strategies, such as cognitive restructuring to less negative and more neutral or even positive thoughts, may result in symptom reduction. Meta-analytic findings suggest that CBT does result in improvements in negative self-talk and negative thinking for both youth anxiety and depression (Luo & McAloon, 2021; Bell *et al.*, 2023).

Parenting behaviors have been directly targeted in youth-focused, parent-focused, and multisystemic interventions for behavioral treatment of ADHD, disruptive behaviors in younger children, mild and more severe conduct problems in adolescents, and substance use. Targeting parenting behaviors relevant to increased supervision, youth rewards and consequences, and skills to improve the parent–youth relationship, may be involved in mechanisms of behavior change for youth with ADHD and behavioral problems, across many different types of EBT (Mestre *et al.*, 2022).

Moderators of treatment: for whom does treatment work?

While a mediator is proposed to be malleable to change in treatment, a moderator is a pretreatment variable that is present prior to randomization and interacts with treatment condition (i.e., treatment effects depend on the level of the moderator). A variety of moderators have been tested in youth interventions, including youth characteristics (demographics such as gender, age, and race/ethnicity, symptom severity of the targeted problem, diagnostic comorbidity), caregiver characteristics (e.g., parenting behaviors at baseline, caregiver stress, or psychopathology), and occasionally broader contextual factors (e.g., socioeconomic status). Some studies have explored whether treatment components moderate treatment for a specific mental health problem (e.g., involving caregivers in youth treatment versus not; caregiver versus youth as treatment recipient). Identifying moderators of treatment response may clarify *for whom* specific treatments might be most helpful.

Meta-analytic findings have been mixed in regards to treatment moderators for specific mental health problems in youth, likely because of the significant heterogeneity in measurement of treatment outcomes and reporter (youth, caregiver, clinician; Weisz *et al.*, 2013a). Some of the more consistent (although not ubiquitous) findings suggest that youth may have poorer CBT response if at baseline they have higher symptom severity and/or co-occurring disorders across youth anxiety and depression (Kunas *et al.*, 2021), co-occurring ADHD and behavior problems in treatment of anxiety (Levy *et al.*, 2022; Luo & McAloon 2021), co-occurring anxiety in treatment of OCD (Turner *et al.*, 2018), and a full PTSD diagnosis in treatment of trauma symptoms (Szota *et al.*, 2023). Some data also suggest that parental psychopathology (Kunas *et al.*, 2021), and possibly parental depression specifically (Szota *et al.*, 2023), may negatively impact youth outcomes in CBT. Moreover, in the United States (U.S.), better parental mental health and parenting skills at pretreatment may lead to less delinquency for youth participating in multisystemic therapy (MST), an intensive home- and community-based treatment program (most often used with high-risk youth with severe behavioral concerns) that includes the youth, their family, and often schools and community partners (van der Stouwe *et al.*, 2014).

Parent-focused treatment and parent involvement in youth treatment have also emerged as moderators of treatment response, although findings may be disorder- and age-specific. For example, involving parents in treatment results in better CBT outcome for youth disruptive behavior problems (Baumel *et al.*, 2021; Boldrini *et al.*, 2023), and PTSD (Somers *et al.*, 2022). In family treatment, protocols that include more components to target a larger number of family factors or teach a broader set of parenting skills (and not just those specific to the youth's mental health concern) can also improve outcome in OCD family treatment (McGrath & Abbott, 2019), callous-unemotional traits in youth with disruptive behavior problems (Perlstein *et al.*, 2023), and adolescent alcohol use (Bo *et al.*, 2018). The data on parent-focused interventions for anxious and depressed youth are mixed. For example, parent-focused interventions and those that add parent components to CBT for children do not consistently outperform individual CBT for youth where parent involvement is not specifically formalized; this may be because there is a mismatch between the skills taught to parents in treatment compared to the parenting behaviors and youth–parent interactions that may contribute to the development and maintenance of anxiety (Peris *et al.*, 2021). Similarly, some data suggest that parental involvement may improve youth depression treatment outcome (Oud *et al.*, 2019), but results differ and the literature is small.

One important caveat for these parenting findings is that some individual studies and meta-analyses explicitly examine baseline parenting stress/psychopathology or parenting behaviors as a moderator. In contrast, other studies use less clear language that suggests measurement of parent involvement and behaviors as they unfold over the course of therapy, which suggests a treatment process (i.e., potential mediator) and not a baseline variable (i.e., moderator). Nonetheless, the two sets of findings converge. Together, these data provide important avenues for future research: youth with more symptoms/diagnoses might benefit from earlier or more intensive treatment; treatment that targets multiple problem domains rather than a disorder-specific protocol; and formally involving parents in treatment should be pursued in future research to clarify whether and how involving parents for specific youth mental health concerns is beneficial.

Although less studied, some work has identified that the intersection of youth and their ecosystem (e.g., systemic racism) may moderate treatment response. For example, some evidence suggests that youth from minority racial/ethnic backgrounds do worse in treatment for anxiety (Levy *et al.*, 2022) and disruptive behavior (Perlstein *et al.*, 2023) than White counterparts. Moreover, psychotherapy may be less effective for Black youth in states with higher anti-Black racism when treatment studies do not specifically recruit Black samples (Price *et al.*, 2022); this may be because treatment components to address coping with and responding to systemic racism have not historically been included in mental health interventions for disorder-specific problems. This is clearly an urgent priority for additional research.

The field faces challenges in its attempts to assess treatment mediators and moderators for several reasons. First, there are significant measurement and methodologic issues that have limited progress in the field. Many of the above-referenced mediator and moderator investigations have found that the relevant variable–outcome relationship differs based on who reports on symptom improvement (i.e., parent, child, clinician). There is currently no consensus for any mental health problem about which measures are ideal and how to resolve reporter discrepancies. Additionally, the time course of measurement when testing mediators is often not tied to clear theory or data on how we would expect change to occur temporally (i.e., When, in CBT, do we expect cognitions to change? Immediately after learning cognitive restructuring, after X number of weeks of practice? After combining this skill with other skills over time?). Relatedly, some variables are proposed as both mediators and moderators (e.g., parental involvement), others are tested as moderators but may reflect changes in treatment process (e.g., number of skills parents learn in treatment), and both types of tests do not consider interactions between and across these relevant treatment variables (which would require tremendous sample sizes but without this measurement we may miss important information).

A second major challenge is when and how to consider the clinical practice context in treatment development, tests of mediation, and understanding of moderators. Historically, treatments have been developed and tested in efficacy trials, and tests of mediation and moderation have also been within this well-controlled context. While tightly controlled RCTs provide many methodological benefits, the findings of these studies may not generalize, and there may be important restriction-of-range issues on critical variables (e.g., not finding moderating effects of income in an academic medical center sample that does not include uninsured families; failure to identify reductions in caregiver stress as a mediating variable in parent training). Further, some variables are omitted entirely unless an effectiveness or dissemination/implementation design is used; aspects of care settings (e.g., level of clinician support, organizational climate, copay service costs) cannot be tested as moderators of treatment effects if these variables are optimized in a "well-designed" efficacy RCT.

Child intervention innovations in the last decade

So, what has happened to improve psychological intervention research and clinical practice in the last decade? Here, we discuss four advances in youth psychotherapy that address scientific (i.e., mechanism tests, intervention potency) and practical (i.e., reducing family and clinician burden, efficacy, and implementation tests in community settings) aspects of the research–practice gap.

Transdiagnostic and modular treatments

Rigorous tests (including in real-world settings with efficacy studies) have been conducted with both transdiagnostic and modular treatments (see Chapter 9). A transdiagnostic treatment is one that uses a few core skills that target processes *across* two or more mental health problems. For example, anxiety and depression have several common core elements, including negative or threat-focused thinking and behavioral avoidance/withdrawal. Transdiagnostic treatments for anxiety and depressive disorders such as the Brief Behavioral Therapy program (Weersing *et al.*, 2021) and the Unified Protocol for Children and Adolescents (Ehrenreich-May & Bilek, 2012) target anxiety, depression, and their comorbidity in youth. Such transdiagnostic treatment packages demonstrate effects comparable to single-disorder treatments, even when clinicians are not experts in child CBT and even when implemented in practice settings such as pediatric primary care (Weersing *et al.*, 2017). While more work needs to be done to move transdiagnostic treatments into clinical practice settings for long-term sustainment and determine their impact on more severe symptom presentations for youth, the efficiency of this approach may make it especially applicable to practice settings where clinicians and youth may have limits to learning multiple treatment strategies or distinguishing which strategies might address which symptoms.

In a similar fashion, modular treatments have been developed whereby providers select from a variety of evidence-based strategies for anxiety, mood, behavior problems, and trauma, again in real-world community and school settings (Chorpita *et al.*, 2017). Such an approach may be suited for clinicians working with youth with a variety of mental health concerns, including co-occurring mental health problems. A current challenge with the modular approach is that is relies heavily on clinical judgment and decision-making, with little data on how to make decisions based on youth and family characteristics, presenting problems, and setting/insurer constraints (Venturo-Conerly *et al.*, 2023b). Both transdiagnostic and modular approaches aim to improve practical aspects of intervention implementation, such as increasing access and reducing provider burden.

A different strategy is to develop interventions for maladaptive transdiagnostic mechanisms or behaviors, without regard to presenting diagnosis (or lack of any diagnosis). In the last decade, interventions have been developed that target problems cutting across youth diagnoses. For example, treatments for serious mood dysregulation and irritability (Breaux *et al.*, 2023), as well as treatments for suicidality and safety (Robinson *et al.*, 2018), have been developed and tested in youth irrespective of mood diagnoses (see Chapter 64 for additional details). Most of this work has been conducted in well-controlled efficacy RCTs in specialty settings.

Third-wave and family intervention tests

Efforts have also been made to improve the armamentarium of EBTs by testing "third-wave" interventions (e.g., acceptance and commitment therapy, dialectical behavior therapy) with youth, either as stand-alone treatments or, more commonly, augmenting CBT with mindfulness. While the first wave of therapies utilized behavioral principles (i.e., classical and operant conditioning), and the second wave of therapies utilized both cognitive and behavioral principles (i.e., CBT), third-wave interventions focus on mindfulness and acceptance. Recent meta-analyses suggest that third-wave approaches, such as dialectical behavior therapy, improve youth eating disorder (Buerger *et al.*, 2021), and anxiety and depression (Perkins *et al.*, 2023) symptoms. Additionally, some specialty clinical settings have begun to add these third-wave approaches, particularly mindfulness, as a supplemental strategy to CBT (e.g., Guo *et al.*, 2020). Similarly, investigators have begun to augment CBT with packaged family-focused interventions to improve family functioning as it relates to specific mental health concerns (e.g., Peris *et al.*, 2017). While there is not yet enough data to consider these approaches as well-established EBTs for youth yet, the data available support continued investigation.

Technology-based interventions

Even before the COVID-19 pandemic, but especially in its context and aftermath, EBTs for youth have been translated into Internet, computerized, and other "user-friendly" packages that increase access and reduce burden on youth and families (Christ *et al.*, 2020; Fedele *et al.*, 2017). Similarly, researchers and practicing clinicians alike have increased their use of telehealth and other digital strategies (e.g., text interventions, freestanding web-based portals with information for youth and families to peruse on their own time). Early data suggest that telehealth is acceptable and shows promise for the evidence-based treatment of both emotional (anxiety, mood) and behavioral (ADHD, conduct) disorders in youth (Ros-DeMarize *et al.*, 2021). See Chapter 49 for details on digital assessment and treatment.

Dissemination, implementation, and effectiveness in practice

National funding agencies (e.g., National Institutes of Health in the U.S.) have made a concerted effort to promote research on the effectiveness of interventions in practice and on "implementation science," or the study of the diffusion, uptake, and sustainment of interventions into practice (Estabrooks *et al.*, 2018; Beidas *et al.*, 2022). There have been policy efforts to disseminate EBTs for youth, developed in efficacy trials, into practice contexts (e.g., parent–child interaction therapy (PCIT); Beveridge *et al.*, 2015). This work has spawned theoretical models for analyzing contextual factors impacting intervention uptake (e.g., Consolidated Framework For Implementation Research (CFIR); Damschroder *et al.*, 2009), measure development (e.g., Implementation Climate Scale; Ehrhart *et al.*, 2014), and a host of studies that examine implementation outcomes (e.g., therapist, including nonpsychologist, training; Frank *et al.*, 2020), as the main target of intervention research rather than focusing exclusively on youth clinical outcomes.

In addition to studying implementation of existing EBTs that have been developed and tested originally in traditional efficacy RCTs, there has been a significant increase in studies that develop and implement treatments in real-world settings early (often referred to as deployment-focused treatment development). When selecting treatment targets and components, these models closely fit to the settings in which child mental health care is provided (e.g., primary care) and system-level factors that may influence service access (e.g., number of sessions likely to receive insurer reimbursement) (Weisz *et al.*, 2013b). As such, youth psychotherapy RCTs have begun to focus not only on youth symptom/diagnostic outcomes, but also factors such as initial training of nonpsychologist clinicians, the ability to provide reduced supervision to those clinicians over time, and how to use feedback from stakeholders for long-term sustainment of the implemented treatment model. The Brief Behavioral Therapy transdiagnostic (Weersing *et al.*, 2017) and modular MATCH (Chorpita *et al.*, 2017) interventions discussed previously are only two such interventions; a growing number of others have begun to take a deployment focus in testing interventions in their real-world contexts and, most relevant to the interventions' intended applications, early in the treatment development process.

Current challenges: a need to further innovate interventions

Despite these innovation advances, the research–practice gap still remains and even well-established interventions tested in carefully controlled efficacy trials leave a proportion of youth in the clinically impaired range at post-treatment. Indeed, a systematic review and meta-analysis (Weisz *et al.*, 2019) examined changes over time in treatment effects for anxiety, depression, ADHD, and conduct problems for youth of ages 4–18. Treatment effects for anxiety and ADHD did not change over the decades, suggesting little to no improvement in interventions for these problem domains. More concerning, depression and conduct treatments appear to be *less* efficacious in recent years. This set of findings is both surprising and concerning—it would be expected that as intervention science improves over the years, we should see larger effect sizes across treatments and disorders for youth over time. However, one important contextual factor may clarify these findings. In youth psychotherapy trials before the 2000s, the typical comparison condition was no-treatment or a wait list control, which has increasingly become an unethical and inappropriate option as we now have well-established EBT options. In contrast, RCTs now often compare treatments to those that have already been demonstrated as well-established, probably efficacious, or the standard treatment-as-usual in community practice. As such, Weisz's 2019 findings (Weisz *et al.*, 2019) do not necessarily suggest that treatments are getting worse, but perhaps that early studies decades ago (and their design features) may have led to an initial overestimation of efficacy.

Across these findings and the meta-analytic results presented earlier, we see three opportunities to improve youth psychological interventions. These three opportunities are obviously not exhaustive; rather, they highlight fruitful areas for immediate investigation to reduce the research–practice gaps referenced throughout this chapter. We first discuss avenues to study optimal identification of core treatment ingredients and mechanisms of change that may improve intervention potency. Next, we turn to intervention testing and modification for diverse youth and families who receive services in real-world settings. And finally, we acknowledge the tension that exists between these first two areas for innovation by discussing how researchers might balance between treatment personalization based on youth characteristics and identified treatment mechanisms versus service access and delivery challenges. Addressing these challenges collectively may provide paths forward for intervention deployment to sustained implementation in the real world.

Better methods for probing treatment mechanisms

Although there is some knowledge about core treatment ingredients and mechanisms of symptom change in youth interventions research, there is room for improvement. Until recently, most efficacy and effectiveness RCTs have only measured potential treatment mechanisms at pre- and post-treatment, which precludes the ability to test whether the possible mechanism changes before symptoms change, a necessary step in determining that changes in the mechanism are responsible for and drive symptom reduction (e.g., Scott, 2016). There are two approaches that may address this need for a clearer understanding of treatment mechanisms: treatment dismantling strategies with measurement of both mechanisms and symptoms at multiple time points during treatment, and new intervention discovery within an experimental framework.

Dismantling studies are those that either randomly assign participants to one of two or more treatment components in order to directly compare those components, or randomize participants to sequenced components of treatment in order to examine changes in outcome following each component. While numerous adult studies provide models for dismantling interventions (e.g., Pompoli *et al.*, 2018; Furukawa *et al.*, 2021), only a handful of such studies have been conducted in youth, primarily as a secondary analysis rather than deliberately and *a priori* determining which treatment components will be compared. For example, one meta-analysis compared child anxiety and OCD studies that incorporated relaxation before exposure therapy versus those that did not, finding that more time spent in exposure led to larger effects on treatment outcome (Ale *et al.*, 2015). In contrast, one study deliberately compared CBT to CBT + parent reinforcement of skills and CBT + parents' relationship skills with their child in anxiety. Youth who received CBT with any type of parent involvement experienced greater anxiety reduction than youth who received CBT alone (Silverman *et al.*, 2022). A combination of dismantling studies with measurement of candidate treatment mediators in youth intervention RCTs may confirm some of the previously suggested treatment mediators and clarify extant mixed findings. Moreover, examination of treatment "dose" (e.g., number of sessions, number and type of skills taught) may also clarify how much of a treatment mechanism is required to result in symptom change.

Novel experimental approaches

"Experimental therapeutics" is a relatively novel intervention discovery approach initiated by the National Institutes of Mental Health (Insel, 2015) to identify and manipulate risk factors for specific disorder groupings as potential causal processes. The hope is that directly targeting and manipulating the putative process may reduce symptoms downstream. For example, there is some data that youth and adults with a variety of mental health concerns exhibit cognitive biases (i.e., threat-focused thinking) compared to peers without those problems (e.g., Pergamin-Hight *et al.*, 2015; Stuijfzand *et al.*, 2018). Computerized interventions that aim to directly target and modify cognitive biases to be more neutral or even positive have demonstrated some support in reducing symptoms, although the data are currently mixed (Jones & Sharpe, 2017; Fodor *et al.*, 2020). These studies provide early models for selecting a process that may underlie a specific mental health problem in youth, attempting to directly modify it, and testing whether changes in the process precede and predict symptom reduction.

The experimental therapeutic approach differs from a full psychotherapy package in that the former focuses on one single process (e.g., threat-focused thinking) whereas even a single psychotherapy skill (e.g., cognitive restructuring) may influence multiple processes (i.e., threat-focused thinking, behavior, therapeutic alliance) and therefore it may be difficult to determine which underlying mechanism(s) are impacted. Use of the experimental therapeutic approach with brain-based, biological, cognitive, and psychophysiological processes identified as disorder correlates in youth may lead to improvements in our ability to directly and quickly target the underlying causal and maintaining factors of mental health problems.

Experimental therapeutics thus far have relied primarily on efficacy trials and, as described above, there is a need to consider how to balance between rigorous laboratory tests and receipt of services in real-world settings. Broadly, with this approach both discovery and replication (possibly utilizing the same criteria for psychological interventions in regards to well-established approaches) is and will continue to be necessary before applying experimental therapeutics on a large scale because, at the time of this writing, these experimental efforts have not yet definitively identified malleable mechanistic treatment targets for youth.

Better representation of and treatment development for all youth

Next, most intervention RCTs have been comprised of youth who are primarily White and middle/upper class as a function of the typical catchment areas surrounding research laboratories and specialty clinics at universities and research hospitals (e.g., Pina *et al.*, 2019). Intervention adaptation for diverse youth in the U.S. and internationally may (Compton *et al.*, 2014; Arora *et al.*, 2021) or may not (e.g., Weersing *et al.*, 2017) be necessary; for example, some findings suggest that interventions developed nonlocally in low- and middle-income countries are more effective than those developed locally (Venturo-Conerly *et al.*, 2023a), raising questions about when and what type of adaptations will improve treatment effects. (See Chapter 33 for details on parenting interventions that show differential support in the U.S. versus other countries, and Chapter 46 for details on psychotherapy in low-resource settings.) Simultaneously, antiracist and affirming practices must be prioritized across settings and services to support all youth (Alvarez *et al.*, 2022; Price *et al.*, 2022), and these have not historically been considered in development and efficacy treatment RCTs.

Recent efforts to adapt evidence-based interventions and develop them from the ground up for youth from a variety of diverse backgrounds, including racial/ethnic minority, LGBTQIA+ identity, refugee, war-exposed, those in the justice system, those whose caregivers have military status, and so forth, are under way (for reviews, see Arora *et al.*, 2021; Huey *et al.*, 2023). However, up to 80% of youth with mental health problems never receive services (Weisz *et al.*, 2017). This service access gap is even more pronounced for racial/ethnic minority youth and those in underresourced settings (Hodgkinson *et al.*, 2017), even with the proliferation and normalization of telehealth during the COVID-19 pandemic (Venturo-Conerly *et al.*, 2021). Moreover, when underresourced and minority youth *do* access care, they are much less likely to receive evidence-based care (Hodgkinson *et al.*, 2017). Even when care is provided and labeled as evidence-based, it is not often implemented with sufficient fidelity to be considered scientifically supported (Park *et al.*, 2015). Efforts to improve service access, particularly for underserved and minoritized youth, and quality of services are both critical.

Sustained implementation of evidence-based interventions in delivery settings

The above-described implementation science and deployment frameworks have started to consider how to make interventions a better fit for frontline practitioners in their settings. For example, combining what we know about psychopathology and EBTs with a social determinant of health framework (Dopp & Lantz, 2020) may make treatments fit better for youth services in community settings. Similarly, consideration of how best to train and provide organizational support to providers and systems to implement EBTs will increase uptake and long-term sustainment. The field already has examples of this—many settings have begun to regularly and successfully screen for symptoms at wellness visits and even implement interventions in primary care. Development of a feedback loop from real-world settings back to intervention science (Figure 31.2) may close some of these gaps in accessible delivery methods for active intervention components. And although practice settings are often constrained with regard to time, integration of some core features of efficacy RCTs (e.g., clearly defined intervention targets and outcomes, agreed-upon standardized measures, and mechanisms tests when possible) may further advance implementation science for youth (Williams & Beidas, 2019).

Balancing between rigorous clinical science and service delivery access

Because of this research–practice gap, the two challenges described previously—more rigorous intervention tests to determine for whom and under what circumstances EBTs work versus problems with service delivery—can seem at odds with

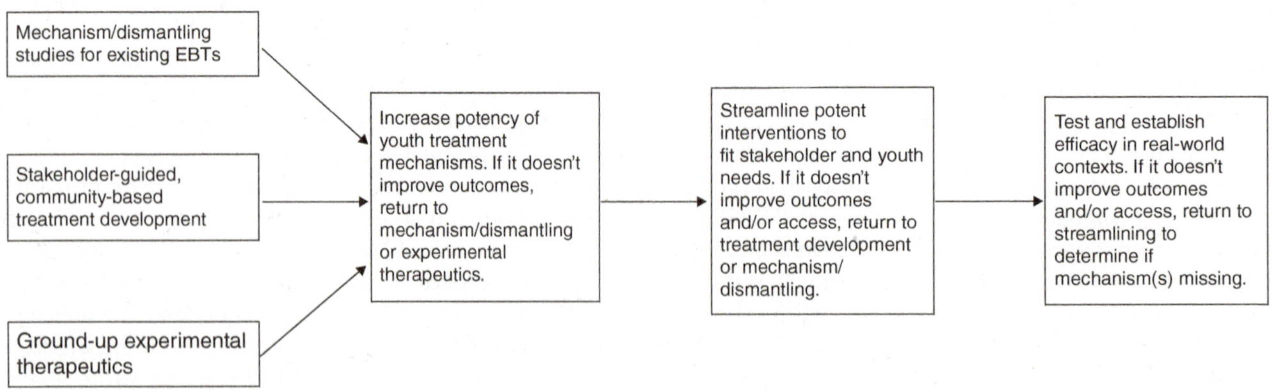

Figure 31.2 Where do we go from here? A potential process for stakeholder-informed, mechanism-focused research for effective psychotherapeutics. While the processes outlined in this diagram occur in cyclical fashion, with each step informing others, they are presented in a linear fashion in this figure to depict how the findings may ultimately lead to development of effective psychotherapeutics based on stakeholder-informed, mechanism-focused research. *Note:* EBT = evidence-based treatment.

one another. However, one method that may help to achieve a balance is to consider translation, uptake, and sustainment into settings even when intervention development is in its infancy. While there is no single path forward, Figure 31.2 outlines some aspects of three relevant paths: mediation and dismantling studies for existing EBTs; stakeholder-guided, community-based treatment development; and ground-up experimental therapeutics with novel treatment targets. There are already a few examples of implementation efforts and experimental therapeutic efficacy RCTs that involve the perspectives of youth and families, providers, and systems stakeholders to participate in the development and dissemination of interventions (e.g., Schleider, 2023). Systems- and policy-level change and deliberate actions on the part of youth intervention developers to collaborate with the possible settings where the intervention might ultimately be deployed will reduce the research–practice gap.

Long term, it will be critical to address these areas in concert for future innovation in a way that incorporates both the precision medicine approach (Insel, 2015) and simultaneously focuses on intervention application in real-world settings. This is complicated to do in a field that has established interventions with unknown processes, novel interventions that have not been tested in large-scale fashion, and need for new intervention development, particularly for underrepresented groups. In both research and clinical practice, current foci for youth psychotherapy are on how treatments work and how we can increase this potency for real-world effective delivery.

References

Ale, C.M. *et al.* (2015) Components of cognitive behavioral therapy related to outcome in childhood anxiety disorders. *Clinical Child and Family Psychology Review* **18**(3), 240–251.

Alvarez, K. *et al.* (2022) Review: structural racism, children's mental health service systems, and recommendations for policy and practice change. *Journal of the American Academy of Child and Adolescent Psychiatry* **61**(9), 1087–1105.

Arora, P.G. *et al.* (2021) Cultural adaptations to youth mental health interventions: a systematic review. *Journal of Child and Family Studies* **30**(10), 2539–2562.

Baumel, A. *et al.* (2021) Psychosocial interventions for children with externalized behavior problems: an updated meta-analysis of moderator effects. *Journal of Child and Family Studies* **30**(1), 65–86.

Beidas, R.S. *et al.* (2022) Promises and pitfalls in implementation science from the perspective of US-based researchers: learning from a pre-mortem. *Implementation Science* **17**(1), 55.

Bell, I.H. *et al.* (2023) The effect of psychological treatment on repetitive negative thinking in youth depression and anxiety: a meta-analysis and meta-regression. *Psychological Medicine* **53**(1), 6–16.

Beveridge, R.M. *et al.* (2015) State-wide dissemination and implementation of parent–child interaction therapy (PCIT): application of theory. *Children and Youth Services Review* **48**, 38–48.

Bo, A. *et al.* (2018) Parent-based interventions on adolescent alcohol use outcomes: a systematic review and meta-analysis. *Drug and Alcohol Dependence* **191**, 98–109.

Boldrini, T. *et al.* (2023) Systematic review and meta-analysis: psychosocial treatments for disruptive behavior symptoms and disorders in adolescence. *Journal of the American Academy of Child and Adolescent Psychiatry* **62**(2), 169–189.

Breaux, R. *et al.* (2023) Systematic review and meta-analysis: pharmacological and nonpharmacological interventions for persistent nonepisodic irritability. *Journal of the American Academy of Child and Adolescent Psychiatry* **62**(3), 318–334.

Buerger, A. *et al.* (2021) Third-wave interventions for eating disorders in adolescence: systematic review with meta-analysis. *Borderline Personality Disorder and Emotion Dysregulation* **8**(1), 1–14.

Chorpita, B.F. *et al.* (2017) Child STEPs in California: a cluster randomized effectiveness trial comparing modular treatment with community implemented treatment for youth with anxiety, depression, conduct problems, or traumatic stress. *Journal of Consulting and Clinical Psychology* **85**(1), 13–25.

Christ, C. *et al.* (2020) Internet and computer-based cognitive behavioral therapy for anxiety and depression in adolescents and young adults: systematic review and meta-analysis. *Journal of Medical Internet Research* **22**(9), e17831.

Cohen, J. (1988) *Statistical Power Analysis for the Behavioural Science*, 2nd edn. Lawrence Erlbaum, Hillsdale, NJ.

Compton, S.N. *et al.* (2014) Predictors and moderators of treatment response in childhood anxiety disorders: results from the CAMS trial. *Journal of Consulting and Clinical Psychology* **82**(2), 212–224.

Damschroder, L.J. *et al.* (2009) Fostering implementation of health services research findings into practice: a consolidated framework for advancing implementation science. *Implementation Science* **4**(1), 1–15.

Dopp, A.R. & Lantz, P.M. (2020) Moving upstream to improve children's mental health through community and policy change. *Administration and Policy in Mental Health and Mental Health Services Research* **47**(5), 779–787.

Ehrenreich-May, J. & Bilek, E.L. (2012) The development of a transdiagnostic, cognitive behavioral group intervention for childhood anxiety disorders and co-occurring depression symptoms. *Cognitive and Behavioral Practice* **19**(1), 41–55.

Ehrhart, M.G. *et al.* (2014) Assessing the organizational context for EBP implementation: the development and validity testing of the Implementation Climate Scale (ICS). *Implementation Science* **9**, 1–11.

Estabrooks, P.A. *et al.* (2018) Dissemination and implementation science for public health professionals: an overview and call to action. *Preventing Chronic Disease* **15**(12).

Fedele, D.A. *et al.* (2017) Mobile health interventions for improving health outcomes in youth a meta-analysis. *JAMA Pediatrics* **171**(5), 461–469.

Fitzpatrick, O.M. *et al.* (2022) Empirically supported principles of change in youth psychotherapy: exploring codability, frequency of use, and meta-analytic findings. *Clinical Psychological Science* **11**(2), 326–344.

Fodor, L.A. *et al.* (2020) Efficacy of cognitive bias modification interventions in anxiety and depressive disorders: a systematic review and network meta-analysis. *The Lancet Psychiatry* **7**(6), 506–514.

Frank, H.E. *et al.* (2020) Therapist training in evidence-based interventions for mental health: a systematic review of training approaches and outcomes. *Clinical Psychology: Science and Practice* **27**(3), e12330.

Furukawa, T.A. *et al.* (2021) Dismantling, optimising, and personalising internet cognitive behavioural therapy for depression: a systematic review and component network meta-analysis using individual participant data. *The Lancet Psychiatry* **8**(6), 500–511.

Guo, S. *et al.* (2020) Flexible adaptation of evidence-based treatment principles and practices in an intensive outpatient setting for pediatric OCD. *Evidence-Based Practice in Child and Adolescent Mental Health* **5**(3), 301–321.

Hodgkinson, S. *et al.* (2017) Improving mental health access for low-income children and families in the primary care setting. *Pediatrics* **139**(1), e20151175.

Huey, S.J. *et al.* (2023) Culturally responsive cognitive behavioral therapy for ethnically diverse populations. *Annual Review of Clinical Psychology* **19**(1), 51–78.

Insel, T.R. (2015) The NIMH experimental medicine initiative. *World Psychiatry* **14**(2), 151–153.

Jones, E.B. & Sharpe, L. (2017) Cognitive bias modification: a review of meta-analyses. *Journal of Affective Disorders* **223**, 175–183.

Kazdin, A.E. (2017) Addressing the treatment gap: a key challenge for extending evidence-based psychosocial interventions. *Behaviour Research and Therapy* **88**, 7–18.

Kunas, S.L. *et al.* (2021) Psychological predictors of cognitive-behavioral therapy outcomes for anxiety and depressive disorders in children and adolescents: a systematic review and meta-analysis. *Journal of Affective Disorders* **278**, 614–626.

Levy, H.C. *et al.* (2022) Research review: a meta-analysis of relapse rates in cognitive behavioral therapy for anxiety and related disorders in youth. *Journal of Child Psychology and Psychiatry and Allied Disciplines* **63**(3), 252–260.

Luo, A. & McAloon, J. (2021) Potential mechanisms of change in cognitive behavioral therapy for childhood anxiety: a meta-analysis. *Depression and Anxiety* **38**(2), 220–232.

Martin, F. & Oliver, T. (2019) Behavioral activation for children and adolescents: a systematic review of progress and promise. *European Child and Adolescent Psychiatry* **28**(4), 427–441.

McGrath, C.A. & Abbott, M.J. (2019) Family-based psychological treatment for obsessive compulsive disorder in children and adolescents: a meta-analysis and systematic review. *Clinical Child and Family Psychology Review* **22**(4), 478–501.

Mestre, J.M. *et al.* (2022) Theories of change and mediators of psychotherapy effectiveness in adolescents with externalising behaviours: a systematic review. *Frontiers in Psychiatry* **12**, 2172.

Oud, M. *et al.* (2019) Effectiveness of CBT for children and adolescents with depression: a systematic review and meta-regression analysis. *European Psychiatry* **57**, 33–45.

Park, A.L. *et al.* (2015) Integrity of evidence-based practice: are providers modifying practice content or practice sequencing? *Administration and Policy in Mental Health and Mental Health Services Research* **42**(2), 186–196.

Pergamin-Hight, L. *et al.* (2015) Content specificity of attention bias to threat in anxiety disorders: a meta-analysis. *Clinical Psychology Review* **35**, 10–18.

Peris, T.S. *et al.* (2017) Targeted family intervention for complex cases of pediatric obsessive-compulsive disorder: a randomized controlled trial. *Journal of the American Academy of Child & Adolescent Psychiatry* **56**(12), 1034–1042.

Peris, T.S. *et al.* (2021) Family intervention for child and adolescent anxiety: a meta-analytic review of therapy targets, techniques, and outcomes. *Journal of Affective Disorders* **286**, 282–295.

Perkins, A.M. *et al.* (2023) The effectiveness of third wave cognitive behavioural therapies for children and adolescents: a systematic review and meta-analysis. *British Journal of Clinical Psychology* **62**(1), 209–227.

Perlstein, S. *et al.* (2023) Treatment of childhood disruptive behavior disorders and callous-unemotional traits: a systematic review and two multilevel meta-analyses. *Journal of Child Psychology and Psychiatry and Allied Disciplines* **64**, 1372–1387.

Pilling, S. *et al.* (2020) Long-term outcomes of psychological interventions on children and young people's mental health: a systematic review and meta-analysis. *PLoS One* **15**(11), e0236525.

Pina, A.A. *et al.* (2019) Evidence-based psychosocial interventions for ethnic minority youth: the 10-year update. *Journal of Clinical Child and Adolescent Psychology* **48**(2), 179–202.

Pompoli, A. *et al.* (2018) Dismantling cognitive-behaviour therapy for panic disorder: a systematic review and component network meta-analysis. *Psychological Medicine* **48**(12), 1945–1953.

Price, M.A. *et al.* (2022) Meta-analysis: are psychotherapies less effective for black youth in communities with higher levels of anti-black racism? *Journal of the American Academy of Child and Adolescent Psychiatry* **61**(6), 754–763.

Rith-Najarian, L.R. *et al.* (2019) Durability of cognitive behavioral therapy effects for youth and adolescents with anxiety, depression, or traumatic stress: a meta-analysis on long-term follow-ups. *Behavior Therapy* **50**(1), 225–240.

Robinson, J. *et al.* (2018) What works in youth suicide prevention? A systematic review and meta-analysis. *EClinicalMedicine* **4–5**, 52–91.

Ros-DeMarize, R. *et al.* (2021) Pediatric behavioral telehealth in the age of COVID-19: brief evidence review and practice considerations. *Current Problems in Pediatric and Adolescent Health Care* **51**(1), 100949.

Schleider, J.L. (2023) The fundamental need for lived experience perspectives in developing and evaluating psychotherapies. *Journal of Consulting and Clinical Psychology* **91**(3), 119–121.

Schopf, K. *et al.* (2020) The role of exposure in the treatment of anxiety in children and adolescents: protocol of a systematic review and meta-analysis. *Systematic Reviews* **9**(1), 1–6.

Scott, S. (2016) Commentary: finding out the best way to tailor psychological interventions for children and families—a commentary on Ng and Weisz (2016). *Journal of Child Psychology and Psychiatry, and Allied Disciplines* **57**(3), 237–240.

Silverman, W.K. & Hinshaw, S.P. (2008) The second special issue on evidence-based psychosocial treatments for children and adolescents: a 10-year update. *Journal of Clinical Child and Adolescent Psychology* **37**(1), 1–7.

Silverman, W.K. *et al.* (2022) Does training parents in reinforcement skills or relationship skills enhance individual youths' cognitive behavioral therapy for anxiety? Outcome, specificity, and mediation. *Clinical Psychological Science* **10**(2), 355–373.

Somers, K. *et al.* (2022) Identifying effective moderators of cognitive behavioural trauma treatment with caregiver involvement for youth with PTSD: a meta-analysis. *European Child and Adolescent Psychiatry* **33**(7), 1–15.

Southam-Gerow, M.A. & Prinstein, M.J. (2014) Evidence base updates: the evolution of the evaluation of psychological treatments for children and adolescents. *Journal of Clinical Child and Adolescent Psychology* **43**(1), 1–6.

Stuijfzand, S. *et al.* (2018) Research review: is anxiety associated with negative interpretations of ambiguity in children and adolescents? A systematic review and meta-analysis. *Journal of Child Psychology and Psychiatry, and Allied Disciplines* **59**(11), 1127.

Szota, K. *et al.* (2023) Interventions involving caregivers for children and adolescents following traumatic events: a systematic review and meta-analysis. *Clinical Child and Family Psychology Review* **26**(1), 17–32.

Turner, C. *et al.* (2018) Moderators and predictors of response to cognitive behaviour therapy for pediatric obsessive-compulsive disorder: a systematic review. *Psychiatry Research* **261**, 50–60.

van der Stouwe, T. *et al.* (2014) The effectiveness of multisystemic therapy (MST): a meta-analysis. *Clinical Psychology Review* **34**(6), 468–481.

Venturo-Conerly, K.E. *et al.* (2021) Effectiveness of youth psychotherapy delivered remotely: a meta-analysis. *American Psychologist* **77**(1), 71–84.

Venturo-Conerly, K.E. *et al.* (2023a) Meta-analysis: the effectiveness of youth psychotherapy interventions in low- and middle-income countries. *Journal of the American Academy of Child and Adolescent Psychiatry* **62**(8), S0890–S8567.

Venturo-Conerly, K.E. *et al.* (2023b) Personalizing youth psychotherapy: a scoping review of decision-making in modular treatments. *Clinical Psychology: Science and Practice* **30**(1), 45–62.

Weersing, V.R. *et al.* (2017) Brief behavioral therapy for pediatric anxiety and depression in primary care: a randomized clinical trial. *JAMA Psychiatry* **74**(6), 571–578.

Weersing, V.R. *et al.* (2021) *Brief Behavioral Therapy for Anxiety and Depression in Youth: Therapist Guide*. Oxford University Press, New York.

Weisz, J.R. *et al.* (2013a) Performance of evidence-based youth psychotherapies compared with usual clinical care: a multilevel meta-analysis. *JAMA Psychiatry* **70**(7), 750–761.

Weisz, J.R. *et al.* (2013b) Evidence-based youth psychotherapy in the mental health ecosystem. *Journal of Clinical Child and Adolescent Psychology* **42**(2), 274–286.

Weisz, J.R. *et al.* (2017) What five decades of research tells us about the effects of youth psychological therapy: a multilevel meta-analysis and implications for science and practice. *American Psychologist* **72**(2), 79–117.

Weisz, J.R. *et al.* (2019) Are psychotherapies for young people growing stronger? Tracking trends over time for youth anxiety, depression, attention-deficit/hyperactivity disorder, and conduct problems. *Perspectives on Psychological Science* **14**(2), 216–237.

Whiteside, S.P.H. *et al.* (2020) A meta-analysis to guide the enhancement of CBT for childhood anxiety: exposure over anxiety management. *Clinical Child and Family Psychology Review* **23**(1), 102–121.

Williams, N.J. & Beidas, R.S. (2019) Annual research review: the state of implementation science in child psychology and psychiatry: a review and suggestions to advance the field. *Journal of Child Psychology and Psychiatry and Allied Disciplines* **60**(4), 430–450.

CHAPTER 32

Prevention of mental, emotional, and behavioral disorders and promotion of well-being

Nathaniel R. Riggs[1] and Brittany Rhoades Cooper[2]

[1]Department of Human Development and Family Studies, Colorado State University, Fort Collins, CO, USA

[2]Department of Human Development, Washington State University, Pullman, WA, USA

This chapter covers the broad area of prevention science (see Video 32.1 on the companion website for this book for an introduction to prevention science; https://www.youtube.com/watch?v=P1NqouyANss&t=2s), focusing on universal and selective prevention. While space limitations prevent a comprehensive review of mental health prevention and promotion, we have selected issues and challenges affecting researchers and practitioners. The chapter is divided into sections on (i) epidemiology and the role of developmental theory in prevention and promotion, (ii) defining the levels of prevention, (iii) Type I translational research and exemplar prevention programs and policies for children and families, (iv) Type II translational research, and (v) key issues in current prevention research. We conclude with recommendations to address the global challenges faced by research and practice in implementing effective preventive interventions.

Epidemiology and the role of developmental theory in prevention

In 2019, 970 million people lived with a mental disorder, with depression and anxiety being the most common (Institute of Health Metrics and Evaluation, 2023). A striking 50% of adult mental disorders have an onset during or before adolescence (Belfer, 2008) and one in five US adolescents report at least one mental health problem (Mojtabai & Olfson, 2020). Therefore, preventing mental, emotional, and behavioral disorders (MEBDs) in childhood and adolescence is key to reducing the human toll and economic burden of MEBDs. This is not only because childhood problems predict adult mental health and substance use disorders, but also because they serve as risk factors for many other poor health outcomes in adolescence and adulthood.

One hallmark of prevention science is that it is steeped in developmental theory, which spans and integrates related fields including public health, epidemiology, neuroscience, behavioral genetics, and developmental psychopathology (e.g., Bradshaw *et al.*, 2012; Toth & Gravener, 2012). Developmental theory is conceived broadly to include multilevel, biopsychosocial ecological, and systems science perspectives which incorporate layered contexts interacting dynamically to influence risk and resilience (Sameroff, 2010). This richness in theoretical breadth and depth provides a powerful framework for understanding the etiology of MEBDs and serves as the basis for conceptualizing, designing, and implementing preventive interventions that target their theoretically and empirically supported precursors.

Decades of epidemiological research have identified that adult MEBDs have a developmental etiology in empirically supported risk and protective factors that emerge in childhood and adolescence. Risk factors increase the likelihood of the incidence of an MEBD. Current theory and research have contributed to several observations regarding the relation of risk factors to MEBDs. First, due to the complex nature of human development, it is likely that few MEBDs are due to a single cause, or risk factor, residing in the child alone (Michelini *et al.*, 2021). Rather the development of MEBDs is often the result of multiple accumulated risks across time and contexts, potentially exhibiting a nonlinear (i.e., exponential) relationship with developmental outcomes (Sameroff, 2010). Second, not all children who experience any given risk factor, or set of risk factors, will develop adjustment problems, suggesting that children vary in their resilience in the face of adversity (MacPhee *et al.*, 2015). Third, developmental epidemiology findings indicate that there are multiple pathways to most psychological disorders, there are different combinations of risk factors that may lead to the same disorder (i.e., equifinality), and that risk

Rutter's Child and Adolescent Psychiatry and Psychology, Seventh Edition.

Edited by Anita Thapar, Daniel S. Pine, Samuele Cortese, Cathy Creswell, Tamsin J. Ford, James F. Leckman, and Argyris Stringaris.

Companion website: www.wiley.com/go/thapar/rutterspsych7

factors are rarely disorder-specific (i.e., multifinality) (Kretschmer *et al.*, 2015). Thus, upstream prevention efforts that focus on reducing multiple interacting risk factors—especially those known to be related to multiple MEBDs—early in development may have direct effects on diverse downstream outcomes.

Protective factors reduce the likelihood of maladaptive outcomes under conditions of risk and thus build resilience. Protective factors operate in the same contexts as risk factors and moderate the relationship between risk factors and MEBDs. By specifying links between protective factors, positive outcomes, and reduced problem behaviors, prevention researchers may more successfully identify relevant targets for intervention (Fagan *et al.*, 2007) and nurture environments central to positive mental, emotional, and behavioral health, averting MEBDs (Biglan *et al.*, 2012). The field of prevention science translates this basic developmental research into prevention programs, practices, and policies, henceforth referred to as preventive interventions, that target malleable risk and protective factors known to affect future health and well-being (Type I translational research). By altering these malleable factors earlier in life, preventive interventions can prevent the development of MEBDs later in life.

New and complementary approaches to preventing MEBDs also include strength-based models such as social-emotional learning (SEL) and positive youth development. For example, the Collaborative for Academic and Social-Emotional Learning (CASEL) approach to preventing mental health problems promotes self-regulation, self-awareness, social awareness, positive peer relationships, and responsible decision-making as components of social-emotional competence (Mahoney *et al.*, 2021). Research shows that proficiency in each of these five domains of social competence is related to positive academic, behavioral, and mental health outcomes (Weissberg, 2019).

A second complementary approach to focusing on risk and protective factors is to leverage individual, family, and community assets, or strengths, that manifest as resilience through exposure to stressful (i.e., risky) contexts (Ellis *et al.*, 2017). Resilience-focused interventions take issue with the deficit-focused assertion that children and families from high-stress backgrounds are "at risk" for academic and behavioral health problems and that the goal of interventions should be to prevent, reduce, or repair the damage resulting from risk. Instead, a resilience approach to prevention leverages unique strengths and abilities that develop among individuals, families, and communities in response to high-stress environments (Ellis *et al.*, 2017). For example, resilience-focused preventive interventions may work with individuals and families faced with adversity on strategies for promoting conscious control of emotions or repairing relationships (MacPhee *et al.*, 2015).

Defining the levels of prevention

Prevention programs can take several forms depending on community needs and capacity (Figure 32.1). The Institute of Medicine has placed preventive interventions within a broader mental health intervention framework that differentiates prevention from treatment (National Academies of Sciences, Engineering, and Medicine, 2019). Due to their diversity, it is helpful to classify preventive interventions based on their focus, scope, and delivery contexts, among other factors.

Universal prevention programs

Universal preventive interventions are implemented for entire youth populations, regardless of risk status, recognizing that all youth can benefit from the content. For example, SEL programs, implemented across grade levels, schools, or school districts,

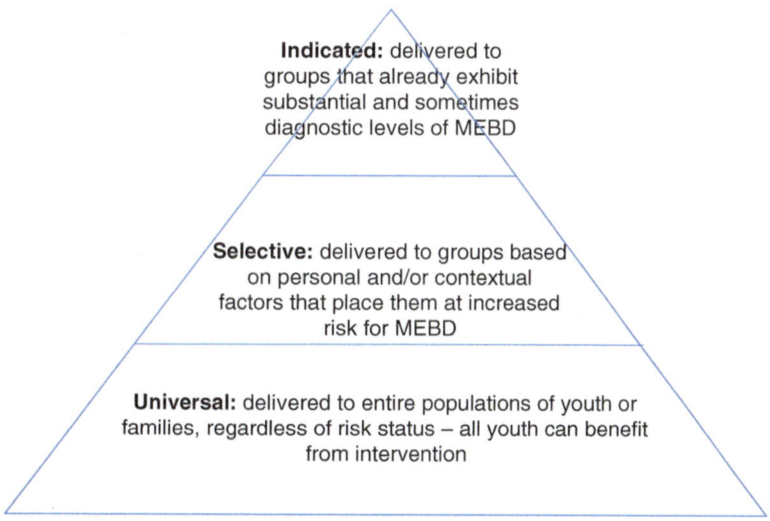

Figure 32.1 Levels of prevention. (MEBD = mental, emotional, and behavioral disorders.)

provide all youth opportunities to practice social competency skills. Among the advantages of this approach are that universal prevention programs are nonstigmatizing and focus on positive and adaptive coping and resilience for all participants.

Universal preventive interventions also promote protective factors and reduce risk factors associated with the onset of several downstream MEBDs and therefore may reduce or prevent multiple, potentially unmeasured, behavioral health problems that share overlapping risk and protective factors, increasing their potential for public health impact (Kretschmer *et al.*, 2015). For example, SEL curricula teach young people self-awareness, self-management, social awareness, relationship skills, and responsible decision-making, all of which are protective factors against the development of downstream MEBDs including conduct problems and bullying, substance use and misuse, and sexual risk-taking (e.g., Greenberg *et al.*, 2017).

Selective preventive interventions

Selective preventive interventions are delivered to groups of youth based on personal and/or contextual factors that place them at relatively greater risk for later problems. However, although the biological, psychological, social, or environmental contexts within which that group exists elicit risk, individuals in selective preventive interventions may, or may not, demonstrate maladjustment or health behavior problems at the time of intervention. Two broad classes of selective interventions include those based on risk characteristics of the child, family, or community (e.g., poverty, the children of parents who are depressed, children with social skills difficulties) and children or families who have experienced a stress-triggered event that increases their risk for maladjustment (e.g., divorce, loss of a parent through death, moving to a new school, other traumas) (Wolchik *et al.*, 2007). Selective interventions often involve specialized services such as family or peer group interventions, mentoring, or motivational interviewing techniques that promote youth development. Among the advantages of selective interventions is that effort and resources are focused on children and youth who are at elevated risk for developing future health behavior problems. Thus, selective interventions often provide greater precision, intensity, and focus for children in high-risk contexts.

Indicated preventive interventions

Indicated prevention is directed to children or families already showing substantial and sometimes even diagnostic levels of difficulty. These programs usually occur after a child has had substantial difficulties (e.g., has received psychiatric diagnoses or has been arrested). Such interventions are intensive and expensive but may be cost-effective given the high-cost and long-term effects of such experiences (Lee *et al.*, 2012). Indicated prevention can be distinguished from treatment in that indicated prevention focuses on youth who have symptoms of a disorder, but do not yet meet the disorder's diagnostic criteria, whereas treatment is generally provided for those with a diagnosable MEBD. As this chapter is focused on universal and selective models, the reader is referred to other sources for further review (Greenberg & Lippold, 2013).

Universal and selective interventions may employ multiple components that target school, family, and community factors. Given their extra cost, multicomponent interventions are more often utilized with selective interventions, or with universal models in high-risk neighborhoods or schools. Universal preventive interventions are likely to be most effective when implemented as part of a comprehensive, potentially tiered, approach to prevention (Greenberg *et al.*, 2001), an example of which is the Seattle Social Development Project (Hawkins *et al.*, 2005).

A relative advantage of universal prevention is that selective and indicated approaches are not sensitive to a large percentage of MEBDs that develop later in life. Durlak (1995) points out that if only 8% of well-adjusted children go on to have serious adjustment problems as adults (as opposed to 30% of children with early signs of dysfunction), the well-adjusted children will represent 50% more of the population of maladjusted adults. This follows Rose's maxim that "a large number of people exposed to a small risk may generate many more cases than a small number exposed to a high risk." It may then be beneficial to provide universal preventive interventions regardless of the low prevalence rate of childhood psychopathology (Rose, 1985). Thus, when dealing with a common and costly disorder such as depression or conduct disorder, there may be justification for preventive efforts that are universal and provided at the population level (Shamblen & Derzon, 2009).

There are also "trade-offs" between universal and targeted (i.e., selective or indicated) approaches. A potential disadvantage of universal programs is if used in contexts with low prevalence of psychopathology, substantial effort will be spent on children who may not develop mental health problems. Further, universal preventive interventions might not provide sufficient duration or intensity to alter the developmental pathways of children at most risk. The implementation of universal interventions in schools also poses challenges. First, they require the approval of schools that are often burdened with other priorities. They require multiple levels of approval from administrators, community partners, and local authorities. Generally, universal interventions are likely to be most effective when they have sufficient duration and intensity, target the development of protective factors related to multiple disorders, or target problems with high prevalence (e.g., bullying, early alcohol use).

Type I translational research and exemplar preventive interventions for children and families

Type I translational research translates basic research in developmental science to preventive interventions, targeting malleable risk and protective factors known to affect future health and well-being. Type I translational research in the form of randomized controlled trials (RCTs) aimed at determining the efficacy and effectiveness of interventions has generated numerous evidence-based (i.e., empirically supported) preventive interventions that can be delivered within several community contexts (e.g., schools, social service agencies, mental health treatment facilities, assisted care facilities, online, media) (Sandler *et al.*, 2014). It is important to note that "evidence-based" should be considered along a continuum of confidence as depicted in Figure 32.2.

Preventive interventions with strong evidence of positive or negative outcomes from rigorous evaluations (like those described above) fall on the two ends of the continuum where there is enough information to feel confident that they are either harmful or effective. Those that fall on the right (effective) end of the continuum include "research-based" programs that are based on sound theory and informed by research but have yet to be rigorously evaluated. At the right-hand end of the scale, "evidence-based" programs are those with strong evidence from rigorous (e.g., RCTs) efficacy and effectiveness evaluations empirically demonstrating consistent improvement in participant outcomes (Gottfredson *et al.*, 2015). Importantly, evidence-based interventions (EBIs) also demonstrate minimal risk for harmful or iatrogenic effects, unlike those that fall on the far left (harmful) end of the continuum. These "harmful or iatrogenic" programs have been rigorously evaluated, like evidence-based programs, but have been shown to be harmful, whereas "ineffective" programs have been evaluated and shown to have null effects—in other words, no positive or negative effects.

Preventive interventions with less evidence fall somewhere in the middle (i.e., we have less confidence in our ability to determine their effectiveness). Here, "promising approaches" are like other effective programs (e.g., they are theoretically based or may have preliminary evidence of their positive impact), and "discouraged approaches" include programs like other ineffective or harmful programs (e.g., include known ineffective/harmful components). However, in these cases, the research is not conclusive enough to consider them evidence-based or iatrogenic.

Reviews of EBIs, those we have the most confidence in based on empirical evidence, provide support for the ability of preventive interventions to reduce an array of mental and behavioral health problems (e.g., Durlak *et al.*, 2011), substance misuse (Hennessey *et al.*, 2019), and promote school readiness and academic proficiency (Durlak *et al.*, 2011), and physical health (Schembre *et al.*, 2018). Registries of EBIs are also now widely available for community prevention stakeholders to search, identify, and select preventive interventions with the most rigorous empirical support for efficacy and effectiveness that are also responsive to their community's unique characteristics, context, and culture (e.g., Blueprints for Healthy Youth Development, https://www.blueprintsprograms.org; the Cochrane Library, https://www.cochranelibrary.com/cdsr/reviews; the Campbell Collaboration, https://www.campbellcollaboration.org).

The state of the science in the prevention of specific mental, emotional, and behavior disorders

Conduct problems and aggression

The prevention of conduct problems and aggression has dominated early prevention trials. A meta-analysis examining 249 experimental studies designed to prevent aggressive and disruptive behavior yielded a significant mean effect size on aggression of 0.21 (Wilson & Lipsey, 2007). Within these studies, there were somewhat larger effects for younger children and those of lower socioeconomic status (SES). The effect size for selected and indicated interventions was 0.29; among the targeted students, those who showed greater problems also showed greater improvements. In addition, behavioral strategies were more effective than cognitively-oriented models. There was a significant impact of the quality of implementation on outcome with higher quality implementation related to greater effect size. The authors concluded that these effects are not only

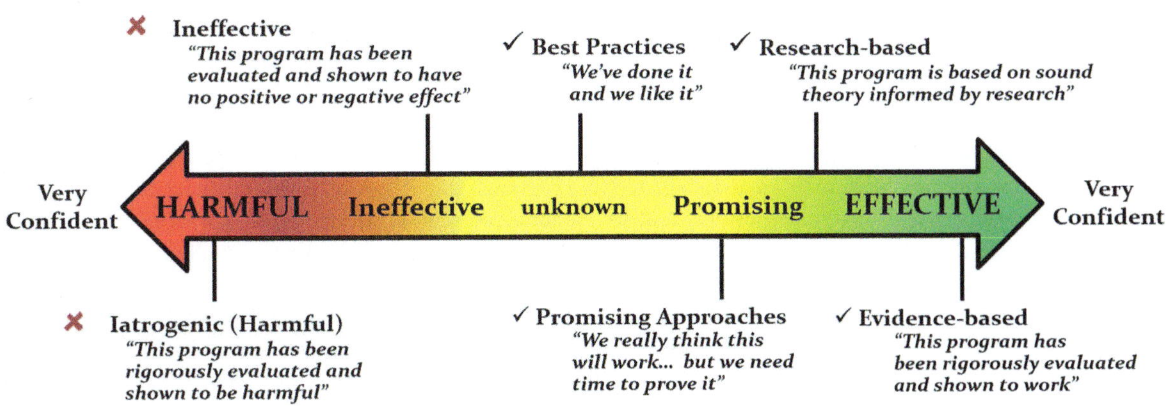

Figure 32.2 Continuum of confidence for effective interventions.

statistically significant but also of practical significance and they forecast that such programs would lead to a 25–33% reduction in the base rate of aggressive problems in an average school.

Burkey *et al.* (2018) reviewed 26 RCTs of 28 (universal, selective, indicated, and treatment) psychosocial interventions aimed at reducing disruptive behavior problems among children in low- and middle-income countries (LMICs). For the prevention programs (universal and selective), their findings were strikingly similar to Wilson and Lipsey (2007) with a significant mean effect size of 0.25 for the prevention of child behavior problems. The universal interventions in the Burkey *et al.* (2018) review were delivered to general populations whereas selective interventions were delivered to populations with increased risk for disruptive behaviors based on exposure to poverty or trauma, for example. They also reported that child-focused and parent-focused interventions were similarly effective. In another meta-analysis of 31 high-quality RCTs and quasi-experimental studies of early childhood programs, Schindler *et al.* (2015) found that programs with clear and intensive focus on child social skills training or caregiver behavioral management training showed significant reductions in externalizing behaviors with an average effect size of 0.50. Taken together, this evidence indicates strong support for the effectiveness of preventive interventions aimed at reducing child conduct problems and aggression by targeting children and/or their caregivers in Western, high-income countries (Wilson & Lipsey, 2007) as well as in LMICs (Burkey *et al.*, 2018).

Depression

There has been a dramatic increase in the development and evaluation of both universal and targeted depression prevention models since the 2010s. Although meta-analyses show some inconsistency in findings, in general, the results show substantial effects of selective programs; however, effects vary by population and there is a need for further replication in school settings (e.g., Stice *et al.*, 2009). They also show promise due to the absence of the need for screening, the potential benefits of non-depressed peers as models, and the role universal programs can play in reducing mental health stigma (Horowitz *et al.*, 2007).

One recent meta-analysis of 50 RCTs examined the effectiveness of indicated interventions where participants have some depression symptoms but do not meet full criteria, and selective interventions where participants are at higher risk for depression based on membership in an at-risk group, e.g., children of depressed parents. Overall, these preventive interventions, which were delivered to participants without a depression diagnosis at baseline, found a 19% reduction in risk of developing depression 1 year following the intervention (Cuijpers *et al.*, 2021). The findings for the effectiveness of school-based depression prevention programs are weaker (Caldwell *et al.*, 2019). The Penn Resiliency Program (PRP; Gillham *et al.*, 2008), which includes cognitive restructuring, problem-solving, and social skills training, has been among the most widely researched depression prevention programs. A meta-analysis of 17 studies showed consistent small, but significant, effects at 6- and 12-month follow-ups in both universal implementations and selective implementations where youth have a known risk factor for developing depression (Brunwasser *et al.*, 2009). A more recent meta-analysis of 38 RCT studies of resilience-oriented cognitive behavioral interventions (including PRP) aimed at preventing depression in adolescents found similar findings with a small overall effect size at post-intervention (Ma *et al.*, 2020). Subgroup analyses showed that selective interventions (i.e., delivered to students identified as having known risk factors for depression or who had elevated symptoms of depression), interventions based on PRP, interventions delivered by professional interventionists (not school personnel), and those with homework had significant effect sizes at 6 months. Whereas those interventions delivered to universal samples, interventions based on the Resourceful Adolescent Program (Shochet & Osgarby, 1999), interventions delivered by school personnel, and those without homework had nonsignificant effect sizes at 6 months.

Anxiety

Anxiety disorders are the most frequent psychiatric disorders in adolescents, yet only recently have they been a focus for preventive interventions. Although there are relatively few studies that have examined preventive interventions for anxiety disorders, these programs appear quite promising (Neil & Christensen, 2009; see also Chapter 8 for a description of interventions for behaviorally inhibited temperament to prevent anxiety disorders). Both universal and indicated interventions have been conducted with populations from preschoolers through early teens and have shown significant reductions at post-test (e.g., Moreno-Peral *et al.*, 2017; Howes Vallis *et al.*, 2020), with some effects maintained as long as 2–3 years after intervention. Initial studies have, in some cases, shown the largest impact on girls (although the impact on boys is also reported) and on children around ages 11 and 12. Teubert and Pinquart (2011) conducted a meta-analysis of 65 trials. They reported small but significant effects on anxiety at post-test (effect size; symptoms = 0.22, diagnosis = 0.23) and follow-up (effect size; symptoms = 0.19, diagnosis = 0.32). Intervention effects at post-test varied by type of prevention. As expected, selective programs showed larger effects than universal programs, but it is worth noting that Stockings *et al.* (2016) conducted a multivariate meta-analysis examining the efficacy of preventive interventions on depression and anxiety outcomes separately, and the joint efficacy on both disorders combined. According to their meta-regression results examining heterogeneity in findings, reductions in internalizing symptoms occurred up to 12 months post-intervention for universal prevention; however, reductions only occurred in the shorter term for selective and indicated prevention.

Early substance use

Spoth *et al.* (2008) reviewed 127 reports of prevention studies with alcohol-specific outcome measures. Most studies were in schools, taught social, cognitive, and peer resistance skills, and fell into three age groups (below 10, 10–15, 16–20+). They classified interventions as "most promising evidence," "mixed or emerging evidence," and "insufficient or no evidence of impact." Twelve interventions met the criteria for "most promising" and 28 met the criteria for "mixed or emerging." A meta-analysis focused on universal school-based interventions promoting resilience found an overall intervention effect on rates of illicit substances (in some cases, including cannabis use) (Hodder *et al.*, 2017). The 2016 report on addiction from the United States (U.S.). Department of Health and Human Services, Office of the Surgeon General identified 42 evidence-based substance misuse prevention programs, including universal, selective, and indicated programs targeting young children through adolescents and young adults, some of which are highlighted in the following section on exemplary programs.

Promotion of social and emotional competence

Several recent meta-analyses have demonstrated the effectiveness of universal SEL curricula to improve various social-emotional outcomes across various populations (e.g., preschool, adolescents, young adults). A recent report by the Learning Policy Institute summarized findings from 12 independent meta-analyses from 6 continents examining the effects of SEL programs in preschool through grade 12 schools in studies published from 2011 to 2022. They found consistent medium to large effect sizes for the following outcomes: social and emotional competencies, prosocial behaviors and positive relationships with others, disruptive behaviors, and learning engagement (Greenberg, 2023).

Evidence-based interventions that prevent multiple mental, emotional, and behavior disorders

The following section highlights successful programs included in many of the reviews discussed above. However, it should be noted that positive intervention effects are not universally found despite well-reasoned theory, fidelity of implementation, and rigorous evaluation design. Thus, the following successful programs should be viewed within the context of other preventive interventions that have demonstrated effects limited to subsamples of participants or null effects on all or some MEBD outcomes (e.g., Scott *et al.*, 2010). It should also be noted that most evidence-based preventive interventions have only been tested in the United States (U.S.). However, several of the following six programs have been tested outside of the U.S. including PATHS (Ireland, United Kingdom (UK), Turkey), Triple P (Australia), and The Incredible Years (New Zealand, UK).

Table 32.1 summarizes the six exemplary universal, selective, and indicated EBIs described in this section that represent a variety of populations and delivery contexts—and highlights those that target and/or have evidence of reducing more than one of the MEBD outcomes that are a focus of this chapter. All six programs are currently rated as Model+, Model, or Promising according to Blueprints for Health Youth Development (see website: https://www.blueprintsprograms.org). Only one (LifeSkills Training) of the six programs is rated Model+ indicating it has been evaluated in at least one independent replication.

Parenting or family-focused interventions

Preventive interventions that focus on enhancing parenting skills and/or family connection and bonding have been shown to prevent or reduce MEBD outcomes for youth (Vermeulen-Smit *et al.*, 2015; Burkey *et al.*, 2018) (see also Chapter 33). Below are three such programs delivered to parents of children from infancy through adolescence.

The Incredible Years (IY) BASIC Parent Training is an exemplary selective intervention designed to reduce child behavior problems through parent training, which focuses on improving parent competencies, parent involvement in school, and effective management of child behavior problems (Webster-Stratton & Reid, 2010). Although initially used and evaluated with clinical populations (i.e., referred based on evidence of children's conduct problems and/or elevated risk based on economic disadvantage), numerous studies in the U.S. and other countries (e.g., Baker-Henningham *et al.*, 2012) have shown its effectiveness in improving parenting and reducing child behavior problems across different levels of family disadvantage (Gardner *et al.*, 2019), and with selective samples including those at risk for maltreatment (Hurlburt *et al.*, 2013).

The Triple P Positive Parenting Program (Sanders, 2008) uses a five-level comprehensive model using media that provide basic information, advice, and support from health workers, selective parenting groups, and treatment. One evaluation of this program employed a community-level "workforce development strategy" to deliver the program across diverse family-helping agencies and showed countywide reductions in child abuse and neglect (Prinz *et al.* 2009). This model, which originated in Australia, has shown evidence of positive social-emotional competence outcomes for children in numerous countries (Sanders *et al.*, 2014). In a population-level study in 20 communities in Brisbane, Sydney, and Melbourne there were greater reductions in emotional problems for intervention children and their parents as compared to "care as usual" control communities (Sanders *et al.*, 2008).

Family Foundations is a universal, eight-session intervention for expectant parents delivered before and after birth by childbirth education departments (Feinberg, 2010). The program prepares couples for parenthood by fostering attitudes and skills related to positive parenting teamwork (called "coparenting"). Through age 3, effects include reduced parental

Table 32.1 Evidence-based interventions that prevent youth mental, emotional, and behavioral disorders.

Name and website	Brief description	Level(s) of prevention U: universal S: selective I: indicated	Outcomes			
			Conduct problems	Depression/ anxiety	Substance use	Social-emotional competence
Parenting or family-focused interventions						
The Incredible Years: BASIC parent training www.incredibleyears.com Blueprints rating: promising	Based in cognitive social learning, modeling, and attachment theories, parents of babies, toddlers, preschoolers, or school-age children learn about key developmental milestones and age-appropriate parenting that promotes children's social competence and reduces behavior problems.	U, S, I	X	X		X
Triple P Positive Parenting Program https://www.triplep.net/glo-en/home Blueprints rating: promising	Five intervention levels (each additional level increases intensity and narrows focus on subpopulation of parents with increased risk) aimed at providing a comprehensive system supporting parents with children between birth-12 years old. The universal component uses a media campaign to normalize parenting challenges and reduce stigma.	U, S				X
Family Foundations www.famfound.net Blueprints rating: model	Four 2-hour prenatal and four 2-hour postnatal sessions delivered to couples expecting their first child aim to enhance coparenting quality to improve young children's emotional and behavioral outcomes.	U	X	X		
Youth-focused, school-based interventions						
Blues Program https://bluesprogram.org Blueprints rating: model	Six weekly 1-hour cognitive behavioral group sessions aimed at high school students with symptoms of or at risk of depression. Home practice assignments reinforce and encourage application of skills taught during the group sessions.	I, S		X	X	
LifeSkills Training www.lifeskillstraining.com Blueprints rating: model+	Includes 30 classroom-based lessons taught to middle-school students over 3 years focused on personal self-management skills, social skills, and drug use resistance skills.	U	X		X	
PATHS Program https://pathsprogram.com Blueprints rating: model	Developmentally targeted lessons for each grade (K–6) focused on teaching self-control, emotional understanding, positive self-esteem, relationships, and interpersonal problem-solving skills.	U	X	X		X

stress, depression, and harsh parenting, and improved child social competence. A study examining the long-term effects followed children as they entered school (average age of 6 years old) also found significantly lower teacher-reported internalizing symptoms for children whose parents participated in the program prior to their birth (Feinberg *et al.*, 2014).

Youth-focused, school-based interventions

Schools are common settings for preventive interventions since most of the youth attend school from early childhood through late adolescence. Increasingly, schools see their mission as extending beyond academic instruction to supporting the broader health and well-being of their students and therefore integrate preventive interventions focused on reducing or preventing MEBDs into their curricula (also see Chapter 38). Below are three such programs delivered to youth in a school setting.

The Blues Program is a group-based cognitive behavioral indicated preventive intervention aimed at teens with elevated depression symptoms. It consists of 6 1-hour weekly group sessions with home practice assignments and is often implemented in school settings. Rohde *et al.* (2018) conducted an individual patient data meta-analysis from four separate RCTs (2 with high school students and 2 with college students). Compared to a brochure control group, teens in the intervention groups were 7 times less likely to be diagnosed with major depressive disorder at post-test and were 3 times less likely to be diagnosed at 3- and 6-month follow-up. These positive findings, however, were not maintained at 12- or 24-month follow-up indicating lack of sustained effects.

LifeSkills Training (LST) is a 15-session universal school-based program with additional booster sessions that has been widely studied and implemented (Botvin *et al.*, 2006). The curriculum, delivered primarily by classroom teachers, provides students with training in personal self-management, social skills, and resistance skills specifically related to drug use. RCTs of LST have demonstrated short- and long-term (up to 10-year follow-up) effects on life skills knowledge, substance use knowledge, substance use, violence, and HIV risk behaviors. LST program effects have also been shown to generalize across ethnic groups and SES.

PATHS Program (Greenberg *et al.*, 1995) is a school-based SEL curriculum aimed at reducing aggression and behavior problems by promoting social-emotional competence in children during the elementary school years. PATHS places particular attention on neurocognitive models of development related to youth self-regulation, social relationships, and effective decision-making (Riggs *et al.*, 2006). The curriculum promotes SEL by implementing a set of developmentally appropriate lessons for specific K-5th grade (e.g., K-5th grade) and providing environmental prompts that allow youth to practice conscious strategies for self-control, prosocial peer interactions, and making healthy choices. Several RCTs have demonstrated the effectiveness of PATHS, including research demonstrating intervention effects on youth externalizing and internalizing behavior problems, through the curriculum's ability to promote SEL and enhance neurocognitive (i.e., executive function (EF)) processing (Riggs *et al.* 2006). A recent study also demonstrated the importance of sufficient doses by showing stronger outcomes for those youth exposed to at least 67% of specified PATHS lessons for the identified grade (Panayiotou *et al.*, 2019).

Type II translational research: adoption, implementation, sustainability, and scale-up of preventive interventions

As can be seen from the numerous EBIs described above, the past few decades have witnessed an increasingly robust empirical base in the field of prevention science (National Academies of Sciences, Engineering, and Medicine, 2019). According to Brown et al. (2017), efficacy and effectiveness studies like those cited above help us answer the questions "Could this program work?" and "Does this program work?" (Figure 32.3). This helps set the stage for Type II translational research where the emphasis is on dissemination and implementation studies that improve our understanding of "making the program work." We know there is often a significant gap between the availability of EBIs and their widespread, high-quality implementation across communities and nations, thus necessitating systematic studies of the dissemination and implementation process under real-world conditions (Glasgow *et al.*, 2003; Rhoades *et al.*, 2012).

Type II translational research investigates the complex processes and systems through which EBIs are adopted, implemented, and sustained on a large scale, as well as devising empirically driven strategies for increasing their population impact. Spoth *et al.* (2013b) proposed a heuristic model, the Translation Science to Population Impact (TSci Impact) Framework, to conceptualize research and practice issues related to the four phases of preadoption, adoption, implementation, and sustainability.

In the preadoption phase, there are numerous issues including how information on EBIs is diffused by governments and nongovernmental organizations, and understanding the communication channels used by prospective adopters. One strategy for assisting the diffusion process is to provide agencies, schools, and communities with guidelines and recommendations for choosing among EBIs. Numerous best-practice guidelines and reports have been published in the U.S. (e.g., CASEL Program Guide; https://pg.casel.org), in Europe (Fundacion Marcelino Botin, 2008), and in the UK (Allen, 2011). However, the lack of well-standardized criteria for selecting "model" or "effective" programs can confuse prospective adopters, including whether these guides and registries provide information on EBIs' dissemination readiness (Buckley *et al.*, 2020).

Selecting evidence-based prevention strategies is just the first step to achieving widespread, high-quality, and sustained prevention programming. Once selected, adopters require expert training and technical assistance to ensure high-fidelity

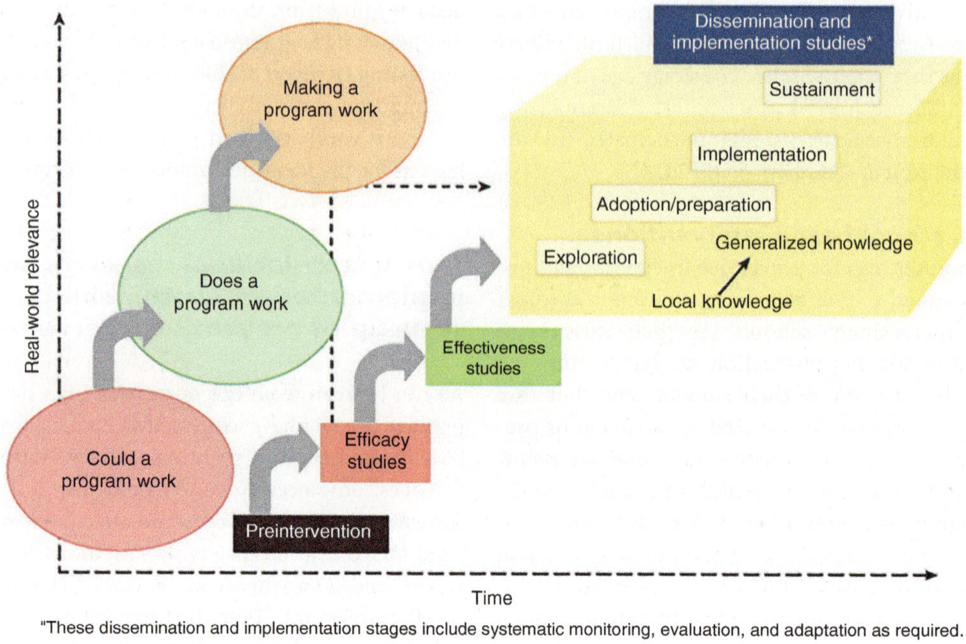

Figure 32.3 Traditional translational pipeline (Brown *et al.* 2017/with permission of Annual Reviews).

implementation. Adopters must ensure that they are faithfully replicating the core intervention components and ongoing monitoring and technical assistance are necessary to ensure that implementation is congruent with the core principles associated with program success (Kemp, 2016). Finally, to achieve population-level outcomes, communities must learn how to effectively recruit intervention participants via large-scale media or marketing campaigns. Implementation challenges will inevitably occur, and communities will be more successful when they increase their capacity for effective implementation and are provided with proactive technical assistance to carefully monitor program needs. A key issue in implementation is the need to adapt EBIs to create a better fit with the nature of public mental health and social service systems. This requires that public systems and program developers work together to understand scaling issues as they design, test, and implement new interventions. To achieve long-term success, organizations need to enhance their internal capacity to support preventive interventions (Fagan *et al.*, 2019).

As effective programs become more widely adopted, the need for strategies to enhance their long-term sustainability becomes increasingly important. Program sustainability can be threatened by many causes, including implementation challenges, loss of funding, changes in priorities among key players, and low resources in most of the world, including high-income countries. Moving from funding based on discretionary, short-term grants to more stable funding streams is a substantial challenge. Research regarding the conditions that facilitate or undermine sustainability has ramped up recently resulting in frameworks outlining the outer and inner contextual factors, processes, and characteristics of the interventions and interventionists needed for sustainability (Shelton *et al.*, 2018). Empirical research shows that long-term sustainability is associated with strong levels of staff and leaders' support; widespread belief in the benefits of the innovation; and a strong integration between the EBI and the agency's mission, schedule of services, staffing profile, and organizational capacity (Cooper *et al.*, 2022). These factors also promote the adoption and quality implementation of new programs, indicating that efforts to increase organizational capacity for prevention can increase the likelihood of widespread, high-quality, and sustained prevention programming.

Strong collaborations between researchers, practitioners, and governments are necessary to increase the general and specific capacity of local communities to undertake successful prevention. One model is to develop an intermediary organization between the government and local communities to support quality implementation and sustainability (Rhoades *et al.*, 2012). In the U.S., models have also been developed to create community-level infrastructure to facilitate prevention efforts including the Communities That Care (CTC) and The PROmoting School-community-university Partnerships to Enhance Resilience (PROSPER) models (Catalano *et al.*, 2012). CTC includes structured training workshops and proactive technical assistance for communities when conducting needs assessments, and selecting and implementing EBIs that address these needs. The PROSPER model seeks to increase community capacity by explicitly linking community stakeholders with university faculty and researchers who undertake prevention activities in local schools (Spoth *et al.*, 2013a). Both CTC and PROSPER have been successful in enhancing community collaboration to undertake prevention activities, reducing rates of problem behaviors among youth, and sustaining prevention activities over time (Kuklinski *et al.*, 2021; Spoth *et al.*, 2022).

Key issues in current prevention research

Developmental neuroscience

Advances in developmental neuroscience have recently enhanced traditional theories of prevention science. Developmental neuroscience research has demonstrated the importance of executive attention systems and EF (Blair & Raver, 2016). There has been an expansion of knowledge regarding the development of EF skills, the growth and differentiation of the prefrontal area of the brain, and the effects of poverty and stress on EF development (Blair & Raver, 2016). In turn, there has been progress in the development of school-based curricula, mindfulness, and physical activity training programs to promote self-regulation and EF skills (Takacs & Kassai, 2019). For example, Riggs and colleagues demonstrated that program effects of the PATHS Program on childhood externalizing and internalizing behaviors were partially mediated by inhibitory control, one EF process (Riggs *et al.*, 2006). Recent meta-analyses have demonstrated support for the efficacy of some EF interventions, but that benefits can be moderated by age, comorbid conditions, baseline level of functioning, and outcome measures (e.g., Jacob & Parkinson, 2015). Furthermore, many studies contained design flaws that limited the ability to draw causal inferences or demonstrate the long-term sustainability of program effects.

Assessing the cost, cost–benefit, and efficiency of prevention

Evidence has accumulated since the 2010s confirming the positive economic impact of prevention relative to its cost. This evidence has come in the form of peer-reviewed economic analyses and legislative (i.e., Washington State Institute of Public Policy [WSIPP]) efforts to catalog the cost-effectiveness of existing prevention programs. Peer-reviewed cost–benefit analyses suggest that EBIs are generally low-cost and cost-effective (Lee *et al.*, 2012). WSIPP provides a publicly accessible database that researchers and practitioners can search for information related to EBI cost and benefit–cost (https://www.wsipp.wa.gov/BenefitCost). Here, WSIPP lists benefits to taxpayers and nontaxpayers, costs, benefits minus costs, benefit-to-cost ratios, and the percent chance that benefits will exceed costs across 11 areas including public health and prevention, which is further categorized into school-based, home- or family-based, community-based, and population-level policies. One caveat is that WSIPP's cost–benefit analyses are calculated based on some Washington State-specific parameters, which require adjustment outside of Washington. For example, several states have adapted WSIPP's model by adjusting for state-specific tax structures, among other parameters.

Addressing the potential for iatrogenic harm resulting from ineffective prevention programs

Although evidence suggests that theoretically informed, well-designed, and effectively implemented preventive interventions can yield positive effects on youth well-being and development, there is the potential for ill-conceived (e.g., scare tactics, moralistic appeals, solely information-based approaches without skill-building) and/or ineffectively implemented programs to do harm either to participating youth or the system implementing the program (e.g., schools). For example, Foulkes and Stringaris (2023) caution that although most students want mental health taught in schools and school-based prevention programs can be effective, a growing body of quantitative research indicates that some school-based mental health interventions can cause harm. Preventive interventions may also be effective for some youth, but ineffective or iatrogenic for others based on any number of factors including cognitive differences, developmental stage, or cultural mismatch between the intervention and subgroups of participants. This reinforces the need to test for differences in program effects that may emerge due to participant or contextual characteristics. Finally, if school-based preventive interventions are simply ineffective (i.e., show no positive or negative effects), concerns arise related to lost opportunities to implement more effective approaches to promoting positive youth development and well-being. Implementing EBIs will decrease the likelihood of program failure. However, they can, and often do, fail in practice when there is a lack of fidelity to program implementation protocols, which emphasizes the importance of training facilitators to adhere to implementation fidelity and increase program effectiveness.

Limited study of factors that moderate effects

It is essential to understand the factors that may moderate (i.e., increase or decrease) the magnitude of intervention effects. This is especially important for universal interventions that target all members of a certain population. Is the intervention equally effective for all population members, regardless of their level of risk for mental health problems? Such analyses are necessary as it is unlikely that intervention effects are uniform for participants and information from moderation analyses can inform enhancements to EBIs to increase their effectiveness (Howe & Leijten, 2023).

The need for independent replication studies

Replication is critical for distinguishing false positives from truly efficacious preventive interventions and identifying the robustness of programs and policies across various settings and populations (Chinman *et al.*, 2022). Most Blueprints for Healthy Youth Development certified programs have been tested more than once, up from 13% reported in 2011 (Aos *et al.*, 2011). However, there has been substantial controversy regarding potential publication bias and the lack of independent replication of programs and policies (Axford & Morpeth, 2013). Replication with long-term follow-up is especially important for universal studies as few children in a whole population have, or are at risk for, a disorder. Here, the follow-up period should be sufficiently long to "allow" the control populations to develop symptoms/disorders.

Although replications conducted by program developers can maintain replication rigor by reproducing precise research procedures, providing access to program resources, and ensuring implementation fidelity with proper training, concerns may emerge regarding potential bias introduced by replications that are not independent of program developers (Leadbeater *et al.*, 2018). As desirable as independent replication is to the field of prevention science, some argue that requiring independent replication before scaling up EBIs would impede the widespread diffusion of EBIs (Gottfredson *et al.*, 2015). Regardless, clear standards are needed for judging when a study is truly a replication trial or when substantial program modifications would mean the study no longer qualifies as a replication (Valentine *et al.*, 2011).

The need for prevention research focused on understanding and reducing health disparities, and promoting health equity

For prevention to reduce health disparities and promote health equity, EBIs must be prioritized for dissemination and implementation in culturally responsive ways within diverse populations. As preventive interventions are transported across cultures and contexts, adaptations and modifications are often needed, at least in terms of their surface structure (Moore *et al.*, 2013). Castro and Yasui (2017) describe the "fidelity-adaptation dilemma" wherein a dynamic tension exists between implementing EBIs with strict fidelity versus the liberal adaptation of EBIs to fit community context and culture. Over the past 20 years, several conceptual and practical guidelines for cultural adaptations have been developed and there are numerous examples of such adaptations (e.g., Barrera Jr. *et al.*, 2017; Mejia *et al.*, 2017). However, innovative strategies are needed to examine whether systematically adapting and/or developing new EBIs with cultural fit and health equity goals at the forefront enhances the capacity of prevention to decrease health disparities and reduce inequity (Boyd *et al.*, 2022).

Global integration and translation of prevention models

The vast majority of EBIs have been developed in Western countries. However, given the global toll that MEBDs take on health, social, and economic development, the need to disseminate effective prevention practices is pressing. An essential question is whether a preventive intervention developed in Western technological societies will be transferable (albeit with modifications) to non-Western countries (e.g., LMICs). Among the critical components to supporting the successful implementation of EBIs is strengthening the "culture of prevention" by, among other things, supporting local prevention leadership and integrating cultural and contextual resources (Heikkilä *et al.*, 2021).

Since the 2000s, there has been a substantial rise in the number of preventive interventions focused on mental health in such countries as Tanzania (Hermenau *et al.*, 2012), Iran (Oveisi *et al.*, 2010), Mauritius (Rivet-Duval *et al.*, 2011), and Romania (Stefan and Miclea, 2013). Mejia *et al.* (2017) provide thoughtful discussions of the numerous issues in creating a culture of prevention, program modification, and implementation. Future research should focus on the relative benefits and challenges to the adaptation of existing programs for implementation in non-Western countries (i.e., an etic approach) versus the development of programs developed specifically for local populations (i.e., an emic approach).

Conclusion

During the past few decades, prevention science has emerged as a new multidisciplinary science. Research, primarily in high-income countries, has demonstrated that major mental and behavioral health problems can be moderately reduced through population-level preventive interventions and programs that selectively intervene with children already at risk due to early behavioral risk and experience/context. However, few of these interventions have reached the status of "business-as-usual" or been scaled at the level necessary to have a broad public health impact (Fagan *et al.*, 2019). The expansion and broad use of these interventions will require changes in policy and practice, as well as further demonstrations of cost-effectiveness. New research is needed to understand for whom these interventions are most effective, as well as how to modify interventions to fit cultural circumstances. Policy work is necessary to inform government officials regarding the importance of EBIs, which have the potential to reduce health spending and other social costs. To create widespread adoption in developing countries it is necessary to understand if there are unique risk and protective factors that might lead to new or modified interventions that better suit these contexts. Governments, agencies, schools, and local communities will vary in their capacity to incorporate EBIs into service systems and schools. A future goal of the field is to identify approaches that promote the readiness and capacity of prospective stakeholders to adopt effective interventions in a coordinated manner, implement them effectively, and sustain them over time. Such a systematic process will be necessary to substantially reduce the public health burden of MEBDs and improve community-level well-being.

References

Allen, G. (2011) *Early Intervention: The Next Steps, An Independent Report to Her Majesty's Government*. HM Government, UK. Available: https://www.gov.uk/government/news/graham-allen-launches-second-report-on-early-intervention

Aos, S. *et al.* (2011) Commentary on Valentine, Jeffrey, *et al.* replication in prevention science. *Prevention Science* **12**, 121–122.

Axford, N. & Morpeth, L. (2013) Evidence-based programs in children's services: a critical appraisal. *Children and Youth Services Review* **35**, 268–277.

Baker-Henningham, H. *et al.* (2012) Reducing child conduct problems and promoting social skills a middle-income country: cluster randomised controlled trial. *British Journal of Psychiatry* **201**, 101–108.

Barrera, M., Jr. *et al.* (2017) Directions for the advancement of culturally adapted preventive interventions: local adaptations, engagement, and sustainability. *Prevention Science* **18**, 640–648.

Belfer, M.L. (2008) Child and adolescent mental disorders: the magnitude of the problem across the globe. *Journal of Child Psychology and Psychiatry* **49**, 226–236.

Biglan, A. *et al.* (2012) The critical role of nurturing environments for promoting human well-being. *American Psychologist* **67**, 257–271.

Blair, C. & Raver, C.C. (2016) Poverty, stress, and brain development: new directions for prevention and intervention. *Academic Pediatrics* **16**, S30–S36.

Botvin, G.J. *et al.* (2006) Preventing youth violence and delinquency through a universal school-based prevention approach. *Prevention Science* **7**, 403–408.

Boyd, R.C. *et al.* (2022) Strategic directions in preventive intervention research to advance health equity. *Prevention Science* **1**, 1–20.

Bradshaw, C.P. *et al.* (2012) Infusing developmental neuroscience into school-based preventive interventions: implications and future directions. *Journal of Adolescent Health* **51**, S41–S47.

Brown, C.H. *et al.* (2017) An overview of research and evaluation designs for dissemination and implementation. *Annual Review of Public Health* **38**(1), 1–22.

Brunwasser, S.M. *et al.* (2009) A meta-analytic review of the Penn resiliency program's effect on depressive symptoms. *Journal of Consulting and Clinical Psychology* **77**, 1042–1054.

Buckley, P.R. *et al.* (2020) Making evidence-based interventions relevant for users: a comparison of requirements for dissemination readiness across program registries. *Evaluation Review* **44**(1), 51–83.

Burkey, M.D. *et al.* (2018) Psychosocial interventions for disruptive behaviour problems in children in low- and middle-income countries: a systematic review and meta-analysis. *Journal of Child Psychology and Psychiatry* **59**(9), 982–993.

Caldwell, D.M. *et al.* (2019) School-based interventions to prevent anxiety and depression in children and young people: a systematic review and network meta-analysis. *The Lancet Psychiatry* **6**(12), 1011–1020.

Castro, F.G. & Yasui, M. (2017) Advances in EBI development for diverse populations: towards a science of intervention adaptation. *Prevention Science* **18**, 623–629.

Catalano, R.F. *et al.* (2012) Adolescent health: global application of the prevention science research base. *Lancet* **379**, 1653–1664.

Chinman, M. *et al.* (2022) "What we have here, is a failure to [replicate]": ways to solve a replication crisis in implementation science. *Prevention Science* **23**, 739–750.

Cooper, B.R. *et al.* (2022) Using qualitative comparative analysis to uncover multiple pathways to program sustainment: implications for community-based youth substance misuse prevention. *Implementation Science Communications* **3**(1), 1–12.

Cuijpers, P. *et al.* (2021) Psychological interventions to prevent the onset of depressive disorders: a meta-analysis of randomized controlled trials. *Clinical Psychology Review* **83**, 101955.

Durlak, J.A. (1995) *School-based Prevention Programs for Children and Adolescents*. Sage Publishers, Thousand Oaks, CA.

Durlak, J.A. *et al.* (2011) The impact of enhancing students' social and emotional learning: a meta-analysis of school-based universal interventions. *Child Development* **82**, 405–432.

Ellis, B.J. *et al.* (2017) Beyond risk and protective factors: an adaptation-based approach to resilience. *Perspectives on Psychological Science* **12**, 561–587.

Fagan, A.A. *et al.* (2007) Using community and family risk and protective factors for community-based prevention planning. *Journal of Community Psychology* **35**, 535–555.

Fagan, A.A. *et al.* (2019) Scaling up evidence-based interventions in US public systems to prevent behavioral health problems: challenges and opportunities. *Prevention Science* **20**(8), 1147–1168.

Feinberg, M.E. (2010) Community epidemiology of risk and adolescent substance use: practical questions for enhancing prevention. *American Journal of Public Health* **102**, 457–468.

Feinberg, M.E. *et al.* (2014) Long-term follow-up of a randomized trial of family foundations: effects on children's emotional, behavioral, and school adjustment. *Journal of Family Psychology* **28**(6), 821–831.

Foulkes, L. & Stringaris, A. (2023) Do no harm: can school mental health interventions cause iatrogenic harm? *BJPsych Bulletin* **47**(5), 267–269. doi:10.1192/bjb.2023.9.

Fundacion Marcelino Botin (2008) *Social and Emotional Education: An International Analysis*. Author, Santander, Spain.

Gardner, F. *et al.* (2019) Equity effects of parenting interventions for child conduct problems: a pan-European individual participant data meta-analysis. *The Lancet Psychiatry* **6**(6), 518–527.

Gillham, J.E. *et al.* (2008) Preventing depression in early adolescence: the Penn resiliency program. In: *Handbook of Depression in Children and Adolescents*. (eds J.R.Z. Abela & B.L. Hankin). Guilford Press, New York. pp. 309–322.

Glasgow, R.E. *et al.* (2003) Why don't we see more translation of health promotion research to practice? Rethinking the efficacy-to-effectiveness transition. *American Journal of Public Health* **93**, 1261–1267.

Gottfredson, D.C. *et al.* (2015) Standards of evidence for efficacy, effectiveness, and scale-up research in prevention science: next generation. *Prevention Science* **16**, 893–926.

Greenberg, M.T. (2023) Evidence for social and emotional learning in schools. Learning Policy Institute. Available: https://doi.org/10.54300/928.269 [6 October 2024].

Greenberg, M.T. & Lippold, M.A. (2013) Promoting healthy outcomes among youth with multiple risks: innovative approaches. *Annual Review of Public Health* **34**, 253–270.

Greenberg, M.T. *et al.* (2001) The prevention of mental disorders in school-age children: current state of the field. *Prevention & Treatment* **4**, 1–62.

Greenberg, M.T. *et al.* (1995) Promoting emotional competence in school age children: the effects of the PATHS curriculum. *Development and Psychopathology* **7**, 117–136.

Greenberg, M.T. *et al.* (2017) Social and emotional learning as a public health approach to education. *The Future of Children* **27**, 13–32.

Hawkins, J.D. *et al.* (2005) Promoting positive adult functioning through social development intervention in childhood: long-term effects from the Seattle social development project. *Archives of Pediatrics & Adolescent Medicine* **159**, 25–31.

Heikkilä, H. *et al.* (2021) The United Nations Office on Drugs and Crime's efforts to strengthen a culture of prevention in low- and middle-income countries. *Prevention Science* **22**, 18–28.

Hennessey, E.A. *et al.* (2019) Comparative effectiveness of brief alcohol interventions for college students: results from a network meta-analysis. *Prevention Science* **20**, 715–740.

Hermenau, K. *et al.* (2012) Childhood adversity, mental ill-health and aggressive behavior in an African orphanage: changes in response to trauma-focused therapy and the implementation of a new instructional system. *Child and Adolescent Psychiatry and Mental Health* **5**, 29–38.

Hodder, R.K. *et al.* (2017) Systematic review of universal school-based 'resilience' interventions targeting adolescent tobacco, alcohol or illicit substance use: a meta-analysis. *Preventive Medicine* **100**, 248–268.

Horowitz, J.L. *et al.* (2007) Prevention of depressive symptoms in adolescents: a randomized trial of cognitive–behavioral and interpersonal prevention programs. *Journal of Consulting and Clinical Psychology* **75**, 693–706.

Howe, G. & Leijten, P. (2023) When is it time to revise or adapt our prevention programs? Introduction to special issue on using baseline target moderation to assess variation in prevention impact. *Prevention Science* **24**(2), 199–203.

Howes Vallis, E. *et al.* (2020) Cognitive-behavioural interventions for prevention and treatment of anxiety in young children: a systematic review and meta-analysis. *Clinical Psychology Review* **81**, 101904.

Hurlburt, M.S. *et al.* (2013) Efficacy of The Incredible Years group parent program with families in Head Start who self-reported a history of child maltreatment. *Child Abuse & Neglect* **37**, 531–543.

Institute of Health Metrics and Evaluation (2023) Global Health Data Exchange (GHDx). Available: https://vizhub.healthdata.org/gbd-results/ [10 April 2023].

Jacob, R. & Parkinson, J. (2015) The potential for school-based interventions that target executive function to improve academic achievement: a review. *Review of Educational Research* **85**, 512–552.

Kemp, L. (2016) Adaptation and fidelity: a recipe analogy for achieving both in population scale implementation. *Prevention Science* **17**(4), 429–438.

Kretschmer, T. *et al.* (2015) Multifinality of peer victimization: maladjustment patterns and transitions from early to mid-adolescence. *European Child & Adolescent Psychiatry* **24**, 1169–1179.

Kuklinski, M.R. *et al.* (2021) Long-term impacts and benefit–cost analysis of the communities that care prevention system at age 23, 12 years after baseline. *Prevention Science* **22**(4), 452–463.

Leadbeater, B.J. *et al.* (2018) Ethical challenges in promoting the implementation of preventive interventions: report of the SPR task force. *Prevention Science* **19**, 853–865.

Lee, S. *et al.* (2012) Return on investment: evidence-based options to improve statewide outcomes. April 2012 (Document No. 12-04-1201). Washington State Institute for Public Policy, Olympia, WA.

Ma, L. *et al.* (2020) Resilience-oriented cognitive behavioral interventions for depressive symptoms in children and adolescents: a meta-analytic review. *Journal of Affective Disorders* **270**, 150–164.

MacPhee, D. *et al.* (2015) Resilience as regulation of family and developmental processes. *Family Relations* **64**, 153–175.

Mahoney, J.L. *et al.* (2021) Systemic social and emotional learning: promoting educational success for all preschool to high school students. *American Psychologist* **76**, 1128–1142.

Mejia, A. *et al.* (2017) Different strokes for different folks? Contrasting approaches to cultural adaptation of parenting interventions. *Prevention Science* **18**, 630–639.

Michelini, G. *et al.* (2021) Multiple domains of risk factors for first onset of depression in adolescent girls. *Journal of Affective Disorders* **283**, 20–29.

Mojtabai, R. & Olfson, M. (2020) National trends in mental health care for US adolescents. *JAMA Psychiatry* **77**, 703–714.

Moore, J.E. *et al.* (2013) Examining adaptations of evidence-based programs in natural contexts. *Journal of Primary Prevention* **34**, 147–161.

Moreno-Peral, P. *et al.* (2017) Effectiveness of psychological and/or educational interventions in the prevention of anxiety: a systematic review, meta-analysis, and meta-regression. *JAMA Psychiatry* **74**(10), 1021–1029.

National Academies of Sciences, Engineering, and Medicine (2019) *Fostering Healthy Mental, Emotional, and Behavioral Development in Children and Youth: A National Agenda*. The National Academies Press, Washington, DC.

Neil, A.L. & Christensen, H. (2009) Efficacy and effectiveness of school-based prevention and early intervention programs for anxiety. *Clinical Psychology Review* **29**, 208–215.

Oveisi, S. *et al.* (2010) Primary prevention of parent-child conflict and abuse in Iranian mothers: a randomized-controlled trial. *Child Abuse and Neglect* **34**, 206–213.

Panayiotou, M. *et al.* (2019) Implementation matters: using complier average causal effect estimation to determine the impact of the promoting alternative thinking strategies (PATHS) curriculum on children's quality of life. *Journal of Educational Psychology* **112**, 236–253.

Prinz, R.J. *et al.* (2009) Population-based prevention of child maltreatment: the U.S. Triple P system population trial. *Prevention Science* **10**, 1–12.

Rhoades, B.L. *et al.* (2012) The role of a state-level prevention support system in promoting high-quality implementation and sustainability of evidence-based programs. *American Journal of Community Psychology* **50**, 386–401.

Riggs, N.R. *et al.* (2006) The mediational role of neurocognition in the behavioral outcomes of a social–emotional prevention program in elementary school students: effects of the PATHS curriculum. *Prevention Science* **7**, 91–102.

Rivet-Duval, E. *et al.* (2011) Preventing adolescent depression in Mauritius: a universal school-based program. *Child and Adolescent Mental Health* **16**, 86–91.

Rohde, P. *et al.* (2018) Major depression prevention effects for a cognitive-behavioral adolescent indicated prevention group intervention across four trials. *Behaviour Research and Therapy* **100**, 1–6.

Rose, G. (1985) Sick individuals and sick populations. *International Journal of Epidemiology* **14**, 32–38.

Sameroff, A.J. (2010) A unified theory of development, a dialectical integration of nature and nurture. *Child Development* **81**, 6–22.

Sanders, M. (2008) Triple-P Positive Parenting Program as a public health approach to strengthening parenting. *Journal of Family Psychology* **22**, 506–517.

Sanders, M.R. *et al.* (2008) Every family: a population approach to reducing behavioral and emotional problems in children making the transition to school. *The Journal of Primary Prevention* **29**, 197–222.

Sanders, M.R. *et al.* (2014) The Triple P-Positive Parenting Program: a systematic review and meta-analysis of a multi-level system of parenting support. *Clinical Psychology Review* **34**(4), 337–357.

Sandler, I. *et al.* (2014) Overview of meta-analyses of the prevention of mental health, substance use and conduct problems. *Annual Review of Clinical Psychology* **10**, 243–273.

Schembre, S.M. *et al.* (2018) Just-in-time feedback in diet and physical activity interventions: systematic review and practical design framework. *Journal of Medical Internet Research* **20**, e106.

Schindler, H.S. *et al.* (2015) Maximizing the potential of early childhood education to prevent externalizing behavior problems: a meta-analysis. *Journal of School Psychology* **53**(3), 243–263.

Scott, S. *et al.* (2010) Impact of a parenting program in a high-risk, multi-ethnic community: the PALS trial. *The Journal of Child Psychology and Psychiatry* **51**, 1331–1341.

Shamblen, S.R. & Derzon, J.H. (2009) A preliminary study of the population-adjusted effectiveness of substance abuse prevention programming: towards making IOM program types comparable. *Journal of Primary Prevention* **30**, 89–107.

Shelton, R.C. *et al.* (2018) The sustainability of evidence-based interventions and practices in public health and health care. *Annual Review of Public Health* **39**, 55–76.

Shochet, I. & Osgarby, S. (1999) The resourceful adolescent project: building psychological resilience in adolescents and their parents. *The Australian Educational and Developmental Psychologist* **16**(1), 46–65.

Spoth, R.L. *et al.* (2008) Preventive interventions addressing underage drinking: state of the evidence and steps toward public health impact. *Pediatrics* **121**, S311–S336.

Spoth, R.L. *et al.* (2013a) Longitudinal effects of universal PROSPER community–university partnership delivery system effects on substance misuse through 6 1/2 years past baseline from a cluster randomized controlled intervention trial. *Preventive Medicine* **56**, 190–196.

Spoth, R.L. *et al.* (2013b) Addressing challenges for the next generation of Type 2 translation research: the translation science to population impact framework. *Prevention Science* **14**, 319–351.

Spoth, R. *et al.* (2022) Applying the PROSPER prevention delivery system with middle schools: emerging adulthood effects on substance misuse and conduct problem behaviors through 14 years past baseline. *Child Development* **93**(4), 925–940.

Stefan, C.A. & Miclea, M. (2013) Effects of a multifocused prevention program on preschool children's competencies and behavior problems. *Psychology in the Schools* **50**, 382–402.

Stice, E. *et al.* (2009) A meta-analytic review of depression prevention programs for children and adolescents: factors that predict magnitude of intervention effects. *Journal of Consulting and Clinical Psychology* **77**, 486–503.

Stockings, E.A. *et al.* (2016) Preventing depression and anxiety in young people: a review of the joint efficacy of universal, selective and indicated prevention. *Psychological Medicine* **46**(1), 11–26. doi:10.1017/S0033291715001725.

Takacs, Z.K. & Kassai, R. (2019) The efficacy of different interventions to foster children's executive function skills: a series of meta-analyses. *Psychological Bulletin* **145**, 653–697.

Teubert, D. & Pinquart, M. (2011) A meta-analytic review on the prevention of symptoms of anxiety in children and adolescents. *Journal of Anxiety Disorders* **25**, 1046–1059.

Toth, S. & Gravener, J. (2012) Review: bridging research and practice: relational interventions for maltreated children. *Child and Adolescent Mental Health* **17**, 131–138.

U.S. Department of Health and Human Services (HHS) (2016) Office of the Surgeon General, Facing Addiction in America: The Surgeon General's Report on Alcohol, Drugs, and Health. HHS, Washington, DC.

Valentine, J.C. *et al.* (2011) Replication in prevention science. *Prevention Science* **12**, 103–117.

Vermeulen-Smit, E. *et al.* (2015) The effectiveness of family interventions in preventing adolescent illicit drug use: a systematic review and meta-analysis of randomized controlled trials. *Clinical Child and Family Psychology Review* **18**, 218–239.

Webster-Stratton, C. & Reid, M.J. (2010) The incredible years parents, teachers and children training series: a multifaceted treatment approach for young children with conduct problems. In: *Evidence-based Psychotherapies for Children and Adolescents.* (eds J. Weisz & A. Kazdin), 2nd edn. Guilford Press, New York. pp. 194–210.

Weissberg, R. (2019) Promoting the social and emotional learning of millions of school children. *Perspectives on Psychological Science* **14**, 65–69. doi:10.1177/1745691618817756.

Wilson, S.J. & Lipsey, M.J. (2007) Effectiveness of school-based intervention programs on aggressive behavior: update of a meta-analysis. *American Journal of Preventive Medicine* **33**(Suppl. 2), S130–S143.

Wolchik, S.A. *et al.* (2007) New beginnings: an empirically-based program to help divorced mothers promote resilience in their children. In: *Handbook of Parent Training: Helping Parents Prevent and Solve Problem Behaviors.* (eds J.M. Briesmeister & C.E. Schaefer). Wiley, New York. pp. 25–62.

CHAPTER 33
Parenting programs

Stephen Scott[1] and Frances Gardner[2]
[1]Department of Child and Adolescent Psychiatry, Institute of Psychiatry, Psychology and Neuroscience, King's College London, London, UK
[2]Centre for Evidence-Based Intervention, Department of Social Policy and Intervention, University of Oxford, Oxford, UK

Overview

With over 300 randomized controlled trials (RCTs) showing effectiveness, parenting programs are the most widely proven intervention for children's behavior and attachment problems. Delivered face-to-face, either individually with a therapist or in a group setting, better quality evidence-based programs have moderate to large effect sizes on improving parenting practices and reducing childhood conduct problems, as well as increasing attachment security in young children. However, the evidence on effectiveness for adolescent conduct problems is much more uncertain. The rise of programs delivered over the Internet offers the opportunity to widen access, which in most countries is limited. However, without practitioner support, completion rates of online programs are low. Further research is needed on how to improve outcomes for those who do not respond to parenting programs and on key mediating mechanisms. There is still a long way to go in making effective parenting programs more widely available in both developed and low- and middle-income countries (LMICs), although the evidence base in the latter is growing.

Introduction

A parenting program is a specific intervention designed to improve the overall quality of parenting that a child receives. Parenting programs aim to help the way mothers, fathers, and other caregivers relate to their child primarily by changing their behavior in moment-to-moment interchanges throughout the day, although they also address parental beliefs and feelings. Change is achieved through the training of specific skills, such as collaborative play, selective attention, and praise, to promote sociable behavior and clear rules backed by consistently applied consequences to reduce unwanted behavior. There is a structured sequence of sessions that builds up each of the competencies. This approach to intervention is distinct from counseling, where the emphasis is usually on understanding the parent's views and giving them nondirective general support, but not coaching them (see Chapter 36); it differs from psychoeducation where a parent is informed about the nature of the child's difficulties and given advice on management but not trained in specific skills. In family therapy, the therapist typically addresses the whole family system, often with a primary emphasis on deeper understanding of interpersonal processes and meanings; it is change in understanding, rather than skills, that is postulated to lead to changes in relationships (see Chapter 35).

Parenting programs typically aim to improve child symptoms as well as the quality of the relationship. Where neglectful or abusive parenting has been uncovered, the goal may only be to improve positive parental engagement with the child and reduce harsh emotional and physical practices, whether or not the child is displaying problems (see Chapter 25). In turn, reduced maltreatment is likely to prevent adverse child outcomes in the long term. And where there are child emotional or behavioral problems, parenting programs may help regardless of whether suboptimal parenting has contributed to causing the problem. Thus, programs can help parents to better manage children with problems that are mainly genetically influenced, such as autistic spectrum disorders (ASDs) (see Chapter 51) even though parenting quality is satisfactory at the outset.

Furthermore, where there are child symptoms and parenting is less than optimal, this does not necessarily mean that the parenting caused the child's problems. Parent–child relationships are bidirectional, and more difficult child behavior can elicit harsher parenting. Several lines of evidence show this, from the classic experiment where parents with relatively well-behaved children were asked to look after children with behavioral problems and became harsher and more critical (Anderson

Rutter's Child and Adolescent Psychiatry and Psychology, Seventh Edition.
Edited by Anita Thapar, Daniel S. Pine, Samuele Cortese, Cathy Creswell, Tamsin J. Ford, James F. Leckman, and Argyris Stringaris.

Companion website: www.wiley.com/go/thapar/rutterspsych7

et al., 1986), to experiments showing that where disruptive child behavior, such as attention deficit hyperactivity disorder (ADHD), is reduced by medication parenting quality improves (Schachar *et al.*, 1987). Nonetheless, two areas of child functioning which have been found to be closely linked to parenting are conduct problems and insecure attachment; we concentrate on these domains in this chapter, but refer to others.

Styles of parenting addressed by parenting programs

Because there are many different theories of what constitutes good parenting, there are many different approaches incorporated in intervention programs. We focus here on those dimensions that are well supported empirically and that have led to proven intervention programs.

Dimensions of parenting addressed in interventions derived from social learning theory

Social learning theory evolved from general learning theory and behaviorism (Bandura, 1977). The notion is that children's real-life experiences and exposures directly or indirectly shape behavior; processes underlying this learning can be diverse. Traditionally, social learning theory had a primary focus on externally observable behavior rather than children's inner mental states (Patterson, 1982). Operant behavioral principles of reinforcement and (noncoercive) consequences are applied immediately after the child has acted/responded; there is less emphasis on classical, stimulus-controlled conditioning. Moment-to-moment exchanges are crucial: if a child receives an immediate reward for their behavior, such as getting parental attention or approval, then they are more likely to repeat the behavior, whereas if they are ignored or an unwelcome sanction is applied, then they are less likely to do it again.

Patterson (1982) showed how children's aggressive behaviors were learned from and reinforced by parallel negative behaviors by parents. A negative parenting style appears to have a causal role in leading to conduct problems, even after allowing for intergenerational genetic influences and child effects (Harold *et al.*, 2017). The association has been repeatedly found in: (i) large-scale epidemiological investigations (e.g., Farrington *et al.*, 2023); (ii) intensive observational clinical investigations such as Patterson's work mentioned above; and (iii) numerous naturalistic studies of diverse samples using various methods (e.g., Farrington *et al.*, 2023). The parenting behaviors identified are high criticism and hostility, harsh punishment, inconsistent discipline, low warmth, involvement, and encouragement, and poor supervision.

A further important dimension for older children is monitoring their whereabouts and activities outside the home. Careful monitoring has greater effects in neighborhoods where there are many risks such as drugs and violence (Pettit *et al.*, 1999). Monitoring is not just a matter of parents being good "police," since knowing where a child is depends in part on the child having a good enough relationship with the parent to tell them what they are doing (Vaughan *et al.*, 2022). Therefore, enabling parents to impose effective discipline depends on them also developing a positive relationship with their child, skills addressed in most programs. These elements promote child positive behavior and affect, and provide a more positive relationship context for parental disciplinary interventions. More recently, social learning models have increasingly considered inner cognitive or "mindful" processes such as attributions that underlie parents' behavior (Coatsworth *et al.*, 2015). Beliefs can vary considerably across cultures, with more traditional societies showing more authoritarian views.

Dimensions of parenting addressed in interventions derived from attachment theory

Attachment theory (Fearon & Roisman, 2017; see Chapter 6) focuses on the extent to which the relationship provides the child with protection against harm and a sense of emotional security, resulting in a "secure base" for exploration. The theory proposes that the quality of parental care, particularly "sensitive responding" to the child's emotional needs, promotes a relationship characterized by warm, expressive to-and-fro interchanges ("mutuality"), leading to secure attachment. Evidence shows that sensitive responding is important in promoting attachment security, but less than theorized (see Chapter 6); longitudinal studies confirm that attachment security does not shape development deterministically, but interacts with child and family factors to influence outcome (Sroufe *et al.*, 2010). A particularly harmful parenting style is frightening and abusive parenting, which is associated with "disorganized" attachment patterns—meta-analyses confirm a strong association with maltreatment. Disorganization is associated with many forms of child psychopathology, especially conduct problems (Groh *et al.*, 2017), although it is important to note that it occurs in 15% or more in the general population.

Over time, attachment relationships are internalized and carried forward to influence expectations for other important relationships, by an "internal working model." Since the 2010s, progress has been made in measuring internal working models and shows their continuing importance in adolescence when they are also still related to sensitive parenting (Scott *et al.*, 2011). Indeed, sensitive parenting may be a stronger predictor of outcomes than attachment security. For example, Fraley and Roisman (2015) found that young children exposed to more sensitive responding showed better academic attainment and social outcomes aged 33 years, and Bachmann *et al.* (2022) found it was associated in adolescence with lower service use and economic costs to society.

Child characteristics that may affect susceptibility to the effects of parenting

Some child disorders and traits have high heritability, for example, ADHD, autism, and callous-unemotional (CU) traits, leading some to assume they are less susceptible to intervention efforts. However, this is not always the case.

Inherited characteristics and behavioral phenotypes

The effects of parenting can differ according to the characteristics of children. Adoption studies are one way of investigating this. In a classic follow-up study, Bohman (1996) divided early adopted infants into those whose birth parents had histories of offending or problematic alcohol use, representing higher congenital (genetic plus early environmental) risk, versus those who did not. Adopting parents were categorized the same way, to index more and less favorable child-rearing conditions. Police contact by age 17 was 3% versus 12% for children with low versus high congenital risk favorably reared, suggesting a substantial inherited component under good conditions. For those raised under unfavorable conditions, the rates were 7% and 40% respectively. This study, replicated since, shows that some children have a much greater liability to poorer outcomes under stressful rearing conditions.

More recently, the possibility has been explored that rather than just confer liability to poorer outcomes under stressful rearing, some child characteristics may also confer liability to better outcomes under benign conditions, the so-called differential susceptibility hypothesis (Belsky *et al.*, 2022). Experimentally, Scott and O'Connor (2012) found that antisocial children who were more emotionally dysregulated (tantrums, anger) showed a greater response to improved parenting than those who were disobedient in a more controlled way. However, while differential susceptibility is an exciting theory, more replication of findings (e.g., Chhangur & Belsky, 2023) is necessary to characterize the scope of its impact.

Father involvement

Most literature refers to "parenting" as if it made no difference whether fathers or mothers were involved. While in the majority of cultures it is often mothers who spend most time looking after younger children, fathers have a particular role, which often increases as children become older. When it comes to parenting programs, it should not be assumed that evidence about effectiveness applies equally to mothers and fathers. The amount and quality of father involvement in parenting is beneficial to children's mental health and behavior, so *a priori* it would seem desirable to involve fathers in parenting programs. Gonzalez *et al.* (2023) have carried out a helpful review of strategies that can help to achieve this.

Issues in measuring the effectiveness of parenting programs

A range of methods can be used to assess the effectiveness of parenting programs. Parent-completed questionnaires are relatively quick and easy, but may be subject to attributional bias, for example, seeing only negative aspects of child behavior, thus exaggerating the extent of the child's problems. Vice-versa, after intervention, the parent may generally feel better or overestimate the degree of improvement. Structured interviews are little better since they accept the respondent's ratings. In contrast, semi-structured interviews probe for detailed descriptions of the child's behavior, then the investigator makes the rating. This helps diminish over- and underreporting of problems (see Chapter 28).

Direct observation is often held to be the "gold standard" of measurement since it is free of informant bias (see Chapter 28). It has led to some important revisions of the effectiveness of parenting programs. For example, the meta-analysis of methods used to assess parenting programs by Daley *et al.* (2014) found improvement in both conduct problems and ADHD symptoms on parent report, but on direct observation there was no improvement in ADHD symptoms although conduct problems did reduce, which was nonetheless of considerable benefit to the child and the parents. However, the proviso here is that in nearly all cases the direct observation methodology was over a short time, around 20–30 minutes, in structured tasks and was not typically in the classroom or another more ecological environment such as at home. It is notable that in large reviews of parenting for conduct problems, observational data do not show diminished intervention effects compared to parent report (Beelmann *et al.*, 2022). Prepubertal children typically underreport challenging behavior compared with parent accounts or direct observation, whereas adolescent self-reports are more variable. Police records provide an independent index of delinquent acts, but require the young person to be apprehended.

Application of programs to specific child issues

Conduct problems in children

Parenting programs for conduct problems are almost exclusively based on social learning theory. Characteristics of some of the more widely used programs are given in Table 33.1, the basic content of a typical program in Table 33.2, and the pros and cons of group-based versus individual-based delivery in Table 33.3.

Effectiveness

Programs based on social learning theory have been tested for over 60 years and there is a larger evidence base for this intervention than any other in child mental health, with over 300 RCTs published. Thus, the meta-analysis by Beelmann *et al.* (2022) that included both community and clinical samples found that, overall, the mean effect for parenting programs was moderate-to-large for parent outcomes (effect size = 0.46 SD) and for child conduct problems (effect size = 0.47 SD). They also found higher effects on more proximal parental outcomes such as parental stress, parental competencies, and parent–child interaction. However, more distal outcomes, such as marital satisfaction or parent psychopathology, showed lower effect sizes; to be fair, the interventions were not targeting these outcomes. No adverse effects or harms were recorded. In addition, the link between

Table 33.1 Characteristics of some widely used programs. To choose a program, consider the strength of the evidence (number of trials, appropriateness for the particular population in question, and availability of training and supervision, all of which are covered in the Foundations guidebook [https://guidebook.eif.org.uk]).

Name	Target population	Levels and delivery modes	Evidence	Comments, website, dissemination
The Incredible Years	A series of parent group programs from babyhood to age 12	*Universal*: 6 weeks *Indicated*: Prevention: 14 weeks Treatment: 18–24 weeks	50 randomized controlled trials (RCTs), 10 by developer and 40 independent replications, confirm effects	Developer: Carolyn Webster-Stratton. One of the most intensive programs in clinical process and supervision www.incredibleyears.com
Triple P	A range of programs at all levels and ages	*Universal*: Online; broadcast media *Selective*: short one-off sessions of up to 4 weeks *Indicated*: 6–8 weeks	Over 50 RCTs by developer; 8 independent replications, 2 prevention trials failing to show effects	Developer: Matt Sanders. Comprehensive range of levels https://www.triplep.net/glo-en/home/
Parent–Child Interaction Therapy (PCIT)	Child disruptive and parenting difficulties including maltreatment	Parent–child dyad is live coached by therapist over 12–20 sessions	21 RCTs by developer and independent evaluators show effects	Developer: Sheila Eyberg http://www.pcit.org
Parent Management Training, Oregon, US	Behavioral problems for ages 4–12; parents with mental health problems	Individual program: 19–30 sessions, group program: 14 sessions	7 RCTs by program developer and independents show effects	Developer: Marion Forgatch
Strengthening Families Program	Universal preventive program for ages 10–14	7 2-hour sessions including whole family and separate parent and child groups	2 RCTs by program developer show effects	Developer: Karol Kumpfer http://www.strengtheningfamilies program.org
Nurse–Family Partnership	Preventive for young, disadvantaged first-time mothers	Trained nurses home visit mother during pregnancy and first 24 months	3 RCTs have shown varied and long-lasting effects	Developer: David Olds http://www.nursefamily partnership.org

Table 33.2 Content of a typical social learning program.

Part 1: Promoting a child-centered approach
Play is covered in the first 2–3 sessions. Instead of giving directions, teaching, and asking questions during play, parents are simply instructed to give a running commentary on their child's actions. Parents are asked to practice these techniques for 10 minutes every day.

Part 2: Increasing acceptable child behavior
Praise and rewards The parent is required to praise their child for lots of simple, desirable everyday behaviors such as playing quietly on their own, eating nicely, getting dressed the first time they are asked, and so on. Later sessions go through the use of reward charts.

Part 3: Setting clear expectations
Clear commands Parents are taught to reduce the number of commands, but also to make them much more authoritative. The manner should be forceful (not sitting down, timidly requesting from the other end of the room; instead, standing over the child, fixing him in the eye, and in a clear firm voice giving the instruction). Commands should specify what the parent *wants* the child to do, not what they should *stop* doing ("please speak quietly," rather than "stop shouting").

Part 4: Reducing unacceptable child behavior
Consequences for unacceptable behavior should be applied as soon as possible. They must always be followed through. Simple logical consequences are encouraged: if water is splashed out of the bath, the bath will end; if a child refuses to eat dinner, there will be no pudding; etc.
Ignoring This sounds easy but is a hard skill to teach parents. Whining, arguing, swearing, and tantrums are not dangerous and can usually be safely ignored. The technique is very effective.
Time out from positive reinforcement remains the final "big one" as a sanction for unacceptable behavior. The child is put in some boring place for a previously agreed reason (hitting, breaking things, etc.—not minor infringements) for a short time (say five minutes). However, the child must be quiet for the last minute.

changes in parental outcomes and changes in conduct problems was significant across several outcome types, confirming the general assumption about the mechanism behind parenting programs, although very few studies tested mediation formally.

However, it should be noted that while parenting programs improve behavior at home, they do not have many significant effects at school (Beelmann *et al.*, 2022). To address this, interventions have taught teachers similar methods as used in parent training, with positive outcomes (Ford *et al.*, 2018); see Chapter 38.

The question arises, "For how long do intervention effects last?" Some follow-ups have been notably successful. Thus, Scott *et al.* (2014) found that a parent training program for clinically referred children with conduct problems aged 4–6 years had lasting effects 8 years later, with a reduction of oppositional defiant disorder (ODD) diagnoses to 25% compared to 50% in controls (Figure 33.1), a reduction in CU traits, making the development of later antisocial personality disorder less likely (Figure 33.2), and an improved reading score (Figure 33.3). The meta-analysis by Van Aar *et al.* (2017) of trials with up to a 3-year follow-up found no diminution of effects, suggesting parenting programs can have long-term sustainable effects.

Failure to respond

Unlike some other mental health conditions, such as depression, there is no generally agreed protocol for the 25–50% of children who do not respond to a parenting intervention, or who drop out. Typically, this occurs because parents have become disaffected or have had difficulty in implementing the

Table 33.3 Pros and cons of delivering parenting programs in individual versus group format.

Individual	Group
Case selection	
Can take cases unsuitable for groups: shy parents; failed group parenting programs; high-risk/abusive parents	Can be hard to stop some parents falling behind
Depth of work	
Therapist can go into greater depth while teaching skills	Less detailed due to time constraints and other parents
Can observe parent interacting with child and pick up styles they are unaware of	Restricted to parents' accounts of what goes on with the child
Can adapt the program for particular child needs, e.g., attachment problems, attention deficit/hyperactivity disorder (ADHD) etc.	Can adapt program to special groups, but may be hard to assemble sufficient numbers to start simultaneously
Flexibility	
Flexible order of delivery of program, e.g., *time out* can be given early	Fixed order
Flexible timing to suit parent (within working hours)	Groups held at a fixed time when parent may be busy
Can easily be delivered at home	Parents have to come to clinic or community venue
No need to set up a crèche for child	May need to set up a crèche for child
Support from other parents	
No support from other parents	Other parents can normalize having a child with problems; they can learn from and support each other
Therapists' skills and support	
Can work as a solo therapist	Requires a second group leader plus group management skills
Duration and cost-effectiveness	
Typical program takes around 8 sessions, more complex programs are 10–12 sessions	Triple P level 4 has 4 group sessions plus 4 phone sessions; IY has minimum of 14 sessions, 18–22 sessions are recommended for clinical cases
Typically, cost £2000/€2200/US$2500	Typically, cost £1500/€1700/US$1800

strategies. A theory-driven approach has been proposed by Scott and Dadds (2009), and an RCT is underway to test a personalized approach for those who decline a parenting program or failed to respond, based on a personalized approach matching what parents wish, while maintaining use of the evidence (Senior *et al.*, 2023).

Comparison with nonbehavioral programs

There have been few if any head-to-head comparisons of social learning theory parenting programs with nonbehavioral, humanistic approaches. Studies have found that the humanistic

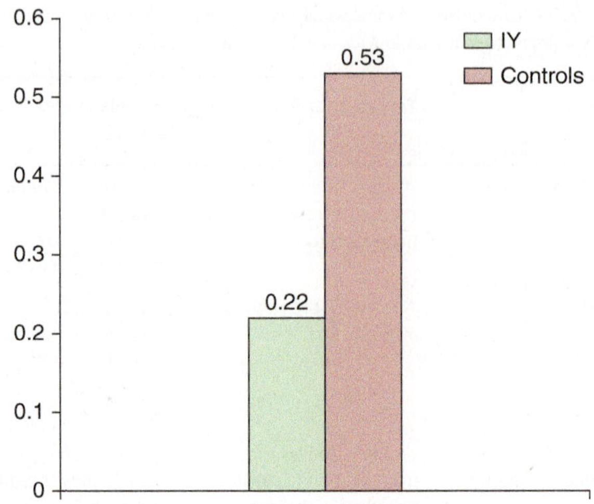

Figure 33.1 Rates of oppositional defiant disorder (ODD) diagnosis at 7–10-year follow-up of clinical referrals treated aged 4–8 years with The Incredible Years (IY), versus controls receiving management as usual ($p < 0.007$). *Source:* Scott *et al.*, 2014/with permission of American Psychiatric Association.

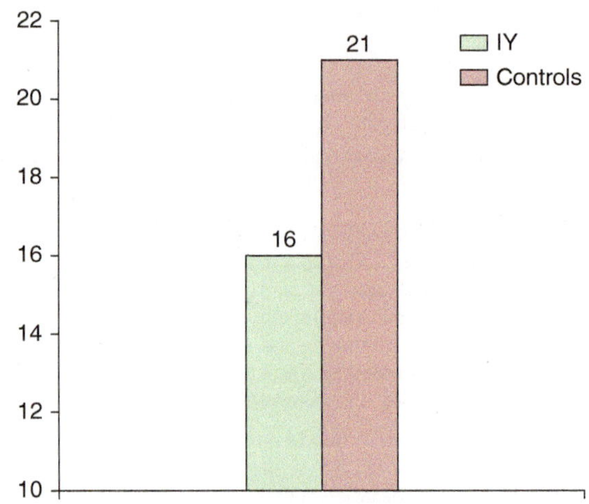

Figure 33.2 Antisocial personality screening device traits ($p < 0.01$).

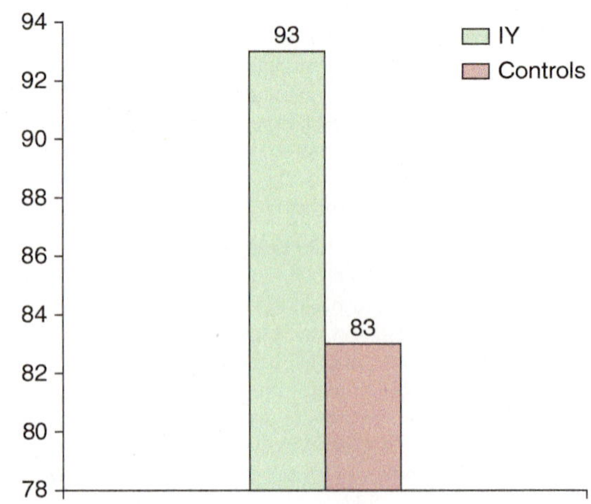

Figure 33.3 Reading score (WORD) ($p < 0.03$).

approach usually had negligible effects. For example, a trial of a parenting program based on primarily on emotional communication (The Family Links Nurturing Programme) for mild-to-moderate antisocial behavior found no significant effects on any outcome (Simkiss *et al.*, 2013). It seems that for child behavior problems, programs with a practical slant and strong focus on parental behavior change are more effective.

Conduct problems in children with callous-unemotional (CU) traits

Despite the not uncommon belief that children with conduct problems who also show CU traits are insensitive to parenting, and to parenting interventions, the evidence suggests that this is by no means the case. Thus, the meta-analysis by Perlstein *et al.* (2023) found that children with disruptive behavior disorders and CU traits showed similar improvements as those without CU traits, although they did start with more severe conduct problems to begin with, which was a predictor of the size of treatment gains. New interventions specially tailored for this group are being developed, for example, Fleming *et al.* (2022) showed that a specially adapted parent–child intervention therapy (PCIT) individual parenting intervention had slightly better effects than the standard form at follow-up.

Conduct problems in adolescents

The meta-analysis by Beelmann *et al.* (2022) suggests somewhat diminished but still significant effects of parenting programs for adolescent antisocial behavior. Many of the trials have been conducted by the program developers' team, for example, Triple P, and need independent replication (Chu *et al.*, 2015). More intense interventions for conduct problems in adolescence mostly use a social learning theory approach delivered through parents, but can include other elements, for example, functional family therapy (FFT) and multisystemic therapy (MST). These are more fully discussed in Chapter 35. However, it is worth noting that independent meta-analyses commissioned by the Campbell Collaboration for both FFT (Littell *et al.*, 2023) and MST (Littell *et al.*, 2021) did not find consistent significant effects outside the United States (U.S.) which practitioners may need to take into account when choosing an intervention.

Attention deficit hyperactivity disorder (ADHD)

Parenting programs have often been recommended as a first line of intervention for ADHD for children under five or older children with ODD/conduct disorder (CD) (NICE, 2019). As noted above, it may be that they are chiefly effective in reducing comorbid conduct problems, but this can still be very useful clinically. Practical issues about implementation in this context have been reviewed by Daley *et al.* (2018) and the meta-analysis by Groenman *et al.* (2022) concluded that, as well as parenting and conduct problems improving, it appeared that ADHD symptoms also improved. Parent training works well in conjunction with stimulant medication for ADHD, for example, the RCT by Sugaya *et al.* (2022) separated out these elements and showed that both components were helpful and worked synergistically.

Depression, anxiety, and other emotional problems

There is clear evidence supporting a link between quality of parent–child relationships and depression, anxiety, and other emotional problems (e.g., somatic complaints, social withdrawal), although smaller than that found for disruptive outcomes. Low warmth, overinvolvement, and control strategies are linked to childhood depression and anxiety (Creswell *et al.*, 2020), and it appears from genetic studies that there may be bidirectional influences from child anxiety to parental control (Eley *et al.*, 2010). The elements of parenting programs aimed primarily at conduct problems can be helpful for children showing emotional symptoms, but should not be the primary approach to intervention, although if there are comorbid conduct problems they may have small but significant effects on child symptoms of depression and anxiety (Kjøbli *et al.*, 2023).

Trials have shown that parent-led cognitive behavior therapy (CBT) for anxiety is effective (Creswell *et al.*, 2020), although, in general, parent involvement in CBT for anxiety does not yield superior effects to child-focused CBT alone. It is likely that if parenting interventions for anxiety were to focus more sharply on known key mechanisms of CBT, namely helping children achieve exposure to their feared situations, then sustained effects on anxiety would be greater. Lawrence *et al.* (2021) argue that there has been a "missed opportunity" to build on learning from the field of parenting interventions to enhance outcomes by involving parents in CBT for depression and anxiety in more targeted ways, based on our recent knowledge of the mechanisms of change. For more information about anxiety see Chapter 59, and on depression see Chapter 63.

Infants

Most programs draw on attachment theory and since the 2000s, several interventions have been developed and validated (see Chapter 6). The more effective interventions for infants typically last 8–20 sessions, videotaping parent–infant interactions and then replaying them to the parent. The great strength of this approach is that: (i) it allows parents to get an accurate picture of what is actually happening (rather than just talking about their perception of their relationship with their infant, as in traditional parent–infant psychotherapies); (ii) it enables them to see for themselves that when they change their behavior, this impacts on their infant; and (iii) it allows simultaneous exploration of the parent's mental state, so that mental blocks to more sensitive responding can be explored and often overcome.

Effectiveness

The meta-analysis by Jeong *et al.* (2021) identified more than 100 RCTs in the 0–3-year-old age group. The results indicated positive benefits of parenting interventions on child cognitive development (effect size 0.32 SD), language development (effect size 0.28 SD), motor development (effect size 0.24 SD), socioemotional development (effect size 0.19 SD), and attachment (effect size 0.29 SD), as well as reductions in behavior problems (effect size −0.13 SD).

An example of a particular, well-researched intervention is that of Video-feedback Intervention to Promote Positive Parenting (VIPP) developed by Van IJzendoorn *et al.* (2023). Meta-analysis of the first 25 RCTs of this intervention (Van IJzendoorn *et al.*, 2023) showed small improvements in positive parenting behavior (effect size 0.18 SD) and attitudes (effect size 0.16 SD), and child attachment security (effect size 0.23 SD), but not for child externalizing behavior.

Programs for specific parental issues and wider social contexts

Parents who maltreat their children

There is good evidence that social learning theory-based programs, with some adaptation and extension, can be effective for parents who maltreat their children (Backhaus *et al.*, 2023), as well as for prevention of maltreatment and some of its risk factors, including harsh parenting, low positive parenting, and parent depression. However, in this population effects may not be long-lasting and follow-up boosters may be necessary (Karjalainen *et al.*, 2021). Decisions about when to recommend a parenting program for seriously abusive or neglectful parents will usually be made by social services agencies, who, if they see potential for change, may refer their family to a parenting program. During this time, they will closely monitor the parents' progress, then take a decision about the best interests of the child which could include removal into foster care if maltreatment continues.

Drug-misusing and depressed parents

The "Parents under Pressure" (PuP) program has shown promising results with drug-misusing parents of children under 3 years of age; the RCT by Barlow *et al.* (2019) showed that child abuse potential was significantly reduced, while controls showed a deterioration, although only about one-third of drug-misusing parents improved their parenting. Better emotional regulation was an important mediator of program effectiveness (Dawe *et al.*, 2021). There are parenting programs specifically addressing parents who are depressed, including incorporating CBT strategies, and the trial by Compas *et al.* (2009) showed good effects on child outcomes. However, such parenting programs should only be used as an adjunct to help the parenting of children of drug-misusing and depressed parents, who should be referred for appropriate individual therapy in their own right.

Nonbiological parents

For children in the foster care system, and for adoptive parents, some trials suggest that parenting interventions aimed at foster carers, can be effective in reducing problem behavior and increasing attachment security in this often very troubled group of young people (Briskman & Scott, 2013). Schoemaker *et al.*'s (2020) meta-analysis showed positive effects for all parent outcomes: sensitive parenting, dysfunctional discipline, parenting knowledge and attitudes, and parenting stress, but while child behavior problems improved, attachment security did not, nor placement disruption frequency. However, placement in foster care away from an abusing or neglectful family is an important parenting intervention in its own right, and Joseph *et al.* (2014) showed that while attachment security to abusive birth parents was very low (0–10%), following six months or more of foster care, security of attachment to foster carers was as good as in normal controls (50% or more).

Grandparents often play a significant role in childcare, and the Triple P and other programs have been adapted specifically for grandparents, and found to be effective (Chan *et al.*, 2019).

Parents who argue about how to bring up children

Strong interparental arguments have harmful effects on children's psychology and biology, as comprehensively reviewed by Harold and Sellers (2018), who also evaluate intervention evidence. Feuerman (2022) offers several very sensible strategies to parents such as talk it out, create rules together, agree on consequences, back each other up, refrain from disagreeing in front of the kids, be flexible, give your partner second chances, and avoid involving children in disagreements.

For separating or divorcing parents, where arguments are common, the New Beginnings program, developed by Sandler and colleagues, has been proven to reduce conflict and improve child outcomes, and to be effective in an online version (Wolchik *et al.*, 2022).

Transportability of parenting programs to different cultures and countries

Parenting programs appear to transport well across cultures, despite different parenting norms and values. Systematic reviews of programs developed in countries, such as the U.S. and Australia, found comparable effect sizes in recipient countries, including those in Europe and Asia (Gardner *et al.*, 2016; Leijten *et al.*, 2016). Surprisingly perhaps, the Gardner *et al.* review found that, on average, "imported" programs were more effective in very different cultural settings (for example, Hong Kong) than in their original setting. These findings are consistent with studies of effects in ethnic minority groups within countries. For example, Reid *et al.* (2001), in a large study of low-income families in the U.S. found no ethnic differences in outcomes, engagement, or satisfaction across four ethnic groups. Similarly, Gardner *et al.* (2019a) found that parenting programs were equally likely to be effective for reducing conduct problems in ethnic minority compared to majority families, in a large individual participant data meta-analysis of trials of The Incredible Years intervention in Europe.

Low- and middle-income countries (LMICs)

Given the high levels of policy concern globally about harsh parenting and violence against children (WHO, 2023), youth crime and violence, and the loss of children's developmental potential due to poverty, poor nutrition, and conflict, it is important to know if parenting programs are effective in LMICs. Recent systematic reviews for a World Health Organization (WHO) guideline on parenting interventions (Backhaus *et al.*, 2023) found over 170 randomized trials in 40 LMICs, a remarkable expansion of the evidence base in the 10 years since the first review was published—a 2013 review found just 12 trials of parenting interventions (Knerr *et al.*, 2013). One of the WHO reviews focused on children and adolescents in LMICs aged 2–17, and found 131 trials, with meta-analyses showing similar beneficial effects on harsh parenting, and child conduct and emotional problems, to those found in high-income countries. Interestingly, it found particularly strong beneficial effects on parent mental health symptoms. There was no evidence of differential effects by child gender or age group, family education, or poverty at either country or family level. As found in high-income countries, children with higher levels of problem behavior showed more benefit from parenting interventions. Parenting interventions were effective even with the most vulnerable groups, such as parents in very low-income, or humanitarian, settings. There was a mix of group-based and single-family interventions, with no evidence of one format being superior to the other. Examples include studies of "Parenting for Lifelong Health," a social-learning theory group-based intervention with young children in low-income communities in South Africa (Ward *et al.*, 2020), and in the conditional cash transfer system in the Philippines (Lachman *et al.*, 2021).

Building on a review by Jeong *et al.* (2021), a WHO review of parenting interventions in the very early years found a further 46 randomized trials in LMICs in the age group 0–2 years. Most of these interventions targeted early child development and stimulation, most were home-based (a minority were group-based), and, overall, they showed positive effects on children's cognitive, social-emotional, and language development (Backhaus *et al.*, 2023). Recently, there has been much innovation in developing and testing digital parenting interventions in LMIC settings, often involving co-creation with vulnerable communities, including those in humanitarian settings (Black *et al.*, 2023), and with careful attention to devising applications that are usable in contexts where families have low-tech, shared phones with limited power and data. Digital applications are covered in a later section on "Online programs."

A particularly vulnerable group in LMICs is children and families in humanitarian settings, given that formal services are often disrupted, and the family may be the only remaining system able to nurture and protect children. Yet parenting may be compromised by parents' trauma and exhaustion, as well as by numerous crises and resettlement-related stressors. The WHO guideline review (Backhaus *et al.*, 2023, 2024) found 23 trials of parenting interventions, typically in post-conflict settings (e.g., Rwanda (Betancourt *et al.*, 2020), Liberia, Bosnia) or areas of conflict-driven migration (e.g., Jordan, Lebanon (Miller *et al.*, 2020), Ethiopia, the Thai–Myanmar border (Puffer *et al.*, 2017)), and in many cases they included components with a focus on child or parent mental health. Meta-analyses based on a dozen or more of these trials found beneficial effects on harsh and positive parenting, and on parent or child mental health symptoms, but not on child conduct problems. Unsurprisingly, there was a great deal of variability between contexts in the outcomes, suggesting further research is needed to delineate the important features of components, context, and implementation factors contributing to success or otherwise. Very few trials were found in the context of natural disasters, although with the climate emergency there is likely to be increasing displacement, conflict, and trauma in the future (Cuartas *et al.*, 2023), and increased need for mental health and family support intervention.

Prevention

In an ideal public health preventive strategy, all parents would learn effective parenting skills, which would help to improve parent–child relationships and child well-being, and reduce the rate of harsh and abusive parenting among the population (see Chapter 26). There would be a tiered set of interventions available in primary care and then in increasingly specialist levels of care, to help those with continuing difficulties. This vision has been well articulated by Sanders (2023), and appropriate programs developed by his group for each level. We have good evidence for the effectiveness of parenting interventions for indicated prevention and for treatment of conduct problems. However, it is less clear whether universal prevention parenting programs work: there have been many successful trials, but also many unsuccessful ones (Simkiss *et al.*, 2013; Averdijk *et al.*, 2016), and, overall, meta-analyses tend to find smaller or no effects of universal—or even selective—interventions (Leijten *et al.*, 2019; Beelmann *et al.*, 2022).

The Fast Track trial selected the children with the worst 10% of conduct problems when they started school and then gave them the multimodal intervention including parenting and social skills training and extra academic support. Despite all this, results were only effective for the most severe cases (Bierman *et al.*, 2017). In contrast the SPOKES trial (Scott *et al.*, 2010) took 4–6-year-old children in the worst 20% of conduct problems and got significant reductions at 2 years, but at a long-term follow-up these findings had washed out as the population had largely reverted to the norm (Scott *et al.*, 2014). Further studies need to understand under which conditions, and using which delivery mechanisms, universal parenting programs can be helpful; if they are not, then the conclusion might be that targeted programs are more useful (see Chapter 32).

What makes parenting programs work?

Moderators of outcome

Moderator analyses are important for understanding for whom interventions are most effective, helping service providers to decide where to best target their efforts, or to decide where different or additional interventions may be needed. They also allow for assessment of the equity effects of interventions, that is, questions about whether interventions are likely to widen or narrow existing inequalities between social groups in mental health outcomes (Gardner *et al.*, 2019a).

Child age and gender

Although earlier interventions are often thought to be more effective, related to a sensitive period for environmental influences in the early years, there is little or no intervention evidence to support this notion (McMahon *et al.*, 2021). For example, a large meta-analysis by Gardner *et al.* (2019b) found no variation in conduct problem outcomes by age across the range 2–10 years, and some have found stronger effects of parenting interventions in older children (Beelmann *et al.*, 2022). There are mixed findings for adolescence versus middle childhood, with some reviews suggesting lower effects in adolescence (Backer *et al.*, 2017; Beelmann *et al.*, 2022). Likewise, across multiple reviews, boys are as likely to improve as girls (McMahon *et al.*, 2021).

Child psychopathology

A consistent finding across the literature is that children with more severe levels of conduct problems at the outset respond better to parenting interventions (McMahon *et al.*, 2021). This has been found whether examining baseline variation in conduct problems at trial level (Beelmann *et al.*, 2022; Backhaus *et al.*, 2023), or at individual level, using data pooled across trials (Leijten *et al.*, 2020). The latter study, however, found no differential effect by level of ADHD. Studies suggest that for conduct problem interventions more generally, comorbidity does not affect outcomes (Ollendick *et al.*, 2008).

Family and demographic factors

Some early reviews found that demographic predictors of outcome, such as single parenthood, lower maternal education, and poverty, have a small negative effect on outcomes; more recent reviews have not found this. Leijten *et al.* (2013), after controlling for confounders, especially initial child problem severity, found no diminished effects of parenting interventions in low socioeconomic status (SES) families, and this is consistent with a larger study using individual participant data meta-analysis (Gardner *et al.*, 2019a), which found no differences by SES, maternal education, or teen or lone parenthood.

There have been mixed findings regarding parental psychopathology, especially maternal depression, as a moderator, but some trials and a well-powered individual participant data meta-analysis (Leijten *et al.*, 2020) found *larger* child improvement with depressed parents.

Mediators and mechanisms of change

Mediation analyses are important in assessing whether interventions work according to their theory of change. Thus, key mechanisms of change in social learning theory-based parenting programs are increases in positive parenting and decreases in harsh parenting. To show mediation the treatment has to (i) change the outcome and (ii) the mediator, (iii) the mediator has to correlate with outcome, and (iv) the effect of treatment on outcome has to reduce or disappear after controlling for the mediator (Kraemer *et al.*, 2002).

Generally, both reductions in harsh parenting and increases in positive parenting mediate change in child conduct problem outcomes (Forehand *et al.*, 2014). Thus, Beauchaine *et al.* (2005) found that changes in critical and ineffective parenting mediated child change in antisocial behavior and Gardner *et al.* (2006) found that it was change in positive parenting skills, rather than confidence in parenting, that predicted change.

Essential components

Parenting interventions usually combine multiple components. Thus, those based on social learning theory focus on parent–child responsive play, praise and reward, rule-setting, and strategies to enforce these such as ignoring, logical consequences, or time out. There are challenges in establishing the causal role of components, particularly where study designs (e.g., meta-analysis of components) are only able to examine correlations between component and outcome. Overall, they suggest that for more minor behavioral difficulties, increasing positive behavior alone has a reasonable effect, but where there are more disruptive child behaviors, then limit setting with consequences are essential (Gubbels *et al.*, 2019; Leijten *et al.*, 2019, 2021).

Implementation and dissemination

Implementation

Generalizability of trials evidence to everyday clinical practice

Most of the trials cited above were carried out using: (i) specially recruited cases rather than clinical referrals; (ii) specially trained research therapists rather than regular clinicians; and (iii) university rather than clinical settings. Indeed, Weisz's studies show that fewer than 5% of psychosocial child mental health trials meet all three "real-life" criteria (see Chapter 37). There is therefore considerable concern as to whether the good effects seen in trials will be replicated in everyday life, where cases have a high degree of comorbid conditions; most therapists do not use evidence-based approaches and do not get skill-specific supervision. Across all therapies for children, trials that compared evidence-based approaches in real life with usual services nonetheless get a clear advantage, by 0.3 SDs (see Chapter 31). The challenge is therefore to disseminate best practice more widely and ensure that it is well implemented.

Therapist effects

Therapist performance can be divided into three elements. (i) The *alliance*, which includes how well client and therapist get on together and agree shared goals. A meta-analysis of youth studies of the alliance found it contributed on average an effect size of 0.18 SD to outcome (Bose *et al.*, 2022). (ii) *Fidelity* or adherence to specific components of a model, that concerns the extent to which the therapist follows the actions prescribed in the manual. The meta-analysis by Collyer *et al.* (2020) found a small but significant relationship between therapist adherence and outcome. There is sometimes a fine line between sticking to a manual which has been proven to work in trials, or being a bit more flexible and personalizing according to perceived parent needs. (iii) The *skill* or competence with which the therapist carries out the tasks, that is how well the therapist performs the actions. Skill can include aspects of the alliance and fidelity. Both Forgatch *et al.* (2005) and Eames *et al.* (2009) found that therapist skill significantly predicted change in independently observed parenting. In summary, there is good evidence that therapist variables make a crucial difference to parenting programs for antisocial behavior.

Dissemination

Although formal data are lacking in most countries, Bachmann *et al.*'s (2024) survey of selected European countries found wide variation in provision of parenting services for children with conduct problems, and, overall, a very low rate of service availability relative to need.

An overarching issue is lack of knowledge by many service providers of what parenting programs can do and which ones to choose for which concerns. There have been several initiatives, therefore, to provide databases to help commissioners evaluate appropriate programs. For example, in the U.S., Blueprints for Healthy Youth Development (https://www.blueprintsprograms.org) has a searchable database of programs for a range of issues from preventive parenting programs targeting infants to intensive programs for delinquents. Likewise, the UK Foundations guidebook (https://guidebook.eif.org.uk) has ratings on a four-point scale of the quality of evidence and cost of parenting programs.

A further issue is the paucity of professionals trained in evidence-based programs. In England, this has been addressed by the Children and Young People's Increasing Access to Psychological Therapies (CYP-IAPT) initiative, which trains staff for a year in evidence-based interventions including parenting programs (Scott, 2017).

Online programs

Given the relative paucity of available services delivering parenting programs alluded to above, the opportunity to deliver them online is an exciting prospect. Considerable progress in developing online programs has been made since the 2010s, accelerated by the COVID-19 pandemic, which made face-to-face interventions unsuitable. Potentially, online programs are cheaper to deliver, with no need for travel, and if therapist involvement is reduced, access can be widened so that parents can engage with the program at a time convenient to themselves, for example, when the children are in bed, at weekends when they are not work, and so on. Variants include doing live individual coaching but using mobile phones and laptops. This can be notably successful, with effect sizes similar to face-to-face therapy (Baumel *et al.*, 2017). A number of programs have been transferred to an online platform (e.g., https://www.triplep-parenting.net/global/about-triple-p/what-is-triple-p/; www.parentingmatters.co.uk) and engaging with these can be supported by a therapist, either individually or in groups. Finally, parents can be offered an online program to do entirely on their own, with no therapist support. This is potentially the cheapest and the most flexible option in terms of times parents can access help, but evidence suggests that the rate of completion in a universal context is only 10% or so (e.g., see Dadds *et al.*, 2018). Completion rates are better for parents of children with significant behavior problems (Dadds *et al.*, 2018) when meta-analyses suggest that self-directed usage, without therapist support, can be effective (effect size 0.47 SD in meta-analysis by Baumel *et al.*, 2017) (Figure 33.4). However, for parents who are socially disadvantaged, which includes the majority with children with significant conduct problems, meta-analysis suggests that without therapist support self-directed programs may be less effective (Harris *et al.*, 2020).

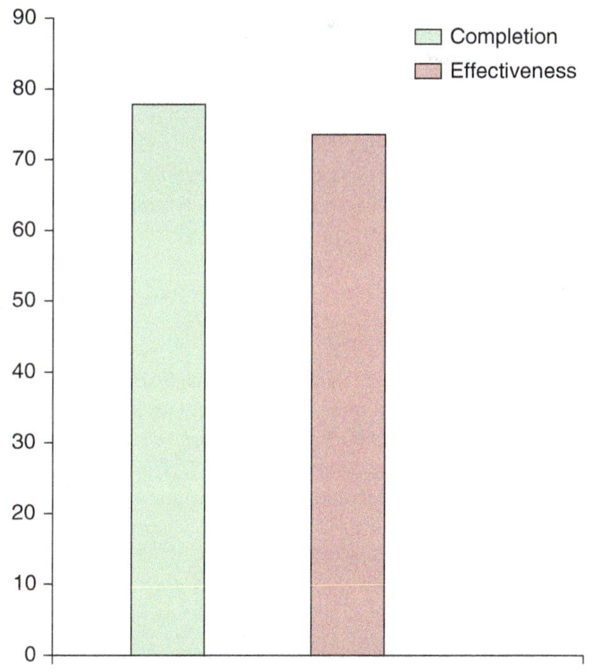

Figure 33.4 Completion rate and effectiveness of supported online parenting programs. Completion = % sessions offered; effectiveness = % of a large effect-size (0.8 SD). *Source:* Baumel *et al.*, 2017/with permission of Physicians Postgraduate Press, Inc.

Conclusions

Parenting programs are among the most effective interventions in children and young people's mental health. This is particularly true for conduct problems, which are one of the most prevalent childhood problems with very poor prognosis if untreated. Future challenges include: (i) finding out how to make programs more effective for adolescents; (ii) making programs more widely available, particularly to parents living in social disadvantage; (iii) developing new programs for those who do not respond to initial intervention; and (iv) understanding how best to deploy online programs, including how much therapist support is needed for which populations.

References

Anderson, K. *et al.* (1986) Mothers' interactions with normal and conduct disordered boys: who affects whom? *Developmental Psychology* **22**, 604–609.

Averdijk, M. *et al.* (2016) Long-term effects of two childhood psychosocial interventions on adolescent delinquency, substance use, and antisocial behavior: cluster RCT. *Journal of Experimental Criminology* **12**, 21–47. doi:10.1007/s11292-015-9249-4.

Bachmann, C. *et al.* (2022) A good investment: longer-term cost savings of sensitive parenting in childhood. *Journal of Child Psychology and Psychiatry* **63**, 78–87. https://acamh.onlinelibrary.wiley.com/doi/epdf/10.1111/jcpp.13461

Bachmann, C.J. *et al.* (2024) Recognition and management of children and adolescents with conduct disorder: a real-world data study from four western countries. *Child and Adolescent Psychiatry and Mental Health* **18**(1), 18.

Backhaus S. *et al.* (2023) WHO guidelines on parenting interventions to prevent maltreatment and enhance parent–child relationships with children aged 0–17 years: Report of the Systematic Reviews of Evidence. World Health Organization, Geneva, Switzerland.

Backhaus, S. *et al.* (2024) The effectiveness of parenting interventions in reducing violence against children in humanitarian settings in low- and middle-income countries: a systematic review and meta-analysis. *Child Abuse & Neglect*, 106850. doi:10.1016/j.chiabu.2024.106850.

Bandura, A. (1977) *Social Learning Theory*. General Learning Corporation, New York.

Barlow, J. *et al.* (2019) A randomized controlled trial and economic evaluation of the parents under pressure program for parents in substance abuse treatment. *Drug and Alcohol Dependence* **194**, 184–194. doi:10.1016/j.drugalcdep.2018.08.044.

Baumel, A. *et al.* (2017) Technology -assisted parent training programs for children and adolescents with disruptive behaviours: a systematic review. *The Journal of Clinical Psychiatry* **78**, 20765.

Beauchaine, T. *et al.* (2005) Mediators, moderators and predictors of 1-year outcomes among children treated for early-onset problems. *Journal of Consulting and Clinical Psychology* **75**, 371–388.

Beelmann, A. *et al.* (2022) Parent training programs for preventing and treating antisocial behavior in children and adolescents: a comprehensive meta-analysis of international studies. *Aggression and Violent Behavior* **68**, 101798. doi:10.1016/j.avb.2022.101798.

Belsky, J. *et al.* (2022) Differential susceptibility 2.0: are the same children affected by different experiences and exposures? *Development and Psychopathology* **34**(3), 1025–1033.

Betancourt, T. *et al.* (2020) Promoting parent-child relationships and preventing violence via home-visiting: cluster RCT among Rwandan families linked to social protection programmes. *BMC Public Health* **20**, 1–11.

Bierman, K. *et al.* (2017) Fast track randomised controlled trial to prevent externalising psychiatric disorders: findings from grades 3 to 9. In: *Effective Interventions for Children in Need.* (eds M. Little & B. Maughan). Taylor and Francis, London, New York. pp. 97–109.

Black, C. *et al.* (2023) Applying human-centered design in global mental health to improve reach among underserved populations in the United States and India. *Global Health: Science and Practice* **11**(1), e2200312.

Bohman, M. (1996) Predisposition to criminality: Swedish adoption studies in retrospect. In: *Genetics of Criminal and Antisocial Behaviour.* (eds G. Bock & J. Goode). Wiley, Chichester, UK. pp. 99–114.

Bose, D. *et al.* (2022) Therapeutic alliance in psychosocial interventions for youth internalizing disorders: a systematic review and preliminary meta-analysis. *Clinical Psychology: Science and Practice* **29**(2), 124.

Briskman, J. & Scott, S. (2013) *Randomised Controlled Trial of Fostering Changes Parenting Groups for Fostered Children.* DfE, London.

Chan, K. *et al.* (2019) The effectiveness of interventions for grandparents raising grandchildren: a meta-analysis. *Research on Social Work Practice* **29**, 607–617.

Chhangur, R. & Belsky, J. (2023) Parents' differential susceptibility to a "micro" parenting intervention: rationale and study protocol for a randomized controlled microtrial. *PLoS One* **18**(3), e0282207.

Chu, J. *et al.* (2015) Parent and adolescent effects of a universal group program for the parenting of adolescents. *Prevention Science* **16**, 609–620.

Coatsworth, J. *et al.* (2015) Integrating mindfulness with parent training: effects of the mindfulness-enhanced strengthening families program. *Developmental Psychology* **51**, 26–35. doi:10.1037/a0038212.

Collyer, H. *et al.* (2020) Systematic literature review and meta-analysis of the relationship between adherence, competence and outcome in psychotherapy for children and adolescents. *European Child & Adolescent Psychiatry* **29**, 417–431. doi:10.1007/s00787-018-1265-2.

Compas, B. *et al.* (2009) Randomized controlled trial of a family cognitive-behavioral preventive intervention for children of depressed parents. *Journal of Consulting and Clinical Psychology* **77**, 1007–1020. doi:10.1037/a0016930.

Creswell, C. *et al.* (2020) Practitioner review: anxiety disorders in children and young people–assessment and treatment. *Journal of Child Psychology and Psychiatry* **61**, 628–643.

Cuartas, J. *et al.* (2023) The climate crisis and violence against children. *The Lancet Child & Adolescent Health* **7**(9), 605–607.

Dadds, M. *et al.* (2018) Keeping parents involved: predicting attrition in a self-directed, online program for childhood conduct problems. *Journal of Clinical Child and Adolescent Psychology.* doi:10.1080/15374416.2018.1485109.

Daley, D. *et al.* (2014) Behavioural interventions in attention deficit/hyperactivity disorder: a meta-analysis of RCTs across multiple outcome domains. *Journal of the American Academy of Child and Adolescent Psychiatry* **53**, 835–847.

Daley, D. *et al.* (2018) Practitioner review: current best practice in the use of parent training and other behavioural interventions in the treatment of children and adolescents with attention deficit hyperactivity disorder. *Journal of Child Psychology and Psychiatry* **59**(9), 932–947.

Dawe, S. *et al.* (2021) Moderators and mediators of outcomes of parents with substance use problems: further evaluation of the parents under pressure programme. *Addiction* **116**, 3206–3218.

Eames, C. *et al.* (2009) Treatment fidelity as a predictor of behaviour change in parents attending group-based parent-training. *Child Care Health and Development* **35**, 603–612.

Eley, T. *et al.* (2010) Does childhood anxiety evoke maternal control? A genetically informed study. *Journal of Child Psychology and Psychiatry* **51**, 772–779.

Farrington, D. *et al.* (2023) *Offending from Childhood to Late Middle Age: Recent Results from the Cambridge Study*, 2nd edn. Springer, New York.

Fearon, R. & Roisman, G. (2017) Attachment theory: progress and future directions. *Current Opinion in Psychology* **15**, 131–136.

Feuerman, M. (2022) Parenting together when you can't agree on a parenting style. *Parents*. Available: https://www.verywellfamily.com/tips-dont-agree-on-parenting-4107372 [8 October 2024].

Fleming, G. *et al.* (2022) Parent training adapted to the needs of children with callous–unemotional traits: a randomized controlled trial. *Behavior Therapy* **53**, 1265–1281.

Ford, T. *et al.* (2018) The effectiveness and cost-effectiveness of the incredible years teacher classroom management programme in primary school children: results of the STARS cluster randomised controlled trial. *Psychological Medicine*, 1–15. doi:10.1017/S0033291718001484.

Forehand, R. *et al.* (2014) Is parenting the mediator of change in behavioral parent training for externalizing problems of youth? *Clinical Psychology Review* **34**, 608–619. doi:10.1016/j.cpr.2014.10.001.

Forgatch, M. *et al.* (2005) Evaluating fidelity: predictive validity for a measure of competent adherence to the Oregon model of parent training. *Behavior Therapy* **36**, 3–13.

Fraley, C. & Roisman, G. (2015) Do early caregiving experiences leave an enduring or transient mark on developmental adaptation? *Current Opinion in Psychology* **1**, 101–106.

Gardner, F. *et al.* (2006) Randomised controlled trial of a parenting intervention in the voluntary sector for reducing child conduct problems: outcomes and mechanisms of change. *Journal of Child Psychology and Psychiatry* **47**(11), 1123–1132.

Gardner, F. *et al.* (2016) Transporting evidence-based parenting programs for child problem behavior (age 3–10) between countries: systematic review and meta-analysis. *Journal of Clinical Child and Adolescent Psychology* **45**, 749–762.

Gardner, F. *et al.* (2019a) Equity effects of parenting interventions for child conduct problems: a pan-European individual participant data meta-analysis. *Lancet Psychiatry* **6**, 518–527.

Gardner, F. *et al.* (2019b) The earlier the better? Individual participant data and traditional meta-analysis of age effects of parenting interventions. *Child Development* **90**, 7–19.

Gonzalez, J. *et al.* (2023) Intervention and implementation characteristics to enhance father engagement: a systematic review of parenting interventions. *Clinical Child and Family Psychology Review* **26**, 445–458.

Groenman, A.P. *et al.* (2022) An individual participant data meta-analysis: behavioral treatments for children and adolescents with attention-deficit/hyperactivity disorder. *Journal of the American Academy of Child & Adolescent Psychiatry* **61**(2), 144–158.

Groh, A. *et al.* (2017) Attachment in the early life course: meta-analytic evidence for its role in socioemotional development. *Child Development Perspectives* **11**, 70–76.

Gubbels, J. *et al.* (2019) The effectiveness of parent training programs for child maltreatment and their components: a meta-analysis. *International Journal of Environmental Research and Public Health* **16**, 2404.

Harold, G. & Sellers, R. (2018) Annual research review: Interparental conflict and youth psychopathology: an evidence review and practice-focused update. *Journal of Child Psychology and Psychiatry* **59**, 374–402. doi:10.1111/jcpp.12893.

Harold, G.T. *et al.* (2017) How can genetically informed research help inform the next generation of interparental and parenting interventions? *Child Development* **88**(2), 446–458.

Harris, M. *et al.* (2020) Technology-assisted parenting interventions for families experiencing social disadvantage: a meta-analysis. *Prevention Science* **21**, 714–727.

Jeong, J. *et al.* (2021) Parenting interventions to promote early child development in the first three years of life: a global systematic review and meta-analysis. *PLoS Medicine* **18**, e1003602.

Joseph, M. *et al.* (2014) The formation of secure new attachments by children who were maltreated: an observational study of adolescents in foster care. *Development and Psychopathology* **26**, 67–80.

Karjalainen, P. *et al.* (2021) Parent- and teacher-reported long-term effects of parent training on child conduct problems in families with child protection services: RCT. *Child and Adolescent Psychiatry and Mental Health* **15**, 7. doi:10.1186/s13034-021-00358-6.

Kjøbli, J. *et al.* (2023) Research review: effects of parenting programs for children's conduct problems on children's emotional problems—a network meta-analysis. *Journal of Child Psychology and Psychiatry* **64**, 348–356.

Knerr, W. *et al.* (2013) Improving positive parenting skills and reducing harsh and abusive parenting in low-and middle-income countries: a systematic review. *Prevention Science* **14**, 352–363.

Kraemer, H. *et al.* (2002) Mediators and moderators of treatment effects. *Archives of General Psychiatry* **59**, 877–883.

Lachman, J. *et al.* (2021) Integrating parent management training within a conditional cash transfer system for low-income families: results from a small-scale randomized trial in the Philippines. *The Lancet Regional Health* **17**, 100279.

Lawrence, P. *et al.* (2021) Supporting the parents of children and young people with anxiety and depressive disorders is an opportunity not to be missed: a scoping review. *The Lancet Psychiatry* **8**, 909–918.

Leijten, P. *et al.* (2013) Does socioeconomic status matter? A meta-analysis on parent training effectiveness for disruptive child behavior. *Journal Clinical Child Adolescent Psychology* **42**, 384–392.

Leijten, P. *et al.* (2016) Transported versus homegrown parenting interventions for reducing disruptive child behavior: a multilevel meta-regression study. *Journal of the American Academy of Child and Adolescent Psychiatry* **55**, 610–617.

Leijten, P. *et al.* (2019) Meta-analyses: key parenting program components for disruptive child behavior. *Journal of the American Academy of Child and Adolescent Psychiatry* **58**, 180–190.

Leijten, P. *et al.* (2021) Optimizing psychological therapy by disentangling intervention effects: a review of research strategies. *Clinical Psychological Science* **9**, 307–322.

Littell, J. *et al.* (2021) Multisystemic Therapy® for social, emotional, and behavioural problems in youth age 10 to 17: an updated systematic review and meta-analysis. *Campbell Systematic Reviews* **17**, e1158. doi:10.1002/cl2.1158.

Littell, J. *et al.* (2023) Functional family therapy for families of youth (age 11–18) with behaviour problems: a systematic review and meta-analysis. *Campbell Systematic Reviews* **19**, e1324. doi:10.1002/cl2.1324.

McMahon, R. *et al.* (2021) Moderators of psychosocial intervention response for children and adolescents with conduct problems. *Journal of Clinical Child and Adolescent Psychology* **50**, 525–533.

Miller, K. *et al.* (2020) Supporting Syrian families displaced by armed conflict: a pilot randomized controlled trial of the caregiver support intervention. *Child Abuse & Neglect* **108**, 104512.

NICE (2019) Recognition, Intervention and Management of Antisocial Behaviour and Conduct Disorders in Children & Young People. Guideline NG87. National Institute for Health and Care Excellence (NICE), London. Available: https://www.nice.org.uk/guidance/ng87 [8 October 2024].

Ollendick, T.H. *et al.* (2008) Comorbidity as a predictor and moderator of treatment outcome in youth with anxiety, affective, ADHD, and ODD/CD. *Clinical Psychology Review* **28**, 1447–1471.

Patterson, G. (1982) *Coercive Family Process*. Castalia, Eugene, OR.

Perlstein, S. *et al.* (2023) Treatment of childhood disruptive behavior disorders and callous-unemotional traits: a systematic review and two multilevel meta-analyses. *Journal of Child Psychology and Psychiatry*. doi:10.1111/jcpp.13774.

Pettit, G. *et al.* (1999) The impact of peer contact on adolescent externalizing problems is moderated by parental monitoring, perceived neighborhood safety, and prior adjustment. *Child Development* **70**, 768–778.

Puffer, E. *et al.* (2017) The impact of a family skills training intervention among Burmese migrant families in Thailand: a randomized controlled trial. *PLoS One* **12**(3), e0172611.

Reid, M. *et al.* (2001) Parent training in HeadStart: a comparison of response among African-American, Asian-American, Caucasian, and Hispanic Mothers. *Prevention Science* **2**, 209–227.

Sanders, M. (2023) The Triple P system of evidence-based parenting support: past, present, and future directions. *Clinical Child and Family Psychology Review* **26**, 880–903. doi:10.1007/s10567-023-00441-8.

Schachar, R. *et al.* (1987) Changes in family functioning and relationships in children who respond to methylphenidate. *Journal of the American Academy of Child and Adolescent Psychiatry* **26**, 728–732.

Schoemaker, N. *et al.* (2020) A meta-analytic review of parenting interventions in foster care and adoption. *Development and Psychopathology* **32**, 1149–1172. doi:10.1017/S0954579419000798.

Scott, S. (2017) A national approach to improving child and adolescent mental health care: the children and young people's improving access to psychological therapies programme in England. In: *Evidence-based Psychotherapies for Children and Adolescents*. (eds J. Weisz & A. Kazdin). Guilford, New York. pp. 415–428.

Scott, S. & Dadds, M. (2009) When parent training doesn't work: theory-driven clinical strategies. *Journal of Child Psychology and Psychiatry* **50**, 1441–1450.

Scott, S. & O'Connor, T. (2012) An experimental test of differential susceptibility to parenting among emotionally dysregulated children. *Journal of Child Psychology and Psychiatry* **53**, 1184–1193.

Scott, S. *et al.* (2010) Randomized controlled trial of parenting groups for child antisocial behavior targeting multiple risk factors: the SPOKES project. *Journal of Child Psychology and Psychiatry* **51**, 48–57.

Scott, S. *et al.* (2011) Attachment in adolescence: overlap with parenting and unique prediction of behavioural adjustment. *Journal of Child Psychology and Psychiatry* **52**, 1052–1062.

Scott, S. *et al.* (2014) Early prevention of antisocial personality: long-term follow-up of two randomized controlled trials comparing indicated and selective approaches. *The American Journal of Psychiatry* **171**, 649–657.

Senior, R. *et al.* (2023) Personalised interventions for parents who have children with behaviour problems: registered trial protocol. *ISRCTN Registry* Available: https://www.isrctn.com/ISRCTN15678369 [8 October 2024].

Simkiss, D. *et al.* (2013) Effectiveness and cost-effectiveness of a universal parenting skills programme in deprived communities: multicentre randomised controlled trial. *BMJ Open* **3**, e002851.

Sroufe, A. *et al.* (2010) Conceptualising the role of early experience: lessons from the Minnesota longitudinal study. *Developmental Review* **30**, 36–51.

Sugaya, L.S. *et al.* (2022) Efficacy and safety of methylphenidate and behavioural parent training for children aged 3–5 years with attention-deficit hyperactivity disorder: a randomised, double-blind, placebo-controlled, and sham behavioural parent training-controlled trial. *The Lancet Child & Adolescent Health* **6**(12), 845–856.

Van Aar, J. *et al.* (2017) Sustained, fade-out or sleeper effects? A systematic review and meta-analysis of parenting interventions for disruptive child behavior. *Clinical Psychology Review* **51**, 153–163.

Van IJzendoorn, M. *et al.* (2023) improving parenting, child attachment, and externalising behaviours: meta-analysis of the first 25 RCTs on the effects of video feedback intervention to promote positive parenting and sensitive discipline. *Development and Psychopathology* **35**, 241–256.

Vaughan, E. *et al.* (2022) Longitudinal associations of parental monitoring and delinquent peer affiliation: the potential influence of parental solicitation and monitoring rules. *Journal of Adolescence* **94**, 656–666. doi:10.1002/jad.12054.

Ward, C. *et al.* (2020) Parenting for lifelong health: randomized trial of a parenting program in South Africa to prevent harsh parenting and child conduct problems. *Journal of Child Psychology and Psychiatry* **61**, 503–512.

WHO (2023) *WHO Guidelines on Parenting Interventions for Reducing Maltreatment and Enhancing Parent–Child Relationships with Children Aged 0–17 Years*. World Health Organization (WHO), Geneva, Switzerland. https://iris.who.int/bitstream/handle/10665/365814/9789240065505-eng.pdf?sequence=1

Wolchik, S. *et al.* (2022) Effects of an asynchronous, fully web-based parenting-after-divorce program to reduce interparental conflict, increase quality of parenting and reduce children's post-divorce behavior problems. *Family Court Review* **60**(3), 474–491. doi:10.1111/fcre.12620.

CHAPTER 34
Cognitive and behavioral therapies for children and young people

Cathy Creswell[1,2] and Eleanor Leigh[1]

[1] Department of Experimental Psychology, University of Oxford, Oxford, UK
[2] Department of Psychiatry, University of Oxford, Oxford, UK

Cognitive behavioral therapy (CBT) is a family of treatments underpinned by theory centered around the role of thoughts and/or behavioral responses in maintaining psychological difficulties. In this chapter, we provide a brief historical introduction to CBT before highlighting common features of the therapeutic process and core techniques used to bring about change in CBT. Much of the background is informed by work on anxiety disorders in children and young people (CYP) as this is where we have the most extensive evidence. However, we also provide a brief overview of the evidence base for CBT with CYP across different clinical areas. Finally, we consider current challenges and recent developments, including advances in addressing comorbid problems, more developmentally informed CBT models, and increasing access to CBT, with a focus on traditionally underserved groups.

A brief history of cognitive behavioral therapy theory and practice

The behavioral origins of CBT were based on the principles of classical and operant conditioning. Classical conditioning can be described with reference to the well-known example of Pavlov's dog, in which it was noted that food (the unconditioned stimulus) automatically produced salivation (the unconditioned response) and then when food was repeatedly paired with the sound of a bell (the conditioned stimulus) the dog began to salivate in response to the sound of the bell (the conditioned response). This effect could also be extinguished when the bell was repeatedly presented without food ("extinction"). Importantly for the development of behavior therapy, classical conditioning could also be applied to emotional responses such as fear.

Operant conditioning refers to behaviors increasing in frequency because they are followed by positive consequences ("positive reinforcement") or by the absence of expected negative consequences ("negative reinforcement"). In addition, the frequency of behaviors may decrease because they are followed by negative experiences ("punishment") or because of the absence of expected reward ("frustrative nonreward"). Of note, operant models were influential in the development of parenting approaches for child behavior problems (see Chapter 33). Classical and operant conditioning theories were later integrated, for example, in Mowrer's Two-Factor Theory (1960) which proposed that fears may develop through a process of classical conditioning, but are maintained by negative reinforcement associated with avoidance of the aversive conditioned stimuli.

This work underpinned behavioral treatments, particularly for fear-based problems, which involved exposure to feared objects simultaneously accompanied by stimuli that would bring about a stronger alternative response ("reciprocal inhibition"). For example, Wolpe (1958) developed the procedure of gradually working through a hierarchy of feared stimuli while engaging in relaxation exercises, which were thought to reciprocally inhibit the fear response ("systematic desensitization"). It has since been established that exposure to feared situations was the key element for successful anxiety reduction (Davison, 1968), and neither a rigid graded approach nor paired relaxation are necessary for successful outcomes.

As behavior therapy became widely accepted, there was also a growing focus on situations in which behavior therapy did not appear to work. One example was when depressed patients engaged in potentially reinforcing activities but achieved limited benefits as patients would continue to interpret the experience in a negative light, e.g., "I only received praise because they felt sorry

Rutter's Child and Adolescent Psychiatry and Psychology, Seventh Edition.
Edited by Anita Thapar, Daniel S. Pine, Samuele Cortese, Cathy Creswell, Tamsin J. Ford, James F. Leckman, and Argyris Stringaris.

Companion website: www.wiley.com/go/thapar/rutterspsych7

for me." This observation underpinned developments, such as Beck's (1967) influential cognitive model of depression, which highlighted the critical role of negative thoughts in the *maintenance of* depression rather than seeing them solely as a symptom. This model was subsequently extended to a broad range of emotional disorders (Beck, 1976) with a central emphasis on how individuals process information (in terms of biases in memory, attention, and thoughts/beliefs) and how this prevents new, adaptive learning. Discoveries relating to learning through observation were also influential (Bandura, 1977), leading to inclusion of strategies such as modeling and role-play within treatment.

Since the development of cognitive theories and therapy, much research has continued to improve our understanding of the cognitive and behavioral processes that maintain psychological difficulties and how to best address them. Since the 2000s, we have also seen the emergence of "third wave" CBT approaches, such as dialectical behavior therapy (DBT), acceptance and commitment therapy (ACT), and mindfulness-based cognitive therapy (MBCT). As an example, DBT was developed to treat individuals with "borderline personality disorder." In common with other "third-wave" approaches, the focus of DBT is on recognizing and accepting difficult thoughts and feelings in addition to attempting to modify them as one would in traditional CBT (see Chapter 67 on Personality Disorders).

Cognitive and/or behavioral?

As can be seen from our brief history, CBT is not one treatment approach but rather a family of interventions. Today, we see the application of behavior therapy, cognitive therapy, and an integration of the two approaches with varying degrees of emphasis on cognitive and behavioral aspects (CBT, including third-wave CBT). CBT with CYP has traditionally had a strong behavioral component, often accompanied by strategies to encourage engagement and tolerability of behavioral approaches, such as exposure in the treatments of anxiety and related disorders. This emphasis on exposure has been supported by several studies. For example, Peris *et al.* (2015) found that the introduction of exposure was associated with an acceleration in reductions in anxiety symptom severity during a course of CBT, and in a meta-analysis Whiteside *et al.* (2020) found that a greater amount of in-session exposure was associated with larger treatment effects. Notably, this review also indicated that treatments that included relaxation training have *smaller* treatment effects. It is not clear whether this reflects a tendency for interventions that include relaxation to de-emphasize other important treatment elements, or whether relaxation actively inhibits exposure effects. However, what is clear from wider studies is that the delivery of exposure without preparatory anxiety management strategies appears to be safe, tolerable, and may improve treatment efficiency and outcomes (Whiteside *et al.*, 2015).

Identifying what promotes and impedes adaptive learning from exposure is a critical question for a CBT therapist to address through case formulation and treatment. The development of cognitive models of, for example, social anxiety disorder (SAD) in adults were driven by a careful analysis of why SAD doesn't "self-correct" despite often repeated exposure to social experiences (e.g., Clark & Wells, 1995). Notably, the techniques that have been developed to target cognitions typically involve a focus on behaviors, for example, experimenting to see what happens when exposure takes place without safety behaviors (things that an individual does to try to minimize threat when they enter a fear-inducing situation, e.g., avoiding eye contact; Leigh *et al.*, 2021).

In parallel, learning theory-based approaches have examined the contexts and conditions required to optimize exposure (e.g., Craske *et al.*, 2008), moving exposure practice away from a reliance on habituation (i.e., a decrease in response after repeated presentations of a stimuli) and toward boosting opportunities for inhibitory learning (i.e., developing new nonthreatening associations that overshadow previously held threatening associations). While there has been far less conclusive research on this with CYP, recent studies highlight the potential to boost outcomes through strategies such as dropping safety behaviors (Plaisted *et al.*, 2021) and other techniques to maximize learning consolidation (Teunisse *et al.*, 2022).

Ultimately, whether an intervention is considered cognitive and/or behavioral will depend on the conceptualization of the presenting problem rather than the specific techniques used, given a general recognition that changing behaviors can be a powerful way to change beliefs, and vice versa. The individual case formulation then guides treatment as we discuss below.

The therapeutic process in cognitive behavioral therapy

Across the family of CBTs, there are a number of therapeutic processes that we would always expect to see. First, CBT is a time-limited approach that works toward explicitly agreed goals that are meaningful to the CYP. In fact, all parts of treatment, not only goals, are made transparent so that the therapist and CYP, and/or parent (see section on "Involving parents"), can work collaboratively together. This approach is facilitated through a clear structure and agreed agenda. CBT is an active approach, where the key task is to create opportunities for new, adaptive learning in the here and now, both within and beyond therapy sessions. Learning is supported through an empirical process of guided discovery, supported by explicitly testing out assumptions and measuring changes in both mechanisms (e.g., negative cognitions) and outcomes (e.g., depression symptoms). Homework is important to ensure that CYP have the opportunity to apply and extend their learning beyond the therapy sessions.

A final point to emphasize is that there is often an assumption that CBT does not consider a CYP's wider environment. However, it is critical to consider how the wider environment may prevent adaptive learning. If a CYP is worried about social situations because they are being bullied, or worried about making mistakes due to an undetected learning difficulty, these will likely contribute to the maintenance of the problem and it is critical that they be addressed.

Core change techniques

Below we describe a selection of change techniques that are used with varying frequency across forms of CBT and clinical conditions. Some CBTs are delivered to parents and much of what is described here in relation to CYP would also apply to work with them.

Psychoeducation

Psychoeducation involves providing information about the CYP's clinical condition, prognosis, and how CBT works. It aims to inform and empower the CYP to better understand and manage their symptoms and to engage as fully as possible in treatment. The stance of the therapist should therefore be one of curiosity and openness, actively encouraging the CYP to ask questions and articulate doubts. Ideally, psychoeducation begins early in the assessment phase (see Chapter 29 on Psychological Assessment in the Clinical Context).

Providing information about the condition aims to answer the "why me" question that many CYP have at the start of therapy. The etiology of the condition is explained using a biopsychosocial model, the range of common symptoms are outlined, and we might list well-known people who experience the same condition to help normalize the CYP's experience. Common myths and misconceptions can be explained. Providing information about prognosis and treatment outcomes can enhance motivation to engage in therapy.

Psychoeducation about CBT involves socializing the CYP to the therapeutic approach and ways of working (see the earlier section on "The therapeutic process in cognitive behavioral therapy"). We find it particularly important to do this with CYP who may look to their therapist as a teacher rather than collaborator.

Formulation

A formulation is a version of the maintenance model personalized to the CYP. The aim is threefold: to ensure the CYP and therapist have a shared understanding of the main problem and agreed focus; to help the CYP notice unhelpful patterns of thinking and behavior; and to provide a springboard and rationale for treatment.

A personalized formulation is typically mapped out in the first session. The therapist will ask the CYP to think of a recent, typical instance when they experienced problematic symptoms (such as feeling anxious or low). The CYP is asked about the thoughts, feelings, and behaviors they experienced at the time and the links between them, and these are mapped out on a whiteboard or paper. Other relevant cognitive and behavioral processes specified in the model (such as mental imagery, attentional processes, or memory features) are identified. The idiosyncratic model may be revisited throughout treatment when new information comes to light or to recap on the treatment rationale.

Different CBT maintenance models, and therefore individual formulations, vary in their emphasis and in how richly specified they are. Figures 34.1 and 34.2 illustrate two formulations, both describing maintenance of social anxiety for a CYP.

Exposure to feared situations

The aim of exposure is to help a CYP to confront and overcome fears, but there are different approaches to this. Some are based on *habituation principles* whereby CYP are encouraged to incrementally face feared situations on a graded hierarchy and remain in the situation until anxiety reduces. CYP are asked to rate their anxiety regularly on a scale (e.g., 0–10), via subjective units of distress (SUDS) ratings. *Inhibitory learning approaches* involve testing a prediction in an exposure task, while maximizing the element of surprise and reducing use of safety behaviors. In *cognitive approaches*, exposure to feared situations is undertaken within behavioral experiments, whereby CYP test their predictions while minimizing cognitive and behavioral processes that impede learning, and then reflect and generalize learning. Typically, there is less of a focus on SUDS ratings in cognitive approaches. Figure 34.3 illustrates the different approaches to exposure to feared situations with a CYP with panic disorder.

Behavioral activation

Behavioral activation (BA) aims to help reduce depression symptoms by increasing engagement in positive and rewarding activities. As a stand-alone treatment it has been found to have equivalent outcomes to CBT in the treatment for adolescent depression (McCauley *et al.*, 2016). There is an emphasis on understanding the function or purpose of avoidance behaviors in a given context; certain cognitive and behavioral responses make sense given the environment but may have unintended and unhelpful consequences, leading to maintenance of depression. Avoidance can be behavioral, e.g., declining invitations, not speaking, or it can be cognitive, e.g., thought suppression, rumination. The therapist helps the CYP use alternative "approach" behaviors in line with their values (what is meaningful and important in their life). For example, in therapy, a depressed CYP might discover that when faced with lots of homework (environmental trigger), they tend to feel overwhelmed and hopeless (symptoms of depression), and climb into bed and think about how rubbish they are (responses). The responses are understandable but unhelpful, and the CYP is supported to identify and practice alternative "approach" behaviors. These might include getting the support of a parent and teacher, breaking the homework into small chunks, texting a friend, and building in breaks and rewards. These help a young person align with their value of doing well in school.

Cognitive restructuring

Cognitive restructuring involves identifying and modifying negative and distorted thoughts and patterns of thinking. It is core to CBT for depression but used in many forms of CBT.

The first step in cognitive restructuring is to identify problematic automatic negative thoughts. Examples include "I always mess up," "I'm useless." It is often difficult for CYP to identify

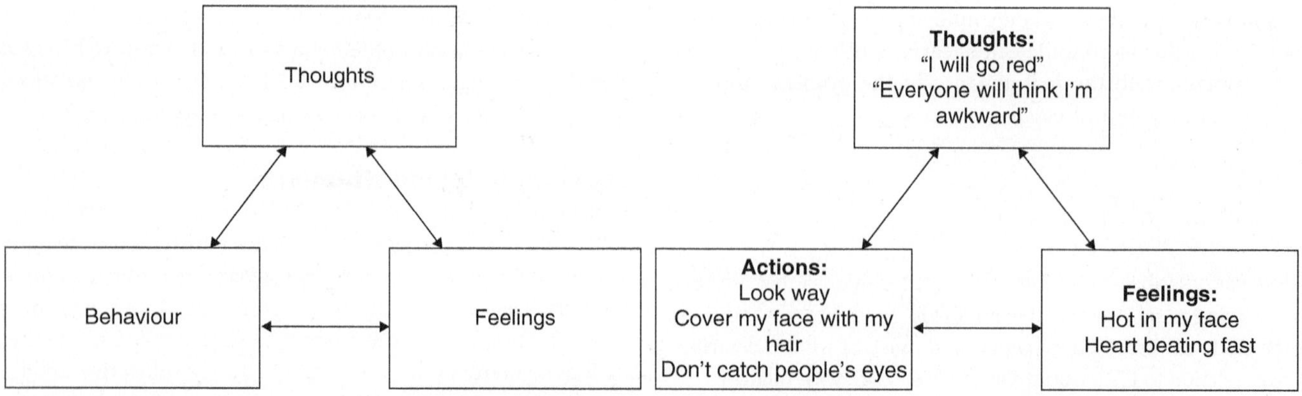

Figure 34.1 Left-hand side: broad-based cognitive behavioral therapy (CBT) model. Right-hand side: personalized version of the model for children and young people (CYP) with social anxiety.

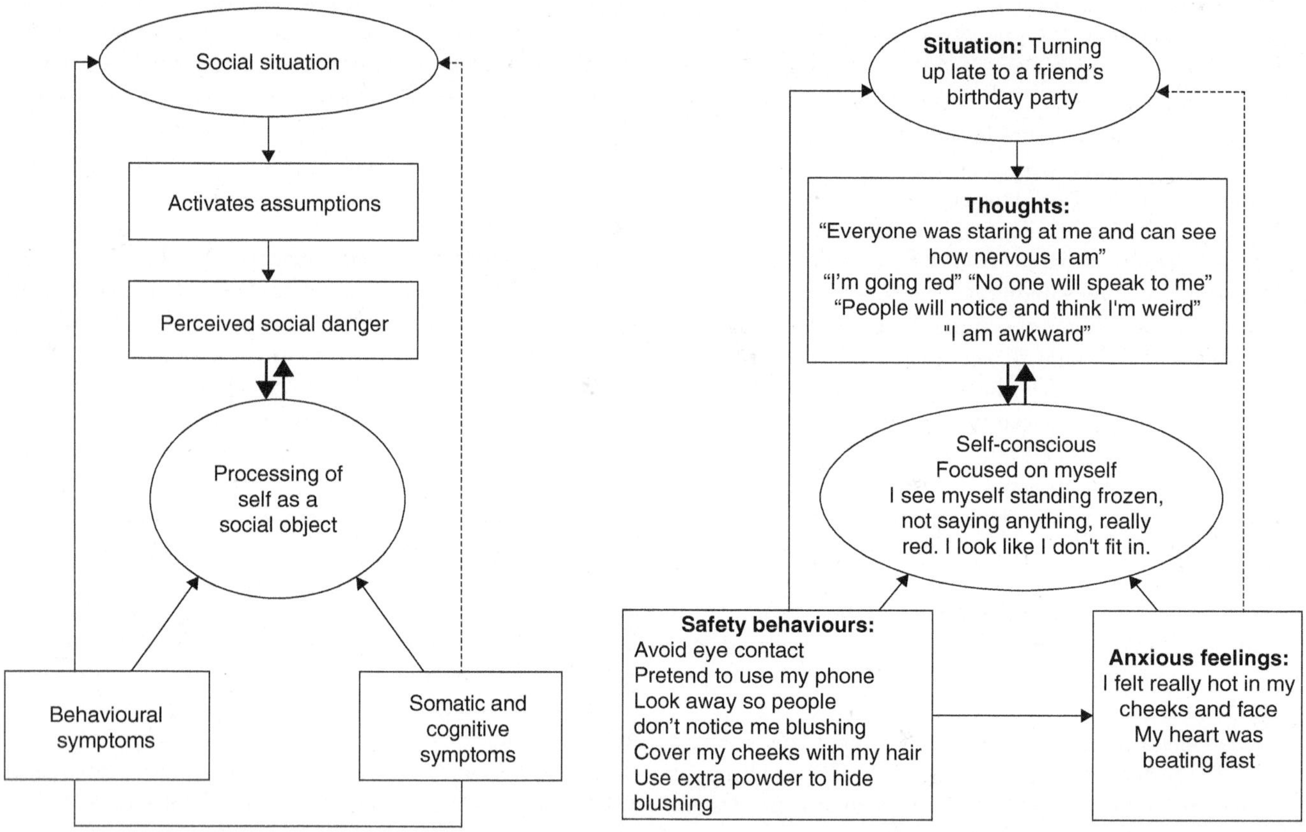

Figure 34.2 Left-hand side: Clark and Wells cognitive model of social anxiety (Clark & Wells, 1995/with permission of American Psychological Association). Right-hand side: personalized version for children and young people (CYP) with social anxiety.

negative thoughts at first because they are habitual, automatic, and unquestioned. One of the most fruitful strategies is to follow the emotion. In session, if the therapist notices the CYP seems to experience a sudden drop in mood, this is often a sign that the CYP is experiencing a negative automatic thought, even if they had not been aware of it. As homework, CYPs are encouraged to look out for shifts in their mood, identify the thoughts, and note these down in a thought tracker (Figure 34.4). With practice, the aim is that the individual notices negative automatic thoughts when they occur, which then provides an opportunity to question the thought and consider alternative perspectives.

The second step in cognitive restructuring is to evaluate the evidence for and against the negative thoughts. This may involve asking questions such as "What evidence do I have to support

Habituation-based exposure task

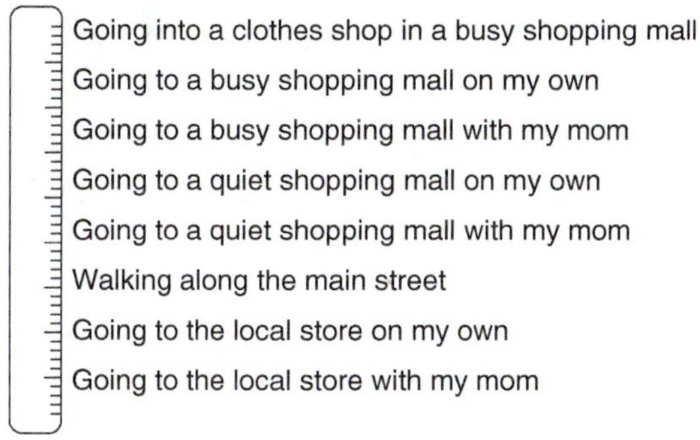

Fear ladder

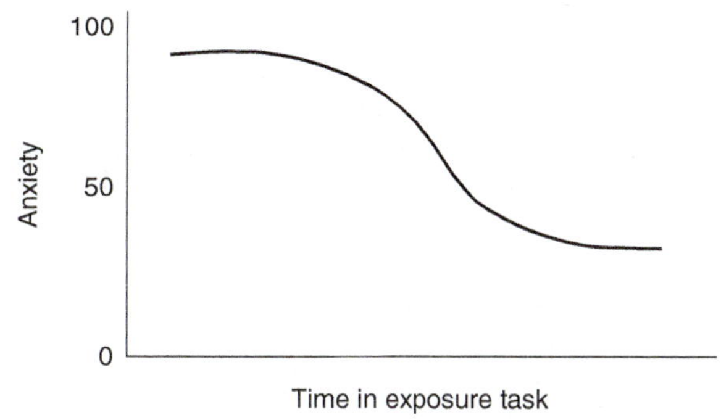

Anxiety ratings for an exposure task.

Inhibitory learning-based exposure task

Before exposure	
Goal	Run around the park
What are you most worried will happen?	My heart will stop and I'll die
On scale of 0–100% how likely does this seem?	75%
After exposure	
Did what you were most worried about occur?	No
How did you know?	I didn't die.
What did you learn?	Just because my heart races doesn't mean I will have a heart attack.

Cognitive exposure task (behavioural experiment)

Focus	Situation	Prediction	Experiment	Outcome	Learning and next steps
My heart stopping	Doing exercise	If my heart rate gets high it means my heart will stop and I'll die. Belief rating: 75%	I will run around the park with my therapist. I won't do my safety behaviours: I won't slow down when my heart rate increases, sip water, or try to control my heartbeat.	I did the experiment and my heart was racing but nothing happened. I was fine. Re-rating belief: 25%	A high heart rate is a sign your heart is working well, not that it is going to stop. It isn't anything to be scared of. I will do this as homework. I will push myself in PE lessons.

Figure 34.3 Examples of different approaches to exposure tasks for children and young people (CYP) with panic disorder.

Thought tracker		
Situation	Feeling	Thought
At home after school, dad has a go at me for not tidying my room.	Angry and sad	"He is always having a go at me" "I never do anything right"

Figure 34.4 Example thought tracker completed by a teenager with depression.

this thought?" and "What evidence do I have that contradicts this thought?" CYP can be encouraged to imagine they are putting their thought "in the dock." Once the evidence has been evaluated, the CYP and therapist work together to generate alternative, more balanced thoughts that can then be tested out in experiments. A teenager with generalized anxiety disorder (GAD) may spend a day making decisions by rolling a dice, to test out the idea that "I can cope with the unexpected."

A common obstacle encountered with this technique is that CYP can feel the therapist is somehow discounting their view. To minimize this, the therapist's stance should be genuinely curious, interested, and unbiased. Another common issue is the head–heart lag, whereby a CYP might intellectually understand that a fear is not realistic and yet continue to feel it to be true. Indeed, while cognitive restructuring can be very helpful in loosening a belief, it is often necessary to then test ideas in action through experiments in order to "feel" the learning.

Imagery techniques

Negative thoughts are often experienced as mental images as well as verbal cognitions. There is increasing appreciation of the relevance and importance of mental imagery across psychopathology. For example, images are experienced in the form of flashbacks and intrusive images in post-traumatic stress disorder (PTSD), as excessively negative self-images of looking foolish in social anxiety, as perceived defects in body dysmorphic disorder (BDD), and as memories of distressing events from the past or suicide-related images of the future in depression.

Imagery techniques can be used from the start of therapy to aid assessment, for example, imaginal reliving of a situation to elicit negative thoughts that are elusive. It is worth noting that CYPs will typically not spontaneously describe experiencing mental images so it is important to explicitly ask about them. Imagery techniques to shift excessively negative imagery linked to distressing memories include imaginal reliving (Ehlers & Clark, 2000; Smith *et al.*, 2007) and imagery rescripting (Arntz & Weertman, 1999). Video feedback with careful verbal preparation is used to correct negative observer perspective images in cognitive therapy for SAD (Warnock-Parkes *et al.*, 2017). Imaginal exposure, involving imagining a fear in vivid detail, is used in various forms of CBT. For example, in GAD (Perrin *et al.*, 2019), worries about being told off in school may be underpinned by the fear that "I am stupid and I'll never get anywhere in life." The CYP is encouraged to describe their fear verbally or in writing in the first person, present tense, with an emphasis on sensory detail, without tempering the emotional intensity. CYP are then encouraged to read or listen back to the account a number of times.

Problem-solving

Problem-solving is found in many forms of CBT. It typically involves two elements: encouraging a positive attitude to problem-solving and teaching systematic problem-solving skills. The steps involved are shown in Figure 34.5. Repeated practice increases skills and improves CYP's confidence in their ability to overcome the obstacles they face.

1. Define the problem
2. Brainstorm possible solutions
3. Evaluate the possible solutions and select one
4. Test it out and reflect on the outcome

Move through steps again if needed

Figure 34.5 Problem-solving steps.

Techniques to scaffold change

Across different forms of CBT, various therapeutic techniques are used to scaffold change that run alongside and support delivery of the core change techniques described above.

In-session tasks

Most CBT sessions involve in-sessions tasks in which individuals test out ideas in real-life situations. They are valuable for a number of reasons. First, they help CYP overcome common obstacles such as low motivation and anxiety. Second, the therapist can encourage a CYP to be more ambitious than they might be alone. Third, the therapist can model certain behaviors for the CYP. This can include the therapist performing certain feared behaviors and giving the CYP the opportunity to see the real-world consequences before trying it out for themselves. For example, when treating a socially anxious teenager who fears shaking, the therapist may intentionally shake and drop their money in a busy shop while the teenager watches. Fourth, the therapist can spot when a CYP is engaging in subtle safety behaviors that they may not have noticed themselves but which can impact on progress.

Involving parents

Evidence on the nature of and outcomes from involvement of parents in CBT for CYP is inconsistent (Lawrence *et al.*, 2021). However, most therapies for CYP will involve parents to some degree, with greater involvement with younger groups, and some forms of CBT being delivered via parents without involving CYP directly (e.g., Creswell *et al.*, 2022). At a minimum, it can be helpful to meet parents at the start of therapy, to understand their perspective on the problem, provide some psychoeducation, and to identify any particular needs in the family that may need addressing such as untreated parental mental illness. Additionally, parents may provide practical support for attending sessions, and completing homework and questionnaires. At other times parents may need to be engaged more directly in therapy, for example, where (typically understandable) parental responses to the child's anxiety may inadvertently be maintaining the problem.

Rewards

While some CYP come to therapy of their own volition, many do not, and this is especially true for younger children and for those with certain conditions, such as separation anxiety. Even those who are motivated may struggle to engage in challenging therapy tasks. One aims to create therapeutic tasks that are aligned with a young person's goals so that they are inherently rewarding. For example, a behavioral experiment for a teenager with panic disorder may revolve around going to a shop which stocks their favorite clothing brand. However, this is not always possible and sometimes judicious use of rewards is helpful to motivate, with the aim of enabling CYP to engage in tasks from which they can learn something new. Rewards should be planned in advance (with agreement of parents) and be explicitly tethered to the CBT task. Stickers or activity-based rewards are typically chosen over financial rewards.

Empirical support for cognitive behavioral therapy: considerations and review

This brief overview of the state of the evidence base for CBT in CYP is in no way comprehensive. We direct interested readers to relevant chapters in Part IV for the evidence base for CBT for different conditions.

Randomized controlled trials (RCTs) are generally considered to be the gold standard for evaluating the effectiveness of interventions such as CBT, but there are a host of design and methodological issues that can impact on validity and reliability of results. A notable example is the choice of comparator. Many psychotherapy trials adopt a waitlist comparator (e.g., James *et al.*, 2020) and effects will inevitably be larger than when compared to active comparisons (e.g., Cuijpers *et al.*, 2023) (and potentially even when compared to observation alone ("nocebo"); Furukawa *et al.*, 2014). It is also worth bearing in mind that the majority of CBT trials are conducted in research settings, making it difficult to draw direct comparisons with the wider body of CBT research and highlighting the need for trials in routine practice. While CBT is broadly well-tolerated, like any other form of therapy that may benefit some individuals, others may experience adverse effects such as a short-term increase in emotional distress. The quality of adverse event reporting in psychological therapy trials is inconsistent and generally low quality with little evidence of improvement in reporting of adverse effects over time (Hayes & Za'ba, 2022).

CBT is well-established for the treatment of anxiety disorders (James *et al.*, 2020, and see Chapter 59), most commonly in a broad-based form designed to treat all common anxiety presentations (e.g., "Coping Cat"; Kendall, 1994). The treatment seems to work similarly well across a range of demographics, including gender, age, ethnicity, and socioeconomic status (Bertie & Hudson, 2021). However, presence of SAD is a consistent predictor/moderator of poorer response (Evans *et al.*, 2021a) and this has motivated the development of SAD specific treatments, including behaviorally focused interventions such as social effectiveness therapy for children (SET-C) (Beidel *et al.*, 2000) and treatments with a cognitive emphasis, such as cognitive therapy for social anxiety disorder (e.g., Leigh & Clark, 2023).

CBT is the most evidence-based treatment for obsessive–compulsive disorder (OCD) (Öst *et al.*, 2016), BDD (Mataix-Cols *et al.*, 2015), and PTSD (Mavranezouli *et al.*, 2020) (see Chapters 60, 61, 58 respectively).

Despite intense research interest spanning decades, effect sizes for CBT for depression in CYP have remained stubbornly small in magnitude (e.g., Eckshtain *et al.* (2020), Weisz *et al.* (2006)). When examining the effectiveness of CBT for depression across the life span, outcomes appear worse for children and adolescents compared to adults (Cuijpers *et al.*, 2020). The findings suggest further work is needed to improve treatment outcomes for depression in CYP, particularly given the burden of the disorder. New directions within CBT interventions have included an enhanced focus on BA (Jenness *et al.*, 2023). Consistent with this, those CBT interventions that have evidenced better outcomes in trials have emphasized BA rather than cognitive restructuring (March *et al.*, 2004; Emslie *et al.*, 2010). In parallel, there has been growing interest in the use of interpersonal psychotherapy for adolescents (IPT-A; Mufson *et al.* (2004)) (see Chapter 36 "Relationship based treatments").

Pharmacotherapy is the first line treatment for bipolar disorder (Brickman & Fristad, 2022; and see Chapter 62), but psychological therapy incorporating psychoeducation and CBT techniques is often provided to alleviate residual symptoms and/or enhance treatment compliance (e.g., Miklowitz *et al.*, 2004). Similarly, the first line treatment for psychosis is medication and there are very few trials of CBT for psychosis in CYP (Stafford *et al.*, 2015), but those that have been published suggest it may be helpful as an adjunctive treatment (Morrison *et al.*, 2020; Müller *et al.*, 2020) (see Chapter 56).

A number of CBT-informed treatments for oppositional and conduct disorders have been developed including parent training programs and child-focused interventions with some evidence of modest effects (Bakker *et al.*, 2017; and see Chapter 65). Stimulant medication is the mainstay treatment of attention deficit hyperactivity disorder (ADHD) and related impairment (DuPaul *et al.*, 2020), but of the psychological interventions, behavioral approaches, such as parent training programs, have the most support in reducing behavioral problems and impairment (Daley *et al.*, 2018), although they appear to have little effect on ADHD symptoms (see Chapter 54).

Evidence is very limited for the use of CBT for eating disorders in CYP but it may be helpful for the treatment of adolescents with bulimia nervosa. However, most of the evidence is for the use of family-based treatments for eating disorders in adolescents, such as the Maudsley Model (Lock & La Via, 2015; and see Chapter 69).

Key challenges and recent developments

Addressing co-occurring mental health problems

Co-occurrence of mental health problems is extremely common among treatment-seeking CYP (e.g., Kendall *et al.*, 2010). While some studies have identified poorer treatment outcomes for those with co-occurring mood and "externalizing" (i.e., conduct disorder (CD), oppositional defiant disorder (ODD), or ADHD) disorders (Hudson *et al.*, 2015) others have not found clear evidence of impaired outcomes (e.g., Kunas *et al.*, 2021).

Notably, however, CBT focused on a primary anxiety disorder can also bring about reductions in symptoms of co-occurring anxiety disorders (Ollendick *et al.*, 2010), depression, and "externalizing" problems (Mahdi *et al.*, 2019). This may reflect the shared applicability of some core components of treatment across disorders, the targeting of potentially shared mechanisms (e.g., threat overestimation, self-efficacy), and/or a direct causal relationship between the disorders (e.g., depression due to impact of social anxiety). This may suggest it is important to focus CBT on targeting one problem and doing it well, while monitoring symptoms and interference associated with co-occurring problems to determine whether further more targeted treatment is required.

An alternative approach with some promising evidence is modular treatment, such as the STEPS program which uses clinical algorithms to guide flexible allocation of treatment components for CYP with anxiety, depression, post-traumatic stress, or conduct problems (Chorpita & Weisz, 2009). An initial RCT indicated that STEPS was associated with a significantly greater rate of improvement than both single disorder-focused CBT and usual care (Weisz *et al.*, 2012), although outcomes were not significantly different to single disorder-focused CBT at two-year follow-up (Chorpita *et al.*, 2013). However, in a more recent trial, STEPS was not superior to usual care which the authors attributed to factors associated with implementation (Weisz *et al.*, 2020).

Modifying cognitive behavioral therapy to account for age and development

Evaluations of CBT have commonly included CYP across broad age ranges, e.g., 7–18 years. While individual therapists undoubtably modify how they deliver treatments to fit the age and development of the CYP they are working with, there has been little direct research examining how CBT should differ to optimize outcomes across childhood and adolescence. Two key areas of adaptation have been highlighted: adaptations to *how* CBT is delivered to ensure it is accessible given a child's cognitive and emotional development (e.g., using visual activities such as cartoons and thought bubbles) and adaptations to the *content* given the different cognitive and behavioral processes that might maintain a disorder at different stages of development (Garber *et al.*, 2016).

Currently, CBT models of psychopathology have limited developmental nuance. However cognitive and behavioral processes implicated in the maintenance of psychopathology, such as children's capacity to see themselves as others see them (Cole *et al.*, 2001), are likely to differ in their effects with age and development. In line with this, some findings suggest that some adult CBT models of psychopathology may fit better for adolescents than younger children (e.g., Fialko *et al.* (2012) for cognitive models of worry; Evans *et al.* (2021b) for cognitive models of SAD). Changing social influences through development are also important to consider (Cole *et al.*, 2001; Blakemore, 2012). In summary, it is important to consider age and development when determining the specific maintenance processes to target in CBT as well as who the treatment is delivered with, to maximize engagement, opportunities for learning through action, and outcomes.

Increasing access

Unfortunately, few CYP who could benefit from CBT access it. Barriers that apply across therapeutic approaches relate to help seeking, problem identification, and accessing professionals (e.g., Radez *et al.*, 2021), but specific CBT barriers can include lack of suitably trained professionals (Baker & Waite, 2020) and capacity to deliver full treatment protocols within stretched services. This is exemplified by studies in the United Kingdom and Australia where the majority of families of CYP with anxiety disorders that had sought help had not received CBT (Reardon *et al.*, 2020; Gandhi *et al.*, 2022).

Recent developments to increase access to CBT have included efficient CBT protocols including single-session interventions and therapist-guided brief interventions, such as remotely delivered forms. The most extensive evidence for single-session interventions for treatment of disorders is likely to be for specific phobias. This approach involves condensed *in vivo* exposure in one prolonged session (up to three hours) and is effective compared to waitlist and active controls (Ollendick *et al.*, 2009). A recent study conducted across real-world child mental health settings found that one session treatment (OST) was noninferior to a full course of CBT (Wright *et al.*, 2023) and was associated with significantly reduced costs (Wang *et al.*, 2022).

Other relatively brief forms of intervention include guided self-help with telephone support, where good outcomes have been achieved for anxiety disorders (Lyneham & Rapee, 2006) and OCD (Turner *et al.*, 2014), and parent-led CBT in which parents are supported by a therapist to apply CBT strategies within their child's day to day life. Parent-led CBT has been applied predominantly with preadolescent children with anxiety problems. Meta-analyses have indicated clinical effectiveness (Jewell *et al.*, 2022) and health economic analyses have indicated cost-effectiveness compared to an alternative brief psychological therapy (Creswell *et al.*, 2017).

In recent years, we have also seen extensive developments in digitally augmented forms of CBT, including for broad anxiety problems (Grist *et al.*, 2019), SAD (Leigh & Clark, 2023), PTSD (Smith *et al.*, 2022), OCD (Babiano-Espinosa *et al.*, 2019), and depression (Grist *et al.*, 2019); see Chapter 49. Here, typically, CBT is delivered via a website or app, with remote therapist support to provide encouragement, personalize content, and troubleshoot. Of particular note, at least two studies have provided good clinical and cost-effectiveness evidence for the integration of digitally augmented therapies as the first step in a CBT-based stepped-care model of treatment delivery (Chatterton *et al.*, 2019; Aspvall *et al.*, 2021), i.e., a treatment delivery model in which the least restrictive treatment is offered first but patients are "stepped up" to more intensive treatments if required (Bower & Gilbody, 2005). Together, these studies highlight the potential to increase CBT efficiency without compromising patient outcomes through brief and digital approaches integrated in service delivery models that capitalize on these efficiencies.

The majority of studies of brief and low-intensity CBT approaches have been conducted in high-income countries. However, the challenges of access to CBT are amplified in low- and middle-income countries (LMICs), where the lack of trained professionals is particularly stark (Saxena *et al.*, 2007). A growing number of trials have demonstrated the effectiveness of CBTs in LMICs (Ribeiro *et al.*, 2023), but there is a clear need to promote implementation at scale. Examples include the development of manuals that can be used by inexperienced personnel (Yule *et al.*, 2013). For example, in a recent trial in India, a school-based lay counselor-delivered problem-solving intervention for adolescents with diverse mental health problems was superior to unguided problem-solving (Michelson *et al.*, 2020).

Cognitive behavioral therapy with vulnerable and underserved children and young people

Evaluations of CBT have predominantly underrepresented groups of CYP who are known to be at particular risk of mental health problems, including ethnic minority CYP, those with experience of the care system, refugees and asylum seekers, sexual or gender minority youth, and neurodiverse CYP. However, there is growing evidence for the effectiveness of CBT among many previously underserved groups.

In a recent systematic review, Pina *et al.* (2019) concluded that CBT for anxiety is now well-established for Hispanic/Latino CYP, although outcomes may be compromised when there is no consideration of cultural contextual factors; but few other CBT programs could be described as "well-supported" specifically with ethnic minority CYP due to a lack of evidence. Clearly, there remains a huge amount of work to ensure equal access and outcome optimization for CYP regardless of their ethnicity.

Despite high rates of mental health problems among CYP who have experienced out-of-home care, professionals seem less likely to deliver recommended treatments for PTSD (e.g., trauma-focused cognitive therapy) for these CYP (McGuire *et al.*, 2022). However, Hiller *et al.* (2021) have found strong evidence for the applicability of cognitive models of PTSD among CYP in out-of-home care, and there is consistent evidence that trauma-focused CBT is an effective treatment for PTSD in maltreated CYP (Bennett *et al.*, 2021). Although studies are limited, trauma-focused CBT also appears to be effective for refugee CYP (Chipalo, 2021).

In relation to neurodiversity, there is now substantial evidence that CBT is effective for anxiety disorders in autistic CYP, at least in the short term (Sharma *et al.*, 2021). These trials have typically modified CBT to better meet the needs of autistic CYP (Walters *et al.*, 2016). Indeed, a recent trial highlighted additional advantages of specifically adapted CBT over more standard CBT, with adaptations including enhanced parental involvement, additional focus on social engagement, and use of "special interests" as an asset (Wood *et al.*, 2020).

Research to examine the application of CBT with lesbian, gay, bisexual, and transgender (LGBT) youth is limited. However, there is promising support for affirmative-CBT (A-CBT) which uses the CBT framework to explore and validate the positive expression of LGBT identities while recognizing the effects of discrimination on young people's mental health (Craig *et al.*, 2019).

This section is far from comprehensive and we would refer you to a number of other chapters that address the needs of particular groups of CYP in greater detail. However, we are keen to emphasize that, while there is evidence to support CBT adaptations to maximize engagement and outcomes by meeting individual CYP's particular needs, it is also evident that ruling out CBT (in the absence of evidence for an alternative therapeutic approach) because of someone's individual characteristics or circumstances risks withholding evidence-based treatment from CYP who have traditionally experienced marked health disparities.

Conclusions and future directions

We now have robust evidence that CBT is effective for a range of psychological disorders in CYP when compared to waitlist, along with some evidence of clinical and/or cost-effectiveness benefits when compared to alternative treatments. Overall, there remains little consistency in research on predictors of treatment response from CBT, which should encourage clinicians to feel comfortable offering CBT to CYP with any of the conditions where an evidence base has been established. The main challenge we currently face is increasing access to CBT. Given the established benefits for a range of disorders, it is imperative that we develop new models of service delivery to enable widespread delivery in ways that continue to achieve good outcomes for CYP.

References

Arntz, A. & Weertman, A. (1999) Treatment of childhood memories: theory and practice. *Behaviour Research and Therapy* **37**, 715–740.

Aspvall, K. *et al.* (2021) Effect of an internet-delivered stepped-care program vs in-person cognitive behavioral therapy on obsessive-compulsive disorder symptoms in children and adolescents: a randomized clinical trial. *JAMA* **325**, 1863–1873.

Babiano-Espinosa, L. *et al.* (2019) Acceptability, feasibility, and efficacy of internet cognitive behavioral therapy (iCBT) for pediatric obsessive-compulsive disorder: a systematic review. *Systematic Reviews* **8**, 284.

Baker, H.J. & Waite, P. (2020) The identification and psychological treatment of panic disorder in adolescents: a survey of CAMHS clinicians. *Child and Adolescent Mental Health* **25**, 135–142.

Bakker, M.J. *et al.* (2017) Practitioner review: psychological treatments for children and adolescents with conduct disorder problems—a systematic review and meta-analysis. *Journal of Child Psychology and Psychiatry* **58**, 4–18.

Bandura, A. (1977) Self-efficacy: toward a unifying theory of behavioral change. *Psychological Review* **84**, 191–215.

Beck, A. (1967) *Cognitive Therapy and the Behavioral Disorders.* Meridian, New York.

Beck, A. (1976) *Cognitive Therapy and the Emotional Disorders.* Meridian, New York. pp. 306–310.

Beidel, D.C. *et al.* (2000) Behavioral treatment of childhood social phobia. *Journal of Consulting and Clinical Psychology* **68**, 1072–1080.

Bennett, R.S. *et al.* (2021) A systematic review of controlled-trials for PTSD in maltreated children and adolescents. *Child Maltreatment* **26**, 325–343.

Bertie, L.-A. & Hudson, J.L. (2021) CBT for childhood anxiety: reviewing the state of personalised intervention research. *Frontiers in Psychology* **12**.

Blakemore, S.-J. (2012) Development of the social brain in adolescence. *Journal of the Royal Society of Medicine* **105**, 111–116.

Bower, P. & Gilbody, S. (2005) Stepped care in psychological therapies: access, effectiveness and efficiency: narrative literature review. *The British Journal of Psychiatry* **186**, 11–17.

Brickman, H.M. & Fristad, M.A. (2022) Psychosocial treatments for bipolar disorder in children and adolescents. *Annual Review of Clinical Psychology* **18**, 291–327.

Chatterton, M.L. *et al.* (2019) Economic evaluation of stepped care for the management of childhood anxiety disorders: results from a randomised trial. *The Australian and New Zealand Journal of Psychiatry* **53**, 673–682.

Chipalo, E. (2021) Is trauma focused-cognitive Behavioral therapy (TF-CBT) effective in reducing trauma symptoms among traumatized refugee children? A systematic review. *Journal of Child & Adolescent Trauma* **14**, 545–558.

Chorpita, B.F. & Weisz, J.R. (2009) *MATCH-ADTC: Modular Approach to Therapy for Children with Anxiety, Depression, Trauma, or Conduct Problems.* PracticeWise, Satellite Beach, FL.

Chorpita, B.F. *et al.* (2013) Long-term outcomes for the child STEPs randomized effectiveness trial: a comparison of modular and standard treatment designs with usual care. *Journal of Consulting and Clinical Psychology* **81**, 999.

Clark, D.M. & Wells, A. (1995) A cognitive model of social phobia. In: *Social Phobia: DIAGNOSIS, Assessment, and Treatment.* (eds R.G. Heimberg, *et al.*). Guilford Press, New York. pp. 69–93.

Cole, D.A. *et al.* (2001) Social origins of depressive cognitions: a longitudinal study of self-perceived competence in children. *Cognitive Therapy and Research* **25**, 377–395.

Craig, S.L. *et al.* (2019) Cognitive–behavioral therapy for sexual and gender minority youth mental health. In: *Handbook of Evidence-Based Mental Health Practice with Sexual and Gender Minorities.* (eds J.E. Pachankis, *et al.*). Oxford University Press, New York. pp. 25–50.

Craske, M.G. *et al.* (2008) Optimizing inhibitory learning during exposure therapy. *Behaviour Research and Therapy* **46**, 5–27.

Creswell, C. *et al.* (2017) Clinical outcomes and cost-effectiveness of brief guided parent-delivered cognitive behavioural therapy and solution-focused brief therapy for treatment of childhood anxiety disorders: a randomised controlled trial. *The Lancet Psychiatry* **4**, 529–539.

Creswell, C. *et al.* (2022) Parent-led cognitive behaviour therapy for child anxiety problems: overcoming challenges to increase access to effective treatment. *Behavioural and Cognitive Psychotherapy*, 1–21.

Cuijpers, P. *et al.* (2020) Psychotherapy for depression across different age groups: a systematic review and meta-analysis. *JAMA Psychiatry* **77**(7), 694–702.

Cuijpers, P. *et al.* (2023) Cognitive behavior therapy vs. control conditions, other psychotherapies, pharmacotherapies and combined treatment for depression: a comprehensive meta-analysis including 409 trials with 52,702 patients. *World Psychiatry* **22**, 105–115.

Daley, D. *et al.* (2018) Practitioner review: current best practice in the use of parent training and other behavioural interventions in the treatment of children and adolescents with attention deficit hyperactivity disorder. *Journal of Child Psychology and Psychiatry* **59**, 932–947.

Davison, G.C. (1968) Systematic desensitization as a counterconditioning process. *Journal of Abnormal Psychology* **73**, 91.

Dupaul, G.J. *et al.* (2020) Future directions for psychosocial interventions for children and adolescents with ADHD. *Journal of Clinical Child & Adolescent Psychology* **49**, 134–145.

Eckshtain, D. *et al.* (2020) Meta-analysis: 13-year follow-up of psychotherapy effects on youth depression. *Journal of the American Academy of Child & Adolescent Psychiatry* **59**, 45–63.

Ehlers, A. & Clark, D.M. (2000) A cognitive model of posttraumatic stress disorder. *Behaviour Research and Therapy* **38**, 319–345.

Emslie, G.J. *et al.* (2010) Treatment of resistant depression in adolescents (TORDIA): week 24 outcomes. *The American Journal of Psychiatry* **167**(7), 782–791.

Evans, R. *et al.* (2021a) Are young people with primary social anxiety disorder less likely to recover following generic CBT compared to young people with other primary anxiety disorders? A systematic review and meta-analysis. *Behavioural and Cognitive Psychotherapy* **49**, 352–369.

Evans, R. *et al.* (2021b) Safety behaviours in social anxiety: an examination across adolescence. *Behaviour Research and Therapy* **144**, 103931.

Fialko, L. *et al.* (2012) Applicability of a cognitive model of worry to children and adolescents. *Behaviour Research and Therapy* **50**, 341–349.

Furukawa, T.A. *et al.* (2014) Waiting list may be a nocebo condition in psychotherapy trials: a contribution from network meta-analysis. *Acta Psychiatrica Scandinavica* **130**, 181–192.

Gandhi, E. *et al.* (2022) Receipt of evidence-based care for children and adolescents with anxiety in Australia. *The Australian and New Zealand Journal of Psychiatry* **56**, 1463–1476.

Garber, J. *et al.* (2016) Developmental demands of cognitive behavioral therapy for depression in children and adolescents: cognitive, social, and emotional processes. *Annual Review of Clinical Psychology* **12**, 181–216.

Grist, R. *et al.* (2019) Technology delivered interventions for depression and anxiety in children and adolescents: a systematic review and meta-analysis. *Clinical Child and Family Psychology Review* **22**, 147–171.

Hayes, D. & Za'ba, N. (2022) What metrics of harm are being captured in clinical trials involving talking treatments for young people? A systematic review of registered studies on the ISRCTN. *Counselling and Psychotherapy Research* **22**, 108–129.

Hiller, R.M. *et al.* (2021) A longitudinal study of cognitive predictors of (complex) post-traumatic stress in young people in out-of-home care. *Journal of Child Psychology and Psychiatry* **62**, 48–57.

Hudson, J.L. *et al.* (2015) Clinical predictors of response to cognitive-behavioral therapy in Pediatric anxiety disorders: the genes for treatment (GxT) study. *Journal of the American Academy of Child & Adolescent Psychiatry* **54**, 454–463.

James, A.C. *et al.* (2020) Cognitive behavioural therapy for anxiety disorders in children and adolescents. *Cochrane Database of Systematic Reviews*.

Jenness, J.L. *et al.* (2023) Behavioral activation as a principle-based treatment: developments from a multi-site collaboration to advance adolescent depression treatment. *Evidence-Based Practice in Child and Adolescent Mental Health* **8**, 55–72.

Jewell, C. *et al.* (2022) The impact of parent-only interventions on child anxiety: a systematic review and meta-analysis. *Journal of Affective Disorders* **309**, 324–349.

Kendall, P.C. (1994) Treating anxiety disorders in children: results of a randomized clinical trial. *Journal of Consulting and Clinical Psychology* **62**, 100–110.

Kendall, P.C. *et al.* (2010) Clinical characteristics of anxiety disordered youth. *Journal of Anxiety Disorders* **24**, 360–365.

Kunas, S.L. *et al.* (2021) Psychological predictors of cognitive-behavioral therapy outcomes for anxiety and depressive disorders in children and adolescents: a systematic review and meta-analysis. *Journal of Affective Disorders* **278**, 614–626.

Lawrence, P.J. *et al.* (2021) Supporting the parents of children and young people with anxiety and depressive disorders is an opportunity not to be missed: a scoping review. *The Lancet Psychiatry* **8**, 909–918.

Leigh, E. & Clark, D.M. (2023) Internet-delivered therapist-assisted cognitive therapy for adolescent social anxiety disorder (OSCA): a randomised controlled trial addressing preliminary efficacy and mechanisms of action. *Journal of Child Psychology and Psychiatry* **64**, 145–155.

Leigh, E. *et al.* (2021) Self-focused attention and safety behaviours maintain social anxiety in adolescents: an experimental study. *PLoS One* **16**, e0247703.

Lock, J. & La Via, M.C. (2015) American Academy of Child and Adolescent Psychiatry (AACAP) Committee on Quality Issues (CQI). Practice parameter for the assessment and treatment of children and adolescents with eating disorders. *Journal of the American Academy of Child and Adolescent Psychiatry* **54**(5), 412–425.

Lyneham, H.J. & Rapee, R.M. (2006) Evaluation of therapist-supported parent-implemented CBT for anxiety disorders in rural children. *Behaviour Research and Therapy* **44**, 1287–1300.

Mahdi, M. *et al.* (2019) Cognitive behavioral therapy for childhood anxiety disorders: what happens to comorbid mood and behavioral disorders? A systematic review. *Journal of Affective Disorders* **251**, 141–148.

March, J. *et al.* (2004) Fluoxetine, cognitive-behavioral therapy, and their combination for adolescents with depression: treatment for adolescents with depression study (TADS) randomized controlled trial. *JAMA* **292**(7), 807.

Mataix-Cols, D. *et al.* (2015) A pilot randomized controlled trial of cognitive-behavioral therapy for adolescents with body dysmorphic disorder. *Journal of the American Academy of Child & Adolescent Psychiatry* **54**, 895–904.

Mavranezouli, I. *et al.* (2020) Psychological and psychosocial treatments for children and young people with post-traumatic stress disorder: a network meta-analysis. *Journal of Child Psychology and Psychiatry* **61**, 18–29.

McCauley, E. *et al.* (2016) The Adolescent Behavioral Activation Program: adapting behavioral activation as a treatment for depression in adolescence. *Journal of Clinical Child and Adolescent Psychology* **45**(3), 291–304.

McGuire, R. *et al.* (2022) Differences in the diagnosis and treatment decisions for children in care compared to their peers: an experimental study on post-traumatic stress disorder. *British Journal of Clinical Psychology* **61**, 1075–1088.

Michelson, D. *et al.* (2020) Effectiveness of a brief lay counsellor-delivered, problem-solving intervention for adolescent mental health problems in urban, low-income schools in India: a randomised controlled trial. *The Lancet Child & Adolescent Health* **4**, 571–582.

Miklowitz, D.J. *et al.* (2004) Family-focused treatment for adolescents with bipolar disorder. *Journal of Affective Disorders* **82**, S113–S128.

Morrison, A.P. *et al.* (2020) Antipsychotic medication versus psychological intervention versus a combination of both in adolescents with first-episode psychosis (MAPS): a multicentre, three-arm, randomised controlled pilot and feasibility study. *The Lancet Psychiatry* **7**, 788–800.

Mowrer, O. (1960) *Learning Theory and Behavior*. John Wiley & Sons Inc., New York.

Mufson, L. *et al.* (2004) A randomized effectiveness trial of interpersonal psychotherapy for depressed adolescents. *Archives of General Psychiatry* **61**, 577–584.

Müller, H. *et al.* (2020) Cognitive behavioral therapy in adolescents with early-onset psychosis: a randomized controlled pilot study. *European Child & Adolescent Psychiatry* **29**, 1011–1022.

Ollendick, T.H. *et al.* (2009) One-session treatment of specific phobias in youth: a randomized clinical trial in the United States and Sweden. *Journal of Consulting and Clinical Psychology* **77**, 504.

Ollendick, T.H. *et al.* (2010) Comorbidity in youth with specific phobias: impact of comorbidity on treatment outcome and the impact of treatment on comorbid disorders. *Behaviour Research and Therapy* **48**, 827–831.

Öst, L.-G. *et al.* (2016) Cognitive behavioral and pharmacological treatments of OCD in children: a systematic review and meta-analysis. *Journal of Anxiety Disorders* **43**, 58–69.

Peris, T.S. *et al.* (2015) Trajectories of change in youth anxiety during cognitive-behavior therapy. *Journal of Consulting and Clinical Psychology* **83**, 239–252.

Perrin, S. *et al.* (2019) GAD-specific cognitive behavioral treatment for children and adolescents: a pilot randomized controlled trial. *Cognitive Therapy and Research* **43**, 1051–1064.

Pina, A.A. *et al.* (2019) Evidence-based psychosocial interventions for ethnic minority youth: the 10-year update. *Journal of Clinical Child & Adolescent Psychology* **48**, 179–202.

Plaisted, H. *et al.* (2021) Optimising exposure for children and adolescents with anxiety, OCD and PTSD: a systematic review. *Clinical Child and Family Psychology Review* **24**, 348–369.

Radez, J. *et al.* (2021) Why do children and adolescents (not) seek and access professional help for their mental health problems? A systematic review of quantitative and qualitative studies. *European Child & Adolescent Psychiatry* **30**, 183–211.

Reardon, T. *et al.* (2020) Seeking and accessing professional support for child anxiety in a community sample. *European Child & Adolescent Psychiatry* **29**, 649–664.

Ribeiro, W.S. *et al.* (2023) A systematic review of evidence-based interventions for child and adolescent mental health problems in low- and middle-income countries. *Comprehensive Psychiatry* **121**, 152358.

Saxena, S. *et al.* (2007) Resources for mental health: scarcity, inequity, and inefficiency. *The Lancet* **370**, 878–889.

Sharma, S. *et al.* (2021) Cognitive behavioural therapy for anxiety in children and young people on the autism spectrum: a systematic review and meta-analysis. *BMC Psychology* **9**, 151.

Smith, P. *et al.* (2007) Cognitive-behavioral therapy for PTSD in children and adolescents: a preliminary randomized controlled trial. *Journal of the American Academy of Child & Adolescent Psychiatry* **46**, 1051–1061.

Smith, P. *et al.* (2022) Therapist-supported online cognitive therapy for post-traumatic stress disorder (PTSD) in young people: protocol for an early-stage, parallel-group, randomised controlled study (OPTYC trial). *BMJ Open* **12**, e054852.

Stafford, M.R. *et al.* (2015) Efficacy and safety of pharmacological and psychological interventions for the treatment of psychosis and schizophrenia in children, adolescents and young adults: a systematic review and meta-analysis. *PLoS One* **10**, e0117166.

Teunisse, A.K. *et al.* (2022) A scoping review investigating the use of exposure for the treatment and targeted prevention of anxiety and related disorders in young people. *JCPP Advances* **2**, e12080.

Turner, C.M. *et al.* (2014) Telephone cognitive-behavioral therapy for adolescents with obsessive-compulsive disorder: a randomized controlled non-inferiority trial. *Journal of the American Academy of Child & Adolescent Psychiatry* **53**, 1298–1307.e2.

Walters, S. *et al.* (2016) A systematic review of effective modifications to cognitive behavioural therapy for Young people with autism spectrum disorders. *Review Journal of Autism and Developmental Disorders* **3**, 137–153.

Wang, H.-I. *et al.* (2022) Cost and effectiveness of one session treatment (OST) for children and young people with specific phobias compared to multi-session cognitive behavioural therapy (CBT): results from a randomised controlled trial. *BMC Psychiatry* **22**, 547.

Warnock-Parkes, E. *et al.* (2017) Seeing is believing: using video feedback in cognitive therapy for social anxiety disorder. *Cognitive and Behavioral Practice* **24**, 245–255.

Weisz, J.R. *et al.* (2006) Effects of psychotherapy for depression in children and adolescents: a meta-analysis. *Psychological Bulletin* **132**, 132–149.

Weisz, J.R. *et al.* (2012) Testing standard and modular designs for psychotherapy treating depression, anxiety, and conduct problems in youth: a randomized effectiveness trial. *Archives of General Psychiatry* **69**, 274–282.

Weisz, J.R. *et al.* (2020) Testing robustness of child STEPs effects with children and adolescents: a randomized controlled effectiveness trial. *Journal of Clinical Child & Adolescent Psychology* **49**, 883–896.

Whiteside, S.P. *et al.* (2015) The feasibility of improving CBT for childhood anxiety disorders through a dismantling study. *Behaviour Research and Therapy* **73**, 83–89.

Whiteside, S.P.H. *et al.* (2020) A meta-analysis to guide the enhancement of CBT for childhood anxiety: exposure over anxiety management. *Clinical Child and Family Psychology Review* **23**, 102–121.

Wolpe, J. (1958) *Psychotherapy by Reciprocal Inhibition*. Stanford University Press, Redwood City, CA. p. 239.

Wood, J.J. *et al.* (2020) Cognitive behavioral treatments for anxiety in children with autism spectrum disorder: a randomized clinical trial. *JAMA Psychiatry* **77**, 474–483.

Wright, B. *et al.* (2023) One session treatment (OST) is equivalent to multi-session cognitive behavioral therapy (CBT) in children with specific phobias (ASPECT): results from a national non-inferiority randomized controlled trial. *Journal of Child Psychology and Psychiatry* **64**, 39–49.

Yule, W. *et al.* (2013) Children and war: the work of the children and war foundation. *European Journal of Psychotraumatology* **4**, 18424.

CHAPTER 35

Systemic family therapy

Mark Rivett[1,2], Hannah Sherbersky[2,3] and Rick Miller[4]

[1] Systemic Family Psychotherapist, South Wales, UK
[2] CEDAR, University of Exeter, Exeter, UK
[3] Association for Family Therapy and Systemic Practice, Warrington, UK
[4] School of Family Life, Brigham Young University, Provo, UT, USA

Introduction

If one of the most significant factors in the development and maintenance of young people's mental health is their family, then one of the most significant clinical interventions must be with their families. The range of therapeutic approaches termed "family interventions" is broad. It includes low-intensity interventions with families (Frost *et al.*, 2003) through to family-based treatments and systemic family psychotherapy. After distinguishing these approaches, this chapter will focus on systemic family therapy. The chapter includes theoretical and conceptual principles and skills for family therapy, the evidence base, and introduces how a systemic framework can highlight health inequalities and shape how we work with marginalized groups.

As societal norms and our global relationships change, so does our definition and understanding of "the family." Reproductive technology has dramatically changed over the past 10 years, challenging assumptions about how parental and family relationships are constituted. This has ethical and legal significance for clinicians. Contemporary understanding of the family includes families where those who live in the same household have a biological connection. However, in this chapter, we take a wide view and see "family" to mean any group of people who define themselves as such. When referring to families, we include blended and stepfamilies, adopted and single-parent families, multigenerational families, same-sex parents, and children born into families through assisted reproduction. We need to recognize how different cultures will conceptualize the term "family" in different ways, and we acknowledge the changing structures of the global family as well as the concept of "the family of choice." The consistent assumption in the treatment of these systems, is that the psychopathology of the individual arises from, or is exacerbated or maintained by, patterns of interactions within a family or wider system.

It is equally important to acknowledge that the contemporary clinical field emphasizes the resources of a family rather than specific "dysfunctions." Along with this emphasis comes a strength-based approach where the etiology of the pathology becomes less significant and collaboration becomes central. Theoretically, this has been represented by attention to "family maintaining" factors for mental health difficulties rather than "family causative" factors (Eisler, 2005). Such a focus has the potential to depathologize and destigmatize both the individual and the family system.

There are a number of ways of typologizing family interventions depending on theoretical orientation, the professional qualifications of the clinician and the kinds of involvement being asked of the family. One such typology (Rivett & Street, 2009) suggests that family intervention can be considered in four interlocking ways:

- **A "family friendly" approach.** Here, family members are informed and involved in the treatment of a family member but are not necessarily seen as central to the work, e.g., a clinician meets a young person for therapy and routinely also meets their parents to update them about progress.
- **A "family containment" approach.** Here, the clinician may do some direct work with family members but the intention is to allow the individual work to proceed. For example, such an approach might involve a clinician using cognitive behavioral therapy (CBT) with a young person. In this instance a parent might be interacting with their child in a way that inadvertently reinforces the child's negative cognitions. The clinician therefore needs to meet the parent to explain the treatment, provide some psychoeducation, and ask for support for the work.
- **A "family involvement" approach.** Here, the family are seen as aides to the therapeutic treatment and are co-opted as therapeutic assistants, e.g., a young person with obsessive-compulsive disorder (OCD) is being taught to use exposure

Rutter's Child and Adolescent Psychiatry and Psychology, Seventh Edition.
Edited by Anita Thapar, Daniel S. Pine, Samuele Cortese, Cathy Creswell, Tamsin J. Ford, James F. Leckman, and Argyris Stringaris.

Companion website: www.wiley.com/go/thapar/rutterspsych7

and response prevention in their therapy and the clinician meets family members to help them practice such techniques with the young person (see, e.g., Chapter 60).

- **A "family systems" approach**, which includes systemic family therapy (variously called family psychotherapy/systemic psychotherapy). Here, the clinician regards the relational patterns in the family (not solely or exclusively) as potentially predisposing, precipitating, and perpetuating the psychological difficulties of children and young people, e.g., a young person is depressed and it is clear that one of their parents also suffers from depression. Here, the treatment is focused on family patterns (beliefs, emotions, and behaviors) rather than the "depression" per se (Diamond *et al.*, 2014).

Unfortunately, researchers and clinicians are not always clear about which type of "family intervention" they are using, promoting, or researching. Indeed, some research reviews are rather broad in the way they define "family intervention." These typologies are, of course, not mutually exclusive. Nor is the intention of delineating them designed to regard one as superior to any other. Thus, some CBT interventions may indeed become systemic ones, *if the locus of treatment is the relational pattern around a problem*. This assumption, a core principle of systems theory, is the topic of the next section.

Principles of systemic work

In this section, we summarize the principles of the theoretical basis for some approaches to working with families: what is called "systems theory."

There are many versions of how systems theory became a theoretical basis for family treatments. Indeed, it has often been said that these different versions have created many "family therapies" rather than one family therapy (Rivett & Street, 2009). The usual history argues that the anthropologist, Gregory Bateson (1972), applied *general systems theory* and *cybernetics* (a more "mechanical" approach to systems) to human relationships in the intellectual and technological maelstrom that followed the World War II. In reality, although Bateson is credited with being the "father" of family psychotherapy, his focus on family relationships and family interactive patterns was by no means unique. For instance, some psychoanalysts had followed Harry Stack Sullivan, the American psychiatrist and psychoanalyst, and the group analytic tradition into a similar territory (Skynner & Cleese, 1983) and, of course, the *anti-psychiatry* movement (Laing & Esterson, 1964) firmly placed the family as the source of psychopathology.

General systems theory argues that human beings are social creatures who influence and are influenced by each other in often circular and recursive ways (e.g., one person influences another who then influences the first person *ad infinitum*). Most languages are littered with axioms that demonstrate this phenomenon, for example, "two heads are better than one." Other cultures have equivalents: in Albania there is a saying that "no problem is an orphan."[1] The implication is that when human beings are in relationships, they experience their own lives within that stream of relationship, and whatever they do, they are in some kind of communication with each other. When this is applied to family relationships, it means that parents and children are constantly influencing each other.

Systems theory further proposes that these processes settle into "patterns." That is, they become habituated and routine. Such patterns and routines are inevitable in the complex nexus of relationships: systems theory does not say these are bad or good. What it proposes is that some of these habitual relational patterns help family members thrive and some may prevent this.

Systems theory suggests that these relationships make up a larger system which can be measured and described. The classic phrase "the whole is greater than the sum of its parts" encapsulates this idea (Rivett & Street, 2003). Thus, the focus of systems theory and, by implication, systemic therapy is on the way individual people come to behave within a human system. A human system can be understood as having a structure (who does what, with whom, when, who is closest to whom, etc.); a process of communication (what can be said, who says it to whom); a "meaning system" (what do relationships mean and what does behavior in those relationships mean); and an emotional component (what emotions can be expressed, what cannot be talked about). Each aspect of these "systemic properties" can be addressed in therapy as a way of helping the system change the patterns between people. Human systems also have a history: they develop, atrophy, and change through time. Systemic therapists, for instance, talk about "family scripts" often influencing what happens between family members, e.g., human beings behave, think, and feel in families in ways they learnt to behave, think, and feel in their own families.

From a systemic perspective, change occurs in the space *between* people. Like all other psychotherapies, this change could be behavioral, emotional, or "meaning" based. It is not enough for one member of a system to change: this has to be expanded into the relational space. Furthermore, because most of our relational processes are habituated, relational change may be hampered. In systemic terms, although development and the passage of time lead all human systems to constantly change ("morphogenesis"), humans also try to adjust to changes and *stay the same* ("homeostasis"). This process can be summed up in the joke about the woman who asks for help after 20 years, because her male partner thinks he is a chicken. When asked why she didn't ask for help earlier, she replies "I needed the eggs."

This joke foregrounds one of the more contentious aspects of systems theory (Priest, 2021). Because it argues that relational patterns are where "problems" lie, it also suggests that often a "problem" serves a relational function. Systemic therapists might therefore talk about "the function of the symptom." There

[1] We are indebted to Rainela Xhmollari for this phrase.

are a number of ways of understanding this phrase. One is that there are "secondary gains" for all members of the system, when one member is troubled. Another is that the problem might function as a way of keeping the family system intact. Last, it might be that the problem actually *creates* a system around it that didn't exist prior to its arrival.

Throughout the history of systemic family therapy, the status and interpretation of systems therapy has been variously debated, resisted, and revised (Rivett & Street, 2003; Priest, 2021). This conversation has occurred within a wider cultural context where the idea of professional expertise, as well as the nature of Western, White, and patriarchal theories of knowledge, have been challenged (McGoldrick & Hardy, 2019). At the same time, systemic family therapy has been influenced by the social constructionist movement (McNamee & Gergen, 1992) which has led to a more collaborative practice where therapists seek humility, uncertainty, and cultural sensitivity in their work (McGoldrick & Hardy, 2019).

Contemporary systemic family therapy practice within children's mental health settings has therefore changed dramatically from the earlier "expert systems diagnosticians." Contemporary practice is largely integrational (Rivett & Buchmüller, 2018) and shares many features with other psychotherapies. Relational formulations about the problem are collaboratively constructed with families and colleagues (Dallos & Stedmon, 2014). Attention is focused on interactional cycles between family members which may be influenced by intergenerational family scripts or by intergenerational trauma. Outcomes are measured by one or other family instrument (Stratton *et al.*, 2010). Also, clinicians are increasingly welcoming the intervention of Experts by Experience to balance their work and to engrain a sense of therapeutic humility into their practice.

Some psychological commentators argue that almost all contemporary psychotherapies have incorporated aspects of systemic therapy into their cannon (Lebow, 2014). Thus, concepts originally described by early family therapists, such as "enmeshed families" or "the function of the symptom," are often used in generic therapeutic parlance. The influence of systemic approaches is not limited to this adoption by other psychotherapies. Systemic therapists have also widened their work from families to schools (Vennum & Goodcase, 2020), to organizations (Fredman *et al.*, 2018), to supervisory relationships (Butler *et al.*, 2021), and to global mental health services (Charlés, 2021). This has led to significant growth in systemic family therapy posts within children's mental health services.

Systems theory highlights that family therapy seeks to help families change family relationships and family patterns rather than focus directly on the "symptom." The assumption is that by targeting *how things are done* in the family, the young person's mental health will improve. As such, the key skill brought into children's mental health services by the systemic approach is the skill of *how to work with families*. Indeed, we might be more specific: the key skill is *how to engage the wider family in helping their young person*. With this skill come important engagement, intervention, and collaborating techniques, which are the subject of the next section.

Systemic family therapy skills and practice

This section describes skills and techniques frequently used by those working with families, both in low-intensity family work settings, and more intensive systemic family therapy. These will be divided into "engaging skills" and "intervention skills." It is important to note, however, that the family therapist may be involved not just in the direct application of these skills in the therapeutic work with the family, but also in providing a systemic understanding for the wider multidisciplinary team.

The service context and the therapist will determine who needs to be seen in the initial family sessions: whether the whole family is brought together in a conjoint (e.g., altogether) session from the outset, or whether different subsystems or individuals would benefit in being seen separately. The therapist needs to consider issues around confidentiality, capacity, and the age of any children and young people involved. None of this negates the importance of assessing risk in the various child and adolescent mental health (CAMH) presentations but this can be assessed systemically and relationally (Flemons & Gralnik, 2013).

Engagement skills

Joining and assessment

One of the unique skills for all family interventions is the requirement to develop and manage multiple therapeutic relationships in the room. This may include holding in mind other family members who might not be present. This requirement is often described by those new to family work as being its most challenging aspect. One study conducted in the United States (U.S.) in a very culturally specific context, demonstrated that clinicians using a systemic framework were often particularly adept at keeping families in treatment and at marshaling family resources toward recovery (Crane & Christenson, 2014).

The importance of the therapeutic alliance has been emphasized in systemic family therapy as it has in other interventions. The System for Observing Family Therapy Alliances (SOFTA) (Friedlander *et al.*, 2006) has provided rich empirical data about how "engaging" works in family interventions. SOFTA is an observational and self-rating measure which divides the alliance into four categories: emotional connection between family members and the clinician; family engagement in the therapeutic task; safety in the family therapeutic system; and a shared sense of purpose within the family. SOFTA provides not only a way of measuring the alliance in family interventions but also guidance on what therapists can do to increase positive scores on each of these dimensions. Families will often attend therapy with very different views of "the problem" or the identified patient, so the first task for the family therapist is to engage the whole family in a way which makes their involvement relevant to all family members. Thus, possibly the most important task is to help the family reach a *shared sense of purpose* about the therapy.

A fundamental way in which family clinicians engage the whole family is to value the perspectives of every family member. One of the early pioneers of family therapy, Boszormenyi-Nagy, used the concept of multidirectional partiality (Boszormenyi-Nagy & Spark, 1984) to explain this process. This position acknowledges the importance of considering multiple perspectives and viewpoints in understanding and addressing issues within the family system. It seeks to empower families to better understand their issues by recognizing each person's unique perspective and experience. The Milan Associates (Rivett & Buchmüller, 2018) used the term neutrality to mean something quite similar, e.g., that the therapist has to align with everyone and no one at the same time. It is within this context, that the clinician engages in a "family assessment" which will include: individual relationships to each other, to the "problem," to the therapy, and to the experience of being helped. The therapist explores how the "problem" has impacted on the family as a whole and each family member individually, and what the interactional maintaining factors for the problem might be. From the outset, the therapist is also required to reflect on how the family impacts on the self of the therapist. This bidirectional flow of information becomes part of the therapeutic process.

Family engagement achieves its systemic goal when the therapist helps the family members (preferably all of them) to recognize how they can be part of the solution to the difficulty that a family member has. Assessment is therefore an intervention. The goal is to achieve a change from "our young person has a problem" to "we can help our young person resolve this problem and maybe there is something we do/have done that hasn't helped them with the problem."

Systemic formulation and hypotheses

The practice of psychological assessment and formulation are core skills for most psychotherapists. Systemic family therapy is no exception (Dallos & Stedmon, 2014). Formulation becomes systemic if it describes a person's difficulties in the context of their relationships, social circumstances, and life events. A systemic formulation is dynamic and understood as a conceptual map, comprised of several working hypotheses that can be tested. Sharing the formulation with the family forms an important part of the therapy, as a starting point for collaboration around setting goals for therapy and as an attempt to convey that the family remains the greatest resource for recovery and resilience.

Intervention skills

In systemic theory and practice, assessment, engagement, and intervention are constantly interconnecting, circular processes. For instance, the initial "family reframe" (the family are the resource for healing) is both an engagement task *and* an intervention. The same is true for all the intervention skills that we itemize below. All of these skills can be learnt and adopted quite easily by family practitioners within CAMH settings whatever model of family intervention they are working within.

Reframing behavior, thoughts, or emotions as relational

Family interventions start by engaging family members. In this engagement various types of "relational reframing" may be undertaken. Reframing is the process in which the clinician gives a relational interpretation to a piece of behavior (Rivett & Buchmüller, 2018) which may not be present in the original description. This interpretation may naturally arise in the conversation, coming from family members, or it may be introduced by the therapist. An example would be where a parent describes the difficult behavior of a child as "attention-seeking." The clinician then proceeds to ask the parent why they think the child needs their attention so much. Here the "locus of control" moves from the child to the parent–child relationship. In attachment-based family therapy (ABFT) (Diamond *et al.*, 2014) a central reframe is to ask the young person (in front of their parents) why they could not turn to their parents when they were so distressed/depressed. Once more, the reframe moves the distress/depression from an intrapersonal (within a person) to an interpersonal (between people) problem.

Emphasizing the circular nature of interaction and problem formation (circularities)

Tracking circularities is a fundamental process in systemic family therapy. Here the clinician and the family identify interactional patterns that influence one another and create a circular feedback loop that may be maintaining the family or individual's difficulties. By describing, or turning these interactions into a diagrammatic form, options for breaking these cycles can emerge. Although these patterns may be held in mind implictly during the conversation, drawing them out provides additional opportunities to track meanings, attributions, and explanations of an individual's behaviour. Furthermore, the 'problems' can also be more easily externalized (White and Epston 1990; Rivett and Buchmüller 2018), giving a greater sense of agency to the family. Here we can note the overlap with Cognitive Behavioural Therapy, where thoughts, behaviours and feelings can be specifically addressed (Reibstein and Sherbersky 2022) although in family therapy there is particular emphasis on how they are understood interactionally and how this can provide new information and levels of empathic understanding between family members (Figure 35.1).

Circular questions

The use of circular questions is relatively unique to systemic family therapy. Their function is to elicit circular connections between family members and to encourage perspective taking within the family. Many authors have described typologies of circular questions (Tomm, 1988). Thus, some questions connect one person's thoughts, behaviors, or feelings to another family member's thoughts, behaviors, or feelings, e.g., "How do you understand your child's tears right now?" (to father). Others project relationships into an imagined future, e.g., "If you have

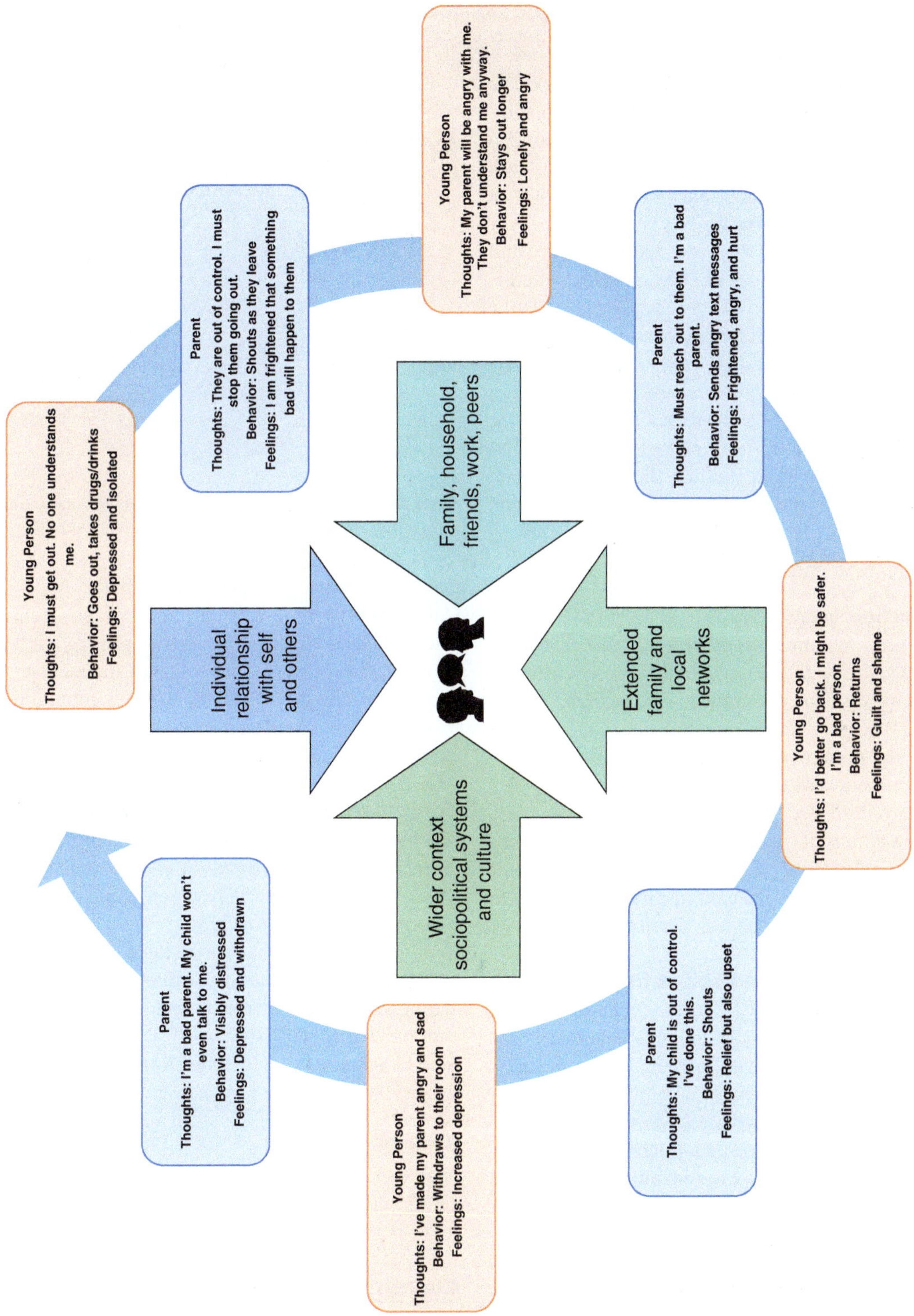

Figure 35.1 Tracking circularities and demonstrating wider context.

children, what kind of a relationship would you like with your Mum then?" (to adolescent). Yet other circular questions bring in triadic relationships, e.g., "If you and your child argued, what do you think your partner would notice?"

Genograms, sculpting, and other interventive techniques

Drawing out the family genogram (family tree) can provide a wealth of information about the context of the family, in addition to offering a practical way of engaging the whole family in a systemic approach. The genogram can be understood as both an assessment tool and intervention in and of itself (McGoldrick *et al.*, 2008). Family members can be actively engaged in the process, enabling them to reflect on their own family identity, and highlighting family strengths and resilience, as well as interactional patterns and family history. Care needs to be given to the therapeutic timing of the genogram: if a loved family member has died, for example, remembering relationships may evoke distress. The therapist may decide to embark on the genogram only once a therapeutic alliance has been established or start the process in the first session as a way of building an alliance. Completing a cultural genogram for the therapist and team (Hardy & Laszloffy, 1995) may also provide the clinician and team with the opportunity to reflect on the similarities and differences of their own cultural backgrounds.

Creative and "action" techniques

Therapists may draw on numerous other techniques that elucidate interactional patterns and behaviors, such as inviting family members to role-play, sculpt, or engage in an enactment (Rivett & Buchmüller, 2018). Here, family members enact interactional patterns within the therapy session. The therapist invites the family to experiment with alternative transactions (also described as going into the "avoided interaction"). This is a unique opportunity for the family and therapist to use the immediacy of the relationship within therapy. There is some evidence that changes in relational patterns first created in such techniques continue into "everyday life" (Hardy *et al.*, 2020).

The self of the therapist and self-reflexivity

Systemic family therapy shares with other psychotherapies an awareness of the self of the therapist (Aponte & Kissil, 2016). This process is called "self-reflexivity" or "relational reflexivity" (Burnham, 2005) in systemic therapy. The importance of the therapist being aware of their own biases and assumptions dates from the development of what is called *second order cybernetics*, which argued that therapists do not see a family objectively but only through the lens they apply to it. Such an orientation is crucial when it is understood that therapists are as affected by cultural contexts such as sexism, racism, and disablism, as are the families they work with. In the United Kingdom (UK), this idea is encapsulated by the mnemonic Social GGRRAAACCEEESSS (more simply Social Graces) (Burnham, 2012) which highlights that in any therapeutic encounter, the clinician should be aware of how the social construction of differences, such as Gender,

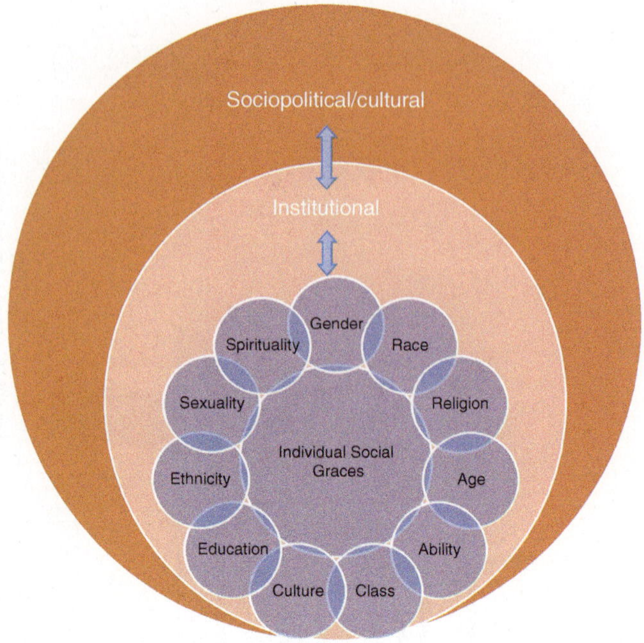

Figure 35.2 Power, intersectionality, and politics—interacting layers of privilege and oppression.

Geography, Race, Religion, Age, Ability, Appearance, Class, Culture, Ethnicity, Education, Employment, Sexuality, Sexual orientation, and Spirituality, may be playing out in the circular relational processes of the therapeutic interaction (Figure 35.2). Systemic family therapists will always account for these factors in their formulations and, in varying degrees, will share their experiences with the families they encounter.

Complexities and contraindications

Inviting families to come together to explore complex and painful feelings will inevitably result in conflict at times. The therapist needs to assess the suitability of convening the whole family and be alert to the impact that hostility and power imbalances in the room may have on what can be talked about. Family therapists and systemic practitioners pride themselves on the ability to manage the tension between multiple perspectives by taking the "both/and" rather than the "either/or" position (Sherbersky, 2016). But it must be acknowledged that sometimes this perspective is unhelpful in situations of abuse and power imbalances within the family. For instance, care must be taken when working in situations of abuse (child or domestic). Models for working in these contexts often include systemic attention to safety plans and close interagency working is important (Vetere & Cooper, 2005).

Current evidence base

The pioneers of systemic family therapy built their theories on many hours of observation of family interaction. Nevertheless, some consider family therapists to be tardy in engaging in empirical research into their field. This is, in part, similar to some other psychotherapies and is connected to the researcher/clinician divide described in many areas of clinical practice (Barkham *et al.*, 2010). Some systemic family therapists have also appeared to doubt the role of empirical research because of a belief that it "simplified" complex interactive processes. However, there has been an exponential growth in statistical ways of mapping relationships between different actors in systems (Miller, 2020). Thus, there is no longer an argument that empirical studies cannot capture the complexity of relational interactions. Other commentators have argued for a nuanced understanding of "evidence" which takes into account more than the "gold standard" randomized controlled trial (RCT) (Sexton *et al.*, 2008). Indeed, qualitative studies (Sprenkle & Piercy, 2005), including conversational analyses, have contributed to understanding the process of systemic family therapy.

At the risk of simplifying the evidence, we describe studies that have evaluated the effectiveness of systemic family therapy for symptom resolution in CAMH contexts. Potential issues with evaluation methodologies are highlighted elsewhere (see Chapter 15). However, a particularly relevant issue in the context of systemic family therapy is *what is being evaluated*. To be concordant with systemic theory, evaluation should include more than the symptom by encompassing relational well-being as well. Indeed, RCTs that have evaluated the effect of family therapy on symptom reduction among children and adolescents have consistently found that the treatment also improved family functioning (Von Sydow *et al.*, 2013; McFarlane, 2016). This evidence is not only important in validating the mechanisms of change in family therapy, but also points to added benefits that extend beyond the primary symptoms of a child.

Table 35.1 provides a summary of the research evidence for the effectiveness of family therapy in treating psychological disorders that are common in childhood and adolescence. Findings had to be based on RCTs in order to be included as evidence. In addition, the treatment protocol had to be based specifically on the principles of systems theory. Many reviews of family therapy, especially those conducted in the U.S., include interventions based on behavioral theory because the protocol involved family members beyond the symptomatic child. However, the practice in Europe has been to include only family therapy RCTs that were explicitly based on family systems theory (Retzlaff *et al.*, 2013). Consequently, the RCTs included in the evaluation of evidence for family therapy in Table 35.1 were based on family systems theory. RCTs that were based on behavioral models of family therapy were excluded. Behaviorally based family intervention models are reviewed in Chapter 33.

Although most RCTs in Table 35.1 tested the effectiveness of systemic family therapy as a "stand-alone" treatment, there are exceptions. For example, family therapy-anorexia nervosa (FT-AN) is usually used in conjunction with some individual work (often eating disorder focused). Also, family treatments for psychosis universally include medication as part of the treatment model. RCTs of family treatments for psychosis include antipsychotic medication in both the treatment and control groups. Although medication leads to improved functioning of persons suffering from psychosis as a "stand-alone" treatment, RCTs have found that the inclusion of family therapy in treatment has a demonstrable additive effect on reducing relapse and rehospitalization. Specifically, research shows that the improvement in individual functioning from combining family therapy with antipsychotic medication, compared to medication alone, is about the same as the difference between medication and taking a placebo (McFarlane, 2016). One other exception to the pattern of family therapy being used as a "stand-alone" treatment is that one of the three RCTs on family therapy with attention deficit hyperactivity disorder (ADHD) (Zhu & Lian, 2009) included medication in both the family therapy treatment group and the control group.

One feature of the effectiveness research of family therapy with children and adolescents is that as the research has matured, it has expanded from its U.S.-centric origins to other research sites around the world. This is a positive development. However, it has created some nuances in the family therapy effectiveness literature. A prime example is the research on family therapy with adolescents struggling with conduct disorders (CDs). For many years, substantial research out of the U.S. found that family therapy treatment models, such multisystemic therapy (MST) and functional family therapy (FFT), were effective. They have long been considered to be empirically supported treatments in the U.S. (Henggeler & Schaeffer, 2016; Robbins *et al.*, 2016). However, more recent research in Europe has not found support for these therapies (Humayun *et al.*, 2017; Fonagy *et al.*, 2018). Von Sydow (2013) suggests that the difference in findings between the U.S. and Europe is probably due to differences in the treatment as usual (TAU) groups (also, see Chapters 33 and 65). When reviewing the results of an RCT that found significant differences between the MST treatment and TAU groups in a U.S. sample, but not in a Swedish sample, Von Sydow *et al.* (2013) found that the improvement from pre- to post-treatment was the same for the treatment groups in the U.S. and Sweden samples. However, the TAU group also improved significantly over the course of the study in the Swedish sample, while there was no improvement in the TAU group in the U.S. sample. As a result, based on a comparison between the treatment and control groups at post-test, MST was found to be effective in the U.S. sample, but not in the Swedish sample.

As indicated in Table 35.1, systemic family therapy has been found to be effective in treating ADHD, based on three RCTS from different countries. Multiple RCTS have found systemic family therapy to be an effective treatment for eating disorders, depression, substance abuse, and psychosis. Family therapy has considerable evidence for being an

Table 35.1 Illustrative examples of randomized controlled trial (RCT) evidence for family therapy.

Diagnostic category of identified child and adolescent problem	Major review papers	Significant conclusions	Limitations
Attention deficit hyperactivity disorder (ADHD)	Babinski & Sibley (2022) Von Sydow *et al.* (2013)	Although most models involving family members are based on behavioral principles, three RCTs of systemic therapy found positive results in reducing ADHD symptoms, including studies in the U.S., Germany, and China. The study in China included medication in both the treatment and control groups. In addition, there is evidence that family therapy improves family functioning in families with a child who has ADHD.	The majority of RCTs examine effectiveness of behaviorally based treatments for ADHD. More RCTs of family therapy based on systems theory are needed.
Eating disorders	Eisler *et al.* (2016) Jewell *et al.* (2016) Blessitt *et al.* (2020) Datta *et al.* (2023)	Family therapy is recommended by NICE for treating adolescent anorexia nervosa and bulimia nervosa. In particular, the Maudsley model, which is an integration of systemic principles, has received substantial empirical support.	Little research has examined the effectiveness of family therapy in the treatment of other disorders, such as binge eating.
Conduct disorders (CDs) (also termed "disruptive behaviors")	Von Sydow *et al.* (2013) Wampler & Whitehead (2020) Sheidow *et al.* (2022)	There are three well-established programs that have a systemic family therapy core: multisystemic therapy (MST; Henggeler & Schaeffer, 2016); functional family therapy (FFT; Robbins *et al.*, 2016); and Treatment Foster Care (Astrom *et al.*, 2020), with all three models demonstrating effectiveness in reducing acting out behaviors. These therapies, especially MST and FFT, have been found to be effective in a number of countries across the globe, including in Europe, China, Australia, and Israel.	Although these family therapy models have considerable evidential support in the U.S., and other non-European countries, recent RCTs in Europe have found fewer positive results. Scholars suggest that this is because treatment-as-usual (TAU) groups in Europe are more beneficial than TAU groups in the U.S. and other countries. Thus, similar levels of improvement from family therapy interventions in Europe are less distinguished from TAU control groups, where study participants also improve.
Depression, self-harm, and suicidality	Retzlaff *et al.* (2013) Diamond *et al.* (2016) Krauthamer Ewing *et al.* (2020) Wittenborn *et al.* (2022)	Attachment-based family therapy (ABFT), which is based on systemic principles, has significant evidence to support its effectiveness for depression among 12–18-year-olds compared to waitlist controls. Other RCTs have shown systemic integrated family therapy to have similar outcomes to established treatments for depression in 8–15-year-olds.	Although there is good evidence for family therapy effectively treating depression, evidence that family therapy is effective in treating self-harm and suicidality is lacking.
Substance abuse	Patton *et al.* (2020) Hogue *et al.* (2022)	Two well-researched systemic models for the treatment of adolescent substance misuse are multidimensional family therapy (Liddle, 2016) and brief strategic family therapy (Szapocznik *et al.*, 2016). Many RCTs have found these models to be significantly more effective than TAU in reducing substance abuse.	Much of this research has been conducted in the U.S., although with diverse samples. However, RCTs conducted in Europe have found multidimensional family therapy to be effective for European participants. Research has focused on adolescents, with very little research on younger children.
Adolescent severe mental illnesses (psychosis and bipolar disorder)	Claxton *et al.* (2017) Carr (2020) Rodolico *et al.* (2022)	Over a dozen RCTs of family therapy, using systemic principles, have found that it is effective in treating adolescent first episode psychosis alongside medication—a best practice standard in psychosocial treatments of psychosis. This combination has been found to be more effective than medication alone and medication combined with individual treatment. Family therapy is based on reducing expressed emotion in families, which refers to hostile interactions and intrusiveness between family members.	There is no evidence from RCTs that family therapy is successful in treating bipolar disorder among children and adolescents.

effective treatment for CDs in the U.S. and other non-European countries.

Clinicians are often interested in *process research* (e.g., what therapist activities make a difference), as well as *outcome research*. Once again, systemic family therapy has explored this area of practice with numerous and varied research methods. Table 35.2 summarizes a number of key findings which have relevance for all clinicians working with families.

Table 35.2 Summary of findings about the process for successful family intervention[a].

Process theme	Evidence	General findings	Reviews	Clinical significance
Alliance with the family and within the family.	A range of alliance scores have been used to assess how the alliance is created and developed. The most well-researched is the System for Observing the Family Therapy Alliances (SOFTA).	A good alliance strongly correlates with a good outcome (Friedlander *et al.*, 2006). Alliances with individual family members need to be balanced by an alliance with the whole family. A split alliance (widely divergent scores by family members) correlates with poorer outcomes (Friedlander *et al.*, 2006). Clinicians often overrate the positivity of the alliance (Robbins *et al.*, 2000).	Karam & Blow (2020) Hardy *et al.* (2020)	The research guides clinicians in how to maintain and increase the alliance with family members.
The expression of blame and hostility are negative indicators for progress in family intervention.	In a number of the evidence- based models and in the studies of the alliance, this has been an important process finding (Robbins *et al.*, 2000).	This hypothesis has been supported in studies of functional family therapy (FFT); brief strategic family therapy, and multisystemic therapy (MST).	Hardy *et al.* (2020)	When blame or hostility emerge in family intervention, the clinician has a responsibility to work with it and ameliorate it. In the literature, a number of techniques have been proposed to achieve this.
How does working with relational patterns create change?	Process research has examined this using self-report and observational methods.	Key processes that have emerged: helping families change how they relate to each other either by behaving differently, by understanding each other better, or by thinking about the problem differently. The research has also highlighted the significance of ethnicity and ethnic matching in improving outcomes.	Hardy *et al.* (2020)	Clinicians need to learn how to challenge established family patterns and guide families to new ways of relating to each other.
There is consistent evidence that a range of systemic family therapy skills (Rivett & Buchmüller, 2018) are effective in enabling change to occur.	Complex sequential behavioral analysis and various methods of conversational analysis have demonstrated that there are three key skills that connect to changed family interactions.	*Circular questions* have been shown to elicit "other" understanding, as well as "self-involvement" (Diorinou & Tseliou, 2014). *Reframing* the intentions of family members leads to an interactional understanding (Robbins *et al.*, 2000). The technique of *enactment* also leads to changes in family understanding and to change in relational patterns (Diamond *et al.*, 2016).	Hardy *et al.* (2020)	There are a range of guidelines that enable clinicians to learn these skills. Most of them are integrated within the evidence-based models of systemic family therapy.
Keeping families in treatment.	A significant number of studies across the life span have demonstrated that working with relationship patterns increases commitment from families and reduces drop out.	This evidence relates to many of the evidence-based models including FFT and MST (McAdams *et al.*, 2018).	Hardy *et al.* (2020)	There are a range of explanations about how this occurs, significantly giving all family members (including those not present) a voice. Another is building a collaborative problem-solving approach with all family members.
Improving therapist performance.	There has been a growing awareness that some clinicians get better results than others. This has resulted in *deliberate practice* (Blow *et al.*, 2023) within systemic family therapy.	One of the central pieces of evidence from the *deliberate practice* research is that working with client/family feedback can improve outcomes (Tilden & Wampold, 2017).	Blow *et al.* (2023)	Routine feedback is now an important aspect of systemic family therapy practice (Tilden & Wampold, 2017). Interestingly, this empirical practice is now embraced by systemic family therapists from all perspectives (Rober, 2017).

[a] The studies referred to have often been ancillary to outcome studies (Table 35.1) and include a range of research methods: observational, self-report, qualitative, conversational analyses, and some statistical designs. At best, these studies provide moderate evidence for specific clinical behavior with families.

Power, privilege, and working with marginalized groups

We know that oppressive social conditions and social inequalities are significant contributors to mental health difficulties (World Health Organization, 2014). Equally, as a modality that privileges the concept of "context," it is unsurprising that systemic family therapy, and family interventions more broadly, have been hugely influenced by the context in which they function. Changes in societal norms, the feminist movement, Black Lives Matter, and other social justice issues have all had a significant impact on the evolving theory and delivery of family interventions.

Systemic family therapy posits the notion that language and narratives are constructed versions of our social world and language is "constitutive" rather than neutral. As such, power dynamics between family and therapist, in addition to the wider institutional power of the psychiatric system, need to be considered. Many family therapists consider it is essential to use their position to highlight oppressive practice, to attend to unconscious bias, and to be alert to the Western, White, male, hetero, and cisnormative discourses that surround their clinical contexts. The social GGRRAAACCEEESSS (Burnham, 2012) were developed to recognize the different aspects of self, as well as "the other" within the context of understanding difference in the therapeutic process. However, this and other models which privilege a single category approach, have been critiqued and are being updated to take into account the intersectional "categories of self" (Crenshaw, 1991) to obviate the possibility of increasing marginalization. Therefore, systemic family practice focuses on the importance of taking an intersectional view of the clinicians, their context, *and* the work. Understanding how power, oppression, and discrimination can not only occur simultaneously around but also *within* relationships is a central task (Figure 35.2).

The future for family interventions and systemic family therapy

Many emerging themes within systemic family therapy foreshadow the future. One is the inevitable and continuing role of research in the development of the field. As we have highlighted, there remains much that we still do not know about how family relational interventions change presenting mental health problems for young people and their families. Fruitful collaboration could emerge between family clinicians and family researchers. For instance, to ensure that evaluations are conducted in ways that are in keeping with systemic principles, while also meeting the robust research standards that are required for recommendations to be made. This will also enable further understanding of mediators and moderators of family therapy outcomes, which can ultimately drive improvements in treatment outcomes. Manualization of family therapy approaches might help both systematic evaluation and dissemination. However, it is also clear that some models of family intervention are more easily adapted to manuals and outcome measures than others (Mariotti *et al.*, 2021). Most certainly the "evidence-based" movement has created a context in which family practitioners in CAMH services, seek to be "evidence-based" or "evidence-informed" in their practice. But the translation of this into changed clinical practice is never straightforward and the continuing researcher/clinician divide acts as a brake on the influence research has on the practice of family intervention.

The second theme highlights the limited amount of new research, especially in contexts outside the U.S., despite increases in funding. Yet family interventions are a global phenomenon (Charlés, 2021). This raises the question about the nature of knowledge in the mental health field. In this chapter, we have highlighted the "Western" nature of many of the systemic family therapy models, the knowledge upon which they are based, and the way these models have been implemented. However, the "family" (in its many cultural interpretations) is a global human phenomenon. Many cultures have historically recognized that families need help and this help has often been unique to the society within which it is embedded (Sim & Sim, 2020). In the 21st century, it is not surprising that non-Western cultures have absorbed some of the ideas of systemic family therapy, redesigned them for their own contexts, and then started making contributions to the global family intervention field. Sim and Sim (2020) call this process one of "indigenization or localization" and a number of research papers have emerged to support this transformation of systemic family therapy. Charlés (2021) is one of a series of family therapists who has not only worked on developing culturally sensitive ways of using systemic family therapy as an intervention for children's mental health difficulties, but has also adapted its skills to work in low- and middle-income countries (LMICs). Indeed, the World Health Organization has also supported these kinds of interventions (World Health Organization, 2008). These developments suggest that during this century, systemic family therapy will cease to be predominantly a Western family intervention model but will bloom into a diverse and varied intervention for families across a range of nations, cultures, and contexts. It may therefore be that systemic family therapy in the 21st century will have truly "left its home" in the Western world.

Conclusion

This chapter has described the essential features of systemic family therapy for CAMH difficulties. It has highlighted that this approach to treatment seeks to change patterns of relationship as a way of improving CAMH. The chapter has also highlighted the social justice aspects of this intervention model and its value to families, children, and societies across the globe. Integrating systems thinking and the application of systemic skills in all types of family intervention can be transformative, both for the family and clinical practitioner alike.

References

Aponte, H. & Kissil, K. (2016) *The Person of the Therapist.* Routledge, New York.

Astrom, T. *et al.* (2020) Treatment Foster Care Oregon for delinquent adolescents: a systemic review and meta-analysis. *Research on Social Work Practice* **30**, 355–367.

Babinski, D. & Sibley, M. (2022) Family based treatments for attention-deficit/hyperactivity disorder: a review of family functioning outcomes in randomised controlled trials from 2010-2019. *Journal of Marital and Family Therapy* **48**, 83–106.

Barkham, M. *et al.* (2010) *Developing and Delivering Practice-based Evidence.* Wiley-Blackwell, Chichester, UK.

Bateson, G. (1972) *Steps to an Ecology of Mind.* Ballantine, New York.

Blessitt, E. *et al.* (2020) Eating disorders in children, adolescents and young adults. In: *The Handbook of Systemic Family Therapy.* (ed K. Wampler). John Wiley & Sons, Hoboken, NJ. pp. 397–427.

Blow, A. *et al.* (2023) *Deliberate Practice in Systemic Family Therapy.* American Psychological Association, Washington, DC.

Boszormenyi-Nagy, I. & Spark, G. (1984) *Invisible Loyalties.* Routledge, New York.

Burnham, J. (2005) Relational reflexivity: a tool for socially constructing therapeutic relationships. In: *The Space Between: Experience, Context, and Process in the Therapeutic Relationships.* (eds C. Flaskas, *et al.*). Karnac, London. pp. 1–18.

Burnham, J. (2012) Developments in social GRRRAAACCEEESSS: visible-invisible and voiced-unvoiced. In: *Culture and Reflexivity in Systemic Psychotherapy: Mutual Perspectives.* (ed J.B. Krause). Karnac, London. pp. 139–160.

Butler, C. *et al.* (2021) Systemic supervision, the last frontier: towards a scale that measures systemic supervision. *Journal of Family Therapy* **43**, 828–851.

Carr, A. (2020) Evidence for the efficacy and effectiveness of systemic family therapy. In: *The Handbook of Systemic Family Therapy.* (ed K. Wampler), Vol. *1.* John Wiley & Sons, Hoboken, NJ. pp. 119–146.

Charlés, L. (2021) *International Family Therapy.* Routledge, New York.

Claxton, M. *et al.* (2017) Do family interventions improve outcomes in early psychosis? A systematic review and meta-analysis. *Frontiers in Psychology* **8**, 371.

Crane, D.R. & Christenson, J.D. (2014) A summary report of cost-effectiveness: recognizing the value of family therapy in health care. In: *Medical Family Therapy: Advanced Applications.* (eds J. Hodgson, *et al.*). Springer, Cham, Switzerland. pp. 419–436.

Crenshaw, K. (1991) Mapping the margins: intersectionality, identity politics and violence against women of colour. *Stanford Law Review* **43**, 1241–1299. doi:10.2307/1229039.

Dallos, R. & Stedmon, J. (2014) Systemic formulation. In: *Formulation in Psychology and Psychotherapy.* (eds L. Johnstone & R. Dallos). Routledge, New York. pp. 67–95.

Datta, N. *et al.* (2023) Evidence based update on psychosocial treatments for eating disorders in children and adolescents. *Journal of Clinical Child & Adolescent Psychology* **52**, 159–170.

Diamond, G. *et al.* (2014) *Attachment-based Family Therapy for Depressed Adolescents.* American Psychological Association, Washington, DC.

Diamond, G. *et al.* (2016) Attachment based family therapy: a review of the empirical support. *Family Process* **55**, 595–610.

Diorinou, M. & Tseliou, E. (2014) Studying circular questioning "in situ": discourse analysis of a first systemic family therapy session. *Journal of Marital and Family Therapy* **40**, 106–121.

Eisler, I. (2005) The empirical and theoretical base of family therapy and multiple family day therapy for adolescent anorexia nervosa. *Journal of Family Therapy* **27**, 104–131.

Eisler, I. *et al.* (2016) Treating adolescents with eating disorders. In: *Handbook of Family Therapy.* (eds T. Sexton & J. Lebow). Routledge, New York. pp. 387–406.

Flemons, D. & Gralnik, L. (2013) *Relational Suicide Assessment.* Norton & Co, New York.

Fonagy, P. *et al.* (2018) Multisystemic therapy versus management as usual in the treatment of adolescent antisocial behaviour (START): a pragmatic, randomised controlled, superiority trial. *The Lancet Psychiatry* **5**, 119–133.

Fredman, G. *et al.* (2018) *Collaborative Consultation in Mental Health.* Routledge, Abingdon, UK.

Friedlander, M. *et al.* (2006) *Therapeutic Alliances in Couple and Family Therapy.* American Psychological Association, Washington, DC.

Frost, N. *et al.* (2003) *Companion to Family Support.* Russell House Publishing, Lyme Regis, UK.

Hardy, K. & Laszloffy, T. (1995) The cultural genogram: key to training culturally competent family therapists. *Journal of Marital and Family Therapy* **21**, 227–237.

Hardy, N. *et al.* (2020) The process of change in systemic family therapy. In: *The Handbook of Systemic Family Therapy.* (ed K. Wampler). John Wiley & Sons, Hoboken, NJ. pp. 171–204.

Henggeler, S.W. & Schaeffer, C.M. (2016) Multisystemic therapy®: clinical overview, outcomes, and implementation research. *Family Process* **55**, 514–528.

Hogue, A. *et al.* (2022) Couple and family therapy for substance misuse disorders: evidence based update 2010-2019. *Journal of Marital and Family Therapy* **48**, 178–203.

Humayun, S. *et al.* (2017) Randomized controlled trial of functional family therapy for offending and antisocial behavior in UK youth. *Journal of Child Psychology and Psychiatry* **58**, 1023–1032.

Jewell, T. *et al.* (2016) Family therapy for child and adolescent eating disorders: a critical review. *Family Process* **55**, 577–594.

Karam, E. & Blow, A. (2020) Common factors underlying systemic family therapy. In: *The Handbook of Systemic Family Therapy.* (ed K. Wampler). John Wiley & Sons, Hoboken, NJ. pp. 147–170.

Krauthamer Ewing, E.S. *et al.* (2020) Youth suicide: risk, prevention and treatment. In: *The Handbook of Systemic Family Therapy.* (ed K. Wampler). John Wiley & Sons, Hoboken, NJ. pp. 343–368.

Laing, R. & Esterson, A. (1964) *Sanity, Madness and the Family.* Penguin, Harmondsworth, UK.

Lebow, J. (2014) *Couple and Family Therapy: An Integrative Map of the Territory.* American Psychological Association, Washington, DC.

Liddle, H. (2016) Multidimensional family therapy. In: *Handbook of Family Therapy.* (eds T. Sexton & J. Lebow). Routledge, New York. pp. 231–249.

Mariotti, M. *et al.* (2021) *Handbook of Systemic Approaches to Psychotherapy Manuals.* Springer, Cham, Switzerland.

McAdams, C. *et al.* (2018) In session therapist actions for improving client retention in family therapy: translating empirical research into clinical practice. *Journal of Family Psychotherapy* **29**, 142–160.

McFarlane, W.R. (2016) Family interventions for schizophrenia and the psychoses: a review. *Family Process* **55**, 468–482.

McGoldrick, M. & Hardy, K. (2019) *Re-visioning Family Therapy.* Guilford Press, New York.

McGoldrick, M. *et al.* (2008) *Genograms: Assessment and Intervention.* Norton & Co, New York.

McNamee, S. & Gergen, K. (1992) *Therapy as Social Construction.* Sage Publishers, London.

Miller, R. (2020) An introduction to a new generation of clinical statistical approaches. *Journal of Marital and Family Therapy* **46**, 577–581.

Patton, R. *et al.* (2020) Systemic approaches to adolescent substance misuse. In: *The Handbook of Systemic Family Therapy.* (ed K. Wampler). John Wiley & Sons, Hoboken, NJ. pp. 297–320.

Priest, J. (2021) *The Science of Systems Theory.* Routledge, New York.

Reibstein, J. & Sherbersky, H. (2021) Manualising the Exeter model: couple therapy for depression—a behavioural-systemic approach. In: *Handbook of Systemic Approaches to Psychotherapy Manuals.* (eds

M. Mariotti, *et al.*), European Family Therapy Association Series. Springer, Cham, Switzerland.

Retzlaff, R. *et al.* (2013) The efficacy of systemic therapy for internalizing and other disorders of childhood and adolescence: a systematic review of 38 randomized trials. *Family Process* **52**, 619–652.

Rivett, M. & Buchmüller, J. (2018) *Family Therapy: Skills and Techniques in Action*. Routledge, London.

Rivett, M. & Street, E. (2003) *Family Therapy in Focus*. Sage Publishers, London.

Rivett, M. & Street, E. (2009) *Family Therapy: 100 Key Points and Techniques*. Routledge, London.

Robbins, M. *et al.* (2000) Disrupting defensive family interactions in family therapy with delinquent adolescents. *Journal of Family Psychology* **14**, 688–701.

Robbins, M.S. *et al.* (2016) Evolution of functional family therapy as an evidence-based practice for adolescents with disruptive behavior problems. *Family Process* **55**(3), 543–557.

Rober, P. (2017) *In Therapy Together: Family Therapy as Dialogue*. Palgrave, London.

Rodolico, A. *et al.* (2022) Family interventions for relapse prevention in schizophrenia: a systematic review and network meta-analysis. *The Lancet* **9**, 211–221.

Sexton, T. *et al.* (2008) Beyond the single standard: levels of evidence approach for evaluating marriage and family therapy research and practice. *Journal of Family Therapy* **30**, 386–398.

Sheidow, A. *et al.* (2022) Family based treatments for disruptive behavior problems in childhood and adolescents: an updated review of rigorous studies (2014–2020). *Journal of Marital and Family Therapy* **48**, 56–82.

Sherbersky, H. (2016) Family therapy and fundamentalism: one family therapist's exploration of ethics and collaboration with religious fundamentalist families. *Clinical Child Psychology and Psychiatry* **21**(3), 381–396.

Sim, T. & Sim, C. (2020) Global contexts for the profession of systemic family therapy. In: *The Handbook of Systemic Family Therapy*. (ed K. Wampler). John Wiley & Sons, Hoboken, NJ. pp. 51–78.

Skynner, R. & Cleese, J. (1983) *Families and How to Survive Them*. Methuen, London.

Spenkle, D. & Piercy, F. (2005) Pluralism, diversity and sophistication in family therapy research. In: *Research Methods in Family Therapy*. (eds D.H. Sprenkle & F.P. Piercy). Guilford, New York. pp. 3–18.

Stratton, P. *et al.* (2010) Developing an indicator of family function and a practicable measure for systemic family and couple therapy: the SCORE. *Journal of Family Therapy* **32**, 232–258.

Szapocznik, J. *et al.* (2016) Brief strategic family therapy treatment for behavior problem youth. In: *Handbook of Family Therapy*. (eds T. Sexton & J. Lebow). Routledge, New York. pp. 286–304.

Tilden, T. & Wampold, B. (2017) *Routine Outcome Monitoring in Couple and Family Therapy*. Springer, Cham, Switzerland.

Tomm, K. (1988) Interventive questioning: intending to ask lineal, circular, strategic or reflexive questions? *Family Process* **27**, 1–15.

Vennum, A. & Goodcase, E. (2020) Interventions for challenges encountered in childcare and school settings. In: *The Handbook of Systemic Family Therapy*. (ed K. Wampler). John Wiley & Sons, Hoboken, NJ. pp. 571–594.

Vetere, A. & Cooper, J. (2005) *Domestic Violence and Family Safety*. Whurr, London.

Von Sydow, K. *et al.* (2013) The efficacy of systemic therapy for childhood and adolescent externalizing disorders: a systematic review of 47 RCT. *Family Process* **52**, 576–618.

Wampler, R. & Whitehead, M. (2020) Disordered behavior and behavior disorders. In: *The Handbook of Systemic Family Therapy*. (ed K. Wampler). John Wiley & Sons, Hoboken, NJ. pp. 265–296.

White, M. & Epston, D. (1990) *Narrative Means to Therapeutic Ends*. Norton, New York.

Wittenborn, A. *et al.* (2022) Couple and family interventions for depressive and bipolar disorders: evidence base update (2010-2019). *Journal of Marital and Family Therapy* **48**, 129–153.

World Health Organization (2008) *Mental Health Gap Action Programme: Scaling Up Care for Mental, Neurological and Substance Use Disorders*. World Health Organization (WHO), Geneva, Switzerland. https://www.who.int/publications/i/item/9789241596206

World Health Organization (2014) *Social Determinants of Mental Health*. World Health Organization (WHO), Geneva, Switzerland. https://www.who.int/publications/i/item/9789241506809

Zhu, Z. & Lian, P. (2009) Effect of structural family therapy on ADHD children with oppositional defiant disorder. *Journal of Taishan Medical College* **30**, 440–442.

CHAPTER 36
Relationship-based treatments

Jonathan Green[1,2] and Nick Midgley[3,4]
[1] Division of Psychology and Mental Health, University of Manchester, Manchester, UK
[2] Royal Manchester Children's Hospital, Manchester, UK
[3] Research Department of Clinical, Educational and Health Psychology, University College London, London, UK
[4] Child Attachment and Psychological Therapies Research Unit (ChAPTRe), Anna Freud, London, UK

Introduction

"Relationship-based treatments" are defined in this chapter as those that have, as their prime aim, either the improvement of a child or adolescent's key relationships or else treatments that use relationships as a core mechanism through which they are delivered and generate psychological and behavior change.

The chapter covers three main areas: (i) interventions that aim to improve the relationship between children and significant caregivers in early childhood; (ii) the relationship between therapist and child or parent in the process of treatment; and (iii) specific treatment modalities used with those in middle childhood and adolescence that either have a particular focus on improving interpersonal relationships or are defined by the use of the relationship between the therapist and the young person as a major mechanism for effecting change. Treatments are included for discussion if they are informed by modern developmental science and/or have an evidence base for the treatment itself or core components. Not covered here are treatments marked by a more cognitive or social learning focus that are specifically addressed in other chapters, such as parent training (see Chapter 33), cognitive behavioral therapy (CBT; see Chapter 34), and systemic family therapy (see Chapter 35).

Treatments targeted at the early parent–child relationship

The quality of a child's early relational environment matters centrally for centrally a range of child developmental outcomes, including language and communication, social competency, attachment security, self-regulation, and behavior adjustment. Interventions have aimed to improve early dyadic caregiver–infant and caregiver–child relationships (see Chapters 6 and 7). They tend to focus on either: (i) known *caregiver vulnerabilities*, such as unresolved previous trauma or mental illness; or (ii) *child vulnerabilities* such as early maltreatment, or temperamental or neurodevelopmental differences.

Context of parental vulnerability

Early meta-analysis (Bakermans-Kranenburg *et al.*, 2003) found that developmentally conceptualized, brief (<16 sessions) individualized interventions, often using video-aided techniques, were more effective in optimizing attachment-related parental behaviors than general parental support or longer-term psychotherapy. The subsequent literature has tended to support these early findings; brief focused therapies, particularly using video feedback techniques, emerge as the strongest intervention option. In these interventions, caregivers typically review videotapes with the therapist of their naturalistic interactions with their infant (the infant is not worked with directly). The focus on real-time learning through videotape is a powerful way of increasing parental awareness, sensitivity, and enjoyment with their infant. Recent meta-analysis of a range of such interventions (O'Hara *et al.*, 2019) found overall positive effects on parental sensitivity (SMD 0.34, 95% CI 0.20–0.49) but not on child attachment outcomes. The best outcomes from a specific example of this approach is video-feedback intervention to promote positive parenting (VIPP; Juffer *et al.*, 2008), in which a recent meta-analysis of the first 25 randomized controlled trials (RCTs) testing VIPP (van IJzendoorn *et al.*, 2023) found by contrast a combined positive effect size on parenting behavior and sensitivity (Cohen's $d = 0.37$) and also on childhood attachment security ($d = 0.47$). No intervention effect, however, was found to improve "downstream" generalized child externalizing behaviors, although this should remain the goal of an early intervention aiming to impact children's lives in the longer term.

Parent–infant psychotherapy (PIP) has also been evaluated in the context of parental vulnerability. A 2015 Cochrane review

Rutter's Child and Adolescent Psychiatry and Psychology, Seventh Edition.
Edited by Anita Thapar, Daniel S. Pine, Samuele Cortese, Cathy Creswell, Tamsin J. Ford, James F. Leckman, and Argyris Stringaris.

Companion website: www.wiley.com/go/thapar/rutterspsych7

(Barlow *et al.*, 2015, 2016), defines PIP as "a psychodynamic intervention with parent–infant dyads, designed to address regulatory disturbances in infancy and problems in the parent–infant relationship." This review included eight studies focused on work with dyads in which mothers had postpartum depression, anxious or insecure attachment, or were imprisoned, including mentalization-based interventions (Minding the Baby), a mothers and toddlers program (New Beginnings), and PIP. The overall quality of evidence was rated low to very low. There was some evidence that the PIP model may have shown improved effects on attachment security compared to other types of treatment, but no differences were found in parental mood or relationship-based outcomes.

Context of child disability or developmental difference

Video-aided, parent-mediated approaches have also been used successfully to improve attachment and relatedness in infants who are vulnerable due to extreme or difficult temperaments (van den Boom, 1994; Cassidy *et al.*, 2011), and to optimize development in children with neurodiversity and developmental disability. In autism, for instance, developmental interventions work in a targeted way with parents (or for older children, teaching assistants, or peers), often using video-aided methods, to enhance parental awareness and understanding and their dyadic responses to the child's different communication style and thus dyadic communication; postulating consequent more generalized positive effects into other contexts and over time (Figure 36.1).

Early dyadic social communication interventions of this kind are currently the only 'consider' recommendation from the UK National Institute for Health and Care Excellence (NICE) (2013, 2021) for developmental features of autism, and two such interventions have reported long-term child developmental impact. Gulsrud *et al.* (2014) showed the greater effect of a 3-month preschool joint attention, symbolic play, engagement, and regulation (JASPER) intervention, compared to play- or behaviorally focused interventions, in improving 5-year follow-up growth trajectories in attention and language up to the age of 8 years. JASPER uses parent coaching and modeling, and direct work with the child to increase joint engagement between parent and child. Pickles *et al.* (2016) showed sustained effect from an 18-session (12-month) preschool pediatric autism communication therapy (PACT) in significantly reduced autistic behaviors for 6 years into middle childhood (mean 10.5 years). PACT uses video-feedback therapy with parents to increase their awareness and understanding of their neurodiverse child's communication differences; it improves the attunement and synchrony of their response to the child and the child's consequent engagement with the parent. Mechanistic studies showed that it was treatment improvement in this *reciprocal relatedness in the dyad* that mediated, respectively, the JASPER language outcomes at 2 years (Gulsrud *et al.*, 2016), and the PACT autistic outcomes at endpoint (Pickles *et al.*, 2015) and 6-year follow-up (Carruthers *et al.*, 2023). These mechanistic findings thus illuminate the equivalent importance of relational development for neurodiverse children as for children with neurotypical development; and provide a model of early relational support for neurodiversity compared to interventions targeting discrete child autistic behaviors (see Chapter 50). Similar approaches have been used earlier, in preemptive care for infants at raised likelihood of an autism trajectory. In these studies, a parent-mediated

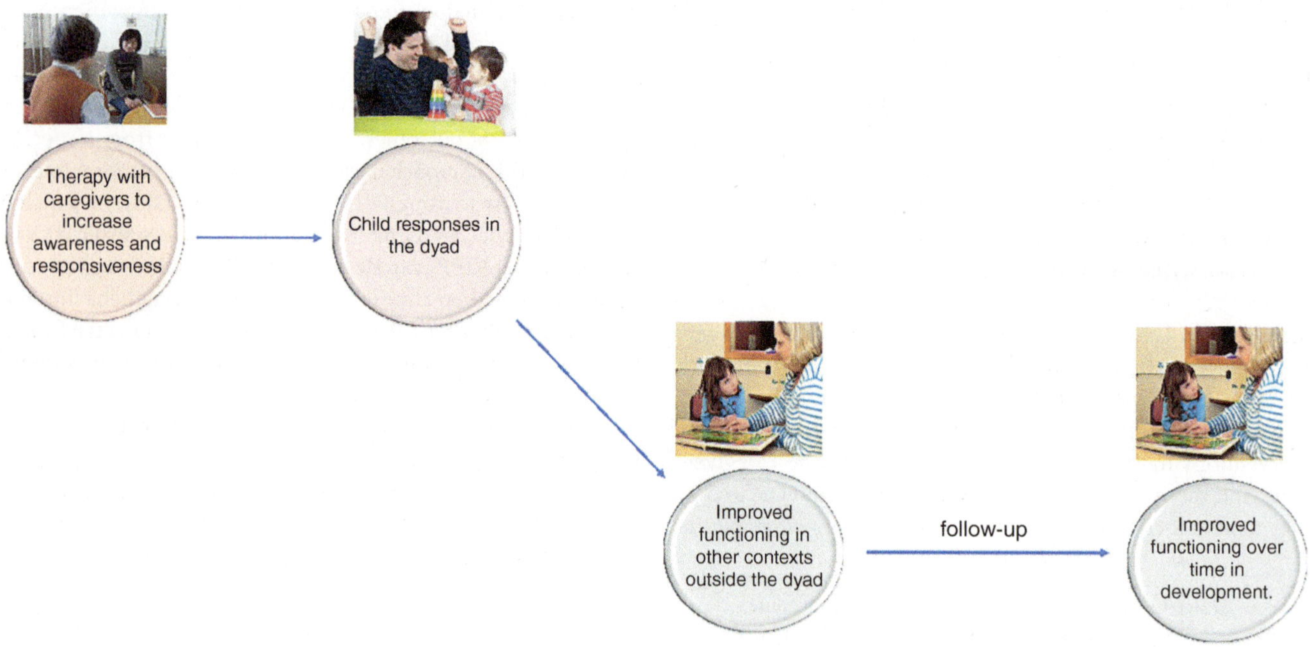

Figure 36.1 Logic model of dyadic interaction therapies.

dyadic intervention (iBASIS) shows effects on emerging autism phenotype expression (Green *et al.*, 2017) leading to reduced 3-year diagnoses in one trial (while the children retain other developmental difficulties; Whitehouse *et al.*, 2021). These findings have clinical and policy implications for preemptive care in autism: for instance, modeling shows health economic benefits of this preemptive approach in relation to downstream service use (Segal *et al.*, 2023), and its health system-wide implementation is being tested in Western Australia. Group approaches to developmental intervention of this kind have obvious attractions in the peer support for caregivers and efficiency for therapists; however, despite those benefits, they have shown an absence of efficacy for child outcomes compared to individualized approaches (Carter *et al.*, 2011).

Conceptually similar approaches have been advocated in another neurodevelopmental condition, attention deficit/hyperactivity disorder (ADHD). Association has been reported between poor quality of early parent–child interaction and relatedness in ADHD children and later oppositional defiant disorder (ODD; Johnston & Jassy, 2007), and longer-term outcomes with high expressed emotion parenting (Keown, 2012); but such studies cannot determine the direction of effects. However, less experimental intervention work along these lines has been done for children with ADHD compared to autism; a 2011 review (Zwi *et al.*, 2011) found little work, generally of poor methodological quality, from which they felt no clinical inferences on efficacy could be made.

Early years relationship-based interventions in low- and middle-income countries (LMICs) and low-resource settings

A recent systematic review (Pedersen *et al.*, 2019) describes accelerating efforts on the part of health professionals to develop or adapt and test early parent- or family-focused interventions in low-resource settings; 65% using "task-shifting" to nonspecialist deliverers. The most common intervention elements used were psychoeducation and coping strategies for parents. The reviewers note methodological limitations in the design and sample sizes of these studies. They advocate more rigorous studies of promising approaches, and highlight the value there would be in mechanistic studies to identify the "active ingredients" for mediating effectiveness, within an intervention or shared across different interventions. Identifying these "active ingredients" would efficiently clarify the key elements that need to be adapted into new delivery contexts (Marchette & Weisz, 2017). As an example, a "task-shifted" adaptation of a UK-tested autism intervention for nonspecialist delivery in India and Pakistan (Parent-mediated intervention for Autism Spectrum Disorder in South Asia (PASS); Divan *et al.*, 2015) was able to replicate the active mechanistic effect of the original UK model, as well as demonstrate family acceptability, delivery and fidelity in the new cultural context (Rahman *et al.*, 2016). Baumann *et al.* (2019) provide a valuable discussion of the principles of scaling up evidence-based practice in parenting programs into low- and middle-income countries (LMICs) and low-resource settings; emphasizing the need for community engagement, judicious use of experience from high-income settings, the centrality of partnerships based on mutuality, trust, and equity of power, and innovative trial designs to preserve rigor in demanding settings. They also point to a bidirectional reciprocity in knowledge sharing; lessons learned in LMICs will be increasingly valuable to stretched high-income health settings.

The therapist–patient relationship and its role in treatment

Focus on the therapist–patient relationship as a mechanism of therapeutic change is not new and is a central feature of various traditions in psychotherapy. This includes transference work in psychoanalysis and the "secure base" ideas from attachment theory, as well as the emphasis on the provision of "unconditional positive regard" in the humanistic tradition, for instance. Construed as the "therapeutic alliance," it has been increasingly understood and studied as a nonspecific therapeutic factor operating across different kinds of psychological therapy.

The therapeutic alliance

The therapeutic alliance is a term encompassing a variety of relational variables between patient and therapist (Green, 2006; Cirasola & Midgley, 2023). Although definitions vary, it is broadly recognized as including a focus on collaboration (especially in terms of agreement on the tasks and goals of treatment) and on the bond between therapist and patient or client. The impact of the therapeutic alliance is observed across many different types of interventions, extending well beyond psychotherapy, including nursing, social work, school counseling, and medicine (see Wampold & Flückiger, 2023). Meta-analytic studies in child and adolescent psychotherapy (Karver *et al.*, 2018; Bose *et al.*, 2022) have, overall, found a robust, albeit modest, association between alliance quality and outcome; $r = 0.20$ across 43 studies of differing methodology, independent of child age and type of treatment. Levels of therapeutic alliance have been found to be comparable in online therapies to those delivered face-to-face (Probst *et al.*, 2019). Alliance is, however, a complex phenomenon—especially in the case of children, where the caregiver–therapist alliance must also be taken into account—and there are methodological limitations with many of these reports (Cirasola & Midgley, 2023).

Therapist qualities, such as active listening, accurate empathy, and commitment, as well as the ability to provide a clear rationale about the treatment and promote collaborative planning, all showed a moderate to strong association with alliance quality in a meta-analysis of 49 studies (Karver *et al.*, 2006). More recent work has also suggested that perceived cultural competence in therapists is associated with higher alliance and reduced dropout (Anderson *et al.*, 2019). Drawing on the work of Safran and Muran (2006), a "second generation" of alliance researchers has moved beyond viewing the alliance as a static variable. They now recognize that alliance is something which fluctuates from moment to moment, with frequent microruptures likely to be taking place between therapist and patient or client. Rather than focusing on the general capacity to build an alliance, this research focuses on the need for effective therapists to be able to identify and repair these ruptures, as and when they happen.

A meta-analytic review of studies examining the impact of rupture and repair in the therapeutic alliance indicates that successful in-session repair of alliance ruptures is associated with improved treatment outcomes (Eubanks *et al.*, 2018). In a review, Muran and Eubanks (2020) identified three core pathways to repairing alliance ruptures (Figure 36.2), all of which are most likely to be effective when they are carried out with humility, compassion, curiosity, and patience.

When it comes to children and adolescents, few empirical studies have evaluated the impact of alliance rupture and repair on outcomes, but studies to date do suggest that repairing such ruptures may be associated with better treatment outcomes (for a review, see Cirasola & Midgley, 2023). How therapists may repair alliance ruptures with young people is still relatively unexamined in the empirical literature, and studies to date have mostly been adaptations "downwards" of the adult models (Nof *et al.*, 2019; Cirasola *et al.*, 2022).

The evidence thus supports the modest but important impact of the quality of the therapist–patient alliance relationship on outcomes across many intervention types, but we still do not know exactly how the alliance impacts on outcome. It may be that the alliance is a necessary but not sufficient element of successful treatment with children and adolescents; and that the capacity to identify and repair ruptures throughout treatment is the most significant clinical capacity for treatment engagement and outcomes. We await experimental trials of whether specific methods to enhance the alliance alone would be as effective as specific intervention protocols (a key question). Notwithstanding this, there is enough evidence to say that promotion of the alliance, and repairing alliance ruptures, should be core features of professional training and intervention development.

Children and young people's experience of the therapeutic relationship

Research that examines young peoples' experiences of therapy highlights the important role of therapeutic relationships. Although there are some differences in how different types of therapy are experienced, what is common is a recognition of certain key features which make the therapeutic relationship effective. That applies to outpatient or inpatient settings (Hartley *et al.*, 2022), or therapies as apparently different as CBT (e.g., Wilmots *et al.*, 2020) and short-term psychoanalytic psychotherapy (e.g., Housby *et al.*, 2021).

While only a small number of studies have examined younger children's experiences of therapy (e.g., Núñez *et al.*, 2022), a number of studies have examined the experience of therapy among adolescents. Across these studies, young people consistently identified a need to give time for the therapeutic relationship to develop, with the young person sometimes setting "tests" of whether the therapist could really be trusted (Stige *et al.*, 2021). Where a relationship could be established, adolescents identified confidence, warmth, empathy, trust, transparency, and support from their therapist as central to what made change possible. Particular importance was given to the therapist being unshockable and nonjudgmental, especially if the adolescent disclosed "weird" thoughts or problematic behavior (e.g., Løvgren *et al.*, 2019; Stige *et al.*, 2021). Adolescents emphasized the importance of having some control over how sessions happened (e.g., by being allowed to make decisions about the format and focus of meetings), having their autonomy respected, and hope for a therapeutic relationship which is not overly formal or hierarchical, to address some of the perceived power imbalances; they typically spoke about the importance of an encounter in which the therapist was experienced as "genuine" (often demonstrated by disclosing certain information about themselves, or by going the extra mile), and not only acting as a professional who was just "doing a job" (Gibson *et al.*, 2016; Løvgren *et al.*, 2019). These priorities appeared to be equally true when young people described their experience of internet-based treatments as when speaking about face-to-face therapy (Gibson & Cartwright, 2014; Lindqvist *et al.*, 2022; MacKean *et al.*, 2023). As Hartley *et al.* (2022) concluded, the therapeutic

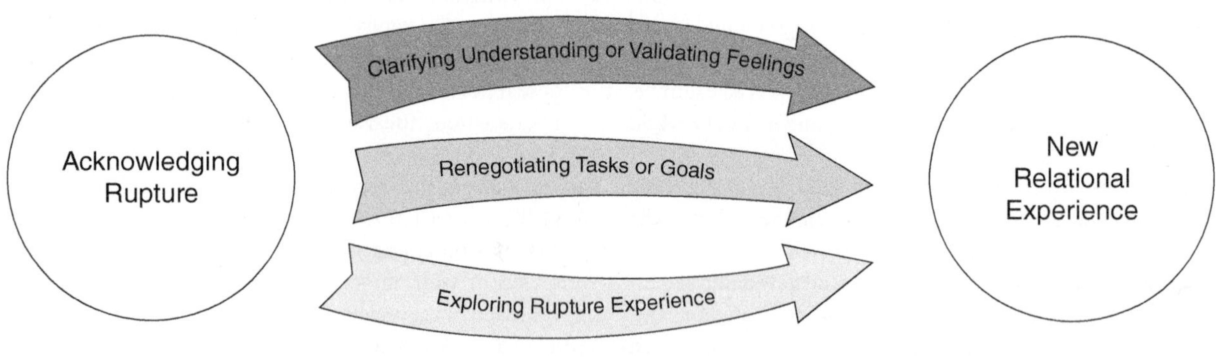

Figure 36.2 Strategies for rupture repair. *Source*: Adapted from Muran and Eubanks (2020).

relationship is not simply a facilitator of therapeutic care; for young people, therapeutic relationships "were seen as key: *they are the treatment*" (2022, p.21).

Engagement and disengagement in treatment

Depending on how "dropout" has been defined, studies estimate that between 40–70% of children and adolescents drop out of therapy (de Haan *et al.*, 2013), and relational factors are likely to be central to this. One study of 344 children (7–18 years) attending community mental health clinics in the United States (Garcia & Weisz, 2002) found that premature ending of treatment was more associated with problems in the therapeutic relationship than lack of family motivation, practical difficulties, time concerns, or perceived lack of symptom improvement. In their review, Becker and Chorpita (2023) argue that the issue of low engagement is the single most ubiquitous challenge facing youth mental health services, especially for those young people with the most severe mental health difficulties, as well as for underserved populations, including young people of color (e.g., Cook *et al.*, 2013).

In studies that have examined the experience of therapy among those who disengaged or who were dissatisfied with treatment, a consistent finding is a feeling among the young people that their therapists did not understand—or did not truly care—for them (e.g., von Below, 2020); that they were not really able to form an "emotional connection" to their therapist (O'Keeffe *et al.*, 2019; Mehta *et al.*, 2023); and that the therapist was experienced as "mechanical," being overly rigid in their approach to therapy, not being transparent or open with the young person, and failing to understand the young person's perspective (Stige *et al.*, 2021).

One approach to enhancing the therapist–patient alliance and relatedness in treatment is motivational interviewing (MI). This approach was first developed in the context of substance misuse in adults, but the principles have been generalized to child and adolescent work (Baer & Peterson, 2002; Naar-King & Suarez, 2011). The interpersonal therapeutic stance in MI pays great attention to the details of the therapists' communication. This includes working to enhance alliance and to identify discrepancies between the young person's current situation or behavior and their own values or wishes, thus eliciting and reinforcing the seeds of a motivation toward change. In keeping with a respect for the young person's autonomy, "resistance to change" is considered in interpersonal terms as a meaningful reaction to external pressure or demand; the therapist sidesteps this by not suggesting or imposing change themselves but rather by using a pattern of reflective questioning to identify and reinforce "change talk" or elements of change behaviors emerging in the young person. MI theorists stress that this is not just a set of "techniques"; rather it is a sustained interpersonal stance, which reflects, questions, and affirms the young person's control of the path toward change. The stance is well adapted to the sensitivities of childhood and adolescence in which young people have often not actively chosen to seek treatment and experience external family or social pressure.

To date there have been few empirical studies of the effectiveness of MI in childhood and adolescence. In anorexia nervosa, a large RCT comparing outpatient CBT plus MI with standard outpatient and inpatient care for 12–18-year-olds (Gowers *et al.*, 2007), found motivation for the therapy improved after the initial MI session and the MI + CBT arm as more cost-effective than the comparators. When examining outpatient attendance for adolescents at a psychiatric service, MI demonstrated an increase of approximately 10% in attendance at scheduled follow-up appointments and a decrease of approximately 4% in cancellations and no-show appointments (Chiappetta *et al.*, 2018).

Relationship-based psychotherapeutic treatments for children and adolescents

All forms of therapy include some kind of therapeutic relationship; but there are also some types of therapy which may be considered "relationship-based treatments." This might be either because they have, as their prime aim, the improvement of a child or adolescent's key relationships; or else they use relationships as a core mechanism through which they are delivered and attempt to generate psychological and behavior change. In this section, we focus on three such relational therapies—psychodynamic psychotherapy, mentalization-based treatment (MBT), and interpersonal therapy (IPT)—because each of them illustrates such a focus well.

Psychodynamic psychotherapy

Psychodynamic psychotherapy is a broad label, which refers to a wide range of psychotherapies which have their roots in the psychoanalytic tradition. Kufferath-Lin *et al.* (2022, pp. 148–149) describe the key features of psychodynamic psychotherapy with children and adolescents to be: (i) the centrality of play as a means of communication and a therapeutic intervention for children; (ii) the notion of unconscious feelings, wishes, and conflicts which contribute to psychological distress; (iii) the concept of defense mechanisms which help to manage this distress; (iv) the idea that observable behaviors have more than one meaning, not all of which we may be consciously aware of; (v) the existence of internal representations of significant people which shape expectations for future relationships; (vi) a non-judgmental and exploratory therapeutic stance which follows the child's lead; and (vii) an emphasis on the therapeutic relationship as an agent of change.

The body of empirical evidence for the effectiveness of psychodynamic psychotherapy with children and adolescents is smaller than that for CBT or even family therapy, and there have been previous concerns about its methodological quality. To date, only one meta-analytic review has been conducted, which focused specifically on short-term psychodynamic psychotherapy (STPP) with adolescents (Abbass *et al.*, 2013). This meta-analysis included 11 RCTs or quasi-experimental studies (total cases, n = 655) with a mean child age of 11.3 years (SD = 2.7) and a session dose of 10–40 sessions (M = 20.0, SD = 10.4). Studies varied greatly in size and quality was classed as moderate, overall. Groups investigated included those with emotional disorders, mixed disorders, anxiety disorders, and personality problems. Seven studies compared STPP to another type of psychotherapy, three to treatment as usual, and three to minimal contact or waitlist controls. Overall, there were generally high within-group effects in both arms of studies but very few between-group differences separating STPP from comparators.

The most recent systematic narrative review of the evidence base for psychodynamic psychotherapies with children and adolescents, including both short- and long-term treatments (Midgley *et al.*, 2021a), included 82 distinct studies. The review noted that both the quality and quantity of empirical papers had increased over time, with increased use of treatment manuals in recent trials (e.g., Cregeen *et al.*, 2017; Göttken & von Klitzing, 2018), as well as better-designed trials; however, a range of methodological limitations (small sample sizes, lack of control groups) remain, and still only 22 out of the 82 studies were RCTs.

The most rigorous evaluation of a STPP to date was a large-scale, three parallel-arm RCT in the UK of the treatment of moderate to severe depression. The Improving Mood with Psychoanalytic and Cognitive Behavioral Therapies (IMPACT) trial found large within-group effect sizes but no statistically significant between-group differences in clinical- or cost-effectiveness between a manualized model of STPP, a manualized CBT, or a manualized brief psychosocial intervention (Goodyer *et al.*, 2017; Loades *et al.*, 2023). Additionally, a therapist-guided, internet-based psychodynamic therapy (iPDT) has recently been evaluated in two clinical trials in Sweden (Lindqvist *et al.*, 2020; Mechler *et al.*, 2022), with iPDT found to be noninferior to internet-based cognitive behavioral therapy (iCBT) in terms of change in depression for the treatment of adolescents with depression.

Although these studies have demonstrated the noninferiority or equivalence of STPPs to other evidence-based treatments, such as CBT, these clinical trials do not in themselves examine whether the defining features of STPP contribute to effectiveness. To begin to address this, Ulberg *et al.* (2021) conducted a study in which they examined the effectiveness of STPP for depressed adolescents, using the same treatment manual as Goodyer *et al.* (2017), and compared it with a "dismantled" version excluding the defining transference work (the latter version involved the therapists working in a psychodynamic way, but being required (and monitored) to not actively discuss the therapeutic relationship, unless the adolescent brought it up themselves). The study found no statistically significant differences in outcome between the two approaches on the primary outcome measures (depressive symptoms and psychodynamic functioning at the end of treatment), but did find benefits for STPP including transference work in terms of greater reduction in depressive symptoms in the period from mid-treatment to one-year follow up. Across the whole literature, further mechanistic studies of this kind will be essential to distinguish treatment-specific from nonspecific, shared psychotherapy treatment effects.

Mentalization-based treatment (MBT)

A further elaboration of the therapeutic relationship in treatment is found in MBT, a contemporary treatment model building on the "secure-base" attachment therapy of Bowlby (Bowlby, 1988) and psychodynamic principles. Like CBT, the therapist and patient or client in MBT occupy a shared empirical stance, but whereas in CBT the object of common regard is the pattern of cognition in relation to affect and behavior, in MBT (as in psychodynamic psychotherapy) an important focus is the therapeutic relationship itself and a capacity to reflect on the mental states (thoughts, feelings, and beliefs) arising within it. In MBT, the therapist models in real time within the therapy how action, reflection, and insight have to be worked for with honesty.

MBT has been adapted in a number of different settings for work with children, adolescents, and families (Midgley & Vrouva, 2012; Midgley *et al.*, 2017; Rossouw *et al.*, 2021). MBT—whether in individual or group format—seems to be especially helpful for young people who struggle with interpersonal relationships and emotion regulation. For example, in an RCT with adolescents who self-harm, MBT was compared with treatment as usual, which was predominantly CBT and counseling intervention (n = 80; Rossouw & Fonagy, 2012). MBT was delivered in weekly individual sessions with monthly family-based sessions focused on affect regulation and mentalization. A moderate effect size in favor of MBT was found in both self-reported and interview-based self-harm estimates after 1 year of treatment, most strikingly in numbers reporting no self-harm over 3 months (chi^2 5, p = 0.01; NNT (number needed to treat) 3.66). This study needs replication on larger samples (there was considerable treatment dropout in both arms) but provides an important preliminary result given the lack of treatment effect found over many years in other interventions for the important problem of adolescent self-harm (Ougrin, 2012; see Chapter 64).

Overall, the emerging evidence base for MBT is now growing (Malda-Castillo *et al.*, 2019), although the evidence base for MBT with children, young people, and families is still at an early stage (Byrne *et al.*, 2020). However, a number of clinical trials of MBT with children and young people are currently underway (e.g., Dalgaard *et al.*, 2023), which should lead to a better understanding of the effectiveness of this type of relationship-based treatment in the coming years. There have also been some interesting adaptations of MBT, e.g., for parenting programs, especially for carers of children in foster care, as well as for schools, hospitals, and inpatient settings (for a review, see Midgley *et al.*, 2021b).

Interpersonal psychotherapy (IPT)

IPT is a manualized psychotherapy for depression that focuses on the reciprocal relationship between mood state and the patient or client's current real-world social relationships; it is pragmatic rather than theory-driven in its focus on disruption in interpersonal relationships as an antecedent for mood change and improvement of relationships as a route into improving mood (Weissman *et al.*, 2000). IPT has two key principles: that depression is a treatable condition and not the patient's fault; and that there is a reciprocal relationship between depression and interpersonal problems (Rose-Clarke *et al.*, 2020). In the standard format of interpersonal therapy for adolescents (IPT-A), it is time-limited (12–16 weekly sessions). IPT has also been adapted to be delivered in groups (IPT-G; Mufson *et al.*, 2004), as well as in briefer formats as a preventative intervention in schools, in the form of IPT adolescent skills training (IPT-AST; Young *et al.*, 2006).

Influenced by the work of Harry Stack Sullivan and Adolf Meyer on interpersonal relationships, in IPT there is less emphasis than in psychodynamic psychotherapy or MBT on the interpersonal relationship between the therapist and patient or client during treatment, although the establishment of the therapeutic alliance is incorporated into the therapy process as a central element (Mufson *et al.*, 2011). In the assessment phase of IPT, a review of current relationships takes place, identifying how mood problems interact with these and the relationship features associated with the onset of mood disorder. This allows the selection of a focus for therapeutic work from a number of typical areas of difficulty in depression, such as grief after the loss of a loved one, conflict in significant relationships, difficulties adapting to changes in relationships or life circumstances, or difficulties stemming from social isolation. In the adaptation of IPT for adolescents, additional areas are included such as development of romantic relationships and initial experience with the death of a relative or friend (Mufson *et al.*, 2011). IPT-A aims to help the adolescent identify and develop more adaptive methods for dealing with the interpersonal issues associated with the onset or maintenance of their depression. Compared to the work with adults, IPT-A places greater emphasis on developing skills to manage current and future interpersonal difficulties that impact, or are impacted by, low mood. Although the treatment involves primarily individual sessions with the teenager, parents are asked to participate in a few sessions to receive education about depression, to address any relationship difficulties that may be occurring between the adolescent and their parents, and to help support the adolescent's treatment.

IPT-A has a promising evidence base for adolescent depression, where it has been evaluated in community settings. In their systematic review and meta-analysis of IPT-A for adolescents with depression, Duffy *et al.* (2019) identified 20 studies, half of which were RCTs. Although study quality was variable, and several of the studies were quite small-scale, IPT-A demonstrated significant improvements in depression symptoms post-intervention, with some evidence that these improvements were maintained for up to 1 year. When compared to other treatments for adolescent depression, IPT-A was shown to be "non-inferior" to CBT, and "superior" to less structured interventions, in terms of reducing depressive symptoms. On this basis, IPT-A is listed as an effective treatment in most treatment guidelines for the treatment of adolescent depression. However, the systematic review noted that there was no difference to other active interventions in terms of reduction in interpersonal problems. This may be surprising given the particular focus of the intervention and highlights the need for further investigation of the underlying mechanisms of change.

IPT is also different from psychodynamic psychotherapy and MBT, in so far as considerable work has been done to adapt the intervention for use with young people in LMICs. Rose-Clarke *et al.* (2020) identify a number of challenges to implementing many types of psychological psychotherapy in LMIC settings, including the lack of trained personnel, potential stigma regarding mental health, and lack of resources to provide individual therapy; in addition, most psychological psychotherapies have been developed in Western societies, and have cultural assumptions embedded within them which may not be applicable in other cultural contexts. There is some evidence that psychological psychotherapies developed in Western countries are more effective when implemented in LMICs if they first go through a process of cultural adaptation (Hall *et al.*, 2016). When it comes to young people, adaptations of IPT have been tried in settings as varied as Iran, Uganda, Ethiopia, and Nepal, as well as with low-income Latino adolescents in the U.S. In Nepal, for example, Rose-Clarke *et al.* (2020) describe how the country's context of civil war, major earthquakes, and socioeconomic deprivation creates a context in which there is a high level of adolescent depression but a scarcity of mental health provision. As part of a feasibility study, IPT was considered to be an appropriate model for adaptation. Nevertheless, considerable adaptations were required as part of the shift to a Nepalese context, including adapting the model to be delivered in schools by school nurses, and adding additional components to promote parental engagement and support. Attention was also paid to language, to ensure that locally acceptable terms for mental illness were used to destigmatize treatment. However, the fundamental IPT focus on enhancing social support, decreasing interpersonal stress, and improving interpersonal skills remained unchanged. Although the study suggests that the adapted intervention is appropriate and could be beneficial in Nepal, evaluation of the effectiveness of the intervention has yet to be reported.

Treatment selection

When considering treatment selection, both theory and evidence suggest that decisions may usefully be informed by assessing the client's quality of prior relationship experience and capacity for social functioning, as well as their current presentation. Therapeutic alliance is usually found to be independent of baseline symptom severity itself, but clinical theory suggests that the patient or client's prior capacity to form general social relationships of collaboration and trust may influence their specific capacity to form a productive therapeutic alliance in the therapy setting (Bowlby, 1988; Green, 2006). Some evidence supports this; for instance, an effect of child pretreatment social competence and intellectual functioning on early treatment alliance was found in an RCT for child behavior problems (Kazdin & Durbin, 2012), and pretreatment personality disorder independently predicted both alliance and outcome in an RCT of adolescents with repeated self-harm (Ayodeji *et al.*, 2015). But equally, attention to the *actual* quality of early engagement around treatment decisions during the formation of the initial "task alliance" will give a more immediate guide to likely later alliance and thus outcomes—and thus influence treatment selection. Such considerations are made implicitly in practice and are in line with emerging guidance on sequencing treatments (NICE, 2019). This is in line with the principles of clinical decision-making, themselves informed by the principles of shared decision-making (Verbist *et al.*, 2020; Hayes *et al.*, 2023). When a positive prior relationship formation history suggests that a positive therapeutic alliance is likely, then it is possible that a variety of therapeutic modalities may have a good chance of effectiveness, with little current evidence that one therapeutic modality has an advantage over another except in regard to preference. This would be consistent with therapeutic effect often being reported for multiple different therapies for the same condition.

For cases with disrupted or vulnerable prior relationships, however, therapeutic alliance may well be harder and clinical experience suggests that specific techniques may be needed (Bowlby, 1988). For example, cases presenting with motivational conflict in relation to change may need more sophisticated techniques to establish a therapeutic alliance, such as MI or IPT. Finally, there are cases with evidence of a disorganized relational history, inconsistent relationships, and unstable mental state, often with a history of unresolved trauma, such as young people with borderline personality development, severe relational disturbance, or self-harm. Here, much attention needs to be paid to the establishment (and ongoing repair) of the therapeutic alliance and this may be where intensive relationship-based approaches, such as psychodynamic psychotherapy or MBT, could be prioritized, where treatment attends directly and explicitly to the "here and now," so that the young person can have direct experience of addressing interpersonal disruptions and building and maintaining relationships.

Much could be done in future trial design to strengthen the evidence behind such critical treatment selection decisions. First, there is a need for more equivalence trials in our discipline, comparing different interventions for the same condition so as to illuminate differential effects. These, moreover, will be most illuminating when combined with a greater mechanistic focus on "active processes" within therapy rather than just efficacy outcomes (Marchette & Weisz, 2017), particularly in this context with baseline measurement of social functioning and process measures including ongoing therapeutic alliance (Kazdin & Nock, 2003; Green, 2006). In this way the relational aspects of therapeutic work identified in this chapter would become more deeply and valuably embedded in the guiding intervention science literature.

Considerations for therapy in low- and middle-income countries (LMICs)

Most of the specific interventions described in this chapter (with the exception of PASS and IPT-A) were developed and evaluated in Western, industrialized countries, as treatments to be delivered by highly specialist mental health staff. And yet a disproportionate number of young people live in LMICs and it is a priority for the global health agenda to address early development and mental health in these countries (Collins *et al.*, 2011). Recent reviews (Pedersen *et al.*, 2019) have identified some adaptation of early relationship-focused interventions to LMICs, and there is some evidence that family-based youth mental health interventions can be delivered in LMICs by nonspecialist providers (Healy *et al.*, 2018). There should be no reason why the therapeutic alliance and relationship-based work should not form as central a part of mental health provision in LMICs as in high-income countries and there is an urgent need to adapt, test, and deliver evidence-based interventions to LMICs, preserving rigor and equity in doing so (Baumann *et al.*, 2019). Relationship-based techniques—building alliance, establishing a secure base—and the more complex differentiated skills in MBT and MI are robust core skill sets with an evidence base that could be incorporated into systematic training of child mental health professionals in LMIC contexts.

Conclusion

This chapter has provided an overview of relationship-based treatments, with a particular focus on three main areas: interventions to improve the relatedness between children and significant caregivers in early childhood; relationship factors that operate across different forms of therapy with children and adolescents; and interventions in middle childhood and adolescence that either have a particular focus on improving social relationships or are defined by the use of the therapist–patient relationship as a major mechanism for effecting change.

Increasing evidence supports models of intervention to improve early caregiver–child interaction and relationships. In the context of both parent and child developmental vulnerabilities particularly, this involves briefer focused interventions using specific techniques such as video-feedback. Aspects of these relationships can be reliably improved in this way in the short term; the conversion of this into long-term measurable benefits for the child's social and mental health development is less consistently found, although there is emerging evidence that this is possible.

Recent work has strengthened our understanding of the components of the therapeutic alliance and its repair, especially in adolescence. The quality of the therapist–patient relationship within the therapeutic alliance shows consistent modest effects on treatment outcome for children and adolescents across a number of types of therapy. Alliance is affected by prior social and psychological functioning as well as therapist behaviors, and more recent research suggests that the most crucial factor may be the ongoing repair of ruptures in the therapeutic relationship, rather than viewing alliance as a more global, static entity. Exploring young people's own experiences of treatment, as well as examining when young people disengage from treatment, or treatment breaks down, also throws light on what makes a therapeutic relationship helpful or unhelpful.

Relationship-based therapies have a role to play in the treatment of child and adolescent mental health problems. Systematic testing of psychodynamic approaches to working with children and adolescents is still relatively rare compared to studies of CBT and the evidence is more preliminary, but there are indications that a focus on working directly on the therapeutic relationship is helpful for some young people. Contemporary integrative approaches, such as MBT, have retained the psychodynamic focus on working with the therapeutic relationship directly, but have moved from framing this in terms of transference toward the way in which mentalizing breaks down, and can be recovered, in the context of the therapeutic setting. IPT-A, in contrast, has a simpler style and is focused on approaches that optimize social functioning and interpersonal relating. It has a growing evidence base for relatively uncomplicated depressive disorders and has been adapted for use with groups and as a preventative intervention.

Traditionally, the types of psychotherapy reviewed in this chapter have been considered as less evidence-based and potentially expensive; however, the difficulty of helping the increasingly complex cases that access child mental health services and the success of some of these approaches in tackling such difficulties provide a counterbalancing argument for their value. Further high-quality evaluation, including of cost-effectiveness, is necessary in order to proceed with more confidence.

Acknowledgments

Jonathan Green is National Institute for Health Research (NIHR) senior investigator (NIHR NF-SI-0617-10168) and Fellow of the Academy of Medical Sciences. The views expressed in this article are those of the authors and not necessarily those of the UK National Health Service (NHS), the NIHR, or the Department of Health and Social Care.

References

Abbass, A. *et al.* (2013) Psychodynamic psychotherapy for children and adolescents: a meta-analysis of short-term psychodynamic models. *Journal of the American Academy of Child and Adolescent Psychiatry* **52**(8), 863–875. doi:10.1016/j.jaac.2013.05.014.

Anderson, K.N. *et al.* (2019) Therapeutic alliance, cultural competence and minority status in premature termination of psychotherapy. *American Journal of Orthopsychiatry* **89**(1), 104–114. doi:10.1037/ort0000342.

Ayodeji, E. *et al.* (2015) The influence of personality disorder on outcome in adolescent self-harm. *British Journal of Psychiatry* **207**(4), 313–319. doi:10.1192/bjp.bp.113.138941.

Baer, J.S. & Peterson, P.L. (2002) Motivational interviewing with adolescents and young adults. In: *Motivational Interviewing: Preparing People for Change*. (eds W.R. Miller & S. Rollnick), 2nd edn. Guilford Press, New York. pp. 217–250.

Bakermans-Kranenburg, M.J. *et al.* (2003) Less is more: meta-analyses of sensitivity and attachment interventions in early childhood. *Psychological Bulletin* **129**(2), 195–215. doi:10.1037/0033-2909.129.2.195.

Barlow, J. *et al.* (2015) Parent-infant psychotherapy for improving parental and infant mental health. *Cochrane Database of Systematic Reviews* **2015**(1). doi:10.1002/14651858.CD010534.pub2.

Barlow, J. *et al.* (2016) Parent–infant psychotherapy: a systematic review of the evidence for improving parental and infant mental health. *Journal of Reproductive and Infant Psychology* **34**(5), 464–482. doi:10.1080/02646838.2016.1222357.

Baumann, A.A. *et al.* (2019) Parenting programs for underserved populations in low- and middle-income countries: issues of scientific integrity and social justice. *Global Social Welfare* **6**(3), 199–207. doi:10.1007/s40609-018-0121-0.

Becker, K.D. & Chorpita, B.F. (2023) Future directions in youth and family treatment engagement: finishing the bridge between science and service. *Journal of Clinical Child & Adolescent Psychology* **52**(2), 284–309. doi:10.1080/15374416.2023.2169926.

Bose, D. *et al.* (2022) Therapeutic alliance in psychosocial interventions for youth internalizing disorders: a systematic review and preliminary meta-analysis. *Clinical Psychology: Science and Practice* **29**(2), 124–136. doi:10.1037/cps0000052.

Bowlby, J. (1988) *A Secure Base: Clinical Applications of Attachment Theory*. Routledge, London.

Byrne, G. *et al.* (2020) Mentalization-based treatments with children and families: a systematic review of the literature. *Clinical Child Psychology and Psychiatry* **25**(4), 1022–1048. doi:10.1177/1359104520920689.

Carruthers, S. *et al.* (2023) Mediation of 6-year mid-childhood follow-up outcomes after pre-school social communication (PACT) therapy for autistic children: randomised controlled trial. *Journal of Child Psychology and Psychiatry*. doi:10.1111/jcpp.13798.

Carter, A.S. *et al.* (2011) A randomized controlled trial of Hanen's 'More Than Words' in toddlers with early autism symptoms. *Journal of Child Psychology and Psychiatry* **52**(7), 741–752. doi:10.1111/j.1469-7610.2011.02395.x.

Cassidy, J. *et al.* (2011) Enhancing infant attachment security: an examination of treatment efficacy and differential susceptibility. *Development and Psychopathology* **23**(1), 131–148. doi:10.1017/S0954579410000696.

Chiappetta, L. *et al.* (2018) Motivational interviewing to increase outpatient attendance for adolescent psychiatric patients. *Journal of Psychosocial Nursing and Mental Health Services* **56**(6), 31–35. doi:10.3928/02793695-20180212-04.

Cirasola, A. & Midgley, N. (2023) The alliance with young people: where have we been, where are we going? *Psychotherapy* **60**(1), 110–118. doi:10.1037/pst0000461.

Cirasola, A. *et al.* (2022) Alliance ruptures and resolutions in short-term psychoanalytic psychotherapy for adolescent depression: an empirical case study. *Psychotherapy Research* **32**(7), 951–968. doi:10.1080/10503307.2022.2061314.

Collins, P.Y. *et al.* (2011) Grand challenges in global mental health. *Nature* **475**(7354), 27–30. doi:10.1038/475027a.

Cook, B.L. *et al.* (2013) Racial/ethnic disparity trends in children's mental health care access and expenditures from 2002 to 2007. *Health Services Research* **48**(1), 129–149. doi:10.1111/j.1475-6773.2012.01439.x.

Cregeen, S. *et al.* (2017) *Short-term Psychoanalytic Psychotherapy for Adolescents with Depression: A Treatment Manual.* Karnac, London.

Dalgaard, N.T. *et al.* (2023) Holding a foster child's mind in mind: study protocol for a cluster-randomized controlled trial of mentalization-based therapy (MBT) for foster families. *BMC Psychology* **11**(1), 62. doi:10.1186/s40359-023-01103-8.

de Haan, A.M. *et al.* (2013) A meta-analytic review on treatment dropout in child and adolescent outpatient mental health care. *Clinical Psychology Review* **33**(5), 698–711. doi:10.1016/j.cpr.2013.04.005.

Divan, G. *et al.* (2015) Adapting an evidence-based intervention for autism spectrum disorder for scaling up in resource-constrained settings: the development of the PASS intervention in South Asia. *Global Health Action* **8**(1), 27278. doi:10.3402/gha.v8.27278.

Duffy, F. *et al.* (2019) Review: the effectiveness of interpersonal psychotherapy for adolescents with depression—a systematic review and meta-analysis. *Child and Adolescent Mental Health* **24**(4), 307–317. doi:10.1111/camh.12342.

Eubanks, C.F. *et al.* (2018) Alliance rupture repair: a meta-analysis. *Psychotherapy* **55**(4), 508–519. doi:10.1037/pst0000185.

Garcia, J.A. & Weisz, J.R. (2002) When youth mental health care stops: therapeutic relationship problems and other reasons for ending youth outpatient treatment. *Journal of Consulting and Clinical Psychology* **70**(2), 439–443.

Gibson, K. & Cartwright, C. (2014) Young people's experiences of mobile phone text counselling: balancing connection and control. *Children and Youth Services Review* **43**, 96–104. doi:10.1016/j.childyouth.2014.05.010.

Gibson, K. *et al.* (2016) What young people want: a qualitative study of adolescents' priorities for engagement across psychological services. *Journal of Child and Family Studies* **25**(4), 1057–1065. doi:10.1007/s10826-015-0292-6.

Goodyer, I.M. *et al.* (2017) Cognitive-behavioural therapy and short-term psychoanalytic psychotherapy versus brief psychosocial intervention in adolescents with unipolar major depression (IMPACT): a multicentre, pragmatic, observer-blind, randomised controlled trial. *Health Technology Assessment* **21**(12), 1–93. doi:10.3310/hta21120.

Göttken, T. & von Klitzing, K. (2018) *Manual for Short-Term Psychoanalytic Child Therapy (PaCT).* Routledge, London. doi:10.4324/9780429477041.

Gowers, S.G. *et al.* (2007) Clinical effectiveness of treatments for anorexia nervosa in adolescents. *British Journal of Psychiatry* **191**(5), 427–435. doi:10.1192/bjp.bp.107.036764.

Green, J. (2006) Annotation: the therapeutic alliance—a significant but neglected variable in child mental health treatment studies. *Journal of Child Psychology and Psychiatry* **47**(5), 425–435. doi:10.1111/j.1469-7610.2005.01516.x.

Green, J. *et al.* (2017) Randomised trial of a parent-mediated intervention for infants at high risk for autism: longitudinal outcomes to age 3 years. *Journal of Child Psychology and Psychiatry* **58**(12), 1330–1340. doi:10.1111/jcpp.12728.

Gulsrud, A.C. *et al.* (2014) Two to ten years: developmental trajectories of joint attention in children with ASD who received targeted social communication interventions. *Autism Research* **7**(2), 207–215. doi:10.1002/aur.1360.

Gulsrud, A.C. *et al.* (2016) Isolating active ingredients in a parent-mediated social communication intervention for toddlers with autism spectrum disorder. *Journal of Child Psychology and Psychiatry* **57**(5), 606–613. doi:10.1111/jcpp.12481.

Hall, G.C.N. *et al.* (2016) A meta-analysis of cultural adaptations of psychological interventions. *Behavior Therapy* **47**(6), 993–1014. doi:10.1016/j.beth.2016.09.005.

Hartley, S. *et al.* (2022) Therapeutic relationships within child and adolescent mental health inpatient services: a qualitative exploration of the experiences of young people, family members and nursing staff. *PLoS One* **17**(1), e0262070. doi:10.1371/journal.pone.0262070.

Hayes, D. *et al.* (2023) A systematic review of shared decision making interventions in child and youth mental health: synthesising the use of theory, intervention functions, and behaviour change techniques. *European Child & Adolescent Psychiatry* **32**(2), 209–222. doi:10.1007/s00787-021-01782-x.

Healy, E.A. *et al.* (2018) Family-based youth mental health interventions delivered by nonspecialist providers in low- and middle-income countries: a systematic review. *Families, Systems & Health* **36**(2), 182–197. doi:10.1037/fsh0000334.

Housby, H. *et al.* (2021) What contributes to good outcomes? The perspective of young people on short-term psychoanalytic psychotherapy for depressed adolescents Taubner, S. (ed.). *PLOS ONE* **16**(9), e0257334. doi:10.1371/journal.pone.0257334.

Johnston, C. & Jassy, J.S. (2007) Attention-deficit/hyperactivity disorder and oppositional/conduct problems: links to parent-child interactions. *Journal of the Canadian Academy of Child and Adolescent Psychiatry = Journal de l'Academie canadienne de psychiatrie de l'enfant et de l'adolescent* **16**(2), 74–79.

Juffer, F. *et al.* (2008) *Promoting Positive Parenting: An Attachment-based Intervention.* Lawrence Erlbaum, New York.

Karver, M.S. *et al.* (2006) Meta-analysis of therapeutic relationship variables in youth and family therapy: the evidence for different relationship variables in the child and adolescent treatment outcome literature. *Clinical Psychology Review* **26**(1), 50–65. doi:10.1016/j.cpr.2005.09.001.

Karver, M.S. *et al.* (2018) Meta-analysis of the prospective relation between alliance and outcome in child and adolescent psychotherapy. *Psychotherapy* **55**(4), 341–355. doi:10.1037/pst0000176.

Kazdin, A.E. & Durbin, K.A. (2012) Predictors of child–therapist alliance in cognitive–behavioral treatment of children referred for oppositional and antisocial behavior. *Psychotherapy* **49**(2), 202–217. doi:10.1037/a0027933.

Kazdin, A.E. & Nock, M.K. (2003) Delineating mechanisms of change in child and adolescent therapy: methodological issues and research recommendations. *Journal of Child Psychology and Psychiatry* **8**, 1116–1129. doi:10.1111/1469-7610.00195.

Keown, L.J. (2012) Predictors of boys' ADHD symptoms from early to middle childhood: the role of father-child and mother-child interactions. *Journal of Abnormal Child Psychology* **40**(4), 569–581. doi:10.1007/s10802-011-9586-3.

Kufferath-Lin, T. *et al.* (2022) Psychodynamic therapy in children and adolescents. In: *Comprehensive Clinical Psychology.* (ed G.J.G. Asmundson). Elsevier, Amsterdam. pp. 148–174. doi:10.1016/B978-0-12-818697-8.00039-X.

Lindqvist, K. *et al.* (2020) Affect-focused psychodynamic internet-based therapy for adolescent depression: randomized controlled trial. *Journal of Medical Internet Research* **22**(3), e18047. doi:10.2196/18047.

Lindqvist, K. *et al.* (2022) "I didn't have to look her in the eyes"—participants' experiences of the therapeutic relationship in internet-based psychodynamic therapy for adolescent depression. *Psychotherapy Research*, 1–15. doi:10.1080/10503307.2022.2150583.

Loades, M.E. *et al.* (2023) In context: lessons about adolescent unipolar depression from the improving mood with psychoanalytic and cognitive therapies trial. *Journal of the American Academy of Child & Adolescent Psychiatry*. doi:10.1016/j.jaac.2023.03.017.

Løvgren, A. *et al.* (2019) How do adolescents with depression experience improvement in psychodynamic psychotherapy? A qualitative study. *BMC Psychiatry* **19**(1), 95. doi:10.1186/s12888-019-2080-0.

MacKean, M. *et al.* (2023) 'I've started my journey to coping better': exploring adolescents' journeys through an internet-based psychodynamic therapy (I-PDT) for depression. *Journal of Child Psychotherapy*, 1–22. doi:10.1080/0075417X.2023.2173271.

Malda-Castillo, J. *et al.* (2019) Mentalization-based treatment and its evidence-base status: a systematic literature review. *Psychology and Psychotherapy: Theory, Research and Practice* **92**(4), 465–498. doi:10.1111/papt.12195.

Marchette, L.K. & Weisz, J.R. (2017) Practitioner review: empirical evolution of youth psychotherapy toward transdiagnostic approaches. *Journal of Child Psychology and Psychiatry* **58**(9), 970–984. doi:10.1111/jcpp.12747.

Mechler, J. *et al.* (2022) Therapist-guided internet-based psychodynamic therapy versus cognitive behavioural therapy for adolescent depression in Sweden: a randomised, clinical, non-inferiority trial. *The Lancet Digital Health* **4**(8), e594–e603. doi:10.1016/S2589-7500(22)00095-4.

Mehta, A. *et al.* (2023) Understanding treatment non-responders: a qualitative study of depressed adolescents' experiences of 'unsuccessful' psychotherapy. *Psychology and Psychotherapy: Theory, Research and Practice*. doi:10.1111/papt.12448.

Midgley, N. & Vrouva, I. (2012) *Mentalization-based Interventions with Children, Young People, and Families*. Routledge, London.

Midgley, N. *et al.* (2017) *Mentalization-based Treatment for Children: A Time-Limited Approach*. American Psychological Association, Washington, DC.

Midgley, N. *et al.* (2021a) The evidence-base for psychodynamic psychotherapy with children and adolescents: a narrative synthesis. *Frontiers in Psychology* **12**. doi:10.3389/fpsyg.2021.662671.

Midgley, N. *et al.* (2021b) Mentalization-based interventions for children aged 6-12 and their carers: a narrative systematic review. *Journal of Infant, Child, and Adolescent Psychotherapy* **20**(2), 169–189. doi: 10.1080/15289168.2021.1915654.

Mufson, L. *et al.* (2004) A group adaptation of interpersonal psychotherapy for depressed adolescents. *American Journal of Psychotherapy* **58**(2), 220–237. doi:10.1176/appi.psychotherapy.2004.58.2.220.

Mufson, L.H. *et al.* (2011) *Interpersonal Psychotherapy for Depressed Adolescents*, 2nd edn. Guilford Press, New York.

Muran, J.C. & Eubanks, C.F. (2020) *Therapist Performance Under Pressure: Negotiating Emotion, Difference, and Rupture*. American Psychological Association, Washington, DC. doi:10.1037/0000182-000.

Naar-King, S. & Suarez, M. (2011) *Motivational Interviewing with Adolescents and Young Adults*. Guilford Press, New York.

National Institute for Health and Care Excellence (NICE) (2013) Autism spectrum disorder in under 19s: support and management.*Clinical guideline [CG170]*. Available: www.nice.org.uk/guidance/CG170 [30 August 2023].

National Institute for Health and Care Excellence (NICE) (2019) *Depression in Children and Young People: Identification and Management*. Available: https://www.nice.org.uk/guidance/ng134 [16 October 2024].

National Institute for Health and Care Excellence (NICE) (2021) Autism spectrum disorder in under 19s: support and management. *Clinical guideline [CG170]*. Available: https://www.nice.org.uk/guidance/cg170/resources/autism-spectrum-disorder-in-under-19s-support-and-management-pdf-35109745515205 [28 October 2024].

Nof, A. *et al.* (2019) If you believe that breaking is possible, believe also that fixing is possible: a framework for ruptures and repairs in child psychotherapy. *Research in Psychotherapy: Psychopathology, Process and Outcome* **22**(1). doi:10.4081/ripppo.2019.364.

Núñez, L. *et al.* (2022) The therapeutic relationship as a change mechanism in child psychotherapy: a qualitative study of children, parents', and therapists' views in different moments of the process. *Studies in Psychology* **43**(3), 666–687. doi:10.1080/02109395.2022.2127233.

O'Hara, L. *et al.* (2019) Video feedback for parental sensitivity and attachment security in children under five years. *Cochrane Database of Systematic Reviews* **2019**(11). doi:10.1002/14651858.CD012348.pub2.

O'Keeffe, S. *et al.* (2019) 'I just stopped going': a mixed methods investigation into types of therapy dropout in adolescents with depression. *Frontiers in Psychology* **10**. doi:10.3389/fpsyg.2019.00075.

Ougrin, D. (2012) Commentary: self-harm in adolescents: the best predictor of death by suicide?—reflections on Hawton et al. (2012). *Journal of Child Psychology and Psychiatry* **53**(12), 1220–1221. doi:10.1111/j.1469-7610.2012.02622.x.

Pedersen, G.A. *et al.* (2019) A systematic review of the evidence for family and parenting interventions in low- and middle-income countries: child and youth mental health outcomes. *Journal of Child and Family Studies* **28**(8), 2036–2055. doi:10.1007/s10826-019-01399-4.

Pickles, A. *et al.* (2015) Treatment mechanism in the MRC preschool autism communication trial: implications for study design and parent-focussed therapy for children. *Journal of Child Psychology and Psychiatry* **56**(2), 162–170. doi:10.1111/jcpp.12291.

Pickles, A. *et al.* (2016) Parent-mediated social communication therapy for young children with autism (PACT): long-term follow-up of a randomised controlled trial. *The Lancet* **388**(10059), 2501–2509. doi:10.1016/S0140-6736(16)31229-6.

Probst, G.H. *et al.* (2019) The alliance-outcome relation in internet-based interventions for psychological disorders: a correlational meta-analysis. *Verhaltenstherapie*, 1–12. doi:10.1159/000503432.

Rahman, A. *et al.* (2016) Effectiveness of the parent-mediated intervention for children with autism spectrum disorder in South Asia in India and Pakistan (PASS): a randomised controlled trial. *The Lancet Psychiatry* **3**(2), 128–136. doi:10.1016/S2215-0366(15)00388-0.

Rose-Clarke, K. *et al.* (2020) Culturally and developmentally adapting group interpersonal therapy for adolescents with depression in rural Nepal. *BMC Psychology* **8**(1), 83. doi:10.1186/s40359-020-00452-y.

Rossouw, T.I. & Fonagy, P. (2012) Mentalization-based treatment for self-harm in adolescents: a randomized controlled trial. *Journal of the American Academy of Child & Adolescent Psychiatry* **51**(12), 1304–1313. doi:10.1016/j.jaac.2012.09.018.

Rossouw, T. *et al.* (2021). In: *Mentalization-based Treatment for Adolescents: A Practical Treatment Guide*. (eds T. Rossouw, *et al.*). Routledge, New York.

Safran, J.D. & Muran, J.C. (2006) Has the concept of the therapeutic alliance outlived its usefulness? *Psychotherapy: Theory, Research, Practice, Training* **43**(3), 286–291. doi:10.1037/0033-3204.43.3.286.

Segal, L. *et al.* (2023) Estimated therapy costs and downstream cost consequences of iBASIS–video interaction to promote positive parenting intervention vs usual care among children displaying early behavioral signs of autism in Australia. *JAMA Network Open* **6**(4), e235847. doi:10.1001/jamanetworkopen.2023.5847.

Stige, S.H. *et al.* (2021) Barriers and facilitators in adolescent psychotherapy initiated by adults—experiences that differentiate adolescents' trajectories through mental health care. *Frontiers in Psychology* **12**. doi:10.3389/fpsyg.2021.633663.

Ulberg, R. *et al.* (2021) The first experimental study of transference work–in teenagers (FEST–IT): a multicentre, observer- and patient-blind, randomised controlled component study. *BMC Psychiatry* **21**(1). doi:10.1186/s12888-021-03055-y.

van den Boom, D.C. (1994) The influence of temperament and mothering on attachment and exploration: an experimental manipulation of sensitive responsiveness among lower-class mothers with irritable infants. *Child Development* **65**(5), 1457–1477. doi:10.1111/j.1467-8624.1994.tb00829.x.

van IJzendoorn, M.H. *et al.* (2023) Improving parenting, child attachment, and externalizing behaviors: meta-analysis of the first 25 randomized controlled trials on the effects of video-feedback intervention to promote positive parenting and sensitive discipline. *Development and Psychopathology* **35**(1), 241–256. doi:10.1017/S0954579421001462.

Verbist, A.N. *et al.* (2020) A review of treatment decision-making models and factors in mental health practice. *Families in Society: The Journal of Contemporary Social Services* **101**(4), 444–455. doi:10.1177/1044389420921069.

von Below, C. (2020) "We just did not get on". Young adults' experiences of unsuccessful psychodynamic psychotherapy—a lack of meta-communication and mentalization? *Frontiers in Psychology* **11**. doi:10.3389/fpsyg.2020.01243.

Wampold, B.E. & Flückiger, C. (2023) The alliance in mental health care: conceptualization, evidence and clinical applications. *World Psychiatry* **22**(1), 25–41. doi:10.1002/wps.21035.

Weissman, M.M. *et al.* (2000) *Comprehensive Guide to Interpersonal Psychotherapy*. Basic Books, New York.

Whitehouse, A.J.O. *et al.* (2021) Effect of preemptive intervention on developmental outcomes among infants showing early signs of autism. *JAMA Pediatrics* **175**(11), e213298. doi:10.1001/jamapediatrics.2021.3298.

Wilmots, E. *et al.* (2020) The therapeutic relationship in cognitive behaviour therapy with depressed adolescents: a qualitative study of good-outcome cases. *Psychology and Psychotherapy: Theory, Research and Practice* **93**(2), 276–291. doi:10.1111/papt.12232.

Young, J.F. *et al.* (2006) Efficacy of interpersonal psychotherapy-adolescent skills training: an indicated preventive intervention for depression. *Journal of Child Psychology and Psychiatry* **47**(12), 1254–1262. doi:10.1111/j.1469-7610.2006.01667.x.

Zwi, M. *et al.* (2011) Parent training interventions for attention deficit hyperactivity disorder (ADHD) in children aged 5 to 18 years. *Cochrane Database of Systematic Reviews*. doi:10.1002/14651858.CD003018.pub3.

CHAPTER 37
Educational interventions for children's learning difficulties

Charles Hulme[1], Enrica Donolato[2] and Monica Melby-Lervåg[2]
[1] School of Psychology, Social Work and Public Health, Oxford Brookes University, Oxford, UK
[2] Department of Special Needs Education and CREATE, University of Oslo, Oslo, Norway

This chapter examines evidence for the efficacy of educational interventions for learning disorders in children. We consider interventions for reading disorders (dyslexia and reading comprehension impairment), mathematics disorders, developmental learning disorders (Intellectual Disability, ID) and developmental coordination disorder (DCD) or dyspraxia. In addition to interventions designed for specific disorders, we consider evidence for some recent approaches that claim to have quite general effects on cognitive functioning in diverse groups of children. We also consider possible adaptations of interventions for children with comorbid disorders. Finally, we discuss some limitations and directions for future studies in this area.

Conceptual and methodological issues

It is important to emphasize that educational or psychological interventions, whatever they are for, should be based on sound principles. Preferably, interventions should be based on a theory of the nature and causes of a disorder that the intervention is designed to help. It is worth emphasizing that the fields of education and special education are plagued by interventions that lack a sound theoretical rationale. It is always possible that such interventions will have effects, but we should expect very high levels of evidence to convince us that interventions that are not based on a sound theoretical foundation really are effective.

We would emphasize that clinicians should evaluate claims for the effectiveness of new educational treatments with caution. For any proposed treatment, a clinician should ask two basic questions: (i) Is the proposed intervention theoretically plausible (i.e., does the intervention directly target a skill that is deficient in a given population, or target a process which has been identified as a likely cause of a disorder)? (ii) If the answer to question (i) is positive, is there evidence from one or more randomized controlled trials (RCTs) to indicate that the intervention has beneficial effects? RCTs are the only the type of study that allow for unbiased conclusions about effectiveness (see Chapters 13 and 14 on causal inference and epidemiology). Given randomization of children to a control group and treatment group any differences between the groups before intervention must reflect chance. Randomization thus controls for preexisting differences between groups—not only known variables (e.g., pretest scores on an outcome measure) but also on unknown variables (e.g., hypothetical genetic differences between individuals that might affect their response to intervention). Figure 37.1 shows an overview of a typical RCT.

Conclusions about effectiveness must include the effect size associated with the intervention; typically computed as the difference between the control group and treatment group after intervention expressed in terms of standard deviation units. This is referred to as Cohen's *d* (or sometimes as Hedges', a very similar measure). Figure 37.2 shows an outline of what an effect size expressed in standard deviation units means.

The definition of a "reasonable effect size" is open to debate. Based on the distribution of 1942 effect sizes from 747 RCTs evaluating education interventions with standardized test outcomes, Kraft (2020) suggested the following benchmarks: a *d* of less than 0.05 is *small*, 0.05 to less than 0.20 is *medium*, and 0.20 or greater is *large*. According to earlier guidelines from the What Works Clearinghouse (2014), an effect size of 0.25 standard deviations or larger was considered "substantially important" and should have consequences for educational practice. In summary, earlier guidelines, combined with Kraft's (2020) more recent review, suggest that effect sizes (*d* or *g*) of 0.20 or larger should be seen as important and clinically relevant. It is important to note that the type of control group used may influence the size of effects obtained. For instance, it is well known that active control groups often lead to smaller effect

Rutter's Child and Adolescent Psychiatry and Psychology, Seventh Edition.
Edited by Anita Thapar, Daniel S. Pine, Samuele Cortese, Cathy Creswell, Tamsin J. Ford, James F. Leckman, and Argyris Stringaris.

Companion website: www.wiley.com/go/thapar/rutterspsych7

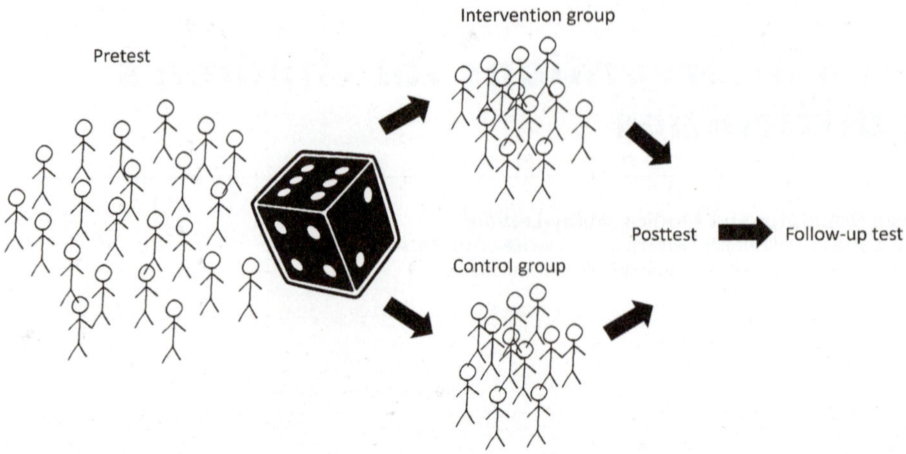

Figure 37.1 A diagram explaining the design of a randomized controlled trial (RCT).

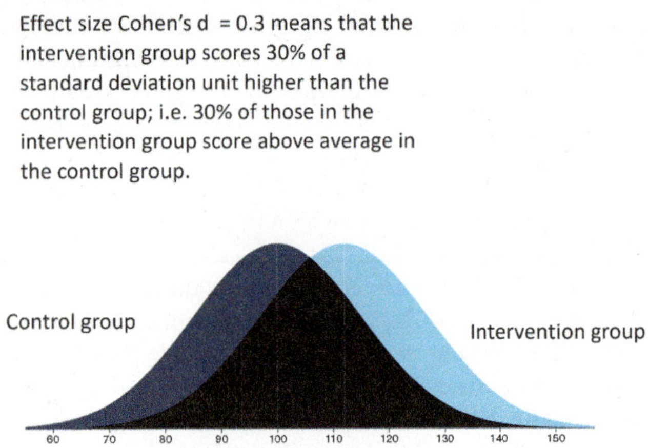

Figure 37.2 Cohen's *d* (standardized mean difference) as a measure of effect size in intervention studies.

sizes than business-as-usual control groups, because active controls account for nonspecific intervention effects such as increased attention or motivation (Melby-Lervåg *et al.*, 2016). Most studies of educational interventions have used business-as-usual control groups, which should be considered when interpreting the effect sizes obtained.

In this chapter, we will concentrate on interventions for which there is good evidence of effectiveness. In general, we will not focus on interventions for which we believe evidence is lacking. Two examples of such interventions would be the Dore program which focused on training balance skills (see Reynolds *et al.*, 2003) and the use of colored overlays or lenses, both of which appear to be ineffective as treatments for dyslexia (Snowling & Hulme 2003; Henderson *et al.* 2013). The omission of these interventions (and many others that lack a sound theoretical rationale) reflects our judgment that adequate evidence for their efficacy is simply lacking. However, we discuss some recent interventions that have received much attention, but where it turns out that evidence is also lacking. Using such interventions is unfortunate for several reasons, including the fact that they take time away from other interventions that might be more effective. Educational interventions are costly and expenditure in schools accounts for a large proportion of the costs related to pediatric mental disorders (see also Chapter 17).

Although methodological issues have been dealt with elsewhere, we believe it is important to emphasize the types of evidence that can establish that interventions "work" (see also Chapters 15 "Establishing the clinical effectiveness of interventions and implementations" and 16 "What clinicians need to know about statistical methods"). In the following sections, we will summarize a great deal of evidence, mostly from RCTs. However, evidence from all studies, including RCTs, may have limitations because of factors such as small sample sizes, lack of implementation fidelity, or other methodological problems. Therefore, meta-analyses of RCTs are often considered to provide the highest quality evidence. If possible, we will use meta-analyses in this review. This evidence shows that a range of educational interventions are effective for children who have difficulties in developing key educational skills including reading accuracy and fluency, reading comprehension, and arithmetic (see Chapter 51 for evidence for treatments for language disorders). The studies usually involve specialist teaching delivered either to individual children or children in small groups. The duration of the educational interventions varies a great deal, typically between 4 and 20–30 weeks, which will potentially be related to the size of the effects obtained. We will therefore explore specifically how duration of intervention, when reported, is related to the effect sizes obtained. Some technical terms used here are defined in Figure 37.3.

Dyslexia and decoding impairments

The nature and causes of dyslexia and decoding impairments

Dyslexia, a severe difficulty in learning to read (in the sense of recognizing printed words accurately and fluently), is a relatively common disorder (see Chapter 52 for a detailed

Experimental design	• Random assignment of participants to conditions • Includes a control group • Helps to establish cause and effect • Considered the most rigorous type of research design (gold standard)
Quasi-experimental design	• No randomization of participants to conditions • May include a control group • Unable to assure causal relationships between variables
Intervention	• Intervention is when the researcher assigns participants to receive a particular treatment for the purpose of the study
Outcome variables	• The outcome (or predicted or dependent) variable defines the skills the intervention aims to develop and change
Pretest, posttest, and follow-up	• Outcome variables are assessed through tests, questionnaires, observation schedules, and checklists to collect data before the intervention (pretest or baseline), right after the intervention (posttest) and after some time from the intervention (follow-up)

Figure 37.3 Main technical constructs in the chapter.

account). Historically, it was typically defined using a discrepancy definition whereby a child's reading attainment needed to be out of line with their age and IQ (e.g., Rutter & Yule, 1975). Such a definition, though still widely used, has fallen from favor, and the *Diagnostic and Statistical Manual of Mental Disorders*, 5th edition (DSM-5; American Psychiatric Association, 2013) makes no explicit reference to this (see Chapter 52 for further discussion). For children within the normal range of intellectual ability (IQs above 70) IQ appears only weakly correlated with reading accuracy, and there is little evidence that IQ is predictive of variations in children's responses to instruction to improve decoding skills (e.g., Hatcher & Hulme, 1999).

Dyslexia is typically diagnosed when a person has severe difficulties with reading accuracy as assessed by a well-standardized test. Given that reading skills have a continuous distribution in the population, the cutoff for defining "dyslexia" is inherently arbitrary. Epidemiological studies suggest that, depending on where the diagnostic cutoff is set, dyslexia affects approximately 3–8% of children (Peterson & Pennington, 2012).

Extracting meaning from text is the overall goal of reading. According to "the simple view of reading," reading comprehension is the product of decoding and language comprehension (Gough & Tunmer, 1986). The "simple view of reading" is outlined in Figure 37.4. This theory has ample support from several studies (García & Cain, 2014; Foorman *et al.*, 2015a; Foorman

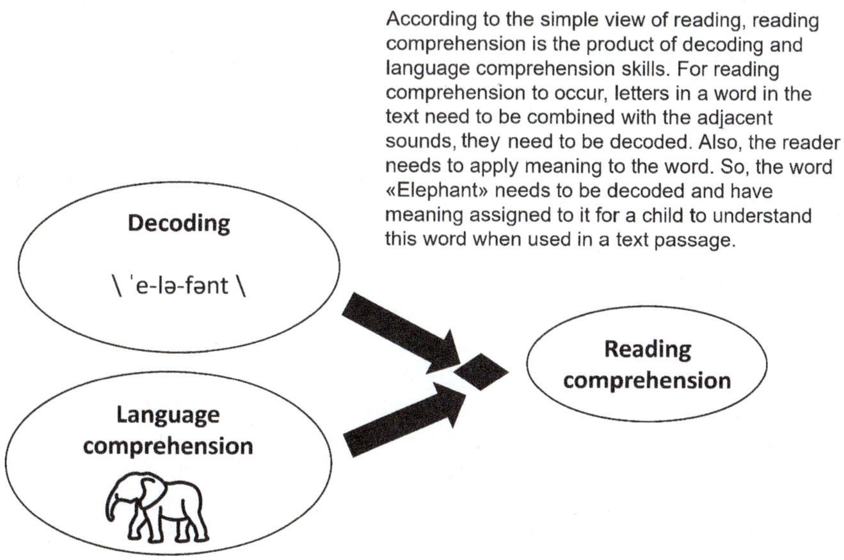

Figure 37.4 The simple view of reading.

et al., 2015b; Lervåg *et al.*, 2018; Hjetland *et al.*, 2020). According to the "simple view," decoding problems do not only affect the ability to read single words accurately but also impair reading fluency and reading comprehension (Hulme & Snowling, 2009, Chapter 2).

The currently accepted view is that the most powerful causal risk factor for dyslexia is a phonological deficit (i.e., a problem in representing the sound structure of spoken words, see Chapter 52). More specifically, phonemic skills (being able to identify and manipulate the constituent sounds in spoken words) measured in children at the earliest stages of learning to read are closely related to the growth in children's word-reading skills (Melby-Lervåg *et al.*, 2012). On this basis, it has been argued that the core problem in dyslexia is a difficulty in creating well-specified phonemic representations of speech (Hulme & Snowling, 2009, see Chapter 2). These findings have important applied implications because they suggest that the early teaching of reading, and the remedial teaching given to children with dyslexia, should emphasize the direct teaching of phonemic skills.

However, another key problem for children with dyslexia is learning letter–sound correspondences, and poor letter–sound knowledge is another longitudinal predictor of learning to read (Lervåg *et al.*, 2009). Furthermore, analysis from an intervention designed to improve decoding skills in children at risk of reading difficulties showed that improvements in phonemic skills and letter–sound knowledge at the end of the intervention were two key mediators of subsequent increases in word-level reading skills (Hulme *et al.*, 2012). This suggests that children with weak word-reading skills require help targeting phonemic awareness and letter–sound knowledge. However, to be maximally effective, such interventions also need to be coupled with direct instruction in word reading, and practice reading texts (Hatcher *et al.*, 1994).

Interventions targeting phonology

Meta-analyses of treatment studies

Several meta-analyses have been published summarizing the effectiveness of phonological interventions designed to improve reading skills in children with reading difficulties (Bus & van Ijzendoorn 1999; Ehri *et al.*, 2001; Lonigan *et al.*, 2008; McArthur *et al.*, 2018; Hall *et al.*, 2022). The most recent meta-analysis of children with, or at family risk of, dyslexia, showed that interventions with a phonological awareness component in addition to decoding had a sizeable effect size ($d = 0.38$, $k = 38$) (Hall *et al.*, 2022). This training taught children to identify phonemes in spoken words (i.e., to match words with the same initial sound) or to manipulate phonemes in spoken words (i.e., combine sounds to form words, segment or delete parts of words) and was typically combined with phonic reading instruction (either training letter knowledge or some aspect of decoding). However, decoding interventions that did not include phonological awareness training also demonstrated improvements in reading, albeit with a smaller effect size ($d = 0.22$, $k = 16$). The interventions were typically given in addition to any instruction children were already receiving, and usually the control group received whatever was typical teaching in their preschool or kindergarten.

The results from this recent meta-analysis are in line with a previous meta-analysis focusing exclusively on children and adults with reading difficulties, which showed that phonic reading instruction (teaching that focuses on getting children to understand letter–sound rules), with or without phonological awareness training, had positive effects on word decoding ($d = 0.51$, $k = 11$), word-reading fluency ($d = 0.45$, $k = 4$), and nonword-reading fluency ($d = 0.39$, $k = 3$) for those with poor reading skills (McArthur *et al.*, 2018). Thus, interventions targeting phonology along with letter–sound training and phonic reading instruction have clear and positive effects on children's reading and phonological skills.

Moderators of treatment

The meta-analysis by Hall *et al.* (2022) suggests that the best effects are obtained when phonological awareness training is combined with teaching related to letter knowledge or phonically based reading instruction. Also, notably, previous meta-analyses have shown that phonological awareness training seemed to be more effective when focusing on smaller units in language such as phonemes (say the sounds in the word CAT -> /k/ /ae/ /t/) rather than larger units such as rimes (a rime unit is the part of a spoken syllable that follows the initial consonant so the rime unit in CAT is /at/) or syllables (Lonigan *et al.*, 2008; see also Melby-Lervåg *et al.*, 2012).

Interventions targeting reading fluency

Meta-analyses of treatment studies

In older children with dyslexia, basic decoding skills may be mastered but reading often remains dysfluent (slow and labored). Poor reading fluency can be a significant impediment to success in formal education. A recent meta-analysis examined the effectiveness of interventions to improve reading fluency in children with reading problems (Zimmerman *et al.*, 2021). The interventions all involved some form of repeated oral reading which involves pupils reading texts with similar levels of difficulty under teacher guidance, until a prespecified level of proficiency was met. The interventions involved reading texts with similar levels of difficulty (not simply repeatedly reading the same text). The studies included children from kindergarten to 17 years with reading difficulties and measured reading fluency. The results (from 8 studies) showed improvements in reading fluency for children receiving intervention compared with controls ($d = 0.18$, $k = 8$). This is somewhat smaller than in previous meta-analyses of reading fluency interventions. For instance, Samuels *et al.* (2000) showed large effects from reading fluency interventions (decoding fluency $d = 0.44$, word recognition $d = 0.55$, and reading comprehension $d = 0.35$) and Therrien (2004) found substantial effects of repeated reading practice on measures of reading fluency ($d = 0.83$) and comprehension ($d = 0.67$). One reason for the differences between these two earlier meta-analyses (Samuels *et al.*, 2000; Therrien, 2004) and the more recent one (Zimmerman *et al.*, 2021), could be that the latter had stricter design criteria for inclusion and only included studies that did not involve rereading the same texts.

Moderators of treatment

Zimmerman *et al.* (2021) found larger effects on comprehension outcomes compared with fluency outcomes, although this difference was not significant ($d = 0.24$ versus $d = 0.11$).

Summary

Interventions for children who have decoding problems are well developed and there is now strong evidence from many RCTs that interventions that target phoneme awareness and letter–sound knowledge, in the context of structured phonic teaching, are highly effective in improving decoding skills. There is also evidence that interventions involving repeated oral reading practice can help to improve reading fluency in children with reading problems. Clinically, it is widely believed that maintaining an interest in reading, and ensuring that children with dyslexia engage in frequent reading practice, are important for helping to reduce the reading fluency problems that are common in this group of children.

Reading comprehension impairment

The nature and causes of reading comprehension impairment

Children with reading comprehension impairment decode words accurately, but nevertheless have problems understanding the meaning of texts they can read accurately (Hulme & Snowling, 2009, 2011). Such children may often go unnoticed in school because they read aloud normally. Reading comprehension difficulties have been much less studied than dyslexia.

Reading comprehension impairment is typically diagnosed if a child shows a large (at least 1 SD) discrepancy between reading accuracy and reading comprehension on a well-standardized test, coupled with a reading comprehension standard score of 90 or below. In a standardization of a reading test involving a nationally representative sample of 1324 UK primary-school children 3.3% of the sample met these diagnostic criteria (Hulme & Snowling, 2011).

A great deal of evidence points to the conclusion that the cause of reading comprehension problems seems to be a language comprehension deficit (Hulme & Snowling, 2011). This implies that interventions targeting language comprehension skills are likely to reduce these children's reading comprehension difficulties.

Interventions targeting reading comprehension impairment

Meta-analyses of treatment studies

Several different meta-analyses have examined interventions to improve children's reading comprehension (Stahl & Fairbanks, 1986; Edmonds *et al.*, 2009; Elleman *et al.*, 2009; Swanson *et al.*, 2011). However, only one meta-analysis specifically targets poor comprehenders and distinguishes them from children with other kinds of reading problems (Lee & Tsai, 2017). This meta-analysis synthesized findings from 14 intervention studies that selected poor comprehenders (i.e., those with specific difficulties with reading comprehension). The 14 studies used eight different types of intervention. The intervention with the largest effect size ($d = 0.86$, $k = 6$) was reciprocal teaching where students practice four reading comprehension strategies (making predictions, seeking clarification, generating questions, and summarizing). For the other types of interventions there were only one or two studies in each category and so it is difficult to draw any firm conclusions. It should be noted that there were relatively few studies in this meta-analysis, and that some of them had weak designs.

Another meta-analysis by Rogde *et al.* (2019), examined the effects on standardized measures of reading comprehension from interventions that target language comprehension skills. Studies in this meta-analysis had to employ either a pretest–posttest control group design, posttest control with randomization, or quasi-experimental design with baseline control. The overall effect size from language comprehension intervention on reading comprehension was close to zero ($d = 0.05$), with evidence of heterogeneity in the effect sizes. At follow-up, the effect size was larger, ($d = 0.33$), but this was based on only four effect sizes.

Moderators of treatment

Rogde *et al.* (2019) found that the three studies that used instruction in small groups found larger effects of intervention than programs where instruction was delivered to whole classes.

Summary

There are far fewer studies of interventions for reading comprehension impairment than for dyslexia. The assessment of reading comprehension skills is inherently much more complex than the assessment of reading accuracy, as are the teaching methods required for improving reading comprehension. The results overall indicate large effects from reciprocal teaching in which students practice reading comprehension strategies. However, the meta-analysis of poor comprehenders included few studies, with typically small samples and variable quality.

There are promising effects from studies of the effects of language comprehension intervention on reading comprehension (Clarke *et al.*, 2010; Brinchmann *et al.*, 2016). After the meta-analysis by Rogde *et al.* (2019) another RCT showed an effect of $d = 0.29$ on a latent variable of reading comprehension from a 20-week decoding and language comprehension intervention (Clarke *et al.*, 2017). Notably, there is also another randomized trial showing no effects on standardized measures of reading comprehension that do not contain the trained language comprehension elements (Jiang & Logan, Language and Reading Research Consortium, 2019). However, in this study, the effect from training on reading comprehension was mediated through gains in language comprehension, but as mentioned, there was no overall effect for the training on the sample as a whole. In conclusion, there are promising effects of interventions to improve language comprehension on reading comprehension, but the effects seem stronger when interventions involve small groups and are of longer duration.

Mathematics disorder

The nature and causes of mathematics disorder

There have been great advances in research on mathematical development and performance since the 2000s, although evidence in this area remains more limited than in the case of reading disorders. The diagnostic criteria for mathematics disorder in DSM-IV (American Psychiatric Association, 1994), was based on a discrepancy definition in which mathematics abilities, as measured by a standardized test, need to be substantially below that expected given chronological age, measured intelligence, and age-appropriate education. However, in DSM-5 (American Psychiatric Association, 2013) mathematics disorder is conflated with other forms of difficulty under the rubric of specific learning disorders, and a discrepancy definition is not used (the use of such a broad category seems unfortunate—see also Chapter 52 for further discussion of the utility of a general category of specific learning disorders).

Mathematics disorder, like the other disorders considered here, is relatively common. Lewis *et al.* (1994) assessed reading, arithmetic, and nonverbal ability in all 9- and 10-year-old children in a single school district in the UK. Using a cutoff of a mathematics standard score of 85 or less, coupled with normal nonverbal ability (at or above a standard score of 90), some 3.6% of children were classified as having mathematics disorder (of these children, roughly two-thirds also had a reading disorder diagnosed in an analogous way).

The main theoretical framework explaining mathematical development is the "triple code model" (Dehaene, 1992). According to this model there are three domains of representation involved in mathematics: a quantitative magnitude system, a language-based system, and a written number system. A deficiency in one or more of these systems can cause problems in the development of mathematical skills. It has also been suggested that learning the mappings between the different forms of representation in the triple code model may be a critical determinant of acquiring arithmetic skills (Malone *et al.*, 2019). The model is displayed in Figure 37.5 and has support both from neuroscience and behavioral studies (Dehaene *et al.*, 1993, 2003; LeFevre *et al.*, 2010; Sowinski *et al.*, 2015; Träff *et al.*, 2018).

A discussion in the field has been whether the core deficit for mathematical problems is in the abstract approximate number sense system (Dehaene, 1997; Butterworth *et al.*, 2011), or whether it is the result of a more general deficit in working memory or visuospatial abilities (e.g., Geary, 2004), or perhaps whether it is a verbally based deficit that involves problems in learning counting skills (Hulme & Snowling, 2009; Chapter 5). Arguably, to date, there has been little linkage between debates about the causes of mathematics disorder and interventions for these children.

Interventions targeting mathematics disorder

Meta-analyses of treatment studies

There has been an increase in the number of intervention studies for mathematics disorder in the last 10 years.

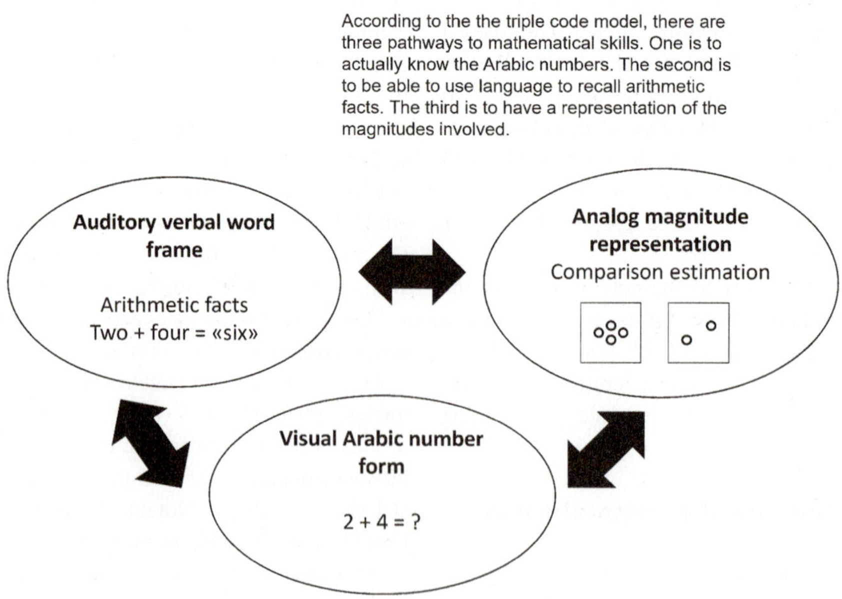

Figure 37.5 The triple code model for mathematical skills.

Interventions for children in preschool and early elementary grades showed large effects (d = 0.64) in the meta-analysis of Nelson and McMaster (2019). The interventions variously targeted number skills, relational skills, and numerical operation skills. One limitation to this meta-analysis is that not all studies involved random assignment to a group.

Another meta-analysis summarized effects from mathematical interventions in children in secondary school with mathematical difficulties (Jitendra *et al.*, 2018). The interventions included varied widely in their content, ranging from computer-based arithmetic interventions to strategy training and training relationships between numbers and their concrete referents, and were delivered in both whole class and special education settings. Nineteen experiments and well-controlled quasi-experiments met the inclusion criteria. The interventions had large effects on mathematics outcomes (d = 0.37).

Finally, a meta-analysis summarized mathematical interventions from grade 4 through 12 (9–17 years) (Stevens *et al.*, 2018). The results from the 25 studies that met the inclusion criteria showed a large effect size (d = 0.49 after adjusting for small-study effects). Studies were included if they used an experimental design, a quasi-experimental design, or a multiple treatment design (i.e., studies comparing treatments rather than a treatment with a business-as-usual group). The authors, however, point out that the findings are limited by variability between studies and the lack of standardized outcome measures of mathematical ability.

Moderators of treatment

Nelson and McMaster (2019) found that interventions to improve mathematical skills had larger effects in younger children, in children at lower risk of mathematics disorders, and if the interventions included counting and were 8 weeks or shorter. However, some of these effects are artifacts of differences in children's age between the studies. Jitendra *et al.* (2018) found that interventions with a duration of 10 hours or more were associated with larger effects than those with less than 10 hours. Stevens *et al.* (2018) found that studies with more than 15 hours of treatment and with a focus on fractions were associated with larger effects than other studies.

Summary

The results from interventions to improve mathematical skills show relatively large effects that are stronger in younger children and in studies where interventions last longer.

The effectiveness of educational interventions for children with general learning difficulties

So far, we have concentrated on interventions for children with specific learning difficulties. There have been several experimental and quasi-experimental studies that have evaluated the effectiveness of interventions for children with general learning difficulties (IDs in U.S. terminology); all of these studies concentrate on reading (or reading and language) skills.

Allor *et al.* (2010b) evaluated the effectiveness of a phonic reading program with 28 children with moderate IDs (IQs 40–79). Children were randomly assigned to daily small group reading instruction or "typical special education" (N = 16 intervention, N = 12 control). The program was delivered for between 1 and 1.5 years and produced large effect sizes on a standardized measure, the Test Of Word Reading Efficiency (TOWRE d = 0.72) and nonword-reading efficiency (TOWRE d = 1.00); these tests simply assess how many words or nonwords a child can read aloud in 90s.

In a similar study with a larger sample, Allor *et al.* (2010a) evaluated the effectiveness of a comprehensive reading program that involved teaching phonological and phonemic awareness, oral language skills, letter knowledge, word reading, vocabulary, reading fluency, and comprehension. Fifty-nine children with moderate IDs (IQs 40–79) were randomly assigned to either the treatment or a business-as-usual control group. Teaching for the intervention children was delivered in daily small group sessions across 2–3 school years. The intervention group showed greater gains, with large effect sizes, on measures of phoneme awareness (d = 0.53–0.66), nonword reading (d = 0.49–0.58), and word reading (d = 0.26–0.51).

In another small-scale RCT, Finnegan (2012) investigated methods of teaching reading to children with IDs. Here 52 children (mean age 8.6 years; mean IQ 56 for those children tested) were randomly assigned to three groups: synthetic phonics, an analogy-based phonic reading program, or an untreated control. The synthetic phonics program involved teaching children to "sound out" unknown words on a letter-by-letter basis and blend the sounds together to form the word. The analogy-based phonics program focused on larger segments of spoken words when trying to decode them (for example, given the word HAT the child might be asked to think of other words that share the same ending (CAT, SAT) or the same initial letter (HIT, HIS) and work out from this the pronunciation of HAT). Teaching only involved 12 sessions. Both phonics programs resulted in improvements in children's ability to read words taught in the program (d = 0.54, and 0.52), and on a measure of transfer to untaught words there was also an advantage for the synthetic phonics group compared to the control group (d = 0.33). Clearly, this study has low power but suggests that phonic reading instruction can be beneficial for children with general ID.

Other studies have specifically aimed at improving reading and language skills in children with Down syndrome. Burgoyne *et al.* (2012) reported a randomized trial evaluating the effects of an integrated reading and language intervention program for children with Down syndrome aged between 5 and 10 years. The intervention involved a highly structured phonic reading program (comparable to that used by Bowyer-Crane *et al.*, 2008) coupled with vocabulary instruction, and was delivered by teaching assistants in 40 minute sessions on each school day over 20 weeks. After 20 weeks of teaching, the intervention group (N = 28) showed significantly greater progress than the waiting control group (N = 26) (with large effect sizes) on measures of single word reading (d = 0.23), letter–sound knowledge (d = 0.42), phoneme blending (d = 0.54), and knowledge of word meanings taught in the program (d = 0.47). However, there was no generalization to skills not directly taught (nonword reading, spelling, standardized expressive and receptive vocabulary, expressive information, and grammar).

Another study by Sepúlveda *et al.* (2013) involved an intervention targeting grammar; 20 individuals with Down syndrome between 6 and 14 years (mean age 10 years; mean IQ 44.8) were randomly assigned to the intervention (N = 10) and control group (N = 10). The training included inflection for number in nouns (e.g., "chair" and "chairs") and other types of grammar-related tasks for nouns, and correct use of pronouns and adjectives (2 sessions), as well as work on verb tenses for the present, past, and future (4 sessions). The training was divided between working on sentence structures and dialogs. The activities were delivered through 30 individual sessions lasting 30 minutes each provided by speech and language therapists twice per week over 3.5 months. The children in the experimental group showed larger gains compared to the control group in the areas of syntax (the arrangement of words and phrases in sentences) (d = 1.54), morphology (knowledge about the internal structure in words) (d = 1.40), and semantics (the meaning of a word, phrase, or text) (d = 1.36), but not in pragmatics (the socially appropriate use of language), where both groups improved to the same extent.

A recent study by Baxter *et al.* (2022) examined the effectiveness of a past tense intervention (PaTI) that was designed to teach the use of the regular simple past tense to 7–11-year-old children with Down syndrome. This RCT study was delivered on an individual basis in daily 20 min sessions for 10 weeks in the children's schools by trained teaching assistants. While the intervention group (N = 26) received the intervention immediately, the control group waited and received the intervention later (N = 26). Immediately after the intervention, the intervention group made significantly greater gains than controls on the regular simple past tense verb forms (composite score d = 1.63) and the Renfrew Action Picture Test Grammar measure (d = 0.24), with generalization to untrained verbs (d = 2.37) and over-regularization errors to irregular verbs (d = 1.45) but not to other measures of expressive grammar (irregular past tense or third person singular) or measures of the amount of information and/or detail used in expressive language. Importantly, the gains made by the intervention group were maintained at follow-up some 12–14 weeks after the intervention had been completed.

Summary

These studies of children with general learning difficulties are typically small scale, and hence suffer from limited statistical power. Nevertheless, the results are consistent in suggesting that reading accuracy problems in this population can be ameliorated by phonically based reading instruction coupled with phonological (phonemic) awareness training. In short, the same approach to teaching reading to children with dyslexia also appears to be effective for children with general learning difficulties. In addition, it appears that children with general learning difficulties (including children with Down syndrome) can learn to improve their vocabulary and grammatical skills given suitable highly structured teaching. Having said this, a clear limitation of the findings from studies with these populations is that typically directly taught skills show improvements, while it is difficult to find evidence of generalization to skills not directly taught. Nevertheless, the evidence suggests that regular structured interventions have clearly beneficial effects for these populations.

The effectiveness of educational interventions for children with developmental coordination disorder (dyspraxia)

DCD refers to children whose motor skills are substantially worse than expected for their age. Difficulties may involve both gross motor skills (large body movements and balance) and fine motor skills (skills involving hand control such as drawing and writing). The DSM-5 definition of DCD refers to "the acquisition and execution of coordinated motor skills being substantially below that expected ... for ... age" (American Psychiatric Association, 2013). To qualify for a diagnosis of DCD motor difficulties should arise early in life, be persistent, and interfere with daily life.

Compared to the other forms of specific learning disorder considered so far there is much less research into the nature, causes, and treatment of DCD. The disorder is best thought of as perceptual-motor problem (Hulme & Snowling, 2009), i.e., a problem in using perceptual information to guide actions in space (hence, earlier terminology such as developmental apraxia (movement disorder) and agnosia (perceptual disorder)). Interventions for this disorder, however, appear to be largely unrelated to cognitive theories about the nature of the underlying difficulties in this group of children.

There have been two recent meta-analyses of treatments for DCD: Smits-Engelsman *et al.* (2018) included 19 studies of children with DCD aged between 4 and 12 years of age; only 10 of the studies were RCTs and these were of varying quality. The studies had to include a measure of motor skill as an outcome measure. The review found that activity-oriented interventions (aimed at directly training a skill) and body function-oriented interventions (aimed at training component skills such as strength, balance, and oculo-motor coordination) had the best evidence for effectiveness. The improvements found on standardized measures of motor skill were large (d = 1.06) but highly variable. The authors suggest that "activity-oriented" approaches should be used (i.e., approaches that involve direct training of skills that children find difficult).

Yu *et al.* (2018) reported another meta-analysis which included 18 studies with participants diagnosed as having DCD who ranged in age between 3–17 years. Just 12 of these studies were RCTs. The treatments were categorized as process-oriented (interventions targeting underlying processes such as balance; this appears to be more or less synonymous with the category of "body function-oriented" interventions identified by Smits-Engelsman *et al.*, 2018) or task-oriented (interventions training specific motor skills, equivalent to the term "activity-oriented" used by Smits-Engelsman *et al.* 2018). They reported large effects of intervention on motor performance (Hedges' = 0.63) with both dose and frequency of intervention being moderators of outcome. They did not separate the effects of different types of intervention when computing effect sizes.

Summary

Studies of interventions for DCD are typically small in scale, of short duration, and with only short-term follow-up. Nevertheless, it appears that direct training of specific motor tasks can be effective for children with DCD. Advances in this area will likely depend on more clearly articulated theories, which can lead to interventions that test out alternative theoretical positions concerning the nature of these children's difficulties (as is in the case of studies of children's reading disorders, where research is more advanced).

The effectiveness of interventions targeting general cognitive functions

In recent years, strong claims have been made for interventions that aim to enhance language and reading skills by training more general cognitive capacities (e.g., Merzenich & Jenkins, 1998; Klingberg, 2010). One such category of interventions aims to train working memory capacity, a cognitive system that is claimed to provide an all-purpose "work-space" for diverse cognitive functions such as reading, language, mathematics, and general attentional abilities. It has been claimed that working memory impairment is a contributory cause to many different forms of learning difficulty including language impairment, dyslexia, reading comprehension impairment, mathematics disorder, and attention deficit (see Melby-Lervåg *et al.*, 2012; Melby-Lervåg & Hulme, 2013). According to such a theory, if working memory capacity can be increased through training, this would have diverse effects on people's ability to perform cognitive tasks, such reading and language comprehension, arithmetic, and reasoning.

Since the 2000s, several studies have examined the effects from working memory training. The meta-analysis of Melby-Lervåg and Hulme (2013) summarized the effects from such training in studies that used a design with a pretest and posttest, and a control group (both randomized and nonrandomized studies, and studies with both trained and untrained control groups). Twenty-three studies with 30 group comparisons met the criteria for inclusion. The studies involved clinical samples and samples of typically developing children and adults. Meta-analyses showed that the working memory programs produced reliable short-term improvements in working memory skills. However, there was no evidence of generalization from working memory training to other skills (nonverbal and verbal ability, inhibitory processes in attention, word decoding, and arithmetic).

These conclusions were confirmed and extended in a subsequent meta-analysis by Melby-Lervåg *et al.* (2016) who found no evidence that working memory training produced improvements on measures such as reading or language skills when compared to active control conditions. These programs appear to produce short-term, specific training effects that do not generalize to skills that are important for children with learning difficulties. This pattern was also confirmed in a recent well-controlled study with adults (Redick *et al.*, 2013) and for the Cogmed training program in a further meta-analysis (Hulme & Melby-Lervåg, 2012).

A second category of interventions based on an approach that seeks to train general cognitive skills derives from a theory that language and literacy learning difficulties in children arise from problems related to rapid auditory temporal processing (Tallal, 2004). According to this theory, a basic deficit in perceiving rapidly changing auditory signals results in problems in perceiving speech, which in turn leads to language learning difficulties. It has been claimed that neuroplasticity means that training of auditory processing skills can lead to improvements in underlying neural systems and thereby ameliorate children's language and reading problems (Merzenich & Jenkins, 1998). One such training program is called Fast ForWord which is marketed by the Carnegie Learning Corporation in the U.S. In this program, children are trained with computer-modified speech in which critical cues in speech are slowed down in order to make them more discriminable to children with auditory temporal processing impairments. Strong *et al.* (2011) examined the effects of the Fast ForWord training programs in a meta-analysis. Six papers met the inclusion criteria of RCTs or matched group comparison studies with baseline equivalence published in refereed journals. The results showed that there was no significant effect of Fast ForWord on language and reading measures when the training groups were compared with active or untreated control groups. Thus, Fast ForWord cannot be recommended for treating language and reading problems.

Another set of educational interventions that has received extensive attention are growth mindset interventions (Dweck, 2006). The theory behind these interventions is that if you believe that your cognitive abilities are fixed, and that there is little you can do to enhance them, you are less likely to improve your academic skills than if you believe your abilities are malleable (Dweck, 2006). This theory is highly controversial, and several studies have been conducted to evaluate it (Yeager & Dweck, 2020).

The two most recent meta-analyses yield conflicting conclusions. One meta-analysis based on 63 studies found an overall small effect size ($d = 0.05$) on academic achievement, which was nonsignificant after correcting for potential publication bias (Macnamara & Burgoyne, 2022). The authors then moved over to examine only studies that showed improvements in children's beliefs about growth mindset as intended. The results from these studies were disappointing and show effects close to zero on academic achievement ($d = 0.04$, $k = 13$). Similarly, studies that were rated as of the highest methodological quality also yielded effects on academic achievement close to zero ($d = 0.04$, $k = 6$). Perhaps disturbingly, the only moderator of outcome in these studies that was significant was whether the authors of the study potentially benefitted from positive results, which showed larger effects than other studies.

Another recent meta-analysis took a different approach. Because of the heterogeneity between studies this meta-analysis chose not to interpret overall mean effect sizes, but focused instead on the results from moderator analyses (Burnette *et al.*, 2022). This is an unusual and controversial approach. Two moderators of outcome were suggested to be important: (i) implementation quality, and (ii) whether a study had examined children at risk, who might be expected to show the largest gains. They found that studies of "at risk" populations with high fidelity had small to moderate effects ($d = 0.14$) on academic achievement. However, the number of studies this analysis is based on is not clear, and it is important to remember that the moderator analyses here are basically bivariate correlations controlling for one confounder. Thus, the studies with at risk samples and high fidelity might have other things in common that can explain why they yielded slightly larger effect sizes than other studies.

Finally, a meta-analysis has also questioned the measurement method used in many of the growth mindset studies (Scherer & Campos, 2022). Most studies in this area are based on the premise that fixed and growth mindsets are mutually exclusive. Thus, it is common to measure one type of mindset, and then reverse the scale to represent the other. However, a meta-analysis of 32 studies using meta-structural equation modeling showed that the two mindsets were not mutually exclusive but instead correlated constructs. This conclusion creates uncertainty regarding the methodology that many of these studies rest on. In summary, there is little evidence that interventions to improve "growth mindset" produce meaningful improvements in educational outcomes.

The effectiveness and adaptations of interventions with comorbid conditions

It is now well recognized that comorbidities between the disorders considered in this chapter are very common (see also Chapter 3 "Neurodevelopmental disorders"). Learning disorders in language, reading, and mathematics frequently co-occur both with attention deficit hyperactivity disorder (ADHD) and autism. For instance, depending on where cutoffs are set, reading disorder and ADHD typically have a co-occurrence rate of 20–50% (Willcutt & Pennington, 2000; Hendren *et al.*, 2018). There is also a considerable overlap between language disorders and autism (Bishop, 2010). Typically, however, children only receive treatment for one disorder (a child with both dyslexia and ADHD may be more likely to receive intervention for dyslexia than ADHD) and this may prevent the child from realizing the maximum benefit of intervention (Kotkin *et al.*, 2001). To date we have little evidence to guide us in adapting interventions for one disorder to account for the possible effects of comorbidities. Future studies will need to address this issue, but the complexity of the questions, and the sample sizes needed to address them rigorously, are daunting.

Conclusions and future directions for clinical practice and research

We have presented evidence for the efficacy of educational interventions for reading disorders (dyslexia and reading comprehension impairment), mathematics disorder, and general learning difficulties. It is clear that research on dyslexia is most advanced, and we have good evidence that phonics reading instruction coupled with oral phoneme awareness training works relatively well as a way of reducing the severity of these children's reading problems. However, problems with reading fluency appear to be more difficult to remediate in this population. There is encouraging evidence that interventions for young children with weak oral language skills can be effective, and that such interventions have knock-on effects to improve reading comprehension skills. Work on interventions for mathematical difficulties is perhaps least advanced, but there is evidence for moderate effects for two published intervention programs.

However, an increasing number of studies show that the effects of 10-week long interventions when targeting academic achievement can be short-lived and often fade out over time (Bailey *et al.*, 2017; Abenavoli, 2019). This is perhaps not surprising given that such interventions typically involve a very limited number of hours, and that the genetic and environmental factors (home and school environment) that drive the development of disorders tend to be highly stable. One obvious way of dealing with this is to construct interventions of longer duration and with a more flexible structure than the traditional "three times a week for 10 weeks" interventions. This has shown promising results so far, and effects have lasted at least 6–8 months (Clarke *et al.*, 2010, 2017; Hagen *et al.*, 2017). However, it is also important to be realistic about what we can expect interventions to achieve for children with learning disorders. It is particularly critical that the universal instruction provided to these children is of high quality, so that any interventions offered for such children can build on a sound foundation.

It may be worth emphasizing some limitations to the evidence considered. First, nearly all the studies considered have fairly liberal criteria for including children to be treated and we have rather little evidence about the effectiveness of the interventions reviewed for children with severe difficulties. Second, nearly all the studies reviewed here involve interventions of quite short duration with only short-term follow-up. A third issue that needs more evidence is the cost-effectiveness of the interventions considered. However, given that a number of effective interventions can be delivered by trained teaching assistants with small groups of children, they are potentially highly cost-effective. Finally, it is notable that most intervention studies focus on evaluating the direct effects that a given intervention has on a given area of educational attainment (reading, language, or mathematics skills). For interventions with demonstrated effectiveness on such measures, it would be useful to have longer-term studies that included broader outcome measures, since clinically it is often claimed that effective educational interventions can have quite broad effects on well-being and self-esteem.

References

Abenavoli, R.M. (2019) The mechanisms and moderators of "fade-out": towards understanding why the skills of early childhood program participants converge over time with the skills of other children. *Psychological Bulletin* **145**(12), 1103–1127. doi:10.1037/bul0000212.

Allor, J.H. *et al.* (2010a) Comprehensive reading instruction for students with intellectual disabilities: findings from the first three years of a longitudinal study. *Psychology in the Schools* **47**, 445–466. doi:10.1002/pits.20482.

Allor, J.H. *et al.* (2010b) Teaching students with moderate intellectual disabilities to read: an experimental examination of a comprehensive reading intervention reading instruction for students with intellectual disabilities. *Education and Training in Autism and Developmental Disabilities* **45**, 3–22.

American Psychiatric Association (1994) *Diagnostic and Statistical Manual of Mental Disorders*, 4th edn. American Psychiatric Association, Washington, DC.

American Psychiatric Association (2013) *Diagnostic and Statistical Manual of Mental Disorders*, 5th edn. American Psychiatric Association, Washington, DC.

Bailey, D. *et al.* (2017) Persistence and fadeout in the impacts of child and adolescent interventions. *Journal of Research on Educational Effectiveness* **10**(1), 7–39. doi:10.1080/19345747.2016.1232459.

Baxter, R. *et al.* (2022) The nature and causes of children's grammatical difficulties: evidence from an intervention to improve past tense marking in children with Down syndrome. *Developmental Science*. doi:10.1111/desc.13220.

Bishop, D.V. (2010) Overlaps between autism and language impairment: phenomimicry or shared etiology? *Behavior Genetics* **40**, 618–629.

Bowyer-Crane, C. *et al.* (2008) Improving early language and literacy skills: differential effects of an oral language versus a phonology with reading intervention. *Journal of Child Psychology and Psychiatry* **49**, 422–432. doi:10.1111/j.1469-7610.2007.01849.x.

Brinchmann, E.I. *et al.* (2016) Lexical quality matters: effects of word knowledge instruction on the language and literacy skills of third- and fourth-grade poor readers. *Reading Research Quarterly* **51**(2), 165–180.

Burgoyne, K. *et al.* (2012) Efficacy of a reading and language intervention for children with Down syndrome: a randomized controlled trial. *Journal of Child Psychology and Psychiatry* **53**(10), 1044–1053. doi:10.1111/j.1469-7610.2012.02557.x.

Burnette, J.L. *et al.* (2022) A systematic review and meta-analysis of growth mindset interventions: for whom, how, and why might such interventions work? *Psychological Bulletin*. doi:10.1037/bul0000368.

Bus, A.G. & van IJzendoorn, M.H. (1999) Phonological awareness and early reading: a meta-analysis of experimental training studies. *Journal of Educational Psychology* **91**, 403–414. doi:10.1037/0022-0663.91.3.403.

Butterworth, B. *et al.* (2011) Dyscalculia: from brain to education. *Science* **332**(6033), 1049–1053. doi:10.1126/science.1201536.

Clarke, P. *et al.* (2010) Ameliorating children's reading-comprehension difficulties: a randomized controlled trial. *Psychological Science* **21**(8), 1106–1116. doi:10.1177/0956797610375449.

Clarke, P.J. *et al.* (2017) Reading intervention for poor readers at the transition to secondary school. *Scientific Studies of Reading* **21**(5), 408–427. doi:10.1080/10888438.2017.1318393.

Dehaene, S. (1992) Varieties of numerical abilities. *Cognition* **44**(1–2), 1–42. doi:10.1016/0010-0277(92)90049-N.

Dehaene, S. (1997) *The Number Sense: How the Mind Creates Mathematics*. Oxford University Press, New York.

Dehaene, S. *et al.* (1993) The mental representation of parity and number magnitude. *Journal of Experimental Psychology: General* **122**(3), 371–396. doi:10.1037/0096-3445.122.3.371.

Dehaene, S. *et al.* (2003) Three parietal circuits for number processing. *Cognitive Neuropsychology* **20**(3–6), 487–506. doi:10.1080/02643290244000239.

Dweck, C.S. (2006) *Mindset: The New Psychology of Success*. Random House, New York.

Edmonds, M.S. *et al.* (2009) A synthesis of reading interventions and effects on reading comprehension outcomes for older struggling readers. *Review of Educational Research* **79**, 262–300. doi:10.3102/0034654308325998.

Ehri, L.C. *et al.* (2001) Phonemic awareness instruction helps children learn to read: evidence from the national reading panel's meta-analysis. *Reading Research Quarterly* **36**(3), 250–287.

Elleman, A. *et al.* (2009) The impact of vocabulary instruction on passage-level comprehension of school-age children: a meta-analysis. *Journal of Research on Educational Effectiveness* **2**, 1–44. doi:10.1080/19345740802539200.

Finnegan, E.G. (2012) Two approaches to phonics instruction: comparison of effects with children with significant cognitive disability. *Education and Training in Autism and Developmental Disabilities* **47**, 269–279.

Foorman, B.R. *et al.* (2015a) The structure of oral language and reading and their relation to comprehension in Kindergarten through Grade 2. *Reading and Writing* **28**, 655–681.

Foorman, B.R. *et al.* (2015b) Examining general and specific factors in the dimensionality of oral language and reading in 4th–10th grades. *Journal of Educational Psychology* **107**(3), 884–899.

García, J.R. & Cain, K. (2014) Decoding and reading comprehension: a meta-analysis to identify which reader and assessment characteristics influence the strength of the relationship in English. *Review of Educational Research* **84**(1), 74–111. doi:10.3102/0034654313499616.

Geary, D.C. (2004) Mathematics and learning disabilities. *Journal of Learning Disabilities* **37**(1), 4–15. doi:10.1177/00222194040370010201.

Gough, P.B. & Tunmer, W.E. (1986) Decoding, reading, and reading disability. *Remedial and Special Education* **7**(1), 6–10. doi:10.1177/074193258600700104.

Hagen, Å.M. *et al.* (2017) Improving language comprehension in preschool children with language difficulties: a cluster randomized trial. *Journal of Child Psychology and Psychiatry* **58**(10), 1132–1140. doi:10.1111/jcpp.12762.

Hall, C. *et al.* (2022) Forty years of reading intervention research for elementary students with or at risk for dyslexia: a systematic review and meta-analysis. *Reading Research Quarterly* **58**(2), 285–312. doi:10.1002/rrq.477.

Hatcher, P.J. & Hulme, C. (1999) Phonemes, rhymes, and intelligence as predictors of children's responsiveness to remedial reading instruction: evidence from a longitudinal intervention study. *Journal of Experimental Child Psychology* **72**, 130–153. doi:10.1006/jecp.1998.2480.

Hatcher, P.J. *et al.* (1994) Ameliorating early reading failure by integrating the teaching of reading and phonological skills: the phonological linkage hypothesis. *Child Development* **65**, 41–57. doi:10.1111/j.1467-8624.1994.tb00733.x.

Henderson, L.M. *et al.* (2013) Questioning the benefits that coloured overlays can have for reading in students with and without dyslexia. *Journal of Research in Special Educational Needs* **13**(1), 57–65. doi:10.1111/j.1471-3802.2012.01237.x.

Hendren, R.L. *et al.* (2018) Recognizing psychiatric comorbidity with reading disorders. *Frontiers in Psychiatry* **9**. doi:10.3389/fpsyt.2018.00101.

Hjetland, H.N. *et al.* (2020) Preschool pathways to reading comprehension: a systematic meta-analytic review. *Educational Research Review*. doi:10.1016/j.edurev.2020.100323.

Hulme, C. & Melby-Lervåg, M. (2012) Current evidence does not support the claims made for Cogmed working memory training. *Journal of Applied Research in Memory and Cognition* **1**(3), 197–200. doi:10.1016/j.jarmac.2012.06.006.

Hulme, C. & Snowling, M. (2009) *Developmental Cognitive Disorders*. Blackwell-Wiley, Oxford, UK.

Hulme, C. & Snowling, M. (2011) Children's reading comprehension difficulties: nature, causes, and treatments. *Psychological Science* **20**(3). doi:10.1177/0963721411408673.

Hulme, C. *et al.* (2012) The causal role of phoneme awareness and letter-sound knowledge in learning to read: combining intervention studies with mediation analyses. *Psychological Science* **23**(6), 572–577. doi:10.1177/0956797611435921.

Jiang, H., Logan, J., & Language and Reading Research Consortium (2019) Improving reading comprehension in the primary grades: mediated effects of a language-focused classroom intervention. *Journal of Speech, Language, and Hearing Research* **62**(8), 2812–2828.

Jitendra, A.K. *et al.* (2018) Mathematical interventions for secondary students with learning disabilities and mathematics difficulties: a meta-analysis. *Exceptional Children* **84**(2), 177–196. doi:10.1177/0014402917737467.

Klingberg, T. (2010) Training and plasticity of working memory. *Trends in Cognitive Sciences* **14**, 317–324. doi:10.1016/j.tics.2010.05.002.

Kotkin, R.A. *et al.* (2001) Comorbid ADHD and learning disabilities: diagnosis, special education, and intervention. In: *Research and Global Perspectives in Learning Disabilities*. (eds D.P. Hallahan & B.K. Keogh). pp. 43–63.

Kraft, M.A. (2020) Interpreting effect sizes of education interventions. *Educational Researcher* **49**(4), 241–253. doi:10.3102/0013189X20912798.

Lee, S.H. & Tsai, S.F. (2017) Experimental intervention research on students with specific poor comprehension: a systematic review of treatment outcomes. *Reading and Writing* **30**, 917–943. doi:10.1007/s11145-016-9697-x.

LeFevre, J.A. *et al.* (2010) Pathways to mathematics: longitudinal predictors of performance. *Child Development* **81**(6), 1753–1767. doi:10.1111/j.1467-8624.2010.01508.x.

Lervåg, A. *et al.* (2009) The cognitive and linguistic foundations of early reading development: a Norwegian latent variable longitudinal study. *Developmental Psychology* **45**(3), 764–781. doi:10.1037/a0014132.

Lervåg, A. *et al.* (2018) Unpicking the developmental relationship between oral language skills and reading comprehension: it's simple, but complex. *Child Development* **89**(5), 1821–1838. doi:10.1111/cdev.12861.

Lewis, C. *et al.* (1994) The prevalence of specific arithmetic difficulties and specific reading difficulties in 9 to 10-year-old boys and girls. *Journal of Child Psychology and Psychiatry*. doi:10.1111/j.1469-7610.1994.tb01162.x.

Lonigan, C.J. *et al.* (2008) Impact of code-focused interventions on young children's early literacy skills. In: *Developing Early Literacy: SREE Spring 2012 Conference Abstract Template A-1Report of the National Early Literacy Panel*. National Institute for Literacy, Washington, DC. pp. 107–151.

Macnamara, B.N. & Burgoyne, A.P. (2022) Do growth mindset interventions impact students' academic achievement? A systematic review and meta-analysis with recommendations for best practices. *Psychological Bulletin* **149**(3–4), 133–173. doi:10.1037/bul0000352.

Malone, S.A. *et al.* (2019) Learning correspondences between magnitudes, symbols and words: evidence for a triple code model of arithmetic development. *Cognition* **187**, 1–9. doi:10.1016/j.cognition.2018.11.016.

McArthur, G. *et al.* (2018) Phonics training for English-speaking poor readers. *Cochrane Database of Systematic Reviews*. doi:10.1002/14651858.CD009115.pub3.

Melby-Lervåg, M. & Hulme, C. (2013) Is working memory training effective? A meta-analytic review. *Developmental Psychology* **49**(2), 270–291. doi:10.1037/a0028228.

Melby-Lervåg, M. *et al.* (2012) Phonological skills and their role in learning to read: a meta-analytic review. *Psychological Bulletin* **138**(2), 322–352. doi:10.1037/a0026744.

Melby-Lervåg, M. *et al.* (2016) Working memory training does not improve performance on measures of intelligence or other measures of "far transfer" evidence from a meta-analytic review. *Perspectives on Psychological Science* **11**(4), 512–534. doi:10.1177/1745691616635612.

Merzenich, M.M. & Jenkins, W.M. (1998) Cortical plasticity, learning, and learning dysfunction. In: *Maturational Windows and Adult Cortical Plasticity*. (eds B. Julesz & I. Kovacs). Addison-Wesley Publishing, New York. pp. 247–272.

Nelson, G. & McMaster, K.L. (2019) The effects of early numeracy interventions for students in preschool and early elementary: a meta-analysis. *Journal of Educational Psychology* **111**(6), 1001–1022. doi:10.1037/edu0000334.

Peterson, R.L. & Pennington, B.F. (2012) Developmental dyslexia. *The Lancet* **379**, 1997–2007. doi:10.1016/S0140-6736(12)60198-6.

Redick, T.S. *et al.* (2013) No evidence of intelligence improvement after working memory training: a randomized, placebo-controlled study.

Journal of Experimental Psychology: General **142**(2), 359–379. doi:10.1037/a0029082.

Reynolds, D. *et al.* (2003) Evaluation of an exercise-based treatment for children with reading difficulties. *Dyslexia* **9**(1), 48–71. doi:10.1002/dys.235.

Rogde, K. *et al.* (2019) The effect of linguistic comprehension instruction on generalized language and reading comprehension skills: a systematic review. *Campbell Systematic Reviews* **15**(4), e1059. doi:10.1002/cl2.1059.

Rutter, M. & Yule, W. (1975) The concept of specific reading retardation. *Journal of Child Psychology and Psychiatry* **16**(3), 181–197. doi:10.1111/j.1469-7610.1975.tb01269.x.

Samuels, S.J. *et al.* (2000) Fluency. In: *National Reading Panel, Teaching Children to Read: An Evidence-based Assessment of the Scientific Research Literature on Reading and its Implications for Reading Instruction.* National Institutes of Health, Washington, DC, pp. 3-1–3-35. https://www.nichd.nih.gov/sites/default/files/publications/pubs/nrp/Documents/report.pdf

Scherer, R. & Campos, D.G. (2022) Measuring those who have their minds set: an item-level meta-analysis of the implicit theories of intelligence scale in education. *Educational Research Review* **37**, 100479. doi:10.1016/j.edurev.2022.100479.

Sepúlveda, E.M. *et al.* (2013) Can individuals with Down syndrome improve their grammar? *International Journal of Language & Communication Disorders* **48**(3), 343–349. doi:10.1111/1460-6984.12002.

Smits-Engelsman, B. *et al.* (2018) Evaluating the evidence for motor-based interventions in developmental coordination disorder: a systematic review and meta-analysis. *Research in Developmental Disabilities* **74**, 72–102. doi:10.1016/j.ridd.2018.01.002.

Snowling, M.J. & Hulme, C. (2003) A critique of claims from Reynolds, Nicolson & Hambly (2003) that DDAT is an effective treatment for children with reading difficulties–'lies, damned lies and (inappropriate) statistics?'. *Dyslexia* **9**(2), 127–133. doi:10.1002/dys.245.

Sowinski, C. *et al.* (2015) Refining the quantitative pathway of the pathways to mathematics model. *Journal of Experimental Child Psychology* **131**, 73–93. doi:10.1016/j.jecp.2014.11.004.

Stahl, S.A. & Fairbanks, M.M. (1986) The effects of vocabulary instruction: a model based meta-analysis. *Review of Educational Research* **56**(1). doi:10.3102/00346543056001072.

Stevens, E.A. *et al.* (2018) Mathematics interventions for upper elementary and secondary students: a meta-analysis of research. *Remedial and Special Education* **39**(6), 327–340. doi:10.1177/0741932517731887.

Strong, G.K. *et al.* (2011) A systematic meta-analytic review of evidence for the effectiveness of the 'Fast ForWord' language intervention program. *Journal of Child Psychology and Psychiatry* **52**(3), 224–235. doi:10.1111/j.1469-7610.2010.02329.x.

Swanson, E. *et al.* (2011) A synthesis of read-aloud interventions on early reading outcomes among preschool through third graders at risk for reading difficulties. *Journal of Learning Disabilities* **44**, 258–275. doi:10.1177/0022219410378444.

Tallal, P. (2004) Improving language and literacy is a matter of time. *Nature Reviews Neuroscience* **5**, 721–728.

Therrien, W. (2004) Fluency and comprehension gains as a result of repeated reading: a meta-analysis. *Remedial and Special Education* **25**(4), 252–261. doi:10.1177/07419325040250040801.

Träff, U. *et al.* (2018) Cognitive mechanisms underlying third graders' arithmetic skills: expanding the pathways to mathematics model. *Journal of Experimental Child Psychology* **167**, 369–387. doi:10.1016/j.jecp.2017.11.010.

What Works Clearinghouse (2014) *Procedures and Standards Handbook* (Version 3.0). U.S. Department of Education, Institute of Education Sciences, National Center for Education Evaluation and Regional Assistance, Washington, DC. Available: http://ies.ed.gov/ncee/wwc/documentsum.aspx?sid=19 [16 October 2024].

Willcutt, E.G. & Pennington, B.F. (2000) Comorbidity of reading disability and attention-deficit/hyperactivity disorder: differences by gender and subtype. *Journal of Learning Disabilities* **33**(2), 179–191. doi:10.1177/002221940003300206.

Yeager, D.S. & Dweck, C.S. (2020) What can be learned from growth mindset controversies? *American Psychologist* **75**(9), 1269–1284. doi:10.1037/amp0000794.

Yu, J.J. *et al.* (2018) Motor skill interventions in children with developmental coordination disorder: a systematic review and meta-analysis. *Archives of Physical Medicine and Rehabilitation* **99**(10), 2076–2099.

Zimmermann, L.M. *et al.* (2021) A meta-analysis of non-repetitive reading fluency interventions for students with reading difficulties. *Remedial and Special Education* **42**, 78–93. doi:10.1177/0741932519855058.

CHAPTER 38

School-based mental health interventions

Hiran Thabrew and Sally Merry

Department of Psychological Medicine, The University of Auckland, Auckland, New Zealand

Introduction

Children and young people spend a large amount of time at school, with net global school attendance rates reported as 89% for primary students (aged 5–12) and 66% for secondary students (aged 13–17) (Kuzik *et al.*, 2022). While designed for education, schools are valuable settings for promoting well-being and safeguarding of students, identifying mental health issues, and supporting those in need (Figure 38.1). Conversely, school-related academic and social demands may precipitate and perpetuate mental health problems. School closures (e.g., during COVID-19 pandemic-related lockdowns) can also adversely impact mental health and academic outcomes (Viner *et al.*, 2021). In this chapter, we explore the role of school-based health teams and review interventions for preserving well-being, addressing common mental health problems, and meeting the needs of specific groups. We also summarize issues associated with implementation and make recommendations for working with schools.

Types of school-based interventions

School-based interventions may be delivered in either a *universal* or *targeted* manner. Universal interventions are usually delivered to the whole school via the curriculum, have wide reach, are associated with less stigma, and can tackle community-wide factors associated with mental health problems. Targeted interventions may be delivered in a *selective* manner to subgroups at elevated risk of developing mental health problems or an *indicated* manner to individuals with detectable levels of symptoms (Stockings *et al.*, 2016). They are usually focused on specific issues, more cost-effective, and yield larger effect sizes (ES) during studies than their universal counterparts (Hayes *et al.*, 2023). Universal and targeted interventions may be combined into *integrated approaches* to increase specific or multipronged effects (Fazel *et al.*, 2014a). Technology is also increasingly being used to deliver both types of interventions (Sakellari *et al.*, 2021), albeit with challenges of program uptake (familiarity of schools with what is available) and completion (students' need for support) (Lattie *et al.*, 2019); see Chapter 49. Although the involvement of parents can augment the effects of many school-based interventions, it is not often undertaken for practical reasons (Shucksmith *et al.*, 2010).

School culture, climate, and connectedness can also have an impact on student well-being, mental health, and academic achievement. *School culture* refers to the way in which a school incorporates beliefs, and written and unwritten rules, as well as balancing academic and recreational time (Jerald, 2006). The *school climate* (Freiberg, 1999) includes psychosocial aspects of educational experience, such as teacher affiliation, conflict, and social facilitation, as well as the experiences of staff and others who engage with schools. *School connectedness* refers to the experience by students that staff and peers care about them and want to see them thrive (Page *et al.*, 2021). It is associated with reduced rates of depression, bullying, and risky behaviors such as substance use and self-harm (Duggins *et al.*, 2016; Weatherson *et al.*, 2018; Raniti *et al.*, 2022), and is protective against mental health problems (Jones *et al.*, 2022).

Schools vary in the way they address mental health problems, with socioeconomic status, geography, political stability, religion, and culture all having an impact. International efforts to improve the consistency of school-based well-being and mental health interventions include policy-based World Health Organization (WHO) initiatives such as "Health Promoting Schools" (Sawyer *et al.*, 2021); the United Nations Educational, Scientific and Cultural Organization (UNESCO)'s "Education for All" movement (Power, 2014); and International Alliance for Child and Adolescent Mental Health and Schools (INTERCAMHS) strategies for promoting student well-being (Weist *et al.*, 2017). To address disparities in program availability for low- and middle-income countries (LMICs), an operational resource for developing and

Rutter's Child and Adolescent Psychiatry and Psychology, Seventh Edition.
Edited by Anita Thapar, Daniel S. Pine, Samuele Cortese, Cathy Creswell, Tamsin J. Ford, James F. Leckman, and Argyris Stringaris.

Companion website: www.wiley.com/go/thapar/rutterspsych7

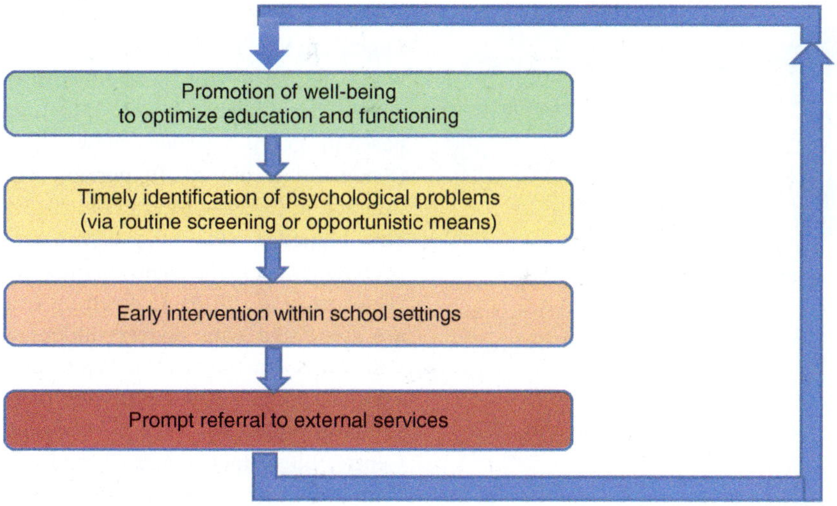

Figure 38.1 Goals of school-based mental health.

implementing mental health programs in diverse settings has also been developed by an International Association for Child and Adolescent Psychiatry and Allied Professions (IACAPAP), World Psychiatric Association (WPA), and WHO-led Child Mental Health Awareness Task Force (Wei & Kutcher, 2012).

School-based health teams

School-based health teams may be loosely configured or formally defined, depending on the school's needs, resources, and wider health system. They typically include school nurses, counselors, and members of the pastoral care team; less often, teachers, visiting psychologists, and general practitioners (GPs). Although no ideal configuration exists, role clarification, team supervision, and maintaining good relationships with external mental health services can optimize their outcomes (Figure 38.2).

Schools and mental health services

Active integration of service provision between school-based health teams, community-based, nonspecialist, and specialist child and adolescent mental health services (CAMHS) and community pediatric services is necessary to provide students with a seamless continuum of care. Precise roles within this joined-up system will depend on available resources in each part (Figure 38.3). From student-centric and economic points of view, mild to moderate issues should ideally be addressed by adequately resourced school or nonspecialist services, and more severe or enduring issues by specialist services. Connections between schools and mental health services may be achieved by routine and opportunistic means. The former includes provision of consultation and/or integration of specialist health professionals within school-based health teams (see Chapter 45). Opportunistic means of strengthening connections between schools and mental

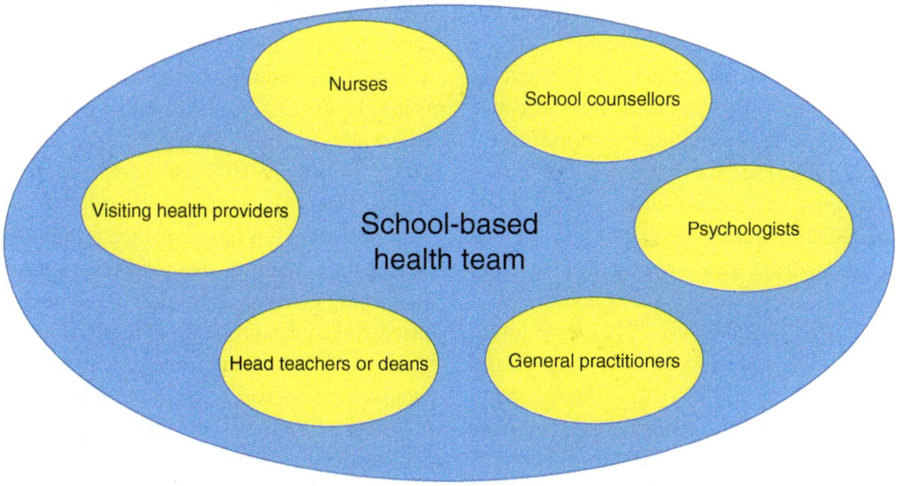

Figure 38.2 School-based health teams.

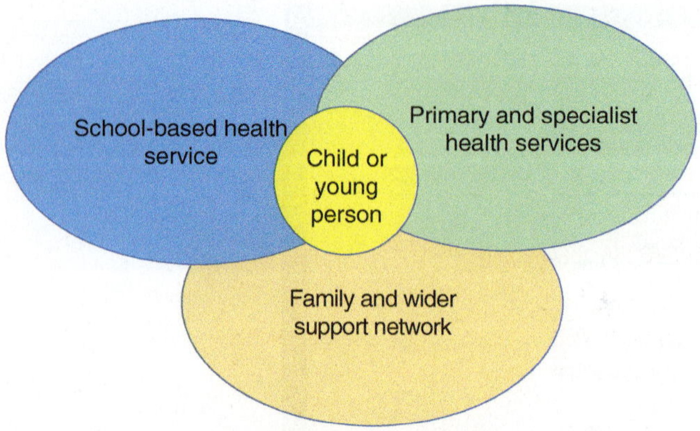

Figure 38.3 School-based mental health in a wider context.

health services include crisis-based sharing of information, prioritizing referrals from schools, and specialists consulting to schools, especially following student suicides, homicides, and natural disasters (Knox & Roberts, 2005).

Interventions for preservation of well-being

Historically construed as merely the absence of illness, *well-being* is now defined by the WHO as a state in which an individual realizes his or her own abilities, can cope with the normal stresses of life, can work productively, and is able to make a contribution to his or her community. Well-being is related to resilience (Wald *et al.*, 2006), social emotional learning (Bridgeland *et al.*, 2013), mental health literacy (Kutcher *et al.*, 2016), and growth mindsets (Yeager & Dweck, 2012). Multiple reviews of school-based well-being interventions have demonstrated mixed results, partly due to heterogeneity of well-being definitions and outcome measures. Currently, positive psychology interventions (Cilar *et al.*, 2020) appear to be most beneficial, albeit with small ES (Mackenzie & Williams, 2018). Some targeted at students at greatest risk (Martínez-García, 2022) and others, that include all students, and are longer, more structured, and focused on multiple components of positive emotions, have been found to be particularly effective (Chuecas *et al.*, 2022). Despite earlier reviews of mindfulness interventions (Felver *et al.*, 2016) identifying positive effects, a large UK-based trial of universal school-based mindfulness (Montero-Marin *et al.*, 2022) recently demonstrated limited benefit and potential harm from this approach. Two large reviews of classroom-based social-emotional learning (SEL) programs (Durlak *et al.*, 2011; Sklad *et al.*, 2012) have found moderate improvements in SEL skills (ES 0.57, 0.48–0.67) and academic performance (ES 0.27, 0.15–0.39), and three reviews of mental health literacy interventions (Salerno, 2016; Nobre *et al.*, 2021; Ma *et al.*, 2022) have identified short-term benefits.

Attempts to identify and modularize common elements of universal well-being programs (e.g., Managing and Adapting Practice [MAP]) have been made, but not widely evaluated. Digital approaches to increasing teacher knowledge and student well-being have been more effective when integrated into the curriculum (Sakellari *et al.*, 2021). Indirectly, physical activity-based programs have been shown to benefit student well-being (Andermo *et al.*, 2020), possibly via self-image and social interaction (Monshouwer *et al.*, 2013). Teacher well-being has also benefited (ES 0.07, 0.02–0.12), mediated by teacher presenteeism and the quality of the student–teacher relationship (Harding *et al.*, 2019). Conversely, teacher stress and burnout are associated with poorer student well-being and learning (Gibson & Carroll, 2021). While uncertainty remains about which specific well-being interventions to recommend, evidence-based guidance is available via the Anna Freud Centre, Blueprints programs, and others. Although research from LMICs is limited, well-being approaches can be developed in line with the WHO's Health Promoting Schools framework (see also Chapter 32).

Identification of mental health problems in schools

School-based screening for mental health problems has been advocated by the United States (U.S.) Preventive Services Task Forces for Depression (Siu *et al.*, 2016) and Anxiety (Mangione *et al.*, 2022) on the basis of these problems being common among school-aged children and earlier identification resulting in more timely and possibly less stigmatizing intervention (Siceloff *et al.*, 2017). However, in other countries, there has been less enthusiasm to endorse this approach due to the inadequacy of evidence to support its acceptability, effectiveness, and feasibility (King, 2021). Recently, there has been greater openness in the United Kingdom (UK) for trialing screening for anxiety in conjunction with school-based intervention. Definitive results of these trials are awaited (Williamson *et al.*, 2022). Screening for suicidal ideation has been recommended by the U.S. Substance Abuse and Mental Health Services Administration (SAMHSA) (Singer *et al.*, 2019) and recent results from the large European Saving and Empowering Young Lives (SEYLE) study show that it may be associated with higher service use (OR [Odds Ratio] 2.7, SE [Standard Error] 1.02, p[p-value] < 0.01) and lower suicidality at 1-year follow-up (OR 0.51, SE 0.11, $p < 0.01$) (Kaess *et al.*, 2020).

A recent review has identified feasibility (including staff time to support screening and follow-up; communication with, and organizing consent from, parents) and cost of primarily paper-based questionnaires (£5–200 per student) as being the main barriers to effective implementation of universal screening programs (Soneson *et al.*, 2020). Electronic screening may help to overcome some of these limitations and multimodal psychosocial screeners, such as YouthCHAT (Thabrew *et al.*, 2019), are showing promise in this regard. Few studies have examined the risk of adverse effects related to school-based screening. The review by Soneson *et al.* found no increased risk of distress or suicidal ideation following universal screening during two studies.

Interventions for problems/disorders

Anxiety and depression

While anxiety and depression have different presentations and trajectories, they are frequently comorbid. Most school-based anxiety and depression interventions are based on cognitive behavior therapy (CBT) or interpersonal therapy (IPT) principles. Universal interventions are delivered to whole classes and targeted interventions are more typically of an *indicated* nature (for students with elevated symptoms who are identified by screening) than *selective* (such as for students affected by bereavement). More recently, computer- or mobile phone-delivered interventions have been investigated with variable success (Jones *et al.*, 2023). For milder symptoms of mental distress, school-based counseling has been shown to be effective (ES 0.81, 0.76–0.86) in high-income countries (Cooper, 2009) and lay counseling has been shown to be helpful in LMIC settings (Michelson *et al.*, 2020). However, there is wide variability in counseling (from humanistic to CBT-based approaches) and the relative efficacy of these approaches has not yet been evaluated.

Although the rationale for prevention and early intervention for anxiety and depression using school-based programs is clear, a number of large, well-conducted meta-analyses have concluded that the size of the effect on reduction of symptoms is generally small and short-term (Stockings *et al.*, 2016; Caldwell *et al.*, 2019; Bradshaw *et al.*, 2021; Werner-Seidler *et al.*, 2021). Due to the high prevalence of these conditions, such small effects may still be of significance at a population health level. For instance, it is estimated that around 21% of new cases of depression can be prevented by existing programs and that the number needed to treat (NNT) to prevent a case of depression is 22 (Werner-Seidler *et al.*, 2021). While targeted interventions usually have larger ES, universal interventions have also been found to benefit both students at high and low risk of anxiety and depression (Stockings *et al.*, 2016). Although there is emerging evidence of the cost-effectiveness of school-based prevention programs for anxiety (Chatterton *et al.*, 2020) and depression (Lee *et al.*, 2021), more research is required before they can be clearly supported, especially for younger children and in LMICs (Bradshaw *et al.*, 2021). While there has been limited research into the extension of school-based approaches to tertiary education settings, a recent review suggests that CBT and mindfulness delivered via digital means may be useful for reducing anxiety and depression among university students (Worsley *et al.*, 2022).

School absenteeism

School absenteeism may be the result of truancy (unexcused, illegal, surreptitious absences), school refusal (difficulty attending school associated with emotional distress), or school phobia (difficulty attending school because of a specific phobia) (Elliott & Place 2019). As chronic absenteeism is often driven by overlapping medical, individual, family, and social factors, contemporary approaches to its management involve addressing these factors rather than focusing on the type of absenteeism (Allen *et al.*, 2018). Interventions for addressing school absenteeism include: CBT (ES 0.54, 0.22–0.86), anxiolytic medication, mentoring, and developmental support-based programs to address individual factors; parent education and support for treatment of parent health problems to address family factors; and school-based antibullying and mental health programs, school nurse interventions, and assistance with safe and reliable transportation to address social factors. Although multiple formal programs have been developed for addressing truancy (https://ojjdp.ojp.gov/taxonomy/term/truancy), criteria for choosing such programs remain unclear and some attention to the way the school system addresses the needs of individual students is important (Rimmington, 2023). Students with chronic illness need to be supported to optimize their medical care via medication support and action plans. For students with significant anxiety or mental health problems, graded return to the classroom and support from health school teachers are usually recommended. Although collaborative, multimodal approaches are generally favored over piecemeal interventions, evidence for the effectiveness of either remains limited (Maynard *et al.*, 2018).

Attention deficit hyperactivity disorder (ADHD)

Children with ADHD experience behavioral issues, lower grades, and worse social relationships in the school environment. These are rarely adequately addressed by medication alone. Nonpharmacologic approaches to management may be broadly classified into behavioral, academic, and self-regulation strategies. Behavioral strategies include the use of clear rules, close monitoring by teachers, nonverbal responses to undesired behavior, appropriate pacing of activities, regular study breaks, and daily report cards. Academic strategies include the use of brief instructions, supported participation, and continuous assessment of understanding. Self-regulation strategies include student recording and rating of unwanted behavior, usually alongside teacher reinforcement of desired behavior (DuPaul, 2007). Multicomponent interventions, such as the Challenging Horizons Program (Evans *et al.*, 2011), have been shown to be effective for middle- and high-school students (DuPaul *et al.*, 2021). Two systematic reviews of school-based ADHD interventions have found widely variable ES (ES 0.2–0.8). Both concluded that contextual factors, including the nature of the classroom environment, stigma, and student, parent, and teacher attributions of ADHD, moderate the implementation and effectiveness of interventions (Richardson *et al.*, 2015; Moore *et al.*, 2019). As such, education about ADHD and relationship building with schools is likely to be critical for the success of any type of intervention.

Disruptive behavior disorders (DBDs)

School-based approaches to preventing and managing DBDs, including oppositional defiant disorder (ODD) and conduct disorder (CD), vary according to the age of students, but in general are focused on promotion of SEL for younger children, positive reinforcement of prosocial behavior and problem-solving for older children, and more complex combinations of behavioral, cognitive, and family strategies for young people (Garland *et al.*, 2008).

Of the many formal school-based programs available, the most formally evaluated include:

- **The Good Behavior Game (GBG)**: Primarily aimed at 6–11-year-olds, the GBG employs increasingly sophisticated team-oriented and reward-based games. Multiple trials in different countries have demonstrated positive effects on aggression, attention, and academic engagement (Kellam *et al.*, 2011). Better effects in males than females (Poduska *et al.*, 2008) are possibly due to differences in traditionally female forms of aggression (e.g., being ignored/left out/subject to nasty rumors).
- **Promoting Alternative THinking Strategies (PATHS)**: A universal, teacher-delivered curriculum aimed at improving emotional and social competencies and reducing aggression. Targeted at children aged 6–11, it includes a suite of developmentally based lessons and materials organized around 5 units (self-control, understanding, positive self-esteem, relationships, and interpersonal solving skills) that can be flexibly used over a 5-year period to target specific goals (Greenberg, 1998). An enhanced version for 6–15-year-olds, The Fast Track Project, includes parent training, home visits, social skills training, and academic tutoring to address multiple risk and protective factors and has been shown to reduce rates of all DBDs including CD (Conduct Problems Prevention Research Group, 2011).
- **The Seattle Social Development Project (SSDP)**: A universal multicomponent intervention for decreasing problem behavior in children aged 6–12. The enhanced version, known as Raising Healthy Children, includes teacher training to support establishment of clear behavioral expectations and frequent, specific, and contingent encouragement and praise for effort; social and emotional skill training for students; and parent training. It has been shown to lead to reduced antisocial behavior and increased social competence (Catalano *et al.*, 2004).
- **The Incredible Years (IY)**: A set of three comprehensive, multicomponent, developmentally based curricula for parents, teachers, and children. Aimed at promoting social competencies in younger children, the IY Training for Children or "Dinosaur School" has been shown to reduce disruptive behavior at school and home by teacher, parent, and independent report (Webster-Stratton *et al.*, 2008). The classroom version of the IY Dinosaur curriculum (The Incredible Years Teacher Classroom Management (IY-TCM) program) specifically designed for children aged 3–8, including regular lessons and small group activities, has been shown to produce small, short-term improvement to student mental health, especially for those already struggling (Ford *et al.*, 2019).
- ***Check-in/Check-out***: A targeted intervention during which students meet with teachers at the start of the day to set expectations of behavior and achievement and again at the end of the day to receive feedback and review their performance (Crone *et al.*, 2010). A recent meta-analysis (Drevon *et al.*, 2019) confirmed positive effects on behavior (ES 1.16) and academic engagement (ES 1.53).

Reviews of school-based programs for preventing and managing disruptive behavior have found generally positive effects on behavior (ES −0.23 to 16.27) and academic engagement (Mytton *et al.*, 2006; Hahn *et al.*, 2007; Wilson & Lipsey, 2007; Matjasko *et al.* 2012; Alperin *et al.*, 2023). However, they remain underused due to cost and teacher time, and are underresearched in LMIC settings. Despite lower student-to-teacher ratios and more individualized approaches (Tobin & Sprague, 1999), alternative education for students whose behavior cannot be managed in typical classrooms has not been shown to produce beneficial outcomes (Ballard & Bender, 2022).

Bullying

Antibullying programs include: global school approaches that encourage and support the value of all individuals; classroom-based strategies targeting behaviors, SEL, and student attitudes and beliefs; the role of bystanders; and increased playground supervision. One of the best-known school-based bullying prevention programs is the Finnish KiVa program (Box 38.1).

Antibullying programs have been shown to reduce bullying perpetration by 19–20% and victimization by 15–16% (Gaffney *et al.*, 2019a). Despite some inconsistency, examination of program components suggests that inclusion of informal peer involvement and use of multiple approaches are associated with greater effectiveness (Gaffney *et al.*, 2021). Regardless of the established relationship between bullying and internalizing disorders, antibullying programs have only been shown to have very small effects on reducing anxiety (ES 0.08; 95% CI; 0.011–0.158) and depression (ES 0.06; 95% CI; 0.014–0.107) (Guzman-Holst *et al.*, 2022). School-based anti-cyberbullying programs

Box 38.1 The KiVa program

The teacher-led KiVa program targets children aged 7–15 through structured lessons about social skills and how to identify and address bullying. Parental involvement is facilitated through online resources. Multiple randomized controlled trials (RCTs) have demonstrated positive effects on rates of bullying and victimization (Kärnä *et al.*, 2013; Nocentini & Menesini, 2016; Green *et al.*, 2020; Huitsing *et al.*, 2020) and academic engagement (Salmivalli *et al.* 2012). Although less favorable results were obtained during a Welsh RCT (Axford *et al.*, 2020), a UK multicenter cluster RCT is underway (Clarkson *et al.*, 2022).

have shown lower effectiveness than those for traditional forms of bullying for bullying perpetration (9–15%) and victimization (14–15%) (Gaffney *et al.*, 2019b).

Substance use disorders

Universal school-based resilience programs have been shown to be effective by some reviews (Hodder *et al.*, 2017), but not others (Bahramnejad *et al.*, 2020), for preventing substance use disorders. Interactive lecture-oriented programs that increase personal coping and interpersonal skills have been shown to be more effective than noninteractive versions stressing drug knowledge and affective development (Tobler *et al.*, 2000; Conrod, 2016). A positive school climate has also been associated with reduced initiation of substance use (Daily *et al.*, 2020). Although a few culturally oriented interventions based on indigenous beliefs, values, language, images, and worldviews have been developed, evidence for their effectiveness remains limited (Okamoto *et al.*, 2020; Smith *et al.*, 2022). Despite previous reviews of digital preventative approaches having mixed results (Das *et al.*, 2016; Champion *et al.*, 2019), a recent study of Australian universal (Climate Schools) and targeted (Preventure) web-based interventions showed that both were effective at reducing alcohol use and related harms at 7-year follow-up (Newton *et al.*, 2022). For those with identified issues, brief interventions (BI) and provision of information about substance use problems have both been shown to be more effective than no intervention at short-term and long-term follow-up (Carney *et al.*, 2016). Computerized BI has also been shown to be as effective as BI delivered by school nurses (Gryczynski *et al.*, 2021).

Eating disorders

Although no specific school-based eating disorder prevention programs have been robustly evaluated or widely implemented, current research suggests that interactive programs with content relevant to participants (Torres-Castaño *et al.*, 2022) may be more acceptable, and that those delivered to targeted groups (i.e., those perceived to be at greater risk) may be more effective (del Pino Sedeño *et al.* 2021). Educational programs also appear more likely to succeed when boys are included, so they better understand pressures faced by girls and are less likely to engage in weight- and appearance-related bullying (Wilksch & Wade 2009). Trained teachers who have ongoing relationships with students may also increase the effectiveness of interventions (Berger *et al.*, 2014). One potential concern is that universal prevention education programs can increase weight-related concerns and body dissatisfaction (Torres-Castaño *et al.*, 2022). These risks may be minimized by focusing programs on personal skill development, empowerment, and self-esteem (O'Dea & Abraham, 2000).

Trauma and post-traumatic stress disorder (PTSD)

Traumatic events may be associated with no discernible effects (most commonly), post-traumatic growth, or, in a third of cases, post-traumatic stress disorder (PTSD) (del Pino Sedeño *et al.*, 2021). PTSD symptoms, such as mood dysregulation, hypervigilance, and avoidance, may be misinterpreted in the school environment as inattention or problematic behavior (van der Kolk, 2009). They may also be associated with academic underachievement and other mental health problems, especially depression, substance use problems, and suicidal ideation (McLaughlin *et al.*, 2018). While older reviews of school-based interventions for PSTD suggested greatest benefits for trauma-focused CBT (TF-CBT) and eye movement desensitization and reprocessing (EMDR) therapy, more recent findings indicate small to medium mean-weighted ES (d = 0.41) and less discernible differences between intervention types (du Mello Kenyon & Schirmer, 2020).

For children living in poverty, political conflict, and natural disaster-affected environments, as well as those affected by interpersonal violence, it may also be possible to improve symptoms of PTSD and anxiety using CBT-oriented interventions (Higgen *et al.*, 2022; Wichmann *et al.*, 2023). For those who have recently experienced disasters such as school shootings, proximity to the trauma, peritraumatic dissociation, post-traumatic emotional regulation difficulties, social support (including parent/sibling reactions), and flexibility of coping style may predict psychological sequelae (Travers *et al.*, 2018). The use of trauma-informed approaches, crisis management plans, and psychological first aid is recommended by the US National Child Traumatic Stress Network and National Centre for PTSD. For further details on PTSD see Chapter 58.

Self-harm and suicide

There are four broad approaches to preventing self-harm and suicide in schools: promoting student well-being; educating staff to recognize and address these problems; screening for suicidal thoughts and behaviors (STBs); and directly addressing STBs with students. Promoting school connectedness and minimizing exposure to bullying, violence, and substance use can also reduce the risk of STBs. While most suicide prevention is undertaken in secondary schools, there is some evidence that primary school-based interventions, such as the previously described GBG, can reduce suicide attempts in the long term (Wilcox *et al.*, 2008).

"Gatekeeper training" includes providing staff with information on STBs, risk factors, warning signs, and how to respond appropriately when risk is identified. Popular examples include Question, Persuade, Respond (QPR) (Wyman *et al.*, 2008); Applied Suicide Intervention Skills Training (ASIST) (Ewell-Foster *et al.*, 2017); and Pathway for Assisting Life (PAL) (Shannonhouse *et al.*, 2017). Despite their popularity, studies of gatekeeper training programs have primarily produced evidence of staff knowledge improvement rather than change in student behavior (Pistone *et al.*, 2019) and one has found increased suicidal ideation among recipients (Sareen *et al.*, 2013).

Screening for suicide may be undertaken using paper-based questionnaires such as the Columbia Suicide Screen (Scott *et al.*, 2009), screening teams (Brown & Grumet, 2009), or composite electronic screeners (Thabrew *et al.*, 2019). Although shown that it is safe to ask students about suicide (Ayer *et al.*, 2022), limited evidence exists for the effectiveness of each of these approaches (e.g., Wasserman *et al.*, 2015), and feasibility of administration with appropriate follow-up in the school setting is a common barrier to their use. Targeting students through the curriculum is controversial. Better known universal programs include the action plan-oriented Signs of Suicide (SOS) (Schilling *et al.*, 2016) and the Youth Aware of Mental Health program (YAM). The former has been shown to reduce suicide attempts, but not ideation in the short term, and the latter to be better than gatekeeper training and screening in reducing short-term suicidal ideation and attempts (Wasserman *et al.*, 2015),

Systematic reviews and meta-analyses have reported increases in staff awareness and understanding of STBs but only small effects in the reduction of self-harm, and suicidal ideation and attempts from school-based prevention studies (Brann *et al.*, 2021; Pierret *et al.*, 2022; Walsh *et al.*, 2023). Few studies have been undertaken in LMICs (Doty *et al.*, 2022) and concerns have been raised about the rigor of conducted research (Kutcher *et al.*, 2017). Based on current evidence, a multitiered approach (e.g., Ayer *et al.*, 2022) may be most effective for prevention and management of self-harm and suicide.

Schools will sometimes have to deal with the aftermath of the suicide of one of their pupils and staff should be trained in how to deal with these events, and appropriate protocols put in place. School-based "postvention" should include strategies to reduce contagion (Diefendorf *et al.*, 2022). Because of the known phenomenon of cluster suicides, schools are encouraged not to sensationalize suicide, to restrict the amount of detail about methods, and to avoid glorifying or condemning victims. Identification and follow-up of vulnerable students and providing support for students, staff, families, and the community are vital components of the school response.

Useful resources for schools can be found on the websites of: SAMHSA; the Suicide Prevention Resource Centre; the New Zealand Ministry of Education: Headspace Australia; and the Anna Freud Centre.

Interventions for specific groups

LGBTQ+ students

Four school-based strategies for improving the well-being of LGBTQ+ students have been developed: (i) policies that identify LGBTQ+ students and create supportive contexts (including programs that reduce bullying); (ii) student access to information and support related to sexual orientation and gender identity or expression (SOGIE); (iii) education of staff; and (iv) student-led clubs and organizations such as gender-sexuality alliances (GSAs) (Russell *et al.*, 2021; Marraccini *et al.*, 2022). To date, there is limited research evidence for the effectiveness of these strategies, with a recent review suggesting lower effects for boys, gender minority students, and bisexual students (Schlief *et al.*, 2023). Academic outcomes and absenteeism have been shown during one study to be improved by student–mentor relationships (Fruiht & Wray-Lake, 2013). Although LGBTQ+ inclusive curricula have been supported by educators in principle, they have neither frequently been used nor shown to lead to substantial change (Bouldin, 2021). As the number of LGBTQ+ students increases, valuable toolkits for supporting their inclusion have been developed by the National Education Union, Proud Trust, and others. Comprehensive trans-specific resources are also available from multiple sources including the British Safe Schools Alliance and Think2Speak.

Refugees

Preventative approaches for refugee students, such as psychological first aid and taught skills for psychological recovery, have shown little evidence of effectiveness (Brymer *et al.*, 2008). Creative expression workshops, art therapy, and drama therapy have demonstrated some positive effects on well-being (Nosè *et al.* 2017). PTSD-focused interventions including TF-CBT, EMDR, and narrative exposure therapy (NET) are useful when delivered in specialist settings (Fazel & Betancourt 2018). Although it has been suggested that training of host communities may increase receptiveness and support, no trials have ever been reported. Overall, there is currently insufficient evidence with which to recommend school-based mental health interventions for prevention or treatment in this population.

Autistic students

School-based interventions trialed for supporting autistic students have been of two broad types: those aimed at improving social skills, behavior, and functioning, and those aimed at reducing anxiety. Positive effects are reported for a range of the former (Dean & Chang 2021), without any clearly superior model. In contrast, a recent review of school-delivered anxiety interventions has found CBT-based programs most effective, with a moderate overall ES ($g = -0.58$) (Perihan *et al.*, 2022).

Implementation of school-based interventions

While universal interventions may be more sustainably delivered via teachers, teacher-supported digital means, or lay counselors (Shinde *et al.*, 2020), targeted interventions may be more effectively delivered by external providers with specific expertise. Establishment of good relationships between CAMHS and schools via in-reach, timely response to crisis referrals, regular liaison, and provision of staff training and appealing resources are all likely to support effective implementation of school-based well-being interventions (Fazel *et al.*, 2014a). Further tips are provided in the following list:

- Make sure you have talked to all the relevant people, e.g., principal, school-based health team.

- Establish relationships with key people by visiting schools in the area served by your service.
- Use technology to work with schools and maintain relationships.
- Be active about communication—check on progress at school and have a strategy to keep schools informed about what is happening in your service.
- Check you have a shared understanding about what happens.
- Understand that there may be a different culture within the education sector around confidentiality, parental involvement, and consent. This needs to be balanced with your professional responsibilities as a mental health clinician or researcher.
- Take the school year into account, including the term structure. You may need to work around particularly busy times such as exams and major school activities.
- Plan ahead: It is often easier to start things at the beginning of a school year, which requires action well before the end of the previous year.

Numerous toolkits for implementing student well-being and mental health, including the Schools in Mind website and the Targeted Mental Health in Schools (TaMHS) website, are also available.

Areas of uncertainty

While there are many school-based interventions from which to choose, the quality of supporting evidence for their use varies widely and is hard to navigate via health and education databases. Few studies of magnitude, with a focus on harm (Foulkes & Stringaris, 2023) or addressing the needs of students in LMICs (Fazel *et al.*, 2014b), have ever been conducted and there is mixed evidence for the cost-effectiveness of interventions (Anderson *et al.*, 2019; Le *et al.*, 2021) leaving educators and health professionals uncertain about which to implement (Thabrew *et al.*, 2023). Despite modest research ES, it is important to note that even small shifts at a population level can result in significant societal benefits (Tanner-Smith *et al.*, 2018).

Conclusion

Schools offer multiple opportunities for preserving student well-being and identifying and managing mental health problems when they arise in a universal, targeted, or selected manner. While a wide range of effective interventions currently exist, they remain underutilized due to cost, staff time, and school uncertainty about which interventions to implement. Few have also been studied in LMICs. With improved research and combined guidance from health and education organizations, the potential of school-based interventions may gradually be achieved.

References

Allen, C.W. *et al.* (2018) School absenteeism in children and adolescents. *American Family Physician* **98**(12), 738–744.

Alperin, A. *et al.* (2023) School-based interventions for middle school students with disruptive behaviors: a systematic review of components and methodology. *School Psychology Review* **52**(2), 180–205.

Andermo, S. *et al.* (2020) School-related physical activity interventions and mental health among children: a systematic review and meta-analysis. *Sports Medicine-Open* **6**(1), 1–27.

Anderson, J.K. *et al.* (2019) A systematic review of effectiveness and cost-effectiveness of school-based identification of children and young people at risk of, or currently experiencing mental health difficulties. *Psychological Medicine* **49**(1), 9–19.

Axford, N. *et al.* (2020) The effectiveness of the KiVa bullying prevention program in Wales, UK: results from a pragmatic cluster randomized controlled trial. *Prevention Science* **21**(5), 615–626.

Ayer, L. *et al.* (2022) Effective suicide prevention and intervention in schools. In: *Youth Suicide Prevention and Intervention: Best Practices and Policy Implications*. (eds J.P. Ackerman & L.M. Horowitz). Springer International Publishing, Cham, Switzerland. pp. 31–40.

Bahramnejad, A. *et al.* (2020) Universal school-based intervention for increasing resilience, and its effect on substance use. *Children and Youth Services Review* **118**, 105378.

Ballard, S.C. & Bender, S.L. (2022) A systematic review of social, emotional, and behavioral interventions and outcomes for students in alternative education. *Preventing School Failure: Alternative Education for Children and Youth* **66**(2), 136–149.

Berger, U. *et al.* (2014) Effectiveness of reducing the risk of eating-related problems using the German school-based intervention program, "Torera" for preadolescent boys and girls. *Prevention Science* **15**(4), 557–569.

Bouldin, M. (2021) *Effective interventions to support LGBTQ+ youth*. Master's Thesis, Northwestern College, Orange City, IA.

Bradshaw, M. *et al.* (2021) Universal school-based mental health programmes in low- and middle-income countries: a systematic review and narrative synthesis. *Preventive Medicine* **143**, 106317.

Brann, K.L. *et al.* (2021) A meta-analysis of suicide prevention programs for school-aged youth. *Children and Youth Services Review* **121**, 105826.

Bridgeland, J. *et al.* (2013) The Missing Piece: A National Teacher Survey on How Social and Emotional Learning Can Empower Children and Transform Schools. A Report for CASEL. Civic Enterprises, Institute of Education Sciences, Washington, DC.

Brown, M.M. & Grumet, J.G. (2009) School-based suicide prevention with African American youth in an urban setting. *Professional Psychology: Research and Practice* **40**(2), 111.

Brymer, M.J. *et al.* (2008) Acute interventions for refugee children and families. *Child and Adolescent Psychiatric Clinics of North America* **17**(3), 625–640.

Caldwell, D.M. *et al.* (2019) School-based interventions to prevent anxiety and depression in children and young people: a systematic review and network meta-analysis. *The Lancet Psychiatry* **6**(12), 1011–1020.

Carney, T. *et al.* (2016) Brief school-based interventions and behavioural outcomes for substance-using adolescents. *Cochrane Database of Systematic Reviews* **2016**(1), CD008969.

Catalano, R.F. *et al.* (2004) The importance of bonding to school for healthy development: findings from the social development research group. *Journal of School Health* **74**, 252–261.

Champion, K.E. *et al.* (2019) Effectiveness of school-based eHealth interventions to prevent multiple lifestyle risk behaviours among adolescents: a systematic review and meta-analysis. *The Lancet Digital Health* **1**(5), e206–e221.

Chatterton, M.L. *et al.* (2020) Cost-effectiveness of preventing child internalising problems: results from the translational trial of Cool Little Kids at school entry. *Journal of Anxiety Disorders* **70**, 102191.

Chuecas, M.J. *et al.* (2022) A systematic narrative review of subjective well-being promotion intervention programmes in the school setting. *Review of Education* **10**(1), e3345.

Cilar, L. *et al.* (2020) Effectiveness of school-based mental well-being interventions among adolescents: a systematic review. *Journal of Advanced Nursing* **76**(8), 2023–2045.

Clarkson, S. *et al.* (2022) The UK stand together trial: protocol for a multicentre cluster randomised controlled trial to evaluate the effectiveness and cost-effectiveness of KiVa to reduce bullying in primary schools. *BMC Public Health* **22**(1), 608.

Conduct Problems Prevention Research Group (2011) The effects of the fast track preventive intervention on the development of conduct disorder across childhood. *Child Development* **82**(1), 331–345.

Conrod, P.J. (2016) Personality-targeted interventions for substance use and misuse. *Current Addiction Reports* **3**, 426–436.

Cooper, M. (2009) Counselling in UK secondary schools: a comprehensive review of audit and evaluation data. *Counselling and Psychotherapy Research* **9**(3), 137–150.

Crone, D.A. et al. (2010) *Responding to Problem Behavior in Schools: The Behavior Education Program*, 2nd edn. Guilford Press, New York.

Daily, S.M. *et al.* (2020) School climate as a universal intervention to prevent substance use initiation in early adolescence: a longitudinal study. *Health Education & Behavior* **47**(3), 402–411.

Das, J.K. *et al.* (2016) Interventions for adolescent mental health: an overview of systematic reviews. *Journal of Adolescent Health* **59**(4), S49–S60.

Dean, M. & Chang, Y.C. (2021) A systematic review of school-based social skills interventions and observed social outcomes for students with autism spectrum disorder in inclusive settings. *Autism* **25**(7), 1828–1843.

del Pino Sedeño, T. *et al.* (2021) Efectividad y coste-efectividad de la prevención universal de los trastornos de la conducta alimentaria en población infantil, preadolescente y adolescente escolarizada. Ministerio de Sanidad. Servicio de Evaluación del Servicio Canario de la Salud, Informe deEvaluación de Tecnologías Sanitarias.

Diefendorf, S. *et al.* (2022) Understanding suicide bereavement, contagion, and the importance of thoughtful postvention in schools. In: *Youth Suicide Prevention and Intervention: Best Practices and Policy Implications.* (eds J.P. Ackerman & L.M. Horowitz). Springer International Publishing, Cham, Switzerland. pp. 51–60.

Doty, B. *et al.* (2022) Systematic review of suicide prevention studies with data on youth and young adults living in low-income and middle-income countries. *BMJ Open* **12**(9), e055000.

Drevon, D.D. *et al.* (2019) A meta-analytic review of the evidence for check-in check-out. *Psychology in the Schools* **56**(3), 393–412.

du Mello Kenyon, G. & Schirmer, J. (2020) Common practice elements of school-based trauma interventions for children and adolescents exhibiting symptoms of post-traumatic stress disorder: a systematic review. *Journal of Psychologists and Counsellors in Schools* **30**(2), 112–128.

Duggins, S.D. *et al.* (2016) Aggression among adolescent victims of school bullying: protective roles of family and school connectedness. *Psychology of Violence* **6**(2), 205.

DuPaul, G.J. (2007) School-based interventions for students with attention deficit hyperactivity disorder: current status and future directions. *School Psychology Review* **36**(2), 183–194.

DuPaul, G.J. *et al.* (2021) School-based intervention for adolescents with attention-deficit/hyperactivity disorder: effects on academic functioning. *Journal of School Psychology* **87**, 48–63.

Durlak, J.A. *et al.* (2011) The impact of enhancing students' social and emotional learning: a meta-analysis of school-based universal interventions. *Child Development* **82**(1), 405–432.

Elliott, J.G. & Place, M. (2019) Practitioner review: school refusal: developments in conceptualisation and treatment since 2000. *Journal of Child Psychology and Psychiatry* **60**(1), 4–15.

Evans, S.W. *et al.* (2011) Effectiveness of the challenging horizons after-school program for young adolescents with ADHD. *Behavior Therapy* **42**(3), 462–474.

Ewell Foster, C.J. *et al.* (2017) Identification, response, and referral of suicidal youth following applied suicide intervention skills training. *Suicide and Life-Threatening Behavior* **47**(3), 297–308.

Fazel, M. & Betancourt, T.S. (2018) Preventive mental health interventions for refugee children and adolescents in high-income settings. *The Lancet Child & Adolescent Health* **2**(2), 121–132.

Fazel, M. *et al.* (2014a) Mental health interventions in schools in high-income countries. *The Lancet Psychiatry* **1**(5), 377–387.

Fazel, M. *et al.* (2014b) Mental health interventions in schools in low-income and middle-income countries. *The Lancet Psychiatry* **1**(5), 388–398.

Felver, J.C. *et al.* (2016) A systematic review of mindfulness-based interventions for youth in school settings. *Mindfulness* **7**, 34–45.

Ford, T. *et al.* (2019) The effectiveness and cost-effectiveness of the Incredible Years® Teacher Classroom Management programme in primary school children: results of the STARS cluster randomised controlled trial. *Psychological Medicine* **49**(5), 828–842.

Foulkes, L. & Stringaris, A. (2023) Do no harm: can school mental health interventions cause iatrogenic harm? *BJPsych Bulletin* **47**(5), 1–3.

Freiberg, H.J. (ed) (1999) *School Climate: Measuring, Improving, and Sustaining Healthy Learning Environments*. Psychology Press, UK.

Fruiht, V.M. & Wray-Lake, L. (2013) The role of mentor type and timing in predicting educational attainment. *Journal of Youth and Adolescence* **42**, 1459–1472.

Gaffney, H. *et al.* (2019a) Evaluating the effectiveness of school-bullying prevention programs: an updated meta-analytical review. *Aggression and Violent Behavior* **45**, 111–133.

Gaffney, H. *et al.* (2019b) Are cyberbullying intervention and prevention programs effective? A systematic and meta-analytical review. *Aggression and Violent Behavior* **45**, 134–153.

Gaffney, H. *et al.* (2021) What works in anti-bullying programs? Analysis of effective intervention components. *Journal of School Psychology* **85**, 37–56.

Garland, A.F. *et al.* (2008) Identifying common elements of evidence-based psychosocial treatments for children's disruptive behavior problems. *Journal of the American Academy of Child & Adolescent Psychiatry* **47**(5), 505–514.

Gibson, S. & Carroll, C. (2021) Stress, Burnout, Anxiety and Depression: How They Impact on Mental Health and Wellbeing of Teachers and on Learner Outcomes. Education Support. Available: https://www.educationsupport.org.uk/media/qeupkgep/literature-review-stress-anxiety-burnout-and-depression-impact-on-teachers-and-on-learner-outcomes.pdf [18 October 2024].

Green, V.A. *et al.* (2020) An evaluation of the KiVa anti-bullying program in New Zealand. *International Journal of Bullying Prevention* **2**, 225–237.

Greenberg, M.T. (1998) *Promoting Alternative Thinking Strategies (PATHS)*. Center for the Study and Prevention of Violence, Institute of Behavioral Science, University of Colorado at Boulder, Boulder, CO.

Gryczynski, J. *et al.* (2021) Computer-vs. nurse practitioner-delivered brief intervention for adolescent marijuana, alcohol, and sex risk behaviors in school-based health centers. *Drug and Alcohol Dependence* **218**, 108423.

Guzman-Holst, C. *et al.* (2022) Research review: do antibullying interventions reduce internalizing symptoms? A systematic review, meta-analysis, and meta-regression exploring intervention components, moderators, and mechanisms. *Journal of Child Psychology and Psychiatry* **63**(12), 1454–1465.

Hahn, R. *et al.* (2007) Effectiveness of universal school-based programs to prevent violent and aggressive behavior: a systematic review. *American Journal of Preventive Medicine* **33**(2), S114–S129.

Harding, S. *et al.* (2019) Is teachers' mental health and wellbeing associated with students' mental health and wellbeing? *Journal of Affective Disorders* **242**, 180–187.

Hayes, D. *et al.* (2023) The impact of universal, school based, interventions on help seeking in children and young people: a systematic literature review. *European Child & Adolescent Psychiatry* **33**(9), 1–18.

Higgen, S. *et al.* (2022) Universal mental health interventions for young students in adverse environments: a systematic review of evaluated interventions. *Child and Adolescent Mental Health* **27**(3), 281–293.

Hodder, R.K. *et al.* (2017) Systematic review of universal school-based 'resilience' interventions targeting adolescent tobacco, alcohol or illicit substance use: a meta-analysis. *Preventive Medicine* **100**, 248–268.

Huitsing, G. *et al.* (2020) A large-scale replication of the effectiveness of the KiVa antibullying program: a randomized controlled trial in the Netherlands. *Prevention Science* **21**, 627–638.

Jerald, C.D. (2006) *School Culture*. Center for Comprehensive School Reform and Improvement, Institute of Education Sciences, Washington, DC.

Jones, S.E. *et al.* (2022) Mental health, suicidality, and connectedness among high school students during the COVID-19 pandemic—adolescent behaviors and experiences survey, United States, January–June 2021. *MMWR Supplements* **71**(3), 16.

Jones, R.B. *et al.* (2023) Digital technologies to support adolescents with depression and anxiety. *BJPsych Advances* **29**(4), 1–15.

Kaess, M. *et al.* (2020) Twelve-month service use, suicidality and mental health problems of European adolescents after a school-based screening for current suicidality. *European Child & Adolescent Psychiatry* **31**(2), 1–10.

Kärnä, A. *et al.* (2013) Effectiveness of the KiVa antibullying program: grades 1–3 and 7–9. *Journal of Educational Psychology* **105**(2), 535–555.

Kellam, S.G. *et al.* (2011) The good behavior game and the future of prevention and treatment. *Addiction Science & Clinical Practice* **6**(1), 73.

King, K. (2021) Screening children for mental health difficulties in school settings. *British Journal of Child Health* **2**(6), 275–287.

Knox, K.S. & Roberts, A.R. (2005) Crisis intervention and crisis team models in schools. *Children & Schools* **27**(2), 93–100.

Kutcher, S. *et al.* (2016) Mental health literacy: past, present, and future. *The Canadian Journal of Psychiatry* **61**(3), 154–158.

Kutcher, S. *et al.* (2017) School-and community-based youth suicide prevention interventions: hot idea, hot air, or sham? *The Canadian Journal of Psychiatry* **62**(6), 381–387.

Kuzik, N. *et al.* (2022) School-related sedentary behaviours and indicators of health and well-being among children and youth: a systematic review. *International Journal of Behavioral Nutrition and Physical Activity* **19**(1), 1–32.

Lattie, E.G. *et al.* (2019) Technology and college student mental health: challenges and opportunities. *Frontiers in Psychiatry* **10**, 246.

Le, L.K.D. *et al.* (2021) Cost-effectiveness evidence of mental health prevention and promotion interventions: a systematic review of economic evaluations. *PLoS Medicine* **18**(5), e1003606.

Lee, Y.Y. *et al.* (2021) The cost-effectiveness of delivering universal psychological interventions in schools to prevent depression among Australian adolescents: a model-based economic evaluation. *Mental Health & Prevention* **24**, 200213.

Ma, K.K.Y. *et al.* (2022) School-based interventions to improve mental health literacy and reduce mental health stigma—a systematic review. *Child and Adolescent Mental Health* **28**, 230–240.

Mackenzie, K. & Williams, C. (2018) Universal, school-based interventions to promote mental and emotional well-being: what is being done in the UK and does it work? A systematic review. *BMJ Open* **8**(9), e022560.2.

Mangione, C.M. *et al.* (2022) Screening for anxiety in children and adolescents: US preventive services task force recommendation statement. *JAMA* **328**(14), 1438–1444.

Marraccini, M.E. *et al.* (2022) The roles of school in supporting LGBTQ+ youth: a systematic review and ecological framework for understanding risk for suicide-related thoughts and behaviors. *Journal of School Psychology* **91**, 27–49.

Martínez-García, A. (2022) Contributions of universal school-based mental health promotion to the wellbeing of adolescents and preadolescents: a systematic review of educational interventions. *Health Education* **122**(5), 564–583.

Matjasko, J.L. *et al.* (2012) A systematic meta-review of evaluations of youth violence prevention programs: common and divergent findings from 25 years of meta-analyses and systematic reviews. *Aggression and Violent Behavior* **17**(6), 540–552.

Maynard, B.R. *et al.* (2018) Treatment for school refusal among children and adolescents: a systematic review and meta-analysis. *Research on Social Work Practice* **28**(1), 56–67.

McLaughlin, K. *et al.* (2018) Posttraumatic stress disorder in children and adolescents: epidemiology, pathogenesis, clinical manifestations, course, assessment, and diagnosis. *Geological Society, London, Special Publications* **372**(1), 473–494.

Michelson, D. *et al.* (2020) Effectiveness of a brief lay counsellor-delivered, problem-solving intervention for adolescent mental health problems in urban, low-income schools in India: a randomised controlled trial. *The Lancet Child & Adolescent Health* **4**(8), 571–582.

Monshouwer, K. *et al.* (2013) Possible mechanisms explaining the association between physical activity and mental health: findings from the 2001 Dutch health behaviour in school-aged children survey. *Clinical Psychological Science* **1**(1), 67–74.

Montero-Marin, J. *et al.* (2022) School-based mindfulness training in early adolescence: what works, for whom and how in the MYRIAD trial? *BMJ Mental Health* **25**(3), 117–124.

Moore, D.A. *et al.* (2019) Non-pharmacological interventions for ADHD in school settings: an overarching synthesis of systematic reviews. *Journal of Attention Disorders* **23**(3), 220–233.

Mytton, J.A. *et al.* (2006) School-based secondary prevention programmes for preventing violence. *Cochrane Database of Systematic Reviews* **2006**(3), CD004606.

Newton, N.C. *et al.* (2022) The 7-year effectiveness of school-based alcohol use prevention from adolescence to early adulthood: a randomized controlled trial of universal, selective, and combined interventions. *Journal of the American Academy of Child & Adolescent Psychiatry* **61**(4), 520–532.

Nobre, J. *et al.* (2021) Promotion of mental health literacy in adolescents: a scoping review. *International Journal of Environmental Research and Public Health* **18**(18), 9500.

Nocentini, A. & Menesini, E. (2016) KiVa anti-bullying program in Italy: evidence of effectiveness in a randomized control trial. *Prevention Science* **17**, 1012–1023.

Nosè, M. *et al.* (2017) Psychosocial interventions for post-traumatic stress disorder in refugees and asylum seekers resettled in high-income countries: systematic review and meta-analysis. *PLoS One* **12**(2), e0171030.

O'Dea, J.A. & Abraham, S. (2000) Improving the body image, eating attitudes, and behaviors of young male and female adolescents: a new educational approach that focuses on self- esteem. *International Journal of Eating Disorders* **28**(1), 43–57.

Okamoto, S.K. *et al.* (2020) The implementation of a culturally grounded, school-based, drug prevention curriculum in rural Hawai'i. *Journal of Community Psychology* **48**(4), 1085–1099.

Page, A. *et al.* (2021) Fostering school connectedness online for students with diverse learning needs: inclusive education in Australia during the COVID-19 pandemic. *European Journal of Special Needs Education* **36**(1), 142–156.

Perihan, C. *et al.* (2022) Assessment and treatment of anxiety in children with autism spectrum disorder in school settings: a systematic review and meta-analysis. *School Mental Health* **14**(1), 153–164.

Pierret, A.C. *et al.* (2022) Education and training interventions, and support tools for school staff to adequately respond to young people who disclose self-harm–a systematic literature review of effectiveness, feasibility and acceptability. *Child and Adolescent Mental Health* **27**(2), 161–172.

Pistone, I. *et al.* (2019) The effects of educational interventions on suicide: a systematic review and meta-analysis. *International Journal of Social Psychiatry* **65**(5), 399–412.

Poduska, J.M. *et al.* (2008) Impact of the Good Behavior Game, a universal classroom-based behavior intervention, on young adult service use for problems with emotions, behavior, or drugs or alcohol. *Drug and alcohol dependence* **95**, S29–S44.

Power, C. (2014) *The Power of Education: Education for All, Development, Globalisation and UNESCO*, Vol. 27. Springer, Cham, Switzerland.

Raniti, M. *et al.* (2022) The role of school connectedness in the prevention of youth depression and anxiety: a systematic review with youth consultation. *BMC Public Health* **22**(1), 2152.

Richardson, M. *et al.* (2015) Non-pharmacological interventions for attention-deficit/hyperactivity disorder (ADHD) delivered in school settings: systematic reviews of quantitative and qualitative research. *Health Technology Assessment* **19**(45), 1.

Rimmington, M. (2023) Square pegs—inclusivity, compassion and fitting in: a guide for schools. Author: Fran Morgan with Ellie Costello. Editor: Ian Gilbert. *International Journal of Positive Behavioural Support* **13**(1), 61–62.

Russell, S.T. *et al.* (2021) Promoting school safety for LGBTQ and all students. *Policy Insights from the Behavioral and Brain Sciences* **8**(2), 160–166.

Sakellari, E. *et al.* (2021) Mental health and wellbeing at schools: health promotion in primary schools with the use of digital methods. *Children* **8**(5), 345.

Salerno, J.P. (2016) Effectiveness of universal school-based mental health awareness programs among youth in the United States: a systematic review. *Journal of School Health* **86**(12), 922–931.

Salmivalli, C. *et al.* (2012) KiVa anti-bullying program: Implications for school adjustment. In: *Peer Relationships and Adjustment at School.* (eds A.M. Ryan & G.W. Ladd). Information Age Publishing, Charlotte, NC. pp. 279–305.

Sareen, J. *et al.* (2013) Gatekeeper training for suicide prevention in First Nations community members: a randomized controlled trial. *Depression and Anxiety* **30**(10), 1021–1029.

Sawyer, S.M. *et al.* (2021) Making every school a health-promoting school. *The Lancet Child & Adolescent Health* **5**(8), 539–540.

Schilling, E.A. *et al.* (2016) The SOS suicide prevention program: further evidence of efficacy and effectiveness. *Prevention Science* **17**, 157–166.

Schlief, M. *et al.* (2023) A rapid realist review of universal interventions to promote inclusivity and acceptance of diverse sexual and gender identities in schools. *Nature Human Behaviour* **7**, 1–12.

Scott, M.A. *et al.* (2009) School-based screening to identify at-risk students not already known to school professionals: the Columbia suicide screen. *American Journal of Public Health* **99**(2), 334–339.

Shannonhouse, L. *et al.* (2017) Suicide intervention training for college staff: program evaluation and intervention skill measurement. *Journal of American College Health* **65**(7), 450–456.

Shinde, S. *et al.* (2020) A multicomponent secondary school health promotion intervention and adolescent health: an extension of the SEHER cluster randomised controlled trial in Bihar, India. *PLoS Medicine* **17**(2), e1003021.

Shucksmith, J. *et al.* (2010) The role of parental involvement in school-based mental health interventions at primary (elementary) school level. *Advances in School Mental Health Promotion* **3**(1), 18–29.

Siceloff, E.R. *et al.* (2017) Universal behavioral/emotional health screening in schools: overview and feasibility. *Report on Emotional & Behavioral Disorders in Youth* **17**(2), 32.

Singer, J.B. *et al.* (2019) School-based suicide prevention: a framework for evidence-based practice. *School Mental Health* **11**, 54–71.

Siu, A.L. & US Preventive Services Task Force (2016) Screening for depression in children and adolescents: US preventive services task force recommendation statement. *Annals of Internal Medicine* **164**(5), 360–366.

Sklad, M. *et al.* (2012) Effectiveness of school-based universal social, emotional, and behavioral programs: do they enhance students' development in the area of skill, behavior, and adjustment? *Psychology in the Schools* **49**(9), 892–909.

Smith, L.H. *et al.* (2022) A scoping review of school-based prevention programs for indigenous students. *Educational Psychology Review* **34**(4), 2783–2824.

Soneson, E. *et al.* (2020) Feasibility of school-based identification of children and adolescents experiencing, or at-risk of developing, mental health difficulties: a systematic review. *Prevention Science* **21**, 581–603.

Stockings, E.A. *et al.* (2016) Preventing depression and anxiety in young people: a review of the joint efficacy of universal, selective and indicated prevention. *Psychological Medicine* **46**(1), 11–26.

Tanner-Smith, E.E. *et al.* (2018) Empirically based mean effect size distributions for universal prevention programs targeting school-aged youth: a review of meta-analyses. *Prevention Science* **19**, 1091–1101.

Thabrew, H. *et al.* (2019) Comparison of YouthCHAT, an electronic composite psychosocial screener, with a clinician interview assessment for young people: randomized trial. *Journal of Medical Internet Research* **21**(12), e13911.

Thabrew, H. *et al.* (2023) O is for awesome: national survey of New Zealand school-based well-being and mental health interventions. *School Mental Health* **15**, 1–17.

Tobin, T. & Sprague, J. (1999) Alternative education programs for at-risk youth: issues, best practice, and recommendations. *Oregon School Study Council Bulletin* **42**(4), n4.

Tobler, N.S. *et al.* (2000) School-based adolescent drug prevention programs: 1998 meta-analysis. *Journal of Primary Prevention* **20**, 275–336.

Torres-Castaño, A. *et al.* (2022) Universal programs to prevent eating disorders in children and adolescents: a scoping review of ethical, legal, organizational and social impacts. *European Eating Disorders Review* **30**(6), 706–722.

Travers, Á. *et al.* (2018) Youth responses to school shootings: a review. *Current Psychiatry Reports* **20**, 1–9.

Van der Kolk, B.A. (2009) Developmental trauma disorder: towards a rational diagnosis for chronically traumatized children. *Praxis der Kinderpsychologie und Kinderpsychiatrie* **58**(8), 572–586.

Viner, R. *et al.* (2021) Impacts of school closures on physical and mental health of children and young people: a systematic review. *MedRxiv* **176**(4), 400–409.

Wald, J. *et al.* (2006) *Literature review of concepts: psychological resiliency.* [Final Report: W7711-057959/A]. University of British Columbia, Vancouver, BC.

Walsh, E.H. *et al.* (2023) A systematic review of school-based suicide prevention interventions for adolescents, and intervention and contextual factors in prevention. *Prevention Science* **24**(2), 365–381.

Wasserman, D. *et al.* (2015) School-based suicide prevention programmes: the SEYLE cluster-randomised, controlled trial. *The Lancet* **385**(9977), 1536–1544.

Weatherson, K.A. *et al.* (2018) The protective effects of school connectedness on substance use and physical activity. *Journal of Adolescent Health* **63**(6), 724–731.

Webster-Stratton, C. *et al.* (2008) Preventing conduct problems and improving school readiness: evaluation of The Incredible Years teacher and child training programs in high-risk schools. *Journal of Child Psychology and Psychiatry* **49**(5), 471–488.

Wei, Y. & Kutcher, S. (2012) International school mental health: global approaches, global challenges, and global opportunities. *Child and Adolescent Psychiatric Clinics* **21**(1), 11–27.

Weist, M.D. *et al.* (2017) School mental health promotion and intervention: experiences from four nations. *School Psychology International* **38**(4), 343–362.

Werner-Seidler, A. *et al.* (2021) School-based depression and anxiety prevention programs: an updated systematic review and meta-analysis. *Clinical Psychology Review* **89**, 102079.

Wichmann, M.L. *et al.* (2023) School-based interventions for child and adolescent victims of interpersonal violence. *Trauma, Violence, & Abuse* **24**(3), 1743–1762.

Wilcox, H.C. *et al.* (2008) The impact of two universal randomized first-and second-grade classroom interventions on young adult suicide ideation and attempts. *Drug and Alcohol Dependence* **95**, S60–S73.

Wilksch, S.M. & Wade, T.D. (2009) Reduction of shape and weight concern in young adolescents: a 30-month controlled evaluation of a media literacy program. *Journal of the American Academy of Child & Adolescent Psychiatry* **48**(6), 652–661.

Williamson, V. *et al.* (2022) School-based screening for childhood anxiety problems and intervention delivery: a codesign approach. *BMJ Open* **12**(6), e058089.

Wilson, S.J. & Lipsey, M.W. (2007) School-based interventions for aggressive and disruptive behavior: update of a meta-analysis. *American Journal of Preventive Medicine* **33**(2), S130–S143.

Worsley, J.D. *et al.* (2022) Supporting mental health and wellbeing of university and college students: a systematic review of review-level evidence of interventions. *PLoS One* **17**(7), e0266725.

Wyman, P.A. *et al.* (2008) Randomized trial of a gatekeeper program for suicide prevention: 1-year impact on secondary school staff. *Journal of Consulting and Clinical Psychology* **76**(1), 104.

Yeager, D.S. & Dweck, C.S. (2012) Mindsets that promote resilience: when students believe that personal characteristics can be developed. *Educational Psychologist* **47**(4), 302–314.

CHAPTER 39

Pharmacological treatments, dietary-based interventions, and neuromodulation therapies

Samuele Cortese[1,2,3,4] and David Coghill[5]

[1] Centre for Innovation in Mental Health, School of Psychology, Faculty of Environmental and Life Sciences, University of Southampton, Southampton, UK
[2] Hampshire and Isle of Wight Healthcare NHS Foundation Trust, Southampton, UK
[3] University of Bari "Aldo Moro", Italy
[4] Department of Child and Adolescent Psychiatry, NYU Grossman School of Medicine, New York, USA
[5] Departments of Paediatrics and Psychiatry, University of Melbourne, Melbourne, Victoria, Australia

Chapter overview

In this chapter, after a brief historical note and an overview of pharmacoepidemiological trends and regulatory issues, we discuss general practical aspects related to medications for child and youth mental health conditions. This is followed by specific sections presenting a summary of the evidence base, alongside specific practical guidance, for key mental health conditions. We conclude with an overview of neuromodulation therapies and dietetic interventions.

Historical notes

The serendipitous discovery by Dr. Charles Bradley in 1937 of the positive effects of benzedrine sulphate, an amphetamine, on symptoms of what we would nowadays label as attention deficit hyperactivity disorder (ADHD) is considered by many as the official start of modern pediatric psychopharmacology (Rapoport, 2013).

Despite this early work, pediatric psychopharmacology was viewed negatively by many clinicians until later in the 20th century. Rigorous randomized controlled trials (RCTs) in the 1990s contributed to an evidence base that then changed clinical practice (Vitiello & Davico, 2018). Some have argued that the acceptance and uptake of pharmacotherapy for children and young people with mental conditions over this time was too fast and somewhat acritical (Rapoport, 2013), leading to inappropriately high rates of prescribing, but, overall, evidence shows both over- and underprescription of medications (Vitiello & Davico, 2018).

Despite the increasing amount of evidence from RCTs, concerns remain around adverse effects, particularly longer-term safety, of these medications in real-world practice. These concerns are beginning to be addressed through increasingly sophisticated epidemiological studies such as the within-subject case control design, where outcomes of interest are assessed in the same individual during periods on and off medication, thus avoiding confounding by indication (e.g., Man *et al.*, 2023).

Alongside medications, dietary interventions have been proposed for some of the mental health conditions in children and young people, with the first studies appearing in the 1970s–1980s (e.g., Goyette *et al.*, 1978), but, since then, the evidence base for the use of dietary interventions has remained limited and controversial.

Likewise, modern neurostimulation approaches such as repetitive transcranial magnetic stimulation (rTMS), transcranial electrical stimulation (tES), transcranial alternating current stimulation (tACS), and transcranial direct current stimulation (tDCS) were first tested in young people in the late 1990s, but their role in mental health conditions in youth deserves further investigation.

Pharmacoepidemiological trends

Overall, international pharmacoepidemiological data describe significant increases in the use of psychotropic medications for children and adolescents since the 2000s. In a study across 65 countries, the total psychotropic medicines sales for children and adults increased from 2008 to 2019, with a relatively average annual increase of around 4% (Brauer *et al.*, 2021b).

When reporting data on changes in medication use over time the focus is usually on relative change. It is, however, important to also consider to what extent the prevalence of prescribing matches the expected rates based on the prevalence of the condition and guideline recommendations. ADHD provides

Rutter's Child and Adolescent Psychiatry and Psychology, Seventh Edition.
Edited by Anita Thapar, Daniel S. Pine, Samuele Cortese, Cathy Creswell, Tamsin J. Ford, James F. Leckman, and Argyris Stringaris.

Companion website: www.wiley.com/go/thapar/ruttерspsych7

a useful case study here. All international guidelines agree that medication should be considered as part of the treatment plan for most children and adolescents receiving a diagnosis of ADHD. ADHD medication consumption has been reported to have increased across 64 countries by nearly 10% per year, from 2015 to 2019, with important differences across geographical locations (Chan *et al.*, 2023). However, the prevalence of medication prescription rate was still lower, across many countries, compared to the estimated prevalence of ADHD (around 5%). Indeed, according to a meta-analysis (Massuti *et al.*, 2021) in the United States(U.S.), for each person using medication without a formal ADHD diagnosis, there would be three patients with a formal diagnosis who might benefit from medication but do not receive it.

General considerations when prescribing medications for child and youth mental health conditions

In child and adolescent mental health (CAMH), psychological therapies are generally acknowledged as the primary course of treatment for many disorders, with medication considered as a second line. However, for certain conditions, such as ADHD, bipolar disorder, and schizophrenia, pharmacological treatment can legitimately be considered as a first-line treatment approach.

Most conditions that benefit from medication primarily affect older children and adolescents (Table 39.1). It is uncommon to prescribe psychotropic medications to preschool-aged children. The response of these very young children to such medications is considerably less predictable and is associated with higher rates of adverse effects compared to older children and adolescents, who themselves are also more susceptible to adverse effects than adults. Additionally, it is worth noting that certain psychotropic medications have demonstrated lasting developmental changes on the immature brain through animal studies, although no one specific medication or class is singled out and the implications for humans remain uncertain. It is therefore strongly recommended that clinicians exercise great caution when considering the use of any medications mentioned in this chapter for children under the age of five.

Developmental considerations for pharmacokinetics

Although the concept of children being distinct from adults has long been recognized, most pediatric dosages are still derived from studies conducted on adults. Childhood and adolescence are clearly associated with significant growth and development, not just of the body but also the brain. This leads to considerable variations in the way the medications used to treat mental health disorders are processed (their pharmacokinetics).

Table 39.1 Summary of the main medications used in child and adolescent mental health (CAMH) disorders.

Class	Main medicines within class used in children/ adolescents	Main indications
Stimulants	Methylphenidate Amphetamines Lisdexamfetamine	Attention deficit/ hyperactivity disorder (ADHD) Binge-eating disorder
Nonstimulant ADHD medications	Atomoxetine Viloxazine (U.S.)	ADHD
Alpha-2 agonists	Guanfacine Clonidine	ADHD Tics and Tourette syndrome Sleep disorders
Serotonin reuptake inhibitors		
Selective (SSRIs)	Citalopram Escitalopram Fluoxetine Fluvoxamine Paroxetine Sertraline	Depression Anxiety Obsessive–compulsive disorder (OCD)
Less selective	Clomipramine	OCD
Other antidepressants	Bupropion Venlafaxine	ADHD Treatment-resistant depression
Atypical antipsychotics	Risperidone Aripiprazole Quetiapine Olanzapine Lurasidone Brexpiprazole	Schizophrenia Mania Tourette's Irritability, aggression (in autism spectrum disorder (ASD) and intellectual disability (ID))
Mood stabilizers	Carbamazepine Valproate Lithium Lamotrigine Gabapentin Topiramate	Mania, bipolar disorder Irritability, mood instability, aggression
Other medicines	Melatonin	Sleep disorders

Absorption

As most cases of prescribing for mental health disorders will commence after infancy, absorption is not generally an issue. By early childhood, absorption profiles for most medications are similar for children, adolescents, and adults. However, ionized medicines, many of which are weak acids, may be less well absorbed from a child's less acidic stomach.

Distribution

The distribution of medicines within the body changes throughout childhood as the balance between fat and water stores varies. Infants and younger children have a higher proportion of extracellular water, while body fat increases as they grow. Depending on whether a medicine is fat or water soluble, these changes in distribution can impact a medicine's half-life, necessitating adjustments up or down in dosing intervals. As rates of obesity rise, it is also important to note that while limited dosing information is available for children with obesity, most pediatric texts recommend to calculate the dose based on the ideal, rather than actual, body weight, with the dose further adjusted based on clinical response. The rationale for this is that using actual weight to calculate the dose puts them at a higher risk of toxicity from medicines which do not distribute into fat. Specific to psychotropic medications, the greater permeability of the blood–brain barrier in children compared to adults may mean a greater than predicted effect.

Metabolism

Young livers are in general more active than those of adults. For example, the cytochrome P450 (CYP) enzymes that are involved in the metabolism of many medicines (e.g., atomoxetine, many selective serotonin reuptake inhibitors (SSRIs), antipsychotics and dexamphetamine) already demonstrate activity during fetal development and undergo considerable changes during the first few months of life. Their levels gradually reach or surpass adult levels by approximately 2 years of age, while most enzymes experience increased activity during the initial months. This means that for many medicines, including those metabolized by the CYP enzymes, there is less bioavailability in children than adults and therefore a need for a higher dose in mg/kg terms during childhood. While it is now possible to conduct genetic testing to identify CYP fast and slow metabolizers, the link between CYP status and clinical effects is not yet well established and most, but not all, authorities do not advise routine testing.

Elimination

Excretion plays a crucial role in the complete elimination of medicines and their metabolites from the body. This process relies on the proper functioning of the kidneys and liver, which develop gradually over time. In contrast to the differences in hepatic function noted above, glomerular filtration rates, which are an indicator of renal function, reach levels comparable to those of adults by approximately 2 years of age.

Recommended dosing for the psychotropic medications in children and adolescents

Currently, there are no general rules that can help determine which people with a specific condition will respond to any medication. Nor are there any accurate ways to predict what the optimal dose will be for any individual. This means that age, sex, height, weight, and severity of the condition *do not* accurately predict the optional dose for any of the mental health conditions treated with medication. For example, there is considerable interpersonal variability in optimal dosing for psychostimulants and weight-based dosing does not help predict the optimal dose.

Table 39.2 Suggested starting doses for commonly used psychotropic medications[a] in children and adolescents.

Medicine	Starting dose	Comment
Fluoxetine	10 mg	Adjust dose according to response and adverse effects
Citalopram	10 mg	
Escitalopram	5 mg	
Sertraline	25–50 mg	
Risperidone	0.25–0.5 mg	
Olanzapine	2.5–5 mg	Consider using plasma levels to determine maintenance dose
Aripiprazole	2 mg	
Clozapine	6.25–12.5 mg	Use plasma levels to determine maintenance dose
Lithium	100–200 mg/day lithium carbonate Note: Preparations vary widely in bioavailability so changing the preparation requires the same precautions as initiation of treatment	Dose adjusted according to serum-lithium concentration. Doses are initially divided throughout the day, but once serum-lithium concentration is stabilized, daily administration is preferred

[a] Attention deficit hyperactivity disorder (ADHD) medications have not been included to avoid overgeneralization due to the many different preparations available.

Titration according to clinical response is therefore generally preferable to weight-based dosing for most medications and suggested doses mostly indicate a general range rather than a specific mg/kg calculation. Table 39.2 gives an indication of usual starting doses for some commonly prescribed medications.

Potential medicine–medicine and medicine–condition interactions

Despite a lack of evidence to support it, there has been an increasing trend in some regions to prescribe multiple psychotropic medications together. While this is not inherently wrong—it is, for example, often easier to vary pharmacological actions independently when each action is targeted by a separate medicine—polypharmacy does come with some increased risk of adverse effects. Perhaps most prominent, and least well recognized by most prescribers, is the risk of medicine–medicine interactions. These can make one or both medicines less effective, cause unexpected side effects, or increase the action of a particular medicine. Examples of potentially problematic medicine–medicine interactions include several second-generation antipsychotics (including olanzapine, risperidone, quetiapine, and clozapine) and fluoxetine, paroxetine, and fluvoxamine, and also benzodiazepines and fluvoxamine as well as grapefruit juice. Importantly, there are no recorded interactions between the SSRIs and the stimulants.

Medicine–condition interactions occur when an existing medical condition makes the use of certain medicines potentially harmful, for example, if someone with preexisting high blood pressure is prescribed a psychostimulant for ADHD. There are two general rules that clinicians should follow to reduce the risks for their patients. First, it is wise to develop a deep familiarity with at least one medicine, but more helpfully two, of each main class. This would include not only information about dosing, duration of action, and time to response but also knowledge of likely medicine–medicine and medicine–condition interactions. Second, become familiar with one of the manuals or websites that list interactions (e.g., Drugs.com, 2024, https://www.drugs.com/drug_interactions.html).

General aspects of good prescribing practice

Prescribers should always ensure that the decision to prescribe is well-founded, the target symptoms are clearly defined and appropriate, the most suitable medication is selected and offered at the correct dosage, the measurable outcomes can be monitored, and the patient, along with their family if applicable, is fully informed about the potential risks and benefits of the treatment options and agrees with the treatment plan. Although it may be tempting to bypass these preparatory steps, neglecting to adhere to them is likely to have detrimental effects on treatment outcomes.

The four important stages of prescribing highlighted by Coombes et al. (2011) are detailed in the following subsections.

Information gathering

This phase requires the skills and opportunity to gather pertinent patient information. Modern approaches to child mental health treatment are beginning to emphasize the benefits of measurement-based care (MBC). MBC involves the systematic administration of symptom rating scales and use of the results to drive clinical decision-making at the level of the individual patient. For MBC to be effective it is necessary to gather baseline ratings, not only of core symptoms but also potential adverse effects (e.g., sleep difficulties, appetite).

Clinical decision-making and treatment planning

This requires the clinician to integrate their pharmacological knowledge in conjunction with the diagnosis, clinical presentation, demographic information, and developmental factors to determine the most suitable medication and appropriate dosing protocol for each individual patient. During this process, it is crucial to also consider non-pharmacological treatments and provide sufficient information to the patient and their family, enabling them to participate in collaborative decision-making. This collaborative approach has the potential to significantly enhance adherence to treatment and improve patient outcomes. Additionally, the prescriber should consistently value and consider the perspectives and preferences of the patient and their caregivers throughout the decision-making process.

Another key aspect of treatment planning is to carefully choose the treatment targets. Traditionally, medication treatments focus on symptoms rather than disorders. However, it is increasingly acknowledged that it may be more helpful to also think about the effects of treatment on quality of life, functioning, and cognition (e.g., Adamo *et al.*, 2015). Once the targets are chosen, they should be measured using appropriate instruments and integrated into the MBC approach.

Communication

Prior to initiating treatment, it is essential to consider and obtain clear consent. The specific rules for consent will differ across countries but it is essential to recognize that children may not have the capacity to make decisions regarding medication, and in such cases, their parents or legal guardians make decisions on their behalf. However, even if children's views are a secondary consideration, their assent should still be sought and their opinions respected. The amount of information provided should be tailored to the individual, particularly with children at the cusp of maturity, who should be included in the decision-making. The minimum information necessary for consent is summarized in Box 39.1. A particularly important situation is where parents are separated but retain legal rights to oversee the child. Again, rules differ between countries. It is, however, good practice to obtain consent from both parents in this situation.

The agreed management plan should be clearly outlined and include specific triggers for review in the event of any serious or unexpected adverse events. Furthermore, the prescriber should discuss monitoring requirements, potential adverse effects, and contingency plans with the patient. One key issue to bear in mind is that we need to be realistic about the treatment aims and likely outcomes. This ensures that we keep expectations grounded and do not overpromise. It is helpful to be open and honest about what we do not know as well as what we do. This can be challenging at times but is ultimately in the best interest of patients and their families.

Many factors contribute to problems with adherence to treatment (Sebate, 2003) (Table 39.3). Addressing potential barriers to treatment adherence is a key part of this early communication. It is not uncommon for young people, and even adults, to feel ambivalent about taking medication regularly. However, for many children and adolescents, the idea of taking medication may be perceived as an unwelcome imposition, or stigmatizing, particularly if the decision to start has been made solely based

Box 39.1 Information required for consent

- The condition to be treated
- The nature of proposed treatment
- The nature and probability of material risks of the medication
- Expected benefits
- The prescriber's inability to predict results
- Irreversibility (if applicable)
- Likely results of no treatment
- Likely risks/benefits of alternatives

(Based on the findings of the case of *Hamish v Children's Medical Center 1982*.)

Table 39.3 Dimensions of adherence—example of attention deficit hyperactivity disorder (ADHD).

Dimension	Factors related to poorer adherence
Health system/health care team factors	Poor training Poor organization Overworked Lack of focus Lack of structure Ambivalence toward treatment Cost
Condition-related factors	Memory problems Poor organization Less baseline symptoms (probably related to lower initial response) Conduct problems/oppositional defiant disorder (ODD) (although presence of other comorbidities may increase adherence)
Patient-related factors	Increased age Strained family relationships Caucasian boys > African-American boys and girls and Caucasian girls Belief that ADHD is biological disorder leads to increased adherence Perceived stigma
Therapy-related factors	Stimulants better than nonstimulants Experience of adverse effects Preexisting beliefs about medications Single daily dose better than multiple doses Embarrassment of taking pills in front of others
Socioeconomic status-related factors	Not well studied in ADHD with contradictory findings

Source: Adapted from Chacko *et al.* (2010) and Sebate (2003).

on discussions with parents. Improved adherence over the long term can be facilitated by the clinician engaging in individual discussions with the child or young person at the beginning of treatment. These discussions should focus on the principles of psychoeducation, explaining why the medication is being prescribed, discussing potential benefits, informing about expected adverse effects, providing a timeline for when positive effects may be observed, and outlining the anticipated duration of treatment. It is important to note that people tend to remember only a small portion of what is said during clinical discussions. Therefore, the use of developmentally appropriate handouts that describe the prescribed medication can be very helpful, likely more than the data sheets supplied by the manufacturers.

It is not uncommon for children to face difficulties in swallowing tablets and capsules, and liquid preparations may not always be available. In such cases, it may be necessary to teach the child how to swallow a tablet, for example, using a graded series of small cake decorations and sweets, gradually progressing to the actual medication. It is crucial to ensure that swallowing a solid item is always followed by a drink to aid swallowing.

Furthermore, it is vital to emphasize the importance of keeping medications safe and secure. This is particularly critical for controlled medicines, such as stimulants, which require extra precautions to prevent misuse or accidental ingestion.

Initiating medication, monitoring, and review

Titrating medication

The well-known principle of "start low go slow" emphasizes the importance of starting medication treatment at a low dosage and gradually increasing it to achieve optimal response while minimizing adverse effects. However, it is crucial to strike a balance between starting too low or going too slow and achieving an adequate dosage, as excessively cautious approaches can increase the risk of undertreatment and result in patients discontinuing treatment due to a perceived lack of response. The process of titration, or dosage adjustment, becomes a balancing act aimed at finding the optimal therapeutic response with the fewest adverse effects.

Off-label use

Off-label prescription is currently the norm rather than the exception in the pharmacological management of mental health conditions in children and young people. Off-label prescribing refers to medication use outside marketing authorization in relation to one or more of the following: (i) the type of disorder being treated, (ii) the age of the patient, (iii) the dosage being prescribed as well as the route of administration, and (iv) the duration of treatment (Sharma *et al.*, 2016). Prescribing a medication which is contraindicated would also constitute off-label use, although this is clearly inappropriate prescribing and conceptually different from the other four conditions, all of which can be appropriate. "Unlicensed prescribing" refers to prescribing of a medicine or formulation of medicines that has not yet received marketing authorization for any indication or prescribing a medicine when marketing authorization has been withdrawn.

Prescribing within the licensed framework does not always guarantee the safety or effectiveness of the compound. For instance, haloperidol, which is licensed for tics/Tourette syndrome, is neither safer nor more effective than alternative nonlicensed options. Therefore, the prescriber should always ensure that they are aware of the most up-to-date evidence base for all medications they use, regardless of whether they have marketing authorization.

Measurement-based care (MBC)

There is now clear evidence demonstrating that satisfaction with care and clinical outcomes can be improved through the recurrent assessment of clearly measurable outcomes, particularly when these are seen as desirable by patients, families, and providers. This should come as no surprise as it is well recognized within somatic medicine. Currently, within mental health the main evidence relates to the routine use of valid and reliable symptom rating scales. However, despite the availability of a wide range of such scales, only a minority of mental health clinicians routinely administer these to their patients. This is necessary as, based on clinical judgment alone, mental health providers detect deterioration for only around 20% of their patients who experience increased symptom severity, and rates are even worse for patients whose symptoms are not only deteriorating but are also not improving as expected (Hatfield *et al.*, 2010). These failures contribute significantly to clinical inertia—not changing a treatment plan despite a lack of improvement. The use of MBC provides an important opportunity for clinicians to self-reflect on what is and is not working and hone their clinical skills over time. To be clinically effective the symptom severity feedback must be clinically actionable and perceived by providers to have a direct benefit to patients, and the instruments used to measure symptom severity must be both reliable (consistent across repeated measurements when there is no actual change in severity) and sensitive to change (able to detect clinically meaningful changes in actual severity). The rating scale data must also be current, interpretable, and readily available during the clinical encounter. Changes in symptom severity should be classified into clinically meaningful categories (response, remission, nonresponse, relapse, and recurrence) and the clinician must be able to compare current symptom severity to past symptom severity. Coghill and Seth (2015) demonstrated the potential benefits of MBC within a busy publicly funded ADHD clinic setting (Coghill & Seth, 2015) and provide a detailed account of how MBC can be applied in routine clinical care. Ongoing work is looking to extend this model to other conditions and settings and to broaden the outcomes beyond improving symptoms to embrace broad functional outcomes and quality of life.

Identifying and managing adverse effects

The utilization of structured approaches for measuring adverse effects is still limited both in clinical trials and routine clinical practice. This is a significant concern, particularly as medications are being used more frequently and for longer durations.

The use of antipsychotics in the management of nonpsychotic disorders, such as aggressive behaviors associated with autism, intellectual disability (ID), ADHD, and conduct disorder (CD), exemplifies the need. Initially, these interventions are often intended to be brief, but the absence of a planned exit strategy frequently leads to prolonged treatment. While newer medications have fewer extrapyramidal side effects compared to older typical antipsychotics, like haloperidol, there is a higher prevalence of obesity, diabetes mellitus, and metabolic and cardiovascular side effects in younger patients than in adults (Fraguas *et al.*, 2011). Developmental factors can further amplify the impact of certain adverse events. For instance, hypogonadism resulting from elevated prolactin levels may have more severe long-term consequences for younger individuals who have not yet reached peak bone density (Haddad & Wieck, 2004). Notably, while there is clear guidance about the need to closely monitor for these serious adverse effects, few clinics have a clear protocol for doing so.

Both clinicians and researchers need to make greater efforts in routinely measuring baseline and follow-up data.

Understanding the evidence base

Medications for specific conditions

In this section we first describe the current evidence for efficacy/effectiveness, based on one umbrella review (UR; i.e., a quantitative synthesis of available meta-analyses) encompassing pharmacological and nonpharmacological interventions in youth, including a total of 187 pairwise meta-analyses and 14 network meta-analyses (Correll *et al.*, 2021), and on another UR focusing on tolerability (9 network meta-analyses, 39 meta-analyses, 90 individual RCTs, and 8 cohort studies) (Solmi *et al.*, 2020). A more in-depth discussion of the treatment of each disorder is reported in the related specific chapters.

Attention deficit hyperactivity disorder (ADHD)

Evidence review

In the UR by Correll *et al.* (2021), compared to placebo, amphetamines had the largest effect size (ES), in terms of efficacy, based on the clinician-rated primary efficacy outcome (large ES), and led to significantly lower discontinuation rates due to inefficacy (large ES).

Methylphenidate had a medium-to-large ES regarding the primary efficacy outcome versus placebo across different raters and was superior to placebo in terms of cognitive outcomes (small-to-medium ES), overall symptoms improvement (large ES), quality of life (medium ES), and acceptability (small ES), and showed significantly lower discontinuation due to inefficacy (medium ES), without significant differences concerning discontinuation due to intolerability.

Clonidine, guanfacine, and atomoxetine were also efficacious compared to placebo, regarding the primary efficacy outcome, but with less consistent results across raters. Guanfacine and clonidine were an effective augmentation strategy when added to stimulants versus placebo (small ES).

In head-to-head comparisons, amphetamines were better than methylphenidate, which outperformed bupropion and atomoxetine on the primary efficacy outcome. Amphetamines were superior to methylphenidate for aggressive behavior and had lower rates of discontinuation due to inefficacy compared to atomoxetine. Methylphenidate was superior to atomoxetine regarding acceptability (i.e., dropout due to any cause), and to guanfacine in terms of less discontinuation due to intolerability.

Regarding tolerability/safety, in the UR by Solmi *et al.* (2020), when compared to placebo: worse appetite reduction was seen for atomoxetine, d-amphetamine, lisdexamfetamine, methylphenidate, and modafinil; insomnia with d-amphetamine, lisdexamfetamine, methylphenidate, and modafinil; weight loss with atomoxetine, methylphenidate, and modafinil; abdominal pain with methylphenidate and guanfacine; hypertension with atomoxetine and lisdexamfetamine; sedation with clonidine and guanfacine; and QT prolongation with guanfacine.

Practical prescribing

Guidelines are consistent in recommending that stimulants are usually the first-choice medications with nonstimulants reserved for those with contraindications to stimulants, who have either not responded to an adequate trial of both stimulant classes (methylphenidate and amphetamines) or not tolerated stimulants. As we cannot predict who will respond to which stimulant, choices are often based on practical issues such as cost and availability.

Probably more important than which stimulant one starts with is how they are titrated and monitored. Adopting the approach to titration and monitoring used in the influential Multimodal Treatment Study of Children with ADHD, Coghill and Seth demonstrated that MBC led to significant improvements in outcomes within a publicly funded clinical service in the UK (Coghill & Seth, 2015). This highlights the substantial benefits that can be attained through the implementation of these approaches, not only in ADHD but also in the broader context of CAMH (Liu *et al.*, 2019).

In parallel to optimizing clinical outcomes, it is important to adopt a structured approach when assessing adverse events associated with ADHD medications. The European ADHD Guidelines Group (EAGG) has provided comprehensive guidance in this regard (Cortese *et al.*, 2013). While long-term effects on growth are important, identifying potential cardiac risk factors and managing ongoing cardiovascular adverse effects are of paramount significance. The EAGG recommends routine inquiry into personal history of cardiac disease, history of sudden death in a close relative before the age of 40 years, symptoms suggestive of cardiac disease (such as effort intolerance, frequent palpitations, and frequent syncope, particularly when exercise-induced), and other medications that may pose cardiac risks. Positive findings should prompt consideration of a 24-hour tape or 12-lead electrocardiogram (ECG) if the former is not available. Although the average increases in pulse and blood pressure with ADHD medications are modest, a subset of individuals may experience clinically significant elevations (Cortese *et al.*, 2013) and a heart rate consistently above 120 beats per minute or blood pressure above the 95th centile should be considered abnormal and warrant follow-up.

Depression

Evidence review

In the UR of Correll *et al.* (2021), fluoxetine was the only medication that was superior to placebo on the primary efficacy outcome (medium ES), as well as on response and remission (both with small ES). Venlafaxine increased suicidality (large ES). Solmi *et al.* (2020) found that, compared to placebo, nausea/vomiting was significantly worse with duloxetine, nefazodone, paroxetine, sertraline, and vilazodone; extrapyramidal side effects were associated with clomipramine, imipramine, and paroxetine; sedation with imipramine and nefazodone; diarrhea with duloxetine and sertraline; headache with nefazodone and venlafaxine; anorexia with amitriptyline and venlafaxine; weight gain with escitalopram and sertraline; weight loss with fluoxetine; and suicidality with venlafaxine.

Practical prescribing

Only two antidepressants are approved for the treatment of depression in children and adolescents: fluoxetine, which is approved in several countries, and escitalopram (Cymbalta), approved in the U.S. Guidelines on the treatment of depression vary in their advice about when it is appropriate to consider medication for depression in children and adolescents. In the UK, the National Institute of Health and Care Excellence (NICE) guidelines recommend that antidepressant medications should not be used as the initial independent treatment for depression in children and adolescents. Instead, specific psychological therapies such as cognitive behavioral therapy (CBT) or interpersonal psychotherapy (IPT) are recommended for all patients with moderate to severe depression. However, NICE recommend that a combination of medication treatment with psychological therapy may be considered as an initial treatment for moderate to severe depression in young people aged 12–18 years. The American Academy of Child and Adolescent Psychiatry (AACAP) recommends that children/adolescents with moderate to severe major depression or persistent depression should be treated with CBT, IPT, *and/or* an SSRI.

Support for the use of medication alongside CBT comes from two large publicly funded studies, the Treatment of Adolescents with Depression Study (TADS) (March *et al.*, 2004) in the U.S. and the Adolescent Depression Antidepressants and Psychotherapy Trial (ADAPT) (Goodyer *et al.*, 2008) in the UK. TADS found that both combination treatment and fluoxetine alone were more effective than placebo, with the combination being the most effective. In ADAPT, both the SSRI and SSRI + CBT groups showed improvement, with no significant difference between the two groups (see Chapter 63 for more details).

For those individuals who do not respond to an initial trial of an adequately dosed SSRI treatment, evidence from the Treatment of Resistant Depression in Adolescents (TORDIA) trial (Brent *et al.*, 2008) provides helpful information for clinical decision-making (see Chapter 63). The combination of CBT with a switch to another antidepressant showed a higher rate of clinical response compared to a medication switch alone. Simple switching to another SSRI was as effective as switching to venlafaxine and had fewer adverse effects. Several studies have highlighted the risks of increased suicidal ideation in children and adolescents treated with venlafaxine and paroxetine, and these medications should therefore be avoided in this population. Also, there is strong evidence to indicate that tricyclic antidepressants are ineffective in the treatment of depression in children and adolescents and in view of their poor safety profile they should also be avoided.

Psychotic depression is rare in this age group but, where it does occur, augmentation of antidepressant treatment with second-generation antipsychotic (under specialist supervision) should be considered for children, although the optimum dose and duration of treatment are unknown.

Anxiety disorders

Evidence review

Correll *et al.* (2021) found evidence that three SSRIs (fluoxetine, fluvoxamine, paroxetine) outperformed placebo on the primary efficacy outcome and response (small-to-medium ESs). Fluoxetine was also significantly better than placebo with respect to remission (small ES). Of note, duloxetine carries a Food and Drug Administration (FDA) indication for generalized anxiety disorder.

Practical prescribing

While cognitive and behavioral interventions have high success rates, a significant proportion of individuals still require additional intervention. The UK NICE guidelines (NICE, 2013) do not recommend medication for managing anxiety in children and adolescents, whereas the AACAP practice parameters (Connolly *et al.*, 2007) suggest considering SSRIs for moderate to severe cases and nonresponders to psychological therapies.

While SSRIs are considered the first-choice pharmacological treatment for child and adolescent anxiety disorders, there are no specific recommendations within the clinical guidelines on which medications to use or in which order. Based on the above evidence, fluoxetine and fluvoxamine would generally be recommended over paroxetine in view of the evidence that paroxetine in depression may be associated with an increased signal for suicidality. Of note, escitalopram received approval recently in the U.S. for generalized anxiety disorder (GAD) among children and adolescents. Citalopram, despite a lack of formal evidence, is an alternative. Response rates are reasonable, with data from a Cochrane review reporting pooled treatment response rates of 64% for SSRIs versus 34% for placebo, a number needed to treat (NNT) of 3 and a pooled ES of 0.82 (Ipser *et al.*, 2009). Clinicians should allow at least 3 weeks at an adequate dose before assessing treatment response. In cases of nonresponse, switching to an alternative SSRI is appropriate before considering medications from different classes. Tricyclic antidepressants are not recommended as first-line treatments for pediatric anxiety disorders. Benzodiazepines should only be considered when other pharmacological approaches have failed, and their use should be limited to weeks rather than months. Limited open-label evidence suggests that buspirone, a nonbenzodiazepine anxiolytic, may have similar efficacy to benzodiazepines with fewer adverse events, but controlled data on safety and efficacy are lacking.

Most studies on medication treatments for pediatric anxiety disorders have been short-term trials, lasting up to 16 weeks. The Child/Adolescent Anxiety Multimodal Study investigated the long-term efficacy and persistence of treatment effects over 36 weeks (Walkup *et al.*, 2008). The study included CBT, sertraline, combined therapy (CBT + sertraline), and placebo. Combined therapy showed the highest improvement rate (80.7%), followed by CBT alone (59.7%), and sertraline alone (54.9%). Adverse event rates did not differ significantly between the sertraline and placebo groups. This study emphasizes the importance of a multimodal approach to the management of anxiety in this population. However, a recent trial of the efficacy of CBT for children and young people with anxiety disorders showed that efficacy is not significantly enhanced by combination with a short-term course of antidepressants (Hudson *et al.*, 2023) (for more details on the treatment of anxiety disorders, see Chapter 59).

Obsessive–compulsive disorder (OCD)

Evidence review

In Correll *et al.* (2021), fluoxetine was the psychotropic medication with the broadest efficacy, including primary efficacy outcome, response, and global illness severity, versus placebo (small ES). SSRIs as a class also improved response, remission, and global illness severity, but they were associated with a higher discontinuation rate due to intolerability than placebo. As an augmentation strategy, risperidone had a large ES in individuals with SSRI-refractory OCD versus placebo. Regarding combination treatment, CBT and sertraline were significantly better than placebo (medium ES).

Practical prescribing

In addition to the evidence on CBT, there is strong evidence to support the use of medication for early-onset OCD. Only one study, the Pediatric OCD Treatment Study (POTS) (2004), has directly compared the efficacy of CBT versus SSRI medication in pediatric OCD. POTS found that CBT and sertraline resulted in comparable levels of symptom reduction, but combining CBT and SSRI treatment led to superior outcomes. Subsequent research confirmed that the combination of CBT and medication is more effective than medication alone, but only if a full course of CBT is completed.

Clinical trial data suggest that fluoxetine, sertraline, paroxetine, fluvoxamine, and citalopram are associated with a 29–44% reduction in symptoms and are generally well tolerated and safe. There is limited evidence comparing the efficacy of different SSRIs, and no specific SSRI has been found to be significantly more effective than the others. While clomipramine has also been demonstrated to be effective in pediatric OCD its use is limited due to safety concerns.

SSRIs have been shown to be well tolerated and effective in maintaining improvement over time, with continued symptom reduction for up to 1 year (Cook *et al.*, 2001). However, continuing treatment beyond this period does not appear to yield further improvements. The optimal duration of treatment is unknown, but it is generally recommended to consider stopping medication after 1–1.5 years and restarting if significant symptoms return.

If there is no response to the initial SSRI, it is recommended to trial a second SSRI along with CBT augmentation. Augmentation strategies using antipsychotics, which have shown efficacy in adults with partial response to treatment, have some support, and can be considered in refractory cases of OCD with tics. More details on the treatment of OCD are reported in Chapter 60.

Schizophrenia

Evidence review

Correll *et al.* (2021) found that all investigated antipsychotics, other than ziprasidone, outperformed placebo with a small ES, except for olanzapine and risperidone, which had a large ES. Small ESs were found regarding response (except for asenapine), and all antipsychotics improved overall symptoms severity. Acceptability was superior versus placebo for paliperidone, risperidone, and olanzapine, without differences for the other antipsychotics. Paliperidone and olanzapine were associated with more discontinuation due to intolerability than placebo, while discontinuation due to inefficacy was least evident in paliperidone, olanzapine, risperidone, and ziprasidone. In head-to-head comparisons, risperidone and second-generation antipsychotics outperformed first-generation antipsychotics (large ES), and clozapine was better than olanzapine on the primary efficacy outcome (large ES).

Solmi *et al.* (2020) found that: sedation was associated with the majority of antipsychotics; extrapyramidal side effects with amisulpride, aripiprazole, haloperidol, loxapine, molindone, olanzapine, paliperidone, risperidone, and ziprasidone; weight gain with aripiprazole, asenapine, clozapine, olanzapine, paliperidone, quetiapine, and risperidone; hyperprolactinemia with haloperidol, olanzapine, paliperidone, quetiapine, and risperidone; increased cholesterol with aripiprazole, olanzapine, and quetiapine; and glucose increase/diabetes with asenapine, olanzapine, and risperidone.

Practical prescribing

Based on the evidence detailed in the previous section, the profile of adverse effects plays a significant role in clinical decision-making (Table 39.4). The recent regulatory requirements of the FDA and the European Medicines Agency (EMA) have, however, led to an increasing number of studies for newer antipsychotics with improved adverse effect profiles. Lurasidone, for example, has undergone this process and is now licensed in several countries for the treatment of adolescent schizophrenia.

Regarding the monitoring of adverse effects when using antipsychotic medications in children and adolescents, sensible advice is to adhere to the recommendations provided by the NICE schizophrenia guidelines. Baseline assessments and investigations should be conducted and properly recorded as set out in Box 39.2. Efficacy, along with safety assessments similar to the baseline investigations, should be systematically repeated throughout treatment according to the following schedule: weekly weight measurement for the first 6 weeks, followed by weight measurement at 12 weeks and then every 6 months (plotted on a growth chart); height measurement every 6 months (plotted on a growth chart); waist and hip circumference measurement every 6 months (plotted on a percentile chart); pulse and blood pressure measurement at 12 weeks and then every 6 months (plotted on a percentile chart); and fasting blood glucose, glycosylated hemoglobin (HbA1c), blood lipid, and prolactin level measurement at 12 weeks and then every 6 months. These assessments should be conducted periodically throughout treatment, and any abnormal or negative changes should be addressed promptly.

It is customary to ensure that patients have undergone a sufficient trial period of 6 weeks with an appropriate dosage. If there is no response during this period, it is recommended to try a different antipsychotic medication. In cases of treatment-resistant schizophrenia, clozapine is widely recognized as the most effective medication for adults. While there is limited evidence regarding the use of clozapine in children and adolescents, some studies suggest that it may be more effective than haloperidol and olanzapine in treating both positive and negative symptoms (Kumra *et al.*, 2008). However, serious adverse effects, such as neutropenia and seizures, are not uncommon and necessitate close monitoring and regular blood testing. Clozapine should be reserved for patients who have not responded to at least two adequate trials of other antipsychotic agents, including at least one atypical agent, or who have experienced significant medicine-induced side effects (e.g., tardive dyskinesia).

Bipolar disorder

Evidence review

In Correll *et al.* (2021), quetiapine was not superior to placebo regarding the primary efficacy outcome, separating only on global illness severity (small ES). Concerning mania, aripiprazole was more effective than placebo regarding the primary efficacy outcome (large ES) and response (small ES), and without differences versus placebo regarding acceptability, while being superior regarding less discontinuations for inefficacy. Although not included in the UR, RCT data also support olanzapine, quetiapine, risperidone, and ziprasidone. In contrast to adults, divalproex (sodium valproate) does not appear to be effective and was not significant in meta-analysis, and topiramate and oxcarbazepine (a carbamazepine derivative) have only modestly positive effects. While there is some evidence suggesting that lithium is effective in treating bipolar disorder type 1 (BP I) in children and adolescents, the quality of the evidence is low and findings are mixed.

Solmi *et al.* (2020) reported, compared to placebo, that two mood stabilizers were associated with significantly worse sedation (oxcarbazepine, valproate), and weight gain/increased body mass index (oxcarbazepine, valproate), and one each with weight loss or anorexia (topiramate), thrombocytopenia and leukocytopenia (valproate), and nausea/vomiting (oxcarbazepine).

Practical prescribing

Given the complexity and variability of treatment practice across countries, the reader is invited to consult Chapter 62.

Table 39.4 Adverse effect profiles of second-generation antipsychotics in children and adolescents.

Adverse Effect	Time of onset	Aripiprazole	Clozapine	Lurasidone	Olanzapine	Quetiapine	Risperidone	Ziprasidone
Anticholinergic	Early	–	+++	–	++	–/+	–	–
Acute parkinsonism	Early	+	–	++	+	–	++	+
Akathisia	Early/intermediate	++	+	++	+	+	+	+
Tardive dyskinesia	Late	–/+	–	–/+	–/+	–/+	–/+	–/+
Withdrawal dyskinesia	During switch	++	–	–/+	–/+	–/+	+	+
Diabetes	Late	–/+	+++	–	+++	++	+	–/+
Increased lipids	Early/intermediate	–/+	++	–/+	++	+	+	–/+
Weight gain	Intermediate	+	+++	–	+++	++	++	+
Increased prolactin/ sexual dysfunction	Early	–	–	–	++	–	+++	+
Decreased prolactin	Early	++	–	–	–	–	–	–
Sedation	Early	–/+	+++	++	++	++	+	–/+
Increased QTc	Throughout	–/+	+	–/+	–/+	+	+	++
Postural hypotension	Early	+/–	+++	–/+	++	++	+	–
Neutropenia	Early/intermediate	–/+	++	–/+	–/+	–/+	–/+	–/+

– = not present, –/+ = minimal, + = mild, ++ = moderate, +++ = severe.

Box 39.2 Investigations prior to initiation of an antipsychotic medication and during treatment

- Measurement of weight and height, plotted on a growth chart
- Waist and hip measurement
- Pulse and blood pressure assessment
- Fasting blood glucose or glycosylated hemoglobin (HbA1c) measurement
- Blood lipid and prolactin level assessment
- Evaluation of any movement disorders
- Assessment of nutritional status, diet, and physical activity level

Tics/Tourette syndrome

Evidence review

In Correll *et al.* (2021), antipsychotics (including haloperidol, pimozide, risperidone, and ziprasidone) and guanfacine were superior to placebo regarding the primary efficacy outcome (both moderate ES). No significant difference versus placebo emerged for methylphenidate. A more recent network meta-analysis (Farhat *et al.*, 2023) concluded that antipsychotics are the most efficacious intervention for Tourette syndrome (moderate ES), and that alpha-2 agonists are less efficacious but did outperform placebo (low ES).

Practical prescribing

The waxing and waning patterns of tics pose significant challenges in assessing the effects of treatment interventions, emphasizing the need for meticulous documentation of baseline symptoms and ongoing monitoring before and during medication therapy.

Clearly not everyone with tics requires, or wishes, medication. The European Society for the Study of Tourette Syndrome (ESSTS) guidelines [52] suggest that medication should be considered when tics cause:

- subjective discomfort (e.g., pain or injury)
- sustained social or emotional problems for the patient (e.g., social isolation or bullying)
- functional interference (e.g., impairment of academic achievements).

Based on the evidence of the 2023 network meta-analysis, antipsychotics are supported as a first-line medication treatment for tics/Tourette syndrome. Evidence was provided for aripiprazole, haloperidol, olanzapine, pimozide, and risperidone. The first- and second-generation antipsychotics did not separate in efficacy and we would recommend that medication choice is based on adverse effect profile (Table 39.4).

The alpha-2 agonists, clonidine and guanfacine, could be considered for those who choose not to take an antipsychotic. While evidence supporting their use is less robust, they are associated with fewer long-term adverse effects and may also help to manage coexisting ADHD symptoms.

Disruptive behavior/dissocial/conduct disorders

Evidence review

In Correll *et al.* (2021), risperidone outperformed placebo across different raters regarding the primary efficacy outcome (medium ES), aggressive behavior (medium ES, also in youth with ID), and overall symptom severity (medium ES).

Practical prescribing

This is another area where there is considerable variation in practice. In the UK, NICE makes a clear recommendation that psychological treatments are primary and that pharmacological interventions should not be offered for the routine management of behavioral problems in children and young people with oppositional defiant disorder (ODD) or CD. However, risperidone can be considered for the short-term management of severely aggressive behavior in young people with a CD who have problems with explosive anger and severe emotional dysregulation and who have not responded to psychosocial interventions. We are aware, however, that many clinicians use risperidone and other atypical antipsychotics to manage aggressive behaviors and report positive results. In our view, NICE guidance is sensible and appropriate. The key to appropriate use of medication in these circumstances is that use should be short term, at as low a dose as possible, and with a clear exit strategy.

Safety is a key concern and, as suggested by NICE, we recommend that clinicians clearly inform young people and their parents or caregivers about the potential risks associated with antipsychotics, including metabolic effects such as weight gain and diabetes, extrapyramidal effects like akathisia, dyskinesia, and dystonia, cardiovascular effects involving QT interval prolongation, hormonal effects including increased plasma prolactin levels, and other potential experiences that may be unpleasant. As for all other situations where antipsychotics are used the prescriber should conduct and clearly document the baseline investigations highlighted in Box 39.2. These indicators should be reassessed regularly during treatment. Treatment should be evaluated after 3–4 weeks and discontinued if there is no clinically significant response observed by 6 weeks.

Autism

Evidence review

In Correll *et al.* (2021), aripiprazole was better than placebo in relation to the following outcomes: aggressive behavior, overall noncore symptom severity, and acceptability (all with small ES). Risperidone presented with a similar profile, except for a large ES regarding response. Both aripiprazole and risperidone were not significantly different from placebo concerning discontinuation due to intolerability.

Practical prescribing

There is currently no recognized medication treatment for core autism symptoms. There are, however, several interventions targeting associated troublesome behaviors and comorbid conditions such as self-injury, aggression, tantrums, stereotypies, hyperactivity, impulsivity, and agitation. While evidence for the efficacy and safety of many of these approaches remains limited, it is important for clinicians to be familiar with the existing research to inform their clinical practice.

Irritability and aggression are among the most impairing symptoms in individuals with autism spectrum disorder (ASD) and have been extensively studied in the context of pharmacological interventions. Antipsychotics, mood stabilizers, antidepressants (clomipramine), and other agents (clonidine, amantadine, naltrexone, pentoxifylline) have been investigated for reducing irritability in ASD. Notably, the FDA has approved risperidone (since 2006) and aripiprazole (since 2009) specifically for the treatment of irritability associated with ASD. Risperidone is indicated for children over 5 years of age and a body weight of ≥9.1 kg, while aripiprazole is approved for children older than 6 years. The ES for risperidone is around 1.2 (at doses between 0.5–3.5 mg/day), and for aripiprazole, it is 0.6–0.9 (at doses of 5, 10, 15 mg/day). Adverse effects, such as extrapyramidal side effects, weight gain, dizziness, and somnolence, are commonly associated with these medications. The positive effects on irritability and aggression do not appear to be solely attributable to somnolence.

The management of ADHD symptoms in individuals with ASD is not extensively studied. Limited evidence suggests that treatment should follow similar approaches used for routine cases of ADHD. However, ESs are somewhat lower compared to children and adolescents with ADHD but without ASD, particularly for stimulant medications. Adverse effects are also more likely in the ADHD and ASD group. Therefore, clinicians should adopt a cautious "start low and go slow" approach when prescribing ADHD medications in children and young people with ASD, gradually increasing medication doses while closely monitoring tolerability.

Various medications, including antipsychotics, antidepressants, and mood stabilizers, have been investigated for reducing stereotypies and repetitive behaviors in individuals with ASD. Studies have reported significant improvements in more than 50% of participants treated with aripiprazole and risperidone. Modest improvements have also been observed with fluoxetine, valproic acid, haloperidol, clomipramine, and guanfacine.

In summary, given the limited evidence, selection and administration of medications should be done with caution, closely monitoring both the therapeutic effects and potential adverse effects.

Medications in the pipeline

A recent systematic review (Cortese *et al.*, 2023) explored RCTs in phases 2, 3, and 4 of novel medications, or medications used for unlicensed indications ("off-label"), for child/adolescent mental conditions, alongside RCTs of dietary interventions/probiotics, as well as phase 4 RCTs of agents targeting unlicensed indications for children/adolescents with mental health disorders. The review retrieved 234 ongoing or completed RCTs. The only 2 compounds with evidence of significant effects that were replicated in at least 2 RCTs without any negative RCTs were dasotraline for ADHD (whose developmental program, however, was halted by the manufacturer in 2020) and carbetocin for hyperphagia in Prader-Willi syndrome.

Dietary interventions

A network meta-analysis (Siafis *et al.*, 2022) of 125 RCTs of pharmacological and dietary supplement treatments for autism found inconclusive evidence of efficacy of dietary supplements. In particular, omega-3-fatty-acids could lead to improvement in social-communication difficulties with small ESs, but evidence was of very low-quality and based on 10 studies in children/adolescents. There was inconclusive evidence for carnosine, folinic acid, probiotics, and sulforaphane (broccoli sprout extract). Additionally, both cysteine-rich whey-protein and vitamin-B12 increased the number of responders but were not found to be efficacious for core or associated symptoms. Notably, vitamin-B12 was found to worsen irritability.

A review (Stevenson *et al.*, 2014) of existing meta-analyses on dietary intervention in ADHD found evidence from well-conducted studies for a small effect of supplementation with free fatty acids. Additionally, there was evidence that restricted elimination diets may be efficacious, but large-scale studies are needed on unselected children (i.e., not selected for nutritional deficiencies), using blind assessment and including assessment of long-term outcome. Artificial food color elimination was also found to be a potentially valuable treatment, but its ES and the type of child for whom it is likely to be efficacious are currently poorly understood.

Regarding depression, a meta-analysis (Campisi *et al.*, 2021) in children and adolescents with depressive symptoms failed to find any significant effect when focusing on RCTs, while it reported small-to-medium effects in pre-post studies on depressive symptoms.

Currently, guidelines do not recommend any dietary intervention as part of the general strategy to treat any mental health or neurodevelopmental conditions in youths. However, in the NICE ADHD guidelines (NICE, 2018), it is acknowledged that if caregivers are under the impression that certain foods increase the severity of the symptoms a consultation with a dietitian would provide valuable insights.

Neuromodulation therapies

A large scale UR (Rosson *et al.*, 2022) of RCTs of deep brain stimulation (DBS), TMS, tDCS, and electroconvulsive therapy (ECT) found two meta-analyses including studies of children and/or adolescents. The first one (Brauer *et al.*, 2021a), including 8 RCTs of tDCS, showed small-to-moderate effect on overall ADHD core symptoms, inattention, and impulsivity but not hyperactivity on ADHD (moderate certainty of evidence). The meta-analysis could not assess specific side effects in children. The second meta-analysis, focused on autism, included only

3 RCTs (2 from the same author), showing, overall, a significant improvement in two subdomains of the Autism Treatment Evaluation Checklist (ATEC)—Social, and Health and Behavioral Problems—as well as in the ATEC total score (−0.97, −1.58, −0.36), (very low certainty of evidence). Finally, a systematic review of studies of external trigeminal nerve stimulation (eTNS) (Westwood *et al.*, 2023) found only two studies (from the same group) in children and adolescents, focusing on ADHD. In the first one (McGough *et al.*, 2015), a pilot feasibility open trial in 24 children and young people (aged 7–14 years) with ADHD, significant improvements were noted on parent-rated symptoms and objective test measuring reaction time after 8 weeks of eTNS. In the second one, a double-blind, sham-controlled pilot study in 62 children and young people (aged 8–12 years), eTNS was superior to placebo (ES: 0.5) on the study primary outcome (ADHD symptom severity). No RCTs for ECT were found.

Currently, none of the most used guidelines recommends any neurotherapy for any mental condition in children and young people. However, it should be noted that the FDA approved eTNS for the treatment of ADHD in 2019, based on the only available pilot RCT, which calls for independent replication of results.

Conclusions and future perspectives

The use of medications to treat CAMH conditions is increasing. This increase has been to some degree supported by an improved evidence base that now supports the inclusion of medication as a component of treatment plans for many conditions. There is, however, still a long way to go in generating new knowledge and the risk of clinical practice outstripping the evidence remains a real one. We need further primary evidence about determining which medications work and, particularly in the long term, are safe. We need to better evaluate the efficacy of combined medication and nonmedication treatments. There is very little evidence to aid clinical decision-making as to the best way to sequence pharmacological treatment, nonmedication, and combination treatments. We also need to better understand the role, if any, of nonpharmacological approaches, such as dietary interventions and neurostimulation, on the core symptoms and/or associated impairments of mental health conditions in children and young people.

The aim of personalized medicine is, we believe, ultimately achievable, but it is going to take time and will require close collaboration between researchers working across a wide range of basic and clinical science disciplines (Buitelaar *et al.*, 2022). There are also opportunities for improvements in the design of clinical trials and observational studies (Wong *et al.*, 2019).

From a clinical perspective there is still a lot of work to be done translating current evidence into more effective clinical practice. We have, for example, highlighted the real improvements in clinical outcomes that are associated with MBC.

Finally, for many people stigma continues to be a major hurdle to accessing mental health care. As clinicians we can play a major role in reducing stigma through the accurate and transparent dissemination of evidence and the delivery of better psychoeducation. We also need to ensure that we are neither overpromoting the use of medications nor undermining the potential benefits through ideologies that run counter to the evidence.

References

Adamo, N. *et al.* (2015) Pharmacological treatment of attention-deficit/hyperactivity disorder: assessing outcomes. *Expert Review of Clinical Pharmacology* **8**, 383–397.

Brauer, H. *et al.* (2021a) Transcranial direct current stimulation in attention-deficit/hyperactivity disorder: a meta-analysis of clinical efficacy outcomes. *Progress in Brain Research* **264**, 91–116.

Brauer, R. *et al.* (2021b) Psychotropic medicine consumption in 65 countries and regions, 2008-19: a longitudinal study. *The Lancet Psychiatry* **8**, 1071–1082.

Brent, D. *et al.* (2008) Switching to another SSRI or to venlafaxine with or without cognitive behavioral therapy for adolescents with SSRI-resistant depression: the TORDIA randomized controlled trial. *JAMA* **299**, 901–913.

Buitelaar, J. *et al.* (2022) Toward precision medicine in ADHD. *Frontiers in Behavioral Neuroscience* **16**, 900981.

Campisi, S.C. *et al.* (2021) Do healthy dietary interventions improve pediatric depressive symptoms? A systematic review and Meta-analysis. *Advances in Nutrition* **12**, 2495–2507.

Chacko, A. *et al.* (2010) Improving medication adherence in chronic pediatric health conditions: a focus on ADHD in youth. *Current Pharmaceutical Design* **16**(22), 2416–2423.

Chan, A.Y.L. *et al.* (2023) Attention-deficit/hyperactivity disorder medication consumption in 64 countries and regions from 2015 to 2019: a longitudinal study. *EClinicalMedicine* **58**, 101780.

Coghill, D. & Seth, S. (2015) Effective management of attention-deficit/hyperactivity disorder (ADHD) through structured re-assessment: the Dundee ADHD clinical care pathway. *Child and Adolescent Psychiatry and Mental Health* **9**, 52.

Connolly, S.D. *et al.* (2007) Practice parameter for the assessment and treatment of children and adolescents with anxiety disorders. *Journal of the American Academy of Child and Adolescent Psychiatry* **46**, 267–283.

Cook, E.H. *et al.* (2001) Long-term sertraline treatment of children and adolescents with obsessive-compulsive disorder. *Journal of the American Academy of Child and Adolescent Psychiatry* **40**, 1175–1181.

Coombes, I.D. *et al.* (2011) Pilot of a National Inpatient Medication Chart in Australia: improving prescribing safety and enabling prescribing training. *British Journal of Clinical Pharmacology* **72**(2), 338–349.

Correll, C.U. *et al.* (2021) Efficacy and acceptability of pharmacological, psychosocial, and brain stimulation interventions in children and adolescents with mental disorders: an umbrella review. *World Psychiatry* **20**, 244–275.

Cortese, S. *et al.* (2013) Practitioner review: current best practice in the management of adverse events during treatment with ADHD medications in children and adolescents. *Journal of Child Psychology and Psychiatry* **54**, 227–246.

Cortese, S. *et al.* (2023) The future of child and adolescent clinical psychopharmacology: a systematic review of phase 2, 3, or 4 randomized controlled trials of pharmacologic agents without regulatory approval or for unapproved indications. *Neuroscience and Biobehavioral Reviews* **149**, 105149.

Drugs.com (2024) Drug Interaction Checker. [Online]. Available: https://www.drugs.com/drug_interactions.html [27 October 2024].

Farhat, L.C. *et al.* (2023) Comparative efficacy, tolerability, and acceptability of pharmacological interventions for the treatment of children, adolescents, and young adults with Tourette's syndrome: a systematic review and network meta-analysis. *The Lancet Child & adolescent Health* **7**(2), 112–126.

Fraguas, D. *et al.* (2011) Efficacy and safety of second-generation antipsychotics in children and adolescents with psychotic and bipolar spectrum disorders: comprehensive review of prospective head-to-head and placebo-controlled comparisons. *European Neuropsychopharmacology* **21**, 621–645.

Goodyer, I.M. *et al.* (2008) A randomised controlled trial of cognitive behaviour therapy in adolescents with major depression treated by selective serotonin reuptake inhibitors. The ADAPT trial **12**(14). iii–iv, ix–60

Goyette, G.H. *et al.* (1978) Effects of artificial colors on hyperkinetic children: a double-blind challenge study [proceedings]. *Psychopharmacology Bulletin* **14**, 39–40.

Haddad, P.M. & Wieck, A. (2004) Antipsychotic-induced hyperprolactinaemia: mechanisms, clinical features and management. *Drugs* **64**, 2291–2314.

Hatfield, D. *et al.* (2010) Do we know when our clients get worse? An investigation of therapists' ability to detect negative client change. *Clinical Psychology & Psychotherapy* **17**, 25–32.

Hudson, J.L. *et al.* (2023) Combining CBT and sertraline does not enhance outcomes for anxious youth: a double-blind randomised controlled trial. *Psychological Medicine* **53**, 1741–1749.

Ipser, J.C. *et al.* (2009) Pharmacotherapy for anxiety disorders in children and adolescents. *Cochrane Database of Systematic Reviews*, CD005170.

Kumra, S. *et al.* (2008) Clozapine and "high-dose" olanzapine in refractory early-onset schizophrenia: a 12-week randomized and double-blind comparison. *Biological Psychiatry* **63**, 524–529.

Liu, F.F. *et al.* (2019) Mind the gap: considering disparities in implementing measurement-based care. *Journal of the American Academy of Child and Adolescent Psychiatry* **58**, 459–461.

Man, K.K.C. *et al.* (2023) Long-term safety of methylphenidate in children and adolescents with ADHD: 2-year outcomes of the attention deficit hyperactivity disorder drugs use chronic effects (ADDUCE) study. *The Lancet Psychiatry* **10**, 323–333.

March, J. *et al.* (2004) Fluoxetine, cognitive-behavioral therapy, and their combination for adolescents with depression: Treatment for Adolescents with Depression Study (TADS) randomized controlled trial. *Journal of the American Medical Association* **292**(7), 807–820.

Massuti, R. *et al.* (2021) Assessing undertreatment and overtreatment/misuse of ADHD medications in children and adolescents across continents: a systematic review and meta-analysis. *Neuroscience and Biobehavioral Reviews* **128**, 64–73.

McGough, J.J. *et al.* (2015) An eight-week, open-trial, pilot feasibility study of trigeminal nerve stimulation in youth with attention-deficit/hyperactivity disorder. *Brain Stimulation* **8**, 299–304.

National Institute for Health and Care Excellence (NICE) (2013) *Social anxiety disorder: recognition, assessment and treatment. Treatment for children and young people.* [Online]. Available: www.nice.org.uk/guidance/cg159/ifp/chapter/treatment-for-children-and-young-people [28 October 2024].

National Institute for Health and Care Excellence (NICE) (2018) *Attention deficit hyperactivity disorder: diagnosis and management* [Online]. Available: www.nice.org.uk/guidance/ng87 [19 October 2024].

Pediatric OCD Treatment Study (POTS) (2004) Cognitive-behavior therapy, sertraline, and their combination for children and adolescents with obsessive-compulsive disorder: the pediatric OCD treatment study (POTS) randomized controlled trial. *JAMA* **292**, 1969–1976.

Rapoport, J.L. (2013) Pediatric psychopharmacology: too much or too little? *World Psychiatry* **12**, 118–123.

Rosson, S. *et al.* (2022) Brain stimulation and other biological non-pharmacological interventions in mental disorders: an umbrella review. *Neuroscience and Biobehavioral Reviews* **139**, 104743.

Sabaté, E. (ed) (2003) *Adherence to Long-term Therapies: Evidence for Action.* World Health Organization, Geneva, Switzerland.

Sharma, A.N. *et al.* (2016) BAP position statement: off-label prescribing of psychotropic medication to children and adolescents. *Journal of Psychopharmacology* **30**, 416–421.

Siafis, S. *et al.* (2022) Pharmacological and dietary-supplement treatments for autism spectrum disorder: a systematic review and network meta-analysis. *Molecular Autism* **13**, 10.

Solmi, M. *et al.* (2020) Safety of 80 antidepressants, antipsychotics, anti-attention-deficit/hyperactivity medications and mood stabilizers in children and adolescents with psychiatric disorders: a large scale systematic meta-review of 78 adverse effects. *World Psychiatry* **19**(2), 214–232.

Stevenson, J. *et al.* (2014) Research review: the role of diet in the treatment of attention-deficit/hyperactivity disorder—an appraisal of the evidence on efficacy and recommendations on the design of future studies. *Journal of Child Psychology and Psychiatry* **55**, 416–427.

Vitiello, B. & Davico, C. (2018) Twenty years of progress in paediatric psychopharmacology: accomplishments and unmet needs. *Evidence-Based Mental Health* **21**, e10.

Walkup, J.T. *et al.* (2008) Cognitive behavioral therapy, sertraline, or a combination in childhood anxiety. *The New England Journal of Medicine* **359**, 2753–2766.

Westwood, S.J. *et al.* (2023) Computerized cognitive training in attention-deficit/hyperactivity disorder (ADHD): a meta-analysis of randomized controlled trials with blinded and objective outcomes. *Molecular Psychiatry* **28**(4), 1402–1414.

Wong, I.C.K. *et al.* (2019) Emerging challenges in pharmacotherapy research on attention-deficit hyperactivity disorder-outcome measures beyond symptom control and clinical trials. *The Lancet Psychiatry* **6**, 528–537.

C: Contexts of the clinical encounter and specific clinical situations

CHAPTER 40

Diversity: gender identity and sexual orientation

Tomer Shechner[1] and Aron Janssen[2]

[1] School of Psychological Sciences and the Integrated Brain and Behavior Research Center, University of Haifa, Haifa, Israel

[2] Pritzker Department of Psychiatry and Behavioral Health, Northwestern Feinberg School of Medicine, Ann and Robert H. Lurie Children's Hospital of Chicago, Chicago, IL, USA

Introduction

The study of gender and sexuality has seen significant changes in recent decades, with clinical, scientific, and sociocultural perspectives shifting to reflect new understanding. Taking a developmental perspective, this chapter provides an overview of the changes in how we understand gender and sexuality and the impact of these changes on mental health providers who work with youth. The first part of the chapter covers gender and sexual terminology, development, minority stress, and building resilience and support for LGBTQ (lesbian, gay, bisexual, transgender, queer) youth and their families. The second part focuses on gender dysphoria assessment, co-occurring mental health difficulties, and treatment in children and adolescents. The chapter concludes with a brief discussion on the detrimental effects of recent legislation restricting access to gender-affirming care for transgender and gender-diverse (TGD) youth.

Guiding principles

It is essential for mental health providers working with youth to understand and use appropriate gender and sexuality language. *Biological sex* refers to the anatomical and genetical characteristics that differentiate males from females; these include external and internal genital structures, gonads, hormones, and sex chromosomes. *Assigned sex* refers to the classification of individuals as male, female, or intersex, commonly based on external genitalia after birth. The terminology used in the *Diagnostic and Statistical Manual of Mental Disorders* (DSM-5-TR; American Psychiatric Association, 2022) was recently revised to reflect the changing gender terminology more accurately, with "natal male/natal female" replaced by "individual assigned male/female at birth." *Gender identity* is a psychological term describing an individual's deeply held sense of personal gender, encompassing a range of definitions which can be binary (male, female) or non-binary. *Cisgender* describes individuals who identify as the same gender as their assigned sex, whereas *transgender* is an umbrella term describing incongruency between gender identity and assigned sex. *Gender expression*, also known as sex-typed behavior, describes the external manifestations and behaviors that correspond to what is considered typically masculine or typically feminine in a certain culture. This includes clothing, body language, pronouns, and interests, such as hobbies, activities, and occupational preferences. Finally, *sexual orientation* describes a pattern of emotional, romantic, and/or sexual attraction to people of the opposite gender (heterosexuality), the same gender (homosexuality), both genders (bisexuality), or absence of sexual attraction to any gender (asexuality). Sexual orientation is not limited by a person's gender identity, as individuals of any gender can have any sexual orientation.

Among the different identities (ethnic, cultural, professional, etc.), gender is arguably the most salient cross-culturally and the first to develop. Hence, it has a profound influence on all other developmental aspects, including interests, traits, peer selection, intimate relationships, future aspirations, and many more. However, the relationships among gender identity, gender expression, and societal norms and expectations are likely reciprocal, creating a complex interplay, particularly when considered from a developmental perspective.

Gender development

Gender development is a complex and ongoing process influenced by a combination of biological, psychological, and social factors, as well as interactions with family, peers, school, and culture. As different aspects of sex and gender continue to develop throughout life, it is important to recognize that they may not remain consistent over time.

Rutter's Child and Adolescent Psychiatry and Psychology, Seventh Edition.
Edited by Anita Thapar, Daniel S. Pine, Samuele Cortese, Cathy Creswell, Tamsin J. Ford, James F. Leckman, and Argyris Stringaris.

Companion website: www.wiley.com/go/thapar/rutterspsych7

The biological view of gender development highlights the role of genes, hormones, and brain organization in shaping physical and psychological differences associated with masculinity and femininity. Findings from behavioral genetics indicate the heritability of gender-incongruent identity ranges between 30–60% (Polderman *et al.*, 2018). Male and female primary sex hormones, androgens, and estrogens, influence body and behavioral development. Organizational effects mainly occur prenatally, causing lasting bodily changes, while activational effects arise from hormone fluctuations, causing temporary shifts (Arnold, 2009). Animal studies show altered androgen and estrogen levels impact behaviors: females with increased early-life androgen exhibit more masculine behaviors, and males with decreased androgen show more feminine behaviors (Wallen, 2005; Fuxjager *et al.*, 2017). The type and timing of exposure to sex hormones both play a crucial role in determining behavioral outcomes.

Individuals with disorders of sex development (DSDs) offer a unique opportunity to examine the effects of sex hormones, particularly prenatal and early postnatal androgens, on sex-typed behavior and gender development. For example, females with congenital adrenal hyperplasia (CAH) produce high levels of androgen in early gestation and during prenatal development. After the condition is treated, their androgen levels are usually normal, and they are typically raised as girls/women. Girls with CAH exhibit a stronger interest in traditionally masculine toys and activities than girls without CAH (Berenbaum *et al.*, 1995; Meyer-Bahlburg *et al.*, 2004). As they grow to adulthood, they continue to show an interest in male-typical activities, careers, and sport (Meyer-Bahlburg *et al.*, 2006). While *in utero* androgen exposure plays a role, it is not the exclusive, and likely not the predominant, factor shaping gender identity. A meta-analysis of 250 adults with CAH who were raised as girls found 95% identified as females (Dessens *et al.*, 2005). About 5.2% either identified as male or experienced gender dysphoria. Even though these values are about five times the 0.4–1.2% estimates for transgender identity in individuals assigned female at birth, the majority of the sample identified as female (Winter *et al.*, 2016).

Awareness of gender as a social category forms early in development. During the first year of life, infants develop the ability to distinguish between male and female categories by discriminating between faces and voices. By the end of the first year, they are able to associate male and female faces with gender-typed objects, developing an early ability to form gender stereotypes (Martin & Ruble, 2010). This early associative network develops gradually, and by 3 years, children demonstrate gender stereotypes in domains such as physical appearance, toys, activities, and traits. With development, gender-related stereotypes and sex-typing knowledge expand to include occupations, sports, and other daily roles (King *et al.*, 2021).

Psychological theories offer different explanations of the emergence of gender identity and sex-typical behaviors. According to the *cognitive schema theory*, from a young age, children organize gender-related information in mental frameworks, or schemas, which are networks of associations. These schemas help children make sense of the abundant gender-related information they encounter and thereby influence their thinking and behavior (Martin & Ruble, 2004). The *developmental intergroup theory* highlights children's innate drive to categorize environmental information into significant groups and their proclivity to categorize individuals of their own gender as part of their "in-group" and others as belonging to the "out-group." Engaging with members of the in-group fosters a sense of shared identity and similarities and leads to the adoption of gender roles and expectations associated with that group. In contrast, members of the out-group are perceived as distinct and dissimilar, possibly resulting in the formation of stereotypes and biases (Bigler & Liben, 2006). The *social cognitive theory* of gender development stresses the effect of social and environmental factors on the development of gender identity and expression. Children learn about gender roles and expectations through observation, imitation, and reinforcement from others in their social environment and through the gender-typed feedback they receive (Bussey & Bandura, 1999).

Easy and extensive access to the Internet and social media has allowed youth to encounter diverse, intricate ideas of gender that challenge the traditional binary model. With these historical shifts in the accessibility of information and models of gender diversity, younger individuals are more likely to explore and embrace nontraditional gender identities and expression. Social media are used not only to obtain information, but also to gain support and a sense of community (Hardy, 2021). Sexual and gender minority youth spend more time online than their heterosexual and cisgender peers and are more likely to look for resources related to their community in online than offline environments (McInroy *et al.*, 2019).

Sexual development

Sexual development begins at birth and continues over the life course (Figure 40.1). It manifests in various forms at different stages and includes sexual behaviors, orientation, and identity.

Physical sexual responses are innate. Male infants exhibit erections, while female infants display signs of vaginal lubrication within 24 hours of birth (Masters *et al.*, 1995). At a few months old, infants exhibit sexually related behaviors such as touching their genitals with rhythmic movements. From the ages of 3–7, children show a noticeable increase in sexual curiosity and experimentation, both in self-directed sexual play and in imaginary play with peers of the same age, and develop a greater understanding of their own sexuality. However, as they progress through the elementary school years (ages 6–9), sexual play becomes more discreet, as they start to understand cultural norms and restrictions (Kellogg, 2009). During preadolescence (ages 8–12), children tend to interact and educate themselves about sexuality among same-gender peers. Adolescence is

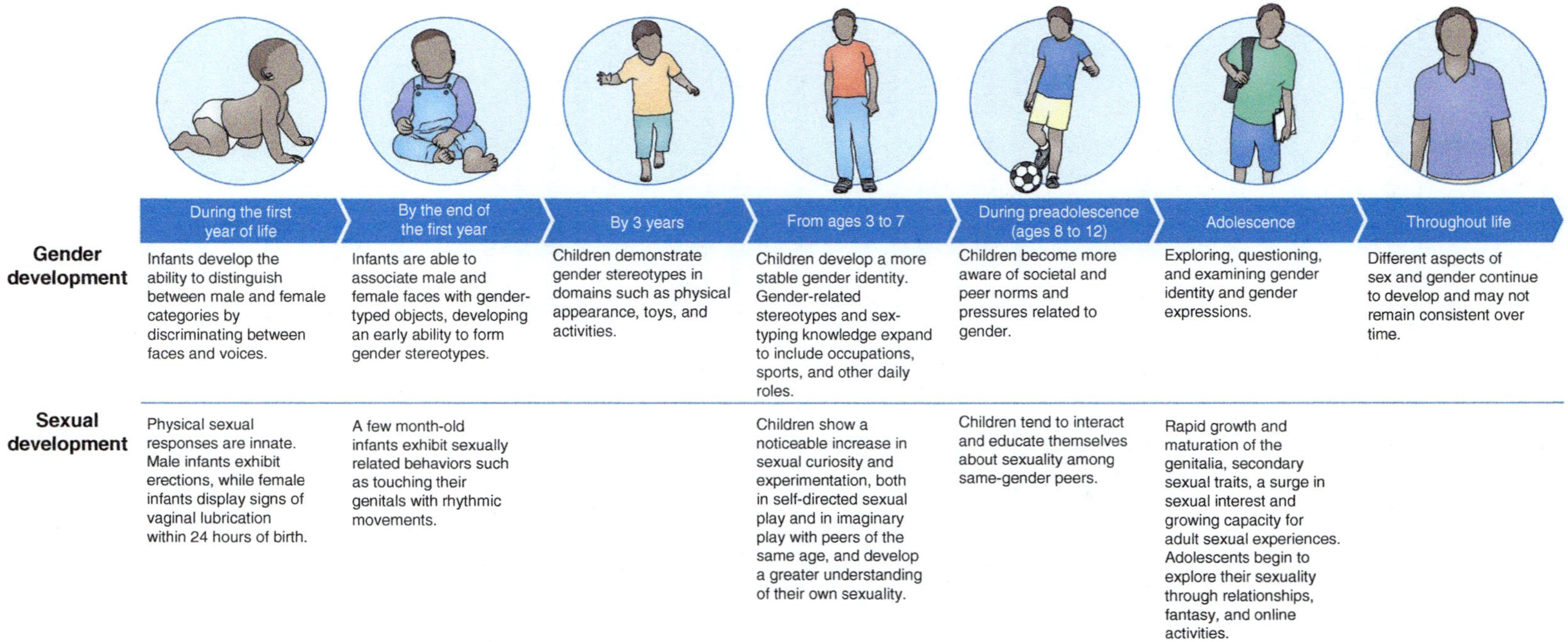

Figure 40.1 Gender and sexual developmental milestones.

marked by the rapid growth and maturation of the genitalia, the development of secondary sexual traits, and a surge in sexual interest due to increased sex hormone levels and a growing capacity for adult sexual experiences. Adolescents begin to explore their sexuality through relationships, fantasy, and online activities, and sexual exploration and sexual attraction become more prominent (Ponton & Judice, 2004).

Sexual orientation constitutes a person's emotional, romantic, and/or sexual attraction toward individuals of the opposite sex (heterosexuality), the same sex (homosexuality), both sexes (bisexuality), or neither sex (asexuality). Its determination is a multifaceted process influenced by a variety of factors, including genetics, hormonal regulation, and neural correlates (for a comprehensive review, see Bogaert & Skorska, 2020). While most research points to the biological origins of sexual orientation, social, cultural, and political factors may influence attitudes to and beliefs about nonheterosexual orientation and may therefore influence its expression. Interestingly, sexual orientation in women seems more related to environmental influences and is less rigid than sexual orientation in men (Diamond *et al.*, 2017).

Sexual orientation identity development involves an individual's changing awareness, exploration, and understanding of personal sexual identity over time, based on patterns of sexual attraction and behavior (Hall *et al.*, 2021). Traditional developmental models of nonheterosexual identity depict these processes as linear and universal. For example, the Cass model outlines a five-stage process: awareness of nonheterosexual feelings followed by confusion and denial, acceptance of being part of the lesbian, gay, or bisexual (LGB) community, involvement with the community, awareness of discrimination, and integration of LGB identity into the self (Cass, 1979).

More contemporary approaches focus on the concept of milestones, significant events marking life changes, or achievements. Milestones for LGB individuals include the recognition of nonheterosexual desires, first same-sex sexual contact, self-identification as LGB, and "coming out" to friends and family. This approach does not assume a single path of development; instead, it stresses the variations among LGB individuals and the factors that influence the timing and sequence of milestones (Calzo *et al.*, 2011; Savin-Williams, 2018). A recent meta-analysis found that, on average, individuals experience attraction and question their orientation during early adolescence; they self-identify as LGB, engage in sexual activity, and come out for the first time in late adolescence; they come out to parents and family members and have a romantic relationship in emerging adulthood (Hall *et al.*, 2021). On average, males reach the milestones of attraction, self-identification, and sexual activity earlier than females. Nonetheless, both genders disclose their sexual orientation and enter their first romantic relationship at similar ages. This study also found interesting differences among generations. The youngest generation (Millennials) reached all five milestones in the shortest time, the middle two generations (Generation X and Baby Boomers) took longer, and the oldest generation (Silent Generation) took the longest time. There was a notable difference in the milestone sequence, with sexual activity following self-identification as LGB for most generations, but sexual activity coming before self-identification as LGB for the youngest generation. Possible reasons for these differences include technological advancements, the ubiquity of social media, and increased acceptance of diverse sexual identities (Andersen & Fetner, 2008; Hall & Rodgers, 2019).

In summary, gender and sexual development are complex, multidimensional concepts shaped by a combination of biological, psychological, and social factors. As a result, societal, clinical, and scientific views on gender and sexual development have evolved, with a decreasing emphasis on the terms "typical" and "atypical" and a growing acknowledgment and acceptance of the diverse expressions within gender and sexuality, thus fostering understanding and support for individuals across the spectrum (Figure 40.1).

Developmental trajectories of gender/sexual minority youth

The Savin-Williams concept suggests LGBTQ youth share many of the same developmental tasks as other youth (Savin-Williams, 2018). They experience similar biological and cultural contexts and navigate age-appropriate developmental milestones. Regardless of their gender identity or sexual orientation, youth must manage and handle social and interpersonal relationships. While the gender of their fantasies and objects of desire may vary, adolescents of almost all sexualities explore and are preoccupied with sexual and emotional intimacy. However, sexual- and gender-minority youth may have developmental trajectories that differentiate them from their heterosexual peers based on biological factors and the social and cultural environments they experience. They may also face unique developmental tasks related to their identity and relationship with their community.

Gender and sexual diversity

Gender dysphoria, a psychiatric diagnosis introduced in DSM-5 (American Psychiatric Association, 2013), pertains to the significant distress or functional impairment experienced by individuals due to a discrepancy between their experienced or expressed gender and their assigned gender. This clinical diagnosis differs from the various terms describing gender identity (transgender, nonbinary, fluid, etc.) which are considered part of human gender diversity and are not pathological. DSM-5's emphasis on the subjective experience of distress represents a substantial shift in the diagnostic understanding of gender diversity. DSM-IV (American Psychiatric Association, 1994) classified all individuals who experienced incongruency between assigned sex and gender identity or expression as having a gender identity disorder. However, the DSM-5 diagnosis of gender dysphoria does not apply to all individuals who identify as TGD. Rather, it is focused on the emotional turmoil and psychological challenges that sometimes arise from the mismatch between gender identity or expression and assigned gender. More recently, DSM-5-TR made further revisions to reflect a more accepting and affirmative stance on gender diversity, marking a significant step forward in societal attitudes to gender identity (American Psychiatric Association, 2022).

Similarly, since the 1950s, DSM classified homosexuality as a mental disorder. However, in 1973, after an extensive review of the scientific literature and input from mental health professionals, the American Psychiatric Association removed homosexuality from the DSM (Spitzer, 1981). This decision was based on accumulating evidence showing homosexuality to represent a normal variation of human sexuality, not a mental illness.

Prevalence

Large population-based surveys in the United States conducted among high school students have found 1.8–2.7% of individuals identify as TGD (Rider *et al.*, 2018; Johns *et al.*, 2019). According to a 2016 international review, an estimated 0.5–1.3% of birth-assigned males and 0.4–1.2% of birth-assigned females are transgender (Winter *et al.*, 2016). More recent surveys based on a broader definition of gender-diverse identity using self-reported discrepancy between current gender identification and assigned sex at birth have reported even higher percentages of gender diversity in youth (~9%) (Kidd *et al.*, 2021).

Referral rates to gender clinics support population-based survey data, indicating a significant increase in referrals of children and adolescents (Chen *et al.*, 2016; Handler *et al.*, 2019; Kaltiala *et al.*, 2020; Segev-Becker *et al.*, 2020). Reports from gender clinics show an uneven ratio of referrals based on assigned sex. Adolescents assigned female at birth seek care 2.5–7.1 times more frequently than those assigned male at birth. This observation has been documented in multiple clinics worldwide (Aitken *et al.*, 2015; Arnoldussen *et al.*, 2020; Kaltiala *et al.*, 2020; Bauer *et al.*, 2021). Birth-assigned females may find it easier to express their transgender feelings because they experience less stigma expressing masculine traits than birth-assigned males displaying feminine traits. In addition, the earlier onset of puberty in birth-assigned females might contribute to an earlier and potentially more prolonged experience of dysphoria related to their physical characteristics and body.

The Youth Risk Behavior Survey (YRBS) is a biennial survey of high-school students conducted by the US Center for Disease Control and Prevention that has allowed a longitudinal view of changes in self-identification of sexual orientation and sexual behavior. Rates of self-identification of LGB youth increased from 8.3% of the sample in 2015 to 11.7% in 2019. It is notable that self-identification of engagement in same-sex behavior has consistently captured a larger percentage of the population than self-identification as LGB, with 11.5% of the 2015 sample and 13.3% of the 2019 sample falling into this category (Rapoport *et al.*, 2021).

Social ecological frame

Children and adolescents are shaped by nested systems, as Bronfenbrenner's ecological theory suggests (Bronfenbrenner, 1979). Their sense of self and their overall functioning are inherently linked to the multiple internal and external factors over which they have differential levels of influence. This theory set the stage for the concept of "spheres of influence" in understanding social health determinants (DeCamp *et al.*, 2020). These spheres represented by individuals (clinicians, parents, teachers) and institutions (hospital systems, schools, religious organizations) help elucidate how internal and external factors shape LGBTQ youth's identity comprehension and experiences. They also inform intervention levels for functional impairments (Wanta *et al.*, 2022). Professionals working with LGBTQ youth should recognize how individual, home, school, community, and clinical factors—along with stigma and bias—affect their navigation of the world.

Minority stress model

The minority stress model describes the detrimental effects of stigma, discrimination, prejudice, and their correlates on the mental health and well-being of LGBTQ individuals (Meyer, 2003). These additional chronic stressors are associated specifically with being a member of a sexual or gender minority marginal group and stem primarily from social/structural forces. The model suggests three main processes impact the mental health of LGBTQ individuals: (i) external, objective stressful events and circumstances; (ii) negative expectations of such events; and (iii) the internalization of negative social attitudes. While the theory was developed to explain associations between sexual orientation and mental health, it has been extended to include physical and mental health disparities associated with gender identity in adults and youth (White Hughto *et al.*, 2015; Delozier *et al.*, 2020). Stigma and minority stress can manifest in individual, interpersonal, and structural domains (Hatzenbuehler & Pachankis, 2016). Individual forms of stigma include internalized homophobia/transphobia, sensitivity to rejection, and concealment of sexual/gender identity. Interpersonal minority stress pertains to overt and covert prejudice and discrimination. Structural stigma encompasses societal-level conditions, cultural norms, and institutional policies that restrict the opportunities, resources, and well-being of the stigmatized group, operating beyond individual and interpersonal interactions. A recent meta-analysis found a medium positive correlation between minority stress and mental health problems in LGB adolescents, with a stronger association between minority stress and depression than between minority

Box 40.1 Ways clinicians can create a safe and nonjudgmental setting

- Use appropriate terminology and inclusive language and ask youth how they prefer to be referred to.
- Ask open-ended questions to avoid assumptions about sexual orientation or gender identity.
- Be aware of unique challenges and stressors faced by LGBTQ youth, such as discrimination, family rejection, and bullying, and ask open-ended questions about their experiences.
- Explore how sexual orientation or gender identity may impact the youth's future goals and aspirations.
- Normalize experiences by acknowledging that coming out and navigating sexual orientation or gender identity can be challenging for anyone, regardless of age or background.
- Display LGBTQ-friendly signage, such as a rainbow flag or sticker, to create a welcoming, inclusive, and safe environment.
- Provide a gender-neutral restroom to make transgender and nonbinary youth feel comfortable and respected.
- Offer LGBTQ-related reading materials like magazines, brochures, or other resources.

stress and general mental health problems or trauma symptoms (Dürrbaum & Sattler, 2020). Other meta-analyses examining youth have previously reported links between peer victimization and suicide and nonsuicidal self-injury (Liu *et al.*, 2019; Hatchel *et al.*, 2021). Additional studies have found links between minority stress and sexual risk behaviors (Rosario *et al.*, 2006), and between elevated internalized transphobic beliefs and diagnostic criteria for major depressive disorder (MDD) and generalized anxiety disorder (GAD) (Chodzen *et al.*, 2019). The minority stress model not only provides a framework to explain the higher physical and mental challenges of LGBTQ youth, but also provides efficient ways to reduce these challenges by tailoring specific interventions. The effects of minority stress on TGD youth's mental health are discussed in a later section of the chapter.

In conclusion, it is crucial to acknowledge the inherent value of listening, understanding, and supporting youth's exploration and articulation of their gender and sexuality. These issues have enormous psychological, personal, and cultural significance to most youth, regardless of their sexual orientation or gender identity. It is essential for clinicians to address gender and sexuality issues in every clinical encounter, interview, and assessment, to ensure youth receive the support they need to thrive. Box 40.1 describes ways for clinicians to create a safe and nonjudgmental setting for youth to explore and articulate their gender and sexuality.

Building family resilience and support

Given the higher rates of suicidality among LGBTQ youth facing rejection by family and the lower rates of suicidality among those accepted by family (Haas *et al.*, 2011; Price & Green, 2023), it is vital to strengthen support for all members of a family involved in the care of children coming to understand themselves as LGBTQ. Unlike many other minoritized identities, sexual and gender identities are often discordant in families, and the LGBTQ child may be reared by a family who lacks awareness of the development processes and has varying degrees of empathy for the LGBTQ community prior to the child/sibling coming out. A prospective cohort study, the Transgender Youth Project, found TGD children who were socially affirmed and accepted by their families had rates of anxiety and depression similar to age-matched controls (Durwood *et al.*, 2017).

However, levels of distress and hardship differ both between families and among individual family members. Clinicians working with LGBTQ youth and their families need to recognize varying levels of family discord and disagreement. For interventions to be effective, clinicians must use their best clinical judgment to provide balanced support to youth, their parents, and their siblings. A recent systematic review (Malpas *et al.*, 2022) provided clinical recommendations for maintaining a balance in support for parents and their TGD youth, addressing prevalent instances of family distress. These recommendations are also broadly applicable to LGBTQ youth and their families:

- Provide caregivers with psychoeducation on gender identity and expression, the range of gender identities, the ways gender identity may be expressed, and the different medical and social interventions available to support the well-being of youth and their families.
- Allow caregivers to process positive and negative emotions. Caregivers may experience a range of emotions in response to their youth coming out, including grief, fear, loss, surprise, sadness, joy, relief, and gratitude. By processing these emotions, caregivers can better support their youth and create a more positive and accepting environment.
- Emphasize family acceptance and engagement as a major protective factor.
- A variety of different interventions can be used flexibly to support TGD youth and their families, including group sessions, and individual sessions for caregivers, siblings, and youth.
- Caregivers can become allies for their youth by accessing resources to learn how to navigate health care, legal, and educational systems.
- Encourage connection with support groups and other community resources.
- Incorporate intersectional and contextual approaches, including race, class, religion, and legal status, in all dimensions of care and services.

Gender dysphoria

This section of this chapter focuses on working with TGD youth and their families. Clinicians caring for TGD youth should be familiar with the World Professional Association for Transgender Health's (WPATH) Standards of Care, 8th version (SOC 8,

Coleman *et al.*, 2022). WPATH is a global, interdisciplinary professional organization dedicated to enhancing transgender health through evidence-based care, education, research, and public policy.

Assessment

When assessing gender issues in children and adolescents, it is pertinent to collect information from various informants using a multimodal approach and to consider societal and cultural contexts, as well as individual characteristics. The general aim is to assess: (i) gender incongruence, identity, expression, and gender dysphoria; (ii) mental health concerns; (iii) child/adolescent resilience, vulnerabilities; and (iv) social support systems, mainly the family.

Prepubertal children

The degree of comprehensiveness required in the assessment process is influenced by the purpose of the family referral. Not all gender-diverse children require an exhaustive evaluation. However, the assessment process could represent a valuable opportunity to enhance the child's and the family's coping mechanisms in the context of the unfamiliar and unique challenges associated with gender diversity and should aim to augment support and acceptance (Coleman *et al.*, 2022).

Prepubertal gender-diverse children are not eligible for medical interventions and are more likely to solely seek psychosocial support. Hence, as per the recommendations of SOC 8 and recent clinical guidelines, a comprehensive assessment should cover: (i) the child's current and past gender identity and gender expression, gender incongruence, and gender dysphoria; (ii) the strengths and challenges of the child, family, peers, and others' beliefs about and attitudes toward gender diversity, acceptance, and support for the child; (iii) the child's and the family's experiences of gender minority stress; (iv) the level of expected support in school, extended family, and faith communities; (v) the child's mental health, communication, cognitive abilities, neurodivergence, and/or any behavioral difficulties causing significant functional impairment; (iv) the child's relevant medical and developmental history; (vii) potential risks to the child, such as exposure to domestic or community violence, maltreatment, history of trauma, victimization, or suicidality; and (viii) the child's mental health and/or behavioral challenges causing functional difficulties for any other family member (Ristori & Steensma, 2016; Janssen & Leibowitz, 2018; Coleman *et al.*, 2022). Examples of questions for the prepubertal child are presented in Box 40.2.

Box 40.2 Interview questions for children and adolescents

For children, use age-appropriate language and simplify the questions as needed to ensure the child can understand them. Examples of questions for children include:

- Can you tell me more about how you feel about being a boy/girl/nonbinary?
- What do you think it means to be a boy/girl/nonbinary?
- Can you tell me about your friends?
- How do you like to spend time with your friends?
- How long have you felt that you are different from other boys/girls?
- How do you feel about your body? Are there any changes you would like to make to your body or appearance to feel more comfortable?
- Have you told anyone about your gender identity/feeling different from other boys/girls?
- Have you experienced any negative responses or bullying because of your gender identity/your feelings about being a boy/girl/nonbinary?

For adolescents, in addition to the suggested questions for children, interviews should focus on different body-related issues and general perceptions of societal gender expression. Examples of questions for adolescents include:

- How do you identify in terms of gender?
- Can you explain why you feel more comfortable as a boy/girl/nonbinary?
- Can you tell me about your relationship to your body?
- How do you feel about the changes that happen during puberty, such as developing breasts or facial hair?
- Are there any aspects of the body of a different gender that you desire? Which ones?
- What are the advantages that men/women/nonbinary experience in society?

Adolescents

Similar to the process for children, the assessment of gender-diverse adolescents should focus on gender-related issues and overall psychological functioning and well-being. Gender identity development can start in early childhood for some, while for others, it may not begin until after pubertal changes have occurred (Steensma *et al.*, 2013). Consequently, there is no set pace, course, or outcome that can be predicted for gender-diverse adolescents. The biopsychological assessment of adolescents seeking gender-affirming care should be comprehensive and include aspects of physical and psychological readiness for medical treatment, such as puberty blockers and gender-affirming hormonal treatment (Leibowitz & de Vries, 2016; Coleman *et al.*, 2022). Adolescents must exhibit sufficient psychological maturity indicating their capacity to give informed consent/assent before any medical intervention. Therefore, assessment should examine youth's ability to understand the nature of the treatment, capacity to weigh the risks and benefits of treatment options, appreciation of the long-term consequences, and ability to communicate their choices effectively (Grootens-Wiegers *et al.*, 2017). The assessment should also determine the presence of any co-occurring psychiatric diagnosis. In line with SOC 8, the existence of a co-occurring mental health diagnosis should not necessarily disqualify an eligible adolescent who meets the criteria for gender dysphoria or gender incongruency from receiving psychological or physical interventions (Coleman *et al.*, 2022). Nonetheless, understanding how co-occurring psychiatric diagnoses relate to gender dysphoria is necessary to choose the most suitable and effective intervention (Leibowitz & de Vries, 2016). Finally, to complement the psychosocial assessment of adolescents seeking medical affirmative treatment, a physical examination is necessary to determine pubertal stage. Please refer to Chapter 30 for a review of the details of the physical exam. Examples of questions for adolescents are presented in Box 40.2.

Co-occurring mental health difficulties

Research suggests a higher prevalence of mental health difficulties among TGD than cisgender youth. They are more likely to report higher psychological distress, particularly depression, anxiety, self-harm, and suicidality (Connolly *et al.*, 2016; Eisenberg *et al.*, 2017; Veale *et al.*, 2017; Becerra-Culqui *et al.*, 2018). They also have higher prevalence of psychiatric disorders than cisgender sexual minority youth (Newcomb *et al.*, 2020). Recent studies indicate that nonbinary treatment-seeking youth are at greater risk of developing anxiety, depression, and low self-esteem than binary transgender youth (Chew *et al.*, 2020). Finally, TGD youth, specifically those with gender dysphoria, experience lower quality of life than their same-age peers (Engel *et al.*, 2023).

Suicidal ideation and attempts are more common among TGD than cisgender youth (Toomey *et al.*, 2018; Kingsbury *et al.*, 2022). Some data show transmasculine and nonbinary youth are particularly at higher risk (Toomey *et al.*, 2018; de Graaf *et al.*, 2022). The lifetime prevalence rate of nonsuicidal self-injury is also higher among gender-minority individuals (46.65%) than among their cisgender counterparts (14.57%), and gender-minority youth are especially vulnerable (Liu *et al.*, 2019). Elevated rates of suicidality among TGD youth have been extensively documented, not just in clinical samples but also in National Violent Death Reports (Ream, 2022), national registries (Erlangsen *et al.*, 2023), population-based surveys (Johns *et al.*, 2019), and a recent meta-analysis on the global prevalence of suicidality among trans individuals (Kohnepoushi *et al.*, 2023).

The prevalence of autism among TGD individuals ranges between 5–26% compared to about 1% in the general population (Wamithi *et al.*, 2015; Cheung *et al.*, 2018). Studies using autism screening tools have identified higher levels of autistic symptoms and traits in gender clinic-referred youth (Akgül *et al.*, 2018). A large recent study (n = 641,860) found TGD individuals are 3.03–6.36 times more likely to have autism and score higher on various autistic traits than cisgender individuals (Warrier *et al.*, 2020). The increased overlap between autism and gender diversity is noted in diverse research samples, but the definitive reasons, whether due to reduced social conformity pressures or shared etiological factors, remain speculative. TGD youth who are also autistic face a heightened risk of experiencing mental health challenges because of the social impairments associated with autism, as well as difficulties with executive functioning, such as planning and effectively communicating their gender-related needs. At the same time, they may struggle with monitoring their gender-affirmative care and have fewer adaptive coping strategies to manage minority stress (Strang *et al.*, 2023).

Other neurodevelopmental disorders and psychiatric conditions are more prevalent among TGD individuals across the life span. Specifically, attention deficit hyperactivity disorder (ADHD), learning disorders, obsessive–compulsive disorder (OCD), bipolar disorder, and schizophrenia were found to be elevated in a large TGD sample compared to a cisgender sample (Warrier *et al.*, 2020). Furthermore, emerging evidence suggests an increased prevalence of eating disorders among TGD adults and youth (Feder *et al.*, 2017; Parker & Harriger, 2020).

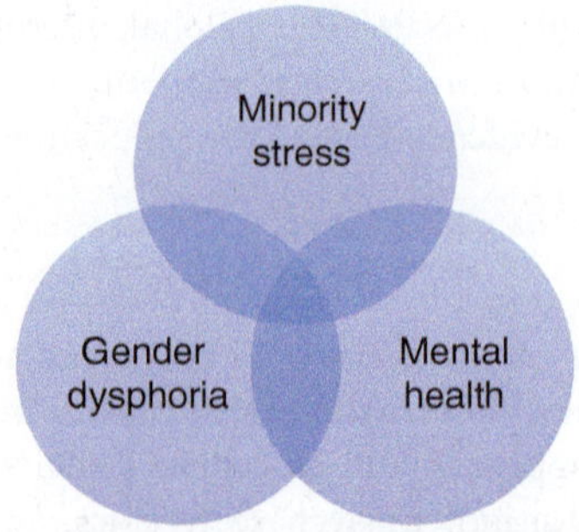

Figure 40.2 Factors explaining co-occurrence of mental health difficulties in transgender and gender-diverse (TGD) youth.

The mental health challenges of TGD youth may stem from three main factors (Janssen & Leibowitz, 2018). These are shown in Figure 40.2. The first is *minority stress* and challenges related to identifying as a member of a marginalized group. Exposure to prejudice and discrimination, along with the long-term effects of internalized transphobia, put TGD youth at heightened psychological risk. The second factor is *gender dysphoria*, such as experiencing discomfort with secondary sex characteristics that do not align with one's gender identity. The third is psychopathology *unrelated to gender identity concerns*. Like cisgender youth, TGD youth might experience a range of mental health conditions impacting how they express and experience their gender. For example, bipolar disorder can impact an individual's self-perception, including gender identity and expression, during manic or depressive episodes. In the past, those with poorly managed psychiatric disorders were often denied access to gender-related psychological or medical care. However, clinical guidelines and case reports suggest individuals with chronic psychotic conditions and gender dysphoria can benefit from concurrent treatment of both conditions (Meijer *et al.*, 2017).

Gender-affirming care

For optimal care and support of TGD youth, interventions should be tailored to their personal needs and sociocultural context. This may involve psychological and supportive interventions for prepubertal children and their families, supplemented by medical interventions if deemed necessary or requested during adolescence (Coleman *et al.*, 2022). To facilitate successful outcomes, health care professionals should prioritize gender-affirming care that seeks to reduce distress related to gender incongruency, bolster resilience factors, and enhance social support (Ehrensaft, 2017). To achieve these objectives, collaborative efforts between the health care provider, the youth, and the family are necessary, and these should be accompanied by interventions that foster long-term well-being and positive mental health.

Supportive therapy gives youth the opportunity to explore and better understand their gender identity, expression, and sexual orientation. Therapy can assist TGD youth in developing adaptive coping mechanisms and address their concerns, such as relationships, intimacy, coming out, social support, minority stress, and anxiety about their future. By providing a supportive and nonjudgmental environment, therapy can help youth process their experiences and emotions, build self-confidence and resilience, and develop the skills they need to navigate challenges related to their gender identity and expression. Therapy can also help youth build a sense of community and develop a support system. This is particularly valuable for those who lack parental support; supportive therapy may offer an opportunity to improve communication and understanding with family, ultimately leading to better coping and resilience (Adelson, 2012; American Psychological Association, 2015).

To better align their gender expression with their gender identity, some youth choose to undergo full or partial social transitioning. This typically involves changing their name, pronouns, clothing, and hairstyle to match their identified gender. Although social transitioning is a reversible and nonpermanent process with no lasting physiological effects, concerns have been raised about the possibility of retransitioning causing distress, particularly for children who may not continue to identify as TGD. However, recent studies suggest retransitioning is rare, and the majority of children who undergo social transitioning at an early age continue to identify as TGD five years later (Olson *et al.*, 2022).

Social transition appears to alleviate negative mental health afflictions. For example, TGD children who have undergone social transitioning show overall comparable levels of depression and anxiety as their siblings and age-matched peers (Durwood *et al.*, 2017). This is a noteworthy difference from the elevated levels of depression and anxiety commonly reported among gender-nonconforming children who have not yet undergone social transitioning. In such cases, refraining from social transitioning should not be considered a neutral position. Creating an adaptable and welcoming environment where children can freely explore their gender is essential. TGD children who are accepted and supported by their families are less likely to experience negative mental health consequences (Olson *et al.*, 2016). Therefore, health care providers often need to educate and work with families on the significance of fostering an affirmative atmosphere.

As adolescents enter puberty, some may opt for medical gender transitioning, which involves hormone therapy and/or surgery (Coleman *et al.*, 2022; Lee & Rosenthal, 2023). This chapter excludes discussion of gender-affirming surgical interventions that are commonly available for individuals at the age of majority, with the exception of a chest muscularization procedure that can be performed in adolescents. Hormone therapy includes either gonadotropin-releasing hormone (GnRH) agonists to suppress puberty or gender-affirming hormones (GAH) to foster secondary sex characteristics congruent with identified gender. In Tanner stage II, puberty suppression hormones, such as GnRH analogs, can be administered to delay natal pubertal development. Puberty blockers are reversible, and discontinuation of treatment leads to resumption of natal puberty. Puberty suppression helps alleviate the distress caused by physical development. Halting pubertal development also gives youth and families more time to consider more invasive and permanent gender-affirming medical interventions. GAH, such as exogenous androgen therapy for transgender males and estrogen therapy for transgender females, can alleviate gender dysphoria by changing the physical appearance to make it more congruent with the identified gender.

Several studies examining the outcomes of GnRH agonists or a combination of GnRH agonists and GAH suggest gender-affirming medical care can have positive effects on the psychosocial well-being of youth (de Vries *et al.*, 2014; Costa *et al.*, 2015; Allen *et al.*, 2019; Achille *et al.*, 2020; Kuper *et al.*, 2020; Tordoff *et al.*, 2022). It is important to note that use of randomized controlled trials (RCTs) for GnRH agonists and GAH are both ethically and pragmatically unfeasible. The impacts of these medications have physically evident effects that are desired by potential participants, which elicit concerns of study participation and completion, adherence, and response bias, as well as exposure to harm of progression of unwanted physical changes that come with puberty (Ashley *et al.*, 2023). The largest multisite longitudinal study to date, with over 300 transgender and nonbinary youth (12–20 years) receiving GAH, found an increase in appearance congruence, positive affect, and life satisfaction, and a decrease in depression and anxiety symptoms over a 2-year period (Chen *et al.*, 2023). Of note, initial levels and rates of change in appearance congruence correlated with psychological outcomes.

Administration of GnRH agonists or GAH presents some risks that must be considered. Specifically, impaired bone mineralization and compromised fertility are recognized as possible concerns. Consequently, a thorough consideration of the potential impact on fertility should be discussed with TGD youth prior to the implementation of GnRH agonist or GAH treatment. Moreover, there is a paucity of empirical evidence on the effects of this type of intervention on brain development (Rosenthal, 2021). Studies examining the effects of GAH and GnRH agonist treatment on metabolic parameters in transgender adolescents and young adults have yielded mixed results. While some found increased insulin resistance and altered body composition in transgender individuals compared to cisgender controls, others reported no clinically significant adverse effects from GAH treatment on a variety of metabolic parameters (Rosenthal, 2021). Long-term adverse medical effects of estrogen treatment may include an increased risk of hypercoagulability and breast cancer. Long-term use of testosterone may increase the risk of skin acne, male pattern baldness, polycythemia, and cardiovascular disease (T'Sjoen *et al.*, 2019).

These risks should be discussed with youth and family, and the treatment plan should be tailored following a careful weighing of risks and benefits.

Politics and law

Across multiple countries, policies and laws have reduced access to medical care for TGD youth, and in some cases, access to medical care for TGD adults as well. Several medical, state, and federal entities have commissioned reports reviewing the state of the evidence in gender-affirming care. The Cass Report, which reviewed the state-of-care of transgender youth in the UK, has received considerable attention. The report elicited extensive discussion among researchers and clinicians, with debates centering less on the quality of the data reviewed or the need for more robust evidence, but rather on the recommended approaches to treatment during the period before such data becomes available. The recent policy changes and laws have generally led to restrictions in access to care, and these new laws and policies ignore the harms associated with prohibiting access to evidence-based care and can cause additional direct distress by targeting a minoritized group of youth already facing overwhelming mental and medical health disparities. Signaling TGD youth specifically as a threat requiring prohibition of care can directly contribute to poorer mental health outcomes (Owen-Smith *et al.*, 2018).

The introduction, debate, and adoption of discriminatory laws and policies negatively affects the mental health of TGD youth. A prospective study with sexual minority populations found that living in states with discriminatory policies was associated with a statistically significant increase in the number of psychiatric disorder diagnoses (Hatzenbuehler *et al.*, 2010) and destructive health behaviors (Du Bois *et al.*, 2018; Cunningham *et al.*, 2022). In a 2022 survey, 86% of transgender and nonbinary youth said exposure to debates about antitransgender bills had negatively impacted their mental health (Trevor Project and Morning Consult, 2023). And a 2022 study, albeit with limitations, found the passage of antitransgender bills was linked with Internet searches related to depression and suicide (Cunningham *et al.*, 2022).

More poignantly, those of us with clinical experience hear from our patients how it feels to be targeted with this kind of legislation. As an example, a transgender patient recently posed the question, "Why does everyone hate me just for existing?" Another simply said, "It's a hard time to be transgender right now."

References

Achille, C. *et al.* (2020) Longitudinal impact of gender-affirming endocrine intervention on the mental health and well-being of transgender youths: preliminary results. *International Journal of Pediatric Endocrinology* **2020**(1), 8. doi:10.1186/s13633-020-00078-2.

Adelson, S.L. (2012) Practice parameter on gay, lesbian, or bisexual sexual orientation, gender nonconformity, and gender discordance in children and adolescents. *Journal of the American Academy of Child and Adolescent Psychiatry* **51**(9), 957–974. doi:10.1016/j.jaac.2012.07.004.

Aitken, M. *et al.* (2015) Evidence for an altered sex ratio in clinic-referred adolescents with gender dysphoria. *The Journal of Sexual Medicine* **12**(3), 756–763. doi:10.1111/jsm.12817.

Akgül, G.Y. *et al.* (2018) Autistic traits and executive functions in children and adolescents with gender dysphoria. *Journal of Sex and Marital Therapy* **44**(7), 619–626. doi:10.1080/0092623X.2018.1437489.

Allen, L.R. *et al.* (2019) Well-being and suicidality among transgender youth after gender-affirming hormones. *Clinical Practice in Pediatric Psychology* 7, 302–311. doi:10.1037/cpp0000288.

American Psychiatric Association (1994) *Diagnostic and Statistical Manual of Mental Disorders*, 4th edn. American Psychiatric Association, Washington, DC.

American Psychiatric Association (2013) *Diagnostic and Statistical Manual of Mental Disorders*, 5th edn. American Psychiatric Association, Washington, DC.

American Psychiatric Association (2022) *Diagnostic and Statistical Manual of Mental Disorders*, 5th edn. text revision edn. American Psychiatric Association, Washington, DC.

American Psychological Association (2015) Guidelines for psychological practice with transgender and gender nonconforming people. *American Psychologist* **70**, 832–864. doi:10.1037/a0039906.

Andersen, R. & Fetner, T. (2008) Cohort differences in tolerance of homosexuality: attitudinal change in Canada and the United States, 1981–2000. *Public Opinion Quarterly* **72**(2), 311–330.

Arnold, A.P. (2009) The organizational-activational hypothesis as the foundation for a unified theory of sexual differentiation of all mammalian tissues. *Hormones and Behavior* **55**(5), 570–578. doi:10.1016/j.yhbeh.2009.03.011.

Arnoldussen, M. *et al.* (2020) Re-evaluation of the Dutch approach: are recently referred transgender youth different compared to earlier referrals? *European Child and Adolescent Psychiatry* **29**(6), 803–811. doi:10.1007/s00787-019-01394-6.

Ashley, F. *et al.* (2023) Randomized-controlled trials are methodologically inappropriate in adolescent transgender healthcare. *International Journal of Transgender Health* **25**(3), 407–418. doi:10.1080/26895269.2023.2218357.

Bauer, G.R. *et al.* (2021) Transgender youth referred to clinics for gender-affirming medical care in Canada. *Pediatrics* **148**(5). doi:10.1542/peds.2020-047266.

Becerra-Culqui, T.A. *et al.* (2018) Mental health of transgender and gender nonconforming youth compared with their peers. *Pediatrics* **141**(5). doi:10.1542/peds.2017-3845.

Berenbaum, S. *et al.* (1995) Early hormonal influences on childhood sex-typed activity and playmate preferences: implications for the development of sexual orientation. *Developmental Psychology* **31**, 31–42. doi:10.1037//0012-1649.31.1.31.

Bigler, R.S. & Liben, L.S. (2006) A developmental intergroup theory of social stereotypes and prejudice. *Advances in Child Development and Behavior* **34**, 39–89. doi:10.1016/s0065-2407(06)80004-2.

Bogaert, A.F. & Skorska, M.N. (2020) A short review of biological research on the development of sexual orientation. *Hormones and Behavior* **119**, 104659. doi:10.1016/j.yhbeh.2019.104659.

Bronfenbrenner, U. (1979) *The Ecology of Human Development: Experiments by Nature and Design*. Harvard University Press, Cambridge, MA.

Bussey, K. & Bandura, A. (1999) Social cognitive theory of gender development and differentiation. *Psychological Review* **106**, 676–713. doi:10.1037/0033-295X.106.4.676.

Calzo, J.P. *et al.* (2011) Retrospective recall of sexual orientation identity development among gay, lesbian, and bisexual adults. *Developmental Psychology* **47**(6), 1658.

Cass, V.C. (1979) Homosexual identity formation. *Journal of Homosexuality* **4**(3), 219–235. doi:10.1300/J082v04n03_01.

Chen, M. *et al.* (2016) Characteristics of referrals for gender dysphoria over a 13-year period. *Journal of Adolescent Health* **58**(3), 369–371. doi:10.1016/j.jadohealth.2015.11.010.

Chen, D. *et al.* (2023) Psychosocial functioning in transgender youth after 2 years of hormones. *New England Journal of Medicine* **388**(3), 240–250. doi:10.1056/NEJMoa2206297.

Cheung, A.S. *et al.* (2018) Sociodemographic and clinical characteristics of transgender adults in Australia. *Transgender Health* **3**(1), 229–238. doi:10.1089/trgh.2018.0019.

Chew, D. *et al.* (2020) Youths with a non-binary gender identity: a review of their sociodemographic and clinical profile. *The Lancet. Child & Adolescent Health* **4**(4), 322–330. doi:10.1016/s2352-4642(19)30403-1.

Chodzen, G. *et al.* (2019) Minority stress factors associated with depression and anxiety among transgender and gender-nonconforming youth. *Journal of Adolescent Health* **64**(4), 467–471. doi:10.1016/j.jadohealth.2018.07.006.

Coleman, E. *et al.* (2022) Standards of care for the health of transgender and gender diverse people, version 8. *International Journal of Transgender Health* **23**(Suppl 1), S1–S259. doi:10.1080/26895269.2022.2100644.

Connolly, M.D. *et al.* (2016) The mental health of transgender youth: advances in understanding. *Journal of Adolescent Health* **59**(5), 489–495. doi:10.1016/j.jadohealth.2016.06.012.

Costa, R. *et al.* (2015) Psychological support, puberty suppression, and psychosocial functioning in adolescents with gender dysphoria. *The Journal of Sexual Medicine* **12**(11), 2206–2214. doi:10.1111/jsm.13034.

Cunningham, G.B. *et al.* (2022) Anti-transgender rights legislation and internet searches pertaining to depression and suicide. *PLoS One* **17**(12), e0279420. doi:10.1371/journal.pone.0279420.

de Graaf, N.M. *et al.* (2022) Suicidality in clinic-referred transgender adolescents. *European Child and Adolescent Psychiatry* **31**(1)), 67–83. doi:10.1007/s00787-020-01663-9.

de Vries, A.L. *et al.* (2014) Young adult psychological outcome after puberty suppression and gender reassignment. *Pediatrics* **134**(4), 696–704. doi:10.1542/peds.2013-2958.

DeCamp, M. *et al.* (2020) Ethics and spheres of influence in addressing social determinants of health. *Journal of General Internal Medicine* **35**(9), 2743–2745. doi:10.1007/s11606-020-05973-1.

Dessens, A.B. *et al.* (2005) Gender dysphoria and gender change in chromosomal females with congenital adrenal hyperplasia. *Archives of Sexual Behavior* **34**(4), 389–397. doi:10.1007/s10508-005-4338-5.

Delozier, A.M. *et al.* (2020) Health disparities in transgender and gender expansive adolescents: a topical review from a minority stress framework. *Journal of Pediatric Psychology* **45**(8), 842–847. doi:10.1093/jpepsy/jsaa040.

Diamond, L.M. *et al.* (2017) Stability of sexual attractions across different timescales: the roles of bisexuality and gender. *Archives of Sexual Behavior* **46**(1), 193–204. doi:10.1007/s10508-016-0860-x.

Du Bois, S.N. *et al.* (2018) Examining associations between state-level transgender policies and transgender health. *Transgender Health* **3**(1), 220–224. doi:10.1089/trgh.2018.0031.

Dürrbaum, T. & Sattler, F.A. (2020) Minority stress and mental health in lesbian, gay male, and bisexual youths: a meta-analysis. *Journal of LGBT Youth* **17**(3), 298–314. doi:10.1080/19361653.2019.1586615.

Durwood, L. *et al.* (2017) Mental health and self-worth in socially transitioned transgender youth. *Journal of the American Academy of Child and Adolescent Psychiatry* **56**(2), 116–123.e112. doi:10.1016/j.jaac.2016.10.016.

Ehrensaft, D. (2017) Gender nonconforming youth: current perspectives. *Adolescent Health, Medicine and Therapeutics* **8**, 57–67. doi:10.2147/ahmt.S110859.

Eisenberg, M.E. *et al.* (2017) Risk and protective factors in the lives of transgender/gender nonconforming adolescents. *Journal of Adolescent Health* **61**(4), 521–526. doi:10.1016/j.jadohealth.2017.04.014.

Engel, L. *et al.* (2023) Assessment of quality of life of transgender and gender-diverse children and adolescents in Melbourne, Australia, 2017-2020. *JAMA Network Open* **6**(2), e2254292. doi:10.1001/jamanetworkopen.2022.54292.

Erlangsen, A. *et al.* (2023) Transgender identity and suicide attempts and mortality in Denmark. *JAMA* **329**(24), 2145–2153. doi:10.1001/jama.2023.8627.

Feder, S. *et al.* (2017) Exploring the association between eating disorders and gender dysphoria in youth. *Eating Disorders* **25**(4), 310–317. doi:10.1080/10640266.2017.1297112.

Fuxjager, M.J. *et al.* (2017) What can animal research tell us about the link between androgens and social competition in humans? *Hormones and Behavior* **92**, 182–189. doi:10.1016/j.yhbeh.2016.11.014.

Grootens-Wiegers, P. *et al.* (2017) Medical decision-making in children and adolescents: developmental and neuroscientific aspects. *BMC Pediatrics* **17**(1), 120. doi:10.1186/s12887-017-0869-x.

Haas, A.P. *et al.* (2011) Suicide and suicide risk in lesbian, gay, bisexual, and transgender populations: review and recommendations. *Journal of Homosexuality* **58**(1), 10–51. doi:10.1080/00918369.2011.534038.

Hall, W.J. & Rodgers, G.K. (2019) Teachers' attitudes toward homosexuality and the lesbian, gay, bisexual, and queer community in the United States. *Social Psychology of Education* **22**, 23–41.

Hall, W.J. *et al.* (2021) Sexual orientation identity development milestones among lesbian, gay, bisexual, and queer people: a systematic review and meta-analysis. *Frontiers in Psychology* **12**, 753954. doi:10.3389/fpsyg.2021.753954.

Handler, T. *et al.* (2019) Trends in referrals to a pediatric transgender clinic. *Pediatrics* **144**(5). doi:10.1542/peds.2019-1368.

Hardy, J. (2021) Queer information literacies: social and technological circulation in the rural Midwestern United States. *Information, Communication and Society* **24**(1), 102–117. doi:10.1080/1369118X.2019.1635184.

Hatchel, T. *et al.* (2021) Suicidal thoughts and behaviors among LGBTQ youth: meta-analyses and a systematic review. *Archives of Suicide Research* **25**(1), 1–37.

Hatzenbuehler, M.L. & Pachankis, J.E. (2016) Stigma and minority stress as social determinants of health among lesbian, gay, bisexual, and transgender youth: research evidence and clinical implications. *Pediatric Clinics of North America* **63**(6), 985–997. doi:10.1016/j.pcl.2016.07.003.

Hatzenbuehler, M.L. *et al.* (2010) The impact of institutional discrimination on psychiatric disorders in lesbian, gay, and bisexual populations: a prospective study. *American Journal of Public Health* **100**(3), 452–459. doi:10.2105/ajph.2009.168815.

Janssen, A. & Leibowitz, S. (2018) *Affirmative Mental Health Care for Transgender and Gender Diverse Youth: A Clinical Guide.* Springer International, Cham, Switzerland. doi:10.1007/978-3-319-78307-9.

Johns, M.M. *et al.* (2019) Transgender identity and experiences of violence victimization, substance use, suicide risk, and sexual risk behaviors among high school students—19 states and large urban school districts, 2017. *Morbidity and Mortality Weekly Report* **68**(3), 67–71. doi:10.15585/mmwr.mm6803a3.

Kaltiala, R. *et al.* (2020) Time trends in referrals to child and adolescent gender identity services: a study in four Nordic countries and in the UK. *Nordic Journal of Psychiatry* **74**(1), 40–44. doi:10.1080/08039488.2019.1667429.

Kellogg, N.D. (2009) Clinical report: the evaluation of sexual behaviors in children. *Pediatrics* **124**(3), 992–998. doi:10.1542/peds.2009-1692.

Kidd, K.M. *et al.* (2021) Prevalence of gender-diverse youth in an urban school district. *Pediatrics* **147**(6). doi:10.1542/peds.2020-049823.

King, T.L. *et al.* (2021) Gender stereotypes and biases in early childhood: a systematic review. *Australasian Journal of Early Childhood* **46**(2), 112–125. doi:10.1177/1836939121999849.

Kingsbury, M. *et al.* (2022) Suicidality among sexual minority and transgender adolescents: a nationally representative population-based study of youth in Canada. *Canadian Medical Association Journal* **194**(22), E767–E774. doi:10.1503/cmaj.212054.

Kohnepoushi, P. *et al.* (2023) Prevalence of suicidal thoughts and attempts in the transgender population of the world: a systematic review and meta-analysis. *Annals of General Psychiatry* **22**(1), 28. doi:10.1186/s12991-023-00460-3.

Kuper, L.E. *et al.* (2020) Body dissatisfaction and mental health outcomes of youth on gender-affirming hormone therapy. *Pediatrics* **145**(4). doi:10.1542/peds.2019-3006.

Lee, J.Y. & Rosenthal, S.M. (2023) Gender-affirming care of transgender and gender-diverse youth: current concepts. *Annual Review of Medicine* **74**(1), 107–116. doi:10.1146/annurev-med-043021-032007.

Leibowitz, S. & de Vries, A.L. (2016) Gender dysphoria in adolescence. *International Review of Psychiatry* **28**(1), 21–35. doi:10.3109/09540261.2015.1124844.

Liu, R.T. *et al.* (2019) Prevalence and correlates of non-suicidal self-injury among lesbian, gay, bisexual, and transgender individuals: a systematic review and meta-analysis. *Clinical Psychology Review* **74**, 101783.

Malpas, J. *et al.* (2022) Family-based interventions with transgender and gender expansive youth: systematic review and best practice recommendations *Transgender. Health* **7**(1), 7–29. doi:10.1089/trgh.2020.0165.

Martin, C.L. & Ruble, D. (2004) Children's search for gender cues: cognitive perspectives on gender development. *Current Directions in Psychological Science* **13**(2), 67–70. doi:10.1111/j.0963-7214.2004.00276.x.

Martin, C.L. & Ruble, D.N. (2010) Patterns of gender development. *Annual Review of Psychology* **61**, 353–381. doi:10.1146/annurev.psych.093008.100511.

Masters, W.H. *et al.* (1995) *Human Sexuality*, 5th edn. HarperCollins College Publishers, New York.

McInroy, L.B. *et al.* (2019) LGBTQ+ youths' community engagement and resource seeking online versus offline. *Journal of Technology in Human Services* **37**(4), 315–333. doi:10.1080/15228835.2019.1617823.

Meijer, J.H. *et al.* (2017) Gender dysphoria and co-existing psychosis: review and four case examples of successful gender affirmative treatment. *LGBT Health* **4**(2), 106–114. doi:10.1089/lgbt.2016.0133.

Meyer, I.H. (2003) Prejudice, social stress, and mental health in lesbian, gay, and bisexual populations: conceptual issues and research evidence. *Psychological Bulletin* **129**, 674–697. doi:10.1037/0033-2909.129.5.674.

Meyer-Bahlburg, H.F.L. *et al.* (2004) Prenatal androgenization affects gender-related behavior but not gender identity in 5–12-year-old girls with congenital adrenal hyperplasia. *Archives of Sexual Behavior* **33**(2), 97–104. doi:10.1023/B:ASEB.0000014324.25718.51.

Meyer-Bahlburg, H.F. *et al.* (2006) Gender development in women with congenital adrenal hyperplasia as a function of disorder severity. *Archives of Sexual Behavior* **35**(6), 667–684. doi:10.1007/s10508-006-9068-9.

Newcomb, M.E. *et al.* (2020) High burden of mental health problems, substance use, violence, and related psychosocial factors in transgender, non-binary, and gender diverse youth and young adults. *Archives of Sexual Behavior* **49**(2), 645–659. doi:10.1007/s10508-019-01533-9.

Olson, K.R. *et al.* (2016) Mental health of transgender children who are supported in their identities. *Pediatrics* **137**(3), e20153223. doi:10.1542/peds.2015-3223.

Owen-Smith, A.A. *et al.* (2018) Association between gender confirmation treatments and perceived gender congruence, body image satisfaction, and mental health in a cohort of transgender individuals. *The Journal of Sexual Medicine* **15**(4), 591–600. doi:10.1016/j.jsxm.2018.01.017.

Olson, K.R. *et al.* (2022) Gender identity 5 years after social transition. *Pediatrics* **150**(2). doi:10.1542/peds.2021-056082.

Parker, L.L. & Harriger, J.A. (2020) Eating disorders and disordered eating behaviors in the LGBT population: a review of the literature. *Journal of Eating Disorders* **8**(1), 51. doi:10.1186/s40337-020-00327-y.

Polderman, T.J.C. *et al.* (2018) The biological contributions to gender identity and gender diversity: bringing data to the table. *Behavior Genetics* **48**(2), 95–108. doi:10.1007/s10519-018-9889-z.

Ponton, L.E. & Judice, S. (2004) Typical adolescent sexual development. *Child and Adolescent Psychiatric Clinics of North America* **13**(3), 497–511, vi. doi:10.1016/j.chc.2004.02.003.

Price, M.N. & Green, A.E. (2023) Association of gender identity acceptance with fewer suicide attempts among transgender and nonbinary youth. *Transgender Health* **8**(1), 56–63. doi:10.1089/trgh.2021.0079.

Rapoport, E. *et al.* (2021) Prevalence of nonheterosexual identity and same-sex sexual contact among high school students in the US from 2015 to 2019. *JAMA Pediatrics* **175**(9), 970–972. doi:10.1001/jamapediatrics.2021.1109.

Ream, G.L. (2022) Trends in deaths by suicide 2014-2019 among lesbian, gay, bisexual, transgender, queer, questioning, and other gender/sexual minority (LGBTQ+) youth. *Journal of Adolescent Health* **71**(5), 609–615. doi:10.1016/j.jadohealth.2022.06.017.

Rider, G.N. *et al.* (2018) Health and care utilization of transgender and gender nonconforming youth: a population-based study. *Pediatrics* **141**(3). doi:10.1542/peds.2017-1683.

Ristori, J. & Steensma, T.D. (2016) Gender dysphoria in childhood. *International Review of Psychiatry* **28**(1), 13–20. doi:10.3109/09540261.2015.1115754.

Rosario, M. *et al.* (2006) A model of sexual risk behaviors among young gay and bisexual men: longitudinal associations of mental health, substance abuse, sexual abuse, and the coming-out process. *AIDS Education and Prevention* **18**(5), 444–460. doi:10.1521/aeap.2006.18.5.444.

Rosenthal, S.M. (2021) Challenges in the care of transgender and gender-diverse youth: an endocrinologist's view. *Nature Reviews. Endocrinology* **17**(10), 581–591. doi:10.1038/s41574-021-00535-9.

Savin-Williams, R.C. (2018) Developmental trajectories and milestones of sexual-minority youth. In: *The Cambridge Handbook of Sexual Development: Childhood and Adolescence.* (eds J. Gilbert & S. Lamb). Cambridge University Press, Cambridge, UK. pp. 156–179. doi:10.1017/9781108116121.009.

Segev-Becker, A. *et al.* (2020) Children and adolescents with gender dysphoria in Israel: increasing referral and fertility preservation rates. *Endocrine Practice* **26**(4), 423–428. doi:10.4158/ep-2019-0418.

Spitzer, R.L. (1981) The diagnostic status of homosexuality in DSM-III: a reformulation of the issues. *American Journal of Psychiatry* **138**(2), 210–215. doi:10.1176/ajp.138.2.210.

Steensma, T.D. *et al.* (2013) Gender identity development in adolescence. *Hormones and Behavior* **64**(2), 288–297. doi:10.1016/j.yhbeh.2013.02.020.

Strang, J.F. *et al.* (2023) In addition to stigma: cognitive and autism-related predictors of mental health in transgender adolescents. *Journal of Clinical Child and Adolescent Psychology* **52**(2), 212–229. doi:10.1080/15374416.2021.1916940.

Toomey, R.B. *et al.* (2018) Transgender adolescent suicide behavior. *Pediatrics* **142**(4), e20174218. doi:10.1542/peds.2017-4218.

Tordoff, D.M. *et al.* (2022) Mental health outcomes in transgender and nonbinary youths receiving gender-affirming care. *JAMA Network Open* **5**(2), e220978–e220978. doi:10.1001/jamanetworkopen.2022.0978.

Trevor Project and Morning Consult (2023) Issue impacting LGBTQ youth. Available: https://www.thetrevorproject.org/wp-content/uploads/2023/01/Issues-Impacting-LGBTQ-Youth-MC-Poll_Public-2.pdf [29 October 2024].

T'Sjoen, G. *et al.* (2019) Endocrinology of transgender medicine. *Endocrine Reviews* **40**(1), 97–117. doi:10.1210/er.2018-00011.

Veale, J.F. *et al.* (2017) Mental health disparities among Canadian transgender youth. *Journal of Adolescent Health* **60**(1), 44–49. doi:10.1016/j.jadohealth.2016.09.014.

Wallen, K. (2005) Hormonal influences on sexually differentiated behavior in nonhuman primates. *Frontiers in Neuroendocrinology* **26**(1), 7–26. doi:10.1016/j.yfrne.2005.02.001.

Wamithi, S. *et al.* (2015) Cross-sectional survey on prevalence of attention deficit hyperactivity disorder symptoms at a tertiary care health facility in Nairobi. *Child and Adolescent Psychiatry and Mental Health* **9**(1), 1. doi:10.1186/s13034-015-0033-z.

Wanta, J.W. *et al.* (2022) Considering 'spheres of influence' in the care of lesbian, gay, bisexual, transgender, and queer-identified youth. *Child and Adolescent Psychiatric Clinics of North America* **31**(4), 649–664. doi:10.1016/j.chc.2022.05.008.

Warrier, V. *et al.* (2020) Elevated rates of autism, other neurodevelopmental and psychiatric diagnoses, and autistic traits in transgender and gender-diverse individuals. *Nature Communications* **11**(1), 3959. doi:10.1038/s41467-020-17794-1.

White Hughto, J.M. *et al.* (2015) Transgender stigma and health: a critical review of stigma determinants, mechanisms, and interventions. *Social Science and Medicine* **147**, 222–231. doi:10.1016/j.socscimed.2015.11.010.

Winter, S. *et al.* (2016) Transgender people: health at the margins of society. *The Lancet* **388**(10042), 390–400. doi:10.1016/s0140-6736(16)00683-8.

CHAPTER 41

Refugee, asylum-seeking, and internally displaced children

Mina Fazel
Department of Psychiatry, University of Oxford, Oxford, UK

Global refugee context

The numbers of children forcibly displaced across the world are ever increasing. The causes of displacement are manifold and include natural disasters, humanitarian crises that range from drought to abject poverty, and upheavals within a country because of war, violence, conflict, or feared persecution. This chapter will focus on children who have been forcibly displaced because of war and persecution as this is the group classified as "refugees." There are a substantial number of internally displaced children (IDP) who have not crossed an international border but might experience similarly precarious conditions who are also included here (see Table 41.1 for definitions). Children in this chapter will refer to children and adolescents under the age of 18 years, unless otherwise specified.

In 2022, there were an estimated 108 million people forcibly displaced because of persecution worldwide, of whom 35 million were officially recognized as refugees, 5.4 million were asylum seekers, 62.5 million were internally displaced, and 5.2 million were "other people in need of international protection" including those from Palestine (UNHCR, 2023b). Forty percent of all forcibly displaced persons were children. Refugees originate from all over the globe, and their countries of origin are constantly shifting, reflecting current global stressors (see Figures 41.1 and 41.2 for maps of countries where IDPs and refugees were residing in 2022 and 2023, respectively; and Figure 41.3 for the major refugee hosting countries for 2022). In 2022, over half of all refugees came from just three countries: Syria, Ukraine, and Afghanistan.

Refugee children are a diverse group (Arakelyan & Ager, 2021). They can range from children that might have experienced relatively limited conflict to those living for many years in unstable and unsafe settings with disrupted families, communities, and education. They might also have a wide variety of different experiences in the journey from a place of conflict to a place of relative safety. They might then settle in countries that can be culturally close or ethnically and culturally very distinct to their countries of origin. Much of the research, therefore, represents a distinct subsection of refugee children—often either by studying a particular postmigration country or one ethnic group. Any conclusions must be interpreted in this light. There are also some high-risk refugee populations, for example, unaccompanied refugee minors, trafficked and undocumented children, former child soldiers, and those with a history of torture, who might need different and tailored mental health support (Arakelyan & Ager, 2021). Furthermore, with increasing numbers of children forcibly displaced across the globe who do not fall under the "refugee" category, understandings garnered from the study of refugee children might be of relevance to these other groups. Many of their postmigration experiences can be similar, even if their premigration stressors might be very different (for example, if leaving because of a natural disaster versus fear of persecution). The latter are discussed in Chapter 18 on global mental health and threats.

It is important to think about the mental health needs of refugee children because their presentation can lie at the intersection of many important risk and protective factors of relevance to mental health and well-being. They carry their unique genetic profiles, but these can intersect with complex family circumstances alongside many other psychosocial changes that result from living in an area of conflict and the numerous problems that can result following forced displacement. A discussion of these factors will be the main focus of this chapter. A search of three databases of all systematic reviews focusing on the mental health of refugee children published in the decade, 2013–2023, was conducted and informs the results presented below.

There are three noteworthy trends that are currently affecting refugee children. The first is that the number of forcibly

Rutter's Child and Adolescent Psychiatry and Psychology, Seventh Edition.
Edited by Anita Thapar, Daniel S. Pine, Samuele Cortese, Cathy Creswell, Tamsin J. Ford, James F. Leckman, and Argyris Stringaris.

Companion website: www.wiley.com/go/thapar/rutterspsych7

Table 41.1 Definitions of displacement.

Term	Description	Estimated global numbers in 2022
Migrant	A person who makes a conscious, voluntary choice to leave their country of origin and who, when they want to, can return home in safety.	41,000,000 children
Refugee	A person who has fled their country due to fear of persecution, and has been granted the legal right to remain in the country of refuge. Refugee status is given to applicants by the United Nations (UN) or by a third-party country.	16,000,000 children
Asylum seeker	A person who has fled their country due to fear of persecution, is seeking international protection, and is applying for refugee status.	1,500,000 children
Internally displaced person	A person living inside the borders of their own country, but unable to safely live in their own home or region.	25,800,000 children
Unaccompanied minor	A child (under 18 years) who has been separated from both parents and other relatives and is not being cared for by an adult who, by law or custom, is responsible for doing so.	41,000–300,000 unaccompanied and separated children
Trafficked person	A person illegally transported or recruited for exploitation by the use of threat, force, fraud, or the abuse of vulnerability.	1,000,000 trafficked annually
Stateless person	A person who does not have a nationality recognized by any country. The exact figure can be difficult to determine because not all stateless individuals are officially registered or recognized.	10,000,000

Source: Mainly taken from United Nations (UN) and United Nations High Commissioner for Refugees (UNHCR) documents (including NSW Government, 2019; Migration Data Portal, 2023; UNHCR, 2023a; UNHCR, 2023c; UNICEF, 2023).

displaced children has been steadily increasing (Figure 41.4) and by 2023 is at the highest number ever recorded. As almost half of all refugees are under the age of 18, in 2022, this amounted to over 17 million child refugees and asylum seekers (UNICEF, 2023).

The second important consideration is that conflicts are increasingly targeting civilian populations (rather than military "combatants") and, concerningly, children. This includes reports of schools being targeted in conflicts, for example, in the Middle East, sub-Saharan Africa, and Europe, as well as increasing recruitment of children into civilian militia. For example, between 30,000 and 300,000 children may have been "stolen" from the Ukraine and taken to Russia as part of a targeted strategy to influence their beliefs (referred to as "Russification") and undermine the Ukrainian population. These can be considered as war crimes, similar to many crimes committed at times of war against children (Ioffe, 2023). Children, especially girls, who have been forced to migrate have been reported to be in situations of physical insecurity, and experience more conflict-related violence, domestic violence, sexual violence, and early and forced marriage (Bennouna *et al.*, 2020; Gordon & Lee-Koo, 2021).

The third relevant consideration is that finding a country of "refuge" is becoming harder. Although there are notable exceptions, such as in the welcome that many Ukrainian refugees experienced in European countries early in the Russian invasion, there are changes in the way refugee children, adolescents, and families are settled and managed in the places in which they arrive. For example, more refugees are being placed in temporary housing, refugee camps in third/transit countries, or detention centers. Furthermore, with the increasing barriers placed in the way of legally reaching countries of refuge, more children are traveling under traffickers, putting their lives at heightened risk.

Conceptualizing refugee children's experiences

A useful way to frame the refugee experience is into pre-, peri-, and postmigration, as described in the Video 41.1 (which can be found on the companion website for this book) introducing this chapter where an unaccompanied minor depicts their journey. The stressors are particularly complicated in each of these different periods and therefore benefit from specific consideration, especially for the refugee child, their family, their community, and educational contexts.

Each refugee context is different and unique. There are important overall trends to be aware of, depending on the conflict and the nature of persecution and threat encountered. Many refugee groups have been predominantly male, usually traveling alone either to escape involvement in armed conflict or being the target of the conflict. Younger males are most likely to be recruited into armies, and so have often been the first to leave many situations, also hoping to either carve the way for their families to later join them or send back financial resources. In these situations, refugee children might have been left without a parental figure in their countries of origin—with or without awareness of their parent's motives. Maintaining a relationship at a distance, if safely possible, and also navigating the complexities of reunification with family members, if this does take place, might require careful consideration of the mental health impacts on both the children and their family

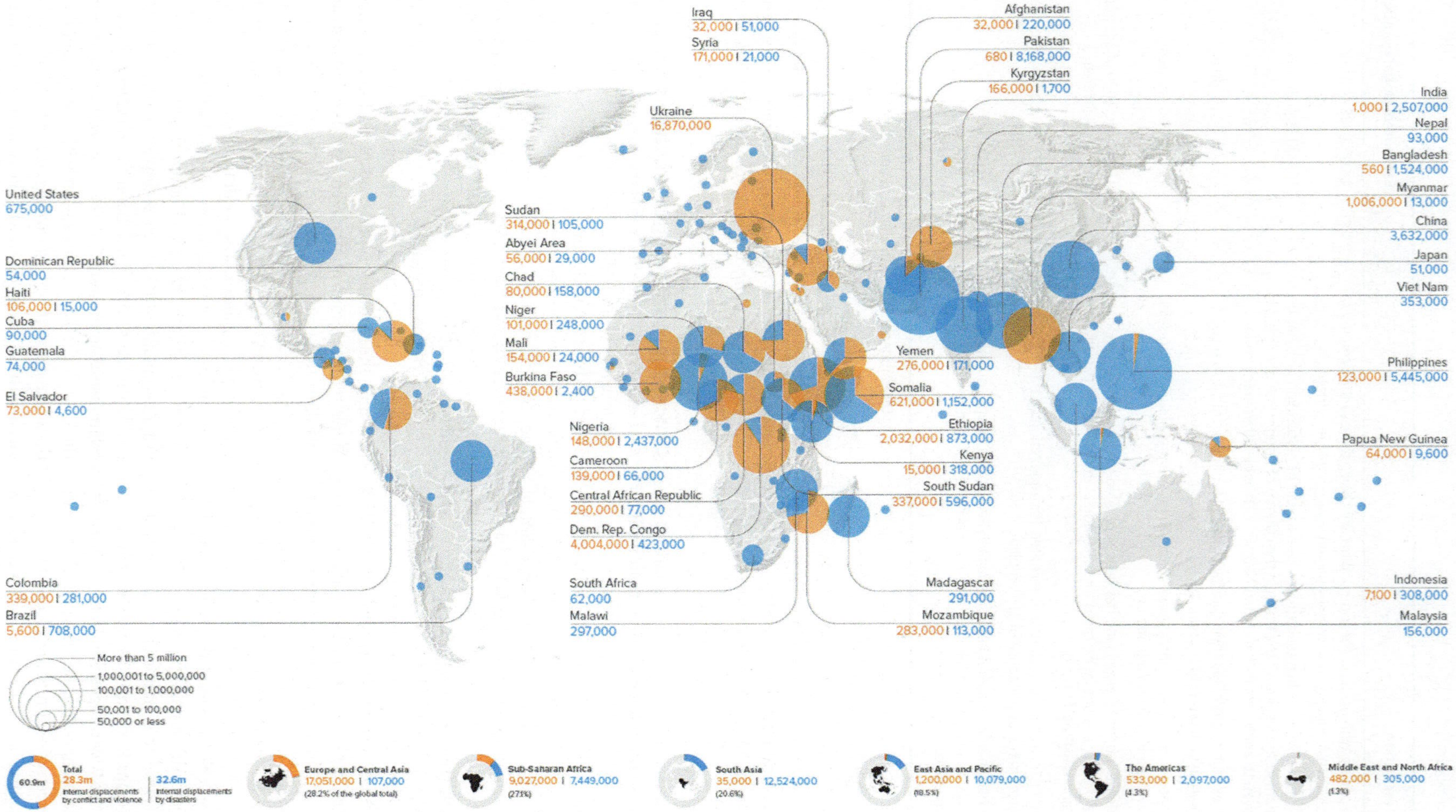

The country and territory names and figures are shown only when the total displacements value exceeds 50,000.
Due to rounding, some totals may not correspond with the sum of the separate figures.

Figure 41.1 Internal displacements by conflict and disaster in 2022. *Source:* .

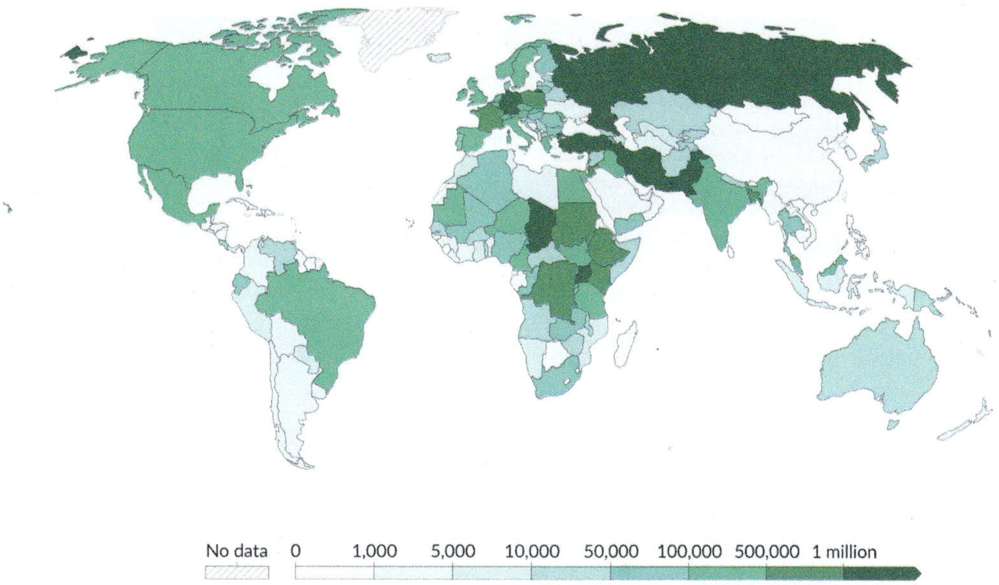

Figure 41.2 Refugee population by country or territory of asylum, 2023. The total number of refugees by country that they are taking asylum in.
Source: UNHCR (2024); OurWorldInData.org/migration

members. In contrast, in the relatively recent Ukrainian refugee situation women and children were the predominant refugees. Therefore, the implications for family and children need to be considered within each of these different contexts. In postmigration nations there will be refugees from very different regions and with different experiences to the host nation. In the United Kingdom (UK) in 2023, there were recent refugee arrivals from Afghanistan, Ukraine, and Iran, alongside legacy communities, under different living, working, and immigration regulations—all of which impact on refugee children.

In the premigration environment, children might have experienced many years of disruption and witnessed, or been injured in, a range of adverse and potentially traumatic events. Their families, education, and communities might have been under stress for a number of years and they might have experienced significant periods without education, felt that their lives were threatened, and experienced complex bereavements. The negative impact of experiencing the threat of harm and prolonged instability at such an important developmental period cannot be underestimated. In a comprehensive review, Arakelyan and Ager (2021) describe the multilevel bioecological factors that influence the mental health and psychosocial well-being of refugee children. They highlight how, given the developmental needs of refugee children, consideration needs to also be taken of the child's sense of agency alongside the sociopolitical context of the countries they are from and currently residing in.

Evidence collated from refugee studies highlights how some might experience multiple atrocities in the premigration phase of forced migration (Arakelyan & Ager, 2021). Common reports include experience of armed conflict, political persecution, financial hardship, homelessness, physical violence, torture or sexual abuse, maltreatment, or bereavement. A dose–response association is often reported whereby children experiencing multiple and prolonged exposures before displacement later present with more severe post-traumatic stress disorder (PTSD), depression, and anxiety. Differences are also identified in relation to type of trauma exposure. Children who suffer physical violence, and witness gunfights and people being killed are more likely to present with more severe PTSD (Arakelyan & Ager, 2021). Please refer to Chapter 58 where trauma-related psychopathology is discussed.

Refugee children can continue to be exposed to many of these stressors in the perimigration or "flight" phase of their journeys with possible exposure to violence, hunger, physical or sexual abuse, detention, forced labor, and homelessness. This might be especially prominent for unaccompanied children at high risk of exploitation by traffickers. In one of the few qualitative studies of such experiences, 19 unaccompanied minors in Italy were interviewed. All reported physical abuse (e.g., being insulted, hit with an object, punished with infliction of pain, tortured, forced to engage in dangerous activity) and more than half had experienced sexual abuse (Longobardi *et al.*, 2017).

Since 2010, the most marked development in the evidence base has been in the improved understanding of the extent and impact of postmigration stressors. Host countries often fall short in providing adequate psychosocial and health care, as well as educational and financial support to refugee children (Arakelyan & Ager, 2021). Dissatisfaction and emotional tensions arising from uncertainty, unmet needs and expectations are linked to a range of persistent psychosocial problems. Again, these experiences are more pronounced for unaccompanied minors, who are variably accommodated in the care system (Jensen *et al.*, 2014; Hirani *et al.*, 2018; see Chapter 42 for the mental health needs of children in the care system). A 2-year

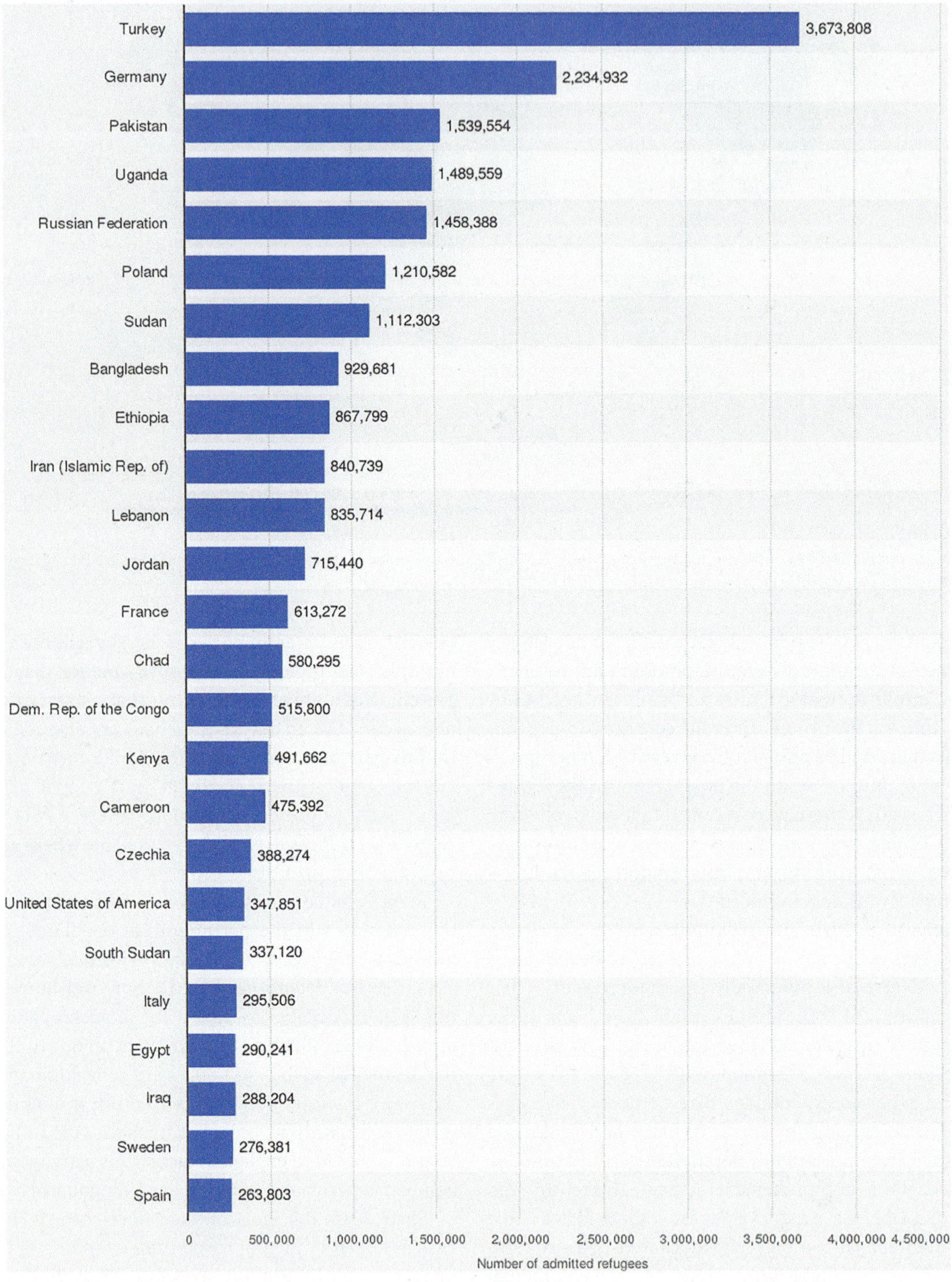

Figure 41.3 Countries hosting the largest numbers of refugees (2022). These are the numbers of refugees that are "currently" under the United Nations High Commissioner for Refugees (UNHCR) mandate. *Source:* Adapted from UNHCR (2022a).

follow-up assessment of unaccompanied refugee children's mental health resettled in Norway showed that psychopathology remained high over time, with 11% scoring high on suicidal ideation (Jensen *et al.*, 2014).

Younger children are generally at greater risk for developing psychopathology in response to war-related adversities (Beiser *et al.*, 2015; Lincoln *et al.*, 2016; Aitcheson *et al.*, 2017). This might be because infants and young children rely heavily on parents (or other caregivers) for food, warmth, shelter, and protection (Smith & Waite, 2019). Provisions of these basic resources can be heavily compromised for refugee families, especially for those in temporary settlements.

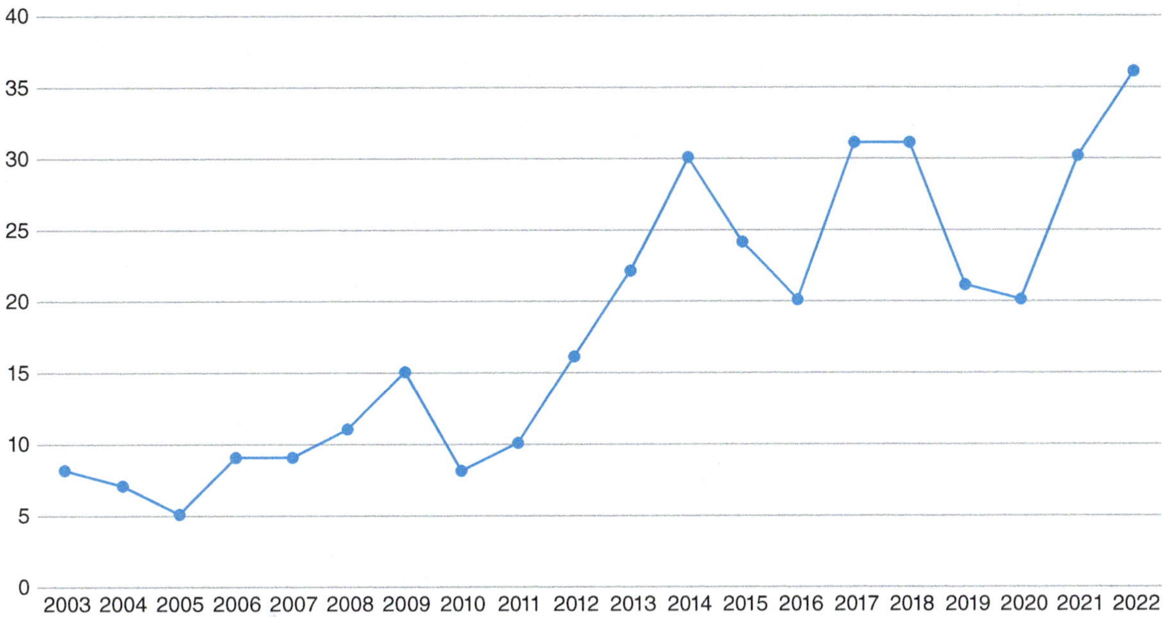

Figure 41.4 Newly displaced persons per minute (2003 to 2022).

Common clinical presentations

Literature review

Despite the increased research attention on the mental health needs of refugee children, the prevalence estimates of mental illness are based on relatively small numbers of studies. Blackmore's systematic review identified only 8 eligible studies for the 15 years up to 2018, involving 779 child and adolescent refugees and asylum seekers, conducted in only 5 countries (Blackmore *et al.*, 2020). The studies were conducted in Turkey, Germany, Sweden, Norway, and Malaysia and were studying refugees from different countries of origin.

Consistent with many other studies, the most prevalent mental illness was PTSD, with an overall prevalence of 22.71% (95% CI 12.79–32.64) (Blackmore *et al.*, 2020). PTSD is also the most studied disorder. The additional classification of complex PTSD has been studied less although is probably highly relevant for this population. The clearest risk factor for PTSD in refugee child populations is the number of previous exposures to potentially traumatic events. These events can take place in any of the stages of migration—pre-, peri-, and postmigration—so careful history taking is essential.

Anxiety disorders and depressive disorders are the next most commonly identified mental illnesses, often having high comorbidity with each other and also with PTSD. In the Blackmore *et al.* review (2020), the prevalence of anxiety disorders was 15.77% (95% CI 8.04–23.50) and of depression was 13.81% (95% CI 5.96–21.67).

A systematic review of migration and age of presentation of psychotic disorders reinforced the long-established risk of migration for psychosis. The risk of psychotic disorder among people who migrate prior to age 18 was identified as nearly twice as high as the native-born population (Anderson & Edwards, 2020). Of note, people who migrate during early adulthood (19–29 years) had a similar risk of psychotic disorder as the native-born population (IRR = 0.93, 95% CI 0.60–1.44). Although this review did not specifically report on child refugee status, there is no reason to suspect that the anticipated rates would be lower and, if anything, might be higher (Fazel *et al.*, 2005).

A number of other disorders have been studied, but less so. These include attention deficit hyperactivity disorder (ADHD), which has a relatively high prevalence when identified of 8.6% (95% CI 1.08-16.12) and oppositional defiant disorder (ODD) at 1.69% (95% CI 0.78–4.16) (Blackmore *et al.*, 2020).

Parental mental health problems are discussed below in the section on "Range of presentations." It is important to be aware of parental mental health problems, including perinatal mental health disorders (Anderson *et al.*, 2017), exacerbated by low social support, minority ethnicity, low socioeconomic status (SES), lack of proficiency in host country language, and refugee or asylum-seeking status. These issues all place migrant parent populations at increased risk of mental illness and especially perinatal mental disorders.

Range of presentations

As discussed, refugee and asylum-seeker children have high rates of PTSD, depression, and anxiety. The presentations of these disorders are likely to have some similarities and differences to host populations. The most important difference will be in the identification of these disorders given the cultural differences that are likely to exist in the understanding of and attitudes toward mental health difficulties. Although mental illness remains one of the most highly stigmatized areas of health, it is possible that many refugees come from societies where mental illness might be less publicly discussed and potentially even more stigmatized. This can impact on attitudes to help-seeking (Box 41.1) and also on willingness to discuss their difficulties—because of this stigma or because of a lack of understanding that the symptoms they are experiencing might be something that is amenable to treatment.

Sleep disturbance is a common presentation for refugee children and also likely to be impaired for most mental illnesses (Richter *et al.*, 2020). In younger refugee populations, psychological problems and disturbed sleep are associated with previous traumatic experiences during their journey to the host country. The sleep difficulties can include acute insomnia, recurrent nightmares, disturbed sleep, and substantial daytime sleepiness.

There are also higher rates of somatic presentations of mental health problems, such as headaches and abdominal pain, in refugee children (Clemente *et al.*, 2022). This can be appreciated given host language difficulties, culturally different presentations of mental illness, and fear of potential stigmatization. Somatization is therefore prominent and should be enquired about in detail.

Finally, the importance of the family context cannot be overestimated. There are innumerable stressors that affect forcibly displaced families, from premigration exposures that can cause post-traumatic symptomatology and/or the complex changes that can take place in relationships and roles following these experiences (Fazel & Betancourt, 2018). There can be greatly enhanced family coherence as a result of their forced displacement experience. It is, however, important to note, there are many difficulties that can arise from fractured relationships and family separation including increased rates of interpersonal conflict and violence, as well as child maltreatment. If mental health difficulties are contributing to these family stressors then it is important for parental mental illness to be identified and treated (see Figure 41.5 for a helpful model of how premigration and postmigration stressors impact on child and adolescent mental health) (Fazel, 2019).

Kelstrup and Carlsson's systematic review of traumatized refugee parents and the mental health impacts on their children (both trauma-exposed and nonexposed) included 12 studies (Kelstrup & Carlsson, 2022). Parenting style was identified as both a potential risk and a protective factor, with most studies emphasizing the negative effects of parental mental illness. There was substantial evidence of an association between parental PTSD and increased risk of psychological problems in offspring. Risk/protective factors at the individual and family level were identified, but small sample sizes and limitations in

Box 41.1 Practice pointers for assessing refugee mental health needs

For mental health services

- Location of provision
  There are many advantages to co-locating mental health services in community settings to enable access for refugee communities. There are examples of services set up in schools, in primary care, and in community centers alongside charities.
- Skill base of staff
  The most common presentations are of anxiety, depression, and PTSD, and many of the needs of these children will lie within the existing skill set of services. There are advantages and disadvantages to setting up special, targeted services (advantages include awareness of the current immigration processes and local service landscape, and developing expertise), while maintaining provision within generic services also has advantages (ensures all members of the mental health services maintain skills, ensures provision remains accessible to all as not all in need are categorized as "refugees").
- Language support
  Interpretation support is essential—either with in-person interpreters or via online or telephone-based support—dependent on location of service and resources available. Some families will not want external interpreters, and when there are ethnic and cultural tensions, it is important to be sensitive about bringing in an individual who might be perceived as threatening.
- Linking with other services and organizations

For individual assessments

The assessment needs to take into account general principles—please refer to Chapter 27 on clinical assessment and Chapter 30 on physical examination. In addition, it is important to find out:

- Displacement History
  This includes a detailed history of the premigration experience and how long the child lived in an area of political and physical insecurity, as well as information about their household, community, and education. The migration experience and journey to their current home, and what might have happened to them and their companions, needs to be sensitively explored. Then, gain an understanding of the myriad complexities of arrival in different postmigration settings.
- Health history
  As many refugees come from lower-resource settings, asking about communicable and noncommunicable diseases is important, as well as obtaining more detailed information if there is any history of exposure to organized violence or torture, including head injury.
- Education history
  There are many disruptions that can take place in education and some of these might have mental health impacts. An understanding of how a child was coping prior to any disruptions to their education and subsequent to their displacement is needed.
- Current living circumstances
  This needs to include who is in their current home, their sense of safety and security, and the mental health of those with whom they are living.
- Broader stressors
  The immigration determination process, the educational (and, for family, occupational) opportunities, and the community around the child, are some of the many potential different stressors that need to be examined.

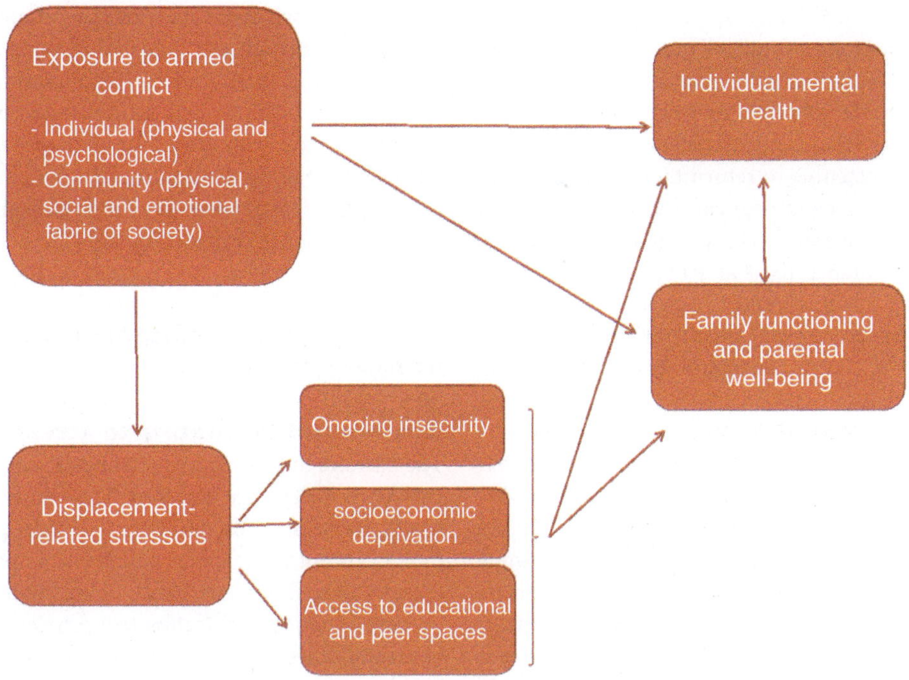

Figure 41.5 Model of stressful exposures and their relationship to mental health for refugee children. *Source:* Adapted from Miller and Rasmussen (2010).

study designs were noted. In another systematic review of adult migrant populations, those exposed to premigration armed conflict had the poorest mental health outcomes (Mesa-Vieira *et al.*, 2022). This is further reinforced by the description by Arakelyan and Ager (2021) of the different ways that family factors can impact on refugee children. They describe the negative impact of persistent exposure to stressors from multilayered developmental contexts on children's emotional well-being and psychosocial adjustment via influences of parental psychopathology (familial factors), interparental conflict (familial factors) and low quality of parent–child interactions (proximal processes) (Arakelyan & Ager, 2021).

Finally, in a systematic review of family-related violence in refugee families (Timshel *et al.*, 2017), the risk and protective factors associated with these families were categorized at the individual, family, societal, and cultural levels. For example, at the individual level, parental trauma experiences/mental illness, substance abuse, and history of child abuse were found to be risk factors. Family-level risk factors included the quality of the parent–child interaction, family structure, and family acculturation stress. At the societal level, low SES was identified as a risk factor. Cultural-level risk factors included patriarchal beliefs. Positive parental coping strategies were a protective factor. They conducted a further ecological analysis of the results highlighting how family-related violence in refugee families could result from accumulating multiple risk factors on the individual, familial, societal, and cultural levels—underlining the importance of multilevel interventions to address the many different stressors being encountered.

Complexity of assessment

The different experiences a refugee child might have had, as well as the range of mental health problems they and their families can present with, makes the assessment of a refugee child a potentially complex and delicate task. This has been discussed in a number of places and, in summary, benefits from cultural and linguistic support, sufficient allocation of time, and an appreciation of the different periods of adversity the child and their family have potentially experienced (Fazel, 2018). There is a marked absence of validated psychometric tools for accurate measurement (Gadeberg *et al.*, 2017), somewhat expected given the number of different cultures refugee communities come from.

Some factors, such as sense of belonging in the host country, can be a risk or protective factor depending on the time point, and their gender and cultural identity. At present, we know much more about risk factors than about protective factors. Knowing more about protective factors may inform the development of interventions to foster them; see Box 41.1 and Chapter 23 on resilience.

Asylum-seeking children including unaccompanied minors

Children who have not yet been granted the permanent right to remain in their host countries, and especially those who are unaccompanied minors (referred to as unaccompanied refugee minors [URM] or unaccompanied asylum-seeking children [UASC]), need special consideration. Their risk for developing mental health difficulties is exacerbated by the instability of their immigration status. Furthermore, policies in some nations, that seem to place deterrence ahead of protection of asylum seekers, can have a particularly negative impact on children. For example, tightening border controls and/or placing children and families in large hostels, detention centers, or offshore processing facilities (or threatening to return them to their countries of origin or to transit countries) can leave these children with little capacity to manage survival needs in the host country. The evidence suggests higher rates of PTSD and depression among older children, but this trend is especially apparent in those who are unaccompanied (who are often in the older child age-bracket (Jensen *et al.*, 2014; Longobardi *et al.*, 2017; Hirani *et al.*, 2018)).

The time taken before an asylum determination decision is made can range from weeks to years, and this period of instability is particularly complex for the mental health of unaccompanied minors. A systematic review by Daniel-Calveras *et al.* (2022) of the mental health of unaccompanied refugee minors in Europe described how a notable proportion of the child refugees entering Europe are unaccompanied. Their review included 23 studies conducted in 9 countries examining 80,651 child and adolescent URM. Afghanistan was the most common country of origin in most studies and >75% were boys. Many of the studies (N = 13, 56.5%) assessed PTSD prevalence. They reported a high prevalence of mental illness, which varied between 4.6–43% for PTSD (with lower rates for accompanied versus unaccompanied minors), 2.9–61.6% for depression, 32.6–38.2% for anxiety, and 4–14.3% for behavioral problems. They also observed higher rates of self-harm in URM compared to the host population. The studies examining risk factors for mental illness suggest that levels of social support in the host country and rearing environment are associated with mental health outcomes.

A synthesis of qualitative studies examining the stressors for URM confirmed that the number of stressful/adverse life events are both the most evaluated and confirmed risk factor for the mental health of URM (Höhne *et al.*, 2020). A stable environment and social support were shown to protect URM from developing poor mental health. Besides that, several other influencing factors were identified, such as type of accommodation, family contact, gender, and cultural competences (described as knowledge and skills about verbal and nonverbal communication and interpersonal behavior patterns to help develop a sense of belonging within both the heritage and the host culture).

Mitra and Hodes (2019) examined factors that enhanced URM resilience in postmigration contexts and showed that URM in more supportive living arrangements, including foster care, had a lower risk of PTSD and lower depressive symptoms compared with those in semi-independent care arrangements (Mitra & Hodes, 2019) (see Chapter 23 on resilience as principles are consistent with observation in refugee populations). URM living in reception facilities that restricted freedom had more anxiety symptoms. Female URM are more vulnerable than males (Mohwinkel *et al.*, 2018), likely due to their smaller numbers, and greater risk of abuse during all phases of migration.

Less is known about the longer-term outcomes for URM (as well as for most refugee children) as there are few longitudinal studies. Vervliet *et al.* studied 103 unaccompanied minors over 18 months in Belgium, and demonstrated that not only did this population have high scores for anxiety, depression, and PTSD but also these levels did not improve over time, highlighting the risk of long-term persistence of mental health problems in refugee populations (Vervliet *et al.*, 2014).

Interventions to support the mental health of refugee children

Barriers and facilitators to accessing care

The barriers to accessing mental health support can be particularly high for refugee children. They do not present to mental health services in the numbers that their predicted psychopathology would indicate, which is important to consider (Fazel, 2018). There are likely to be barriers to accessing care because of poor identification that problems might be indicative of mental illness, lack of understanding of host-country mental health services, especially if these services are different to those from their countries of origin, and worries that accessing care might impact on any ongoing immigration determination decisions. Refugee children accompanied by adult carers are dependent on their carers to be able to access support. If these carers have their own unidentified mental health problems, in particular PTSD, then accessing care might be compounded by the core PTSD symptom of avoidance. Avoidance can make it even harder to access care, if they fear that support will also potentially include discussion of their own previous traumatic exposures (see Chapter 58).

A systematic review highlighted how few URM had good access to mental health services despite high prevalence of psychiatric symptoms (Mitra and Hodes, 2019). One study in the review found that only 30% of URM had foster parents or guardians who could detect a mental health need and URM were less likely than accompanied children to receive trauma-focused interventions, cognitive therapy, or even practical assistance with basic social needs (Mitra & Hodes, 2019). Three studies found cognitive behavioral therapy (CBT) improved PTSD symptoms and mental health outcomes, but in general there are few studies evaluating treatment effectiveness for this group (Mitra & Hodes, 2019).

There are many examples of good practice, including involvement of refugee community members in service provision and making services accessible in community locations, such as schools (Fazel & Betancourt, 2018). Good linguistic support is essential but does complicate access to care—official interpreters might be limited in number and if they come from the same community as the refugee, this might compound problems of access if confidentiality, even if promised, is not actually believed. Consistency of interpreter can assist in the therapeutic relationship, if a refugee child is needing longer-term psychotherapeutic support, but it can be difficult to find an interpreter able to commit to longer-term work, as well as access to the financial resources to pay for it. There are many difficulties in utilizing family members for interpretation—even though these individuals might be better trusted by a refugee child, they might impede a child's decision to share more sensitive information (Patel *et al.*, 2021).

Principles of evidence-based mental health interventions

As demonstrated by the high rates of mental health problems and the difficulties in accessing mental health care, the provision of evidence-based interventions aimed at improving child refugee outcomes is of particular importance. A systematic review and narrative synthesis of 31 studies identified five critical time points for the mental health of asylum seekers and refugees in high-income countries (Giacco, 2019). These five periods could potentially guide the development and selection of well-timed preventive and treatment interventions: (i) before the travel; (ii) during the travel; (iii) at initial settlement in the host country; (iv) when attempting to integrate in the host country; and (v) when the immigration status is challenged or revoked (Giacco, 2019).

It is necessary to focus not only on the refugee child but also on their environment—be that parents, family, community, and school. For adult refugees, there is good evidence of the efficacy and acceptability of psychosocial interventions for asylum seekers and refugees. Psychosocial interventions are broadly defined as interventions with a focus on the interrelation between social circumstances and peoples' thoughts, emotions, and behaviors, and include cognitive and narrative therapies (such as CBT and narrative exposure therapy (NET)), group therapies, family-group interventions, and common elements treatment approaches (CETA) (see Chapters 31–36 on psychological therapies). A review of 26 studies with 1959 participants revealed that psychosocial interventions have a clinically significant beneficial effect on PTSD, depression, and anxiety outcomes (Turrini *et al.*, 2019). Most evidence-supported interventions are based on CBT with a trauma-focused component.

Focusing on parenting interventions to improve child refugee outcomes has an emerging evidence base with emphasis on improving parental mental health and reinforcing parenting skills (Kelstrup & Carlsson, 2022). The Arakelyan and Ager (2021) research review concluded that the greatest impact for the mental health of refugee children would be from multilevel interventions across systems of support and including more family members. These interventions need to address synergies between ecological systems, engaging proximal processes (including parenting programs) and interventions facilitating the agency of the developing refugee child. As they describe: "Refugee families high in interpersonal conflict may become overloaded with stress. Stress can foster more conflict and conflict elevates stress levels in parents." Accumulated tension from parental mental health and interpersonal conflict often spills over into parent–child interactions. This can then manifest in harsh or punitive parenting behaviors (proximal processes), negatively impacting on child psychosocial developmental outcomes. Therefore, addressing the mental health and psychosocial needs of refugee children requires thorough consideration of the mental health cascade across generations and the cumulative adversities that can negatively impact on proximal processes within a family system (Arakelyan & Ager, 2021). Improvements in family cohesion may support psychosocial and mental health outcomes in refugee children (Fazel & Betancourt, 2018; Arakelyan & Ager, 2021). There are, however, few studies on family interventions (Slobodin & de Jong, 2015) or community interventions (Soltan *et al.*, 2022).

In a systematic review examining treatments for depression for refugee children, 16 interventions were identified as meeting the study inclusion criteria (Simenec & Reid, 2022). It is important to note that the interventions were assessed using an ecological framework and findings suggested that interventions including caregivers, involving the child's community, addressing multiple contexts, and that are culturally informed may improve outcomes. This further reinforces the need to design and evaluate interventions across the whole system rather than a siloed approach of targeting and evaluating the child in isolation. A meta-analytic review investigating specific psychosocial treatments for children and adolescents after man-made *and* natural disasters identified 36 relevant studies (Brown *et al.*, 2017). Overall, treatments showed high effect sizes in pre-post comparisons (Hedges' g = 1.34) and medium effect sizes as compared with control conditions (Hedges' g = 0.43). Treatments investigated by at least two studies were CBT, eye movement desensitization and reprocessing (EMDR), NET for children (KIDNET), and classroom-based interventions, which showed similar effect sizes. However, studies were very heterogenous with regard to their outcomes, limiting comparisons.

The postmigration context and belonging

The importance of the postmigration environment has been an increasing focus of research for refugee children, although there remain many areas that are still poorly understood. Many of the pre- and perimigration stressors are less easy to modify for those working in postmigration countries. The postmigration stressors, however, are more tractable, yet most postmigration countries have policies that perpetuate detrimental mental health outcomes through continued stressors. A focus on the prevention of mental health difficulties for refugee children can highlight the many aspects of the postmigration environment which can contribute to mental health outcomes. For example, in a review on preventive mental health interventions, individual and parental therapeutic interventions were discussed alongside the importance of living circumstances, the school and community, and social interactions (Fazel & Betancourt, 2018). Therefore, those working in postmigration settings need to find ways to coordinate and collaborate across sectors to provide support and services to refugee children and their carers, family members, and communities. Furthermore, the importance of enhancing a sense of belonging has been identified as important for maintaining good mental health. Belonging can be experienced in a number of ways—within the school environment (to the school, felt from the teachers and peers), by their families within their communities, and by the postmigration community within society as a whole (Abdi *et al.*, 2023). A serious commitment is therefore needed, not only from health and resettlement services, but also throughout many of the institutions and individuals with which refugee children and their families interact.

One example of a postmigration policy that can seriously compromise the mental health of forcibly displaced children is that of immigration detention. Detention facilities are being utilized in many low-, middle-, and high-income countries, with many also incarcerating children, including children forcibly separated at international borders, such as in the United States (U.S.) (Ataiants *et al.*, 2018; Hampton *et al.*, 2021). There is overwhelming evidence that such treatment is likely to seriously compromise the short-, medium-, and long-term mental health of children experiencing immigration detention, as well as those placed in care when their parents are detained (Fazel *et al.*, 2014). A scoping review of the mental health consequences of such policies identified 22 studies of children detained by 6 countries (Australia, Canada, Hong Kong, Netherlands, the UK, and the U.S.) (Mares, 2021). It provides a rich and consistent picture of the experience and impact of immigration detention on children's well-being, parental mental health, and parenting, compounding perimigration trauma and loss by further adversity while detained.

It is therefore important to provide early support to refugee children to mitigate risk for educational disadvantage and poor social integration in postmigration communities. A growing literature points to challenges within the postmigration context as key determinants of poor mental health. In a systematic review examining "everyday stressors" and postmigration factors, early detection of poor adjustment and interventions to facilitate positive adaptation within refugee communities was identified as a critical public health priority (Hou *et al.*, 2020). Analysis of 59 eligible studies (n = 17,763) revealed that daily stressors were associated with higher psychiatric symptoms and general distress (Hou *et al.*, 2020). Larger effect sizes were observed for mixed daily stressors relative to subjective, interpersonal, and material daily stressors, and for general distress relative to posttraumatic stress symptoms and general well-being. Effect sizes were also larger for children and adolescents relative to adults, confirming the crucial role unfavorable everyday life experiences play and their negative associations with poor mental health among refugees.

In a review of 63 studies examining the postmigration outcomes for refugees (Scharpf *et al.*, 2021), premigration individual (risk: exposure to war-related trauma, female gender) and postmigration family factors (risk: parental mental health problems and impaired parenting; protective: family cohesion) had the strongest evidence base. Postmigration community (protective: school connectedness, support by peers) and sociocultural factors (risk: discrimination and acculturative stress; protective: integrative acculturation) also had some support in high-income settings.

A review of experiences reported by Canadian refugee children also indicated the importance of family involvement, as well as school settings as points of care and services. They recommend that in terms of timing, there should be a focus on the first year following arrival (Guruge & Butt, 2015). The importance of the initial settlement period has further been reinforced in a systematic review synthesizing research about psychosocial interventions for refugee youth during the first year after arrival (Hettich *et al.*, 2020). Seven studies showed positive effects on psychological symptoms of anxiety, PTSD, and depression, as well as on the personal development of adolescents regarding their life satisfaction, hope for the future, and social and cultural integration. Effective elements of interventions were categorized into trauma-related elements (self-efficacy, safety, and connectedness) and elements associated with forced migration (culture, postmigration environment, and support network).

Role of schools

Schools have been identified across refugee studies as a key institution to support the mental health of refugee children (Fazel & Betancourt, 2018; Arakelyan & Ager, 2021). School is a location where refugee children not only access academic opportunities but are also most likely to receive linguistic instruction and potentially build important social, peer, family, and community networks. In a systematic review of academic achievement and psychosocial adjustment, child refugees in the 45 included studies had high rates of academic difficulties and poor psychosocial well-being (Aghajafari *et al.*, 2020). Although early educational deficits often resolved with time spent in the host country, the risks for psychosocial problems persisted.

It can be particularly difficult to identify the education needs of refugee children when they first arrive, especially if their carers have poor language proficiency. Their academic performance will need to be interpreted in the knowledge of the extent of educational disruption before and during migration, and underlying learning difficulties can be complex to identify—especially if there are also mental health problems such as depression, anxiety, or PTSD. Identifying autism spectrum disorder (ASD) is also particularly difficult if the child or parents cannot speak the host-country language and the cultures are very different. In a systematic review of learning problems in refugee children (Graham *et al.*, 2016), 34 included studies showed that refugee youth had similar secondary school outcomes to their native-born peers. There were no data on preschool or primary school outcomes. There was limited prevalence data on learning problems, with single studies informing most estimates and no studies examining specific language disorders or ASD. Major risk factors for learning problems included parental misunderstandings about educational styles and expectations, teacher stereotyping and low expectations, bullying and racial discrimination, premigration and postmigration trauma, and immigration detention. Factors for success included high academic and life ambition, parental involvement in education, family cohesion and a supportive home environment, accurate educational assessment and grade placement, teacher understanding of linguistic and cultural heritage, culturally appropriate school transition, supportive peer relationships, and successful acculturation.

A scoping review of school-based programs for supporting the mental health and psychosocial well-being of adolescent refugees in high-income countries, described the central role schools play for families (Bennouna *et al.*, 2019). The included studies faced similar challenges including school capacity, the need to better adapt to individual needs, and their multiple needs, as well as building trusting partnerships with schools, communities, and students. In the supplementary materials, a refugee mental health toolbox developed for teachers is included. It includes different suggestions about how to support the mental health of refugee children alongside commonly utilized psychotherapeutic techniques including relaxation techniques, sleep advice, and how to manage difficult emotions. Evaluation of this "mental health toolbox" showed how the most commonly utilized "tools" were relaxation techniques and sleep advice (Fazel *et al.*, 2023).

Refugee children in low- and middle-income settings

The highest proportion of forcibly displaced children reside in low- and middle-income countries (LMICs), primarily in their countries of origin, as IDPs, or in countries neighboring their countries of origin. Many of these environments are poorly resourced with poor sanitary, housing, and health availability but might be culturally closer. Whole community structures might be transplanted into these new areas. Refugees might be placed in refugee camps as a way to house large numbers fleeing in acute emergencies, although many camps remain utilized for longer periods of time, with even second- and third-generation refugees born into these settings (Table 41.2).

Physical, psychological, and educational development can be challenging in refugee camp settings (Figure 41.6). However, relative to communities in regions around borders or compared to provision for IDPs, there might be better provision as often humanitarian organizations (United Nations Educational, Scientific and Cultural Organization [UNESCO], United Nations High Commissioner for Refugees [UNHCR], and United Nations Children's Fund [UNICEF]) are involved in psychosocial and education programs. Systematic reviews have demonstrated the weak evidence base regarding the impact of

Table 41.2 Largest refugee camps in 2023.

Location	Name	Estimated population	Country of origin of most inhabitants
Bangladesh	***Kutupalong*** in Cox's Bazar	800,000–960,000	Myanmar (Rohingya)
Kenya	***Kakuma*** Refugee Camp	200,000	South Sudan, Sudan, Somalia, DR Congo, Burundi, Ethiopia, Uganda
Kenya	***Dadaab*** Refugee Complex	200,000–330,000	Somalia
Jordan	***Za'atari*** Refugee Camp	80,000–160,000	Syria

Source: Adapted from WFP (2023).

such interventions. For example, a meta-analysis of the impact of Child Friendly Spaces (CFS), one commonly implemented intervention after humanitarian emergencies (Hermosilla *et al.*, 2019), only identified some inconsistent mental health protective and promotive impacts for younger children but no impact with older children or in connecting children and carers with wider community resources. As some displacement is protracted, these camps have been described as "incinerators of time" placing many lives in limbo—educationally, occupationally, and socially. This questions the very phrasing of "temporary," particularly as one in five refugees live in refugee camps (Qasmiyeh, 2020).

A review of mental health outcomes for youth living in refugee camps described how they face a wide range of difficulties placing them at risk for trauma exposure and negative mental health outcomes; but little is known about specific mental health outcomes (Vossoughi *et al.*, 2018). Twenty studies were included in the review and among these studies, the prevalence of mental health disorders varied greatly, with some studies reporting high prevalence for PTSD. Levels of anxiety, somatic symptoms, depression, and aggression also varied across studies with fairly consistent findings of a range of maladjustment problems. Conducting research in these settings is beset with many difficulties and barriers (Reed *et al.*, 2012).

Psychosocial interventions for refugee children in LMICs draw from a small number of studies. A systematic review of "focused" psychosocial interventions for children in low-resource humanitarian settings (Purgato *et al.*, 2018) demonstrated a beneficial effect of focused psychosocial support on PTSD symptoms (especially for those aged 15–18 years) and benefits for functional impairment. They were also shown to increase hope, coping, and social support.

In a research review of resilience and mental health in children and adolescents living in areas of armed conflict within LMICs, 53 studies were identified (mostly cross-sectional) (Tol *et al.*, 2013). Generally, promotive and protective factors showed gender-, symptom-, and phase of conflict-specific effects on

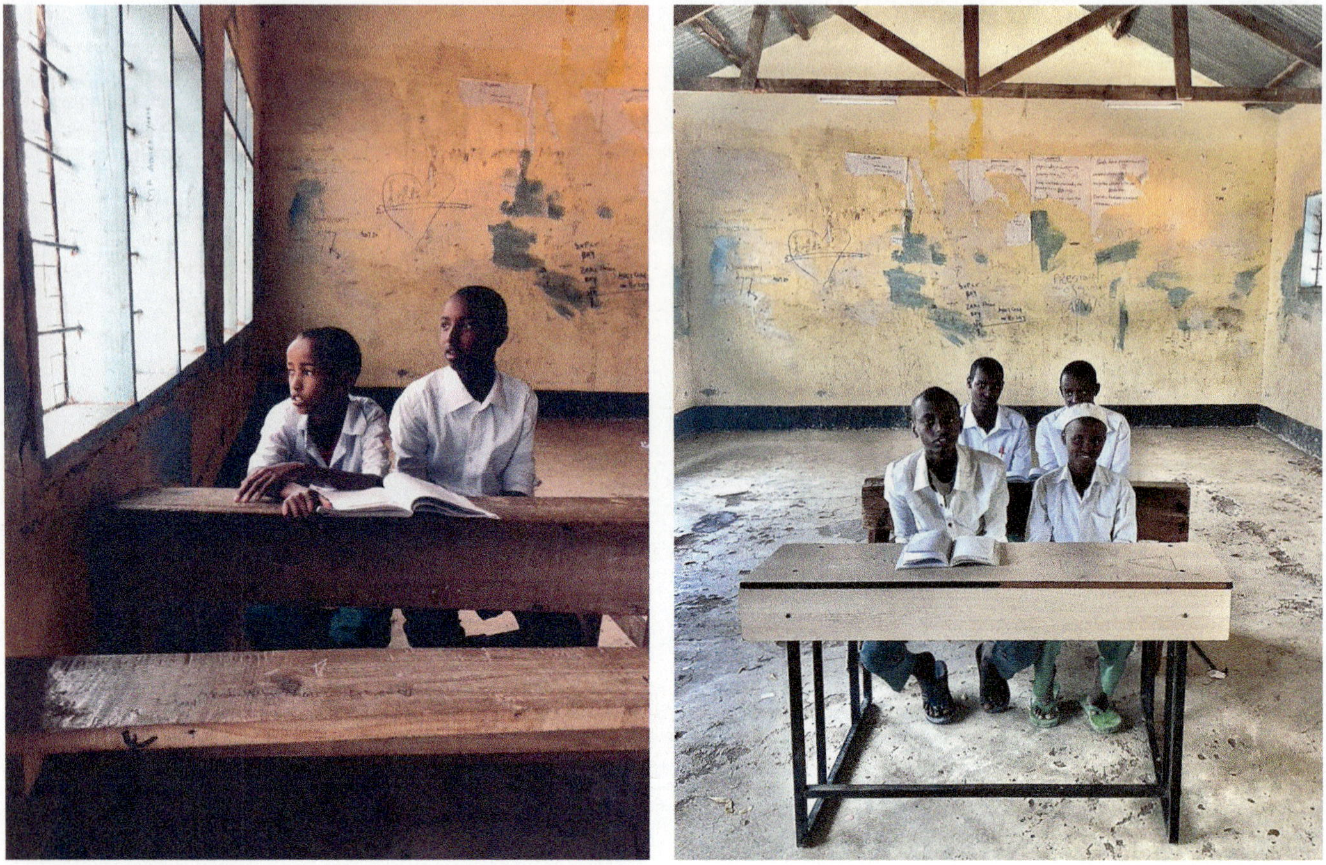

Figure 41.6 Children attending school in a sub-Saharan refugee camp highlighting the limited resources available. *Source:* Courtesy of Jalan Sahba.

mental health outcomes. Refugee child resilience is a complex dynamic process driven by time- and context-dependent variables, rather than a balance between risk and protective factors with known impacts on mental health (for further reading on resilience see Chapter 23). They concluded that resilience-focused interventions would need to be highly tailored to specific contexts.

Consistent with interventions described in higher-resources settings, there remains a need to consider the refugee child's family environment. Considering maternal mental illness, a systematic review of migrant women from LMICs reported that one in three experience symptoms of perinatal depression (Fellmeth *et al.*, 2017). Social support is an important protective factor but little is known about other support available in low-resource settings.

Internally displaced children

IDPs do not officially fall under the definition of "refugee children" although given the many millions of children who have been displaced within their native countries, it is important to consider some of their mental health needs and the complexities of their situations. These children might be displaced many miles from any location that might be familiar to them, they might have moved to an ethnically different community, even if within the same national boundaries, and their displacement might have compromised their socioeconomic and educational opportunities. There are likely to be many children who have been separated from their primary caregivers, if, for example, a parent leaves to try and establish passage for the rest of their family to a different country. These children can be placed at both physical and psychological risk and reviews of primarily adult IDPs highlight how these populations often have the worst health outcomes of any displaced persons (Cantor *et al.*, 2021). They have been described as suffering from a double disadvantage—both experiencing the losses and new hazards of forced displacement (disadvantage relative to the local population) and also not having access to the international protections and resources that refugee status potentially provides as a result of crossing an international border. There is limited research to draw on for IDP children, but crude mortality rates have been shown to be high, possibly driven by poor nutrition, and poor access to health care and sanitation, as well as exposure to many of the adversities that deprivation can lead to (Cantor *et al.*, 2021).

Looking to the future

In summary, the mental health needs of refugee, asylum-seeking, and IDP children are significant and complex. There are increasing numbers of children affected by forced displacement and this therefore raises the importance of considering their needs, enhancing the evidence base from which to draw in support of their mental health, and raising awareness of key policy drivers that can best enable them to thrive in their post-displacement environments.

Integrated models of care hold the greatest promise as they can address the multilevel needs that these children and their families will have and therefore working across health, education, social care, and third-sector organizations is crucial. Greater coproduction of services with refugee children and their families, although potentially requiring greater time and resources, will likely address many of the acceptability and accessibility difficulties that refugee children have experienced to achieve mental health support.

Additional supportive material

Audio 41.1 is a set of audio-supported power-point slides that are available on the companion website for this book. This educational material consists of psychotherapeutic tools to support refugee children in school settings.

References

Abdi, S. *et al.* (2023) Promoting positive development among refugee adolescents. *Journal of Research on Adolescence* **33**, 1064–1084.

Aghajafari, F. *et al.* (2020) Academic achievement and psychosocial adjustment in child refugees: a systematic review. *Journal of Traumatic Stress* **33**, 908–916.

Aitcheson, R.J. *et al.* (2017) Resilience in Palestinian adolescents living in Gaza. *Psychological Trauma: Theory, Research, Practice, and Policy* **9**(1), 36.

Anderson, K.K. & Edwards, J. (2020) Age at migration and the risk of psychotic disorders: a systematic review and meta-analysis. *Acta Psychiatrica Scandinavica* **141**, 410–420.

Anderson, F.M. *et al.* (2017) Prevalence and risk of mental disorders in the perinatal period among migrant women: a systematic review and meta-analysis. *Archives of Women's Mental Health* **20**, 449–462.

Arakelyan, S. & Ager, A. (2021) Annual research review: a multilevel bioecological analysis of factors influencing the mental health and psychosocial well-being of refugee children. *Journal of Child Psychology and Psychiatry* **62**, 484–509.

Ataiants, J. *et al.* (2018) Unaccompanied children at the United States border, a human rights crisis that can be addressed with policy change. *Journal of Immigrant and Minority Health* **20**, 1000–1010.

Beiser, M. *et al.* (2015) Cultural distance and emotional problems among immigrant and refugee youth in Canada: findings from the New Canadian Child and Youth Study (NCCYS). *International Journal of Intercultural Relations* **49**, 33–45.

Bennouna, C. *et al.* (2019) School-based programs for supporting the mental health and psychosocial wellbeing of adolescent forced migrants in high-income countries: a scoping review. *Social Science & Medicine* **239**, 112558.

Bennouna, C. *et al.* (2020) Children and adolescents in conflict and displacement. In: *Child, Adolescent and Family Refugee Mental Health: A Global Perspective.* (eds S.J. Song & P. Ventevogel). Springer, Cham, Switzerland. pp. 17–36.

Blackmore, R. *et al.* (2020) Systematic review and meta-analysis: the prevalence of mental illness in child and adolescent refugees and asylum seekers. *Journal of the American Academy of Child and Adolescent Psychiatry* **59**, 705–714.

Brown, R.C. *et al.* (2017) Psychosocial interventions for children and adolescents after man-made and natural disasters: a meta-analysis and systematic review. *Psychological Medicine* **47**, 1893–1905.

Cantor, D. *et al.* (2021) Understanding the health needs of internally displaced persons: a scoping review. *Journal of Migration and Health* **4**, 100071.

Clemente, N.S. *et al.* (2022) A whole-child, whole-family approach to health assessments for asylum-seeking children. *BMJ Paediatrics Open* **6**(1), e001575.

Daniel-Calveras, A. *et al.* (2022) Mental health of unaccompanied refugee minors in Europe: a systematic review. *Child Abuse & Neglect* **133**, 105865.

Fazel, M. (2018) Psychological and psychosocial interventions for refugee children resettled in high-income countries. *Epidemiology and Psychiatric Sciences* **27**, 117–123.

Fazel, M. (2019) Focusing a lens on refugee families to address layers of avoidance. *The Lancet Public Health* **4**(7), e318–e319.

Fazel, M. & Betancourt, T.S. (2018) Preventive mental health interventions for refugee children and adolescents in high-income settings. *The Lancet Child & Adolescent Health* **2**, 121–132.

Fazel, M. *et al.* (2005) Prevalence of serious mental disorder in 7000 refugees resettled in western countries: a systematic review. *The Lancet* **365**, 1309–1314.

Fazel, M. *et al.* (2014) Detention, denial, and death: migration hazards for refugee children. *The Lancet Global Health* **2**, e313–e314.

Fazel, M. *et al.* (2023) Partnerships at the interface of education and mental health services: the utilisation and acceptability of the provision of specialist liaison and teacher skills training. *International Journal of Environmental Research and Public Health* **20**, 4066.

Fellmeth, G. *et al.* (2017) Migration and perinatal mental health in women from low- and middle-income countries: a systematic review and meta-analysis. *BJOG* **124**, 742–752.

Gadeberg, A.K. *et al.* (2017) Assessing trauma and mental health in refugee children and youth: a systematic review of validated screening and measurement tools. *European Journal of Public Health* **27**, 439–446.

Giacco, D. (2019) Identifying the critical time points for mental health of asylum seekers and refugees in high-income countries. *Epidemiology and Psychiatric Sciences* **29**, e61.

Gordon, E. & Lee-Koo, K. (2021) Addressing the security needs of adolescent girls in protracted crises: inclusive, responsive, and effective? *Contemporary Security Policy* **42**, 53–82.

Graham, H.R. *et al.* (2016) Learning problems in children of refugee background: a systematic review. *Pediatrics* **137**, e20153994.

Guruge, S. & Butt, H. (2015) A scoping review of mental health issues and concerns among immigrant and refugee youth in Canada: looking back, moving forward. *Canadian Journal of Public Health* **106**, e72–e78.

Hampton, K. *et al.* (2021) The psychological effects of forced family separation on asylum-seeking children and parents at the US-Mexico border: a qualitative analysis of medico-legal documents. *PLoS One* **16**, e0259576.

Hermosilla, S. *et al.* (2019) Child friendly spaces impact across five humanitarian settings: a meta-analysis. *BMC Public Health* **19**, 576.

Hettich, N. *et al.* (2020) Psychosocial interventions for newly arrived adolescent refugees: a systematic review. *Adolescent Research Review* **5**, 99–114.

Hirani, K. *et al.* (2018) Identification of health risk behaviours among adolescent refugees resettling in Western Australia. *Archives of Disease in Childhood* **103**(3), 240–246.

Höhne, E. *et al.* (2020) A systematic review of risk and protective factors of mental health in unaccompanied minor refugees. *European Child & Adolescent Psychiatry* **31**, 1–15.

Hou, W.K. *et al.* (2020) Everyday life experiences and mental health among conflict-affected forced migrants: a meta-analysis. *Journal of Affective Disorders* **264**, 50–68.

Ioffe, Y. (2023) Forcibly transferring Ukrainian children to the Russian Federation: a genocide? *Journal of Genocide Research* **25**, 1–37.

Jensen, T.K. *et al.* (2014) Development of mental health problems: a follow-up study of unaccompanied refugee minors. *Child and Adolescent Psychiatry and Mental Health* **8**, 1–10.

Kelstrup, L. & Carlsson, J. (2022) Trauma-affected refugees and their non-exposed children: a review of risk and protective factors for trauma transmission. *Psychiatry Research* **313**, 114604.

Lincoln, A.K. *et al.* (2016) The impact of acculturation style and acculturative hassles on the mental health of Somali adolescent refugees. *Journal of Immigrant and Minority Health* **18**, 771–778.

Longobardi, C. *et al.* (2017) Abuses, resilience, behavioural problems and post-traumatic stress symptoms among unaccompanied migrant minors: an Italian cross-sectional exploratory study. *Psychiatria i Psychologia Kliniczna* **17**, 87–92.

Mares, S. (2021) Mental health consequences of detaining children and families who seek asylum: a scoping review. *European Child & Adolescent Psychiatry* **30**, 1615–1639.

Mesa-Vieira, C. *et al.* (2022) Mental health of migrants with pre-migration exposure to armed conflict: a systematic review and meta-analysis. *The Lancet Public Health* **7**, e469–e481.

Migration Data Portal (2023) *Child and young migrants* [Online]. Available: https://www.migrationdataportal.org/themes/child-and-young-migrants [29 July 2023].

Miller, K.E. & Rasmussen, A. (2010) War exposure, daily stressors, and mental health in conflict and post-conflict settings: bridging the divide between trauma-focused and psychosocial frameworks. *Social Science & Medicine* **70**, 7–16.

Mitra, R. & Hodes, M. (2019) Prevention of psychological distress and promotion of resilience amongst unaccompanied refugee minors in resettlement countries. *Child: Care, Health and Development* **45**, 198–215.

Mohwinkel, L.M. *et al.* (2018) Gender differences in the mental health of unaccompanied refugee minors in Europe: a systematic review. *BMJ Open* **8**, e022389.

NSW Government (2019) Roads to Refuge. [Online]. Available: https://www.roads-to-refuge.com.au/ [22 October 2024].

Patel, P. *et al.* (2021) Communication experiences in primary healthcare with refugees and asylum seekers: a literature review and narrative synthesis. *International Journal of Environmental Research and Public Health* **18**, 1469.

Purgato, M. *et al.* (2018) Focused psychosocial interventions for children in low-resource humanitarian settings: a systematic review and individual participant data meta-analysis. *The Lancet Global Health* **6**, e390–e400.

Qasmiyeh, Y.M. (2020) Writing the camp, writing the camp archive: the case of Baddawi camp in Lebanon. In: *Refuge in a Moving World: Tracing Refugee and Migrant Journeys Across Disciplines*. (ed E. Fiddian-Qasmiyeh). UCL Press, London. pp. 52–73.

Reed, R.V. *et al.* (2012) Mental health of displaced and refugee children resettled in low-income and middle-income countries: risk and protective factors. *The Lancet* **379**, 250–265.

Richter, K. *et al.* (2020) Sleep disorders in migrants and refugees: a systematic review with implications for personalized medical approach. *The EPMA Journal* **11**, 251–260.

Scharpf, F. *et al.* (2021) A systematic review of socio-ecological factors contributing to risk and protection of the mental health of refugee children and adolescents. *Clinical Psychology Review* **83**, 101930.

Simenec, T.S. & Reid, B.M. (2022) Refugee children and interventions for depression: a review of current interventions and implications of the ecological context. *Trauma Violence Abuse* **23**, 877–890.

Slobodin, O. & de Jong, J.T. (2015) Family interventions in traumatized immigrants and refugees: a systematic review. *Transcultural Psychiatry* **52**, 723–742.

Smith, K. & Waite, L. (2019) New and enduring narratives of vulnerability: rethinking stories about the figure of the refugee. *Journal of Ethnic and Migration Studies* **45**(13), 2289–2307.

Soltan, F. *et al.* (2022) Community-based interventions for improving mental health in refugee children and adolescents in high-income countries. *Cochrane Database of Systematic Reviews* **5**.

Timshel, I. *et al.* (2017) A systematic review of risk and protective factors associated with family related violence in refugee families. *Child Abuse & Neglect* **70**, 315–330.

Tol, W.A. *et al.* (2013) Annual Research Review: Resilience and mental health in children and adolescents living in areas of armed conflict—a systematic review of findings in low- and middle-income countries. *Journal of Child Psychology and Psychiatry* **54**, 445–460.

Turrini, G. *et al.* (2019) Efficacy and acceptability of psychosocial interventions in asylum seekers and refugees: systematic review and meta-analysis. *Epidemiology and Psychiatric Sciences* **28**, 376–388.

UNHCR (2022a) *Ranking of the Largest Refugee-Hosting Countries as of 2022*. Statista.

UNHCR (2023a) *Fleeing Unaccompanied: Healing the Suffering of Children Who've Lost Everything*. United Nations High Commissioner for Refugees (UNHCR), Geneva, Switzerland. [Online]. Available: https://www.unhcr.org/hk/en/unaccompanied-children [29 July 2023].

UNHCR (2023b) Refugee Data Finder. United Nations High Commissioner for Refugees (UNHCR), Geneva, Switzerland. [Online]. Available: https://www.unhcr.org/refugee-statistics [22 October 2024].

UNHCR (2023c) *Statelessness Around the World*. United Nations High Commissioner for Refugees (UNHCR), Geneva, Switzerland. [Online]. Available: https://www.unhcr.org/ibelong/statelessness-around-the-world/#:~:text=At%20least%2010%20million%20people%20in%20the%20world%20today%20are%20stateless. [29 July 2023].

UNICEF (2023) *Child Displacement*. United Nations Children's Fund (UNICEF), New York. [Online]. Available: https://data.unicef.org/topic/child-migration-and-displacement/displacement [29 July 2023].

WFP (2023) Hunger in the 4 largest refugee camps in the world [Online]. World Food Programme (WFP), Rome. Available: https://www.wfpusa.org/articles/hunger-largest-refugee-camps-world [29 July 2023].

Vervliet, M. *et al.* (2014) Longitudinal follow-up of the mental health of unaccompanied refugee minors. *European Child & Adolescent Psychiatry* **23**, 337–346.

Vossoughi, N. *et al.* (2018) Mental health outcomes for youth living in refugee camps: a review. *Trauma Violence Abuse* **19**, 528–542.

CHAPTER 42

Residential care, foster care, and adoption

Helen Minnis[1] and Rachel Hiller[2]

[1] School of Health and Wellbeing, University of Glasgow, Glasgow, UK

[2] Department of Clinical, Educational and Health Psychology, University College London, London, UK

This chapter aims to provide clinicians with the best evidence for the assessment, formulation, and treatment of mental health difficulties in children in substitute care. We refer to children who have, for whatever reason, spent a period of time in the care of a child welfare/state care system.

Globally, the most common reason a young person may need to live in substitute care is the experience of abuse and/or neglect. Parental disability, illness or death, natural disasters, or war are other reasons. Exact legal definitions and types of care differ between regions and countries. These includes adoption, foster care, kinship care (e.g., with a relative or friend), or institutional care (all discussed in more detail in this chapter). In many cultures, such care arrangements might occur outside of any state-governed or official requirements or support.

Part 1 provides an overview of the main types of substitute care, what makes for better quality care, and the developmental impact that substitute care can have on a young person. Part 2 provides a summary of what we know about the mental health of care-experienced children, what drives mental health/illness in this group, and strategies for addressing difficulties. At the end of the chapter, we provide examples of useful resources, including animations for young people and brief videos for professionals.

Part 1: Types and impact of substitute care

Substitute care across the world

Lack of parental care is a developmental emergency for any child. Attachment behaviors (see Chapter 6), which bring primary caregivers close and elicit caregiving, are present from birth (Sroufe & Waters, 1977) and ensure infants and young children are protected and nurtured by family members (Ainsworth, 1979). Absent or grossly abnormal parental or family care can have a significant impact on these typical developmental processes, with knock-on effects for many other aspects of development (see Chapters 25 on maltreatment and 57 on attachment disorders).

Lack of adequate or appropriate parental care can stem from a range of contextual factors: parental substance misuse (Russell *et al.*, 2022), illness (Fry & Casey, 2017), natural disaster (Seddighi *et al.*, 2021), extreme poverty, and/or war (Wagstaff *et al.*, 2017). In the UK, the large majority of young people in care will be with a nonbiological foster carer. Rates of children living in foster care globally are unknown due to poor data gathering in most countries (Petrowski *et al.*, 2017). In some circumstances, and predominantly in some cultures, children may be cared for by extended family or friends (informal kinship care) outside of any formal/official state system. Institutional care rates are better documented although there is still huge uncertainty, and it is estimated that between 3.18–9.42 million children are living in institutional care worldwide (Desmond *et al.*, 2020).

When finding or designing substitute care, three main principles need to be borne in mind:

- the child's need for attuned, committed care to be provided as soon as possible;
- the need to prevent or eliminate abuse and neglect; and
- the need to support and maintain the child's wider social relationships, where possible.

Foster care as a child protection intervention

Foster care may include a placement with a nonbiological caregiver or with a relative or friend (a kinship placement). Family-style care has overtaken institutional care in many countries, with a growing awareness that young people need a secure and loving attachment with a caregiver in a family context if they are

Rutter's Child and Adolescent Psychiatry and Psychology, Seventh Edition.
Edited by Anita Thapar, Daniel S. Pine, Samuele Cortese, Cathy Creswell, Tamsin J. Ford, James F. Leckman, and Argyris Stringaris.

Companion website: www.wiley.com/go/thapar/rutterspsych7

to recover and thrive after adversity. The nature of foster care is, however, very variable: some children will enter "emergency" or "short-term" foster care before returning home after what is deemed to be adequate improvement in parenting, while others will move into either adoption or long-term foster care. What constitutes "short-term" and "long-term" care can differ greatly, and long-term care often does not mean permanent (e.g., in the UK, at least one-third of children in care—including those in foster care—have more than one placement in a year).

An ideal foster placement should be one of emotional and physical safety, security, sensitivity, and commitment. Increasingly, research is demonstrating the importance of caregiver commitment in creating this environment. High levels of commitment may be evidenced by foster carer expressions of desire to adopt the child (where appropriate), investment in emotional and physical resources, and integration of the child into the family, while low commitment is conceptualized as relative indifference regarding the child and the relationship (Bernard & Dozier, 2011). Optimum commitment has been associated with fewer reported behavioral problems in children (Lindhiem & Dozier, 2007), more positive expressions of the child–carer relationship from the foster carers point of view (Bernard & Dozier, 2011), and less placement disruption. To support this commitment, it is vital that services are able to adequately support carers—particularly over periods where the young person's behavior may become more challenging. In the UK, most young people enter care from school age (GOV. UK, 2022), while adolescence is the fasting growing age group entering care. Many children are entering foster placements following long periods of instability (and potentially maltreatment), often with preexisting mental health difficulties. Even the most committed and warm caregiver can find these situations difficult to manage, particularly if there is violence or externalizing difficulties. Although the relationship with the foster carer is crucial (especially in young children), it is important that services do not expect foster carers to replace mental health interventions, where such intervention is required.

Institutional or residential care

Occasionally, institutional or residential care is the safest or the only option for the young person in need of substitute care, especially when additional support is not available to help a carer or family manage a child's complex needs or developmental disabilities in the home and/or family care has become impossible (Foster *et al.*, 2019). More often, across the globe, children are placed in institutional care because of poverty, social marginalization, or the social fragmentation that accompanies war, or natural disasters. Worldwide, it is estimated that 80–90% of children placed in orphanages have a living parent (van IJzendoorn *et al.*, 2020). The quality of institutional care varies greatly across and within countries. Common features of these types of settings often include rigid, nonindividualized schedules, rotating shift-work that limits sustained relationships with children, low standards in staff training given the complexity of the role, and insufficient numbers of caregivers to respond to children's individual needs. Extensive reviews have documented the pervasive deleterious effects of institutional rearing on young children's development, across virtually every developmental domain (van IJzendoorn *et al.*, 2020). This includes physical growth, brain structure and functioning, cognitive development and executive functions, language development, disturbances of attachment and social relatedness, emotional problems, and behavioral problems (Baptista *et al.*, 2019; Wade *et al.*, 2022). Much of this evidence comes from two seminal studies: The European Romanian Adoption Studies (ERAS) followed, into adulthood, families of 165 young children adopted from Romania (144 from institutions) into England between 1990 and 1992 (Rutter & Sonuga-Barke, 2010). The Bucharest Early Intervention Project (BEIP; Nelson *et al.*, 2014), involved 136 children aged 6–31 months, recruited from all 6 institutions in Bucharest, and creation of a network of foster homes to which 50% of the children were randomized. Both studies follow children placed in institutional care from very young ages and subject to very poor levels of care. Thus, findings are not necessarily generalizable to the more common situations in places like the UK, where young people are more likely to be placed in group care homes in adolescence (sometimes after periods of time in multiple foster placements). Nevertheless, these seminal studies both showed the major cross-domain effects of institutional care across nearly all domains of a child's development. Group or institutional care should be a last option, or only when absolutely required for the needs of the young person, rather than based on funding or availability issues, or a consequence of a lack of earlier appropriate support.

Part 2: The mental health of care-experienced children

What we know about mental health outcomes for infants, children, and adolescents placed in foster care or adoption

There is a vast amount of evidence on the mental health outcomes of infants, children, and teens with experience of substitute care (van IJzendoorn *et al.*, 2020)—although almost exclusively from Western high-income countries (Engler *et al.*, 2020). The limited longitudinal evidence is that mental health difficulties are most likely to be chronic and pervasive (Tarren-Sweeney & Goemans, 2019; Hiller *et al.*, 2023). That means the process of removal into care, where physical *safety* (usually) improves, does not mean improvements in mental health will automatically follow. Conversely, it is crucial to remember that not all infants, children, or young people who are adopted or in the care system develop mental health problems. Children and teens in care are children first, and their needs should be assessed without assumptions. In particular, children and teens in care often voice frustration with assumptions that any mental health difficulties are caused by their pre-care experiences, when some difficulties may be driven by their experiences since being in care, including their experiences of navigating the care system, further trauma or exploitation (Landers *et al.*, 2021), and experiences of stigma or victimization in school (Dansey *et al.*, 2019).

Meta-analytic reviews show that at least half of young people in substitute care meet criteria for at least one diagnosable psychiatric disorder (Dubois-Comtois *et al.*, 2021), as defined in the *Diagnostic and Statistical Manual of Mental Disorders*, 5th edition (DSM-5; American Psychiatric Association (2013)) or the *International Classification of Diseases* (ICD-11; World Health Organization (2019)). These include: internalizing difficulties (e.g., depression, anxiety), externalizing difficulties (e.g., oppositional defiant and conduct disorders), and trauma-related difficulties (e.g., post-traumatic stress disorder (PTSD), reactive attachment disorder (RAD), disinhibited social engagement disorder (DSED)) (Engler *et al.*, 2020). Mental health needs are often complex, commonly with multiple comorbidities and other complexities (Seim *et al.*, 2022), such as low self-esteem (Seim *et al.*, 2021), self-harm, sleep difficulties, education challenges (Seim *et al.*, 2022), and/or housing or placement instability (Prince *et al.*, 2019). Problems with under- and overnutrition are not uncommon (Sokol *et al.*, 2018). Neurodevelopmental conditions (e.g., attention deficit hyperactivity disorder (ADHD), Autism, and intellectual disabilities) are also far more common in this population than in the general population of young people (Dinkler *et al.*, 2017). A child can have a heritable neurodevelopmental condition *and* experience trauma—indeed having a neurodevelopmental condition such as ADHD, or even a genetic liability for ADHD, is a risk factor for exposure to maltreatment (Zwicker *et al.*, 2020). Dismissing symptoms of neurodevelopmental conditions, such as ADHD, as being "trauma-related," or avoiding appropriate diagnosis because of a trauma history, can deny a child access to evidence-based treatments or support strategies.

How to assess mental health needs

There already exists large numbers of mental health screening tools validated for use with children (see Chapter 28), including following maltreatment. Young people may prefer this method as it requires less personal interaction and less confronting disclosure. Parents and carers are also often happy to complete standardized measures, especially when focusing on problems that are rarely discussed or that they are desperate to seek help with. Instead of services developing their own tools, we strongly suggest offering the completion of standardized measures as routine with all care-experienced young people who access mental health services—both at initial assessment and to monitor progress. In the Resources section, we provide a web link that gives access to various freely available validated screening tools. We also encourage readers to refer to Chapter 28 and disorder-specific chapters for information on other screening tools.

Who should information be collected from?

Where developmentally appropriate, the child should always be involved in the assessment of their own mental health. It is concerning how many services conduct consultations and assessments without inviting the young person to be involved, or without observing infants or young children with their caregiver. Care-experienced children often *underreport* their symptoms, so professionals should be mindful that low scores that seem inconsistent with the child's presentation could reflect a lack of willingness to fully report on their mental health. Report by a caregiver who is familiar with the child is also likely to be hugely helpful. Caregivers may also underreport symptoms, especially if concerned about being seen as unable to cope with a child's difficult behavior (Pritchett *et al.*, 2016). Child and carer reports may be inconsistent—a common phenomenon in any family—and disagreements between child and caregiver reports may provide a useful platform for discussing how each experience and understand the child's needs. Finally, reporting from a teacher or other professional (e.g., social worker) who knows the child may also be helpful.

Do we need new diagnostic criteria?

The continual debate and research on existing diagnostic frameworks is essential for increasing understanding of the needs of young people with very complex needs. But, while these debates continue, we encourage professionals to use current best-evidenced practice, rather than unestablished or undefined labels (e.g., "developmental trauma" as a mental health outcome). Young people in care experiencing mental ill-health are likely to meet criteria for existing recognized mental health conditions, which also provide pathways to evidence-based treatments.

Examples of factors requiring consideration for infants, children, and young people who are adopted or living in foster or residential care

Although care-experienced children have far higher rates of mental illness and neurodivergence than the general population, they do not require a different type of supraspecialist psychiatric assessment. They simply need us to do the basics well, i.e., to offer a comprehensive psychiatric assessment, to work in partnerships with other agencies, and to recommend appropriate (ideally, evidence-based) treatment(s). A short discussion of this important principle is contained in this UK Trauma Council video, which can also be found on the companion website to this book: https://uktraumacouncil.org/research_practice/aces-research.

Far less is known about drivers of negative outcomes in care-experienced children. We discuss some of the factors worth bearing in mind in the following sections.

Adverse prenatal factors

Many children in adoptive or care placements will have experienced high levels of maternal stress, dietary insufficiencies, or exposure to toxins while *in utero*. These often co-occur and although the immature brain cannot simply replace lost brain cells after injury (Bennet *et al.*, 2013), antenatal adversity does not necessarily have entirely negative consequences. Globally, the most important prenatal influence on children's neurodevelopment is malnutrition, including lack of calories, especially protein, or when an otherwise well-nourished mother lacks specific nutrients such as folate (Churuangsuk *et al.*, 2018) or iodine (Bouga *et al.*, 2018). Certain groups within the population, such as mothers with substance misuse problems (Sebastiani *et al.*, 2018) or antenatal depression (Bleker *et al.*, 2019), are at higher risk of micronutrient deficiencies in pregnancy. Many children adopted or in care will have experienced antenatal exposure to drugs or alcohol (Russell *et al.*, 2022). Prenatal exposure to alcohol has a teratogenic effect on the developing fetus. Fetal alcohol syndrome (FAS) is recognizable through a specific constellation of features that includes: short palpebral fissures (i.e., a short distance between the inner and outer edge of the eye); smooth nasal philtrum; thin upper lip vermilion; and, usually, intellectual disability and a small head circumference (Charness, 2022). Fetal alcohol spectrum disorder (FASD) is a broader umbrella term for a range of developmental disabilities presumed to be caused by prenatal alcohol toxicity (McQuire *et al.*, 2020). The prevalence of FASD is thought to be at least 1.8% in the UK general population (McCarthy *et al.*, 2021), although this could well be an underestimate since epidemiology is very challenging to conduct in this area. Diagnosis of FASD is also complicated by the fact that some guidelines (for example, the Scottish Intercollegiate Guidelines Network, SIGN 156) (SIGN, 2019) suggest FASD can be diagnosed without presence of sentinel physical features, and there is no significant neuropsychiatric difference between children with and without the sentinel physical features (Webster *et al.*, 2023). Rates of comorbidity are very high in FASD (94%), and include conduct disorder (91%), ADHD (51%), and depression (35%) (Broccia *et al.*, 2023). It can be challenging to separate prenatal, obstetric (Broccia *et al.*, 2023), environmental, and genetic factors in the etiology of FASD (McQuire *et al.*, 2020): for example, neurodevelopmental conditions such as ADHD are highly heritable, and ADHD in the child's mother would have increased her risk of developing alcohol misuse (see Chapters 3 and 66). In care-experienced children, it is not unusual for the prenatal and early-childhood history to be lost or uncertain, which can make the diagnosis of FASD even more challenging. Evidence-based treatments, such as stimulant treatment for ADHD, are, however, as likely to be successful whether FASD is present or not, so should not be withheld because of doubts about the causal basis for the symptoms (Ozsarfati & Koren, 2015).

Neurodevelopmental factors

As mentioned previously, children who have been abused and neglected are at higher risk, compared to their peers, of also having neurodevelopmental conditions such as ADHD (Stern *et al.*, 2018), Autism (Minnis *et al.*, 2020), and intellectual disability (Lewis *et al.*, 2021). Evidence from both prospective longitudinal cohort studies and twin studies suggests that these neurodevelopmental conditions—and/or the disruptive behaviors that can be associated with them—might have increased these children's risks of experiencing maltreatment (Stern *et al.*, 2018; Lewis *et al.*, 2021). Maltreatment itself might also cause these disorders in certain circumstances (Kennedy *et al.*, 2016) or, at the very least, increase the symptom load (Dinkler *et al.*, 2017). Traumatic brain injury is relatively common in children who have experienced abuse and neglect (Jackson *et al.*, 2022), and ADHD is common in children who have experienced head injury (Asarnow *et al.*, 2021).

Maltreatment and adversity

Although maltreatment is one of the strongest preventable risk factors for mental health problems (see Chapter 25), there is little robust evidence that specific aspects of a young person's trauma history can predict specific mental health outcomes. Therefore, presuming that a child who has experienced X type of abuse will have greater needs than a child who has experienced Y type of abuse, is likely to be inaccurate or misplaced. Caution is warranted in using the type and extent of maltreatment as a means of prioritizing where mental health support should be directed.

Psychological and social drivers of mental health problems

Most care-experienced children and young people, particularly those entering substitute care in later childhood or adolescence, have developed and consolidated their own strategies to cope with their day-to-day experiences of unsafety. At one point in their life, these strategies might have been helpful or even essential. Being hyperaware of signs of danger, avoiding thinking about their experiences, or being indiscriminate in social behavior toward strangers—these are all examples of coping that might have been necessary for that young person's survival. However, once in the relative physical safety of the substitute care system, these same processes can become maladaptive, and can drive or maintain poor mental health. Much of what we know about psychological and social drivers of mental ill-health is extrapolated from the general maltreatment field (see Chapter 20, "Biological mechanisms linking childhood adversity to mental health problems")—which we strongly encourage professionals working with children in care to read. Here we provide a much briefer summary on some key processes likely of relevance to mental health:

Maladaptive cognitions/appraisals

How we think about ourselves and the world around us is fundamental to our mental well-being. It is easy to see why a young person in substitute care might develop entrenched maladaptive or unhelpful cognitions about themselves and the world around them. This is not just due to their potential early life maltreatment and adversity, but often also formed out of their experiences within the substitute care system. Indeed, these are often based on the reality of their experiences—that the world is not safe for them, that people are untrustworthy, that adults will ultimately let them down. Thoughts about themselves like it was their fault, they are to blame, they cannot cope, or are a bad person, can also be common. There is good evidence that maladaptive cognitions drive mental health difficulties in maltreated young people, including those in substitute care. Multiple quantitative studies, including longitudinal work, have demonstrated the strength of these associations—particularly in relation to post-traumatic stress, depression, and anxiety (e.g., Hiller *et al.*, 2021b).

Minimal seeking or accepting of comfort

Understandably, many young children who have been abused and neglected have problems signaling their needs to their adult caregivers. This can manifest as a lack of comfort seeking and/or refusal to accept comfort in a stressful situation such as when the child is hungry or scared. Typically, young children's attachment behaviors involve noise (e.g., crying) and movement (e.g., reaching out to be picked up), and signal the child's needs to the caregiver so that these can be addressed (see Chapter 6). Unfortunately, a *lack* of comfort-seeking is easy to ignore: children who lack comfort-seeking are quiet and still when stressed which does not alert caregivers to the fact that the child has a need which needs to be met. Lack of comfort-seeking behavior is therefore a potentially devastating problem which needs to be urgently addressed because it signals the closing down of the attachment system. When minimal comfort-seeking/acceptance persists into middle childhood or adolescence, it continues to be highly problematic because sensitive caregivers will tend to leave such a young person to their own devices. These young people do not get their needs met—and this is frustrating for parents who wish to offer help but do not feel invited to do so. Some children indiscriminately approach strangers for comfort or support. When these behaviors are entrenched, the child or young person might warrant a diagnosis of RAD or DSED—see Chapter 57.

Threat biases

There is some, albeit inconsistent, evidence that children who experience maltreatment can have heightened sensitivity to threat. This might look like a child seemingly "acting out" in class when a teacher criticizes them or becoming aggressive in a seemingly innocuous social situation. These behaviors can contribute to "social thinning" (McCrory *et al.*, 2022)—i.e., the gradual loss of friends or people in one's support network, that is experienced at a higher rate in those who have experienced maltreatment. This may then further entrench maladaptive cognitions such as "there is no one I can trust," or "nobody cares about me."

Avoidant coping

Following trauma, it is completely natural to want to avoid thinking about or talking about your experiences. Children in care often feel shame or blame about what they (a sibling or parent) have experienced. However, those who endorse greater avoidant coping (avoiding thoughts or feelings, talking about, or reminders of their experience) have greater mental health difficulties. This link is well-established, particularly for internalizing difficulties such as anxiety or post-traumatic stress.

Understanding this is crucial for mental health professionals. No child should be forced to talk about experiences they are not ready to discuss. However, it is likely to be a central job of a mental health professional to support the young person to be comfortable to discuss their experiences.

Social support

Children in substitute care consistently report the need for a consistent adult in their life who cares about them and their needs. Someone who can accept them for who they are, is proud of them, will be there for them even when they make mistakes. Where this is not available, mental health suffers. Unfortunately, many young people in substitute care do not have this person, since placement breakdowns are comment. There is an established cyclical association between placement breakdowns and mental ill-health, whereby children who have more placements also have poorer mental health. Placement breakdowns prevent children maintaining healthy attachments and provide the child with further evidence of their beliefs that they are unworthy or that no one can be trusted—further eroding mental health. Yet mental health difficulties can also make children more difficult to care for, especially when appropriate mental health support for the child or support for the foster family is not available. Yet this group is at particular risk of not being able to access appropriate mental health support, because there is no caregiver to advocate for and support them. Some services still will not provide mental health support until a young person is in a stable placement, so that children requiring the most support are those who miss out, further entrenching layers of inequality.

Children's past experiences of being let down or hurt might mean they are unwilling to seek or access available support options. However, professionals working with a child in substitute care should spend time understanding who is in the child's support network, from the child's own perspective and potentially from adult caregivers. Such information might be an important part of formulation and treatment.

Systemic challenges

Anyone working with care-experienced children will encounter systemic challenges. The way countries and regions support and organize systems around care-experienced children can make a big difference to their outcomes (Prince *et al.*, 2019), e.g., as regards the length of time children are offered support into early adulthood, the degree of support with finances and housing upon leaving care, and attitudes to services crossing geographical boundaries.

Every care-experienced child has, by definition, lived in more than one family or residential context. This can lead to challenges in accessing reliable information about the child's early developmental history, potentially compounded by geographical boundary issues. At the other extreme, a child might be having to navigate relationships with both the current family and the birth family and a lack of scaffolding from a strongly supportive family network can create major challenges (Boddy *et al.*, 2020). Thinking about these systemic issues should be a routine part of any psychiatric assessment for this group of children and young people.

Unfortunately, qualitatively, young people often report that their experiences within social care have been a key driver of their mental health difficulties (Hiller *et al.*, 2021a). In particular, frequent changes of social workers are experienced as highly disruptive and problematic. At a practical level these disruptions can leave young people feeling disempowered and with nowhere clear to turn. At a psychological level, this can further entrench thoughts that adults cannot be trusted and are not sources of support. Changes in social workers are mostly inevitable, especially for those who may spend many years in care. Social work faces one of the highest burnout rates of any profession. However, services should have protocols in place to minimize the negative impact of these changes on young people, particularly via forward planning, handover periods, and open discussion with the young person.

The same can be said for interactions with mental health services. Too often, a child not being ready to talk about their experiences is conflated with an unwillingness to engage in support and a reason to not provide intervention. Care-experienced adults often reflect on experiences in mental health services where they have been actively told *not* to disclose their experiences or where they have had a negative or stigmatizing reaction to disclosures (including not being believed). These messages might be interpreted by the child if the professional tries to change the subject or distract them with another activity. It is crucial that professionals are able to sit with a child's disclosure and sit with their distress. It is okay to be distressed when disclosing very difficult experiences, and it is important that behavior of professionals reflects this. This is also what makes supervision so essential for professionals as it can be very difficult to hear about some of these experiences. Many young people in substitute care (and their caregivers) are dissatisfied with mental health support (Hiller *et al.*, 2021a) and will come into the mental health system presuming they cannot trust anyone or that no one will be able to help them. Building trust, safety, and consistency is a fundamental part of any therapeutic intervention. All mental health services should reflect on their pathways into their service, and consider whether they are accessible to this population of young people (Munson *et al.*, 2020). This includes strict rules around missing sessions (something that should be expected in this group, and not a reason for ceasing treatment), placement stability, and placement moves that might place them out of the "catchment" area for the service (which should not mean a ceasing of treatment).

At the end of this chapter, we provide three timelines that describe typical journeys of children in substitute care, composites of real-life examples, to highlight the kinds of experiences these children (and their caregivers) can face in accessing mental health support, often resulting in many years of oscillation in and out of services without any thorough assessment of need (see Figures 42.1–42.3 for examples).

Information sharing

A key challenge for young people in substitute care is that many do not have a consistent advocate. Thus, where young people do access mental health services it is crucial that systems are in place to ensure accurate reporting of assessments and any management or treatment decisions, and that this information is appropriately shared with the social care system. Additional

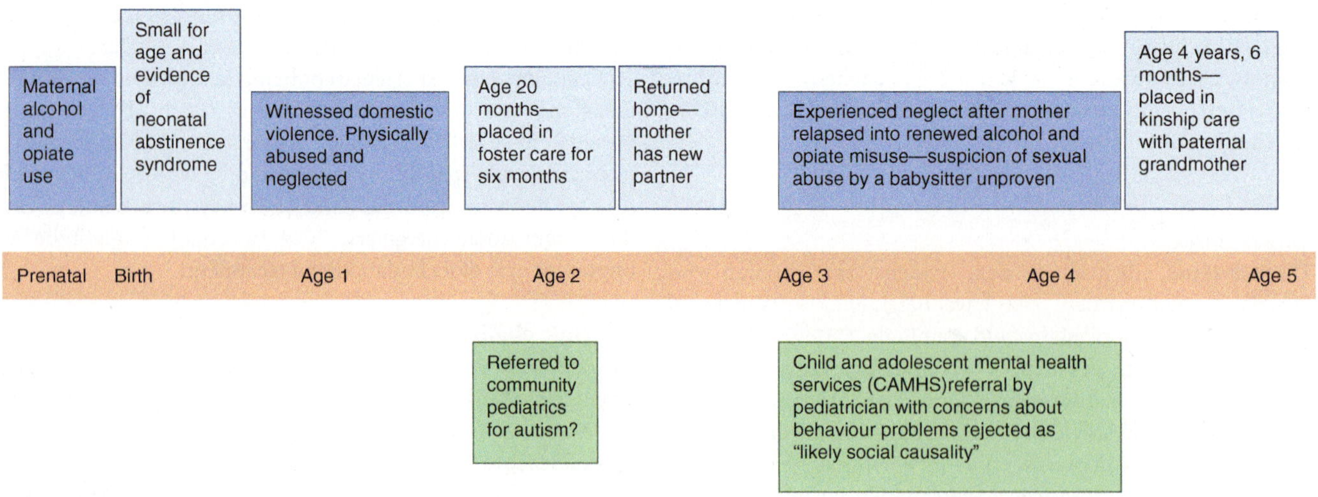

Figure 42.1 Leigh's journey through placement in the preschool years—a fairly typical pattern for a child placed in care under age 5 (blue—care history; green—health history).

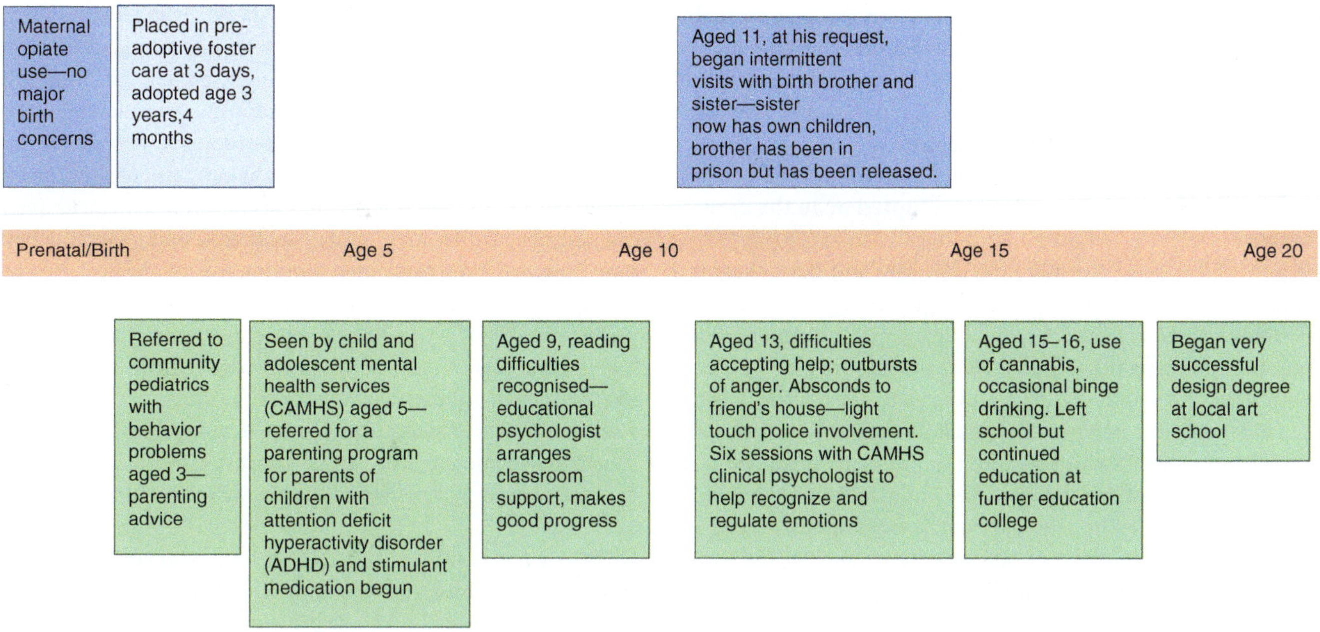

Figure 42.2 Jason's journey through the process of adoption—birth to age 20 (blue—care history; green—health history).

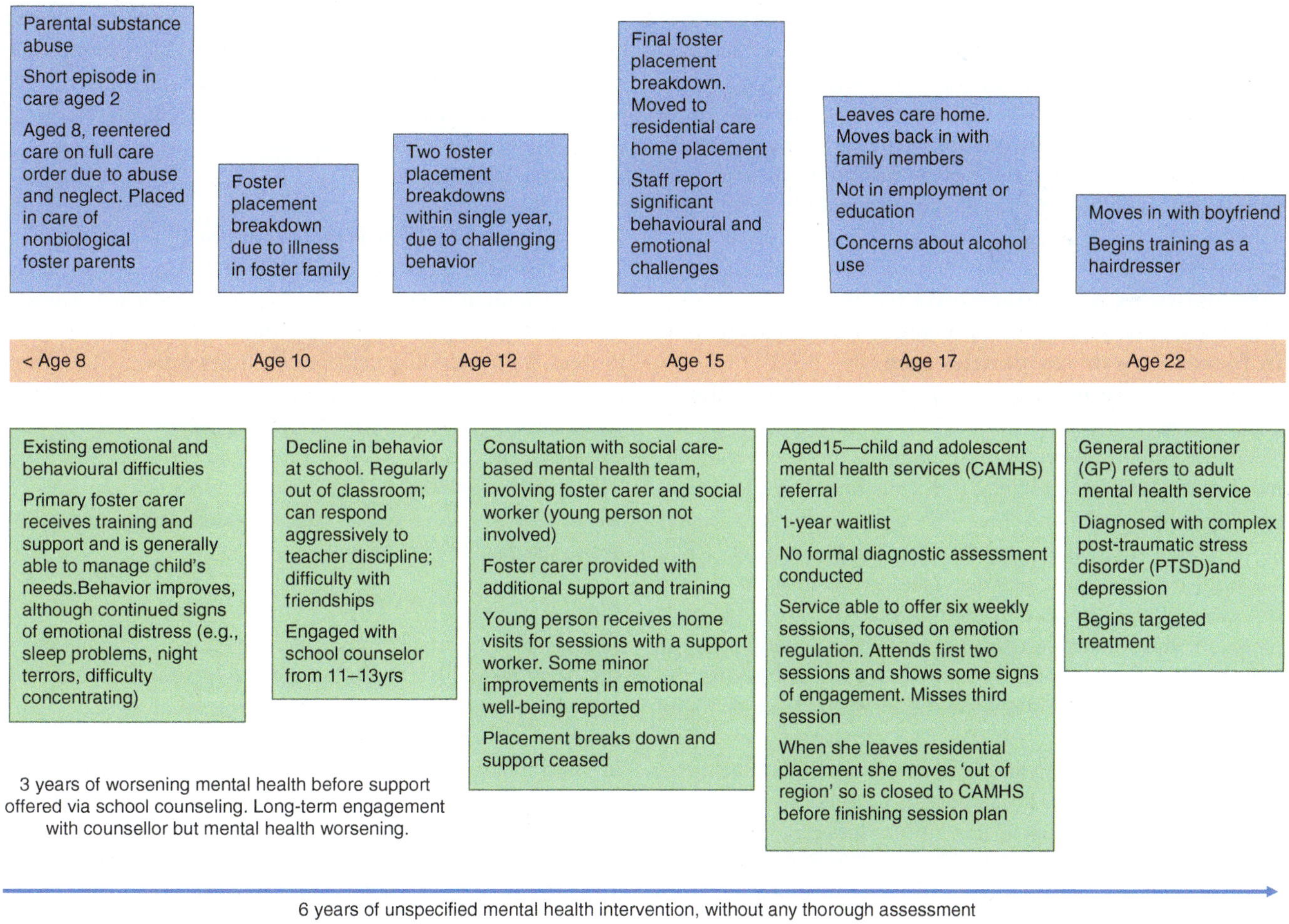

Figure 42.3 Sandra's journey from age 8 to young adulthood (blue—care history; green—health history).

effort may be required to access information across geographical boundaries, so that important knowledge already gathered about a child's developmental or psychiatric history is not lost. Where age-appropriate, it is also essential that young people are aware of how their information is shared.

When to assess children who are adopted or in the care system

If a child has been recently placed in care and has behavioral difficulties, some professionals suggest waiting until the child is stable placement before conducting a mental health assessment on the basis that adjustment problems are likely to settle with time. We would argue that a wait-and-see approach is not sensible because behavioral problems might jeopardize the stability of the placement—and placement breakdown is undoubtedly detrimental for the child. Instead, the child should be offered a holistic psychiatric assessment, investigating neurodevelopmental conditions, internalizing and externalizing difficulties, and trauma and stress-related conditions. Offering a comprehensive formulation of the child's difficulties can help the caregiver understand the nature of the child's difficulties and be supported in providing more targeted support. Once the child is more settled in placement, a further assessment might be required to fully understand the nature of the child's difficulties in the absence of adjustment problems (Pritchett *et al.*, 2016). Ideally, we would argue that all young people in care should have a comprehensive mental health needs assessment within 6-months of entering the care system. At the very least, when a young person is flagged as struggling with their mental health or wellbeing, they should be offered a comprehensive mental health assessment by the service.

Interventions and treatments for infants, children, and young people who are adopted or in foster care or residential care

Interventions for infants and preschool children in the care system

There are some well-evidenced treatments to improve attachment in children with problems signaling their needs, for example, Circle of Security and child–Parent psychotherapy (Tsappis *et al.*, 2022). Attachment and biobehavioural catch-up (ABC) can improve attachment security in children in foster care (Bick & Dozier, 2013). The core intervention in ABC is "gentle challenge" in which foster carers are encouraged to gently offer the child what they need, not simply what they are asking for. Details of these interventions can be found in Chapter 57 on attachment disorders.

Although reactivating an infant or young child's attachment system is clearly a crucially important process, this alone may not result in a resolution in the child's difficulties. First, this group of children is at much higher risk of having neurodevelopmental conditions. Second, when an attachment starts to form, the child's behavior can deteriorate (Turner *et al.*, 2023). Yet placement in nurturing care is clearly associated with excellent longer-term outcomes (Sonuga-Barke *et al.*, 2017). Taken together, this research suggests that an important message to foster carers and adoptive parents might be that "things might get worse before they get better." Adoptive parents and foster carers need support to weather this process, especially during difficult times where placements might be at risk of breakdown. Foster parents of preschoolers may also need support with feeding and sleep difficulties, temper tantrums, and general behavioral support. Preschool interventions for common issues are discussed further in Chapter 7. The provision of a detailed formulation is likely to be helpful and it is appropriate to offer a hopeful message, based on the knowledge that the overwhelming majority of children do very well in nurturing families when placed there in the early years. However, alongside that, it is crucial to take parents' and carers' concerns seriously and offer evidence-based treatment and support when required.

Delivering mental health support and interventions for older children and young people in the care system

The principles described in the previous section apply equally to older care-experienced children and young people so, in this section, we have highlighted additional specific aspects that are important for practitioners not to miss:

General support for mental health: Young people in substitute care are children first. What they need for good mental health does not differ from what any young person might need—it is just often not available. There are core components of supporting good mental health that should be the foundations of addressing need.

Establishing who is in their support network

Young people in substitute care who do not have a consistent and safe adult in their life are most at risk since a lack of availability of safe and consistent day-to-day support is a key risk factor both for mental ill-health and for intervention effectiveness. An integrative care team should have a focus on ensuring a clear understanding of who is in the young person's network, and consideration of how to build this social support. This might best sit at the social care or education level, rather than services, but should be considered as part of understanding the mental health needs of the young person.

Sleep

Sleep is an important, often overlooked, core component of almost all mental health difficulties. Addressing sleep might be experienced as less stigmatizing for young people, and be a pathway into starting to address mental health needs. Adolescence, for both biological and social reasons, is a period where many sleep difficulties develop. An intervention might usefully incorporate psychoeducation about sleep and sleep hygiene, and the regulation of their sleep routine. Sometimes, sleep problems will be so closely linked with their mental health (e.g., nightmares of their traumatic experiences) that it will need addressing as part of the treatment of the broader symptoms.

Risk, dysregulation, and stabilization

Most young people in substitute care, who are accessing mental health services, will be experiencing emotion dysregulation (hence why they/their carer are seeking support). Many will also come with risk and safeguarding issues, such as self-harm and/or suicidality, risk of placement breakdown, disengagement with school, or risk of exploitation and/or homelessness. For many, this may mean a period of therapeutic intervention focused on "stabilizing" their emotional state. This might focus on basic emotion regulation skills—labeling and recognizing emotions, recognizing situations that might "trigger" dysregulation, and coping skills to deal with "big emotions." All of this is likely to be an important part of any treatment approach. Crucially, however, stabilization should not be used to avoid moving into the treatment (particularly trauma work) nor the only aspect of treatment offered.

Interventions to strengthen the relationship with caregivers

Foster placement or adoption breakdown (i.e., unplanned disruption of the placement resulting in the child having to move) is often an extremely negative event for both the child and the family. Preventing placement breakdowns is often a key focus of services. Reviews in the area have shown that certain parenting programs can improve foster carer sensitivity and child behavior. However, there is limited empirical evidence that common programs are effective at preventing placement breakdowns (Schoemaker *et al.*, 2019). Commonly used programs (e.g., Dyadic Developmental Psychotherapy) are only just starting to be assessed via research trials (e.g., http://ClinicalTrials.gov Identifier: NCT04187911). While it is essential that carers receive training and ongoing support for their own well-being and that of the child in their care, this should occur alongside targeted intervention for the young person's mental health needs (discussed in the next section).

Mental health interventions directed toward the young person

If a child in care is experiencing significant emotional distress, they are likely to benefit from direct mental health intervention and it is crucial that services are commissioned in a way that allows this. As with the assessment, there is no supraspecialist intervention that should be used simply because a child is in care. Instead, what they need is access to existing best-evidenced treatments based on the assessment and formulation of their needs. As with any young person with complex mental health needs, a care-experienced child will likely need treatment to last longer. For example, for PTSD (including complex PTSD), the best-evidenced treatment is trauma-focused CBT. However, young people are likely to need more sessions than a child who has experienced a one-off trauma (NICE, 2018). They may need longer on particular sections (e.g., working through their trauma narrative) or addressing maladaptive cognitions or schemas. They may need longer on psychoeducation or coping or to develop trust with their clinician. Further, a child can have both a neurodevelopmental and a mental health condition (or multiple mental health difficulties). In this case, each might sensibly require treatment, and the existing guidelines for each should be followed. Elsewhere in this book are descriptions of treatment approaches for specific mental health needs and we strongly encourage the reader to refer to these sections.

Summary

Children in substitute care have often experienced an accumulation of risk factors, from the prenatal period through to trauma and adversity in early childhood, instability and separation, and potential further risks within the welfare system. They often face instability in their caregiver relationships and in the range of professionals who enter their lives. Their mental health needs can be complex, but are most appropriately categorized using current diagnostic criteria. Thorough assessments, using established screening tools, are essential for this group, as is high-quality formulation. Such work allows stronger information sharing between appropriate parties, improves understanding of the needs of the young person, and supports access to best-evidenced support and interventions.

Acknowledgment

Thanks to Professor Kayoko Ito for her comments on an earlier draft.

References

Ainsworth, M.D.S. (1979) Infant-mother attachment. *American Psychologist* **34**, 932–937.

American Psychiatric Association (2013) *Diagnostic and Statistical Manual of Mental Disorders*, 5th edn. American Psychiatric Association, Washington, DC.

Asarnow, R.F. *et al.* (2021) Association of attention-deficit/hyperactivity disorder diagnoses with pediatric traumatic brain injury: a meta-analysis. *JAMA Pediatrics* **175**, 1009–1016.

Baptista, J. *et al.* (2019) Early family adversity, stability and consistency of institutional care and infant cognitive, language and motor development across the first six months of institutionalization. *Infant Behavior and Development* **57**, 101387.

Bennet, L. *et al.* (2013) Neural plasticity and the Kennard principle: does it work for the preterm brain? *Clinical and Experimental Pharmacology and Physiology* **40**, 774–784.

Bernard, K. & Dozier, M. (2011) This is my baby: foster parents' feelings of commitment and displays of delight. *Infant Mental Health Journal* **32**, 251–262.

Bick, J. & Dozier, M. (2013) The effectiveness of an attachment-based intervention in promoting foster mothers' sensitivity toward foster infants. *Infant Mental Health Journal* **34**, 95–103.

Bleker, L.S. *et al.* (2019) Malnutrition and depression in pregnancy and associations with child behaviour and cognitive function: a review of recent evidence on unique and joint effects. *Canadian Journal of Physiology and Pharmacology* **97**, 158–173.

Boddy, J. *et al.* (2020) Navigating precarious times? The experience of young adults who have been in care in Norway, Denmark and England. *Journal of Youth Studies* **23**, 291–306.

Bouga, M. *et al.* (2018) Contemporary challenges to iodine status and nutrition: the role of foods, dietary recommendations, fortification and supplementation. *Proceedings of the Nutrition Society* **77**, 302–313.

Broccia, M. *et al.* (2023) Heavy prenatal alcohol exposure and overall morbidities: a Danish nationwide cohort study from 1996 to 2018. *The Lancet Public Health* **8**, e36–e46.

Charness, M.E. (2022) Fetal alcohol spectrum disorders: awareness to insight in just 50 years. *Alcohol Research: Current Reviews* **42**, 05.

Churuangsuk, C. *et al.* (2018) Micronutrient intakes and plasma antioxidant micronutrients on low-carbohydrate diets: a systematic review. *The Proceedings of the Nutrition Society* **77**, E37.

Dansey, D. *et al.* (2019) Keeping secrets: how children in foster care manage stigma. *Adoption & Fostering* **43**, 35–45.

Desmond, C. *et al.* (2020) Prevalence and number of children living in institutional care: global, regional, and country estimates. *The Lancet Child & Adolescent Health* **4**, 370–377.

Dinkler, L. *et al.* (2017) Maltreatment-associated neurodevelopmental disorders: a co-twin control analysis. *Journal of Child Psychology and Psychiatry* **58**, 691.

Dubois-Comtois, K. *et al.* (2021) Are children and adolescents in foster care at greater risk of mental health problems than their counterparts? A meta-analysis. *Children and Youth Services Review* **127**, 106100.

Engler, A.D. *et al.* (2020) A systematic review of mental health disorders of children in foster care. *Trauma, Violence, & Abuse* **23**, 255–264.

Foster, C.C. *et al.* (2019) Home health care for children with medical complexity: workforce gaps, policy, and future directions. *Health Affairs* **38**, 987–993.

Fry, D. & Casey, T. (2017) Bringing the global to the local review of global trends in the prevalence and services for child maltreatment in order to inform research, policy and practice in England. National Society for the Prevention of Cruelty to Children (NSPCC), London.

GOV.UK (2022) *Children looked after in England including adoptions* [Online]. OGL. Open Government Licence v3.0. Available: https://explore-education-statistics.service.gov.uk/find-statistics/children-looked-after-in-england-including-adoptions [23 October 2024].

Hiller, R.M. *et al.* (2021a) Coping and support-seeking in out-of-home care: a qualitative study of the views of young people in care in England. *BMJ Open* **11**, e038461.

Hiller, R.M. *et al.* (2021b). A longitudinal study of cognitive predictors of (complex) post-traumatic stress in young people in out-of-home care. *Journal of Child Psychology & Psychiatry* **62**, 48–57.

Hiller, R.M. *et al.* (2023) The development of young peoples' internalising and externalising difficulties over the first three-years in the public care system. *Child Maltreatment* **28**, 141–151.

Jackson, D.B. *et al.* (2022) Adverse childhood experiences and traumatic brain injury among adolescents: findings from the 2016–2018 national survey of children's health. *European Child & Adolescent Psychiatry* **31**, 289–297.

Kennedy, M. *et al.* (2016) Early severe institutional deprivation is associated with a persistent variant of adult attention-deficit/hyperactivity disorder: clinical presentation, developmental continuities and life circumstances in the English and Romanian adoptees study. *Journal of Child Psychology and Psychiatry* **57**, 1113–1125.

Landers, A.L. *et al.* (2021) Abuse after abuse: The recurrent maltreatment of American Indian children in foster care and adoption. *Child Abuse & Neglect* **111**, 104805.

Lewis, S.J. *et al.* (2021) Unravelling the contribution of complex trauma to psychopathology and cognitive deficits: a cohort study. *The British Journal of Psychiatry* **219**, 448–455.

Lindhiem, O. & Dozier, M. (2007) Caregiver commitment to foster children: the role of child behavior. *Child Abuse & Neglect* **31**, 361–374.

McCarthy, R. *et al.* (2021) Prevalence of fetal alcohol spectrum disorder in greater Manchester, UK: an active case ascertainment study. *Alcoholism: Clinical and Experimental Research* **45**, 2271–2281.

McCrory, E. *et al.* (2022) Social thinning and stress generation after childhood maltreatment: a neurocognitive social transactional model of psychiatric vulnerability. *The Lancet Psychiatry* **9**, 828–837.

McQuire, C. *et al.* (2020) The causal web of foetal alcohol spectrum disorders: a review and causal diagram. *European Child & Adolescent Psychiatry* **29**, 575–594.

Minnis, H. *et al.* (2020) Autism and attachment disorder symptoms in the general population: prevalence, overlap, and burden. *Developmental Child Welfare* **2**, 37–51.

Munson, M.R. *et al.* (2020) Mental health management among older youth in foster care: service utilization and preparedness. *Journal of Adolescent Health* **67**, 225–231.

Nelson, C.A. *et al.* (2014) *Romania's Abandoned Children: Deprivation, Brain Development and the Struggle for Recovery*. Harvard University Press, Cambridge, MA.

NICE (2018) *Post-traumatic stress disorder*. National Institute for Health and Care Excellence, London. [Online] Available: www.nice.org.uk/guidance/ng116 [23 October 2024].

Ozsarfati, J. & Koren, G. (2015) Medications used in the treatment of disruptive behavior in children with FASD-a guide. *Journal of Population Therapeutics and Clinical Pharmacology* **22**, e59–e67.

Petrowski, N. *et al.* (2017) Estimating the number of children in formal alternative care: challenges and results. *Child Abuse and Neglect* **70**, 388–398.

Prince, D.M. *et al.* (2019) Effects of individual risk and state housing factors on adverse outcomes in a national sample of youth transitioning out of foster care. *Journal of Adolescence* **74**, 33–44.

Pritchett, R. *et al.* (2016) Challenges of assessing maltreated children coming into foster care. *The Scientific World Journal* **2016**, 5986835.

Russell, L. *et al.* (2022) Gender, addiction and removal of children into care. *Frontiers in Psychiatry* **13**, 887660.

Rutter, M. & Sonuga-Barke, E. (2010) Deprivation-specific psychological patterns: effects of institutional deprivation. *Monographs of the Society for Research in Child Development* **75**, 212–229.

Schoemaker, N.K. *et al.* (2019) A meta-analytic review of parenting interventions in foster care and adoption. *Development and Psychopathology* **32**(3), 1149–1172.

Sebastiani, G. *et al.* (2018) The effects of alcohol and drugs of abuse on maternal nutritional profile during pregnancy. *Nutrients* **10**, 1008.

Seddighi, H. *et al.* (2021) Child abuse in natural disasters and conflicts: a systematic review. *Trauma, Violence, & Abuse* **22**, 176–185.

Seim, A.R. *et al.* (2021) Self-esteem in adolescents with reactive attachment disorder or disinhibited social engagement disorder. *Child Abuse & Neglect* **118**, 105141.

Seim, A.R. *et al.* (2022) Reactive attachment disorder and disinhibited social engagement disorder in adolescence: co-occurring psychopathology and psychosocial problems. *European Child & Adolescent Psychiatry* **31**, 85–98.

SIGN (2019) SIGN 156 children and young people exposed prenatally to alcohol. A national clinical guideline. Health Improvement Scotland. SIGN Evidence-based Clinical Guidelines. NHS Scotland, Edinburgh, UK.

Sokol, R.L. *et al.* (2018) Relationship between child maltreatment and adolescent body mass index trajectories. *Children and Youth Services Review* **93**, 196–202.

Sonuga-Barke, E.J. *et al.* (2017) Child-to-adult neurodevelopmental and mental health trajectories after early life deprivation: the young adult follow-up of the longitudinal English and Romanian adoptees study. *The Lancet* **389**, 1539–1548.

Sroufe, A.L. & Waters, E. (1977) Attachment as an organizational construct. *Child Development* **48**, 1184–1199.

Stern, A. *et al.* (2018) Associations between abuse/neglect and ADHD from childhood to young adulthood: a prospective nationally-representative twin study. *Child Abuse & Neglect* **81**, 274–285.

Tarren-Sweeney, M. & Goemans, A. (2019) A narrative review of stability and change in the mental health of children who grow up in family-based out-of-home care. *Developmental Child Welfare* **1**, 273–294.

Tsappis, E. *et al.* (2022) Promoting secure attachment. *Paediatrics and Child Health* **32**, 191–197.

Turner, F. *et al.* (2023) "I will commit to this child as much as I can for the time that they are with me:" a qualitative examination of how foster carer commitment relates to short-term foster care for young children following abuse and neglect. *Child Abuse & Neglect* **135**, 105983.

Van Ijzendoorn, M.H. *et al.* (2020) Institutionalisation and deinstitutionalisation of children 1: a systematic and integrative review of evidence regarding effects on development. *The Lancet Psychiatry* **7**, 703–720.

Wade, M. *et al.* (2022) The Bucharest Early Intervention Project: adolescent mental health and adaptation following early deprivation. *Child Development Perspectives* **16**, 157–164.

Wagstaff, J. *et al.* (2017) Orphans, Foster Care and Adoption: Global Perspective. Cinahl Information Services, a division of EBSCO Information Services, Ipswich, MA.

Webster, B.M. *et al.* (2023) Evaluating the difference in neuropsychological profiles of individuals with FASD based on the number of sentinel facial features: a service evaluation of the FASD UK National Clinic Database. *Children* **10**, 266.

World Health Organization (2019) *International Statistical Classification of Disease and Related Health Problems*, 11th edn, Geneva, Switzerland.

Zwicker, A. *et al.* (2020) Neurodevelopmental and genetic determinants of exposure to adversity among youth at risk for mental illness. *Journal of Child Psychology and Psychiatry* **61**, 536–544.

CHAPTER 43

Pediatric consultation and psychiatric aspects of somatic disease

Eric P. Hazen[1,2] and Jessica E. Becker[3]

[1]Harvard Medical School, Boston, MA, USA

[2]Pediatric Psychiatry Consultation-Liaison Service, Department of Psychiatry, Massachusetts General Hospital, Boston, MA, USA

[3]Department of Child and Adolescent Psychiatry, NYU Grossman School of Medicine and NYU Langone Health, New York, NY, USA

Introduction

In the medical setting, "pediatric consultation" or "pediatric consultation-liaison" care refers to child psychiatrists, psychologists, or other mental health practitioners providing mental health care to medically ill children, with special attention to biological, psychological, and social mediators of well-being. Here, we refer to the task of the "mental health consultant" as assessment and management of the psychiatric status of the medically ill child, most often in a medical hospital environment.

Mental health consultants assess: (i) children with primary psychiatric illnesses leading to medical conditions, (ii) psychiatric manifestations of medical illnesses, (iii) adjustment to medical illness, and (iv) differential diagnosis of psychosomatic illness. The consultant's scope also may include working with parents, providing liaison work with ward staff, teaching across medical disciplines, and working with hospital leadership to develop more psychologically attuned standard practices.

History

Adult consultation psychiatry arose in general hospitals during the 1930s, with the recognition that psychological issues have an impact on medical illness and treatment (Ortiz, 1997). As the integral role of psychological factors was established in adult medical care, similar attention was focused on the needs of children (Work 1989). While the literature continues to demonstrate the benefits of collaboration between child psychiatrists and pediatric staff (Carter *et al.*, 2003; Fritz, 2003), consultation psychiatry remains a limited resource and may be virtually unavailable in many low- and middle-income countries. While telemedicine has allowed for innovation in consultation practice, funding challenges continue to impact the availability of consultation.

Consultation service models

Consultation service models are determined by the characteristics of the patient group served and the availability of child mental health consultants. Regardless of their training discipline, consultants need an understanding of disease processes and treatments, and skill in a wide range of psychological interventions.

Inpatient consultations may be initiated on a case-by-case basis, by protocol, or both. In the case-by-case model, the pediatrician requests a consultation after assessing an individual patient, while consultation by protocol systematizes consultation for children with certain diagnoses or risk factors. Examples of protocol-driven consultation include routine consultation to patients who are candidates for transplant or who have been admitted after suicide attempts.

Increasingly, pediatric consultation-liaison psychiatrists and psychologists serve a role in the outpatient setting, in both primary care and subspecialty pediatric settings. Outpatient consultation models, often termed integrated behavioral health models, may similarly include mental health providers from various specialties, including social work, psychology, or psychiatry. Integration models vary in scale from co-location to population health management to fully embedded and integrated systems of care.

Rutter's Child and Adolescent Psychiatry and Psychology, Seventh Edition.
Edited by Anita Thapar, Daniel S. Pine, Samuele Cortese, Cathy Creswell, Tamsin J. Ford, James F. Leckman, and Argyris Stringaris.

Companion website: www.wiley.com/go/thapar/rutterspsych7

"Liaison" care

Arguably, no consultation to a hospitalized child can be provided effectively without the integral "liaison" component addressing concerns arising from members of the treatment team. Work with medically ill children is rewarding, but it can also arouse powerful feelings in providers. Pediatric units may seek input from the consultant to address the emotional challenges experienced by the medical team, assist them in their ability to provide the best care for patients, and prevent long-term burnout (Bateman *et al.*, 2012).

The consultation

The following section discusses aspects of evaluation, diagnosis, and formulation in the context of the specific pediatric consultation-liaison setting. For additional details on these topics more generally, please refer to Chapters 2, 24, and 27 of this text.

Approach to consultation requests

The first task for the consultant when responding to a request is to understand: "What is the consultation question?" While the consultation question is sometimes clear, often it is obscured by affect among care providers or with the family or patient. The consultant should speak directly with the consulting provider, listen to the expressed concerns, and ask for elaboration about concerns that appear present but not disclosed. It is important to establish realistic goals and to determine acuity for the initial consultation as early as possible and as part of a step-by-step approach to the consultation (Table 43.1). The medical provider with whom the family already has a relationship should inform the parents of the decision to obtain a psychiatric consultation and obtain appropriate consent. In cases where the family does not understand the referring provider's reasoning, the consultant may be able to explain their role more fully to the family as part of the consent process. If families refuse consultation, the consultant may meet with the team in a liaison capacity and assist the team without directly interviewing the child. If consultation is refused but deemed critical, the pediatrician should seek input from the hospital legal counsel about the appropriate way to proceed within the legal system in which the pediatrician practices.

Prior to meeting with the family and child, the consultant should review relevant medical data, including notes, laboratory and imaging studies, and medication administration reports. The consultant should also review basic information about any specific medical illness and be familiar with planned workup or treatment.

Table 43.1 Top tips for pediatric consultation.

- Review the medical chart and speak with the requesting clinician before the consult to discuss the specific questions or difficulties they are hoping the consultant will address.
- It is often helpful to verify that the patient and family have been informed about the involvement of a psychiatric consultant prior to the assessment. Some providers may benefit from discussion and guidance about how best to introduce the consult.
- For younger children, it can be helpful to bring play or art materials to the initial encounter to engage the child.
- Thought should be given to whether to interview the patient and parents/guardians separately or together, which may depend upon the developmental stage of the child, the consult question, and patient preferences. Generally, it is helpful to spend some time observing a patient and parents/guardians together as this provides helpful insight into their interactions, but, particularly for older children and adolescents, spending some time speaking separately gives both the patient and the parents/guardians an opportunity to convey things that they might not feel comfortable stating in the presence of the other.
- Collateral information can be critical to a thorough assessment. This can include information gathered from outside sources, such as outpatient providers or school contacts, as well as from other members of the multidisciplinary team working closely with the patient.
- After the initial evaluation, direct communication with the requesting clinician is preferable to communication through chart documentation alone, as it assures that all questions and concerns have been considered.
- Regular communication with the medical team is essential to providing ongoing care. In many cases, particularly those with significant medical and psychosocial complexity, multidisciplinary team meetings can be an effective strategy for coordinating care efforts.

Interview of child and family

Depending on the age and circumstances of the child's condition, the consultant will decide whether to meet with the parents first, the child first, or both together. Meeting with older children without a parent present at some point is usually essential. This allows them to voice private concerns and allows for observation of differences in mental status with and without family present. Children under six are often more comfortable meeting with the consultant along with a parent. The parents of young children are likely to want time alone with the consultant to share observations and concerns which are not appropriate to share in the child's presence. Similarly, many parents of older children will find it easier to be candid about their worries in the absence of the child.

No child can be understood independently of his or her family. In the initial evaluation, it is therefore essential to assess the family's level of functioning and their ability to support the child through treatment. Parental anxiety and distress are associated with a child's psychological adjustment and capacity to cope (Wagner *et al.*, 2003). Asking parents to share the history of the current illness, from the first symptoms through to the present hospital stay, allows the consultant to learn about the parents' experience of the medical care. It is helpful to understand the parents' views of medical caregivers as well as their experience of their own role in the child's medical condition. An assessment of the family should include family history of psychiatric illness and questions about the family's past experiences with illness and loss. Helping the parent differentiate the current medical situation from past experiences helps the parent be more attuned to the child's actual needs.

Siblings are often the forgotten sufferers (Alderfer *et al.*, 2010). The sick child is commonly the object of everyone's attention, while siblings often live with disrupted schedules, less attention, and less emotionally available parents. The consultant can model empathy for siblings and help parents find ways of addressing the needs of their well children.

Some parents cannot bear their feelings of helplessness and vent their anger and frustration on hospital staff by being critical and devaluing (Groves & Beresin, 1999). Pediatric hospital staff members may have a harder time working with some parents than the patient. The consultant can help the team understand the family better and feel more empathy for difficult behaviors while setting limits on abusive behavior to staff.

Collateral sources

The consultant should seek information from other members of the treatment team, including nursing and therapeutic staff, who may offer especially valuable observations. After the initial assessment and with parental consent, the consultant may seek input provided by sources outside of the medical arenas such as an outpatient psychotherapist, school professionals, or members of involved social agencies.

Formulation: premorbid medical and psychiatric functioning

When the consultant is assessing a hospitalized child, the consultant is seeing only "a snapshot" of the child's life. Some families will be confronting a new diagnosis or change in prognosis, while others may have had time to develop an ongoing coping strategy in the face of a chronic illness. Assessment should recognize the potential for wide variation in coping at different points in the unfolding medical experience.

Formulation: conceptions of medical illness across child development

Development is an important lens through which a childhood medical illness can be observed. A full review of the interplay of development and medical illness is beyond the scope of this chapter, but a few key developmental points will be highlighted to illustrate common issues. These points are summarized in Table 43.2.

Infants and toddlers cannot understand the gravity of a given diagnosis. They live in the moment experiencing the medical condition and treatment according to the physical limitations and discomforts imposed. Infants rely on key caretakers to hold and soothe them and to make the hospital environment feel safe. It is important for the hospital staff to support the infant–parent attachment, and not allow treatments and technologies to interfere with this developmental cornerstone. Interventions include supporting breast-feeding mothers and allowing rooming-in by parents.

Table 43.2 Developmental considerations in the medically ill child.

Age	Developmental focus as related to health	Interventions in the hospital
0–2	Attachment	Support parents with rooming in and feeding
3–6	Egocentricity, "magical thinking," physical integrity	Understand and correct self-blame regarding illness, prepare for procedures
7–12	Rule-focused, concrete thinking, pride in knowledge	Use simple, clear language to describe illness and treatment
13+ (adolescence)	Abstract thinking, self-consciousness, growing independence	Respect treatment decisions and obtain consent as indicated, support age-appropriate autonomy, support in transition of care from pediatric to adult medicine

Very young children (3–6-year-olds) are egocentric, that is, they understand all events as occurring in relation to them. They have associative logic, which means that for them any two unrelated things can be understood as if one is causing or explaining the other. The combination of egocentricity and associative logic leads to "magical thinking," the weaving together of fantasy and logic to explain how the young child caused something to happen. In the medical setting, it is frequently the child's misconception that having a "bad illness" means they did something wrong and are being punished. It is helpful to get young children (and often older children as well) to elaborate their understanding of the etiology of their medical conditions to uncover self-blaming misconceptions and correct them.

At this age, children cannot localize a medical condition to a specific body part, so they feel particularly physically vulnerable when ill. Faced with needle sticks, intravenous medication, and surgical procedures, they are often fearful. They rely on parents and medical staff to prepare them for procedures so they come to trust that there will not be surprise medical attacks at any moment. The young child is likely to demonstrate the most affect around separations, such as having anxiety about going to sleep at night in his own bed, or wanting a parent to promise to be there when they wake up from surgery.

Older children (approximately 7–12 years of age) can understand simple, functional explanations of medical conditions. Many will pride themselves on mastering the names of medicines, illness-related terminology, and how to use hospital equipment. Children of this age look for simple cause and effect etiologies for illnesses. They can understand viral illnesses being caused by "germs," but are perplexed when there is no clear causal explanation, for example, for why they have cancer without having smoked cigarettes. It is important to explain illness and treatment simply and clearly. In the context of understanding why a treatment plan is being initiated, the medical staff should seek the child's assent to procedures and treatments. This age group is typically rule-bound, and it is troubling to the child that so often medical illness does not follow "the rules" (e.g., a child avoids their asthma triggers and has an asthma attack anyway).

Adolescents (13 and older) generally have abstract thinking and thus are able to understand the chance bad luck of having an uncommon, life-threatening, or chronic illness with the same cognitive complexity of an adult. That said, teens often do not have the maturity to incorporate the healthy behaviors that they know that they should engage in into appropriate changes in lifestyle. Turning cognitive understanding into behavioral change is the common battleground of adolescent and authority figures—parent or physician. The potential impact on medical management is discussed further in the later "Reasons for consultation: psychological distress in medically ill children" section.

Adolescence is a self-conscious time with the emergence of sexual interests and heightened reliance on peer group norms for style and status. Medical illnesses or treatments that affect appearance are particularly difficult such as losing hair with chemotherapy. The medical staff are challenged to find ways to respect the teen's age-appropriate wish to be more independent in the face of illness that so often increases dependency.

As children with chronic illnesses live into adulthood, the transition to young adulthood and understanding associated issues becomes relevant. Young adults are negotiating intimate relationships, career decisions, independence from parents, and sometimes relocation or parenthood. One challenge that the treatment team and patient may face is whether to transition care from a pediatric setting into an adult setting, which often necessitates a new treatment team. This is a particularly vulnerable time with increased risks of nonadherence and loss to follow-up (Garvey *et al.*, 2012). Some patients may prefer to be on an adult ward or waiting room, but may find it very difficult to leave lifelong caretakers and the pediatric model of care.

Mental status examination in the hospitalized or medically ill child

Hospitalized children have many reasons to have an altered mental status including delirium, central nervous system (CNS) changes secondary to medical conditions, effects of medications, and trauma. Thus, a thorough mental status examination is a critical part of the consultation.

Medically ill children may be developmentally delayed or emotionally immature. It is helpful for the consultant to integrate the information from the mental status examination and premorbid school and developmental information to assist the medical team in understanding the child's ability to comprehend medical information.

Presenting recommendations to the team

After meeting with the child and family for the initial assessment, the consultant will share observations and recommendations with the referring provider and write a note in the medical record. The formulation and recommendations should avoid the use of psychiatric jargon. Clear practical recommendations to improve coping, address behavioral problems, treat primary psychiatric disorders, and maintain safety are most helpful. Sharing an understanding of motivations that may underlie maladaptive behaviors can increase empathy for the child and family, but the consultant should also provide concrete, practical suggestions. One should assume that patients and caregivers will read the record, as can hospital staff and insurers. Moreover, consultants may have a role in liaising between families and members of the medical team and may initiate multidisciplinary team meetings as an efficient way to address clinical needs in complex patients.

Reasons for consultation: primary psychiatric illnesses

Depression

Symptoms of depression are common in the hospitalized child. One barrier to the appropriate treatment of depression in hospitalized children is the misconception that depressed mood is an appropriate response to serious illness. Another barrier to treatment is the difficulty of making the diagnosis of depression in a medically ill child given the overlap of somatic symptoms and depressive symptoms (Shemesh *et al.*, 2005). Short-term psychotherapeutic interventions are useful modalities in the hospital setting, with subsequent referral for ongoing treatment after discharge. Medications, including antidepressants, are sometimes used effectively in hospitalized children (Kersun & Elia, 2007). Selective serotonin reuptake inhibitors (SSRIs) are typically the first-line agent of choice as they are well-tolerated, have limited interactions with other medications, and present a lower risk of morbidity in overdose. Additional information on depression is found in Chapter 63.

Anxiety

Anxiety disorders can be preexisting or secondary to the stresses of a medical condition and treatment. Children with preexisting generalized anxiety or specific fear of doctors or needles are likely to have more difficulty adjusting to medical treatment. In addition to the discomfort anxiety causes to children and parents, anxiety can interfere with evaluation and treatment. Age-appropriate explanation of medical interventions for older children, and medical play with explanation for younger children, can decrease anxiety. Many children respond well to coping techniques to help with anxiety-provoking procedures, including distraction, breathing exercises, visualization, or hypnotherapy (Koller & Goldman, 2012). Anxiety may also improve with interventions to address pain, including preparation, relaxation, distraction, use of anesthetic creams before procedures, and treating chronic and acute pain with analgesics (Fein *et al.*, 2012). For young children, painful procedures should occur in a treatment room and not in the child's bed or the playroom. Protecting the child's bed and the playroom as safe havens will help the young child relax in these settings. Additional information on anxiety is found in Chapter 59.

Eating disorders

Pediatric hospitalizations for eating disorders have been increasing in recent years (Zima *et al.*, 2022). Children with different kinds of eating disorders, including anorexia nervosa, bulimia nervosa, and avoidant/restrictive food intake disorder (ARFID) are hospitalized when there has been rapid or profound weight loss, cardiovascular abnormalities, or electrolyte imbalance. The goal of hospitalization is medical stabilization with nutritional replenishment, psychological assessment of the child and family, and recommendation for the level of psychiatric intervention after medical stabilization. Eating disorder protocols provide established guidelines for structuring inpatient clinical care. The protocols are detailed and may include restrictions of activity, observation during and after mealtimes, and bathroom privileges only after weight gain has begun (Sylvester & Forman, 2008). Once the child is medically stable, recommendations about disposition can be initiated. Additional information on feeding and eating disorders is found in Chapter 69.

Somatic symptom and related disorders

Children frequently experience distress through physical symptoms. Somatizing behavior can become a disorder when it begins to interfere in a child's daily functioning, such as attending school or participating in activities. Some children are admitted to pediatric units with intense, persistent somatic complaints such as headaches, abdominal pain, neurologic symptoms, or fatigue. The pediatricians may suspect that the intensity of the symptoms or the combination of complaints exceeds what can be explained by a medical condition and may thus seek a psychiatric consultation for a suspected somatic symptom and related disorder (SSRD). The pediatrician's assessment that psychological factors are influencing the somatic presentation may be at odds with the child and parents' understanding of the etiology of the condition.

While SSRDs can be challenging for patients, families, and medical teams given the complexities with which they can present, it is important for primary teams and consultants to remember that these symptoms often present in children with other known physical health conditions. As such, a unified approach to diagnosis and treatment is crucial, and hospitalization can be an important opportunity for a coordinated care plan addressing psychological and physical issues together. The American Academy of Child and Adolescent Psychiatry (AACAP) has put together a helpful pathway for diagnosing and addressing SSRDs in the inpatient setting (Ibeziako *et al.*, 2019). When SSRDs are suspected by the primary team, early involvement of psychiatry consultation, rather than reactive consultation after an unrevealing medical workup, is critical in helping patients and families understand the real nature of the mind–body connection and the benefit of behavioral strategies in addressing many somatic symptoms (Ibeziako *et al.*, 2019). Coordinated, multidisciplinary messaging to families and regularly scheduled outpatient follow-up with medical teams, mental health providers, and rehabilitation services like physical therapy can help children with SSRDs regain their functioning. Additional information on SSRDs is found in Chapter 70.

Nonadherence

Nonadherence with medical treatments is common. There are many factors contributing to nonadherence, including the medication regimen, family systems, denial, psychiatric illness, and relationships with medical providers. Physicians recognize that education and an alliance with parents and children can improve adherence rates. The consultant's task is to understand why the child is nonadherent and to work with the team to modify aspects of treatments that trouble the child where possible, while working to help the child and family adopt strategies that support clinically important treatments. Treatable psychiatric disorders need to be identified and addressed. Treatment promoting supports, such as disease-specific support groups and psychoeducation groups, can be helpful.

Autism spectrum disorder

Rates of diagnosis of autism spectrum disorder (ASD) in children have been rising steadily, with recent estimates indicating a prevalence as high as 1 in 36 children at age 8 years (Maenner *et al.*, 2023). See Chapter 50 for further discussion of this pattern. Children with ASD have higher rates of medical illness and greater frequency of medical admissions than the general population (Croen *et al.*, 2006; Gurney *et al.*, 2006). The features of ASD make the hospital setting particularly challenging, which may lead to distress, agitation, aggression, or self-injury (Hazen *et al.*, 2020). Difficulties communicating, sensory sensitivities, departure from comforting routines, and the social stress of encountering unfamiliar people can all play a part in these difficulties (Thom *et al.*, 2020a). A consulting psychiatrist can be helpful in reducing the distress experienced by patients with ASD and their families in medical settings. Beginning with a detailed developmental, behavioral, and psychiatric evaluation of the child, the consultant can help the medical team modify their approach to care and implement a behavioral plan that can make a medical admission more tolerable for an individual with ASD (Thom *et al.*, 2019). Thoughtful use of medications to reduce anxiety or manage agitation may also be incorporated into the plan. More information regarding ASD may be found in Chapter 50.

Substance use

The prevalence of substance use in pediatric patients is increasing (Moss *et al.*, 2018) and can be associated with medical illness, either due to risk of accidents or by exacerbation of an existing medical condition. The consulting psychiatrist may assist in guiding substance use screening practices for pediatric units, evaluating patients for possible substance use disorder, initiating treatment in the hospital including management of withdrawal, and referral to outpatient services (Smith *et al.*, 2020). Additional information on substance use can be found in Chapter 66.

Reasons for consultation: emergency consultations

Suicide attempts

Suicide risk assessment is the most common reason for psychiatric consultation to pediatrics. The consultant may be asked to evaluate a patient who has made suicidal statements or engaged in a suicide attempt or self-injurious behavior. The consultant's first priorities in this situation are to assure the child's immediate safety and to perform a thorough assessment of imminent risk of suicide based upon: the patient's thoughts and behavior; information from collateral sources such as parents, outpatient providers, or school personnel; and a careful weighing of risk and protective factors. The consultant then must make recommendations about the most appropriate disposition for the child, such as referral to an inpatient psychiatric unit, as well as measures that are needed to maintain the child's safety in the hospital, which might include provision of a patient observer or limiting access to sharp objects or ligature.

There has been a growing appreciation in recent years of the importance of screening children and adolescents in medical settings for suicide risk, and specific instruments have been developed and demonstrated to be effective for this purpose (Thom *et al.*, 2020b). The psychiatric consultant can assist medical teams in choosing an appropriate instrument and implementing an effective screening program. For additional information on suicidal behavior, see Chapter 64.

Altered mental status

Psychiatry consultation is often sought to assist in the assessment and treatment of altered mental status in hospitalized children.

Delirium

Delirium is commonly encountered in medically ill children and is characterized by: (i) acute onset and waxing and waning course, (ii) cognitive impairment or confusion, and (iii) disturbance of arousal. Delirium can occur either in the setting of an underlying general medical illness or secondary to medications or toxins. Conditions commonly associated with delirium are listed in Table 43.3; infectious and toxic etiologies (including medications) are the most common in the pediatric population. The underlying mechanisms of delirium remain poorly understood, but it is thought to represent derangements in multiple neurotransmitter systems, particularly dysregulation of acetylcholine and dopamine. In addition to confusion, symptoms of delirium commonly include hallucinations, delusions, disorganized behavior, disorientation, and disruptions in memory, mood, affect, and the sleep–wake cycle (Turkel *et al.*, 2006). The nature of the disturbance of arousal in delirium varies. Hyperactive delirium is associated with combativeness and agitation. Hypoactive delirium is a state of quiet confusion and is often overlooked as the symptoms do not interfere with care.

Table 43.3 Conditions commonly associated with delirium.

Condition type	Conditions
Infectious	Encephalitis, meningitis, syphilis, pneumonia, urinary tract infection (UTI)
Withdrawal	Alcohol, benzodiazepines, sedative-hypnotics
Acute metabolic	Acidosis, alkalosis, electrolyte disturbances, liver or kidney failure
Trauma	Heatstroke, burns, post-operative
Central nervous system (CNS) pathology	Abscess, hemorrhage, seizure, stroke, tumor, vasculitis, normal pressure hydrocephalus
Hypoxia	Anemia, carbon monoxide poisoning, hypotension, pulmonary embolus, lung or heart failure
Deficiencies	B12, niacin, thiamine
Endocrinopathies	Hyper- or hypoglycemia, hyper- or hypoadrenocorticism, hyper- or hypothyroidism
Acute vascular	Hypertensive encephalopathy or shock
Toxins or drugs	Medications, pesticides, solvents
Heavy metals	Lead, manganese, mercury

Source: Adapted from Stern *et al.*, (2010)/with permission of ELSEVIER.

Delirium should always be considered in the differential for new-onset psychosis in the hospital setting; moreover, while many patients with new psychotic symptoms will not have impairments of cognition and arousal associated with delirium, all patients with first-episode psychosis should have a thorough workup for medical etiologies of psychosis. More details on the workup of psychotic symptoms can be found in Chapter 56.

Definitive treatment for the delirious patient is identification and treatment of the underlying cause while managing symptoms in order to ensure patient safety. Management incorporates environmental interventions, including reassurance, use of environmental cues, and frequent reorienting to place and familiar people. Pharmacologic interventions, particularly antipsychotic medications, can ease distressing symptoms including psychosis and fear, as well as decrease agitation. Benzodiazepines and medications with anticholinergic properties can compound the core symptoms of confusion and disorientation and should usually be avoided in the delirious patient (with the notable exception of delirium that is due to withdrawal from alcohol or benzodiazepines).

Catatonia

Catatonia, a syndrome of combined motor and mental status changes, has been growing in prevalence in children, yet is still frequently missed or undertreated in pediatric populations

(Becker *et al.*, 2020). While commonly attributed to underlying psychiatric conditions, catatonia frequently occurs in the context of underlying medical illness, such as infections, seizures, or autoimmune illness; additionally, children with certain developmental disorders are at increased risk for developing catatonia, and the signs and symptoms of catatonia can overlap with those of the developmental disorder itself (Becker *et al.*, 2020). Screening scales, such as the Bush-Francis scale or the Pediatric Catatonia Symptom Rating Scale, can be used both to assist in diagnosis of catatonia and in tracking response to treatment. The mainstay of treatment is lorazepam, which is most effective when given intravenously, and high doses may be necessary to lyse the symptoms of catatonia; antipsychotic medications and other D2 receptor antagonists can worsen catatonia symptoms and should be avoided (Becker *et al.*, 2020). In refractory cases, augmentation may include N-methyl-D-aspartate antagonist medications such as amantadine or memantine, or, particularly in the case of concern for life-threatening malignant catatonia, electroconvulsive therapy (ECT) (Becker *et al.*, 2020). Access to ECT may unfortunately be limited, particularly for children, depending on a jurisdiction's regulations.

Autoimmune encephalitis and other neuroimmunologic conditions

In pediatric patients with acute onset of altered mental status, including new symptoms of psychosis or mood lability, autoimmune processes should be a consideration for the primary team and consulting psychiatrist. Autoimmune encephalitis, another increasingly recognized condition, can present solely with psychiatric symptoms and is treatable with immune-modulating agents (Becker *et al.*, 2020). Medical workup for this condition may include electroencephalography and testing for autoantibodies in the serum and spinal fluid. Other immunologic conditions, such as lupus, can present with neuropsychiatric manifestations. As such, it is important that the consulting psychiatrist help the primary team in ensuring a thoughtful medical workup is completed for new psychiatric symptoms and altered mental status.

The challenging family

Parental behavior may be the reason for an urgent referral to the mental health consultant or to the team social worker. Parents may be refusing essential medical treatment for the child, threatening to remove an ill child from the hospital against medical advice, or acting strangely. The reason for the parental actions may remain unclear, or may be explained by beliefs at odds with standard medical practice, mistrust of the hospital staff, psychiatric illness in the parent, or extreme distress. Hostile parents may interfere with critical care by frightening the medical staff.

Often parents who are obstructing needed care for their child are doing so because they are themselves overwhelmed with helplessness and are trying to control what they consider as uncontrollable. By helping the parent to feel that he or she is an essential member of the decision-making process and thus has some control in productive ways, many parents will step out of a combative stance and into a more collaborative one. Specific legal interventions may be implemented when parents prevent a life-sustaining treatment and will be determined by the legal parameters of the place of practice.

Child abuse

Physical abuse, neglect, and sexual abuse may result in emergency consultation and are discussed elsewhere in this book. In the consultation setting, it is appropriate to restate the importance of considering abuse. Without educated suspicion, abuse will often go undetected. Suspicious injuries, implausible or inconsistent stories from caretakers, and inappropriate delay in bringing a child for medical care should raise suspicion. Suspicion of abuse must be reported to the appropriate social agency. It is important to notify authorities of other children known to be in a potentially unsafe home. The pediatric unit may serve as a safe haven for a child while allegations are being investigated.

The pediatric medical unit also may be the primary setting as families or patients seek excessive medical treatment for their reported symptoms/illness, which in extreme cases is considered medical child abuse. One form of medical child abuse involves fabrication of illness by a parent or caregiver, widely known as factitious disorder by proxy (formerly Munchausen syndrome by proxy). The psychiatric consultant may become involved in such cases as the medical team grapples with providing appropriate medical treatment when the history and presentation are inconsistent. When the child suffers harm related to these interventions, regardless of caregiver intent, medical child abuse has occurred. In such cases, early, multidisciplinary team evaluation is crucial, and it can be useful to enlist a hospital's child protection team and legal team. The psychiatric consultant may be able to help assess for trauma and support a child who is the victim of abuse.

Reasons for consultation: psychological distress in medically ill children

Children with medical illnesses serious enough to warrant hospitalization are at increased risk for emotional disorders, with estimates of psychological distress in hospitalized children and adolescents varying from 20% to greater than 35% (Stoppelbein *et al.*, 2005). Medical treatment itself—particularly involving procedures or a stay in the intensive care unit—can be traumatic for some children, with 10–20% of medically ill children estimated to develop post-traumatic stress disorder (Forgey & Bursch, 2013). Tertiary care hospitalizations for children with mental health conditions have been growing steadily in recent years (Zima *et al.*, 2016); compared to children without mental health conditions, medically hospitalized children with comorbid mental health conditions have longer hospital lengths of stay, increased health care utilization, and increased rates of hospital readmissions (Doupnik *et al.*, 2016; Perrin *et al.*, 2019). Official practice parameters released by the AACAP in 2009 offer principles for the assessment, management, and treatment of the medically ill child (DeMaso *et al.*, 2009).

Coping with chronic illness

Chronically ill children should not be defined by their illnesses. To the contrary, chronically ill children have the same range of personalities and coping styles observed in healthy children and are engaged in mastering the developmental milestones and challenges they share with their peers.

Estimates of psychological morbidity associated with chronic illnesses in childhood range between 10–30%, which is only slightly higher than the general pediatric population (Barlow & Ellard, 2006). Greater morbidity is associated with multiple hospitalizations, physical disability and brain dysfunction, pain frequency, younger age, poverty, single-parent family, and increased psychological symptoms in the parents (Geist, 1977; Knapp & Harris, 1998).

Specific illnesses present specific challenges, as discussed in the following sections. That said, innumerable factors influence how problematic any given challenge is for an individual child. It is the consultant's job to understand the unique meaning of the illness to the child and family and to assist in the process of adaptation. The consultant should explore the child's subjective experience of illness, such as the hardest aspects of illness or treatment from the child's perspective, how it affects the child's self-image, and specific worries about the future. Inquiries about the impact on peer interactions or favorite activities, areas of conflict between the child and parent in relation to the illness, and the child's perception of the parents' concerns may be useful.

Asthma

Asthma is one of the most common chronic illnesses of childhood (Pijnenburg & Fleming, 2020). While there have been advances in treatment in recent years, the subset of children with severe asthma tends to have higher health care utilization, comorbidities, and more severe behavioral and emotional symptoms.

Hospitalization is an opportunity to emphasize education. Clear guidelines on when to call the pediatrician can be established while seeking input from the family about barriers to these contacts. Triggers in the home, such as smoking and pets, can be addressed realistically and empathically in light of the exacerbation that led to admission. School-related issues need to be explored from the perspective of the child (e.g., embarrassment associated with going to the school nurse) and the school (e.g., access to inhalers in the classroom). Strategies such as stress management and distress tolerance skills to improve parent and child anxiety and to address parent–child conflicts around adherence are valuable.

Diabetes

Insulin-dependent diabetes presents special medical challenges associated with control of blood sugars and insulin delivery, as well as emotional challenges related to the primary role of food as a source of nurturance and soothing. The acute consequences of blood sugar abnormalities include symptomatic hypoglycemia, hyperglycemia, and ketoacidosis and may lead to hospitalization. The long-term sequelae include effects on vision, renal function, and neuropathy. Symptoms associated with hypoglycemia can be difficult for parents to differentiate from common irritability or anxiety in children. This may lead to either more frequent blood glucose testing or a tendency to keep the blood sugars at a higher level than the physician would recommend. It is key to treat anxiety, mood, and attention deficit hyperactivity disorder (ADHDs) to improve adherence and to recognize emerging eating disorders—including the intentional withholding of insulin—as a factor in nonadherence (Hamilton & Daneman, 2002).

Nonadherence in insulin dependent diabetes can be life-threatening. Blood testing (hemoglobin A1C) enables pediatricians to assess the child's adherence over an extended period and may be considered an appropriate factor for protocol-driven mental health consultation. Technologies including continuous glucose monitors (CGMs) and subcutaneous insulin pumps, which deliver a continuous infusion of rapid-acting insulin at both basal and bolus rates, allow for tighter control of blood sugars when combined with careful tracking of carbohydrate intake. While these potentially life-changing technologies may be especially appealing by allowing greater flexibility in meal and activity planning and more discreet delivery of insulin, they can also come with their own psychosocial challenges, including discomfort or self-consciousness related to being connected to physical devices or anxiety related to frequent checking of CGM readings.

Cancer

Childhood cancer presents numerous challenges to adaptation and development, though studies suggest that most childhood cancer survivors adapt well following treatment (Zeltzer *et al.*, 2009). There are predictable stress points in the course of an illness that often coincide with hospitalization, including diagnosis, initiation of treatment, and treatment completion, as well as, for some, illness recurrence, renewed treatment, and end-of-life care. Psychological support for the child and family is particularly beneficial at these critical points.

Challenges to psychological adaptation include persistent pain, debilitating side effects of treatment such as nausea, alteration in body image, school disruptions, compromised peer relationships, interference with ability to engage in favorite activities, or conflicts in the family (Hockenberry *et al.*, 2011). Adolescents may worry about future health status, sexual function and reproductive capacities, and future career choices (Patenaude & Kupst, 2005). This age group benefits from special attention to their specific developmental needs (Abrams *et al.*, 2007).

During the course of cancer treatment, many children develop strong positive relationships with members of the medical team, experience a special closeness with supportive parents, and maintain key preexisting peer friendships while acquiring new friends in the hospital. Many children will report feeling a special sense of purpose for living as a result of the cancer diagnosis and most will be treated with special status as a result of the illness. Resilience and positive life change are also part of the cancer experience (Phipps *et al.*, 2012).

Organ transplantation

Liver, kidney, heart, and lung transplantation are well-established practices in the pediatric population. Transplantation centers in the United States are required to include psychological assessment in the transplant evaluation process. The serious disease process leading up to transplantation, the risks of surgery, the long-term medical management of organ rejection post-transplantation, and the threat to survival place these children in the highest of high-risk populations. It is noteworthy, therefore, that the data on adjustment to liver and renal transplantation suggests that, overall, these children view themselves as healthy and competent (Tong *et al.*, 2011). Not surprisingly, some children and parents are vulnerable to anxiety and experience distress post-transplant. It is therefore important that transplant centers involve mental health consultants and provide emotional support (Shemesh, 2008).

Inflammatory bowel disease

Crohn's disease and ulcerative colitis, collectively called inflammatory bowel disease (IBD), are distinct disease processes characterized by chronic inflammation of the gastrointestinal tract with relapsing and remitting courses that lead to abdominal pain, bloody diarrhea, and fatigue. Neither Crohn's nor ulcerative colitis has a cure; they are managed through medical and surgical interventions aimed at controlling inflammation. Pain, unpredictability, and functional impairment are among the potential challenges faced by the child with IBD. Treatment with systemic steroids is a mainstay of IBD regimens during acute flares and may lead to derangements in cognitive function, mood, and behavior. Additional stressors include adaptation to the physical sequelae of IBD (e.g., short stature, weight loss, weakness, and delayed puberty), as well as physical sequelae of treatment (e.g., steroid-induced acne, visible feeding tubes, and J-pouches) and embarrassment around frequent use of bathrooms.

Rates of depression among adolescents with IBD have been found to be as high as 25% (Szigethy *et al.*, 2004). Moreover, children with IBD have been found to have increased rates of anxiety, as well as decreased psychosocial health, social functioning, and school functioning (Mackner *et al.*, 2006; Greenley *et al.*, 2010). The mental health consultant is often involved in the care of IBD patients in both inpatient and outpatient settings. Psychosocial interventions (including psychoeducation, school-based services, and support groups), psychotherapy, and psychopharmacology to treat depression, anxiety, and insomnia have all demonstrated efficacy in adults or children with IBD (Szigethy *et al.*, 2011).

Cystic fibrosis

Cystic fibrosis (CF) is the most common life-limiting genetic disorder among Caucasian populations, affecting 1 in 2500 newborns (Davies *et al.*, 2007). CF is a commonly encountered diagnosis in the inpatient pediatric medical setting. Typically diagnosed in infancy or early childhood, CF is caused by a gene defect in the chloride transport protein that leads to complex, multisystem disease, most notably chronic pulmonary inflammation and infection, as well as gastrointestinal sequelae including pancreatic insufficiency with malabsorption and failure to thrive. Treatment advances have enabled many children with CF to live well into adulthood, but it remains a chronic, life-limiting illness. Treatment regimens are demanding and require strict dietary regimens, multiple medications, and vigorous daily physical therapies. For many children, periodic exacerbations of pulmonary disease require repeated hospitalizations for "clean-outs," consisting of long admissions for parenteral antibiotics and aggressive physical therapy.

Despite these staggering demands, most children and families living with CF report high quality of life and have rates of psychopathology similar to cohorts of well peers (Szyndler *et al.*, 2005). Nevertheless, a full range of psychiatric challenges have been reported in children with CF, and studies have shown higher rates of psychopathology, including anxiety, depression, and eating disorders emerging in adolescence (Quittner *et al.*, 2008; Smith *et al.*, 2010). As with other chronic illnesses, nonadherence is a significant issue for adolescents with CF and needs to be monitored closely.

Neurologic illness

Epilepsy is the most common neurologic disorder of childhood, affecting between 0.5–1% of children under age 16 (Shinnar & Pellock, 2002). Psychiatric comorbidity is very common in pediatric epilepsy, with rates ranging between 33–77% (Davies *et al.*, 2003; Plioplys *et al.*, 2007). Epilepsy is associated with ADHD, depression, anxiety disorders, and ASD (Jones *et al.*, 2008). Rarely, interictal psychotic disorders may occur, or psychosis may be a feature of focal seizure semiology. Some antiepileptic drugs may cause poor concentration, impulsivity, or hyperactivity; others have been associated with depressed mood or mood lability. For children with epilepsy who require pharmacologic management of depression or anxiety, SSRIs are the first-line treatment. Prescribers should monitor potential interactions with hepatically metabolized antiepileptic drugs and cytochrome P450 inhibitors. For children with comorbid ADHD, there is mounting evidence that methylphenidate treatment is safe in children with epilepsy and clinical guidelines state that benefits outweigh risks (Davis *et al.*, 2010; Koneski *et al.*, 2011). Additional details on neurological illness can be found in Chapter 26.

Dying in the hospital

The death of a child is an enormous tragedy affecting every member of the child's family. There is no way to protect a child or family from the unique pain of the loss of a child, but sensitive care may serve to lessen regrets and support bereavement (Kreicbergs *et al.*, 2004). Attending to pain, anxiety, and privacy/dignity needs is key. Adapting the medical setting to allow parents to nurture the dying child or facilitating a child's return home to die can play a significant role in the family's experience of the death and the subsequent bereavement (Stevenson *et al.*, 2013). The consultant may work with the primary medical team, palliative care team, and family to elicit and support the child and family's wishes around death and dying.

Consultants may also help ready parents for discussions with their dying child. Asking open-ended questions about worries, inquiring whether the child has questions that they are afraid to say aloud, or asking if they think about peers from the hospital who have died may serve as invitations to begin the dialog. Reminding children that articulating worries does not make them happen may free some children who are worrying silently to speak. Many parents will feel more comfortable embarking on end-of-life conversations with a child if they are told that they can welcome the child's questions warmly without having specific answers. In the role of child mental health consultant, one of the most useful comments in response to questions about death is to tell a child "I don't know what it is like to be dead, because I have never been dead. But, I am always interested to hear children's ideas about it." The emotional impact of a child's death on the medical team also deserves careful attention in order to preserve the team's ability to deliver quality care into the future. The grieving process of the staff warrants recognition. Some units will have staff meetings including the child mental health consultant or other facilitator after a child dies (Bateman *et al.*, 2012).

The consultant should encourage hospital staff to follow up with parents at 6 months to 1 year after the death of a child. Parents are appreciative when staff attend memorial services and funerals, write sympathy cards, and make telephone calls (Macdonald *et al.*, 2005). Telephone calls provide an opportunity to assess the parents' grieving and need for referral.

Consultation lessons learned from the COVID-19 pandemic

The onset of the COVID-19 pandemic in 2020 brought newfound challenges to child development and medical care of children in the hospital. Pediatric psychiatry consultation services saw shifts in service needs, with some hospitals shuttering pediatric care altogether to care for the surge of critically ill adults, and others seeing significant increases in patients with psychiatric needs. Many consultation services saw an initial drop in patient volume, with a subsequent rebound about 6 months into the pandemic (Brahmbhatt *et al.*, 2021; Zima *et al.*, 2022). The clinical severity of psychiatric symptoms appeared overall to increase during the pandemic (Schneider *et al.*, 2023), and certain diagnoses at the intersection of physical and mental health, including eating disorders and functional neurologic disorders, appeared to skyrocket (Zima *et al.*, 2022; Trau *et al.*, 2022). The rapid shift to use of telemedicine services to provide psychiatric consultation in the hospital, initially to minimize physical presence to limit infectious spread in the context of shortages of personal protective equipment, proved to be overall successful, though with limitations, which has implications for expanding access to child psychiatry consultation to rural and resource-limited settings, even in the post-pandemic world (Brahmbhatt *et al.*, 2021; Shapiro *et al.*, 2021; Schneider *et al.*, 2023).

Conclusion

Child mental health consultants must stay attuned to the changes in the field of pediatrics. Advances in pharmacology, genomics, and technology offer new hope and new challenges to psychosocial adaptation. Patterns of access to consultation will need to reflect shorter hospital stays and utilization of outpatient venues. New technology, such as telemedicine, can offer novel access to consultative expertise. Research in adherence, outcomes, efficacy, and quality of life become increasingly important.

However, many of the key features of quality consultation will remain unchanged. The consultant will continue to bring to the multidisciplinary medical team the combined expertise of psychodynamic understanding, psychopharmacology, developmental perspective on the meaning of illness, adaptation to trauma, knowledge of psychiatric conditions, behavioral interventions, and CNS influences in medical illness and as a result of medical treatment. The goal will remain to answer the consultation request in a thoughtful, timely fashion that respects the needs of the child, the family, and the treatment team while facilitating quality of care and quality of life.

Acknowledgment

This chapter is based on the published chapter from the 6th edition of this book, with permission from that version's authors, Doctor Elizabeth Pinsky, Doctor Paula K. Rauch, and Doctor Annah N. Abrams.

References

Abrams, A.N. *et al.* (2007) Psychosocial issues in adolescents with cancer. *Cancer Treatment Reviews* **33**(7), 622–630.

Alderfer, M.A. *et al.* (2010) Psychosocial adjustment of siblings of children with cancer: a systematic review. *Psychooncology* **19**(8), 789–805.

Barlow, J.H. & Ellard, D.R. (2006) The psychosocial well-being of children with chronic disease, their parents and siblings: an overview of the research evidence base. *Child: Care, Health and Development* **32**(1), 19–31.

Bateman, S.T. *et al.* (2012) The wrap-up: a unique forum to support pediatric residents when faced with the death of a child. *Journal of Palliative Medicine* **15**(12), 1329–1334.

Becker, J.E. *et al.* (2020) Pediatric consultation-liaison psychiatry: an update and review. *Psychosomatics* **61**, 467–480.

Brahmbhatt, K. *et al.* (2021) Adaptations made to pediatric consultation-liaison psychiatry service delivery during the early months of the COVID-19 pandemic: a North American multisite survey. *Journal of the Academy of Consultation-Liaison Psychiatry* **62**, 511–521.

Carter, B.D. *et al.* (2003) Inpatient pediatric consultation-liaison: a case-controlled study. *Journal of Pediatric Psychology* **28**(6), 423–432.

Croen, L.A. *et al.* (2006) A comparison of health care utilization and costs of children with and without autism spectrum disorders in a large group-model health plan. *Pediatrics* **118**, 1203–1211.

Davies, S. *et al.* (2003) A population survey of mental health problems in children with epilepsy. *Developmental Medicine and Child Neurology* **45**(5), 292–295.

Davies, J.C. *et al.* (2007) Cystic fibrosis. *BMJ* **335**(7632), 1255–1259.

Davis, S.M. *et al.* (2010) Epilepsy in children with attention-deficit/hyperactivity disorder. *Pediatric Neurology* **42**(5), 325–330.

DeMaso, D.R. *et al.* (2009) Practice parameter for the psychiatric assessment and management of physically ill children and adolescents. *Journal of the American Academy of Child and Adolescent Psychiatry* **48**(2), 213–233.

Doupnik, S.K. *et al.* (2016) Mental health conditions and medical and surgical hospital utilization. *Pediatrics* **138**(6), e20162416.

Fein, J.A. *et al.* (2012) Relief of pain and anxiety in pediatric patients in emergency medical systems. *Pediatrics* **130**(5), e1391–e1405.

Forgey, M. & Bursch, B. (2013) Assessment and management of pediatric iatrogenic medical trauma. *Current Psychiatry Reports* **15**, 340.

Fritz, G.K. (2003) Promoting effective collaboration between pediatricians and child and adolescent psychiatrists. *Pediatric Annals* **32**(6), 383. 387–389

Garvey, K.C. *et al.* (2012) Health care transition in patients with type 1 diabetes: young adult experiences and relationship to glycemic control. *Diabetes Care* **35**(8), 1716–1722.

Geist, R.A. (1977) Consultation on a pediatric surgical ward: creating an empathic climate. *The American Journal of Orthopsychiatry* **47**(3), 432–444.

Greenley, R.N. *et al.* (2010) A meta-analytic review of the psychosocial adjustment of youth with inflammatory bowel disease. *Journal of Pediatric Psychology* **35**(8), 857–869.

Groves, J. & Beresin, E. (1999) Difficult patients, difficult families. *New Horizons* **6**, 331–343.

Gurney, J.G. *et al.* (2006) Parental report of health conditions and health care use among children with and without autism: national survey of children's health. *Archives of Pediatrics and Adolescent Medicine* **160**, 825–830.

Hamilton, J. & Daneman, D. (2002) Deteriorating diabetes control during adolescence: physiological or psychosocial? *Journal of Pediatric Endocrinology & Metabolism* **15**(2), 115–126.

Hazen, E.P. *et al.* (2020) Agitation in patients with autism spectrum disorder admitted to inpatient pediatric medical units. *Pediatrics* **145**(Suppl 1), S108–S116.

Hockenberry, M.J. *et al.* (2011) Managing painful procedures in children with cancer. *Journal of Pediatric Hematology/Oncology* **33**(2), 119–127.

Ibeziako, P. *et al.* (2019) Developing a clinical pathway for somatic symptom and related disorders in pediatric hospital settings. *Hospital Pediatrics* **9**(3), 147–155.

Jones, J.E. *et al.* (2008) Psychiatric disorders in children and adolescents who have epilepsy. *Pediatrics in Review/American Academy of Pediatrics* **29**(2), e9–e14.

Kersun, L.S. & Elia, J. (2007) Depressive symptoms and SSRI use in pediatric oncology patients. *Pediatric Blood & Cancer* **49**(7), 881–887.

Knapp, P.K. & Harris, E.S. (1998) Consultation-liaison in child psychiatry: a review of the past 10 years. Part II: research on treatment approaches and outcomes. *Journal of the American Academy of Child and Adolescent Psychiatry* **37**(2), 139–146.

Koller, D. & Goldman, R.D. (2012) Distraction techniques for children undergoing procedures: a critical review of pediatric research. *Journal of Pediatric Nursing* **27**(6), 652–681.

Koneski, J.A. *et al.* (2011) Efficacy and safety of methylphenidate in treating ADHD symptoms in children and adolescents with uncontrolled seizures: a Brazilian sample study and literature review. *Epilepsy & Behavior* **21**(3), 228–232.

Kreicbergs, U. *et al.* (2004) Talking about death with children who have severe malignant disease. *The New England Journal of Medicine* **351**(12), 1175–1186.

Macdonald, M.E. *et al.* (2005) Parental perspectives on hospital staff members' acts of kindness and commemoration after a child's death. *Pediatrics* **116**(4), 884–890.

Mackner, L.M. *et al.* (2006) Psychosocial functioning in pediatric inflammatory bowel disease. *Inflammatory Bowel Diseases* **12**(3), 239–244.

Maenner, M.J. *et al.* (2023) Prevalence and characteristics of autism spectrum disorder among children aged 8 years—autism and developmental disabilities monitoring network, 11 sites, United States, 2020. *Morbidity and Mortality Weekly Report* **72**(2), 1–14.

Moss, J. *et al.* (2018) State prevalence and ranks of adolescent substance use: implications for cancer prevention. *Preventing Chronic Disease* **15**(170345).

Ortiz, P. (1997) General principles in child liaison consultation service: a literature review. *European Child & Adolescent Psychiatry* **6**(1), 1–6.

Patenaude, A.F. & Kupst, M.J. (2005) Psychosocial functioning in pediatric cancer. *Journal of Pediatric Psychology* **30**(1), 9–27.

Perrin, J.M. *et al.* (2019) Mental health conditions and health care payments for children with chronic medical conditions. *Academic Pediatrics* **19**(1), 44–50.

Phipps, S. *et al.* (2012) Resilience in children undergoing stem cell transplantation: results of a complementary intervention trial. *Pediatrics* **129**(3), e762–e770.

Pijnenburg, M.W. & Fleming, L. (2020) Advances in understanding and reducing the burden of severe asthma in children. *The Lancet Respiratory Medicine* **8**, 1032–1044.

Plioplys, S. *et al.* (2007) 10-year research update review: psychiatric problems in children with epilepsy. *Journal of the American Academy of Child and Adolescent Psychiatry* **46**(11), 1389–1402.

Quittner, A.L. *et al.* (2008) Prevalence and impact of depression in cystic fibrosis. *Current Opinion in Pulmonary Medicine* **14**(6), 582–588.

Schneider, N.M. *et al.* (2023) Pediatric consultation-liaison psychology: insights and lessons learned during the COVID-19 pandemic. *Journal of Clinical Psychology in Medical Settings* **30**, 51–60.

Shapiro, P.A. *et al.* (2021) Report of the academy of consultation-liaison psychiatry task force on lessons learned from the COVID-19 pandemic: executive summary. *Journal of the Academy of Consultation-Liaison Psychiatry* **62**, 377–386.

Shemesh, E. (2008) Assessment and management of psychosocial challenges in pediatric liver transplantation. *Liver Transplantation: Official Publication of the American Association for the Study of Liver Diseases and the International Liver Transplantation Society* **14**(9), 1229–1236.

Shemesh, E. *et al.* (2005) Assessment of depression in medically ill children presenting to pediatric specialty clinics. *Journal of the American Academy of Child and Adolescent Psychiatry* **44**(12), 1249–1257.

Shinnar, S. & Pellock, J.M. (2002) Update on the epidemiology and prognosis of pediatric epilepsy. *Journal of Child Neurology* **17**(Suppl 1), S4–S17.

Smith, B.A. *et al.* (2010) Depressive symptoms in children with cystic fibrosis and parents and its effects on adherence to airway clearance. *Pediatric Pulmonology* **45**(8), 756–763.

Smith, J.R. *et al.* (2020) Literature review: substance use screening and co-morbidity in medically hospitalized youth. *General Hospital Psychiatry* **67**, 115–126.

Stern, T.A. *et al.* (2010) *Massachusetts General Hospital Handbook of General Hospital Psychiatry*, 6th edn. Saunders, Philadelphia, PA.

Stevenson, M. *et al.* (2013) Pediatric palliative care in Canada and the United States: a qualitative metasummary of the needs of patients and families. *Journal of Palliative Medicine* **16**, 566–577.

Stoppelbein, L. *et al.* (2005) Factor analysis of the pediatric symptom checklist with a chronically ill pediatric population. *Journal of Developmental and Behavioral Pediatrics* **26**(5), 349–355.

Sylvester, C.J. & Forman, S.F. (2008) Clinical practice guidelines for treating restrictive eating disorder patients during medical hospitalization. *Current Opinion in Pediatrics* **20**(4), 390–397.

Szigethy, E. *et al.* (2004) Depressive symptoms and inflammatory bowel disease in children and adolescents: a cross-sectional study. *Journal of Pediatric Gastroenterology & Nutrition* **39**(4), 395–403.

Szigethy, E. *et al.* (2011) Inflammatory bowel disease. *Pediatric Clinics of North America* **58**(4), 903–920. x–xi

Szyndler, J.E. *et al.* (2005) Psychological and family functioning and quality of life in adolescents with cystic fibrosis. *Journal of Cystic Fibrosis: Official Journal of the European Cystic Fibrosis Society* **4**(2), 135–144.

Thom, R.P. *et al.* (2019) Challenges in the medical care of patients with autism spectrum disorder: the role of the consultation-liaison psychiatrist. *Psychosomatics* **60**(5), 435–443.

Thom, R.P. *et al.* (2020a) Providing inpatient medical care to children with autism spectrum disorder. *Hospital Pediatrics* **10**(10), 918–924.

Thom, R. *et al.* (2020b) Suicide risk screening in the hospital setting: a review of brief validated tools. *Psychosomatics* **61**(1), 1–7.

Tong, A. *et al.* (2011) Quality of life of adolescent kidney transplant recipients. *The Journal of Pediatrics* **159**(4), 670–675.e2.

Trau, S.P. *et al.* (2022) Creating a patient-based diagnostic checklist for functional tics during the COVID-19 pandemic. *Neurology. Clinical Practice* **12**(5), 365–376.

Turkel, S.B. *et al.* (2006) Comparing symptoms of delirium in adults and children. *Psychosomatics* **47**(4), 320–324.

Wagner, J.L. *et al.* (2003) The influence of parental distress on child depressive symptoms in juvenile rheumatic diseases: the moderating effect of illness intrusiveness. *Journal of Pediatric Psychology* **28**(7), 453–462.

Work, H.H. (1989) The "menace of psychiatry" revisited: the evolving relationship between pediatrics and child psychiatry. *Psychosomatics* **30**(1), 86–93.

Zeltzer, L.K. *et al.* (2009) Psychological status in childhood cancer survivors: a report from the childhood cancer survivor study. *Journal of Clinical Oncology: Official Journal of the American Society of Clinical Oncology* **27**(14), 2396–2404.

Zima, B.T. *et al.* (2016) Psychiatric disorders and trends in resource use in pediatric hospitals. *Pediatrics* **138**(5), e20160909.

Zima, B.T. *et al.* (2022) Use of acute mental health care in U.S. children's hospitals before and after statewide COVID-19 school closure orders. *Psychiatric Services* **73**(11), 1202–1209.

CHAPTER 44

Children with specific sensory impairments

Naomi Dale[1,2] and Fionna Bathgate[1]

[1] Psychological and Mental Health Services, Great Ormond Street Hospital NHS Foundation Trust, London, UK

[2] Developmental Neurosciences, UCL Great Ormond Street Institute of Child Health, London, UK

Visual impairment

Nature and prevalence

Visual impairment (VI) refers to all degrees of vision reduction or impairment, which include vision clarity or "acuity," or field or higher visual processing disorders. The term encompasses children who have partial vision or are sight-impaired and can access the visual environment with additional low vision aids and enlargement modifications. Those who have very severe to profound VI (blindness) require tactile and auditory methods of learning including Braille text and typing. The classification of VI of best-corrected visual acuity (with refracted spectacles if necessary) is divided into "blindness" at 3/60 or less vision, or better levels of vision. This means, for instance, that a person sees at 3 m what a typical sighted person sees at 60 m, or a person sees at 20 ft what a typical sighted person sees at 400 ft (20/400) (United Kingdom [UK], United States [US], respectively). VI is also measured according to the Logarithm of the Minimum Angle of Resolution (logMAR), which is a standard decimal measure of letter optotypes. There are four categories in this classification system: (i) no/mild VI (better than logMAR 0.5), (ii) moderate VI (logMAR 0.5–0.9), (iii) severe VI (logMAR 1.0–1.3), and (iv) blindness (worse than logMAR 1.3 to light perception/no vision).

The two main types of childhood VI are *peripheral or ocular* and *cerebral,* although a "mixed" condition is possible. The former arises from abnormalities of the eye globe (including cornea and lens), retina, or anterior optic nerve, and the latter originates in the brain including the posterior or postchiasmatic optic nerve, optic radiations, and visual and other cortical areas (Figure 44.1).

Peripheral visual disorders can be divided into "simple," where VI is the only known impairment in the pediatric diagnosis, and "complex" with additional known brain involvement in the diagnosis. Estimates of the incidence of severe sight impairment/blindness is 5–6/10,000 infants in the first year, rising to 10/10,000 at 16 years in a higher income country (UK) (Teoh *et al.*, 2021).

Etiology, identification, and visual management

The most common anatomical sites of origin for VI are cerebral visual pathways (48%), the retina (36%), including retinopathy of prematurity, and the optic nerve (28%) in higher income countries (UK) (Teoh *et al.*, 2021). Congenital peripheral visual disorders are associated with rare ophthalmological and pediatric diseases, such as anophthalmia (absence of eyes), microphthalmia (small eyes), Leber's amaurosis (retinal dystrophy), corneal anomalies, and "complex" syndromic conditions like Joubert syndrome (with VI and cerebellar anomalies). More than 350 hereditary eye diseases are now identified, leading to redefinitions of the conditions, e.g., aniridia as a PAX6 disease entity and anophthalmia including SOX2 mutation. Knowledge of the relationship of broader behavioral genotype to phenotype is still lacking and there may be considerable individual variability. Cerebral VI (CVI) has many origins, including unknown and idiopathic to likely or assumed prenatal, perinatal, neonatal, and childhood factors. These include injury, vascular pathology, focal tumors, infections, and some inherited conditions. The majority emerge during the neonatal period or early months of life.

Levels of VI are identified through age-appropriate near detection and acuity measurement in children with peripheral or cerebral VI, whatever their etiology. Visual perceptual testing is undertaken to establish visual perceptual profiles and subgroupings in higher functioning children with cerebral VI (Dale *et al.*, 2022).

Parents first notice that their baby is not looking at them or tracking their movements. Prompt identification and any medical treatment available is essential as infants may have the potential to develop useful functional vision. Early childhood

Rutter's Child and Adolescent Psychiatry and Psychology, Seventh Edition.
Edited by Anita Thapar, Daniel S. Pine, Samuele Cortese, Cathy Creswell, Tamsin J. Ford, James F. Leckman, and Argyris Stringaris.

Companion website: www.wiley.com/go/thapar/rutterspsych7

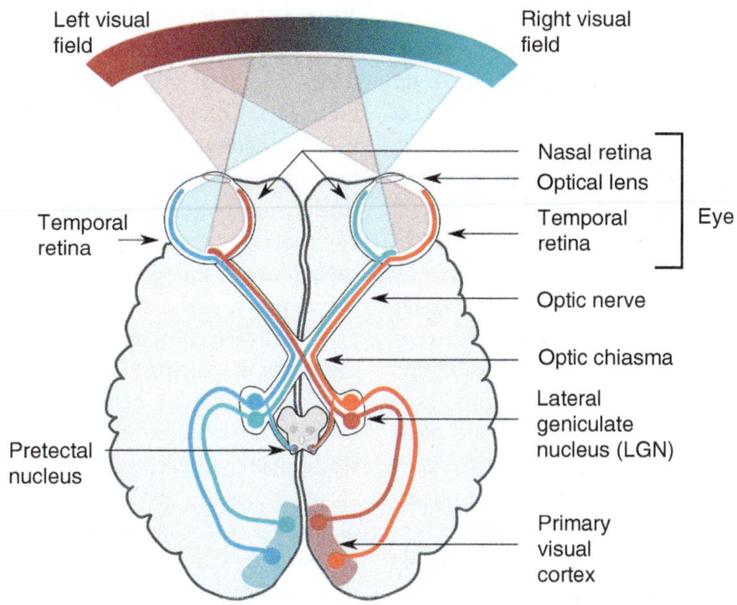

Figure 44.1 The inferior surface of the brain illustrating the visual pathway. *Source*: The University of Texas Health Science Center at Houston/https://nba.uth.tmc.edu/neuroscience/m/s2/chapter15.html, Last accessed 8 April 2024.

intervention including functional vision promotion using a parent-mediated multisensory behavioral method in the first year of life may help accelerate possible vision development; this is crucial as some early "form" vision (nonlight reflecting substance) may accelerate general development (Dale *et al.* 2017).

Early family support and intervention

During the early period of diagnosis, parents may feel isolated and distressed. The infant is generally passive and quiet and lacks social responses, like eye gaze and smiling. This is a "developmental emergency" as the infant is totally dependent on parental interactions in the early months to connect with the external environment. Lack of vision affects all aspects of early development. Infants are reluctant to feel and explore their physical environment, and auditory-directed reaching occurs later than visual-directed reaching. Extensive delay in achieving sensorimotor and cognitive milestones is common, with most vulnerability occurring in those with profound VI (light perception at best). Having some "form" vision (of nonlight reflective substance), however limited, appears protective as infants accelerate their sensorimotor understanding and learning (Dale *et al.*, 2019).

Early language milestones are often delayed, such as recognizing and labelling object concepts or using reverse pronouns in language structure (Mosca *et al.*, 2015). Young children may imitate speech frequently (echolalia) without linking the surface words to underlying meaning. Family environment may play a role; greater maternal responsiveness including sensitivity in late infancy may be positively related to young children's advances in verbal comprehension (Sakkalou *et al.*, 2018). As vocabulary expands, syntax and grammar begin to develop and become more similar or normalized to typical speech. Nevertheless, language may be more "learned" or formulaic with expressive ability outstripping semantic understandings. Pragmatic or social use of language lags behind, with difficulty in adapting to the child's social and communicative context (Tadić *et al.*, 2010; Bathelt *et al.*, 2017).

Parents of infants with a new diagnosis generally face a worrying and unfamiliar pathway, with elevated distress in the parent and high parenting stress found by the end of the first year of life. It may reduce if the child makes steady progress, develops more functional vision, and shows adaptive behavior responses but otherwise it may remain high at two or three years (Sakkalou *et al.*, 2018). Informed developmental guidance will give them a supportive "roadmap" and normative expectations to help them anticipate, celebrate, and optimize their infant's developmental steps in the home environment. Scientific evaluation shows that parenting stress, child behavior and sensory-motor understanding, and language expression are improved if receiving a structured home-based early intervention program, the Developmental Journal for babies and young children with VI (DJVI; Dale *et al.*, 2007; Salt & Dale, 2017; Dale *et al.*, 2019).

Developmental aspects of visual impairment

Educational attainment

By school years, some children with VI reach or exceed the linguistic skills and verbal intelligence level of their typically sighted peers (Tadić *et al.*, 2010). Growing cognitive capacity supports active learning, though children need access to concrete near-vision or tactile experiences to underpin conceptual understanding and semantic meanings. Depending on vision level, children are introduced to Braille or enlarged print (or both) for reading. By 7 years, Braille readers tend to lag behind their sighted peers in reading rate and writing (Harris *et al.*, 2012). Children with low vision levels may read enlarged print more slowly though comprehension can be similar to sighted peers (Mohammed & Omar, 2011). Adolescents may be slower than peers in acquiring advanced attainment skills, including mathematics, though more specialized academic support or helping parents feel confident in supporting their child's reading or mathematics can accelerate progress (e.g., Giesen *et al.*, 2012). Some children may be at risk of a reading and spelling dyslexia based in phonological problems (Greaney *et al.* 2000) or visual perceptual-related problems in cognitively able children with cerebral VI.

The nursery or school environment needs to be carefully structured to enable safe mobility and navigation and a quiet learning environment that is not too auditorily distracting or overwhelming. As children grow up, emphasis is also placed on developing self-help skills, and organization and study skills to enhance independence in the school environment and autonomy. Augmentative materials and approaches, including enlarged font, reading on digital tablets, adapted measurement tools, Braille font and typing, and software links between teacher whiteboard and tablet, are all required to enable the child to access the curriculum. Braille reading, mathematics, and science need specialized teaching.

Neuropsychological processes

School-aged children with VI vary in their "higher order" cognitive processes. Some show particular strengths in working memory and verbal abilities. However, neuropsychological assessment can reveal uneven strengths and weaknesses in individual children (Greenaway *et al.*, 2017). Spatial perception may be strong including the exceptional auditory use of vocal echo to map the environment of some young people (echolocation). Some young people develop exceptional blind sports levels in skiing, blind football, and goal-ball, for instance. Tactile discrimination will also be highly developed, particularly in children with no or very little vision. Weaker spatial perception is found in some children, especially in cerebral VI, which may affect navigation, object search, and haptic (perception and manipulation of objects using touch) orientation (Gori *et al.*, 2010). Those with greater difficulty in attention shifting from one object to another in the preschool years tend to show more rigid behavior patterns (such as obsessional object or topic interests) and weaker executive function (self-planning and initiative) later (Tadić *et al.*, 2009). Although children may succeed in verbal fluency, undertaking behavioral executive functioning and planning and initiative in the everyday environment may be adversely affected in some children (Greenaway *et al.*, 2017; Bathelt *et al.*, 2019).

Neuroplasticity and brain organization

With the posterior visual cortex of the brain underutilized, the brain migrates some nonvisual functions into this area—highlighting the "cross-plasticity" of the visual cortex. Adults with congenital blindness activate the visual cortex for Braille reading and other tactile tasks; auditory motion perception activates visual motion areas of the visual cortex (Sadato *et al.*, 1996). Neuroplasticity and auditory learning may lead to increased capabilities in sound localization, speech processing, biographical memory, and associative learning (Withagen *et al.*, 2013). Some children show exceptional pitch discrimination and singing or music-playing talents.

Changes at brain neural level may be associated with developmental risk. Those with severe visual reduction showed lower white matter integrity in tracts of the visual system, posterior corpus callosum, and lower left thalamus even though they were of average verbal intelligence (Bathelt *et al.*, 2020). Lack of response to the child's own name at electrophysiological level was evident in infancy and later childhood, raising the question of whether this is an early biomarker for social cognitive risk (Bathelt *et al.*, 2017).

Psychological and emotional development and well-being

There has long been concern about the passivity and self-centeredness of the infant with profound VI; this creates challenges for parents who vary in their sensitivity and reciprocity with the infant (Sakkalou *et al.*, 2021). Children can develop affectionate secure, albeit at times delayed, attachment with their parents and others, continuing into adulthood (Ardito *et al.*, 2004).

Beyond infancy, the ability to recognize emotions develops slowly though it is queried whether this is part of a general or specific delay (Dyck *et al.*, 2004). Children lack information about facial expressions which supports emotional learning. In contrast to children with hearing impairment (HI), emotion recognition is more vulnerable than emotion understanding and vocabulary, which are more verbally mediated processes. As language skills develop, parents use "mental state" language during conversation and storytelling to help their child understand other people's emotions, beliefs, and intentions (Tadić *et al.*, 2009). Delay occurs in first order "false belief" tasks, like the Sally Ann task, which are traditionally visual (Green *et al.*, 2004). Advanced theory of mind (ToM) skills, i.e., awareness that other people have beliefs about beliefs, may possibly emerge more similarly to typically sighted children, at least in children with a wider range of severity of VI, and appears associated with age and verbal intelligence (Pijnacker *et al.*, 2012).

Social development and peer relationships

One of the greater challenges for children with VI is social integration. They may desire friends but lack necessary skills and be restricted from playground activities due to fears of safety or bullying. They may experience rejection and exclusion from other children and cannot easily find other children to play with or join in group sport games in the playground. Some children may experience bullying and social anxiety with peers is common. Adolescents may spend more time alone, have smaller social networks, and lower social skills—with further risk if the parents are overprotective or the young person is introverted (Pinquart & Pfeiffer, 2013). They can nonetheless be successful in establishing and maintaining reciprocal intimate best friendships, doing many activities together that were typical of adolescents without disabilities (Rosenblum, 1998). Young people with VI are often resilient, and research suggests that children with VI can develop self-esteem that is similar or higher than in sighted peers (Kef & Deković, 2004; Lifshitz *et al.*, 2007). Inclusive blind sports and music-making, drama, arts, IT clubs, and other communal activities are seen to be protective and highly valued by children with VI and their families.

Visual impairment and complexity

Assessment and diagnosis of neurodevelopmental disorders

Over three-quarters of children with VI in the UK have additional nonophthalmic disorders including intellectual disability (ID), motor or hearing impairment, epilepsy, autism, attention deficit hyperactivity disorder (ADHD), and health impairments (Teoh *et al.*, 2021). There are a growing number of recognized ocular genetic mutations and genetic syndromes involving VI and neurodevelopmental risks. About half of children with cerebral visual disorders have intellectual and neurological difficulties, leading to more complex behavior presentations than in children with "simple" peripheral visual disorders. The rate of ID is estimated to be around 20% in children with "simple" congenital disorders of the peripheral visual system (Dale *et al.*, 2002; Dale *et al.*, 2019). One in 10 children with intellectual and neurodevelopmental disabilities are estimated to have a VI, rising to 22% in those with an IQ under 50 (Nielsen *et al.*, 2007).

A third of infants with profound VI are at risk of regressing or plateauing in their development in their second year of life and showing autism symptomatology, a phenomenon first described as "developmental setback" (Dale *et al.*, 2002; Dale *et al.*, 2019).

Autism and visual impairment

A clinical challenge to differentiating autism spectrum disorder (ASD) in children with VI is that, in the early years, many children with VI show delays in all-round development including some autistic-like difficulties. Behavior features like echolalia, self-directed behavior, stereotypies, communication challenges, failure of developing joint attention, and obsessional restricted interests or compulsive rituals are common in the preschool period (Dale *et al.* 2014). The long-term outlook for children presenting with early ASD features is variable. In some children, the traits reduce significantly as the child develops more adaptive social behavior, language, and communication (Hobson *et al.*, 2010). For a substantial subgroup, significant difficulties continue; it is their continuity and intensity by 4–6 years and older that should alert the clinician to a possible ASD. Even milder presentations can have a severe disabling impact in the context of VI.

Current estimates are of 19% with clinical ASD in heterogeneous populations, with higher incidence in lower IQ and more severe VI—rising to at least 30% in profound VI (Do *et al.*, 2017). The overall risk ratio of ASD is 31 times greater in the VI population compared to in the general population. Skilled specialist ASD assessment teams with expertise in VI are required to undertake the diagnostic assessments. It can be difficult to differentiate whether a social or communicative response is affected by VI or ASD in the child, such as absence of eye contact, facial expression, gestural communication, or symbolic play. A modified ADOS-2® (Module 3) (Lord *et al.*, 2012), which does not require pictorial material or ratings of vision-based behaviors, has been validated for use with children with VI. It requires specialized training in administration and reliable ratings; its new diagnostic algorithm has been developed scientifically (Dale *et al.*, 2024).

Psychological and psychiatric issues

As with known risks from living with a chronic health condition, children with VI may have to cope with multiple hospital treatments and pain and fatigue, appearance-related differences and visibility of impairment, and stigma of disability. They also have the challenges of navigating the physical environment which is not adapted for VI and may be additionally disabling, and a cause for anxiety and fears (Visagie *et al.*, 2013).

A systematic review of mental health in children and young adults found two-thirds of the studies report an increased incidence of emotional problems, with females expressing depression more frequently than males (Augestad, 2017). A recent UK study of 8–11-year-olds, with congenital disorders of the peripheral visual system and no known neurological or intellectual impairment, showed increased risk of psychopathology compared to normative data, with 32% at "high risk" of internalizing disorder and 21% at "high risk" of externalizing disorder (MacKechnie *et al.*, 2018).

There is individual variation with a complex interplay of risk and protective factors identified. Risk factors include having additional intellectual and other disabilities, elevated social communication/ASD difficulties, greater severity of vision reduction, weakness in adaptive functioning, receiving less parental emotional support, being isolated and lacking friends, being female, experiencing bullying, and having lower self-esteem (Harris & Lord, 2016; Augestad, 2017; MacKechnie *et al.*, 2018). As in typically sighted peers, older adolescents are more at risk of psychological difficulties.

Other protective factors for psychological well-being and positive self-esteem include congenital and early blindness compared with later acquired vision loss, network size and satisfaction with social support including peers, independence in mobility, greater locus of control, and enhancement of autonomy (Pinquart & Pfeiffer, 2011, 2013).

Parental well-being and support for parents is an important factor in their ability to cope and support their child's behavior, which may be challenging to manage. Behavior problems in young and older children are a high source of stress in parents, especially if the child has higher caregiving demands and intellectual or multiple disabilities. Nearly a quarter of 2-year-olds with congenital disorders of the peripheral visual system were rated by their parent as having "internalizing" ("withdrawn," "emotionally reactive") difficulties (O'Reilly *et al.*, 2017). This was associated with increased parenting stress on the Difficult Child subscale of the Parenting Stress Index (Sakkalou *et al.*, 2018).

Anxiety disorders can occur across the age range, particularly in children with ASD traits. Young people with VI may be more prone to fears and phobias of potentially harmful situations, such as insect phobia (Ollendick *et al.*, 1985). The high risk for separation anxiety (30% in a higher functioning sample) may be a natural response to fears about the environment and dependency on adult assistance (MacKechnie *et al.*, 2018).

Formulations need to account for the impact of VI on the behavior and well-being of the child (and the family), and relative risk and protective factors. Tailored intervention may include psychoeducation for parents and teachers, environmental restructuring, ensuring educational and social demands match the child's capability, behavioral interventions, and strategies to enhance compensatory function and developmental growth. The shared risk of VI for ASD or ID may warrant a full cognitive and clinical assessment and exploration before formulating an intervention plan. This plan can include managing adaptations of the environment, increasing predictability of explicit structures and routines, promoting the child's effective communication, and supporting their visual, auditory, and tactile sensory needs. Other interventions include goal planning and behavior modification with parents and educators, and also therapeutic approaches including cognitive behavioral therapy (CBT), narrative therapy, or solution-focused therapy with older children and their families (Jackson, 2022). Acceptance and commitment therapy may be helpful for strengthening resilience in children and parents where there is a health risk like deterioration of vision, brain tumor regrowth, or late-acquired retinal dystrophy or other VI condition.

There is also a focus on evaluating programs of social participation including community-based mentoring (Heppe *et al.*, 2021) and healthy normalization programs to enhance self-esteem, and support coping strategies and psychological adjustment in children and young people, and their families. Periods of transition (e.g., entry to school, transition to secondary or higher education or adulthood) are often stress-arousing and are supported by careful planning and structuring with the child and young person and parents, such as ensuring that all teaching support and augmentative modifications are in place.

Sleep disorders are common in children with VI, with a significant impact on the health of the child and causing distress to their caretakers (Ingram *et al.*, 2022) These are more prevalent when there is an accompanying ID. Sleep hygiene and behavioral approaches may be successful, but with unresponsive sleep disorders improved sleep latency with melatonin has been demonstrated.

Septo-optic dysplasia is a complex condition with optic nerve hypoplasia, midline brain defects, and hypopituitarism and other endocrinological abnormalities. Higher levels of ASD, ADHD, impulsivity, mood dysregulation, poor stress and frustration tolerance, obsessional interests, anxiety, and behavioral difficulties are observed. These can be very challenging to manage and benefit from joint psychiatric and psychological interventions (Mann *et al.*, 2023).

Hearing impairment

Nature and prevalence

The two main types of childhood HI are conductive and sensorineural; it is also possible to have a "mixed" loss. The former is usually the result of otitis media with effusion and may be transient. Permanent causes of conductive hearing loss include syndromes resulting in malformations of the middle ear and disorders such as congenital cholesteatoma. Sensorineural hearing loss, the great majority of which is caused by abnormality or poor function of the hair cells of the cochlea, can be congenital, progressive, or of sudden onset due to illness or injury (Figure 44.2). The UK prevalence of permanent hearing impairment of more than 40 dB at 3 years old is 1.07/1000. For children aged 9 to 15 years this is 2.05/1000 (Solutions for Public Health, 2019). More than 90% of deaf children are born to two hearing parents, with implications for their communication mode and educational choices. A third, more recently described hearing disorder, is auditory neuropathy spectrum disorder (Colucci, 2020) in which children characteristically have poor speech-perception abilities relative to their degree of HI. The prevalence is cited at 1 in 7000 neonates (Rance & Starr, 2015). All types of hearing loss, including those resulting from otitis media with effusion (middle ear infection with glue ear), can have a detrimental impact on the development of language skills. However, fewer developmental disadvantages are seen in deaf children of deaf parents who are raised within the Deaf culture and use sign language as their means of communication, depending nevertheless on whether the child has additional disabilities or not. See Table 44.1 for hearing loss categories and Figure 44.3 for an audiogram of hearing levels.

Etiology, identification, and audiological management

The primary cause of permanent HI in children is genetic anomalies, accounting for approximately 60% of cases. In 70–80% of these cases, HI is the only impairment, for example,

1) **Sounds enter the ear canal**
Sound waves move through the ear canal and strike the eardrum.

2) **The eardrum and bones of hearing vibrate**
These sound waves cause the eardrum, and the three bones (ossicles) within the middle ear, to vibrate.

3) **Fluid moves through the inner ear**
The vibrations move through the fluid in the spiral shaped inner ear—known as the cochlea—and cause the tiny hair cells in the cochlea to move. The hair cells detect the movement and change it into the chemical signals for the hearing nerve.

4) **Hearing nerves communicate to the brain**
The hearing nerve then sends the information to the brain with electrical impulses, where they are interpreted as sound.

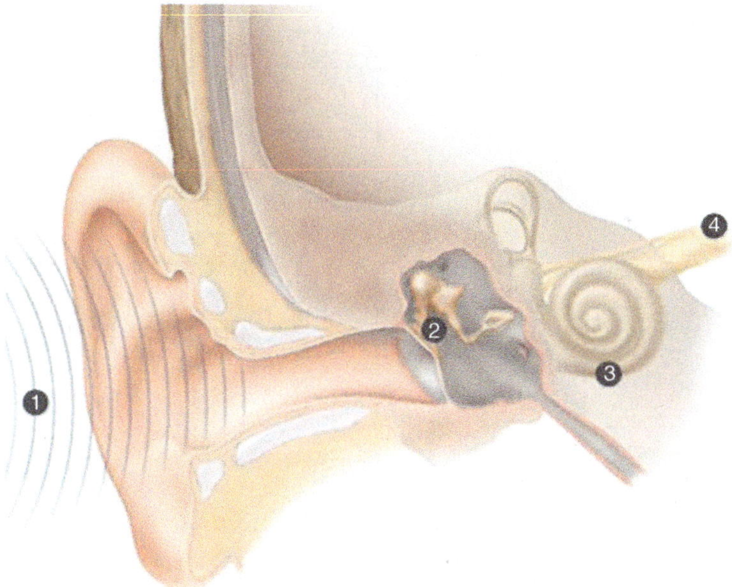

Figure 44.2 How hearing works.

Table 44.1 Hearing loss categories across the world and associated difficulties.

US		UK		Australia[a]		Practical
Level of hearing loss	**Hearing loss range (dB HL)**	**Level of hearing loss**	**Hearing loss range (dB HL)**	**Level of hearing loss**	**Hearing loss range (dB HL)**	
Normal	−10–15	Normal	20	Normal	≤25	No difficulties
Slight	16–25					
Mild	26–40	Mild	25–39	Mild	26–40	You have difficulty following speech in noisy situations
Moderate	41–55	Moderate	40–69	Moderate	41–60	You have difficulty following speech without a hearing aid
Moderately severe	56–70			Severe	61–80	
Severe	71–90	Severe	70–89	Profound	>81	You require powerful hearing aids or a cochlear implant
Profound	91+	Profound	90			You need to rely mainly on lipreading and/or sign language, or a cochlear implant

[a] Degrees of hearing loss (https://www.audika.com.au/hearing-loss/levels).

Connexin 26 mutation. Genetic causes are further subdivided into syndromic versus nonsyndromic categories with up to 30% of genetic HI being syndromic. There are well over a hundred known syndromes, most of which are associated with sensorineural hearing loss. Small proportions of childhood HI are due to various medical issues including severe prematurity or neonatal complications and ototoxic medications. A variety of tests are used in the identification of HI, from shortly after birth (newborn screening) and through early childhood. Once a permanent HI is confirmed, assistive hearing devices aim to optimize access to and clarity of the speech signal; these include hearing aids, cochlear implants, and bone-anchored hearing aids, depending on the nature and severity of the hearing loss. A more recent intervention is an auditory brainstem implant (ABI) for children without cochlear nerves. Initial research indicates that ABI can provide users with an awareness of environmental sound (Puram *et al.*, 2016).

Cochlear implantation is often the treatment of choice for severe to profound congenital HI and also for progressive or

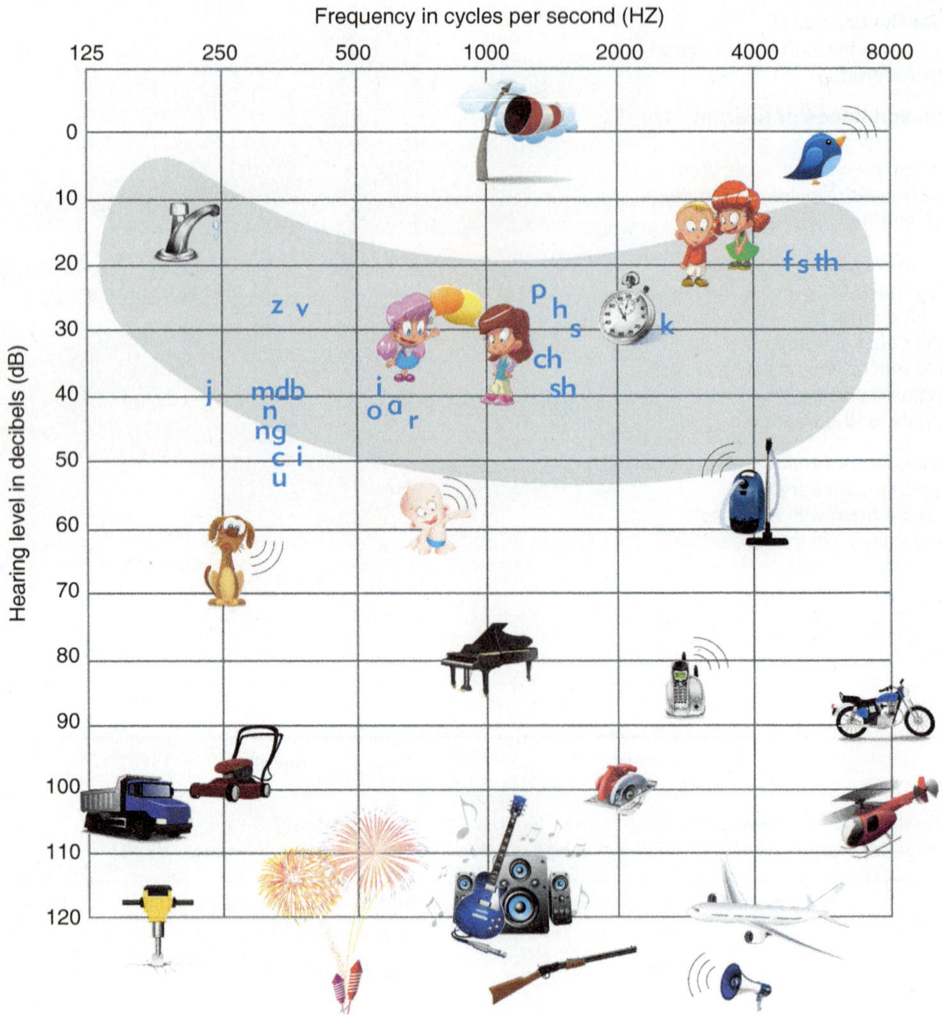

Figure 44.3 Image of an audiogram.

acquired losses after language has developed. Extensive research demonstrates the positive impact of cochlear implantation on speech perception and production, and language and reading skills, including evidence on the benefits of bilateral implantation. Superior outcomes are associated with early implantation, particularly when implanted in the first two years of life (Sharma *et al.*, 2020). However, there remains great variability in outcomes and many children with cochlear implants remain vulnerable to the detrimental effects of HI and other associated factors on development.

Early family support and intervention

Probably the single largest impact on developmental outcomes for children with HI has been early detection. Universal newborn hearing screening was fully implemented across the UK in 2006. There are similar programs in many higher income countries, e.g., early hearing detection and intervention (EHDI) programs in the US. In the UK, the majority of sensorineural hearing loss is identified by two months of age and amplification or implants are introduced promptly. Once permanent HI is identified, family-centered interventions aim to promote optimal development of the child. Early identification and intervention have been associated with better speech, language, and academic outcomes (Fulcher *et al.*, 2012).

Possible language interventions for children with HI range from fully visual-manual to fully auditory-oral, with sign and speech combinations in between (e.g., sign-supported speech, simultaneous communication, cued speech, and total communication) (Stredler-Brown, 2010).

Developmental aspects of hearing impairment

Cognitive and language development

Specific cognitive or information-processing abilities such as memory, attention, verbal rehearsal speed, inhibition, problem-solving, and visuo-motor integration have been found to be adversely affected by HI and appear to be more useful than overall IQ for understanding the difficulties in learning language experienced by many HI children (Marschark *et al.*, 2008).

HI is strongly associated with spoken language delays in receptive and expressive skills (speech perception and production), and speech intelligibility. Most children with HI have smaller vocabularies and poorer use of grammar than their hearing peers, especially in the early years (Blamey, 2003). The rate of spoken language development is not strongly dependent on the degree of hearing reduction because other factors such as age of provision of hearing device, type of educational approach, nonverbal ability, presence of additional disabilities, educational emphasis on oral communication, and family support are all influential.

Attainments: reading, writing, and numeracy

A sound spoken language base in early childhood underlies learning to read and write. While appropriate amplification and early intervention can allow children to acquire early oral language skills that show little difference from children with typical hearing (Geers & Nicholas, 2013), research indicates that these early gains do not lead to comparable gains in academic attainment (Marschark *et al.*; 2015; Breland *et al.*, 2022).

Mathematical attainment has been much less systematically researched, but the evidence suggests it is often significantly compromised (Sarant *et al.*, 2015). Word-based mathematical problem-solving is more reliant on language or reading skills, in comparison with quantity recognition and computational skills, and particularly disadvantages children with HI who are weaker in these areas (Edwards *et al.*, 2013).

Emotional development and psychological well-being

Toddler tantrums in preschool-aged children with HI often extend beyond the expected age period for hearing children, typically because effective age-appropriate communication is lacking and language development is delayed. Some young children with HI appear to be excessively shy and avoid interacting with other adults or children, except within their immediate family. Childhood HI has a significant impact on family communication patterns and dynamics. Most children do develop close attachment relationships with their parents, and deaf children of deaf parents show similar attachment patterns to hearing children of hearing parents in the Strange Situation Paradigm according to Meadow-Orlans *et al.* (1983).

The role of parental stress in the process of attachment has been investigated. Some studies (Pipp-Siegel *et al.*, 2002) indicated no differences in levels of stress in parents of hearing and deaf children, but others indicated that parents of children with HI are significantly more stressed (Quittner *et al.*, 1990). One identified reason for these differences is posited to be the level of support given to parents. Evidence indicates that as a child's level of language and communication increases, so parental stress—which is at its highest at diagnosis—decreases (Weisel *et al.*, 2007).

Yoshinaga-Itano (2003) cites three main social-emotional factors found to be highly related to better language development in deaf children: the extent to which parents are involved in intervention, the resolution of grieving, and mother–child attachment.

In school-aged children with HI, disruptions may occur in the development of empathy, emotion recognition and understanding, and using emotion vocabulary and recognition of facial expressions (Ludlow *et al.*, 2010). Consequently, many children with HI experience difficulties in establishing and maintaining positive reciprocal peer relationships. Social competence and the quality of interactions between children with HI and those with typical hearing are partially dependent on school setting (mainstream versus special education), associated with self-esteem, and often negatively impacted by language and communication delays (Martin *et al.*, 2011). Children with HI are sometimes rejected by their peers and experience victimization or bullying, leading to lowered self-esteem, and emotional and behavioral problems (van Gent *et al.*, 2011).

Stevenson *et al.*'s (2015) review and meta-analysis concludes that children with HI are more likely to show emotional and behavioral difficulties than other children. However, they state that the effect may be less marked than earlier studies indicated and seems to be lowest for children with cochlear implants. Ratings by teachers show the largest effect. There is no indication that HI is related to hyperactivity or ADHD-related behaviors. It is in the area of peer relationships that the most marked behavior difficulties for children with HI are found.

Identity

The hearing world defines deafness as a disability, but the Deaf community consider themselves as a cultural and linguistic minority because they communicate using a language that is not widely understood. Research in this area has focused on the significance of identity on psychological well-being. Glickman (1993) describes the development of four culturally Deaf identities, and Chapman and Dammeyer (2017) emphasize the importance of the level of discrimination felt, as well as identification with a marginalized group, in the role of psychological well-being.

Additionally, attention has turned to hearing children of Deaf adults (CODA). In the US, the distinction is made between CODA and KODA. CODA refers to adult children of Deaf adults, while KODA is used to refer to younger children or kids of Deaf adults. In the UK, the term CODA refers to both children and adult children. The literature focuses on the development of a bicultural identity of typically hearing children in a hearing world and Deaf culture and was given mainstream attention by the Oscar-winning film CODA (2021). See MacDougall (2022) for discussion.

Social-cognitive development

From the earliest days, parent–child interaction shapes the development of prelingual social communicative behaviors such as visual attention and eye contact, joint attention, turn-taking, and the use of facial expressions to support the meaning of verbal information. Research suggests that some, but not all, aspects of these early interactions may develop differently in children with HI and hearing parents (Nowakowski *et al.*, 2009).

Development of mentalizing skills in children with HI is significantly delayed, as in those with VI. Children typically fail to pass first-order ToM tasks, that are characteristically mastered by hearing 3–4-year-olds, until they are aged 13 years and even beyond. The ability is strongly related to the language and communicative competency of the child, whether in spoken or sign language; notably, deaf children of deaf parents do not demonstrate such delays (Meristo *et al.*, 2007). Little or no delay in ToM follows early cochlear implantation when this is associated with improved spoken language proficiency (Remmel *et al.*, 2009). Early conversational input about the beliefs and mental states of others and overall language competency is therefore crucial in fostering adaptive social-cognitive development. Unfortunately, parents of deaf children often find it extremely challenging to modify their use of language and communication to meet the changing needs of their child through infancy and childhood. Compensatory strategies, such as establishing eye contact before speaking, "scaffolding" the child's attempts at producing spoken words or phrases, and using a "sign sandwich" when necessary (saying the target word, signing it, then saying it again), usually need to be explicitly taught to parents, from the earliest days, by teachers of the deaf or speech and language therapists.

Other neuropsychological processes: executive function, attention, and working memory

The "higher-order" cognitive processes comprising executive function abilities are vulnerable in children with HI. Deficits in working memory are consistently found in those with and without cochlear implants (Pisoni *et al.*, 2008). Attention control, particularly visual attention, is altered by hearing reduction; deaf children show deficits in selective attention but enhanced peripheral attention (Dye *et al.*, 2008). Studies exploring other executive functions generally indicate greater impulsivity and difficulties in problem-solving, sequencing, and planning compared with hearing children (Pisoni *et al.*, 2010). The development of all these functions is closely linked with language skills such that the deficits are ameliorated or no longer present once language level is controlled for (Figueras *et al.*, 2008).

Neuroplasticity and brain organization

In the absence of auditory input, thalamo-cortical areas of the brain and the auditory cortex become utilized by other sensory modalities, particularly the visual modality, showing cross-modal plasticity (Gordon *et al.*, 2011). In children with HI, increased capabilities and compensatory skill in nonauditory modalities have been demonstrated, for example, enhanced tactile accuracy, visual attention, and processing of stimuli in the peripheral visual field (Bavelier *et al.*, 2000). In children with normal hearing, synaptic density in the temporal cortex peaks at between 2–4 years of age, with HI resulting in delayed synaptogenesis in the auditory cortex (see Kral *et al.*, 2012 for a review). Auditory stimulation is required for normal development of speech perception and language during a "sensitive period" of higher neuronal plasticity up until the age of about 3.5 years. After the age of 7 years irreversible changes in cortical organization prevent adequate processing of auditory signals.

Kral *et al.* (2016) explain the reciprocal relationship between language, sensory experiences, and neurocognitive outcomes during development in children with cochlear implants: "better sensory functioning from the cochlear implant is related to stronger and more robust language skills; stronger language skills predict better neurocognitive outcomes; and neurocognitive functioning acts to support language." It is this complex and dynamic interdependence that explains the variability in outcomes in children with cochlear implants.

Hearing impairment and complexity

Assessment and diagnosis of neurodevelopmental disorders

Around 40% of children with HI have additional impairments arising from the underlying syndromic etiology including generalized or specific ID, VI, ASD, ADHD, motor, and health impairments. Diagnoses of ASD are more common among HI than hearing children at around 2–4%, and the prevalence appears to be increasing (Szymanski *et al.*, 2012), probably due to greater awareness of ASD in clinicians and the general public. Intellectual or learning disability, with its consequent impact on adaptive behavior, affects around 8–10% of children with HI, and specific learning disability a further 8%. Significant neurodevelopmental motor impairments, e.g., cerebral palsy, affect around 14% of deaf children. Rates of attention and hyperactivity problems are elevated in children with HI compared with their hearing peers, and are largely associated with infectious etiologies of HI (Hindley *et al.*, 1998).

In young children with HI, care must be taken to distinguish between ASD and other social communication difficulties that may arise because of the impact of HI on language and (preverbal) communication. In the former, there is typically a lack of communicative intent and the presence of restrictive, repetitive, and stereotyped patterns of behavior (Edwards *et al.*, 2008a). In the early years, it is not uncommon for very young children with HI to actively avoid eye contact or to show restrictive interests in certain toys or activities. While these may be early warning signs of ASD, for many deaf children they are more transient and as language develops, these behaviors frequently disappear along with the concerns regarding ASD.

To diagnose ASD and other neurodevelopmental impairments, skilled differential diagnosis by multidisciplinary pediatric teams with expertise in HI and neurodisability is required. In children with sensory impairments with cerebral palsy or other significant fine-motor impairments, and those with dual sensory impairment (visual and hearing), assessment of cognitive and language abilities can be very challenging. The motor or visual disabilities may "mask" relatively well-preserved intellectual abilities, with serious consequences for educational placements and expectations for achievement.

Psychological and psychiatric issues

Prevalence and risk factors

There is little epidemiological consistency in the reported prevalence of mental health problems with prevalence rates ranging between 11–60%; this arises from differences in sampling, assessment method, definitions of "disorder," and criteria for clinical "caseness" (Hindley *et al.*, 1994; Cornes *et al.*, 2006). As well as the typical risk factors for psychiatric disorders in children, additional factors to be considered for HI children include low language competency, additional disabilities, severe learning difficulty, communication difficulties with family or peers, being bullied, isolation, and discrimination (Fellinger *et al.*, 2009; Hogan *et al.*, 2011). The overall picture is a higher risk for psychological and psychiatric difficulties in children with HI, though there is considerable individual variation.

Parenting a child with HI has been described by mothers as more stressful than parenting a hearing one (Horsch *et al.*, 1997). However, more recent research indicates that this is not inevitable and is likely related to amount of information and support parents receive as part of early intervention programs (Hintermair, 2006). Parents of children with HI and additional needs report higher levels of stress. Research suggests that the stresses may vary over time and be related to factors such as behavior problems and language delays (Lederberg *et al.*, 2002; Quittner *et al.* 2010).

Behavioral and emotional difficulties

Some of the most common presentations to child mental health services of preschool-aged children with HI are severe noncompliance with adult requests, temper tantrums, and aggressive behavior. Parents typically report that they do not know how to set boundaries and feel helpless in conveying instructions or explanations when the child's language is significantly delayed. Parental attitudes toward childrearing, disability, and personal feelings of guilt or loss may contribute to expectations of the child's appropriate behavior and use of disciplinary strategies. Psychoeducation and behavioral interventions adapted to accommodate the child's communication and language level are effective if implemented in conjunction with support to improve parent–child communication.

School-aged children have an increased referral rate for assessment of ADHD. Delays in language acquisition and deficits in executive function may result in difficulties mastering affect regulation and verbally mediated self-control, with consequent behavioral manifestations of poor attention, impulsivity, and hyperactivity. The assessment and diagnosis of ADHD in children with HI is complicated and controversial; behaviors considered diagnostic in hearing children must be interpreted with caution in those with HI. For example, behaviors such as seeming to not listen when spoken to directly and being distracted by irrelevant visual stimuli are typical of children with HI. They may not be aware that they are being spoken to or are monitoring what is happening around them visually to compensate for the lack of auditory information (Edwards *et al.*, 2008b). Effective management of these difficulties can usually be achieved through psychoeducation of parents and teachers and behavioral strategies, with infrequent necessity for pharmacological treatment.

Anxiety disorders, such as obsessive–compulsive disorder (OCD) and social anxiety disorder (SAD), tend to emerge in older children and adolescents with HI, similar to their hearing peers. High levels of anxiety may be associated with issues around the individual's developing identity and the perception of themself as deaf or hearing (including the issue of cochlear implantation), and their involvement with Deaf culture. Depressive disorders occur more commonly in adolescence and need to be considered in the context of the individual's school setting (whether there is a comparable peer group), emerging personal identity, and the ease of communication within the family in terms of communication mode (Mance *et al.*, 2012).

Assessment and interventions need to consider the child and family's communication preferences and competencies and treatments such as CBT, and family, narrative, or solution-focused therapy will need to be tailored appropriately. Much work has been done in recent years in validating assessment tools for children with hearing impairment (Kronenberger *et al.*, 2014; Niclasen & Dammeyer, 2016) including those delivered in British Sign Language (Roberts *et al.*, 2015; Phillips *et al.* 2022).

Professional approaches for management and care

The management of children with VI or HI (or dual sensory impairment) requires a multidisciplinary care package, with an integrated service comprising health, education, and social services. This includes ophthalmology and a peripatetic teacher of the visually impaired for the infant and young child with VI, and audiology, speech, and language therapy, and a peripatetic teacher of the deaf for the infant and young child with HI. During the early years, children need access to specialist multidisciplinary pediatric teams with expertise in VI or HI. Because of the vulnerabilities of infancy and the early years for the child and parent relationship, early parent-mediated intervention, such as the DJVI (Salt & Dale, 2017), should promote functional vision or hearing (if feasible) and general development across the first three years. A holistic approach to the child should be pursued including monitoring of cognition, communication and language, and behavior. School-aged children continue to need input from specialist teachers for VI or HI within the mainstream or specialist school environment. Close monitoring of progress from all perspectives will need to continue, with occasional review by multidisciplinary specialist services using adapted methods of assessment as required (see Further Reading). Individualized family-centered care, including working with parents in partnership, is important for supporting families.

In all community and specialized services, holistic positive psychology approaches focusing on normalization, quality of life, self-determination, and effective problem-solving and coping abilities may assist young people and their families. The richness and diversity of Blind culture and community, such as blind sports and drama, and Deaf culture and community, with the use of British Sign Language for communication, needs to be fully recognized as part of participation and disability affirmativeness. Nevertheless, the parent, educator, or clinician needs to be alert to possible psychological problems in children and young people with VI or HI, as they would be in typically seeing or hearing peers. There are higher risks for mental health needs. Formulation, diagnostic, and treatment approaches draw on the same principles as with a typical child of similar age and intellectual capacity but need to be informed and tailored to needs arising from living with VI or HI.

Access to pediatric, psychological, and psychiatric services comprising professionals with specialist knowledge and expertise for working with children with VI or HI may be available. These include tertiary developmental vision and cochlear implant services, and VI- and HI-child and adolescent mental health services. Where not available, children may also be seen by pediatric and child development teams and child and adolescent mental health services (CAMHS). Wherever the child is seen, it is essential that their written or communication abilities and preferences are understood and accommodated, using enlarged font, Braille, or sign language interpreters if required.

In all service delivery of any kind, the voice of the child and young person with VI or HI, and their families, needs consideration and advocacy (Tadić *et al.*, 2015). Formulations and intervention should build on personal decision-making, preferences, quality of life, and opportunity to fulfill access, inclusion, and participation within society.

References

Visual impairment

Ardito, R.B. *et al.* (2004) Attachment representations in adults with congenital blindness: association with maternal interactive behaviours during childhood. *Psychological Reports* **95**, 263–274.

Augestad, I.B. (2017) Self-concept and self-esteem among children and young adults with visual impairment: a systematic review. *Cogent Psychology* **4**, 1319652.

Bathelt, J. *et al.* (2017) Event-related potential response to auditory social stimuli, parent-reported social communicative deficits and autism risk in school-aged children with congenital visual impairment. *Developmental Cognitive Neuroscience* **27**, 10–18.

Bathelt, J. *et al.* (2019) Adaptive behaviour and quality of life in school-age children with congenital visual disorders and different levels of visual impairment. *Research in Developmental Disabilities* **85**, 154–162.

Bathelt, J. *et al.* (2020) Brain structure in children with congenital visual disorders and visual impairment. *Developmental Medicine and Child Neurology* **62**(1), 125–131.

Dale, N. *et al.* (2002) Developmental outcome, including setback, in young children with severe visual impairment. *Developmental Medicine & Child Neurology* **44**, 613–622.

Dale, N. *et al.* (2007) Early support developmental journal for children with visual impairment: the case for a new developmental framework for early intervention. *Child: Care, Health and Development* **33**, 684–690.

Dale, N.J. *et al.* (2014) Social communicative variation in 1-3-year-olds with severe visual impairment. *Child: Care, Health and Development* **40**(2), 158–164.

Dale, N. *et al.* (2017) Functional vision and cognition in infants with congenital disorders of the peripheral visual system. *Developmental Medicine and Child Neurology* **59**(7), 725–731.

Dale, N.J. *et al.* (2019) Home-based early intervention in infants and young children with visual impairment using the Developmental Journal: a longitudinal cohort study. *Developmental Medicine and Child Neurology* **61**(6), 697–709.

Dale, N. *et al.* (eds) (2022) *Children with Vision Impairment: Assessment, Development and Intervention: A Clinic Practice Guide.* MacKeith Press, London.

Dale, N. *et al.* (2024) Modification and validation of an autism observational assessment including ADOS-2 for use with children with visual impairment. *Journal of Autism and Developmental Disorders.* doi:10.1007/s10803-024-06514-z.

Do, B. *et al.* (2017) Systematic review and meta-analysis of the association of autism spectrum disorder in visually or hearing impaired children. *Ophthalmic & Physiological Optics* **37**(2), 212–224.

Dyck, M.J. *et al.* (2004) Emotion recognition/understanding ability in hearing or vision-impaired children: do sounds, sights, or words make the difference? *Journal of Child Psychology and Psychiatry* **45**, 789–800.

Giesen, J.M. *et al.* (2012) Academic supports, cognitive disability and mathematics achievement for visually impaired youth: a multilevel modeling approach. *International Journal of Special Education* **27**, 1–10.

Gori, M. *et al.* (2010) Poor haptic orientation discrimination in non-sighted children may reflect disruption of cross-sensory calibration. *Current Biology* **20**, 223–225.

Greaney, J. *et al.* (2000) Braille reading by children: is there a phonological explanation for their difficulties? *British Journal of Visual Impairment* **18**, 35–40.

Green, S. *et al.* (2004) An investigation of first-order false belief understanding of children with congenital profound visual impairment. *British Journal of Developmental Psychology* **22**, 1–17.

Greenaway, R. *et al.* (2017) Neuropsychological presentation and adaptive skills in high-functioning adolescents with visual impairment: a preliminary investigation. *Applied Neuropsychology: Child* **6**(2), 145–157.

Harris, J. & Lord, C. (2016) Mental health of children with visual impairment at 11 years of age. *Developmental Medicine Child Neurology* **58**, 774–779.

Harris, J. *et al.* (2012) *Sight Impaired at Age Seven: Secondary Analysis of the Millennium Cohort Survey.* RSLB, RNIB and NatCen Social Research, London/Northampton, UK.

Heppe, E.C.M. *et al.* (2021) Evaluation of a community-based mentoring program on psychosocial functioning of adolescents with a visual impairment: a randomised controlled trial. *British Journal of Visual Impairment* **39**(3), 251–265.

Hobson, R.P. *et al.* (2010) Reversible autism among congenitally blind children? A controlled follow-up study. *Journal of Child Psychology and Psychiatry* **51**, 1235–1241.

Ingram, D. *et al.* (2022) Sleep challenges and interventions in children with visual impairment. *Journal of Pediatric Ophthalmology and Strabismus* **59**(2), 77–86.

Jackson, C. (2022) Psychological wellbeing, mental health and behaviour. In: *Children with Vision Impairment: Assessment, Development and Management.* (eds N. Dale, *et al.*), MacKeith Practice Guides. MacKeith Press, London. pp. 223–233.

Kef, S. & Deković, M. (2004) The role of parental and peer support in adolescents well-being: a comparison of adolescents with and without a visual impairment. *Journal of Adolescence* **27**, 453–466.

Lifshitz, H. *et al.* (2007) Self concept, adjustment to blindness, and quality of friendship among adolescents with visual impairments. *Journal of Visual Impairment and Blindness* **101**(2), 96–107.

Lord, C. *et al.* (2012) *Autism Diagnostic Observation Schedule, (ADOS-2), Part II: Toddler Module*, 2nd edn. Western Psychological Services, Los Angeles.

MacKechnie, R. *et al.* (2018) Psychopathology profiles in children with congenital visual impairment. Unpublished PhD thesis. Royal Holloway, University of London, London.

Mann, A. *et al.* (2023) Neurodevelopmental impairments in children with septo-optic dysplasia spectrum conditions: a systematic review. *Molecular Autism* **14**, 26.

Mohammed, Z. & Omar, R. (2011) Comparison of reading performance between visually impaired and normally sighted students in Malaysia. *British Journal of Visual Impairment* **29**(3), 196–207.

Mosca, R. *et al.* (2015) Language and communication development in preschool children with visual impairment: a systematic review. *The South African Journal of Communication Disorders* **62**(1), e1–e10.

Nielsen, L.S. *et al.* (2007) Visual dysfunctions and ocular disorders in children with developmental delay. I. prevalence, diagnoses and aetiology of visual impairment. *Acta Ophthalmologica Scandinavica* **85**(2), 149–156.

Ollendick, T.H. *et al.* (1985) Fears in visually-impaired and normally-sighted youths. *Behaviour Research and Therapy* **23**, 375–378.

O'Reilly, M.A. *et al.* (2017) Frontal EEG asymmetry and later behavior vulnerability in infants with congenital visual impairment. *Clinical Neurophysiology* **128**(11), 2191–2199.

Pijnacker, J. *et al.* (2012) Pragmatic abilities in children with congenital visual impairment: an exploration of non-literal language and advanced theory of mind understanding. *Journal of Autism and Developmental Disorders* **42**, 2440–2449.

Pinquart, M. & Pfeiffer, J.P. (2011) Psychological well-being in visually impaired and unimpaired individuals: a meta-analysis. *British Journal of Visual Impairment* **29**(1), 27–45.

Pinquart, M. & Pfeiffer, J.P. (2013) Change in psychological problems of adolescents with and without visual impairment. *European Child and Adolescent Psychiatry* **23**, 571–578.

Rosenblum, L.P. (1998) Best friendships of adolescents with visual impairments: a descriptive study. *Journal of Visual Impairment and Blindness* **92**, 593–608.

Sadato, N. *et al.* (1996) Activation of the primary visual cortex by Braille reading in blind subjects. *Nature* **380**(6574), 526–528.

Sakkalou, E. *et al.* (2018) Parenting stress, anxiety, and depression in mothers with visually impaired infants: a cross-sectional and longitudinal cohort analysis. *Developmental Medicine and Child Neurology* **60**(3), 290–298.

Sakkalou, E. *et al.* (2021) Mother-infant interactions with infants with congenital visual impairment and associations with longitudinal outcomes in cognition and language. *Journal of Child Psychology and Psychiatry* **62**(6), 742–750.

Salt, A. & Dale, N. (2017) Developmental Journal for babies and young children with visual impairment (DJVI). Available: https://xip.uclb.com/product/DJVI_professional [26 October 2024].

Tadić, V. *et al.* (2009) Attentional processes in young children with congenital visual impairment. *British Journal of Developmental Psychology* **27**, 311–330.

Tadić, V. *et al.* (2010) Are language and social communication intact in children with congenital visual impairment at school age? *Journal of Child Psychology and Psychiatry* **51**, 696–705.

Tadić, V. *et al.* (2015) Vision-related quality of life (VQoL) group. Seeing it my way: living with childhood onset visual disability. *Child: Care, Health and Development* **41**(2), 239–248.

Teoh, L.J. *et al.* (2021) Visual impairment, severe visual impairment and blindness in children in Britain (BCVIS2): a national observational study. *The Lancet Child & Adolescent Health* **5**(3), 190–200.

Visagie, L. *et al.* (2013) Comparing fears in South African children with and without visual impairments. *Journal of Visual Impairment and Blindness* **111**, 231–246.

Withagen, A. *et al.* (2013) Short term memory and working memory in blind versus sighted children. *Research in Developmental Disabilities* **34**, 2161–2172.

Hearing impairment

Bavelier, D. *et al.* (2000) Visual attention to the periphery is enhanced in congenitally deaf individuals. *Journal of Neuroscience* **20**(17), RC93.

Blamey, P.J. (2003) Development of spoken language by deaf children. In: *The Oxford Handbook of Deaf Studies, Language, and Education.* (eds M. Marschark & P.E. Spencer), Vol. *1*. Oxford University Press, New York. pp. 478–490.

Breland, L. *et al.* (2022) Disparate oral and written language abilities in adolescents with cochlear implants: evidence from narrative samples. *Language, Speech, and Hearing Services in Schools* **53**(1), 193–212.

Chapman, M. & Dammeyer, J. (2017) The significance of deaf identity for psychological well-being. *The Journal of Deaf Studies and Deaf Education* **22**(2), 187–194.

Colucci, D. (2020) Updates on auditory neuropathy spectrum disorder. *The Hearing Journal* **73**(6), 32–34.

Cornes, A. *et al.* (2006) Reading the signs: impact of signed versus written questionnaires on the prevalence of psychopathology among deaf adolescents. *Australian and New Zealand Journal of Psychiatry* **40**(8), 665–673.

Dye, M.W.G. *et al.* (2008) Visual attention in deaf children and adults. In: *Deaf Cognition: Foundations and Outcomes.* (eds M. Marschark & P.C. Hauser). Oxford University Press, New York. pp. 250–263.

Edwards, L. *et al.* (2008a) Disorders of communication. In: *Psychological Processes in Deaf Children with Complex Needs: An Evidence-based Practical Guide.* (eds L. Edwards & S. Crocker). Jessica Kingsley Publishers, London. pp. 106–131.

Edwards, L. *et al.* (2008b) Behavioural and emotional disorders. In: *Psychological Processes in Deaf Children with Complex Needs: An Evidence-Based Practical Guide.* (eds L. Edwards & S. Crocker). Jessica Kingsley Publishers, London. pp. 40–60.

Edwards, A. *et al.* (2013) The mathematical abilities of children with cochlear implants. *Child Neuropsychology* **19**(2), 127–142.

Fellinger, J. *et al.* (2009) Correlates of mental health disorders among children with hearing impairments. *Developmental Medicine and Child Neurology* **51**(8), 635–641.

Figueras, B. *et al.* (2008) Executive function and language in deaf children. *Journal of Deaf Studies and Deaf Education* **13**(3), 362–377.

Fulcher, A. *et al.* (2012) Listen up: children with early identified hearing loss achieve age-appropriate speech/language outcomes by 3 years-of-age. *International Journal of Pediatric Otorhinolaryngology* **76**(12), 1785–1794.

Geers, A.E. & Nicholas, J.G. (2013) Enduring advantages of early cochlear implantation for spoken language development. *Journal of Speech, Language, and Hearing Research* **56**, 643–655.

Glickman, N.S. (1993) *Deaf Identity Development: Construction and Validation of a Theoretical Model.* University of Massachusetts Amherst, Amherst, MA.

Gordon, K.A. *et al.* (2011) Use it or lose it? Lessons learned from the developing brains of children who are deaf and use cochlear implants to hear. *Brain Topography* **24**(3–4), 201–219.

Hindley, P.A. *et al.* (1994) Psychiatric disorder in deaf and hearing impaired children and young people: a prevalence study. *Journal of Child Psychology and Psychiatry* **35**(5), 917–934.

Hindley, P.A. *et al.* (1998) Theoretical and epidemiological aspects of attention deficit and overactivity in deaf children. *Journal of Deaf Studies and Deaf Education* **3**(1), 64–72.

Hintermair, M. (2006) Parental resources, parental stress, and socioemotional development of deaf and hard of hearing children. *Journal of Deaf Studies and Deaf Education* **11**(4), 493–513.

Hogan, A. *et al.* (2011) Communication and behavioural disorders among children with hearing loss increases risk of mental health disorders. *Australian and New Zealand Journal of Public Health* **35**(4), 377–383.

Horsch, U. *et al.* (1997) Stress experienced by parents of children with cochlear implants compared with parents of deaf children and hearing children. *American Journal of Otology* **18**(6 Suppl), S161–S163.

Kral, A. *et al.* (2012) Developmental neuroplasticity after cochlear implantation. *Trends in Neurosciences* **35**(2), 111–122.

Kral, A. *et al.* (2016) Neurocognitive factors in sensory restoration of early deafness: a connectome model. *The Lancet Neurology* **15**(6), 610–621.

Kronenberger, W.G. *et al.* (2014) Neurocognitive risk in children with cochlear implants. *JAMA Otolaryngology–Head & Neck Surgery* **140**(7), 608–615.

Lederberg, A.R. *et al.* (2002) Parenting stress and social support in hearing mothers of deaf and hearing children: a longitudinal study. *Journal of Deaf Studies and Deaf Education* **7**(4), 330–345.

Ludlow, A. *et al.* (2010) Emotion recognition in children with profound and severe deafness: do they have a deficit in perceptual processing? *Journal of Clinical and Experimental Neuropsychology* **32**(9), 923–928.

MacDougall, J.C. (2022) Dialogue with the deaf: the future role of psychology. *Canadian Psychology/Psychologie Canadienne* **63**(4), 637–650.

Mance, J. *et al.* (2012) Self-perceptions in adolescents with cochlear implants. *Cochlear Implants International* **13**(2), 93–104.

Marschark, M. *et al.* (2008) *Deaf Cognition: Foundations and Outcomes.* Oxford University Press, New York.

Marschark, M. *et al.* (2015) Predicting the academic achievement of deaf and hard-of-hearing students from individual, household, communication, and educational factors. *Exceptional Children* **81**(3), 350–369.

Martin, D. *et al.* (2011) Peer relationships of deaf children with cochlear implants: predictors of peer entry and peer interaction success. *Journal of Deaf Studies and Deaf Education* **16**(1), 108–120.

Meadow-Orlans, K.P. *et al.* (1983) Attachment behaviour of deaf children with deaf parents. *Journal of the American Academy of Child Psychiatry* **22**(1), 23–28.

Meristo, M. *et al.* (2007) Language access and theory of mind reasoning: evidence from deaf children in bilingual and oralist environments. *Developmental Psychology* **43**(5), 1156–1169.

Niclasen, J. & Dammeyer, J. (2016) Psychometric properties of the strengths and difficulties questionnaire and mental health problems among children with hearing loss. *The Journal of Deaf Studies and Deaf Education* **21**(2), 129–140.

Nowakowski, M.E. *et al.* (2009) Establishment of joint attention in dyads involving hearing mothers of deaf and hearing children, and its relation to adaptive social behaviour. *American Annals of the Deaf* **154**(1), 15–29.

Phillips, H. *et al.* (2022) Adapting and validating the autism diagnostic observation schedule version 2 for use with deaf children and young people. *Journal of Autism and Developmental Disorders* **52**, 553–568.

Pipp-Siegel, S. *et al.* (2002) Predictors of parental stress in mothers of young children with hearing loss. *Journal of Deaf Studies and Deaf Education* **7**(1), 1–17.

Pisoni, D.B. *et al.* (2008) Efficacy and effectiveness of cochlear implants in deaf infants. In: *Deaf Cognition: Foundations and Outcomes.* (eds M. Marschark & P.C. Hauser). Oxford University Press, New York. pp. 52–101.

Pisoni, D.B. *et al.* (2010) Executive function, cognitive control, and sequence learning in deaf children with cochlear implants. In: *The Oxford Handbook of Deaf Studies, Language, and Education.* (eds M. Marschark & P.E. Spencer), Vol. 2. Oxford University Press, New York. pp. 439–457.

Puram, S.V. *et al.* (2016) Outcomes following pediatric auditory brainstem implant surgery: early experiences in a North American center. *Otolaryngology—Head and Neck Surgery* **155**(1), 133–138.

Quittner, A.L. *et al.* (1990) Chronic parenting stress: moderating versus mediating effects of social support. *Journal of Personality and Social Psychology* **59**(6), 1266.

Quittner, A.L. *et al.* (2010) Parenting stress among parents of deaf and hearing children: associations with language delays and behaviour problems. *Parenting: Science and Practice* **10**(2), 136–155.

Rance, G. & Starr, A. (2015) Pathophysiological mechanisms of functional hearing consequences of auditory neuropathy. *Brain* **138**(Pt 11), 3141–3158.

Remmel, E. *et al.* (2009) Theory of mind and language in children with cochlear implants. *Journal of Deaf Studies and Deaf Education* **14**(2), 218–236.

Roberts, S. *et al.* (2015) *Translation into British Sign Language and Validation of the Strengths and Difficulties Questionnaire.* NIHR Journals Library, Southampton, UK.

Sarant, J.Z. *et al.* (2015) Academic outcomes for school-aged children with severe–profound hearing loss and early unilateral and bilateral cochlear implants. *Journal of Speech, Language, and Hearing Research* **58**(3), 1017–1032.

Sharma, D.S. *et al.* (2020) Hearing and speech benefits of cochlear implantation in children: a review of the literature. *International Journal of Pediatric Otorhinolaryngology* **133**, 109984.

Solutions for Public Health (2019) Screening for Permanent Hearing Loss in Children at School Entry: External Review Against Programme Appraisal Criteria for the UK National Screening Committee. UK National Screening Committee, London. Available: https://view-health-screening-recommendations.service.gov.uk/document/371/download [27 December 2024].

Stevenson, J. *et al.* (2015) Emotional and behavioural difficulties in children and adolescents with hearing impairment: a systematic review and meta-analysis. *European of Child & Adolescent Psychiatry* **24**, 477–496.

Stredler-Brown, A. (2010) Communication choices and outcomes during the early years: an assessment and evidence-based approach. In: *The Oxford Handbook of Deaf Studies, Language, and Education.* (eds M. Marschark & P.E. Spencer), Vol. *2*. Oxford University Press, New York. pp. 292–315.

Szymanski, C.A. *et al.* (2012) Deaf children with autism spectrum disorders. *Journal of Autism and Developmental Disorders* **42**(10), 2027–2037.

van Gent, T. *et al.* (2011) Self-concept and psychopathology in deaf adolescents: preliminary support for moderating effects of deafness-related characteristics and peer problems. *Journal of Child Psychology and Psychiatry* **52**(5), 720–728.

Weisel, A. *et al.* (2007) Mothers' stress and expectations as a function of time since child's cochlear implantation. *Journal of Deaf Studies and Deaf Education* **12**(1), 55–64.

Yoshinaga-Itano, C. (2003) From screening to early identification and intervention: discovering predictors to successful outcomes for children with significant hearing loss. *The Journal of Deaf Studies and Deaf Education* **8**(1), 11–30.

Further reading

Booth, R. *et al.* (eds) (2022) *Pediatric Neuropsychology within the Multidisciplinary Context.* MacKeith Press, London. For details of cognitive and neuropsychological assessment methods for children with VI, see Chapter 1, or HI, see Chapter 2

CHAPTER 45

Child and youth mental health services in community health care settings

J.L. Henderson[1] and Skye Barbic[2]

[1] Centre for Addiction and Mental Health, Department of Psychiatry, University of Toronto, Toronto, Ontario, Canada

[2] Department of Occupational Science and Occupational Therapy, Faculty of Medicine, The University of British Columbia, Vancouver, British Columbia, Canada

Mental health services (including substance use services) delivered in community health care settings are those delivered through community-based organizations by nonpsychiatrists and nonpsychologists. Community-based organizations include primary care settings, community health centers, community-based child and youth mental health (nonprofit/charitable) organizations, and grassroots organizations or initiatives. Community-based mental health services may be delivered by social workers, peer support workers, primary care physicians, nursing professionals, lay health workers, occupational therapists, community pediatricians, and other nonpsychiatrists. Primary health care services, typically delivered by family physicians or general practitioners (referred to as *primary care physicians* throughout this chapter) and nursing professionals, provide the bulk of health services to children and youth (under 18 years of age) worldwide. These services are designed to identify and treat health conditions, provide health promotion and prevention services, and meet the needs of the communities they serve (World Health Organization, 1978; Boerma, 2006), and are often the first point of contact for mental health concerns. Globally, however, there is substantial variability in primary health care availability, staffing, and funding, with other community-based organizations, public health organizations, and schools playing critical roles in meeting the mental health needs of children and youth. The community health care setting is ideal for delivering child and youth mental health services due to its ease of access and interconnectivity with other services and settings.

This chapter describes prominent considerations for services to address the mental health and substance use (MHSU) needs of children and youth offered in primary health and other community-based health care settings. Specific primary and community-based service models are discussed including primary care physician delivered services, community-based integrated youth services, specific intervention approaches delivered in primary health and other community settings, and broad health provider training considerations for delivering MHSU health services reflective of the needs of children and youth from diverse communities. Global health, culture, and equity considerations are discussed throughout.

The need for primary and other community-based mental health and substance use care for children and youth

While adult psychiatry is considered the "orphan" of the health care system, with inadequate funding relative to the mortality and morbidity associated with psychiatric disorders (Patel *et al.*, 2018), child and youth psychiatry is considered the "orphan of the orphan," with little investment or recognition (Lu *et al.*, 2018) and limited access for many children and youth. Indeed, children and youth with MHSU concerns have among the poorest access to timely, evidence-based, effectively delivered health care services, despite the strong return on investment demonstrated for early MHSU interventions (Malla *et al.*, 2018; McGorry *et al.*, 2022). Further, the underresourcing of MHSU care is not equitably distributed. Racialized, Indigenous, and rural children and youth, and those from limited resource settings in high-income countries have disproportionately poor access to effective MHSU treatment services (Sudak *et al.*, 2020; Castro-Ramirez *et al.*, 2021). Globally, children and youth living in low- or middle-income countries (LMICs)—where the majority of the world's children and youth live (World Health Organization, 2019)—have the poorest access to effective MHSU treatment services, with limited

Rutter's Child and Adolescent Psychiatry and Psychology, Seventh Edition.
Edited by Anita Thapar, Daniel S. Pine, Samuele Cortese, Cathy Creswell, Tamsin J. Ford, James F. Leckman, and Argyris Stringaris.

Companion website: www.wiley.com/go/thapar/rutterspsych7

availability of mental health specialists and low mental health provider resource capacity (Kohrt *et al.*, 2018). Accordingly, MHSU practitioners in primary and other community settings play a critical role in connecting youth to the right MHSU care at the right time (MacDonald *et al.*, 2018).

Barriers and facilitators of child and youth mental health care in primary and other community health care settings

Many global MHSU systems are characterized as fragmented, underresourced, unresponsive, not culturally safe, and not efficient or effective in meeting the needs of youth and families/caregivers (Hetrick *et al.*, 2017; Malla *et al.*, 2018; Mei *et al.*, 2020). Specific barriers to children and youth seeking primary and other community MHSU care have been well documented, though individuals with help-seeking experience are underrepresented in studies, as are children and youth from LMICs (Aguirre Velasco *et al.*, 2020; Radez *et al.*, 2021). Some services impose arbitrary limitations on access, such as excluding youth with multiple diagnoses, leaving youth struggling to navigate a complex system as their needs evolve (Cleverley *et al.*, 2020). Other selected barriers and facilitators to MHSU care are detailed in Table 45.1.

Table 45.1 Selected barriers and facilitators to child and youth community mental health care.

	Barriers	Facilitators
Demand-side (help-seeking)	• *Stigma*, or negative beliefs and attitudes about mental health and substance use (MHSU) services • Negative past experiences with services and historical harm • Distrust • Beliefs that services are not helpful • Limited MHSU literacy and service awareness • MHSU symptoms which impact help-seeking • Confidentiality and lack of autonomy concerns	• Previous positive experiences with services • Strong trusted relationships with gatekeepers (e.g., primary care physicians, teachers, family members, and other health service providers) • Low public stigma • Perceived similarities with service providers (e.g., like-gender, race, ethnicity, age)
Supply-side	• Availability of services • Cost • Wait times • Provider attitudes • Communication challenges • Transportation challenges • Racism in service provision • Lack of cultural sensitivity in service provision	• Strong community engagement • Good MHSU problem recognition • Service providers that respect, listen, and validate youth experiences

Sources: Aguirre Velasco *et al.*, 2020; Sudak *et al.*, 2020; Castro-Ramirez *et al.*, 2021; Radez *et al.*, 2021.

Demand-side, or help-seeking barriers, are especially problematic for children, youth, and families experiencing poverty, racial and other minority groups, and refugee and immigrant populations (Aguirre Velasco *et al.*, 2020; Castro-Ramirez *et al.*, 2021). Children and youth with intersectional experiences, or experiences that are shaped by the intersection of social positions (e.g., race/ethnicity, income status) and reinforced by systems of oppression (Hankivsky, 2014), especially those associated with marginalization, are at high risk of experiencing barriers to effective treatment (Harris *et al.*, 2020).

Interventions that promote help-seeking behaviors among adults have shown positive effects on improved literacy, reduced stigma, and increased help-seeking intentions (Xu *et al.*, 2018; Aguirre Velasco *et al.*, 2020). There has been limited research, however, demonstrating help-seeking behavior improvements among family members, children, or youth (Xu *et al.*, 2018). Some education-based interventions have shown promise among these groups, but more research is needed (Aguirre Velasco *et al.*, 2020).

Core role of primary and other community-based mental health and substance use services

Primary and other community-based MHSU practitioners, such as primary care physicians, community pediatricians, nurse practitioners, mental health counselors, lay health workers, and peer support workers serve a critical role as a first point of contact in the health care system for children and youth with MHSU needs. They have essential roles in health promotion, prevention, early identification, early intervention, referral to MHSU specialist services, and care coordination over time and across physical, mental health, and other needs. Primary and other community health care practitioners are well-positioned to address barriers by providing timely access to MHSU services locally, offering services in the context of established and trusted relationships, and enhancing service integration across health, community, educational, and social services (MacDonald *et al.*, 2018; Duong *et al.*, 2021). Importantly, primary and other community-based MHSU practitioners serve a critical function in reducing MHSU treatment delays for children and youth. Unmet MHSU needs, especially when experienced during development, are associated with significant negative short- and long-term difficulties, including disrupted peer and family relationships, academic/vocational interruptions, symptom exacerbation, increased comorbidity risk, and disruptions in the transition to adulthood (Hetrick *et al.*, 2017; MacDonald *et al.*, 2018). Box 45.1 identifies common treatment delays. Given their essential role in facilitating access to MHSU services and reducing the duration of untreated MHSU needs, primary and other community-based MHSU practitioners need to be adequately resourced, trained, and equipped to: (i) identify difficulties; (ii) provide initial intervention; (iii) determine need for referral; (iv) make referrals; and (v) coordinate care (Xu *et al.*, 2018). Training of care providers will be explored later in this chapter.

Box 45.1 Common mental health and substance use treatment delays

Delays can arise at multiple points in the MHSU treatment seeking process, including:

- Individual and family identification of need and decision-making about seeking help from primary care physicians (or other practitioners)
- Access to primary care physicians (or other practitioners) who can provide early identification, intervention, and referrals to MHSU-specific supports
- Inefficient or inappropriate referrals due to limited awareness of and integration with MHSU-specific treatment services and/or MHSU specialist services
- Lengthy, multivisit pretreatment MHSU processes such as intake, screening, assessment, and treatment planning

Existing and emerging models of mental health care for children and youth in primary and other community health care settings

Global considerations for mental health models of care for children and youth in community health care settings

Given that most children and youth with MHSU needs who receive services will receive primary and other community-based MHSU care, it is essential that practitioners be equipped with evidence-based practices with demonstrated effectiveness in primary and other community-based MHSU care settings. This is especially true in LMIC contexts, where most child and youth MHSU services are delivered in community settings. Given the dominance of the Western approaches in the development of current evidence-based MHSU practices, readers should consider the applicability to some LMIC contexts and the potential for outcome enhancement through integrating local expertise (Weisz *et al.*, 2017; see Chapter 46 for a review of child and youth mental health treatment in low-resource settings). Moreover, future development and implementation of primary and other community-based child and youth MHSU innovations present critical opportunities to integrate a broader range of cultural approaches and perspectives. See Box 45.2 for an abbreviated list of key considerations for developing and implementing primary and other community MHSU services for children and youth living in LMIC settings.

Box 45.2 Key considerations for developing and implementing community mental health and substance use services for children and youth living in low- and middle-income country settings

- Codevelop and test new services with local communities, including youth and families
- Integrate local expertise into the service model
- Ensure services are culturally appropriate and involve service providers with local cultural expertise
- Ensure models and services reflect local resource availability
- Ensure new models or services address the social determinants of mental health, inequities, and exposure to war or other forms of conflict and trauma
- Plan to implement in partnership with community-based organizations, particularly nonmedical organizations

Sources: Castillo et *al.*, 2019; Pedersen et *al.*, 2019; Rose-Clarke et *al.*, 2019; Barbui et *al.*, 2020.

Child and youth mental health and substance use services delivered in primary health care settings

Core roles of primary care physicians and other practitioners in health promotion, prevention, and intervention

Primary health care plays a crucial role in addressing child and youth MHSU needs and improving transitions of youth from pediatric to adult health care (Bhawra *et al.*, 2016; Mulvaney-Day *et al.*, 2018; Rojas *et al.*, 2019). This care includes health promotion, prevention, early intervention, and continuous care across the life span (O'Brien *et al.*, 2016; Mulvaney-Day *et al.*, 2018; Rojas *et al.*, 2019). In health promotion, primary care physicians and other primary health care providers promote mental health and well-being by educating children, youth, and their families/caregivers about healthy lifestyles and positive mental health practices (Rojas *et al.*, 2019; Mathias *et al.*, 2021). Primary care physicians and other primary health care providers may also offer guidance on maintaining adequate sleep, stress management, and healthy coping mechanisms, including encouraging participation in education and play (Mulvaney-Day *et al.*, 2018). For MHSU prevention, primary care providers play an important role identifying and mitigating risk factors, together with children, youth, and families (Rojas *et al.*, 2019). Ideally, primary care physicians and other primary health care providers conduct routine screening to detect early signs of MHSU issues, such as anxiety or depression, conduct assessments where needed, and provide timely and appropriate initial interventions to prevent progression of MHSU difficulties (Correll *et al.*, 2018; Mulvaney-Day *et al.*, 2018, Rojas *et al.*, 2019; Fusar-Poli *et al.*, 2021; Habayeb *et al.*, 2022;). Services may also include referring children and youth to other community-based or specialized MHSU services for peer support, counseling, assessment, diagnosis, and treatments. Globally, gaps in standardized tools and training to support early identification and intervention in primary health care, as well as MHSU service availability, have been identified as barriers to fulsome implementation (Fusar-Poli *et al.*, 2021). Evidence shows that screening in primary care settings delivers valuable information to improve resource planning and mapping, and engages children and youth in MHSU services who may otherwise be missed (Habayeb *et al.*, 2022).

When MHSU problems become more pronounced, primary care physicians, community pediatricians, and other primary health care providers can also play a vital MHSU service role by delivering evidence-based MHSU interventions that are adapted for implementation in primary care (Asarnow *et al.*, 2015; Rojas *et al.*, 2019). They may collaborate with MHSU specialists to develop, implement, and coordinate comprehensive and multidisciplinary treatment plans, prescribe and monitor medications, provide therapy or counseling, support school accommodations, and coordinate care with other professionals. Care coordination is a crucial primary care role to provide ongoing support and guidance to the child, youth, and their families/caregivers and ensure comprehensive and integrated care for children and youth (Bhawra *et al.*, 2016; Rojas *et al.*, 2019; Habayeb *et al.*, 2022;).

Screening, assessment, diagnosis, and measurement-based care in primary health care settings

Screening, assessment, diagnosis, and measurement-based care (MBC) are essential processes for addressing child and youth MHSU concerns in primary health care settings (Van Cleave *et al.*, 2012). Routine screening within primary care services involves use of brief questionnaires, interviews, observations, or other tools by primary care physicians or other primary care practitioners as an initial service step to identify individuals at risk for MHSU disorders and determine if further assessment is needed (Sarvet, 2020). Validated and reliable screening tools designed for youth MHSU (e.g., the Pediatric Symptom Checklist [PSC], Adverse Childhood Event Questionnaire [ACE-Q], Strengths and Difficulties Questionnaire [SDQ], or Patient Health Questionnaire for Adolescents [PHQ-A]) are recommended for use (Flynn *et al.*, 2015; Pardee *et al.*, 2017; Mulvaney-Day *et al.*, 2018). Positive screening results usually suggest a need for more comprehensive evaluation (assessment and/or diagnosis) by the primary care practitioner or an MHSU specialist (Van Cleave *et al.*, 2012; Flynn *et al.*, 2015; Mulvaney-Day *et al.*, 2018). While jurisdictions vary in the extent to which primary care physicians and community pediatricians assess, diagnose, and prescribe medications for MHSU needs, some MHSU needs, for example, the presence of depression and anxiety, are more commonly assessed and treated (including with medication) by primary care physicians than psychiatrists in many jurisdictions, including the US (Kroenke & Unutzer, 2017). Integrated or collaborative care models of mental health services implemented in primary care settings, however, have been shown to outperform usual primary care services in patient experience, outcomes, and quality of life (Reed *et al.*, 2016). These models involve MHSU specialists supporting primary care physicians and other primary care practitioners to deliver high-quality MHSU services. Notably, a key component of collaborative care is MBC (Kroenke & Unutzer, 2017), which is also increasingly identified as essential for delivering patient-centered services, including to youth (Sarvet, 2020). MBC involves routine use of patient-reported outcome measures over time to identify initial MHSU needs, including suicide-related needs, determine MHSU areas of improvement or challenges over the course of intervention, and guide intervention plan adjustments to more-or-less specialized MHSU services (Van Cleave *et al.*, 2012; Sarvet, 2020;). MBC also facilitates primary care physician identification of interactions between physical and mental health, and communication with MHSU specialists (Kroenke & Unutzer, 2017; Sarvet, 2020).

Community-based integrated youth services: an example of an expanding community-based, nonspecialist model for youth with mental health and substance use needs

These integrated services are co-located into a "one-stop shop" model of service delivery, with visible, youth-friendly branding and physical spaces (McGorry *et al.*, 2022). Integrated youth services (IYS) emphasize equitable and inclusive access to evidence-informed services for youth (Box 45.3; Mathias *et al.*, 2021; Henderson *et al.*, 2023).

IYS, as a community-based service model for children and youth, initially emerged in Australia in the mid-2000s to address the unmet mental health needs of youth by offering integrated youth primary mental health care in a program known as *headspace* (McGorry *et al.*, 2022). Emphasizing early identification and intervention, *headspace* built upon emerging evidence on the value of early intervention in psychosis (McGorry *et al.*, 2022). These services also aligned with the World Health Organization's calls for a primary care-based approach to mental health service delivery (Funk & Ivbijaro, 2008).

While integration of mental health services into conventional primary care settings was the initial focus of primary mental health care efforts for youth globally, in Australia this approach did not adequately address barriers to help-seeking (e.g., service awareness, youth friendliness, adequate service availability). Accordingly, the *headspace* model enhanced the traditional primary care service model by emphasizing codesign with youth, as well as service accessibility and youth friendliness (e.g., nonjudgmental, respectful, empowering services), grounding these services in the community (McGorry *et al.*, 2022).

Since 2010, various versions of the IYS model have been implemented in more than 300 communities in several high-income countries, including France, Ireland, the US, and Canada. IYS typically offer services to youth aged 12–25 years, distinct from services for children and adults over 25 years old (McGorry *et al.*, 2022). These services are intentionally designed to facilitate timely access to MHSU services in the community,

Box 45.3 Integrated youth services (IYS)

Integrated youth services (IYS) have emerged to overcome chronic mental health and substance use (MHSU) service shortcomings and to support child and youth MHSU outcomes in many parts of the world. IYS are dynamic, community-embedded, evidence-based multidisciplinary services, and include:

- MHSU support;
- physical health, including sexual health care;
- peer support;
- education, employment, and vocational services;
- social services; and
- other developmentally appropriate services.

through walk-in or drop-in access to service and integration of care navigation into IYS. Diagnostic assessment is de-emphasized while youth needs, goals, and strengths are the focus (Hetrick *et al.*, 2017; Settipani *et al.*, 2019).

Some later IYS initiatives (e.g., Canada, U.S.) have been created with integration of higher intensity services into the model, such as early psychosis interventions, to address challenges faced by earlier model versions (McGorry *et al.*, 2022; Henderson *et al.*, 2023). Typical IYS roles in health systems in high-income contexts include stigma reduction, mental health literacy enhancement, health promotion and prevention, early identification and intervention, and delivery of specific evidence-based interventions. Peer support and care navigation services are also common (Hetrick *et al.*, 2017; Settipani *et al.*, 2019). Services are delivered by a wide range of service providers including peer support workers, lay health workers, youth workers, nursing professionals, primary care physicians, cultural leaders, and vocational specialists, as well as MHSU specialists.

Similar to primary care, screening, assessment, and MBC are essential aspects of IYS provision. Screening in IYS includes the identification of MHSU needs, as well as other social, vocational, and housing needs, to facilitate the provision of early intervention, service matching, and resource allocation across these domains. IYS also involves the regular and standardized assessment of symptoms, functioning, quality of life, goal achievement, treatment progress, and service experience. In IYS, MBC is used to systematically measure and track outcomes and experiences of care (Rickwood *et al.*, 2023). Tracked outcomes may not only be related to symptoms (e.g., improvements in anxiety, depression), but also to developmentally and culturally specific goals identified as meaningful by youth, including participation in school, improved confidence in social relationships, and decreased use of MHSU services over time (Barbic *et al.*, 2018). While MBC is viewed as essential to optimizing IYS care quality, like many areas of child and youth MHSU care, actual use continues to be a challenge (Barbic *et al.*, 2018; Hickie *et al.*, 2019; Krishna *et al.*, 2020).

Also similar to other system-wide child and youth MHSU services (e.g., specialist child and youth MHSU services), IYS outcome evaluations rely heavily on evidence supporting each of the service components (e.g., evidence-based psychotherapies, medication, care navigation, sexual health services) and evidence from pre-post changes in core outcome measures. For example, Rickwood *et al.*, (2023) demonstrated significant improvement on a combination of three outcomes—distress, functioning, and quality of life—for the majority of more than 58,000 youth who received *headspace* services. In addition, analyses from a pragmatic randomized controlled trial comparing adolescent MHSU services offered through hospital-based outpatient psychiatry services to community-based collaborative care services (Henderson *et al.*, 2017), are nearing completion and will contribute to the IYS evidence base.

Interventions and treatments for children and youth in primary and other community health care settings

Universal and selective interventions to promote good mental health among children and adolescents in primary and other community settings

Within child and youth mental health, there has been considerable attention on the potential value of promoting good mental health as part of healthy development and universal and selective interventions to promote good mental health have been extensively explored (Fusar-Poli *et al.*, 2021; see Chapter 32 for detailed discussion). Specifically relevant to children and youth receiving services in primary and other community-based MHSU services, like children and youth with MHSU needs in LMIC contexts, it is important to note that current conceptualizations of "good mental health" largely reflect Western cultural contexts, and there are calls to expand this concept to reflect additional cultural perspectives (Fusar-Poli *et al.*, 2021). In addition, primary and other community-based MHSU services have an important role to play in addressing social determinants of health as an MHSU prevention strategy. In particular, Harris *et al.* (2020) have highlighted the importance of interventions that support the development of safe and stable family relationships, and address food security, community safety, access to health care, access to quality education, family violence, parental employment, and social isolation.

Psychological treatments for children and youth in primary and other community health care settings

Schools are common settings for children and youth to receive MHSU services. School-based services can include delivery of psychological treatments across a range of MHSU areas (e.g., attentional, behavioral, anxiety, and mood difficulties; see Chapter 38 for a review). Primary health care settings are also ideally positioned to deliver psychological treatments to address child and youth MHSU needs. A meta-analysis of integrated primary and mental health care as compared to primary care as usual for child and adolescent mental health revealed promising effects for anxiety, depression, and behavior, when mental health treatments including cognitive behavioral therapy (CBT), parenting interventions, and other evidence-based interventions were integrated with primary care (Asarnow *et al.*, 2015). Strongest effects were found for collaborative care interventions that combined medication algorithms and CBT for depression or behavior problems. In the context of depression specifically, Oud *et al.* (2019) reviewed evidence on the effectiveness of CBT for children and adolescents across 31 studies, with 71.4% of interventions delivered in home, school, or community settings. The authors found positive but modest effects for reducing depressive symptoms. Combined behavioral activation and aspects of cognitive restructuring (challenging thoughts) were associated with more favorable outcomes, as was caregiver involvement, particularly for children under 12 years old.

Peer support for children and youth

A notable, emerging community-based nonspecialist intervention approach to supporting children and youth with MHSU concerns is the peer support service model. Peer support workers intentionally draw on their lived experience with MHSU concerns to support children and youth to achieve positive MHSU outcomes. In a systematic review of 24 studies, de Beer *et al.* (2022) identify engagement, providing emotional support, supporting navigating and planning, advocating, and supporting research and/or education as key aspects of the peer support worker role. de Beer and colleagues also highlight that offering youth peer support services requires a careful and multilayered approach to planning, and requires consideration of differences in power among peer support and other staff, and adequate resourcing to provide ongoing meaningful training and supervision. Peer support services have been shown to enhance MHSU understanding, provide validation for youth, and reduce feelings of isolation (Wolpert *et al.*, 2019; King & Fazel, 2021; de Beer *et al.*, 2022). In the context of peer-led parenting interventions, results have shown these interventions to significantly decrease child behavior problems, improve child health outcomes, and increase parents perceived self-competence (Day *et al.*, 2012; Sheidow *et al.*, 2022).

The number of studies of peer support models remains sparse, however, and the findings suggest that the benefits of participation for those who are trained peers exceed the benefits to those who receive peer support (King & Fazel, 2021).

Culturally specific community-based treatments for children and youth

Culturally specific and contextually specific treatments for children and youth have been growing in prominence but additional innovation, research, and implementation trials are required, especially trials of treatments that emphasize specific cultures, as opposed to comparing Western versus non-Western models. In addition, more studies in LMICs are needed. There is, however, sufficient evidence for a number of authors to have conducted relevant systematic reviews. For example, in some LMICs, context-specific interventions (e.g., children and youth in war situations) are used to support children and youth. Kohrt *et al.* (2018) in their meta-review of community components of mental health care in LMICs described that in armed conflict situations arts-based programing, traditional/cultural ceremonies, restoration of traditional beliefs and practices, mobilization for social action, and support for family reintegration of child soldiers have been implemented to support child and youth mental health outcomes (Kohrt *et al.*, 2018). For culturally specific treatments in child and youth mental health generally, most of the evidence to date focuses on cultural adaptation of existing evidence-based practices. Culturally adapted MHSU health treatments demonstrate positive treatment effects and outperform nonadapted interventions, though few rigorous head-to-head comparisons exist (Kumpfer *et al.*, 2017; Rathod *et al.*, 2018; Contreras-Perez *et al.*, 2023). Adaptations typically occur in content and process, and across multiple domains, for example, content, language, delivery/implementation, family involvement, team practice, setting/context, training, and treatment goals (Kumpfer *et al.*, 2017; Rathod *et al.*, 2018; Weeks, 2022). Based on their study of family evidence-based interventions implemented in 36 countries, Kumpfer *et al.* (2017) recommend nine steps for culturally adapting evidence-based interventions, derived from the United Nations Office of Drugs and Crime (UNODC)'s recommendations for cultural adaptation of family-based, evidence-based interventions:

- engage a culturally appropriate advisory group
- assess specific needs
- conduct language translation
- hire individuals from the culture to implement
- develop culturally adapted training
- cautiously make adaptations over repeated implementations
- rigorously and continuously monitor outcomes
- develop local partnerships, as well as international collaborations
- secure sustainable funding

These steps align with key components of typical frameworks for culturally adapting treatments, though most adaptation frameworks have been developed for immigrant or minority populations in Western contexts, potentially limiting their applicability in other contexts (Rathod *et al.*, 2018). Clinicians and system decision-makers are encouraged to partner with local cultural leaders, experts (including youth and caregivers), and organizations to understand local needs and approaches.

Training of health providers to support mental health and substance use assessment and treatment of children and youth

Emphasis on equity-informed training to support MHSU service delivery has been growing recently. At the structural level, it has been argued that more diverse voices, especially those with experiences of marginalization, need to be meaningfully integrated into decision-making processes in governmental and academic institutions where system and service design, resource allocation, research, and training decisions are made (Castro-Ramirez *et al.*, 2021). The need for more diverse trainees and faculty to be recruited and resourced to be successful has been identified - "whom we train is equally important as how we train" (Sudak *et al.*, 2020, p. 564).

Significant shifts are also proposed in the training of all health care providers, researchers, and administrators in community care settings (Box 45.4). Health equity scholars have argued that health care professionals need to be trained in the exclusionary and discriminatory history of psychiatry and psychology and the ways in which these influences continue to be

Box 45.4 Training of health providers to support mental health and substance use assessment and treatment of children and youth

Training all health providers, including primary care physicians and other primary and community health care practitioners, to support the assessment and treatment of children and youth promotes positive health outcomes and experiences.

- Training equips health providers with the necessary knowledge, skills, and tools to effectively identify, evaluate, and address the developmentally specific physical, mental, and emotional health needs of children and youth, in their contexts.
- Training empowers health providers with tools and strategies to deliver more effective, personalized, and evidence-based care.

Sources: Godoy *et al.*, 2019; Russet *et al.*, 2019; Castro-Ramirez *et al.*, 2021.

present in current practices, contributing to inequities. Training should also include how power and privilege influence interactions with clients/patients and the value of cultural humility (Harris *et al.*, 2020; Sudak *et al.*, 2020; Rafla-Yuan *et al.*, 2022). At the level of day-to-day practice, health care providers need to be trained to work with lay health workers and interpreters, deliver trauma-informed care (see Raja *et al.*, 2015), and attend to the impacts of language conventions in MHSU. They also need to be trained to recognize the potential biases and limitations of current assessment approaches and tools, including the harms associated with conceptualizing the consequences of exposure to trauma and inequity as psychopathology. Last, training of health care providers should include how to appropriately and effectively consider the influence of structural barriers and determinants of health (e.g., transportation, hours of service, financial resources, food security, housing), as well as cultural context and intersectional experiences on child and youth MHSU. At a system level, health care providers need to be trained to recognize inequities, advocate for change, supervise and mentor diverse trainees effectively, and identify and address policy drivers of inequities (Harris *et al.*, 2020; Sudak *et al.*, 2020; Castro-Ramirez *et al.*, 2021; Rafla-Yuan *et al.*, 2022).

Conclusions and future directions for community-based care for children and youth

This chapter highlights the important role that primary health and other community-based MHSU practitioners have in identifying and addressing the MHSU needs of children and youth. Primary health and other community-based MHSU services for children and youth can support enhanced access to care, as well as the coordination of care across systems and developmental stages. With the increasing roles of primary health care settings and community-based integrated youth service models, specific aspects of these models, such as MBC, hold the potential to guide global reform to ensure that effective interventions and practices are experienced by more children and youth. Moreover, to enhance further MHSU equitable service access and outcomes for children and youth, primary health and other community-based health care settings will need to continue to develop their capacity to reflect the social, developmental, and cultural contexts of children and youth. The critical role of health care provider training is also discussed, identifying key future directions for enhanced child and youth MHSU care across settings.

References

Aguirre Velasco, A. *et al.* (2020) What are the barriers, facilitators and interventions targeting help-seeking behaviours for common mental health problems in adolescents? A systematic review. *BMC Psychiatry* **20**(1), 293. doi:10.1186/s12888-020-02659-0.

Asarnow, J.R. *et al.* (2015) Integrated medical-behavioral care compared with usual primary care for child and adolescent behavioral health: a meta-analysis. *JAMA Pediatrics* **169**(10), 929–937. doi:10.1001/jamapediatrics.2015.1141.

Barbic, S.P. *et al.* (2018) The problem of patient-centred outcome measurement in psychiatry: why metrology hasn't mattered and why it should. *Journal of Physics: Conference Series* **1044**(1), 1–6.

Barbui, C. *et al.* (2020) Efficacy of psychosocial interventions for mental health outcomes in low-income and middle-income countries: an umbrella review. *The Lancet Psychiatry* **7**(2), 162–172.

de Beer, C.R.M. *et al.* (2022) A systematic review exploring youth peer support for young people with mental health problems. *European Child & Adolescent Psychiatry* **33**, 2471–2484. doi:10.1007/s00787-022-02120-5.

Bhawra, J. *et al.* (2016) Primary care interventions to improve transition of youth with chronic health conditions from paediatric to adult healthcare: a systematic review. *BMJ Open* **6**(5), e011871. doi:10.1136/bmjopen-2016-011871.

Boerma, W. (2006) Coordination and integration in European primary care. In: *Primary Care in The Driver's Seat? Organizational Reform in European Primary Care.* (eds R.B. Saltman, *et al.*). Open University Press, Maidenhead, UK. pp. 534–546.

Castillo, E.G. *et al.* (2019) Community interventions to promote mental health and social equity. *Current Psychiatry Reports* **21**(5), 35. doi:10.1007/s11920-019-1017-0.

Castro-Ramirez, F. *et al.* (2021) Racism and poverty are barriers to the treatment of youth mental health concerns. *Journal of Clinical Child and Adolescent Psychology* **50**(4), 534–546. doi:10.1080/15374416.2021.1941058.

Cleverley, K. *et al.* (2020) Identifying core components and indicators of successful transitions from child to adult mental health services: a scoping review. *European Child & Adolescent Psychiatry* **29**(2), 107–121. doi:10.1007/s00787-018-1213-1.

Contreras-Perez, M.E. *et al.* (2023) Culturally sensitive treatment for underrepresented adolescents with substance use: a systematic review. *Journal of Evidence-Based Social Work* **20**(3), 404–424.

Correll, C.U. *et al.* (2018) Comparison of early intervention services vs treatment as usual for early-phase psychosis: a systematic review, meta-analysis, and meta-regression. *JAMA Psychiatry* **75**(6), 555–565. doi:10.1001/jamapsychiatry.2018.0623.

Day, C. *et al.* (2012) Evaluation of a peer led parenting intervention for disruptive behaviour problems in children: community based randomized controlled trial. *BMJ* **344**, 1107.

Duong, M.T. *et al.* (2021) Rates of mental health service utilization by children and adolescents in schools and other common service settings: a systematic review and Meta-analysis. *Administration and Policy in Mental Health* **48**, 420–439. doi:10.1007/s10488-020-01080-9.

Flynn, A.B. *et al.* (2015) Primary care interventions to prevent or treat traumatic stress in childhood: a systematic review. *Academic Pediatrics* **15**(5), 480–492. doi:10.1016/j.acap.2015.06.012.

Funk, M. & Ivbijaro, G. (2008) *Integrating Mental Health into Primary Care: A Global Perspective.* World Health Organization/WONCA, Geneva, Switzerland.

Fusar-Poli, P. *et al.* (2021) Preventive psychiatry: a blueprint for improving the mental health of young people. *World Psychiatry* **20**(2), 200–221. doi:10.1002/wps.20869.

Godoy, L. *et al.* (2019) Increasing mental health engagement from primary care: the potential role of family navigation. *Pediatrics* **143**(4), e20182418. doi:10.1542/peds.2018-2418.

Habayeb, S. *et al.* (2022) Mental health screening in pediatric primary care: factors associated with screening completion and elevated scores. *Clinical Pediatrics (Phila)* **1**, 99228221139983. doi:10.1177/00099228221139983.

Hankivsky, O. (2014) *Intersectionality 101. Institute for Intersectionality Research & Policy.* Simon Fraser University, Vancouver, Canada.

Harris, T.B. *et al.* (2020) Achieving mental health equity: children and adolescents. *The Psychiatric Clinics of North America* **43**(3), 471–485. doi:10.1016/j.psc.2020.06.001.

Henderson, J.L. *et al.* (2017) Integrated collaborative care teams to enhance service delivery to youth with mental health and substance use challenges: protocol for a pragmatic randomised controlled trial. *BMJ Open* **7**(2), e014080. doi:10.1136/bmjopen-2016-014080.

Henderson, J.L. *et al.* (2023) Youth wellness hubs Ontario: development and initial implementation of integrated youth services in Ontario, Canada. *Early Intervention in Psychiatry* **17**(1), 107–114.

Hetrick, S.E. *et al.* (2017) Integrated (one-stop shop) youth health care: best available evidence and future directions. *The Medical Journal of Australia* **207**(10), S5–S18. doi:10.5694/mja17.00694.

Hickie, I.B. *et al.* (2019) Right care, first time: a highly personalised and measurement-based care model to manage youth mental health. *The Medical Journal of Australia* **211**(Suppl 9), S3–S46. doi:10.5694/mja2.50383.

King, T. & Fazel, M. (2021) Examining the mental health outcomes of school-based peer-led interventions on young people: a scoping review of range and a systematic review of effectiveness. *PLoS One* **16**(4), e0249553. doi:10.1371/journal.pone.0249553.

Kohrt, B.A. *et al.* (2018) The role of communities in mental health care in low-and middle-income countries: a meta-review of components and competencies. *International Journal of Environmental Research and Public Health* **15**(6), 1279.

Krishna, R. *et al.* (2020) Implementing measurement-based care in various practice settings. *Child and Adolescent Psychiatric Clinics of North America* **29**(4), 573–586. doi:10.1016/j.chc.2020.06.007.

Kroenke, K. & Unutzer, J. (2017) Closing the false divide: sustainable approaches to integrating mental health services into primary care. *Journal of General Internal Medicine* **32**(4), 404–410. doi:10.1007/s11606-016-3967-9.

Kumpfer, K. *et al.* (2017) Cultural adaptation and implementation of family evidence-based interventions with diverse populations. *Prevention Science* **18**(6), 649–659. doi:10.1007/s11121-016-0719-3.

Lu, C. *et al.* (2018) Global child and adolescent mental health: the orphan of development assistance for health. *PLoS Medicine* **15**(3), e1002524. doi:10.1371/journal.pmed.1002524.

MacDonald, K. *et al.* (2018) Pathways to mental health services for young people: a systematic review. *Social Psychiatry and Psychiatric Epidemiology* **53**, 1005–1038. doi:10.1007/s00127-018-1578-y.

Malla, A. *et al.* (2018) Youth mental health should be a top priority for health Care in Canada. *Canadian Journal of Psychiatry/Revue Canadienne de Psychiatrie* **63**(4), 216–222. doi:10.1177/07067437 18758968 7.

Mathias, S. *et al.* (2021) Foundry: early learnings from the implementation of an integrated youth service network. *Early Intervention in Psychiatry* **16**(4), 410–418. doi:10.1111/eip.13181.

McGorry, P.D. *et al.* (2022) Designing and scaling up integrated youth mental health care. *World Psychiatry* **21**(1), 61–76. doi:10.1002/wps.20938.

Mei, C. *et al.* (2020) Global research priorities for youth mental health. *Early Intervention in Psychiatry* **14**(1), 3–13. doi:10.1111/eip.12878.

Mulvaney-Day, N. *et al.* (2018) Screening for behavioral health conditions in primary care settings: a systematic review of the literature. *Journal of General Internal Medicine* **33**(3), 335–346. doi:10.1007/s11606-017-4181-0.

O'Brien, D. *et al.* (2016) Barriers to managing child and adolescent mental health problems: a systematic review of primary care practitioners' perceptions. *The British Journal of General Practice* **66**(651), e693–e707. doi:10.3399/bjgp16X687061.

Oud, M. *et al.* (2019) Effectiveness of CBT for children and adolescents with depression: a systematic review and meta-regression analysis. *European Psychiatry* **57**, 33–45. doi:10.1016/j.eurpsy.2018.12.008.

Pardee, M. *et al.* (2017) Current state of screening high-ACE youth and emerging adults in primary care. *Journal of the American Association of Nurse Practitioners* **29**(12), 716–724. doi:10.1002/2327-6924.12531.

Patel, V. *et al.* (2018) The Lancet Commission on global mental health and sustainable development. *The Lancet* **293**, 1553–1598.

Pedersen, G.A. *et al.* (2019) A systematic review of the evidence for family and parenting interventions in low-and middle-income countries: child and youth mental health outcomes. *Journal of Child and Family Studies* **28**, 2036–2055.

Radez, J. *et al.* (2021) Why do children and adolescents (not) seek and access professional help for their mental health problems? A systematic review of quantitative and qualitative studies. *European Child & Adolescent Psychiatry* **30**(2), 183–211. doi:10.1007/s00787-019-01469-4.

Rafla-Yuan, E. *et al.* (2022) Striving for equity in community mental health: opportunities and challenges for integrating care for BIPOC youth. *Child and Adolescent Psychiatric Clinics of North America* **31**(2), 295–312. doi:10.1016/j.chc.2021.11.007.

Raja, S. *et al.* (2015) Trauma informed care in medicine: current knowledge and future research directions. *Fam Community Health.* **38**(3), 216–226. doi: 10.1097/FCH.0000000000000071. PMID: 26017000.

Rathod, S. *et al.* (2018) The current status of culturally adapted mental health interventions: a practice-focused review of meta-analyses. *Neuropsychiatric Disease and Treatment*, 165–178.

Reed, S.J. *et al.* (2016) Effectiveness and value of integrating behavioral health into primary care. *JAMA Internal Medicine* **176**(5), 691–692. doi:10.1001/jamainternmed.2016.0804.

Rickwood, D. *et al.* (2023) Sixteen years of innovation in youth mental healthcare: outcomes for young people attending Australia's headspace centre services. *PLoS One* **18**(6), e0282040. doi:10.1371/journal.pone.0282040.

Rojas, L.M. *et al.* (2019) Evidence-based prevention programs targeting youth mental and behavioral health in primary care: a systematic review. *Preventive Medicine* **120**, 85–99. doi:10.1016/j.ypmed.2018.12.009.

Rose-Clarke, K. *et al.* (2019) Peer-facilitated community-based interventions for adolescent health in low- and middle-income countries: a systematic review. *PLoS One* **14**(1), e0210468–e0210468. doi:10.1371/journal.pone.0210468.

Russet, F. *et al.* (2019) Training of adult psychiatrists and child and adolescent psychiatrists in Europe: a systematic review of training characteristics and transition from child/adolescent to adult mental health services. *BMC Med Education* **19**(1), 204. doi:10.1186/s12909-019-1576-0.

Sarvet, B. (2020) Measurement-based care in the pediatric primary care setting. *Child and Adolescent Psychiatric Clinics of North America* **29**(4), 691–702. doi:10.1016/j.chc.2020.06.009.

Settipani, C.A. *et al.* (2019) Key attributes of integrated community-based youth service hubs for mental health: a scoping review. *International Journal of Mental Health Systems* **13**, 52. doi:10.1186/s13033-019-0306-7.

Sheidow, A.J. *et al.* (2022) Family-based treatments for disruptive behavior problems in children and adolescents: an updated review of rigorous studies (2014-April 2020). *Journal of Marital and Family Therapy* **48**(1), 56–82. doi:10.1111/jmft.12567.

Sudak, D.M. *et al.* (2020) Training psychiatrists to achieve mental health equity. *The Psychiatric Clinics of North America* **43**(3), 555–568. doi:10.1016/j.psc.2020.05.003.

Van Cleave, J. *et al.* (2012) Interventions to improve screening and follow-up in primary care: a systematic review of the evidence. *Academic Pediatrics* **12**(4), 269–282. doi:10.1016/j.acap.2012.02.004.

Weeks, A. (2022) Culturally adapting evidence-based and informed practices to meet client population needs and ensure appropriate allocation of scarce resources: a systematic review. *Human Service Organizations: Management, Leadership & Governance* **46**(3), 238–263.

Weisz, J.R. *et al.* (2017) What five decades of research tells us about the effects of youth psychological therapy: a multilevel meta-analysis and implications for science and practice. *American Psychologist* **72**(2), 79.

Wolpert, M. *et al.* (2019) Strategies not accompanied by a mental health professional to address anxiety and depression in children and young people: a scoping review of range and a systematic review of effectiveness. *The Lancet Psychiatry* **6**(1), 46–60. doi:10.1016/s2215-0366(18)30465-6.

World Health Organization (1978) *Declaration of Alma-Ata: International Conference on Primary Health Care*. World Health Organization (WHO), Geneva, Switzerland.

World Health Organization (2019) *Adolescent Mental Health: Time for Action. Knowledge Summary: Women's, Children's, and Adolescent's Health No 36*. World Health Organization (WHO), Geneva, Switzerland.

Xu, Z. *et al.* (2018) Effectiveness of interventions to promote help-seeking for mental health problems: systematic review and meta-analysis. *Psychological Medicine* **48**(16), 2658–2667. doi:10.1017/s0033291718001265.

CHAPTER 46
Working in low-resource settings

Dan J. Stein[1] and Lauren Franz[1,2]

[1] Department of Psychiatry and Mental Health, University of Cape Town, Cape Town, South Africa

[2] Department of Psychiatry and Behavioral Sciences, Duke University, School of Medicine, Duke University, Durham, NC, USA

Considerations in low-resource settings

In this chapter, we focus on child and adolescent mental health (CAMH) in low-resource settings. We consider how low-resource settings impact youth mental health, emphasize the mental health care treatment gap for youth, and detail strategies to strengthen health care systems to increase access to care (Figure 46.1). In this first section of the chapter, we detail the social determinants of CAMH to better understand factors that affect risk, resilience, and ultimately the prevalence and severity of CAMH conditions in low-resource settings Figure 46.1.

Globally, it is estimated that 14% of 10–19-year-olds have a mental health condition (Institute for Health Metrics and Evaluation, 2019). While prevalence estimates range from 12.8% in low-income to 18.3% in high-income countries, the proportion of children and adolescents actually represented by available prevalence data is extremely limited outside of high-income countries (Erskine *et al.*, 2016). This significantly affects the accuracy of youth mental health prevalence estimates currently available in low-resource settings globally. There is, however, strong evidence that youth experiencing social adversity are at greater risk for developing mental health conditions (Arango *et al.*, 2018). Furthermore, a range of factors found in low-resource settings, including increased rates of infectious diseases, food insecurity, and trauma exposure, may lead to differences in the profile of youth mental health conditions in these settings. For example, children living in poverty or in food-insecure homes may be more likely to experience anxiety and/or depressive symptoms (OR: 1.79, 95% CI 1.15–2.79), and exhibit behaviors consistent with attention deficit hyperactivity disorder (ADHD) (OR: 3.06, 95% CI 1.68–5.55) (Melchior *et al.*, 2012).

The World Health Organization (WHO) defines the social determinants of health as "the conditions in which people are born, grow, work, live, and develop, and the wider set of forces, including economic policies, social norms, and political systems, that shape the conditions of daily life and impact health outcomes" (World Health Organization, 2023b). These determinants include economic stability, education and health care access and quality, neighborhoods and built environments, and social and community contexts (U.S. Department of Health and Human Services, 2023b). Social determinants of health influence access, quality, and availability of health care services, so directly affect disease burden and life expectancy in individuals and communities.

The *social determinants of mental health* include adverse economic and social circumstances, such as poverty, income inequality, and interpersonal and community violence, that directly impact the prevalence and severity of mental disorders across the life course (Lund *et al.*, 2018). Social determinants influence the developmental trajectories of children and adolescents as their cognitive, emotional, social, and physical development occur at a time when they are embedded within specific contexts, dependent on their caregivers for their well-being, and have limited control over larger societal forces (Cotton & Shim, 2022). Differences in exposure to social determinants can affect mental health outcomes at an individual and community level, resulting in health disparities.

National-level classifications of low, lower-middle, upper-middle, and high-income, are based on a country's gross domestic product (GDP) (The World Bank, 2023a). While high-income countries spend the greatest amount on child and adolescent mental health services (CAMHS), community-level capacity to provide adequate care to those in need, and contextual factors that impact health outcomes are dependent upon more than just national-level health care expenditure. Rather, health outcomes depend on multiple interrelated factors, including genetic vulnerabilities, experiences of discrimination, *and* the social determinants of health (World Health Organization, 2023b). Disparities in CAMH outcomes also occur in high-income countries with culturally and linguistically diverse

Rutter's Child and Adolescent Psychiatry and Psychology, Seventh Edition.
Edited by Anita Thapar, Daniel S. Pine, Samuele Cortese, Cathy Creswell, Tamsin J. Ford, James F. Leckman, and Argyris Stringaris.

Companion website: www.wiley.com/go/thapar/rutterspsych7

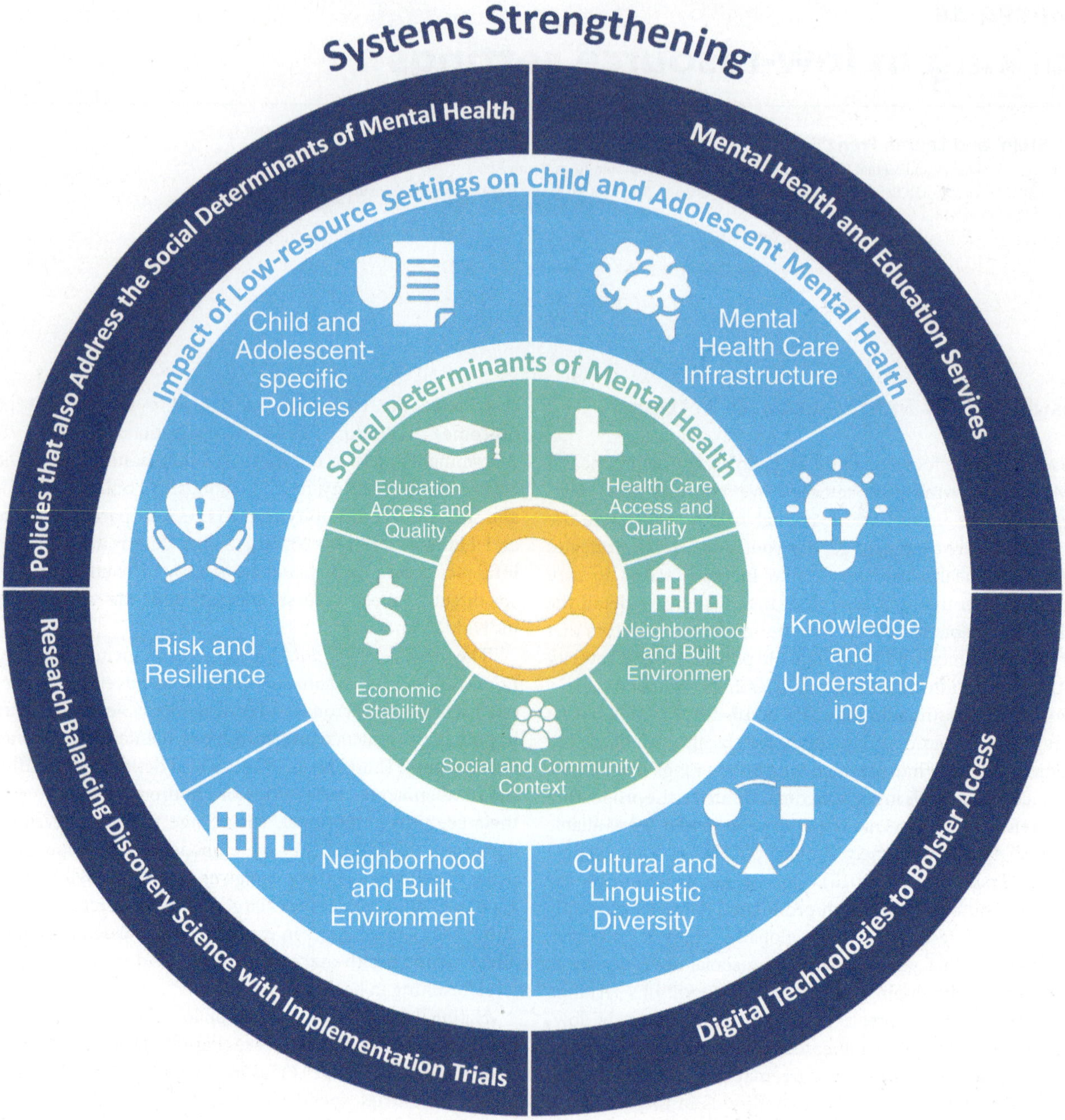

Figure 46.1 Strategies to strengthen systems to increase access to child and adolescent mental health (CAMH) care.

"minority" populations who may live in communities with limited access to high-quality services (Monroe *et al.*, 2023).

Country-level classifications based on GDP do not sufficiently describe or quantify individual and community-level factors that affect service-delivery and health outcomes. The term *low-resource settings* may better describe specific contexts across countries that affect CAMH (van Zyl *et al.*, 2021). To ensure that knowledge transfer from one low-resource setting to another can occur, including low-resource settings in high-income countries, it is important to adequately understand contextual factors influencing health care and outcomes. This may in turn allow for initiation and scale-up of effective interventions, which are much needed in CAMH globally.

In low-resource settings, the social determinants of health form an interconnected network of resource limitations that affect individual well-being and health outcomes at multiple levels (World Health Organization, 2023b). Although low-resource settings are quite heterogeneous, they may have a number of characteristics in common, including particular types of social determinants of health. Here we consider five such determinants (Figure 46.1).

First, economic instability can negatively affect the overall well-being of communities. At an individual level, economic instability can lead to caregiver unemployment or underemployment resulting in low total household income and family poverty. It can also result in limited caregiver resources, with food and housing insecurity (Morrissey *et al.*, 2020). Caregiver poverty can act as a significant service access barrier to mental health care, as families often need to prioritize basic needs over mental health or developmental concerns for their child (Lund *et al.*, 2010; Knifton & Inglis, 2020). Economic instability can also cause financial disadvantage at the community level, resulting in limited employment opportunities and unaffordable housing (Hardy *et al.*, 2019). At the national level, economic instability can result in limited government spending on education, health care, and research to improve education and health care services.

Second, limited access to and quality of education impacts society at multiple levels (The Lancet Public Health, 2020). Education provides tools needed to find employment, develop the skills to build strong communities, and develop financial resources to live in safe built environments and neighborhoods. Low education levels impact language and literacy skills, and result in knowledge gaps, including gaps in health literacy. Low education levels can also result in an education and health care workforce that lacks adequate skills and knowledge, further compounding clinical and research gaps. Access to quality education from early childhood onward provides the opportunity for individuals to shift their socioeconomic trajectories, moving themselves and their families out of poverty, and reducing the risk for negative health outcomes (Zajacova & Lawrence, 2018).

Third, suboptimal health care services can exacerbate access barriers and worsen outcomes (U.S. Department of Health and Human Services, 2023a). Human resource limitations in health care, including a lack of sufficiently trained CAMH care professionals, can result in a heavy burden of care for existing staff, staff burnout, and significant gaps in system coverage. For example, in low-income countries there are 0.01 CAMH care workers per 100,000 people, who for the most part are located in urban centers, highlighting significant service access limitations in these regions of the world (World Health Organization, 2020). Furthermore, limitations in skills and knowledge of both clinical and nonclinical health care staff responsible for individual and public health interventions, result in suboptimal health care quality.

Fourth, in terms of neighborhoods and built environments, lack of basic infrastructure, such as water, sanitation, electrical supply, transportation networks, and telecommunications including broadband access, exacerbate existing challenges related to effective delivery of services (Gelormino *et al.*, 2015). In some low-resource communities, underdeveloped infrastructure with lack of basic services is a direct result of unjust structural policies at a national level. For example, structurally racist government-sanctioned policies, such as redlining in the United States and apartheid in South Africa, resulted in residential segregation with poor-quality housing and lack of basic services (Mayosi & Benatar, 2014; Rothstein, 2017). These types of historical policies continue to affect communities, resulting in intergenerational poverty and continued high levels of community violence and health disparities.

Finally, social and community contexts can affect health outcomes at multiple levels. At the individual level, limited social resources, including social support, material resources, and family involvement, may negatively affect caregiver well-being. Communities in low-resource settings may also be impacted by high rates of interpersonal and community violence, child abuse and neglect, and caregiver mental health and substance use disorders (Peek-Asa *et al.*, 2011; Mercy *et al.*, 2017). These factors affect communities in high-resource settings, but rates are generally greater in low-resource contexts. At the same time, traditional and Indigenous beliefs are more common in low-resource communities, and may contribute to increased social capital (United Nations, 2019; Aluaq Daniel *et al.*, 2022). Such beliefs may also directly influence perceptions of available services, health care-seeking behaviors, and health care practices. Differences between traditional and Indigenous beliefs and health care system practices may decrease uptake of health care recommendations.

Low-resource settings can be socially, structurally, environmentally, and culturally complex. Each low-resource setting is a unique reflection of numerous interrelated factors, which influence individuals and systems at multiple levels. Understanding the impact of social determinants of mental health on a particular low-resource setting may allow for more in-depth analysis of how these factors influence service provision, epidemiology of mental health conditions, and youth mental health outcomes. Furthermore, improved understanding and assessment of how low-resource contexts affects CAMH may support development of innovative approaches to support service delivery and community well-being.

Impact of low-resource settings on child and adolescent mental health care

In this section of the chapter, we focus on the treatment gap for children and adolescents with mental health conditions in low-resource settings, exploring why this gap exists. Despite the development of evidence-based psychotherapies and pharmacotherapies for CAMH disorders, the majority of the world's youth live in low-resource settings and do not receive appropriate preventive or therapeutic interventions (Kieling *et al.*, 2011). The specific reasons for the treatment gap in low-resource settings illustrate several characteristics of such settings, and how these characteristics may impact CAMH disorders. Here we outline six such reasons (Figure 46.1):

First, low-resource settings often lack specific CAMH policies (Zhou *et al.*, 2020). Where mental health policies exist, the primary focus is most often on adults. Countries with child-specific mental health policies often lack policy implementation plans (Mokitimi *et al.*, 2018). In low- and middle-income countries (LMICs), where children and adolescents make up at least half of the population, the lack of youth mental health policies is particularly problematic (United Nations—Population Division, 2022). This is also an underresearched area. A recent systematic review on CAMH policies in LMICs, identified only nine publications on the topic (Zhou *et al.*, 2020). CAMH policies are critically important because they can mandate government financial investment, set research priorities, identify service sectors and providers responsible for mental health care delivery, and support intersectorial collaboration (Shatkin & Belfer, 2004). The lack of policy development and implementation negatively affects governance and leadership in CAMH. It also contributes to community-level services that are unresponsive to the needs of children and adolescents, their caregivers, and service providers.

Second, communities often have limited access to dedicated youth mental health care infrastructure, including inpatient and outpatient services, mental health clinicians, and treatment options (Simelane & de Vries, 2021). In low-resource settings, while youth mental health services may be present at the tertiary level, there are limited services embedded within community settings (see Box 46.1 for an example). Significant limitations also exist in terms of human capital—members of the CAMH workforce who have the experience, knowledge, and skills. For example, the ratio of CAMH practitioners to population level is 44 times greater in high-income than in low-income countries (Rathod *et al.*, 2017). Furthermore, treatment options, including psychotropic medication, are limited. This, in part, is due to lack of inclusion of many psychotropic medications for youth mental health conditions on ministry of health lists of essential medication (Ortega & Müller, 2020). Currently, over 155 countries create national lists of essential medication that align with the WHO Model List of Essential Medicines for Children (World Health Organization, 2021). A current example of a notable omission on this WHO list is methylphenidate, or any other stimulant medication, for ADHD (Storebø & Gluud, 2020). The lack of CAMH care infrastructure also affects the ability of low-resource settings to conduct research, with less than 10% of global trials in mental health specifically focusing on the needs of 90% of the world's youth who live in lower income countries (Kieling *et al.*, 2011). While the evidence base for CAMH treatment in low-resource settings is increasing, the quality of this evidence remains variable, contributing to the research gap. Two recent reviews summarize the treatment evidence base in LMICs (Barbui *et al.*, 2020; Ribeiro *et al.*, 2023). In the first, an umbrella review of meta-analyses of randomized controlled trials (RCTs) of psychosocial interventions conducted in LMICs, authors identified 19 meta-analyses. Seven focused on youth with disruptive behavior, post-traumatic stress disorder (PTSD), anxiety, depression, or psychological distress (Barbui *et al.*, 2020). Four of these seven meta-analyses included studies conducted in humanitarian settings, and three included studies that focused on refugee populations. The authors concluded that for PTSD outcomes in youth in humanitarian settings, and for children with disruptive behavior, psychosocial interventions were supported by "suggestive" evidence of efficacy, at best. In the second a systematic review published in 2023, the authors summarized findings from RCT and quasi-experimental studies for a range of mental health interventions for 6–18-year-olds in LMICs (Ribeiro *et al.*, 2023). Overall, authors identified 107 studies, and noted a 60% increase in the number of published intervention trials over the past decade. The authors identified nine different intervention approaches: psychopharmacology, psychotherapy, psychoeducation, neurocognitive, neuromodulation, meditation, dietary supplements, physical activity, and combined interventions. These interventions were used to treat 19 mental health conditions. While 79% of identified studies were RCTs, over half reported no study procedures that related to blinding of participants, assessors, or other study staff. Furthermore, just under half of comparators in the RCTs were "no intervention," and only one-third of included studies were found to be at low risk of bias. Overall, one-third of interventions were superior to control, with psychoeducation and psychotherapy having the greatest number of positive trials (55% and 50% respectively). Interventions for PTSD and depression had the highest proportion of positive results (63% and 57% respectively). Psychotherapy was the most common intervention approach evaluated, with over half of effective psychotherapies evaluated including cognitive behavioral approaches. Twenty percent of studies assessed psychopharmacological interventions, with most finding no difference between intervention and comparator. Seventy percent of these psychopharmacological trials included in the review targeted ADHD. Schools were the most common intervention setting. Intervention delivery format was most often one-on-one or in groups. Intervention delivery agents were most commonly specialist providers, such as psychologists and psychiatrists. While 26 LMICs were included in the systematic review, half of the studies came from Iran, suggesting a concentration of the evidence base in one specific geographic region.

Third, there is limited knowledge about youth mental issues at an individual, community, and national level in low-resource settings (Renwick *et al.*, 2022). This may impede access to existing services, with mental health or developmental conditions misdiagnosed or missed completely

Box 46.1 Limited services embedded within community settings

> A South African study conducted in 2010 reported that less than 2% of outpatient mental health services catered to children and adolescents (Kleintjes *et al.*, 2010). A recent situational analysis conducted in 2018 found little improvement in youth mental health service capacity, with only 4% of primary, and 7% of secondary mental health care visits being for children and adolescents (Mokitimi *et al.*, 2018). Of note, this study found that there was no separation in clinical space between child and adolescent and adult patients at the primary and secondary care level.

(Juengsiragulwit, 2015), and only the most severe cases with the highest levels of acuity being identified (Galagali & Brooks, 2020). This may in turn further increase mental health stigma and compound service access barriers. For example, a review article that synthesized the evidence pertaining to youth mental health literacy in LMICs including attitudes, knowledge, and beliefs, identified low levels of knowledge and recognition of mental health conditions, ubiquitous levels of stigma, and low levels of confidence in available services (Renwick *et al.*, 2022). Limited provider knowledge may also result in inappropriate treatment recommendations. In particular, lack of provider training and knowledge of psychosocial treatments, which are often first-line for child and adolescent mental disorders, may result in overreliance on medication. Lack of knowledge at the national level can result in limited government, health care and education system recognition of child and adolescent mental disorders as specific conditions that require targeted services, and result in underinvestment in appropriate health care infrastructure.

Fourth, in low-resource settings there is significant cultural and linguistic diversity, in addition to traditional and Indigenous beliefs and practices. As previously noted, the CAMH evidence base has predominantly been developed in "WEIRD" (White, Educated, Industrialized, Rich, and Democratic) populations (Henrich *et al.*, 2010; Kieling *et al.*, 2011). Sampling biases, which have strongly favored the inclusion of these WEIRD populations in youth mental health studies, may result in "gold standard" screening protocols, diagnostic guidelines, symptom measures, and intervention approaches not being relevant in low-resource contexts (Nielsen *et al.*, 2017). For example, disparities in age of autism diagnosis in the United States, is thought to at least in part be due to the differential accuracy of screening tools for children from underrepresented groups, and those who are exposed to languages other than English (Guthrie *et al.*, 2019). While the evidence base for youth mental health treatment in low-resource settings is increasing, much remains to be done to ensure the development of appropriate diagnostic and therapeutic approaches in this context (Leijten *et al.*, 2016; Burkey *et al.*, 2018). Alignment of CAMH treatment approaches with community beliefs and practices, can impact the interpretation of symptoms and treatment-seeking behaviors, and whether the individual experiences stigmatization or exclusion from their community (O'Keefe *et al.*, 2021). In low-resource settings, it is therefore particularly important to leverage existing strengths, such as social capital, including networks of community relationships, and use a strengths-based treatment approach to facilitate child and adolescent well-being (Fogarty *et al.*, 2018).

Fifth, neighborhoods and built environments in low-resource settings may increase the likelihood of children and adolescents developing mental health and neurodevelopmental conditions (Grantham-McGregor *et al.*, 2007; Cotton & Shim, 2022). In low-resource neighborhoods, access to reliable transportation, green spaces, and sufficient and healthy food options are often limited. Children and adolescents are more prone to environmental exposures including industrial toxic waste from landfills, high levels of carbon monoxide emissions from heavy traffic, and heavy metals from contaminated drinking water (Burton *et al.*, 2013). Neighborhoods may have high levels of interpersonal and community violence, with children and adolescents exposed to adverse childhood experiences (ACEs) (Hillis *et al.*, 2016). ACEs have been linked to mental health conditions that may impact individuals across their life span (Nelson *et al.*, 2020). The social determinants of mental health, including poverty, food insecurity, and toxic exposures, can negatively impact a child's developing cognitive abilities, emotional self-regulation, social abilities, and physical development (Lund *et al.*, 2010; Knifton & Inglis, 2020; Mezzina *et al.*, 2022).

Finally, contextual differences in risk and resilience factors in low-resource settings result in different profiles of mental health conditions. Understanding such variations should inform efforts to strengthen youth mental health services. For example, across low-resource settings, infectious diseases such as HIV/AIDS are more common (Olashore *et al.*, 2023). HIV-infected youth may experience neurocognitive complications that increase risk-taking behaviors such as substance use (Vreeman *et al.*, 2017). Services and supports focused on understanding and mitigating neuropsychiatric sequelae in HIV-infected youth would be contextually appropriate in low-resource settings impacted by this condition. Critically, exposure to risk factors in low-resource settings, including risk factors related to the social determinants outlined here, does not necessarily mean there will be negative mental health outcomes for children and adolescents. Protective factors may support resilience at the individual, family, and community level. Resilience is an individual's capacity to adapt to stressful or traumatic events, and mitigates the risk of mental disorders (Rutter, 1985, 2012; Southwick *et al.*, 2014; Mesman *et al.*, 2021). Examples of protective factors that support resilience include a positive self-identity, an inner sense of confidence, social support from nuclear and extended family, effective parenting, and cohesive neighborhoods (Li *et al.*, 2007). There is, however, relatively little research on resilience in youth in low-resource settings, and a focus on resilience should not obscure the need to identify and intervene with those who are struggling. Quantifying the links between social determinants and positive aspects of CAMH is an important future goal (Dray, 2021; Mesman *et al.*, 2021). For more in-depth information about psychosocial adversity resilience in CAMH, please refer to Chapters 22 and 23.

The way forward

This section of the chapter focuses on systems strengthening. Systems strengthening is defined by the WHO as "the process of identifying and implementing the changes in policy and practice in a country's health system, so that the country or region can respond better to its health and health system challenges" (World

Health Organization, 2007). Systems strengthening includes an "array of initiatives and strategies that improves one or more of the functions of the health system and that leads to better health through improvements in access, coverage, quality, or efficiency." In CAMH, particularly in low-resource settings, it is critical that systems strengthening be viewed through a broader lens than just health systems, as the social determinants of mental health affect outcomes (Lund *et al.*, 2018; Cotton & Shim, 2022). Furthermore, there may be intersections between interventions outside the health system and mental health outcomes (Lund *et al.*, 2011). Here we cover four key areas: in systems strengthening policy, mental health services, digital technology, and research (Figure 46.1). These key areas of systems strengthening pertain to low-resource settings in general, including low-resource settings in high-income countries. We consider each of the four key areas of systems strengthening next.

First, a stand-alone CAMH policy, accompanied by a dedicated budget is a critical step in systems strengthening (Zhou *et al.*, 2020). Furthermore, while the development of a national-level policy is key, detailed plans to enact the policy at the state or provincial and local level are critical (Box 46.2). In terms of process, policy development and implementation should be collaborative. When policymakers work alongside researchers, clinicians, and individuals with lived experience, key stakeholders buy into the process, which supports development, and implementation and uptake of contextually relevant policies (Erismann *et al.*, 2021). Access to quality mental health and education services, development and maintenance of health care and education infrastructure, and adequate financial commitment by government, specific to CAMH, should be a central focus in policy documents (Toyama *et al.*, 2017). Furthermore, to develop policies that improve CAMH, the specific implementation context should to be considered, so that policies address contextually relevant social determinants of mental health (Lund *et al.*, 2018; Shah *et al.*, 2021; Mezzina *et al.*, 2022). Policies may, for example, emphasize affordable high-quality childcare and universal health coverage (Armstrong, 2020; Jones *et al.*, 2020; World Health Organization, 2022). Policies may also target stigma reduction to promote inclusion of youth with mental health conditions within their families, schools, and communities (Hartog *et al.*, 2020).

Box 46.2 Example of developing policy at the local level

> In South Africa, policymakers and mental health advocates are paying increased attention to child and adolescent mental health (CAMH) at the local level. The Western Cape Provincial Department of Health recently appointed a CAMH provincial coordinator who leads a team dedicated to strengthening the CAMH care system in primary care (Simelane & de Vries, 2021).

Second, system strengthening should focus on increasing the availability of high-quality mental health services. This can be accomplished by increasing the number of trained mental health care professionals, and developing innovative approaches to mental health care delivery. In stepped care, the least resource-intensive, yet effective, service is delivered first, by the most accessible and least expensive provider (Figure 46.2) (Richards *et al.*, 2012; Ho *et al.*, 2016). Task sharing, with nonspecialist mental health care practitioners delivering first-line treatments, is a core principle of the stepped care approach (Hoeft *et al.*, 2018; Devassy *et al.*, 2022; Prina *et al.*, 2023). Task sharing occurs when activities usually conducted by specialist mental health providers, such as psychiatrists, are redistributed to nonspecialist mental

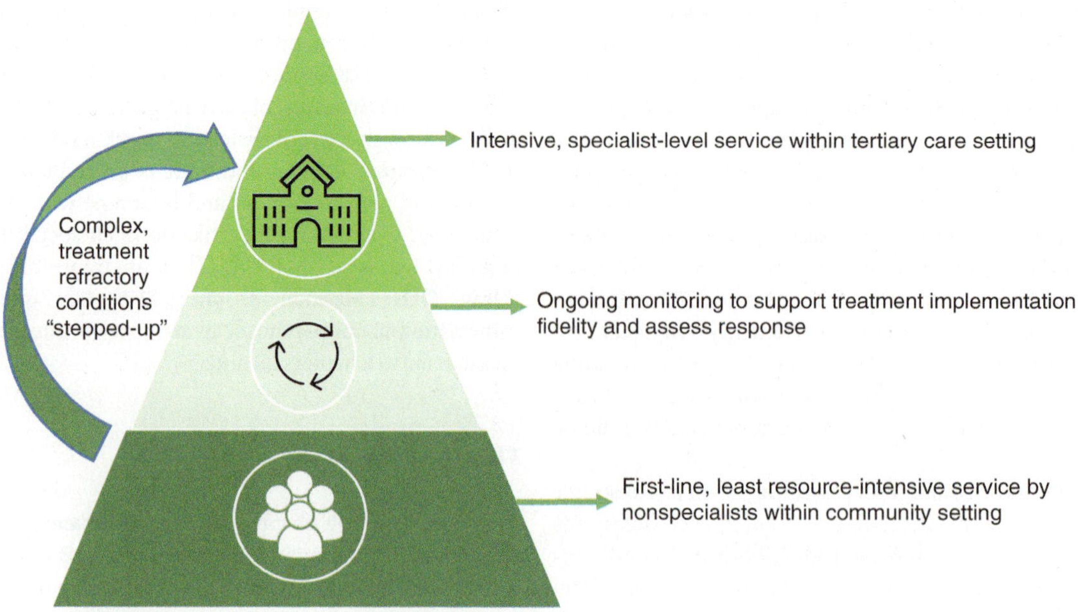

Figure 46.2 Stepped care to service delivery.

health providers who have limited formal training, such as community health workers. While task sharing has emerged as a key strategy of global mental health efforts to address the treatment gap impacting low-resource settings, it has mainly been implemented and evaluated in LMICs with adult populations (Patel *et al.*, 2018). Nonspecialists require training, supervision, and ongoing monitoring by specialist providers to ensure implementation fidelity, which may be supported by a collaborative care framework that integrates mental health services into primary care settings (Härter *et al.*, 2018; Schlesinger *et al.*, 2023). While nonspecialists can fill important service access gaps, there are limitations to their roles and abilities. In the stepped-care approach, more complex, treatment refractory conditions are first identified and then "stepped-up" to more intensive, and expensive, specialist-level providers. Therefore, for stepped-care models to function, it is critical that a sufficient number of specialists are available to train and supervise nonspecialists, and to provide services for more complex cases. Ongoing financial and human resource investment is therefore required to ensure that stepped care is a viable option in low-resource settings. To increase the relevance of mental health services to culturally and linguistically diverse populations in low-resource settings, systems strengthening efforts should aim to build a workforce of nonspecialist providers, as well as expert clinicians and researchers who reflect the diversity of the populations they serve (Jackson & Gracia, 2014). The Mental Health Gap Action Program (mhGAP) is a stepped-care approach that provides clinical guidelines for nonspecialist delivery of mental health treatment within primary care (World Health Organization, 2023a). The mhGAP intervention guide has been translated into more than 20 languages and implemented in over 100 countries. Box 46.3 describes results from a recent systematic review focused on mhGAP (Petagna *et al.*, 2023). Importantly, innovative treatment approaches developed in LMICs may well be relevant to low-resource settings in high-income countries (McKenzie *et al.*, 2004).

Third, digital technologies should be a key component of systems strengthening. Digital technologies can increase access, reduce costs, and improve the quality of mental health services (National Institute of Mental Health, 2021). Mobile phone use, in particular, is widespread globally, including in low-resource environments (The World Bank, 2023b). Mobile phones can be used to access psychoeducational materials and telehealth services, including personalized intervention through text messaging, and voice or video calls (Fedele *et al.*, 2017). Smartphones can run applications (apps) which provide screening and mental health interventions. Box 46.4 describes one example of a screening app, administered on a smartphone, to identify young children at high likelihood for autism (Chang *et al.*, 2021; Krishnappa Babu *et al.*, 2023; Perochon *et al.*, 2023). While digital technologies show promise in helping to address the treatment gap, and studies suggest digital approaches may be feasible and acceptable, there is currently limited evidence of the efficacy of digital mental health interventions in LMICs (Carter *et al.*, 2021). This highlights the need for continued evaluation of digital technology implementation in low-resource settings. As new digital technologies are developed in low-resource settings, including individuals with lived experience and front-line providers in their design and implementation process will help ensure that they are culturally and contextually appropriate, facilitating integration into existing services (Farao *et al.*, 2020). The digital divide also needs to be a considered. The digital divide—the gap between those who have access to digital technologies and the Internet, and those who do not—is an important consideration because it disproportionately affects communities in low-resource settings (The World Bank, 2016). For example, more than 21 million Americans in low-resource communities lack adequate broadband access with those living on tribal lands and in rural communities being particularly impacted (Federal Communications Commission, 2017). Furthermore, gender-based difference in mobile phone and Internet access exists, whereby women, who are usually the primary caregivers, having less access to mobile phones than men in low-resource settings (Organisation for Economic Co-operation and Development, 2018). Concerted efforts to increase equitable access to digital technologies and stable Internet connections are key to ensuring that digitization of mental health services does not further exacerbate existing inequity (United Nations, 2016). For more in-depth information about digital technology-assessment and treatment in CAMH, please refer to Chapter 49.

Fourth, research should be a key component of systems strengthening, with research capacity building in both discovery science and implementation science (Stein *et al.*, 2015; Stein & Wegener, 2017). Research that balances and integrates these approaches will decrease the treatment gap and provide

Box 46.3 Systematic review focused on the Mental Health Gap Action Program (mhGAP)

> A systematic review of the Mental Health Gap Action Program (mhGAP) found that while the approach increased provider knowledge, it did not change clinical practice, and limited evidence of impact on youth mental health outcomes was detected (Petagna *et al.*, 2023). Factors that affected mhGAP implementation included the size of the mental health workforce, provider workload, patient–provider hierarchies, and the cultural relevance of materials. Limited implementation of mhGAP in educational settings was also noted in the review.

Box 46.4 Example of a screening app to identify young children at high likelihood for autism

> A mobile app (SenseToKnow) has been developed, where a brief collection of developmentally appropriate and engaging movies is shown to a young child on a smartphone while their behavior is recorded using the frontal camera of the device. The app uses computer vision analysis and machine learning to elicit and objectively quantify a wide range of early autism-related behaviors, including social attention, facial expressions, head movements, response to name, and motor skills (Chang *et al.*, 2021; Krishnappa Babu *et al.*, 2023; Perochon *et al.*, 2023).

important lessons that apply across low-resource settings. Research capacity building can develop and strengthen a workforce with the skillset needed to move discoveries from bench to bedside and from bedside, beyond (da Silva *et al.*, 2019). Building and strengthening sustainable research capacity within low-resource settings will also help to ensure that the research agenda aligns with local needs. In terms of implementation and scale-up of effective services, important questions remain regarding the degree to which approaches developed in "WEIRD" populations should be adapted to low-resource communities, or whether a ground-up approach to assessment and intervention development should be the way forward (Leijten *et al.*, 2016; Hamdani *et al.*, 2022) While it is possible to strip down complex assessments and interventions to their core components, assessments and interventions should include appropriate cultural and contextual adaptations to improve fit with the implementation context (Movsisyan *et al.*, 2019; Moore *et al.*, 2021). Following adaptation, further research to evaluate effectiveness in real-world, low-resource contexts is needed (Chambers & Norton, 2016). Qualitative research can support a greater understanding of existing beneficial practices and societal strengths (Guler *et al.*, 2018). Hybrid effectiveness-implementation research designs are particularly well suited to studying both the implementation context and the adapted assessment and/or intervention. (Curran *et al.*, 2012). Box 46.5 describes different types of Hybrid effectiveness-implementation designs. Cost-effectiveness analyses should be included in studies testing new approaches in low-resource settings (Ho *et al.*, 2016; Le *et al.*, 2021). This is critical because governments need costing information to make decisions about resource allocation and scale-up. Finally, there are important opportunities in low-resource settings to increase synergy between research on discovery science, and the social determinants of mental health (Stein *et al.*, 2015; Stein & Wegener, 2017). Understanding the contribution of genes, environments, and interactions between genes and environments will advance our understanding of the neurobiology and neuroplasticity of child and adolescent development, and of the etiology of youth mental health disorders across the globe. To date, the vast majority of research in genetics and neuroscience has been conducted in populations of European ancestry, and a great deal of research on social determinants has been done in high-income countries, but research in lower income countries may have global lessons (Patel, 2007; Singla *et al.*, 2017; Sirugo *et al.*, 2019; Kopal *et al.*, 2023). Specifically, the significant genetic diversity seen in many LMICs may contribute to our global understanding of disease mechanisms, and innovative task-sharing approaches developed in these contexts may well have applicability to low-resource settings in high-income countries. There is significant scope for expanding neuroscience and psychosocial research across the globe; this may further our ability to delineate phenotypes, identify biomarkers, and improve treatment options.

Box 46.5 Hybrid effectiveness–implementation designs

> Hybrid type 1 designs primarily aim to determine intervention effectiveness, with the secondary aim to better understand the implementation context (Curran *et al.*, 2012). Hybrid type 2 designs have co-primary aims of assessing the effectiveness of the approach and testing implementation strategies that support uptake and scaling. In Hybrid type 3 designs, the primary aim is to test implementation strategies, with the secondary aim of assessing clinical outcomes. The choice of hybrid design depends upon the level of current evidence supporting the approach—with Hybrid type 1 designs testing new interventions, and type 3 testing implementation of established best practices.

Conclusion

In low-resource settings, the social determinants of mental health form a web of multilevel exposures that influence child and adolescent development and well-being. Health disparities between communities can result from differential exposure to such social determinants. While evidence-based interventions have been developed for youth mental health conditions, a significant treatment gap affects the majority of the world's children who live in low-resource settings. To decrease the treatment gap, systems strengthening in key areas is required. First, systems strengthening should support a stand-alone CAMH policy that focuses on the development and strengthening of youth mental health services, and on the social determinants of mental health. This policy should be accompanied by a dedicated budget and an actionable implementation plan. Second, strengthening the quality and availability of CAMHS can occur through embracing innovative approaches that increase access while reducing costs, including stepped-care models and task sharing. Nevertheless, it remains critical that sufficient specialists are trained, as they are responsible for ongoing supervision and monitoring of front-line providers, and management of complex conditions. Third, digital technology should be part of systems strengthening efforts. These efforts should align with local, national, and global efforts to increase equitable digital access. Finally, building sustainable research capacity in CAMH within low-resource settings will support the development of a contextually relevant research agenda that matches local needs. Integrating discovery neuroscience research with implementation public health research may ultimately be particularly impactful.

References

Aluaq Daniel, R. *et al.* (2022). What is "Indigenous Knowledge" And Why Does It Matter? Integrating Ancestral Wisdom and Approaches into Federal Decision-Making. The White House. Available: https://www.whitehouse.gov/ostp/news-updates/2022/12/02/what-is-indigenous-knowledge-and-why-does-it-matter-integrating-ancestral-wisdom-and-approaches-into-federal-decision-making October 2024].

Arango, C. *et al.* (2018) Preventive strategies for mental health. *The Lancet Psychiatry* **5**(7), 591–604. doi:10.1016/S2215-0366(18)30057-9.

Armstrong, S. (2020) Universal access to quality childcare is good policy and a positive determinant of health. Let's invest. *Paediatrics & Child Health* **26**(2), 82–84. doi:10.1093/pch/pxaa054.

Barbui, C. *et al.* (2020) Efficacy of psychosocial interventions for mental health outcomes in low-income and middle-income countries: an umbrella review. *The Lancet Psychiatry* **7**(2), 162–172. doi:10.1016/S2215-0366(19)30511-5.

Burkey, M.D. *et al.* (2018) Psychosocial interventions for disruptive behaviour problems in children in low- and middle-income countries: a systematic review and meta-analysis. *Journal of Child Psychology and Psychiatry* **59**(9), 982–993. doi:10.1111/jcpp.12894.

Burton, L.M. *et al.* (2013) Inequality, family processes, and health in the "new" rural America. *American Behavioral Scientist* **57**(8), 1128–1151. doi:10.1177/0002764213487348.

Carter, H. *et al.* (2021) The emergence of digital mental health in low-income and middle-income countries: a review of recent advances and implications for the treatment and prevention of mental disorders. *Journal of Psychiatric Research* **133**, 223–246. doi:10.1016/j.jpsychires.2020.12.016.

Chambers, D.A. & Norton, W.E. (2016) The adaptome: advancing the science of intervention adaptation. *American Journal of Preventive Medicine* **51**(4, Suppl 2), S124–S131. doi:10.1016/j.amepre.2016.05.011.

Chang, Z. *et al.* (2021) Computational methods to measure patterns of gaze in toddlers with autism spectrum disorder. *JAMA Pediatrics* **175**(8), 827–836. doi:10.1001/jamapediatrics.2021.0530.

Cotton, N.K. & Shim, R.S. (2022) Social determinants of health, structural racism, and the impact on child and adolescent mental health. *Journal of the American Academy of Child and Adolescent Psychiatry* **61**(11), 1385–1389. doi:10.1016/j.jaac.2022.04.020.

Curran, G.M. *et al.* (2012) Effectiveness-implementation hybrid designs. *Medical Care* **50**(3), 217–226. doi:10.1097/MLR.0b013e3182408812.

Devassy, S.M. *et al.* (2022) Task sharing and stepped referral model for community mental health promotion in low- and middle-income countries (LMIC): insights from a feasibility study in India. *Pilot and Feasibility Studies* **8**(1), 192. doi:10.1186/s40814-022-01159-0.

Dray, J. (2021) Child and adolescent mental health and resilience-focussed interventions: a conceptual analysis to inform future research. *International Journal of Environmental Research and Public Health* **18**(14), 7315. doi:10.3390/ijerph18147315.

Erismann, S. *et al.* (2021) How to bring research evidence into policy? Synthesizing strategies of five research projects in low-and middle-income countries. *Health Research Policy and Systems* **19**(1), 29. doi:10.1186/s12961-020-00646-1.

Erskine, H.E. *et al.* (2016) The global coverage of prevalence data for mental disorders in children and adolescents. *Epidemiology and Psychiatric Sciences* **26**(4), 395–402. doi:10.1017/S2045796015001158.

Farao, J. *et al.* (2020) A user-centred design framework for mHealth. *PLoS One* **15**(8), e0237910. doi:10.1371/journal.pone.0237910.

Fedele, D.A. *et al.* (2017) Mobile health interventions for improving health outcomes in youth. *JAMA Pediatrics* **171**(5), 461–469. doi:10.1001/jamapediatrics.2017.0042.

Federal Communications Commission (2017) *Connect2HealthFCC—Mapping Broadband Health in America 2017*. Available: https://www.fcc.gov/reports-research/maps/connect2health/#ll=40 [30 October 2024].

Fogarty, W. *et al.* (2018) *Deficit Discourse and Strengths-based Approaches*. Available: https://www.lowitja.org.au/wp-content/uploads/2023/05/deficit-discourse-strengths-based.pdf [30 October 2024].

Galagali, P.M. & Brooks, M.J. (2020) Psychological care in low-resource settings for adolescents. *Clinical Child Psychology and Psychiatry* **25**(3), 698–711. doi:10.1177/1359104520929741.

Gelormino, E. *et al.* (2015) From built environment to health inequalities: an explanatory framework based on evidence. *Preventive Medicine Reports* **2**, 737–745. doi:10.1016/j.pmedr.2015.08.019.

Grantham-McGregor, S. *et al.* (2007) Developmental potential in the first 5 years for children in developing countries. *The Lancet* **369**(9555), 60–70. doi:10.1016/S0140-6736(07)60032-4.

Guler, J. *et al.* (2018) The importance of context in early autism intervention: a qualitative South African study. *Autism: The International Journal of Research and Practice* **22**(8), 1005–1017. doi:10.1177/1362361317716604.

Guthrie, W. *et al.* (2019) Accuracy of autism screening in a large pediatric network. *Pediatrics* **144**(4), e20183963. doi:10.1542/peds.2018-3963.

Hamdani, S.U. *et al.* (2022) Feasibility and acceptability of a multicomponent, group psychological intervention for adolescents with psychosocial distress in public schools of Pakistan: a feasibility cluster randomized controlled trial (cRCT). *Child and Adolescent Psychiatry and Mental Health* **16**, 47. doi:10.1186/s13034-022-00480-z.

Hardy, B. *et al.* (2019) Strengthening social programs to promote economic stability during childhood. *Social Policy Report* **32**(2), 1–36. doi:10.1002/sop2.4.

Härter, M. *et al.* (2018) Guideline-based stepped and collaborative care for patients with depression in a cluster-randomised trial. *Scientific Reports* **8**, 9389. doi:10.1038/s41598-018-27470-6.

Hartog, K. *et al.* (2020) Stigma reduction interventions for children and adolescents in low- and middle-income countries: systematic review of intervention strategies. *Social Science & Medicine* **246**, 112749. doi:10.1016/j.socscimed.2019.112749.

Henrich, J. *et al.* (2010) Most people are not WEIRD. *Nature* **466**(7302), 29–29. doi:10.1038/466029a.

Hillis, S. *et al.* (2016) Global prevalence of past-year violence against children: a systematic review and minimum estimates. *Pediatrics* **137**(3), e20154079. doi:10.1542/peds.2015-4079.

Ho, F.Y.-Y. *et al.* (2016) The efficacy and cost-effectiveness of stepped care prevention and treatment for depressive and/or anxiety disorders: a systematic review and meta-analysis. *Scientific Reports* **6**, 29281. doi:10.1038/srep29281.

Hoeft, T.J. *et al.* (2018) Task sharing approaches to improve mental health care in rural and other low resource settings: a systematic review. *The Journal of Rural Health: Official Journal of the American Rural Health Association and the National Rural Health Care Association* **34**(1), 48–62. doi:10.1111/jrh.12229.

Institute for Health Metrics and Evaluation (2019) *Global Burden of Disease Study 2019*. Available: https://www.healthdata.org/research-analysis/gbd [12 November 2024].

Jackson, C.S. & Gracia, J.N. (2014) Addressing health and health-care disparities: the role of a diverse workforce and the social determinants of health. *Public Health Reports* **129**(Suppl 2), 57–61.

Jones, C.M. *et al.* (2020) Identifying and preventing adverse childhood experiences. *JAMA* **323**(1), 25–26. doi:10.1001/jama.2019.18499.

Juengsiragulwit, D. (2015) Opportunities and obstacles in child and adolescent mental health services in low- and middle-income countries: a review of the literature. *WHO South-East Asia Journal of*

Public Health **4**(2), 110. Available: https://journals.lww.com/wsep/fulltext/2015/04020/opportunities_and_obstacles_in_child_and.2.aspx. [30 October 2024].

Kieling, C. *et al.* (2011) Child and adolescent mental health worldwide: evidence for action. *The Lancet* **378**(9801), 1515–1525. doi:10.1016/S0140-6736(11)60827-1.

Kleintjes, S. *et al.* (2010) Mental health care user participation in mental health policy development and implementation in South Africa. *International Review of Psychiatry* **22**(6), 568–577. https://doi.org/10.3109/09540261.2010.536153

Knifton, L. & Inglis, G. (2020) Poverty and mental health: policy, practice and research implications. *BJPsych Bulletin* **44**(5), 193–196. doi:10.1192/bjb.2020.78.

Kopal, J. *et al.* (2023) The end game: respecting major sources of population diversity. *Nature Methods* **20**(8), 1122–1128. doi:10.1038/s41592-023-01812-3.

Krishnappa Babu, P.R. *et al.* (2023) Complexity analysis of head movements in autistic toddlers. *Journal of Child Psychology and Psychiatry, and Allied Disciplines* **64**(1), 156–166. doi:10.1111/jcpp.13681.

Lancet Public Health, The (2020) Education: a neglected social determinant of health. *The Lancet Public Health* **5**(7), e361. doi:10.1016/S2468-2667(20)30144-4.

Le, L.K.-D. *et al.* (2021) Cost-effectiveness evidence of mental health prevention and promotion interventions: a systematic review of economic evaluations. *PLoS Medicine* **18**(5), e1003606. doi:10.1371/journal.pmed.1003606.

Leijten, P. *et al.* (2016) Transported versus homegrown parenting interventions for reducing disruptive child behavior: a multilevel meta-regression study. *Journal of the American Academy of Child and Adolescent Psychiatry* **55**(7), 610–617. doi:10.1016/j.jaac.2016.05.003.

Li, S.T. *et al.* (2007) Risk and protective factors for urban African-American youth. *American Journal of Community Psychology* **39**(1–2), 21–35. doi:10.1007/s10464-007-9088-1.

Lund, C. *et al.* (2010) Poverty and common mental disorders in low and middle income countries: a systematic review. *Social Science & Medicine* **71**(3), 517–528. doi:10.1016/j.socscimed.2010.04.027.

Lund, C. *et al.* (2011) Poverty and mental disorders: breaking the cycle in low-income and middle-income countries. *The Lancet* **378**(9801), 1502–1514. doi:10.1016/S0140-6736(11)60754-X.

Lund, C. *et al.* (2018) Social determinants of mental disorders and the sustainable development goals: a systematic review of reviews. *The Lancet Psychiatry* **5**(4), 357–369. doi:10.1016/S2215-0366(18)30060-9.

Mayosi, B.M. & Benatar, S.R. (2014) Health and health care in South Africa—20 years after Mandela. *New England Journal of Medicine* **371**(14), 1344–1353. doi:10.1056/NEJMsr1405012.

McKenzie, K. *et al.* (2004) Learning from low income countries: mental health. *BMJ* **329**(7475), 1138–1140. doi:10.1136/bmj.329.7475.1138.

Melchior, M. *et al.* (2012) Food insecurity and children's mental health: a prospective birth cohort study. *PLoS One* **7**(12), e52615. doi:10.1371/journal.pone.0052615.

Mercy, J.A. *et al.* (2017) Interpersonal violence: global impact and paths to prevention. In: *Injury Prevention and Environmental Health.* (eds C.N. Mock, *et al.*), 3rd edn. The International Bank for Reconstruction and Development/The World Bank, Washington, DC. doi:10.1596/978-1-4648-0522-6_ch5.

Mesman, E. *et al.* (2021) Resilience and mental health in children and adolescents: an update of the recent literature and future directions. *Current Opinion in Psychiatry* **34**(6), 586–592. doi:10.1097/YCO.0000000000000741.

Mezzina, R. *et al.* (2022) Social vulnerability and mental health inequalities in the "syndemic": call for action. *Frontiers in Psychiatry* **13**, 894370. doi:10.3389/fpsyt.2022.894370.

Mokitimi, S. *et al.* (2018) Child and adolescent mental health policy in South Africa: history, current policy development and implementation, and policy analysis. *International Journal of Mental Health Systems* **12**, 36. doi:10.1186/s13033-018-0213-3.

Monroe, P. *et al.* (2023) Racial/ethnic differences in social determinants of health and health outcomes among adolescents and youth ages 10–24 years old: a scoping review. *BMC Public Health* **23**(1), 410. doi:10.1186/s12889-023-15274-x.

Moore, G. *et al.* (2021) Adapting interventions to new contexts—the ADAPT guidance. *BMJ* **374**, n1679. doi:10.1136/bmj.n1679.

Morrissey, T.W. *et al.* (2020) Household economic instability: constructs, measurement, and implications. *Children and Youth Services Review* **118**, 105502. doi:10.1016/j.childyouth.2020.105502.

Movsisyan, A. *et al.* (2019) Adapting evidence-informed complex population health interventions for new contexts: a systematic review of guidance. *Implementation Science* **14**(1), 105. doi:10.1186/s13012-019-0956-5.

National Institute of Mental Health (2021). Technology and the Future of Mental Health Treatment. National Institute of Mental Health (NIMH). Available: https://www.nimh.nih.gov/health/topics/technology-and-the-future-of-mental-health-treatment [October 2024].

Nelson, C.A. *et al.* (2020) Adversity in childhood is linked to mental and physical health throughout life. *BMJ* **371**, m3048. doi:10.1136/bmj.m3048.

Nielsen, M. *et al.* (2017) The persistent sampling bias in developmental psychology: a call to action. *Journal of Experimental Child Psychology* **162**, 31–38. doi:10.1016/j.jecp.2017.04.017.

O'Keefe, V.M. *et al.* (2021) Increasing culturally responsive care and mental health equity with indigenous community mental health workers. *Psychological Services* **18**(1), 84–92. doi:10.1037/ser0000358.

Olashore, A.A. *et al.* (2023) Psychiatric disorders in adolescents living with HIV in Botswana. *AIDS Research and Therapy* **20**(1), 2. doi:10.1186/s12981-022-00490-z.

Organisation for Economic Co-operation and Development (2018). Bridging the Digital Gender Divide—Include, Upskill, Innovate. Organisation for Economic Co-operation and Development (OECD). Available: https://www.oecd.org/digital/bridging-the-digital-gender-divide.pdf [October 2024].

Ortega, F. & Müller, M.R. (2020) Global mental health and pharmacology: the case of attention deficit and hyperactivity disorders in Brazil. *Frontiers in Sociology* **5**. doi:10.3389/fsoc.2020.535125.

Patel, V. (2007) Closing the 10/90 divide in global mental health research. *Acta Psychiatrica Scandinavica* **115**(4), 257–259. doi:10.1111/j.1600-0447.2007.01012.x.

Patel, V. *et al.* (2018) The Lancet Commission on global mental health and sustainable development. *The Lancet* **392**(10157), 1553–1598. doi:10.1016/S0140-6736(18)31612-X.

Peek-Asa, C. *et al.* (2011) Rural disparity in domestic violence prevalence and access to resources. *Journal of Women's Health* **20**(11), 1743–1749. doi:10.1089/jwh.2011.2891.

Perochon, S. *et al.* (2023) A tablet-based game for the assessment of visual motor skills in autistic children. *npj Digital Medicine* **6**(1), 17. doi:10.1038/s41746-023-00762-6.

Petagna, M. *et al.* (2023) Mental health gap action programme intervention guide (mhGAP-IG) for child and adolescent mental health in low- and middle-income countries (LMIC): a systematic review. *Community Mental Health Journal* **59**(1), 192–204. doi:10.1007/s10597-022-00981-3.

Prina, E. *et al.* (2023) Task-sharing psychosocial interventions for the prevention of common mental disorders in the perinatal period in low- and middle-income countries: a systematic review and meta-analysis. *The International Journal of Social Psychiatry* **69**(7). doi:10.1177/00207640231174451.

Rathod, S. *et al.* (2017) Mental health service provision in low- and middle-income countries. *Health Services Insights* **10**. doi:10.1177/1178632917694350.

Renwick, L. *et al.* (2022) Mental health literacy in children and adolescents in low- and middle-income countries: a mixed studies systematic review and narrative synthesis. *European Child & Adolescent Psychiatry* **33**, 961–985. doi:10.1007/s00787-022-01997-6.

Ribeiro, W.S. *et al.* (2023) A systematic review of evidence-based interventions for child and adolescent mental health problems in low- and middle-income countries. *Comprehensive Psychiatry* **121**, 152358. doi:10.1016/j.comppsych.2022.152358.

Richards, D.A. *et al.* (2012) Delivering stepped care: an analysis of implementation in routine practice. *Implementation Science* **7**(1), 3. doi:10.1186/1748-5908-7-3.

Rothstein, R. (2017) *The Color of Law*. Liveright Publishing Corporation, New York.

Rutter, M. (1985) Resilience in the face of adversity: protective factors and resistance to psychiatric disorder. *The British Journal of Psychiatry: the Journal of Mental Science* **147**, 598–611. doi:10.1192/bjp.147.6.598.

Rutter, M. (2012) Resilience as a dynamic concept. *Development and Psychopathology* **24**(2), 335–344. doi:10.1017/S0954579412000028.

Schlesinger, A. *et al.* (2023) Clinical update: collaborative mental health care for children and adolescents in pediatric primary care. *Journal of the American Academy of Child & Adolescent Psychiatry* **62**(2), 91–119. doi:10.1016/j.jaac.2022.06.007.

Shah, N. *et al.* (2021) National or population level interventions addressing the social determinants of mental health: an umbrella review. *BMC Public Health* **21**(1), 2118. doi:10.1186/s12889-021-12145-1.

Shatkin, J.P. & Belfer, M.L. (2004) The global absence of child and adolescent mental health policy. *Child and Adolescent Mental Health* **9**(3), 104–108. doi:10.1111/j.1475-3588.2004.00090.x.

da Silva, A.T.C. *et al.* (2019) Enhancing mental health research capacity: emerging voices from the National Institute of Mental Health (NIMH) global hubs. *International Journal of Mental Health Systems* **13**, 21. doi:10.1186/s13033-019-0276-9.

Simelane, S. & de Vries, P.J. (2021) Child and adolescent mental health services and systems in low and middle-income countries: from mapping to strengthening. *Current Opinion in Psychiatry* **34**(6), 608–616. doi:10.1097/YCO.0000000000000740.

Singla, D.R. *et al.* (2017) Psychological treatments for the world: lessons from low- and middle-income countries. *Annual Review of Clinical Psychology* **13**, 149–181. doi:10.1146/annurev-clinpsy-032816-045217.

Sirugo, G. *et al.* (2019) The missing diversity in human genetic studies. *Cell* **177**(1), 26–31. doi:10.1016/j.cell.2019.02.048.

Southwick, S.M. *et al.* (2014) Resilience definitions, theory, and challenges: interdisciplinary perspectives. *European Journal of Psychotraumatology* **5**(1). doi:10.3402/ejpt.v5.25338.

Stein, D.J. & Wegener, G. (2017) Discovery versus implementation research on mental disorders in low- and middle-income countries. *Acta Neuropsychiatrica* **29**(4), 191–192. doi:10.1017/neu.2017.25.

Stein, D.J. *et al.* (2015) Global mental health and neuroscience: potential synergies. *The Lancet Psychiatry* **2**(2), 178–185. doi:10.1016/S2215-0366(15)00014-0.

Storebø, O.J. & Gluud, C. (2020) Methylphenidate for ADHD rejected from the WHO Essential Medicines List due to uncertainties in benefit-harm profile. *BMJ Evidence-Based Medicine* **26**(4), 172–175. doi:10.1136/bmjebm-2019-111328.

Toyama, M. *et al.* (2017) Peruvian mental health reform: a framework for scaling-up mental health services. *International Journal of Health Policy and Management* **6**(9), 501–508. doi:10.15171/ijhpm.2017.07.

U.S. Department of Health and Human Services (2023a) Health Care Access and Quality—Healthy People 2030. U.S. Department of Health and Human Services, Washington, DC. Available: https://health.gov/healthypeople/objectives-and-data/browse-objectives/health-care-access-and-quality [30 October 2024].

U.S. Department of Health and Human Services (2023b) Healthy People 2030. U.S. Department of Health and Human Services, Washington, DC. Available: https://health.gov/healthypeople/objectives-and-data/social-determinants-health [30 October 2024].

United Nations (2016) *The Sustainable Development Goals Report*. United Nations (UN), New York. Available: https://unstats.un.org/sdgs/report/2016/the%20sustainable%20development%20goals%20report%202016.pdf [30 October 2024].

United Nations (2019) Indigenous people's traditional knowledge must be preserved, valued globally, speakers stress as permanent forum opens annual session. United Nations (UN), New York. Available: https://press.un.org/en/2019/hr5431.doc.htm [30 October 2024].

United Nations—Population Division (2022) *World Population Prospects*. United Nations (UN), New York. Available: https://population.un.org/wpp [30 October 2024].

Vreeman, R.C. *et al.* (2017) Mental health challenges among adolescents living with HIV. *Journal of the International AIDS Society* **20**(Suppl 3), 21497. doi:10.7448/IAS.20.4.21497.

World Bank, The (2016) *World Development Report 2016: Digital Dividends*. World Bank, Washington, DC. Available: https://www.worldbank.org/en/publication/wdr2016 [30 October 2024].

World Bank, The (2023a) *World Bank Country and Lending Groups—Country Classification*. World Bank, Washington, DC. Available: https://datahelpdesk.worldbank.org/knowledgebase/articles/906519 [30 October 2024].

World Bank, The (2023b) World Bank Open Data. World Bank, Washington, DC. Available: https://data.worldbank.org [30 October 2024].

World Health Organization (2007) *Everybody's Business: Strengthening Health Systems to Improve Health Outcomes: WHO's Framework for Action*. World Health Organization (WHO), Geneva, Switzerland. Available: https://www.who.int/publications/i/item/everybody-s-business----strengthening-health-systems-to-improve-health-outcomes [30 October 2024].

World Health Organization (2020) *Mental Health Atlas 2020*. World Health Organization (WHO), Geneva, Switzerland. Available: https://www.who.int/publications-detail-redirect/9789240036703 [30 October 2024].

World Health Organization (2021) *World Health Organization Model List of Essential Medicines for Children—8th list, 2021*. World Health Organization (WHO), Geneva, Switzerland. Available: https://www.who.int/publications-detail-redirect/WHO-MHP-HPS-EML-2021.03 [30 October 2024].

World Health Organization (2022) Universal health coverage (UHC). World Health Organization (WHO), Geneva, Switzerland. Available:

https://www.who.int/news-room/fact-sheets/detail/universal-health-coverage-(uhc) [30 October 2024].

World Health Organization (2023a) Mental Health Gap Action Programme (mhGAP). World Health Organization (WHO), Geneva, Switzerland. Available: https://www.who.int/teams/mental-health-and-substance-use/treatment-care/mental-health-gap-action-programme [30 October 2024].

World Health Organization (2023b) Social determinants of health. World Health Organization (WHO), Geneva, Switzerland. Available: https://www.who.int/health-topics/social-determinants-of-health [30 October 2024].

Zajacova, A. & Lawrence, E.M. (2018) The relationship between education and health: reducing disparities through a contextual approach. *Annual Review of Public Health* **39**, 273–289. doi:10.1146/annurev-publhealth-031816-044628.

Zhou, W. *et al.* (2020) Child and adolescent mental health policy in low- and middle-income countries: challenges and lessons for policy development and implementation. *Frontiers in Psychiatry* **11**. doi:10.3389/fpsyt.2020.00150.

van Zyl, C. *et al.* (2021) Unravelling 'low-resource settings': a systematic scoping review with qualitative content analysis. *BMJ Global Health* **6**(6), e005190. doi:10.1136/bmjgh-2021-005190.

CHAPTER 47
Forensic child and adolescent psychiatry

Alexandra Lewis[1,2], Seena Fazel[3,4] and Rohan Borschmann[3,4,5]
[1] Cambridge & Peterborough NHS Foundation Trust, Cambridge, UK
[2] Health & Justice Team, NHS, England, London, UK
[3] Department of Psychiatry, The University of Oxford, Oxford, UK
[4] Oxford Health NHS Foundation Trust, Oxford, UK
[5] The University of Melbourne (Centre for Mental Health and Community Wellbeing), Melbourne, Victoria, Australia

Overview

Forensic child and adolescent psychiatry refers to legal aspects of child and adolescent mental health (CAMH).

In the United Kingdom (UK), Europe, and Australasia, it primarily refers to the mental health of young people in contact with, or who are at risk of contact with, the criminal justice system (CJS). It involves consideration of both clinical and criminogenic aspects of a young person's presentation, relating to criminal law. Civil law also affects young people, but such issues are not usually described as forensic child and adolescent psychiatry in these countries. Contrastingly, in the United States (U.S.), any area of law relating to young people tends to be described as forensic child and adolescent psychiatry.

This chapter focuses on the interface between criminal law and CAMH. Civil law issues are addressed in Chapter 19.

This chapter uses "justice-involved young people" in preference to more stigmatizing terms (e.g., "young offenders"). Justice-involved young people may be charged with offenses but subsequently be acquitted, meaning "offender" descriptions are inaccurate. Furthermore, most young people's CJS contact is time-limited, but the stigmatizing labels acquired often persist. These can adversely affect self and societal perceptions, impairing community reintegration and limiting life chances (Tran *et al.*, 2018).

The chapter has the following sections:

- introduction covering international guidance/treaties, minimum age of criminal responsibility and models of youth justice;
- physical and mental health of justice-involved adolescents;
- developmental correlates of CJS involvement;
- mental health provision in CJS settings;
- assessments;
- interventions; and
- professional considerations.

Introduction

There is considerable international variation regarding the minimum age of criminal responsibility and differences between countries regarding what constitutes a criminal offense. This makes establishing the global prevalence of youth crime difficult.

Rates of recorded youth crime are reducing in many countries—although the accuracy of and explanations for this are debated (Griffiths & Norris, 2020). Rates of adolescent offending by males consistently exceed that of females for all offenses. Information regarding the numbers of Indigenous and minority group young people in the CJS is unavailable for many countries but, globally, it appears that these populations are overrepresented.

Countries vary regarding the age at which children are held responsible for offending (the "minimum age of criminal responsibility"—MACR). The global median MACR is 12 years old (Penal Reform International, 2013), but there remains wide variation (e.g., 7 years old in some U.S. states, 10 years old in England, Wales, and Australia, and 18 years old in Brazil), meaning children in different parts of the world may receive different consequences for similar classes of offenses.

The concept of a MACR is consistent with accumulating neurodevelopmental evidence of how brain maturity affects decision-making (Steinberg & Icenogle, 2019). However, the exact cutoff age remains controversial. The lack of nonlinearities in brain development make it hard to use neuroscience to justify selecting one age over another as a cutoff point (see Chapter 12). Some have highlighted inconsistencies within countries between the age at which an adolescent is deemed to have capacity in civil law and the age at which they are regarded as having capacity to understand criminal law (Noroozi *et al.*, 2019).

Rutter's Child and Adolescent Psychiatry and Psychology, Seventh Edition.
Edited by Anita Thapar, Daniel S. Pine, Samuele Cortese, Cathy Creswell, Tamsin J. Ford, James F. Leckman, and Argyris Stringaris.

Companion website: www.wiley.com/go/thapar/rutterspsych7

Some countries have the rebuttable principle of *doli incapax* that applies to children between certain ages charged with criminal offenses. This means children in this age range are presumed not to have capacity to form criminal intent, but this may be overturned if the prosecution can produce evidence proving otherwise. Psychiatrists and psychologists may be asked to contribute expert opinions in such cases. Some argue (Hamer & Crofts, 2023) that *doli incapax* fits well with scientific evidence demonstrating lack of uniformity of neurodevelopment. Despite this, many countries including the UK, Canada, and Ireland have abolished it.

Further heterogeneity exists in the extent to which young people are treated differently from adults. Some countries divert young people out of the CJS completely, others manage them within youth-only justice systems, and some treat them identically to adults.

These differences mean that the characteristics and needs of children in contact with the international CJS vary widely, which can make generalization from the literature challenging. It should further be noted that most published research has been undertaken from Western cultural perspectives and in high-income countries, which may further limit generalizability.

International guidance and treaties

Core principles regarding children and young people are enshrined in the United Nations Convention on the Rights of the Child (UNCRC) (United Nations, 1990a). The African Charter on the Rights and Welfare of the Child (Organization of African Unity, 1990) is complementary to the UNCRC but is tailored for children in Africa. The Arab Charter on Human Rights (League of Arab States, 1994) is not fully compliant with UNCRC, as it permits the imposition of the death penalty on children.

The UNCRC stipulates that States Parties should establish a MACR, although an age is not specified in the Convention. However, criticism has occurred of member states with an age of less than 12 (United Nations, 2007), with recent recommendations to increase to at least 14 years old (United Nations, 2019a).

Additional guidance issued by the United Nations (UN) relates to the management of children and adolescents within the CJS:

- Standard Minimum Rules for the Administration of Juvenile Justice (the "Beijing Rules") address issues such as privacy, the need for special training of police regarding working with young people, and due process guarantees, and advocate for the diversion of young people from judicial proceedings (United Nations, 1986).
- Guidelines for the Prevention of Juvenile Delinquency (the "Riyadh Guidelines") emphasize the importance of early intervention and avoiding premature criminalization of children (United Nations, 1990b).
- Rules for the Protection of Juveniles Deprived of their Liberty (the "Havana Rules") require independent inspection of facilities where young people are detained and place an explicit onus on medical staff (Rule 73) to participate in "evaluating compliance with the rules concerning hygiene, accommodation, food, exercise and medical services as well as any other issues that may affect the ... health of juveniles" (United Nations, 1990c).
- Rules for the Treatment of Women Prisoners and Non-Custodial Measures for Women Offenders (the "Bangkok Rules") also apply to girls (United Nations, 2010).

Despite the above well-intentioned treaties and guidelines, most are not, or are only partly, legally binding on signatory states and not all UN members have ratified them (notably the U.S. has not). In many countries, children are still held in secure settings alongside adults, where there are safety risks and fewer age-appropriate services.

Youth justice approaches

Youth justice approaches have historically been divided into "justice-centered" and "welfare-centered" models. The justice-centered model focuses on the offense, accountability, identifying and addressing factors thought to be driving offending, and deterrence, and is characterized by procedural formality. The welfare-centered model primarily focuses on identifying the unmet needs, including clinical needs, of the child and adopting a more informal approach, often involving diversion away from the CJS, underpinned by the belief that addressing unmet needs will reduce recidivism.

Meta-analyses suggest that diverted young people may be less likely to reoffend than those receiving punitive interventions alone, which may have contributed to increased adoption of the welfare-centered type of approach. No single diversion model has been identified as superior (Wilson *et al.*, 2018). Unequally distributed community diversion resources limit the feasibility and effectiveness of diversion (Baldry *et al.*, 2017).

Most countries have a CJS that is a blend of both approaches.

Since the 1990s, a heightened focus on risk has played a central role in the delivery of youth justice. This actuarial-informed approach is based on the belief that the presence of certain factors increases the probability of a young person offending and should be the focus of interventions (Farrington, 2002). Many risk assessment tools have been developed to facilitate this approach. While considerable support persists for this approach (Barboni *et al.*, 2023), doubts have been expressed by some about both the validity of these tools and the value of such a narrow risk-focused approach (Koh *et al.*, 2020; Senior *et al.*, 2021). Recently, broader and more contextualized approaches, such as "trauma-informed" (the understanding that trauma exposure can affect neurological, biological, psychological, and social development), "public health," and "child first, offence second" concepts, have been proposed as preferable (Case & Browning, 2021; Day, 2022; Klose & Gordon, 2023).

Restorative justice (RJ) approaches have become prominent in youth justice since the early 2000s. RJ views offending as harm against victims and communities and seeks to repair damage and restore the victim and environment back to their original state, rather than punish the perpetrator (Liebmann, 2007). Admission of guilt is a prerequisite. Dialogue between stakeholders is key. In some countries, RJ approaches have been adopted as a way of diverting young people out of the CJS completely. New Zealand was the first to incorporate RJ approaches, through the introduction of the Family Group Conference (FGC), but such approaches have become widespread. However, more rigorous testing of the effectiveness of different RJ approaches and with different types of offenders is needed to establish effectiveness.

Mental and physical health of adolescents in the criminal justice system

There is considerable evidence that justice-involved young people shoulder a disproportionate burden of adolescent morbidity and mortality.

They experience elevated rates of mental disorder (Fazel *et al.*, 2008; Beaudry *et al.*, 2021a), self-harm (Borschmann *et al.*, 2014), suicidal behavior (Hawton *et al.*, 2014), substance dependence (Kinner *et al.*, 2015), neurodevelopmental disorders (NDDs; Hughes *et al.*, 2015), noncommunicable diseases (Feinstein *et al.*, 1998), and sexually transmitted and blood-borne viral infections (Kinner *et al.*, 2018). These health problems frequently co-occur, meaning complex multimorbidity is the norm.

Many underutilize primary and preventive care in the community (Abram *et al.*, 2008) and CJS contact (particularly detention) provides opportunities to identify their mental health needs and initiate treatments (Fazel & Baillargeon, 2011). Most detained adolescents return to the community after detention, and poorer mental health is associated with higher rates of recidivism (Kinner & Wang, 2014). Identification and provision of mental health care while detained has the potential to improve mental health outcomes and reduce rates of reincarceration.

A global scoping review (Borschmann *et al.*, 2020) compared rates of psychiatric, substance use, and NDDs reported by adolescents in youth justice detention with their community-based peers. Detained young people were consistently found to have poorer mental health (Table 47.1). One U.S.-based review of the health of detained adolescents (Barnert *et al.*, 2016) reported that two in three males and three in four females met the diagnostic criteria for at least one mental disorder, depression and behavioral disorders being most prevalent. The point prevalence of any anxiety disorder (including post-traumatic stress disorder—PTSD), psychotic disorders, and major depressive disorder were all higher in detained adolescents. Similar patterns were observed for behavioral disorders, including conduct disorder (CD) and oppositional defiant disorder (ODD).

"Self-harm" refers to any intentional self-poisoning or self-injury. A high prevalence of self-harm across the lifetime was reported (ranging between 17–42%), including a past-year prevalence of up to 20% of all detained adolescents. The prevalence of a reported suicide attempt across the lifetime ranged between 4–51%, including 13–35% during the past year and 2–7% during the past month. Suicidal behavior during detention was common, with prevalence ranging between 5–23%. This was considerably higher than previously reported among adolescents in the general population. Detained adolescents with a history of self-harm and/or suicidal behaviors are a particularly vulnerable group, with high rates of mental and substance use disorders, and social risk factors (Borschmann *et al.*, 2014). As impulsivity is a common precursor to both self-harm and offending behavior, they may benefit from targeted mental health interventions specifically designed to address impulsivity while in detention, as well as transitional mental health care and post-release support.

Table 47.1 Prevalence of mental disorders in adolescents in detention and in the general population.

	Point prevalence (%) in detained adolescents Median (interquartile range); range		Lifetime prevalence in detained adolescents (%)	Lifetime prevalence in adolescents in the general population (%)
	Males	Females		
Mood disorder (any)	10.1; 0.4–36.0	26.6; 0.0–63.0	7.0–82.0	14.3
Major depressive disorder (MDD)	10.8; 0.9–14.0	–; 7.4–36.0	4.7–40.4	1.3
Anxiety disorder (any)	17.8; 3.4–31.5	30.3; 20.9–59.0	9.0–56.3	6.5
Post-traumatic stress disorder (PTSD)	14.1; 0.0–53.0	20.0; 13.0–65.1	11.0–48.9	5.0
Obsessive-compulsive disorder (OCD)	4.9%; 0.4–9.0%	–; 2.0–7.4	0.4–9.0	0.3–4.0
Conduct disorder (CD)	73.5 (53.9–79.8); 26.0–95.0	53.8 (43.1–77.5); 17.0–91.0	13.9–100	2.1
Oppositional defiant disorder (ODD)	19.3 (14.5–48.0); 8.0–51.0	39.7 (25.0–46.4); 17.5–62.0	7.6–22.4	3.6
Schizophrenia spectrum disorders	2.0; 0.8–2.2	1.9; –	2.2–4.0	0.5–1.5

Source: Adapted from Borschmann *et al.* (2020).

A large proportion of detained adolescents reported using illicit substances during the past year, in addition to alcohol and tobacco (Balogun *et al.*, 2018). The reported prevalence of lifetime substance use disorder ranged between 22–96% for detained adolescents, while this figure ranged between 7–11% for adolescents in the general population (Zhou *et al.*, 2012, Elgar *et al.*, 2003). Many established risk factors for substance use are more common among detained adolescents than among their community peers (Loeber & Farrington, 2000).

The reported prevalence of a range of NDDs was higher among detained adolescents than their community peers.

Rates of attention deficit hyperactivity disorder (ADHD) in the general population of children and adolescents are estimated to be between 3% and 9% (National Collaborating Centre for Mental Health, 2009). In detained adolescents, rates ranged between 2–49% (Borschmann *et al.*, 2020), with a pooled prevalence of around 17% (Beaudry et al., 2021a). While there was some evidence of higher rates of autism spectrum disorders (ASDs) among detained adolescents than in the general population (Ali, 2018), many previous studies used selected samples, making true prevalence difficult to establish.

Canadian and Australian studies found rates of fetal alcohol spectrum disorders (FASDs) of 11–36% in detained adolescents (Rojas & Gretton, 2007; Smith *et al.*, 2013; Bower *et al.*, 2018), compared with an estimated 2–5% of children in Western countries (May *et al.*, 2009). Particularly high rates were noted among detained Indigenous adolescents (19–47%), which likely reflects wider health inequalities and disparities between Indigenous and non-Indigenous young people.

Impact of detention on mental and physical health

While it is commonly asserted that detention has a deleterious impact on an individual's mental and physical health, few studies have attempted to generate empirical evidence to support this claim. One matched cohort study from the Netherlands (Dirkzwager *et al.*, 2021) linked national data on all people detained nationally in 2014–2015 to electronic health records of a representative sample of general practitioners, and calculated prevalence rates of health problems in the year before and after detention. Detained adults were characterized by complex health profiles both before and after detention, and poor health post-release could not be attributed causally to the experience of detention. Although this study did not establish a health-depleting effect of detention, it did not show any benefit. It supports the notion that people entering prisons are already in relatively poor health (Dirkzwager *et al.*, 2021).

A systematic review examined the impact of incarceration on health outcomes in adults (Shuttleworth, 2022) finding considerable parallels between factors associated with health status prior to, and following, incarceration. These include structural, health care-related, behavioral, and psychosocial factors (Table 47.2). The review suggested poor health observed following detention may instead reflect the continuity of health disparities experienced by people passing through the CJS. Currently, no definitively causal relationship between detention and poor health outcomes has been established.

Developmental correlates of criminal justice system involvement

Morbidity in young people is concentrated in marginalized subgroups. Typical young people in contact with the CJS have life trajectories characterized by instability, abuse, neglect, low educational attainment, poverty, and entrenched disadvantage (Barnert *et al.*, 2016; Hughes *et al.*, 2020). A *Lancet Commission* (Patton *et al.*, 2016) highlighted the extreme vulnerability of justice-involved young people globally, and the urgent need for better health data in this population. Data, especially from low- and middle-income settings, is urgently needed to inform targeted, evidence-based preventive strategies addressing the social and structural drivers of adolescent criminal behavior, and to provide timely health care to this vulnerable group. As the social and structural drivers of criminal behavior overlap with the determinants of morbidity and mortality, it is likely that strategies to address these factors could help to reduce both rates of adolescent detention and adolescent health inequalities (Borschmann *et al.*, 2020).

While considerable research attention has been devoted to the health of young people who come into contact with the CJS, fewer studies have focused on difficulties associated with health and development which can increase the risk of a young person first becoming exposed to the CJS. Factors which have the potential to impact developmental processes relevant to the risk of criminal behavior (Hughes *et al.*, 2020) include NDDs, traumatic brain injury (TBI), and trauma and adversity (i.e., adverse childhood experiences—ACEs).

Traumatic brain injury (TBI)

TBI is a risk factor for earlier, more violent offending, and is linked to poor engagement in treatment, in-custody infractions, and higher rates of reconviction (Williams *et al.*, 2018). TBI can result in functional difficulties affecting behavior (Hughes, 2015) including deficits in cognition, social communication, impulse control, empathy, and responding to others' emotions (Hughes *et al.*, 2020). It can contribute to poorer responses to rehabilitation (Williams *et al.*, 2018). A meta-analysis of studies involving TBIs in young people convicted of crimes (Farrer *et al.*, 2013) found the proportion with TBI was approximately 30%, markedly higher than observed in the general population. This proportion increased to 32–50% when restricted to adolescents in detention (Hughes *et al.*, 2020).

Neurodevelopmental influences

The prevalence of NDDs is higher among young people in contact with the CJS than in the general population (Borschmann *et al.*, 2020). A population-based Swedish study compared the

Table 47.2 Factors associated with health in people who have experienced incarceration in the U.S.

	Pre-incarceration	Incarceration	Post-incarceration
Structural	• Socioeconomic position • Racism • Exposure to violence • Educational attainment • Exposure to police stops	• Exposure to incarceration policies, institutional violence, and trauma • Guaranteed shelter and food • Congregate living quarters and low-quality food • Overcrowding • Correctional oversight of health care	• Lower socioeconomic position • Racism • Exposure to violence • Collateral consequences • Parole and probation supervision
Health care	• Limited/no access to primary care and insurance • High use of emergency department	• Guaranteed health care • Monitored medication adherence • Newly diagnosed chronic disease • Limited access to medications for addiction • Correctional system involvement in health care • Co-payments exceeding many days' worth of work	• Limited/no access to primary care and insurance • Poor transitions in care • Medical system discrimination • High use of emergency department
Behavioral	• Smoking and substance use • Poor diet and low physical activity • High-risk sexual behavior	• Limited access to smoking, alcohol, and other drugs • Little control over diet and variable physical activity • Limited access to condoms	• Return to smoking and/or other substance use • More control over diet and physical activity • High-risk sexual behavior
Psychosocial	• Adverse childhood experiences (ACEs) • Chronic stress and trauma • Family/social ties • Perceived discrimination • Housing or food insecurity	• Acute and/or chronic stress • Social isolation • Lack of autonomy and low self-efficacy	• Acute and/or chronic stress • Improved self-efficacy • Altered family or social ties • Perceived discrimination • Housing or food insecurity

Source: Adapted from Puglisi and Wang (2021).

risk of violent offending in children with NDDs, with the risk of matched controls without such disorders (Lundström *et al.*, 2014). They found children with ADHD were at increased risk of committing violent crimes compared with their peers, though no association was observed between ASDs and such crimes. Cognitive, communicative, or socio-emotional difficulties associated with NDDs can increase the risk of engaging in criminal behavior (Hughes, 2015). Failure to identify NDDs will decrease understanding of an important influence on antisocial behavior and is potential cause of poor engagement in rehabilitation (National Collaborating Centre for Mental Health, 2009).

Rates of specific learning difficulties among detained adolescents reported in the literature have varied between 10–32%, reflecting varied definitions and assumptions (Borschmann *et al.*, 2020). These rates are still considerably higher than those reported in general population studies (McKay & Neal, 2009).

Research suggests the majority of detained adolescents have some language difficulty that significantly affects their day-to-day functioning (Gregory & Bryan, 2015). This may affect the young person's ability to communicate with police and/or lawyers and reduce their ability to benefit from verbally mediated interventions (Snow & Powell, 2011).

Adverse childhood experiences (ACEs)

Research has demonstrated potential adverse effects on long-term neurological development from ACEs (Shonkoff *et al.*, 2012; Hughes *et al.*, 2020). ACEs can disrupt brain development and functioning, reduce the ability to regulate impulses, and increase the likelihood of a young person engaging in maladaptive behaviors such as aggression and delinquency, and, ultimately, of contact with the CJS during adolescence (Hughes *et al.*, 2020) (Figure 47.1).

Comprehensive forensic child and adolescent mental health services covering the whole pathway through the criminal justice system

Some young people's involvement with mental health services may pre-date their contact with the CJS. Others may only have their mental health needs recognized after they become justice-involved.

Mental health vulnerabilities may become visible at multiple points during a young person's pathway through the CJS. Interventions may be important to ensure fair process and justice, as well as being necessary for the young person's mental health.

Some countries have developed comprehensive forensic child and adolescent services covering the whole pathway through the CJS. They may additionally work in the pre-criminal space. These services aim to identify mental health needs and provide specialist interventions and adjustments, as required (Figure 47.2).

However, such comprehensive and specialized child and adolescent mental health services (CAMHS) are unusual. It is more common for provision to be restricted to certain points of the CJS only.

Most countries have no specialist forensic CAMH professionals. Instead, general CAMH professionals, who may have no forensic training, or adult mental health professionals, who may have no training in CAMH or forensic issues, are tasked with identifying and addressing issues in the forensic child and adolescent population.

Key points where mental health interventions may be required are explored in the following sections.

Police interview

Typically, the first point of contact with the CJS involves an interaction with the police. Suspects are formally interviewed and the consequences may be serious.

At the start of a police interview, a statement (known as the caution or "Miranda") is read to the interviewee informing them of their rights, including the right to remain silent and to have legal representation. However, research demonstrates that these statements are difficult for children to understand, and they may waive their rights without fully understanding the implications (Smalarz *et al.*, 2016; Sharf *et al.*, 2017; Kemp & Watkins, 2022). Young justice-involved people have been demonstrated to have higher levels of communication difficulties (Snow, 2019) and those with developmental language disorders have, unsurprisingly, been found to be at heightened risk of misunderstanding these statements (Lieser *et al.*, 2019).

The implications of waiving the right to legal representation is especially concerning as young people have been demonstrated to be more likely than adults to make false confessions

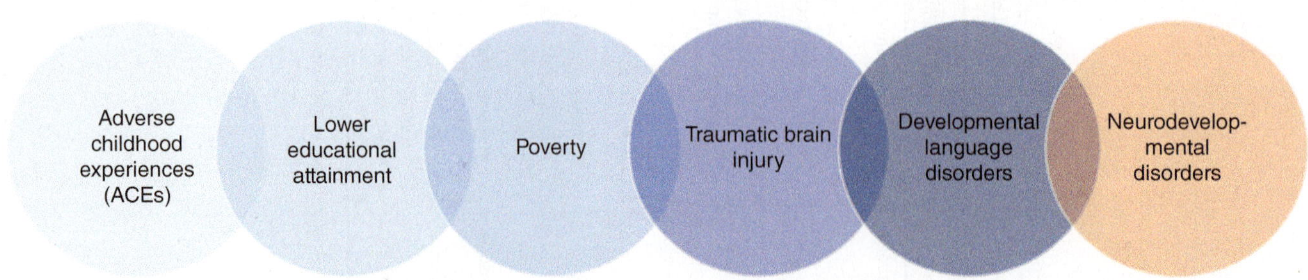

Figure 47.1 Developmental correlates of youth criminal justice system involvement.

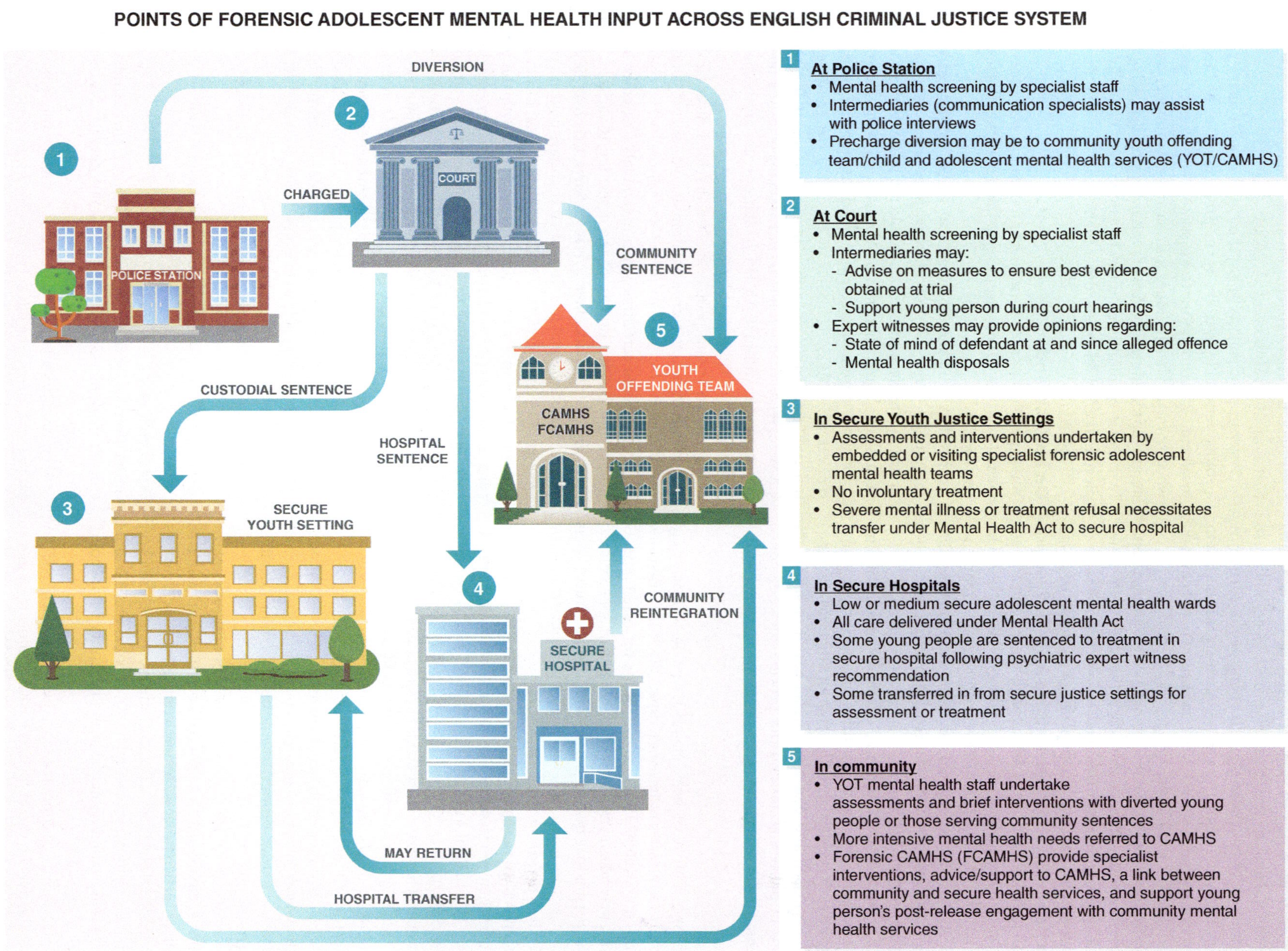

Figure 47.2 Summary of mental health provision across youth criminal justice system in England.

(Haney-Caron *et al.*, 2018). Mental health issues (including neurodevelopmental factors/disorders) have been found to increase the risk of false confession in young people further. A self-report study found that young people with mental health issues were more likely to make false confessions in police interviews (Gudjonsson *et al.*, 2006).

These findings emphasize the importance of young people being provided with additional support at this stage in the criminal justice process. Some jurisdictions require young people to be interviewed by police in the presence of an adult, even if a young person declines legal representation (e.g., the "appropriate adult" (AA) scheme in the UK). However, the adult is not required to be a mental health or legal professional and could be a parent or lay volunteer. The effectiveness of AAs in supporting young people is underresearched, but there is a suggestion that AAs are more passive than expected from the guidelines (Farrugia & Gabbert, 2019).

Police officers need child mental health awareness training so they are able to recognize potential vulnerability in young suspects and seek appropriate help. Some jurisdictions have specialist youth liaison and diversion mental health professionals who work in police stations and can provide advice if police have mental health concerns.

Court

Young people who have been charged with an offense may attend court for a series of hearings, especially if the offense is serious or complicated. This is to allow time for case preparation, which may take many months. Between court appearances, the young person may be bailed to a community address (often with conditions such as a curfew or reporting requirements) or remanded into detention.

Guidelines have been developed in some countries to help courts adapt their processes to meet the needs of young defendants better (Council of Europe, 2010; The Advocates Gateway, 2017; Liefaard, 2020).

Many courts have specialist mental health clinics attached to them which may provide another route to identifying mental health needs in newly charged adolescents about whom there are concerns. Often these clinics experience a mismatch between resource and demand, and provision of in-depth mental health assessments is not possible. However, helpful mental health screening with onward signposting for more detailed assessments is possible.

It is particularly important for queries about fitness to plead or communication issues to be flagged up as early as possible in the criminal justice process, so that appropriate interventions can be organized. For those with acute mental illness, diversion to community or inpatient mental health services may be indicated, with stabilization of mental health necessary before court proceedings can start.

Support by a communication specialist, such as an Intermediary, may be useful for those with significant vulnerabilities or communication deficits to facilitate full participation in court proceedings, although more evidence is needed regarding the cost–benefit of these schemes (Cooper & Mattison, 2017; Howard *et al.*, 2020).

Forensic psychiatrists or psychologists may be instructed by a young person's legal team, by the prosecution, or by the court to provide expert opinions to assist the court when considering whether mental health issues may have some influence over fitness to plead, culpability, risk of reoffending, or disposal options. Psychiatric opinion is required by law to determine fitness to plead in the UK and many other high-income jurisdictions.

On bail/remand

Young people may start their court proceedings with preexisting mental health needs or may develop them over the course of the proceedings.

If bailed, they should be able to access primary care and community-based CAMHS like any other child. Being subject to criminal justice proceedings should not mean they are denied health care. Some countries have developed multidisciplinary community-based forensic child and adolescent mental health services (FCAMHS) (Hindley *et al.*, 2017) but these tend to function as an adjunct, rather than replacement for general CAMHS. It could be argued that fast-tracking of justice-involved young people within CAMHS is appropriate, given the high stakes nature of contact with the CJS.

Remanded young people may be detained in a variety of placements including secure children's homes, secure youth justice or hospital facilities, or mixed-age prisons. Many countries undertake health screening when individuals first enter justice placements, but the quality of the screening is variable, often occurring without adequate privacy. Individuals may be reluctant to disclose mental health issues if they have concerns about the possible consequences of doing so. Any mental health information elicited in a court clinic should travel with the young person to be shared with health staff on arrival. If mental health conditions are identified in screening, onward referral for specialist input should occur. However, the extent of mental health provision varies widely between placements and countries, from an embedded full time multidisciplinary CAMHS to a visiting single practitioner such as a psychiatrist or general practitioner.

Globally, justice-involved young people are at increased risk of suicide attempts and dying by suicide, whether detained (Gallagher & Dobrin, 2006a) or nondetained (Kemp *et al.*, 2016). Processes to improve identification of suicidality at first point of court contact have been described (Kemp *et al.*, 2022) and screening for suicidality within 24 hours of arriving in custody may reduce incidence of suicide attempts (Gallagher & Dobrin, 2006b).

Sentencing

Internationally, there has been a trend away from custodial sentences for young people, and most adolescents receive community sentences.

Community sentences may formally require a young person to engage with mental health services. This means that, if they do not, there is the possibility that they will be viewed as having "breached" the terms of their order and return to court where further sanctions may be imposed. Alternatively, contact with CAMHS/FCAMHS may be recommended but not be mandated.

Detention remains a possibility, especially for violent or other serious offenses. Internationally, at least 410,000 children are detained in remand centers and prisons every year (United Nations, 2019b). These placements range from small secure children's home environments and secure schools, to large placements more akin to a prison. Many countries hold young people in custodial placements separately from adults, but not all. Detaining young people in establishments alongside adults is associated with higher levels of mental health disorders for young people, in addition to raising safeguarding and developmental issues (Woolard *et al.*, 2005; Ng *et al.*, 2011).

Some larger establishments have separate mental health units, where more intensive care can be provided. However, these units rarely provide the equivalent standard of care as delivered in a hospital. Different legislation may also apply in respect to enforced mental health treatment compared with that used in hospitals. Despite these differences, the facilities may be misleadingly referred to as the "prison hospital" or "hospital wing."

With the elevated prevalence of NDDs among justice-involved young people, concerns have been expressed that this cohort may struggle disproportionately when detained, as prisons and police custodial settings are often noisy, bright, and busy. In response, some establishments have adapted their environments and processes to become more responsive to the needs of neurodiverse individuals (Lewis *et al.*, 2015).

For detained mentally disordered young people whose mental health needs cannot be met within criminal justice placements, it may be possible to transfer them to a secure mental health hospital in the community for a period of treatment.

If serious mental health issues are evident at the point of sentencing, some countries may sentence an individual to detention in a secure mental health hospital instead of in a justice setting. Such sentences are a form of mental health diversion. These orders are often indeterminate in length, with the end point being influenced by the individual's mental health, response to treatment, and residual risk.

Reintegration into the community

Relatively little attention has been paid to what happens to the health of young people once their contact with the CJS ends (Wilson & Tully, 2009). Contact with the CJS can be associated with identification and treatment of previously overlooked health issues, but these gains may not be sustained once justice involvement ends. This is especially true for young people who have been detained in facilities some distance from their home location.

Plans to ensure continuity of care and community linkages should begin far in advance to avoid breaks in medication or loss of mental health support. In some countries (e.g., England), regional community FCAMHS are actively involved in release planning of detained young people and support the transfer of care to local health care providers.

Assessment issues

Assessments undertaken within a criminal justice context have many similarities with assessments of young people in any context (see Chapter 27).

Those assessing justice-involved children should have training in working with children but, if not, assessments should demonstrate an understanding that presentations of mental health conditions may differ and be less clear-cut than in adults, and a recognition that children are still developing and so can grow out of difficulties as well as into them.

Many justice-involved young people experience multiple assessments by different professionals, necessitating reiteration of histories which are often characterized by trauma. Reading preexisting records and reports prior to seeing the young person allows the assessor to learn about the child in advance, enabling anticipation of sensitive areas and highlighting any inconsistencies and discrepancies that should be explored.

Safety issues should be considered before undertaking an assessment, especially where there is a history of violence. Seeking advice from carers and reviewing records is recommended.

Assessments could, if feasible, include interviewing a parent or carer. Detained young people may be located away from their families but interviews can be undertaken by telephone or virtually. Difficulties in obtaining collateral information might arise if family members are victims of the (alleged) offense.

Given the high rates of neurodiversity and communication disorders in this population, particular care should be taken in assessing for these conditions.

Assessments of (alleged) offending behavior will be influenced by the legal context. They will differ depending on whether the young person:

- is considered at risk of offending and is being seen preemptively,
- has been charged with an offense and is awaiting trial, or
- has been convicted and is participating in rehabilitation.

It is important to caution young people regarding confidentiality limits if assessing pre-trial, so they understand that anything they disclose about the offense could be entered as evidence.

Assessment of violence risk often forms part of assessments. Structured approaches to assessing risk of dangerousness have been advocated. This involves using tools incorporating a set of risk markers or predictors associated with criminal and violent outcomes. Historically, these have been predominantly actuarial tools, which provide a probability score for future risk, or structured clinical (or professional) judgment (SCJ/SPJ) instruments, where a list of risk factors is used as a framework by which a professional makes a risk categorization (e.g., high or low), allowing for some formulation of risk based on these factors and their imminence. This is a false dichotomy—no actuarial risk tools should be used in isolation from professional decision-making. Rather, they should be used to support, complement, and enhance professional judgment. Newer tools have focused on protective and resilience factors—a more positive framing of risk assessment—but often rely on factors that are simply the inverse of risk factors.

Guidelines exist recommending a minimum set of characteristics for risk assessment tools to be evidence-based (Fazel & Wolf 2018). External validation is the key test of whether a tool can accurately predict outcomes. Development samples tend to overestimate performance. Reporting the accuracy of tools is often poorly done. Sensitivity (the proportion of people who have the outcome and scored high risk by a tool) is one key metric to consider (which relies on a cutoff), alongside calibration and overall discrimination. Evaluating tools on the basis of one performance measure should be avoided.

A review of risk assessment studies for young people found that few reported multiple performance measures, making new tools difficult to appraise (Senior *et al.*, 2021). A 2011 meta-analysis found one tool, the Structured Assessment of Violence Risk in Youth (SAVRY), had higher measures of discrimination (area under the curve [AUC] and classification) than other tools at the time, but comparative performance research needs updating (Singh *et al.*, 2011).

These systematic reviews of risk assessment tools suggest caution is needed in evaluating claims about the evidence for individual tools. Almost all studies fail to report key measures of accuracy, the development of tools is not transparent, and internal and external validations are of low quality and underpowered.

However, as a support to clinical and professional decision-making, they have a role in highlighting key risk factors, provide consistency to assessment, anchor decision-making in empirical evidence, and counter the overreliance on recent events and low sensitivity (i.e., too many false negatives) that seems to characterize unstructured clinical risk assessment for violence (Whiting *et al.*, 2023).

Time spent on risk assessment must be balanced by resources allocated to treatment and management. Many current tools, especially the SCJ ones, are probably too time-consuming for new services given the lack of empirical evidence of their added value. Ultimately, trials are needed to show that a particular risk assessment tool, if introduced to a service, reduces offending outcomes and improves health.

Assessors must also remember that adolescents may simultaneously present a risk to others and be vulnerable to harm, and ensure that safeguarding issues are adequately addressed.

Interventions

Forensic mental health evaluations often rely on before-and-after studies, which are limited in their ability to account for other factors that may explain any change in outcomes, including time and nonspecific effects of a change in therapeutic culture in a particular setting.

Many trauma-based therapies have been introduced based on this type of evidence, but they require randomized controlled trials (RCTs) to demonstrate their effectiveness, particularly if they are resource-intensive. Despite its wholescale adoption in many parts of the CJS, there is currently no RCT evidence that any trauma-based treatment for detained young people improves mental health (Yoon *et al.*, 2017) or recidivism outcomes (Beaudry *et al.*, 2021b).

Other treatments being trialed in adolescent forensic mental health include mindfulness-based treatments, and multisystemic and action-based (e.g., sport, drama) therapies.

One recent RCT for ADHD medication found no benefits for intra-institutional outcomes and symptom scores in detained young people, but the inclusion criteria meant many people without clinical ADHD were included (Asherson *et al.*, 2023), diluting any effects. Others reported, in both smaller randomized trials and large observational studies, clear protective effects of ADHD medication in people with confirmed clinical diagnoses (Lichtenstein *et al.*, 2012).

One challenge is the assessment of treatment needs. In England, NHS England's Framework for Integrated Care has been developed to inform interventions for young people in secure settings, and aims to promote consistent, trauma-informed, formulation-driven, evidence-based care. An independent evaluation suggested that the Framework's formulation-driven approach improved communication, assisted with shared goal setting'(Anna Freud, 2022; Jacob *et al.*, 2024).

Interventions to reduce suicidal risk within criminal justice populations (Marzano *et al.*, 2016) found assessment and treatment are required throughout the various pathways, including before being admitted to forensic services or prison.

On discharge, continuity of treatment and linkage between services is key. Practical considerations relating to interventional work include information sharing, sequencing of interventions, consideration of who delivers treatments (including youth workers, who have most contact but may have limited training), maintenance of gains from forensic to community settings, and possible family involvement.

Professional considerations

Young people within the CJS often have multiple challenges and many agencies involved in their care. It is important that mental health professionals working in this field maintain clarity of purpose and have a good understanding of how their work and skills contribute to the overall management of each young person, while maintaining effective and harmonious relationships with colleagues.

Forensic adolescent mental health involves dealing with high levels of complexity and can raise ethical dilemmas (Eastman & McInerny, 1997; Kaltiala-Heino & Eronen, 2015). Mental health practitioners should maintain high standards of integrity and professionalism and ensure their practice is concordant with relevant professional guidelines. Acute ethical challenges arise in jurisdictions where children can be subject to the death penalty and psychiatrists may be called on to certify them "competent for execution." The World Psychiatric Association's Declaration on the Participation of Psychiatrists in the Death Penalty (World Psychiatric Association, 1989) states that work of this nature is a violation of professional ethics.

Many forensic CAMH professionals work in disciplinary isolation. Participation in regular peer discussion groups (possibly virtually) with others from the same discipline may provide a valuable forum in which to reflect on challenging and sometimes distressing issues and reduce the risk of drift in standards of practice. Resources such as the UK Royal College of Psychiatrists' e-modules in forensic adolescent psychiatry may provide further opportunities for skills development and professional benchmarking (Hales & Lewis, 2022a; Hales & Lewis, 2022b).

In addition to direct therapeutic work with young people, many forensic child and adolescent professionals undertake expert witness work, providing reports and testimony to courts to assist them in understanding clinical matters. These reports may address pre-trial issues, such as fitness to plead and the need for special measures for effective participation, or psychiatric defenses, mitigations, opinions on risk, or recommendations about disposal.

Psychiatrists or psychologists who undertake expert witness work with young people should aim to demonstrate competence, experience, and up-to-date expertise of working with children so they are able to provide developmentally nuanced opinions.

Expert witness opinions should be objective, supported by facts, within the limits of the expert's sphere of competence and be uninfluenced by whether they have been instructed by defense or prosecution. It is unwise for professionals to provide reports about patients with whom they are directly working, as their objectivity may be compromised by the preexisting therapeutic relationship. Expert witnesses continue to have a duty of care to those they are assessing and should be responsive to safeguarding issues that may be identified in the course of this work.

Expert Witness Standards and Guidance have been developed in the UK (British Psychological Society, 2021; Royal College of Psychiatrists, 2023) and skills development courses are becoming widespread.

Conclusions

Forensic CAMH is an important subspeciality, providing the opportunity for meaningful intervention at pivotal moments in a young person's life—often with long-term effects for the individual and society. It is ethically, intellectually, and clinically challenging and involves working across an interesting range of clinical and justice settings.

References

Abram, K.A. *et al.* (2008) Perceived barriers to mental health services among youths in detention. *Journal of the American Academy of Child and Adolescent Psychiatry* **47**, 301–308.

Ali, S. (2018) Autistic spectrum disorder and offending behaviour—a brief review of the literature. *Advances in Autism* **4**, 109–121.

Anna Freud (2022) The Framework for Integrated Care (SECURE STAIRS). Anna Freud, London. Available: https://www.annafreud.org/research/past-research-projects/the-framework-for-integrated-care-secure-stairs/ [8 December 2024].

Asherson, P. *et al.* (2023) Randomised controlled trial of the short-term effects of osmotic-release oral system methylphenidate on symptoms and behavioural outcomes in young male prisoners with attention deficit hyperactivity disorder: CIAO-II study. *The British Journal of Psychiatry* **222**(1), 7–17. doi:10.1192/bjp.2022.77.

Baldry, E. *et al.* (2017) 'Cruel and unusual punishment': an inter-jurisdictional study of the criminalisation of young people with complex support needs. *Journal of Youth Studies* **21**(5), 636–652.

Balogun, T. *et al.* (2018) Does juvenile detention impact health? *Journal of Correctional Health Care* **24**, 137–144.

Barboni, L. *et al.* (2023) Predictive validity of the structured assessment of violence risk in youth (SAVRY) on the recidivism of juvenile offenders: a systematic review. *Psychology, Crime and Law* **30**(10), 1508–1534. doi:10.1080/1068316X.2023.2214661.

Barnert, E.S. *et al.* (2016) Juvenile incarceration and health. *Academic Pediatrics* **16**, 99–109.

Beaudry, G. *et al.* (2021a) An updated systematic review and meta-regression analysis: mental disorders among adolescents in juvenile detention and correctional facilities. *Journal of the American Academy of Child and Adolescent Psychiatry* **60**, 46–60.

Beaudry, G. *et al.* (2021b) Effectiveness of psychological interventions in prison to reduce recidivism: a systematic review and meta-analysis of randomised controlled trials. *The Lancet Psychiatry* **8**(9), 759–773. doi:10.1016/s2215-0366(21)00170-x.

Borschmann, R. *et al.* (2014) Self-harm in young offenders. *Suicide and Life-threatening Behavior* **44**, 641–652.

Borschmann, R. *et al.* (2020) The health of adolescents in detention: a global scoping review. *The Lancet Public Health* **5**, e114–e126.

Bower, C. *et al.* (2018) Fetal alcohol spectrum disorder and youth justice: a prevalence study among young people sentenced to detention in Western Australia. *BMJ Open* **8**, e019605.

British Psychological Society (2021) Psychologists as Expert Witnesses. Best Practice Guidelines for Psychologists. Available at: https://explore.bps.org.uk/content/report-guideline/bpsrep.2021.rep157 [15 July 2023].

Case, S. & Browning, A. (2021) Child First Justice: The Research Evidence-base. [online]. Available at: https://hdl.handle.net/2134/14152040.v1 [9 July 2023].

Cooper, P. & Mattison, M. (2017) Intermediaries, vulnerable people and the quality of evidence. *The International Journal of Evidence & Proof* **21**(4), 351–370.

Council of Europe (2010) Guidelines of the Committee of Ministers of the Council of Europe on child-friendly justice. Council of Europe, Strasbourg, France. Available: https://rm.coe.int/16804b2cf3 [9 July 2023].

Day, A.-M. (2022) It's a hard balance to find': the perspectives of youth justice practitioners in England on the place of 'risk' in an emerging 'child-first'. *World Youth Justice* **23**(1), 58–75.

Dirkzwager, A.J. *et al.* (2021) Mental and physical health problems before and after detention: a matched cohort study. *The Lancet Regional Health—Europe* **8**, 100154.

Eastman, N. & McInerny, T. (1997) Psychiatrists and the death penalty: ethical principles and analogies. *The Journal of Forensic Psychiatry* **8**(3), 583–601.

Elgar, F.J. *et al.* (2003) Behavioural and substance use problems in rural and urban delinquent youths. *The Canadian Journal of Psychiatry* **48**, 633–636.

Farrer, T.J. *et al.* (2013) Prevalence of traumatic brain injury in juvenile offenders: a meta-analysis. *Child Neuropsychology* **19**, 225–234.

Farrington, D. (2002) Developmental criminology and risk focused prevention. In: *The Oxford Handbook of Criminology*. (eds M. Maguire, *et al.*), 3rd edn. Oxford University Press, Oxford, UK. pp. 657–701.

Farrugia, L. & Gabbert, F. (2019) The 'appropriate adult': what they do and what they should do in police interviews with mentally disordered suspects. *Criminal Behaviour and Mental Health* **29**(3).

Fazel, S. & Baillargeon, J.G. (2011) The health of prisoners. *The Lancet* **377**, 956–965.

Fazel, S. & Wolf, A. (2018) Selecting a risk assessment tool to use in practice: a 10-point guide. *Evidence-Based Mental Health* **21**(2), 41–43. doi:10.1136/eb-2017-102861.

Fazel, S. *et al.* (2008) Mental disorders among adolescents in juvenile detention and correctional facilities: a systematic review and meta-regression analysis of 25 surveys. *Journal of the American Academy of Child & Adolescent Psychiatry* **47**, 1010–1019.

Feinstein, R.A. *et al.* (1998) Medical status of adolescents at time of admission to a juvenile detention center. *The Journal of Adolescent Health* **22**, 190–196.

Gallagher, C.A. & Dobrin, A. (2006a) Deaths in juvenile justice residential facilities. *Journal of Adolescent Health* **38**, 662–668.

Gallagher, C.A. & Dobrin, A. (2006b) Facility-level characteristics associated with serious suicide attempts and deaths from suicide in juvenile justice residential facilities. *Suicide and Life Threatening Behaviors* **36**, 363–375.

Gregory, J. & Bryan, K. (2015) Speech and language therapy intervention with a group of persistent and prolific young offenders in a non-custodial setting with previously undiagnosed speech, language and communication difficulties. *International Journal of Language & Communication Disorders*, 1–14.

Griffiths, G. & Norris, G. (2020) Explaining the crime drop: contributions to declining crime rates from youth cohorts since 2005. *Crime Law and Social Change* **73**, 25–53.

Gudjonsson, G. *et al.* (2006) Custodial interrogation, false confession and individual differences: a national study among Icelandic youth. *Personality and Individual Differences* **41**, 49–59.

Hales, H. & Lewis, A. (2022a) Introduction and Structure. CPD e-module Royal College of Psychiatrists. Royal College of Psychiatrists, London. Available: https://elearninghub.rcpsych.ac.uk/product?catalog=004_CORE_LM_Ad_For_Psych_2021 [13 July 2023].

Hales, H. & Lewis, A. (2022b) Adolescent forensic psychiatry: Part 2—Assessment and Treatment. Royal College of Psychiatrists, London. Available: https://elearninghub.rcpsych.ac.uk/product?catalog=242_CORE_LM_Ad_For_Psych2_2022 [Accessed 13 July 2023].

Hamer, D. & Crofts, T. (2023) The logic and value of the presumption of *Doli Incapax* (failing that, an incapacity defence). *Oxford Journal of Legal Studies* **43**(3), 546–571.

Haney-Caron, E. *et al.* (2018) Self-perceived likelihood of false confession: a comparison of justice-involved juveniles and adults. *Criminal Justice and Behavior* **45**(12), 1955–1976.

Hawton, K. *et al.* (2014) Self-harm in prisons in England and Wales: an epidemiological study of prevalence, risk factors, clustering, and subsequent suicide. *The Lancet* **383**(9923), 1147–1154.

Hindley, N. *et al.* (2017) Forensic mental health services for children and adolescents: rationale and development. *BJPsych Advances* **23**(1), 36–43.

Howard, K. *et al.* (2020) What is communication assistance? Describing a new and emerging profession in the New Zealand youth justice system. *Psychiatry, Psychology and Law*, 1–15.

Hughes, N. (2015) Understanding the influence of neurodevelopmental disorders on offending: Utilizing developmental psychopathology in biosocial criminology. *Criminal Justice Studies* **28**, 39–60.

Hughes, N. *et al.* (2015) The prevalence of traumatic brain injury among young offenders in custody: a systematic review. *Journal of Head Trauma Rehabilitation* **30**, 94–105.

Hughes, N. *et al.* (2020) Health determinants of adolescent criminalisation. *The Lancet Child and Adolescent Health* **4**, 151–162.

Jacob, J. *et al.* (2024) "I'm not just some criminal, I'm actually a person to them now": the importance of child-staff therapeutic relationships in the children and young people secure estate. *International Journal of Forensic Mental Health* **23**(1), 24–36. doi:10.1080/14999013.2023.2167893.

Kaltiala-Heino, R. & Eronen, M. (2015) Ethical issues in child and adolescent forensic psychiatry: a review. *The Journal of Forensic Psychiatry & Psychology* **26**(6), 759–780.

Kemp, K. *et al.* (2016) Suicidal ideation and attempts among court-involved, nonincarcerated youth. *Journal of Forensic Psychology Practice* **16**(3), 169–181.

Kemp, K. *et al.* (2022) Suicide screening among youth at first court contact. *Archives of Suicide Research* **26**(2), 748–760. doi:10.1080/13811118.2020.1833795.

Kemp, V. & Watkins, D. (2022) Exploring children's understanding of the legal rights of suspects in England and Wales. *Youth Justice* **22**(3), 320–338. doi:10.1177/14732254211030597.

Kinner, S.A. & Wang, E.A. (2014) The case for improving the health of ex-prisoners. *American Journal of Public Health* **104**, 1352–1355.

Kinner, S.A. *et al.* (2015) Substance use and risk of death in young offenders: a prospective data linkage study. *Drug and Alcohol Review* **34**(1), 46–50.

Kinner, S.A. *et al.* (2018) Age-specific global prevalence of hepatitis B, hepatitis C, HIV, and tuberculosis among incarcerated people: a systematic review. *Journal of Adolescent Health* **62**, S18–S26.

Klose, H. & Gordon, F. (2023) Public health approaches to youth involvement in violence: examining stakeholders' perspectives in Australia and the United Kingdom. *Journal of Criminology* **56**(1), 98–115.

Koh, L.L. *et al.* (2020) The predictive validity of youth violence risk assessment tools: a systematic review. *Psychology, Crime & Law* **26**, 1–21.

League of Arab States (1994) *Arab Charter on Human Rights*. League of Arab States, Cairo. Available: https://www.refworld.org/docid/3ae6b38540.html [8 July 2023].

Lewis, A. *et al.* (2015) Development and implementation of autism standards for prisons. *Journal of Intellectual Disabilities and Offending Behaviour* **6**(2), 68–80.

Lichtenstein, P. *et al.* (2012) Medication for attention deficit-hyperactivity disorder and criminality. *The New England Journal of Medicine* **367**(21), 2006–2014. doi:10.1056/NEJMoa1203241.

Liebmann, M. (2007) *Restorative Justice: How It Works.* Jessica Kingsley Publishers, London; Philadelphia, PA.

Liefaard, T. (2020) Child-friendly justice and procedural safeguards for children in criminal proceedings: new momentum for children in conflict with the Law? *Bergen Journal of Criminal Law & Criminal Justice* **8**(1), 17.

Lieser, A.M. *et al.* (2019) You have the right to remain silent: the ability of adolescents with developmental language disorder to understand their legal rights. *Journal of Communication Disorders* **82**, 105920.

Loeber, R. & Farrington, D.P. (2000) Young children who commit crime: epidemiology, developmental origins, risk factors, early interventions, and policy implications. *Development and Psychopathology* **12**, 737–762.

Lundström, S. *et al.* (2014) Childhood neurodevelopmental disorders and violent criminality: a sibling control study. *Journal of Autism and Developmental Disorders* **44**, 2707–2716.

Marzano, L. *et al.* (2016) Prevention of suicidal behavior in prisons: an overview of initiatives based on a systematic review of research on near-lethal suicide attempts. *Crisis* **37**(5), 323–334.

May, P.A. *et al.* (2009) Prevalence and epidemiologic characteristics of FASD from various research methods with an emphasis on recent in-school studies. *Developmental Disabilities Research Reviews* **15**, 176–192.

McKay, J. & Neal, J. (2009) Diagnosis and disengagement: exploring the disjuncture between SEN policy and practice. *Journal of Research in Special Educational Needs* **9**, 164–172.

National Collaborating Centre for Mental Health (2009) *Attention Deficit Hyperactivity Disorder: Diagnosis and Management of ADHD in Children, Young People and Adults.* National Collaborating Centre for Mental Health, London.

Ng, I.Y. *et al.* (2011) Incarcerating juveniles in adult prisons as a factor in depression. *Criminal Behaviour and Mental Health* **21**(1), 21–34.

Noroozi, M. *et al.* (2019) Evaluation of the minimum age for consent to mental health treatment with the minimum age of criminal responsibility in children and adolescents: a global comparison. *BMJ Mental Health* **21**, 82–86.

Organization of African Unity (1990) *African Charter on the Rights and Welfare of the Child.* Organization of African Unity (OAU), Addis Ababa. Available: https://www.refworld.org/docid/3ae6b38c18.html [8 July 2023].

Patton, G.C. *et al.* (2016) Our future: a Lancet Commission on adolescent health and wellbeing. *The Lancet* **387**, 2423–2478.

Penal Reform International (2013) The Minimum Age of Criminal Responsibility. [online]. Penal Reform International, London. Available: https://cdn.penalreform.org/wp-content/uploads/2013/05/justice-for-children-briefing-4-v6-web_0.pdf [31 October 2024].

Puglisi, L.B. & Wang, E.A. (2021) Health care for people who are incarcerated. *Nature Reviews Disease Primers* **7**, 50.

Rojas, E.Y. & Gretton, H.M. (2007) Background, offence characteristics, and criminal outcomes of aboriginal youth who sexually offend: a closer look at aboriginal youth intervention needs. *Sexual Abuse* **19**, 257–283.

Royal College of Psychiatrists (2023) *Responsibilities of Psychiatrists Who Provide Expert Evidence to Courts and Tribunals.* College Report CR193, Royal College of Psychiatrists, London. Available: www.rcpsych.ac.uk/docs/default-source/improving-care/better-mh-policy/college-reports/college-report-cr193.pdf?sfvrsn=c0381b24_2 [11 July 2023].

Senior, M. *et al.* (2021) Prediction models for child and adolescent mental health: a systematic review of methodology and reporting in recent research. *JCPP Advances* **9**(3), e12034.

Sharf, A.J. *et al.* (2017) Reasoning your way out of Miranda rights: how juvenile detainees relinquish their fifth amendment protections. *Translational Issues in Psychological Science* **3**(2), 121–130.

Shonkoff, J.P. *et al.* (2012) The lifelong effects of early childhood adversity and toxic stress. *Pediatrics* **129**, e232–e246.

Shuttleworth, R. (2022) The impact of incarceration on health outcomes: a global systematic review. Unpublished MPH thesis; The University of Melbourne, Australia.

Singh, J.P. *et al.* (2011) A comparative study of violence risk assessment tools: a systematic review and metaregression analysis of 68 studies involving 25,980 participants. *Clinical Psychology Review* **31**(3), 499–513.

Smalarz, L. *et al.* (2016) Miranda at 50: a psychological analysis. *Current Directions in Psychological Science* **25**, 455–460.

Smith, A. *et al.* (2013) *Time Out III: A Profile of BC Youth in Custody.* McCreary Centre Society, Vancouver, BC.

Snow, P.C. (2019) Speech-language pathology and the youth offender: epidemiological overview and roadmap for future speech-language pathology research and scope of practice. *Language, Speech, and Hearing Services in Schools* **50**(2), 324–339.

Snow, P.C. & Powell, M.B. (2011) Oral language competence in incarcerated young offenders: links with offending severity. *International Journal of Speech-Language Pathology* **13**, 480–489.

Steinberg, L. & Icenogle, G. (2019) Using developmental science to distinguish adolescents and adults under the Law. *Annual Review of Developmental Psychology* **1**(1), 21–40.

The Advocate's Gateway (2017) *Effective participation of young defendants* (Toolkit 8). The Advocate's Gateway, London. Available: https://www.ohchr.org/en/instruments-mechanisms/instruments/united-nations-standard-minimum-rules-administration-juvenile [6 December 2024]

Tran, N.T. *et al.* (2018) Words matter: a call for humanizing and respectful language to describe people who experience incarceration. *BMC International Health and Human Rights* **18**, 41. doi:10.1186/s12914-018-0180-4.

United Nations (1986) *United Nations Standard Minimum Rules for the Administration of Juvenile Justice (The Beijing Rules).* United Nations, New York. Available: https://www.ohchr.org/en/instruments-mechanisms/instruments/united-nations-standard-minimum-rules-administration-juvenile [11 July 2023].

United Nations (1990a) *United Nations Convention on the Rights of the Child.* United Nations, New York. Available: https://www.unicef.org/child-rights-convention/convention-text [8 July 2023].

United Nations (1990b) *Guidelines for the Prevention of Juvenile Delinquency (The Riyadh Guidelines).* United Nations, New York. Available: https://www.ohchr.org/en/instruments-mechanisms/

instruments/united-nations-guidelines-prevention-juvenile-delinquency-riyadh [10 July 2023].

United Nations (1990c) *Rules for the Protection of Juveniles Deprived of their Liberty (the 'Havana Rules')*. United Nations, New York. Available: https://www.ohchr.org/en/instruments-mechanisms/instruments/united-nations-rules-protection-juveniles-deprived-their-liberty [10 July 2023].

United Nations (2007) *General Comment 10: Children's Rights in Juvenile Justice*. United Nations, New York. Available: https://www2.ohchr.org/english/bodies/crc/docs/CRC.C.GC.10.pdf [8 July 2023].

United Nations (2010) *Rules for the Treatment of Women Prisoners and Non-custodial Measures for Women Offenders (Bangkok Rules)*. United Nations, New York. Available: https://www.ohchr.org/sites/default/files/Documents/ProfessionalInterest/BangkokRules.pdf [10 July 2023].

United Nations (2019a) *General Comment No. 24: Children's Rights in the Child Justice System*. United Nations, New York. Available: https://www.ohchr.org/en/documents/general-comments-and-recommendations/general-comment-no-24-2019-childrens-rights-child [8 July 2023].

United Nations (2019b) *Global Study on Children Deprived of Liberty*. United Nations, New York. Available:https://www.ohchr.org/en/treaty-bodies/crc/united-nations-global-study-children-deprived-liberty [7 July 2023].

Whiting, D. *et al.* (2023) Assessing violence risk in first-episode psychosis: external validation, updating and net benefit of a prediction tool (OxMIV). *BMJ Mental Health* **26**, e300634.

Williams, W.H. *et al.* (2018) Traumatic brain injury: a potential cause of violent crime? *The Lancet Psychiatry* **5**(10), 836–844.

Wilson, A. & Tully, P. (2009) Reintegrating young offenders into the community through discharge planning: a review of interventions and needs of youth in secure care. *Australian Journal of Primary Health* **15**(2), 166.

Wilson, D.B. *et al.* (2018) Police-initiated diversion for youth to prevent future delinquent behavior: a systematic review. *Campbell Systematic Reviews* **14**(1), 1–88.

Woolard, J.L. *et al.* (2005) Juveniles within adult correctional settings: legal pathways and developmental considerations. *International Journal of Forensic Mental Health* **4**(1), 1–18.

World Psychiatric Association (1989) *Declaration on the Participation of Psychiatrists in the Death Penalty*. Worl Psychiatric Association (WPA), Geneva Switzerland. Available: https://www.wpanet.org/declaration-on-the-participation-of [11 July 2023].

Yoon, I.A. *et al.* (2017) Outcomes of psychological therapies for prisoners with mental health problems: a systematic review and meta-analysis. *Journal of Consulting and Clinical Psychology* **85**(8), 783–802.

Zhou, J. *et al.* (2012) Psychiatric disorders in adolescent boys in detention: a preliminary prevalence and case–control study in two Chinese provinces. *Journal of Forensic Psychiatry and Psychology* **23**, 664–675.

CHAPTER 48

Intensive community services, day units, and inpatient services

Andy Cotgrove[1], Bernadka Dubicka[2,3,4] and Gabrielle A. Carlson[5]

[1] Formerly Consultant in Adolescent Psychiatry, Cheshire and Wirral Partnership NHS Foundation Trust, UK

[2] Hull York Medical School, University of Hull/University of York, Kingston upon Hull/York, UK

[3] Greater Manchester Mental Health NHS Foundation Trust, Prestwich, UK

[4] Manchester Academic Health Science Centre, University of Manchester, Manchester, UK

[5] Renaissance School of Medicine at Stony Brook University, Stony Brook, NY, USA

Introduction

Historically, the delivery of intensive interventions has been centered around inpatient services. While most accept there will always be a role for beds in the management of the highest risk children and young people (CYP) and those with the most complex and severe mental health needs, increasingly we are seeing the development of community-based alternative modalities of intervention. This is driven, at least in part, by a recognition that alongside the benefits of admission, for some, it can be harmful.

Research in intensive community alternatives to admission suggests that many of these alternatives provide at least as good clinical outcomes, if not better, but with fewer risks and harms, as well as being more cost-effective.

There is no generally accepted definition for intensive intervention services. However, they share some common features:

- manage CYP presenting with high levels of severity, complexity, and risk
- multimodal interventions
- delivered on a frequent basis
- delivered by professionals with specialist skills and working with a small caseload
- often cover larger geographical areas, compared to standard community services

While some intensive services described in this chapter are disorder specific, others treat a range of severe disorders. We review the key principles underpinning the design of intensive services and outline available evidence on a range of service delivery models. We describe different models of service delivery, namely community models of intensive services, day programs, and inpatient models, to reflect increasing intensity and level of restriction. We will review some of the key current challenges including workforce shortages, ensuring quality, and developing a robust evidence base to guide future service developments.

We acknowledge that there are wide variations in service delivery, both within and between countries, and the available evidence needs to be reviewed within the context in which it was conducted.

Key principles and considerations

Forms and functions of intensive services

The form of a service should be designed to fulfill a clear and specific function. The following factors to be considered:

- the size of the population,
- the needs of that population, and
- the functions (or interventions) that are required to address those needs.

For example, a service for CYP with eating disorders may cover a total population of 1 million, from which you estimate how many will have an eating disorder. Criteria for accessing this service should be set, which may relate to severity, and then the functions (treatments and interventions) that are delivered to meet the needs of these CYP should be decided upon. The form of the service should be determined by the functions required to meet the need. This may be outpatient services, home-based treatments, or day or inpatient services. Form should follow function, rather than follow what is available (e.g., inpatient services) or what is funded. It should be noted that the needs of a population will differ by place and by time. For example, there was an increased prevalence of eating disorders after the COVID-19 pandemic.

Rutter's Child and Adolescent Psychiatry and Psychology, Seventh Edition.
Edited by Anita Thapar, Daniel S. Pine, Samuele Cortese, Cathy Creswell, Tamsin J. Ford, James F. Leckman, and Argyris Stringaris.

Companion website: www.wiley.com/go/thapar/rutterspsych7

When reviewing or designing services, professionals, families, and CYP should be involved and work together following the principles of "coproduction" or "participation." A "values-based" approach should be followed where what is important to all stakeholders is considered (Royal College of Psychiatrists, 2016). Services and interventions should be delivered according to the available evidence base.

Criteria for accessing intensive services

Box 48.1 Summary of functions of intensive services and criteria for access

1. Risk management
2. Intensive intervention not available in other services
3. Intensive or specialist assessment

Risk management

Risk management covers high levels of risk secondary to suicidal thoughts or behaviors, self-neglect, or disordered/abnormal thinking, and/or danger to others due to a mental health disorder (or suspected disorder), beyond the capacity of the family and routine community-based services to manage. The intervention used should be expected to reduce this risk.

Intensive intervention not available in other services

This is commonly the case when a disorder is severe, complex, associated with other psychosocial difficulties and/or comorbid disorder, and resulting in difficulties pervading all aspects of the CYP's life and multimodal interventions are required.

Intensive or specialist assessment

Most specialist assessments, such as cognitive and neurodevelopmental assessments, or physical investigations, can and should be carried out in the community. Occasionally, inpatient assessments can add to this by providing 24-hour observation of behavior and interactions with others, or observing the effects of a specific intervention such as the use of medication.

Assessment procedure

Decisions regarding the most appropriate intervention are based on information gathered from a biopsychosocial assessment and diagnostic formulation (see Chapters 27 and 28). Multiple sources should be used, and duplication avoided, but there is still a need for clinicians to carry out a direct assessment to start engaging the child or young person, assess motivation, and clarify aims and objectives with them and their family. Enhancing motivation will improve outcomes. Clear aims and objectives can be helpful in clarifying motivation for change and to gauge progress during treatment.

Inpatient services must be able to respond immediately to CYP in crisis. However, accepting admissions without a comprehensive biopsychosocial preadmission assessment and clear, agreed aims can result in admissions that could have been better managed with intensive community interventions. Crisis admissions can lead to an escalation and/or reinforcement of risky and other unhelpful behaviors, resulting in negative outcomes for the CYP.

The completed assessment needs to guide the intervention providing the:

- least restrictive environment needed to address the identified mental health problems,
- best patient experience and CYP centered intervention,
- best support for parents and carers,
- service closest to home,
- safest intervention (including therapeutic risk-taking, e.g., not admitting to avoid the associated risks of admission, see Box 48.5),
- most clinically effective, evidence-based intervention, and
- appropriate interagency/multisystem involvement, collaboration, and equality of access.

These principles were first clearly articulated in the US Child and Adolescent Service System Program (CASSP) (National Institute of Mental Health, 1983).

Structured assessment tools, such as The Child and Adolescent Service Intensity Instrument (CASII) (Fallon *et al.*, 2006), can provide a multidimensional systematic process for assessing the degree of intensity of services needed (risk of harm, functional status, co-occurring conditions, recovery environment, resilience, and involvement of services).

Collaborative working across systems and agencies

Multiagency collaboration is vital for CYP with complex needs to ensure their care and educational needs are met alongside mental health needs, as well as facilitating timely discharge from inpatient services. There is a wealth of qualitative evidence on what factors facilitate or act as barriers to effective multiagency working, but little research that shows definitively that multiagency working improves outcomes (as opposed to the individual components of a multiagency intervention). Cooper *et al.* (2016) found the factors most commonly identified as facilitating interagency collaboration were good communication, joint training, understanding and mutual valuing across agencies, senior management support, protocols on interagency collaboration, and a named link person.

International context

Most of the evidence cited in this chapter is based on research carried out in high-income countries (HICs). There is less published from low- and middle-income countries (LMICs, see Chapter 46). However, many of the studies from around the world are relevant internationally. With inpatient units often being the most expensive service provision, evidence to support intensive community provision is particularly useful for LMICs with more limited resources. While inpatient facilities are much needed for severe mental health conditions in LMICs, early interventions using transdiagnostic, task-shifting approaches in primary health care systems are potentially more feasible, scalable, and cost-effective (Hamdani *et al.*, 2021). Potentially cost-effective systems of care have been reported in LMICs utilizing volunteers in villages, outreach medical practitioners with skills across a range of specialties, and creative use of hospital beds in wards for physical as well as mental health difficulties. In addition, many CYP with mental health problems in LMICs may seek help first from traditional and religious healers because that is what is available and affordable, or driven by local belief systems that mental illness is a spiritual problem. Collaborations between psychiatrists and traditional healers can help to improve outcomes. Despite significant differences in resources and services, the principles of care and use of evidence base is relevant to both HICs and LMICs.

Perhaps more surprising are the differences between HICs. For example, the mean average length of stay can range from 9 days in Australia and Sweden to 125 days in England (NHS Benchmarking Network, 2022). Lengths of stay can also vary between facilities within a country, and there is little evidence of agreement around admission and discharge criteria (Evans *et al.*, 2020). With quite different funding arrangements, services may be configured according to finance rather than function as perhaps most starkly illustrated by the differences between the US and the UK. In the US services are funded predominantly through insurance, with a safety net of minimal provision funded by a state and federal program (Medicaid). Insurance companies determine what they will fund, often based on diagnosis. This can result in excessive diagnoses of disorders attracting the most funding. In the UK, by contrast, most funding for intensive services comes from the state via the National Health Service (NHS), even if some providers of care are privately run. Interventions are based on perceived need, not diagnosis. For example, CYP in the UK admitted with suicidal behaviors may be diagnosed with a borderline personality disorder, but in the US this diagnosis would not entitle them to inpatient treatment, although a diagnosis of depression would.

Service models

Box 48.2 Summary of key service models

Intensive community interventions:
- intensive crisis interventions
- targeted community interventions designed to treat specific disorders:
  - multisystemic therapy (MST)
  - dialectical behavior therapy (DBT)
  - treatment foster care
  - eating disorder services
- other models of intensive community or home treatment:
  - case management and wraparound
  - intensive home-based treatment

Day patient treatment and partial hospitalization

Inpatient treatment
- general purpose units for children and young people (CYP)
- specialist units, e.g., eating disorder units
- intensive care, secure, and forensic units
- supported discharge and step-down care

Intensive community interventions

Intensive community interventions broadly fall into three categories, with different service models within each category:
- intensive crisis services
- targeted community interventions for specific disorders or symptoms (e.g., eating disorder, self-harm)
- other intensive community home-based interventions effective for a range of psychosocial difficulties and mental health disorders

There are a number of randomized controlled trials (RCTs) across different disorders comparing intensive interventions to inpatient treatment as alternatives to admission, sometimes described as hospital-at-home. Systematic reviews report that intensive community interventions are associated with clinical improvements similar to inpatient care in most studies (e.g., Clisu *et al.*, 2022). Where differences in clinical outcome exist, they tend to favor intensive community treatment. Intensive community services are associated with shorter hospitalizations, lower costs, and greater patient satisfaction.

Until recently, the drive has been to show that an intensive community intervention is at least as good as, if not better than, an inpatient treatment before resources are diverted from inpatient care into intensive community services. Given the high cost and potential harms that can be associated with inpatient treatment (Hannigan *et al.*, 2015; Cotgrove & Northover, 2021), it is now more appropriate to suggest that inpatient treatment is only justified if we have good evidence that it results in better outcomes than intensive community treatment.

Rather than provide intensive services separately, delivering them with an integrated team can offer significant benefits. For example, a single integrated team may offer crisis interventions, planned therapy, and case management/wraparound (services wrapped around the CYP and their family). This is more likely to be clinically and cost effective, reducing the risk of unnecessary referrals between services, avoiding duplication of assessments and delays, and improving the patient experience.

Community-based intensive crisis intervention services

The aim is to deliver rapid assessment and intervention for CYP in a mental health crisis who may otherwise be admitted to hospital, with the intention of offering comprehensive acute care out of hospital. The service should be available 24 hours a day and provide four key components (NHS England, 2020):
- support, advice, and triage to identify those that can be signposted to a more appropriate service, or require a face-to-face assessment;
- crisis assessment including a biopsychosocial assessment;
- brief crisis support; and
- access to longer term intensive community or home treatment.

There are different ways in which urgent and emergency mental health services for CYP can be configured to deliver a comprehensive age-appropriate 24/7 service. Many crisis services are delivered from child and adolescent mental health services (CAMHS), some operate as part of an all-age model and can include collaboration between a number of community CAMHS across geographical areas. There is limited RCT evidence supporting any particular service model, however, Clisu *et al.* (2022) found that in most studies a timely intervention reduced the subsequent risk or duration of admission. Many CYP prefer to receive support in a crisis without the need to go to hospital, sometimes reporting traumatic experiences in emergency departments. Alternative settings for them to be seen and assessed should be available.

Although research remains limited, there is good reason to ensure that intensive community-based crisis services are provided for CYP in need of emergency and urgent care.

Examples of targeted intensive community interventions

Multisystemic therapy

Multisystemic therapy (MST) is an intensive approach to working with young offenders presenting with serious antisocial behaviors, at risk of being placed out-of-home (see Chapter 65). Clinicians work with the young person in their community and are on call 24/7, working intensively with caregivers.

Initial studies showed MST to be effective and superior to inpatient treatment for antisocial behavior. A review (Henggeler & Sheidow, 2012) concluded that the positive findings of early efficacy studies had been sustained in subsequent research; however, a subsequent large UK RCT (Fonagy *et al.*, 2020) showed no reduction in offending in the MST group compared to treatment as usual (TAU) at either 18 months or 5 years. This may be partly due to the effectiveness of TAU in the UK, which rarely involves admission. This is not the case in the US or other countries where admission is more common and a less effective comparator. These findings have resulted in the decommissioning of many UK MST services, emphasizing the importance of culture- and systems-specific research. A further review has confirmed these international differences (Littell *et al.*, 2021). Most trials compared MST to TAU, and, at 1 year, MST reduced out-of-home placements and arrests in the US, but not in other countries. In fact, at 2.5 years, there was evidence of small *increases* in arrest rates and substance use outside the US. These findings emphasize the need to review the context of an intervention when evaluating outcomes.

Intensive services based on dialectical behavior therapy for adolescents who self-harm

There is limited evidence that admissions reduce self-harm; in fact, prolonged admissions may increase self-harm (Ougrin *et al.*, 2021), although admission may still be required if risk is high. Current guidelines recommend dialectical behavior therapy (DBT) adapted for adolescents (DBT-A) for young people with significant emotional dysregulation and frequent self-harm, with some evidence of effectiveness (Kothgassner *et al.*, 2021) (see also Chapter 64).

A DBT program typically might include weekly individual therapy and weekly group work in which young people learn adaptive ways of dealing with emotional crises, how to cope with distress and pain, how to manage healthy relationships, mindfulness meditation, and mentalization. Multifamily work, telephone coaching, outreach strategies, and a weekly consultation team meeting help keep the program on track (see also Chapter 67 on personality disorders). In addition to using DBT as an intensive community-based intervention, it has been adapted for use in many inpatient services.

Interventions for children and young people in care or adopted

For CYP who are in substitute care (see Chapter 42), it is essential that carers receive support for their own well-being, as well as interventions for the CYP's mental health needs. Reviews show that parenting programs can improve carer sensitivity, as well as improving child behavior. However, there is limited evidence that these programs are effective at preventing placement breakdowns (Schoemaker *et al.*, 2020). A review of CYP in foster care reported that of 18 interventions only 3 had some limited evidence of effectiveness (Bergström *et al.*, 2020) (see Chapter 42).

Intensive community eating disorder services

Many CYP with severe eating disorders, in particular anorexia nervosa, require an intensive intervention (see Chapter 69). Gowers conducted a three-arm RCT comparing specialist outpatient treatment vs general outpatient treatment vs inpatient treatment. They found no significant differences in clinical outcomes, but the specialist outpatient intervention resulted in fewer inpatient nights and was more cost-effective (Gowers *et al.*, 2010). A subsequent study compared treatment outcomes for young people who received treatment in a specialist eating disorder service vs generic CAMHS, and also found that treatment was less expensive, with significantly less need for inpatient admissions in the specialist service (House *et al.*, 2012). Outcomes appear to be similar with hospitalizations for medical stabilization or weight restoration when combined with family therapy, suggesting that shorter admissions may also be more cost-effective (Madden *et al.*, 2015).

In recent years, a range of more intensive community treatment options has emerged for this group of young people, including brief intensive outpatient treatments, intensive group-based multifamily treatment interventions, and day programs, as well as residential treatments, with emerging evidence of effectiveness.

Intensive case management and wraparound

The case management model originated as assertive outreach in the US in the 1960s: a "hospital without walls" for adult patients. It can be used for people with a range of different presentations, which are usually severe and/or complex. Case management has been adopted in the US, the UK, several other European countries, and Australia. A range of intensive community services have been developed and expert consensus suggests that these should provide at least some out-of-hours support, and a minimum of 90% of CYP should be supported at least twice per week, with a maximum caseload of around 5 clients per full-time equivalent mental health professional (Keiller *et al.*, 2023). The three main models of case management are assertive outreach, intensive case management, and wraparound. Assertive outreach employs a flexible approach to engaging and working with severely unwell young people in their own community, offering a potentially more accessible service than traditional mental health service provision. Intensive case management shares many key features with assertive outreach, but case managers are more likely to "broker" services rather than provide them directly. Wraparound services deliver an individually tailored package of care with an emphasis on family strengths. Services are provided through teams that link children, families, and carers and their support networks with child welfare (social care), health, mental health, education, and criminal justice services to develop and implement comprehensive support plans.

The evidence base for case management approaches is generally positive but with some mixed findings. A review of youth assertive outreach concluded that the current literature is limited but promising (Vijverberg *et al.*, 2017). There were indications that youth assertive outreach is effective in reducing severity of symptoms, improving functioning, and reducing duration and frequency of admissions. A meta-analysis of wraparound youth services found moderate effects for costs, residential outcomes, and school functioning; with smaller effects for mental health symptoms and functioning (Olson *et al.*, 2021).

Intensive home-based treatment

Intensive home-based treatment (IHBT) covers many of the service models already described. Much of the research is focused on antisocial behavior (see Chapter 65), but IHBT is also commonly used for serious emotional disorder (SED). While these interventions are less well-researched for SED (Moffett *et al.*, 2018), attempts are being made to try to identify the common elements that are effective between the different models in order to define a set of quality standards that can be used to aid future service developments and research (Bruns *et al.*, 2021). Components identified include competent staff, leadership, a defined practice model, organizational support, engagement with the CYP and family, cultural competence of staff, collaborative planning, care coordination, skills building for the young person and parents, use of therapies, and transition planning.

Day patient treatment and partial hospitalization

Day programs were developed in the 1940s and remain part of CYP mental health provision, especially in North America, but in many LMICs they are scarce or nonexistent. In the last decade, the development of community-based intensive services has put pressure on day programs to justify their existence and focus their role more tightly.

What do day programs offer?

Increasingly, day programs offer step-up, step-down support and transition between community services or an inpatient unit. They may be a separate provision or linked to an inpatient service, offering a nonresidential option. Intensive family work may be offered within a weekly 5-day program, as well as problem-specific targeted packages of care, e.g., for eating disorders or psychosis.

Day programs have several advantages and disadvantages compared to admission. Day services work around school or college timetables, can offer family appointments early or late in the day more easily, and individually tailor interventions to CYP's needs. School-aged prepubertal children are rarely admitted to inpatient units so day programs are one option for providing detailed observation, assessment, and treatment. The partial "therapeutic milieu" facilitates close liaison with families and schools and increases the likelihood of learning transferring across settings. However, traveling each day to and from the day program may be tiring and anxiety-provoking for CYP and the costs of travel and loss of income from taking time off work may be substantial for families.

The wide range of these programs makes effectiveness studies difficult to interpret. Research has focused on day programs for specific disorders, with mixed findings. For example, a meta-analysis of the multiple family therapy (MFT) treatment model (several families receiving treatment together) suggests that MFT might have some beneficial effects for families dealing with adult schizophrenia. But no effects were found on mood or conduct problems (van Es *et al.*, 2023).

Studies looking at the use of day hospitals for the treatment of anorexia nervosa are promising. Herpertz-Dahlmann *et al.* (2014) showed day hospital treatment to have similar clinical outcomes to inpatient treatment but to be more cost-effective. Zanna *et al.* (2021), in a pilot study, reported improved weight gain and a significant improvement in other outcomes from a day treatment package when compared to inpatient treatment. A scoping review by Baudinet and Simic (2021) concluded that day programs are an effective alternative to inpatient treatment that can lead to sustained improvements.

Inpatient treatment

Types of inpatient unit

There is significant international variation in usage and models of care for inpatient services. Within Europe there is a wide heterogeneity in the provision of beds (Signorini *et al.*, 2017).

Inpatient units can be freestanding, part of a general hospital or pediatric hospital, or government-run or privately funded. Within general psychiatric units, services are usually divided by age, catering to differing developmental needs. Children's units will often admit from the age of 5 until about 12, and adolescent units from 13–14 up to 16–18 years.

Specialized units treat specific disorders such as eating disorders, or offer a specialist intervention or environment, for example, acute or planned admission units, intensive care units, secure units, and forensic units. General purpose units may cater for all these needs.

In some countries, particularly those in Scandinavia and northern Europe, child psychiatric units include residential facilities for families with an emphasis upon family and parental involvement.

In the US and the UK, the use of inpatient units has increased over the last three decades (O'Herlihy *et al.*, 2007; Blader, 2011; Northover, 2022), but this is changing. For example, between 2014–2021, New York closed 32% of its state-run hospital beds for CYP, cutting the total from 460 to 314. The number of mental health emergency room visits by young people on New York's Medicaid program increased by nearly 25% (Kramer *et al.*, 2023).

In the UK, as in other countries, the number of psychiatric beds for younger children (5–12-year-olds) has decreased substantially since the 2000s with over half of inpatient units closing (Northover, 2022). The latter may not only reflect the increased provision of community services and a reluctance to separate children from families, but also a drive to reduce costs.

While there is accumulating evidence for better outcomes for eating disorders with specialized community and day-patient eating disorder services, there is no such evidence for adolescent eating disorder inpatient units. Indeed, in the UK, they are associated with longer lengths of stay (Northover, 2022) and do not appear to offer a cost-effective alternative to general units or intensive community treatments. Although admissions of CYP with eating disorders is common in some countries such as the UK, it is rarer in countries such as the US and Finland (Woody *et al.*, 2019, Kronström *et al.*, 2021). Even within the UK, there is a large variation in bed use, with some areas managing to avoid admissions altogether (Northover, 2022).

Adolescent intensive care or secure units for violent and/or persistently disruptive behaviors, as well as serious self-harming behaviors and persistent suicide attempts, are organized to cover large populations, across large geographical areas. While many modern adolescent units may incorporate purpose-built intensive care suites, it is sometimes considered useful to provide longer-term secure care in purpose-built units where security can be more easily maintained and where there is access to additional purpose-built resources such as sports facilities. Patients admitted to such units must be under the 1983 Mental Health Act (Department of Health, 2015) in the UK or other statutory provisions (see Chapter 19). Severely disturbed adolescents or those who have committed offenses in the context of mental illness may be referred to adolescent forensic inpatient services in the UK (see Chapter 47).

CYP with mild to moderate intellectual disabilities (IDs) and/or autism can usually be catered for in general purpose inpatient units with consultation from learning disability services and by employing dually trained staff. Those with severe IDs and/or severe autism require separate provision because of their specialized needs and communication difficulties (see Chapters 50–53).

While this section refers mostly to the provision of dedicated mental health beds, it is worth noting that a significant number of CYP with mental health difficulties spend some time in medical or pediatric wards. It is common practice in the UK, particularly for those aged under 16 years, to admit CYP who have taken an overdose or seriously self-harmed to a pediatric bed for up to 24 hours (National Institute for Health and Care Excellence, 2022). This is to allow for medical treatment and a biopsychosocial assessment involving multiple agencies, if appropriate, before a decision to discharge is made. It is also common to admit CYP with serious medical consequences of anorexia nervosa to a pediatric or medical bed. Intensive specialist interventions from eating disorder services liaising with pediatricians have been shown to reduce the need for subsequent psychiatric admissions (Street *et al.*, 2016).

Types of admission

Accepting emergency referrals and admissions on a 24-hour basis, 7 days per week, has been shown to be effective (Cotgrove, 1997; Corrigall & Mitchell, 2002; Cotgrove *et al.*, 2007). To ensure the availability of an emergency bed, a well-integrated community service, including a psychiatric crisis team with in-reach is necessary.

While referrals should not be delayed, a well-timed, planned intervention allowing for therapeutic engagement and development of aims may result in better outcomes than an unplanned crisis admission without a therapeutic alliance (Green *et al.*, 2007). If a young person does require a crisis admission, the UK Far Away from Home Study reported that young people and carers experienced distress and uncertainty with limited or no involvement in decision-making processes and a lack of available information; being placed far away from home posed additional challenges, such as access to family visits and continuity of care.

General inpatient units have come under increasing pressure to manage both acute and planned admissions within the same environment. CYP admitted by these different routes often have quite different and mutually exclusive needs. For example, a young person experiencing an acute psychotic episode may need immediate admission and benefit from a safe, containing, low-stimulus environment. Those with an eating disorder or severe self-harm and suicidality have better outcomes if admission is planned and an active, stimulating, and motivating therapeutic program is provided. In addition, the frequent introduction of acute admissions can destabilize the ward milieu and attract more staff attention, potentially leaving the longer-stay patients feeling neglected (Hazell, 2021). With these challenges in mind many general units separate acute from planned admissions.

Access criteria and assessment procedures

The criteria for accessing inpatient treatment are the same as outlined above for accessing any intensive treatment service (Box 48.1).

If, after a full assessment, an alternative to admission is considered safe and as effective, this should be preferred due to known potential harms associated with admission. Risk alone should not be considered an indication for admission (Northover, 2022). Admission should only be considered when there is a clear beneficial intervention that is only available in an inpatient setting.

Assessments should be focused on the utility of admission (Box 48.3):

Standardized assessments may not be routinely carried out in community services, which can lead to a lack of recognition of important diagnostic categories and appropriate treatment. Structured assessments could pick up diagnoses earlier, resulting in more optimal treatments, and potentially reducing crises.

Social factors tend to play a significant additional role in influencing who is admitted. For example, CYP with social care needs are overrepresented in inpatient populations (Laukkanen *et al.*, 2013), and lack of community support may be a factor in driving these admissions. Family difficulties are common, with parents often having personality or psychological difficulties of their own (Sunseri *et al.*, 2019; Edgcomb *et al.*, 2020). Addressing these social care needs is not ideal in the context of an inpatient service and alternative interventions will usually be preferrable. Good collaboration with social and welfare services is vital to have the best chance of supporting a young person with both mental health and social needs.

Crucially, there is evidence that Black youth are overrepresented in mental health hospital settings: a UK study found that young Black people with psychosis were more likely to have an involuntary hospitalization than young White people with psychosis, which implies that this decision could somehow be influenced by racial biases (Corrigall & Bhugra, 2013). Also, a systematic review and meta-analysis (Walker *et al.*, 2021) reported that involuntary hospitalization was associated with being from a Black rather than a White ethnic group. Further research into the systemic factors underlying these health care inequalities and the barriers to accessing less coercive psychiatric treatment is urgently required, as well as greater training and awareness of potential racial biases that may be held by clinicians (Ayodeji *et al.*, 2021).

Box 48.3 Assessment procedure questions

- Is admission desirable?
- Are the presenting problems likely to be helped by admission?
- Is there motivation to change?
- Are there any suitable alternatives?
- Could admission cause more harm than good?

Source: McDougall and Cotgrove (2013)/Taylor & Francis Group.

Evidence of effectiveness

The research evidence for the comparative efficacy of inpatient treatment is limited. Given that safety is often a major reason for admission it is challenging to design an RCT comparing inpatient treatment with alternatives (see Chapter 65 for evidence on MST).

In Germany, one RCT compared outcomes among 100 children and adolescents who receive home treatment vs inpatient admission (Boege *et al.*, 2015); follow-up data were available for 76 patients—both treatment groups showed a comparable increase in psychosocial functioning, as well as a comparable decrease in level of impairment which remained stable after 8.4 months. After 4.3 years, 51 families were retained at follow-up; 70% of the parents in the home treatment intervention group reported satisfaction with treatment, vs only 36.8% of parents in the control group (Boege *et al.*, 2021).

A small number of nonrandomized trials examining inpatient treatment have been carried out in the US and the UK, generally showing positive outcomes. Green *et al.* (2001, 2007), compared admission with a waiting list control and found significant improvements in global functioning, psychopathology, and "cardinal problem" measures for the inpatient group at discharge, which were maintained at 1-year follow-up. This compared with a much smaller (although still significant) improvement while on the waiting list.

Gowers *et al.* (2000) used the Health of the Nation Outcome Scales for Children and Adolescents (HoNOSCA), a clinician-rated outcome measure, on 35 consecutive admissions to an adolescent unit in England showing significant reductions in scores between admission and discharge. Similar positive findings were made in a subsequent study with larger numbers (137 admissions) by van Niekirk and Cotgrove (2012).

Predictors of outcome

A number of studies have shown factors that are consistently associated with outcome (Box 48.4).

Family characteristics and involvement

These are some of the strongest predictors of outcome and so should be a focus for intervention. Research has demonstrated the benefits of the therapeutic alliance between the young person and their family with the inpatient team, family

Box 48.4 Predictors of positive outcomes from admission

- family involvement and access to multimodel family-based treatment
- collaborative and tailored care planning
- access to specialist interventions with care provided by a multidisciplinary team
- supportive peer relationships established while receiving inpatient care
- early discharge planning and post-discharge support
- multiagency collaboration
- diagnosis of mood disorder or psychosis

participation in the therapeutic process, and the impact of preadmission family functioning (e.g., Pfeiffer & Strzelecki, 1990; Green *et al.*, 2001, 2007). Family problems are often cited as a reason for admission (Bobier & Warwick, 2005) and harsh parental discipline has been found to be a predictor for readmission (Blader, 2004). In Australia, the New South Wales systematic review (NSW Government, 2022) cited other studies confirming these findings and adding more detail. CYP living outside a family have higher rates of readmission compared to children living in families (Edgcomb *et al.*, 2020). There is also evidence that parental mental health difficulties impact negatively on outcomes (Behare *et al.*, 2017).

Care planning

Individual treatment plans developed collaboratively with the young person and their family are associated with improved outcomes (NSW Government, 2022). Some suggest that parents should be admitted with their child, although there is no research evidence to show that this improves outcomes (Cousins & Holmes, 2021). Developing robust safety plans has been shown to reduce length of stay (Sams *et al.*, 2022) and reduce readmissions.

Provision of specialist interventions

Care should be provided by a multidisciplinary team with competencies to treat the range of mental health disorders (Woody *et al.*, 2019; Northover, 2022; NSW Government, 2022). Intensive therapeutic interventions such as cognitive behavioral therapy (CBT) and family-based interventions have been shown to improve a range of outcomes including suicidal ideation and readmission rates (McBee-Strayer *et al.*, 2019).

Peer relationships

Peer relationships can have both positive and negative impacts on outcomes. Potential negative effects are noted in the later section on "Potential harms and risks from admission," but Green *et al.* (2007) and Kennedy *et al.* (2020) identified that the establishment of supportive peer relationships during admission was a significant predictor of positive change during admission and that a failure to engage with treatment and a deterioration in peer relationships were associated with poor outcomes.

Discharge planning and post-discharge support

There is good evidence to support the importance of both early planning for discharge and providing effective post-discharge support. A review by Woody *et al.* (2019) highlighted a number of key features that are common to many services and should be considered to optimize discharge outcomes. These include a commitment to collaborative care planning, close involvement and engagement with families, and a focus on facilitating integration with community-based services. Transitional arrangements and ongoing support are critical to achieving positive outcomes and should begin early and occur in consultation with young people, families, and the broader community, such as schools and other community services. (Ougrin *et al.*, 2018; Woody *et al.*, 2019).

Multiagency collaboration

Woody *et al.* (2019) identified a number of components of effective service delivery, including the importance of multiagency collaboration. Mental health, education, and housing services working together can improve outcomes such as independent living. See also the earlier section on "Collaborative working across systems and agencies."

Length of stay

The effects of length of stay on outcomes is uncertain. Some studies have found that found that outcomes improved with longer stays (Pfeiffer & Strzelecki, 1990; Green *et al.*, 2007); others report that longer stays were associated with increased readmissions (James et al., 2010), or an increase in self-harm (Ougrin et al., 2018). Sams *et al.* (2022) found that brief admissions for young people in crisis receiving additional support (rapid stabilization) had similar readmission rates to those receiving longer, TAU admissions. These inconsistences are not surprising given the existence of variables such as severity and different models of care, including whether CYP are admitted in crisis or for planned treatment. With increasing awareness of the risks and potential harms of admission, and the availability of intensive community treatments, inpatient units generally aim for as short a stay as possible.

Diagnosis

There is consistent evidence that CYP with behavioral disorders are likely to have poorer clinical outcomes and higher readmission rates following inpatient psychiatric care compared to CYP with other mental disorders (NSW Government, 2022). Van Niekirk and Cotgrove (2012) examined HoNOSCA outcome scores for 137 admissions to an adolescent unit. Scores for young people with psychotic disorders or mood disorders improved by 53%; by 35% for those with other emotional disorders, mixed behavioral and emotional disorders, developmental disorders, or eating disorders; and by 25% for those with emerging personality disorders.

Potential harms and risks from admission

Alongside increasing attention to intensive community-based interventions as an alternative to inpatient treatment, there has been a growing awareness of the potential harms from admission (Edwards *et al.*, 2015; Hannigan *et al.*, 2015; Reavey *et al.*, 2017; Cotgrove & Northover, 2021; Box 48.5).

One way of conceptualizing potential harms is to think of admission resulting in a series of unhelpful losses and unhelpful gains (Evans, 2017; NSW Government, 2022). Loss of normal contact and support from family and friends, disruptions to education, loss of freedoms, and gaining institutional dependence, learning unhelpful behaviors from peers, especially in relation to self-harm, and exposure to a distressing environment.

Box 48.5 Potential Harms and Risks from Admission

- separation from family and friends
- risk of dependence and "institutionalization"
- disruption to education
- adverse influences from peers, including risk of increased self-harm (contagion)
- exposure to an environment where there are high levels of disturbance causing distress and compounding their difficulties.
- families and young people feeling disconnected, deskilled, and disempowered
- CYP are over 5 times more likely to be physically restrained than their adult counterparts in the same area

In addition:

- inpatient treatments are expensive and resources may be better deployed to intensive community interventions

Therapeutic environment

To improve outcomes and mitigate against potential harms it is essential that inpatient units have well-trained, competent, and experienced staff that can provide a coherent, consistent, and containing therapeutic environment or milieu (Health Education England, 2021). Working with CYP as a group and supporting positive relationships between CYP and staff should be seen as an essential therapeutic aspect of inpatient treatment (Pfeiffer & Stzelecki, 1990; Green *et al.*, 2007). The staff team need to work together to build a clear structure and routine that maintains consistency and provides an environment that feels predictable and safe (Box 48.6).

Individual interventions and treatments

Inpatient units should provide a range of individualized interventions and evidence-based treatments such as those outlined in the UK's National Institute for Health and Care Excellence (NICE) guidance. These would usually include CBT, psychopharmacology, and family-based therapy delivered by trained and experienced staff, as well as creative and nature-based interventions where evidence is developing (e.g., Hunt *et al.*, 2022). While there is no evidence that these interventions are any more or less effective in an inpatient setting, there may be an opportunity to deliver them in a more intensive way with close observation of their impact.

Management of risk

A systematic approach to risk management is needed. Clinical judgment, a detailed history, corroborative evidence, and observation are at the heart of a risk assessment. Risk assessment is a dynamic process and will need to be constantly reviewed. Routine questionnaires can supplement the clinical risk assessment for self-harm but cannot replace it. Clinical judgment can help predict violence toward others (Phillips *et al.*, 2012). Semistructured assessments such as the Structured Assessment of Violence Risk in Youth (SAVRY) have good predictive validity (Singh *et al.*, 2011) and should be considered routinely for the assessment of violence.

Box 48.6 Key features of a therapeutic environment (milieu)

A therapeutic social environment or milieu aims to help CYP practice new ways of coping through interactions with others (including peers and staff) in a safe, supportive environment, and is characterized by:

- treating the ward as a social community
- providing a clear structure with scheduled routines (e.g., daily activities, free time) and staff-led input (individual and group)
- communicating behavioral expectations with a clear rationale that are not overly restrictive, and limits that are consistently maintained (though balanced with individual need)
- helping CYP understand what will be expected of them and what they can expect from others
- helping CYP cooperate and support each other in making day-to-day decisions about ward functioning, and staff developing a sense of shared responsibility and mutual respect with CYP
- providing regular opportunities for staff and CYP to spend positive, playful time together and engage in "normal" activities and conversations
- maintaining consistent interpersonal boundaries in which staff behave predictably and reliably, and model positive behaviors
- staff are able to move flexibly between positions of "professional helper" and "being human" in response to CYP needs

Source: Adapted from Health Education England (2021).

Management of aggression and restrictive practice

Physical aggression during admission is common, occurring in up to 77% of child inpatients (Carlson *et al.*, 2020) and 28% of adolescent inpatients (Baeza *et al.*, 2013). Factors that predict persistent physical aggression include a history of aggression and use of medication at presentation. Persistent aggression is also associated with increased length of stay, but not necessarily a worse outcome. Behavioral management programs can lead to a reduction in aggression (Carlson *et al.*, 2020; Sorter *et al.*, 2022) emphasizing the importance of an organizational approach to managing aggressive behavior. Inpatient staff exposure to aggression is common, experienced by over 84% of staff in one study (Dean *et al.*, 2010). The impact on staff is considerable with staff absence, difficulty with recruitment and retention, and other emotional and professional sequelae, highlighting the need for a cohesive staff group and regular training and support to deal with violence.

The use of seclusion and other restrictive practices has been a focus of attention in recent years in the UK, as well as other countries. These practices are defined as follows:

- **Seclusion** is defined in the 1983 Mental Health Act Code of Practice (26.103) (Department of Health, 2015) in England and Wales as "the supervised confinement and isolation of a patient, away from other patients, in an area from which the patient is prevented from leaving, where it is of immediate necessity for the purpose of containment of severe behavioural disturbance which is likely to cause harm to others." This should be carried out in a purpose-built area and should be for brief periods only in order to achieve de-escalation.

- **Segregation** is sometimes used on a longer-term basis to prevent a patient mixing freely with other patients on the unit.
- **Restraint** refers to a physical intervention, either through therapeutic holding by a caregiver/staff member, or, as in certain countries, through mechanical restraining tools.

Reasons for seclusion and restraint include threats (73%), agitation (63%), and physical aggression (63%) (Delaney & Fogg, 2005). A review showed that the use of both seclusion and restraint are reduced after behavioral interventions (Carlson *et al.*, 2020) and use of the correct existing legislation is observed. Of concern, international data shows that, on average, use of restraint is approximately 5 times higher in CYP units compared to adult units, and there is a wide variation in the use of restraint between countries (NHS Benchmarking, 2022). Restraint can have severe consequences including trauma for the individual and a reactivation of prior traumatic experiences, and serious physical side effects such as asphyxia, trauma, and even death. One US study (Nunno *et al.*, 2006) reported 45 fatalities related to restraints in CYP psychiatric facilities between 1993–2003.

In certain cases, aggression or disturbed behavior may be managed using medication. Rapid tranquillization techniques involve the administration of short acting benzodiazepines or antipsychotics intramuscularly or via rapidly absorbed oral preparations. While such procedures are relatively safe if there is a clear protocol and regular and frequent physical monitoring by trained staff, there are no data to support the effectiveness of this intervention (Baker & Carlson, 2022; Carlson *et al.*, 2022).

The built environment

The physical environment can play an important part in enriching the experience of CYP, families, staff, and visitors. Improvements to the environment can help reduce anxiety and incidents of challenging behavior, which in turn can improve outcomes and reduce lengths of stay. An Austrian study found that after structural modernization, which included amplifying space, significantly fewer young people were managed by mechanical restraint and the use of coercive measures (Czernin *et al.*, 2024). When designing new facilities, it is essential that CYP experts by experience, families, clinicians, and managers are involved in the coproduction of the building, working with architects and builders. The building design will need to be safe and developmentally appropriate. It will consider any particular special needs, such as intensive care or levels of security. In England, the Department of Health has produced guidance for building inpatient facilities (Department of Health, 2017).

Post-discharge and step-down services

Discharge is a time of potential risk. The death rate within 1 year of discharge from an adolescent inpatient service is 6 times higher than that in the general population of the same age. The suicide rate is highest in the year after inpatient admission with a Korean study showing that the standardized mortality ratio (SMR) among former adolescent inpatients was 14.2 (Park *et al.*, 2013). Among the different diagnostic groups, patients with personality disorders, schizophrenia, or affective disorders had the highest risk for suicide.

Access to aftercare services reduces the risk of readmission. Cheng *et al.* (2017) found a 32% reduction in readmission for CYP receiving aftercare after discharge. Coordination and holistic support following discharge can minimize future issues and assist with successful reintegration into the community (NSW Government, 2022).

Ougrin *et al.* (2018) found that an intensive supportive discharge service, or step-down service, resulted in similar clinical and functional outcomes compared to inpatient TAU, and was more cost-effective, as well as leading to reduced levels of self-harm, reduced lengths of stay, and improved educational reintegration. In the study by Boege *et al.* (2021), long-term benefits were reported from a supportive early discharge package involving intensive home treatment with similar clinical and functional outcomes to admission, but better parental satisfaction.

Summary

The key components of effective inpatient services are summarized in Box 48.7.

Workforce issues and developing a competent workforce

Without an adequately trained, multidisciplinary workforce in adequate numbers to address the complex problems posed by psychiatric disorders, effective delivery of intensive interventions is not possible. Child and adolescent psychiatrists, social workers,

Box 48.7 Summary of key components of effective inpatient services

- thorough preadmission assessment and formulation (Box 48.3) applying clear criteria (Box 48.1) for admission in liaison with referring community teams
- separate units for children and adolescents
- specialist units according to need (e.g., secure, intellectual level)
- separate acute from longer-term admissions
- multiagency collaboration
- family engagement and involvement
- collaborative care planning
- multidisciplinary team
- adequate workforce with competent, trained, and experienced staff
- a program of ongoing staff support, training, and supervision
- specialist interventions provided according to the evidence base
- active measures to mitigate the potential harms of admission (Box 48.5)
- establish a consistent therapeutic environment (milieu) with a clear model of care (Box 48.6)
- physical environment is enriching, safe, and developmentally appropriate
- early discharge planning
- step-down care

psychologists, speech and language therapists, occupational therapists, physiotherapists, family therapists, psychotherapists, and teachers all have important roles in delivering intensive interventions. Unfortunately, there are shortages of appropriately trained staff in many countries, for example, there is an average 19% vacancy level in UK inpatient units. Better levels of staffing reduce length of stay (Northover, 2022).

An alternative approach to recruiting specific professions, is to focus on staff skills and competences through training. Health Education England (2021) have developed a Competence Framework, not reliant on professional groupings, that can be used as a basis for a training needs analysis of staff skills. Key messages are the importance of attitudes, values, and style of interaction; a commitment to human rights, shared decision-making, and coproduction; balancing "being oneself" while offering clinical expertise and holding professional boundaries; and being consistently open, responsive, and receptive (and not critical or blaming).

Quality improvement

We cannot improve what we cannot measure. However, measuring the quality of mental health care is challenging (Kilbourne *et al.*, 2018), and can depend on organizational structures, as well as available resources, including the professional burden required for data collection. Structure, process, and outcome measures are all important for standard setting and quality improvement (QI). Structure measures create the infrastructure for reporting, whereas process measures can assess whether evidence-based practices are being implemented. The use of outcome measures for evaluating quality of care requires risk adjustment approaches to control for factors which can impact outcomes, such as severity of illness and socio-demographic factors. However, this is challenging, due to typically limited available data (Kilbourne *et al.*, 2018). CYP's and carer's experiences and self-reported outcomes are therefore essential to better understand the quality of care being delivered, and should be part of any QI program developed in conjunction with service users and carers.

A national QI program in England reviewed CYP's inpatient units and concluded that there were significant discrepancies in admission costs with no clear association with outcomes or quality, although a relationship was identified between fewer staff, especially psychologists, and longer lengths of stay (Northover, 2022). The review noted that only 23% of CYP in contact with services had paired outcome measures.

An example of a QI framework is the UK Royal College of Psychiatrists' Quality Network for Inpatient Child and Adolescent Mental Health Services (QNIC). These standards have been developed for multidisciplinary, peer-led unit reviews and accreditation, and are regularly reviewed (Box 48.8). The majority of UK units are members, however, the network also includes international units.

Box 48.8 Quality Network for Inpatient Child and Adolescent Mental Health Services standards

- Environment and Facilities
- Staffing and Training
- Access, Admission, and Discharge
- Care and Treatment
- Information, Consent, and Confidentiality
- Young People's Rights and Safeguarding Children
- Clinical Governance

Conclusions

The provision of intensive services is changing. After decades of expanding inpatient beds, these are now reducing in some countries, replaced by intensive community services. These services are generally at least as clinically effective as admission, have fewer risks and harms, and are usually cheaper. When inpatient services are still required, they should be staffed by a highly skilled multidisciplinary team ensuring good engagement with families, carers, and CYP, and providing a range of evidence-based interventions in a therapeutic environment.

Further research and evidence are needed to better support guideline development and to identify valid and useful CYP reported outcomes, adjusted for relevant risk factors in all intensive services. Data-driven QI needs to be embedded within existing services, necessary infrastructure, and leadership, as well as in the overall culture of treatment, with appropriate staff support and training. In light of the costs of admission, further studies are needed to examine the relative cost-effectiveness of alternative treatment pathways, including risks/benefits to different groups of CYP.

References

Ayodeji, E. *et al.* (2021) Editorial perspective: mental health needs of children and young people of Black ethnicity. Is it time to reconceptualise racism as a traumatic experience? *Child and Adolescent Mental Health* **26**(3), 265–266.

Baeza, I. *et al.* (2013) Frequency, characteristics and management of adolescent inpatient aggression. *Journal of Child and Adolescent Psychopharmacology* **23**(4), 271–281.

Baker, M. & Carlson, G.A. (2022) What do we really know about PRN use in agitated children with mental health conditions: a clinical review. *Evidence-Based Mental Health* **21**(4), 166–170.

Baudinet, J. & Simic, M. (2021) Adolescent eating disorder day programme treatment models and outcomes: a systematic scoping review. *Frontiers in Psychiatry* **12**, 539.

Behare, A.P. *et al.* (2017) Effects of family structure on mental health of children: a preliminary study. *Indian Journal of Psychological Medicine* **39**(4), 457–463.

Bergström, M. *et al.* (2020) Interventions in foster family care: a systematic review. *Research on Social Work Practice* **30**(1), 3–18.

Blader, J. (2004) Symptom, family and service predictors of children's psychiatric rehospitalization within one year of discharge. *Journal of American Academy of Child and Adolescent Psychiatry* **43**(4), 440–451.

Blader, J.C. (2011) Acute inpatient care for psychiatric disorders in the United States, 1996 through 2007. *Archives of General Psychiatry* **68**, 1276–1283.

Bobier, C. & Warwick, M. (2005) Factors associated with readmission to adolescent psychiatric care. *Australian & New Zealand Journal of Psychiatry* **39**, 600–606.

Boege, I. *et al.* (2021) Long-term outcome of intensive home treatment for children and adolescents with mental health problems—4 years after a randomized controlled. *Child and Adolescent Mental Health* **26**(4), 310–319.

Boege, I. *et al.* Cost-effectiveness of intensive home treatment enhanced by inpatient treatment elements in child and adolescent psychiatry in Germany: a randomised trial. *European Psychiatry* **30**(5), 583–589.

Bruns, E. *et al.* (2021) Defining quality standards for intensive home-based treatment programs for youth with serious emotional disorders. *Administration and Policy in Mental Health and Mental Health Services Research* **48**, 1065–1088.

Carlson, G.A. *et al.* (2020) Behavior modification is associated with reduced psychotropic medication use in children with aggression in inpatient treatment: a retrospective cohort study. *Journal of the American Academy of Child & Adolescent Psychiatry* **59**(5), 632–641.

Carlson, G.A. *et al.* (2022) Does pro re nata oral medication shorten outburst duration in children? *Journal of the American Academy of Child & Adolescent Psychiatry* **61**(2), 111–114.

Cheng, C. *et al.* (2017) Effects of outpatient aftercare on psychiatric rehospitalization. *Psychiatric Services* **68**(7), 696–703.

Clisu, D.A. *et al.* (2022) Alternatives to mental health admissions for children and adolescents experiencing mental health crisis: a systematic review of the literature. *Clinical Child Psychology and Psychiatry* **27**(1), 35–60.

Cooper, M. *et al.* (2016) Interagency collaboration in children and young people's mental health: a systematic review of outcomes, facilitating factors and inhibiting factors. *Child: Care, Health and Development* **42**(3), 325–342.

Corrigall, R. & Bhugra, D. (2013) The role of ethnicity and diagnosis in rates of adolescent psychiatric admission and compulsory detention: a longitudinal case-note study. *Journal of the Royal Society of Medicine* **106**, 190–195.

Corrigall, R. & Mitchell, B. (2002) Service innovations: rethinking in-patient provision for adolescents: a report from a new service. *Psychiatric Bulletin* **26**(10), 388–392.

Cotgrove, A. (1997) Emergency admissions to a regional adolescent unit: piloting a new service. *Psychiatric Bulletin* **21**(10), 604–608.

Cotgrove, A. & Northover, G. (2021) The future of inpatient units—do we need them? *Child and Adolescent Mental Health* **26**(2), 178–179.

Cotgrove, A. *et al.* (2007) The ability of adolescent units to accept emergency admissions. *Psychiatric Bulletin* **31**(12), 457–459.

Cousins, L. & Holmes, J. (2021) Making the case for the family model in in-patient child and adolescent mental healthcare. *BJPsych Bulletin* **45**(5), 272–274.

Czernin, K. *et al.* (2024) Space for youth mental health: coercive measure use before and after architectural innovation at a department of child and adolescent psychiatry. *Child and Adolescent Mental Health* **29**, 333–339. doi:10.1111/camh.12690.

Dean, A.J. *et al.* (2010) Exposure to aggression and the impact on staff in a child and adolescent inpatient unit. *Archives of Psychiatric Nursing* **24**, 15–26.

Delaney, K.R. & Fogg, L. (2005) Patient characteristics and setting variables related to use of restraint on four inpatient psychiatric units for youths. *Psychiatric Services* **56**, 186–192.

Department of Health (2015) Mental Health Act 1983: Code of Practice. Department of Health, London.

Department of Health (2017) *Health Building Note 03-02: Facilities for Child and Adolescent Mental Health Services*. Department of Health, London.

Edgcomb, J.B. *et al.* (2020) Psychiatric readmissions of children and adolescents: a systematic review and meta-analysis. *Psychiatric Services* **71**(3), 269–279.

Edwards, D. *et al.* (2015) What do we know about the risks for young people moving into, through and out of inpatient mental health care? *Child and Adolescent Psychiatry and Mental Health* **9**, 1–7.

Evans, N. (2017) Using the nominal group technique to involve young people in an evidence synthesis which explored "risk" in inpatient mental health. *Research Involvement and Engagement* **3**(1), 1–11.

Evans, N. *et al.* (2020) Admission and discharge criteria for adolescents requiring inpatient or residential mental health care: a scoping review. *JBI Evidence Synthesis* **18**(2), 275–308.

Fallon, T. *et al.* (2006) CASII—a level of care instrument for children's systems of care: construction, reliability and validity. *Journal of Child and Family Studies* **15**, 140–152.

Fonagy, P. *et al.* (2020) Multisystemic therapy versus management as usual in the treatment of adolescent antisocial behaviour (START): 5-year follow-up of a pragmatic, randomised, controlled, superiority trial MST follow up study. *The Lancet Psychiatry* **7**, 420–430.

Gowers, S. *et al.* (2000) The health of the nation outcome scales for child and adolescent mental health (HoNOSCA). *Child Psychology and Psychiatry Review* **5**, 50–56.

Gowers, S.G. *et al.* (2010) A randomised controlled multicentre trial of treatments for adolescent anorexia nervosa including assessment of cost-effectiveness and patient acceptability: the TOuCAN trial. *Health Technology Assessment* **14**, 1–98.

Green, J. *et al.* (2001) Health gain and outcome predictors during inpatient and related day treatment in child and adolescent psychiatry. *Journal of the American Academy of Child and Adolescent Psychiatry* **40**, 325–332.

Green, J. *et al.* (2007) Inpatient treatment in child and adolescent psychiatry: a prospective study of health gain and costs. *Journal of Child Psychology and Psychiatry* **48**, 1259–1267.

Hamdani, S. *et al.* (2021) Child and adolescent mental health services in Pakistan: do we need in-patient mental health facilities for children and young people? *Child and Adolescent Mental Health* **26**(2), 182–183.

Hannigan, B. *et al.* (2015) An evidence synthesis of risk identification, assessment and management for young people using tier 4 inpatient CAMHS. *Health Services Delivery Research, 3.22.* NIHR Journals Library, Southampton, UK

Hazell, P. (2021) Inpatient units must enhance the system of care. *Child and Adolescent Mental Health* **26**, 176–177.

Health Education England (2021) Delivering inpatient children and young people's mental health care; a multidisciplinary competence framework. Health Education England, London.

Henggeler, S.W. & Sheidow, A.J. (2012) Empirically supported family-based treatments for conduct disorder and delinquency in adolescents. *Journal of Marital & Family Therapy* **38**, 30–58.

Herpertz-Dahlmann, B. *et al.* (2014) Day-patient treatment after short inpatient care versus continued inpatient treatment in adolescents with anorexia nervosa (ANDI): a multicentre, randomised, open-label, non-inferiority trial. *The Lancet* **383**(9924), 1222–1229.

House, J. *et al.* (2012) Comparison of specialist and nonspecialist care pathways for adolescents with anorexia nervosa and related eating disorders. *International Journal of Eating Disorders* **45**(8), 949–956.

Hunt, D.F. *et al.* (2022) Bringing nature into CAMHS inpatient services: reflections for the implementation and integration of training into practice. *International Review of Psychiatry* **34**(5), 546–552.

James, S. *et al.* (2010) Post-discharge services and psychiatric rehospitalization among children and youth. *Administration and Policy in Mental Health and Mental Health Services Research* **37**, 433–445.

Keiller, E. *et al.* (2023) Intensive community care services for children and young people in psychiatric crisis: an expert opinion. *BMC Medicine* **21**(1), 303.

Kennedy, J. *et al.* (2020) Predictors of change in global psychiatric functioning at an inpatient psychiatric unit: a decade of experience. *Clinical Child Psychology and Psychiatry* **25**(2), 995–998.

Kilbourne, A.M. *et al.* (2018) Measuring and improving the quality of mental health care: a global perspective. *World Psychiatry* **17**, 30–38.

Kothgassner, O.D. *et al.* (2021) Efficacy of dialectical behavior therapy for adolescent self-harm and suicidal ideation: a systematic review and meta-analysis. *Psychological Medicine* **51**(7), 1057–1067.

Kramer, A. *et al.* (2023) "We're at a crisis point": NT attorney gen hearing spotlights child mental health care failures. *The City*, New York. Available: https://urldefense.com/v3/__https://www.thecity.nyc/2022/06/23/child-mental-health-letitia-james/*:*:text=From*202014*20to*202021*2C*20New,down*20to*2092*20in*202021__;I34lJSUlJSUlJSU!!PDiH4ENfjr2_Jw!BxJUdrkrhooxr6GJt2otzeR0Jb-utp1PARDKGSfHHsqajhbZbFtX80WlWziXBfwuLJ4IjkrdTIVTCGCCnpUqyKxQcOntRqkewnmoLWH-Kqk1QuDZuSrK$ [31 October 2023].

Kronström, K. *et al.* (2021) Multi-center nationwide study on pediatric psychiatric inpatients 2000-2018: length of stay, recurrent hospitalization, functioning level, suicidality, violence and diagnostic profiles. *European Child & Adolescent Psychiatry* **32**, 835–846.

Laukkanen, M. *et al.* (2013) Does the use of health care and special school services, prior to admission for psychiatric inpatient treatment, differ between adolescents housed by child welfare services and those living with their biological parent(s)? *Community Mental Health Journal* **49**, 528–539.

Littell, J. *et al.* (2021) Multisystemic therapy for social, emotional, and behavioural problems in youth age 10 to 17: an updated systematic review and meta-analysis. *Campbell Systematic Reviews* **17**, e1158.

Madden, S. *et al.* (2015) A randomized controlled trial of in-patient treatment for anorexia nervosa in medically unstable adolescents. *Psychological Medicine* **45**(2), 415–427.

McBee-Strayer, S.M. *et al.* (2019) Intensive crisis intervention for adolescent ideation and behavior—an open trial. *Child and Adolescent Mental Health* **24**, 345–349.

McDougall, T. & Cotgrove, A. (2013) *Specialist Mental Healthcare for Children and Adolescents*. Routledge, Abingdon, UK/New York. Available: https://www.taylorfrancis.com/books/edit/10.4324/9781315857503/specialist-mental-healthcare-children-adolescents-tim-mcdougall-andy-cotgrove [27 June 2024].

Moffett, S. *et al.* (2018) Intensive home-based programs for youth with serious emotional disturbances: a comprehensive review of experimental findings. *Child and Youth Services Review* **85**, 319–325.

National Institute for Health and Care Excellence (2022) Self-harm: assessment, management and preventing recurrence. NICE guideline [NG225]. National Institute for Health and Care Excellence (NICE), London.

National Institute of Mental Health (1983) *Program Announcement: Child and Adolescent Service System Program*. Office of State and Community Liaison, National Institute of Mental Health (NIMH), Rockville, MD.

NHS Benchmarking Network (2022) *International Mental Health Benchmarking*. National Health Service (NHS) Benchmarking Network, London.

NHS England (2020) *Urgent and Emergency Mental Health Care for Children and Young People*. Resource Pack, National Health Service (NHS) England, UK.

Northover, G. (2022) *Getting It Right First Time (GIRFT) Report*. National Health Service (NHS), London.

NSW Government (2022) Accessing inpatient mental health care for children and adolescents. NSW Government, Sydney.

Nunno, M.A. *et al.* (2006) Learning from tragedy: a survey of child and adolescent restraint fatalities. *Child Abuse & Neglect* **30**, 1333–1342.

O'Herlihy, A. *et al.* (2007) Provision of child and adolescent mental health in-patient services in England between 1999 and 2006. *Psychiatric Bulletin* **31**(12), 454–456.

Olson, J.R. *et al.* (2021) Systematic review and meta-analysis: effectiveness of wraparound care coordination for children and adolescents. *Journal of the American Academy of Child & Adolescent Psychiatry* **60**(11), 1353–1366.

Ougrin, D. *et al.* (2018) Comparison of effectiveness and cost-effectiveness of an intensive community supported discharge service versus treatment as usual for adolescents with psychiatric emergencies: a randomised controlled trial. *The Lancet Psychiatry* **5**, 477–485.

Ougrin, D. *et al.* (2021) Supported discharge service versus inpatient care evaluation (SITE): a randomised controlled trial comparing effectiveness of an intensive community care service versus inpatient treatment as usual for adolescents with severe psychiatric disorders: self-harm, functional impairment, and educational and clinical outcomes. *European Child & Adolescent Psychiatry* **30**, 1427–1436.

Park, S. *et al.* (2013) Unnatural causes of death and suicide among former adolescent psychiatric patients. *Journal of Adolescent Health* **52**, 207–211.

Pfeiffer, S.I. & Strzelecki, S.C. (1990) Inpatient psychiatric treatment of children and adolescents: a review of outcome studies. *Journal of the American Academy of Child and Adolescent Psychiatry* **29**, 847–853.

Phillips, N.L. *et al.* (2012) Risk assessment of self- and other-directed aggression in adolescent psychiatric inpatient units. *Australian and New Zealand Journal of Psychiatry* **46**, 40–46.

Reavey, P. *et al.* (2017) The ward as emotional ecology: adolescent experiences of managing mental health and distress in psychiatric inpatient settings. *Health & Place* **46**, 210–218.

Royal College of Psychiatrists (2016) *What Really Matters in Children and Young People's Mental Health: Summary Document*. Values-based Child and Adolescent Mental Health System Commission. Royal College of Psychiatrists, London. Available: https://valuesbasedpractice.org/wp-content/uploads/2015/04/Values-Based-summary.pdf [4 November 2024].

Sams, D. *et al.* (2022) The rapid stabilization pathway: impact of a brief inpatient intervention on the length of stay and readmissions among psychiatrically hospitalized adolescents. *Child and Adolescent Mental Health* **28**, 481–487.

Schoemaker, N. *et al.* (2020) A meta-analytic review of parenting interventions in foster care and adoption. *Development and Psychopathology* **32**(3), 1149–1172.

Signorini, G. *et al.* (2017) Architecture and functioning of child and adolescent mental health services: a 28-country survey in Europe. *The Lancet Psychiatry* **4**, 715–724.

Singh, J.P. *et al.* (2011) A comparative study of violence risk assessment tools: a systematic review and metaregression analysis of 68 studies involving 25,980 participants. *Clinical Psychology Review* **31**, 499–513.

Sorter, M. *et al.* (2022) Management of emotion dysregulation and outbursts in children and adolescents. *Current Psychiatry Reports* **24**(3), 213–226.

Street, K. *et al.* (2016) Structured, supported feeding admissions for restrictive eating disorders on paediatric wards. *Archives of Disease in Childhood* **101**, 836–838.

Sunseri, P. *et al.* (2019) Hidden figures: is improving family function a key to better outcomes for seriously mentally ill children? *Residential Treatment for Children* **37**(1), 1–19.

Van Es, C.M. *et al.* (2023) The effect of multiple family therapy on mental health problems and family functioning: a systematic review and meta-analysis. *Family Process* **62**, 499–514.

Van Niekirk, L. & Cotgrove, A. (2012) Outcomes in a tier 4 general purpose adolescent inpatient unit—5-year case series. RCPsych C&A Faculty Annual Conference.

Vijverberg, R. *et al.* (2017) The effect of youth assertive community treatment: a systematic PRISMA review. *BMC Psychiatry* **17**(1), 284.

Walker, S. *et al.* (2021) Clinical and social factors associated with involuntary psychiatric hospitalisation in children and adolescents: a systematic review, meta-analysis, and narrative synthesis. *The Lancet Child & Adolescent Health* **5**(7), 501–512.

Woody, C. *et al.* (2019) Review of services to inform clinical frameworks for adolescents and young adults with severe, persistent and complex mental illness. *Clinical Child Psychology and Psychiatry* **24**(3), 503–528.

Zanna, V. *et al.* (2021) Improvements on clinical status of adolescents with anorexia nervosa in inpatient and day hospital treatment: a retrospective pilot study. *Frontiers in Psychiatry* **12**, 653482.

CHAPTER 49

Digital technology: assessment and treatment

Chris Hollis[1], Maria Loades[2] and Charlotte L. Hall[1]

[1] NIHR MindTech Health Research Centre, School of Medicine, Institute of Mental Health, University of Nottingham, Nottingham, UK

[2] Department of Psychology, University of Bath, Bath, UK

Introduction

Globally, the majority of young people with mental health disorders receive no treatment, and the burgeoning demand for assessment and intervention far exceeds provision via traditional models of mental health care (Saxena *et al.*, 2007). Digital mental health interventions offer potentially scalable solutions to close this growing needs-provision gap (Roland *et al.*, 2020).

In this chapter, we summarize the emerging application of digital technologies for the assessment, management, and treatment of common child and adolescent mental health (CAMH) disorders. We provide a broad conceptual framework of digital mental health interventions (henceforth referred to as "digital interventions"), which we then apply to the clinical uses and existing evidence for digital interventions using illustrative examples. We identify key issues for clinical practice and implementation, describe where the evidence base is strongest, and highlight important knowledge gaps. We discuss the essential features of a well-designed evaluation of a digital intervention to support the critical interpretation of existing and emerging evidence. We identify future directions for the next generation of digital interventions and the types of research required. Throughout, we focus primarily on the application of digital interventions to common CAMH disorders, including emotional disorders (anxiety and depression) and neurodevelopmental disorders (NDDs) (attention deficit hyperactivity disorder (ADHD), autism spectrum disorder (ASD), and tic disorders). Due to the large number of digital interventions in the field and rapid emergence and turnover of products, we highlight a small sample of existing and emerging digital interventions as exemplars of the conceptual framework and underlying principles for developing, evaluating, and implementing digital interventions for children and young people (CYP).

This chapter focuses on digital interventions with the intended purpose to improve mental health outcomes through assessment and/or treatment of mental health conditions. We do not include digital health technologies applied in the following domains: (i) neuroimaging, biomarker tests/devices, neurostimulation/modulation; (ii) wellness apps and nonpersonalized information to improve lifestyle; (iii) administrative information technologies and databases such as electronic health records; (iv) standardized/nonstandardized questionnaires and tests, which have been translated to an online/digital format; and (v) primary prevention.

What are digital mental health interventions for children and young people?

Digital interventions are defined as the combination of software programs and digital devices, including smartphones, computers, and wearables, that are designed to directly improve the mental health of the user by providing or augmenting clinical assessment, monitoring, and/or treatment. The number of digital interventions aimed at CYP is growing rapidly, and the COVID-19 pandemic has accelerated the widespread adoption of telehealth, remote digital consultations and digitally mediated treatment within CYP's mental health services (Santosh *et al.*, 2023).

Digital interventions encompass many different forms of digitally mediated provision (see Table 49.1 for a glossary of common terms used in digital mental health). Teleconsultation is most similar to traditional face-to-face delivery (i.e., remote consultation delivered in real-time with a health care professional), and its adoption in practice using videoconferencing platforms increased during the COVID-19 pandemic. Emerging in the early 2000s, computerized/digital cognitive behavioral therapy (CBT) was initially designed to be used as a tool within therapist-delivered interventions using a desktop

Rutter's Child and Adolescent Psychiatry and Psychology, Seventh Edition.
Edited by Anita Thapar, Daniel S. Pine, Samuele Cortese, Cathy Creswell, Tamsin J. Ford, James F. Leckman, and Argyris Stringaris.

Companion website: www.wiley.com/go/thapar/rutterspsych7

Table 49.1 Glossary of common terms in digital mental health.

Term (common abbreviation)	Definition
App-based: mental health apps (MHapps)	• Packages of software designed to do specific tasks which are downloaded and stored on a digital device • Aim to improve mental health/well-being by: (i) delivering self-help treatment; (ii) aiding self-monitoring
Artificial intelligence (AI) and machine learning (ML)	• Broad terms, focusing on computational systems that perform cognitive processes characteristic of humans (e.g., learning, problem-solving, predictive inference) • Uses include: (i) AI-based chatbots which are virtual-human therapists and assistants; (ii) remote tracking algorithms to predict clinical status and outcomes
Augmented reality (AR)	• Overlays digital (virtual) information on top of real objects to enhance reality • Enhances the virtual and real world • Allows the therapist to project and control a virtual object in a controlled setting (e.g., therapy room)
Avatar	• Computerized digital human representation of the user within a digital application
Blended approach (also referred to as "digitally enabled therapy")	• Integrates some form of human therapist contact (face-to-face or messaging) with online or digital resources
Chatbots/virtual-human assistants	• Computer programs that simulate human conversation through voice commands and/or text chats • May be driven by AI systems
Computerized cognitive behavioral therapy (cCBT) Internet-delivered CBT (iCBT) Digital CBT	• CBT provided through a digital device where the therapeutic content is contained within a software program • Delivery may be self-guided (without therapist support) or guided (asynchronous therapist support)
Digital health intervention (DHI); digital mental health intervention (DMHI)	• Software that provides assessment/monitoring/therapeutic input for mental health problems via a digital device
Digital therapeutic (DTx)	• Software-driven, evidence-based product which claims to prevent/manage/treat a mental health condition
eHealth (electronic health)	• Internet-based health care delivery, or anything health-related that uses information and communications technology
Extended reality (XR)	• Encompasses all real-and-virtual combined environments and human–machine interactions generated by computer technology and wearables
Mobile-delivered health (mHealth)	• Sub-branch of eHealth • Health care-related information, interventions, and monitoring delivered through portable electronic/mobile devices
Online therapy/treatment: internet counseling, e-counseling, web therapy, teletherapy, remote therapy	• Therapeutic content is delivered by a human therapist • Can be synchronous (in real time and via videoconferencing) or asynchronous (user and therapist not necessarily online at the same time, delivered through text-based messaging/e-mail)
Remote measurement technology (RMT)	• Allows real-time clinically relevant data (e.g., mood) to be logged and shared with a clinician to support assessment/management
Remotely delivered	• Interventions and monitoring delivered outside of the clinic setting and without in-person contact
Self-help; self-guided/self-directed therapy	• Digital therapy conducted without therapist support
Serious games: gamification; applied games	• Game-like features in digital intervention programs designed to educate or change behavior through game play • Primary purpose is therapeutic not enjoyment/fun
Smartphones	• A mobile phone that performs many of the functions of a computer • Capable of running apps
Social media therapy	• Interactive technologies that create a platform for creating and sharing ideas and information through virtual communities (e.g., Instagram, Facebook)
Tele: telehealth, telemedicine, teleconsultation	• *Telehealth*: referring to delivery of health services via telecommunications technology (e.g., videoconferencing, text messaging, e-mail) • *Telemedicine*: focuses solely on clinical care, including consultations, monitoring, and case management • *Teleconsultation*: refers to the remote delivery of clinical services in real time

Table 49.1 (Continued)

Term (common abbreviation)	Definition
Therapist-aided; therapist-supported; therapist-assisted	• Work through an online/digital intervention with synchronous or asynchronous therapist support
Virtual reality (VR)	• Computer modeling and simulation of an entirely virtually created environment that enables a person to interact with an artificial three-dimensional visual simulation • Often used to allow people to test out therapeutic strategies
Wearables	• Includes devices which have sensors that either passively collect data related to mental health (e.g., sleep, activity) or actively collect data inputted by the user (e.g., mood questionnaires) • Remote
Web-based	• Computerized program or service delivered through the Internet

computer. Subsequently, advances in mobile device technology, and growth in device ownership and Internet-delivered CBT (iCBT) has expanded the possibility of delivering mental health interventions remotely "anytime and anyplace." Newer innovations use extended reality technologies, both virtual reality (VR) and augmented reality (AR), harnessing increasingly affordable consumer headsets. Looking forward, rapid advances in artificial intelligence (AI) and machine learning (ML) may one day make it possible to assess mood and emotions in clinical practice through analyzing facial expression and voice, via AI-driven conversational agents (e.g., chatbots, avatars) (Denecke *et al.*, 2021). These technologies are emerging as the next generation of emotionally intelligent virtual (near) human assistants supporting digital intervention users and CYP's mental health care delivery. In the area of assessment and prediction, remote measurement technology (RMT) uses data from wearable devices and smartphones to predict clinical status and outcomes such as risk of relapse and adverse effects of treatment.

Why use digital technology?

Digital interventions have the potential to transform health care delivery by improving treatment effectiveness, service efficiency, and accessibility. A summary of the strengths and limitations of digital interventions is presented in Figure 49.1.

Availability and accessibility

Access to evidence-based interventions delivered face-to-face is curtailed by a limited number of trained mental health care professionals and by their geographical location. This service delivery challenge disproportionately affects low-and-middle-income countries (LMICs) where traditional health care infrastructure lags far behind access to digital devices (e.g., smartphones). Hence, digital interventions are

Advantages

- Reduces travel
- Access at convenient time and location
- Reduces waiting room fears
- Improves access and reach
- Scalability
- High fidelity of therapeutic content when contained within the software program
- Creates service efficiencies
- Reduces therapist time and skill required
- Children and young people comfortable with using technology
- Ability to personalize approach (i.e., specific avatars, emojis)
- Ability to collect real-time measurements

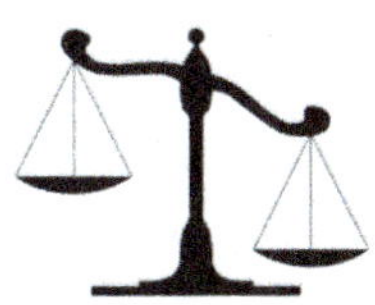

Limitations

- Technology failure
- High attrition rates with self-directed interventions
- Digital divide
- Cost to develop and maintain the technology
- Ensuring the intervention is evidence-based
- Integrating the technology within traditional health care settings (which may have limited technology infrastructure)
- Maintaining engagement with the intervention
- Establishing a therapeutic alliance or therapeutic credibility
- Concerns with managing risk

Figure 49.1 Advantages and limitations of digital interventions. *Note:* Key references—Andersson & Titov (2014); Hollis *et al.* (2017); Liverpool *et al.* (2020); Balcombe & De Leo (2021).

likely to increase access, particularly in hard-to-reach (e.g., remote) areas.

Acceptability

Digital interventions offer users the flexibility to engage with the intervention at a convenient time and location, such as outside traditional working hours, minimizing disruption to school lessons and reducing travel costs and burden (Shah *et al.*, 2019). Digital interventions are intuitively attractive for young people, who are ubiquitous users of technology (e.g., over 80% of 12–15-year-olds in the UK own a smartphone (Bergin & Davies, 2020)). Thus, digital interventions offer a convenient and familiar medium and may help to reduce the anxiety and stigma associated with attending traditional mental health services. Deploying digital interventions has generally led to high levels of user engagement and satisfaction (Little *et al.*, 2018; Valentine *et al.*, 2020), and young people and parents report feeling more relaxed with online delivery (Shah *et al.*, 2019).

Service efficiency and scalability

Digital interventions offer a way to provide "expert therapist" content in a standardized way with high fidelity, with potentially less highly trained human supporters (e.g., entry-level health care professionals) offering problem-solving guidance and encouraging adherence. Given that some digital interventions can be delivered with less (or no) synchronous therapist involvement compared to face-to-face interventions, they potentially enable more efficient provision of evidence-based treatments at scale and reduced cost. Digital interventions offer the flexibility of briefer appointments, which may lead to more timely therapeutic input (Suess *et al.*, 2016), potentially resulting in cost savings. The few studies that have reported economic impact have evidenced time and travel cost savings (Shah *et al.*, 2019), and are, generally, cheaper to provide than face-to-face services (Suess *et al.*, 2016), especially when used as a replacement adjunct to face-to-face treatment (Valentine *et al.*, 2021).

Remote assessment, real-time monitoring, and intervention fidelity

Traditional methods of assessment and monitoring are limited by cross-sectional "snapshots" using subjective measures. Remote measurement technologies have the potential to track symptoms, behavior, and outcomes in real time outside the clinic, which may improve detection of both adverse and beneficial treatment effects, as well as predicting and preventing deterioration and relapse. Therapeutic intervention fidelity and outcomes may also be enhanced by digital interventions as "expert level" therapeutic content is written into the software program and therefore avoids intertherapist variability in skill level associated with traditional delivery.

However, digital interventions also have limitations and drawbacks. One major concern is the *digital divide*, i.e., the gap between those who have *access* to technology and can afford the cost of devices and Internet data access, and those who do not/cannot. Some digital interventions also require particular operating systems or functionality (e.g., a prerequisite is having a smartphone).

A consistently reported frustration for young people is *technology failure*, which ranges from loss of signal, battery power, and data security breaches to the digital service provider/app closing down suddenly (Wallisch *et al.*, 2019). Many users are also concerned about privacy, given the potentially sensitive nature of personal data captured within a digital intervention. Ensuring adequate data security, supported by regulation and industry standards, is essential to build trust and confidence in digital mental health interventions.

In addition, many digital interventions have limited or no *evidence base* of safety and effectiveness, particularly for CYP. In terms of *usage*, low levels of adherence and retention are commonly problematic for many self-directed (unsupported) digital interventions (Khan *et al.*, 2019; Valentine *et al.*, 2020). Overall, evidence suggests that "therapist-guided" digital interventions supported by asynchronous contact with a (para-)professional to encourage engagement and motivation have greater adherence and are more clinically effective (Lehtimaki *et al.*, 2021).

Finally, there is a concern that digital interventions may be offered by health providers as a cost-saving "second best" alternative to face-to-face provision. This is problematic when digital intervention provision is not well integrated with existing care pathways, creating potentially risky "silos" of stand-alone digital interventions or services, with inadequate escalation signposting, monitoring, and follow-up of those who disengage or fail to benefit from the digital intervention.

In summary, digital interventions should not be considered "second best" so long as they (i) have an evidence-base and (ii) are fully integrated/"blended" into routine clinical care to enhance efficiency and outcomes.

Conceptual framework

Currently, there is no accepted conceptual framework, or taxonomy, within which to organize and classify digital interventions. This is problematic for two reasons: (i) without a taxonomy it is very difficult to group sufficiently similar digital interventions together for the purposes of synthesizing evidence in meta-analyses to draw conclusions about effectiveness and provide meaningful head-to-head comparisons; and (ii) it is important to understand the dimensions on which digital interventions differ and how this variation may contribute to clinical outcomes, as well as safety standards and regulatory requirements.

The National Institute for Health and Care Excellence (NICE) is an independent public body that provides national guidance and advice to improve health and social care in England (NICE, 2022). The NICE Evidence Standards Framework (ESF) for Digital Health Technologies (DHTs) is designed to inform the evaluation of digital technology for use in the UK National Health Service (NHS) and social care system (NICE, 2022), and provides a helpful framework to guide the development, evaluation, and deployment of digital interventions in practice.

In Figure 49.2, we present a conceptual framework organized around two key dimensions on which digital interventions vary.

The first dimension (vertical axis) depicts "*digital complexity*." Digital interventions with low digital complexity use digital platforms as an adjunctive or delivery tool (e.g., therapy delivery, data recording) without therapeutic content written into software or data processing functions. Examples of low-complexity digital interventions include teleconsultation via videoconferencing software and electronic diaries (e.g., mood monitoring apps).

These low-complexity digital interventions would broadly map onto Tiers A and B of the NICE ESF for DHTs classification (NICE, 2022). Medium- and high-complexity digital interventions (corresponding to NICE classification Tier C) are designed to assess and/or treat mental health conditions, or guide diagnostic or treatment decisions. An example of a medium-complexity digital intervention is a digital CBT program, which delivers cognitive behavioral therapeutic content through the software. High-complexity digital interventions include personalization of therapeutic content adapted to the user's characteristics/preferences and driven by personal data. Examples include AI-driven therapy chatbots, and RMT with built-in, just-in-time interventions (Wang & Miller, 2020).

The second dimension (horizontal axis) describes the *level of clinician/human support and service integration*. At the right (lowest level of support) end of the axis, no clinician support is provided with fully self-directed digital interventions (e.g., stand-alone mental health apps). Medium levels of clinician support occur with digital CBT programs (where an online therapist provides prompts and motivational support but does not deliver core therapeutic content), and clinician decision aids such as the QbTest computerized assessment for ADHD (Hollis *et al.*, 2018). In these forms of digitally enabled care, the clinician would generally spend less time delivering patient care when using a digital intervention than is typically needed to perform similar functions in standard face-to-face care. The highest level of clinician support/involvement occurs where all components of the intervention and all content are delivered live in real time via a digital platform, such as videoconferencing.

Some key domains of the NICE ESF are outlined below, with exemplar evaluation:

- *Design factors*: Does the intervention meet technical standards for safety and reliability? Have young people and clinicians (end-users) been meaningfully involved in design?
- *Describing value*: Who is the intended recipient and beneficiary? What is the intended purpose and target population? What are the intended benefits and how will these be realized and measured?
- *Demonstrating performance*: Is the intervention acceptable and engaging for the user (e.g., uptake and completion rates)? Is the technology clinically and cost effective? Does the technology deliver clinical utility and acceptable accuracy?

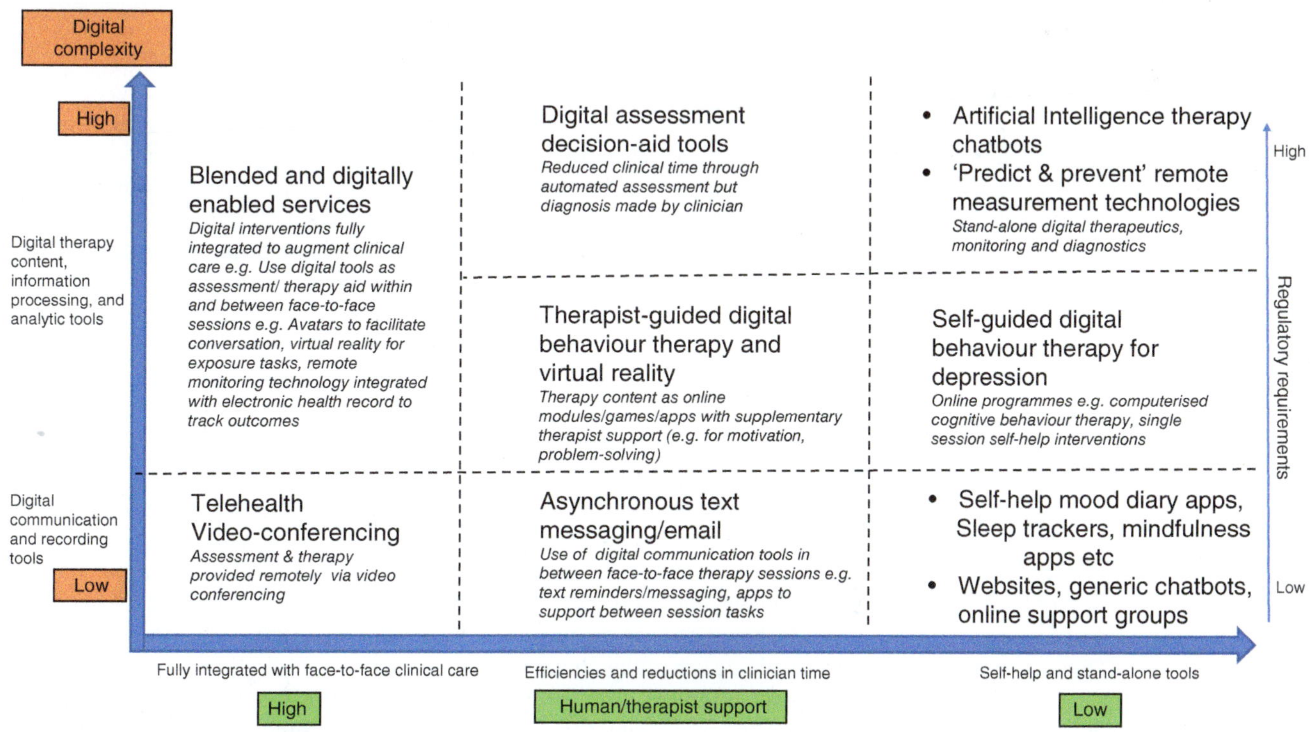

Figure 49.2 Conceptual model of digital mental health interventions.

- *Deployment considerations*: How will the intervention be integrated into existing care pathways? What aspects of existing care will be changed or replaced? What hardware/devices are required to deliver the intervention? What level of clinician support/training is required? How will the intervention be made scalable? How will usage and effectiveness be reported? (Lipschitz *et al*., 2022).

Clinical application and evidence for digital interventions

Anxiety and depression

Assessment and monitoring

As digital interventions evolve, the capacity to use remote measurement technologies to proactively identify individuals with symptoms is increasing. For example, the Artemis-A app is a digital intervention designed to assess mental health difficulties (including anxiety and depression symptoms) at scale in secondary schools, using adaptive testing technology to shorten the length of the overall assessment (Burn *et al*., 2022). The capacity to passively track early warning signs of emotional difficulties, such as step count, geolocation data, and mobile phone screen use, could potentially improve prediction and prevention of clinical episodes in adolescents who are at risk for clinical depression and self-harm (Cao *et al*., 2020). While mood monitoring per se is not necessarily therapeutic (and could pose risks such as negative cognitive ruminations), these extra assessment activities could potentially improve outcome measurement and the precision and personalization of therapeutic digital interventions, supporting engagement and adherence. Furthermore, the distinction between remote tracking assessment and interventions is likely to become increasingly blurred with the use of just-in-time interventions (Wang & Miller, 2020). Passive tracking needs to be used cautiously and consideration needs to be given to responding to signs of deterioration in a timely fashion.

Therapeutic interventions

Depression and anxiety in young people are the most common clinical targets for digital interventions (Hollis *et al*., 2017). A systematic review of 13 trials pooled the outcomes of iCBT for depression and anxiety in young people aged 11–19 and found that there were small, significant benefits reported for depression (effect size = 0.23) and anxiety (effect size = 0.21) (Wickersham *et al*., 2022). However, the quality of study reporting was poor and little is known about cost-effectiveness. Compared to waiting list controls, there is growing evidence of the relative effectiveness of digital interventions based on CBT for: adolescent depression, e.g., SPARX which is gamified (guided) self-help (Fleming *et al*., 2012; Merry *et al*., 2012); childhood anxiety, e.g., OSI (therapist-supported online parent-led CBT targeting primary/elementary school children aged 5–12 (Hill *et al*., 2022), and iCBT for childhood anxiety which is a combined parent–child intervention consisting of 11 modules with written messages and feedback sent from a therapist (Vigerland *et al*., 2016); and adolescent social anxiety disorder, e.g., OSCA (Leigh & Clark, 2023), which is a 14-week treatment via modules online, with a 15-minute phone call each week with a therapist. There is promise of effectiveness for other digital interventions, including gaming interventions, web-based programs, and mental health apps for adolescents with depression and anxiety (Lehtimaki *et al*., 2021). Furthermore, effects seem to be larger when skill-building is facilitated (Venturo-Conerly *et al*., 2022) and the positive effects of iCBT for depression are larger when human support/supervision is provided (Garrido *et al*., 2019). However, for both depression and anxiety, more work is needed to elucidate how digital interventions compare to active control conditions.

Given the number of young people with anxiety and depression, digital interventions, even those that result in small treatment effects, could provide a scalable solution which is time and cost saving, and have considerable public health impact (Carey *et al*., 2023). For example, for CYP with anxiety disorders, iCBT (BRAVE for Teenagers online program) with minimal therapist contact (brief e-mail feedback after each online session and a phone call after the fifth session) was as effective as clinic-based CBT delivered face-to-face by registered psychologists over 10 sessions and 5 parent sessions (Spence *et al*., 2011). However, when trialed in a routine clinical care setting in the UK, these effects were not replicated (Waite *et al*., 2019).

Neurodevelopmental disorders

Assessment and monitoring

Autism spectrum disorder

Given that individuals with ASD often struggle with in-person/face-to-face communication, offering assessment and therapy online may reduce anxiety and increase engagement with clinical services. Initial research comparing in-person versus telehealth assessment for ASD has found that diagnostic accuracy was comparable (Reese *et al*., 2015; Juárez *et al*., 2018) and digital assessment can reduce time to diagnosis in ASD by 11–12 months (Stainbrook *et al*., 2019). However, this research is in its early stages and requires further investigation.

Attention deficit hyperactivity disorder

Computerized cognitive tests, e.g., continuous performance tests (CPTs), which measure attention and impulsivity, have long been used in the assessment of ADHD. The evidence for their use to support clinical assessment is promising and warrants continued investigation to confirm its utility. A systematic review reported mixed findings with contrasting evidence on the ability of CPTs to support clinical decision-making (Hall *et al*., 2016b), and concluded that combining CPTs and with objective measures of activity could be useful and worthy of further research. One such digital intervention, the QbTest (www.qbtech.com), designed to aid clinical assessment in ADHD, combines a CPT with an infrared motion detector to record activity. In a randomized controlled trial (RCT; AQUA trial), when the QbTest was added to standard clinical assessment it increased the speed to diagnostic decision-making (with fewer clinician appointments needed to make a diagnostic decision on ADHD) and increased clinician confidence with no loss of diagnostic accuracy (Hall *et al.*, 2016a; Hollis *et al.*, 2018), resulting in cost savings to the service. On average, clinicians required one less appointment to make a diagnostic decision, and participants whose clinician had access to a QbTest report were 44% more likely, during the study period, to receive a diagnostic decision compared with those who received assessment as usual without the QbTest report. Furthermore, the QbTest has demonstrated good acceptability, including improving communication between families and clinicians and helping families understand how a diagnostic decision was reached (Hall *et al.*, 2017). NICE has produced a Diagnostics Guidance for QbTest (https://www.nice.org.uk/guidance/dg60). NICE Guidance supports use of QbTest to help diagnose ADHD in children aged 6 to 16 alongside clinical assessment. Recently, behavioral tracking and remote tracking has been applied to ADHD to monitor treatment response and adverse events (Denyer *et al.*, 2022).

Therapeutic interventions

Autism spectrum disorder

Digital interventions specifically designed for CYP with ASD are primarily for pre-adolescent children and often incorporate computer game-based formats aimed at training and improving core deficits in social understanding, empathy, and emotional recognition. While these games appear popular (particularly with parents), trials have failed to show consistent benefits and limited skills transfer beyond the specific context of the game to affect core ASD symptoms and deficits (Hollis *et al.*, 2017). Less attention has been given to digital interventions that target associated symptoms and behaviors in ASD such as anxiety and challenging behavior. Given that these symptoms may be more amenable to intervention than core deficits of ASD, and trials show that these interventions work face-to-face, digital adaptations would be welcome.

Attention deficit hyperactivity disorder

A systematic review of cognitive training programs for ADHD, including computer-delivered working memory training, found that while some improvements occurred in trained cognitive functions (e.g., working memory), there was no evidence of reduced ADHD symptoms when blinded ratings were used (Cortese *et al.*, 2015). Similarly, a systematic review evaluating digital interventions (including video game programs or computer programs) aimed at improving ADHD outcomes found that there was no consistent indication of benefit (Hollis *et al.*, 2017). The latter review concluded that interventions targeting broader cognitive functions may have greater effects. A recent large RCT (STARS-ADHD) studied a video game-like intervention (AKL-T01) for children with ADHD (aged 8–12), targeting divided attention and cognitive control, and played at home for 25 minutes/day, 5 days/week, for 4 weeks. There was a small significant improvement in attention (Kollins *et al.*, 2020), but no effect on core ADHD symptoms. This suggests that gamified digital interventions like AKL-T01 may not be sufficient as stand-alone interventions for ADHD but could potentially augment traditional medication or psychosocial therapies, and this approach warrants further study. Despite this limitation, the AKL-T01 was approved by the intervention by the Food and Drug Administration (FDA) in the United States. This occurrence likely reflects FDA rules that allow such approvals for interventions that are deemed to be safe even when data on their possible clinical benefit are weak. Online parenting programs for ADHD are also under development with several evaluations ongoing (Kostyrka-Allchorne *et al.*, 2022).

Tic disorders

The needs-provision gap is particularly severe for CYP with tic disorders, given the lack of tic behavioral therapists and, hence, digital behavioral therapy for tics offers a potentially scalable solution to address this clinical unmet need. A large RCT (ORBIT trial; Hall *et al.*, 2019; Hollis *et al.*, 2021) found that a 10-week, therapist-supported online exposure and response prevention (ERP) behavioral therapy for CYP with tic disorders (age 7–17 years) resulted in clinically meaningful improvement in tics. Importantly, these benefits were maintained for up to 18 months (Hollis *et al.*, 2021; Hollis *et al.*, 2022). Engagement with the intervention was excellent, possibly due to both the asynchronous therapist support and parallel modules targeted at parents, enabling them to support the young person's therapy. More generally, offering a parent component within a digital intervention (e.g., actively involving the parent may help to promote engagement and treatment adherence, particularly with younger children) may result in better therapy adherence and outcomes (Khan *et al.*, 2019).

Summary

We highlight digital interventions that have promising research evidence to support their use within CYP's mental health services. However, technologies with the strongest evidence base for assessment or treatment may not be readily available in routine clinical practice. This is due to the translational gap between best research and best practice. Conversely, commercial digital interventions and services available in clinical practice may have a very limited evidence base. Furthermore, the mechanisms required to embed the technology within the care pathway and the cost of doing so are often poorly understood. Figure 49.3 shows a summary of key considerations for clinicians when integrating a digital intervention into their care pathway. We discuss this further in the section "Key issues for practice and implementation."

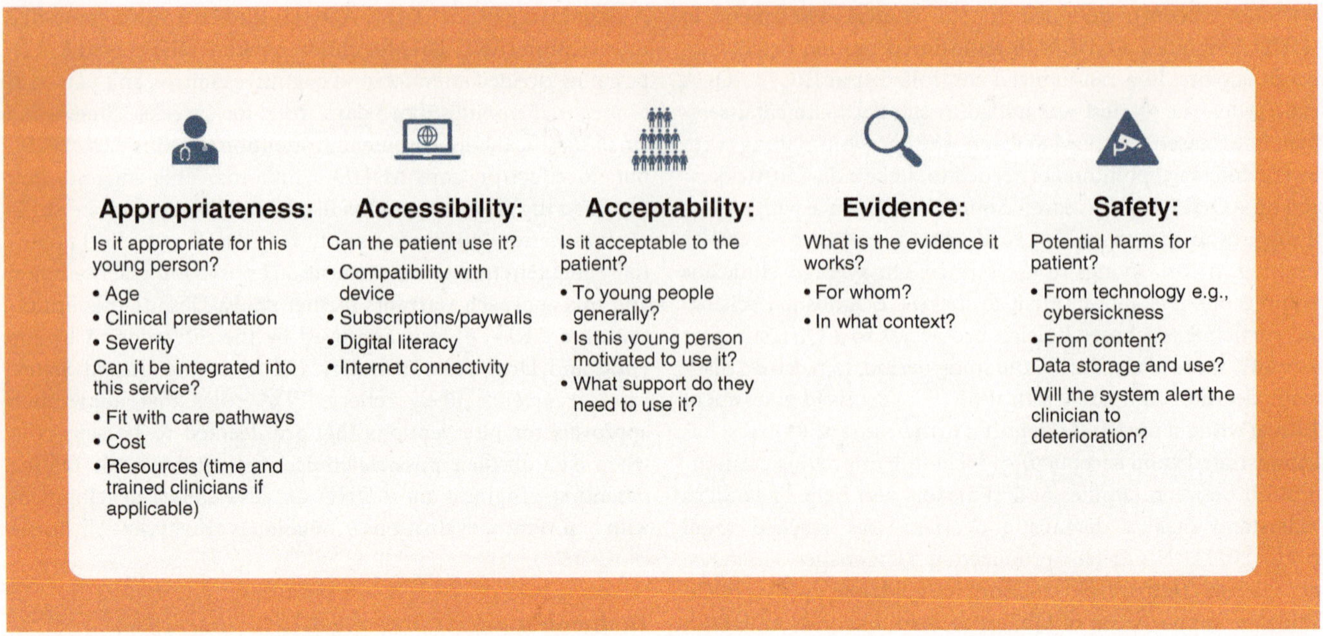

Figure 49.3 Considerations when using a digital health intervention.

Key issues for practice and implementation

Enhancing uptake and engagement

Realizing the potential of digital interventions depends on adequate uptake and engagement in real-world settings. Young people report positive experiences with digital interventions (McCashin *et al.*, 2019); they value the anonymity which digital interventions, such as mobile apps, offer (Garrido *et al.*, 2019) and favor digital interventions which increase their sense of social connection (Liverpool *et al.*, 2020; Borghouts *et al.*, 2021). However, they also report barriers to using digital interventions, which include overreliance on reading and writing skills and technological issues or access, and prefer content which can be personalized, or standardized/over-general content (McCashin *et al.*, 2019), which raises potential challenges for maintaining intervention fidelity. Emerging evidence suggests that that parental feedback, uptake, and engagement with parent-focused digital interventions is also favorable (Hill *et al.*, 2022).

In general, uptake, adherence, and completion tend to be much higher with human-supported digital interventions than with unsupported/self-help apps (Garrido *et al.*, 2019). Similarly, uptake and adherence is also generally higher in research studies (which often offer a mix of tangible and social reinforcers for participation such as shopping vouchers for completion and regular researcher contact) than when the same digital interventions are rolled out in practice settings (March *et al.*, 2018; Liverpool *et al.*, 2020; Cohen & Schleider, 2022). Codesigning digital interventions with intended users from the outset and attending to user experience within the development and implementation phases may particularly aid engagement.

Practitioner digital competence

Competencies required by practitioners delivering digital interventions need consideration. Competence working clinically face-to-face may not equate to competence to support CYP using digital interventions. Hence, specific competencies in the domains of communication skills, risk management (including security and data privacy), confidentiality and ethics, knowing what technology is suitable, and managing a therapeutic relationship may be needed (Pote *et al.*, 2021; Schueller *et al.*, 2022).

Quality control and risk issues

Regulation

Given the global market for most digital interventions, it is important to have universally recognized and endorsed approaches to regulation and quality control. An additional complexity is variation in data privacy laws, making data sharing and global spin-out of technologies complex. Regulation is further complicated by the lack of clarity about whether a specific digital intervention should be classified as a "medical device" (i.e., to treat symptoms, aid diagnosis) or a "wellness aid" (which would not require regulation as a medical device). This has important implications for safety and ensuring the products are fit-for-purpose. Furthermore, the development of new technology typically outpaces the speed in which new regulatory frameworks are developed and implemented, creating risk that regulatory standards may lag behind the latest technology developments.

Digital interventions are broadly developed by two groups; (i) the industry/commercial sector or (ii) the academic/clinical sector, each of which have different skill sets, incentives, and challenges with device regulation. For example, industry (typically small- and medium-sized enterprises) may struggle with end-user (clinician and patient) engagement and clinical evidence generation, and may focus predominantly on the product's business case, value proposition, and route to market. Meanwhile, academic/clinical groups may be unfamiliar with the commercialization and regulatory processes and may focus primarily on generating high-quality clinical evidence of efficacy and safety. Organizations such as MindTech (https://www.mindtech.org.uk/) in the UK and Black Dog Institute in Australia (www.blackdoginstitute.org.au) have been established to bridge the commercial–academic divide, supporting greater collaboration and a more efficient pipeline for digital interventions.

Finally, it is important that the regulation is proportional to risk to ensure a balance between safety and innovation, and a shift to a more risk-based approach has been suggested (ABHI, 2021).

Data security

Digital intervention use may involve the capture and transfer of identifiable and nonidentifiable data, including between the clinician and the user. The capacity to transfer and store information can be critical to using the digital intervention for clinical purposes, for example, sharing resources via a cloud-based system or accessing remotely collected data to aid assessment. However, this has clear implications for data privacy and has raised concerns around confidentiality and data security breaches, which are potentially greater than those associated with face-to-face delivery. Specific risks include human error (communicating with the wrong person), e-mail phishing or hacking an account, messages from the clinician being read by other people other than the intended recipient (e.g., a mobile phone left in a shop, or being viewed by the user's family/friend), or lack of privacy when engaging in remote therapy. For CYP, this also raises issues regarding parental involvement. Whereas young children may require parental support to engage in sessions/technology, older children may want to minimize parental involvement. Despite being frequent users of technology (including, but not limited to, frequent information-sharing on social media), CYP have expressed concerns about data protection and security regarding digital intervention (Hollis *et al.*, 2017). It is possible that these concerns may be a barrier in participation or limit the amount of information sharing a child or young person is willing to disclose. The clinician needs to discuss and agree this with those involved before the start of treatment.

For a digital intervention to pass regulatory approval, the manufacturer will have had to submit technical files assuring the regulatory board that necessary and essential data safety and security regulations have been satisfied. However, it is also important that clinicians inform young people and families about the risks and any limitations to data confidentiality and security so that they can make informed choices.

For telehealth/videoconference sessions, providers should ensure that they have considered with the user the appropriateness of the space available to them from which they engage in the treatment to ensure that it feels sufficiently private, confidential, and comfortable. Providers should also ensure that they understand the privacy and security features and data-sharing arrangements of the platform they are using to provide therapy.

Managing risk and assessing harm/adverse effects

Assessing and monitoring risk is of key importance, given that digital interventions may present unique risks; for example, potential absence of trained staff to support emotional processing, explain the treatment content, or help CYP to safely engage with the technology. Crucially, to make a judgment about any intervention, we must understand any potential harm as well as the potential benefits. However, evidence indicates that harms in digital intervention may currently be underrecorded (Gómez Bergin *et al.*, 2023). Risks can be addressed in various ways, including digitized brief symptom checklists that can send automated alerts when a user meets a symptom threshold. Users should be informed about the frequency with which messages to a clinician will be picked up, the limits of the service for providing in-crisis or immediate support, and escalation signposting should be available should the users of the digital intervention wish to seek more help.

The gap between evidence and implementation in practice

Digital interventions present particularly important opportunities to scale up health care access in LMICs, where high-speed Internet connectivity has progressed rapidly. Thus, digital interventions could better meet mental health needs than traditional face-to-face clinic provision, particularly where stigma is high and numbers of trained professionals are very low.

It is crucial that digital interventions are designed and tested in local contexts to ensure cultural relevance and sensitivity (Groen *et al.*, 2022). The Shamiri intervention is a therapeutic digital intervention developed for anxiety and depression symptoms in Kenyan adolescents where mental health stigma is high. Shamiri (meaning "thrive" in Swahili) includes growth mindset, gratitude, and value affirmation components, and was specifically designed to be nonstigmatizing and nonpathologizing in the language used. Originally developed with local experts by experience to be delivered by lay providers in community settings, a digital, single-session self-help version, Shamiri-Digital, has been trialed (Osborn *et al.*, 2020), with reductions in depression symptoms similar to full-length, face-to-face psychological therapies. With regard to digital interventions for assessment, an innovative global project, MINDKIND, is codesigning a novel mental health databank with young people from India, South Africa, and the UK. The project focuses on establishing whether an app which collects this data would be feasible and acceptable across the world, including in different cultural contexts (Sieberts *et al.*, 2022).

Key ingredients for good research design for digital technology

Research priorities and methodological issues

While the number of digital interventions for CYP's mental health is growing rapidly, evidence of efficacy, cost-effectiveness, usability, uptake, and mechanisms of action has lagged well behind. One factor that has held back progress is the bimodal innovation landscape, in which invention and implementation largely take place in two parallel tracks: (i) academically-driven innovations backed by rigorous evidence of efficacy in trials but disappointing levels of implementation; and (ii) commercially driven innovations with (in some cases) often weak evidence that they actually work.

In this section, we consider research priorities and methodological issues for developing and evaluating digital interventions that address the following three research questions (see also Chapter 15):

- Is the intervention engaging and usable? (Engagement, uptake, and adherence)
- Does the intervention work? (Efficacy, safety, and cost-effectiveness)
- How does the intervention work? (Active components and mechanisms of action)

Is the intervention engaging and usable?

There are two approaches to increase uptake and engagement with digital interventions.

Codesigning digital interventions with children and young people

Codesign aims to create user-centered digital interventions, designed "with" rather than "for" young people and thereby improve engagement, adherence, and potential effectiveness (Bevan Jones *et al.*, 2020). Critically, digital interventions for CYP should not merely be adaptations from adult programs. A developmental or age-appropriate approach is needed regarding the content and design of a program, accounting for the range of interests and tastes of young people. In the UK, the NICE provides best-practice recommendations and guidance for health care practitioners and recommends incorporating intended user group acceptability in the design of digital health technologies (NICE, 2022).

Providing (human) support and personalization in digital interventions

Taken as a whole, the evidence suggests that the provision of human support for therapeutic digital interventions increases uptake, engagement, and clinical effectiveness (Rickwood & Bradford, 2012; Hollis *et al.*, 2017; Lehtimaki *et al.*, 2021). However, the type and level of support and who provides it (peer, professional, or parent), as well as the age and preferences of the individual young person may make important differences. Hence, an important research question concerns the impact of human support on both adherence and outcomes for digital interventions with children and in young people and whether the effects differ (and if so, why) across different conditions and ages. Another unanswered question concerns how and when parental involvement in the digital intervention is helpful.

Support may not have to be a "real person" but could be automated through the digital intervention itself. When asked about their "ideal app" for managing their condition, young people and adults with ADHD highlighted the need for a virtual "coach" or "mentor" to provide support and encouragement (Simons *et al.*, 2016). Developments in VR, AI, and ML are creating "virtual human" chatbots that, in the next generation of digital interventions, could act as automated, interactive coaches to support personalized delivery of digital interventions (Valstar *et al.*, 2014).

The Turing test, originally called the imitation game by Alan Turing in 1950, is a test of a machine's ability to exhibit intelligent behavior equivalent to, or indistinguishable from, that of a human. Although AI-driven chatbots could potentially pass the Turing test, ethically the user should be told when using a digital intervention whether they are interacting with a human supporter or a machine, which in turn may affect the user's engagement and therapeutic alliance (Tong *et al.*, 2022). Digital interventions with personalization functionality tend to facilitate engagement and adherence (Rasing *et al.*, 2020). For instance, even without human support, branching logic within the digital intervention can match a user's main problem(s) with the information and activities they subsequently see. AI can be leveraged to enable a digital intervention to become increasingly accurate over time as it learns the characteristics of the user's voice (Mahlous & Okkali, 2022).

Does the intervention work?

Efficacy and cost-effectiveness

An important challenge is the capacity of traditional RCTs to keep pace with the rapid growth of in the number of digital interventions, the speed of technology development, and the iteration of products (Schueller *et al.*, 2013). However, online "digital" trials can be conducted efficiently and quickly (Hall *et al.*, 2020). Looking forward, digital trials that compare multiple active interventions simultaneously against each other ("head-to-head") and to a single control group (so-called "platform trials") may offer significant advantages and efficiencies for evaluating digital interventions over more traditional trial designs (Gold *et al.*, 2022). Furthermore, more data on the cost-effectiveness of digital interventions is needed, and it is important to demonstrate that the addition of digital interventions into care pathways is cost-effective relative to standard care (Hollis *et al.*, 2022).

It is equally as critical that digital interventions are robustly assessed for safety and that these findings are considered along with clinical and cost-effectiveness. For further details on safety and adverse events, please see the earlier section on "Managing risk and assessing harm/adverse effects."

Choosing appropriate comparators/control groups

Comparators used in trials of digital interventions significantly influence the size and interpretation of therapeutic effects. In general, effects are largest when digital interventions are compared to nonactive (e.g., waitlist or no treatment) controls, and differences are smallest when there is an active comparator (Hollis *et al.*, 2017; Garrido *et al.*, 2019).

When the aim is to determine the effectiveness of a new digital intervention compared to current best practice (e.g., "pragmatic trials"), the trial design is typically testing the "noninferiority" of the digital intervention compared to either a "gold standard" (e.g., protocol delivered face-to-face CBT) or standard care typically described as "treatment-as-usual" (e.g.,(Taylor *et al.*, 2022). In efficacy trials of digital interventions where the aim is to determine the causal effect of a specific therapeutic intervention/component the comparator is typically an active digital control (e.g., online psychoeducation; Hall *et al.*, 2019).

How does the intervention work?

Identifying active components

Understanding which components of a digital intervention are the active ingredients that actually have the predicted impact on the outcome, and whether and how components interact, is critical to digital intervention development and evaluation. Most digital interventions are highly complex, containing multiple components, so the development process needs to include a period of optimization. This entails evaluating the performance of individual components of the intervention, and how they interact with one another (Collins *et al.*, 2014). Here, the term "component" is broadly defined, and may refer to: aspects of the content of the intervention; the type of technical platform; variables and decision rules used to tailor intervention strategy, content, or intensity to individuals; or any other aspect of an intervention that can profitably be separated out for examination (Murray *et al.*, 2016).

An important gap in the field is the lack of an agreed taxonomy for specifying the different components of digital interventions. This would support replication of trial results and comparison between digital interventions, synthesizing data across trials in systematic reviews and meta-analyses.

Tailoring and personalization

In health behavior change interventions, "tailoring" typically refers to how targeted are the health messages being sent to users. For example, "generic" communication reflects messages that are not individualized to the recipient's specific needs, but they may be "personalized" by adding a user characteristic to the messages (e.g., the user's name). "Targeted" communication is used to provide messages to a specific group, such as those of a specific age or who screen for a specific risk of developing a health problem (Noar *et al.*, 2007; Musiat *et al.*, 2012). Tailoring may also mean that an intervention has different user "pathways" depending on, for example, the user's baseline symptoms (Chiauzzi *et al.*, 2008), or allows users to choose the modules or content that is most relevant to their presenting problem (Andersson *et al.*, 2011).

The SPARX intervention team (gamified CBT for adolescent depression) describe the process of "personalization" of SPARX among rural Australian adolescents (Cheek *et al.*, 2014). The personalization of the intervention focused mainly on the ability of the user to choose the gender of the "guide" avatar, which they reported led to improved relatability. This aspect was also highlighted and praised by LGBQ+ adolescents, who felt that allowing them to personalize the avatar's gender and appearance reflected their real-world experience of challenging gender expectations (Lucassen *et al.*, 2013). Furthermore, this research team has analyzed qualitative data from studies of SPARX to understand how users' perceptions and elements of the intervention map onto the autonomy, competence, and relatedness aspects of self-determination theory, which in turn have been theorized as key factors influencing engagement and adherence to digital interventions (Cheek *et al.*, 2015).

Conclusions and future directions

Digital interventions have the potential to transform CYP's mental health services through improved access to evidence-based resources and interventions, and by automating parts of diagnostic, monitoring, and treatment pathways. They can connect young people with peers, mentors, and therapists, potentially closing the mental health treatment gap through novel, tailored, flexible, and less stigmatizing treatments. Effective, usable, and accessible digital innovations could also redress the imbalance of global health inequalities and ensure that evidence-based interventions reach the CYP who need them most. However, this potential is still largely unrealized in practice. Many commercially developed digital interventions available in the marketplace have a minimal evidence base and some could even be harmful. Meanwhile, academic-led evidence-based digital interventions are available, but few, if any, have shown sustained uptake and deployment in real-world settings, and many are not available to the public. The challenge is to close this academic–commercial divide and research-to-practice gap, creating an efficient pipeline of usable and effective digital interventions that address clinical unmet needs, reduce health inequalities, and can be deployed at scale in real-world settings to improve service efficiency and CYP's mental health outcomes.

Key reviews

Hollis, C. *et al.* (2017) Annual research review: digital health interventions for children and young people with mental health problems—a systematic and meta-review. *Journal of Child Psychology and Psychiatry* **58**(4), 474–503. doi:10.1111/jcpp.12663.

Khan, K. *et al.* (2019) The effectiveness of web-based interventions delivered to children and young people with neurodevelopmental disorders: systematic review and meta-analysis. *Journal of Medical Internet Research* **21**(11), e13478. doi:10.2196/13478.

Lehtimaki, S. *et al.* (2021) Evidence on digital mental health interventions for adolescents and young people: systematic overview. *JMIR Mental Health* **8**(4), e25847.

Valentine, A.Z. *et al.* (2020) A systematic review evaluating the implementation of technologies to assess, monitor and treat neurodevelopmental disorders: a map of the current evidence. *Clinical Psychology Review* **80**, 101870. doi:10.1016/j.cpr.2020.101870.

Valentine, A.Z. *et al.* (2021) Implementation of telehealth services to assess, monitor, and treat neurodevelopmental disorders: systematic review. *Journal of Medical Internet Research* **23**(1), e22619.

References

ABHI (2021) *ABHI White Paper: Digital Health Regulatory Concepts*. Association of British HealthTech Industries (ABHI), London.

Andersson, G. & Titov, N. (2014) Advantages and limitations of Internet-based interventions for common mental disorders. *World Psychiatry* **13**(1), 4–11.

Andersson, G. *et al.* (2011) Can the patient decide which modules to endorse? An open trial of tailored Internet treatment of anxiety disorders. *Cognitive Behaviour Therapy* **40**(1), 57–64. doi:10.1080/16506073.2010.529457.

Balcombe, L. & De Leo, D. (2021) Digital mental health challenges and the horizon ahead for solutions. *JMIR Mental Health* **8**(3), e26811.

Bergin, A. & Davies, E.B. (2020) Technology matters: mental health apps–separating the wheat from the chaff. *Child and Adolescent Mental Health* **25**(1), 51.

Bevan Jones, R. *et al.* (2020) Practitioner review: co-design of digital mental health technologies with children and young people. *Journal of Child Psychology and Psychiatry* **61**(8), 928–940.

Borghouts, J. *et al.* (2021) Barriers to and facilitators of user engagement with digital mental health interventions: systematic review. *Journal of Medical Internet Research* **23**(3), e24387.

Burn, A.-M. *et al.* (2022) Developing a web-based app to assess mental health difficulties in secondary school pupils: qualitative user-centered design study. *JMIR Formative Research* **6**(1), e30565.

Cao, J. *et al.* (2020) Tracking and predicting depressive symptoms of adolescents using smartphone-based self-reports, parental evaluations, and passive phone sensor data: development and usability study. *JMIR Mental Health* **7**(1), e14045.

Carey, E. *et al.* (2023) When is a "small effect" actually large and impactful? *PsyArXiv*. January, 18.

Cheek, C. *et al.* (2014) Views of Young people in rural Australia on SPARX, a fantasy world developed for New Zealand youth with depression. *JMIR Serious Games* **2**(1), e3. doi:10.2196/games.3183.

Cheek, C. *et al.* (2015) Integrating health behavior theory and design elements in serious games. *JMIR Mental Health* **2**(2), e11. doi:10.2196/mental.4133.

Chiauzzi, E. *et al.* (2008) MyStudentBody-stress: an online stress management intervention for college students. *Journal of Health Communication* **13**(6), 555–572.

Cohen, K.A. & Schleider, J.L. (2022) Adolescent dropout from brief digital mental health interventions within and beyond randomized trials. *Internet Interventions* **27**, 100496.

Collins, L.M. *et al.* (2014) Optimization of behavioral dynamic treatment regimens based on the sequential, multiple assignment, randomized trial (SMART). *Clinical Trials* **11**(4), 426–434. doi:10.1177/1740774514536795.

Cortese, S. *et al.* (2015) Cognitive training for attention-deficit/hyperactivity disorder: meta-analysis of clinical and neuropsychological outcomes from randomized controlled trials. *Journal of the American Academy of Child & Adolescent Psychiatry* **54**(3), 164–174.

Denecke, K. *et al.* (2021) Artificial intelligence for chatbots in mental health: opportunities and challenges. In: *Multiple Perspectives on Artificial Intelligence in Healthcare: Opportunities and Challenges*. (eds M. Househ, *et al.*). Springer, Cham Switzerland. pp. 115–128.

Denyer, H. *et al.* (2022) ADHD remote technology study of cardiometabolic risk factors and medication adherence (ART-CARMA): a multi-centre prospective cohort study protocol. *BMC Psychiatry* **22**(1), 1–13.

Fleming, T. *et al.* (2012) A pragmatic randomized controlled trial of computerized CBT (SPARX) for symptoms of depression among adolescents excluded from mainstream education. *Behavioural and Cognitive Psychotherapy* **40**(5), 529–541.

Garrido, S. *et al.* (2019) What works and what doesn't? A systematic review of digital mental health interventions for depression and anxiety in young people. *Frontiers in Psychiatry* **10**, 759.

Gold, S.M. *et al.* (2022) Platform trials and the future of evaluating therapeutic behavioural interventions. *Nature Reviews Psychology* **1**(1), 7–8.

Gómez Bergin, A.D. *et al.* (2023) Identifying and categorizing adverse events in trials of digital mental health interventions: narrative scoping review of trials in the international standard randomized controlled trial number registry. *JMIR Mental Health* **10**, e42501.

Groen, G. *et al.* (2022) Development of a mobile application for detection of adolescent mental health problems and feasibility assessment with primary health care workers. *Issues in Mental Health Nursing* **43**(11), 1046–1055.

Hall, C.L. *et al.* (2016a) Innovations in practice: an objective measure of attention, impulsivity and activity reduces time to confirm attention deficit/hyperactivity disorder diagnosis in children - a completed audit cycle. *Child and Adolescent Mental Health* **21**(3), 175–178. doi:10.1111/camh.12140.

Hall, C.L. *et al.* (2016b) The clinical utility of the continuous performance test and objective measures of activity for diagnosing and monitoring ADHD in children: a systematic review. *European Child & Adolescent Psychiatry* **25**(7), 677–699. doi:10.1007/s00787-015-0798-x.

Hall, C.L. *et al.* (2017) Study of user experience of an objective test (QbTest) to aid ADHD assessment and medication management: a multi-methods approach. *BMC Psychiatry* **17**(1), 66. doi:10.1186/s12888-017-1222-5.

Hall, C.L. *et al.* (2019) Investigating a therapist-guided, parent-assisted remote digital behavioural intervention for tics in children and adolescents-'Online Remote Behavioural Intervention for Tics' (ORBIT) trial: Protocol of an internal pilot study and single-blind randomised controlled trial. *BMJ Open* **9**(1), e027583. doi:10.1136/bmjopen-2018-027583.

Hall, C.L. *et al.* (2020) Opportunities and challenges of delivering digital clinical trials: lessons learned from a randomised controlled trial of an online behavioural intervention for children and young people. *Trials* **21**(1), 1–13.

Hill, C. *et al.* (2022) Online Support and Intervention for child anxiety (OSI): development and usability testing. *JMIR Formative Research* **6**(4), e29846.

Hollis, C. *et al.* (2017) Annual research review: digital health interventions for children and young people with mental health problems—a systematic and meta-review. *Journal of Child Psychology and Psychiatry* **58**(4), 474–503. doi:10.1111/jcpp.12663.

Hollis, C. *et al.* (2018) The impact of a computerised test of attention and activity (QbTest) on diagnostic decision-making in children and young people with suspected attention deficit hyperactivity disorder: single-blind randomised controlled trial. *Journal of Child Psychology and Psychiatry* **59**(12), 1298–1308. doi:10.1111/jcpp.12921.

Hollis, C. *et al.* (2021) Therapist-supported online remote behavioural intervention for tics in children and adolescents in England (ORBIT): a multicentre, parallel group, single-blind, randomised controlled trial. *The Lancet Psychiatry* **8**(10), 871–882. doi:10.1016/S2215-0366(21)00235-2.

Hollis, C. *et al.* (2022) Long term clinical and cost-effectiveness of a therapist-supported online remote behavioural intervention for tics (ORBIT) in children and adolescents: extended 12 and 18-month follow-up of a single-blind randomised controlled trial. *Journal of Child Psychology and Psychiatry* **64**, 941–951.

Juárez, A.P. *et al.* (2018) Early identification of ASD through telemedicine: potential value for underserved populations. *Journal of Autism and Developmental Disorders* **48**(8), 2601–2610.

Khan, K. *et al.* (2019) The effectiveness of web-based interventions delivered to children and young people with neurodevelopmental disorders: systematic review and meta-analysis. *Journal of Medical Internet Research* **21**(11), e13478. doi:10.2196/13478.

Kollins, S.H. *et al.* (2020) A novel digital intervention for actively reducing severity of paediatric ADHD (STARS-ADHD): a randomised controlled trial. *The Lancet Digital Health* **2**(4), e168–e178.

Kostyrka-Allchorne, K. *et al.* (2022) Online Parent Training for the Initial Management of ADHD referrals (OPTIMA): the protocol for a randomised controlled trial of a digital parenting intervention implemented to support parents and children on a treatment waitlist. *Trials* **23**(1), 1003.

Lehtimaki, S. *et al.* (2021) Evidence on digital mental health interventions for adolescents and young people: systematic overview. *JMIR Mental Health* **8**(4), e25847.

Leigh, E. & Clark, D.M. (2023) Internet-delivered therapist-assisted cognitive therapy for adolescent social anxiety disorder (OSCA): a randomised controlled trial addressing preliminary efficacy and mechanisms of action. *Journal of Child Psychology and Psychiatry* **64**(1), 145–155.

Lipschitz, J.M. *et al.* (2022) Digital mental health interventions for depression: scoping review of user engagement. *Journal of Medical Internet Research* **24**(10), e39204.

Little, L.M. *et al.* (2018) Acceptability and cost comparison of a telehealth intervention for families of children with autism. *Infants & Young Children* **31**(4), 275–286.

Liverpool, S. *et al.* (2020) Engaging children and young people in digital mental health interventions: systematic review of modes of delivery, facilitators, and barriers. *Journal of Medical Internet Research* **22**(6), e16317.

Lucassen, M.F.G. *et al.* (2013) The views of lesbian, gay and bisexual youth regarding computerised self-help for depression: an exploratory study. *Advances in Mental Health* **12**(1), 22–33. doi:10.5172/jamh.2013.12.1.22.

Mahlous, A.R. & Okkali, B. (2022) A digital mental health intervention for children and parents using a user-centred design. *Advances in Human-Computer Interaction* **2022**(1), 4322177. doi:10.1155/2022/4322177.

March, S. *et al.* (2018) Large-scale dissemination of internet-based cognitive behavioral therapy for youth anxiety: feasibility and acceptability study. *Journal of Medical Internet Research* **20**(7), e9211.

McCashin, D. *et al.* (2019) Qualitative synthesis of young people's experiences with technology-assisted cognitive behavioral therapy: systematic review. *Journal of Medical Internet Research* **21**(11), e13540.

Merry, S.N. *et al.* (2012) The effectiveness of SPARX, a computerised self help intervention for adolescents seeking help for depression: randomised controlled non-inferiority trial. *BMJ* **344**, e2598. doi:10.1136/bmj.e2598.

Murray, E. *et al.* (2016) Evaluating digital health interventions: key questions and approaches. *American Journal of Preventative Medicine* **51**, 843–851.

Musiat, P. *et al.* (2012) Personalised computerised feedback in E-mental health. *Journal of Mental Health* **21**(4), 346–354. doi:10.3109/09638237.2011.648347.

NICE (2022) *Evidence Standards Framework for Digital Health Technologies*. National Institute for Health and Care Excellence (NICE), London. Available: www.nice.org.uk/corporate/ecd7 [2 March 2023].

Noar, S.M. *et al.* (2007) Does tailoring matter? Meta-analytic review of tailored print health behavior change interventions. *Psychological Bulletin* **133**(4), 673–693. doi:10.1037/0033-2909.133.4.673.

Osborn, T.L. *et al.* (2020) Single-session digital intervention for adolescent depression, anxiety, and well-being: outcomes of a randomized controlled trial with Kenyan adolescents. *Journal of Consulting and Clinical Psychology* **88**(7), 657.

Pote, H. *et al.* (2021) Workforce challenges in digital health implementation: how are clinical psychology training programmes developing digital competences? *Digital Health* **7**, 2055207620985396.

Rasing, S.P. *et al.* (2020) Is digital treatment the holy grail? Literature review on computerized and blended treatment for depressive disorders in youth. *International Journal of Environmental Research and Public Health* **17**(1), 153.

Reese, R.M. *et al.* (2015) Brief report: use of interactive television in identifying autism in young children: methodology and preliminary data. *Journal of Autism and Developmental Disorders* **45**(5), 1474–1482.

Rickwood, D. & Bradford, S. (2012) The role of self-help in the treatment of mild anxiety disorders in young people: an evidence-based review. *Psychology Research and Behavior Management* **5**, 25–36.

Roland, J. *et al.* (2020) *The digital mental health revolution: Transforming care through innovation and scale-up*. World Innovation Summit for Health, 2020, Doha, Qatar.

Santosh, P. *et al.* (2023) Remote assessment of ADHD in children and adolescents: recommendations from the European ADHD guidelines group following the clinical experience during the COVID-19 pandemic. *European Child & Adolescent Psychiatry*, 1–15.

Saxena, S. *et al.* (2007) Resources for mental health: scarcity, inequity, and inefficiency. *The Lancet* **370**(9590), 878–889.

Schueller, S.M. *et al.* (2013) Realizing the potential of behavioral intervention technologies. *Current Directions in Psychological Science* **22**(6), 478–483.

Schueller, S.M. *et al.* (2022) An introduction to core competencies for the use of mobile apps in cognitive and behavioral practice. *Cognitive and Behavioral Practice* **29**(1), 69–80.

Shah, R. *et al.* (2019) Participating from homes and offices: proof-of-concept study of multi-point videoconferencing to deliver group parent training intervention for attention-deficit/hyperactivity disorder. *Asian Journal of Psychiatry* **41**, 20–22.

Sieberts, S.K. *et al.* (2022) Young people's data governance preferences for their mental health data: MINDKIND study findings from India, South Africa, and the United Kingdom. *medRxiv*. doi:10.1101/2022.12.19.22283679.

Simons, L. *et al.* (2016) Developing mHealth remote monitoring technology for attention deficit hyperactivity disorder: a qualitative study eliciting user priorities and needs. *JMIR mHealth and uHealth* **e5009**.

Spence, S.H. *et al.* (2011) A randomized controlled trial of online versus clinic-based CBT for adolescent anxiety. *Journal of Consulting and Clinical Psychology* **79**(5), 629.

Stainbrook, J.A. *et al.* (2019) Measuring the service system impact of a novel telediagnostic service program for young children with autism spectrum disorder. *Autism* **23**(4), 1051–1056.

Suess, A.N. *et al.* (2016) Preliminary evidence on the use of telehealth in an outpatient behavior clinic. *Journal of Applied Behavior Analysis* **49**(3), 686–692.

Taylor, L. *et al.* (2022) A randomised controlled trial to compare clinical and cost-effectiveness of an online parent-led treatment for child anxiety problems with usual care in the context of COVID-19 delivered in child and adolescent mental health services in the UK (co-CAT): a study protocol for a randomised controlled trial. *Trials* **23**(1), 942.

Tong, F. *et al.* (2022) Digital therapeutic alliance with fully automated mental health smartphone apps: a narrative review. *Frontiers in Psychiatry* **13**, 819623.

Valentine, A.Z. *et al.* (2020) A systematic review evaluating the implementation of technologies to assess, monitor and treat neurodevelopmental disorders: a map of the current evidence. *Clinical Psychology Review* **80**, 101870. doi:10.1016/j.cpr.2020.101870.

Valentine, A.Z. *et al.* (2021) Implementation of telehealth services to assess, monitor, and treat neurodevelopmental disorders: systematic review. *Journal of Medical Internet Research* **23**(1), e22619.

Valstar, M., *et al.* (2014) AVEC 2014: 3D Dimensional Affect and Depression Recognition Challenge. Unpublished paper presented at the Proceedings of the 4th International Workshop on Audio/Visual Emotion Challenge. Orlando, FL, USA.

Venturo-Conerly, K.E. *et al.* (2022) Effectiveness of youth psychotherapy delivered remotely: a meta-analysis. *American Psychologist* **77**(1), 71.

Vigerland, S. *et al.* (2016) Internet-delivered cognitive behavioural therapy for children with anxiety disorders: a randomised controlled trial. *Behaviour Research and Therapy* **76**, 47–56. doi:10.1016/j.brat.2015.11.006.

Waite, P. *et al.* (2019) A randomized controlled trial of internet-delivered cognitive behaviour therapy for adolescent anxiety disorders in a routine clinical care setting with and without parent sessions. *Child and Adolescent Mental Health* **24**(3), 242–250.

Wallisch, A. *et al.* (2019) Parent perspectives of an occupational therapy telehealth intervention. *International Journal of Telerehabilitation* **11**(1), 15.

Wang, L. & Miller, L.C. (2020) Just-in-the-moment adaptive interventions (JITAI): a meta-analytical review. *Health Communication* **35**(12), 1531–1544.

Wickersham, A. *et al.* (2022) Computerized cognitive behavioral therapy for treatment of depression and anxiety in adolescents: systematic review and meta-analysis. *Journal of Medical Internet Research* **24**(4), e29842.

PART IV

Clinical syndromes: neurodevelopment, emotional, behavior, somatic/body–brain

A: Neurodevelopment

CHAPTER 50
Autism

Peter Szatmari[1,2,3], Stephanie H. Ameis[2,3,4] and Meng-Chuan Lai[3,4,5]
[1]Department of Psychiatry, Temerty Faculty of Medicine, University of Toronto, Toronto, Ontario, Canada
[2]Cundill Centre for Child and Youth Depression, Campbell Family Mental Health Research Institute, Centre for Addiction and Mental Health, Toronto, Ontario, Canada
[3]Neurosciences & Mental Health and Department of Psychiatry, The Hospital for Sick Children, Toronto, Ontario, Canada
[4]Department of Psychiatry and Institute of Medical Science, Temerty Faculty of Medicine, University of Toronto, Toronto, Ontario, Canada
[5]The Margaret and Wallace McCain Centre for Child, Youth & Family Mental Health and Azrieli Adult Neurodevelopmental Centre, Campbell Family Mental Health Research Institute, Centre for Addiction and Mental Health, Toronto, Ontario, Canada

Autism, currently termed "autism spectrum disorder" in the *Diagnostic and Statistical Manual of Mental Disorders*, 5th edition, text Revision (DSM-5-TR; American Psychiatric Association, 2022) and *International Classification of Diseases*, 11th Revision (ICD-11; World Health Organization, 2019a), is a categorical neurodevelopmental diagnosis (see Chapter 3) that is diagnosed nowadays at an average population prevalence of 1–2% (Salari *et al.*, 2022; Zeidan *et al.*, 2022). This chapter starts with a brief introduction to the nosological evolution of the diagnosis, as this is central to understanding the evolving diagnostic concept and its clinical relevance. We then introduce clinical and epidemiological features, which serve as the foundation for assessments. Etiological and neurocognitive bases are illustrated to enhance a developmental understanding of autism. Unique considerations regarding co-occurring psychiatric conditions are highlighted to facilitate tailored care. Finally, the current evidence for support and intervention is discussed.

Diagnostic conceptualization

The diagnosis as a lens of understanding

The definition of autism has evolved greatly over the past century since it was first described as a syndrome (Frankl, 1943; Kanner, 1943; Asperger, 1944; Ssucharewa & Wolff, 1996; Simmonds & Sukhareva, 2020). Evolving nosology reflects efforts to optimize reliability while maintaining reasonable validity. Autism as a diagnostic construct has practical value but is a moving target (Hacking, 2007) rather than an objective entity "independent of its embodiment in particular individuals" (Verhoeff, 2012). Clinicians should be aware of the conceptual evolution of the diagnostic construct and consider intersections with medical and social models of disability.

From the prototypical case series to the diagnostic manual definitions

It is often cited that Leo Kanner (1894–1981) and Hans Asperger (1906–1980) were the first to describe the profiles shaping what is now encapsulated as autism. Kanner's report of 11 children (8 boys, 3 girls) was published in English in 1943 (Kanner, 1943) and Asperger's report of 4 boys published in German in 1944 (Asperger, 1944). Asperger's account was eventually introduced into the English-speaking literature in the 1980s by Lorna Wing (Wing, 1981a). Yet earlier in 1926, Grunya Sukhareva (1891–1981) had already published her observations of 6 boys and 5 girls in two German papers (Ssucharewa & Wolff, 1996; Simmonds & Sukhareva, 2020), with profiles that match current depictions of autism.

From Kanner's depictions in the 1940s–1960s, "extreme self-isolation" and "obsessive insistence on the preservation of sameness" were considered the two defining features; language-speech problems were not considered core but "derivatives of the basic disturbance in human relatedness" (Eisenberg & Kanner, 1956). During the 1960s–1980s, the earliest epidemiological (Lockyer & Rutter, 1969) and cognitive studies (Frith, 1970) reshaped the understanding of autism from emphasizing affective withdrawal as the essential feature toward abnormal language and cognitive-perceptual global integration defects as primary features (Verhoeff, 2013). These findings contributed to Michael Rutter's 1978 "childhood autism" criteria with four essential early developmental features: onset before 30 months, impaired social development, delayed and deviant language development,

Rutter's Child and Adolescent Psychiatry and Psychology, Seventh Edition.
Edited by Anita Thapar, Daniel S. Pine, Samuele Cortese, Cathy Creswell, Tamsin J. Ford, James F. Leckman, and Argyris Stringaris.

Companion website: www.wiley.com/go/thapar/rutterspsych7

and insistence on sameness (Rutter, 1978). This conceptualization was reflected in the first operationalization of autism in DSM-III in 1980 (American Psychiatric Association, 1980).

Meanwhile, Lorna Wing introduced Asperger's depictions as part of the concept of an autism spectrum (Wing, 1981a). Her epidemiological work demonstrated the widely distributed nature of autistic features across developmental disabilities (Wing, 1981b). Wing noted the continuity between Kanner's autism and less marked forms and suggested that the core features were "the triad of impairment on social interaction, communication, and imagination," including difficulties understanding and using "unwritten rules of social behaviour" (Wing, 1981b). This enriched and broadened conceptualization of autism was reflected in DSM-III-R (American Psychiatric Association, 1987). Thereafter, DSM-IV/DSM-IV-TR (harmonized with ICD-10; American Psychiatric Association, 1994, 2000; World Health Organization, 1993) reduced the criteria items to be more succinct from a psychometric perspective and introduced subtypes, including the commonly used, yet inconsistently defined, Asperger's disorder/syndrome. Owing to reliability and validity concerns and a conceptual reorganization of features (Lord & Jones, 2012), DSM-5 (American Psychiatric Association, 2013) and ICD-11 (World Health Organization, 2019a) removed subtypes; new historical evidence on Hans Asperger's involvement in the Nazi regime also questioned the appropriateness of the eponym Asperger's syndrome (Czech, 2018). The label "autism spectrum disorder" is used currently to cover a range of clinical manifestations. Core features include two domains and language is considered a separate construct (see the section "Phenomenology"). Illustrations of subtler presentations (Lai *et al.*, 2022) have also been incorporated in DSM-5-TR (American Psychiatric Association, 2022).

The fuzzy boundary and heterogeneity

Accompanying these evolving conceptualizations are ongoing debates on the boundary of autism with other neurodevelopmental conditions and typical development. This debate is important despite the good test–retest reliability of the DSM-5 criteria (Regier *et al.*, 2013), given the multilevel heterogeneity of autism (Georgiades *et al.*, 2017; Lombardo *et al.*, 2019; Parellada *et al.*, 2023). This heterogeneity and the increasing prevalence (see the section "Epidemiology") can be viewed as a natural consequence of the recognition of the spectrum's dimensionality, and the diverse presentations of autism, highlighting the need for individualized approaches to diagnosis and care (Lai & Baron-Cohen, 2015). Meanwhile, there are concerns that broadening the construct could lead to a poorer mechanistic understanding of autism (Mottron, 2021).

These ongoing reflections should be understood alongside two conceptual lenses. First, some view autism as a qualitatively distinct category (the *categorical* view) and some view it at the extreme of a continuous distribution of traits (the *dimensional* view); psychometric work suggests that both are true and the combination (the *hybrid* view) improves the fit to data (Wittkopf *et al.*, 2023). Second, neurodevelopmental conditions tend to co-occur across diagnoses and symptoms/traits (Thapar *et al.*, 2017). A *transdiagnostic* approach that moves beyond categories and focuses on cross-cutting dimensions may improve mechanistic clarification and care innovation (Astle *et al.*, 2022; Pacheco *et al.*, 2022).

Harmonizing the medical and social models of disability

There are risks for insensitive care when a clinician relies solely on a medical (i.e., disability reflects disorders/impairments existing within the person) or social model (i.e., disability is caused by barriers imposed to the person by society) of disability to understand autism (e.g., overmedicalization of behaviors or overlooking impairments). Disability originates from person–environment interactions, and a neurodiversity approach harmonizes diverging views (Dwyer, 2022). *Neurodiversity* refers to the collective diversity of human minds, a biological phenomenon of the variation of neurocognitive functioning (Walker, 2021). The *neurodiversity movement* is a social justice movement stemming from the disability rights movement and upholds the *neurodiversity paradigm* (Walker, 2021), which does not reject the idea of disability but challenges a narrow medical conceptualization of autism (Kapp *et al.*, 2013; Dwyer, 2022). The neurodiversity paradigm asserts neurodiversity to be a natural and valuable form of human variation, and emphasizes that social dynamics construct the idea of a "normal" or "healthy" mind (Walker, 2021; Pellicano & den Houting, 2022). Autism is viewed as an example of *neurodivergence*, a *neurotype* that functions in ways that diverge substantially from the dominant societal norms. Harmonizing the medical and social models of disability related to autism involves affirming both differences and disabilities (Kapp *et al.*, 2013; Lai *et al.*, 2020), recognizing diagnostic processes as socially situated activities (Hayes *et al.*, 2022), appreciating person–environment fit (Lai & Baron-Cohen, 2015), reconciling autistic self-advocacy with clinical evidence (Schuck *et al.*, 2022), and developing neurodivergence-informed practice (Doherty *et al.*, 2023; Lai, 2023). The neurodiversity paradigm also calls for clinicians to respect a person's identity in relation to autism (e.g., use of identity-first and/or person-first language), to balance the focus between challenges and strengths, and to avoid assumptions that perpetuate stigmatization (Dwyer *et al.*, 2022). Preferred terminology may be evolving, differ by sociolinguistic contexts, and should be based on the best interests and preferences of the autistic person (Dwyer *et al.*, 2022).

Phenomenology

DSM-5-TR and ICD-11 both define "autism spectrum disorder" (ASD) by two core domains: (i) social-communication: persistent deficits in "the ability to initiate and to sustain reciprocal social interaction and social communication" (ICD-11) or "social communication and social interaction across multiple contexts" (DSM-5-TR); and (ii) restricted and repetitive behaviors (RRB): "a range of restricted, repetitive, and inflexible patterns of behavior, interests or activities that are clearly atypical or excessive for the individual's age and sociocultural context" (ICD-11) or "restricted, repetitive patterns of behavior, interests, or activities" (DSM-5-TR). DSM-5-TR categorizes the social-communication domain into three subdomains (social–emotional reciprocity; nonverbal communicative behaviors used for social interaction; and developing, maintaining, and understanding relationships) and requires all three subdomains be met, currently or by history, to warrant a diagnosis. RRB is categorized into four subdomains (stereotyped or repetitive motor movements, use of objects, or speech; insistence on sameness, inflexible adherence to routines, or ritualized patterns of verbal or nonverbal behavior; highly restricted, fixated interests that are abnormal in intensity or focus; hyper- or hyporeactivity to sensory input or unusual interest in sensory aspects of the environment) and at least two subdomains need to be met, currently or by history, for an autism diagnosis. ICD-11 lists seven exemplar manifestations in each of the social-communication and RRB domains, without specifying numbers of features to be met (World Health Organization, 2019b).

These features should be present during early development, typically in early childhood, but may not become fully manifest until later in life when social demands exceed capacities. This acknowledgment offers a principled way for clinicians to diagnose autism beyond childhood, especially for the first time in adolescence or adulthood (Lai & Baron-Cohen, 2015). The features noted in DSM-5-TR and ICD-11 range from prototypical manifestations (e.g., no initiation of social interaction, lack of joint attention and shared social play, hand flapping, distress at small environmental changes, strong attachment to unique objects, extreme noise sensitivity, and echolalia) to subtle presentations that become apparent when contextual demands exceed capacity. Autistic individuals can have any kind of intellectual functioning and language abilities, which can modify their autistic presentations and developmental courses (see the section "Longitudinal outcomes"). A clinical ASD diagnosis (different from an autistic identity of a person) is only adequate when there are significant impairments associated with these features in neurotypical contexts and/or when there are exceptional efforts of the person to minimize impairments and to function (ICD-11).

Specifiers that highlight associated features that reflect heterogeneity include intellectual and functional language abilities (DSM-5-TR and ICD-11), loss of previously acquired skills (ICD-11), catatonia (DSM-5-TR), association with a known genetic or other medical condition or environmental factor (DSM-5-TR), association with a neurodevelopmental, mental, or behavioral problem (DSM-5-TR), and level of support needs (DSM-5-TR).

Epidemiology

Prevalence refers to the number of persons with a certain condition per unit of the population, usually at a single point in time. The condition can be defined based on self-identification, reaching diagnostic criteria on a measure, or via administrative databases where diagnosed individuals are registered. Prevalence should be understood in the sampling and measurement contexts. Sampling is key and ideally should be from a representative subset of the general population. As the diagnostic criteria have evolved (see the section "Diagnostic conceptualization"), when criteria become more inclusive the prevalence estimates increase. In addition, prevalence estimates derived from administrative databases are likely higher in regions with more resource-intensive health services—the easier it is to access a diagnostic center, the more diagnosed individuals there are in a register (O'Donnell *et al.*, 2022).

Recent meta-analyses show pooled autism prevalence estimates are at 1–2% (Salari *et al.*, 2022; Zeidan *et al.*, 2022). However, there is significant variation in estimates by method of diagnosis, whether the country is a high-income country (HIC) or low- and middle-income country (LMIC), sampling methods, screening tools, and autism diagnostic criteria (Salari *et al.*, 2022). A meta-analysis of studies during 2012–2019 across 35 countries reported a mean age of autism diagnosis at 60.48 months (95% CI 50.12–70.83) and at 43.18 months (95% CI 39.79–46.57) for studies including only children ≤10 years of age (van 't Hof *et al.*, 2021). Mean age estimates do not provide information about when identification is most likely and are influenced by the sample age range, which may not include the full age range for when a diagnosis is possible. A recent time-to-event analysis (that minimizes bias in estimating age at identification) using data from two national surveys in the United States (US) during 2009–2012 indicated that one-third to one-half of children receive an autism diagnosis after 6 years of age (Sheldrick *et al.*, 2017).

The sex assigned at birth ratio is 3–4:1 male to female. The largest meta-analysis shows an overall ratio of 4.20:1 (95% CI 3.84–4.60); studies with high-quality methodologies show a ratio of 3.32:1 (95% CI 2.88–3.84), studies screening the general population show a ratio of 3.25:1 (95% CI 2.93–3.62), and both are different from registry-based samples that have a higher ratio of 4.56:1 (95% CI 4.10–5.07) (Loomes *et al.*, 2017). In infants with increased likelihood of developing autism (i.e., those with an older sibling diagnosed with autism), the male-to-female ratio for those diagnosed with autism at 3 years-old is 3.18:1 (Messinger *et al.*, 2015). These findings suggest an underrecognition of autism in females in daily practice (Lai *et al.*, 2023), though the recognition is improving in countries such as the UK (Russell *et al.*, 2022) and the US (Maenner *et al.*, 2023). The prevalence also seems higher in children as opposed to adolescents or adults, although adult diagnosis has been increasing in some countries (Russell *et al.*, 2022) to comparable rates of 1.1% (Brugha *et al.*, 2016). There has been a secular increase in prevalence such that recent studies provide higher rates than older studies, reflective of the combined effects of increasing community awareness, better identification, the impact of more recent diagnostic criteria, and the greater availability of services (Zeidan *et al.*, 2022).

Longitudinal outcomes

A meta-analysis of diagnostic stability over at least a 12-month period for those aged 7 months–16.5 years using the Autism Diagnostic Observation Schedule (ADOS), a widely used instrument to support autism diagnostics, demonstrated that there was no significant change in ADOS scores for the samples overall, but 18% shifted their classification from "autism" to milder "autism spectrum" (Bieleninik *et al.*, 2017). However, there is considerable variation between studies.

A systematic review of adolescent outcomes for autistic children without intellectual disabilities (ID) reported that although IQ scores and ASD diagnosis overall were quite stable, roughly 20% no longer met criteria for ASD during this developmental phase (Rosello *et al.*, 2021). High rates of co-occurring psychiatric diagnoses, including anxiety and depression, were apparent and represented an additional source of impairment. There was improvement across theory of mind (i.e., the ability to understand other people by ascribing mental states to them), executive function, and central coherence (i.e., the tendency to draw together diverse information to construct higher-level meaning in context), but only executive function was an outcome predictor.

For adulthood outcomes, many studies used combined metrics of socialization, occupational status, and independent living (Magiati *et al.*, 2014). Considering that these studies sampled individuals who were diagnosed more than 20 years ago, with a high proportion of them having ID or borderline intelligence, 50% of these autistic adults remained dependent on their families. With some reduction in autism symptoms, diagnostic stability remained high and language skills remained low. IQ was largely stable or showed a slight decline with age. There were some improvements in daily living skills and communication, more so than in socialization. There were high rates of co-occurring anxiety and depression. The two most important early predictors of adulthood outcomes were baseline IQ and language ability. Again, findings show a high degree of variability between studies and between autistic individuals. Newer studies have demonstrated better outcomes, suggesting secular changes and differences in the characteristics of the autistic individuals, likely due to changes in diagnostic criteria and including fewer individuals with ID.

An underaddressed issue is heterogeneity in change. These systematic reviews have focused on studies that assume variation in the outcome domain is quantitative rather than qualitative (e.g., all autistic children change at the same rate and differ by the same amount at inception and at outcome). Qualitative variation would allow for different subgroups to change at different rates and in different directions (i.e., some improving and some worsening). The concept of *chronogeneity*, an emerging theme of recent studies (Pender *et al.*, 2020; Gentles *et al.*, 2024), describes the variation in the rate of change of different domains within the autism phenotype between individuals and within the same person at different developmental stages (Georgiades *et al.*, 2017). For example, in a Canadian inception cohort of autistic children, between 2 and 6 years of age there were at least three trajectories of adaptive functioning, and two trajectories of ADOS scores (Szatmari *et al.*, 2015). The trajectories associated with each domain were not "yoked" together: children with a rapid decrease in ADOS scores were not necessarily in the highest adaptive functioning group. This finding illustrates how heterogeneity between autistic individuals over time exists but that even within a person, different developmental domains change over time at their own rate.

Assessment

A clinical autism diagnosis can be reliably made by 18–24 months, and early features (e.g., differences in attention, prelinguistic communication, social engagement, and sensorimotor processing) can be seen in infancy (Dawson *et al.*, 2023). Two systematic reviews of English-language Clinical Practice Guidelines published during 2000–2022 concluded that the 2011 UK National Institute for Health and Care Excellence (NICE) guidance (updated in 2017) provides the highest quality evidence to guide best practice for the screening and assessment of autism (Penner *et al.*, 2018; Amer *et al.*, 2022).

Surveillance and screening

Most guidance recommends that primary care providers conduct routine systematic monitoring of early development of all children (i.e., developmental surveillance) to provide opportunities for parents to express concerns and identify children requiring secondary screening for autism when developmental, behavioral, or mental health concerns are raised (e.g., language delay, not responding to name, or lack of pointing to show interest) (U.S. Preventive Services Task Force, 2016; National Institute for Health and Care Excellence, 2017; Yuen *et al.*, 2018; Hyman *et al.*, 2020; Ministry of Disabled People, 2022). Of note, the American Academy of Pediatrics recommends standardized universal autism screening (in addition to developmental surveillance) at 18 and 24 months using the parent-reported Modified Checklist for Autism in Toddlers (M-CHAT) (Hyman *et al.*, 2020). M-CHAT has adequate pooled sensitivity (0.83, 95% CI 0.77–0.88) and specificity (0.94, 95% CI 0.89–0.97) (Wieckowski *et al.*, 2023) especially in children aged 24–30 months-old referred for developmental-behavioral or psychiatric concerns (Yuen *et al.*, 2018).

Assessment components

Initial assessment should include the review of perinatal and prenatal history, developmental presentation, presence of regression, possible etiological correlates (see the section "Factors associated with emergence"), and co-occurring developmental, medical, and psychiatric problems. It is of value to review school reports, any material related to the child's early development, and interventions trialed (including complementary and alternative treatment). Once primary care providers collect this initial information and concerns are maintained, a referral should be made for a specialized autism assessment to: (i) clarify an autism diagnosis; (ii) identify co-occurring conditions; (iii) determine an individual's adaptive functioning to clarify strengths, challenges, and support needs; and (iv) develop an individualized longitudinal care plan (National Institute for Health and Care Excellence, 2017; Lord *et al.*, 2022). A family-centered approach is essential to the diagnostic assessment. Sociocultural and linguistic barriers in assessment should be considered, and approaches modified to support family engagement and facilitate the assessment.

Most available guidelines recommend a multidisciplinary team approach to autism assessment to support diagnostic accuracy based on clinical consensus, provide a comprehensive needs assessment, and reduce the burden on families of sequential assessments (Penner *et al.*, 2018). The comprehensive assessment should cover multiple sources of information (Table 50.1) (National Institute for Health and Care Excellence, 2017; Brian *et al.*, 2019; Hyman *et al.*, 2020; Manickam *et al.*, 2021; Ministry of Disabled People, 2022). While a multidisciplinary team approach is recommended, it is important for clinicians to be aware of the limited access to specialized teams that is a reality in many care settings, such as in LMICs or HICs where plans may preclude reimbursement of multiple providers, and that high demand for such teams can lead to prolonged wait times for assessment (Brian *et al.*, 2019; Lord *et al.*, 2022). So as not to delay access to interventions, recent guidance suggests that a trained health care provider comfortable with the application of autism clinical criteria can make an initial autism diagnosis, particularly when the diagnosis is uncomplicated (Brian *et al.*, 2019; Hyman *et al.*, 2020). Ongoing diagnostic clarification with a multidisciplinary approach should follow when resources allow.

Table 50.1 Assessment at a glance.

- A full review of medical and relevant records (e.g., health history, developmental history, and family history)
- Physical examination (e.g., congenital anomalies, skin conditions, head circumference, height, and weight)
- Clinical interviewing of an individual (if appropriate based on age and ability to engage) and their caregivers and/or other informants (e.g., collateral information from teachers and others involved in care) to obtain clinical history and concerns across settings
- Direct observation and interaction, ideally include direct observation in everyday settings
- Tailored etiological evaluation based on clinical presentations:
  - exome and genome sequencing in the presence of congenital anomalies, developmental delay, or intellectual disability (ID)
  - electroencephalography (EEG) with a suspicion of epilepsy
  - magnetic resonance imaging (MRI) in the case of regression, macro/microcephaly, or abnormal neurological findings
  - specialist consultation for metabolic or mitochondrial disorders with atypical developmental regression, based on family history or other presentations (e.g., cyclic vomiting, lethargy, seizures)
  - in North American jurisdictions, chromosomal microarray and fragile X analysis are routinely recommended for children diagnosed with autism
- Assessments to clarify strengths, needs, and co-occurring diagnoses to create tailored and individualized longitudinal treatment plans:
  - cognitive testing to clarify intellectual profile
  - audiology assessment to rule out hearing impairment
  - communication and mental health assessments to clarify co-occurring diagnoses
- A feedback session (Figure 50.1)

Standardized instruments

There are a number of instruments available to support diagnostic assessment across ages (Figure 50.2), more established for children (Randall *et al.*, 2018) than youth and adults (Wigham *et al.*, 2019). A recent Cochrane review of six diagnostic tools enabled meta-analyses to determine pooled sensitivity and specificity, of the ADOS, the Childhood Autism Rating Scale (CARS), and the Autism Diagnostic Interview-Revised (ADI-R) for children ≤6 years of age. All tools had similar specificity and the ADOS had the highest summary sensitivity (Randall *et al.*, 2018), underlining the usefulness of the ADOS/ADOS-2 in clinical settings. Reliability of diagnosis across settings and time improves when caregiver report and clinical observation is collected alongside standardized information (Zander *et al.*, 2015). While current recommendations emphasize that a best-estimate clinical diagnosis should be based on multiple convergent sources of information rather than a specific instrument, clinicians should use at least one standardized instrument to document autism features to support diagnosis and for comparison with later assessments (Lord *et al.*, 2022).

Age, developmental level, sex/gender, and socioecological considerations

There are several factors that can influence whether an individual receives an autism diagnosis, such as race-ethnicity, immigrant status, and socioeconomic disadvantage. In North America and Europe, children from non-white backgrounds, especially females assigned at birth (Roman-Urrestarazu *et al.*, 2022), tend to be less often diagnosed (Habayeb *et al.*, 2022) or diagnosed later (Constantino *et al.*, 2020) with autism than their white peers. Epidemiological data show a potential underrecognition of autism in females in clinical settings (Loomes *et al.*, 2017). The historical stereotypes that autism in females is associated with neurological and cognitive impairments might render those without such presentations as less noticeable (Bölte *et al.*, 2023), resulting in later diagnosis (Russell *et al.*, 2022). A fulsome consideration of how behaviors diverge from same-sex/gender peers and are shaped by gender socialization is important to capturing subtle autism presentations (Lai *et al.*, 2023). Co-occurring conditions such as attention deficit hyperactivity disorder (ADHD) may delay autism diagnosis (Kentrou *et al.*, 2019). Diagnostic clarification can be particularly difficult in younger children (<24 months), adolescents and adults, those with co-occurring conditions, and when an informant of early developmental history is not available.

To overcome these difficulties, clinicians should collect information across multiple contexts, such as school and home

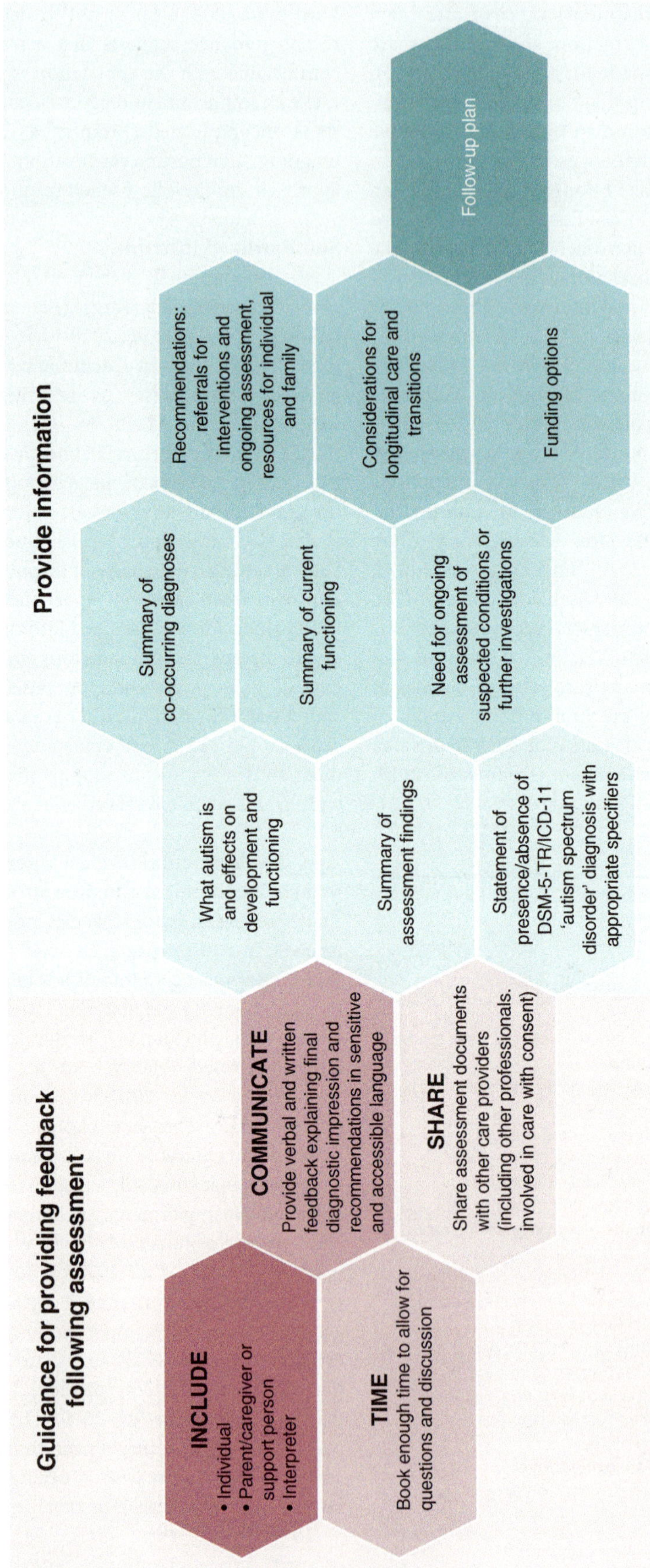

Figure 50.1 Components of assessment feedback.

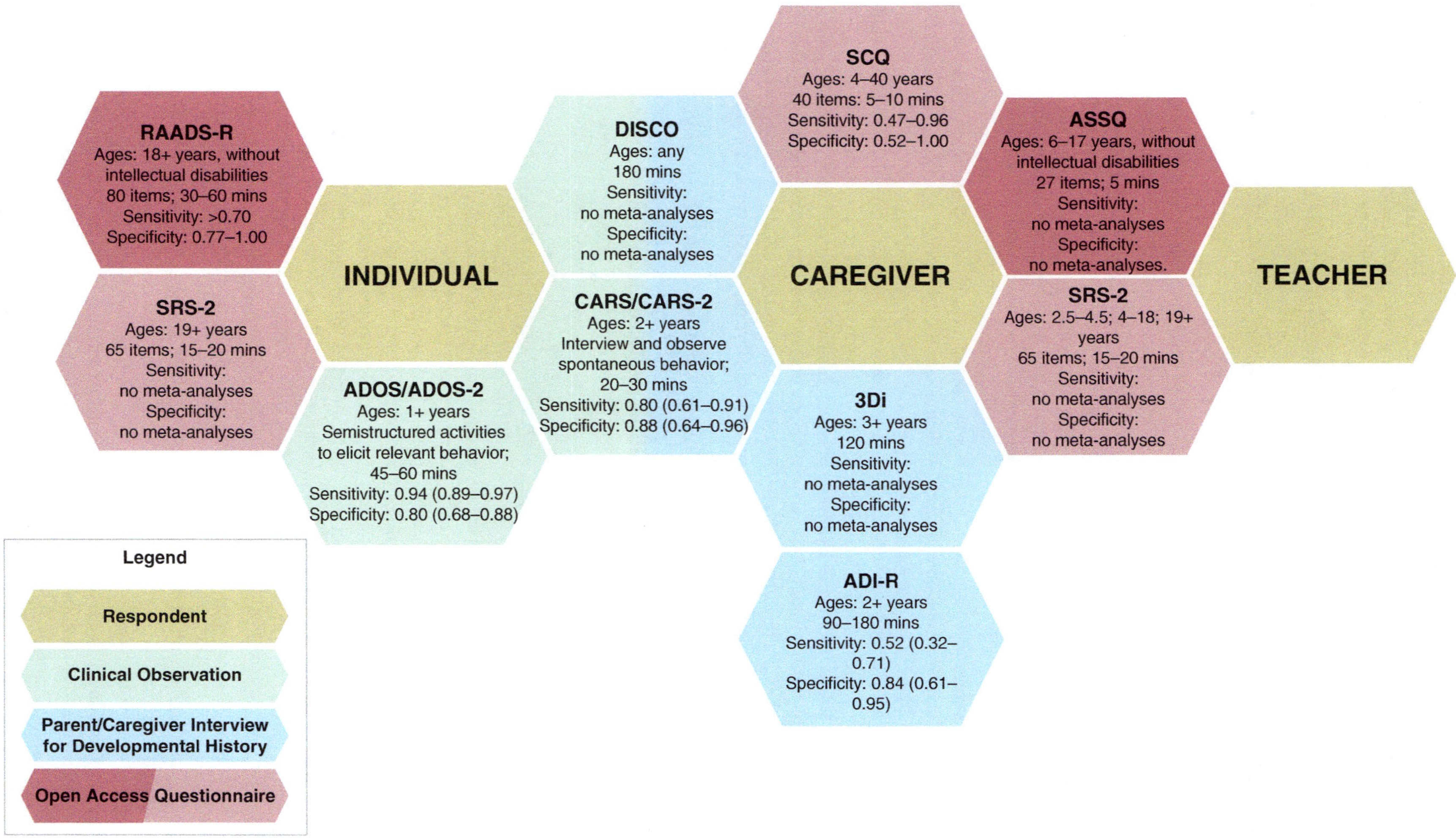

Figure 50.2 Commonly used and validated standardized instruments: Ritvo Autism Asperger Diagnostic Scale–Revised (RAADS-R); Social Responsiveness Scale, 2nd edition (SRS-2); Autism Diagnostic Observation Schedule, 1st/2nd edition (ADOS/ADOS-2); Diagnostic Interview for Social and Communication Disorders (DISCO); Childhood Autism Rating Scale, 1st/2nd edition (CARS/CARS-2); Social Communication Questionnaire (SCQ); Developmental, Dimensional, and Diagnostic Interview (3Di); Autism Diagnostic Interview–Revised (ADI-R); Autism Spectrum Screening Questionnaire (ASSQ).

(rather than based on a one-off observation), including childhood observers and the person themselves. A developmental lens is needed to understand the person's coping experiences in their unique socioecology (i.e., the interplay between individual, relationship, community, and societal factors), and to adequately capture subtle presentations and their functional impact. So-called masking, compensation, or camouflaging experiences (Zhuang *et al.*, 2023) may be present in older children and adolescents and can be identified through a developmental lens, but they are not diagnostic nor specific to autism (Lai *et al.*, 2022). This socioecological diagnostic formulation is especially informative for the planning of personalized and neurodivergence-informed care (see the section "Support and intervention").

Factors associated with emergence

Genetic and environmental factors

Autism can run in the family and the diagnostic outcome can be relevant for genetic counseling (see Chapter 21). The increased occurrence rates in families with one autistic individual also cut across neurodevelopmental and psychiatric diagnoses (Baselmans *et al.*, 2021). Individuals with a first-degree relative diagnosed with autism, compared to those without, have an elevated likelihood of being diagnosed with autism themselves (risk ratio 8.7) (Baselmans *et al.*, 2021). Population-based data that estimate *heritability* (i.e., variance of the phenotype "explained" by genetics) provide strong evidence for the role of genetic factors. A meta-analysis of twin studies published before 2015 found substantial heritability (64–91%) and significant shared environmental effects (7–35%) for autism (Tick *et al.*, 2016). Later large-scale studies confirm that the heritability, by narrow (autistic disorder) or broad (ASD) criteria, is around, or larger than, 80% (Bai *et al.*, 2019; Taylor *et al.*, 2020).

Molecular and clinical genetic studies suggest that the genetic etiology of autism comes from the joint effects of a diverse set of genes, and there is substantial heterogeneity regarding the contributing genetic loci; two autistic individuals can have very different genetic backgrounds leading to a similar autism presentation (i.e., *equifinality*). Autism-associated genetic factors can be categorized into two sets: changes that are *rare* and have strong effects in eliciting autism phenotypes but have low population rates, and *common* genetic variants that each have small effects but jointly contribute to autism phenotypic traits (see Chapter 21).

For rare variants, *de novo* (i.e., not inherited from parents) mutations play strong etiological roles but with high interindividual variability in the genetic loci involved. Recent exome sequencing data show there are at least 72 genes specifically associated with autism that are functionally disrupted by these variants in the forms of protein-truncating variants, damaging missense variants, and copy number variants (CNVs), with CNVs conferring the greatest relative risk, alongside at least 373 genes associated with both autism and developmental delay (Fu *et al.*, 2022). The continuing discovery of rare genetic variants via exome and genome sequencing offers the possibility of a finite (but regularly updating) gene list for examination when autism is diagnosed and/or suspected (Schaaf *et al.*, 2020). This can inform holistic health care as many rare variants have pleiotropic (i.e., multiple) effects with variable penetrance (Fu *et al.*, 2022), associated with other health outcomes. Exome and genome sequencing is currently only clinically recommended for a subset of autistic individuals, such as those with congenital anomalies, developmental delay, or ID (Manickam *et al.*, 2021).

The prevalence rates of autism phenotypes are also substantially high in several genetic syndromes characterized by large structural changes (see Chapter 21), such as Rett's syndrome (61%, only females), Cohen's syndrome (54%), Cornelia de Lange syndrome (43%), tuberous sclerosis complex (36%), Angelman's syndrome (34%), CHARGE syndrome (30%), fragile X syndrome (22%; 30% in males), neurofibromatosis type 1 (18%), Down syndrome (16%), Noonan's syndrome (15%), Williams' syndrome (12%), and 22q11.2 deletion syndrome (11%) (Richards *et al.*, 2015).

For small-effect common genetic variants, studies so far might be underpowered to pinpoint specific single nucleotide polymorphisms (Grove *et al.*, 2019). However, polygenic scores (PGS, summary measures from genome-wide association studies) demonstrate joint effects of common variants and show complementary roles to rare variants in autism emergence, and, in contrast to rare variants, are less associated with developmental delay (Antaki *et al.*, 2022; Warrier *et al.*, 2022). Like the pleiotropic effects of rare variants, effects of autism-related common variants are shared with other human traits. Autism-related PGS correlate with PGS for several later-occurring psychiatric illnesses (i.e., schizophrenia, mood disorders, substance use) as well as higher intelligence and educational attainment (Grove *et al.*, 2019; Abdellaoui & Verweij, 2021).

While genetic factors account for the most variance associated with the autism phenotype, there are also important roles of environmental factors. Factors operating preconceptionally and prenatally (Lord *et al.*, 2020) that are likely associated with an increased probability of autism include: advanced parental age (>40 years for maternal and >50 years for paternal age), short (<12 months) interpregnancy interval, valproate use during pregnancy, gestational diabetes mellitus, maternal obesity, preterm birth, and neonatal hypoxia. Plausible factors but with inconclusive evidence include: prenatal air pollution exposure (especially fine inhalable particles $\leq 2.5\,\mu m$, PM2.5 (Dutheil *et al.*, 2021)), prenatal pesticides exposure, summer birth, and labor epidural analgesia exposure (very weak evidence due to a lack of cumulative dose–response effect (Hung *et al.*, 2023)). Factors with evidence clearly *not* supporting a role in autism emergence include: child vaccination (e.g., MMR), prolonged labor, premature rupture of membrane, assisted vaginal delivery, cesarean section, conception through assisted reproductive technologies, prenatal smoking, and hypertensive disease of pregnancy. Adequate maternal intakes of folic acid, Vitamin D, and multivitamins during pregnancy are associated with reduced autism emergence in the child (Zhong *et al.*, 2020). Although maternal use of selective serotonin reuptake inhibitors (SSRIs) and serotonin norepinephrine reuptake inhibitors (SNRIs) during pregnancy has been linked to increased likelihood of autism in the offspring, similar association found for SSRIs/SNRIs use prior to pregnancy suggests important confounding factors and thus a causal link cannot be assumed (Leshem *et al.*, 2021).

Baby-sibling studies

The age of onset/emergence of autism has been the subject of great interest. Retrospective reports of phenotypic autism onset have not offered definitive findings. Baby-sibling studies provide a prospective lens by sampling families with an older autistic child and at least one newborn baby. By following the baby's development with precise measurements over time, the emerging patterns of autistic features could be delineated. About 20% of the younger siblings of older autistic children develop autism themselves by around 3 years of age (Szatmari *et al.*, 2016). Autistic features emerge on average around 12 months but may not be apparent until 18 months of age (Dawson *et al.*, 2023). The domains of atypical early development involve differences in attention, prelinguistic and nonverbal communication, social orientation, joint attention and engagement, and sensorimotor processing (Dawson *et al.*, 2023). Among baby-siblings, almost all autistic children will be diagnosed by 24 months old. In addition, a substantial proportion of baby-siblings not diagnosed with autism develop language delay, ADHD, learning disabilities, or challenges in social interaction (Johnson *et al.*, 2015). Neuroimaging studies in baby-siblings have identified predictive features of emerging autism, such as cortical surface area hyperexpansion, excessive cerebrospinal fluid in the subarachnoid space, and white matter network inefficiencies in low-level sensory processing regions in the first year (Molnar-Szakacs *et al.*, 2021), suggesting an active brain developmental process in the beginning of life prior to the emergence of behavioral signs.

Neurocognitive processes

Neurobiological hypotheses

Convergence in findings across molecular genetics to animal model systems (Parker, 2022; Crawley, 2023) indicates that autism-associated genes involve the developing excitatory neurons in the human mid-gestational prefrontal cortex, and pathways impacting neurogenesis, chromatin modification, and synaptic function (Willsey *et al.*, 2022). While several promising neurobiological models and hypotheses are being examined (presented in the following subsections), small sample sizes and demographic, clinical (e.g., medication exposure), and methodological heterogeneity remain key challenges. So far, across candidate biomarkers correlated with autism behavioral phenotypes, including molecular biomarkers (e.g., cytokines), neurotransmitters and hormones (e.g., oxytocin, vasopressin), and neurophysiology and neuroimaging markers, none of them is ready for use to inform clinically oriented research and clinical care (Parellada *et al.*, 2023).

Excitation–inhibition balance

The excitation–inhibition (E:I) balance hypothesis posits that increased excitation relative to inhibition during neurodevelopment contributes to circuit hyperexcitability and altered differentiation of physiological processes that impede optimal language and social development (Rubenstein & Merzenich, 2003). Several developmental processes are implicated in E:I imbalance (e.g., synaptic plasticity and connectivity, neuronal morphology, excitatory–inhibitory neuron interplay, and neuronal or network excitability) (Lee *et al.*, 2017; Culotta & Penzes, 2020). E:I imbalance as a final common pathway to autism is conceivably consistent with its heterogeneity (e.g., involving various brain systems), and could explain the high co-occurrence with epilepsy and altered sensitivity to external stimuli (Rubenstein & Merzenich, 2003). While this hypothesis is supported by animal and stem cell studies (Lee *et al.*, 2017; Sohal & Rubenstein, 2019; Culotta & Penzes, 2020), human neuroimaging findings indexing E:I balance (e.g., magnetic resonance spectroscopy, MRS) remain inconsistent (Port *et al.*, 2019).

Maternal immune activation, microglial activation, and sex steroid-immune mechanisms

The maternal immune activation (MIA) hypothesis postulates that *in utero* exposure to inflammatory perturbations shapes the developing fetal brain, influencing later emergence of autism and other neurodevelopmental phenotypes (Han *et al.*, 2021). MIA animal models show that environmental exposures can activate pro-inflammatory cytokines and placental immune activation, resulting in upregulation of genes involved in microglial and astrocyte-related inflammation in the fetus. Secondary effects on neurogenesis, synaptic pruning, and neural circuits development, including E:I balance (Careaga *et al.*, 2017; Han *et al.*, 2021), could then influence behavioral outcomes that would depend on the timing, intensity, and specificity of the immune response. Animal studies indicate that the immune system also has a role in brain masculinization. Inflammatory factors and the plasticity of the male versus female fetal brain suggest that genetic and environmental factors (such as MIA) might affect the likelihood of autism or other neurodevelopmental conditions differentially by sex (McCarthy & Wright, 2017). No study in humans has yet demonstrated a direct link between MIA and neuroinflammation in newborns (Careaga *et al.*, 2017; Han *et al.*, 2021).

Microbiome–gut–brain axis

The gut microbiome is involved in immune modulation and nervous system development and has been implicated in neuropsychiatric disorders (Andrioaie *et al.*, 2022). Co-occurrence between autism and gastrointestinal problems, differences in gut bacterial communities in autistic individuals, and animal models of autism have led to research examining whether the gut microbiota plays a role in autism emergence (Andreo-Martínez *et al.*, 2022). While animal work has indicated that gut microbiota can produce autism-like features in mice (Sharon *et al.*, 2019), a recent meta-analysis in humans did not show evidence of a relevant association between bacterial phyla and autism (Andreo-Martínez *et al.*, 2022). Furthermore, large-scale stool metagenomics studies in children found negligible direct associations between autism diagnosis and the gut microbiome; rather, autism-related RRB were associated with less diverse diet, reducing microbial taxonomic diversity (Yap *et al.*, 2021).

Brain-level heterogeneity

Collaborative efforts to pool neuroimaging data for large-scale analyses have reported differences in brain structure in autism, such as reduced subcortical volume, altered cortical thickness (van Rooij *et al.*, 2018), asymmetry (Postema *et al.*, 2019), and structural connectivity (Sha *et al.*, 2022). Small effect sizes (Cohen's *d* 0.1–0.2) suggest that mean differences between autistic and nonautistic groups are subtle. Whole-brain resting-state functional MRI (fMRI) data show replicable altered connectivity patterns between neural circuits in autism versus nonautistic controls that have been associated with autistic features (Floris *et al.*, 2021; Ilioska *et al.*, 2023). However, neuroimaging findings remain largely inconsistent (Lombardo *et al.*, 2019) and unreplicated (Parellada *et al.*, 2023), which might in part reflect the heterogeneity inherent to the current classification of autism.

Different brain-level features can be associated with diagnoses with overlapping behavioral phenotypes, such as the associations between enlarged amygdala and autism in contrast to enlarged caudate and fragile X syndrome in infants aged 6–24 months (Shen *et al.*, 2022). Meanwhile, cross-disorder meta-analytic studies have also shown that related conditions (e.g., autism, ADHD, obsessive–compulsive disorder (OCD), depressive disorder, schizophrenia, bipolar disorder) feature diagnosis-specific as well as nondistinct brain characteristics, echoing the diagnostic overlap and heterogeneity within and across diagnoses (Boedhoe *et al.*, 2020; Radonjić *et al.*, 2021; Hettwer *et al.*, 2022). The US National Institute of Mental Health Research Domain Criteria (RDoC) and comparable European initiatives now support transdiagnostic research (i.e., domain-focused and cutting across current diagnostic categories) that shifts away from the conventional group-wise (i.e., "case" versus "control") approach (Kas *et al.*, 2019). This paradigm shift explores whether new subgroups (that may or may not follow current diagnostic boundaries) feature more homogeneous patterns of brain-behavior relations that could relate to distinct neurobiological-etiological pathways (Wolfers *et al.*, 2019). However, large-scale efforts have yet to test, replicate, or validate this concept in autism (Pacheco *et al.*, 2022).

Cognitive features

Historically, the "deficit models" of (i) theory of mind (or mentalizing) impairment, and reduced social orientation and social motivation, (ii) executive dysfunction, and (iii) weak central coherence are used to explain autistic cognitive difficulties (Fletcher-Watson & Happé, 2019). However, autistic people's mentalizing and executive function (but not central coherence) only weakly correlate with social functioning (Bottema-Beutel *et al.*, 2019). Although the primary sociocognitive difficulties experienced by many autistic individuals relate to intuitive mentalizing (Happé & Frith, 2020), such difficulties can be transactional, influenced by nonautistic people's difficulties understanding autistic people (i.e., the "double empathy problem," a breakdown in the communication between autistic and neurotypical people, because of dispositional differences in the representation of the social world (Milton, 2012)). Reduced social orienting in autism happens in the first years, rather than at birth, indicating an autism-related difference from the typical developmental transition from reflex-like to experience-dependent social orienting (Shultz *et al.*, 2018). Accordingly, eye-tracking measurement of social visual engagement has shown promise in aiding early identification of autism (e.g., in children aged 16–30 months) (Jones *et al.*, 2023). Executive dysfunction is not autism-specific and does not link directly to the autism phenotypes, but is a common co-occurring feature impeding adaptive functioning (Astle *et al.*, 2022). An updated view of autistic cognition is that of alternative (instead of impaired) information processing, such as atypical attentional, sensory-perceptual, cognitive processing (e.g., focused attention on a narrow range of interests), and rule-based thinking (Fletcher-Watson & Happé, 2019).

Co-occurring conditions and differential diagnoses

Autism often co-occurs with other neurodevelopmental conditions (e.g., ADHD, tic disorders, developmental coordination disorder (DCD), communication disorders, and ID) (Thapar *et al.*, 2017), psychiatric disorders (Lai *et al.*, 2019) (Figure 50.3), and physical health issues such as epilepsy (Liu *et al.*, 2022), sleep problems (Schreck & Richdale, 2020), sensory impairments, atopy, autoimmune disorders, gastrointestinal problems, and obesity (Rydzewska *et al.*, 2021). Neurodevelopmental co-occurrence extends transdiagnostically to dimensions such as hyperactivity-impulsivity, inattention, social-communication, executive functioning, and phonological processing (Astle *et al.*, 2022). Psychiatrically, the pooled current prevalence estimates from recent meta-analyses are 20% (95% CI 17–23) for anxiety disorders, 13% (9–17) for sleep–wake disorders, 12% (10–15) for disruptive, impulse-control, and conduct disorders, 11% (9–13) for depressive disorders, 9% (7–10) for OCD, 5% (3–6) for bipolar disorders, and 4% (3–5) for schizophrenia spectrum disorders (Lai *et al.*, 2019). Mood and psychotic disorders increase with age (Lai *et al.*, 2019; Mutluer *et al.*, 2022), with high lifetime prevalence by adulthood (e.g., 9.4% for psychotic disorders, 7.5% for bipolar disorders (Varcin *et al.*, 2022), and 37% for depressive disorders (Hollocks *et al.*, 2019)). Other common health issues include feeding and eating problems (e.g., food selectivity, sensory sensitivity, ritualistic eating

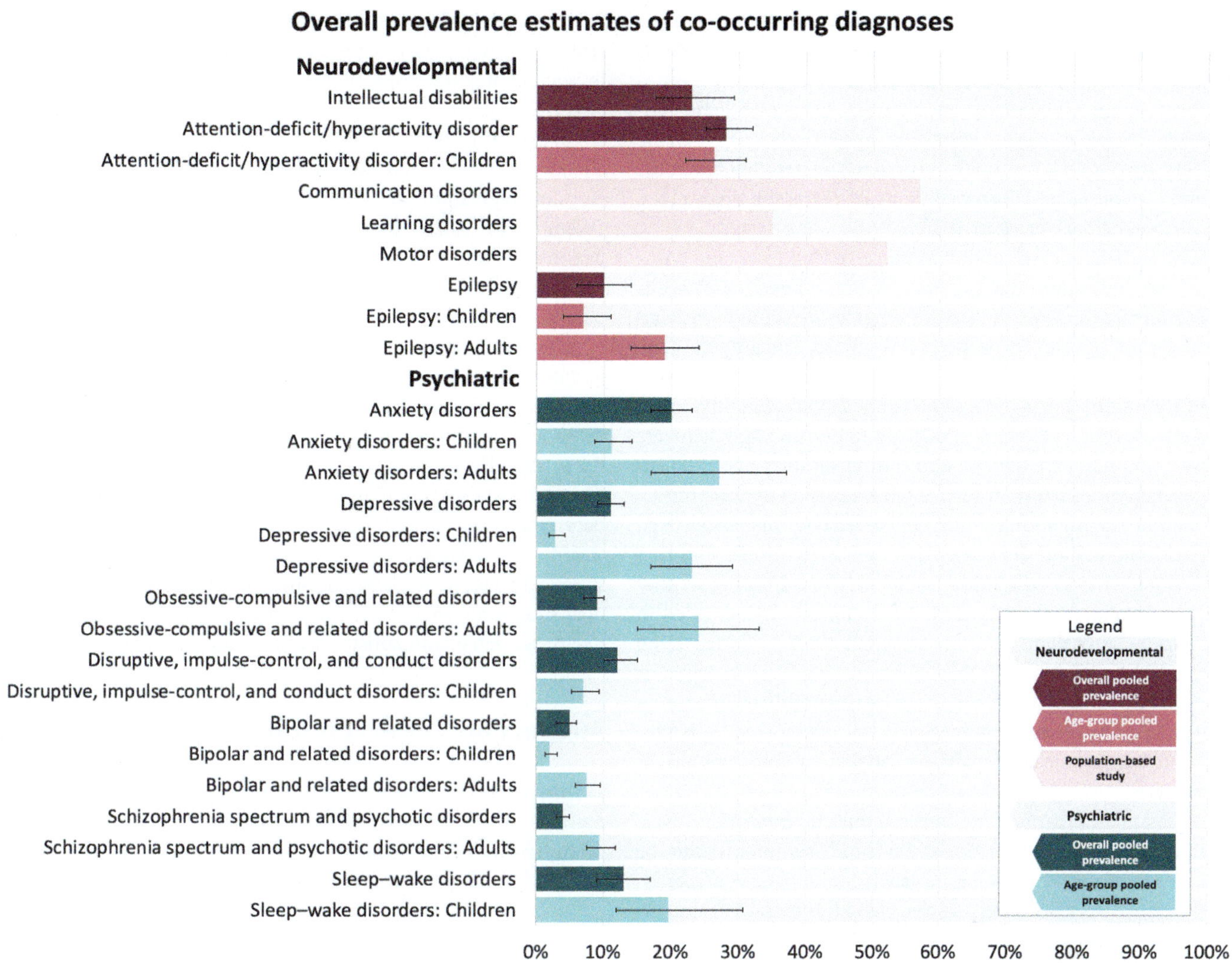

Figure 50.3 Co-occurring diagnoses in autistic people. Estimates come from different meta-analyses and large-scale studies, so they are not directly comparable. Error bars represent 95% CI for meta-analysis-reported estimates.

behaviors, or pica) and disorders (e.g., avoidant/restrictive food intake disorder and anorexia nervosa) (Baraskewich *et al.*, 2021; Bourne *et al.*, 2022), subthreshold psychotic symptoms (Kiyono *et al.*, 2020), trauma-related and stress-related experiences (Ng-Cordell *et al.*, 2022; Trundle *et al.*, 2023), substance use (especially in those with ADHD, anxiety, or depression) (Ressel *et al.*, 2020; Huang *et al.*, 2021; Haasbroek & Morojele, 2022; Roux *et al.*, 2022), suicidal behaviors (Mournet *et al.*, 2022; O'Halloran *et al.*, 2022), and catatonia (Vaquerizo-Serrano *et al.*, 2021). Particularly, 44% of autistic people have experienced some form of victimization (Trundle *et al.*, 2023). In autistic youth, the meta-analytic prevalence rates of suicide-related behaviors are 25.2% (95% CI 18.2–33.8) for suicidal ideation, 8.3% (4.3–15.6) for self-harm or suicide attempts, and 0.2% (0.05–0.52) for death by suicide (O'Halloran *et al.*, 2022). About 10% of autistic individuals have experienced catatonia, often starting during late adolescence (Vaquerizo-Serrano *et al.*, 2021; Hauptman *et al.*, 2023).

Psychiatric symptom trajectories in autistic people are characterized by overall persistence (Stringer *et al.*, 2020) with subgroups showing diverging patterns (McCauley *et al.*, 2020). Psychiatric disorders in autistic people largely manifest similarly as in neurotypical people, but autism, as well as communication and intellectual functioning, can shape the presentations in unique ways (Lai, 2023). They can have unconventional anxiety manifestations beyond traditional categories, including fears of novelty/change, excessive worry about access to focused interests, unusual phobias, and anxiety related to confusion or unpredictability in social situations (instead of a fear of negative social evaluation) (Ng-Cordell *et al.*, 2022). Depressive symptoms can highlight increased irritability, change of focused interests, increased sameness behaviors, sensory alterations, regressive behaviors, and decline in adaptive functioning (Oakley *et al.*, 2021). Differentiating OCD symptoms from autistic RRB is sometimes difficult. In principle, autistic RRB reflect intrinsic sensorimotor inclinations, are mostly egosyntonic, soothing, and pleasurable for autistic individuals (Kapp *et al.*, 2019); on the contrary, although OCD compulsions relieve anxiety (similar to some autistic RRB) and can be temporarily soothing, OCD symptoms are overall distressful and egodystonic (unless with poor or absent insight). While anxiety-driven OCD compulsions reduce anxiety but reinforce themselves, autistic RRB are typically not distressful themselves, yet distress can occur when or after RRB is interrupted.

The autistic person's ability to perceive, delineate, and communicate these emotional experiences, and other people's accurate understanding of the nature of such, determine whether these symptoms can be properly recognized. Alexithymia (i.e., inability to recognize or describe one's emotions) and difficulties with interoception (i.e., senses of one's internal bodily states) and introspection can make it difficult to perceive and delineate these emotional experiences, and communication and intellectual capabilities further influence the expression of emotions.

Despite the high rates of disruptive behavior diagnoses (e.g., oppositional defiant disorder, ODD) given to autistic children and youth (Lai *et al.*, 2019; Mutluer *et al.*, 2022), and that callous-unemotional traits seem more commonly identified in autistic (~22%) than nonautistic youth (~5%) (Carter Leno *et al.*, 2021), it is important that clinicians do not misinterpret or mislabel an autistic child's behaviors because of their differences or a poor person–environment fit (e.g., distress-related behavioral and communication patterns labeled as oppositional or disruptive).

Assessment regarding psychosis should be mindful of overshadowing in both directions. Psychotic symptoms can be underrecognized when being mislabeled as autistic characteristics (e.g., disorganization labeled as idiosyncratic thought-speech, behavioral responses to perceptual changes labeled as representing rich fantasy); meanwhile, autistic characteristics, especially when the person is in distress and/or when seen by a clinician who is not familiar with them, can be mislabeled as psychotic (e.g., autistic thinking-communication patterns labeled as disorganization or positive symptoms, autistic social-communication labeled as negative symptoms, or concrete/literal answers to imprecise questions about perceptual experiences labeled as indicative of positive symptoms) (Lai & Baron-Cohen, 2015; Jutla *et al.*, 2022). Such overshadowing can also occur for bipolar symptoms (e.g., irritability associated with environment-routine changes in autism to be differentiated from pervasive mood fluctuations in bipolar disorders) (Dunalska *et al.*, 2021). Catatonia should be assessed when there is deterioration in motor, speech, or adaptive functioning from one's personalized baseline (Shah, 2020; Hauptman *et al.*, 2023). Clinicians should attend to red-flags that can be confounded with baseline characteristics: worsening of stereotypies, new-onset refusal to eat, new-onset or worsening incontinence, regression in daily living activities, onset or exacerbation of self-injurious behaviors, and purposeless agitation (Hauptman *et al.*, 2023).

Although these co-occurring psychiatric challenges can be partly attributable to shared genetic predispositions (Abdellaoui & Verweij, 2021; Fu *et al.*, 2022) and early environmental factors (Han *et al.*, 2021), autistic people are also particularly vulnerable to sociocontextual risks such as bullying (Park *et al.*, 2020), adverse childhood experiences (Hoover & Kaufman, 2018), and stigmatization (Milton, 2012; Turnock *et al.*, 2022). Cognitive challenges experienced by some autistic people regarding self/emotion regulation (Beck *et al.*, 2021) and executive function (Wong *et al.*, 2023) can further hamper coping with mental health difficulties. A formulation that incorporates these considerations is useful for planning tailored support for autistic people (Lai, 2023).

Most of these co-occurring conditions can be part of the differential diagnoses (Table 50.2), especially when autism has not yet been diagnosed. Differentiation is particularly important for those with seemingly or truly overlapping behavioral presentations (e.g., ID or global developmental delay, communication disorders, ADHD, social anxiety disorder, OCD, psychotic disorders, attachment disorders or other sequelae of trauma or maltreatment). Clarifying the developmental history, the person's stress-response styles, and the onset and longitudinal course of new symptoms against baseline presentations (i.e., those most likely associated with autism) is critical for differentiation.

Support and intervention

Changing the systems of care

Systems of care for autistic individuals and their families, which often involve health, education, social, employment, financial, and social safety-net services, need much advancement (Lord

Table 50.2 Differential diagnoses.

- Neurodevelopmental disorders:
  - specific language delay or disorder
  - a learning (intellectual) disability or global developmental delay
  - developmental coordination disorder (DCD)
  - attention deficit hyperactivity disorder (ADHD)
- Mental and behavioral disorders:
  - mood disorders
  - anxiety disorders
  - attachment disorders
  - oppositional defiant disorder (ODD)
  - conduct disorder (CD)
  - obsessive–compulsive disorder (OCD)
  - psychosis
- Conditions in which there is developmental regression:
  - Rett syndrome
  - epileptic encephalopathy
- Other conditions
  - severe hearing impairment
  - severe visual impairment
  - maltreatment
  - selective mutism

Source: Adapted from National Institute for Health and Care Excellence CG 128 (2017)/ https://www.nice.org.uk/guidance/cg128, last accessed 8 April 2024.

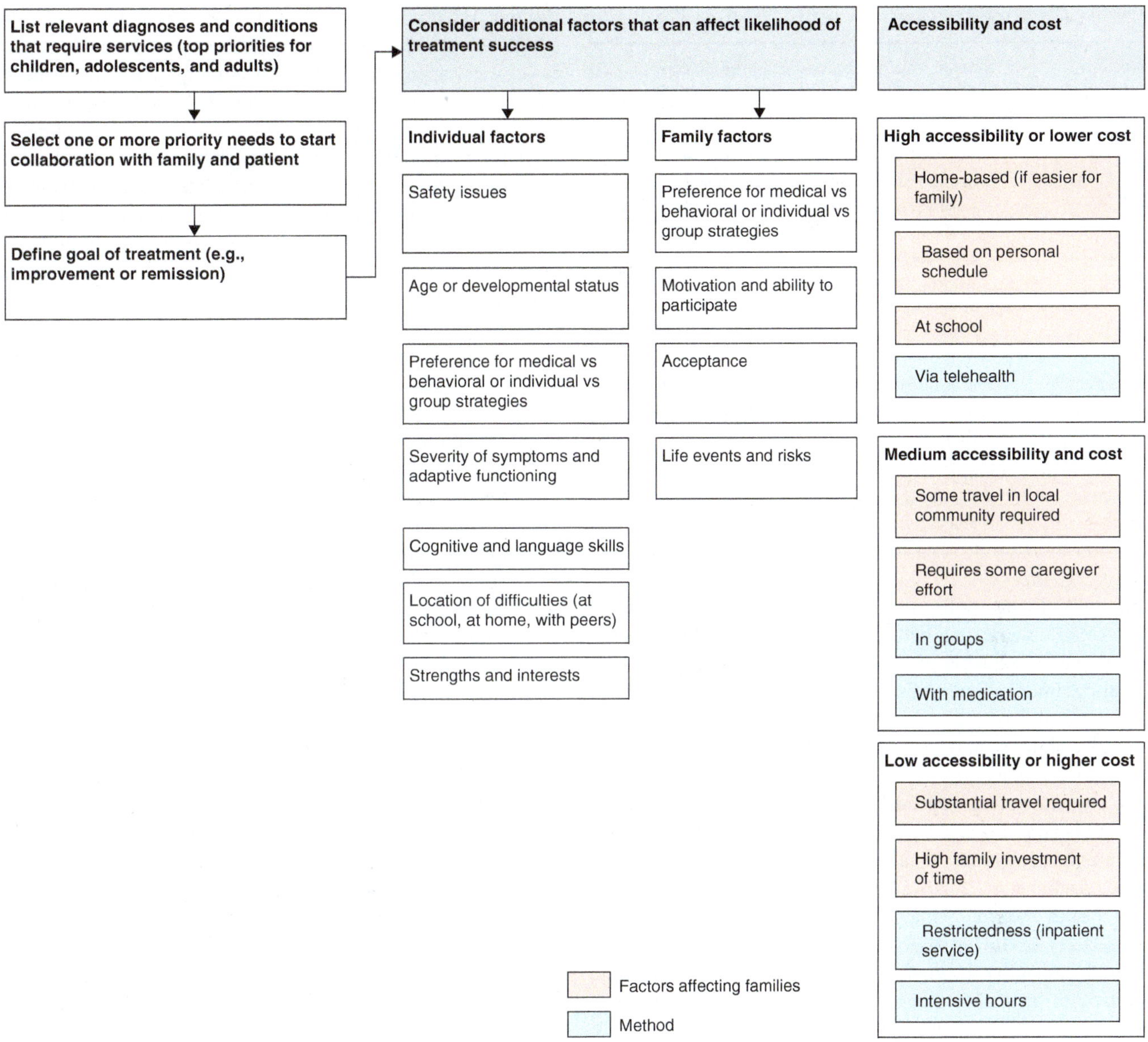

Figure 50.4 A stepped care and personalized health intervention model. *Source:* Lord *et al.* (2022)/with permission of Elsevier.

et al., 2022). Individual needs vary and they change over time; there is no single pathway nor one system of care that suits all autistic individuals across the life span. Improving accessibility and quality can include navigation programs (McBrien *et al.*, 2018), the primary care "medical home" model (Todorow *et al.*, 2018), and a stepped care and personalized health model that emphasizes shared decision-making based on available evidence, and individual and family preferences and resources (Figure 50.4) (Lord *et al.*, 2022). Clinicians serve important roles in supporting the autistic person and their family to navigate the systems and advocating for policy and systems-level changes.

Harmonizing medical and social models of disability as a clinician

There are ongoing debates about what are appropriate interventions (and adequate purposes of intervention), pharmacological or nonpharmacological, for autistic people (Schuck *et al.*, 2022). Several pharmacological agents that had shown promise in altering autism symptom levels or adaptive function failed to show efficacy in large-scale trials (e.g., oxytocin (Sikich *et al.*, 2021) and balovaptan (Hollander *et al.*, 2022)). Since the 1960s, the most widely used interventions are behavioral-educational approaches starting early in life (i.e., "early intervention") to help the autistic child develop social-communication

Table 50.3 Intervention at a glance.

Direction	Most promising approaches based on current clinical evidence and community knowledge
Maximizing potential	• Early childhood: relationship-based intervention involving caregivers, such as the naturalistic developmental behavioral intervention (NDBI) models • Childhood, adolescence, and beyond: Individualized educational support and social skills group programs
Minimizing barriers	• Augmentative and alternative communication systems for those who need them • Screening, prevention, and timely treatment of physical health and psychiatric symptoms and illnesses
Optimizing the person–environment fit	• Reasonable environmental adjustments (e.g., reducing sensory and social overload, increasing predictability, gradually building flexibility) • Support family and caregivers • Reduce stigmatization and prevent victimization • Vocational support • Strength-based approaches

and daily living skills and reduce so-called challenging/problematic/interfering behaviors. Commonly targeted outcomes include reducing autism "core symptoms" (i.e., increasing social-communication skills and decreasing RRB), increasing expressive and receptive language, adaptive functioning, and cognitive abilities, and reducing disruptive behaviors (Gosling *et al.*, 2022). However, some advocates criticize the heavy reliance on behaviorism approaches targeting autistic characteristics (Pellicano & den Houting, 2022); others emphasize truly meaningful outcomes to autistic people and their families (McConachie *et al.*, 2020), such as skill-building across the life span, health and well-being, and accessibility to services (Roche *et al.*, 2021). Reducing disability of autistic people can be done via both reshaping the environment (e.g., reducing stigma and barriers to inclusion) and supporting an individual (e.g., increasing adaptive skills) (Dwyer, 2022). Accordingly, evidence-informed interventions can be summarized in three directions (Table 50.3) (Lai *et al.*, 2020). Although the evidence base continues to grow, current autism intervention science findings, especially those in nonpharmacological trials, are still substantially hampered by low replicability, study design biases, insufficient examination and reporting of harm, and underdisclosure of potential conflicts of interest (Bottema-Beutel *et al.*, 2021a, 2021b; Sandbank *et al.*, 2023). While these evidence gaps are being addressed, clinicians should always try to harmonize the medical and social models of disability in developing and implementing an intervention plan.

Maximizing potential

Early intervention to support development

Early intensive behavioral intervention has been used since the 1960s for young children diagnosed with autism. This broad approach uses applied behavior analysis (ABA) principles and discrete trial training, one-on-one, with an adult therapist, using a highly structured, intensive (20–40 hours/week) and long-term (1–4 years) approach. However, traditional ABA interventions have scarcer support from the randomized controlled trial (RCT) literature compared with the naturalistic developmental behavioral intervention (NDBI) models (Sandbank *et al.*, 2023), which not only adopt some behaviorism principles (as in ABA) but also uniquely incorporate developmental science and developmentally oriented interventions. NDBIs emphasize supporting a child's initiative and spontaneity, engaging the child via emotionally meaningful interactions, and connecting new learning opportunities with current abilities within developmentally appropriate sequences, in naturalistic contexts (Schreibman *et al.*, 2015). NDBIs include examples such as pivotal response treatment and its derivatives, the Early Start Denver Model, and joint attention symbolic play engagement and regulation (JASPER) (Sandbank *et al.*, 2023). The most rigorously conducted meta-analyses of RCTs show that traditional ABA interventions improve caregiver perception of challenging behavior and child social-emotional functioning, technology-based interventions improve specific social-communication and social-emotional skills, developmental interventions improve social-communication, and NDBIs improve core challenges associated with autism, particularly social-communication. When outcomes were restricted to examine only those not subject to high risk of detection bias, the only significant effect was for NDBIs on reducing autism diagnostic characteristics (i.e., scores on diagnostic assessments). Overall, intervention effects were larger for context-bound outcomes (i.e., behaviors measured within interactions similar to the context of intervention) and for directly taught behaviors compared with skills not directly targeted, indicating challenges with the generalization of skills to other settings/contexts (Sandbank *et al.*, 2023).

Increasing evidence suggests caregiver-mediated NDBIs that focus on caregiver–child synchrony, joint attention, and engagement, as a kind of relationship-based treatment (see Chapter 36), improve these targeted developmental domains (Green & Garg, 2018). Meta-analytic evidence indicates that caregiver-mediated interventions might reduce disruptive behaviors and increase adaptive skills in autistic children, though data quality concerns warrant the need for further research (Conrad *et al.*, 2021). Enhancing caregivers' understanding of and joining the child in naturalistic settings cultivates the individual child's agency and optimizes early person–environment fit, and thus can be aligned with the neurodiversity paradigm (Lai *et al.*, 2020; Schuck *et al.*, 2022).

Later targeted intervention to build skills

When an autistic person enters the school systems, educational support becomes integral to the child's daily living, self-regulation, organization, social interaction, and academic skills-building. In some jurisdictions, this is supported by an individualized education plan (e.g., from the UK's National Autistic Society (n.d.)). On top of these educational supports that usually focus on concrete targets, social skills group programs also show promise in supporting socialization needs and social-communication of autistic school-age children, adolescents, and young adults, although most studies have high risk of bias in design (Gosling *et al.*, 2022; Afsharnejad *et al.*, 2024).

Minimizing barriers

Reducing communication barriers

Despite early intervention, ~30% of autistic individuals are "minimally verbal" beyond early childhood—those whose spoken language expression is absent or limited to a restricted set of words or phrases (Schaeffer *et al.*, 2023). This is a heterogenous group with some having profound cognitive impairments and others with average intelligence (Bal *et al.*, 2016). Access to assistive technology, such as the augmentative and alternative communication systems (e.g., devices for expressive and receptive communication via non-speech means), should be offered to reduce communication barriers (Brignell *et al.*, 2018; Morin *et al.*, 2018). Assistive technology for autistic individuals is a flourishing field that awaits rigorous trials to establish evidence for appropriate personalization (Lord *et al.*, 2022), such as how speech-generating devices may augment current interventions to improve communication (Kasari *et al.*, 2014).

Coping with sensory experiences

Interfering sensory experience (e.g., hyperresponsivity) can be a significant source of distress (Williams *et al.*, 2021) and is a focus of occupational therapy to enhance daily functioning (Ismael *et al.*, 2018). Sensory-based interventions show little evidence to improve language outcomes (Sandbank *et al.*, 2020), but some short-term approaches that show promise (all with low strength of evidence) include sensory integration-based approaches (i.e., interventions using combinations of sensory and kinetic components to ameliorate sensory challenges) to improve sensory and motor skills, environmental enrichment with sensory stimulation to enhance tolerance and improve nonverbal cognitive skills, and massage to reduce sensory challenges (Weitlauf *et al.*, 2017).

Treating co-occurring psychiatric manifestations

A key principle to assess psychiatric manifestations in autistic individuals is to first screen for and consider physical health (including dental) problems, communication difficulties, environmental-contextual changes and psychosocial stressors (even seemingly minor), and habitual maladaptive behaviors stemming from poor person–environment fit (McGuire *et al.*, 2016). Environmental adjustments are helpful, such as preventing bullying to reduce suicide risks (O'Halloran *et al.*, 2022), incorporating family in cognitive behavioral therapy (CBT) to reduce anxiety (Wichers *et al.*, 2023), and using universal design (i.e., designs to be accessible and usable by all people) in educational settings (Waisman *et al.*, 2023). Tools supporting health literacy and self-advocacy should be offered (Lai, 2023).

Whether to prescribe new medications for psychiatric manifestations should be carefully thought through as real-world data suggest there is increasing polypharmacy in autistic individuals (Jobski *et al.*, 2017). For impairing irritability and aggressive behaviors, when clinically indicated (McGuire *et al.*, 2016), aripiprazole and risperidone show the strongest efficacy (Salazar de Pablo *et al.*, 2023), but short-term (e.g., extrapyramidal syndrome and sedation) and long-term (e.g., weight gain and metabolic syndrome) risks must be weighed against benefits (Deb *et al.*, 2023). Medications for ADHD show some efficacy in reducing irritability and emotion dysregulation (Salazar de Pablo *et al.*, 2023). Less evidence exists for N-acetylcysteine and clonidine, but they have been recommended because of the preferred safety profile of the former and the long-standing clinical-use experiences of the latter (McGuire *et al.*, 2016; Vasa *et al.*, 2016; Lord *et al.*, 2022). For catatonia, an individualized formulation should guide the prevention of sensory or social overload, removing potential medication causes (e.g., dopamine antagonists), and prompts to keep the autistic person responsive and active (Shah, 2020). Benzodiazepines (e.g., lorazepam) can be used carefully—responses might be less robust in autistic individuals—and electroconvulsive therapy can be considered (Rogers *et al.*, 2023).

Treatment for psychiatric disorders in autistic people should follow the available evidence in the general population in the absence of autism-specific evidence (Linden *et al.*, 2023). Meanwhile, there are specific considerations based on accumulating evidence in autistic people. For ADHD, parent training and classroom interventions should be implemented first, especially for preschool-age children (see Chapter 54); medication treatment can follow meta-analysis-guided recommendations (e.g., methylphenidate as the first choice, followed by second-line choices including amphetamines, atomoxetine, or alpha-2 agonists (guanfacine or clonidine)), noting the potentially less robust responses and greater side effects (especially to stimulants) in autistic individuals (Rodrigues *et al.*, 2021). For sleep problems, improving sleep hygiene is fundamental, and prolonged-release melatonin alone or administered with CBT has been recommended (Williams Buckley *et al.*, 2020; Nogueira *et al.*, 2023). For anxiety and depression, psychotherapeutic interventions should be adapted and individualized (Figure 50.5). Autism-informed adapted CBT (White *et al.*, 2018) and mindfulness-based intervention (Linden *et al.*, 2023) can result in symptom reduction (Wichers *et al.*, 2023), but there is a lack of evidence for those with ID. Although antidepressants are clinically prescribed for anxiety, depression, and OCD in autistic individuals, RCT findings in this population have yet to show group-level benefits (Deb *et al.*, 2021). If clinically indicated, one should start with lower than typical dosage (e.g., one-fourth or half of the typical starting dose), titrate it up slowly, and watch for behavior activation side effects (e.g., increasing activity, impulsivity, insomnia, and disinhibition) that might be more commonly experienced by autistic individuals (Vasa *et al.*, 2016; Lord *et al.*, 2022). Mood stabilizers,

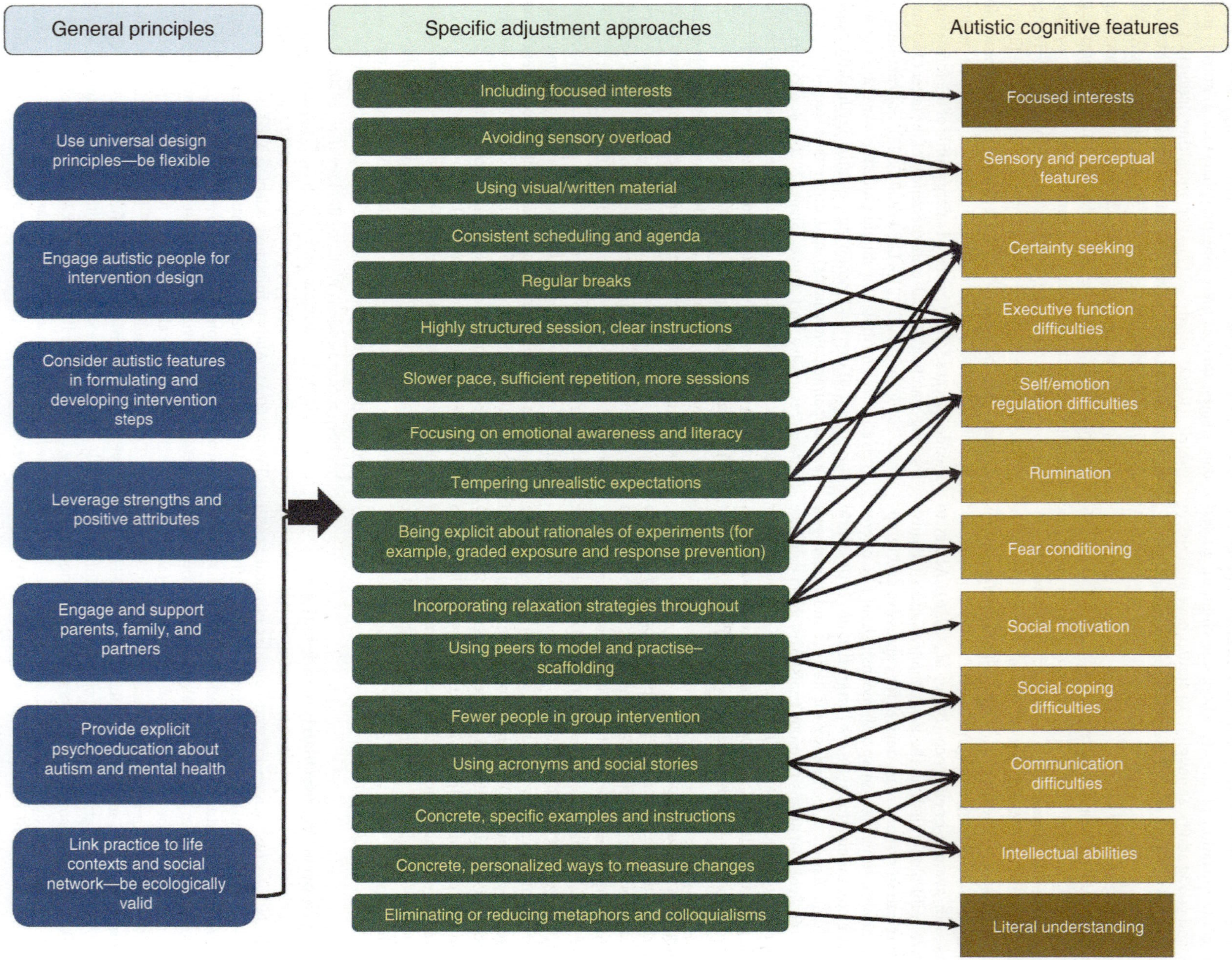

Figure 50.5 Current adaptation principles for psychotherapeutic interventions with autistic people. *Source:* Lai (2023)/with permission of Springer Nature.

especially lithium, should be prioritized for manic/mixed episode and maintenance treatment for bipolar disorders in autistic individuals (Amadori *et al.*, 2022).

Optimizing person–environment fit

Clinicians are important allies of autistic people and their families, and should treat advocacy for autistic people's well-being as an integral part of the care they offer, to enhance holistic care and person–environment fit (Lai *et al.*, 2020; Lord *et al.*, 2022). This socioecologically focused support ranges from care for family members (Yu *et al.*, 2019; Sartore *et al.*, 2021), engaging nonautistic peers (Sutton *et al.*, 2019), and enhancing employment (Baker-Ericzén *et al.*, 2022), to increasing public knowledge of autism and high-quality, frequent contact with autistic people (Kim *et al.*, 2023). Optimizing fit should also consider cultural factors (de Leeuw *et al.*, 2020) and intersectional identities (Mallipeddi & VanDaalen, 2022). For example, considering the increased autism diagnoses in gender-diverse populations and increased gender diversity in autistic children, adolescents, and adults (Kallitsounaki & Williams, 2023), some autistic people have unique gender-related experiences, including gender dysphoria, requiring tailored care that involves contextual supports (Strang *et al.*, 2018; Cooper *et al.*, 2023) (see Chapter 40).

Complementary and alternative treatment

Available data show moderate certainty of evidence for positive effects of music therapy, with no increase in adverse events (Geretsegger *et al.*, 2022). There are potential benefits and acceptable adverse effects for animal-assisted therapy (Rehn *et al.*, 2023), exercise (Ruggeri *et al.*, 2020), massage (Ruan *et al.*, 2022), acupuncture (Lun *et al.*, 2023), and omega-3 fatty acids and vitamin supplementation (Fraguas *et al.*, 2019); such evidence is emerging but insufficient, due to low-quality trial designs, high risk of bias, and high heterogeneity of implementation. No supportive evidence is found for gluten-free and casein-free diets (Piwowarczyk *et al.*, 2018). There are some treatments advertised in the market that are not supported by current evidence, have substantial risk of harm (e.g., chelation, hyperbaric oxygen therapy, secretin, antifungal treatment, leuprorelin), and are overly costly (e.g., stem cell), and hence should not be recommended (Lai *et al.*, 2020; Lord *et al.*, 2022).

Conclusion

Understanding autism as a clinical neurodevelopmental diagnosis as well as an example of neurodivergence, and an identity for some youth, is helpful for clinicians to appreciate the impact and meaning of autism for the family and its impact on a person's functioning, coping, and well-being. A holistic and transdiagnostic approach to understanding a person's development in their unique socioecological contexts, with information collected from multiple sources, is essential for diagnostic assessments and optimizing care. The heterogeneity of autism across clinical and neurobiological levels means that personalized assessment and intervention is essential, although evidence-based approaches for this are still being developed. Future intervention should integrate strength-based approaches, include autistic voices in developing and evaluating intervention models and targets, and redefine intervention effectiveness to incorporate meaningful outcomes endorsed by the autistic communities.

References

Abdellaoui, A. & Verweij, K.J.H. (2021) Dissecting polygenic signals from genome-wide association studies on human behaviour. *Nature Human Behaviour* **5**, 686–694.

Afsharnejad, B. *et al.* (2024) The methodological quality and intervention fidelity of randomised controlled trials evaluating social skills group programs in autistic adolescents: a systematic review and meta-analysis. *Journal of Autism and Developmental Disorders* **54**, 1281–1316.

Amadori, S. *et al.* (2022) Pharmacotherapy for bipolar disorder in adults with high-functioning autism. *Expert Opinion on Pharmacotherapy* **23**, 1753–1760.

Amer, Y.S. *et al.* (2022) AGREEing on clinical practice guidelines for autism spectrum disorders in children: a systematic review and quality assessment. *Children* **9**, 1050.

American Psychiatric Association (1980) *Diagnostic and Statistical Manual of Mental Disorders*, 3rd edn. American Psychiatric Association, Washington, DC.

American Psychiatric Association (1987) *Diagnostic and Statistical Manual of Mental Disorders*, 3rd edn. revised edn. American Psychiatric Association, Washington, DC.

American Psychiatric Association (1994) *Diagnostic and Statistical Manual of Mental Disorders*, 4th edn. American Psychiatric Association, Washington, DC.

American Psychiatric Association (2000) *Diagnostic and Statistical Manual of Mental Disorders*, 4th edn. text revision, edn. American Psychiatric Association, Washington, DC.

American Psychiatric Association (2013) *Diagnostic and Statistical Manual of Mental Disorders*, 5th edn. American Psychiatric Association, Washington, DC.

American Psychiatric Association (2022) *Diagnostic and Statistical Manual of Mental Disorders*, 5th edn. text revision, edn. American Psychiatric Association, Washington, DC.

Andreo-Martínez, P. *et al.* (2022) A meta-analysis of gut microbiota in children with autism. *Journal of Autism and Developmental Disorders* **52**, 1374–1387.

Andrioaie, I.M. *et al.* (2022) The role of the gut microbiome in psychiatric disorders. *Microorganisms* **10**, 2436.

Antaki, D. *et al.* (2022) A phenotypic spectrum of autism is attributable to the combined effects of rare variants, polygenic risk and sex. *Nature Genetics* **54**, 1284–1292.

Asperger, H. (1944) Die "autistichen psychopathen" im kindersalter [Autistic psychopathy in childhood]. *Archive fur Psychiatrie und Nervenkrankheiten* **117**, 76–136.

Astle, D.E. *et al.* (2022) Annual research review: the transdiagnostic revolution in neurodevelopmental disorders. *Journal of Child Psychology and Psychiatry* **63**, 397–417.

Bai, D. *et al.* (2019) Association of genetic and environmental factors with autism in a 5-country cohort. *JAMA Psychiatry* **76**, 1035–1043.

Baker-Ericzén, M.J. *et al.* (2022) Current status of evidence-based practices to enhance employment outcomes for transition age youth and adults on the autism spectrum. *Current Psychiatry Reports* **24**, 161–170.

Bal, V.H. *et al.* (2016) Understanding definitions of minimally verbal across instruments: evidence for subgroups within minimally verbal children and adolescents with autism spectrum disorder. *Journal of Child Psychology and Psychiatry* **57**, 1424–1433.

Baraskewich, J. *et al.* (2021) Feeding and eating problems in children and adolescents with autism: a scoping review. *Autism* **25**, 1505–1519.

Baselmans, B.M.L. *et al.* (2021) Risk in relatives, heritability, SNP-based heritability, and genetic correlations in psychiatric disorders: a review. *Biological Psychiatry* **89**, 11–19.

Beck, K.B. *et al.* (2021) Assessment and treatment of emotion regulation impairment in autism spectrum disorder across the life span: current state of the science and future directions. *The Psychiatric Clinics of North America* **44**, 95–110.

Bieleninik, L. *et al.* (2017) Tracing the temporal stability of autism spectrum diagnosis and severity as measured by the Autism Diagnostic Observation Schedule: a systematic review and meta-analysis. *PLoS One* **12**, e0183160.

Boedhoe, P.S.W. *et al.* (2020) Subcortical brain volume, regional cortical thickness, and cortical surface area across disorders: findings from the ENIGMA ADHD, ASD, and OCD working groups. *The American Journal of Psychiatry* **177**, 834–843.

Bölte, S. *et al.* (2023) Sex and gender in neurodevelopmental conditions. *Nature Reviews. Neurology* **19**, 136–159.

Bottema-Beutel, K. *et al.* (2019) A systematic review and meta-regression analysis of social functioning correlates in autism and typical development. *Autism Research* **12**, 152–175.

Bottema-Beutel, K. *et al.* (2021a) Adverse event reporting in intervention research for young autistic children. *Autism* **25**, 322–335.

Bottema-Beutel, K. *et al.* (2021b) Research review: conflicts of interest (COIs) in autism early intervention research—a meta-analysis of COI influences on intervention effects. *Journal of Child Psychology and Psychiatry* **62**, 5–15.

Bourne, L. *et al.* (2022) Avoidant/restrictive food intake disorder and severe food selectivity in children and young people with autism: a scoping review. *Developmental Medicine and Child Neurology* **64**, 691–700.

Brian, J.A. *et al.* (2019) Standards of diagnostic assessment for autism spectrum disorder. *Paediatrics & Child Health* **24**, 444–460.

Brignell, A. *et al.* (2018) Communication interventions for autism spectrum disorder in minimally verbal children. *Cochrane Database of Systematic Reviews* **11**, CD012324.

Brugha, T.S. *et al.* (2016) Epidemiology of autism in adults across age groups and ability levels. *The British Journal of Psychiatry* **209**, 498–503.

Careaga, M. *et al.* (2017) Maternal immune activation and autism spectrum disorder: from rodents to nonhuman and human primates. *Biological Psychiatry* **81**, 391–401.

Carter Leno, V. *et al.* (2021) Callous-unemotional traits in youth with autism spectrum disorder (ASD): replication of prevalence estimates and associations with gaze patterns when viewing fearful faces. *Development and Psychopathology* **33**, 1220–1228.

Conrad, C.E. *et al.* (2021) Parent-mediated interventions for children and adolescents with autism spectrum disorders: a systematic review and meta-analysis. *Frontiers in Psychiatry* **12**, 773604.

Constantino, J.N. *et al.* (2020) Timing of the diagnosis of autism in African American children. *Pediatrics* **146**, e20193629.

Cooper, K. *et al.* (2023) Phenomenology of gender dysphoria in autism: a multiperspective qualitative analysis. *Journal of Child Psychology and Psychiatry* **64**, 265–276.

Crawley, J.N. (2023) Twenty years of discoveries emerging from mouse models of autism. *Neuroscience and Biobehavioral Reviews* **146**, 105053.

Culotta, L. & Penzes, P. (2020) Exploring the mechanisms underlying excitation/inhibition imbalance in human iPSC-derived models of ASD. *Molecular Autism* **11**, 32.

Czech, H. (2018) Hans Asperger, National Socialism, and "race hygiene" in Nazi-era Vienna. *Molecular Autism* **9**, 29.

Dawson, G. *et al.* (2023) Prediction of autism in infants: progress and challenges. *The Lancet Neurology* **22**, 244–254.

de Leeuw, A. *et al.* (2020) A conceptual framework for understanding the cultural and contextual factors on autism across the globe. *Autism Research* **13**, 1029–1050.

Deb, S. *et al.* (2021) Randomised controlled trials of antidepressant and anti-anxiety medications for people with autism spectrum disorder: systematic review and meta-analysis. *BJPsych Open* **7**, e179.

Deb, S. *et al.* (2023) Randomised controlled trials of antipsychotics for people with autism spectrum disorder: a systematic review and a meta-analysis. *Psychological Medicine* **53**(16), 7964–7972.

Doherty, M. *et al.* (2023) Autistic SPACE: a novel framework for meeting the needs of autistic people in healthcare settings. *British Journal of Hospital Medicine* **84**, 1–9.

Dunalska, A. *et al.* (2021) Comorbidity of bipolar disorder and autism spectrum disorder—review paper. *Psychiatria Polska* **55**, 1421–1431.

Dutheil, F. *et al.* (2021) Autism spectrum disorder and air pollution: a systematic review and meta-analysis. *Environmental Pollution* **278**, 116856.

Dwyer, P. (2022) The neurodiversity approach(es): what are they and what do they mean for researchers? *Human Development* **66**, 73–92.

Dwyer, P. *et al.* (2022) First do no harm: suggestions regarding respectful autism language. *Pediatrics* **149**, e2020049437N.

Eisenberg, L. & Kanner, L. (1956) Childhood schizophrenia; symposium, 1955. VI. Early infantile autism, 1943-55. *The American Journal of Orthopsychiatry* **26**, 556–566.

Fletcher-Watson, S. & Happé, F. (2019) *Autism: A New Introduction to Psychological Theory and Current Debate.* Routledge, London, New York.

Floris, D.L. *et al.* (2021) Towards robust and replicable sex differences in the intrinsic brain function of autism. *Molecular Autism* **12**, 19.

Fraguas, D. *et al.* (2019) Dietary interventions for autism spectrum disorder: a meta-analysis. *Pediatrics* **144**, e20183218.

Frankl, G. (1943) Language and affective contact. *Nervous Child* **2**, 251–262.

Frith, U. (1970) Studies in pattern detection in normal and autistic children. II. Reproduction and production of color sequences. *Journal of Experimental Child Psychology* **10**, 120–135.

Fu, J.M. *et al.* (2022) Rare coding variation provides insight into the genetic architecture and phenotypic context of autism. *Nature Genetics* **54**, 1320–1331.

Gentles, S.J. *et al.* (2024) Trajectory research in children with an autism diagnosis: a scoping review. *Autism* **28**(3), 540–564.

Georgiades, S. *et al.* (2017) Editorial perspective: longitudinal research in autism—introducing the concept of 'chronogeneity'. *Journal of Child Psychology and Psychiatry* **58**, 634–636.

Geretsegger, M. *et al.* (2022) Music therapy for autistic people. *Cochrane Database of Systematic Reviews* **5**, CD004381.

Gosling, C.J. *et al.* (2022) Efficacy of psychosocial interventions for autism spectrum disorder: an umbrella review. *Molecular Psychiatry* **27**, 3647–3656.

Green, J. & Garg, S. (2018) Annual research review: the state of autism intervention science: progress, target psychological and biological mechanisms and future prospects. *Journal of Child Psychology and Psychiatry* **59**, 424–443.

Grove, J. *et al.* (2019) Identification of common genetic risk variants for autism spectrum disorder. *Nature Genetics* **51**, 431–444.

Haasbroek, H. & Morojele, N. (2022) A systematic literature review on the relationship between autism spectrum disorder and substance use among adults and adolescents. *Review Journal of Autism and Developmental Disorders* **9**, 1–20.

Habayeb, S. *et al.* (2022) Still left behind: fewer black school-aged youth receive ASD diagnoses compared to white youth. *Journal of Autism and Developmental Disorders* **52**, 2274–2283.

Hacking, I. (2007) Kinds of people: moving targets. *Proceedings of the British Academy, Volume 151, 2006 Lectures*. Oxford University Press, Oxford, UK.

Han, V.X. *et al.* (2021) Maternal immune activation and neuroinflammation in human neurodevelopmental disorders. *Nature Reviews. Neurology* **17**, 564–579.

Happé, F. & Frith, U. (2020) Annual research review: looking back to look forward—changes in the concept of autism and implications for future research. *Journal of Child Psychology and Psychiatry* **61**, 218–232.

Hauptman, A.J. *et al.* (2023) Catatonia in neurodevelopmental disorders: assessing catatonic deterioration from baseline. *The Lancet Psychiatry* **10**, 228–234.

Hayes, J. *et al.* (2022) Autism diagnosis as a social process. *Autism* **26**, 488–498.

Hettwer, M.D. *et al.* (2022) Coordinated cortical thickness alterations across six neurodevelopmental and psychiatric disorders. *Nature Communications* **13**, 6851.

Hollander, E. *et al.* (2022) Balovaptan vs placebo for social communication in childhood autism spectrum disorder: a randomized clinical trial. *JAMA Psychiatry* **79**, 760–769.

Hollocks, M.J. *et al.* (2019) Anxiety and depression in adults with autism spectrum disorder: a systematic review and meta-analysis. *Psychological Medicine* **49**, 559–572.

Hoover, D.W. & Kaufman, J. (2018) Adverse childhood experiences in children with autism spectrum disorder. *Current Opinion in Psychiatry* **31**, 128–132.

Huang, J.S. *et al.* (2021) Risk of substance use disorder and its associations with comorbidities and psychotropic agents in patients with autism. *JAMA Pediatrics* **175**, e205371.

Hung, K.C. *et al.* (2023) Association of labor epidural analgesia exposure with long-term risk of autism spectrum disorder in offspring: a meta-analysis of observational studies. *Autism* **27**, 1177–1189.

Hyman, S.L. *et al.* (2020) Identification, evaluation, and management of children with autism spectrum disorder. *Pediatrics* **145**, e20193447.

Ilioska, I. *et al.* (2023) Connectome-wide mega-analysis reveals robust patterns of atypical functional connectivity in autism. *Biological Psychiatry* **94**, 29–39.

Ismael, N. *et al.* (2018) Relationship between sensory processing and participation in daily occupations for children with autism spectrum disorder: a systematic review of studies that used Dunn's sensory processing framework. *The American Journal of Occupational Therapy* **72**, 1–9.

Jobski, K. *et al.* (2017) Use of psychotropic drugs in patients with autism spectrum disorders: a systematic review. *Acta Psychiatrica Scandinavica* **135**, 8–28.

Johnson, M.H. *et al.* (2015) Annual research review: infant development, autism, and ADHD—early pathways to emerging disorders. *Journal of Child Psychology and Psychiatry* **56**, 228–247.

Jones, W. *et al.* (2023) Eye-tracking-based measurement of social visual engagement compared with expert clinical diagnosis of autism. *JAMA* **330**, 854–865.

Jutla, A. *et al.* (2022) Autism spectrum disorder and schizophrenia: an updated conceptual review. *Autism Research* **15**, 384–412.

Kallitsounaki, A. & Williams, D.M. (2023) Autism spectrum disorder and gender dysphoria/incongruence: a systematic literature review and meta-analysis. *Journal of Autism and Developmental Disorders* **53**, 3103–3117.

Kanner, L. (1943) Autistic disturbances of affective contact. *Nervous Child* **2**, 217–250.

Kapp, S.K. *et al.* (2013) Deficit, difference, or both? Autism and neurodiversity. *Developmental Psychology* **49**, 59–71.

Kapp, S.K. *et al.* (2019) People should be allowed to do what they like': autistic adults' views and experiences of stimming. *Autism* **23**, 1782–1792.

Kas, M.J. *et al.* (2019) A quantitative approach to neuropsychiatry: the why and the how. *Neuroscience and Biobehavioral Reviews* **97**, 3–9.

Kasari, C. *et al.* (2014) Communication interventions for minimally verbal children with autism: a sequential multiple assignment randomized trial. *Journal of the American Academy of Child and Adolescent Psychiatry* **53**, 635–646.

Kentrou, V. *et al.* (2019) Delayed autism spectrum disorder recognition in children and adolescents previously diagnosed with attention-deficit/hyperactivity disorder. *Autism* **23**, 1065–1072.

Kim, S.Y. *et al.* (2023) A systematic review and meta-analysis of associations between primarily non-autistic people's characteristics and attitudes toward autistic people. *Autism Research* **16**, 441–457.

Kiyono, T. *et al.* (2020) The prevalence of psychotic experiences in autism spectrum disorder and autistic traits: a systematic review and meta-analysis. *Schizophrenia Bulletin Open* **1**(1), sgaa046.

Lai, M.C. (2023) Mental health challenges faced by autistic people. *Nature Human Behaviour* **7**, 1620–1637.

Lai, M.C. & Baron-Cohen, S. (2015) Identifying the lost generation of adults with autism spectrum conditions. *The Lancet Psychiatry* **2**, 1013–1027.

Lai, M.C. *et al.* (2019) Prevalence of co-occurring mental health diagnoses in the autism population: a systematic review and meta-analysis. *The Lancet Psychiatry* **6**, 819–829.

Lai, M.C. *et al.* (2020) Evidence-based support for autistic people across the lifespan: maximising potential, minimising barriers, and optimising the person-environment fit. *The Lancet Neurology* **19**, 434–451.

Lai, M.C. *et al.* (2022) Towards equitable diagnoses for autism and attention-deficit/hyperactivity disorder across sexes and genders. *Current Opinion in Psychiatry* **35**, 90–100.

Lai, M.C. *et al.* (2023) Improving autism identification and support for individuals assigned female at birth: clinical suggestions and research priorities. *The Lancet Child & Adolescent Health* **7**, 897–908.

Lee, E. *et al.* (2017) Excitation/inhibition imbalance in animal models of autism spectrum disorders. *Biological Psychiatry* **81**, 838–847.

Leshem, R. *et al.* (2021) Selective serotonin reuptake inhibitors (SSRIs) and serotonin norepinephrine reuptake inhibitors (SNRIs) during pregnancy and the risk for autism spectrum disorder (ASD) and attention deficit hyperactivity disorder (ADHD) in the offspring: a true effect or a Bias? A systematic review & meta-analysis. *Current Neuropharmacology* **19**, 896–906.

Linden, A. *et al.* (2023) Benefits and harms of interventions to improve anxiety, depression, and other mental health outcomes for autistic people: a systematic review and network meta-analysis of randomised controlled trials. *Autism* **27**, 7–30.

Liu, X. *et al.* (2022) Prevalence of epilepsy in autism spectrum disorders: a systematic review and meta-analysis. *Autism* **26**, 33–50.

Lockyer, L. & Rutter, M. (1969) A five- to fifteen-year follow-up study of infantile psychosis. *The British Journal of Psychiatry* **115**, 865–882.

Lombardo, M.V. *et al.* (2019) Big data approaches to decomposing heterogeneity across the autism spectrum. *Molecular Psychiatry* **24**, 1435–1450.

Loomes, R. *et al.* (2017) What is the male-to-female ratio in autism spectrum disorder? A systematic review and meta-analysis. *Journal of the American Academy of Child and Adolescent Psychiatry* **56**, 466–474.

Lord, C. & Jones, R.M. (2012) Annual research review: re-thinking the classification of autism spectrum disorders. *Journal of Child Psychology and Psychiatry* **53**, 490–509.

Lord, C. *et al.* (2020) Autism spectrum disorder. *Nature Reviews. Disease Primers* **6**, 5.

Lord, C. *et al.* (2022) The Lancet Commission on the future of care and clinical research in autism. *The Lancet* **399**, 271–334.

Lun, T. *et al.* (2023) Acupuncture for children with autism spectrum disorder: a systematic review and meta-analysis. *Medicine (Baltimore)* **102**, e33079.

Maenner, M.J. *et al.* (2023) Prevalence and characteristics of autism spectrum disorder among children aged 8 years—autism and developmental disabilities monitoring network, 11 sites, United States, 2020. *MMWR Surveillance Summaries* **72**, 1–14.

Magiati, I. *et al.* (2014) Cognitive, language, social and behavioural outcomes in adults with autism spectrum disorders: a systematic review of longitudinal follow-up studies in adulthood. *Clinical Psychology Review* **34**, 73–86.

Mallipeddi, N.V. & VanDaalen, R.A. (2022) Intersectionality within critical autism studies: a narrative review. *Autism in Adulthood* **4**, 281–289.

Manickam, K. *et al.* (2021) Exome and genome sequencing for pediatric patients with congenital anomalies or intellectual disability: an evidence-based clinical guideline of the American college of medical genetics and genomics (ACMG). *Genetics in Medicine* **23**, 2029–2037.

McBrien, K.A. *et al.* (2018) Patient navigators for people with chronic disease: a systematic review. *PLoS One* **13**, e0191980.

McCarthy, M.M. & Wright, C.L. (2017) Convergence of sex differences and the neuroimmune system in autism spectrum disorder. *Biological Psychiatry* **81**, 402–410.

McCauley, J.B. *et al.* (2020) Trajectories of co-occurring psychopathology symptoms in autism from late childhood to adulthood. *Development and Psychopathology* **32**, 1287–1302.

McConachie, H. *et al.* (2020) What is important in measuring quality of life? Reflections by autistic adults in four countries. *Autism in Adulthood* **2**, 4–12.

McGuire, K. *et al.* (2016) Irritability and problem behavior in autism spectrum disorder: a practice pathway for pediatric primary care. *Pediatrics* **137**(Suppl 2), S136–S148.

Messinger, D.S. *et al.* (2015) Early sex differences are not autism-specific: a baby siblings research consortium (BSRC) study. *Molecular Autism* **6**, 32.

Milton, D. (2012) On the ontological status of autism: the 'double empathy problem'. *Disability & Society* **27**, 883–887.

Ministry of Disabled People (2022) Aotearoa New Zealand Autism Guideline: Third Edition [Online]. Available: https://www.whaikaha.govt.nz/about-us/policy-strategies-and-action-plans/NZ-autism-guideline [7 November 2024].

Molnar-Szakacs, I. *et al.* (2021) Neuroimaging markers of risk and pathways to resilience in autism spectrum disorder. *Biological Psychiatry. Cognitive Neuroscience and Neuroimaging* **6**, 200–210.

Morin, K.L. *et al.* (2018) A systematic quality review of high-tech AAC interventions as an evidence-based practice. *Augmentative and Alternative Communication* **34**, 104–117.

Mottron, L. (2021) A radical change in our autism research strategy is needed: back to prototypes. *Autism Research* **14**, 2213–2220.

Mournet, A.M. *et al.* (2022) A systematic review of predictors of suicidal thoughts and behaviors among autistic adults: making the case for the role of social connection as a protective factor. *Clinical Psychology Review* **99**, 102235.

Mutluer, T. *et al.* (2022) Population-based psychiatric comorbidity in children and adolescents with autism spectrum disorder: a meta-analysis. *Frontiers in Psychiatry* **13**, 856208.

National Autistic Society (n.d.) *Individual education plans*. National Autistic Society, London. Available: www.autism.org.uk/advice-and-guidance/topics/education/extra-help-at-school/northern-ireland/individual-education-plans. [16 November 2024].

National Institute for Health and Care Excellence (2017) Autism spectrum disorder in under 19s: recognition, referral and diagnosis. Nice Institute forHealth and Care Excellence (NICE), London [Online]. Available: www.nice.org.uk/guidance/cg128 [7 November 2024].

Ng-Cordell, E. *et al.* (2022) Anxiety and trauma-related disorders in children on the autism spectrum. *Current Psychiatry Reports* **24**, 171–180.

Nogueira, H.A. *et al.* (2023) Melatonin for sleep disorders in people with autism: systematic review and meta-analysis. *Progress in Neuro-Psychopharmacology & Biological Psychiatry* **123**, 110695.

Oakley, B. *et al.* (2021) Autism and mood disorders. *International Review of Psychiatry* **33**, 280–299.

O'Donnell, S. *et al.* (2022) Accuracy of administrative database algorithms for autism spectrum disorder, attention-deficit/hyperactivity disorder and fetal alcohol spectrum disorder case ascertainment: a systematic review. *Health Promotion and Chronic Disease Prevention in Canada* **42**, 355–383.

O'Halloran, L. *et al.* (2022) Suicidality in autistic youth: a systematic review and meta-analysis. *Clinical Psychology Review* **93**, 102144.

Pacheco, J. *et al.* (2022) Annual research review: the contributions of the RDoC research framework on understanding the neurodevelopmental origins, progression and treatment of mental illnesses. *Journal of Child Psychology and Psychiatry* **63**, 360–376.

Parellada, M. *et al.* (2023) In search of biomarkers to guide interventions in autism spectrum disorder: a systematic review. *The American Journal of Psychiatry* **180**, 23–40.

Park, I. *et al.* (2020) Prevalence of and factors associated with school bullying in students with autism spectrum disorder: a cross-cultural meta-analysis. *Yonsei Medical Journal* **61**, 909–922.

Parker, K.J. (2022) Leveraging a translational research approach to drive diagnostic and treatment advances for autism. *Molecular Psychiatry* **27**, 2650–2658.

Pellicano, E. & den Houting, J. (2022) Annual research review: shifting from 'normal science' to neurodiversity in autism science. *Journal of Child Psychology and Psychiatry* **63**, 381–396.

Pender, R. *et al.* (2020) The longitudinal heterogeneity of autistic traits: a systematic review. *Research in Autism Spectrum Disorders* **79**, 101671.

Penner, M. *et al.* (2018) Systematic review of clinical guidance documents for autism spectrum disorder diagnostic assessment in select regions. *Autism* **22**, 517–527.

Piwowarczyk, A. *et al.* (2018) Gluten- and casein-free diet and autism spectrum disorders in children: a systematic review. *European Journal of Nutrition* **57**, 433–440.

Port, R.G. *et al.* (2019) Revisiting the excitation/inhibition imbalance hypothesis of ASD through a clinical lens. *The British Journal of Radiology* **92**, 20180944.

Postema, M.C. *et al.* (2019) Altered structural brain asymmetry in autism spectrum disorder in a study of 54 datasets. *Nature Communications* **10**, 4958.

Radonjić, N.V. *et al.* (2021) Structural brain imaging studies offer clues about the effects of the shared genetic etiology among neuropsychiatric disorders. *Molecular Psychiatry* **26**, 2101–2110.

Randall, M. *et al.* (2018) Diagnostic tests for autism spectrum disorder (ASD) in preschool children. *Cochrane Database of Systematic Reviews* **7**, CD009044.

Regier, D.A. *et al.* (2013) DSM-5 field trials in the United States and Canada, part II: test-retest reliability of selected categorical diagnoses. *The American Journal of Psychiatry* **170**, 59–70.

Rehn, A.K. *et al.* (2023) The effectiveness of animal-assisted therapy for children and adolescents with autism spectrum disorder: a systematic review. *Complementary Therapies in Clinical Practice* **50**, 101719.

Ressel, M. *et al.* (2020) Systematic review of risk and protective factors associated with substance use and abuse in individuals with autism spectrum disorders. *Autism* **24**, 899–918.

Richards, C. *et al.* (2015) Prevalence of autism spectrum disorder phenomenology in genetic disorders: a systematic review and meta-analysis. *The Lancet Psychiatry* **2**, 909–916.

Roche, L. *et al.* (2021) Research priorities of the autism community: a systematic review of key stakeholder perspectives. *Autism* **25**, 336–348.

Rodrigues, R. *et al.* (2021) Practitioner review: pharmacological treatment of attention-deficit/hyperactivity disorder symptoms in children and youth with autism spectrum disorder: a systematic review and meta-analysis. *Journal of Child Psychology and Psychiatry* **62**, 680–700.

Rogers, J.P. *et al.* (2023) Evidence-based consensus guidelines for the management of catatonia: recommendations from the British Association for Psychopharmacology. *Journal of Psychopharmacology* **37**, 327–369.

Roman-Urrestarazu, A. *et al.* (2022) Autism incidence and spatial analysis in more than 7 million pupils in English schools: a retrospective, longitudinal, school registry study. *The Lancet Child & Adolescent Health* **6**, 857–868.

Rosello, R. *et al.* (2021) Developmental outcomes in adolescence of children with autism spectrum disorder without intellectual disability: a systematic review of prospective studies. *Neuroscience and Biobehavioral Reviews* **126**, 590–603.

Roux, A.M. *et al.* (2022) A national profile of substance use disorder among Medicaid enrollees on the autism spectrum or with intellectual disability. *Disability and Health Journal* **15**, 101289.

Ruan, H. *et al.* (2022) Medicine insufficient evidence for the efficacy of massage as intervention for autism spectrum disorder: a systematic review. *Evidence-based Complementary and Alternative Medicine* **2022**, 5328320.

Rubenstein, J.L. & Merzenich, M.M. (2003) Model of autism: increased ratio of excitation/inhibition in key neural systems. *Genes, Brain, and Behavior* **2**, 255–267.

Ruggeri, A. *et al.* (2020) The effect of motor and physical activity intervention on motor outcomes of children with autism spectrum disorder: a systematic review. *Autism* **24**, 544–568.

Russell, G. *et al.* (2022) Time trends in autism diagnosis over 20 years: a UK population-based cohort study. *Journal of Child Psychology and Psychiatry* **63**, 674–682.

Rutter, M. (1978) Diagnosis and definition of childhood autism. *Journal of Autism and Childhood Schizophrenia* **8**, 139–161.

Rydzewska, E. *et al.* (2021) Umbrella systematic review of systematic reviews and meta-analyses on comorbid physical conditions in people with autism spectrum disorder. *The British Journal of Psychiatry* **218**, 10–19.

Salari, N. *et al.* (2022) The global prevalence of autism spectrum disorder: a comprehensive systematic review and meta-analysis. *Italian Journal of Pediatrics* **48**, 112.

Salazar de Pablo, G. *et al.* (2023) Systematic review and meta-analysis: efficacy of pharmacological interventions for irritability and emotional dysregulation in autism spectrum disorder and predictors of response. *Journal of the American Academy of Child and Adolescent Psychiatry* **62**, 151–168.

Sandbank, M. *et al.* (2020) Project AIM: autism intervention meta-analysis for studies of young children. *Psychological Bulletin* **146**, 1–29.

Sandbank, M. *et al.* (2023) Autism intervention meta-analysis of early childhood studies (Project AIM): updated systematic review and secondary analysis. *BMJ* **383**, e076733.

Sartore, G.M. *et al.* (2021) Peer support interventions for parents and carers of children with complex needs. *Cochrane Database of Systematic Reviews* **12**, CD010618.

Schaaf, C.P. *et al.* (2020) A framework for an evidence-based gene list relevant to autism spectrum disorder. *Nature Reviews. Genetics* **21**, 367–376.

Schaeffer, J. *et al.* (2023) Language in autism: domains, profiles and co-occurring conditions. *Journal of Neural Transmission* **130**, 433–457.

Schreck, K.A. & Richdale, A.L. (2020) Sleep problems, behavior, and psychopathology in autism: inter-relationships across the lifespan. *Current Opinion in Psychology* **34**, 105–111.

Schreibman, L. *et al.* (2015) Naturalistic developmental behavioral interventions: empirically validated treatments for autism spectrum disorder. *Journal of Autism and Developmental Disorders* **45**, 2411–2428.

Schuck, R.K. *et al.* (2022) Neurodiversity and autism intervention: reconciling perspectives through a naturalistic developmental behavioral intervention framework. *Journal of Autism and Developmental Disorders* **52**, 4625–4645.

Sha, Z. *et al.* (2022) Subtly altered topological asymmetry of brain structural covariance networks in autism spectrum disorder across 43 datasets from the ENIGMA consortium. *Molecular Psychiatry* **27**, 2114–2125.

Shah, A. (2020) Catatonia. In: *A Clinician's Guide to Mental Health Conditions in Adults with Autism Spectrum Disorders: Assessment and Interventions.* (eds E. Chaplin, *et al.*). Jessica Kingsley Publishers, London, UK. pp. 186–198.

Sharon, G. *et al.* (2019) Human gut microbiota from autism spectrum disorder promote behavioral symptoms in mice. *Cell* **177**, 1600–1618.

Sheldrick, R.C. *et al.* (2017) Age at first identification of autism spectrum disorder: an analysis of two US surveys. *Journal of the American Academy of Child and Adolescent Psychiatry* **56**, 313–320.

Shen, M.D. *et al.* (2022) Subcortical brain development in autism and fragile X syndrome: evidence for dynamic, age- and disorder-specific trajectories in infancy. *The American Journal of Psychiatry* **179**, 562–572.

Shultz, S. *et al.* (2018) Neonatal transitions in social behavior and their implications for autism. *Trends in Cognitive Sciences* **22**, 452–469.

Sikich, L. *et al.* (2021) Intranasal oxytocin in children and adolescents with autism spectrum disorder. *The New England Journal of Medicine* **385**, 1462–1473.

Simmonds, C. & Sukhareva, G.E. (2020) The first account of the syndrome Asperger described? Part 2: the girls. *European Child & Adolescent Psychiatry* **29**, 549–564.

Sohal, V.S. & Rubenstein, J.L.R. (2019) Excitation-inhibition balance as a framework for investigating mechanisms in neuropsychiatric disorders. *Molecular Psychiatry* **24**, 1248–1257.

Ssucharewa, G.E. & Wolff, S. (1996) The first account of the syndrome Asperger described? Translation of a paper entitled "die schizoiden Psychopathien im Kindesalter" by Dr. G.E. Ssucharewa; scientific assistant, which appeared in 1926 in the Monatsschrift fur Psychiatrie und Neurologie 60:235-261. *European Child & Adolescent Psychiatry* **5**, 119–132.

Strang, J.F. *et al.* (2018) Initial clinical guidelines for co-occurring autism spectrum disorder and gender dysphoria or incongruence in adolescents. *Journal of Clinical Child and Adolescent Psychology* **47**, 105–115.

Stringer, D. *et al.* (2020) Trajectories of emotional and behavioral problems from childhood to early adult life. *Autism* **24**, 1011–1024.

Sutton, B.M. *et al.* (2019) A systematic review of school-based interventions targeting social communication behaviors for students with autism. *Autism* **23**, 274–286.

Szatmari, P. *et al.* (2015) Developmental trajectories of symptom severity and adaptive functioning in an inception cohort of preschool children with autism spectrum disorder. *JAMA Psychiatry* **72**, 276–283.

Szatmari, P. *et al.* (2016) Prospective longitudinal studies of infant siblings of children with autism: lessons learned and future directions. *Journal of the American Academy of Child and Adolescent Psychiatry* **55**, 179–187.

Taylor, M.J. *et al.* (2020) Etiology of autism spectrum disorders and autistic traits over time. *JAMA Psychiatry* **77**, 936–943.

Thapar, A. *et al.* (2017) Neurodevelopmental disorders. *The Lancet Psychiatry* **4**, 339–346.

Tick, B. *et al.* (2016) Heritability of autism spectrum disorders: a meta-analysis of twin studies. *Journal of Child Psychology and Psychiatry* **57**, 585–595.

Todorow, C. *et al.* (2018) The medical home for children with autism spectrum disorder: an essential element whose time has come. *Current Opinion in Pediatrics* **30**, 311–317.

Trundle, G. *et al.* (2023) Prevalence of victimisation in autistic individuals: a systematic review and meta-analysis. *Trauma Violence Abuse* **24**, 2282–2296.

Turnock, A. *et al.* (2022) Understanding stigma in autism: a narrative review and theoretical model. *Autism in Adulthood* **4**, 76–91.

U.S. Preventive Services Task Force. 2016. Autism Spectrum Disorder in Young Children: Screening U.S. Preventive Services Task Force, Rockville, MD. [Online]. Available: https://www.uspreventiveservicestaskforce.org/uspstf/recommendation/autism-spectrum-disorder-in-young-children-screening [7 November 2024].

van Rooij, D. *et al.* (2018) Cortical and subcortical brain morphometry differences between patients with autism spectrum disorder and healthy individuals across the lifespan: results from the ENIGMA ASD working group. *The American Journal of Psychiatry* **175**, 359–369.

van 't Hof, M. *et al.* (2021) Age at autism spectrum disorder diagnosis: a systematic review and meta-analysis from 2012 to 2019. *Autism* **25**, 862–873.

Vaquerizo-Serrano, J. *et al.* (2021) Catatonia in autism spectrum disorders: a systematic review and meta-analysis. *European Psychiatry* **65**, e4.

Varcin, K.J. *et al.* (2022) Occurrence of psychosis and bipolar disorder in adults with autism: a systematic review and meta-analysis. *Neuroscience and Biobehavioral Reviews* **134**, 104543.

Vasa, R.A. *et al.* (2016) Assessment and treatment of anxiety in youth with autism spectrum disorders. *Pediatrics* **137**(Suppl 2), S115–S123.

Verhoeff, B. (2012) What is this thing called autism? A critical analysis of the tenacious search for autism's essence. *BioSocieties* **7**, 410–432.

Verhoeff, B. (2013) Autism in flux: a history of the concept from Leo Kanner to DSM-5. *History of Psychiatry* **24**, 442–458.

Waisman, T.C. *et al.* (2023) Learning from the experts: evaluating a participatory autism and universal design training for university educators. *Autism* **27**, 356–370.

Walker, N. (2021) *Neuroqueer Heresies: Notes on the Neurodiversity Paradigm, Autistic Empowerment, and Postnormal Possibilities.* Autonomous Press, Fort Worth, TX.

Warrier, V. *et al.* (2022) Genetic correlates of phenotypic heterogeneity in autism. *Nature Genetics* **54**, 1293–1304.

Weitlauf, A.S. *et al.* (2017) Interventions targeting sensory challenges in autism spectrum disorder: a systematic review. *Pediatrics* **139**, e20170347.

White, S.W. *et al.* (2018) Psychosocial treatments targeting anxiety and depression in adolescents and adults on the autism spectrum: review of the latest research and recommended future directions. *Current Psychiatry Reports* **20**, 82.

Wichers, R.H. *et al.* (2023) Psychotherapy for co-occurring symptoms of depression, anxiety and obsessive-compulsive disorder in children and adults with autism spectrum disorder: a systematic review and meta-analysis. *Psychological Medicine* **53**, 17–33.

Wieckowski, A.T. *et al.* (2023) Sensitivity and specificity of the modified checklist for autism in toddlers (original and revised): a systematic review and meta-analysis. *JAMA Pediatrics* **177**, 373–383.

Wigham, S. *et al.* (2019) Psychometric properties of questionnaires and diagnostic measures for autism spectrum disorders in adults: a systematic review. *Autism* **23**, 287–305.

Williams, Z.J. *et al.* (2021) A review of decreased sound tolerance in autism: definitions, phenomenology, and potential mechanisms. *Neuroscience and Biobehavioral Reviews* **121**, 1–17.

Williams Buckley, A. *et al.* (2020) Practice guideline: treatment for insomnia and disrupted sleep behavior in children and adolescents with autism spectrum disorder: report of the Guideline Development, Dissemination, and Implementation Subcommittee of the American Academy of Neurology. *Neurology* **94**, 392–404.

Willsey, H.R. *et al.* (2022) Genomics, convergent neuroscience and progress in understanding autism spectrum disorder. *Nature Reviews. Neuroscience* **23**, 323–341.

Wing, L. (1981a) Asperger's syndrome: a clinical account. *Psychological Medicine* **11**, 115–129.

Wing, L. (1981b) Language, social, and cognitive impairments in autism and severe mental retardation. *Journal of Autism and Developmental Disorders* **11**, 31–44.

Wittkopf, S. *et al.* (2023) Conceptualization of the latent structure of autism: further evidence and discussion of dimensional and hybrid models. *European Child & Adolescent Psychiatry* **32**, 2247–2258.

Wolfers, T. *et al.* (2019) From pattern classification to stratification: towards conceptualizing the heterogeneity of autism spectrum disorder. *Neuroscience and Biobehavioral Reviews* **104**, 240–254.

Wong, O.W.H. *et al.* (2023) Executive function as a generalized determinant of psychopathology and functional outcome in school-aged autism spectrum disorder: a case-control study. *Psychological Medicine* **53**, 4788–4798.

World Health Organization (1993) *International Statistical Classification of Disease and Related Health Problems*, 10th edn. World Health Organization, Geneva, Switzerland.

World Health Organization (2019a) *International Statistical Classification of Disease and Related Health Problems*, 11th edn. World Health Organization, Geneva, Switzerland.

World Health Organization (2019b) Autism spectrum disorder. In: *International Statistical Classification of Disease and Related Health Problems*, 11th edn. World Health Organization, Geneva, Switzerland. Available: https://icd.who.int/browse/2024-01/mms/en#437815624. [16 November 2024].

Yap, C.X. *et al.* (2021) Autism-related dietary preferences mediate autism-gut microbiome associations. *Cell* **184** (5916–5931).

Yu, Y. *et al.* (2019) Effects of caregiver-focused programs on psychosocial outcomes in caregivers of individuals with ASD: a meta-analysis. *Journal of Autism and Developmental Disorders* **49**, 4761–4779.

Yuen, T. *et al.* (2018) Assessing the accuracy of the modified checklist for autism in toddlers: a systematic review and meta-analysis. *Developmental Medicine and Child Neurology* **60**, 1093–1100.

Zander, E. *et al.* (2015) The added value of the combined use of the autism diagnostic interview-revised and the autism diagnostic observation schedule: diagnostic validity in a clinical Swedish sample of toddlers and young preschoolers. *Autism* **19**, 187–199.

Zeidan, J. *et al.* (2022) Global prevalence of autism: a systematic review update. *Autism Research* **15**, 778–790.

Zhong, C. *et al.* (2020) Maternal dietary factors and the risk of autism spectrum disorders: a systematic review of existing evidence. *Autism Research* **13**, 1634–1658.

Zhuang, S. *et al.* (2023) Psychosocial factors associated with camouflaging in autistic people and its relationship with mental health and well-being: a mixed methods systematic review. *Clinical Psychology Review* **105**, 102335.

CHAPTER 51
Developmental language disorders

Courtenay Norbury
Division of Psychology and Language Sciences, University College London, London, UK

Overview

Language is a uniquely human accomplishment that underpins academic and economic success (Conti-Ramsden *et al.*, 2018), societal participation (McLeod, 2018), and well-being (Eadie *et al.*, 2018). For most children, language is easily acquired through rich social interactions with caregivers. However, a substantial number of children have language disorders that disrupt their ability to learn from the usual language input (Bishop *et al.*, 2016). Relative to other neurodevelopmental conditions with similar prevalence and severity, there is less awareness, less research, and fewer services for these vulnerable children (McGregor, 2020). This is surprising given that children with language disorder are at substantially increased risk for social, emotional, and mental health challenges (Yew & O'Kearney, 2013).

This chapter begins with an overview of the language system and recent consensus decisions on terminology and diagnostic criteria for language disorders. Box 51.1 presents a case history that illustrates both key characteristics and the functional impact of language disorder from the perspective of a young person with lived experience. I will then discuss the long-term impacts of language disorder, with particular reference to the association between language disorder and mental health. I will summarize current evidence for language interventions, and highlight strategies and techniques that practitioners can use to facilitate communication in clinical settings.

Terminology and key diagnostic features of developmental language disorders

Terminology

Bishop (2010) searched the literature to 2010 and found that 130 different terms for language difficulties had been used at least once in a publication, and 33 distinct forms (e.g., specific language impairment [SLI], language delay, language disability, language disorder, or developmental language disorder) had been used 600 times or more. In contrast, other diagnostic terms (e.g., autism or attention deficit hyperactivity disorder [ADHD]) have remained relatively stable over time. A decade later, McGregor (2020) concluded that inconsistent terminology was a barrier to public understanding of language disorder, with negative consequences for research and practice.

To address this issue, the international CATALISE consortium invited key stakeholders (families, speech-language pathologists, researchers, teachers, etc.) to review evidence and agree on terminology and diagnostic criteria (Bishop *et al.* 2017). CATALISE recommended the term "developmental language disorder" (DLD) for a condition in which language is not developing as expected, but no other associated biomedical condition is present.

DLD supersedes the term "SLI," previously used in research but not in formal diagnostic frameworks such as the *Diagnostic and Statistical Manual of Mental Disorders*, 5th edition, text revision (DSM-5-TR; American Psychiatric Association, 2022) or the *International Classification of Diseases*, 11th edition (ICD-11; World Health Organization, 2019). DLD is a more inclusive term—all children with SLI would meet criteria for DLD, but DLD also includes children with lower nonverbal cognitive ability scores (an exclusion criterion for SLI). For individuals with DLD, language is the primary presenting concern, and the origin of the language deficit is unknown. During the assessment process, DLD is distinguished from "language disorder," the term used when language difficulties are associated with other neurodevelopment conditions such as autism or intellectual disabilities (ID; Box 51.2).

DLD represents a subset of wider *speech, language,* and *communication* needs (Figure 51.1, Bishop *et al.*, 2017). These three often go together, though not always, although challenges with one may well influence development of competencies in another.

Rutter's Child and Adolescent Psychiatry and Psychology, Seventh Edition.
Edited by Anita Thapar, Daniel S. Pine, Samuele Cortese, Cathy Creswell, Tamsin J. Ford, James F. Leckman, and Argyris Stringaris.

Companion website: www.wiley.com/go/thapar/ruttерspsych7

Box 51.1 Case study

Maggie is a 13-year-old girl who tries hard to cover up her development language disorder (DLD). Her speech is clear, but she speaks slowly and it takes a long time to find the words she wants to say. Often, she does not understand what other people are saying to her, but smiles and nods so they do not ask her a question. She is very keen to have friends, but she cannot keep up with conversations with other girls. She says it is like "experiencing everything on catch-up"—by the time she has figured out what they are talking about, they have moved on to a new topic. School is even worse—she struggles with reading and has problems with the complex vocabulary and sentences used in lessons. Lots of information she is expected to know is not even explicitly stated and it takes a long time to process even short texts. Lessons are confusing because the words and phrases mean more than one thing. Yesterday in science was a typical example. The topic was "The Greenhouse Effect" and even though she was listening as hard as she could, Maggie was still confused. When she asked "Sir, where is the greenhouse?" everyone in the class laughed. The teacher told her to stop daydreaming and pay attention. Maggie feels that all the other students think she is stupid. Increasingly, she does not want to go to school because she feels so anxious about getting things wrong. Her mother took her to see a clinical psychologist, but the psychologist had never heard of DLD before and did not know any strategies for supporting her. They spent the whole session talking about feelings and the events at school that led Maggie to feel anxious, both topics that Maggie finds really difficult to talk about. Her mom had to make an additional appointment to explain DLD to the psychologist and discuss ways to support communication, for example, using visual aids and taking a photo of key points on Maggie's phone, so they could discuss the session when they got home

Source: Adapted from https://www.youtube.com/RADLD/last accessed 8 April 2024.

Box 51.2 Differential diagnosis differentiating conditions, risk factors, and co-occurring conditions

In trying to navigate the complexities of diagnostic terminology, the CATALISE consortium (Bishop *et al.* 2017) made a threefold distinction among *differentiating conditions, risk factors*, and *co-occurring conditions*.

Differentiating conditions

Differentiating conditions are biomedical conditions in which language impairment is one of a complex set of symptoms, as in autism or Down syndrome. In these cases, the term "language disorder associated with X" was advocated to highlight the child's language profile and the associated functional impacts, and indicate the need to target language directly in intervention. Examples of differentiating conditions are given below.

Language disorder associated with autism

The "structural" language skills (phonology, semantics, syntax) of autistic individuals are hugely variable, ranging from minimally verbal to exceptional. Language skills at age 5 are a prognostic indicator of a range of adult outcomes (Howlin *et al.*, 2004). Presence of language regression is not typical of developmental language disorder (DLD) and should therefore prompt further investigation for autism and/or neurological investigation for acquired epileptic aphasia (Pickles *et al.*, 2022). Pragmatic skills, especially inferencing, figurative language, and ambiguity resolution, are closely aligned with structural language competence (Saul *et al.* 2023). Clinical observations and investigations should focus on whether and how children communicate with peers and how they repair communication (through use of gesture, rewording) when it breaks down. In sum, the key indicators to differentiate autism and DLD are: (i) restricted and repetitive interests and behaviors—these are indicative of autism, not DLD; (ii) differences in social reciprocity—-children with DLD may show more interest in peers, but may have difficulty accessing interaction because of language issues; and (iii) language regression—indicative of autism, not DLD. Detailed language profiles are useful for planning education support and intervention for autistic children and their families.

Language disorder associated with intellectual disability

Most conditions associated with intellectual disability (ID; e.g., Down syndrome, Fragile X) are characterized by language difficulties. In cases in which the cause of ID is unknown, the differential diagnosis should be based on both standardized tests and measures of adaptive behavior. Language tends to be more severely impaired in individuals with ID and may, in some instances, require alternative or augmentative forms of communication.

Language disorder associated with trauma

DLD has a biological basis but extreme forms of environmental deprivation and trauma may also give rise to difficulties with language that are similar to those seen in DLD. Children experiencing trauma or other adverse childhood experiences are more likely than peers to have difficulties acquiring grammar (Selin *et al.*, 2022), narratives (Ciolino *et al.*, 2021), and pragmatic language (Di Sante *et al.*, 2019). The ability to recognize and express emotion and mental states, and regulate emotion, is also challenging for children experiencing trauma and is posited as a key mechanism linking early deprivation to later psychopathology (Wade *et al.*, 2022).

Risk factors

Risk factors are preexisting biological or environmental exposures that have a weak statistical association with language outcome. For language disorder these may include:

- parent concern (language, behavior, social responsiveness)premature birth
- family history of language, literacy, or learning difficulties
- delays in acquiring first words and word combinations
- delays in gross motor or general cognitive skills

language regression (child stops using words previously acquired)

Co-occurring conditions

Co-occurring conditions are conditions like attention deficit hyperactivity disorder (ADHD) or dyslexia that are seen in children with DLD at a much higher rate than expected given their prevalence in the general population (for example, dyslexia has a population prevalence of ~5% but as many as 50% of children with DLD are likely to have difficulty learning to read (Adlof & Hogan, 2018). However, we cannot be sure what the direction of the causal relationships between these co-occurring conditions might be. For this reason, children presenting with reading disorders and/or behavioral difficulties should have a language assessment to determine if support for language is warranted.

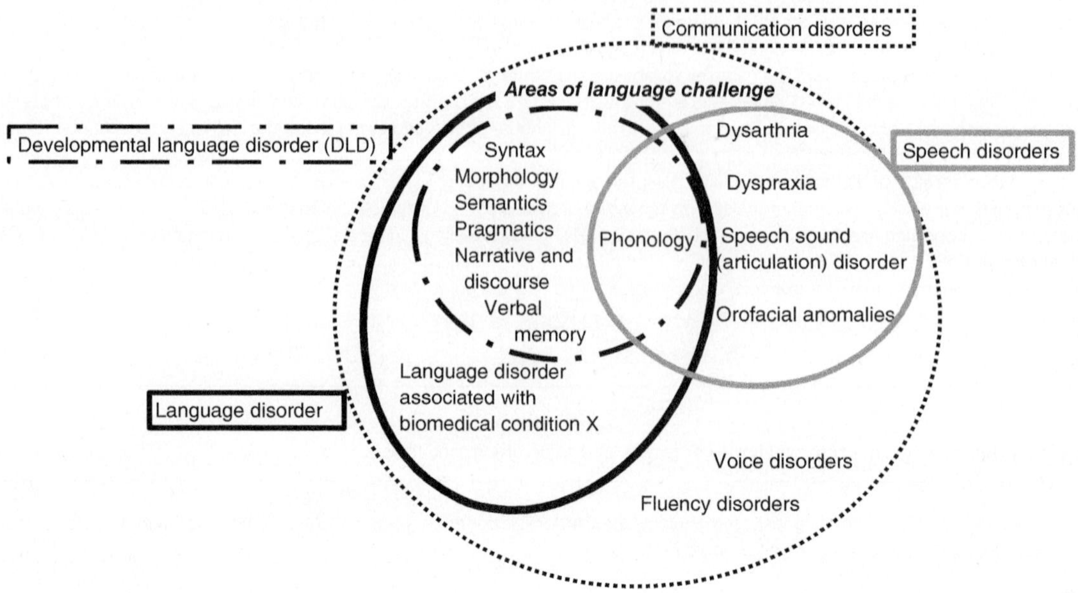

Figure 51.1 Venn diagram of how developmental language disorder (DLD) fits within the broader spectrum of speech, language, and communication needs. *Source:* Bishop *et al.* (2017)/John Wiley & Sons/CC BY - 4.0.

Communication is an overarching term for the transmission of information (a message) between a source and a receiver, using a common signaling system. Animals communicate. For example, birdsong is a species-typical signal used to attract mates and, like human speech, is learned in social contexts through exposure to vocalizations during sensitive periods in development. Humans communicate using a variety of means including body language, tone of voice, facial expressions, or gestures, as well as conventional symbols and signals (e.g., an alarm to signal danger, or more recently, emojis).

Language is a powerful mode of communication. It is a complex system that takes a finite number of units (sounds, words) that can be combined in rule-governed ways to convey an infinite number of meanings. Human language can be conveyed through writing or manual signs, or most commonly, through speech.

Speech is a particular way of expressing language through orally produced units of sounds combined to form words. A child with speech sound disorder (SSD) typically produces a restricted range of speech sounds, rendering spoken output unintelligible. For example, a child with SSD may substitute one speech sound for others (saying "tate" for "Kate" or "gate"), omit sounds ("cool" instead of "school") or syllables ("puter" for "computer"), or reverse sounds and syllables ("pesgetti" instead of "spaghetti"). Children with dyspraxia have motor planning issues that make speech errors more variable and less consistent. Dysarthria is typically caused by neurological conditions that affect the muscles of the mouth and face and disrupt the precision and quality of articulation. SSDs, dyspraxia, and dysarthria are likely to affect the child's ability to communicate, because conversational partners may not understand what the child is trying to say. Nevertheless, the child may have age-appropriate language skills, in that they understand what other people say and can use grammatically complex sentences in stories and conversation. They may also have a typical drive to communicate, supplementing unintelligible speech with gestures and reformulating utterances in order to make themselves understood.

A child with *language* disorder may produce speech sounds accurately, but communication may be limited by poor understanding of what others say to them, impoverished vocabulary, and reliance on simple or immature sentence structures. However, they may use these limited language skills to share their thoughts and experiences with others. In contrast, some children may have perfect articulation, exceptional vocabularies, and express themselves using long and grammatically-complex sentences, yet their *communication* is limited by tangential speech, repetitive words or phrases, and a reduced ability to repair breakdowns in conversation. This communication profile is more common in autistic children. Researchers and practitioners often draw distinctions among speech, language, and communication in order to highlight a particular child's strengths and challenges.

Diagnostic criteria

Language criteria

CATALISE criteria for DLD are closely aligned to the criteria for language disorder described in DSM-5-TR (American Psychiatric Association, 2022) and ICD-11 (World Health Organization, 2019). Both diagnostic frameworks require:

- Persistent difficulties in the acquisition, comprehension, production, and/or use of language across modalities (i.e., spoken, written, sign language).
- Measured language abilities are below age expectations.

- Differences in language lead to functional impacts in communication, social participation, academic achievement, and/or occupational performance.
- Language difficulties are evident early in development and are not the consequence of an acquired pathology (e.g., traumatic brain injury, stroke, tumor).
- Difficulties with language are not attributable to sensory impairment, motor difficulties, or another medical or neurological condition, and are not better explained by ID.

The language differences indicative of DLD may manifest in any area of language in isolation or in combination (Figure 51.2):

Phonemes

The speech sounds of our language are the building blocks of morphemes (prefixes and suffixes) and words. For example, /k/ is a sound made at the back of the throat that can be realized in written English by various letters (e.g., c̲at, k̲ey, tac̲k̲). In general, children with DLD do not have difficulties producing phonemes (<2% meet criteria for SSD, Wren *et al.*, 2016), but may have challenges acquiring and deploying the rules that allow us to flexibly combine speech sounds to create new words or morphemes. Phonemic awareness is important for making the transition to literacy and notably, the co-occurrence of DLD and dyslexia is extremely high (see Chapter 52).

Morphemes

These are the smallest units of meaning. Morphemes may be base words or affixes that can be combined and recombined to create new meanings (e.g., clean, *un*clean, clean*er*, *un*clean*able*, clean*liness*) or signal grammatical information such as number or tense (e.g., we walk, she walk*s*, he walk*ed* to the park, she is walk*ing* there now). Children with DLD are noted for challenges with grammatical morphology. For example, English-speaking children with DLD are likely to omit markers of case and tense ("him walk_ to school yesterday"), subject–verb agreement ("her walk_ to school and he run__"), auxiliary verbs ("She [is] reading"; "He [can] help"), and articles ("[the] book"; "[an] apple"; "[a] teddy bear").

Semantics (vocabulary)

Words can refer to tangible objects, or abstract and imaginary constructs, including thoughts and emotions. Children with DLD are frequently slow to acquire first words, and as they grow older, their vocabularies are limited in both breadth (the number of words they know) and depth (nuanced information about those words) (McGregor *et al.*, 2013). Limitations in semantic knowledge may contribute to difficulties with flexible word use, for example, understanding multiple meanings (e.g., "she is *cold*") or making inferences (e.g., "he *pedaled* to school" means he went on his bike).

Syntax (grammar)

Grammar comprises the rules that govern how we combine words to form sentences. Grammar allows us to represent relations between people, feelings, actions, and consequences, making explicit the links between our internal states and our actions in the world. While children typically start producing multiword utterances at 18–24 months of age, children with DLD are often 2 ½–4 years old before word combinations start to appear. They persist in using shorter, simpler sentences and have particular difficulty with passives (e.g., "the boy *was kissed* by the girl"), complement clauses (e.g., "she thinks *that the train is canceled*"), and relative clauses (e.g., "she messaged the boy *[who was] wearing the green socks*"; "they will stop for a cup of tea *when they get tired of walking*"). Complex grammar is more common in books (Nation *et al.*, 2022) and is therefore important for literacy and academic attainment.

Narratives (stories)

are collections of words and sentences that connect people, their internal states, and external events. Personal narratives are the stories we tell about ourselves and our experiences, and are a key means by which we make sense of the world and share social and emotional conventions (Westby & Culatta, 2016). Fictional narratives bridge oral language and more literate language forms. Both are challenging for young people with DLD, who are likely to produce stories that contain fewer and less complex utterances and leave out essential information, including the mental or emotional states of story characters (Winters *et al.*, 2022).

Discourse

Conversation requires us to use a common language system to facilitate social interaction and affiliation. Conversational discourse can be a strength for children with DLD, but success may depend on the ability of conversational partners to modify their language and give the young person with DLD plenty of time to process what has been said and formulate a response. Some young people with DLD may avoid conversation in order to "mask" their communication difficulties (Hobson & Lee, 2022).

Pragmatics

Pragmatics refers to the various ways in which we use language for social communication. It may include aspects of narrative and discourse in that we must tailor the language we use to meet the needs of our communication partners, a skill that requires children to represent someone else's knowledge state (e.g., theory of mind). It often involves going beyond the explicit linguistic form to make an inference, understand ambiguous words and phrases (e.g., a river *bank* versus a financial *bank*), and figurative expressions such as similes (e.g., "my love *is like* a red, red rose"), metaphors (e.g., "she's *under the weather*"), and verbal humor. These pragmatic skills draw heavily on linguistic context and therefore pose considerable challenges for young people with language disorders.

Other criteria

In addition to language criteria, CATALISE made three other significant recommendations (Bishop *et al.*, 2016). First, diagnosis requires evidence of persistence and likely poor prognosis.

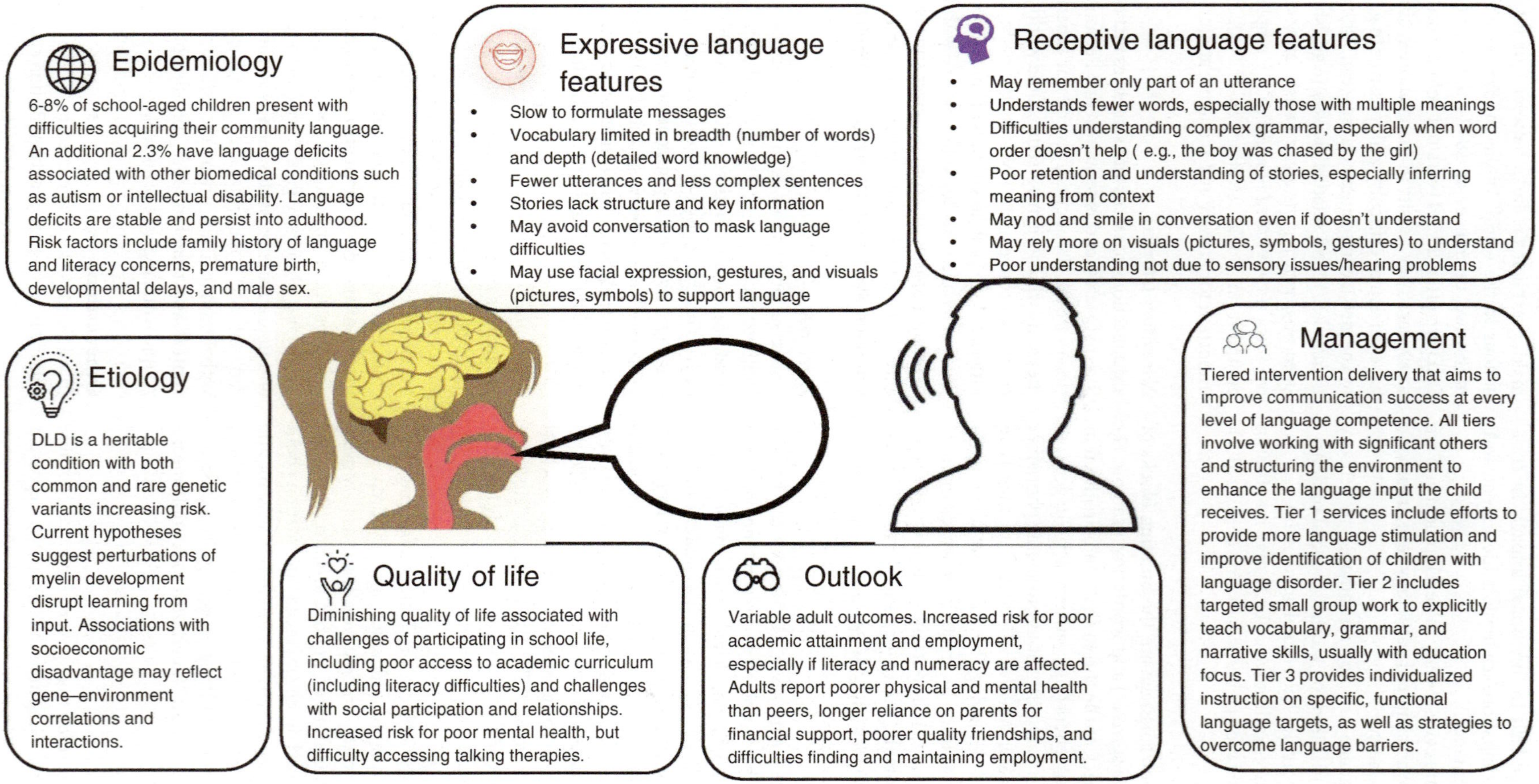

Figure 51.2 Developmental language disorder (DLD) at a glance.

Second, nonverbal cognitive abilities are not referenced for diagnosis or access to specialist services. Finally, current evidence does not support identification of specific subtypes of language disorder. These issues are considered in more detail below.

Delay versus disorder

Diagnosis of DLD prior to the age of five is challenging as many late talkers (children with limited expressive vocabulary at 18–24 months) catch up without any additional special help (Wake *et al.*, 2011). Children at greatest risk of persisting problems have poor language comprehension, poor use of gesture, and/or family risks such as socioeconomic disadvantage, poor maternal mental health and lower levels of maternal education, and family history of language or literacy difficulties (Eadie *et al.*, 2021). Nevertheless, even with these indicators, prediction of outcomes for individual children is unreliable. CATALISE therefore recommended reassessment after 6 months before making a clinical diagnosis of DLD (Bishop *et al.*, 2016). This does not preclude guidance and support for parents and/or a period of intervention, which may in turn inform diagnosis.

Nonverbal cognitive abilities

For years, diagnosis of "SLI" required children to have age-appropriate nonverbal cognitive abilities and a marked discrepancy between verbal and nonverbal IQ scores (see Bishop *et al.* (2017) for discussion). Thus, a child with a nonverbal IQ score of 90 and a language score of 75 would be diagnosed with DLD, but one with a nonverbal IQ score of 80 and a language score of 75 would not, limiting access to speech-language therapy services for children with cognitive deficits. These decisions were based on assumptions that a child with a mismatch between language and nonverbal skills is qualitatively different or has a different etiology from one whose poor language is commensurate with nonverbal ability and that nonverbal cognitive ability limits the potential for learning, thus limiting the potential to benefit from therapy.

CATALISE questioned these assumptions, highlighting arbitrary cutoffs on what are continuous distributions of nonverbal and language test scores. In addition, many linguistically able children use verbal strategies to help them reason about the answers to nonverbal tests, putting the child with DLD at a distinct disadvantage. More recently, Griffiths *et al.* (2022) demonstrated that over time, language predicted change in nonverbal IQ scores to the same extent that nonverbal IQ scores predicted change in language. This indicates that nonverbal ability does not necessarily "cap" language potential and suggests that improvements in language could benefit cognition. Direct comparison of children meeting criteria for "SLI" and those with nondiscrepant language difficulties also failed to identify qualitative differences in the severity of language issues, academic performance, or the percentage of children with social, emotional, or behavioral difficulties (Norbury *et al.*, 2016). However, a more severe presentation was evident in children with a co-occurring biomedical condition.

Subtypes of language disorder

Historically, a child may have been described as having an "expressive language disorder" or a "receptive–expressive language disorder." However, recent analyses have tested the underlying dimensionality of language and shown that assessments in either modality tend to go together (Bornstein *et al.*, 2018). Statistical tests of language dimensions (vocabulary, syntax, discourse) have shown interesting developmental trends; early on, all three tend to form one single underlying construct of language (e.g., Bornstein *et al.* 2018). However, as children get older, vocabulary, syntax, and discourse skills become more distinct although they remain highly correlated with one another (Language and Reading Research Consortium [LARRC], 2017). The CATALISE consortium (Bishop *et al.*, 2017) therefore decided against identifying "subtypes" of language disorder and advocate using DLD as the diagnostic label, with qualifiers to highlight specific areas of strength and challenge at a given assessment point.

Impact of disorder on functioning and quality of life

Tomblin (2006) argued that functional impact should consider society's values and expectations. Under this perspective, a language "difference" becomes a disorder when the child's level of language results in unacceptable risk for undesirable outcomes, now or in the future.

Impact on quality of life

Many young people with DLD report challenges with social relationships, emotions, classroom participation, school achievement, independence, and a lack of appropriate support, all of which negatively impact quality of life (Figure 51.3). As many as 60% of children with low language scores at age 4 show a pattern of declining quality of life to age 13 (Le *et al.*, 2020). This declining profile likely reflects pronounced difficulties at school, in accessing language for learning and in forming and maintaining supportive social relationships. Hobson and Lee (2022) describe a range of "camouflaging" behaviors that children engage in to mask their difficulties at school, for example, trying to copy others, smiling and nodding when not understanding, avoiding situations that involve speaking and listening, and disruptive behavior. Parents report that the effort involved in masking and the impact of these masking behaviors on the perceptions of other people (i.e., that the child is difficult or noncompliant) left their children with DLD exhausted, with negative impacts on self-esteem and well-being.

Impact on mental health

Language can impact mental health through its role in social-emotional development. Language provides a framework for organizing variable input from the environment into nuanced concepts that become increasing granular over time, allowing more precision in identification and understanding of our own and other's emotional states (Nook, 2021). Griffiths *et al.* (2020)

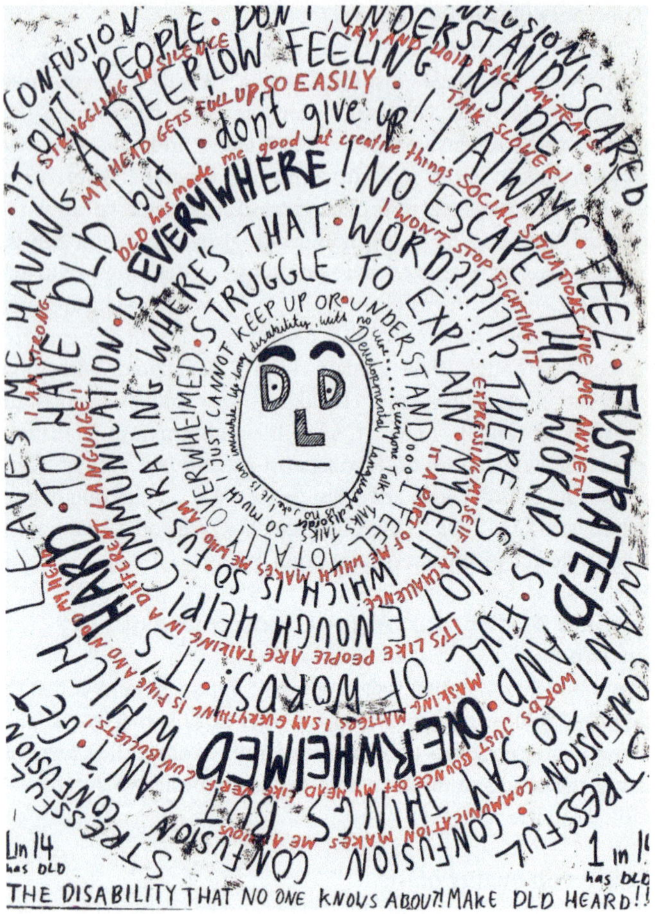
1 in 14
has DLD
1 in 14
has DLD
THE DISABILITY THAT NO ONE KNOWS ABOUT!! MAKE DLD HEARD!!

Figure 51.3 My experience of developmental language disorder (DLD). *Source:* With permission of Siouxsie Webster.

reported that language skills at 5 years predicted emotion recognition from faces and voices at age 10–11, while nonverbal cognitive skills did not. Increased rates of alexithymia (difficulty labeling one's internal states) are associated with DLD (Hobson *et al.*, 2019).

Language is also important for emotion regulation via the use of verbal strategies, or "self-talk." For example, considering how a negative event that happens today will be experienced in the future attenuates the emotional response; young people with language disorders have reported that this kind of future/hypothetical thinking is challenging, making it difficult to use these verbal strategies to regulate emotion (Griffiths *et al.*, 2021). Furthermore, early language appears to predict later task success, even when current language skills are accounted for (Griffiths *et al.* 2021), suggesting a role for language in learning how to use self-talk for emotion regulation.

Impact on academic success

Education outcomes are variable, though as a group, young people with DLD have lower levels of academic attainment and pass fewer statutory examinations (Conti-Ramsden & Durkin, 2012). They are also more likely to leave school early, with a smaller proportion of young people with DLD completing high school or university (Dubois *et al.*, 2020).

Summary and conclusions

The field has achieved consensus on terminology and diagnostic criteria for DLD. Given the important role that language plays in societal participation, DLD, and language disorder associated with other developmental conditions can have profound and far-reaching impacts on young people's quality of life, including education opportunities and mental health.

Epidemiology of developmental language disorders

Incidence and prevalence, economic burden

We currently do not have robust data on the incidence of DLD. Prevalence estimates vary depending on child age and diagnostic algorithms employed. The first prevalence study to employ CATALISE criteria identified 7.58% of children as having DLD in the first year of school (5–6 years) (Norbury *et al.*, 2016); 4.8% met traditional criteria for "SLI" in that they had nonverbal IQ scores of 85 or greater, and 2.78% had nonverbal IQ scores between 70–85. A further 2.34% of children met criteria for Language Disorder associated with another biomedical condition, such as autism or ID. As a group, these children had more severe language, cognitive, academic, and behavioral challenges (Norbury *et al.*, 2016).

DLD places an increasing burden on health, education, and welfare systems as children move through school and require more intensive special education provision and clinical services (Cronin *et al.*, 2017). DLD also impacts future earning potential, as a result of low levels of literacy and numeracy that affect employment. In addition, carers of children with DLD work fewer paid hours, and mothers of children with severe DLD are less likely to be employed (Cronin *et al.*, 2017).

Global and time variations

Comparison of prevalence estimates is complicated by varying diagnostic criteria. Beitchman *et al.* (1986) identified language impairment in children scoring −1SD below the mean on an omnibus test of oral language with nonverbal IQ scores in the expected range for age. This algorithm yielded a prevalence estimate of 12.6% of 5-year-old children in Ottawa. A decade later, Tomblin *et al.* (2020) identified children scoring −1.25SD on 2 out of 5 language composite scores with nonverbal IQ standard scores above 87 as having SLI, yielding a prevalence estimate in the United States (US) of 7.4%. Norbury *et al.* (2016) used a similar assessment procedure and reported a near identical prevalence estimate of 7.58% of children in the United Kingdom (UK) aged 5–6 years. However, this cohort had more severe language deficits (−1.5SD on 2 out of 5 composite scores), and lower nonverbal IQ scores (standard scores of 70 or above). Norbury directly compared different diagnostic algorithms and found that CATALISE criteria were more closely aligned with functional impact (measured by academic attainment), and were highly predictive of language status 2 years later (*Norbury et al.*, 2017).

More recent epidemiological studies in Australia and China, yielded similar prevalence estimates (e.g., Australia, 6.4%: Calder *et al.*, [2022]; Shanghai, 8.6%: Wu *et al.*, [2023]), while retrospective reporting of DLD by adults in a large Danish population sample yielded lower prevalence estimates of 3.36–3.70% (Nudel *et al.*, 2023). Here, DLD was associated with higher rates of literacy and learning disorder, and poorer physical and mental health.

It is worth noting that the language a child is exposed to will have implications for how language disorder manifests (Leonard & Schroeder, 2023). For example, in languages in which grammatical morphemes are syllabic and stressed (and therefore more salient, like Italian), grammatical errors are rare. Some languages, like Cantonese, have flexible grammatical structures in which producing all elements of a sentence is optional. Therefore, omitting words or morphemes is not regarded as a problem, and may mask underlying disorder. More universal signs of language disorder include delays in the acquisition of first words and phrases, difficulties with comprehension and verbal memory, and slow and effortful language production.

Public health implications

Traditionally, speech-language therapists (SLTs) have focused on diagnosing and remediating language disorder via an individualized therapeutic service. Increasingly, however, language disorder is viewed as a public health issue, given the socioeconomic circumstances that are associated with poor language and the need to address these social, as opposed to individual, challenges (Law *et al.*, 2013). In addition, many children with clinically significant language deficits go unrecognized and undiagnosed, and therefore do not access available interventions (McGregor, 2020). Universal provision of language enrichment activities, perhaps targeted in areas of socioeconomic disadvantage, could aid prevention of negative impact by removing barriers to language support (cf. Law *et al.*, 2013). This has been realized in some countries as a move away from individualized speech-language therapy to a more "consultative" service, in which clinicians advise nursery or school staff on language stimulation techniques (Ebbels *et al.*, 2019).

However, we currently lack robust evidence that such approaches reduce the prevalence or impact of language disorder (Ebbels *et al.*, 2019), with potential opportunity costs in reduced individualized services and threats to professional competencies. While a public health strategy for language development is much needed, Norbury *et al.* (2019) questioned whether this should be the purview of individual SLT teams. Drawing parallels with other public health issues such as obesity, Norbury *et al.* (2019) noted that specialist clinical services are still required for young people with the most significant needs and challenges and that this should sit alongside public health approaches. In other countries, "response to intervention" methods have been implemented in which specialist clinical services are only offered to those who do not make expected progress from universal or targeted interventions. However, in one evaluation the prevalence rates of language disorder increased, rather than decreased, within the community (Hall-Mills, 2019). There is an urgent need for more robust clinical trials to determine optimal methods of service delivery that improve outcomes for young children with language disorder.

Screening

To improve early identification and timely treatment, many have called for universal screening (Adlof & Hogan, 2019). However, for under-5s, universal screening is not recommended given the low levels of screen accuracy, high rates of spontaneous recovery, and lack of evidence indicating positive benefits of screening on later language outcomes (see Bishop *et al.* [2017] for discussion). For school-aged children, language skills tend to become more stable, and screening followed by intervention can yield at least short-term positive benefits for children with low language proficiency (West *et al.*, 2021). It is unclear whether screening reduces prevalence or incidence of DLD; the possibility remains that it may be better to focus intervention efforts on those for whom there are language concerns.

Summary and conclusions

Prevalence estimates across the globe have settled around 6–8% of school-aged children, making DLD a very common, but often unrecognized condition. DLD is a global public health issue and policymakers will need to plan for long-term health, education, and social support, combining universal efforts to improve oral language skills in the population with access to specialist services for those with the most severe language needs.

Assessment of language disorders

Core aspects to consider at assessment

The evaluation of children suspected of language disorder is generally undertaken by SLTs, specialists trained in the anatomy, psychology, linguistics, education, and remediation of language disorder. Given the prevalence of language disorder in other neurodevelopmental conditions (see Chapter 3), SLTs would ideally be core members of any multidisciplinary team involved in diagnosis and management.

Delays in acquiring first words and phrases are often the earliest signs that prompt parents to seek help and advice concerning their child's development (Rannard *et al.*, 2005). For young children, general practitioners (GPs) and health visitors are the professionals most likely to make referrals to specialist SLT services; however, parents report that often professionals underestimate language concerns and assume that most children will spontaneously improve, leading to inappropriate advice and delays in seeking SLT support

(Rannard *et al.*, 2005). For school-aged children, teachers are the primary agents of referral, though here again there is considerable underidentification, often because language difficulties are overshadowed by other issues such as behavior regulation, challenges with learning and literacy, or social-emotional difficulties (McGregor, 2020).

Assessment and diagnosis as hypothesis testing

Although diagnosis will be carried out predominantly by SLTs, Box 51.3 gives an overview of issues GPs, psychologists, and psychiatrists may like to probe. In the first instance, asking parents about their concerns and any contact with SLT services can be a useful way to discover if DLD is suspected, and what strategies families use that could facilitate communication during the assessment. A case history of early developmental milestones will indicate whether there is broader involvement of cognitive, sensory, or motor systems, and will highlight the child's motivation to communicate and interact with others. The clinician will also want to know what language(s) the child is exposed to at home, and should ask about family history of language, literacy, or learning difficulties.

Language difference versus disorder

English as an additional language

In multicultural societies it can be difficult to determine whether a child has a language disorder, or simply a language difference that arises from limited exposure to the societal language. Ideally, we would assess language competencies in all the languages a child speaks, but we often lack valid and reliable tools or the people to perform such assessments. This is exacerbated by a lack assessment instruments that have been normed on bilingual children, though recent initiatives through the European Union are addressing this clinical gap (https://www.bi-sli.org/litmus-tools).

Diagnosis therefore requires integration of information from various sources, including family and teacher report, a sample of

Box 51.3 Assessment at a glance

Formal diagnostic assessment should be carried out by a speech-language therapist (SLT). The following are strategies and measures that psychologists, psychiatrists, and general practitioners (GPs) could use to facilitate assessment and inform referral decisions. If parents raise concerns about language or DLD, ask about strategies used to facilitate communication.

- **General strategies for interviewing individuals with language disorder**
  - sit next to, rather than opposite the child
  - slow your rate of speech
  - simplify language, for instance, give one instruction at a time (e.g., "put your bag down. Good, now choose a book" instead of "put your book down and then grab a book to read")
  - use gestures (point to the chair when saying "sit next to me")
  - use visuals (symbols or pictures, write down key points)
  - give the child extra time to formulate a response
  - give choices where possible (instead of "what would you do in this situation?" ask "would you do X or Y?")
- **Case history (red flags or "risk factors")**
  - parent concern (language, behavior, social responsiveness)
  - premature birth
  - family history of language, literacy, or learning difficulties
  - delays in acquiring first words and word combinations
  - delays in gross motor or general cognitive skills
  - language regression (child stops using words previously acquired)
- **Observations**
  - child takes longer to respond to verbal instructions
  - child only follows part of an instruction (seemingly forgetting the rest) versus child follows simple/complex instructions
  - child uses shorter sentences and says less overall
  - child relies more on nonverbal strategies to communicate (e.g., facial expression, gestures)
  - child interest in exploring the environment
  - child initiates interaction with caregivers (pointing, showing objects of interest)
  - child responds to name
  - child engages in conversation, can give a reasonable account of a recent vacation, holiday, or school experience (appropriate for age)
  - how child attempts to repair communication if not understood
- **Rating scales/screening**
  - Children's Communication Checklist-2 *(CCC-2)* (Bishop, 2003). Parent report measure of language used in everyday situations. Suitable for young people aged 4–16, includes subscales tapping structural and pragmatic aspects of language, and interests and social behaviors indicative of autism.
- **Measures of functional impact**
  - academic attainment, including literacy
  - social, emotional, or behavioral challenges (e.g., Strengths and Difficulties Questionnaire, Goodman, 1997)
  - quality of life, preferably with focus on language, communication, and participation (e.g., Eadie *et al.*, 2018)
- **Standardized tests of receptive/expressive language**
  - will be completed by SLTs and should include areas of language and communication summarized in section on "Diagnostic criteria"

expressive language, and observation of classroom learning (Castilla-Earls *et al.*, 2020). Formal assessment is also recommended, using culturally fair, process-oriented tasks such as nonsense word repetition (which taps the phonological memory and encoding skills thought to underlie word learning), dynamic assessment and/or fast mapping (in which children are taught and asked to retain new word labels or word meanings), or rapid automatic naming (such as saying all the days of the week in rapid sequence).

Persistent low levels of English language proficiency over time, despite regular exposure to English in school, may be more indicative of an underlying language disorder than low scores at any one point in time (Whiteside & Norbury, 2017). Notably, exposure to more than one language does not cause or exacerbate language disorder, and parents should be encouraged to continue talking to their child in whatever language they themselves are most comfortable and fluent in speaking.

Neurodiversity

Children with DLD may also be considered neurodivergent (see Chapter 3). According to this view, individual differences in a range of human traits, including language, are a natural and valuable aspect of human experience, not necessarily pathological. Some argue that we should avoid using terms such as "disorder" because "there is no objective reason why a condition should be defined by its disadvantageous elements instead of its advantageous elements" (Astle & Fletcher-Watson, 2020, p. 435).

Others consider that the term "disorder" could be appropriate when individual differences confer disadvantage for the individual within society (Tomblin, 2006). As noted, there is substantial evidence that limited language skills prevent individuals from full participation in society, compromise well-being, and limit self-advocacy (Snow, 2021). Thus, both strengths and challenges associated with language disorder should be acknowledged and addressed to maximize future opportunities.

Common approaches to assessment

Case history

Possible "red flags" for language disorder include parent concern, a positive family history of language, literacy, or learning difficulties, poor understanding of what others say, and functional impact at home or at school. Additional red flags that warrant onward referral include prematurity, language regression, broader health, or developmental concerns (motor, cognition, sensory), lack of social engagement, socioeconomic disadvantage, and/or adverse childhood experiences.

Clinical observations

Informal observation during the assessment session can be an invaluable way to establish how the child currently communicates and use of compensatory strategies. The clinician will be noting whether the child produces single words or phrases or sentences, the accuracy of speech sounds or other vocalizations, how they respond to their name or follow simple verbal instructions, and how they use gestures or pointing, or show, point, or talk about new things in the environment with caregivers. Informal conversation samples, in which the child and clinician engage in talk around objects or topics of interest to the child, can provide more detail about the level and quality of the child's expressive language, including speech sound production, utterance length and complexity, fluency, and vocal quality.

In general, children with DLD say less, use simple grammar, may take longer to respond to what has been said or to express themselves, may seem to forget what has been said or only follow part of an instruction, may need more repetition, may use more general vocabulary ("doing the scissors" instead of "cutting"), and may leave out key pieces of information in recounting an event. They may also rely more on nonverbal strategies to communicate, including the use of gestures or pictures/symbols.

Standardized assessment of comprehension and expression

While an estimate of expressive language is possible from informal assessment, it can be more challenging to accurately gauge a child's level of understanding. Standardized assessments carried out by SLTs can provide important information about the child's comprehension and expressive language skills in each of the language domains outlined in the section "Diagnostic criteria," relative to peers of the same age and from the same language community.

There remains limited consensus as to precise cutoffs that are associated with language disorder (Bishop *et al.*, 2016). The most commonly used cutoff for research diagnosis is −1.25 SD below the normative mean, while a cutoff of −1.5 SD on a composite language score was most closely aligned with functional impact on early academic attainment (Norbury *et al.*, 2016).

Rating scales

Standardized tests provide an estimate of language abilities in optimal speaking and listening conditions. However, we are often more interested in how children use language in everyday contexts, and rely on parent and teacher rating scales to inform us. The CCC-2 (Bishop, 2003) provides an overview of structural (speech, syntax, vocabulary) and pragmatic (coherence, initiation, nonverbal communication, use of context) language skills, with two additional subscales tapping potential autism characteristics related to social relationships and specific interests. Low scores on the pragmatic subscales of the CCC-2 are associated with both academic underachievement and increased rates of social, emotional, and behavioral concerns in a population sample; however, these pragmatic deficits usually co-occur with limitations in structural language competence and/or an increase in autism behaviors (Saul *et al.*, 2023). The CCC-2 can usefully signpost the clinician to potential areas of concern that require further evaluation.

Co-occurring conditions of relevance

Social, emotional, and behavioral problems, and mental health

Between 50–80% of adolescents identified as having social-emotional concerns (Hollo *et al.*, 2014), or referred to tertiary mental health services, are found to have language deficits on assessment, many of which have been previously undiagnosed (Cohen *et al.*, 2013). Similarly, young children with language disorder are at 1.5–2 times the risk of anxiety/depression and behavioral/attention disorders by adolescence relative to peers (Yew & O'Kearney, 2013; Donolato *et al.*, 2023). Mental health symptoms in language disorder are more common in those with a family history of poor mental health (Conti-Ramsden & Botting, 2008), and reflect, at least in part, shared genetic risk factors (Newbury *et al.*, 2019).

Despite increased risk, there is a paucity of research investigating the mechanisms that underpin the relationship between language and mental health. Challenges with language and communication may predispose children to a range of environmental experiences that also increase risk for adverse mental health. For example, young people with language disorders are more likely than peers to be involved in youth offending (Snow, 2019), to be bullied and/or victimized by peers (Van Den Bedem *et al.*, 2018), and, in extreme cases, to experience maltreatment and sexual abuse (Brownlie *et al.*, 2017). Language disorder may have more direct effects on mental health via its role in emotion recognition (Griffiths *et al.*, 2020), alexithymia (Hobson *et al.*, 2019), emotion regulation (Griffiths *et al.*, 2021), and access to mental health interventions (Hobson *et al.*, 2022).

Specific learning disorders

Educational outcomes for young people with language disorder are heterogeneous, though there is little doubt that as a group they underachieve academically in all areas of the curriculum (Conti-Ramsden *et al.*, 2018). Interventions that target oral language can have positive impacts on reading and reading comprehension (see Chapter 52), especially when delivered in combination with systematic phonics instruction to support word decoding. Language is a medium through which we communicate, represent, and retrieve mathematics knowledge, as well as facilitating working memory and reasoning during mathematics performance and learning (see Chapter 52).

Social (pragmatic) communication disorder

The introduction of social (pragmatic) communication disorder (SPCD) to DSM-5-TR (American Psychiatric Association, 2022) provided an opportunity to formalize identification and support needs for individuals who struggle to use language in socially appropriate ways, but do not meet conventional criteria for autism. Nevertheless, DSM-5-TR inclusion and exclusion criteria generated considerable clinical and theoretical debate about the validity of this diagnosis, in particular, the presence of social (pragmatic) communication deficits in the absence of structural (vocabulary, grammar, phonology) language difficulties. ICD-11 did not include SPCD as a distinct diagnostic entity; instead, pragmatic challenges are specified under a diagnosis of DLD, "with impairment of mainly pragmatic language" (code 6A01.22). Like DSM-5-TR, however, use of this qualifier stipulates that pragmatic language impairments are not better explained by autism, or deficits in receptive and expressive language.

In reality, structural and pragmatic language skills are intimately related and can be difficult to tease apart. In a population sample, selective social (pragmatic) difficulties were extremely rare, affecting <1% of the population (Saul *et al.*, 2023). More typically, social-pragmatic difficulties were accompanied by low language scores and/or autistic traits and were associated with academic underachievement and elevated symptoms of behavioral difficulty. Therefore, any child presenting with social (pragmatic) deficits should have a thorough language assessment.

Hearing loss and auditory processing

Hearing assessment by an audiologist should be part of every evaluation, in order to rule out hearing loss as a potential cause of language difficulties. In high-income countries, universal neonatal hearing screening coupled with early intervention has improved language outcomes for infants with permanent childhood hearing loss (Pimperton & Kennedy, 2012). Conductive hearing losses associated with bouts of otitis media with effusion are extremely common, though the causal relationship with poor language is unclear. Prospective, epidemiological studies have indicated that in otherwise healthy children, episodes of otitis media with hearing loss have little to no impact on language development (Feldman *et al.*, 2003).

Diagnosis of central auditory processing disorder (APD), in which problems with listening, comprehension, and attention occur despite normal peripheral hearing, remains controversial. One reason is that APD is typically assessed and diagnosed using verbal materials (e.g., comprehending speech in noise), leading many to argue that, "most if not all cases of childhood 'APD' are better characterized by more commonly recognized learning disorders, especially language disorder (Moore, 2018, p. 617)" and that "such a diagnosis could even be harmful if it prevents children receiving evidence-based and soundly reasoned diagnosis and treatment (Moore, 2018, p. 618)."

Assessment summary and conclusions

DLD is frequently underidentified by parents and teachers and virtually unheard of in mental health settings, in part because it may be overshadowed by concerns about behavior, reading, or academic learning. Assessment on more than one occasion is warranted, especially in multilingual populations, as progress may be more informative for diagnosis than a snapshot of language skills at any one point in time. Tools such as the CCC-2, that incorporate information about pragmatics as well as structural aspects of language, can signpost further assessment needs.

Longitudinal outcome

Language stability and change

Longitudinal analyses have demonstrated impressive stability of language, with similar rates of progress across the spectrum of ability throughout the school years (Norbury *et al.*, 2017). Thus, children identified as having language disorder at school entry continue to be about 2–3 years behind their peers in language scores throughout their education. Language stability has been reported for children with a range of developmental concerns and biological and social risks (Bornstein *et al.*, 2018).

Adult outcomes

There are relatively few studies of adult outcomes for individuals with DLD, and those that exist highlight heterogeneous outcomes in every area of functioning (Dubois *et al.*, 2020).

Employment

In general, young people with DLD experience higher rates of unemployment and part-time working relative to peers. At the age of 19, young people with DLD were twice as likely as peers to be not in education, employment, or training (NEET; Conti-Ramsden & Durkin, 2012)). When employment is found, the majority (90%) of individuals with DLD have jobs in nonmanagerial occupational categories and are more likely to be working in service, catering, trade, construction, and mechanical services (Conti-Ramsden *et al.*, 2018). By the time they are in their 30s more than 25% of those in work are on low incomes (Dubois *et al.*, 2020). Adult men with a history of severe language disorder experience more prolonged periods of unemployment and higher rates of dismissal relative to siblings and peers (Clegg *et al.*, 2005).

Challenges with language and literacy make finding and keeping a job difficult; young people report that the interview process is a major barrier to employment as they require extra time to process questions, formulate responses, and have difficulty understanding questions or thinking of relevant examples (Mathrick *et al.*, 2017). Despite recognizing these challenges, very few (15%) ask for reasonable adjustments to support them through the interview process (Conti-Ramsden *et al.*, 2018). Following instructions, working independently and to deadlines, problem-solving, and engaging in social chat with coworkers create additional barriers to employment success.

Independence and community engagement

Individuals with DLD are just as likely as peers to participate in social groups and activities, but often require more support from family and close friends to access these activities (Dubois *et al.*, 2020). For example, adults with DLD may have poor financial literacy skills and considerable issues managing finances, relying on parents for financial support for longer periods of time. In addition, fewer young people with DLD have driving licenses, limiting opportunities to attend social or work activities. Participants from population cohorts do not report increased risk of negative integration within the community, for example, lawbreaking. Nevertheless, a high percentage of young people involved in youth justice services have clinically significant language disorders (Snow, 2019).

Social relationships

Many adults with DLD do enjoy meaningful social relationships, and rates of marriage do not differ for adults with DLD relative to peers (Dubois *et al.*, 2020). However, some adults report difficulties with friendships, associated with lower levels of social confidence and self-esteem. In the few studies that have measured this, parenthood has come earlier for individuals with DLD, including higher rates of teenaged pregnancy. Individuals with severe childhood DLD report fewer friendships as adults, and are less likely to be involved in romantic relationships or living with a romantic partner relative to siblings (Clegg *et al.*, 2005).

Summary and conclusions

Many adults with DLD continue to rely on family members to help them navigate adult society. There are few services for adults with DLD but it is increasingly evident that such services are needed to mitigate the long-term negative impacts of poor language on adult outcomes.

Biological and environmental bases of developmental language disorder

Genetic influences on language and developmental language disorder

Clinicians and researchers have known for some time that DLD tends to run in families, and twin studies have established that DLD is highly heritable (Verhoef *et al.*, 2021). Heritability estimates increase with age, perhaps reflecting gene x environment correlations, in which children select and modify their experiences in accordance with their genotype. For example, children with language disorders may select more solitary activities that not only make fewer demands on verbal skills, but also offer fewer opportunities to learn or use language in social contexts. Few consistent associations have emerged from language-related genome-wide association studies, and the consensus is that common language disorders are usually influenced by multiple common and rare genetic variants, each one of small effect (Mountford *et al.*, 2022).

Neuroimaging studies of developmental language disorder

Unlike cases of adult stroke, there are no gross lesions of neurological structures in the left hemisphere for children with DLD. A long-standing hypothesis is that DLD might reflect a failure to establish normal lateralization of language in the left hemisphere. However, a large study using functional transcranial Doppler (fTCD) sonography, found that rates of atypical lateralization in the DLD group were similar to rates in the typically developing group (Wilson & Bishop, 2018). Investigators have recently proposed that subcortical structures, such as the striatum and the hippocampus, and/or aberrant development of the white matter that connects different brain regions, might disrupt learning networks and give rise to language disorder (Krishnan *et al.*, 2016).

Environmental influences on developmental language disorder

The association between socioeconomic disadvantage and lower levels of language proficiency is well known and likely reflects differences in parent education and language input, differences in child physical/neural development, reduced resources available for child learning activities or family support, and increased family stress and discord (Pace *et al.*, 2017). However, children are active learners who influence opportunities for caregiver interaction. For example, a child who is exploring her environment and pointing at unfamiliar objects is likely to elicit more words from adults than a child who is sitting quietly and playing repetitively with the same object. The environment can also have substantial influences on biological mechanisms; for example, Romeo *et al.* (2021) demonstrated that a family-focused intervention increased adult–child conversational turns, and that changes in turn-taking were associated with cortical thickening in language relevant brain regions.

Summary and conclusions

Language disorders have a biological basis, though precise neurobiological pathways have yet to be fully specified and we are a long way from genetic or neuroimaging assessments that are predictive at the individual level. Limited maternal/paternal education, lower incomes, and reduced language input are associated with DLD, but may reflect parental challenges with language and literacy. Therefore, language disorder in the context of socioeconomic disadvantage should alert clinicians and educators to the need for careful monitoring and support for parents.

Intervention approaches

General approaches to language intervention

Intervention goals may vary according to the age and needs of the child, but normalization of language is rarely a realistic therapy goal. Instead, clinicians and educators may focus on teaching language forms, providing the children with strategies to minimize the impact of language differences on communication and participation, and working with significant others to facilitate communication.

Interventions structure language input so that it is easier for the child with language disorder to learn. "Implicit" approaches target language structures in naturalistic situations and emphasize joint attention (so that adult language input is aligned with the child's focus of attention) and multiple repetitions of language targets (so the child has multiple exposures to the language and the referent) (Baron & Arbel, 2022). Implicit approaches are favored for preschool children and are usually delivered by parents. For older children, "explicit" approaches are more common, in which language goals are known to the child, definitions or grammatical rules are made explicit and usually accompanied by visual cues, and there is a specific requirement for children to practice producing or making judgments about language target (Baron & Arbel, 2022). While the evidence base for language interventions is growing (Box 51.4), there are very few high-quality, adequately powered trials with long-term follow-up to determine which approaches to language intervention are most efficacious (Donolato *et al.*, 2023).

Tiered approaches to language intervention

In many high-income countries, language interventions are increasingly delivered using a multitiered system of support, which includes *universal*, *targeted*, and *specialist* interventions (Ebbels *et al.*, 2019). *Universal* approaches are designed to benefit all children and are aligned with a public health perspective on language promotion. Continuing professional development (Markussen-Brown *et al.*, 2017), whole-class instruction, and manualized curricula (Dobinson & Dockrell, 2021) are thought to enhance the quality of language instruction and thus benefit those with language disorder. The evidence suggests that one-to-one coaching and/or joint session planning is more effective than short-term professional training sessions alone (Markussen-Brown *et al.*, 2017). Whole-class initiatives have negligible effects that generally fade out over time, with limited evidence that they reduce the need for later language support (cf. Bailey *et al.*, 2020).

Targeted interventions are short-term, manualized intervention programs delivered by school staff to small groups of children with the ultimate goal of normalizing language trajectories and reducing the need for future intervention. Their appeal is that they are more scalable and therefore able to reach more children. In general, these programs show small-to-medium effects relative to business as usual, and these benefits are retained 6–12 months post-treatment, though very few studies monitor longer-term maintenance of treatment effects (Rogde *et al.*, 2019).

Specialist interventions are more typically delivered by SLTs, usually one-to-one or in small groups, and are individualized to a particular child's language and learning needs. At this level, the intervention seeks to improve particular aspects of language that are functionally important to the child. A systematic review and meta-analysis by Donolato *et al.* (2023) considered specialist language interventions across a range of neurodevelopment

Box 51.4 Treatment and management at a glance

- Parent-mediated (Heidlage *et al.*, 2020): focus on enhancing parent–child interaction by coaching parents to:
  - establish joint attention and provide commentary on child's interests
  - recognize child communicative cues (e.g., vocalizations, eye gaze, pointing, child initiation)
  - respond contingently to child communicative cues and simplify adult language to align with child's language level
  - use gestures, objects, and other nonverbal means alongside spoken language
- Shared book reading (Dowdall *et al.*, 2020): introduce language through book reading, exposing the child to more complex talk about events removed from the here and now:
  - pointing and labeling in response to the child's focus of interest
  - open-ended questions to engage the child
  - "decontextualized talk" going beyond the storybook to concepts that are novel and unfamiliar to the child
- Universal (Tier 1) interventions (Markussen-Brown *et al.*, 2017; Dobinson & Dockrell, 2021): focused training for educators to provide high-quality communication environments:
  - minimize background noise
  - create language learning opportunities through book reading and conversation
  - get down to child's physical level and adapt to child's language level
  - appropriate pacing of talk
  - mix of questions (open-ended) and comments
  - use of gesture/objects/pictures/symbols to support spoken language
- Targeted (Tier 2) oral language interventions (Rogde *et al.*, 2019): typically, interventions delivered to small groups of children with low language proficiency that provide explicit instruction in:
  - listening and listening comprehension
  - vocabulary and figurative expressions
  - grammar and morphology
  - storytelling
  - phonological awareness
- Specialist (Tier 3) interventions (Donolato *et al.*, 2023): individualized interventions delivered under guidance of specialist clinician (usually a speech-language therapist):
  - focuses on specific language targets (e.g., past tense, -ed; idioms)—these should be agreed with families and young people and should be functionally relevant
  - makes use of visuals to support spoken language (Balthazar *et al.*, 2020)
  - may involve augmentative or alternative forms of communication (Barton-Hulsey *et al.*, 2021) (e.g., picture exchange communication systems)
- Adaptations and adjustments advocated by young people with lived experience of developmental language disorder (DLD):
  - support me to ask questions in class
  - do not put me on the spot by asking a question in front of everyone
  - give me extra time to respond to what you say
  - slow down your talking
  - use visuals, colors, simple bullet points, signs, and gestures
  - teach new words before the lesson
  - repeat new information over and over again
  - write things down or take a picture so I can remember what's been said

conditions. Overall, these interventions have modest treatment effects, at least in the short term. However, most studies were underpowered and there was clear evidence of publication bias. When these issues were statistically controlled, the effect of intervention was significantly attenuated.

Challenges of accessing mental health interventions for children with language disorders

Mental health interventions, such as cognitive behavioral therapy (CBT), are verbally mediated and include discussion of thoughts and feelings, use of verbal strategies, and planning for future scenarios, all of which present major obstacles to participation for young people with language disorder. To date, there are no known studies investigating the efficacy or effectiveness of school-based (Clarke *et al.*, 2021) or clinical (James *et al.*, 2020) mental health interventions on young people with language disorder. Families, SLTs, and mental health practitioners all report that "talking therapies" are inaccessible and ineffective for young people with language disorder (Hancock *et al.*, 2022; Hobson *et al.*, 2022). Blended therapy approaches (combining psychological and language therapies) are advocated by clinicians but, as yet, are untested in clinical trials (Hancock *et al.*, 2022). Evidence-based adaptations to CBT for young people with autism (Ung *et al.*, 2015) may provide insights to improving intervention for young people with DLD.

Mediators and moderators of treatment effects

Dosage is inevitably tied to time-, resource-, and cost-efficiency constraints, yet few studies have experimentally manipulated dosage to determine optimal treatment parameters (Frizelle *et al.*, 2021). Preliminary evidence suggests that when session dosage is high (i.e., number of learning opportunities per session), frequency of intervention sessions may be reduced (Frizelle *et al.*, 2021). Session duration and the overall length of the intervention (number of weeks) are positively associated with treatment effect sizes (Donolato *et al.*, 2023).

Implementation is also of interest as language interventions are frequently delivered by family members, teachers, or trained teaching/therapy assistants rather than qualified SLTs. Implementation quality is consistently found to be an important moderator of treatment effects (Rogde *et al.*, 2019); treatment effects are negligible in studies with poor implementation, but educationally important (g = 0.24) in studies reporting high-quality implementation. This is echoed in the moderating effects of who delivers the intervention; the treatment effect doubled when intervention was delivered by nonschool staff (Rogde *et al.*, 2019). This likely reflects the number of intervention sessions school staff are able to provide; they provide, on average, half of the expected sessions, with diminishing effects on child language outcomes.

Where it has been reported, child factors such as age, sex, and nonverbal IQ do not moderate treatment effects (Rogde *et al.*, 2019; Donolato *et al.*, 2023). Initial language severity has more mixed outcomes, though children with more severe language disorders tend to experience larger treatment effects than those with mild difficulties (Donolato, *et al.*, 2023). These results are encouraging in demonstrating that interventions can have modest, positive impacts on children with varying degrees of language and developmental challenge.

Summary and conclusions

The evidence base for language interventions is growing, but there is an urgent need for more robust, adequately powered randomized controlled trials (RCTs) to evaluate intervention at different levels of support. These should include long-term follow-up and systematic evaluation of the impact of language interventions on other outcomes, such as mental health. Age, nonverbal ability, and socioeconomic factors do not appear to moderate treatment outcomes, but dosage and implementation quality do. Current mental health interventions are unlikely to be suitable for young people with DLD.

Conclusions

DLD is highly prevalent, persistent, and very common in referrals to tertiary child and adolescent mental health services. Furthermore, language skills are highly predictive of academic and employment outcomes, vital to societal participation, and critical to the cognitive, social, and emotional development of children, whatever their primary diagnosis. Given the overlaps with mental health, future work should explicitly test language intervention as a potential protective factor for mental health, and, more urgently, seek to test adaptations to currently recommended mental health interventions to ensure that young people with language disorders are able to access these treatments. Clinicians should be alert to signs of language disorder, and work together with families, and health and education partners to facilitate the most appropriate education and treatment pathways.

References

Adlof, S.M. & Hogan, T.P. (2018) Understanding dyslexia in the context of developmental language disorders. *Language, Speech, and Hearing Services in Schools* **49**, 762–773. doi:10.1044/2018_LSHSS-DYSLC-18-0049.

Adlof, S.M. & Hogan, T.P. (2019) If we Don't look, we Won't see: Measuring language development to inform literacy instruction. *Policy Insights from the Behavioral and Brain Sciences* **6**, 210–217. doi:10.1177/2372732219839075.

American Psychiatric Association (2022) 5th edn. *text revision*, American Psychiatric Association, Washington, DC. doi:10.1176/appi.books.9780890425787.

Astle, D.E. & Fletcher-Watson, S. (2020) Beyond the core-deficit hypothesis in developmental disorders. *Current Directions in Psychological Science* **29**, 431–437. doi:10.1177/0963721420925518.

Bailey, D.H. *et al.* (2020) Persistence and fade-out of educational-intervention effects: mechanisms and potential solutions. *Psychological Science in the Public Interest* **21**, 55–97. doi:10.1177/1529100620915848.

Balthazar, C.H. *et al.* (2020) Explicit grammatical intervention for developmental language disorder: three approaches. *Language, Speech, and Hearing Services in Schools* **51**, 226–246. doi:10.1044/2019_LSHSS-19-00046.

Baron, L.S. & Arbel, Y. (2022) An implicit–explicit framework for intervention methods in developmental language disorder. *American Journal of Speech-Language Pathology* **31**, 1–17. doi:10.1044/2022_AJSLP-21-00172.

Barton-Hulsey, A. *et al.* (2021) Augmentative and alternative communication supports for language and literacy in preschool: considerations for down syndrome and autism Spectrum disorder. *Seminars in Speech and Language* **42**, 345–362. doi:10.1055/s-0041-1730996.

Beitchman, J.H. *et al.* (1986) Prevalence of speech and language disorders in 5-year-old kindergarten children in the Ottawa-Carleton region. *Journal of Speech and Hearing Disorders* **51**, 98.

Bishop, D.V.M. (2003) *The Children's Communication Checklist*, 2nd edn. The Psychological Corporation, London.

Bishop, D.V.M. (2010) Which neurodevelopmental disorders get researched and why? *PLoS One* **5**, e15112. doi:10.1371/journal.pone.0015112.

Bishop, D.V.M. *et al.* (2016) CATALISE: a multinational and multidisciplinary Delphi Consensus Study. Identifying language impairments in children. *PLoS One* **11**, e0158753. doi:10.1371/journal.pone.0158753.

Bishop, D.V.M. *et al.* (2017) Phase 2 of CATALISE: a multinational and multidisciplinary Delphi consensus study of problems with language development: terminology. *Journal of Child Psychology and Psychiatry* **58**, 1068–1080. doi:10.1111/jcpp.12721.

Bornstein, M.H. *et al.* (2018) Stability of core language skill from infancy to adolescence in typical and atypical development. *Science Advances* **4**, eaat7422. doi:10.1126/sciadv.aat7422.

Brownlie, E.B. *et al.* (2017) Language disorder and retrospectively reported sexual abuse of girls: severity and disclosure. *Journal of Child Psychology and Psychiatry* **58**, 1114–1121. doi:10.1111/jcpp.12723.

Calder, S.D. *et al.* (2022) The prevalence of and potential risk factors for Developmental Language Disorder at 10 years in the Raine Study. *Journal of Paediatrics and Child Health* **58**(11), 2044–2050. doi:10.1111/jpc.16149.

Castilla-Earls, A. *et al.* (2020) Beyond scores: using converging evidence to determine speech and language services eligibility for dual language learners. *American Journal of Speech-Language Pathology* **29**, 1116–1132. doi:10.1044/2020_AJSLP-19-00179.

Ciolino, C. *et al.* (2021) Narrative and other pragmatic language abilities of children with a history of maltreatment. *Perspectives of the ASHA Special Interest Groups* **6**, 230–241. doi:10.1044/2020_PERSP-20-00136.

Clarke, A. et al. (2021) Adolescent Mental Health: A Systematic Review on The Effectiveness of School-based Interventions. Early Intervention Foundation, London.

Clegg, J. *et al.* (2005) Developmental language disorders - a follow-up in later adult life. Cognitive, language and psychosocial outcomes. *Journal of Child Psychology and Psychiatry* **46**, 128–149. doi:10.1111/j.1469-7610.2004.00342.x.

Cohen, N.J. *et al.* (2013) Higher order language competence and adolescent mental health. *Journal of Child Psychology and Psychiatry* **54**, 733–744. doi:10.1111/jcpp.12060.

Conti-Ramsden, G. & Botting, N. (2008) Emotional health in adolescents with and without a history of specific language impairment (SLI). *Journal of Child Psychology and Psychiatry* **49**, 516–525. doi:10.1111/j.1469-7610.2007.01858.x.

Conti-Ramsden, G. & Durkin, K. (2012) Postschool educational and employment experiences of young people with specific language impairment. *Language, Speech, and Hearing Services in Schools* **43**, 507–520. doi:10.1044/0161-1461(2012/11-0067).

Conti-Ramsden, G. *et al.* (2018) Education and employment outcomes of young adults with a history of developmental language disorder. *International Journal of Language & Communication Disorders* **53**, 237–255. doi:10.1111/1460-6984.12338.

Cronin, P. *et al.* (2017) The impact of childhood language difficulties on healthcare costs from 4 to 13 years: Australian longitudinal study. *International Journal of Speech-Language Pathology* **19**, 381–391. doi:10.1080/17549507.2016.1216599.

Di Sante, M. *et al.* (2019) The pragmatic language skills of severely neglected 42-month-old children: results of the ELLAN Study. *Child Maltreatment* **24**, 244–253. doi:10.1177/1077559519828838.

Dobinson, K.L. & Dockrell, J.E. (2021) Universal strategies for the improvement of expressive language skills in the primary classroom: a systematic review. *First Language* **41**, 527–554. doi:10.1177/0142723721989471.

Donolato, E. *et al.* (2023) Oral language interventions can improve language outcomes in children with neurodevelopmental disorders: a systematic review and meta-analysis. *Campbell Systematic Reviews* **19**(4), e1368. Available: https://onlinelibrary.wiley.com/doi/10.1002/cl2.1368 [16 November 2024].

Dowdall, N. *et al.* (2020) Shared picture book Reading interventions for child language development: a systematic review and Meta-analysis. *Child Development* **91**, e383–e399. doi:10.1111/cdev.13225.

Dubois, P. *et al.* (2020) Young adults with developmental language disorder: a systematic review of education, employment, and independent living outcomes. *Journal of Speech, Language, and Hearing Research* **63**(11), 3786–3800.

Eadie, P. *et al.* (2018) Quality of life in children with developmental language disorder: Quality of life in children with DLD. *International Journal of Language & Communication Disorders* **53**, 799–810. doi:10.1111/1460-6984.12385.

Eadie, P. *et al.* (2021) Predictors in infancy for language and academic outcomes at 11 years. *Pediatrics* **147**. doi:10.1542/peds.2020-1712.

Ebbels, S.H. *et al.* (2019) Evidence-based pathways to intervention for children with language disorders. *International Journal of Language & Communication Disorders* **54**, 3–19. doi:10.1111/1460-6984.12387.

Feldman, H.M. *et al.* (2003) Parent-reported language skills in relation to otitis media during the first 3 years of life. *Journal of Speech, Language, and Hearing Research* **46**, 273–287. doi:10.1044/1092-4388(2003/022).

Frizelle, P. *et al.* (2021) The influence of quantitative intervention dosage on oral language outcomes for children with developmental language disorder: a systematic review and narrative synthesis. *Language, Speech, and Hearing Services in Schools* **52**, 738–754. doi:10.1044/2020_LSHSS-20-00058.

Goodman, R. (1997) The Strengths and Difficulties Questionnaire: a research note. *Journal of Child Psychology and Psychiatry* **38**, 581–586. doi:10.1111/j.1469-7610.1997.tb01545.x.

Griffiths, S. *et al.* (2020) Early language competence, but not general cognitive ability, predicts children's recognition of emotion from facial and vocal cues. *PeerJ* **8**, e9118. doi:10.7717/peerj.9118.

Griffiths, S. *et al.* (2021) Relationship between early language competence and cognitive emotion regulation in adolescence. *Royal Society Open Science* **8**, 210742. doi:10.1098/rsos.210742.

Griffiths, S. *et al.* (2022) Mutualistic coupling of vocabulary and non-verbal reasoning in children with and without language disorder. *Developmental Science* **25**. doi:10.1111/desc.13208.

Hall-Mills, S. (2019) A comparison of the prevalence rates of language impairment before and after response-to-intervention implementation. *Language, Speech, and Hearing Services in Schools* **50**, 703–709. doi:10.1044/2019_LSHSS-18-0144.

Hancock, A. *et al.* (2022) Speech, language and communication needs and mental health: the experiences of speech and language therapists and mental health professionals. *International Journal of Language & Communication Disorders*. doi:10.1111/1460-6984.12767.

Heidlage, J.K. *et al.* (2020) The effects of parent-implemented language interventions on child linguistic outcomes: a meta-analysis. *Early Child Research Quarterly* **50**, 6–23. doi:10.1016/j.ecresq.2018.12.006.

Hobson, H.M. & Lee, A. (2022) Camouflaging in developmental language disorder: the views of speech and language pathologists and parents. *Communication Disorders Quarterly*, 152574012211209. doi:10.1177/15257401221120937.

Hobson, H. *et al.* (2019) The role of language in alexithymia: moving towards a multiroute model of alexithymia. *Emotion Review* **11**, 247–261. doi:10.1177/1754073919838528.

Hobson, H. *et al.* (2022) Supporting the mental health of children with speech, language and communication needs: the views and experiences of parents. *Autism Developmental Language Disorder* **7**, 239694152211011. doi:10.1177/23969415221101137.

Hollo, A. *et al.* (2014) Unidentified language deficits in children with emotional and behavioral disorders: a meta-analysis. *Exceptional Children* **80**, 169–186. doi:10.1177/001440291408000203.

Howlin, P. *et al.* (2004) Adult outcome for children with autism. *Journal of Child Psychology and Psychiatry* **45**, 212–229. doi:10.1111/j.1469-7610.2004.00215.x.

James, A.C. *et al.* (2020) Cognitive behavioural therapy for anxiety disorders in children and adolescents. *Cochrane Database of Systematic Reviews* **2020**. doi:10.1002/14651858.CD013162.pub2.

Krishnan, S. *et al.* (2016) Neurobiological basis of language learning difficulties. *Trends in Cognitive Sciences* **20**, 701–714. doi:10.1016/j.tics.2016.06.012.

Language and Reading Research Consortium (LARRC) (2017) Oral language and listening comprehension: same or different constructs? *Journal of Speech, Language, and Hearing Research* **60**, 1273–1284. doi:10.1044/2017_JSLHR-L-16-0039.

Law, J. *et al.* (2013) Child speech, language and communication need re-examined in a public health context: a new direction for the speech and language therapy profession: child speech, language and communication need in the context of public health. *International Journal of Language & Communication Disorders* **48**, 486–496. doi:10.1111/1460-6984.12027.

Le, H.N.D. *et al.* (2020) Health-related quality of life, service utilization and costs of low language: a systematic review. *International Journal of Language & Communication Disorders* **55**, 3–25. doi:10.1111/1460-6984.12503.

Leonard, L.B. & Schroeder, M.L. (2023) The study of children with developmental language disorder beyond English: a tutorial. *Language Acquisition*, 1–19. doi:10.1080/10489223.2023.2197891.

Markussen-Brown, J. *et al.* (2017) The effects of language- and literacy-focused professional development on early educators and children: a best-evidence meta-analysis. *Early Child Research Quarterly* **38**, 97–115. doi:10.1016/j.ecresq.2016.07.002.

Mathrick, R. *et al.* (2017) Evaluation of an interview skills training package for adolescents with speech, language and communication needs. *International Journal of Language & Communication Disorders* **52**, 786–799. doi:10.1111/1460-6984.12315.

McGregor, K.K. (2020) How we fail children with developmental language disorder. *Language, Speech, and Hearing Services in Schools* **51**, 981–992. doi:10.1044/2020_LSHSS-20-00003.

McGregor, K.K. *et al.* (2013) Children with developmental language impairment have vocabulary deficits characterized by limited breadth and depth. *International Journal of Language & Communication Disorders* **48**, 307–319. doi:10.1111/1460-6984.12008.

McLeod, S. (2018) Communication rights: fundamental human rights for all. *International Journal of Speech-Language Pathology* **20**, 3–11. doi:10.1080/17549507.2018.1428687.

Moore, D.R. (2018) Guest editorial: auditory processing disorder. *Ear and Hearing* **39**, 617–620. doi:10.1097/AUD.0000000000000582.

Mountford, H.S. *et al.* (2022) The genetic and molecular basis of developmental language disorder: a review. *Children* **9**, 586. doi:10.3390/children9050586.

Nation, K. *et al.* (2022) Book language and its implications for children's language, literacy, and development. *Current Directions in Psychological Science*, 096372142211032. doi:10.1177/09637214221103264.

Newbury, D.F. *et al.* (2019) Using polygenic profiles to predict variation in language and psychosocial outcomes in early and middle childhood. *Journal of Speech, Language, and Hearing Research* **62**, 3381–3396. doi:10.1044/2019_JSLHR-L-19-0001.

Nook, E.C. (2021) Emotion differentiation and youth mental health: current understanding and open questions. *Frontiers in Psychology* **12**, 700298. doi:10.3389/fpsyg.2021.700298.

Norbury, C.F. *et al.* (2016) The impact of nonverbal ability on prevalence and clinical presentation of language disorder: evidence from a population study. *Journal of Child Psychology and Psychiatry* **57**, 1247–1257. doi:10.1111/jcpp.12573.

Norbury, C.F. *et al.* (2017) Language growth in children with heterogeneous language disorders: a population study. *Journal of Child Psychology and Psychiatry* **58**, 1092–1105. doi:10.1111/jcpp.12793.

Norbury, C.F. *et al.* (2019) Public health approaches still have room for individualized services: response to commentaries on 'evidence-based pathways to intervention for children with language disorders.' *International Journal of Language & Communication Disorders* **54**, 28–29. doi:10.1111/1460-6984.12436.

Nudel, R. *et al.* (2023) Developmental language disorder: A comprehensive study of more than 46,000 individuals. *Psychiatry Research* **323**, 115171. doi:10.1016/j.psychres.2023.115171.

Pace, A. *et al.* (2017) Identifying pathways between socioeconomic status and language development. *Annual Review of Linguistics* **3**, 285–308. doi:10.1146/annurev-linguistics-011516-034226.

Pickles, A. *et al.* (2022) Predictors of language regression and its association with subsequent communication development in children with autism. *Journal of Child Psychology and Psychiatry* **63**, 1243–1251. doi:10.1111/jcpp.13565.

Pimperton, H. & Kennedy, C.R. (2012) The impact of early identification of permanent childhood hearing impairment on speech and language outcomes. *Archives of Disease in Childhood* **97**, 648–653. doi:10.1136/archdischild-2011-301501.

Rannard, A. *et al.* (2005) Parent concerns and professional responses: the case of specific language impairment. *The British Journal of General Practice* **55**, 710–714.

Rogde, K. *et al.* (2019) The effect of linguistic comprehension instruction on generalized language and reading comprehension skills: a systematic review. *Campbell Systematic Reviews* **15**, e1059. doi:10.1002/cl2.1059.

Romeo, R.R. *et al.* (2021) Neuroplasticity associated with changes in conversational turn-taking following a family-based intervention. *Developmental Cognitive Neuroscience* **49**, 100967. doi:10.1016/j.dcn.2021.100967.

Saul, J. *et al.* (2023) Prevalence and functional impact of social (pragmatic) communication disorders. *Journal of Child Psychology and Psychiatry* **64**, 376–387. doi:10.1111/jcpp.13705.

Selin, C. *et al.* (2022) Adversity exposure, syntax, and specific language impairment: an exploratory Study. *Journal of Speech, Language, and Hearing Research* **65**, 3471–3490. doi:10.1044/2022_JSLHR-21-00578.

Snow, P.C. (2019) Speech-language pathology and the youth offender: epidemiological overview and roadmap for future speech-language pathology research and scope of practice. *Language, Speech, and Hearing Services in Schools* **50**, 324–339. doi:10.1044/2018_LSHSS-CCJS-18-0027.

Snow, P.C. (2021) SOLAR: The science of language and reading. *The Child Language and the Teacher* **37**, 222–233. doi:10.1177/0265659020947817.

Tomblin, J.B. (2006) A normativist account of language-based learning Disability1,2. *Learning Disabilities Research and Practice* **21**, 8–18. doi:10.1111/j.1540-5826.2006.00203.x.

Tomblin, J.B. et al. (2020) Prevalence of specific language impairment in kindergarten children. *J Speech Lang Hear Res* [Internet 1997 Dec] **40**(6), 1245–1260. Available from http://pubs.asha.org/doi/10.1044/jslhr.4006.1245.

Ung, D. *et al.* (2015) A systematic review and meta-analysis of cognitive-behavioral therapy for anxiety in youth with high-functioning autism spectrum disorders. *Child Psychiatry and Human Development* **46**, 533–547. doi:10.1007/s10578-014-0494-y.

Van Den Bedem, N.P. *et al.* (2018) Victimization, bullying, and emotional competence: longitudinal associations in (pre)adolescents with and without developmental language disorder. *Journal of Speech, Language, and Hearing Research* **61**, 2028–2044. doi:10.1044/2018_JSLHR-L-17-0429.

Verhoef, E. *et al.* (2021) The developmental origins of genetic factors influencing language and literacy: associations with early-childhood vocabulary. *Journal of Child Psychology and Psychiatry* **62**, 728–738. doi:10.1111/jcpp.13327.

Wade, M. *et al.* (2022) The effects of early life adversity on children's mental health and cognitive functioning. *Translational Psychiatry* **12**, 244. doi:10.1038/s41398-022-02001-0.

Wake, M. *et al.* (2011) Outcomes of population based language promotion for slow to talk toddlers at ages 2 and 3 years: let's learn language cluster randomised controlled trial. *BMJ* **343**, d4741–d4741. doi:10.1136/bmj.d4741.

West, G. *et al.* (2021) Early language screening and intervention can be delivered successfully at scale: evidence from a cluster randomized controlled trial. *Journal of Child Psychology and Psychiatry* **62**, 1425–1434. doi:10.1111/jcpp.13415.

Westby, C. & Culatta, B. (2016) Telling tales: personal event narratives and life stories. *Language, Speech, and Hearing Services in Schools* **47**, 260–282. doi:10.1044/2016_LSHSS-15-0073.

Whiteside, K.E. & Norbury, C.F. (2017) The persistence and functional impact of English language difficulties experienced by children learning English as an additional language and monolingual peers. *Journal of Speech, Language, and Hearing Research* **60**, 2014–2030. doi:10.1044/2017_JSLHR-L-16-0318.

Wilson, A.C. & Bishop, D.V.M. (2018) Resounding failure to replicate links between developmental language disorder and cerebral lateralisation. *PeerJ* **8**(6), e4217. doi:10.7717/peerj.4217.

Winters, K.L. *et al.* (2022) Investigating narrative performance in children with developmental language disorder: a systematic review and meta-analysis. *Journal of Speech, Language, and Hearing Research* **65**, 3908–3929. doi:10.1044/2022_JSLHR-22-00017.

World Health Organization (2019) *International Statistical Classification of Diseases and Related Health Problems*, 11th edn. World Health Organization, Geneva, Switzerland.

Wren, Y. *et al.* (2016) Prevalence and predictors of persistent speech sound disorder at eight years old: findings from a population cohort Study. *Journal of Speech, Language, and Hearing Research* **59**, 647–673. doi:10.1044/2015_JSLHR-S-14-0282.

Wu, S. *et al.* (2023) Prevalence, co-occurring difficulties, and risk factors of developmental language disorder: first evidence for Mandarin-speaking children in a population-based study. *The Lancet Regional Health West Pacific* **34**, 100713. doi:10.1016/j.lanwpc.2023.100713.

Yew, S.G.K. & O'Kearney, R. (2013) Emotional and behavioural outcomes later in childhood and adolescence for children with specific language impairments: meta-analyses of controlled prospective studies: SLI and emotional and behavioural disorders. *Journal of Child Psychology and Psychiatry* **54**, 516–524. doi:10.1111/jcpp.12009.

CHAPTER 52

Specific learning disorders

Margaret J. Snowling[1,2] and Charles Hulme[1,3]

[1] Department of Experimental Psychology, University of Oxford, Oxford, UK

[2] St. John's College, Oxford, UK

[3] School of Psychology, Social Work and Public Health, Oxford Brookes University, Oxford, UK

Introduction

Problems of literacy and numeracy are common and may greatly hinder educational attainment and career opportunities. Less researched and arguably less recognized are problems with motor coordination which may hinder learning to write and spell and can affect performance in school, self-esteem, and confidence.

The more recent *Diagnostic and Statistical Manual of Mental Disorders*, 5th edition, text revision (DSM-5-TR), like its forerunner, DSM-5 (American Psychiatric Association, 2013), classifies reading disorders (RD), mathematical disorders (MD), and disorders of written expression under one overarching diagnosis: specific learning disorder (SLD). It also emphasizes the developmental nature of SLD as: "a type of Neurodevelopmental Disorder that impedes the ability to learn or use specific academic skills (e.g., reading, writing, or arithmetic), which are the foundation for other academic learning." Along similar lines, the *International Classification of Diseases*, 11th edition (ICD-11; World Health Organization, 2019) uses the term "developmental learning disorder" to encompass significant and persistent difficulties in learning academic skills, which may include reading, writing, or arithmetic. Developmental coordination disorder (DCD), sometimes referred to as "dyspraxia," is a disorder of motor learning; it is included here because DCD often co-occurs with SLDs, and it may also have adverse effects on children's educational attainment.

Conceptual issues

Two important issues have dominated the field of SLDs in recent years. The first is the extent to which learning to read depends upon IQ. One significant difference between ICD-11 and DSM-5 is that the requirement for reading (or spelling) to be below expectation given age and intellectual ability (the so-called discrepancy definition) is only included in ICD-11. This difference is unfortunate and leads different jurisdictions to use different diagnostic criteria. From a theoretical stance, the discrepancy definition has fallen out of use because the underlying cognitive deficits underpinning poor reading are similar regardless of IQ level (Stanovich & Siegel 1994). We argue that the discrepancy definition should be abandoned and that there is no basis for withholding intervention from some children based on their IQ.

The second issue is where to set the boundary between "typical" and "atypical" development. Since variations in reading, numerical, and motor skills represent continuous dimensions, the severity, persistence, and degree of difficulty caused to an individual in everyday functioning needs to be considered when formulating "diagnoses." Traditionally learning disorders, such as dyslexia and MD, have been considered modular and causal explanations formulated at different levels of explanation: biological, cognitive, or environmental. However, in common with other neurodevelopmental disorders (NDDs), SLDs tend to co-occur with other disorders, or at least, they share traits with them, perhaps most commonly deficits in executive function (EF) (see Chapter 3). Comorbidity rates between RD and other NDDs range between 11–70% for RD and MD (e.g., Moll *et al.*, 2014), 20–50% for RD with attention deficit hyperactivity disorder (ADHD) and conduct disorder (e.g., Hendren *et al.*, 2018), and 9–29% for RD and anxiety disorder (e.g., Margari *et al.*, 2013). Much less studied is the comorbidity between SLD and developmental language disorder (DLD) but this is likely to be high given that both reading and mathematics draw on language skills.

Rutter's Child and Adolescent Psychiatry and Psychology, Seventh Edition.
Edited by Anita Thapar, Daniel S. Pine, Samuele Cortese, Cathy Creswell, Tamsin J. Ford, James F. Leckman, and Argyris Stringaris.

Companion website: www.wiley.com/go/thapar/rutterspsych7

Reading disorders

Literacy development: a framework

Reading comprehension is the product of decoding and language comprehension (Gough & Tunmer, 1986). Thus, when considering the demands of learning to read, it is essential to make a clear distinction between the ability to translate printed words into speech (decoding) and the ability to read for meaning (to understand what has been decoded); both of these are dimensional skills. They are also related—if a child cannot decode a text, they cannot comprehend it.

This dimensional view of reading underlies the differences between two commonly occurring forms of RD in children. Dyslexia is a difficulty in decoding print. Children with dyslexia typically read slowly and inaccurately and, in most cases, also have spelling difficulties. Reading comprehension impairment, in contrast, refers to children who can read aloud accurately but have difficulty understanding what they read (Cain, 2022). This reading profile reflects an underlying language comprehension problem and is frequently observed in children with autism spectrum disorder (ASD) and in communication disorders, such as DLD (Adlof *et al.*, 2022).

Learning to read proceeds in tandem with learning to spell but the two processes are not simply the reciprocal of one another. Reading can sometimes proceed using partial cues, especially when there is context, but spelling requires recall of the precise letter sequences of words. Learning to spell depends critically on phoneme awareness, specifically the ability to segment the sounds of spoken words, and letter-sound knowledge (the rules mapping phonemes in speech to letters). However, proficient spelling requires more than good phonology: the quality of the orthographic representations built up during reading provide a critical foundation for spelling; awareness of the morphological structure of words, such as how spellings represent grammatical information, is also important. For further information on language terms see Box 52.1.

Individual differences in learning to read across languages

A key question is whether the skills required for reading and spelling differ across writing systems (orthographies). In alphabetic systems, there are fine-grained mappings between symbols (letters) and sounds (phonemes). However, languages differ in the size of the mappings, for example, mappings are at the level of the syllable in the Japanese Kana, and Chinese has mappings between meaning units (morphemes) and orthography. Languages also vary in the size of the symbol set to be learned, with English being one of the smallest, having 44 letter-sound correspondences.

It follows that the demands of learning to read differ between languages. Nevertheless, converging evidence shows that the core skills required (and hence the deficits in dyslexia) are similar, at least across alphabetic languages (Caravolas *et al.*, 2012). Turning to nonalphabetic writing systems, such as Chinese (Cantonese and Mandarin), there is a stronger role for morphological and visual skills than for English and learning to read places significant demands on semantic, morphological (meaning), and visual skills (McBride *et al.*, 2022). Nevertheless, phonological skills remain important predictors of individual differences. This is also the case in visually complex orthographies, such as Kannada from southern India (an alphasyllabary), which depends on both phonological and visual skills (Nag & Snowling, 2012).

In summary, although orthographic differences affect the rate of reading development, the key predictors of learning in all alphabetic languages are awareness of the sound structure of spoken words (phonology), knowledge of symbol-sound associations and rapid automatized naming (RAN) skills—a triple

Box 52.1 Glossary of terms

Alphasyllabary
An alphasyllabary is an orthographic system which, like an alphabetic system, maps symbols to sounds but at the level of the syllable (consonant vowel sequences).

Approximate number system (ANS)
The ANS is one of three systems for processing numbers according to the Triple Code model of Dehaene (1999); it is the nonverbal system used for estimating magnitudes and numerosity.

Logographic
A logographic writing system (orthography) is one in which whole words are represented and connected to word pronunciations (in contrast to an alphabetic system in which mappings are at the level of phonemes to graphemes—letters and letter combinations).

Morpheme
The parts of words that carry meaning. There are two types of morphemes: grammatical and derivational. "Cat" is a monomorphemic word (contains one morpheme). The plural "cats" contains two morphemes: the stem (cat) and the grammatical morpheme signaling the plural -s. A derivational morpheme changes the meaning or the class of a word. The morpheme "ness" cannot stand alone but changes the main word: happy -> happiness; sad -> sadness, etc.

Orthographic
The "orthography" is the writing system and the conventions or rules for writing a language. English is a "deep" orthography that contains many exceptions to the rules. Other alphabetic languages, such as Spanish or Finnish, have a "shallow" or transparent orthography because the rules are mostly applied consistently. The term "orthographic" is used to describe the skills used to read and write in the orthography.

Phoneme
The smallest speech sound in a word. "Cat" has three phonemes: /k/-/a/-/t/.

Rime
The vowel and final consonant in a syllable. The rime in "cat" is /at/.

foundation dependent on oral language. The same predictors are also important in nonalphabetic orthographies (such as Chinese) although here other skills such as semantics (knowledge of word meanings) may assume greater importance.

Nature and prevalence of reading disorders

It is generally understood that the cutoff between typical reading and RD depends upon context and estimates of prevalence vary between 2–20% across studies. Although the label "dyslexia" continues to be controversial, it remains important to identify significant and persistent reading difficulties if appropriate support and intervention is to follow (Wagner *et al.*, 2020).

In line with this view, DSM-5-TR (American Psychiatric Association, 2022) states that for diagnosis of a SLD, the affected skill (reading, writing, or arithmetic) must have been significantly impaired relative to age expectation for at least six months despite intervention, and the onset must have been in the school years (though the manifestation may change over time). It recommends adding a specifier to the diagnosis of "reading disorder" to indicate whether accuracy, fluency, and/or reading comprehension are affected. Two working definitions also require evidence of phonological processing deficits (Rose, 2009; Tunmer & Greaney, 2010). In addition, Rose (2009) notes the frequent presence of co-occurring conditions but states "they are not themselves markers of dyslexia." In none of these definitions is a diagnosis of learning disorder appropriate in the presence of intellectual impairment or adverse factors affecting education, including not being proficient in the language of instruction.

Prevalence

Given the conceptual issues surrounding the identification of SLDs, including the different cutoffs, estimates of prevalence must be interpreted with care. In a large representative sample of German children in Grades 3 and 4, Moll *et al.* (2014) reported the prevalence of RD and spelling disorder, both as single disorders and/or in combination with each other and/or with arithmetic disorder. Using a criterion of −1.5SD to define a disorder, they report prevalence rates of 7.4% for RD and 8.9% for spelling disorder. In contrast to English, where most individuals with RD also have spelling deficits, these two disorders often dissociate in German speakers. They also found that arithmetic disorder often co-occurred with spelling disorder.

Di Folco *et al.* (2022) estimated the prevalence of RD in a large representative sample of French children in Grade 6 (N = 25,000) comparing estimates that used the criteria for DSM-5 (below age expectation in reading) and for ICD-11 (below expectation given nonverbal IQ), using a range of different cut points (from −1SD to −2SD). When using a criterion of −1.5SD and operationalization of the ICD-11 criteria, the prevalence was 3.5%. Relaxing the IQ criterion raised prevalence to 7.9%, comparable to the German study (Moll *et al.*, 2014). They also report the concordance between the two definitions using the −1.5SD for reading severity (and school attainment <−0.5SD), DSM-5 classifying twice as many individuals as RD.

Epidemiological studies of children reading in nonalphabetic orthographies are rare. An exception is a study of 2955 Chinese children aged 7–12 years (Lin *et al.*, 2020) who were assessed according to DSM-5 criteria for dyslexia, corroborated by performance on the Chinese Reading Ability Test. The reported prevalence rate for dyslexia was 5.4%. As expected, the children with dyslexia scored poorly on measures of phonological awareness, morphological awareness, RAN, and orthographic awareness.

Assessing reading comprehension is labor intensive and therefore few studies report the prevalence of reading comprehension impairment. Importantly, however, reading comprehension impairment is quite a common disorder but often goes undetected. Hulme and Snowling (unpublished), using data from the standardization of a reading test, reported that 10% of the sample had reading comprehension scores that were 1SD below their reading accuracy scores, and 3.3% of the sample satisfied a more restrictive definition of a reading comprehension impairment with a 1SD discrepancy, coupled with a reading comprehension standard score below 90 and a reading accuracy score above 90. Many children with reading comprehension impairment have wide-ranging oral language impairments but develop good phonological decoding skills enabling them to mask their reading difficulties.

Sex ratio

Epidemiological studies have tended to report more boys than girls with RD; this sex difference increases along with the severity of reading difficulties (Arnett *et al.*, 2017). How universal this finding is across languages is not clear. Among European languages, Moll *et al.* (2014) reported a nearly equal number of boys and girls affected with RD in Germany; Di Folco *et al.* (2022) using the same criterion in France, reported 1.6 boys:1 girl affected. An issue of clinical concern is lack of agreement between research criteria and school-based identification procedures: Quinn and Wagner (2015) reported that only about 20% of children identified as having reading problems using objective tests were identified as learning disabled by schools and it was females who were less likely to be identified.

Causal risk factors for reading disorders

For many years, the dominant approach to research on SLDs was to study individuals with a clinical diagnosis. One problem with this approach is that such samples are likely to include cases with a wide range of deficits, some of which may be secondary consequences or co-occurring features (comorbidities). At the same time, some studies in this tradition have included only individuals who fulfill the IQ-discrepancy definition of dyslexia. An alternative, and arguably more appropriate, approach, given that reading skills are dimensional, is to study SLDs by reference to longitudinal studies investigating individual differences in representative samples. This approach enables the identification of risk factors for disorders, free of referral bias.

Cognitive and perceptual impairments

There have been various hypotheses regarding the causes of RD, including putative impairments in phonological, visual, auditory, and motor domains. Acknowledging that dyslexia and other SLDs are typically the outcome of multiple risk factors, here we focus on the main causal hypotheses.

Phonological deficits

The predominant theoretical view is that difficulties with reading accuracy and fluency (RD/dyslexia) arise from difficulties with phonological processing. Following a meta-analysis of case-control studies, Melby-Lervåg *et al.* (2012) reported a large effect size ($d = -1.37$) for differences between groups with RD and typical readers on tasks tapping phoneme awareness relative to children of the same age; in a stricter comparison with younger children reading at the same level, the effect size was also substantial ($d = -0.57$). Group differences in rime awareness and in verbal short-term memory were smaller but significant. RAN of familiar objects and digits, a skill requiring the rapid retrieval of phonological information, is also associated with reading skill and appears to be a useful measure for differentiating children with language disorders who will develop dyslexia from those who can learn to decode normally (Ramus *et al.*, 2013).

Particularly strong evidence for the importance of phonological deficits in dyslexia comes from studies that show such difficulties exist before reading instruction begins. Data from a large-scale longitudinal study of children at risk of dyslexia (Snowling *et al.*, 2019) showed that children who went on to reach criterion for dyslexia at 8 years of age showed deficits in the preschool period on tests of nonword repetition (a measure of phonological memory) and in RAN of objects; their letter-sound knowledge was also slow to develop.

Auditory and speech processing deficits

Where measures of auditory processing have been included in longitudinal studies, findings confirm the importance of phonological processing to reading development but several also suggest a role for auditory processing (e.g., Hämäläinen *et al.*, 2012; Carroll *et al.*, 2016).

A prominent hypothesis has been that auditory processing problems might predispose a child to problems with speech perception which cascade to affect the development of phonological awareness (Tallal, 1980). Contrary to this view, O'Brien *et al.* (2018) reported findings from a study of speech perception in dyslexia using two phoneme categorization tasks. While there were group differences between the children with dyslexia and controls, it appeared that lapses of attention—which were more common in those with dyslexia—could explain group differences (see also Schulte-Körne and Bruder (2010)). Further, the relationship between speech categorization and reading was not mediated by phonological awareness, refuting the auditory deficit hypothesis of poor reading.

Visual processing deficits

Visual processing deficits have been reported in dyslexia, particularly in the magnocellular visual system responsible for rapid temporal processing and motion detection; these could in principle affect the development of orthographic representations which depends upon the ability to process letters within words in parallel (Grainger *et al.*, 2016). Manning *et al.* (2022) investigated visual motion processing in dyslexia, modeling the different stages in the decision-making process. Children aged 8–14 judged the direction of motion in two discrimination tasks (motion coherence and direction integration) using a "drift diffusion" paradigm. Children with dyslexia had general problems extracting global motion information in both tasks and they accumulated sensory evidence more slowly than controls. As a result, they were slower to make decisions. However, why such deficits should compromise reading remains unclear. One of the few longitudinal studies to investigate the putative causal role of visual processing in reading development was conducted by Valdois *et al.* (2019) who reported a significant effect of visual attention span in kindergarten on measures of word, nonword, and text reading fluency in Grade 1 when letter knowledge and phonological awareness were controlled. However, the measure of visual attention involved digit processing and, arguably, therefore tapped verbal processing.

Profiles of deficits in cases of dyslexia

Several studies have investigated the relative frequency of phonological and visual deficits in the etiology of dyslexia. Saksida *et al.* (2016) assessed a large sample of French-speaking children aged 8–13 years, examining their performance on tasks tapping visual stress (the experience of visual distortions when reading text), visual attention, and phonological skills. Problems of visual stress were more common in the control than the group with dyslexia; 28% of the dyslexic group showed reduced visual attention span but, importantly, each of these children also had phonological deficits. Indeed, difficulties in phonological skills were widespread, affecting over 90% of the group (Figure 52.1).

In a similar vein, O'Brien and Yeatman (2021) assessed different hypotheses about deficits in dyslexia but came to a slightly different conclusion. In their study, tasks tapping motion detection using the drift diffusion paradigm revealed several different profiles of impairment associated with reading skill: reduced

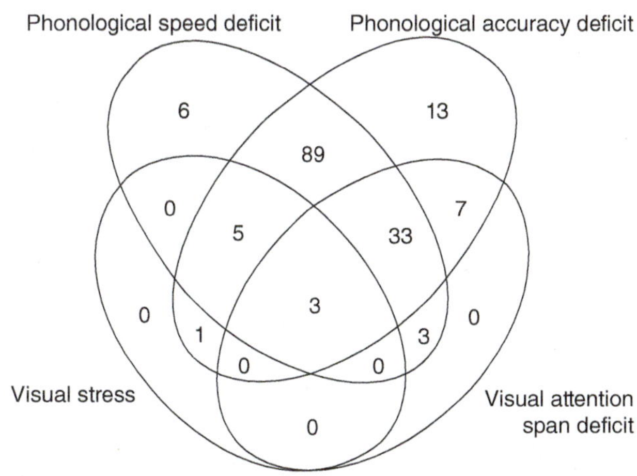

Figure 52.1 Heterogeneity in dyslexia. The Venn diagram shows the number of cases who show deficits in accuracy on phonological awareness tasks, in speed of completing such tasks, or in visual attention, or experience visual stress. There is considerable overlap, with phonological skills the most commonly affected. *Source*: Reproduced from Saksida *et al.* (2016), with permission of American Psychological Association.

ability to encode and integrate visual information, setting a "conservative" criterion for decisions about motion that would ensure accuracy, and variability in terms of the time taken to gather evidence and/or execute a decision. Modeling these data together with measures of phonological processing indicated that each contributed independent variance to individual differences in reading. Thus, they suggest it is possible that underlying sensory impairments play a significant role in the etiology of dyslexia (see Pennington *et al.* (2012) for a similar argument).

Summary

There is a voluminous literature on the cognitive and perceptual processing deficits associated with dyslexia. In addition to the studies we have reviewed, separate lines of research have pursued domain-general hypotheses that aim to integrate findings of dyslexic difficulties across modalities. These include theories that posit speed-of-processing deficits (Araújo & Faísca, 2019; cf. Bonifacci & Snowling, 2008), problems in implicit procedural or statistical learning (Ullman & Pullman, 2015; cf. West *et al.*, 2018; Schmalz *et al.*, 2019), or problems in automaticity (Nicolson & Fawcett, 1990; cf. Rochelle & Talcott, 2006). However, many of the studies lack statistical power, longitudinal studies are rare, and failures to replicate confound interpretation.

Current evidence indicates that the most robust findings are those that point to phonological processing deficits in dyslexia, with performance on speeded tasks being the most affected, persistent across the age range and across orthographies. Notwithstanding this, an emerging view is that, while there are causal relationships between phonological skills and learning to read, this causal pathway does not explain reading failure in all cases. There is a need to understand why some children with adequate phonological skills fail to become fluent readers and, conversely, why a minority of children with poor phonology read well. Promising areas of research are in studies investigating aspects of visual attentional processing where longitudinal studies are badly needed.

Genetic risk factors and brain correlates of reading disorders

Heritability of reading and language skills

It is well established that reading skills, and the phonological skills that underpin them, are highly heritable (Christopher *et al.*, 2015; Little *et al.*, 2017; Tosto *et al.*, 2017). However, heritability estimates are based on group data and tell us little about the risk to an individual of developing an RD.

There have now been several studies of the molecular genetics of dyslexia focusing on the identification of genetic linkages and gene loci associated with the disorder (Paracchini (2022) for review). While the use of genome-wide association (GWAS) methods has provided important leads, few of these are well-powered and therefore findings are not robust. An exception is a GWAS study by Gialluisi *et al.* (2019) of some 8000 European individuals which also incorporated an investigation of associations with polygenic risk scores (PGSs) for other NDDs. Such scores are derived by aggregating genetic effects across SNPs associated with specific traits within an individual (a weighted average of many different alleles associated with that trait). Findings revealed significant associations with two gene loci in this sample: LOC388780 (20p13), the function of which is uncertain and VEPH1 (3q25), a gene implicated in brain development. There were also significant associations of dyslexia risk with PGSs for ADHD, bipolar disorder, and schizophrenia as well as educational attainment (a proxy for reading skill) and intelligence. In addition, an association with cortical thickness in the region of the temporal lobe converges with findings from studies of the brain bases of dyslexia.

Familial risk of dyslexia

One way of elucidating how genetic risk factors, in addition to gene–environment correlations, are related to the risks for poor reading is to study children at family risk of dyslexia. A meta-analytic review of family risk studies in children learning to read in English, Danish, Dutch, Finnish, and Chinese confirmed an elevated risk of dyslexia in the children of parents with reading problems, with a mean prevalence rate of 45%, compared with 12% for children not at risk (Snowling & Melby-Lervåg, 2016). Analysis of precursor skills showed that children who go on to be diagnosed with dyslexia have significant language difficulties in the preschool years, including phonological difficulties, and problems at the age of school entry in acquiring the triple foundation of decoding (letter knowledge, phonological awareness, and RAN). Many children with language difficulties also have speech problems; however, speech difficulties per se only seem to be associated with reading difficulties when they are persistent (Hayiou-Thomas *et al.*, 2017).

Brain bases of dyslexia

The neural pathways involved in reading are now understood to build on the circuits used for processing spoken language, connecting them with the "visual word form area" (VWFA), an area concerned with visual processing. Taylor *et al.* (2013) reported a meta-analysis of 36 brain-imaging studies in which they examined the validity of cognitive models of reading for predicting the neural processing of words versus nonwords, and regular versus irregular words. They found that reading print depended upon activation of left-hemisphere clusters, the precise pathways depending upon word-type. Moreover, different regions were involved in different stages of the reading process from visual (orthographic) analysis through semantic processing or spelling-sound conversion to phonological output.

With studies such as these as a backdrop, meta-analyses have investigated findings of studies imaging the brain in "dyslexia." Paulesu *et al.* (2014) analyzed peaks of activations across multiple studies of adults and children with dyslexia; these analyses revealed 193 clusters that confirm reduced activation of the left occipito-temporal cortex in dyslexia during reading and visual-phonological tasks. More recently, studies have investigated whether this "brain signature" is the same across orthographies. A synthesis by Richlan (2020) comparing alphabetic, syllabic, and logographic writing systems reported universal underactivation of the left-hemisphere reading network in dyslexic readers relative to typical readers, specifically, within the occipito-temporal, temporo-parietal, and inferior frontal cortex. Abnormalities specific to different orthographies primarily related to the degree and spatial extent of under- and overactivation clusters. In similar vein, a meta-analysis by Devoto *et al.* (2022) reported that across European (alphabetic) writing systems, the core neural correlate of dyslexia was the underrecruitment of the middle portion of the fusiform gyrus, that is the VWFA.

According to Yeatman (2022) these functional differences between the brains of dyslexic and typical readers, and structural differences in brain connectivity may predate literacy acquisition (see Vandermosten *et al.* (2016) for review). One of the first studies to relate early measures of brain structure and function to reading was reported by Hoeft *et al.* (2011) who followed children with dyslexia for some 2.5 years. Importantly, those who made most progress in reading had greater white matter integrity in the right arcuate fasciculus (a pathway linking parieto-temporal and frontal regions). Myers *et al.* (2014) went on to examine the structure of the left and right arcuate fasciculus in children followed from preschool to Grade 3. In this study, measures of preliteracy and a measure of change in white matter density in the left arcuate fasciculus over time accounted for significant variance in reading in Grade 3 (56%). In fact, growth of this "temporal" pathway continued to predict individual differences in reading when measures of prereading in kindergarten, socioeconomic status (SES), and home literacy were controlled. Similarly, Preston *et al.* (2016) found that the co-activation of regions involved in processing speech and print across the left hemisphere's reading network in beginner readers predicted reading 2 years later when pretest reading scores and general activation in each region alone were controlled.

Building on this evidence, Huber *et al.* (2018) used diffusion magnetic resonance imaging (MRI) data to monitor changes in brain connectivity in children undergoing an intensive reading intervention. Large-scale changes in a collection of white matter tracts paralleled increases in reading skill, whereas other tracts involved in reading did not change. Although this was only a short intervention, findings suggest there may be fiber tracts that show rapid structural changes following reading practice, while other structures that may be causally related to learning to read are less malleable following intervention.

Environmental risk factors

Home and school background

A strong correlation between socioeconomic background and children's reading skills reflects multiple influences including family, home, and school factors (Jerrim, *et al.*, 2015; Lervåg *et al.*, 2019). More specifically, the home environment is particularly important for literacy development and shared reading with adults is a vehicle for honing prereading skills (Sénéchal & LeFevre, 2014). However, the quantity and quality of such "shared reading" is influenced by characteristics of the parent and child: parents with low literacy have fewer books in the home (a passive gene–environment influence) and children with reading difficulties may seek out fewer literacy-related opportunities (an active gene–environment influence) (Little & Hart, 2022).

Since adults with dyslexia tend to read less it might be expected that children at family risk of dyslexia experience a different home environment to controls. However, after controlling for maternal language and literacy skills, Puglisi *et al.* (2017) found no direct effect of measures of the informal home literacy environment on child outcomes and suggested these effects may instead reflect genetic risk factors. Consistent with this, Chow *et al.* (2017) reported, in a sample of Cantonese-speaking twins aged 3–11 years, that both the SES and the home literacy environment had effects on reading and language development, but these factors did not moderate genetic influences. Regarding wider environmental influences, there are school-level differences in the reading attainment of pupils (e.g., Sammons *et al.*, 1993), as well as national differences in literacy levels.

Beyond the early years, an important predictor of reading fluency is the amount of reading a child does "for pleasure." Van Bergen *et al.* (2018) extracted data from the Netherlands Twin Register to estimate genetic and environmental influences on reading ability. Direction of causality models suggested that reading skill was the driver of how much children read and not vice versa. A clear implication is that poor readers need to be encouraged to practice reading as they are more likely to avoid doing so at home and elsewhere.

Cultural and cross-linguistic factors

Studies of research on dyslexia in non-English-speaking countries has burgeoned in recent years. Whereas in English poor reading and spelling accuracy are primary behavioral markers of dyslexia, in languages such as German or Finnish, which are more regular than English, reading difficulties are identified by a slow reading rate with few reading errors. European languages have small symbol sets that are relatively easy to acquire. In contrast, mastering the symbol set can be a protracted process in scripts with large character sets, especially for poor readers (McBride *et al.*, 2022, for Chinese; Nag, 2022, for alphasyllabic scripts).

Beyond orthography, home learning environments and school curricula are deeply embedded in the culture (Nag *et al.*, 2024). While many children in Western countries are monolingual, it is not unusual for children in low- and middle-income countries to live in bilingual or multilingual communities, and for many families, levels of literacy are low and this may have both a direct and indirect impact on the educational attainments of their children. Indeed, children who are raised in multilingual environments confront difficulties if the language of school differs from the home language, and dialectical difference between

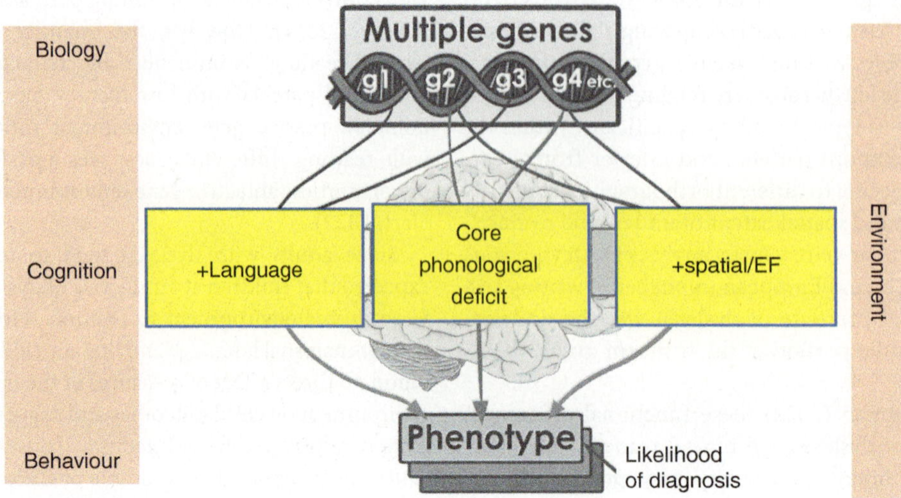

Figure 52.2 Schematic diagram showing risk factors for reading disorder/dyslexia at different levels of explanation.

home and school may also be associated with educational under-attainment (Washington, 2001).

In summary, theories of RD need to take account of a wide range of both genetic and environmental risk factors which affect learning to read. Figure 52.2 is a schematic representation of the different influences on learning to read and the probabilistic risk factors for dyslexia. The figure shows that at the cognitive level, the primary deficit is in phonological skills; the likelihood of diagnosis will depend not only on the severity of this deficit but also the co-occurrence of deficits shared with other NDDs and the presence of adverse environmental factors. While understanding of how these different factors interact over time remains limited, findings serve to remind us that the proximal environment during the early years of development provides a critical foundation for later educational attainment and schooling may be particularly valuable as compensation for poorer home circumstances.

Mathematics disorders

Definition and prevalence of mathematical disorders

As noted in the "Reading disorders" section, DSM-5-TR (American Psychiatric Association, 2022) classifies MD with other educational difficulties, under the category of SLDs. An alternative term that is sometimes used is dyscalculia, usually defined as a difficulty learning mathematics which is out of line with other aspects of a child's development (particularly IQ). In practice, the diagnosis typically reflects difficulties with basic arithmetic skills, rather than difficulties with higher-level mathematical abilities, such as algebra and geometry.

The prevalence of mathematics difficulties appears similar to that for reading difficulties. Morsanyi *et al.* (2018) in a study of over 2000 children reported that approximately 6% of the sample satisfied DSM-5 (American Psychiatric Association, 2013) criteria for SLD in mathematics (SLDM; equivalent to MD) with no appreciable difference in rates for boys and girls. Similarly, Moll *et al.* (2019) reported that 5.4% of Grade 3 children had below average arithmetic fluency and some 22% also showed deficits of similar magnitude on a measure of literacy (reading and spelling), a rate of comorbidity that is over 4 times that expected by chance.

The profile of children with mathematics disorder

Children with MD typically show patterns of performance on simple arithmetic tasks that are characteristic of much younger children. Frequently, they experience problems learning to count—a foundational skill for mastering basic arithmetic skills which requires understanding a set of abstract principles as well as verbal skills. Once at school, children are taught arithmetic formally, and master (in roughly the following order), addition (single digit addition then multidigit), subtraction, multiplication, and division. Children with mathematical difficulties show delays in mastering addition and subtraction, and often tend to rely on the "count-on" strategy for longer than typically developing children when solving simple addition problems (Gilmore *et al.*, 2018). With more complex addition problems, they guess more often and less accurately than their peers and, while they use the same strategies as age-matched controls, they differ in the speed and skill of strategy execution, can retrieve fewer number facts from memory, are poor at monitoring their counting and detecting computational errors (Geary, 2004).

Risk factors for mathematics disorder

The dominant theoretical framework for MD posits three domains of representation involved in mathematics: a quantitative magnitude system, a language-based system, and a written number system (Dehaene, 1992). If one or more of these systems are deficient this can cause problems in the development of mathematical skills. Here we consider several possible cognitive explanations for the development of MD within this framework.

Magnitude representation

Dehaene (1992) has argued that the basis of numerical cognition is an innate "approximate number sense" (ANS)—a preverbal system involving the ability to understand physical magnitudes and numerical quantities. The precision of coding within the ANS is typically assessed by tasks that measure the accuracy and speed of discriminating groups of objects based on their numerosity (see Figure 52.3 for an example). The difficulty of such discriminations varies in proportion to the ratio between the numerosities to be judged and there are large individual differences in the precision of the ANS within an age group (Castronovo & Göbel, 2012).

In support of the hypothesis that representations in the ANS may provide a critical underpinning for understanding numbers, Malone *et al.* (2019) found that children's ability to learn associations between arrays of dots of differing magnitudes and spoken nonwords or abstract visual symbols were both predictors of variations in children's arithmetic skills. In addition, there is evidence suggesting that variations in nonsymbolic number judgment skill (using stimuli like those in Figure 52.3) measured at roughly 5.5 years of age are predictive of later number ordering skills, which in turn predict arithmetic skill some 2 years later (Malone *et al.*, 2021).

Number knowledge

Formal arithmetic depends upon having intact representations of numbers represented as both verbal codes (the spoken word "three") and visual codes (the Arabic numeral "3") and the ability to translate between them. Concretely, a young child presented with the sum 3 + 2 may be heard to say aloud the digit names and then count to generate an answer (3, 4, 5—before saying the correct answer of 5). There is very good evidence that measures of number knowledge, such as the ability to read and write numbers, are very strong predictors of formal arithmetic skill in young children (Göbel *et al.*, 2014; Malone *et al.*, 2020). Problems in learning Arabic numerals therefore appear to be another critical foundation for learning arithmetic (just as learning letter–sound relationships is critical for learning to read and write).

Number ordering (ordinal number knowledge)

A distinct aspect of number knowledge is understanding the ordinal relationship between numbers (e.g., that 5 comes later than 3 in the count sequence) and the association of this with arithmetic skill appears to increase with age (Lyons *et al.*, 2014). Malone *et al.* (2021), showed that ordinal number knowledge was underpinned by the ANS and this, in turn, supports the development of formal arithmetic skills.

General processing constraints

Beyond the number system, general cognitive resources are required to develop proficiency in arithmetic, not least because mathematics requires the storage and manipulation of information in working memory, and problem-solving often requires the comprehension of problems cast in words.

Executive function

EF is typically described as a set of higher-order cognitive processes important for planning and problem-solving. These skills include working memory, cognitive flexibility, attention, and inhibitory control and it has been suggested that these disparate skills may be subsumed under a factor for general cognitive ability (Himi *et al.*, 2021)

There is good evidence that measures of EF are predictors of arithmetic (Nesbitt *et al.*, 2015; Halverson *et al.*, 2021; see Cragg & Gilmore (2014) for a review), and it has been suggested that EF supports the manipulation of numerical information in mind, suppression of distractions, and engagement in flexible thinking. A critical issue is whether EF is a unique predictor of arithmetic development after accounting for other

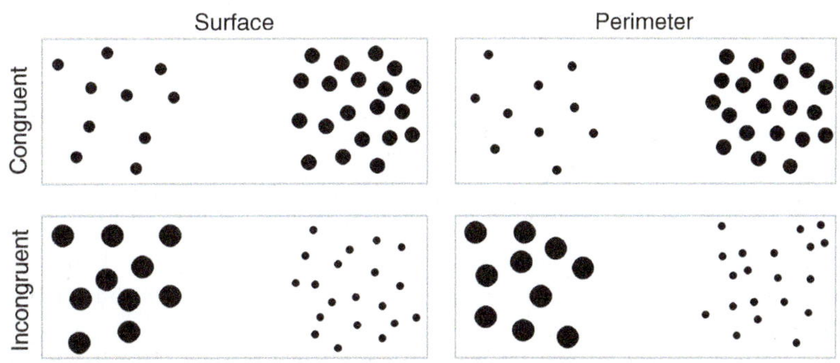

Figure 52.3 Examples of a task to assess magnitude representation. The child decides which of the two displays (in each row) contain more dots (here physical size does not provide a clue). Reaction time is measured. *Source:* Soltész *et al.* (2010)/Springer Nature/CC BY-4.0.

skills. Clinically, it is likely to be more useful to focus on proximal skills (such as number knowledge) when assessing and providing interventions for MD rather than assessing EF skills.

Language skills

Arithmetic is at least partly a verbal skill and measures of arithmetic ability typically correlate moderately to highly with measures of both reading and oral language skills. There appear to be quite specific links between knowledge of math-specific vocabulary and numeracy skills, with the relationship between general language skills and numeracy skills in preschool children being fully mediated by measures of their math language skills (Purpura & Reid, 2016). Furthermore, training math language skills directly in a dialogic reading intervention improved preschool children's numeracy skills (Purpura *et al.*, 2017).

Summary

To summarize, mathematical skills depend upon a complex interplay between nonverbal and verbal cognitive systems, and mathematical skills are arguably more diverse and more complex than reading skills. It seems likely from a cognitive perspective that mathematical difficulties result from several underlying cognitive deficits, some of which may be specific to MD and others shared with co-occurring disorders. Possible specific deficits include early impairments in nonverbal magnitude representations (the ANS), as well as the creation of links between such magnitude representations and the verbal and written representations of number.

Genetic risk factors and brain correlates of mathematics disorder

Heritability of mathematical abilities

There appear to be substantial genetic influences on the development of mathematical skills, and the findings of a small-scale study of parent-adopted offspring supports this view: the mathematical skills of birth parent–offspring pairs were high whereas those between adoptive mother and child were low (Borriello *et al.*, 2020). In an earlier large-scale UK twin study, Kovas *et al.* (2005) found evidence for substantial heritability for variations in mathematical skill in the general population and substantial overlaps between the genes responsible for arithmetic and general intelligence, and arithmetic and reading. Focusing on mathematical difficulties (as opposed to normal variations in mathematical skills), Oliver *et al.* (2004) reporting a heritability estimate of 0.65. Together, these results are compatible with the same genetic influences operating across the range of individual differences in mathematical skills observed within the population (Plomin & Kovas, 2005). To date, there has been little progress in identifying the genetic markers that are involved; extant studies (e.g., Ludwig *et al.*, 2013; Pettigrew *et al.*, 2015) have low power and are hence inconclusive.

There have been fewer studies of the brain correlates of mathematics than of reading. According to a review of brain-imaging studies by Peters and De Smedt (2018), a network of interconnected brain regions is involved including prefrontal, posterior parietal, occipito-temporal, and hippocampal areas. An area that has generated considerable research interest is the left horizontal intra-parietal sulcus (HIPS), since Isaacs *et al.* (2001) reported a specific reduction in grey matter in this region in a group of adolescents with mathematical difficulties (without reading problems). An influential hypothesis is that networks in this area specializing in spatial processing overlap with networks subserving number processing and create a kind of "mental blackboard" for mathematical operations. The role of these parietal circuits in operations requiring magnitude estimation seems particularly important (Hawes & Ansari, 2020). Consistent with this, Roell *et al.* (2021), found a correlation between measures of HIPS anatomy (the extent to which there were perpendicular branches sectioning the HIPS in the right and the left hemisphere), math fluency, and number comparison ability but not nonsymbolic (dot patterns) number judgment. Similarly, studies in adults using repetitive transcranial magnetic stimulation (rTMS) to disrupt the functioning of this area of the brain led to problems with judgments requiring number comparison (Göbel *et al.*, 2004) and with simple addition and subtraction (Montefinese *et al.*, 2017).

Environmental risk factors

Mathematics, like all aspects of learning, is subject to environmental influences. While likely to reflect genetic influences, aspects of the home numeracy environment, such as activities involving counting objects, identifying written numbers, and playing board games that involve counting, are considered important for developing a foundation for number skills (LeFevre *et al.*, 2009). Such measures correlate positively with children's arithmetic skills both concurrently (Kleemans *et al.*, 2012) and longitudinally (Skwarchuk *et al.*, 2014; Casey *et al.*, 2018). One recent experimental study (Gibson *et al.*, 2020) found improvements in 2–4-year-old children's understanding of numbers after an intervention in which parents read books that involved counting objects to their children once a day for 4 weeks (parents in a control condition read books that did not involve counting objects). Clearly more randomized experiments, over a longer duration, will be necessary to establish the role of different influences of the home environment on the development of early number skills.

Developmental coordination disorder

Definitions and characteristics

The ICD-11 criteria for diagnosis of DCD is "a significant delay in the acquisition of gross and fine motor skills and impairment in the execution of coordinated motor skills that manifest in clumsiness, slowness, or inaccuracy of motor performance. Coordinated motor skills are markedly below that expected given the individual's chronological age and level of intellectual functioning" (World Health Organization, 2019). Onset of coordinated motor skills difficulties occurs during the developmental period and is typically apparent from early childhood. Additionally, as in DSM-5, such difficulties need to be of a severity such that they interfere with "daily living or academic achievement" and they should not be due to a general medical condition (e.g., cerebral palsy, hemiplegia, or muscular dystrophy).

In practice, the symptoms of DCD vary considerably (Wilson *et al.*, 2017). They may include gross motor difficulties, such as problems running, hopping, jumping, catching a ball, postural control, and balancing, and fine motor difficulties including a lack of manual dexterity, and difficulty in doing up buttons and laces, in dressing, and in using scissors or cutlery. Speech-motor skills can be affected and problems of pencil control are widespread.

Population estimates of the incidence of DCD vary widely (from 1.8% to 8%) (Biotteau *et al.*, 2020) and a sex ratio of between 2:1 and 3:1 of boys to girls with DCD has been reported (Wright & Sugden, 1996). A mistaken view is that children with DCD grow out of their difficulties; follow-up studies are rare but evidence suggests that such children remain less physically competent throughout adolescence and adulthood. Difficulties in secondary school include problems with handwriting and the presentation of work, and difficulties in science, art, design, and technology. A small-scale study by Hill *et al.* (2017) suggests that young people with DCD are prone to anxiety, are vulnerable to bullying and loneliness, and school refusal is common. More generally, individuals with DCD may become increasingly reluctant to take part in physical activity, placing them at risk of obesity and cardiovascular disease (Tal-saban *et al.*, 2012).

Etiology and co-occurring features

There is evidence that low birth weight or prematurity increases the risk of developing DCD (Jongmans *et al.*, 1996). Furthermore, clinical examination may reveal neurological symptoms such as choreiform movements of unsupported limbs in such children. More generally, the comorbidity of DCD with impairments of reading and language, as well as with ADHD and ASD, suggests shared genetic risk with these other developmental disorders.

Several twin studies have assessed the genetic contribution to DCD. The heritability estimates range from 0.44 (Moruzzi *et al.*, 2010) to 0.7 (Lichtenstein *et al.*, 2010) and there appears to be substantial shared genetic influence on DCD and ADHD (Martin *et al.*, 2006). Mountford *et al.* (2021) used data from the Avon Longitudinal Study of Parents and Children (ALSPAC) to conduct a GWAS of motor coordination and motor disorders, but the findings are inconclusive. Like other NDDs, it seems likely that the genetic contribution to DCD will involve a combination of both rare genes (e.g., 22q11.2 deletion) that affect a number of NDDs (Cunningham *et al.*, 2018), and common gene variants.

Abnormal maturation of several brain regions has been implicated in DCD including the cerebellum, basal ganglia, and parietal and frontal lobes. Functional imaging studies confirm anomalies in these areas, as well as cingulate cortex and lingual gurus, suggesting the involvement of an extensive brain network (Biotteau *et al.*, 2016; Wilson *et al.*, 2017) but no clear brain signature.

Explanations for development coordination disorder

The normal development of motor skills is heavily dependent on maturational changes. Most crucially, however, most motor actions depend on visual information to initiate and guide movements. It has been proposed that guidance of movements in space depends upon a sensorimotor map that serves to translate visually perceived locations to spatially appropriate action patterns (Held & Hein, 1963) and deficits in this sensorimotor map may provide a unifying cognitive explanation for many of the problems seen in motor control in children with DCD.

Recent meta-analyses have revealed deficits of large effect size when comparing individuals with DCD with controls across a range of perceptual, motor, and EF tasks (Wilson *et al.*, 2017). While a dearth of longitudinal studies makes it difficult to ascertain the significance of such deficits, there are four main hypotheses regarding the causes of DCD (Biotteau *et al.*, 2020).

First, there is strong evidence for an association between visual perceptual problems and motor disorders (in the absence of problems with visual acuity) in DCD, with the greatest deficiency being observed in visuospatial tasks which have a motor component. For example, children with DCD have difficulty in imitating gestures. The deficit, which is thought to affect one-third of children with DCD appears to primarily involve perception–action coupling and motor learning is compromised as a result.

Second, it has been hypothesized that children with DCD have deficits in procedural learning. At least three stages are involved in learning new motor tasks: fast learning, slower consolidation, and, finally, automation (in which the skill can be performed without attention). Children with DCD are unable to automate skills or transfer them to a new domain. This means that they have difficulty in adapting motor movements by building on past experiences and in such situations show more variable and error-prone performance than typically developing children.

A third likely causal explanation for DCD is a problem with the internal modeling of motor movements, that is with neural mechanisms that allow movements to be predicted and corrected before sensorimotor feedback becomes available. A meta-analysis of 48 studies investigating the operation of this mechanism revealed deficits of predictive control across all "effector" systems: in visuospatial attention and oculomotor control, control of manual action, and dynamic postural control (Adams *et al.*, 2014).

Finally, executive deficits have been identified in children and in adults with DCD affecting cognitive processes such as working memory, fluency, and planning, as well as self-regulation. These deficits have been offered as explanations for problems with personal organization and time management. However, studies have not typically excluded children with comorbid ADHD and therefore the extent to which these impairments are causally linked with DCD remains unclear. Nonetheless, they remain stable over time and may have adverse consequences for quality of life in adulthood.

Comorbidities of learning disorders

A shift from models of NDDs that regard them as "specific" and "selective" to multifactorial theories has led to a better understanding of the nature and causes of SLDs (McGrath *et al.*, 2020). Multiple-deficit approaches recognize that the behavioral profiles of NDDs result from interactions between biological, cognitive, and environmental risk and protective factors (Pennington *et al.*, 2012). Within this conceptualization, there is a distinction between specific and shared risk factors for disorders—comorbidity is the outcome when risk factors are shared between two (or more) disorders. For example, early language difficulties are a shared risk factor for both reading and mathematical impairments (Snowling *et al.*, 2021). Notwithstanding this, different disorders have different core deficits, and these are likely to be weighted more strongly than other deficits in determining outcomes.

Shared and common cognitive risk factors for reading and mathematics disorders

The comorbidity between RD and MD is well researched. There is little doubt that this reflects shared genetic risk factors for both conditions—so call "generalist" genes that predispose an individual to experience problems of neural development (Plomin & Kovas, 2005). At a cognitive level, domain-general risk factors which have been associated with both disorders include working memory impairments, EF deficits, attention problems, and slow processing speed—factors that also suggest possible comorbidity with ADHD, as well as with DLD (Viesel-Nordmeyer *et al.*, 2023). A schematic summary of specific and shared risk factors between RD and MD is shown in Figure 52.4.

Comorbidity between specific learning disorders, and emotional and behavioral disorders

The causal relationships between educational attainment, behavior, and emotion are complex, and the presence of comorbidities complicates the developmental course of SLDs. While there is an established association between reading difficulties and psychiatric symptoms (e.g., Carroll *et al.*, 2005; Francis *et al.*, 2019), few studies focus on mathematics, excepting research on "math anxiety" (e.g., Dowker *et al.*, 2016).

Margari *et al.* (2013) examined the presence of emotional and behavioral disorders in children and young people aged 7–16 years with SLDs, including reading, writing, and MDs. SLD was comorbid with ADHD in 33% of the sample, anxiety disorder in 28.8%, DCD in 17.8%, language disorder in 11%, and mood disorder in 9.4% of patients. Sex appears to be an important moderating factor, especially in relation to the link between poor reading and low mood: Willcutt and Pennington (2000) reported heightened levels of depression in girls, whereas Carroll *et al.* (2005) found that self-reported low mood was more common in boys than girls.

Along similar lines, Visser *et al.* (2020) investigated the prevalence of comorbid emotional and behavioral problems in German children with SLD in reading, spelling, and/or arithmetic from Grades 3 and 4. The study sample was assessed using web-based tests of reading, spelling, arithmetic, and intelligence,

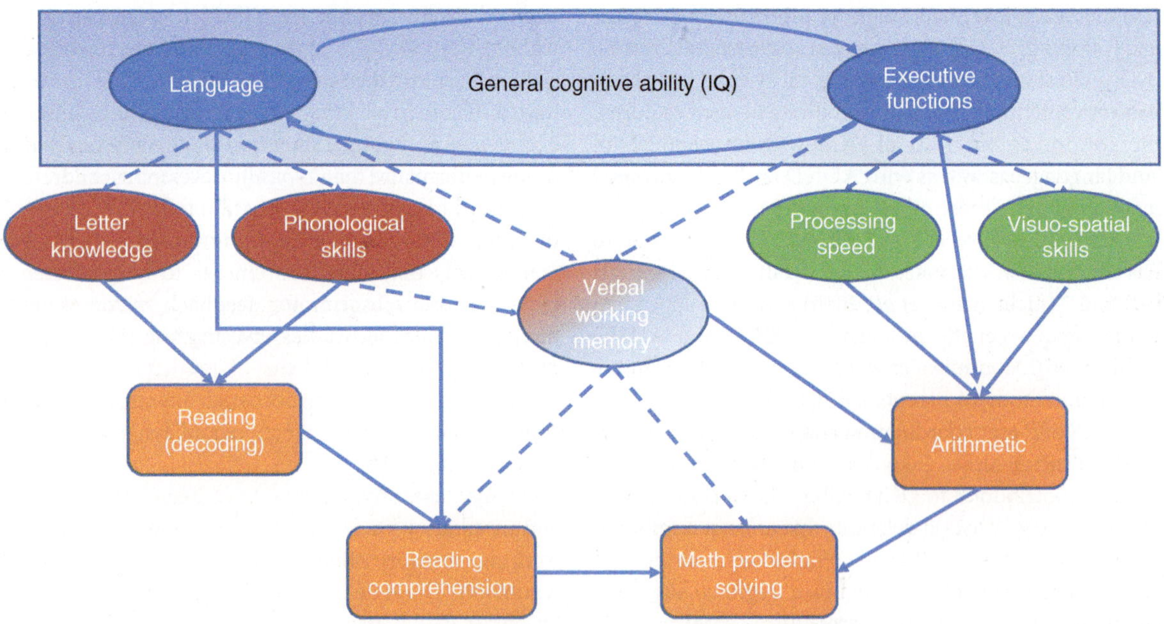

Figure 52.4 Schematic diagram showing causal risk factors (solid lines) for reading disorders (RD) and mathematics disorders (MD), and correlated skills (dotted lines).

and parents completed questionnaires tapping psychiatric symptoms. There were high rates of anxiety disorder, depression, ADHD, and conduct disorder in the sample (respectively 21%, 28%, 28%, and 22%) and children with deficits in multiple learning domains had more psychiatric comorbidities.

Drawing together these findings, Donolato *et al.* (2022) report a meta-analysis of the associations between language and learning disorders and internalizing and externalizing disorders. In this study, internalizing disorders included anxiety and/or depression, and externalizing problems included aggressive behaviors, rule-breaking, and conduct and oppositional difficulties. In line with previous findings, children with learning disorders showed elevated rates of both types of disorder. The size of effects was moderated by primary disorder: children with DLD showed the highest rates of internalizing disorders and girls were more prone to internalizing than boys, whereas the moderators of externalizing disorders were less clear-cut.

Finally, reviewing the relationship between dyslexia and mental health, Deighton *et al.* (2020) suggest the need to better understand three key pathways: (i) common risk factors; (ii) reading difficulties leading to mental health problems via low self-esteem, stigma, and bullying; and (iii) mental health problems exacerbating the impact of reading difficulties through mechanisms such as low motivation linked with expectation of failure, especially where symptoms of depression and anxiety are present.

Turning to DCD, Piek *et al.* (2010) reported a weak but significant association between gross motor performance across preschool and symptoms of both anxiety/depression and anxiety at 6 and 12 years. The data confirm clinical reports of heightened levels of anxiety among children with DCD although for many, psychosocial outcomes are reasonably good with low self-esteem restricted to the motor domain (Losse *et al.*, 1991).

In summary, an important area for future research is the course of emotional and behavioral adjustment in individuals with learning disorders and sources of resilience (e.g., Haft *et al.*, 2016), not least because many children with specific difficulties in literacy, numeracy, or motor skills are relatively free of mental health problems.

Longitudinal outcomes of specific learning disorders

There is stability in literacy skills from an early age and although there has been discussion of "compensated" dyslexia, most poor readers continue to have problems of reading fluency, spelling, and phonological awareness through into the adult years (Maughan *et al.*, 2009). There is also evidence that educational attainment is strongly predicted by literacy skills (Snowling *et al.*, 2001). Furthermore, it is likely that the effects of reduced reading experience are cumulative, causing differences in reading competence to become magnified over time; in turn career prospects are restricted. Despite this, Maughan and Hagell (1996) reported that many adult poor readers had gained employment, albeit in roles where there were restricted literacy demands and hence their reading problems were no longer of functional significance. However, young women with a history of specific reading retardation were at increased risk of psychiatric disorder, possibly related to a high rate of relationship breakdown. Male poor readers, in contrast, had more difficulty in gaining independence, though these difficulties were the consequence of difficulties with peer relationships rather than reading problems.

Clinical assessment

Children with SLDs will rarely be referred to child and adolescent mental health services unless such difficulties have contributed to emotional or behavioral difficulties. However, it may be easy to miss a specific language or learning difficulty in a child with a mental health problem. Here we outline an approach to assessment, beginning with a set of questions a clinician might ask about development and educational progress, before outlining the components of a comprehensive assessment battery.

The first step to diagnosing an SLD is via clinical review of an individual's developmental, medical, educational, and family history (Figure 52.5). Risk signs evident from the history include late talking, speech difficulties, delayed motor development, and a slow start in learning the names of colors, letters, and numbers. A family history of reading or math difficulties or an affected older sibling are noteworthy signs. In the case of DCD, tell-tale signs will include significant problems with gross and fine motor coordination and often balance.

Most clinicians will have access to educational data and school reports and a simple questionnaire asking for teacher ratings of reading, spelling, and math can be very helpful. Documentation of whether the child's additional learning needs are recognized, the history of interventions received including speech and language therapy, and any special support currently in place is important. Some simple tests may also aid in determining whether the child needs further assessment.

For dyslexia, these might include asking the child to: repeat some difficult words, such as "preliminary," "philosophical," "statistical," and some nonwords ("bagmivishent," "turnadulatical") to assess whether they do less well than might be expected for their age; to complete a short reading test; and, if mathematical difficulties are noted, a math screener (Box 52.2). For DCD, a questionnaire is useful and often the Strengths and Difficulties Questionnaire (SDQ; Goodman, 1999) will also have been completed and can provide information as to whether the child has issues with attention control, and if they may be at risk of emotional or behavioral difficulties. If problems with language or communication are suspected, then a questionnaire completed by carers or teachers can highlight the need for further assessment.

Together the findings will enable the clinical team to decide:

- Does the child's school have sufficient resources to support the child without further educational assessment?

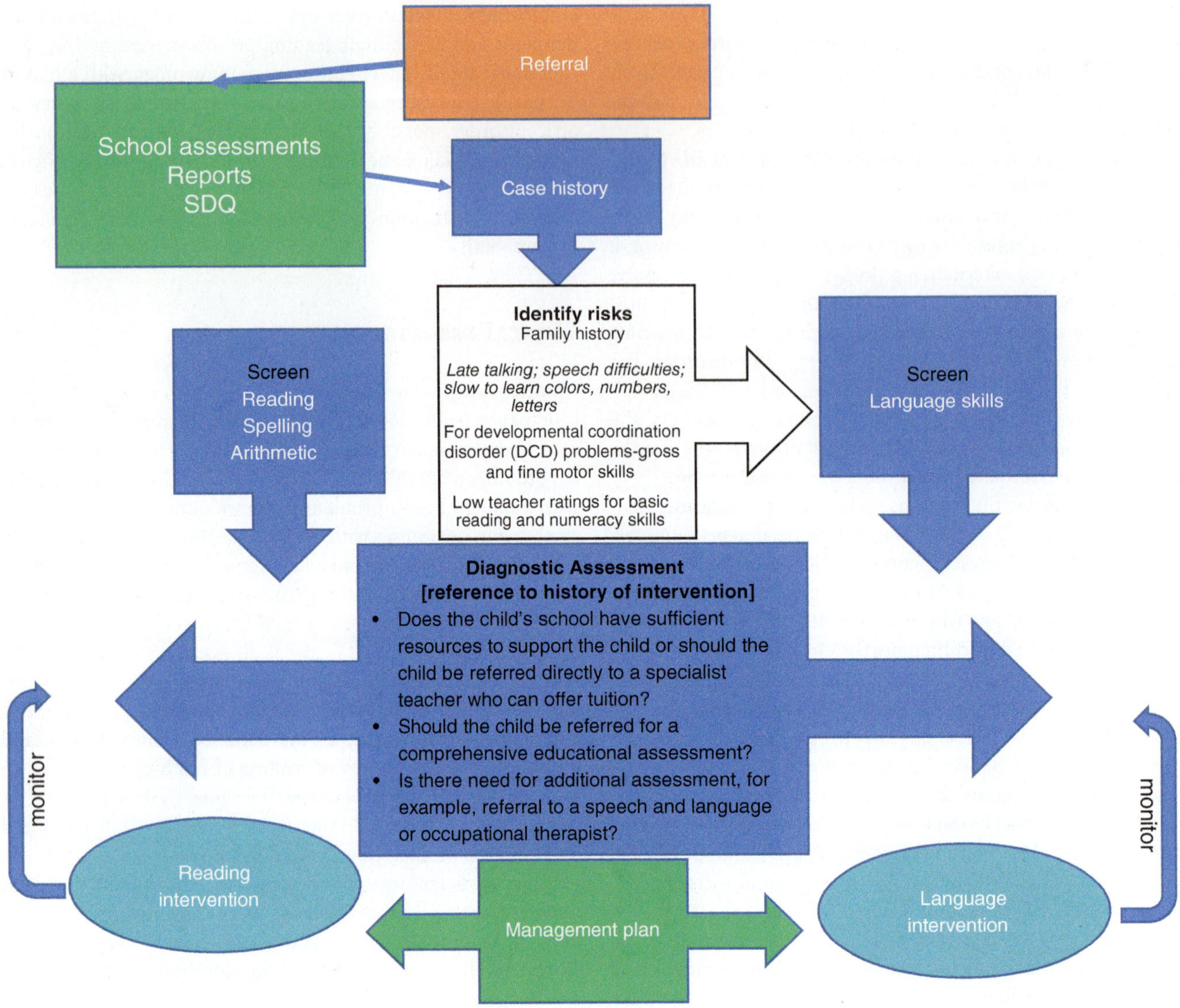

Figure 52.5 Flowchart for clinician.

- Should the child be referred directly to a specialist teacher who can offer tuition?
- Should the child be referred for a comprehensive educational assessment (see the following section "Diagnostic assessment")?
- Is there a need for additional assessment, for example, referral to a speech and language therapist or, in the case of motor incoordination, to an occupational therapist?

Diagnostic assessment

While it is common for an educational or school psychologist to undertake a diagnostic assessment of educational needs, in the UK and US, a dyslexia assessment can normally be undertaken by a specialist teacher. To provide a preliminary picture of whether an SLD is present, this should include tests of single word and nonword reading and spelling alongside assessments of phonological awareness and RAN, and a test of arithmetic skills. If, as the result of this brief assessment, it is suspected that a child has broader language difficulties, then tests of sentence and nonword repetition can confirm whether referral to a speech and language therapist is necessary.

In practice, to provide a comprehensive picture of a child's learning problems and teaching needs, an assessment should include measures of single word reading and spelling, reading comprehension, and expressive writing skills. Measures of phonological awareness, RAN, and verbal short-term memory are usually included because of their value as concurrent predictors of dyslexia. The Comprehensive Test of Phonological Processing 2 (Wagner *et al.*, 2013) provides a robust assessment of these processing skills. The assessment will have more value if it proceeds to assess the reading strategies the child is using (phonic strategies versus guessing from context) and the nature of spelling errors (phonetically accurate or not) with a view to prescribing

Box 52.2 Screening in child and adolescent mental health services at a glance

Case history

- Risk signs for SLDs:
  - family history or an affected older sibling
  - late talking, speech difficulties
  - slow start in learning the names of colors, letters, and numbers
- Risk signs for DCD:
  - motor milestones delayed
  - problems with gross and fine motor coordination
- Educational data
  - teacher ratings of reading, spelling, and math below age expectation
  - weak oral language skills
  - does not recognize letters, characters, or digits
  - does not know sounds and/or names of letters/symbols/characters
  - less proficient in phonics than peers
  - makes spelling errors that are not phonetically accurate
  - does not know numbers sequence or cannot count
  - poor pencil control and handwriting
  - poor coordination; does not like physical education or games
- History of interventions
  - speech and language therapy
  - reading intervention/extra phonics
  - private tuition

Examples of screening tests

- For reading fluency: Test of Word Reading Efficiency (TOWRE-2; Wagner *et al.*, 2011); takes 90 seconds.
- For basic arithmetic: One-minute math test of addition and subtraction—several freely available on the internet, e.g., https://cpb-ap-se2.wpmucdn.com/global2.vic.edu.au/dist/f/57644/files/2015/05/One_Minute_Basic_Facts_Test_-_Instructions_for_Administration-p68k9z.pdf.
- For dyslexia: the following website explains the rationale for assessing nonword repetition and provides a demo, https://www.leadersproject.org/non-word-repetition-tasks.

Questionnaires for completion by carers/teachers

- For DCD: Developmental Coordination Disorder Questionnaire (DCDQ; Green *et al.*, 2005), https://www.dcdq.ca for children aged 5–15 years.
- For attention and psychosocial difficulties: Strengths and Difficulties Questionnaire (SDQ; Goodman, 1999)
- For problems with language or communication: Children's Communication Checklist, www.pearsonclinical.com.au/store/auassessments/en/Store/Professional-Assessments/Speech-%26-Language/Children%27s-Communication-Checklist---Second-Edition/p/P100010033.html.

appropriate intervention. Given the substantial overlap between reading and mathematical difficulties, an assessment of mathematical performance using standardized tests of arithmetic, as well as mathematical problem-solving, should ideally be part of a comprehensive assessment. The Wechsler Individual Assessment Test provides measures of mathematical skills, as well as reading and oral language skills (Wechsler, 2016). The field is divided as to the importance of a test of general cognitive ability. Used judiciously, this can provide useful insights, not only to the profile of strengths and weaknesses but also the individual's language skills and approach to problem-solving.

A diagnosis of DCD normally requires input from an interdisciplinary team. Following medical examination to rule out any neurological involvement, diagnosis should preferably be made following administration of a standardized test of motor skill—the Movement Assessment Battery for Children, 2nd edition (MABC-2) being the most widely used (Henderson *et al.*, 2007). This would usually be accompanied by a test of handwriting skill (e.g., DASH, Barnett, *et al.*, 2007) and by parent and teacher reports of functional difficulties at home and at school—the MABC-2 checklist is useful in this regard (Banátová & Psotta, 2022). Since DCD is commonly comorbid with other developmental disorders, such as language impairment (Hill, 2001), a full psychometric assessment is valuable and the overlap between DCD, autism, and attention problems warrants investigation. In addition, some children will require an orthoptic examination.

It can be challenging for clinicians to provide parents with the answer to the question often foremost in their mind "Is my child dyslexic?" or perhaps "Does my child have dyscalculia?" Current diagnostic practice varies considerably, and although the terms "dyslexia" and "dyscalculia" are more widely accepted in educational circles than in the past, the term "SLD" tends to be preferred. As with all NDDs, clinicians need to emphasize to families the dimensional nature of dyslexia; it can vary from mild to severe, there may be individuals who show some but not all symptoms (likely in families with dyslexia), and the problems that the child experiences may change through development with compensation possible in favorable circumstances.

Treatment for specific learning disorders

Evidence-based interventions for reading, mathematical, and motor impairments are reviewed by Hulme, Donolato, and Melby-Lervag (see Chapter 37). See Table 52.1 for a summary of interventions.

Here, we focus on principles which guide the management of SLDs.

In the preschool and early school years, children are in receipt of a mainstream curriculum and, for many, this is the time when problems in learning will first come to light. Children who enter school with poor language are at high risk of reading and mathematical problems, and parents and teachers need to be alert to these emerging problems so that appropriate interventions can be put into place. Depending on the nature and the severity of the problems, interventions for language, reading, or mathematics will be prioritized, and ideally advice should be given as to how parents can support their child's learning. However, it is important to be mindful that many children with language learning impairments may make a good start in learning to read but fail later as literacy demands increase. Careful

Table 52.1 Summary of interventions for specific learning disorders (SLDs).

Type of learning disorder	Intervention target	Content	Evidence
Reading	Decoding skill	Phoneme awareness and letter training; phonics reading instruction	Strong Large effect size; many studies
	Reading fluency	Repeated reading practice	Moderate effect size
	Reading comprehension	Teaching in small groups training strategies: clarification of text, predicting what happens next, asking questions about the text; summarizing the text	Strong Large effect size in meta-analysis
		Oral language training: vocabulary, narrative; metaphor, etc.	Moderate; few studies
Writing	Spelling	Systematic structured approaches; teaching meaning (morphemic) relationships between words, e.g., "less" in helpless, useless, thoughtless	Few robust studies; most common remediation in clinical practice
	Free writing	Spoken and written narrative; teaching prompts (e.g., when, where, why) and story grammar (structures)	Few robust studies
Mathematics	Arithmetic	Number skills; numerical operations	Strong
	Mathematics	Strategy training; relationships between numbers	Moderate
Developmental coordination disorder	Motor movements	Activity-oriented (training tasks); body-orientated (focusing on body movements)	Few studies; mostly direct training; dosage effects

Source: Hulme *et al.*, Chapter 37.

monitoring of progress is therefore important throughout the primary school years.

Some children with significant SLDs may be slow to respond even to the most effective teaching approach, perhaps because co-occurring problems are impeding progress and require further assessment and management. Aside from this, for children who do not respond to conventional treatments, the best advice is to consider more intensive interventions, including placement in alternative education provision, even if only for a short time. Education technology applications (ed tech apps), for example an app for improving reading fluency—https://www.aisforapp.eu, and other assistive technologies have a lot to offer though few have been subject to robust evaluation.

Ideally, students with SLDs should be taught to become fluent keyboard users, with special instruction in the use of a spell-checker, and voice-recognition software as an aid to written work. In formal assessments and examinations, people with SLDs are normally eligible for special arrangements.

Finally, all who work with children with SLDs are aware of the effort and motivation required to circumvent a learning difficulty during the school years, and to cope with its impact. There is a growing interest in the contribution of cognitive and emotional resilience to the educational outcomes of individuals with SLDs and professionals have a key role to play.

Conclusions and future directions

Understanding of the nature and causes of specific learning difficulties is well advanced and there is a growing body of evidence as to how these can be managed. Mental health professionals have a role to play in identifying SLDs and making appropriate decisions concerning future referrals, interventions, and management. Cognitive models of reading and numeracy development have enabled progress in understanding the nature of dyslexia and dyscalculia, and how they can be assessed. Furthermore, an understanding of the cognitive profile of disorders can foster understanding of links between genes, brain, and behavior. Future research is needed to better understand how comorbidity changes the developmental course and outcomes of SLDs and the implications for mental health.

References

Adams, I.L. *et al.* (2014) Compromised motor control in children with DCD: a deficit in the internal model? A systematic review. *Neuroscience & Biobehavioral Reviews* **47**, 225–244. doi:10.1016/j.neubiorev.2014.08.011.

Adlof, S.M. *et al.* (2022) Learning to read with a language or hearing impairment. In: *The Science of Reading: A Handbook.* (eds M.J. Snowling, *et al.*), 2nd edn. Wiley-Blackwell, Oxford, UK. pp. 460–486.

American Psychiatric Association (2013) *Diagnostic and Statistical Manual of Mental Disorders*, 5th edn. American Psychiatric Association, Washington, DC.

American Psychiatric Association (2022) *Diagnostic and Statistical Manual of Mental Disorders*, 5th edn. text revision edn. American Psychiatric Association, Washington, DC.

Araújo, S. & Faísca, L. (2019) A meta-analytic review of naming-speed deficits in developmental dyslexia. *Scientific Studies of Reading* **23**(5), 349–368. doi:10.1080/10888438.2019.1572758.

Arnett, A.B. *et al.* (2017) Explaining the sex difference in dyslexia. *Journal of Child Psychology and Psychiatry* **58**(6), 719–727. doi:10.1111/jcpp.12691.

Banátová, K. & Psotta, R. (2022) The MABC-2 checklist: a review of the psychometric properties of a screening tool for developmental coordination disorder. *Journal of Occupational Therapy, Schools, & Early Intervention* **15**(1), 72–89. doi:10.1080/19411243.2021.1934228.

Barnett, A. *et al.* (2007) *The Detailed Assessment of Speed of Handwriting (DASH): Manual.* Pearson, London.

Biotteau, M. *et al.* (2016) Neural signature of DCD: a critical review of MRI neuroimaging studies. *Frontiers in Neurology* **7**, 227. doi:10.3389/fneur.2016.00227.

Biotteau, M. *et al.* (2020) Developmental coordination disorder. *Handbook of Clinical Neurology* **174**, 3–20. doi:10.1016/b978-0-444-64148-9.00001-6.

Bonifacci, P. & Snowling, M.J. (2008) Speed of processing and reading disability: a cross-linguistic investigation of dyslexia and borderline intellectual functioning. *Cognition* **107**(3), 999–1017. doi:10.1016/j.cognition.2007.12.006.

Borriello, G.A. *et al.* (2020) The intergenerational transmission of mathematics achievement in middle childhood: a prospective adoption design. *Developmental Science* **23**(6), e12974. doi:10.1111/desc.12974.

Cain, K. (2022) Children's reading comprehension difficulties. In: *The Science of Reading: A Handbook.* (eds M.J. Snowling, *et al.*), 2nd edn. Wiley-Blackwell, Oxford, UK. pp. 298–322.

Caravolas, M. *et al.* (2012) Common patterns of prediction of literacy development in different alphabetic orthographies. *Psychological Science* **23**(6), 678–686. doi:10.1177%2F0956797611434536.

Carroll, J. *et al.* (2005) Literacy difficulties and psychiatric disorders: evidence for co-morbidity. *Journal of Child Psychology & Psychiatry* **46**, 524–532. doi:10.1111/j.1469-7610.2004.00366.x.

Carroll, J.M. *et al.* (2016) Predicting dyslexia using prereading skills: the role of sensorimotor and cognitive abilities. *Journal of Child Psychology and Psychiatry* **57**(6), 750–758. doi:10.1111/jcpp.12488.

Casey, B.M. *et al.* (2018) Maternal support of children's early numerical concept learning predicts preschool and first-grade math achievement. *Child Development* **89**(1), 156–173. doi:10.1111/cdev.12676.

Castronovo, J. & Göbel, S.M. (2012) Impact of high mathematics education on the number sense. *PLoS One* **7**(4), e33832. doi:10.1371/journal.pone.0033832.

Chow, B.W.Y. *et al.* (2017) Home environmental influences on children's language and reading skills in a genetically sensitive design: are socioeconomic status and home literacy environment environmental mediators and moderators? *Scandinavian Journal of Psychology* **58**(6), 519–529. doi:10.1111/sjop.12397.

Christopher, M.E. *et al.* (2015) Genetic and environmental etiologies of the longitudinal relations between prereading skills and reading. *Child Development* **86**(2), 342–361. doi:10.1111%2Fcdev.12295.

Cragg, L. & Gilmore, C. (2014) Skills underlying mathematics: the role of executive function in the development of mathematics proficiency. *Trends in Neuroscience and Education* **3**(2), 63–68. doi:10.1016/j.tine.2013.12.001.

Cunningham, A.C. *et al.* (2018) Developmental coordination disorder, psychopathology and IQ in 22q11. 2 deletion syndrome. *The British Journal of Psychiatry* **212**(1), 27–33. doi:10.1192%2Fbjp.2017.6.

Dehaene, S. (1992) Varieties of numerical abilities. *Cognition* **44**(1–2), 1–42. doi:10.1016/0010-0277(92)90049-n.

Dehaene, S. (1999) *The Number Sense: How the Mind Creates Mathematics.* Penguin, London.

Deighton, J. *et al.* (2020) *Dyslexia and Allied Reading Difficulties and Their Relationship with Mental Health Problems: A rapid Review of Evidence.* Children and Families Policy Research Unit (CPRU)/University College London, London. Available: https://www.ucl.ac.uk/children-policy-research/sites/children_policy_research/files/cpru_dyslexia_and_mental_health_june_2020.pdf [11 November 2024].

Devoto, F. *et al.* (2022) A meta-analysis of functional neuroimaging studies on developmental dyslexia across European orthographies: the ADOD model. *Language, Cognition and Neuroscience* **37**(3), 285–314. doi:10.1080/23273798.2021.1970200.

Di Folco, C. *et al.* (2022) Epidemiology of reading disability: a comparison of DSM-5 and ICD-11 criteria. *Scientific Studies of Reading* **26**(4), 337–355. doi:10.1080/10888438.2021.1998067.

Donolato, E. *et al.* (2022) Research review: language and specific learning disorders in children and their co-occurrence with internalizing and externalizing problems: a systematic review and meta-analysis. *Journal of Child Psychology and Psychiatry* **63**(5), 507–518. doi:10.1111/jcpp.13536.

Dowker, A. *et al.* (2016) Mathematics anxiety: what have we learned in 60 years? *Frontiers in Psychology* **7**, 508. doi:10.3389%2Ffpsyg.2016.00508.

Francis, D.A. *et al.* (2019) The association between poor reading and internalising problems: a systematic review and meta-analysis. *Clinical Psychology Review* **67**, 45–60. doi:10.1016/j.cpr.2018.09.002.

Geary, D.C. (2004) Mathematics and learning disabilities. *Journal of Learning Disabilities* **37**(1), 4–15. doi:10.1177/00222194040370010201.

Gialluisi, A. *et al.* (2019) Genome-wide association scan identifies new variants associated with a cognitive predictor of dyslexia. *Translational Psychiatry* **9**(1), 77. doi:10.1038/s41398-019-0402-0.

Gibson, D.J. *et al.* (2020) Causal effects of parent number talk on preschoolers' number knowledge. *Child Development* **91**(6), e1162–e1177. doi:10.1111/cdev.13423.

Gilmore, C. *et al.* (2018) *An Introduction to Mathematical Cognition.* Routledge, London/New York.

Göbel, S.M. *et al.* (2004) Response-selection-related parietal activation during number comparison. *Journal of Cognitive Neuroscience* **16**(9), 1536–1551. doi:10.1162/0898929042568442.

Göbel, S.M. *et al.* (2014) Children's arithmetic development: it is number knowledge, not the approximate number sense, that counts. *Psychological Science* **25**(3), 789–798. doi:10.1177/0956797613516471.

Goodman, R. (1999) The extended version of the strengths and difficulties questionnaire as a guide to child psychiatric caseness and consequent burden. *The Journal of Child Psychology and Psychiatry and Allied Disciplines* **40**(5), 791–799. doi:10.1111/1469-7610.00494.

Gough, P.B. & Tunmer, W.E. (1986) Decoding, reading, and reading disability. *Remedial and Special Education* **7**(1), 6–10. doi:10.1177/074193258600700104.

Grainger, J. *et al.* (2016) A vision of reading. *Trends in Cognitive Sciences* **20**(3), 171–179. doi:10.1016/j.tics.2015.12.008.

Green, D. *et al.* (2005) Is questionnaire-based screening part of the solution to waiting lists for children with developmental coordination disorder? *British Journal of Occupational Therapy* **68**(1), 2–10. doi:10.1177/030802260506800102.

Haft, S.L. *et al.* (2016) Socio-emotional and cognitive resilience in children with reading disabilities. *Current Opinion in Behavioral Sciences* **10**, 133–141. doi:10.1016/j.cobeha.2016.06.005.

Halverson, K.K. *et al.* (2021) Executive functioning with the NIH EXAMINER and inference making in struggling readers. *Developmental Neuropsychology* **46**(3), 213–231. doi:10.1080/87565641.2021.1908291.

Hämäläinen, J.A. *et al.* (2012) Basic auditory processing deficits in dyslexia: systematic review of the behavioral and event-related potential/field evidence. *Journal of Learning Disabilities* **46**(5), 413–427. doi:10.1177/0022219411436213.

Hawes, Z. & Ansari, D. (2020) What explains the relationship between spatial and mathematical skills? A review *of evidence from brain and behavior. Psychonomic Bulletin & Review* **27**, 465–482. doi:10.3758/s13423-019-01694-7.

Hayiou-Thomas, M.E. *et al.* (2017) When does speech sound disorder matter for literacy? The role of disordered speech errors, co-occurring language impairment and family risk of dyslexia. *Journal of Child Psychology and Psychiatry* **58**(2), 197–205. doi:10.1111/jcpp.12648.

Held, R. & Hein, A. (1963) Movement-produced stimulation in the development of visually guided behavior. *Journal of Comparative and Physiological Psychology* **56**(5), 872–876. doi:10.1037/h0040546.

Henderson, S.E. *et al.* (2007) Movement Assessment Battery for Children-2 [Database record]. *APA PsycTests*. doi:10.1037/t55281-000.

Hendren, R.L. *et al.* (2018) Recognizing psychiatric comorbidity with reading disorders. *Frontiers in Psychiatry* **101**. doi:10.3389/fpsyt.2018.00101.

Hill, E.L. (2001) Non-specific nature of specific language impairment: a review of the literature with regard to concomitant motor impairments. *International Journal of Language & Communication Disorders* **36**(2), 149–171. doi:10.1080/13682820010019874.

Hill, E. *et al.* (2017) Motor and coordination difficulties in children with emotional and behavioural difficulties. *Emotional and Behavioural Difficulties* **22**(4), 293–302. doi:10.1080/13632752.2017.1287400.

Himi, S.A. *et al.* (2021) Advancing the understanding of the factor structure of executive functioning. *Journal of Intelligence* **9**(1), 16. doi:10.3390/jintelligence9010016.

Hoeft, F. *et al.* (2011) Neural systems predicting long-term outcome in dyslexia. *Proceedings of the National Academy of Sciences* **108**(1), 361–366. doi:10.1073/pnas.1008950108.

Huber, E. *et al.* (2018) Rapid and widespread white matter plasticity during an intensive reading intervention. *Nature Communications* **9**(1), 2260. doi:10.1038/s41467-018-04627-5.

Isaacs, E.B. *et al.* (2001) Calculation difficulties in children of very low birthweight: a neural correlate. *Brain* **124**(9), 1701–1707. doi:10.1093/brain/124.9.1701.

Jerrim, J. *et al.* (2015) The socio-economic gradient in children's reading skills and the role of genetics. *British Educational Research Journal* **41**(1), 6–29. doi:10.1002/berj.3143.

Jongmans, M. *et al.* (1996) How local is the impact of a specific learning difficulty on premature children's evaluation of their own competence? *Journal of Child Psychology and Psychiatry* **37**(5), 563–568. doi:10.1111/j.1469-7610.1996.tb01442.x.

Kleemans, T. *et al.* (2012) Child and home predictors of early numeracy skills in kindergarten. *Early Childhood Research Quarterly* **27**(3), 471–477. doi:10.1016/j.ecresq.2011.12.004.

Kovas, Y. *et al.* (2005) 'Generalist genes' and mathematics in 7-year-old twins. *Intelligence* **33**(5), 473–489. doi:10.1016/j.intell.2005.05.002.

LeFevre, J.A. *et al.* (2009) Home numeracy experiences and children's math performance in the early school years. *Canadian Journal of Behavioural Science* **41**(2), 55–66. doi:10.1037/A0014532.

Lervåg, A. *et al.* (2019) Socioeconomic background, nonverbal IQ and school absence affects the development of vocabulary and reading comprehension in children living in severe poverty. *Developmental Science* **22**(5), e12858. doi:10.1111/desc.12858.

Lichtenstein, P. *et al.* (2010) The genetics of autism spectrum disorders and related neuropsychiatric disorders in childhood. *American Journal of Psychiatry* **167**(11), 1357–1363. doi:10.1176/appi.ajp.2010.10020223.

Lin, Y. *et al.* (2020) The prevalence of dyslexia in primary school children and their Chinese literacy assessment in Shantou, China. *International Journal of Environmental Research and Public Health* **17**(19), 7140. doi:10.3390/ijerph17197140.

Little, C.W. & Hart, S.A. (2022) Genetic and environmental influences on learning to read. In: *The Science of Reading: A Handbook*. (eds M.J. Snowling, *et al.*), 2nd edn. Wiley-Blackwell, Oxford, UK. pp. 515–532.

Little, C.W. *et al.* (2017) Cross-study differences in the etiology of reading comprehension: a meta-analytical review of twin studies. *Behavior Genetics* **47**(1), 52–76. doi:10.1007%2Fs10519-016-9810-6.

Losse, A. *et al.* (1991) Clumsiness in children-do they grow out of it? A 10-year follow-up study. *Developmental Medicine and Child Neurology* **33**(1), 55–68. doi:10.1111/j.1469-8749.1991.tb14785.x.

Ludwig, K.U. *et al.* (2013) A common variant in *Myosin-18B* contributes to mathematical abilities in children with dyslexia and intraparietal sulcus variability in adults. *Translational Psychiatry* **3**(2), e229–e229. doi:10.1038/tp.2012.148.

Lyons, I.M. *et al.* (2014) Numerical predictors of arithmetic success in grades 1–6. *Developmental Science* **17**(5), 714–726. doi:10.1111/desc.12152.

Malone, S.A. *et al.* (2019) Learning correspondences between magnitudes, symbols and words: evidence for a triple code model of arithmetic development. *Cognition* **187**, 1–9. doi:10.1016/j.cognition.2018.11.016.

Malone, S.A. *et al.* (2020) Number knowledge and the approximate number system are two critical foundations for early arithmetic development. *Journal of Educational Psychology* **112**(6), 1167. doi:10.1037/edu0000426.

Malone, S.A. *et al.* (2021) Separable effects of the approximate number system, symbolic number knowledge, and number ordering ability on early arithmetic development. *Journal of Experimental Child Psychology* **208**, 105120. doi:10.1016/j.jecp.2021.105120.

Manning, C. *et al.* (2022) Visual motion and decision-making in dyslexia: reduced accumulation of sensory evidence and related neural dynamics. *Journal of Neuroscience* **42**(1), 121–134. doi:10.1523%2FJNEUROSCI.1232-21.2021.

Margari, L. *et al.* (2013) Neuropsychopathological comorbidities in learning disorders. *BMC Neurology* **13**(1), 1–6. doi:10.1186/1471-2377-13-198.

Martin, N.C. *et al.* (2006) DCD and ADHD: a genetic study of their shared aetiology. *Human Movement Science* **25**(1), 110–124. doi:10.1016/j.humov.2005.10.006.

Maughan, B. & Hagell, A. (1996) Poor readers in adulthood: psychosocial functioning. *Development and Psychopathology* **8**(2), 457–476. doi:10.1017/S0954579400007197.

Maughan, B. *et al.* (2009) Persistence of literacy problems: spelling in adolescence and at mid-life. *Journal of Child Psychology and Psychiatry* **50**(8), 893–901. doi:10.1111/j.1469-7610.2009.02079.x.

McBride, C. *et al.* (2022) Reading and reading disordered in Chinese. In: *The Science of Reading: A Handbook*. (eds M.J. Snowling, *et al.*), 2nd edn. Wiley-Blackwell, Oxford, UK. pp. 354–370.

McGrath, L.M. *et al.* (2020) The multiple deficit model: progress, problems, and prospects. *Scientific Studies of Reading* **24**(1), 7–13. doi:10.1080/10888438.2019.1706180.

Melby-Lervåg, M. *et al.* (2012) Phonological skills and their role in learning to read: a meta-analytic review. *Psychological Bulletin* **138**(2), 322. doi:10.1037/a0026744.

Moll, K. *et al.* (2014) Specific learning disorder: prevalence and gender differences. *PLoS One* **9**(7), e103537. doi:10.1371/journal.pone.0103537.

Moll, K. *et al.* (2019) Understanding comorbidity of learning disorders: task-dependent estimates of prevalence. *Journal of Child Psychology and Psychiatry* **60**(3), 286–294. doi:10.1111/jcpp.12965.

Montefinese, M. *et al.* (2017) Causal role of the posterior parietal cortex for two-digit mental subtraction and addition: a repetitive TMS study. *NeuroImage* **155**, 72–81. doi:10.1016/j.neuroimage.2017.04.058.

Morsanyi, K. *et al.* (2018) The prevalence of specific learning disorder in mathematics and comorbidity with other developmental disorders in primary school-age children. *British Journal of Psychology* **109**(4), 917–940. doi:10.1111/bjop.12322.

Moruzzi, S. *et al.* (2010) Clumsiness and psychopathology: causation or shared etiology? A twin study with the CBCL 6–18 questionnaire in a general school-age population sample. *Human Movement Science* **29**(2), 326–338. doi:10.1016/j.humov.2010.01.005.

Mountford, H.S. *et al.* (2021) Genome-wide association study of motor coordination. *Frontiers in Human Neuroscience* **286**. doi:10.3389/fnhum.2021.669902.

Myers, C.A. *et al.* (2014) White matter morphometric changes uniquely predict children's reading acquisition. *Psychological Science* **25**(10), 1870–1883. doi:10.1177/0956797614544511.

Nag, S. (2022) Reading the Akshara writing system. In: *The Science of Reading: A Handbook*. (eds M.J. Snowling, *et al.*), 2nd edn. Wiley-Blackwell, Oxford, UK. pp. 372–389.

Nag, S. & Snowling, M.J. (2012) Reading in an alphasyllabary: implications for a language universal theory of learning to read. *Scientific Studies of Reading* **16**(5), 404–423. doi:10.1080/10888438.2011.576352.

Nag, S. *et al.* (2024) Home learning environments and children's language and literacy skills: a meta-analytic review of studies conducted in low- and middle-income countries. *Psychological Bulletin* **150**(2), 132. doi:10.1037/bul0000417.

Nesbitt, K.T. *et al.* (2015) Executive function skills and academic achievement gains in prekindergarten: contributions of learning-related behaviors. *Developmental Psychology* **51**(7), 865. doi:10.1037/dev0000021.

Nicolson, R.I. & Fawcett, A.J. (1990) Automaticity: a new framework for dyslexia research? *Cognition* **35**(2), 159–182. doi:10.1016/0010-0277(90)90013-a.

O'Brien, G. & Yeatman, J.D. (2021) Bridging sensory and language theories of dyslexia: toward a multifactorial model. *Developmental Science* **24**(3), e3039. doi:10.1111/desc.13039.

O'Brien, G.E. *et al.* (2018) Reading ability and phoneme categorization. *Scientific Reports* **8**(1), 16842. doi:10.1038/s41598-018-34823-8.

Oliver, B. *et al.* (2004) A twin study of teacher-reported mathematics performance and low performance in 7-year-olds. *Journal of Educational Psychology* **96**(3), 504. doi:10.1037/0022-0663.96.3.504.

Paracchini, S. (2022) The genetics of dyslexia: learning from the past to shape the future. In: *The Science of Reading: A Handbook*. (eds M.J. Snowling, *et al.*), 2nd edn. Wiley-Blackwell, Oxford, UK. pp. 491–514.

Paulesu, E. *et al.* (2014) Reading the dyslexic brain: multiple dysfunctional routes revealed by a new meta-analysis of PET and fMRI activation studies. *Frontiers in Human Neuroscience* **8**, 830. doi:10.3389/fnhum.2014.00830.

Pennington, B.F. *et al.* (2012) Individual prediction of dyslexia by single versus multiple deficit models. *Journal of Abnormal Psychology* **121**(1), 212. doi:10.1037/a0025823.

Peters, L. & De Smedt, B. (2018) Arithmetic in the developing brain: a review of brain imaging studies. *Developmental Cognitive Neuroscience* **30**, 265–279. doi:10.1016/j.dcn.2017.05.002.

Pettigrew, K.A. *et al.* (2015) Lack of replication for the myosin-18B association with mathematical ability in independent cohorts. *Genes, Brain and Behavior* **14**(4), 369–376. doi:10.1111/gbb.12213.

Piek, J.P. *et al.* (2010) Do motor skills in infancy and early childhood predict anxious and depressive symptomatology at school age? *Human Movement Science* **29**(5), 777–786. doi:10.1016/j.humov.2010.03.006.

Plomin, R. & Kovas, Y. (2005) Generalist genes and learning disabilities. *Psychological Bulletin* **131**(4), 592. doi:10.1037/0033-2909.131.4.592.

Preston, J.L. *et al.* (2016) Print-speech convergence predicts future reading outcomes in early readers. *Psychological Science* **27**(1), 75–84. doi:10.1177/0956797615611921.

Puglisi, M.L. *et al.* (2017) The home literacy environment is a correlate, but perhaps not a cause, of variations in children's language and literacy development. *Scientific Studies of Reading* **21**(6), 498–514. doi:10.1080/10888438.2017.1346660.

Purpura, D.J. & Reid, E.E. (2016) Mathematics and language: individual and group differences in mathematical language skills in young children. *Early Childhood Research Quarterly* **36**, 259–268. doi:10.1016/j.ecresq.2015.12.020.

Purpura, D.J. *et al.* (2017) Causal connections between mathematical language and mathematical knowledge: a dialogic reading intervention. *Journal of Research on Educational Effectiveness* **10**(1), 116–137. doi:10.1080/19345747.2016.1204639.

Quinn, J.M. & Wagner, R.K. (2015) Gender differences in reading impairment and in the identification of impaired readers: results from a large-scale study of at-risk readers. *Journal of Learning Disabilities* **48**(4), 433–445. doi:10.1177/0022219413508323.

Ramus, F. *et al.* (2013) Phonological deficits in specific language impairment and developmental dyslexia: towards a multidimensional model. *Brain* **136**(2), 630–645. doi:10.1093/brain/aws356.

Richlan, F. (2020) The functional neuroanatomy of developmental dyslexia across languages and writing systems. *Frontiers in Psychology* **11**, 155. doi:10.3389/fpsyg.2020.00155.

Rochelle, K.S. & Talcott, J.B. (2006) Impaired balance in developmental dyslexia? A meta-analysis of the contending evidence. *Journal of Child Psychology and Psychiatry* **47**(11), 1159–1166. doi:10.1111/j.1469-7610.2006.01641.x.

Roell, M. *et al.* (2021) Sulcation of the intraparietal sulcus is related to symbolic but not non-symbolic number skills. *Developmental Cognitive Neuroscience* **51**, 100998. doi:10.1016/j.dcn.2021.100998.

Rose, J. (2009) *Identifying and Teaching Children and Young People with Dyslexia and Literacy Difficulties.* The Dyslexia-SpLD Trust, UK Available: https://www.thedyslexia-spldtrust.org.uk/media/downloads/inline/the-rose-report.1294933674.pdf [15 August 2023].

Saksida, A. *et al.* (2016) Phonological skills, visual attention span, and visual stress in developmental dyslexia. *Developmental Psychology* **52**(10), 1503. doi:10.1037/dev0000184.

Sammons, P. *et al.* (1993) Differential school effectiveness: results from a reanalysis of the Inner London Education Authority's Junior School Project Data. *British Educational Research Journal* **19**(4), 381–405. doi:10.1080/0141192930190407.

Schmalz, X. *et al.* (2019) Is statistical learning ability related to reading ability, and if so, why? *Scientific Studies of Reading* **23**(1), 64–76. doi: 10.1080/10888438.2018.1482304.

Schulte-Körne, G. & Bruder, J. (2010) Clinical neurophysiology of visual and auditory processing in dyslexia: a review. *Clinical Neurophysiology* **121**(11), 1794–1809. doi:10.1016/j.clinph.2010.04.028.

Sénéchal, M. & LeFevre, J.A. (2014) Continuity and change in the home literacy environment as predictors of growth in vocabulary and reading. *Child Development* **85**(4), 1552–1568. doi:10.1111/cdev.12222.

Skwarchuk, S.L. *et al.* (2014) Formal and informal home learning activities in relation to children's early numeracy and literacy skills: the development of a home numeracy model. *Journal of Experimental Child Psychology* **121**, 63–84. doi:10.1016/j.jecp.2013.11.006.

Snowling, M.J. & Melby-Lervåg, M. (2016) Oral language deficits in familial dyslexia: a meta-analysis and review. *Psychological Bulletin* **142**(5), 498. doi:10.1037/bul0000037.

Snowling, M.J. *et al.* (2001) Educational attainments of school leavers with a preschool history of speech-language impairments. *International Journal of Language & Communication Disorders* **36**(2), 173–183. doi:10.1080/13682820120976.

Snowling, M.J. *et al.* (2019) Developmental outcomes for children at high risk of dyslexia and children with developmental language disorder. *Child Development* **90**(5), e548–e564. doi:10.1111/cdev.13216.

Snowling, M.J. *et al.* (2021) Language difficulties are a shared risk factor for both reading disorder and mathematics disorder. *Journal of Experimental Child Psychology* **202**, 105009. doi:10.1016/j.jecp.2020.105009.

Soltész, F. *et al.* (2010) Relationships between magnitude representation, counting and memory in 4-to-7-year-old children: a developmental study. *Behavioral and Brain Functions* **6**, 1–14. doi:10.1186/1744-9081-6-13.

Stanovich, K.E. & Siegel, L.S. (1994) Phenotypic performance profile of children with reading disabilities: a regression-based test of the phonological-core variable-difference model. *Journal of Educational Psychology* **86**(1), 24. doi:10.1037/0022-0663.86.1.24.

Tallal, P. (1980) Auditory temporal perception, phonics, and reading disabilities in children. *Brain and Language* **9**(2), 182–198. doi:10.1016/0093-934x(80)90139-x.

Tal-Saban, M. *et al.* (2012) The functional profile of young adults with suspected developmental coordination disorder (DCD). *Research in Developmental Disabilities* **33**(6), 2193–2202. doi:10.1016/j.ridd.2012.06.005.

Taylor, J.S.H. *et al.* (2013) Can cognitive models explain brain activation during word and pseudoword reading? A meta-analysis of 36 neuroimaging studies. *Psychological Bulletin* **139**, 766. doi:10.1037/a0030266.

Tosto, M.G. *et al.* (2017) The genetic architecture of oral language, reading fluency, and reading comprehension: a twin study from 7 to 16 years. *Developmental Psychology* **53**(6), 1115. doi:10.1037/dev0000297.

Tunmer, W. & Greaney, K. (2010) Defining dyslexia. *Journal of Learning Disabilities* **43**(3), 229–243. doi:10.1177/0022219409345009.

Ullman, M.T. & Pullman, M.Y. (2015) A compensatory role for declarative memory in neurodevelopmental disorders. *Neuroscience & Biobehavioral Reviews* **51**, 205–222. doi:10.1016/j.neubiorev.2015.01.008.

Valdois, S. *et al.* (2019) Visual attention modulates reading acquisition. *Vision Research* **165**, 152–161. doi:10.1016/j.visres.2019.10.011.

van Bergen, E. *et al.* (2018) Why do children read more? The influence of reading ability on voluntary reading practices. *Journal of Child Psychology and Psychiatry* **59**(11), 1205–1214. doi:10.1111/jcpp.12910.

Vandermosten, M. *et al.* (2016) Integrating MRI brain imaging studies of pre-reading children with current theories of developmental dyslexia: a review and quantitative meta-analysis. *Current Opinion in Behavioral Sciences* **10**, 155–161. doi:10.1016%2Fj.cobeha.2016.06.007.

Viesel-Nordmeyer, N. *et al.* (2023) Cognitive profiles of children with isolated and comorbid learning difficulties in reading and math: a meta-analysis. *Educational Psychology Review* **35**(1), 34. doi:10.1007/s10648-023-09735-3.

Visser, L. *et al.* (2020) Comorbidities between specific learning disorders and psychopathology in elementary school children in Germany. *Frontiers in Psychiatry* **292**. doi:10.3389%2Ffpsyt.2020.00292.

Wagner, R. *et al.* (2011) Test of Word Reading Efficiency—Second Edition (TOWRE-2). Available: https://www.pearsonclinical.co.uk/store/ukassessments/en/Store/Professional-Assessments/Speech-%26-Language/Test-of-Word-Reading-Efficiency-%7C-Second-Edition/p/P100009057.html?srsltid=AfmBOop3imXQLm1KN0wwzJ21pTLBuAzX1KwLWhu9U54yisem5WK3OQnm [26 November 2024].

Wagner, R.K. *et al.* (2013) *Comprehensive Test of Phonological Processing (CTOPP2).* Pearson, London.

Wagner, R.K. *et al.* (2020) The prevalence of dyslexia: a new approach to its estimation. *Journal of Learning Disabilities* **53**(5), 354–365. doi:10.1177%2F0022219420920377.

Washington, J.A. (2001) Early literacy skills in African–American children: research considerations. *Learning Disabilities Research & Practice* **16**(4), 213–221. doi:10.1111/0938-8982.00021.

Wechsler, D. (2016) Wechsler Individual Achievement Test - Third UK Edition (WIAT-III UK). Pearson, London. Available: https://www.pearsonclinical.co.uk/store/ukassessments/en/Store/Professional-Assessments/Academic-Learning/Reading/Wechsler-Individual-Achievement-Test---Third-UK-Edition/p/P100009274.html?srsltid=AfmBOopOtdqXD4HjNheA8nBo5psMDuWhERdzZjj70pABNmj4Uzurxx3Q [11 November 2024].

West, G. *et al.* (2018) The procedural learning deficit hypothesis of language learning disorders: we see some problems. *Developmental Science* **21**(2), e12552. doi:10.1111/desc.12552.

Willcutt, E. & Pennington, B. (2000) Psychiatry co-morbidity in children and adolescents with reading disability. *Journal of Child Psychology & Psychiatry* **41**, 1039–1048. doi:10.1111/1469-7610.00691.

Wilson, P.H. *et al.* (2017) Cognitive and neuroimaging findings in developmental coordination disorder: new insights from a systematic review of recent research. *Developmental Medicine and Child Neurology* **59**(11), 1117–1129. doi:10.1111/dmcn.13530.

World Health Organization (2019) *International Statistical Classification of Disease and Related Health Problems*, 11th edn, Geneva, Switzerland.

Wright, H.C. & Sugden, D.A. (1996) A two-step procedure for the identification of children with developmental co-ordination disorder in Singapore. *Developmental Medicine and Child Neurology* **38**(12), 1099–1105. doi:10.1111/j.1469-8749.1996.tb15073.x.

Yeatman, J.D. (2022) The neurobiology of literacy. In: *The Science of Reading: A Handbook*. (eds M.J. Snowling, *et al.*), 2nd edn. Wiley-Blackwell, Oxford, UK. pp. 533–555.

CHAPTER 53

Intellectual disability

Emily Simonoff[1] and Maria Rogdaki[2]

[1] Department of Child and Adolescent Psychiatry, Institute of Psychiatry, Psychology and Neuroscience, King's College London, London, UK

[2] Department of Psychosis Studies, Institute of Psychiatry, Psychology and Neuroscience, King's College London, London, UK

Terminology and classification

Intellectual disability (ID) refers to the presence of significant global and functionally impairing deficits in intellectual functioning that have commenced in early life and persist with development. ID is a descriptive diagnosis with many identified causes, but in many individuals no single cause has been identified. Over the past century, terminology for ID has varied widely including both "learning disability" and "learning difficulties" in the United Kingdom (UK) and, till recently, "mental retardation." Current terminology is Intellectual Disability or Intellectual Developmental Disorder in the *Diagnostic and Statistical Manual of Mental Disorders*, 5th Edition, text revision (DSM-5-TR) and Disorders of Intellectual Development in the *International Classification of Diseases*, 11th Revision (ICD-11). Here we will use the generic term ID.

Diagnostic criteria for ID have two mandatory elements: substantially below average intellectual function, as measured on tests of intelligence quotient (IQ), and significant impairment in adaptive functioning. IQ is typically, but not invariably, expected to be more than two standard deviations below the mean, i.e., <70. Both classification systems now emphasize adaptive functioning. Impairments can occur in communication, social skills, personal independence, and school or work functioning and, where these are substantial, IQ scores of up to 75 are considered consistent with the diagnosis. ID is a developmental disorder, and impairments should be evident in childhood. While the latter makes good sense with respect to etiological differences, it can become a barrier to accessing services when impairment was not noted early on or for people functioning in the ID range with a later acquired condition such as head injury or encephalitis.

The degree of ID is subclassified according to the extent of combined impairment in IQ and adaptive behavior as measured with appropriately normed and standardized tests, or based on clinical indicators if no tests are available. Both DSM-5-TR and ICD-11 provide severity specifiers or behavior indicators, respectively. The boundaries are not firmly fixed and serve as a guide. Mild ID is associated with an IQ of 50–69, moderate ID 35–49, severe ID 20–35, and profound ID below 20. In contrast to clinicians, researchers often distinguish only two groups, referred to as mild ID (IQ 50–69) and severe ID (IQ below 50). This terminology is based on the "two-group" theory of the etiology of ID, discussed in the section "Risk factors for intellectual disability."

While adaptive function correlates moderately well with IQ at a group level (Papazoglou *et al.*, 2013), there are considerable individual differences. In general, people with autism spectrum disorders (ASDs), fragile X, and Williams syndrome perform more poorly on measures of adaptive functioning than would be expected on the basis of their IQ, while those with neurofibromatosis type 1 and Down syndrome show relative strengths in adaptive functioning (Charman *et al.*, 2011). Individual circumstances may also influence the level of adaptive function; family stress and adversity may reduce adaptive function (Koskentausta *et al.*, 2007), while engagement in daily living activities appropriate for developmental level may enhance functioning (Brown *et al.*, 2013).

Neurodiversity and intellectual disability

The concept of neurodiversity was first introduced in relation to autistic traits (Singer, 1999). A neurodiversity perspective argues that cognitive and behavioral differences, alongside the underpinning differences in brain structure and function,

Rutter's Child and Adolescent Psychiatry and Psychology, Seventh Edition.
Edited by Anita Thapar, Daniel S. Pine, Samuele Cortese, Cathy Creswell, Tamsin J. Ford, James F. Leckman, and Argyris Stringaris.

Companion website: www.wiley.com/go/thapar/rutterspsych7

reflect a continuum in which biological and cultural diversity should be valued characteristics. The broader model also argues the social and mental health disadvantages experienced by neurodiverse individuals arise because the environment is configured for the majority neurotypical population. More generally, the neurodiversity movement promotes the use of nonstigmatizing language in everyday life and a focus on individual strengths rather than impairments (Baron-Cohen, 2017). The neurodiversity model contrasts to the biopsychosocial disease model, whose most extreme form conceptualizes neurodevelopmental disorders (NDDs) as conditions to be eradicated through prevention and intervention (Sonuga-Barke & Thapar, 2021). While some aspects of prevention and intervention may be universally welcomed, in its extreme form this latter perspective was responsible for the deplorable eugenics movement which included the forced sterilization and prohibition of marriage for people with ID. This has contributed to lasting sensitivities about research, such as the elucidation of genetic risk factors, whose results might enable the implementation of social policies designed to reduce the number of people born with ID. More broadly, people with ID remain disadvantaged within society and have limited opportunities for employment, community participation, and support to live full lives. Possibly more than any other group, they have been excluded from relevant patient, public, and policy involvement, despite recent advances in strategies to elicit the views of those with limited or no spoken communication. While a distinction between diversity and disorder can ensure appropriate services are available for the most vulnerable in society (Nelson, 2021), a neurodiversity approach may promote a focus on strengths, individual choice, and functional goals.

Epidemiology of intellectual disability

Prevalence rates of ID vary widely; recent studies of administrative or parent-reported prevalence rates range between 0.05–1.55% globally (McKenzie *et al.*, 2016). This heterogeneity can be attributed to methodological differences, case definition, study settings, and age groups (Cuypers *et al.*, 2021). Prevalence rates for severe ID (IQ < 50) are consistently reported as 2–5/1000 with variation greatest for mild ID (McKenzie *et al.*, 2016). Severe ID is more likely to be identified regardless of study methods, while accurate detection of mild ID is more dependent on direct measurement. Studies directly measuring IQ in adolescent populations showed rates ranging between 3.2–8.6%, with the majority having milder levels of ID that had not been formally identified by services (Simonoff *et al.*, 2006; Platt *et al.*, 2019,). Many studies have used IQ as the sole criterion, and these tend to report higher rates than those also measuring adaptive function (Maulik *et al.*, 2011). Studies of children and adolescents report substantially higher rates than those of adults. This finding is confounded with methodological factors, but decreased life expectancy likely plays a role.

Factors influencing the prevalence of intellectual disability

Sex

The male excess reported in the prevalence of ID arises from studies relying on administrative prevalence (Zablotsky *et al.*, 2019; Dalsgaard *et al.*, 2020), and those focusing on mild ID directly estimated in the population do not support this (Simonoff *et al.*, 2006; Platt *et al.*, 2019,). The male excess observed in severe ID is likely accurate and mainly due to X-linked genetic disorders affecting males (Neri *et al.*, 2018).

Socioeconomic factors

Socioeconomic adversity is mainly associated with milder ID although one study in a low- to middle-income setting reported an association with both mild and severe ID, possibly suggesting different risk mechanisms (Durkin & Yeargin-Allsopp, 2018). In high-income countries (HICs), raising a child with ID confers direct and opportunity costs on the family, which can increase socioeconomic disadvantage (Arora *et al.*, 2020). The mechanisms for these associations are likely multiple, including not only familial low IQ and diminished psychosocial stimulation but also poorer pre- and perinatal health care and screening alongside, possibly, occupational exposure to toxins (Hunter *et al.*, 2013).

Ethnicity

Ethnicity can be a risk factor for ID through several mechanisms. Studies in the United States (US) (Croen *et al.*, 2001) and Australia (O'Rance, 2007) show that ethnic minorities are more likely to have ID. The relationship is likely mainly through social disadvantage as the link is with minority status rather than specific ethnicities and the effect is largely accounted for when social disadvantage is considered (Yeargin-Allsopp *et al.*, 1995). Immigrant status has been linked to higher rates of autism with ID (but not autism alone); and the risk may be limited to births around the time of migration hence pointing to pre- and perinatal factors.

Some ethnic groups who have intermarried for many generations may have elevated rates of deleterious genetic mutations (Arcos-Burgos & Muenke, 2002). Consanguinity is more common in certain ethnic groups and has also been associated with autosomal recessive disorders leading to ID (Harlalka *et al.*, 2013).

Geographical differences

Higher rates of ID exist in low- and medium-income countries (LMICs) compared with HICs, with one meta-analysis reporting comparative rates of 16, 15.9, and 9.2/1000, respectively (Maulik *et al.*, 2011). More recent studies in LMICs are lacking, so it is unclear whether improvements in health care may have reduced these disparities. Genetic disorders (and the failure to detect them), maternal factors such as poor nutrition, infectious diseases, pregnancy at early or late age, lack of awareness or access to preventative measures, and poor health care are all modifiable risks that contribute to higher rates of ID in LMICs (Durkin & Yeargin-Allsopp, 2018).

Risk factors for intellectual disability

The two-group theory of ID was first proposed by Lewis (Lewis, 1933) and Penrose (Penrose *et al.*, 1938) and subsequently elaborated by Zigler (Zigler, 1967) to distinguish between "pathological" and "sociocultural/familial" mechanisms for ID, respectively linked to severe versus mild ID. Pathological factors included individually relatively rare medical or genetic and extreme environmental events where exposure almost invariably led to ID. In contrast, the sociocultural/familial form of ID was postulated to be caused by common adverse family- and socially based risk factors, including low parental IQ, lack of environmental stimulation, and social deprivation. Pathological factors were also thought to cause severe ID, with IQ <50, while sociocultural/familial factors were associated with mild ID and borderline intelligence. Recent support for the theory comes from large population genetic studies, discussed below. It is helpful, clinically to differentiate individuals based on the severity of intellectual impairment, in determining investigations, planning interventions, and guiding longer-term prognosis. However, the dichotomy is overrestrictive in applying a threshold to a truly continuous trait. There is great variability in intellectual ability in individuals with genetic disorders, such as Down syndrome and fragile X, and the same applies for environmental factors such as prematurity. Similarly, families with high rates of ID and socioenvironmental adversity may have members with severe, as well as mild, ID (Broman *et al.*, 1987). However, despite the limitations of the two-group theory, causes and severity of ID are linked, and it is often helpful to consider different etiologies in the context of the degree of intellectual impairment, as well as other factors such as associated physical, cognitive, and behavioral features. Figure 53.1 summarizes the risk factors of ID.

Genetic factors

IQ is a heritable trait, and both molecular genetic (Reichenberg *et al.*, 2016) and family (Lichtenstein *et al.*, 2022) studies have shown that similar genetic variants influence mild ID and IQ within the normal range in the rest of the population. In contrast, severe ID is linked with a range of genetic mechanisms and different genes, many of which are very strongly associated with ID. Current evidence suggests that there are over than 1500 genes associated with ID (https://panelapp.genomicsengland.co.uk/panels/285/) (Jansen *et al.*, 2023), and up to 20% of individuals with neurodevelopmental conditions including ID have a known genetic condition (Donnelly *et al.*, 2023). In Table 53.1 we describe the most common genetic factors associated with ID.

Other medical disorders associated with intellectual disability

A host of disorders that affect brain structure or function are associated with ID. Epilepsy is more common in people with ID, with a dose–response relation to severity, occurring in 7% of children with mild ID versus 35% with severe ID (van Ool *et al.*, 2016). Cerebral palsy is another disorder associated with ID with a prevalence of 12/1000 in high-income settings and again being more common in those with severe ID (Cummins *et al.*, 2021). Meningo-encephalitis can lead to reduced IQ and ID (Christie *et al.*, 2017).

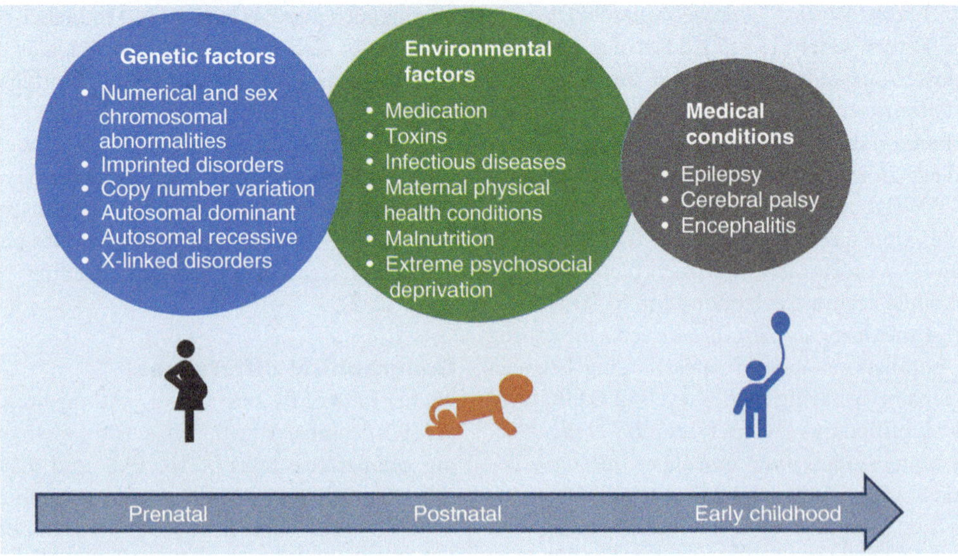

Figure 53.1 Causes of intellectual disability (ID) and their interplay. Genetic, environmental, and medical factors and their interaction are the main causes of ID.

Table 53.1 Genetic risks associated with intellectual disability (ID).

Genetic mechanisms associated with ID	Genetic abnormality	Prevalence	Clinical phenotype
Numerical/chromosomal abnormalities			
Down syndrome (DS)	Trisomy 21	6–8% of ID cases	• Hypotonia, cardiac abnormalities, leukemia, and early onset Alzheimer's disease • One-third of individuals with DS live to over 40 years of age • Mortality rate is greater than other causes of ID
Edwards syndrome	Trisomy 18	1/8000 live births	• Psychomotor and cognitive impairment, malformation, and growth deficiency in infants • 5–10% of children affected survive past the first year of life
Sex chromosome anomalies			
A: Klinefelter syndrome	XXY	1–2/1000	• IQ in the low normal range • Impairments in nonverbal cognitive skills, executive functioning, and language and social development • Strengths in verbal abilities
B: Turner syndrome	XO	1/2500 in female infants	
Copy number variants (CNVs)	Duplications or deletions of small segments of DNA	25% of ID cases can be attributed to CNVs	For CNV examples, see Table
Mendelian inheritance			
Autosomal recessive	–	13–24% of ID cases are due to autosomal recessive mutations	• 2500 autosomal recessive genes are associated with ID • Overrepresentation in ID autosomal recessive disorders in regions with higher rates of consanguinity such as Africa, the Middle East, and South Asia
Autosomal dominant	–	–	Examples of autosomal dominant ID: neurofibromatosis, tuberous sclerosis, myotonic dystrophy, Duchenne muscular dystrophy, Noonan-spectrum disorders
X-linked disorders			
Fragile X syndrome	>200 trinucleotide (CCG) repeat sequence in the region of the fragile X mental retardation 1 (FMR1) gene	• 1/5000 males • 1/4000 to 1/8000 in females	Please see details on Table
Imprinted disorders	The process where only one copy of a gene (either paternal or maternal) is expressed, while the other one is suppressed. This does not affect the DNA sequence itself, but can have significant consequences on fetal growth, placenta development, and clinical phenotype.	–	Examples include Prader-Willi and Angelman syndromes that are described in detail in Table

Environmental factors

Diverse environmental risk factors during the antenatal, perinatal, and postnatal period are linked to ID in offspring. Although it is often not detected by inexperienced clinicians, fetal alcohol spectrum disorder (FASD) is the most common cause of noninherited ID, with an estimated global prevalence of 14.6/10,000 cases, although prevalence varies widely among populations reflecting differences in socioeconomic status and drinking patterns (Popova *et al.*, 2017). Cognitive and language impairments and ID are highly variable in this population. History of prenatal exposure of alcohol, growth retardation, facial dysmorphic features, central nervous system dysfunction, or neurodevelopmental conditions should prompt clinicians to consider FASD (Denny *et al.*, 2017). Prenatal exposure to cocaine, opioids, cannabis, and methamphetamine is also associated with reduced IQ and behavior problems (Nashed *et al.*, 2020, Kunkler *et al.*, 2022).

In relation to prescribed drugs, use of anti-epileptics, including valproate, carbamazepine, oxcarbamazepine, and lamotrigine, during pregnancy are all associated with developmental problems including ID in offspring, although the strength of effect varies according to drug (Daugaard *et al.*, 2020). Early studies suggesting causal relationships between offspring ID and drugs prescribed for maternal psychiatric conditions, including antipsychotics, antidepressants, benzodiazepines, and hypnotics such as Zolpidem, have not been supported in more rigorously controlled studies (Jensen *et al.*, 2022).

There is a dose–response relationship between exposure to heavy metals such as arsenic, lead, and mercury during pregnancy and/or childhood and degree of cognitive impairment (Hsueh *et al.*, 2017).

Prenatal maternal infections linked to ID include rubella, toxoplasma gondii, and cytomegalovirus (Bopegamage *et al.*, 2012). Numerous maternal physical health conditions are linked to higher rates of offspring ID. These include obesity preceding pregnancy, asthma, hypertension, urinary tract infections, pregestational and gestational diabetes, and malnutrition. Other important risk factors include advanced maternal age, preterm birth, a history of previous miscarriages, and low birth weight. The underpinning mechanisms are various, often poorly understood, and likely to be indirect in many instances. For example, preterm birth is itself often associated with maternal infections (Brynge *et al.*, 2022), but can itself also lead to brain damage.

As described above, socioeconomic adversity is associated with increased rates of ID, but the mechanisms are complex and bidirectional. Severe, chronic social deprivation, often associated with malnutrition, is a cause of ID and other NDDs (Sonuga-Barke *et al.*, 2017). In low-income settings, early childhood psychosocial stimulation has shown medium- and long-term benefits for growth-retarded children and was more effective than nutritional supplementation in improving both cognition and behavior (Grantham-McGregor *et al.*, 2014).

Biological–environmental interplay

As with other behavioral and cognitive phenotypes, many risk factors for ID increase susceptibility but are not deterministic. For example, parenting interventions in LMICs improved outcomes in children's cognitive and language development (Zhang *et al.*, 2021). Poorer cognitive outcome following preterm birth is related to lower maternal education (Sentenac *et al.*, 2022). A better understanding of the environmental mediators and moderators of biological risk has the potential to improve interventions for high-risk groups.

Assessment and diagnosis of intellectual disability

Early identification of ID provides the possibility for children to receive appropriate support and planning from education, health, and social services. Parents often find a diagnosis aids their understanding of their child, especially if strengths as well as impairments are identified. If a genetic cause for ID is identified, it may influence family planning as well as guide additional investigations and management. In general, severe ID is identified early in life while mild ID may go unrecognized, particularly in the absence of additional medical problems. Therefore, clinicians should be alert to subtle indicators, such as school nonattendance, poor academic performance, and immaturity of interests and behavior. School reports with information about attainments and behavior can be helpful. A common clinical error is to misattribute these warning signs to adverse early experience, family stress, or other risk factors, and to fail to consider ID. Also, clinicians may not consider ID in a "chatty" child, although a more in-depth dialogue would likely identify impairments in comprehension.

History

History-taking should determine if there are impairments in intellectual functioning and adaptive behavior that have an onset during the developmental period, and identify possible causes of ID and co-occurring conditions. Global developmental delay in the early milestones of language, communication, motor, and social skills is present in many but not all children who go on to receive a later diagnosis of ID. Clinicians should be aware that parental recollection of milestones is often inaccurate and, if important to establish, contemporaneous developmental records should be sought. With increasing age, the gap between the achievements of average intelligence children and those with ID become more apparent, and parents of children with mild ID are often only aware of differences after their child starts school. Loss of language skills or stasis in development during the first three years is common in autism. However, a clear history of loss of skills after the age of three years should trigger referral to a pediatric neurologist for further investigation.

A comprehensive approach to assessment should follow that outlined in Chapter 27, with a detailed account of the prenatal, perinatal, and early developmental periods, and considering the risk factors discussed above. ID is strongly associated with autism and the developmental history should consider social communication and patterns of restricted and repetitive behavior (see Chapter 50). Associated physical disorders are more common and a full medical history should identify any neurological, neuromuscular, or brain-based conditions such as epilepsy, cerebral palsy, or muscular dystrophy. Red flags suggestive of metabolic disorders are particularly important as some conditions are treatable. These include episodic life-threatening illness, lethargy/somnolence, vomiting, seizures, poor feeding, failure to thrive, and signs of hyper/hypotonia or movement disorder, enlarged liver, and dysmorphic features on examination (Belanger & Caron, 2018). General health problems, including hearing and visual impairments, are more common in people with ID and more likely to be overlooked.

ID-specific elements of the family history include a three-generation pedigree for NDDs and history of consanguinity. ID may not have been formally diagnosed in the wider family, but there may be a history of attending specialist schools, requiring extra academic help, or limited attainments.

Educational history should include parental account of schools attended including specialist placement. A school report can determine academic levels achieved and whether the child receives additional support. For older adolescents, plans for extended education and training should be identified.

Psychological assessment

In making the diagnosis of ID, a cognitive assessment is required, as described in Chapter 29. Care should be taken to ensure assessment is valid, and with more behaviorally disturbed children, flexibility in approach is important, which may mean administering subtests out of their usual order, with more breaks and with behavioral reinforcers. In using standardized measures among those with severe ID, the possibility of "floor" effects may necessitate the use of tests standardized for younger children to get an estimate of what the child can (rather than cannot) do. Even when the diagnosis of ID is clear from the history and observation, a cognitive assessment establishes the level of impairment and identifies strengths within the profile, which aids in planning educational strategies and behavioral management. Impairment in adaptive function is often evident from the history and presentation but a structured review should focus on everyday functioning in the domains of communication, conceptual understanding, motor skills, self-care, and independence. Several standardized measures are recommended for quantifying the profile of skills and estimating the functional level of the child or young person (Harrison & Oakland, 2015, Sparrow *et al.*, 2016). In Box 53.1, we summarize the process of the assessment.

Box 53.1 Assessment of ID at a glance

History
- Prenatal, perinatal, and developmental history, including history of miscarriages, and maternal drug and alcohol use
- Medical history
- Family history including three-generation pedigree and consanguinity
- Social history (current living arrangements, potential stressors/supports, and family coping mechanisms)
- Educational history

Psychological assessment
- Cognitive assessment
- Adaptive functioning

Physical examination and investigations

Physical examination

The role of the child psychiatrist in undertaking a physical examination and organizing investigations varies across health care systems. Regardless of local arrangements, child and adolescent mental health services may be the first to identify ID and, at a minimum, they have responsibility for arranging for examination and investigations, whose aim is to identify possible causes of ID and co-occurring conditions.

Box 53.2 Physical examination and investigations for intellectual disability

Physical examination
- Multisystem examination
- Dysmorphology examination (e.g., craniofacial dysmorphisms, skin abnormalities)
- Anthropometry measures including height, weight, head/chest/abdominal circumference

Investigations
- Routine
  - Hearing and eye tests
  - Genetic testing (different methods used depending on guidelines available)
- Specific indications
  - Specific genetic tests recommended by regional clinical geneticists if normal microarrays and testing for fragile X
  - Metabolic and biochemical testing
    - full blood count
    - urea and electrolytes
    - creatine kinase
    - thyroid function
    - lead, urate
    - ferritin
    - biotinidase

    (full blood count to biotinidase: UK and US recommendations)
    - screening for inborn errors of metabolism (amino acids, homocysteine, acylcarnitine profile, organic acids, purines and pyrimidines, mucopolysaccharides, and oligosaccharides)
  - Magnetic resonance imaging (MRI) (when neurological signs present)

The general approach to physical examination is described in detail in Chapter 30, and here, and in Box 53.2, we discuss components most important in ID. These include a dysmorphology examination for signs of birth defects and genetic syndromes, such as minor physical anomalies and craniofacial dysmorphisms (Toriello, 2008). Coarse facial features may indicate a metabolic disorder. Common skin abnormalities of note include *café au lait* spots in neurofibromatosis and areas of depigmentation, detected by Wood's lamp, in tuberous sclerosis. Delayed motor coordination with some degree of clumsiness is common and may represent a nonspecific developmental immaturity but specific neurological signs should be investigated. Other clinical features that should lead to consideration of specialist referral include presence of a muscle disorder, muscle pain or weakness, and cognitive/behavioral deterioration associated with possible seizures (Mithyantha *et al.*, 2017). This detailed examination should be undertaken alongside a systematic general examination that is aimed at common co-occurring conditions.

Physical investigations

The methods for identifying genetic disorders are constantly advancing, and present recommendations will quickly become out of date. Clinicians should consult their genetic services about which tests to order and the interpretation and feedback of any positive results. In high-income settings, all children presenting with global developmental delay or ID of unknown cause should receive genetic testing, including comparative genomic hybridization (Savatt & Myers, 2021). Investigation is recommended for fragile X for all children with ID of unknown etiology in the US (Siegel *et al.*, 2020), and in the UK for those with moderate to profound ID (Mithyantha *et al.*, 2017) or where other features are suggestive of the diagnosis (Moeschler & Shevell, 2014). When these tests are normal, individuals with moderate to profound ID, dysmorphic features, strong family history of ID, regression, or specific neurological findings should be assessed by a clinical geneticist to ensure the appropriate evaluation. Second-line investigations include routine karyotyping, sequencing specific genes or panels of genes, or exome sequencing. As discussed in Chapter 21, the results of genetic investigations can reveal unexpected findings with wider clinical and ethical implications, so informed consent is essential.

Routine metabolic and biochemical tests currently recommended in the UK are urea and electrolytes, creatine kinase, thyroid function, lead, urate, full blood count, ferritin, and biotinidase (Mithyantha *et al.*, 2017). US guidance also recommends screening for inborn errors of metabolism for all individuals with ID of unknown etiology, including amino acids, homocysteine, acylcarnitine profile, organic acids, purines and pyrimidines, mucopolysaccharides, and oligosaccharides as detailed in (Moeschler & Shevell, 2014).

Structural brain imaging reveals nonspecific abnormalities in up to 30% of children with ID but provides etiologically relevant information in less than 2.5% (Belanger & Caron, 2018). Guided by a pediatric neurologist, neuroimaging should be undertaken when there are neurological signs, micro- or macrocephaly, and some instances of epilepsy.

Longitudinal course and prognosis of intellectual disability

Although ID involves a life-persistent diminution in cognitive function, it is not static and there is considerable variability in the course and adaptive outcomes of individuals. The degree of cognitive impairment and adaptive skills will change over time as environmental demands change. Parents and carers frequently become more concerned about a young person's ability to function independently in adolescence, when it becomes clearer that there is not going to be a "catch up" (Siegel *et al.*, 2020).

Over and above the age-related widening gap in cognition and skills, several disorders, including Down syndrome, fragile X, and Williams syndrome, show a relative decline in IQ from childhood through adolescence and early adult life. In Down syndrome, this may be related to the onset of dementia (Grieco *et al.*, 2015), but for all syndromes this may also reflect greater impairments in the conceptual reasoning that takes on greater importance in adolescence. Neurofibromatosis type 1 is different, with decline in cognitive skills observed in males, but not in females (Fisch *et al.*, 2010).

Life expectancy is decreased, particularly in those with severe to profound ID, with an overall 19-year reduction compared to the general population (Hirvikoski *et al.*, 2021). ID-related conditions, such as central nervous system disorders and congenital anomalies, and nonspecific and potentially modifiable conditions, such as obesity and cardiovascular disorder, all play a role, some of which are modifiable with improved health care (Tyrer *et al.*, 2019).

Behavioral phenotypes

The term "behavioral phenotype" refers to a relatively predictable set of behavioral and sometimes cognitive characteristics that occur in individuals with a known genetic abnormality (Skuse, 2000). The individual features of behavioral phenotypes may be common or rare; what distinguishes these conditions is the *combination* of features and their association with a particular condition. This is useful for clinicians in predicting behaviors and preventing negative consequences, such as compulsive overeating with severe obesity in Prader-Willi syndrome. Conversely, observing a characteristic pattern of behaviors may provoke specific genetic testing, leading to a diagnosis that is relevant to other family members. No behavioral phenotype is invariant; for example, schizophrenia occurs in only ~25% of people with 22q11.2 deletion syndrome (Van *et al.*, 2017); however, no other single risk factor is so strongly associated with psychosis. Researchers are particularly interested in behavioral phenotypes because they can shed light on the biological pathways involved in gene–cognition–behavior links. Table 53.2 describes the most well-known behavioral phenotypes and their underlying etiologies.

Psychiatric and neurodevelopmental disorders in children and adolescents with intellectual disability

Co-occurring psychiatric and NDDs are increased in children with ID, with period prevalence rates around 40% (Totsika *et al.*, 2022) and lifetime prevalence of 65% by adolescence (Platt

Table 53.2 Behavioral phenotypes.

Name of condition	Genetic abnormality	Behavioral/cognitive features	Physical and other features
Angelman syndrome	~70% maternal deletions involving chromosome 15q11.2-q13 (same region as Prader-Willi syndrome); ~2% paternal uniparental disomy, 2–3% result from imprinting defects. Some of the remaining due to UBE3A gene mutations. Protein ligase E3A gene (UBE3A; mutations in the MECP2 gene can present a similar phenotype.601623).	Usually severe to profound intellectual disability (ID) with absence of speech, episodic paroxysmal laughter	• Features include ataxia, hypotonia, epilepsy, unusual large mandible and open-mouthed expression revealing the tongue. • Frequent depigmentation relative to family members.
Cornelia de Lange syndrome	Marked genetic heterogeneity: 50% of cases with mutation in NIPBL gene and also cases with mutations in X-linked genes SMC1A, SMC3, CDLS4, RAD21, and HDAC8. All involved in two systems pathways.	• Typically, severe ID but variable IQ into normal range • Self-injurious behavior • Communication relatively impaired compared to adaptive function	• Multiple and variable abnormalities but typical facial features include low anterior hairline, arched eyebrows, anteverted nares, maxillary prognathism, long philtrum, thin lips, and "carp" mouth • Parental and postnatal growth retardation • Ptosis, nystagmus, and high myopia • Microcephaly • Gastroesophageal reflux in ~60%, hypothesized to be a cause of behavior that challenges
Fragile X syndrome	See Table	• Variable level of ID (average IQ in males ≈40; normal to moderate ID in females) • Variable behavioral manifestations include hyperactivity and attention deficit hyperactivity disorder (ADHD), poor eye contact and autistic features	Notable features include long face, large ears, prominent jaw, and macroorchidism, typically post-pubertally
Lesch–Nyhan syndrome	X-linked mutation in hypoxanthine-guanine phosphoribosyltransferase gene	Low average to mild ID is typical, severe self-injurious behavior, typically compulsive biting of fingers and lips	Spastic cerebral palsy, choreoathetosis, uric acid urinary stones
Prader-Willi syndrome	• Deletion or disruption of a gene or several genes on paternal chromosome 15 or maternal uniparental of same region • Overlapping clinical phenotype in chromosome 15q11-q13 duplication syndrome	• Mild ID/borderline IQ • Excessive appetite in which food-seeking behavior can cause behavior that challenges • Excessive daytime sleepiness with sleep architecture abnormalities • Delayed motor milestones and speech difficulties • Skin-picking.	• Features include diminished fetal activity, neonatal hypotonia, subsequent obesity, muscular hypotonia, short stature, hypogonadotropic hypogonadism, and small hands and feet • Depigmentation compared to family members
Rett syndrome	X-linked mutation in MECP2 gene, affecting girls only as lethal in males	• Normal early development with abnormalities beginning toward end of first year • Some autistic symptoms, compulsive hand movements, hyperventilation • Often stabilizes in mid to late childhood with no further progression, bruxism • Profound ID	• Deceleration of head growth leading to microcephaly, short stature • Constipation and gastroesophageal reflux, prolonged QT interval on electrocardiogram (ECG) • Spasticity, seizures, ataxia
Rubenstein-Taybi syndrome	Deletion at the 16p13.3 chromosome	Mild to moderate ID, anxiety, OCD, self-stimulatory and challenging behavior, autism spectrum disorder (ASD)	Slow development of height and weight, microcephaly, dysmorphic facial features, broad thumbs, congenital heart diseases, renal malformations, immune deficiencies, hypothyroidism

(Continued)

Table 53.2 (Continued)

Name of condition	Genetic abnormality	Behavioral/cognitive features	Physical and other features
Smith-Magenis syndrome	Deletion at the 17p11 chromosome	• Severe ID is usual, often with additional speech delay • Typically includes severe self-injurious behavior, disruptive/aggressive outbursts, sleep disturbance, possibly with absence of rapid eye movement (REM) sleep • Hyperactivity and ADHD may occur	Common features include broad flat face, brachycephaly, midface hypoplasia, prognathism, hoarse voice, peripheral neuropathy
Williams syndrome	Deletion in chromosome 7q11	• Moderate ID to borderline IQ • Language acquisition delayed but subsequent superficially good expressive language, with high sociability but a failure of social flexibility • Often anxious despite friendliness	• Supravalvular aortic stenosis is common • Distinctive facies involve broad forehead, medial eyebrow flare, periorbital fullness, strabismus, stellate iris pattern, flat nasal bridge, malar flattening, full cheeks and lips, long smooth philtrum, pointed chin, wide mouth and dental deformities • Infantile hypercalcaemia is frequent as is a harsh, brassy voice
22q11.2 deletion syndrome	Deletion at chromosome 22q11	• Mild ID to borderline IQ is typical • Childhood features include ADHD, autistic features. Mood swings are also common • In adolescence/adulthood, ~25% develop schizophreniform psychosis	• Highly variable but main features include cleft palate and cardiac anomalies • Typical facies involve narrow palpebral fissures, square nasal root • Less frequent features included microcephaly, short stature, slender hands and digits, minor auricular anomalies, and inguinal hernia
22q11.2 duplication	Duplication at chromosome 22q11.2	Borderline to mild ID, ASD, ADHD	Hypotonia, congenital heart abnormalities, kidney anomalies, facial dysmorphic features—hypertelorism, broad nasal bridge, epicanthal folds, high forehead, downslanting palpebral fissures
16p11.2 deletion syndrome	Deletion at chromosome 16q11.2	Mild ID, developmental coordination disorder, phonological processing disorder, language disorders, and ASD	Webbed toes, obesity, seizures, scoliosis, hearing loss
16p11.2 duplication syndrome	Duplication at chromosome 16q11.2	Borderline to mild ID, language and speech delay, ADHD, ASD, increased risk for schizophrenia	Gastrointestinal problems (gastroesophageal reflux, constipation, diarrhea), microcephaly, underweight, kidney malformations, epilepsy, heart conditions (atrial septal defects, ventricular septal defects, Shone's complex, and tetralogy of Fallot)

et al., 2019). The increased risk is greatest for other NDDs, with rates of ASD ranging between 30–50% and of attention deficit hyperactivity disorder (ADHD) between 29–39%. Risk for psychiatric disorders shows a less profound increase: anxiety disorders 7–34%, depressive disorders 3–5%, and conduct and externalizing disorders 3–21% (Totsika *et al.*, 2022). Psychosis rates are uncertain in childhood and adolescence but rise to 3.7–5.3% in adulthood (Morgan *et al.*, 2008). We focus in the following sections on considerations that are relatively specific to ID and readers should refer to other chapters on assessment, intervention, and specific disorders to gain a comprehensive account.

Differences in psychiatric presentation among children with intellectual disability

As the degree of intellectual impairment increases, the risk for both ASD and ADHD increases (Simonoff *et al.*, 2007; McClain *et al.*, 2017). At the same time, differentiating specific psychiatric disorders becomes more challenging, and eliciting a history and/or mental state that fulfills diagnostic criteria can be difficult. First, it may be difficult to identify symptoms that require the behavior to be inappropriate for developmental age, such as ASD or ADHD, in those with severe or profound ID. Second, a mental state is more difficult to obtain in people with severe communication impairments, and informants may have limited insight into internal experiences. Third, some disorders include symptoms that require higher cognitive processes, such as hopelessness and helplessness in depression. For all these reasons, there has been a movement for a separate psychiatric classification with modified criteria for people with severe to profound ID and at least one system has been proposed for adults (Fletcher *et al.*, 2018). While this alternative classification has not been widely adopted, these considerations influence the approach to assessment, discussed below.

The syndrome of "behavior that challenges": a distinct condition?

The terms "behavior that challenges," "problem behavior," or "maladaptive behavior" are frequently used to describe a syndrome of problematic behavior that is relatively specific to people with ID and associated NDDs such as autism (Kurtz *et al.*, 2020). It refers to aggression directed at others or self, severe temper tantrums, destruction of property and high levels of noncompliance. Studies report rates of some form of challenging behavior in about 50% of individuals with ID and 5–10% present with severe behavior that challenges (Kurtz *et al.*, 2020). The role of biological factors is demonstrated by high rates in certain genetic conditions, such as Prader-Will and Cornelia de Lange syndromes, and tuberous sclerosis. Although there is no association with family adversity, it appears to show person-specific correlates, including male sex, lower adaptive functioning, and poor communication skills (Crawford *et al.*, 2019).

Behavior that challenges is also related to a wide range of psychiatric and NDDs such as ADHD, anxiety, depression and psychosis, poor impulse control (Davies & Oliver, 2016), subdiagnostic traits such as low mood (Vos *et al.*, 2013), and repetitive/stereotyped behaviors (Oliver *et al.*, 2012). Any condition causing pain or discomfort may cause behavior that challenges, including chronic physical disorders, acute infection or inflammation, and adverse effects of treatments (Oliver *et al.*, 2017). Moreover, self-injury occurring in the context of behavior that challenges typically lacks the intentions associated with suicidal behavior or deliberate self-harm and often has stereotyped (e.g., head-banging) and/or sensory (e.g., picking or biting) elements (Kurtz *et al.*, 2020).

Clinicians find the term useful because it highlights the need for different types of assessment and interventions. Applied behavior analysis (ABA) conceptualizes behavior that challenges in relation to learning theory, with maladaptive behaviors arising for a host of reasons and being reinforced, often inadvertently (Cooper & Heron, 2007).

Risk factors for psychiatric and neurodevelopmental disorders in intellectual disability

Because genetic, medical, and environmental risk factors are often shared in NDDs, they will be present at higher rates in ID compared to general populations and hence increase the likelihood of these co-occurring conditions. Shared genetic factors are particularly linked to co-occurring NDDs (Wolstencroft *et al.*, 2022). Medical disorders are linked to both neurodevelopmental and emotional and behavioral disorders, while environmental factors appear to have the strongest associations with psychiatric disorders (Platt *et al.*, 2019; Totsika *et al.*, 2022; Wolstencroft *et al.*, 2022).

Conditions affecting brain structure and/or function such as epilepsy, cerebral palsy, and acquired brain injury predispose to both ID and psychiatric disorders. As highlighted above, clinicians should also consider common illnesses and pain, especially as a cause of emotional and behavioral problems. Psychosocial adversity is also linked to parental IQ, raising questions about the strength of the direct environmental mechanism.

ID itself may increase the risk of psychiatric disorders. Impairments in cognition, adaptive behavior, and language can decrease the ability of individuals with ID to communicate their needs, understand the environment, and respond flexibly to varying situations, which can lead to anxiety or oppositional, noncompliant behavior (Siegel *et al.*, 2020). The timing of risk factors varies across the life span, as depicted in Figure 53.2.

Assessment of psychiatric disorders in people with intellectual disability

Most aspects of assessment and treatment overlap with those discussed in relation to individual disorders and here we highlight the distinct considerations for children with ID. Box 53.3 describes the overarching approach to assessment in this population. The cognitive assessment should provide a good understanding of a child's cognitive level and adaptive function. Because inappropriate environmental expectations can trigger or exacerbate psychiatric problems, it is important to

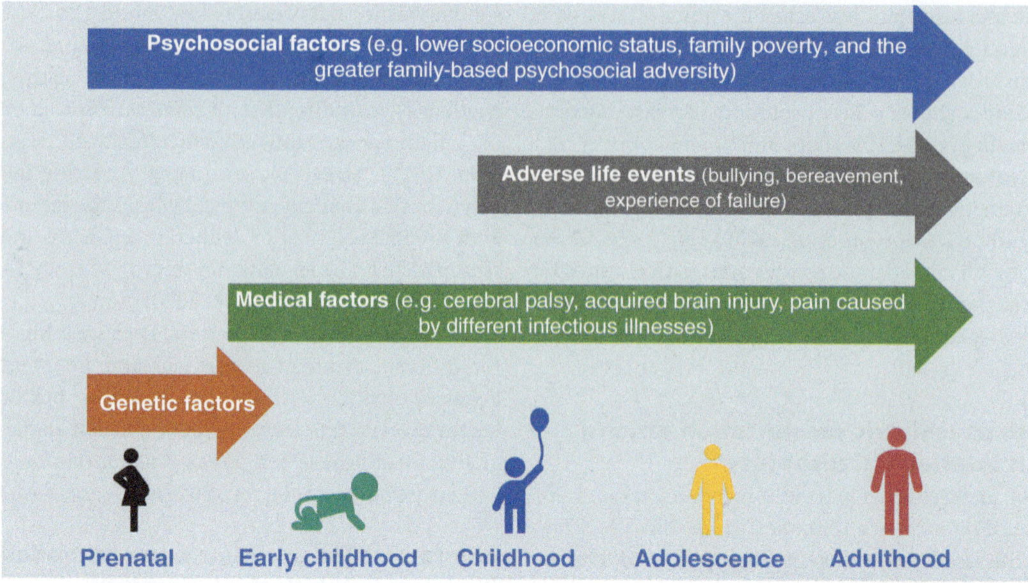

Figure 53.2 Factors that increase the risk for the development of psychiatric and other neurodevelopmental disorders (NDDs) in intellectual disability (ID). Genetics and obstetric complications are the first factors that increase the risk. Medical and psychosocial factors are present across the life span and contribute significantly increased risk.

Box 53.3 Approach to accurate diagnosis of neurodevelopmental and psychiatric disorders in children with intellectual disability

Are "symptoms" developmentally appropriate?

- Consider behaviors in the context of a child's IQ and developmental age
- Is the child's environment adapted for their developmental level?
- Are home and school expectations appropriate?

Avoiding risk of diagnostic overshadowing

- Comprehensive and systematic inquiry for all children
- Do not use cutoffs on screening instruments to exclude from further diagnostic consideration
- Elicit behavioral descriptions of symptoms, including from children—always check children's understanding of your questions by asking for examples
- Account of acute stressors/life events/environmental changes—small changes can be significant and the child may not volunteer information
- Consider atypical presentations, including behavioral manifestations of emotional symptoms
- Consider whether somatic conditions, including pain and/or medication could cause/exacerbate psychiatric symptoms

enquire about the parent/carer's understanding of the child's level of functioning, to observe the pattern and complexity of their communication with the child, and to ascertain the appropriateness of the educational placement. As psychiatric symptoms may manifest in atypical ways, inquiry should always elicit specific descriptions. Emotional symptoms may be more difficult to identify when the child's communication ability is significantly impaired, and in such instances, observable features of emotional disorders are more important. On the other hand, care should be taken not to inappropriately ascribe psychiatric symptoms to ID itself, the well-documented process of "diagnostic overshadowing" (Mason & Scior, 2004). Diagnostic overshadowing is likely to play an important role in the underreferral and underdiagnosis of psychiatric disorders in children with ID. This can be avoided by eliciting accounts of behavior in different contexts. Those working in specialist settings, such as schools for children with ID, may not see psychiatric or neurodevelopmental symptoms as atypical, as they may be present in many children, and therefore staff fail to raise these concerns. The personal interview and/or direct observation of the child needs to take account of their verbal skills, communication style, and interests, using simpler language and considering play-based materials even into adolescence. Judgments about the presence of symptoms should be made in the context of developmental (rather than chronological) age.

While the assessment should aim to identify psychiatric disorders as treatment targets, it should not exclude other causes of disturbed behavior, as described under behavior that challenges. The assessment should ascertain the presence of eating/feeding and sleeping problems, and the role of coexisting physical disorders, especially brain-based disorders and conditions or treatments that may cause pain. Wider inquiry includes the presence of parental learning problems/ID and parental stress, psychosocial adversity, and support from statutory and voluntary services.

Assessing behavior in its context

A key element in the evaluation of behavior that challenges is the assessment of triggers or precipitants and reinforcement of maladaptive behaviors. Alongside the rigorous approach of applied behavioral analysis used by specialists, all clinicians can use functional behavior assessment to generate hypotheses about triggers that may provoke and consequences that reinforce behaviors. This involves obtaining a history of the antecedents and context, a detailed description of the behaviors and the response of others, both immediate and longer term. Clinicians should consider that sanctions usually effective in typically developing groups, such as time-out, may be positive experiences for some children with ID. Different behaviors should be evaluated separately. Information should include the effect of different settings, whether the onset was acute or insidious, and the relation to environmental changes or life events, as well as whether there has been a change over time and, if so, whether it has been gradual or abrupt. When behavioral changes are sudden, particular consideration should be given to environmental alterations, life events, physical conditions causing pain, and adverse effects of medication.

Assessment instruments for psychiatric and neurodevelopmental symptoms and disorders in intellectual disability

There are few structured or semistructured instruments validated for children and adolescents with ID, and those developed for people with ID are not organized according to diagnostic systems. Therefore, while such instruments may be valuable in structuring information gathering, results should be treated cautiously, and cutoffs developed for non-ID populations should not be used to determine diagnosis or access to care. A general approach is to use questionnaires for the non-ID population in children with mild ID and more specialized instruments in those with more severe ID. Eliciting self-reports is important, and, where structured instruments are used, we recommend administration in person utilizing open-ended follow-up questions to assess the child's understanding. Clinicians should not make the error of assuming that when children give a closed response they have understood the question, and eliciting descriptions increases confidence in the information gathered and promotes rapport with the child. Table 53.3 provides examples of instruments specifically developed for people with ID that may be useful in assessment.

Table 53.3 Assessment tools for neurodevelopmental and psychiatric disorders in individuals with moderate to severe intellectual disability (ID).

Type of instrument	Measure
Interviews	Challenging Behavior Interview (Oliver *et al.*, 2003) Disability Adjustment Scale (DAS) (Tsakanikos *et al.*, 2011) PAS-ADD and Mini PAS-ADD (Moss *et al.*, 1998) Questions about Behavioral Function (Paclawskyj *et al.*, 2000)
Questionnaires	Aberrant Behavior Checklist (Aman, 1986) Developmental Behavior Checklist (DBC) (Einfeld & Tonge, 1995) Nisonger Child Behavior Rating Form (Aman *et al.*, 1996) Profile of Neuropsychiatric Disorders (PONS) (Santosh *et al.*, 2015)

Physical examination and investigations

If ID has not previously been diagnosed, the examination should include those elements that may identify an underlying cause, which may also shed light on psychopathology as described above. With respect to behavior that challenges, examination should look for possible causes of pain and adverse drug effects. The examination also provides an opportunity to identify possible contraindications to pharmacological interventions.

Interventions

Clinicians should take a goal-based and symptom-oriented approach in selecting treatment targets and deciding how response will be judged. Goals should be generated with children and young people where appropriate, as well as their parents, and should prioritize areas of functioning that are most distressing and/or impairing, as well as those that are most likely to respond to intervention. A strengths-based approach, which views disability as natural differences that contribute to positive characteristics and identifies individual strengths, is an important component of positive psychology approaches but has been little used with people with ID. The cognitive and adaptive function assessment will inform this approach.

In general, there is a dearth of evidence on mental health interventions in children with ID, who are often excluded from studies of pertinent treatments (Totsika *et al.*, 2022). Children with ID are more likely to experience adverse effects and show lower levels of positive effects from interventions (although the latter may also reflect measurement difficulties in this population). In the following sections we discuss ID-specific evidence and readers should consider the wider literature for children with average IQ and specific conditions.

Nonpharmacological interventions

Psychological interventions

Modifications of psychological interventions should simplify language, reduce the need for abstract thinking, include visual materials, and review progress more regularly. Greater involvement of parents/carers is usually needed. In children with severe to profound ID or a developmental age under about seven years, behavioral interventions that are delivered by parents/carers and other adults are likely to be more effective. Principles should include clearly described, visually depicted expectations and reinforcers that are activated immediately when the behavior occurs, usually with short-term effects. It is important to identify reinforcers for the individual child, rather than relying on more generally used rewards and sanctions. For behaviors that occur in multiple settings a consistent approach should be adopted in all domains, because this group of children have more difficulties with generalization.

Parents' needs should be addressed as parenting stress and mental health problems are increased and there is a likely reciprocal relationship between child psychopathology and parental mental health and stress (Smith *et al.*, 2012). Psychoeducation should be standard. Impact on siblings should also be considered (Neece *et al.*, 2010).

Environmental modifications are important for enhancing adaptive, communication, and learning skills, and improving behaviors in different settings. Changing the setup of a room, having a sensory room, modifying materials or equipment, simplifying tasks in terms of duration or difficulty, and use of special equipment are some examples that may help to reduce anxiety or behavior that challenges (Casson *et al.*, 2021).

Pharmacological intervention

The choice of psychotropic medication should follow recommendations based on evidence-based pharmacology for children and young people with ID if available, or of average intellectual ability if not, as described in Chapter 39.

There is currently no evidence that ID itself changes the mechanism of action of psychotropic medication. However, it is possible that physical health comorbidities and brain differences may alter efficacy and increase adverse effects. As multiple psychiatric problems/disorders are frequent in people with ID, polypharmacy is common (Torelli *et al.*, 2022). However, it should be avoided whenever possible because of increased susceptibility to adverse drug effects. Several steps may help minimize the use of multiple drugs. First, the target symptoms should be carefully identified, prioritized for treatment, and linked to an underlying psychiatric disorder or evidence-based intervention. Second, baseline information on severity, frequency, and duration should be obtained, using either a standardized or bespoke measure. Regular monitoring of change should use the same scale, along with a systematic enquiry about adverse effects. If no or inadequate response occurs, adherence should first be checked, and consideration given to whether the dose can be increased. In evaluating possible adverse effects, the clinician needs to balance the increased susceptibility of this population against variation in the child's behavior; certain potential adverse effects, such as irritability, aggression, and mood changes, may reflect variation in the child's behavior for other reasons. Drug initiation at low doses with gradual increases will reduce early and unwarranted cessation of medication due to possible adverse effects. When treatment response remains inadequate despite therapeutic doses, the diagnostic hypothesis should be reviewed before initiating an alternative medication.

Attention deficit hyperactivity disorder

Randomized controlled trials (RCTs) on methylphenidate (Aman *et al.*, 2003, Simonoff *et al.*, 2013a, Simonoff *et al.*, 2013b) report reduced but significant effect sizes (~0.4–0.5) and higher rates of adverse effects. Children with co-occurring autism may be particularly sensitive to adverse effects but nevertheless can also experience benefit (Simonoff *et al.*, 2013b). One trial on clonidine in children and young people with ID reported benefits (Agarwal *et al.*, 2001), but no studies have looked into the efficacy of atomoxetine or guanfacine in the ID population, despite their use in autistic populations with ADHD. There is also some evidence that atypical antipsychotics, either as monotherapy or augmentation to stimulants, can improve symptoms of hyperactivity or inattention (Aman *et al.*, 2004), although this would not be considered first line. Given the antipsychotic side-effect profile, these drugs should be reserved for instances when all other medications are not tolerated and/or ineffective and symptoms remain highly impairing.

Anxiety/depression

Over the last 20 years, there have been no pharmacological studies of the efficacy and safety of antidepressants in this population. Selective serotonin reuptake inhibitors (SSRIs) are usually used for the treatment of anxiety and depression, as per guidance, in typically developing children and young people (Bushnell *et al.*, 2018).

Psychosis

Although there is lack of evidence for management of psychosis in youth with ID, atypical compared to typical antipsychotics are usually preferred as they have fewer extrapyramidal side effects.

Irritability/aggressive behavior

RCTs in this population provide some evidence of efficacy of risperidone (Findling *et al.*, 2004) and aripiprazole (Deb *et al.*, 2014) in the management of irritability. One trial of autistic children with and without ID, comparing risperidone alone and with parent training, showed that the combined intervention led to the use of lower doses of medication and slightly greater behavioral improvement than risperidone alone (Scahill *et al.*, 2012). However, antipsychotics have been associated with side effects; therefore, nonpharmacological interventions should be considered first line.

Other interventions

Other nonspecific elements of intervention for children with ID include enhancement of communication, adaptive function, and social skills, which in adults can improve community participation and reduce behaviors that challenge (Walker & Snell, 2013). Clinicians should liaise with schools so they can support the recommended interventions. All children with ID and a psychiatric disorder should have some additional educational support. The overwhelming majority of children with severe/profound ID will be best placed in specialist schools catering for their educational and mental health needs. The needs of children and their families for respite care organized through social services vary widely but families should be aware of the range of options. Often voluntary organizations, including disorder-specific societies, offer information and support for both parents and children. Social care and voluntary agencies may also help by increasing access to community activities for children and young people with ID.

Mental health services for children and adolescents with intellectual disability

The successful delivery of mental health services for children and adolescents with ID depends not only on the expertise of mental health clinicians within that service but also on the configuration of supporting health, education, and social services. Different models operate across and within national boundaries and there is an absence of research that identifies the most effective service models (Casanova Dias *et al.*, 2020).

"De-institutionalization" of people with ID living in large facilities occurred between 1960 and 2000 in most HICs, returning large numbers of adults to their communities with clear benefits. However, despite many attempts to completely close such establishments, there remains a very small proportion of people with ID, including children and adolescents, whose needs extend beyond current community provision, and they have been cared for in specialist placements. In many instances, these provide positive experiences for both children and their families (Karni-Visel *et al.*, 2023). However, there continue to be troubling accounts of inappropriate treatment and abuse in these settings, which have not been resolved despite many government reviews. Ultimately, the most promising approach to this stubborn problem will be early and more effective interventions that reduce behaviors that challenge.

The COVID-19 pandemic demonstrated the vulnerability of service provision for people with disabilities, including ID, who were disproportionately adversely affected by the withdrawal of services and, in some instances, experienced reduced access to routine health care such as COVID testing and intensive hospital care (Oakley *et al.*, 2021). Furthermore, adaptations to care, such as videoconferencing, may disadvantage people with ID who have greater need for the in-person multisensory therapeutic environment (Pinkerton *et al.*, 2022).

Some principles can be distilled to guide service organization. First, the rights of people with disability to equal access to services (among other rights) has been established in a large number of international policies and legal frameworks, including the UK Human Rights Act and the World Report on Disability. Second, children with ID account for ~15% of the those presenting with mental health problems (Emerson & Hatton, 2007). Thus, mainstream mental health services may want to consider their practice in identifying mild ID and adapting care for this group of children. In contrast, there is a much smaller group of children who require highly specialist mental health services, including those with significant communication problems, severe or profound ID, unusual behavioral phenotypes, and high levels of behavior that challenges. Multidisciplinary clinics for specific genetic syndromes can provide comprehensive care and, more generally, mental health services for children with ID should collaborate with services in physical health, education, and social services as well as adult mental health (both with respect to transitional arrangements for adolescents and also to provide services for parents). Consideration should be given to inpatient psychiatric care and ensuring the availability of professional skills and an appropriate environment for those with ID. In units without these qualities, children and adolescents are often misdiagnosed, e.g., as having a psychotic disorder when their communication is idiosyncratic or difficult to understand. While there are no agreed standards, mental health services should include professionals from a range of backgrounds trained to work with children and adolescents with ID; psychiatry, psychology, and psychiatric nursing are essential and there should be access to team members with the skills to work with families, and speech/language and occupational therapists. The model of care often practiced in mental health services, in which treatment for an episode of illness is followed by discharge, may not be optimal for children with ID, whose mental health problems can be chronic. Some children and their families may benefit from predictable reviews, especially around key transition points, even if these are infrequent.

Transition to adult mental health services

Effective communication between child and adolescent and adult mental health services, as well as clarity of responsibilities, is important to ensure there is no gap in service provision. Difficulties can arise when ID has not been clearly established, or where ID is mild, as some adult services may exclude those with mild ID. Adult services may be configured differently and identifying the "best fit" and future care objectives may delay access to the appropriate adult service (Royal College of Psychiatrists, 2016).

Special issues in mental health and intellectual disability

Children and adolescents with intellectual disability and the criminal justice system

The rate of individuals with ID in the criminal justice system is unknown, with prevalence rates across studies varying too widely to combine (Munoz Garcia-Largo *et al.*, 2020) (see Chapter 47). Arson and sex offending have been found to be the most common offence types (Barron *et al.*, 2004). Males with ID may have lower rates of recidivism (Alexiou *et al.*, 2023). Systematic studies of young people in the criminal justice system report that youth with mild ID and borderline IQs are overrepresented (Haysom *et al.*, 2014), although rates of identification vary widely (see Chapter 47). It appears that those with more severe ID are protected by greater levels of community supervision, a reduced range of activities and social interaction, and also by intervention from carers when they come into contact with the criminal justice system (Worthington & Rossetti, 2020). They are also more likely to be perceived as unfit to stand trial (Young *et al.*, 2018). Factors associated with ID that may increase the likelihood of juvenile offending include behavioral problems, autistic symptoms (Yu *et al.*, 2021), and the increased likelihood of detection. Young people with ID are also more likely to be the victims of crime (Anstis & Thomas, 2022) and other forms of maltreatment (Christoffersen, 2019). They are perceived as more suggestible and poor witnesses (Manzanero *et al.*, 2015), which may influence the willingness of authorities to prosecute when they have been victims.

Parents with intellectual disability and their parenting

With changing attitudes to disability, deinstitutionalization, and the UK Human Rights Act, many societies now recognize the desire of adults with ID to become parents and are beginning to investigate their needs and those of their children. Estimated rates of ID among parents vary widely and formal identification is likely to prove an underestimate with the majority of parents having borderline to mild ID and not being formally registered (Brown *et al.*, 2018). Most research involves families who have come to the attention of services, so generalizability of the findings is uncertain. These studies indicate increased risk of neglect among their children (Powell & Parish, 2017). Parents with ID have high rates of psychopathology and experience of previous childhood abuse and trauma, as well as socioeconomic disadvantage (Llewellyn & Hindmarsh, 2015), and these factors are linked to professional concerns about their parenting (Rebbe *et al.*, 2021). Mothers with ID may also be more prone to have antisocial (often without ID) male partners which may increase concerns about parenting and the home environment (McGaw *et al.*, 2010). Once concerns have reached the judicial system, children of parents with ID are more likely to be removed from their birth parents and subsequently placed for adoption (Booth *et al.*, 2005). Recent modifications of parent training programs to meet the needs of these parents have been evaluated and early results are promising (Feldman & Aunos, 2020).

Multisensory impairment in individuals with intellectual disability

Multisensory impairment is a rare condition referring to the combination of vision and hearing impairments, and characterized by different types and severity (Aitken *et al.*, 2013). Children and young people with multisensory impairment commonly present with severe or profound cognitive impairment, and significant difficulties in communication, social interaction, and movement control (Kamenopoulou *et al.*, 2021). Given the complexity in their presentation, it is essential that specialist support is provided from early years to address their needs across all aspects, including education, and physical and mental health.

Future developments and necessary research

Research and clinical advances in ID have lagged behind those in other areas of child and adolescent psychiatry. There has been a tendency to assume "one size fits all" and that clinical advances in other areas can be directly applied to children with ID; where the evidence is available, this is not at always the case. Substantial work is required in all domains to reach the same level of care for this population, but key priorities can be identified.

Prenatal and newborn screening

The introduction of amniocentesis in the 1970s enabled the identification of women at increased risk of giving birth to an infant with chromosomal abnormalities. Advanced maternal age was initially the only eligibility criterion; subsequent quantification of fetal risk based on blood-based markers and ultrasound resulted in the incorporation of screening into routine prenatal care for all pregnant women. In 2011, cell-free DNA screening became widely available. This noninvasive prenatal test is based on the analysis of a blood sample of the pregnant woman, also containing fragments of fetal DNA. It has increased the detection of the three most common trisomies: Down, Edwards, and Patau syndromes. However, the test has both false positives and false negatives, leading to ongoing challenges in its implementation as a screening tool (Taylor-Phillips *et al.*, 2016). Regardless of the type of prenatal screening test, decisions about potential termination of pregnancy following an abnormal genetic result must be nuanced and centered around personal beliefs and preferences. Furthermore, there are wide variations in legal frameworks around termination of pregnancies that should be considered when planning the timing of prenatal screening.

Newborn screening tests for serious but treatable conditions, whose course can be modified if detected early, have been implemented in high-income settings. Phenylketonuria (PKU) is one such example, in which a diet excluding phenylalanine can almost completely remove the risk of developing what would otherwise be severe ID. Countries vary in the number of conditions for which they screen, depending on the prevalence of individual disorders and the perception of cost–benefit (Downie *et al.*, 2021). As the cost of testing reduces, many countries will likely extend their screening programs.

Service development in low- and middle-income countries

While considerable progress has been made in HICs in prevention and early intervention to reduce the incidence of ID, many of these advances have not been translated into care in poorer countries due to financial and cultural obstacles, including stigma. To address all these issues, the World Psychiatric Association Action Plan came into effect in 2020 with an ambition to improve care for people with ID in LMICs focusing on empowering young people and their families, developing mental health services for people with ID, improving training and support to mental health professionals, and partnering with other professional organizations and nongovernmental organizations (Roy *et al.*, 2021).

Improved tools for assessing mental disorder in intellectual disability and quantifying outcome

There are few available validated measures of psychopathology for those with ID which limits other clinical and scientific advances. The problem is most acute in relation to self-report measures, for unusual behaviors, and in measuring outcomes. Furthermore, many of the currently available measures do not map well to recognized mental disorders and therefore are less helpful in guiding intervention. Effort should be made to include developing and modifying instruments that are aligned with recognized conditions and allow evaluation of treatment response (Shields *et al.*, 2023). An important advance would be alternative measures, such as digital or biological markers, that are more sensitive to change.

Interventions: How far away are we?

Children and adolescents with ID are underrepresented in clinical trials and current evidence in terms of interventions remains limited (Efron *et al.*, 2020). Pharmacological trials of psychotropic medication indicate reduced effect sizes for conventional interventions in children with ID, but the reasons for this are unclear. More experimental approaches to pharmacological trials (e.g., different treatments, adaptive trial designs) can help understand this phenomenon. Nonpharmacological interventions, behavioral modifications, have rarely been rigorously evaluated in children with ID. High-quality interventional research involving children with ID is an imperative need (Baumer *et al.*, 2022).

The genetic advances since the 2000s have been immense in identifying causes of ID and gaining more understanding of biological pathways. Studies have shown that genes associated with ID are implicated in brain development (differentiation and maturation of neurons) and synaptic function (the prerequisites for effective communication between neurons) (Maynard & Stein, 2012), and can now be targeted using advanced gene-editing techniques. Animal models of syndromic ID have found alterations in gene expression at critical developmental periods which can subsequently lead to abnormalities of the brain architecture and networks (Quach *et al.*, 2021). Advances in our understanding of the mechanisms that underly these alterations during these critical developmental windows have the potential to reveal new approaches for pharmacological intervention and gene targets. A great example of this approach that was translated to treatment is trofinetide, a promising drug that was developed for the treatment of rare childhood NDDs, and has been recently approved in the US for Rett syndrome (Keam, 2023).

The COVID-19 pandemic in 2019 has had a formidable global impact on every aspect of society, including mental and physical health (Holmes *et al.*, 2020). It remains unclear what the effects will be for the generations to come. Previous studies have shown that maternal activation of the immune system leads to an inflammatory response that continues during postnatal life and has significant effects on fetal brain development, increasing the risk for NDDs and ID (Choi *et al.*, 2016). Therefore, modeling this process in the laboratory can advance our understanding of the neurobiological pathways between infection and mental health outcomes. Given that COVID-19, among other viruses, can elicit this immune response, it will be important for longitudinal studies to explore this (McAlonan *et al.*, 2020).

References

Agarwal, V. *et al.* (2001) Double-blind, placebo-controlled trial of clonidine in hyperactive children with mental retardation. *Mental Retardation* **39**, 259–267.

Aitken, S. *et al.* (2013) *Teaching Children Who are Deafblind: Contact Communication and Learning*. David Fulton Publishers, London.

Alexiou, E. *et al.* (2023) Criminal recidivism of patients in Swedish forensic psychiatry: a register-based comparison study. *International Journal of Law and Psychiatry* **88**, 101884.

Aman, M. (1986) *Aberrant Behavior Checklist - Community*. Slosson Educational Publications, Inc, New York.

Aman, M.G. *et al.* (1996) The Nisonger CBRF: a child behavior rating form for children with developmental disabilities. *Research in Developmental Disabilities* **17**, 41–57.

Aman, M.G. *et al.* (2003) Methylphenidate treatment in children with borderline IQ and mental retardation: analysis of three aggregated studies. *Journal of Child and Adolescent Psychopharmacology* **13**, 29–40.

Aman, M.G. *et al.* (2004) Risperidone effects in the presence/absence of psychostimulant medicine in children with ADHD, other disruptive behavior disorders, and subaverage IQ. *Journal of Child and Adolescent Psychopharmacology* **14**, 243–254.

Anstis, S. & Thomas, S.D.M. (2022) Exploring the victim offender overlap among people with an intellectual disability. *Journal of Applied Research in Intellectual Disabilities* **35**, 789–799.

Arcos-Burgos, M. & Muenke, M. (2002) Genetics of population isolates. *Clinical Genetics* **61**, 233–247.

Arora, S. *et al.* (2020) Societal cost of childhood intellectual disability in Australia. *Journal of Intellectual Disability Research* **64**, 524–537.

Baron-Cohen, S. (2017) Editorial perspective: neurodiversity—a revolutionary concept for autism and psychiatry. *Journal of Child Psychology and Psychiatry* **58**, 744–747.

Barron, P. *et al.* (2004) Offenders with intellectual disability: a prospective comparative study. *Journal of Intellectual Disability Research* **48**, 69–76.

Baumer, N.T. *et al.* (2022) Conducting clinical trials in persons with down syndrome: summary from the NIH INCLUDE down syndrome clinical trials readiness working group. *Journal of Neurodevelopmental Disorders* **14**, 22.

Belanger, S.A. & Caron, J. (2018) Evaluation of the child with global developmental delay and intellectual disability. *Paediatrics & Child Health* **23**, 403–419.

Booth, T. *et al.* (2005) The prevalence and outcomes of care proceedings involving parents with learning difficulties in the family courts. *Journal of Applied Research in Intellectual Disabilities* **18**, 7–17.

Bopegamage, S. *et al.* (2012) Outcome of challenge with Coxsackievirus B4 in young mice after maternal infection with the same virus during gestation. *FEMS Immunology and Medical Microbiology* **64**, 184–190.

Broman, S.H. *et al.* (1987) *Retardation in Young Children: A Developmental Study of Cognitive Deficit*. Routledge, UK.

Brown, I. *et al.* (2013) Quality of life indicators for individuals with intellectual disabilities: extending current practice. *Intellectual and Developmental Disabilities* **51**, 316–332.

Brown, H.K. *et al.* (2018) Maternal intellectual or developmental disability and newborn discharge to protective services. *Pediatrics* **142**, 12.

Brynge, M. *et al.* (2022) Maternal infection during pregnancy and likelihood of autism and intellectual disability in children in Sweden: a negative control and sibling comparison cohort study. *The Lancet Psychiatry* **9**, 782–791.

Bushnell, G.A. *et al.* (2018) Treating pediatric anxiety: initial use of SSRIs and other antianxiety prescription medications. *The Journal of Clinical Psychiatry* **79**, 16m11415.

Casanova Dias, M. *et al.* (2020) Are we training psychiatrists to develop skills in intellectual disability psychiatry? Current European context and future directions. *European Psychiatry* **63**, e99.

Casson, J. *et al.* (2021) Housing design and modifications for individuals with intellectual and developmental disabilities and complex behavioral needs: scoping review. *Journal of Policy and Practice in Intellectual Disabilities* **18**, 217–228.

Charman, T. *et al.* (2011) IQ in children with autism spectrum disorders: data from the Special Needs and Autism Project (SNAP). *Psychological Medicine* **41**, 619–627.

Choi, G.B. *et al.* (2016) The maternal interleukin-17a pathway in mice promotes autism-like phenotypes in offspring. *Science* **351**, 933–939.

Christie, D. *et al.* (2017) Impact of meningitis on intelligence and development: a systematic review and meta-analysis. *PLoS One* **12**, e0175024.

Christoffersen, M.N. (2019) Violent crime against children with disabilities: a nationwide prospective birth cohort-study. *Child Abuse & Neglect* **98**, 104150.

Cooper, J.O. & Heron, T.E. (2007) *Applied Behavior Analysis*. Pearson, Harlow, UK.

Crawford, H. *et al.* (2019) The persistence of self-injurious and aggressive behavior in males with fragile X syndrome over 8 years: a longitudinal Study of prevalence and predictive risk markers. *Journal of Autism and Developmental Disorders* **49**, 2913–2922.

Croen, L.A. *et al.* (2001) The epidemiology of mental retardation of unknown cause. *Pediatrics* **107**, E86.

Cummins, D. *et al.* (2021) Risk factors for intellectual disability in children with spastic cerebral palsy. *Archives of Disease in Childhood* **106**, 975–980.

Cuypers, M. *et al.* (2021) Linking national public services data to estimate the prevalence of intellectual disabilities in the Netherlands: results from an explorative population-based study. *Public Health* **195**, 83–88.

Dalsgaard, S. *et al.* (2020) Incidence rates and cumulative incidences of the full Spectrum of diagnosed mental disorders in childhood and adolescence. *JAMA Psychiatry* **77**, 155–164.

Daugaard, C.A. *et al.* (2020) Association of prenatal exposure to valproate and other antiepileptic drugs with intellectual disability and delayed childhood milestones. *JAMA Network Open* **3**, e2025570.

Davies, L.E. & Oliver, C. (2016) Self-injury, aggression and destruction in children with severe intellectual disability: incidence, persistence and novel, predictive behavioural risk markers. *Research in Developmental Disabilities* **49-50**, 291–301.

Deb, S. *et al.* (2014) The effectiveness of aripiprazole in the management of problem behaviour in people with intellectual disabilities, developmental disabilities and/or autistic spectrum disorder: a systematic review. *Research in Developmental Disabilities* **35**, 711–725.

Denny, L. *et al.* (2017) Fetal alcohol syndrome and fetal alcohol Spectrum disorders. *American Family Physician* **96**, 515–522.

Donnelly, N. *et al.* (2023) Identifying the neurodevelopmental and psychiatric signatures of genomic disorders associated with intellectual disability: a machine learning approach. *Molecular Autism* **14**, 19.

Downie, L. *et al.* (2021) Principles of genomic newborn screening programs: a systematic review. *JAMA Network Open* **4**, e2114336.

Durkin, M.S. & Yeargin-Allsopp, M. (2018) Socioeconomic status and pediatric neurologic disorders: current evidence. *Seminars in Pediatric Neurology* **27**, 16–25.

Efron, D. *et al.* (2020) Does cannabidiol reduce severe behavioural problems in children with intellectual disability? Study protocol for a pilot single-site phase I/II randomised placebo controlled trial. *BMJ Open* **10**, e034362.

Einfeld, S.L. & Tonge, B.J. (1995) The Developmental Behavior Checklist: the development and validation of an instrument to assess behavioral and emotional disturbance in children and adolescents with mental retardation. *Journal of Autism and Developmental Disorders* **25**, 81–104.

Emerson, E. & Hatton, C. (2007) Mental health of children and adolescents with intellectual disabilities in Britain. *The British Journal of Psychiatry* **191**, 493–499.

Feldman, M.A. & Aunos, M. (2020) Recent trends and future directions in research regarding parents with intellectual and developmental disabilities. *Current Developmental Disorders Reports* **7**, 173–181.

Findling, R.L. *et al.* (2004) Long-term, open-label study of risperidone in children with severe disruptive behaviors and below-average IQ. *The American Journal of Psychiatry* **161**, 677–684.

Fisch, G.S. *et al.* (2010) The course of cognitive-behavioral development in children with the FMR1 mutation, Williams-Beuren syndrome, and neurofibromatosis type 1: the effect of gender. *American Journal of Medical Genetics. Part A* **152A**, 1498–1509.

Fletcher, R.J. *et al.* (2018) *DM-ID-2: Diagnostic Manual, Intellectual Disability: A textbook of Diagnosis of Mental Disorders in Persons with Intellectual Disability*. NADD Press, Kingston, NY.

Grantham-Mcgregor, S.M. *et al.* (2014) Effects of integrated child development and nutrition interventions on child development and nutritional status. *Annals of the New York Academy of Sciences* **1308**, 11–32.

Grieco, J. *et al.* (2015) Down syndrome: cognitive and behavioral functioning across the lifespan. *American Journal of Medical Genetics Part C: Seminars in Medical Genetics* **169**, 135–149.

Harlalka, G.V. *et al.* (2013) Mutation of HERC2 causes developmental delay with Angelman-like features. *Journal of Medical Genetics* **50**, 65–73.

Harrison, P.L. & Oakland, T. (2015) *Adaptive Behavior Assessment System*, Third edn. Pearson, Oxford, UK.

Haysom, L. *et al.* (2014) Intellectual disability in young people in custody in New South Wales, Australia: prevalence and markers. *Journal of Intellectual Disability Research* **58**, 1004–1014.

Hirvikoski, T. *et al.* (2021) Association of intellectual disability with all-cause and cause-specific mortality in Sweden. *JAMA Network Open* **4**, e2113014.

Holmes, E.A. *et al.* (2020) Multidisciplinary research priorities for the COVID-19 pandemic: a call for action for mental health science. *The Lancet Psychiatry* **7**, 547–560.

Hsueh, Y.M. *et al.* (2017) Association of blood heavy metals with developmental delays and health status in children. *Scientific Reports* **7**, 43608.

Hunter, J.E. *et al.* (2013) The association of low socioeconomic status and the risk of having a child with Down syndrome: a report from the National Down Syndrome Project. *Genetics in Medicine* **15**, 698–705.

Jansen, S. *et al.* (2023) The genetics of intellectual disability. *Brain Sciences* **13**.

Jensen, A.G. *et al.* (2022) Prenatal exposure to benzodiazepines and the development of the offspring: a systematic review. *Neurotoxicology and Teratology* **91**, 107078.

Kamenopoulou, L. *et al.* (2021) Multi–sensory impairment: convenient label or recipe for confusion? A scoping review of research conducted in England (2001-20). *Journal of Research in Special Educational Needs* **21**, 98–110.

Karni-Visel, Y. *et al.* (2023) Family quality of life in children with severe or profound disability: home versus residential care. *Journal of Developmental and Behavioral Pediatrics* **44**, e32–e40.

Keam, S.J. (2023) Trofinetide: first approval. *Drugs* **83**, 819–824.

Koskentausta, T. *et al.* (2007) Risk factors for psychiatric disturbance in children with intellectual disability. *Journal of Intellectual Disability Research* **51**, 43–53.

Kunkler, C. *et al.* (2022) Methamphetamine exposure during pregnancy: a meta-analysis of child developmental outcomes. *Neuroscience and Biobehavioral Reviews* **138**, 104714.

Kurtz, P.F. *et al.* (2020) Behavioral approaches to assessment and early intervention for severe problem behavior in intellectual and developmental disabilities. *Pediatric Clinics of North America* **67**, 499–511.

Lewis, E.O. (1933) Types of mental deficiency and their social significance. *Journal of Mental Science* **79**, 298–304.

Lichtenstein, P. *et al.* (2022) Familial risk and heritability of intellectual disability: a population-based cohort study in Sweden. *Journal of Child Psychology and Psychiatry* **63**, 1092–1102.

Llewellyn, G. & Hindmarsh, G. (2015) Parents with intellectual disability in a population context. *Current Developmental Disorders Reports* **2**, 119–126.

Manzanero, A.L. *et al.* (2015) (The null) importance of police experience on intuitive credibility of people with intellectual disabilities. *Research in Developmental Disabilities* **36c**, 191–197.

Mason, J. & Scior, K. (2004) 'Diagnostic Overshadowing' amongst clinicians working with people with intellectual disabilities in the UK. *Journal of Applied Research in Intellectual Disabilities* **17**, 85–90.

Maulik, P.K. *et al.* (2011) Prevalence of intellectual disability: a meta-analysis of population-based studies. *Research in Developmental Disabilities* **32**, 419–436.

Maynard, K.R. & Stein, E. (2012) DSCAM contributes to dendrite arborization and spine formation in the developing cerebral cortex. *The Journal of Neuroscience* **32**, 16637–16650.

McAlonan, G.M. *et al.* (2020) Multidisciplinary: research priorities for the COVID-19 pandemic. *The Lancet Psychiatry* **7**, e35.

McClain, M.B. *et al.* (2017) Inattention and hyperactivity/impulsivity among children with attention-deficit/hyperactivity-disorder, autism spectrum disorder, and intellectual disability. *Research in Developmental Disabilities* **70**, 175–184.

McGaw, S. *et al.* (2010) Predicting the unpredictable? Identifying high-risk versus low-risk parents with intellectual disabilities. *Child Abuse & Neglect* **34**, 699–710.

McKenzie, K. *et al.* (2016) Systematic review of the prevalence and incidence of intellectual disabilities: current trends and issues. *Current Developmental Disorders Reports* **3**, 104–115.

Mithyantha, R. *et al.* (2017) Current evidence-based recommendations on investigating children with global developmental delay. *Archives of Disease in Childhood* **102**, 1071–1076.

Moeschler, J.B. & Shevell, M. (2014) Comprehensive evaluation of the child with intellectual disability or global developmental delays. *Pediatrics* **134**, e903–e918.

Morgan, V.A. *et al.* (2008) Intellectual disability co-occurring with schizophrenia and other psychiatric illness: population-based study. *The British Journal of Psychiatry* **193**, 364–372.

Moss, S. *et al.* (1998) Reliability and validity of the PAS-ADD checklist for detecting psychiatric disorders in adults with intellectual disability. *Journal of Intellectual Disability Research* **42**, 173–183.

Munoz Garcia-Largo, L. *et al.* (2020) Intellectual disability rates among male prison inmates. *International Journal of Law and Psychiatry* **70**, 101566.

Nashed, M.G. *et al.* (2020) Prenatal cannabinoid exposure: emerging evidence of physiological and neuropsychiatric abnormalities. *Frontiers in Psychiatry* **11**, 624275.

Neece, C.L. *et al.* (2010) Impact on siblings of children with intellectual disability: the role of child behavior problems. *American Journal on Intellectual and Developmental Disabilities* **115**, 291–306.

Nelson, R.H. (2021) A critique of the neurodiversity view. *Journal of Applied Philosophy* **38**, 335–347.

Neri, G. *et al.* (2018) X-linked intellectual disability update 2017. *American Journal of Medical Genetics Part A* **176**, 1375–1388.

Oakley, B. *et al.* (2021) COVID-19 health and social care access for autistic people: European policy review. *BMJ Open* **11**, e045341.

Oliver, C. *et al.* (2003) Assessing the severity of challenging behaviour: psychometric properties of the challenging behaviour interview. *Journal of Applied Research in Intellectual Disabilities* **16**, 53–61.

Oliver, C. *et al.* (2012) The association between repetitive, self-injurious and aggressive behavior in children with severe intellectual disability. *Journal of Autism and Developmental Disorders* **42**, 910–919.

Oliver, C. *et al.* (2017) Self-injurious behaviour in people with intellectual disability and autism spectrum disorder. *Current Opinion in Psychiatry* **30**, 97–101.

O'Rance, L. (2007) Intellectual disability in Australia's Aboriginal and Torres Strait Islander peoples. *Journal of Intellectual & Developmental Disability* **32**, 222–225.

Paclawskyj, T.R. *et al.* (2000) Questions About Behavioral Function (QABF): a behavioral checklist for functional assessment of aberrant behavior. *Research in Developmental Disabilities* **21**, 223–229.

Papazoglou, A. *et al.* (2013) Sensitivity of the BASC-2 Adaptive Skills Composite in detecting adaptive impairment in a clinically referred sample of children and adolescents. *The Clinical Neuropsychologist* **27**, 386–395.

Penrose, L.S. *et al.* (1938) *A Clinical and Genetic Study of 1280 Cases of MENTAL DEFECT*. H.M.S.O., London.

Pinkerton, L.M. *et al.* (2022) Therapy service delivery for children with disabilities during COVID-19: parent perceptions and implementation recommendations. *Journal of Community Psychology* **51**, 2430–2441.

Platt, J.M. *et al.* (2019) Intellectual disability and mental disorders in a US population representative sample of adolescents. *Psychological Medicine* **49**, 952–961.

Popova, S. *et al.* (2017) Estimation of national, regional, and global prevalence of alcohol use during pregnancy and fetal alcohol syndrome: a systematic review and meta-analysis. *The Lancet Global Health* **5**, e290–e299.

Powell, R.M. & Parish, S.L. (2017) Behavioural and cognitive outcomes in young children of mothers with intellectual impairments. *Journal of Intellectual Disability Research* **61**, 50–61.

Quach, T.T. *et al.* (2021) Intellectual disability: dendritic anomalies and emerging genetic perspectives. *Acta Neuropathologica* **141**, 139–158.

Rebbe, R. *et al.* (2021) Prevalence of births and interactions with child protective services of children born to mothers diagnosed with an intellectual and/or developmental disability. *Maternal and Child Health Journal* **25**, 626–634.

Reichenberg, A. *et al.* (2016) Discontinuity in the genetic and environmental causes of the intellectual disability spectrum. *Proceedings of the National Academy of Sciences of the United States of America* **113**, 1098–1103.

Roy, A. *et al.* (2021) Setting priorities for people with intellectual disability/intellectual developmental disorders across the lifespan: a call to action by the World Psychiatric Association. *BJPsych International* **18**, 54–57.

Royal College of Psychiatrists (2016) Psychiatric services for young people with intellectual disabilities. CR200, College Report, Royal College of Psychiatrists, London.

Santosh, P.G. *et al.* (2015) Development and psychometric properties of the parent version of the Profile of Neuropsychiatric Symptoms (PONS) in children and adolescents. *BMC Paediatrics* **15**, 1–8.

Savatt, J.M. & Myers, S.M. (2021) Genetic testing in neurodevelopmental disorders. *Frontiers in Pediatrics* **9**, 526779.

Scahill, L. *et al.* (2012) Effects of risperidone and parent training on adaptive functioning in children with pervasive developmental disorders and serious behavioral problems. *Journal of the American Academy of Child and Adolescent Psychiatry* **51**, 136–146.

Sentenac, M. *et al.* (2022) Maternal education and cognitive development in 15 European very-preterm birth cohorts from the RECAP preterm platform. *International Journal of Epidemiology* **50**, 1824–1839.

Shields, R.H. *et al.* (2023) Sensitivity of the NIH toolbox to detect cognitive change in individuals with intellectual and developmental disability. *Neurology* **100**, e778–e789.

Siegel, M. *et al.* (2020) Practice parameter for the assessment and treatment of psychiatric disorders in children and adolescents with intellectual disability (intellectual developmental disorder). *Journal of the American Academy of Child and Adolescent Psychiatry* **59**, 468–496.

Simonoff, E. *et al.* (2006) The Croydon Assessment of Learning study: prevalence and educational identification of mild mental retardation. *Journal of Child Psychology & Psychiatry* **47**, 828–839.

Simonoff, E. *et al.* (2007) ADHD symptoms in children with mild intellectual disability. *Journal of the American Academy of Child and Adolescent Psychiatry* **46**, 591–600.

Simonoff, E. *et al.* (2013a) The persistence and stability of psychiatric problems in adolescents with autism spectrum disorders. *Journal of Child Psychology and Psychiatry* **54**, 186–194.

Simonoff, E. *et al.* (2013b) Randomized controlled double-blind trial of optimal dose methylphenidate in children and adolescents with severe attention deficit hyperactivity disorder and intellectual disability. *Journal of Child Psychology and Psychiatry* **54**, 527–535.

Singer, J. (1999) Why can't you be normal for once in your life? From a problem with no name to the emergence of a new category of difference. In: *Disability Discourse*. (eds M. Corker, *et al.*). Open University Press, Buckingham, UK.

Skuse, D.H. (2000) Behavioural phenotypes: what do they teach us? *Archives of Disease in Childhood* **82**, 222–225.

Smith, L.E. *et al.* (2012) Developmental trajectories in adolescents and adults with autism: the case of daily living skills. *Journal of the American Academy of Child and Adolescent Psychiatry* **51**, 622–631.

Sonuga-Barke, E. & Thapar, A. (2021) The neurodiversity concept: is it helpful for clinicians and scientists? *The Lancet Psychiatry* **8**, 559–561.

Sonuga-Barke, E.J.S. *et al.* (2017) Child-to-adult neurodevelopmental and mental health trajectories after early life deprivation: the young adult follow-up of the longitudinal English and Romanian Adoptees study. *The Lancet* **389**, 1539–1548.

Sparrow, S.S. *et al.* (2016) *Vineland Adaptive Behavior Scales, Third Edition (Vineland-3)*. Pearson, Oxford, UK.

Taylor-Phillips, S. *et al.* (2016) Accuracy of non-invasive prenatal testing using cell-free DNA for detection of Down, Edwards and Patau syndromes: a systematic review and meta-analysis. *BMJ Open* **6**, e010002.

Torelli, J.N. *et al.* (2022) A systematic review of direct assessments to evaluate psychotropic medication effects for children with disabilities. *American Journal on Intellectual and Developmental Disabilities* **127**, 103–124.

Toriello, H.V. (2008) Role of the dysmorphologic evaluation in the child with developmental delay. *Pediatric Clinics of North America* **55**(1085–1098), xi.

Totsika, V. *et al.* (2022) Mental health problems in children with intellectual disability. *The Lancet Child Adolescent Health* **6**, 432–444.

Tsakanikos, E. *et al.* (2011) Psychometric properties of the Disability Assessment Schedule (DAS) for behavior problems: an independent investigation. *Research in Developmental Disabilities* **32**, 653–658.

Tyrer, F. *et al.* (2019) Multimorbidity and lifestyle factors among adults with intellectual disabilities: a cross-sectional analysis of a UK cohort. *Journal of Intellectual Disability Research* **63**, 255–265.

Van, L. *et al.* (2017) Update on the 22q11. 2 deletion syndrome and its relevance to schizophrenia. *Current Opinion in Psychiatry* **30**, 191–196.

Van Ool, J.S. *et al.* (2016) A systematic review of neuropsychiatric comorbidities in patients with both epilepsy and intellectual disability. *Epilepsy & Behavior* **60**, 130–137.

Vos, P. *et al.* (2013) Investigating the relationship between observed mood and emotions in people with severe and profound intellectual disabilities. *Journal of Intellectual Disability Research* **57**, 440–451.

Walker, V.L. & Snell, M.E. (2013) Effects of augmentative and alternative communication on challenging behavior: a meta-analysis. *Augmentative and Alternative Communication* **29**, 117–131.

Wolstencroft, J. *et al.* (2022) Neuropsychiatric risk in children with intellectual disability of genetic origin: IMAGINE, a UK national cohort study. *The Lancet Psychiatry* **9**, 715–724.

Worthington, R.E. & Rossetti, S. (2020) Attitudes towards offenders with intellectual disability. *Journal of Criminological Research, Policy and Practice* **7**, 93–111.

Yeargin-Allsopp, M. *et al.* (1995) Mild mental retardation in black and white children in metropolitan Atlanta: a case-control study. *American Journal of Public Health* **85**, 324–328.

Young, J.T. *et al.* (2018) Severity of cognitive disability and mental health court determinations about fitness to stand trial. *Journal of Intellectual Disability Research* **62**, 126–139.

Yu, Y. *et al.* (2021) Young adults with autism Spectrum disorder and the criminal justice system. *Journal of Autism and Developmental Disorders* **51**, 3624–3636.

Zablotsky, B. *et al.* (2019) Prevalence and trends of developmental disabilities among children in the United States: 2009-2017. *Pediatrics* **144**, e20190811.

Zhang, L. *et al.* (2021) Supporting child development through parenting interventions in low- to middle-income countries: an updated systematic review. *Frontiers in Public Health* **9**, 671988.

Zigler, E. (1967) Familial mental retardation: a continuing dilemma. *Science* **155**, 292–298.

CHAPTER 54

Attention deficit hyperactivity disorder

Samuele Cortese[1,2,3,4] and Luis Augusto Rohde[5,6,7]

[1] Centre of Innovation in Mental Health, School of Psychology, Faculty of Environmental and Life Sciences, University of Southampton, Southampton, UK

[2] Hampshire and Isle of Wight Healthcare NHS Foundation Trust, Southampton, UK

[3] University of Bari "Aldo Moro", Italy

[4] Department of Child and Adolescent Psychiatry, NYU Grossman School of Medicine, New York, USA

[5] ADHD Outpatient Program and Development Psychiatry Program, Hospital de Clínicas de Porto Alegre, Porto Alegre, Brazil

[6] Department of Psychiatry, Universidade Federal do Rio Grande do Sul, Porto Alegre, Brazil

[7] Advisory Council, Medical School, UNIEDUK, Indaiatuba, Brazil

Overview of the chapter

In this chapter we provide a comprehensive overview of key clinically relevant issues related to one of the most prevalent child mental conditions, attention deficit hyperactivity disorder (ADHD). Diverse facets of the disorder are described, including the evolution of the concept, its phenomenology, and cultural contextualization, key elements for assessment and diagnosis, epidemiological data, developmental trajectories and outcomes, the impact of the disorder, etiological factors, neurobiological correlates, and evidence-based management strategies. Current limitations and challenges for the future in each of these areas are addressed.

Characterizing the condition

Evolution of the concept and controversies

Although there are some claims that descriptions of what we currently recognize as ADHD can be traced to the Greek philosopher Theophrastus in the 4th century BCE (Victor *et al.*, 2018), most have identified the first reports of an ADHD syndrome in German, French and Scottish textbooks in the second half of the 18th century (Figure 54.1). The first report describing the phenomenology, potential etiology, and course of a condition that resembles ADHD in a medical journal was presented by Still in 1902 (Still, 1902). After Still's description, ADHD was named *minimal brain damage* due to the assumption that it was associated with brain lesions (Hohman, 1922; Kahn & Cohen, 1934). In 1937, Bradley reported that benzedrine, a stimulant, could decrease hyperactivity and improve attention and academic performance (Bradley, 1937). Later, recognizing that children might not have brain lesions, the syndrome was renamed *minimal brain dysfunction* (Clements & Peters, 1962). Hyperactivity was the symptom used to name the disorder when first included in the *International Classification of Diseases*, 9th edition (ICD-9) in 1975 as "hyperkinetic syndrome of childhood" (subsequently called "hyperkinetic disorder" in ICD-10 in 1995) and in the *Diagnostic and Statistical Manual of Mental Disorders*, 2nd edition (DSM-2) ("hyperkinetic reaction of childhood"), also in the 1970s. It was only in 1980 that the role of inattention was recognized, and the disorder renamed "attention-deficit disorder with or without hyperactivity" (DSM-III). This was the first time operational criteria for the disorder were introduced. Subsequently, DSM-III-R and DSM-IV renamed the disorder as "Attention deficit hyperactivity disorder," equilibrating the relevance of both inattentive and hyperactive/impulsive symptoms. In 2013, DSM-5 made some operational criteria adjustments and adapted the description of symptoms to older adolescents and adults. ICD-11, for the first time, changed the nomenclature from *Hyperkinetic Disorder* to *Attention Deficit Hyperactivity Disorder*, abandoning more structured operational criteria and the requirement for a specific number of symptoms. The milestones characterizing the history of the ADHD concept are described in Figure 54.1. Overall, this history portrays the evolution of the ADHD concept as a medical condition. However, controversies on this conceptualization of ADHD, first raised in the 1960s, still persist. Indeed, some authors from social science claim that there is an excessive medicalization of the concept of ADHD, making variations of human behavior pathological (Bergey *et al.*, 2018).

Nonetheless, currently ADHD is mainly defined as a neurodevelopmental condition characterized by age-inappropriate, frequent and/or extreme, pervasive, and impairing inattention and/or hyperactivity/impulsivity symptoms (American Psychiatric Association, 2022).

Rutter's Child and Adolescent Psychiatry and Psychology, Seventh Edition.
Edited by Anita Thapar, Daniel S. Pine, Samuele Cortese, Cathy Creswell, Tamsin J. Ford, James F. Leckman, and Argyris Stringaris.

Companion website: www.wiley.com/go/thapar/rutterspsych7

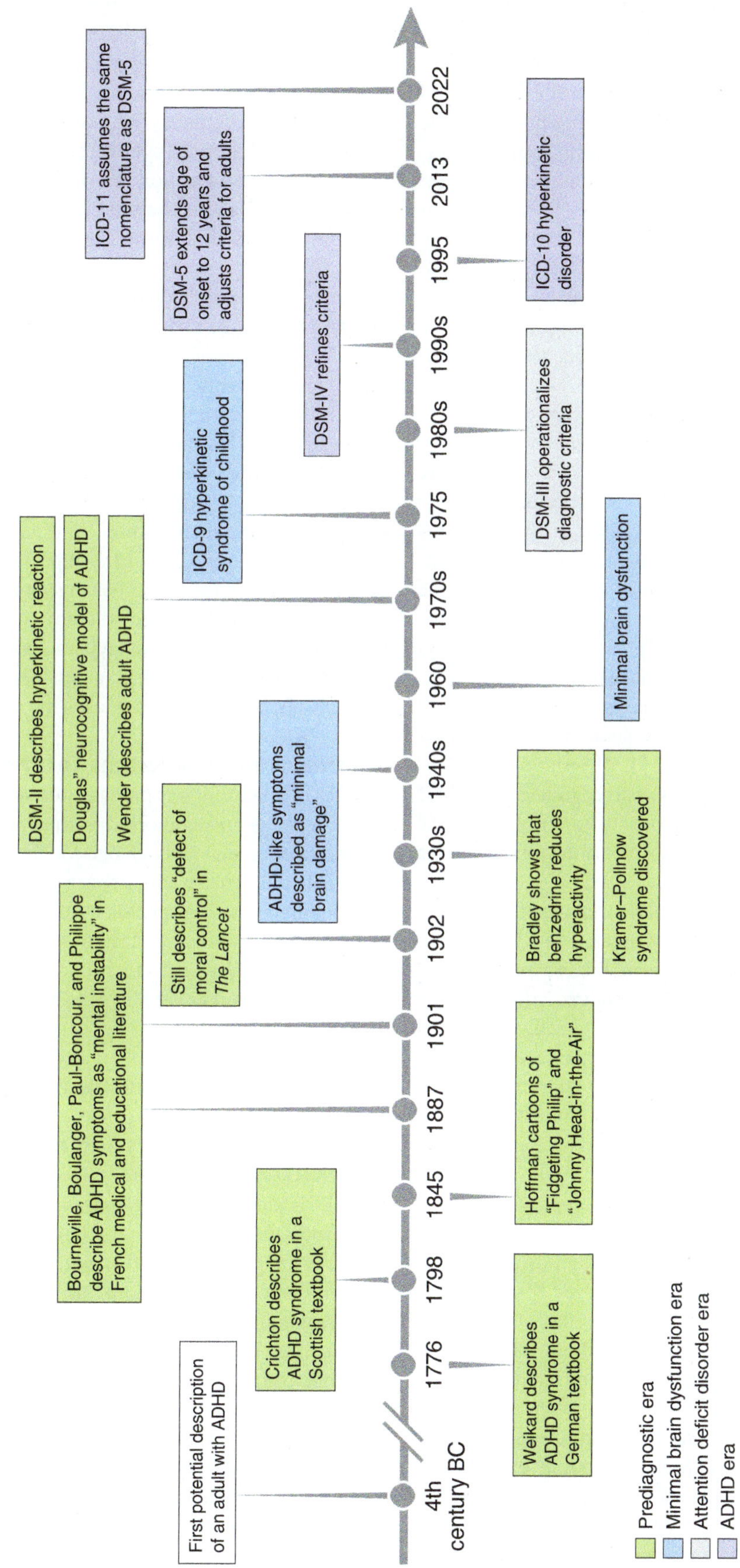

Figure 54.1 Milestones characterizing the history of the attention deficit hyperactivity disorder (ADHD) concept.

Current conceptualization of attention deficit hyperactivity disorder as a neurodevelopmental disorder

ADHD was conceptualized in DSM-5 as a neurodevelopmental disorder (NDD) given: (i) its onset in early childhood; (ii) the neurobiological underpinnings associated with brain maturation; and (iii) its trajectory during childhood and adolescence being mostly stable after onset (Bishop, 2011). However, recent evidence challenges this notion. As discussed in the following sections, this evidence includes findings that a proportion of individuals might have the onset in adolescence or young adulthood and that some individuals have a fluctuating course within some developmental stages (Sonuga-Barke *et al.*, 2023).

Attention deficit hyperactivity disorder phenomenology

Like most mental disorders and several medical diseases, there is evidence that symptoms of ADHD lie on a continuum (Posner *et al.*, 2020). However, most health care decisions, like decisions about who should be referred to treatment, involve categorizations (i.e., *yes* or *no*). Thus, classificatory systems, such as the DSM-5, require a threshold associated with impairment (for example, six symptoms of inattention and/or hyperactivity/impulsivity in children). Several investigations suggest that individuals below these thresholds might exhibit significant impairment depending on other circumstances such as context and comorbidities (Kirova *et al.*, 2019). Thresholds of symptoms depend on developmental stage, as recognized by DSM-5 (i.e., adults need fewer ADHD symptoms to have the same level of impairment as children and adolescents), and culture, among other factors.

Heterogeneity is a key factor in ADHD and one of the biggest challenges for investigations on the disorder. The ADHD clinical presentation might depend on several factors including: (i) the polythetic nature of the ADHD diagnostic criteria in the classificatory systems like DSM (i.e., theoretically, there are 116,220 different combinations of symptoms to achieve the DSM-5 threshold); (ii) comorbidity; (iii) the information source; (iv) developmental aspects; and (v) context (i.e., individuals in less demanding settings might present less prominent symptomatology) (Cortese & Rohde, 2019).

ADHD is highly associated with overlapping disorders. Seminal work (Angold *et al.*, 1999) found children with ADHD to be over 10 times more likely to have conduct disorder (CD) or oppositional defiant disorder (ODD), over 5 times more likely to have depression, and 3 times more likely to have any anxiety disorder, compared to children without ADHD. One key strength in this study is the reliance on community data. In addition, ADHD frequently co-occurs with other NDDs such as autism spectrum disorder (ASD), communication and specific learning or motor disorders (e.g., reading disability or developmental coordination disorder), intellectual disability, and tic disorders (Thapar & Cooper, 2016). Moreover, substance use disorders, sleep disorders, and even medical comorbidities like obesity, asthma, and type 2 diabetes co-occur more frequently with ADHD than in the general population (Arrondo *et al.*, 2022). Beyond categorical diagnoses, ADHD has been associated with several other clinically relevant phenotypes like emotional dysregulation, sluggish cognitive tempo, executive dysfunction syndromes, time perceptions distortions, and delay aversion (Sonuga-Barke *et al.*, 2023). The extent to which these phenotypes constitute core ADHD components or correlated features is debated.

Attention deficit hyperactivity disorder in the context of age, sex, and culture

ADHD phenomenology strongly depends on other issues like age or developmental stage (see the later section covering DSM-5-TR criteria), sex, and context. While girls tend to present with more inattention than hyperactivity and impulsivity, their comorbid profile is not substantially different than the one presented by boys. In both sexes, ADHD relates more strongly to comorbid externalizing than internalizing disorders (Tung *et al.*, 2016). Culture shapes the expression and expectations of behaviors and symptoms. For instance, cultures from Latin America tend to be more tolerant than those from Asia of behavioral problems and hyperactivity, especially in boys (Azevêdo *et al.*, 2020). Thus, assessment of ADHD symptoms must always consider cultural aspects.

Summary and challenges for the future

ADHD is a neurodevelopmental dimensional disorder, highly heterogeneous and comorbid with other mental and physical disorders. One major challenge for the field involves reducing ADHD heterogeneity and assessing if more homogeneous phenotypes are related to specific etiologies, trajectories, biological markers, and responses to treatment. Defining boundaries with other disorders in an extremely comorbid condition like ADHD is another relevant area of investigation.

Diagnosis and assessment

Key elements in assessing attention deficit hyperactivity disorder

ADHD is defined by the presence of a persistent and age-inappropriate pattern of inattention and/or hyperactivity–impulsivity that interferes with normal functioning or development. Manifestations of inattention are numerous, including mind-wandering while performing a task, lack of persistence, and disorganization. Hyperactivity manifests as excessive, inappropriate activity, fidgeting, tapping, or talkativeness. Impulsive symptoms include making decisions or actions without thinking or considering consequences, difficulty waiting turns, and social intrusiveness. Of note, these behaviors should not be due to defiance or lack of comprehension (American Psychiatric Association, 2022). Moreover, ADHD symptoms might fail to manifest in health care settings, since the child is in an artificial environment where performance anxiety might alter typical behavior (Rohde *et al.*, 2019).

A persistent pattern of symptoms is essential for making an ADHD diagnosis. While a specific duration of at least six months is suggested in classificatory systems, this is not an evidence-based criterion. ADHD cardinal symptoms are non-specific and may arise as short-term responses to stressors like family problems or higher school demands. Thus, clinicians should discuss each symptom with patients and their families, considering only those that are frequently present in patients' daily lives, as indicative of the disorder. In this assessment, it is essential to set a common understanding with the family on a culturally acceptable definition of what is considered to be frequent.

The symptoms must be inconsistent with the developmental stage of the individual under assessment. Since ADHD symptomatology is dimensionally distributed in the population, any clinical cutoff involves a level of arbitrariness. Thus, clinicians are faced with the difficult task of defining the boundaries separating typical from pathological behavior for each individual. In this scenario, extensive knowledge on normal human development is crucial.

Despite the conceptualization of ADHD as an NDD, no evidence, beyond symptom levels as compared to same-age peers, defines thresholds for the presence of symptoms. Although onset in childhood is frequently found in referred cases, clinicians should be cautious when excluding ADHD based only on onset of symptoms after 12 years of age (Rohde *et al.*, 2019).

Investigation of the pervasiveness of symptoms in different environments is another key aspect for ADHD diagnosis. The underlying rationale is to avoid diagnosis in cases where symptoms manifest only in relation to environment-specific triggers (e.g., only at home due to severe family conflicts; only at school due to material inappropriate for a child's capacities). However, ADHD is one of the few disorders for which operational criteria require symptoms in multiple settings, and few studies have tested the validity of this criterion (Willcutt *et al.*, 2012). Some children who display impairment in only one setting at one point in time may display impairment in multiple settings at a later point when facing more challenging demands. Nonetheless, some children who meet symptom criteria for ADHD may exhibit significant impairment that is truly restricted to one setting. This pattern may be especially common in groups with predominantly inattentive ADHD presentation because this symptomatic presentation is associated more strongly with difficulties in academic domains (Rohde *et al.*, 2019). Thus, caution is needed if symptoms with clinically relevant impairment only occur in one setting.

Another area of assessment considers distinguishing impairment derived from ADHD as opposed to frequent comorbidities. Since ADHD symptoms reflect a dimensional trait in the population, failure to incorporate interference of symptoms in functioning as part of the diagnostic criteria for the disorder results in a substantial increase in prevalence rates.

In the assessment, it is paramount to understand the role of motivation in the manifestations of the symptoms. Children affected by ADHD might be able to remain focused when performing specific tasks such as playing video games. Motivation, relevance, the attractiveness of the task for the child, and the demands of the environment influence symptomatic manifestations. Thus, overconcentration or "hyperfocus" is frequent in individuals with ADHD. ADHD can thus be viewed as an attention dysregulation (rather than deficit) disorder. Many patients with ADHD are capable of concentrating in some contexts, but they cannot deploy concentration at moments when it is needed. Regarding environmental demands, careful parents might provide structured environments and stimulation for their children with ADHD, creating a situation where symptoms only manifest later in adolescence when more autonomy is needed (Rohde *et al.*, 2019; Freitas de Sousa *et al.*, 2020).

The developmental stage of the individual must be considered when characterizing ADHD clinical presentation. In preschoolers, hyperactivity and impulsivity are much more prominent than inattention due to fewer environmental demands requiring focus on the child. ADHD diagnosis is possible and reliable in children as young as three years of age, and these children have clinically significant impairment across all relationships and settings (Shephard *et al.*, 2022). While the combination of inattentive and hyperactive/impulsive symptoms is the most common presentation in clinical samples during school age, inattentive symptoms are more prominent in nonreferred samples. It remains unclear whether high rates of inattentive presentation in these nonreferred samples reflect sex differences in the threshold for referrals or other factors. Since hyperactive/impulsive symptoms decrease more significantly than inattention, the most frequent presentation found in older adolescents and adults is ADHD with predominantly inattentive symptoms. Additionally, the clinical picture in adults might also involve symptoms related to executive dysfunction and emotional impulsivity. Core ADHD symptoms might manifest differently in adults. Thus, hyperactivity in adults often manifests as inner restlessness, or not being able to relax properly. Impulsive behavior might manifest as acting without thinking or in blurting things out, spending too much money or spending it too quickly, carrying out plans immediately, resigning from jobs in a flurry, starting relationships quickly, and not being able to postpone need gratification. Older adolescents and adults frequently report "sensation-seeking," "novelty-seeking," or seeking out excitement (Asherson *et al.*, 2016).

Attention deficit hyperactivity disorder diagnosis in classificatory systems

Diagnostic and Statistical Manual of Mental Disorders, 5th edition, text revision

The list of ADHD symptoms in DSM-5-TR is organized in two dimensions—inattentive and hyperactive/impulsive domains (Box 54.1), based on studies in predominantly school-age children from the United States (US). Thus, this generates some

Box 54.1

Diagnostic criteria for attention deficit hyperactivity disorder

A A persistent pattern of inattention and/or hyperactivity–impulsivity that interferes with functioning or development, as characterized by (1) and/or (2):

1 **Inattention:** Six (or more) of the following symptoms have persisted for at least six months to a degree that is inconsistent with developmental level and that negatively impacts directly on social and academic/occupational activities*:

(a) Often fails to give close attention to details or makes careless mistakes in schoolwork, at work, or during other activities (e.g., overlooks or misses details, work is inaccurate).

(b) Often has difficulty sustaining attention in tasks or play activities (e.g., has difficulty remaining focused during lectures, conversations, or lengthy reading).

(c) Often does not seem to listen when spoken to directly (e.g., mind seems elsewhere, even in the absence of any obvious distraction).

(d) Often does not follow through on instructions and fails to finish schoolwork, chores, or duties in the workplace (e.g., starts tasks but quickly loses focus and is easily sidetracked).

(e) Often has difficulty organizing tasks and activities (e.g., difficulty managing sequential tasks; difficulty keeping materials and belongings in order; messy, disorganized work; has poor time management; fails to meet deadlines).

(f) Often avoids, dislikes, or is reluctant to engage in tasks that require sustained mental effort (e.g., schoolwork or homework; for older adolescents and adults, preparing reports, completing forms, reviewing lengthy papers).

(g) Often loses things necessary for tasks or activities (e.g., school materials, pencils, books, tools, wallets, keys, paperwork, eyeglasses, mobile telephones).

(h) Is often easily distracted by extraneous stimuli (for older adolescents and adults, may include unrelated thoughts).

(i) Is often forgetful in daily activities (e.g., doing chores, running errands; for older adolescents and adults, returning calls, paying bills, keeping appointments).

2 **Hyperactivity and impulsivity:** Six (or more) of the following symptoms have persisted for at least six months to a degree that is inconsistent with developmental level and that negatively impacts directly on social and academic/occupational activities*:

(a) Often fidgets with or taps hands or feet or squirms in seat.

(b) Often leaves seat in situations when remaining seated is expected (e.g., leaves their place in the classroom, in the office or other workplace, or in other situations that require remaining in place).

(c) Often runs about or climbs in situations where it is inappropriate. (Note: In adolescents or adults, may be limited to feeling restless.)

(d) Often unable to play or engage in leisure activities quietly.

(e) Is often "on the go," acting as if "driven by a motor" (e.g., is unable to be, or uncomfortable being, still for extended time, as in restaurants or meetings; may be experienced by others as being restless or difficult to keep up with).

(f) Often talks excessively.

(g) Often blurts out an answer before a question has been completed (e.g., completes people's sentences; cannot wait for turn in conversation).

(h) Often has difficulty waiting their turn (e.g., while waiting in line).

(i) Often interrupts or intrudes on others (e.g., butts into conversations, games, or activities; may start using other people's things without asking or receiving permission; for adolescents and adults, may intrude into or take over what others are doing).

B. Several inattentive or hyperactive–impulsive symptoms were present prior to age 12 years.

C. Several inattentive or hyperactive–impulsive symptoms are present in two or more settings (e.g., at home, school, or work; with friends or relatives; in other activities).

D. There is clear evidence that the symptoms interfere with, or reduce the quality of, social, academic, or occupational functioning.

E. The symptoms do not occur exclusively during the course of schizophrenia or another psychotic disorder, and are not better explained by another mental disorder (e.g., mood disorder, anxiety disorder, dissociative disorder, personality disorder, substance intoxication or withdrawal).

Specify whether:

- **(F90.2) Combined presentation:** If both criterion A1 (inattention) and criterion A2 (hyperactivity–impulsivity) are met for the past six months.
- **(F90.0) Predominantly inattentive presentation:** If criterion A1 (inattention) is met but criterion A2 (hyperactivity–impulsivity) is not met for the past six months.
- **(F90.1) Predominantly hyperactive/impulsive presentation:** If criterion A2 (hyperactivity–impulsivity) is met and criterion A1 (inattention) is not met for the past six months.

Specify if:

- **In partial remission:** When full criteria were previously met, fewer than the full criteria have been met for the past six months, and the symptoms still result in impairment in social, academic, or occupational functioning.

Specify current severity:

- **Mild:** Few, if any, symptoms in excess of those required to make the diagnosis are present, and symptoms result in no more than minor impairments in social or occupational functioning.
- **Moderate:** Symptoms or functional impairment between "mild" and "severe" are present.
- **Severe:** Many symptoms in excess of those required to make the diagnosis, or several symptoms that are particularly severe, are present, or the symptoms result in marked impairment in social or occupational functioning.

***Note:** The symptoms are not solely a manifestation of oppositional behavior, defiance, hostility, or failure to understand tasks or instructions. For older adolescents and adults (aged 17 and older), at least five symptoms are required.

uncertainty about diagnostic performance in different cultures and age ranges (e.g., preschoolers and adults). For the first time, DSM-5 proposed a lower threshold (five symptoms or more) for the diagnosis of ADHD in adults than in youth. This decision reflects previous research demonstrating that adults present significant impairment even with a lower number of symptoms. There is evidence that symptoms like emotional impulsivity and those linked to executive deficits might be very relevant in adults with ADHD (Asherson *et al.*, 2016). Other relevant criteria (pervasiveness, age-of-onset, impairment, exclusionary criterion) appear in Box 54.1.

Notably, DSM-5 removed the exclusion of the diagnosis in the presence of ASD. ADHD and autism frequently co-occur, and the presence of ADHD symptoms in patients with ASD confers distinct problems from those of ASD alone. DSM-5 also changed the nomenclature from ADHD presentations, due to developmental instability across DSM-IV subtypes and weak evidence separating them on neuropsychological grounds.

International Classification of Diseases, 11th revision

ICD-11 replaced the nomenclature used in previous versions, *Hyperkinetic Disorder*, with *ADHD*. Although it does not present strict operational criteria like the DSM-5, the general principles for diagnosing are the same, as well as the three presentations proposed (https://icd.who.int/browse11/l-m/en#/http%3a%2f%2fid.who.int%2ficd%2fentity%2f821852937).

Best practice overview

There are some general principles when conducting an assessment for ADHD. They are:

- Conduct a comprehensive assessment taking into consideration cultural norms of age and gender-appropriate behavior, as well as family values and environmental demands, avoiding rapid evaluations based only on checklists.
- Assess primarily if symptoms are not accounted for by physical conditions like impaired vision or hearing. Although ADHD might relate to sleep disorders, evaluate if ADHD symptoms, especially inattention, manifest independently of sleep problems.
- Search extensively for comorbidities.
- Rely on multiple information sources. It is essential to fully include a child or young person's perspective in the assessment process. Teachers' and parents' reports should be obtained to establish the diagnosis in children and adolescents when available, even if there is evidence of low levels of agreement across teachers on ADHD symptomatology in children (Rohde *et al.*, 2019). In adults, the report of a significant other, family member, or co-worker can provide important additional information.
- There are no ancillary tests or biomarkers with sufficient positive and negative predictive power for the diagnosis of ADHD. No evidence supports the inclusion of neuroimaging exams (e.g., magnetic resonance imaging (MRI), single-photon emission computerized tomography (SPECT), positron emission tomography (PET) scans) or electroencephalogram (EEG) in routine clinical assessment of ADHD, although they can be useful in very specific cases for differential diagnosis (Buitelaar *et al.*, 2022).
- Neuropsychological or IQ and achievement tests are not necessary for diagnosing ADHD, but they might be helpful to estimate intellectual impairment, severe executive function deficits, and potential learning disorders (Rohde *et al.*, 2019).

Tools

For children and adolescents, an extensively used open-access option for screening ADHD symptoms is the SNAP-IV scale (https://www.caddra.ca/wp-content/uploads/SNAP-IV-26.pdf). Although there are some controversies about its psychometric properties in population samples, this scale is helpful for clinicians in: (i) initial screening of ADHD symptoms; (ii) obtaining information from teachers on ADHD symptoms when direct contact is not feasible; and (iii) monitoring symptoms trajectories or during treatment (Rohde *et al.*, 2019). When a shorter screening scale is needed, one option is the Hyperactivity scale of the Strengths and Difficulties Questionnaire (SDQ), an instrument translated into several languages (https://www.sdqinfo.org). For adults, the Adult ADHD Self-Report Scale (ASRS) is an open-access instrument with two versions: (i) a screener version developed by the World Health Organization (WHO) with six items, that is suitable for primary care settings and for a quick screening of ADHD (https://www.hcp.med.harvard.edu/ncs/ftpdir/adhd/6Q_ASRS_English.pdf), translated into various languages; and (ii) a long version with the 18 DSM symptoms, probably more useful for specialized settings (https://novopsych.com.au/assessments/diagnosis/adult-adhd-self-report-scale-asrs/#:~:text=The%20Adult%20ADHD%20Self%2DReport,symptoms%20in%20adults%20(18%2B).). Both versions use wording more appropriate for adults. A short version adapted for DSM-5 is also available (https://psychology-tools.com/test/adult-adhd-self-report-scale#:~:text=The%20tool%20consists%20of%2018,of%20ADHD%20symptoms%20over%20time.).

Several structured and semistructured interviews can be used for diagnosing ADHD and comorbidities, including the Diagnostic Interview Schedule for Children (DISC), the Child and Adolescent Psychiatric Assessment (CAPA), the Development and Well-being Assessment (DAWBA), and the Kiddie Schedule for Affective Disorders and Schizophrenia—present and lifetime version (KSADS-PL) (https://www.pediatricbipolar.pitt.edu/sites/default/files/KSADS_DSM_5_SCREEN_Final.pdf). However, their use tends to be restricted to research settings (Angold *et al.*, 1999). For adults, an instrument for assessing the diagnosis of ADHD is the DIVA 2.0, a semistructured interview based on DSM-IV-TR that can be downloaded in many languages but is not an open-access instrument—a small payment is requested (https://www.advancedassessments.co.uk/resources/ADHD-Screening-Test-Adult.pdf).

Differential diagnosis

Physical and laboratory investigations might help in excluding other clinical conditions (e.g., hyperthyroidism); likewise, it is important to rule out the use of any medicine that might cause inattentive and/or hyperactive/impulsive symptoms. Referral for genetic examination is recommended if there is a clear developmental delay and/or if suggestive phenotypes manifest (i.e., neurofibromatosis type I, fragile X syndrome). Several potentially co-occurring psychiatric disorders must also be considered in the differential diagnosis (i.e., generalized anxiety disorder, bipolar disorder, major depression, sleep disorders, and learning disorders). Although ADHD can be comorbid with post-traumatic stress disorder (PTSD) (Spencer *et al.*, 2016), severe traumatic events might create a clinical picture that resembles ADHD.

In the process of conducting a careful differential diagnosis, some clinical tips might be relevant:

- Consider the age of onset of the ADHD symptoms and of the symptoms from the other psychiatric problems. For example, this might be considered when disentangling inattention as part of ADHD or of a mild chronic depressive disorder (dysthymia). Inattentive symptoms before the onset of any mood symptoms reinforce ADHD diagnosis.
- Examine the trajectory of the symptoms (some disorders, like bipolar disorder, are much more episodic). Thus, strong swings of symptoms might suggest other disorders, like bipolar disorder, where, besides the core manic symptoms, hyperactivity, impulsivity, and irritability are episodic.
- Assess if the symptoms are better explained by the other mental disorder (e.g., inattention only as a consequence of dysfunctional thoughts/rumination related to performance as in generalized anxiety disorder, or mental rituals of counting as in obsessive–compulsive disorder (OCD); inattention and executive deficits following abuse or dependence on marijuana without any previous history of ADHD symptoms; inattention only related to reading in dyslexia) (Rohde *et al.*, 2019).

Relative immaturity might also be considered in the differential diagnosis. Children who are the youngest in the class are more likely to be diagnosed as suffering from ADHD (Caye *et al.*, 2020). Although the reasons for this are unclear, it could be due to: (i) younger (less mature) children being incorrectly diagnosed as having ADHD (false positives); or (ii) younger children with ADHD in the same school grade may have a more severe clinical presentation, making the recognition easier (Gosling *et al.*, 2023).

Summary and challenges for the future

ADHD is a clinical diagnosis requiring a careful and comprehensive assessment. Among challenges for the future, age-of-onset of symptoms is a central issue. More investigation is needed to see if there is sufficient evidence to restrict ADHD diagnosis to cases with clear symptoms onset during childhood. Furthermore, the construct of ADHD in different cultures, in females, and in other age ranges (e.g., preschoolers and adults) should be further investigated.

Box 54.2 summarizes the key elements for the assessment of ADHD.

Epidemiology

Incidence and prevalence

Adequate epidemiological data are essential for service planning. Polanczyk *et al.* (2007) estimated a worldwide ADHD prevalence of 5.29% (95% CI 5.01–5.56). Willcutt *et al.* (2012) found similar results (5.9%) in a subsequent meta-analysis. Moreover, (Polanczyk *et al.*, 2014) found no increase in the prevalence of ADHD in children and adolescents over the previous three decades preceding their meta-analysis. Thus, media claims about an ADHD epidemic are not supported by scientific data. However, large studies in some countries have suggested that ADHD is more likely to have been diagnosed in recent years, probably reflecting changes in administrative and clinical practices (Faraone *et al.*, 2021). Varying prevalence rates across countries are mostly due to methodological differences among studies (i.e., diagnostic criteria used—DSM versus ICD systems,

Box 54.2 Assessment at a glance

Essential for the diagnosis

- Interview with child/young person and parents/carers, including detailed developmental history
- Mental state examination
- Corroborative information from other sources, including school. This information can be gathered via questionnaires/rating scales but please note: questionnaires/rating scales are not diagnostic per se (i.e., scores above clinical thresholds are not necessarily an indication of a diagnosis of attention deficit hyperactivity disorder (ADHD); rather they provide additional information to be integrated within the diagnostic work-up and can allow the clinicians to track the severity of the symptoms over time). School observations can be helpful in cases where information from questionnaires is deemed not reliable or when it is not possible to gather such information.

Not necessary for the diagnosis, but can complement the diagnostic process (even though the specific algorithm to integrate them in the diagnostic process is currently not well established)

- QbTest and its variants (for preschoolers: QbMini; for individuals aged over 12 years: QbTest+[clinic-based])

Not required for the diagnosis, but can provide useful information for the differential diagnosis and management plan

IQ test

Not required for the diagnosis, but can provide useful information for the management plan

- Neuropsychological tests, including continuous performance test (CPT)

Indicated only if clinical characteristics of the child/young person suggest their usefulness to refine the phenotype or for the differential diagnosis with other medical conditions

- Auditory and visual tests
- Blood test (e.g., to rule out anemia or hyperthyroidism)
- Genetic test (if phenotypic characteristics suggest possible genetic syndromes)
- Electroencephalography (EEG) (differential diagnosis with epilepsy)
- Polysomnography (differential diagnosis with sleep disorders)
- Magnetic resonance imaging (MRI) (differential diagnosis with head injuries/brain lesions)

sources of information—parents, teachers, or both, and the requirement of functional impairment for diagnosis) (Posner *et al.*, 2020). Regarding age differences, ADHD incidence rate peaked at age 5–9, in both sexes, with larger figures for males, according to Global Burden of Disease (GBD) data (Cortese *et al.*, 2023a). Prevalence rates then decrease steadily between 10–14 years-of-age. Song *et al.* (2021) found a meta-analytic prevalence rate of ADHD in adults of 2.58%. Interestingly, this rate is more than double the rate when age-of-onset in childhood is not required for diagnosis. Regarding male/female ratio in childhood, previous investigations have suggested that approximately 2.5 times more males than females present with ADHD in population samples. This ratio can be even higher, around 4 times in clinical studies (Faraone *et al.*, 2021; Cortese *et al.*, 2023a). There is growing evidence that this ratio changes substantially from adolescence through adulthood, with an increasingly large proportion of ADHD cases being female (Faraone *et al.*, 2021). In clinical samples, this phenomenon may partly reflect referral bias, involving higher tendencies to refer males in childhood due to hyperactivity and behavior problems, and a greater search for treatment by females in adulthood. Additionally, females might need a more severe presentation to receive an ADHD diagnosis in childhood, due to diagnostic operationalization relying on samples composed mostly of boys. As severity is the main predictor of persistence, this higher severity in females might make persistence into adolescence and adulthood higher for females than for males. Previous beliefs of lower prevalence in minorities are not supported by recent data showing higher ADHD rates in Black individuals than in the general population (14.54%; 95% CI 10.64–19.56) (Cénat *et al.*, 2021). Russell *et al.* (2016) found that children in families of low socioeconomic status (SES) are on average 1.85–2.21 times more likely to have ADHD than their peers in high SES families. This finding may not reflect a causal effect of SES, since we cannot exclude reverse causation (e.g., underemployment that might be an outcome of the disorder could lead to the overrepresentation of socioeconomic disadvantage among ADHD families). In addition, the association might be linked to other confounding factors like parental mental health.

Health economic burden

According to the 2019 GBD data, ADHD accounted for 0.8% of the global mental disorder disability-adjusted life years across age. However, this indicator is probably underestimated, since mortality was set at 0 despite meta-analytic evidence of significantly increased ADHD-related mortality due to unnatural causes (Cortese *et al.*, 2023a). The health costs of individuals with ADHD seem to be at least double those of individuals without ADHD, even in investigations where confounders such as other mental disorders are considered (Faraone *et al.*, 2021). These findings translate into major economic impact. For instance, in the US, a review found overall national annual incremental costs of ADHD ranged between US$143–266 billion, from 1990 to 2011 (Doshi *et al.*, 2012).

Current limitations and challenges for the future

More epidemiological data are needed from low-income countries. We need to better understand reasons for the ADHD male preponderance in childhood and why the male/female proportion decreases along development, as well as other reasons, besides methodological ones, that determine different prevalence rates among countries. The great majority of investigations on health economic burdens associated with ADHD examine only high-income countries. The development of open-access epidemiological measures tuned to diverse cultural environments and translated into many languages is badly needed, as are transparent, calibrated mathematical models for deriving adequate data from screening tools.

Developmental pathways, phenotypes, and outcomes

Onset, offset, persistence, and stability

Two trajectories are traditionally recognized for ADHD: (i) an early childhood onset with a steady course from childhood to adulthood; and (ii) an early childhood onset with a steady course during childhood with clear attenuation of symptoms and/or impairment during adolescence or young adulthood (Sonuga-Barke *et al.*, 2023). Despite marked heterogeneity, most individuals diagnosed with ADHD in childhood still have significant symptoms and/or impairments in adolescence and early adulthood (Sonuga-Barke *et al.*, 2023). In fact, the Multimodal Treatment of ADHD (MTA) study, using data collected at multiple ages across development, suggested that full recovery/sustained remission during the period up to adulthood occurs in less than 10% of ADHD individuals (Sibley *et al.*, 2022). Longitudinal studies have established that hyperactivity is less persistent across development than impulsivity and inattention, both in the general population and in clinical samples (Willcutt, 2012). A meta-analysis of childhood factors predicting ADHD persistence into adulthood found that symptom severity and co-occurrence with CD and major depressive disorder were statistically significant predictors (Caye *et al.*, 2016). ADHD family history also predicts persistent ADHD (Faraone *et al.*, 2015). ADHD polygenic risk scores (PRSs), neuroimaging, and neuropsychological data, although promising, need more investigation. One investigation in three population samples from the UK, Brazil, and the US provided evidence that a risk calculator using clinical and demographic data collected in childhood might perform adequately in predicting ADHD persistence from childhood to young adulthood (see https://www.ufrgs.br/prodah/adhd-calculator) (Caye *et al.*, 2019).

Regarding the effects of sex, while average ADHD traits are consistently lower for females than males during childhood (especially motor hyperactivity) and part of adolescence, males have a more pronounced later decline, decreasing this sex difference. Beyond core symptoms, there are changes in the pattern of co-occurring mental health conditions as individuals grow.

For instance, while in childhood ODD and CD are the most prevalent conditions co-occurring with ADHD; substance use disorders, and mood and anxiety disorders become more common co-occurrences in adulthood (Sonuga-Barke *et al.*, 2023).

Data from several longitudinal investigations have challenged two cornerstones of the ADHD conceptualization as an NDD. First, Moffitt *et al.* (2015) surprisingly found that 90% of individuals with ADHD at 38 years of age lacked a history of childhood ADHD. Similar findings were subsequently confirmed in samples from other countries, but the exact rates of late-onset ADHD are uncertain, with estimates ranging between around 30–87% of those presenting with ADHD in adulthood (Sonuga-Barke *et al.*, 2023). In-depth analysis suggests that individuals with the putative late-onset variant might differ from their childhood-onset counterparts in important ways. They seem to have less severe symptoms and/or a lower genetic liability for ADHD, may have lived in more supportive families during childhood, have a higher IQ, or a combination of these factors (Asherson & Agnew-Blais, 2019). These data suggest clinicians should avoid discarding ADHD simply for not tracing inattentive and/or hyperactive/impulsive symptoms since childhood (Sonuga-Barke *et al.*, 2023).

Second, Sibley *et al.* (2022), assessing data from the MTA naturalistic follow-up, found that ADHD symptoms and impairment frequently fluctuate across time, contradicting the traditional notion that childhood-onset ADHD is a stable condition. Their findings suggest that over 60% of children with ADHD combined type had a fluctuating symptom course with repeated periods of remission and recurrence—even when the former was conservatively defined as lack of (i) substantial ADHD symptoms, (ii) impairment, and (iii) treatment in the last six months. A replication investigation in three cohorts in the US, including the Adolescent Brain Cognitive Development study, has reported similar findings, though with lower rates of this fluctuating course (16.3–29.6%), possibly related to a less frequent reassessment schedule (Norman *et al.*, 2023). This phenotypic profile may reflect the interplay between time-varying environmental demands and underlying genetic vulnerability (Sibley *et al.*, 2022).

Clinical implications and impact of attention deficit hyperactivity disorder

Meta-analytic data suggest that youths with ADHD have a significantly lower quality of life than individuals without the disorder, either by self-report or parent report. In addition, parents of children with ADHD perceive their own quality of life as worse than those of typically developing children. Youths with ADHD are at high risk for school failure, parental and family conflict, social rejection by peers, delinquent behavior, engagement in bullying, being victim of sexual crimes, low self-esteem, and low social skills. In addition, meta-analyses also indicate a higher risk of a range of domestic accidents and traumatic brain injury in youths with the disorder. Although the risk for smoking and substance use disorders seems increased for patients with ADHD, it yet remains unclear if this risk is entirely mediated by comorbidity with CD. In adolescence and young adulthood, ADHD is associated with a higher risk of pregnancy and contraction of sexual transmitted diseases, academic and vocational underachievement, school dropout, reduced occupational functioning and satisfaction, obesity, emotional dysregulation, unemployment, and suicide. Several investigations suggest higher rates of traffic accidents and violations in drivers with ADHD than in those without the disorder. As a result, ADHD is associated with higher rates of mortality than populational rates, although the increase seems to be partially explained by comorbid conditions (Faraone *et al.*, 2021).

Although considerable work emphasizes negative outcomes associated with ADHD, the concept of neurodiversity highlights strengths-based approaches. This perspective notes potential positive aspects of ADHD, like the creative ability to "think out of the box" or the energy, drive, and risk taking required by successful entrepreneurship (Sonuga-Barke *et al.*, 2023).

Current limitations and challenges for the future

Several limitations hinder understandings of ADHD developmental pathways. For instance, it remains unclear whether adding polygenic risk scores (PRSs), early life determinants, or neuropsychological data enhances prediction of ADHD persistence from childhood to adulthood. More work is also needed concerning mechanisms explaining different trajectories and onset, as well as their moderation by biological sex. Similarly, studies are needed on potential positive aspects of ADHD.

Risk and resilience

A biopsychosocial model of interacting developmental risks and protective factors

Early research on the etiology of ADHD focused mainly on genetic risk factors, spurred by evidence on the putative high heritability of the disorder, provided mainly by studies in twins (Langley, 2018). Over time, research increasingly treated ADHD as a multifactorial disorder, resulting from a complex interplay of genetic and environmental factors, each with a small impact, and none of which is necessary or sufficient to cause ADHD alone (Sonuga-Barke, 2018). Importantly, awareness has grown regarding potential gene–gene and gene–environment interactions (Franke, 2018), as well as possible protective factors.

Originating risks

Genes

Estimated heritability

Early family studies (e.g., Biederman *et al.*, 1992) found ADHD to run in families, with parents, siblings, or half-siblings of individuals with ADHD facing a higher risk of having the disorder themselves. However, as family members share both genes and environmental factors, family studies fail to disentangle causal contributions from these factors. In this regard, twin studies are more informative, Studies using a categorical diagnosis of ADHD estimate heritability falling between 77–88%, among the highest for mental disorders (Faraone & Larsson, 2019).

Adoption studies also more strongly implicate genetic than environmental factors in ADHD. This is because risk in adopted children relates more strongly to features of biological than adoptive parents. However, conclusions remain tentative, as the few available adoption studies tend to possess small sample sizes (Langley, 2018).

Molecular genetics

Early genetic research on ADHD examined so-called *candidate genes*. However, experts in genetics suggest that such research possesses little value. Such experts emphasize the importance of findings arising from another approach, referred to as *genome-wide association study* (GWAS), which involves testing common gene variants (single nucleotide polymorphisms (SNPs)) across the genome. The most recent GWAS report in the field of ADHD (Demontis *et al.*, 2023) noted 27 genome-wide significant associations, implicating 76 genes, expressed mainly in early development and in association with several brain-specific neuronal subtypes, including midbrain dopaminergic neurons. However, once again, contributions from each gene are small, and even when combined, overall genetic risk identified by GWAS explains a relatively small portion of the variance of ADHD. While it is likely that larger sample sizes will identify additional genes with small effects, other more rare genetic variants, with a frequency of less than 1% in the general population, also appear to play an important role in the risk for ADHD (Langley, 2018). One such rare form of risk may involve copy number variants (CNVs), which involve deletion or repetitions of segments of DNA larger than 1000 base pairs. Research suggests that a high CNV burden relates to risk for ADHD (Williams *et al.*, 2010). In particular, a 22q11 microdeletion increases the risk of ADHD symptoms. It remains unclear the degree to which different patterns of genetic risk relate to different clinical phenotypes. Furthermore, additional alterations, such as rare protein truncating variants in exome, have been observed in ADHD with similar burden as in ASD (Satterstrom *et al.*, 2019).

Environments

Research on genetic factors suggests that environmental, non-genetic factors might also play a role in the etiology of ADHD. Evidence on putative environmental risk factors is comprehensively summarized in an umbrella review (Kim *et al.*, 2020) that quantitatively synthesized data from reviews/meta-analyses while grading the level of evidence. Drawing on evidence from 63 meta-analyses, there was: convincing evidence (class I) of an association with pre-pregnancy maternal obesity, childhood eczema, hypertensive disorders during pregnancy, pre-eclampsia, and maternal acetaminophen exposure during pregnancy; highly suggestive evidence (class II) for maternal smoking during pregnancy, childhood asthma, and pre-pregnancy overweight; suggestive evidence (class III) for perinatal hypoxia and preterm birth; weak, but significant, (class IV) evidence for parental education level and single parent family. However, correlation does not imply causation. Three possibilities could explain these associations: (i) passive genotype–environment correlation—for instance, mothers with ADHD are more likely to smoke during pregnancy, so smoking is passively correlated with ADHD in children (Skoglund *et al.*, 2014); unmeasured genetic/family factors could confound the association between smoking during pregnancy and ADHD; (ii) evocative genotype–environment correlation, where genetically influenced characteristics of the child evoke a response from the environment, such as a child's behavior evoking hostile parenting (Cartwright *et al.*, 2011); and (iii) environmental factors are indeed causal contributors to ADHD symptoms. This may be the case for severe early adversity, such as the effect of extreme early deprivation in children in institutions in Romania during the Ceauşescu regime, contributing to ADHD. There is evidence of a correlation between the duration of the deprivation and the severity of ADHD symptoms, with children exposed to extended (>6 months) deprivation showing a sevenfold increase in the risk of ADHD symptoms (Sonuga-Barke *et al.*, 2017). However, the extent to which this presentation of ADHD is similar to and shares common neurobiological signatures with classical ADHD is unclear.

Gene–environment interplay

The interplay between gene and environment includes gene–environment correlation, previously discussed, and gene–environment interactions (GxE), which may inflate the high heritability suggested by twin studies (see earlier section on "Estimated heritability"). Several models have been used to describe GxE, including the diathesis-stress model, which suggests that the genetic effects on ADHD appear more evident within the context of high environmental adversity. Indeed, evidence from animal models shows that ADHD-related environmental factors can modify gene expression via DNA methylation (Luo *et al.*, 2014). However, studies in humans have in general been underpowered. Overall, GxE studies in the field of ADHD are still in their infancy and await solid meta-analytic replication.

Causal heterogeneity and overlap with other conditions

As highlighted in the previous subsections, in line with the phenotypic heterogeneity of ADHD, its underlying etiology is heterogeneous. Of note, twin studies have shown a considerable overlap between ADHD and other (neuro)psychiatric conditions such as ASD (Rommelse *et al.*, 2010) or CD (Thapar *et al.*, 2001). Indeed, genome-wide genetic correlations showed ADHD to be closely correlated with autism and depression (Cross-Disorder Group of the Psychiatric Genomics Consortium, 2019). Chapter 23 describes the concepts of multifinality and equifinality, which likely contribute to such causal heterogeneity in ADHD.

Clinical implications

Currently, genetic tests play no role in the routine clinical care of patients with ADHD (Brennan, 2018). A systematic review of candidate diagnostic biomarkers for NDDs, including genetic biomarkers for ADHD, found no biomarker with a specificity and sensitivity of at least 80%—a threshold considered acceptable—from two or more studies from independent research groups (Cortese *et al.*, 2023b). The plethora of common genetic variants that have been found to contribute to ADHD have an effect size which is too small to be used to diagnose ADHD. Likewise, the rare genetic variants that have been found to be associated with ADHD are not sufficiently predictive of case status to be clinically useful. In the past years, there has been an increasing interest in clinical use for polygenic risk scores (PRSs), but current evidence also fails to support their clinical utility (Khera *et al.*, 2019). Therefore, while testing for possible genetic syndromes, prompted by clinical features, is needed for a more comprehensive assessment of the individual with ADHD, a systematic genetic testing for diagnostic purposes is not recommended (please also see Chapter 21).

Brain correlates

Placing neuroscience in the biopsychosocial model

Alterations in the neurochemistry, structure, and function of the brain are considered mediators in pathways between underlying genetic and environmental risks, on the one hand, and behavioral symptoms and related impairment, on the other hand. Therefore, brain alterations represent potential targets for new interventions. Neurobiological correlates of the disorder should be considered within the context of existing models of the disorders, including psychosocial aspects.

Neuroscience of attention deficit hyperactivity disorder

Neurochemistry

While post-mortem analyses are currently lacking in the field of ADHD, evidence of alterations in human neurochemistry mainly derives from studies using PET and magnetic resonance spectroscopy (MRS). Catecholamines, including dopamine (DA) and norepinephrine (NE) relate to ADHD based on *in vivo* receptor binding studies and animal models. Meta-analytic evidence implicates that striatal D2/D3 receptors, as well as the dopamine transporters (DAT), are involved neurocognitive and behavioral dimensions related to ADHD (Wu *et al.*, 2012), such as motivation/reward, impulsive responding, delay aversion, inhibition, attention, and learning (Dalley *et al.*, 2008). PET studies further implicate striatal DA and DAT, as well as limbic DAT and D2/D3 profiles in the amygdala and hippocampus, with their role in motivation/reward (Fusar-Poli *et al.*, 2012; Volkow *et al.*, 2011). Research also shows NE to modulate impulsivity/inhibition (Prince, 2008), but findings are limited by PET radioligand methodology for NE. More recent meta-analytic evidence from spectroscopy studies (Vidor *et al.*, 2022) points to a role of glutamatergic metabolites, which may ultimately hamper neurotrophic activity. Other neurotransmitters may relate to ADHD through their effects on arousal and attention (for acetylcholine, nicotine, gamma-aminobutyric acid (GABA), and histamine-3) or through effects on impulse control (for serotonin). For these chemicals, solid meta-analytic supporting evidence is currently lacking. Likewise, recent interest for the orexin system, involved in a plethora of functions including the regulation of arousal, awaits further rigorous research (Sonuga-Barke *et al.*, 2023).

Brain structure and function

MRI research in ADHD has found possible alterations in brain volume, density, cortical thickness, surface area, and gyrification, as well as structural connectivity. While early studies have been hampered by small sample sizes, recent mega-analyses have provided more solid findings. Data (Hoogman *et al.*, 2017) from the Enhancing Neuro-Imaging Genetics Through Meta-Analyses (ENIGMA) consortium has pointed to smaller global intracranial volume, and smaller volumes of accumbens, amygdala, caudate, hippocampus, and putamen in individuals with ADHD compared to typically developing comparisons. Notably, these differences refer to the group, rather than individual, level; almost all differences manifested primarily in children, typically with small effect sizes between 0.1–0.19. Another ENIGMA report (Hoogman *et al.*, 2019) showed smaller surface areas, particularly in frontal, cingulate, and temporal cortices, and thinner cortex in the fusiform gyrus and temporal pole in children—but not adolescents or adults—with ADHD compared to typically developing controls.

Structural connectivity can be estimated with diffusion tensor imaging (DTI). The most recent systematic review of DTI findings through meta-analysis (Parlatini *et al.*, 2023) showed reduced fractional anisotropy (FA)—a proxy for white matter integrity—in the splenium and body of the corpus callosum, extending to the cingulum, across samples of children and adults. No alterations in FA were found when restricting the analyses to samples of children/adolescents.

With regards to brain function, perhaps the most innovative hypothesis suggested so far relates to the default mode network (DMN), a network of brain areas involved in a broad array of activities including self-referential thoughts and mind-wandering. In 2007, Sonuga-Barke and Castellanos proposed that attentional lapses in ADHD arise from inappropriate intrusion of the DMN into the activity of brain networks involved in tasks that require attention to external stimuli (Sonuga-Barke & Castellanos, 2007). Some meta-analyses (Hart *et al.*, 2012; Norman *et al.*, 2016) supported this hypothesis using data from task-based functional MRI (fMRI) studies and showing reduced ADHD-related control over interoceptive attention orientation and mind-wandering, alongside poor activation of task-relevant networks. However, another large-scale meta-analysis (Samea *et al.*, 2019) of task-based fMRI studies failed to find any significant convergence of results across studies. Likewise, evidence is also mixed from studies using resting-state fMRI (RS-fMRI), which assesses spontaneous activity and intrinsic functional connectivity without any active task. While two meta-analyses of RS-fMRI studies (Gao *et al.*, 2019; Sutcubasi *et al.*, 2020) support the DMN interference hypothesis, another meta-analysis using more conservative statistical methods (Cortese *et al.*, 2021a) failed to find any convergence across studies on multiple intrinsic connectivity metrics.

In addition to MRI, brain function in ADHD has been evaluated mainly via electroencephalography (EEG) and event-related potentials (ERP). Initial reports of excess EEG theta activity, possibly indicative of decreased cortical activation, and reduced alpha and beta activity, have not been confirmed in subsequent studies (Brandeis *et al.*, 2018). Likewise, early work related ADHD to an elevated theta/beta power ratio (TBR), considered a marker of hypoarousal, but such findings did not manifest in meta-analytic evidence (Arns *et al.*, 2013), highlighting the heterogeneous nature of ADHD in terms of EEG correlates. Indeed, as many as nine different EEG subtypes have been described in ADHD (Brandeis *et al.*, 2018). ERP research has provided evidence, overall, of inhibitory control deficits (attenuation of P3, N2 error-related negativity, ERN amplitude), deficient orientating and preparation processes (cue P3 and contingent negative variation, CNV), and perceptual difficulties (reduced mismatch negativity (MMN)) (Brandeis *et al.*, 2018).

Cognition

Meta-analytic evidence links ADHD to cognitive deficits in a broad array of functions, including working memory, inhibition, temporal discounting, decision-making, time estimation, and response time variability, with the strongest and most consistent associations with response inhibition, vigilance, working memory, and planning (Willcutt *et al.*, 2005; Marx *et al.*, 2022), albeit none of these deficits is consistently found across all individuals with ADHD. Importantly, when studies use neuropsychological tests to examine medication-naïve children (Coghill *et al.*, 2014), groups of children with ADHD display worse performance than groups of healthy children, but substantial overlap exists between the groups. Furthermore, only a minority of children with ADHD show deficits in any neuropsychological domain, and around 25% do not show any neuropsychological deficit. Therefore, cognitive deficits are dissociable from ADHD symptoms and may confer additional impairment in subgroups of children with ADHD. As such, the presence of neuropsychological deficits is not required to establish diagnosis of ADHD but can identify additional domains that require attention. Please also see Chapter 29.

Heterogeneity and overlap with other conditions

Overall, reflecting phenotypic, neuropsychological, and etiological overlap, brain studies point to both shared and unique patterns of structural and functional abnormalities between ADHD and other (neuro)psychiatric disorders, albeit disorder specific alterations seem more prominent. For instance, in terms of structural alterations, findings from the ENIGMA consortium (Boedhoe *et al.*, 2020) showed that, despite indications of common reductions in subcortical volumes and cortical thickness in ADHD and ASD during childhood, ADHD in childhood was associated with lower global brain and hippocampal volumes relative to OCD, ASD, and neurotypical controls. OCD was associated with greater striatal and lower limbic volumes in adulthood, but not in childhood or adolescence, and there were no disorder-specific effects on cortical thickness or surface area in childhood. Using an advanced methodology to avoid biased selection of tasks across disorders, a large-scale meta-analysis of task-based fMRI studies (Tamon *et al.*, 2023) found that participants with ADHD and ASD showed both shared and disorder-specific task-independent neural activation abnormalities, although the latter were more prominent.

Clinical implications

Cortese *et al.* (2023a) did not find any neuroimaging, neurophysiological, or neuropsychological candidate biomarker with specificity and sensitivity >80% replicated in at least one additional study. As such, current evidence does not support any neurobiological biomarker as a stand-alone tool to diagnose ADHD. Therefore, clinicians are advised to avoid using any neurobiological measure to replace a full clinical assessment or as a triage system to allocate to assessment waiting-list individuals referred to clinical services. Of note, in 2012 and 2013, respectively, the US Food and Drug Administration (FDA) approved the QB test—a commercially available device combining a continuous performance test (CPT) with an infrared motion tracker—and a TBR-based EEG test (despite uncertain evidence, see earlier section on "Brain structure and function") as tools to aid, rather than replace, the clinical diagnosis of ADHD. Furthermore, in 2024, the National Institute for Health and Care Excellence (NICE) stated, 'Use QbTest as an option to help diagnose attention deficit hyperactivity disorder (ADHD) in people aged 6 to 17 years. It should only be used alongside a standard clinical assessment by a healthcare professional.' (NICE, 2024). How exactly these tools should be used alongside the clinical assessment awaits further evidence and clarification.

Current limitations and challenges for the future

We remain far removed from a comprehensive understanding of the complex and heterogeneous pathophysiology of ADHD. The adoption of novel analytic approaches, such as normative modeling (Oliveira-Saraiva & Ferreira, 2023), will hopefully allow the field to move away from the average patient explored in the case–control paradigm, toward the individual patient. Perhaps, rather than for diagnostic purposes, the main function of neuroscientific studies will be to allow patient stratification toward precision-medicine-grounded treatments.

Treatment

Placing attention deficit hyperactivity disorder treatment in the biopsychosocial model

Several interventions options exist to support individuals with ADHD. These include pharmacological and nonpharmacological therapies (psychological interventions, diet, and neurostimulation). To adequately address each patient's needs, most interventions should be considered as complementary, rather than exclusive and antithetic. Indeed, growing meta-analytic evidence from the past decade shows that different interventions may be effective for different, specific outcomes that include ADHD core symptoms (inattention, hyperactivity, and impulsivity), as well as noncore aspects that may be as or even more relevant than core symptoms per se. This growing body of evidence is progressively reflected in available clinical guidelines (Table 54.1). Importantly, while evidence and associated guidelines inform decision-making, patients' preferences are a crucial component in the definition of the intervention plan. This section details the evidence on pharmacological and nonpharmacological interventions for individuals with ADHD across the life span, as well as key aspects regarding the clinical management. Details on pharmacological (Chapter 39) and nonpharmacological therapies (Chapters 31, 34, 36, 38, 39) can be found elsewhere.

Preschool: early intervention, prevention, and treatment

Current guidelines (Table 54.1) suggest behavior interventions, in the form of parent training, as first-line interventions for preschoolers with ADHD, and pharmacotherapy as an option to consider when nonpharmacological strategies fail to be effective. These recommendations reflect randomized controlled trials (RCTs) testing parent training for ADHD in preschoolers, as well as early evidence (Greenhill *et al.*, 2006), currently challenged, showing that medications for ADHD, in particular stimulants, are generally less effective and less well tolerated in preschoolers as compared to school-age children. More recent meta-analytic evidence (Sugaya *et al.*, 2023) showed a moderate effect size in favor of methylphenidate (0.59, 95% CI 0.41–0.77), with no significantly higher rates of discontinuation compared to placebo, albeit the confidence of estimated effect size was very low. Furthermore, current guidelines do not reflect data from the first, large, well-designed comparative efficacy trial (Sugaya *et al.*, 2022) of methylphenidate and behavioral parent training. This trial showed that preschool children randomized to methylphenidate plus the educational intervention had a significantly greater reduction in the severity of ADHD core symptoms and in global functioning compared to those assigned to a placebo pill plus educational interventions, with moderate (0.55, 95% CI 0.10–0.99) and high (0.8, 95% CI 0.24–1.16) effect size, respectively. Mild adverse events (including appetite decrease), but not moderate or severe adverse events, were more frequent in the methylphenidate plus education group. Should the conclusions of this trial be confirmed in future meta-analytic evidence, and corroborated in longer-term studies, they would provide a compelling rationale to revise current clinical guidelines.

Regarding prevention, a meta-analysis (Shephard *et al.*, 2022) of 28 RCTs encompassing a broad range of interventions (including mainly parent training and cognitive training) showed significant effects on ADHD core symptoms and working memory, respectively, but not on other early domains, such as emotional difficulties and sleep problems, that could be the target of prevention. Most of the RCTs were conducted with preschool-aged children rather than with infants and toddlers, so further evidence is needed to inform whether early intervention can modify precursors of ADHD earlier in development.

Table 54.1 Treatment at a glance. A summary of selected recent clinical guidelines for the management of attention deficit hyperactivity disorder (ADHD) in children/adolescents.

National Institute for Health and Care Excellence (NICE), UK (2018)	American Academy of Pediatrics (2019)	Attention deficit hyperactivity disorder (ADHD) German Guidelines (2018)
Children < 5 years First line: ADHD-focused group parent training program. Medication only after second specialist opinion	***Preschool children 4–6 years*** First line: Parent training and/or behavioral classroom interventions Second line: Methylphenidate	***Children < 6 years*** First line: ADHD-focused group or individual parent or teacher training. Medication only after specialist advice for children >3 years
Children ≥ 5 years and young people ADHD-focused support. Medication (order: (i) methylphenidate; (ii) lisdexamfetamine (or dexamphetamine if lisdexamfetamine not tolerated); (iii) atomoxetine or guanfacine). If symptoms of oppositional defiant disorder (ODD) or conduct disorder (CD): parent training. Cognitive behavioral therapy (CBT) for young people if symptoms still impairing.	***Children 6–11 years*** Food and Drug Administration (FDA)-approved medications (order suggested by evidence: (i) stimulants; (ii) atomoxetine; (iii) extended-release guanfacine; (iv) extended-release clonidine) and parent training and/or behavioral classroom interventions (preferably both) ***Adolescents 12–18 years*** FDA-approved medications. Training and/or behavioral interventions if available. Educational interventions.	***Children ≥ 6 years and young people*** After psychoeducation: *Mild to moderate ADHD:* First line: parent-training or family-based interventions; if needed, patient- and school/workplace-based interventions. Second line: medication (order: (i) stimulants; (ii) atomoxetine or guanfacine) *Moderate to severe ADHD:* First line: medication (order: (i) stimulants; (ii) atomoxetine or guanfacine). Second line: parent training or family-based interventions; if needed, patient- and school/workplace-based interventions.

Childhood/adolescence

Medication

Pharmacotherapy, including stimulants (methylphenidate and amphetamines) and nonstimulants (such as atomoxetine, guanfacine, clonidine, and viloxazine) is an important component of the multimodal treatment of ADHD.

A growing body of evidence informs clinical decision-making in daily practice, in relation to the different phases of pharmacological management. In terms of initial medications, a network meta-analysis (NMA) (Cortese *et al.*, 2018) of 133 RCTs showed that in children and adolescents, based on ratings by clinicians, amphetamines were superior to guanfacine; methylphenidate was superior to atomoxetine; guanfacine and amphetamines were less well tolerated than placebo; and methylphenidate was the only compound with better acceptability than placebo. Of note, the effect sizes of stimulants (in particular, amphetamines) in the short term are not only among the highest in psychiatry, but also among the highest in general medicine (Leucht *et al.*, 2012). Considering both efficacy and tolerability/acceptability, available evidence is consistent with the recommendations from the UK National Institute for Health and Care Excellence (NICE) (www.nice.org.uk/guidance/ng87) suggesting that pharmacotherapy should be first-line treatment, after environmental modifications, and, in youth, methylphenidate should be tried first, followed by lisdexamfetamine or other amphetamines, and then nonstimulants. However, it is important to appreciate that available meta-analytic evidence refers to the group, rather than the individual level, so that some individuals may respond to and tolerate better amphetamines or a nonstimulant. However, as no predictors of response are currently available, the hierarchy suggested by NICE provides a general guide to inform the trial-and-error process to find the best medication for each patient. Other guidelines (Table 54.1) recommend methylphenidate *or* amphetamines as first line, rather than specifying which of the two should be the first choice, but guidelines are in general consistent in recommending stimulants over non-stimulant as first-line choice.

Once a pharmacological treatment is started, it is crucial to optimize, i.e., properly titrate the dose considering the benefit/risk trade-off, and provide an appropriate coverage during the day based on the needs of the patients and their families. Indeed, a meta-analysis (Farhat *et al.*, 2022) showed increased efficacy alongside reduced likelihood of discontinuations for any reason with increasing stimulant doses up opt the maximum licensed dose.

Details on practical prescribing appear in Chapter 39; we report here guidance on the treatment of stimulant refractory cases (Table 54.2), and the management of side effects of stimulants (Table 54.3). Medication choice hierarchy is typically not influenced by comorbidity (i.e., stimulants should also be first line when there is a comorbid anxiety disorder). However, a specific evidence-based algorithm has been proposed for the management of ADHD in individuals with ASD (Figure 54.2), with methylphenidate as first line, followed by atomoxetine, alpha-2 agonists, and amphetamines. With comorbid learning disability (referred to as "disorder of intellectual development" ICD-11),

Table 54.2 Recommendations for the management of stimulant refractory cases.

- Before switching to nonstimulants or adding medications:
  1. Have you titrated properly to the maximum tolerated dose?
  2. Do you need to change the dose or preparation to get a more balanced effect?
  3. Are you targeting the right symptoms and time of day?
  4. Has the patient become tolerant to this medication?
  5. Are any life circumstances contributing to the poor response?
  6. Have I missed any comorbidity?
  7. Is the diagnosis correct?
- Consider second-line medications (e.g., atomoxetine, guanfacine XR)
- Consider augmenting agents (combine stimulants with other immediate release or extended-release stimulants, guanfacine XR or clonidine XR)
- Consider other agents (off-label) under specialistic advice/supervision

Source: Adapted from Cortese *et al.* (2021b).

Table 54.3 Recommendations from the European ADHD Guidelines Group (EAGG) for the management of common side effects of stimulants. *Source:* Adapted from Cortese *et al.* (2013).

Adverse event	Suggested management strategy
Decreased appetite Height and weight gain deficit	• If weight loss of clinical concern: take medication either with or after food, rather than before meals; take additional meals or snacks early in the morning or late in the evening; obtain dietary advice; consume high-calorie foods of good nutritional value; take a planned break from treatment, or change medication • Consider a planned break in treatment over school holidays • Refer to pediatric endocrinologist/growth specialist if height and weight values are below critical thresholds
Increased blood pressure/ heart rate	• If sustained resting tachycardia > 120 beats per minute, arrhythmia, or systolic blood pressure > 95th percentile (or a clinically significant increase) is measured on two occasions, reduce the dose and refer to a specialist • If sustained orthostatic hypotension/fainting with guanfacine, reduce the dose or switch to another attention deficit hyperactivity disorder (ADHD) medication
Sleep disturbance	• If behavioral measures (sleep hygiene) are insufficient and it is not convenient to stop medication: (i) treat Restless Legs Syndrome if present; (ii) if rebound effect with stimulants: add small doses of short-acting stimulants in the evening; (iii) if stimulant is the current treatment: consider reducing dose, alternative classes or formulations of stimulants, or atomoxetine. Consider adding melatonin
Tics	• Monitor tics over a 3-month period before any decision regarding ADHD treatment • If tics are stimulant-related, reduce the stimulant dose, or consider changing to guanfacine (in children aged 5 years and over and young people only), atomoxetine, clonidine, or stopping medication, or add an antipsychotic (please also see Chapter 55)
Psychotic symptoms	• If they occur with therapeutic doses of ADHD medications, reduce the dose or discontinue the ADHD drug • Once the psychotic or manic symptoms resolve, consider a rechallenge with ADHD medications

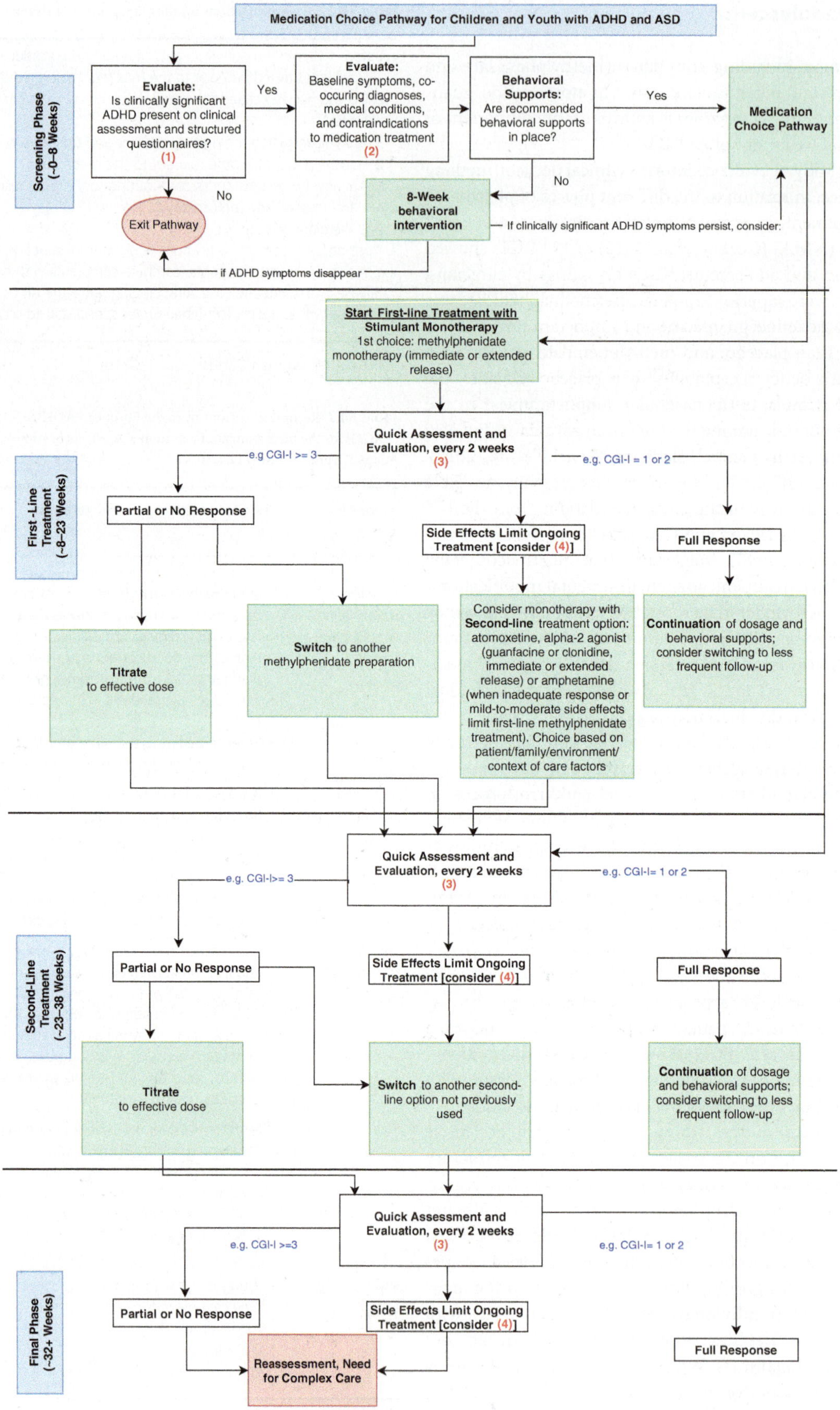

Figure 54.2 Algorithm for the management of attention deficit hyperactivity disorder (ADHD) in individuals with autism spectrum disorder (ASD). *Source:* Rodrigues *et al.*, (2021)/with permission of John Wiley & Sons.

efficacy may be decreased, and titration should be cautious as tolerability may be worse, especially in severe learning disability. There is no evidence of a causal link between use of stimulants and onset of psychotic events, but some individuals may be prone to develop psychotic events after stimulant treatment (Cortese, 2019). Stimulants can be used in individuals with bipolar disorder when mania/depression are stabilized. In terms of possible adverse events, we note that an international naturalistic, longitudinal, controlled study showed relatively small methylphenidate-related pulse and blood pressure changes (increase) after 24 months of treatment, suggesting the need for regular monitoring of these parameters (Man *et al.*, 2023).

Methodological challenges complicate attempts to rigorously assess the longer-term effects of medications. Hence, the extent to what beneficial medications effect persists over time is unclear. Nevertheless, withdrawal RCTs demonstrate persistent effects—albeit with lower effect sizes (around 0.2–0.5) compared to effects in the short term (around 0.8–1.0) after a few years of treatment (Cortese, 2020). Likewise, high-quality evidence on the long-term safety of stimulants is difficult to gather. Of note, a recent long-term, naturalistic, longitudinal, controlled study, has confirmed that the long-term treatment with methylphenidate is safe (Man *et al.*, 2023) and there is no evidence that stimulants increase the risk of substance use disorder (Young *et al.*, 2023). There is no evidence that persistent use of a stimulant significantly alters the brain structure (Cortese, 2020).

Psychosocial, behavioral, and educational treatment

Appraising the large body of evidence on (cognitive) behavioral interventions for ADHD is challenging due to issues around blinding in RCTs and substantial heterogeneity across studies in terms of treatment components (operant reinforcement, social skills, problem-solving, and teacher-directed intervention components), outcome measures, and duration. Meta-analytic evidence shows significant, moderate effects on ADHD core symptoms rated by informants involved in the delivery of the treatment but no significant effects when considering more distal—and hence less biased—raters (Daley *et al.*, 2018). However, behavioral interventions have been found to improve parenting and oppositional behaviors, even when considering ratings from distal informants (Daley *et al.*, 2018). NICE (www.nice.org.uk/guidance/ng87) recommends behavioral interventions only when there is a comorbid oppositional/conduct disorder. Others (Sibley *et al.*, 2023) deem that they can be offered as a first-line intervention when patients and their carers have a strong preference for behavioral intervention over pharmacotherapy. Commonly used behavioral programs for ADHD include The Incredible Years (US, https://incredibleyears.com), the Barkley (US, https://www.russellbarkley.org), and The New Forest Parenting Programme (UK, https://guidebook.eif.org.uk/programme/the-new-forest-parenting-programme).

Alongside parent training (and behavioral interventions for teenagers with ADHD) it is crucial to consider psychoeducation and interventions for teachers. ADHD teacher-training programs have been shown to be effective in initially improving ADHD teachers' knowledge, but there is inconsistent evidence for their efficacy to reduce students' ADHD behavioral symptoms (Ward *et al.*, 2022).

Cognitive behavioral therapy (CBT) may be considered in adolescents to tackle noncore symptoms that are often the consequences of ADHD-related impairment, such as low self-esteem.

Useful psychoeducation material for educators is available at: https://www.caddra.ca/public-information/educators.

Brain-based treatments

In a meta-analysis of RCTs of computer-delivered cognitive training, Westwood *et al.* (2023) found that, when considering "probably blinded" raters, there was no effect on ADHD total or hyperactivity/impulsivity symptoms and only a small improvement in inattention symptoms. Cognitive training improved working memory, not other neuropsychological or academic outcomes. Of note, EndeavorRX, a prescription cognitive training, was cleared by the FDA to improve attention functions rather than ADHD behavioral symptoms (Food and Drug Administration, 2020).

When considering more distal raters, there is no evidence to date that neurofeedback improves ADHD core symptoms nor any neuropsychological function (Westood *et al.*, 2024) and, based on clinicians' reports, the effects of at-home neurofeedback as a stand-alone treatment have been found to be inferior to those of methylphenidate (Purper-Ouakil *et al.*, 2022).

External trigeminal stimulation has been approved by the FDA for ADHD treatment based only on evidence from a pilot RCT (McGough *et al.*, 2019), so that additional RCTs are needed to establish it as an effective treatment for ADHD. To date, there is no evidence to support other types of neurostimulation (transcranial direct current stimulation (tDCS) and transcranial magnetic stimulation (TMS)) for ADHD (Hyde *et al.*, 2022).

Alternative treatments

In a comprehensive systematic review, Sibley *et al.* (2023) concluded that, while there is evidence that mindfulness, supplementation with polyunsaturated fatty acids, if taken for at least three months in sufficient doses (>1 g), and multinutrient supplementation with four or more ingredients have small effects, especially on non-ADHD core symptom outcomes (e.g., global impairment and caregiver behavior), there is insufficient evidence to support other alternative treatments such as body therapies (e.g., acupuncture and massage) and physical activity.

Approaches to support life transitions

Transition from child to adult mental health services is a crucial, and often very challenging moment in the life of an individual with ADHD, especially in those health care systems where provision of services for adult with ADHD is unsatisfactory. Two models have been discussed (Young *et al.*, 2011): (i) a "transition team" that operates independently from child and adolescent mental health services (CAMHS), on the one side, and adult mental health services (AMHS), on the other side, to bridge the gap; and (ii) the use of shared care protocols during which CAMHS and AMHS interact and facilitate a gradual transfer of care. Empirical evidence is needed on the feasibility and effectiveness of these two models.

The national and international context

While the community prevalence of ADHD, after controlling for the methods used for the diagnosis, is fairly stable across countries, there are substantial variations across geographic locations in terms of the administrative prevalence (i.e., the prevalence of the actual diagnoses), as well as of the ways to provide care to an individual with ADHD, based on administrative registries. For instance, while in some US states, the administrative prevalence, and the prevalence of treatment use, is very close to or even higher than the community prevalence, in the UK less than half of children with ADHD are diagnosed and receive treatment (Sayal *et al.*, 2018), and in other countries, such as Italy or France, the administrative prevalence is even lower. This is likely accounted for by several reasons, including historical and sociocultural factors. In relation to the delivery of care, while, for instance, in the UK, the diagnosis is usually made by child and adolescent psychiatry or pediatric specialists within secondary health care, with shared care agreements between primary and secondary care for continuing care, in the US, ADHD is generally managed by primary care pediatricians or child and adolescent psychiatrists in isolation (Sayal *et al.*, 2018).

Differences across countries are also reflected in their clinical guidelines (Table 54.1). While guidelines generally tend to agree on the requirements for the diagnosis, they differ in terms of how they appraise and integrate evidence, the type of recommended treatments, and their sequencing.

Current limitations and challenges for the future

Three key issues will need to be addressed in future research and implemented in clinical practice: (i) stratify the treatment according to the clinical and possibly neurobiological characteristics of each individual; (ii) design and test interventions with long-term, curative action, rather than symptomatic treatments; and (iii) improve adherence to treatment, which will arguably be enhanced by the availability of more effective and especially better tolerated treatments.

An overview of future challenges and opportunities

For decades, reflecting a predominantly medical model, ADHD has been conceptualized as a categorical entity with clear boundaries, both in relation to typically developed individuals and between ADHD and other disorders, caused by dysfunction mainly within the individual (Sonuga-Barke *et al.*, 2023). However, this conceptualization of the disorder has been challenged by a large body of neuroscientific investigation highlighting the dimensional nature of ADHD and the poor specificity of its risk factors. An important challenge for the field will be to balance these findings with the need, from clinicians, for a categorical classification (*yes* or *no*) to address pragmatic issues (treatment versus no treatment). The medical model of ADHD is also being challenged by the relatively recent neurodiversity movement, which considers ADHD as a difference, with important positive aspects, rather than as a disorder. This will likely stimulate the development of research on non-medical models (e.g., systemic model) in ADHD, which have been so far downplayed (Cortese *et al.*, 2022). However, the traditional approach based on clinical assessment and treatment and the neurodiverse approach are not necessarily antithetic (Sonuga-Barke & Thapar, 2021). A challenge for the future will be to integrate them with the ultimate goal of supporting the development and well-being of individuals with ADHD.

References

American Psychiatric Association (2022) *Diagnostic and Statistical Manual of Mental Disorders, 5 text revision*. American Psychiatric Association, Washington, DC.

Angold, A. *et al.* (1999) Comorbidity. *Journal of Child Psychology and Psychiatry* **40**, 57–87.

Arns, M. *et al.* (2013) A decade of EEG theta/beta ratio research in ADHD: a meta-analysis. *Journal of Attention Disorders* **17**, 374–383.

Arrondo, G. *et al.* (2022) Associations between mental and physical conditions in children and adolescents: an umbrella review. *Neuroscience and Biobehavioral Reviews* **137**, 104662.

Asherson, P. & Agnew-Blais, J. (2019) Annual research review: does late-onset attention-deficit/hyperactivity disorder exist? *Journal of Child Psychology and Psychiatry* **60**, 333–352.

Asherson, P. *et al.* (2016) Adult attention-deficit hyperactivity disorder: key conceptual issues. *The Lancet Psychiatry* **3**, 568–578.

Azevêdo, P.V.B. *et al.* (2020) Suggestive diagnosis of attention-deficit/hyperactivity disorder in indigenous children and adolescents from the Brazilian Amazon. *European Child & Adolescent Psychiatry* **29**(3), 373–384.

Bergey, M.F. *et al.* (2018) *Global Perspectives on ADHD: Social Dimensions of Diagnosis and Treatment in Sixteen Countries*. Johns Hopkins University Press, Baltimore, MD.

Biederman, J. *et al.* (1992) Further evidence for family-genetic risk factors in attention deficit hyperactivity disorder: patterns of comorbidity in probands and relatives psychiatrically and pediatrically referred samples. *Archives of General Psychiatry* **49**, 728–738.

Bishop, D.V.M. (2011) Neurodevelopmental disorders: conceptual issues. In: *Rutter's Child and Adolescent Psychiatry*. (eds M. Rutter, *et al.*), 5th edn. Blackwell Publishing, Oxford, UK. pp. 32–41.

Boedhoe, P.S.W. *et al.* (2020) Subcortical brain volume, regional cortical thickness, and cortical surface area across disorders: findings from the ENIGMA ADHD, ASD, and OCD working groups. *The American Journal of Psychiatry* **177**, 834–843.

Bradley, C. (1937) The behavior of children receiving benzedrine. *American Journal of Psychiatry* **94**, 577–588.

Brandeis, D.L. *et al.* (2018) Neurophysiology. In: *Oxford Textbook of Attention Deficit Hyperactivity Disorder*. (eds T. Banasxhewski, *et al.*). Oxford University Press, Oxford, UK. pp. 82–93.

Brennan, Z. (2018) FDA warns against use of unapproved genetic tests. *Regulatory News* [Online]. Available: https://www.raps.org/news-and-articles/news-articles/2018/11/fda-warns-against-use-of-unapproved-genetic-tests [15 November 2024].

Buitelaar, J. *et al.* (2022) Toward precision medicine in ADHD. *Frontiers in Behavioral Neuroscience* **16**, 900981.

Cartwright, K.L. *et al.* (2011) Disentangling child and family influences on maternal expressed emotion toward children with attention-deficit/hyperactivity disorder. *Journal of the American Academy of Child and Adolescent Psychiatry* **50**, 1042–1053.

Caye, A. *et al.* (2016) Predictors of persistence of ADHD into adulthood: a systematic review of the literature and meta-analysis. *European Child & Adolescent Psychiatry* **25**, 1151–1159.

Caye, A. *et al.* (2019) A risk calculator to predict adult attention-deficit/hyperactivity disorder: generation and external validation in three birth cohorts and one clinical sample – ERRATUM. *Epidemiology and Psychiatric Sciences* **29**, e41.

Caye, A. *et al.* (2020) Relative age and attention-deficit/hyperactivity disorder: data from three epidemiological cohorts and a meta-analysis. *Journal of the American Academy of Child and Adolescent Psychiatry* **59**, 990–997.

Cénat, J.M. *et al.* (2021) Prevalence and risk factors associated with attention-deficit/hyperactivity disorder among US black individuals: a systematic review and meta-analysis. *JAMA Psychiatry* **78**, 21–28.

Clements, S.D. & Peters, J.E. (1962) Minimal brain dysfunctions in the school-age child: diagnosis and treatment. *Archives of General Psychiatry* **6**, 185–197.

Coghill, D.R. *et al.* (2014) A comprehensive assessment of memory, delay aversion, timing, inhibition, decision making and variability in attention deficit hyperactivity disorder: advancing beyond the three-pathway models. *Psychological Medicine* **44**, 1989–2001.

Cortese, S. (2019) Psychosis during attention deficit-hyperactivity disorder treatment with stimulants. *The New England Journal of Medicine* **380**, 1178–1180.

Cortese, S. (2020) Pharmacologic treatment of attention deficit-hyperactivity disorder. *The New England Journal of Medicine* **383**, 1050–1056.

Cortese, S. & Rohde, L.A. (2019) ADHD diagnoses: are 116 200 permutations enough? *The Lancet Child & Adolescent Health* **3**, 844–845.

Cortese, S. *et al.* (2013) Practitioner review: current best practice in the management of adverse events during treatment with ADHD medications in children and adolescents. *Journal of Child Psychology and Psychiatry* **54**, 227–246.

Cortese, S. *et al.* (2018) Comparative efficacy and tolerability of medications for attention-deficit hyperactivity disorder in children, adolescents, and adults: a systematic review and network meta-analysis. *The Lancet Psychiatry* **5**, 727–738.

Cortese, S. *et al.* (2021a) Systematic review and meta-analysis: resting-state functional magnetic resonance imaging studies of attention-deficit/hyperactivity disorder. *Journal of the American Academy of Child and Adolescent Psychiatry* **60**, 61–75.

Cortese, S. *et al.* (2021b) A practical, evidence-informed approach to managing stimulant-refractory attention deficit hyperactivity disorder (ADHD). *CNS Drugs* **35**, 1035–1051.

Cortese, S. *et al.* (2022) Half a century of research on attention-deficit/hyperactivity disorder: a scientometric study. *Neuroscience and Biobehavioral Reviews* **140**, 104769.

Cortese, S. *et al.* (2023a) Candidate diagnostic biomarkers for neurodevelopmental disorders in children and adolescents: a systematic review. *World Psychiatry* **22**, 129–149.

Cortese, S. *et al.* (2023b) Incidence, prevalence, and global burden of ADHD from 1990 to 2019 across 204 countries: data, with critical re-analysis, from the global burden of disease study. *Molecular Psychiatry*. 28, 4823–4830.

Cross-Disorder Group of the Psychiatric Genomics Consortium (2019) Genomic relationships, novel loci, and pleiotropic mechanisms across eight psychiatric disorders. *Cell* **179**, 1469–1482.e11.

Daley, D. *et al.* (2018) Practitioner review: current best practice in the use of parent training and other behavioural interventions in the treatment of children and adolescents with attention deficit hyperactivity disorder. *Journal of Child Psychology and Psychiatry* **59**, 932–947.

Dalley, J.W. *et al.* (2008) Neurobehavioral mechanisms of impulsivity: fronto-striatal systems and functional neurochemistry. *Pharmacology, Biochemistry, and Behavior* **90**, 250–260.

Demontis, D. *et al.* (2023) Genome-wide analyses of ADHD identify 27 risk loci, refine the genetic architecture and implicate several cognitive domains. *Nature Genetics* **55**, 198–208.

Doshi, J.A. *et al.* (2012) Economic impact of childhood and adult attention-deficit/hyperactivity disorder in the United States. *Journal of the American Academy of Child and Adolescent Psychiatry* **51**, 990–1002.e2.

Faraone, S.V. & Larsson, H. (2019) Genetics of attention deficit hyperactivity disorder. *Molecular Psychiatry* **24**, 562–575.

Faraone, S.V. *et al.* (2015) Attention-deficit/hyperactivity disorder. *Nature Reviews Disease Primers* **1**, 15020.

Faraone, S.V. *et al.* (2021) The world federation of ADHD international consensus statement: 208 evidence-based conclusions about the disorder. *Neuroscience and Biobehavioral Reviews* **128**, 789–818.

Farhat, L.C. *et al.* (2022) The effects of stimulant dose and dosing strategy on treatment outcomes in attention-deficit/hyperactivity disorder in children and adolescents: a meta-analysis. *Molecular Psychiatry* **27**, 1562–1572.

Food and Drug Administration (2020) Permits marketing of first game-based digital therapeutic to improve attention function in children in ADHD. Food and Drug Administration (FDA), Silver Spring, MD. Available: https://www.fda.gov/news-events/press-announcements/fda-permits-marketing-first-game-based-digital-therapeutic-improve-attention-function-children-adhd [27 November 2024].

Franke, B.B. (2018) Gene-environment interactions. In: *Oxford Textbook of Attention Deficit Hyperactivity Disorder*. (eds T. Banasxhewski, *et al.*). Oxford University Press, Oxford, UK. pp. 35–56.

Freitas de Sousa, A. *et al.* (2020) Attention deficit hyperactivity disorder. In: *Rey's IACAPAP e-Textbook of Child and Adolescent Mental Health*. (eds J.M. Rey & A. Martin). International Association for Child and Adolescent Psychiatry and Allied Professions, e-chapter. pp. 1–28.

Fusar-Poli, P. *et al.* (2012) Striatal dopamine transporter alterations in ADHD: pathophysiology or adaptation to psychostimulants? A meta-analysis. *The American Journal of Psychiatry* **169**, 264–272.

Gao, Y. *et al.* (2019) Impairments of large-scale functional networks in attention-deficit/hyperactivity disorder: a meta-analysis of resting-state functional connectivity. *Psychological Medicine* **49**, 2475–2485.

Gosling, C. *et al.* (2023) Association between relative age at school and persistence of attention-deficit hyperactivity disorder in prospective studies: an individual participant data meta-analysis. *The Lancet Psychiatry*. 10, 922–923

Greenhill, L. *et al.* (2006) Efficacy and safety of immediate-release methylphenidate treatment for preschoolers with ADHD. *Journal of the American Academy of Child and Adolescent Psychiatry* **45**, 1284–1293.

Hart, H. *et al.* (2012) Meta-analysis of fMRI studies of timing in attention-deficit hyperactivity disorder (ADHD). *Neuroscience and Biobehavioral Reviews* **36**, 2248–2256.

Hohman, L. (1922) Post-encephalitic behavior disorder in children. *Johns Hopkins Hospital Bulletin* **33**, 89–97.

Hoogman, M. *et al.* (2017) Subcortical brain volume differences in participants with attention deficit hyperactivity disorder in children and adults: a cross-sectional mega-analysis. *The Lancet Psychiatry* **4**, 310–319.

Hoogman, M. *et al.* (2019) Brain imaging of the cortex in ADHD: a coordinated analysis of large-scale clinical and population-based samples. *The American Journal of Psychiatry* **176**, 531–542.

Hyde, J. *et al.* (2022) Efficacy of neurostimulation across mental disorders: systematic review and meta-analysis of 208 randomized controlled trials. *Molecular Psychiatry* **27**, 2709–2719.

Kahn, E. & Cohen, L.H. (1934) Organic drivenness: a brain stem syndrome and experience. *New England Journal of Medicine* **210**, 748–756.

Khera, A.V. *et al.* (2019) Polygenic prediction of weight and obesity trajectories from birth to adulthood. *Cell* **177**, 587–596.e9.

Kim, J.H. *et al.* (2020) Environmental risk factors, protective factors, and peripheral biomarkers for ADHD: an umbrella review. *The Lancet Psychiatry* **7**, 955–970.

Kirova, A.M. *et al.* (2019) Are subsyndromal manifestations of attention deficit hyperactivity disorder morbid in children? A systematic qualitative review of the literature with meta-analysis. *Psychiatry Research* **274**, 75–90.

Langley, K. (2018) ADHD genetics. In: *Oxford Textbook of Attention Deficit Hyperactivity Disorder*. (eds T. Banasxhewski, *et al.*). Oxford University Press, Oxford, UK. pp. 19–24.

Leucht, S. *et al.* (2012) Putting the efficacy of psychiatric and general medicine medication into perspective: review of meta-analyses. *The British Journal of Psychiatry* **200**, 97–106.

Luo, M. *et al.* (2014) Epigenetic histone modification regulates developmental lead exposure induced hyperactivity in rats. *Toxicology Letters* **225**, 78–85.

Man, K.K.C. *et al.* (2023) Long-term safety of methylphenidate in children and adolescents with ADHD: 2-year outcomes of the attention deficit hyperactivity disorder drugs use chronic effects (ADDUCE) study. *The Lancet Psychiatry* **10**, 323–333.

Marx, I. *et al.* (2022) Meta-analysis: altered perceptual timing abilities in attention-deficit/hyperactivity disorder. *Journal of the American Academy of Child and Adolescent Psychiatry* **61**, 866–880.

McGough, J.J. *et al.* (2019) Double-blind, sham-controlled, pilot study of trigeminal nerve stimulation for attention-deficit/hyperactivity disorder. *Journal of the American Academy of Child and Adolescent Psychiatry* **58**, 403–411.e3.

Moffitt, T.E. *et al.* (2015) Is adult ADHD a childhood-onset neurodevelopmental disorder? Evidence from a four-decade longitudinal cohort study. *The American Journal of Psychiatry* **172**, 967–977.

National Institute for Health and Care Excellence (2018) Attention deficit hyperactivity disorder: diagnosis and management. https://www.nice.org.uk/guidance/ng87

National Institute for Health and Care Excellence [NICE] (2024). Digital technologies for assessing attention deficit hyperactivity disorder (ADHD). https://www.nice.org.uk/guidance/dg60

Norman, L.J. *et al.* (2016) Structural and functional brain abnormalities in attention-deficit/hyperactivity disorder and obsessive-compulsive disorder: a comparative meta-analysis. *JAMA Psychiatry* **73**, 815–825.

Norman, L.J. *et al.* (2023) Longitudinal trajectories of childhood and adolescent attention deficit hyperactivity disorder diagnoses in three cohorts. *EClinicalMedicine* **60**, 10202.

Oliveira-Saraiva, D. & Ferreira, H.A. (2023) Normative model detects abnormal functional connectivity in psychiatric disorders. *Frontiers in Psychiatry* **14**, 1068397.

Parlatini, V. *et al.* (2023) White matter alterations in attention-deficit/hyperactivity disorder (ADHD): a systematic review of 129 diffusion imaging studies with meta-analysis. *Molecular Psychiatry* **28**, 4098–4123. doi:10.1038/s41380-023-02173-1.

Polanczyk, G. *et al.* (2007) The worldwide prevalence of ADHD: a systematic review and metaregression analysis. *The American Journal of Psychiatry* **164**, 942–948.

Polanczyk, G.V. *et al.* (2014) ADHD prevalence estimates across three decades: an updated systematic review and meta-regression analysis. *International Journal of Epidemiology* **43**, 434–442.

Posner, J. *et al.* (2020) Attention-deficit hyperactivity disorder. *The Lancet* **395**, 450–462.

Prince, J. (2008) Catecholamine dysfunction in attention-deficit/hyperactivity disorder: an update. *Journal of Clinical Psychopharmacology* **28**, S39–S45.

Purper-Ouakil, D. *et al.* (2022) Personalized at-home neurofeedback compared to long-acting methylphenidate in children with ADHD: NEWROFEED, a European randomized noninferiority trial. *Journal of Child Psychology and Psychiatry* **63**, 187–198.

Rodrigues, R. *et al.* (2021) Practitioner review: pharmacological treatment of attention-deficit/hyperactivity disorder symptoms in children and youth with autism spectrum disorder: a systematic review and meta-analysis. *Journal of Child Psychology and Psychiatry* **62**, 680–700.

Rohde, L.C.D. *et al.* (2019) ADHD assessment across the life span. In: *The World Federation of ADHD Guide*. (eds L.B.J. Rohde, *et al.*). World Federation of ADHD, Zurich, Switzerland. pp. 42–62.

Rommelse, N.N. *et al.* (2010) Shared heritability of attention-deficit/hyperactivity disorder and autism spectrum disorder. *European Child & Adolescent Psychiatry* **19**, 281–295.

Russell, A.E. *et al.* (2016) The association between socioeconomic disadvantage and attention deficit/hyperactivity disorder (ADHD): a systematic review. *Child Psychiatry and Human Development* **47**, 440–458.

Samea, F. *et al.* (2019) Brain alterations in children/adolescents with ADHD revisited: a neuroimaging meta-analysis of 96 structural and functional studies. *Neuroscience and Biobehavioral Reviews* **100**, 1–8.

Satterstrom, F.K. *et al.* (2019) Autism spectrum disorder and attention deficit hyperactivity disorder have a similar burden of rare protein-truncating variants. *Nature Neuroscience* **22**, 1961–1965.

Sayal, K. *et al.* (2018) ADHD in children and young people: prevalence, care pathways, and service provision. *The Lancet Psychiatry* **5**, 175–186.

Shephard, E. *et al.* (2022) Systematic review and meta-analysis: the science of early-life precursors and interventions for attention-deficit/hyperactivity disorder. *Journal of the American Academy of Child and Adolescent Psychiatry* **61**, 187–226.

Sibley, M.H. *et al.* (2022) Variable patterns of remission from ADHD in the multimodal treatment study of ADHD. *The American Journal of Psychiatry* **179**, 142–151.

Sibley, M.H. *et al.* (2023) Non-pharmacological interventions for attention-deficit hyperactivity disorder in children and adolescents. *The Lancet Child & Adolescent Health* **6**, 415–428.

Skoglund, C. *et al.* (2014) Familial confounding of the association between maternal smoking during pregnancy and ADHD in offspring. *Journal of Child Psychology and Psychiatry* **55**, 61–68.

Song, P. *et al.* (2021) The prevalence of adult attention-deficit hyperactivity disorder: a global systematic review and meta-analysis. *Journal of Global Health* **11**, 04009.

Sonuga-Barke, E. & Thapar, A. (2021) The neurodiversity concept: is it helpful for clinicians and scientists? *The Lancet Psychiatry* **8**, 559–561.

Sonuga-Barke, E.H.G. (2018) Conceptualizing and investigating the role of the environment in ADHD: correlate, cause, consequence, context, and treatment. In: *Oxford Textbook of Attention Deficit Hyperactivity Disorder*. (eds T. Banasxhewski, *et al.*). Oxford University Press, Oxford, UK. pp. 25–34.

Sonuga-Barke, E.J. & Castellanos, F.X. (2007) Spontaneous attentional fluctuations in impaired states and pathological conditions: a neurobiological hypothesis. *Neuroscience and Biobehavioral Reviews* **31**, 977–986.

Sonuga-Barke, E.J.S. *et al.* (2017) Child-to-adult neurodevelopmental and mental health trajectories after early life deprivation: the young adult follow-up of the longitudinal English and Romanian adoptees study. *The Lancet* **389**, 1539–1548.

Sonuga-Barke, E.J.S. *et al.* (2023) Annual research review: perspectives on progress in ADHD science: from characterization to cause. *Journal of Child Psychology and Psychiatry* **64**, 506–532.

Spencer, A.E. *et al.* (2016) Examining the association between posttraumatic stress disorder and attention-deficit/hyperactivity disorder: a systematic review and meta-analysis. *The Journal of Clinical Psychiatry* **77**, 72–83.

Still, G. (1902) Some abnormal psychical conditions in children. *The Lancet*, 163–168.

Sugaya, L.F. *et al.* (2023) Efficacy of stimulants for preschool attention-deficit/hyperactivity disorder: a systematic review and meta-analysis. *JCPP Advances* **3**(3), e12146. doi:10.1002/jcv2.12146.

Sugaya, L.S. *et al.* (2022) Efficacy and safety of methylphenidate and behavioural parent training for children aged 3-5 years with attention-deficit hyperactivity disorder: a randomised, double-blind, placebo-controlled, and sham behavioural parent training-controlled trial. *The Lancet Child & Adolescent Health* **6**(12), 845–856.

Sutcubasi, B. *et al.* (2020) Resting-state network dysconnectivity in ADHD: a system-neuroscience-based meta-analysis. *The World Journal of Biological Psychiatry* **21**, 662–672.

Tamon, H.F. *et al.* (2023) Shared and specific neural correlates in attention-deficit/hyperactivity disorder and autism spectrum disorder: meta-analysis of 251 task-based functional MRI studies. *The American Journal of Psychiatry*. 181, 541–552.

Thapar, A. & Cooper, M. (2016) Attention deficit hyperactivity disorder. *The Lancet* **387**, 1240–1250.

Thapar, A. *et al.* (2001) Examining the comorbidity of ADHD-related behaviours and conduct problems using a twin study design. *The British Journal of Psychiatry* **179**, 224–229.

Tung, I. *et al.* (2016) Patterns of comorbidity among girls with ADHD: a meta-analysis. *Pediatrics* **138**, e20160430.

Victor, M.M. *et al.* (2018) Attention-deficit hyperactivity disorder in ancient Greece: the obtuse man of theophrastus. *The Australian and New Zealand Journal of Psychiatry* **52**, 509–513.

Vidor, M.V. *et al.* (2022) Emerging findings of glutamate-glutamine imbalance in the medial prefrontal cortex in attention deficit/hyperactivity disorder: systematic review and meta-analysis of spectroscopy studies. *European Archives of Psychiatry and Clinical Neuroscience* **272**, 1395–1411.

Volkow, N.D. *et al.* (2011) Motivation deficit in ADHD is associated with dysfunction of the dopamine reward pathway. *Molecular Psychiatry* **16**, 1147–1154.

Ward, R.J. *et al.* (2022) The effects of ADHD teacher training programs on teachers and pupils: a systematic review and meta-analysis. *Journal of Attention Disorders* **26**, 225–244.

Westwood, S.J. *et al.* (2023) Computerized cognitive training in attention-deficit/hyperactivity disorder (ADHD): a meta-analysis of randomized controlled trials with blinded and objective outcomes. *Molecular Psychiatry* **28**, 1402–1414.

Westwood, S.J. *et al.* (2024) Neurofeedback for attention-deficit/hyperactivity disorder: A systematic review and meta-analysis. *JAMA Psychiatry*. doi: 10.1001/jamapsychiatry.2024.3702. Epub ahead of print. PMID: 39661381.

Willcutt, E.G. (2012) The prevalence of DSM-IV attention-deficit/hyperactivity disorder: a meta-analytic review. *Neurotherapeutics* **9**, 490–499.

Willcutt, E.G. *et al.* (2005) Validity of the executive function theory of attention-deficit/hyperactivity disorder: a meta-analytic review. *Biological Psychiatry* **57**, 1336–1346.

Willcutt, E.G. *et al.* (2012) Validity of DSM-IV attention deficit/hyperactivity disorder symptom dimensions and subtypes. *Journal of Abnormal Psychology* **121**, 991–1010.

Williams, N.M. *et al.* (2010) Rare chromosomal deletions and duplications in attention-deficit hyperactivity disorder: a genome-wide analysis. *The Lancet* **376**, 1401–1408.

Wu, J. *et al.* (2012) Role of dopamine receptors in ADHD: a systematic meta-analysis. *Molecular Neurobiology* **45**, 605–620.

Young, S. *et al.* (2023) Identification and treatment of individuals with attention-deficit/hyperactivity disorder and substance use disorder: an expert consensus statement. *World Journal of Psychiatry* **13**, 84–112.

CHAPTER 55

Tic disorders

James F. Leckman and Michael H. Bloch
Child Study Center, Yale University School, New Haven, CT, USA

Introduction

Tic disorders are transient or chronic conditions associated with difficulties in self-esteem, family life, social acceptance, or school or job performance that are directly related to the presence of motor and/or phonic tics. Although tic symptoms have been reported since antiquity, systematic study of individuals with tic disorders dates only from the 19th century with the reports of Itard (1825) and Gilles de la Tourette (1885). Gilles de la Tourette described nine cases characterized by motor "incoordinations" or tics, "inarticulate shouts accompanied by articulated words with echolalia and coprolalia." In addition to identifying the cardinal features of severe tic disorders, his report noted an association between tic disorders and obsessive–compulsive (OC) symptoms, as well as the hereditary nature of the syndrome in some families.

In addition to tics, individuals with tic disorders may present with a broad array of behavioral difficulties including disinhibited speech or conduct, impulsivity, distractibility, motoric hyperactivity, and OC symptoms (Leckman *et al.*, 2022). Scientific opinion has been divided on how broadly to conceive the spectrum of maladaptive behaviors associated with Tourette syndrome (TS) (Shapiro *et al.*, 1988). This controversy is fueled in part by the frustration that parents and educators encounter when they attempt to divide an individual child's repertoire of problem behaviors into those that are "Tourette-related" and those that are not. Population-based epidemiological studies and family-genetic studies have begun to clarify these issues, but much more work remains to be done.

In this chapter, a presentation of the phenomenology and classification of tic disorders precedes a review of the etiology, neurobiological substrates, assessment including differential diagnosis of tics, and management of tic disorders. The general perspective that will be presented is that TS and related disorders are associated with multiple genetic and environmental mechanisms that interact over the course of development to produce a distinctive range of complex syndromes of varying severity. When treating tic symptoms, the goal of treatment is to minimize the impairment associated with tic symptoms and their comorbidities and not to attempt to obliterate the tics given the adverse events and limitations of current treatments and the ephemeral nature of tics experienced by many pediatric patients.

Phenomenology of tics and diagnosis of tic disorders

Phenomenology of tics

A *tic* is a sudden, repetitive movement, gesture, or utterance that typically mimics some aspect or fragment of normal behavior (Leckman *et al.*, 2022). Individual tics rarely last more than a second. Individual tics can occur singly or together in an orchestrated pattern. They vary in their intensity or forcefulness. As depicted in Figure 55.1, motor tics vary from simple abrupt movements such as eye blinking, head jerks, or shoulder shrugs to more complex, apparently purposive, behaviors such as facial expressions or gestures of the arms or head. In extreme cases, these movements can be obscene (coprolalia and copropraxia) or self-injurious, e.g., hitting or biting oneself. Phonic or vocal tics can range from simple throat clearing sounds to more complex vocalizations and speech. In severe cases, coprolalia (obscene or socially unacceptable speech) is present.

By the age of 10 years, most individuals with tics are aware of premonitory urges that may either be experienced as a focal perception in a particular body region where the tic is about to occur (like an itch or a tickling sensation) or as a mental awareness (Leckman *et al.*, 1993). Most patients also report a fleeting sense of relief after a bout of tics has occurred. These premonitory phenomena contribute to an individual's sense that

Rutter's Child and Adolescent Psychiatry and Psychology, Seventh Edition.
Edited by Anita Thapar, Daniel S. Pine, Samuele Cortese, Cathy Creswell, Tamsin J. Ford, James F. Leckman, and Argyris Stringaris.

Companion website: www.wiley.com/go/thapar/rutterspsych7

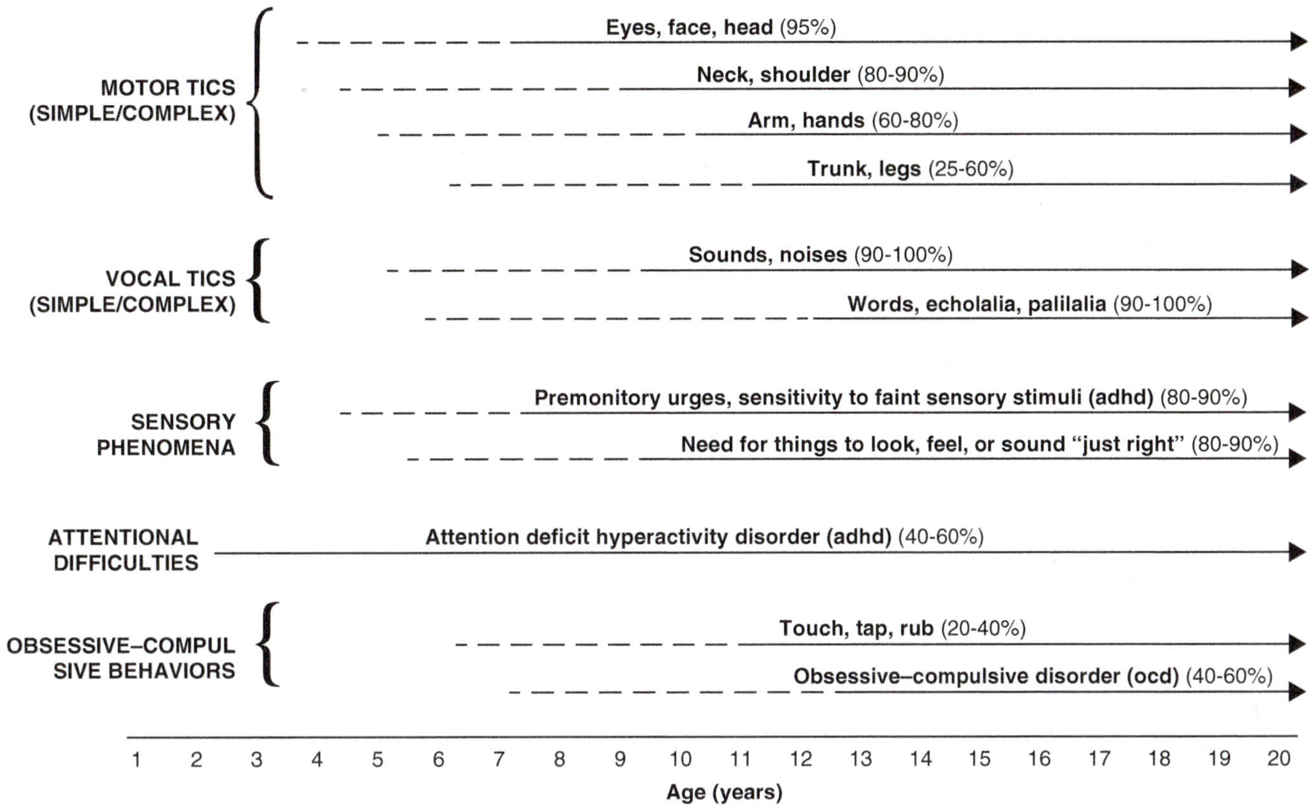

Figure 55.1 Natural history of tics and associated behaviors. The occurrence of motor and oral tics and related behaviors progressing at different ages from transient episodes (broken lines) to sustained periods (solid lines).

tics are a habitual, yet partially intentional, response to unpleasant stimuli. Indeed, most adolescent and adult subjects describe their tics as either "voluntary" or as having both voluntary and involuntary aspects. In contrast, many young children are oblivious to their tics and experience them as wholly involuntary movements or sounds. Most tics can also be consciously suppressed for brief periods of time. The warning given by premonitory urges may contribute to this phenomenon.

Clinicians characterize tics by their anatomical location, number, frequency, and duration. The intensity or "forcefulness" of the tic can also be an important characteristic. Tics vary in terms of their "complexity." Complexity usually refers to how simple or involved a movement or sound is, ranging from brief, meaningless, abrupt fragments (simple tics) to ones that are longer, more involved, and seemingly more goal-directed in character (complex tics). Each of these elements has been incorporated into clinician rating scales that have proven to be useful in monitoring tic severity (Leckman *et al.*, 1989).

Diagnostic categories

Diagnostic categories provide a common basis for discussion and are an essential tool in epidemiological and clinical research. Several widely used diagnostic classifications currently include sections on tic disorders. These include both the *Diagnostic and Statistical Manual of Mental Disorders,* 5th edition, text revision (DSM-5-TR) classification system published by the American Psychiatric Association (2022), and the *International Classification of Disease and Related Health Problems,* 11th Revision (ICD-11) criteria published by the World Health Organization (2021). DSM-5 currently classifies tic disorders as a neurodevelopmental disorder (NDD), whereas ICD-11 does not. Although differences exist, these classification schemes are broadly congruent with each other, containing three major categories: TS or its equivalent; persistent (chronic) motor or vocal tic disorder (CMTD or CVTD) or their equivalents; and transient tic disorder or its equivalent. However, the ICD-11 and DSM-5 diagnostic groupings suffer from uncertainties about how best to categorize conditions that potentially encompass a broad range of symptoms that wax and wane in severity. Since the current nosological boundaries are set by convention and clinical practice, they may not reflect true etiological differences.

Tourette syndrome

The most severe tic disorder is best known by the eponym, "Gilles de la Tourette's Syndrome." Typically, the disorder begins in early childhood with transient bouts of simple motor tics such as eye blinking or head jerks. These tics may initially come and go, but eventually they become persistent and begin to have adverse effects on the child and the family. The repertoire of motor tics can be vast, incorporating virtually any voluntary movement by any portion of the body (Leckman *et al.*, 2022).

Although some patients have a "rostral-caudal" progression of motor tics (head, neck, shoulders, arms, torso), this course is not predictable. As the syndrome develops, complex motor tics may appear. Typically, they accompany simple motor tics. Often, they have a "camouflaged" or purposive appearance, e.g., brushing hair away from the face with an arm, and can only be distinguished as tics by their repetitive character. They can involve dystonic movements. In a small fraction of cases (<5%), complex motor tics have the potential to be self-injurious. These self-injurious symptoms may be relatively mild, e.g., slapping or tapping, or quite dangerous, e.g., punching one side of the face, biting a wrist, or gouging eyes to the point of blindness. On average, phonic tics begin one to two years after the onset of motor symptoms and are usually simple in character, e.g., throat clearing, grunting, and squeaking. More complex vocal symptoms, such as echolalia (repeating another's speech), palilalia (repeating one's own speech), and coprolalia, occur in a minority of cases. Other complex phonic symptoms include dramatic and abrupt changes in rhythm, rate, and volume of speech.

Persistent (chronic) motor or vocal tic disorder

This chronic condition can be observed among children and adults. As with other tic disorders, CMTD is characterized by a waxing and waning course and a broad range of symptom severity. Chronic simple and complex motor tics are the most common manifestations. A majority of tics involve the eyes, face, head, neck, and upper extremities. Although some children may display other developmental difficulties such as attention deficit hyperactivity disorder (ADHD), the disorder can be compatible with an otherwise normal course of childhood. This condition can also appear as a residual state, where a predictable repertoire of tic symptoms may be seen only during periods of heightened stress or fatigue.

Transient tic disorder

Almost invariably a disorder of childhood, transient tic disorder is usually characterized by one or more simple motor tics that wax and wane in severity over weeks to months. The anatomical distribution of these tics is usually confined to the eyes, face, neck, or upper extremities. Transient phonic tics, in the absence of motor tics, can also occur, though more rarely. The age of onset is typically 3–10 years. Boys are at greater risk. The initial presentation may be unnoticed. Family practitioners, pediatricians, allergists, and ophthalmologists are typically the first to see the child. Missed diagnoses are common, particularly as the symptoms may have completely disappeared by the time of the consultation.

Provisional tic disorder

Provisional tic disorder is a diagnosis meant to describe an individual with motor and/or vocal tics that are ongoing and have not been present for long enough to qualify for a diagnosis of a chronic tic disorder or TS. A provisional tic disorder is distinguished from a transient tic disorder by the fact that in provisional tic disorders the tics are still ongoing whereas in transient tic disorders the tic symptoms have resolved.

Other specified tic disorder

This is a diagnosis in DSM-5 utilized to describe individuals with impairing tic symptoms who do not meet the full criteria for the chronic tic disorders or TS described earlier. Specifically, individuals who have new-onset tics after 18 years of age do not meet the age-of-onset criteria for TS. Adults with new-onset tics present with a much larger differential diagnosis than younger children who present with new-onset tics. The differential diagnosis can include stroke, tumors, adverse effects of medication, and other hyperkinetic movement disorders (e.g., chorea, dystonias, and myoclonus). Therefore, the diagnostic workup for adults with new-onset tics is much more extensive than for a typical child presenting with new-onset tics.

Epidemiology

Children are 5–12 times more likely to be identified as having a tic disorder than adults. In fact, transient tics are so common that it is estimated that one in five school-age children will express them if observed closely (Scahill *et al.*, 2014). Although boys are more commonly affected with tic behaviors than girls, the male–female ratio varies considerably from 1 : 1 to 10 : 1. Once thought to be rare, current estimates of the prevalence of TS vary 100-fold, from 2.9/10,000 (Caine *et al.*, 1988) to 299/10,000 (Mason *et al.*, 1998). Methodological differences between studies (parent-report versus direct observation in the classroom versus self-report versus medical diagnosis), age of sample (childhood versus adult), and threshold differences in detection (sampling techniques that require some degree of impairment or distress, as well as the changing of diagnostic criteria and categories over time) likely account for much of the reported variation in prevalence rates. Best estimates from meta-analyses of pediatric studies suggest a prevalence rate of TS was approximately 0.52% (95% CI 0.32–0.85) or 52/10,000 children and a population prevalence that is considerably lower in adults (Scharf *et al.*, 2015; Levine *et al.*, 2019). By contrast, it is estimated that approximately 20% of school-aged children have at least transient tics (Scahill *et al.*, 2014), thus the vast majority of children who display tics will not develop TS or a chronic tic disorder.

Clinical course

Tics typically have an onset between the ages of 4–6 years and reach their worst-ever severity between the ages of 10–12 years (Bloch & Leckman, 2009) (Figure 55.1). On average, tic severity declines during adolescence. By early adulthood, roughly three-quarters of children with TS will have greatly diminished tic symptoms and over one-third will be tic free. As depicted in Figure 55.1, ADHD symptoms are often evident prior to the onset of tics. Other comorbid conditions, such as obsessive–compulsive disorder (OCD) and anxiety and depressive disorders, are more common during the adolescence and early adulthood of individuals with TS than in the general population.

Motor and phonic tics tend to occur in bouts (Leckman *et al.*, 2022). Their frequency ranges from nonstop bursts that are virtually uncountable (>100 tics per minute) to rare events that occur only a few times a week. Single tics may occur in isolation or there may be orchestrated combinations of motor and phonic tics. The forcefulness of motor tics and the volume of phonic tics can also vary from behaviors that are not noticeable (a slight shrug or a hushed guttural noise) to strenuous displays (arm thrusts or loud barking) that are frightening and exhausting. During periods of waxing tic symptoms, clinicians may find themselves under extreme pressure to intervene medically. Factors such as increased stress and poor sleep are known to exacerbate tics. While such interventions may be warranted, it is often the case that the tic symptoms will wane substantially within a few weeks.

By the age of 10, most children and adolescents have some awareness of the premonitory urges that frequently precede both motor and vocal tics (Leckman *et al.*, 2022). These urges add to the subjective discomfort associated with having a tic disorder. They may also contribute to an individual's ability to suppress their tics for longer periods of time.

Although children with TS can be loving and affectionate, maintaining age-appropriate social skills is particularly difficult for many of them (Dykens *et al.*, 1990; Bawden *et al.*, 1998). Whether this is due to the stigmatizing effects of the tics, the patient's own uneasiness, or some more fundamental difficulty linked to the neurobiology of this disorder is unknown.

Relatively few cross-sectional or longitudinal studies of tic disorders have been performed (Leckman *et al.*, 1998). These studies indicate that tic disorders tend to improve in late adolescence and early adulthood (Bloch, 2022). In many instances, the phonic symptoms become increasingly rare or may disappear altogether, and the motor tics may be reduced in number and frequency. Complete remission of both motor and phonic symptoms has also been reported. It remains unclear how many of these adults who "recover" from tic disorders do not experience any tics in adulthood or experience mild tics that cause minimal-to-no discernable distress or impairment (Black *et al.*, 2021). Clinical experience suggests that some adult patients experience a reemergence of tics even after a prolonged disappearance of tics (Black *et al.*, 2021). Regardless, adulthood is also the period when the most severe and debilitating forms of tic disorder can be seen. It is also clear that children with TS are at increased risk for other psychiatric conditions that cause impairment such as depression, OCD, anxiety and substance use (Gorman *et al.*, 2010). The factors that influence the continuity of tic disorders from childhood to adolescence to adulthood are not well understood but likely involve the interaction of normal maturational processes occurring in the central nervous system (CNS) with the neurobiological mechanisms responsible for TS. Certainly, the level of emotional trauma and distress experienced by affected individuals, as well as inappropriate parenting styles, can contribute to a more severe course (Li *et al.*, 2022). In addition, tic disorders may be etiologically separable so that some of these factors, such as activation of the immune system, exposure to heat stress, or exposure to cocaine or anabolic steroids, may influence the pathogenesis and intramorbid course for some individuals but not others.

The natural history of TS has clear implications for the treatment of individuals with this condition. Children with tics have a substantial probability of improvement in both the severity and impact of tic symptoms during adolescence and young adulthood. Given the ephemeral nature of tics in many children, pharmacological treatment should be conservative and focused on reducing functional impairment. Parents, teachers, and peers can benefit from psychoeducational interventions.

Clinical assessment

Assessment instruments

The complex motor, vocal, and behavioral phenotype of TS presents a unique challenge to measurement. Although the visible and audible nature of core TS symptoms allows direct observation, their waxing and waning character, even over the course of the day, present challenges to the clinician. A variety of clinician-, parent-, and self-report rating instruments are available for tics and associated symptoms, for use in clinical practice and/or research settings (Cavanna, 2022; King & Landeros-Weisenberger, 2022). The Yale Global Tic Severity Scale (YGTSS) and the YGTSS-Revised (YGTSS-R) are the most widely used measures of tic severity in TS and other tic disorders (Leckman *et al.*, 1989; McGuire *et al.*, 2018). These measures use a semistructured interview of symptoms over the past week, where the clinician is asked to document the patient's motor and phonic tics. The motor and vocal tics are rated separately based on their number, frequency, intensity, complexity, and interference from 0 (no tic symptoms) to 5 (severe). The tic severity subscore consists of the motor and phonic tic severity scores. This is added to the impairment subscore, which rates the severity of functional impairment from 0 to 50, to produce the total score (0–100). In addition to the YGTSS and the YGTSS-R, the Premonitory Urge for Tics Scale (PUTS) is being increasingly used to characterize individuals with tic disorders. The PUTS is a relatively brief self-report scale designed to quantify the premonitory sensory urges that frequently precede motor and vocal tics (Woods *et al.*, 2005). The PUTS contains 10 descriptions of somatic sensations. The severity of these urges is rated on a 4-point ordinal scale ranging from 1 (not at all true) to 4 (very much true). A wide range of psychometrically

Box 55.1 Assessment at a glance

- Tic disorders, including Tourette syndrome, are a clinical diagnosis that is typically made based solely on a clinical evaluation.
- Laboratory testing (e.g., neuroimaging and blood tests) is typically not recommended for most children with tic disorders.
- Assessment should include a detailed history about tic symptoms examining:
  - The characteristics of current and previous tics (type, location, frequency, severity, age of onset, premonitory urges, suppressibility, exacerbating and alleviating factors).
  - Functional impairment related to tics (difficulties in school, activities that are disrupted, interrupted, or avoided because of tics, peer and family difficulties related to tics).
- Assessment should include screening for common comorbidities including attention deficit hyperactivity disorder (ADHD), obsessive–compulsive disorder (OCD), oppositional behaviors, anxiety, and depression as often these comorbidities cause more impairment than the tics themselves.
- Structured rating scales can be useful for measuring and tracking the severity of tics and premonitory urges:
  - Yale Global Tic Severity Scale (YGTSS) – a 10-item clinician-rated semistructured interview that is the gold standard for measuring the severity of both motor and vocal tics, as well as a total tic score. Additionally, has a tic symptom checklist that is useful in cataloging lifetime tics, as well a rating of impairment (Leckman *et al*., 1989; McGuire *et al*., 2018).
  - Premonitory Urge for Tic Scale (PUTS) – a 9-item self-report measure that measures the presence and severity of physical sensations or urges that commonly precede tic symptoms (Woods *et al*., 2005/with permission of Wolters Kluwer Health, Inc.).

validated clinician- and self-rated measures for ADHD, anxiety, OCD, and depressive symptoms are also available (see Chapters 54, 59, 60, 63, respectively) and they are commonly used in assessing individuals with TS and other tic disorders. As noted in Chapter 27, the potential differences between information gathered from clinicians and patients should always be considered if the assessment is to be considered comprehensive and accurate (Box 55.1).

Prognosis and quality of life

Prospective cohort studies have fairly consistently shown that most children with TS will improve during adolescence (Bloch & Leckman, 2009). Current research indicates that estimates of current tic severity have limited value in terms of long-term prognosis for tic severity. Although lifetime histories of comorbid ADHD and OCD symptoms are associated with poorer adulthood psychosocial functioning in patients with TS, the presence of these comorbid symptoms in childhood has not been found to be associated with higher levels of severity in adulthood (Bloch *et al.* 2006b; Cavanna *et al*., 2012). However, initial studies do suggest that poor performance on standardized tests of fine-motor coordination (dominant hand, Purdue Pegboard test) and smaller caudate nucleus volumes (using volumetric magnetic resonance images [MRIs]) are associated with more severe tic symptoms in adulthood (Bloch *et al*., 2005, 2006a). These initial studies require replication. Careful clinical evaluation is required to understand profiles of strengths and weaknesses in adaptive functioning and to disentangle the relative contributions of tics and co-occurring disorders from other problems with peers, academic functioning, or family life. Whenever possible, clinical interviews should be supplemented by collecting standardized ratings of adaptive functioning.

Comorbid conditions

In both clinical and epidemiological samples TS alone is the exception rather than the rule. Symptoms associated with ADHD and OCD have received the most attention. It is also becoming clear that the more severe the tic disorder the greater the likelihood of detecting coexisting conditions, even in representative, population-based samples.

Both clinical and epidemiological studies vary according to setting and established referral patterns, but it is not uncommon to see reports of 30–50% of children with TS diagnosed with comorbid ADHD (Khalifa & von Knorring, 2005; Rothenberger & Roessner, 2022). TS has the highest rate of ADHD relative to the other lesser variants of tic disorders. Although the etiological relationship between TS and ADHD is in dispute, it is clear that those individuals with both TS and ADHD are at a much greater risk for a variety of untoward outcomes (Carter *et al*., 2000; Peterson *et al*., 2001; Sukhodolsky *et al*., 2003, 2005). They are often regarded as less likeable, more aggressive, and more withdrawn than their classmates (Stokes *et al*., 1991).

More than 40% of individuals with TS experience recurrent OC symptoms (Khalifa & von Knorring, 2005; Ferrão *et al*., 2022). Genetic, neurobiological, and treatment response studies suggest that there may be qualitative differences between tic-related forms of OCD and cases of OCD in which there is no personal or family history of tics. Specifically, tic-related OCD has a male preponderance, an earlier age of onset, a poorer level of response to standard antiobsessional medications, and a greater likelihood of first-degree family members with a tic disorder (Hounie *et al*., 2006). Symptomatically, the most common OC symptoms encountered in TS patients are obsessions concerning a need for symmetry or exactness, repeating rituals, counting compulsions, and ordering/arranging compulsions (Leckman *et al*., 1997). Also, OC symptoms, when present, in children with TS, appear more likely to persist into adulthood than the tics themselves (Bloch *et al.* 2006b). Tics are also thought to represent a moderator of response to pharmacological treatment in patients with OCD in that individuals with tic-related OCD tend to be less responsive to selective serotonin reuptake inhibitor (SSRI) pharmacotherapy and more responsive to antipsychotic augmentation than individuals with OCD but without comorbid tic symptoms (Geller *et al*., 2004; Bloch *et al*., 2006c; March *et al*., 2007).

The co-occurrence of depression and anxiety symptoms with TS are commonplace and may reflect the cumulative psychosocial burden of having tics or shared biological diatheses or both (Coffey *et al.*, 2000; Martino & Leckman, 2022). Antecedent depressive symptoms do predict modest increases in tic severity. Future depression severity is more closely associated with antecedent worsening of psychosocial stress and OC symptoms than it is with future measures of tic severity (Martino & Hedderly, 2019). Nevertheless, individuals diagnosed with tic disorders are at higher risk for suicide (Fernandez de la Cruz *et al.*, 2017).

Children with autism spectrum disorders (ASDs) are also at higher risk for developing TS (Baron-Cohen *et al.*, 1999). A number of medical and neurological disorders also have a higher prevalence in children with TS. These include asthma and allergic disorders, as well as restless legs syndrome, migraine headaches, sleep disorders, and streptococcal infections (Fernandez de la Cruz *et al.*, 2017).

Differentiating tics from other common movement disorders

Tics can typically be easily distinguished from other movement disorders based on clinical history and observation of the movements. However, there are a few common conditions that the examiner is asked to distinguish from tics.

In younger children, stereotypic movements can sometimes be confused with tics. In contrast to tics, stereotypic movements are described as repetitive, patterned, nonpurposeful movements (e.g., body rocking, tapping, hand flapping, arm waving) (Oakley *et al.*, 2015). Stereotypic movements frequently occur in children with intellectual disability (ID) or ASDs but quite commonly affect typically developing children (Martino & Hedderly, 2019). Stereotypic movements are longer in duration, rhythmic, and less variable in type, intensity, severity, and location over time. Stereotypic movements typically have an earlier age of onset than tics (before three years of age), are less likely to interrupt purposeful activities, and are typically not associated with premonitory urges (Oakley *et al.*, 2015; Martino & Hedderly, 2019). Table 55.1 contrasts the characteristics of stereotypic movements and tics.

Stereotypies and tics can often occur in the same child. Children with a range of NDDs are at increased risk for tic disorders. Kurlan and colleagues reported a fourfold increase in the prevalence of tic disorders among children in special educational settings in a single school district in upstate New York (Kurlan *et al.*, 1994). These children did not have an ID but did have significant specific learning problems, and/or other speech or physical impairments. Children with ASDs are also at higher risk for developing TS (Baron-Cohen *et al.*, 1999). However, in many instances the tics go unrecognized and are regarded as stereotypies.

Although functional movements have always been recognized on the differential diagnosis of tic disorders, there was a dramatic rise in both recognition and incidence of these cases during the COVID-19 pandemic. The increase of these functional tic-like behaviors was initially recognized to be related to social media content with particular geographic presentations highly related to topical videos posted by influential social media personalities in the area (Muller-Vahl *et al.*, 2022).

Table 55.2 contrasts the characteristic of functional tic-like behaviors and TS. Functional tic-like behaviors, in contrast to tics in TS, typically have a later age of onset (adolescence to early adulthood), rapid onset of symptoms, increase in the presence of other people, tend to be primarily complex in character, are associated with other functional neurologic symptoms, anxiety, and depression, and are generally more severe and impairing (Berg *et al.*, 2022). Functional tic-like behaviors have been observed to have a strong female predominance in contrast to TS, which has a strong male predominance.

Although investigators have begun to establish characteristics that can most reliably distinguish between cases of functional tics and typical tic disorders, it is important to note that few studies have challenged these criteria in prospective cohorts (and have typically applied factors to retrospective datasets) (Frey *et al.*, 2022). Therefore, it is unclear how well even the most astute neurologist or psychiatrist can readily distinguish these cases. The challenge of differentiating functional tics is made

Table 55.1 Distinguishing tics and stereotypic movements.

Feature	Tics	Stereotypic movements
Age of onset	5–7 years	<3 years
Fluctuation of symptom severity	Waxing and waning	Consistent severity
Timing of movements	Brief, sudden	Rhythmic, continuous, prolonged
Character of movements	Unilateral	Bilateral
Consistency of particular movements over time	Change in character	Relatively constant in character
Common movements	Eye blinking, throat clearing, facial grimace	Arm flapping, rocking
Premonitory urges	Present	Absent
Suppressibility	Temporarily	Rarely
Interruptible?	No	Usually
Impact	Disruptive, bothersome	Comforting, gratifying
Common comorbidities	Attention deficit hyperactivity disorder (ADHD), obsessive–compulsive disorder (OCD)	Autism spectrum disorders (ASDs)
Medication	Antipsychotics, alpha-2 agonists	No evidence-based pharmacologic treatment

Table 55.2 Distinguishing tics from functional movements.

Feature	Tics	Functional tic-like behaviors
Age of onset	5–7 years	Adolescence and early adulthood
Sex distribution	Male predominance	Female predominance
Speed of symptom onset	Variable but typically gradual	Abrupt, explosive
Severity	Variable (typically mild or moderate)	Severe
Impairment	Variable (typically mild or moderate)	Severe
Effect of observation	Often improves when in presence of others	Typically worsens when observed by others
Common motor movements	Eye blinking, facial grimace with more complex tics developing later	Copropraxia, self-injurious behaviors, throwing or hitting objects
Common vocalizations	Throat clearing, sniffing, grunting with more complex vocal tics developing later	Animal noises, coprolalia
Complexity of movements	Begin as simple movements and can increase in complexity over time	Often complex movements from onset
Antecedent phenomenon	Premonitory urges	Anxiety (less common)
Common comorbidities	Attention deficit hyperactivity disorder (ADHD), obsessive–compulsive disorder (OCD)	Anxiety, depression, other functional neurologic symptoms

Table 55.3 Distinguishing tics and tardive dyskinesia.

Feature	Tics	Tardive dyskinesia
Age-of-onset	5–7 years	Any age with exposure
Risk factors	Multifactorial and largely unknown	Specific medication exposure (antipsychotics, metoclopramide)
Severity of symptoms	Waxing and waning	Consistent severity
Timing of movements	Brief, sudden	Rhythmic
Awareness of movements	Increasing awareness with age	Typically unaware
Consistency of particular movements over time	Change in character	Constant in character
Common movements	Eye blinking, throat clearing, facial grimace	Tongue and mouth movements
Premonitory urges	Present	Absent
Suppressibility	Temporarily	Not Suppressible
Pharmacological treatment	Antipsychotics, alpha-2 agonists	Vesicular monoamine transporter type 2 (VMAT2) inhibitors, decreasing antipsychotic exposure

even more difficult by the observation that some patients with TS may have some functional tics or behaviors. Additionally, since these functional tics have been recognized to be highly influenced by social media and peer exposure, the characteristics of functional tics (and functional tic disorders) may (or may not) change as the particularly influential social influences change. Further research is needed to determine the ideal treatment for functional tic-like behaviors and how similar it is compared to other functional neurologic disorders (LaFaver *et al.*, 2021).

In adults and children treated with antipsychotic medications it is sometimes important to distinguish tics from tardive dyskinesia. Tardive dyskinesia is typically characterized by involuntary, spontaneous movements of the tongue and mouth (but can involve other body parts) that are similar in appearance to tics (Caroff, 2022). In contrast to tics, the movements of tardive dyskinesia typically occur outside of the awareness of the individual, remain constant in character and intensity over time and are not associated with premonitory urges. Table 55.3 contrasts the characteristics of tics to the movements of tardive dyskinesia. Risk factors for tardive dyskinesia include treatment with antipsychotic medications (especially first-generation antipsychotics) or, les commonly, other medications such as metoclopramide, as well as several antidepressants, antiepileptics, and antiemetics (Caroff, 2022). It is important to distinguish tardive dyskinesia from tics as tardive dyskinesia movements can be lifelong, even if the offending agent is removed and the pharmacological treatment is typically opposite that of tics (removing or lowering the dose of antipsychotic medications). Vesicular monoamine transporter type 2 (VMAT2) inhibitors, such as valbenazine and deutetrabenazine, are US Food and Drug Administration (FDA)-approved medications with demonstrated efficacy for treating tardive dyskinesia (Artukoglu *et al.*, 2020).

Risk factors

Genetic risk factors

Tic disorders are among the most heritable neuropsychiatric disorders. Twin and family studies provide clear evidence that genetic factors are involved in the vulnerability to TS and related disorders (Mataix-Cols *et al.*, 2015; Abdallah & Fernandez, 2022). The concordance rate for TS among monozygotic twin pairs is greater than 50% while the concordance of dizygotic twin pairs is about 10% (Price *et al.*, 1985; Hyde *et al.*, 1992). First-degree family members of individuals with TS are at substantially higher risk for having TS, CMTD, and OCD than unrelated individuals (Scharf *et al.*, 2013; Yu *et al.*, 2019). That being said, the offspring of individuals with TS have only approximately a 10% chance of developing significant tics (Bloch & Leckman, 2009).

The high heritability of TS has led investigators to investigate specific genetic causes of TS. Efforts to identify susceptibility genes within large multigenerational families, or using affected sibling pairs or genome-wide association designs have met with limited success (Yu *et al.*, 2019; Abdallah & Fernandez, 2022; Jain *et al.*, 2023). However, a recent a genome-wide meta-analysis using data from 6133 individuals with TS and 13,565 ancestry-matched control participants identified a genome-wide significant locus on chromosome 5q15 linked to the NR2F1 gene (Tsetsos *et al.*, 2023). Another report described a two-generation family with nine affected members with TS. They eventually identified a rare functional mutation in the gene encoding L-histidine decarboxylase, the rate-limiting enzyme in histamine biosynthesis (Ercan-Sencicek *et al.*, 2010). These findings point to a role for histaminergic neurotransmission in the mechanism and modulation of TS and tics. Additionally, whole-exome sequencing studies of have also suggested the importance of rare variants in the pathogenesis of TS. Specifically, a study examining whole-exome sequencing in a cohort of over 500 trios with TS, demonstrated an increase in *de novo* likely gene disrupting and damaging variants in patients with TS (Willsey *et al.*, 2017).

Nongenetic risk factors

Twin studies, despite their small size and number, have consistently demonstrated that nongenetic factors play a role in the pathogenesis of TS (Abdallah & Fernandez, 2022). The fact that concordance for monozygotic twins for TS and tic disorders is well below 100% indicates that nongenetic factors are critical in determining the nature and severity of the clinical syndrome. Several nongenetic factors, including obstetric and perinatal complications, psychological stress, and infection, have been studied as risk factors for TS.

Many case–control and cohort studies have examined the association between obstetrics and perinatal complications, and risk for TS and chronic tic disorders. Low Apgar scores at five minutes, low birth weight, maternal smoking during pregnancy, and high levels of maternal stress during pregnancy have been associated with increased risk of tics in individual case–control and cohort studies (Brander *et al.*, 2018; Hoekstra & Dietrich, 2022). Other perinatal adversities have been associated with risk of comorbid OCD and ADHD in these same studies. It remains uncertain whether, how, and how much perinatal environmental influences impact the severity and presence of tic symptoms. Replication of specific findings in prospective studies will help alleviate concerns that recall bias of perinatal risk factors among parents of affected probands or multiple hypothesis testing may be responsible for these associations. Furthermore, proof of a clear association between specific perinatal environmental influence and the presence or severity of tics does not prove causation.

Psychosocial stress is an increasingly recognized risk factor for the emergence and exacerbation of tic symptoms. Tic disorders have long been identified as "stress-sensitive" conditions. Typically, symptom exacerbations follow in the wake of stressful life events. Clinical experience suggests that in some instances a vicious cycle is initiated in which attempts to suppress the symptoms by punishment and humiliation lead to a further exacerbation of symptoms and further increase in stress in the child's interpersonal environment. Unchecked, this vicious cycle can lead to the most severe manifestations of TS. Prospective longitudinal studies have shown that patients with TS experience more stress than matched healthy controls (Findley *et al.*, 2003) and that antecedent stress may play a role in subsequent tic exacerbation (Lin *et al.*, 2007, 2010). Increases in depressive symptoms have also emerged as a significant predictor of future tic severity.

In addition to the intramorbid effects of stress, anxiety, and depression, premorbid stress may also act as a sensitizing agent in the pathogenesis of TS among vulnerable individuals (Leckman *et al.*, 1984). It is likely that the immediate family environment, e.g., parental discord and the coping abilities of family members, plays some role (Leckman *et al.*, 1990), and this may lead to a sensitization of stress-responsive biological systems such as the hypothalamic–pituitary–adrenal axis (Chappell *et al.*, 1994; Leckman *et al.*, 1995).

The potential association between antecedent infections and the emergence and exacerbation of tic symptoms has been the object of much interest and controversy in the study of TS and related conditions (Martino *et al.*, 2022). Initial interest for the potential importance of infection in the pathogenesis of TS originated from the observation that motor and vocal tics, as well as OCD, are common manifestations in Sydenham's chorea. Sydenham's chorea is a known autoimmune disorder following group A beta-hemolytic streptococcus (GABHS) infections. The most compelling evidence of an etiological link between these disorders and GABHS infection comes from a study that found an increased proportion of GABHS infections (odds ratio = 13.6) within the preceding 12 months in children newly diagnosed with TS compared to well-matched controls in a well-conducted epidemiologic study (Mell *et al.*, 2005). However, prospective longitudinal studies have provided little support for the idea that GABHS infections induce future tic exacerbations (Luo *et al.*, 2004). The potential association of antecedent infection and tic symptoms has led to the proposal of multiple potential diagnostic syndromes that may identify potential "post-infection" cases of tics and OCD (Swedo *et al.*, 1998; Chang *et al.*, 2015; Swedo *et al.*, 2017). The validity of these proposed diagnostic syndromes remains unproven and not recognized by the currently utilized diagnostic criteria in psychiatry (Gilbert, 2019). Nonetheless, the link between the emergence of tic disorders and the immune system remains an important area worthy of further study given the increasing evidence from genetic studies and basic science (Hsu *et al.*, 2021).

Pathophysiology

The basal ganglia and their connections—specifically the multisynaptic cortico-striato-thalamo-cortical (CSTC) circuits or loops that link the cerebral cortex with subcortical regions—have

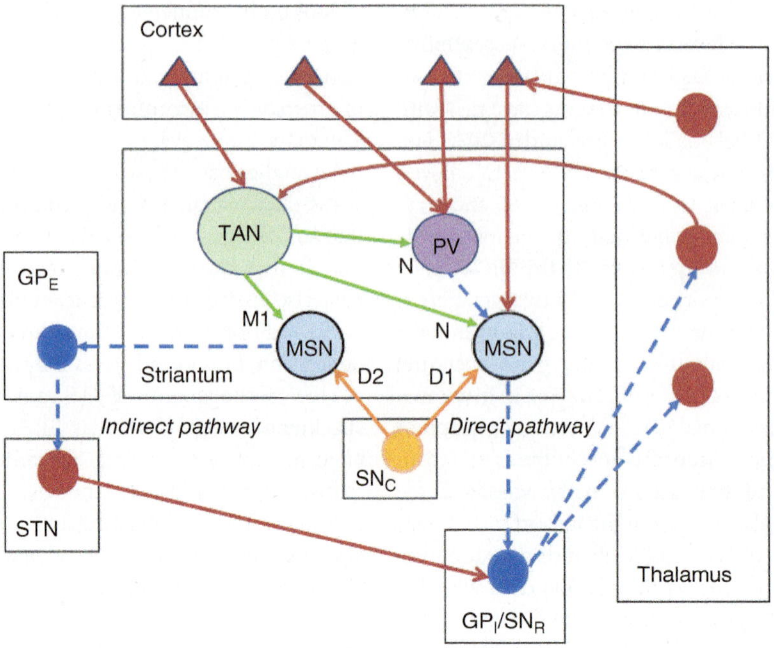

Figure 55.2 Cortico-striato-thalamo-cortical circuitry in Tourette syndrome. Red—excitatory glutamatergic neurons; blue—gamma-aminobutyric acid (GABA)-ergic inhibitory neurons; green—cholinergic tonically active interneurons (TANs); purple—parvalbumin (PV) fast-spiking GABAergic interneurons; and orange—dopaminergic neurons. Parvalbumin (PV) fast-spiking GABAergic interneurons mediate the cortical inhibition upon the medium spiny neurons (MSNs) of the striatopallidal direct pathway, resulting in inhibition of voluntary movements. Cholinergic TANs enhance the responsiveness of the MSNs of the striatopallidal direct pathway, resulting in movement suppression. PVs and TANs also enhance the responsiveness of the MSNs of the striatonigral indirect pathway resulting in movement suppression. PVs and TANs are diminished in number in the brains of adults with severe, persistent Tourette's syndrome (see "Pathophysiology" section). The volume of the striatum, particularly the caudate nuclei, is smaller in both children and adults with Tourette's syndrome. Receptors include: M1 and nicotinic (N) cholinergic receptors; and D1 and D2 dopamine receptors. *Source*: Fasching *et al.* (2022)/with permission of Oxford University Press.

the focus of most neurobiological research on TS (Graybiel & Canales, 2001; Dyke *et al.*, 2022; Greene *et al.*, 2022; Singer & Augustine, 2022). As a whole, structural and functional neuroimaging, as well as neuropathological studies, strongly implicate the importance of CSTC circuits, especially involving motor and supplementary motor circuits, frontal circuits involved in cognitive control, and habit formation in the pathogenesis of TS.

Extensive immunohistochemical studies of the basal ganglia have demonstrated the presence of a wide spectrum of classic neurotransmitters, neuromodulators, and neuropeptides. The most compelling data have implicated central dopaminergic systems in the pathobiology of TS (Figure 55.2). Of the various dopaminergic hypotheses proposed, an alteration of the tonic–phasic neurotransmitter release system appears most viable (Singer & Augustine, 2022).

Neural circuits

CSTC circuits are involved in procedural learning, habit formation, and internally and externally guided motor control (Graybiel & Canales, 2001; Dyke *et al.*, 2022; Singer & Augustine, 2022). As a result, the most widely accepted neuroanatomical model of TS proposes a regional imbalance of the direct versus the indirect pathway within one or more of these CSTC circuits (Albin & Mink, 2006) (Figure 55.2). In the direct pathway, an excitatory glutamatergic signal projects to the striatum, sending an inhibitory gamma-aminobutyric acid (GABA)-ergic signal to the internal part of the globus pallidus. This signal results in a decreased inhibition (disinhibition) of the thalamus and thus an increased excitatory effect on the prefrontal cortex. In the indirect pathway, the striatum projects an inhibitory signal to the external part of the globus pallidus and the subthalamic nucleus, sending an excitatory signal to the internal part of the globus pallidus. The net effect is an increased inhibition of the thalamus and decreased excitation on the prefrontal cortex. It is hypothesized that the direct pathway functions as a self-reinforcing positive feedback loop and contributes to the initiation and continuation of behaviors, whereas the indirect pathway provides a mechanism of negative feedback which is important for the inhibition of behaviors and in switching between behaviors. Based on postmortem studies, as well as structural and functional neuroimaging studies, it appears that an imbalance between these frontal–striatal circuits might mediate tic symptomatology, as well as that of related disorders (Johnson *et al.*, 2023).

Neuropathology

Although neuropathological studies of postmortem TS brains are few in number, a recent stereological study indicates that there is a marked alteration in the number and density of at least two classes of interneurons (parvalbumin(PV)-positive fast-spiking GABAergic interneurons and cholinergic tonically active neurons(TANs)) in the caudate and putamen (Kalanithi *et al.*, 2005; Kataoka *et al.*, 2010; Lennington *et al.*, 2016; Xu *et al.*, 2015). Further studies are needed to confirm and extend these findings. A key question concerns whether these alterations are causal or simply a consequence of having lifelong TS.

Structural brain imaging

Volumetric MRI studies have demonstrated abnormalities in basal ganglia regions, cortical areas, including the prefrontal cortex and motor cortex, that are implicated in executive functions and motor control, as well as white matter tracts connecting different brain regions. For example, in a prospective longitudinal study, clinical status and basal ganglia volumes of 43 children with TS were measured on high-resolution MRIs before age 14 years. Follow-up clinical assessments were conducted after age 16 years, an average of 7.5 years later. Volumes of the caudate nucleus correlated significantly and inversely with the severity of tic and OCD symptoms in early adulthood. However, the caudate volumes did not correlate with the severity of symptoms at the time of the MRI scan (Bloch *et al.*, 2005).

More recent, voxel-based quantitative meta-analyses using activation likelihood estimation have largely confirmed the importance of CSTC circuits in the pathogenesis of TS when combining data from more recent structural neuroimaging studies (Wen *et al.*, 2021). Specifically, a meta-analysis of 6 structural neuroimaging studies, involving 247 TS subjects and 236 unaffected controls, demonstrated significantly increased gray matter volumes in the bilateral thalamus, right hypothalamus, right precentral gyrus, left postcentral gyrus, left inferior parietal lobule, right lentiform nucleus, and left insula in TS subjects compared to controls (Wen *et al.*, 2021). The meta-analysis also demonstrated that gray matter volumes were significantly decreased in the bilateral postcentral gyrus, bilateral anterior cingulate, bilateral insula, left posterior cingulate, and left postcentral gyrus in TS subjects (Wen *et al.*, 2021).

Thinning in sensorimotor cortices has also been detected in children and adults with TS, with a negative correlation between thickness and orofacial tic severity (Sowell *et al.*, 2008; Greene *et al.*, 2022). There is also a striking correspondence between the degree of cortical thinning in sensorimotor cortical regions and the types of tics. Several portions of the brain, including the prefrontal cortex, corpus callosum, amygdala, and hippocampus, have been proposed to constitute a network of neural adaptation to the presence of tics, a network in which compensatory changes help to suppress or modulate the severity of tic symptoms (Plessen *et al.*, 2009). Regional volumes and surface features morphology of the right hippocampus and the right globus pallidus provided the best sensitivity and specificity (Wen *et al.*, 2021).

Functional brain imaging

There are a growing number of studies using functional MRI (fMRI) to study individuals with TS (Greene *et al.*, 2022). One of the first studies compared brain activity in blocks of time during which tics were voluntarily suppressed or not suppressed (Peterson & Leckman, 1998; Peterson *et al.*, 1998a, 1998b). During tic suppression, prefrontal cortical, thalamic, and basal ganglia areas were activated. These activations were inversely correlated with tic severity (i.e., lower activation was associated with higher tic severity). This suggests that a greater ability of basal ganglia to suppress cortical activity might be linked with decreased tic severity, Similar results have been demonstrated in event-related fMRI designs contrasting brain activation patterns preceding tics or voluntary movements (Bohlhalter *et al.*, 2006; Hampson *et al.*, 2009).

Resting-state functional connectivity has also been studied in adolescents and adults with TS. Results have demonstrated increased connectivity within CSTC circuitry involving the basal ganglia, prefrontal cortex, and supplementary motor area (SMA) in TS compared to controls (Church *et al.*, 2009; Worbe *et al.*, 2012). Other studies have suggested aberrant connectivity between CSTC circuits and brain regions involved in emotion regulation and sensory processing (Makki *et al.*, 2009).

Neurophysiology

Sensorimotor gating deficits are hypothesized to play a crucial role in the manifestation of TS. Sensorimotor gating refers to the brain's ability to filter and inhibit irrelevant sensory information and motor responses, allowing for more efficient processing of relevant stimuli. Prepulse inhibition using a startle paradigm is a common experimental technique to measure sensorimotor gating by comparing the degree of reduction in startle reflex magnitude when a subthreshold stimulus precedes it. Prepulse inhibition abnormalities have been demonstrated in TS and are associated with CSTC circuit abnormalities and dopamine dysfunction (Swerdlow *et al.*, 2001). Prepulse inhibition abnormalities are by no means unique to TS, having been observed across a variety of neuropsychiatric populations, including schizophrenia, OCD, Huntington's disease, nocturnal enuresis, ADHD, Asperger's syndrome, and TS, suggesting that some final common pathways mediate abnormal prepulse inhibition in all of these conditions. With respect to TS, these deficits are consistent with the idea that there is diminished ability to appropriately manage or "gate" sensory inputs to motor programs, which are released as tics (Swerdlow & Sutherland, 2006). A second advance has been the investigation of motor system excitability by means of single and paired pulse transcranial magnetic stimulation. Studies of groups of patients with TS have indicated that the cortical silent period (a period of decreased excitability following stimulation) is shortened in TS. This intracortical excitability is frequently seen in children with ADHD comorbid with a tic disorder (Ziemann *et al.*, 1997). This heightened level of cortical excitability may be related to a reduction in the number of GABAergic interneurons in the cortex.

Treatment

Tic disorders are frequently chronic, if not lifelong, conditions. Continuity of care is desirable and should be considered before embarking on a course of treatment. Usual clinical practice focuses initially on educational and supportive interventions. Behavioral treatments for TS are recognized as first-line interventions for children with tics, with pharmacological treatments typically held in reserve. Given the waxing and waning course of the disorders, it is likely that whatever is done (or not done) will lead, in the short term, to some improvement in tic severity. The decision to employ psychoactive medications is usually made after the educational and supportive interventions have been in place for a period of months, and it is clear that the tic symptoms are persistently severe and are themselves a source of impairment in terms of self-esteem, relationships with the family or peers, or school performance (Bloch & Leckman, 2009) (Figure 55.3).

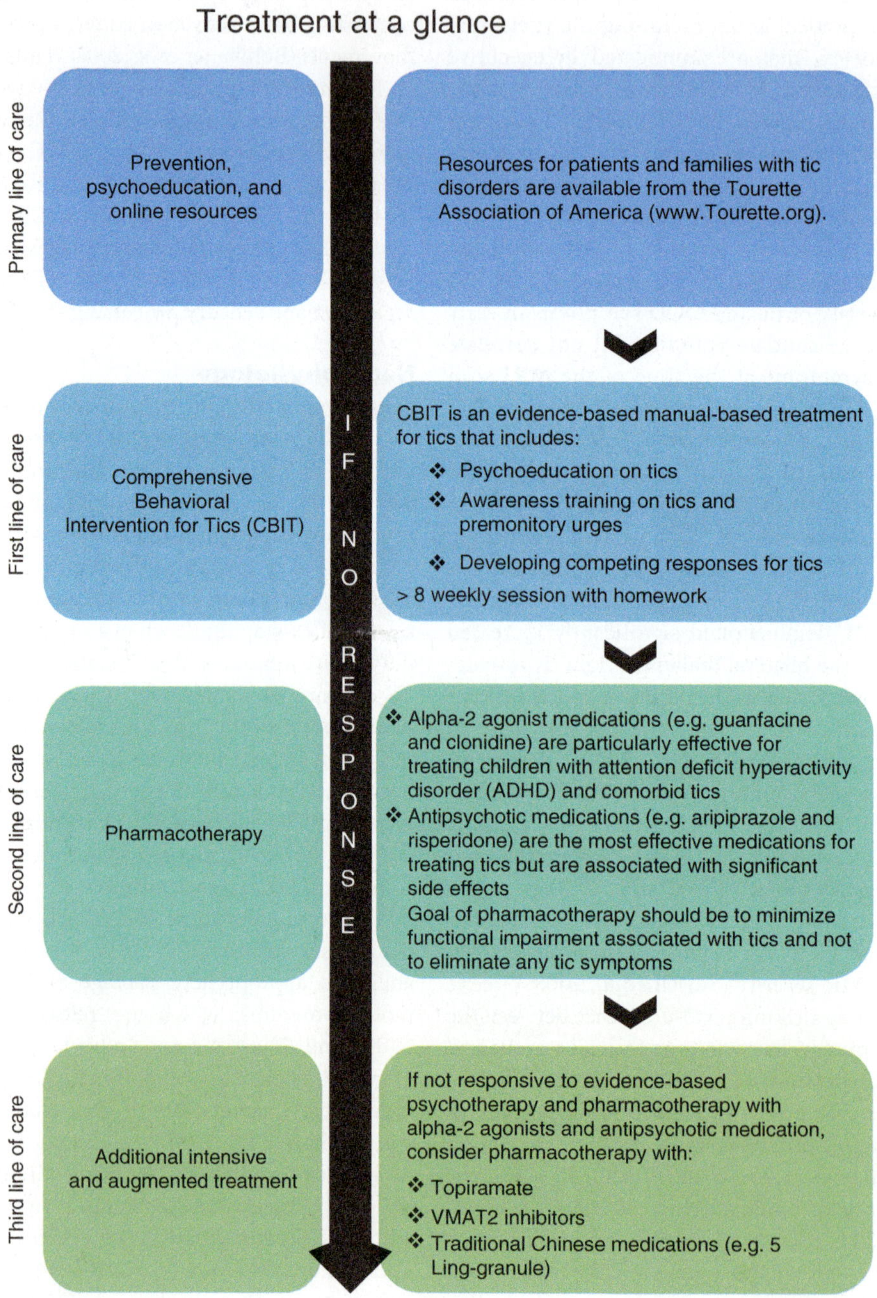

Figure 55.3 Treatment at a glance.

Educational and supportive interventions

Educational activities are among the most important interventions available to clinicians (Lebowitz & Artukoglu, 2022). They should be undertaken first, not only with children with TS but also with those with milder presentations. Although the efficacy of these educational and supportive interventions has not been rigorously assessed, they appear to have positive effects by reshaping familial expectations and relationships (Cohen *et al.*, 1988). This is particularly true when the family and others have misconstrued the tic symptoms as being intentionally provocative. Families also find descriptions of the natural history comforting in that the disorders tend not to be relentlessly progressive and usually improve during adulthood. This information often contradicts the impressions gained from the available lay literature on TS that typically focuses on the most extreme cases. Armed with this knowledge, patients, family members, and others can begin to understand why waiting before beginning medical treatment makes sense. If a child is in the midst of a bad period of tics, it is likely that whether or not a new medication is prescribed, the tics will improve in the near future. This insight will also help children and their families realize why, at times in the past, their medications have suddenly stopped working. These dialogs can be relieving and can interrupt a vicious cycle of recrimination that leads to further tic exacerbation, and it can help parents shift the focus from blame to problem-solving.

By educating the educators, clinicians can make significant progress toward securing a positive and supportive environment in the classroom for the child (Pruitt & Packer, 2022). If possible, teachers need to respond to outbursts of tics with grace and understanding. Repeatedly scolding a child for their tics can be counterproductive. The child may develop a negative attitude to authority figures and may be reluctant to attend school, and classmates may feel freer to tease the child. If tics interfere with a student's ability to receive information in the classroom, it is imperative to find alternative ways to present the material. By helping the student find a way to function, even during periods of severe tics, teachers model problem-solving skills that will foster future self-esteem. It is also important for teachers to know that in unstructured settings, such as the cafeteria, gym, playground, and school bus, peers who tease or taunt tend to take advantage of the lack of adult supervision. The assignment of a paraprofessional aide to accompany the student can be remarkably beneficial—particularly in situations where there is a history of teasing. Other useful strategies that teachers may consider include: providing short breaks out of the classroom to let the tics out in private, allowing students with severe tics to take tests in private so that a child does not have the pressure to suppress tics during the test period, and being flexible with regard to scheduling so that the child is not expected to make an oral presentation at a point when the tics are severe (Bronheim, 1991).

Educated peers are equally important. Many clinicians actively encourage children, families, and teachers to help educate peers and classmates about TS. It is remarkable what can be tolerated in the classroom and on the playground when teachers and peers simply know what the problem is and learn to disregard it. When TS patients, themselves, are uncomfortable educating classmates, teachers, and peers, organizations like the Tourette Association of America help train peer advocates that can assist in providing classroom presentations about tics.

Finally, it is important for clinicians to determine the family's awareness and potential interest in advocacy organizations around the world (Anderson *et al.*, 2022). They include the Tourette Association of America (www.tourette.org), the International OCD Foundation (https://iocdf.org/), and the Children and Adults with Attention Deficit Hyperactivity Disorder (http://www.chadd.org). In the United States, these organizations have made a positive contribution to the lives of many patients and their families by providing support and information. They can also be a valuable outlet for families—to advance research and raise the general level of awareness among health care professionals, educators, and the public at large (Pruitt & Packer, 2022).

Behavioral, cognitive, and other psychotherapeutic treatments

The presence of premonitory urges and the characteristic suppressibility of tic symptoms may have broad implications for behavioral interventions and treatment. Prior to seeking professional consultation, many families will have experimented with a variety of ad hoc behavioral approaches on their own. It is useful to elicit information concerning these efforts and their sequelae.

A variety of cognitive and behavioral approaches have been used with TS. Although success with various techniques, such as assertiveness training, biofeedback, massed practice, time-out, hypnosis, and differential reinforcement, has been reported most of these studies have involved small numbers of poorly characterized participants with no replication (Piacentini & Chang, 2006). To date, only habit reversal training (HRT), known as Comprehensive Behavioral Intervention for Tics (CBIT) when specifically related to tic disorders, has been shown to be efficacious in two large multisite clinical trials involving both children and adults with TS (Deckersbach *et al.*, 2005). Medium effect sizes were found in both the pediatric (ES = 0.68) and the adult (ES = 0.57) trials. CBIT is now considered to be the first-line treatment for children above the age of nine years (McGuire *et al.*, 2022).

CBIT includes a number of techniques: awareness training, self-monitoring, contingency management, inconvenience review, relaxation, and competing responses. For example, awareness training includes: (i) response description, i.e., the patient is trained to describe tic occurrences in detail and to reenact tic movements while looking in a mirror; (ii) response detection, where the therapist helps the patient's ability to detect tics; (iii) an early warning procedure, in which the patient is taught to become aware of the earliest signs of tic occurrence (such as the premonitory urge); and (iv) situation awareness training, in which situations that make tics more likely are identified. When the patient is able to detect the tic and related urges, they are instructed to invoke a competing response at each occurrence of the tic or the urge to tic and to avoid doing the tic until the urge passes (McGuire *et al.*, 2022). Historically, a competing response involved a voluntary act that is physically incompatible with production of a particular motor or vocal tic, e.g., humming instead on making a vocal tic or slightly tilting one's head to the left when the tic involves a sudden tilt to the right. More recent applications have been less strict, deemphasizing tensing of opposite muscles and occasionally selecting unrelated alternative behaviors.

A meta-analysis of 8 randomized controlled trials (RCTs) of individualized behavioral treatments for TS involving 438 participants demonstrated consistent benefit of medium-to-large effect (ES = 0.67) (McGuire *et al.*, 2014). The magnitude of the benefit of behavioral treatments for TS appears similar in magnitude to the most effective pharmacological interventions available for TS. To date, only one study has examined the long-term efficacy of CBIT (Espil *et al.*, 2022). They assessed 80 participants from a child CBIT clinical trial (Piacentini *et al.*, 2010) approximately 11 years later. At follow-up, they found that the CBIT responders (n = 21) in the original trial were more likely (67%) to achieve remission (YGTSS total tic score < 14) at follow-up compared to psychoeducation/supportive therapy responders (n = 6, 0%) on the YGTSS. Fortunately, tic-related impairment decreased across the entire sample, with no significant differences between the treatment groups.

Though the benefits of behavioral therapy for tic disorders have been definitively established, accessibility to patients remains a significant challenge. Recent trials have shown evidence that these behavioral therapies are effective when performed remotely and in a group setting. Most recently, a therapist-supported online remote behavioral intervention trial (ORBIT) demonstrated the efficacy of a therapist-supported online remote behavioral intervention compared to psychoeducational control in a large trial of over 200 children and adolescents with tics in England (Hollis *et al.*, 2021). Trainings in CBIT are readily available to interested providers through the Tourette Association of America. It remains to be established whether and how much the substantial benefits of CBIT and other behavioral treatments for TS are reduced as these treatments are provided by practitioners with less specialized expertise, remotely, and in nonindividualized settings.

Although not indicated for the treatment of tics, individual and family counseling may alleviate secondary symptoms such as low self-esteem, and defiant and disruptive behavior, as well as family conflict. These interventions may also serve to reduce a significant source of psychological stress (McGuire *et al.*, 2014).

Pharmacological treatments

The decision whether or not to use medication is based on the level of symptoms and the clinical presentation of the individual case. Given the waxing and waning of tic symptoms, it is best to withhold psychotropic medications until the tics, even at their best, are a significant source of impairment. Additionally, when possible and consistent with patient preference, it makes sense to try behavioral interventions for tics prior to employing pharmacological treatments. Many cases of TS can be successfully managed without medication. When patients present with coexisting ADHD, OCD, anxiety, or depression, it is often better to treat these comorbid conditions first, as successful treatment of these disorders will often diminish tic severity.

A wide variety of therapeutic agents are now available for the treatment of tics (Scahill *et al.*, 2006). In many instances, pharmacotherapy induces faster tic reduction in comparison to behavioral interventions. Each medication should be selected on the basis of expected efficacy and potential side effects. The goal of pharmacological treatment should be to minimize functional impairment rather than attempting to obliterate the tics out of existence. Efforts to stop the tics completely risk over-medication. Each medication should be selected on the basis of expected efficacy and potential side effects. Table 55.4 describes currently available evidence-based treatments for TS along with side effects and dosing recommendations.

Clonidine and guanfacine are potent alpha-2 receptor agonists that are thought to function by stimulating post-synaptic alpha-2A receptors on dendritic spines of the prefrontal cortical pyramidal cells, and by increasing the functional connectivity of the prefrontal cortical networks. These agents have demonstrated efficacy and are FDA approved to treat ADHD. A meta-analysis of six randomized, placebo-controlled trials demonstrated that alpha-2 agonists had a medium effect size (ES = 0.68) in reducing tic symptoms in trials in which participants also had ADHD. These results were consistent with a large, well-designed, multisite, clinical trial involving 136 subjects with chronic tics or TS that confirmed clonidine's efficacy in the treatment of tics with comorbid ADHD (Tourette's Syndrome Study Group, 2002). However, in the absence of ADHD, the efficacy of these agents was small (ES = 0.15) and nonsignificant (Weisman *et al.*, 2013). Despite the mixed evidence of efficacy for alpha-2 agonists in TS, especially in tic patients without ADHD, they are generally recommended as first-line treatments of TS given their benign side-effect profile compared to other compounds with demonstrated efficacy.

In contrast, antipsychotic medications are the pharmacological intervention with the greatest evidence of efficacy in the acute treatment of tic disorders. Antipsychotics with dopamine D_2 receptor antagonism remain the most predictably effective tic-suppressing agents in the short term. Documentation of haloperidol's effectiveness in the early 1960s was a landmark in the history of TS as it called into question the prevailing view that tics were psychogenic in origin. A recent network meta-analysis suggested that both first-generation antipsychotics (ES = 0.65) and second-generation antipsychotics (ES = 0.71) are similarly effective for the treatment of tics. Several typical antipsychotics (haloperidol, pimozide, and tiapride) and atypical antipsychotics (aripiprazole, ziprasidone, risperidone,

Table 55.4 Evidence-based pharmacological treatments for tics.

Medication	Dosing range	Starting dose	Titration schedule	Advantages	Adverse effects
			Antipsychotics		
			Atypical antipsychotics		
Aripiprazole	5–20 mg daily	2.5–5 mg	Increase by 2.5–5 mg weekly	Most effective pharmacological treatment for tics, fewer extrapyramidal symptoms (EPS) than typicals	Weight gain, metabolic syndrome, EPS, fatigue, galactorrhea, gynecomastia
Risperidone	1–6 mg daily	0.5 mg	Increase by 0.5 mg weekly		
Ziprasidone	5–40 mg daily	5 mg	Increase by 5–10 mg weekly		
			Typical antipsychotics		
Haloperidol	0.5–6 mg daily	0.5 mg	Increase by 0.5 mg weekly	Most effective pharmacological treatment for tics, decreased risk of metabolic side effects compared to atypicals	Tardive dyskinesia, akathisia, parkinsonism, dystonic reaction, weight gain, metabolic syndrome
Pimozide	2–10 mg daily	1–2 mg	Increase by 1–2 mg weekly		
			Alpha-2 agonists		
Clonidine	0.1–0.4 mg total divided BID	0.1 mg nightly	Increase by 0.1 mg q 3–7 days	Effective in treating comorbid attention deficit hyperactivity disorder (ADHD), better tolerated than antipsychotics	Sedation, hypotension, rebound hypertension with discontinuation, constipation
Guanfacine	1–4 mg total divided BID	1 mg nightly	Increase by 1 mg q 3–7 days		

and olanzapine) have been demonstrated to be effective for tic disorders in randomized, placebo-controlled trials (Farhat *et al.*, 2023). There is no strong evidence that any particular antipsychotic is significantly more effective for the treatment of tic disorders than any other. That being said, there is much more supporting evidence of efficacy for several antipsychotics with significant D2 receptor antagonism (e.g., aripiprazole, risperidone, haloperidol, pimozide). We generally use tolerability to select initial treatment among these antipsychotics.

A recent systematic review and network meta-analysis demonstrated several emerging pharmacological agents that deserve additional study for TS (Farhat *et al.*, 2023). Ecopipam, a D1 and D5 receptor antagonist, has demonstrated efficacy against placebo in two randomized, placebo-controlled, multisite trials in children with TS (Gilbert *et al.*, 2018, 2023). In a recent, multisite randomized, placebo-controlled trial of 153 children with TS, ecopipam demonstrated significant benefit compared to placebo, leading to an average improvement of 3.44 YGTSS points (95% CI 0.79–6.09) compared to placebo, which is similar in overall measured effect size compared to antipsychotic medications (Gilbert *et al.*, 2018). Furthermore, ecopipam was associated with significantly less weight gain than placebo. However, ecopipam remains an investigational product which is not clinically available as it has yet to receive FDA approval.

An individual, single-site, randomized, placebo-controlled trial of 29 subjects with TS demonstrated a significant benefit of topiramate compared to placebo (Jankovic *et al.*, 2010). Topiramate was given at a dose of 50–200 mg/day and resulted in a 9-point greater YGTSS reduction when compared to placebo over the 10-week trial (effect size = 0.92). Future investigations should consider replicating this preliminary study in a larger, multisite sample.

The network meta-analysis also identified several traditional Chinese medicine (TCM) remedies which were demonstrated to more efficacious than placebo in RCTs exclusively conducted in China, often with additional TCM inclusion criteria and sometimes only published in the Chinese language literature (Zheng *et al.*, 2016; Farhat *et al.*, 2023). Replication of these findings by studies conducted in the US and/or other Western countries are required to clarify if these findings are generalizable to Western populations and to patients with tic disorders in general.

Substantial clinical experience also suggested that VMAT2 inhibitors, dopamine depleting agents, that are currently FDA-approved for the treatment of tardive dyskinesia and hyperkinetic movement disorders might be beneficial in the treatment of tic disorders. Despite promising results from initial uncontrolled studies, several well-conducted, multisite, randomized, placebo-controlled trials failed to demonstrate a benefit of VMAT2 inhibitors, such as valbenazine and deutetrabenazine, compared to placebo (Behling *et al.*, 2022).

Pharmacotherapy of coexisting attention deficit hyperactivity disorder

Psychostimulant medications are currently recommended as the first-line treatment for ADHD (Brown *et al.*, 2005). However, the use of stimulants in ADHD associated with a tic disorder remains somewhat controversial with stimulant medications in the United States containing a warning that they are contraindicated in patients with tic disorders or a family history of TS. Many patients with both ADHD and a preexisting tic disorder will do well on stimulants. For example, in one large-scale multicenter, randomized, double-blind clinical trial with 136 children with ADHD and a chronic tic disorder, significant improvements in ADHD symptoms occurred for subjects assigned to clonidine alone and those assigned to methylphenidate alone (Tourette's Syndrome Study Group, 2002). Compared with placebo, the greatest benefit occurred with the combination of methylphenidate and clonidine. The proportion of individuals reporting a worsening of tics was no higher in those treated with methylphenidate (20%) than those being administered clonidine alone (26%) or placebo (22%). Sedation was common with clonidine treatment (28% reported moderate or severe sedation), but otherwise the drugs were tolerated well, with no evidence of cardiac toxicity. This trial did not support prior recommendations to avoid methylphenidate in these children because of concerns of worsening tics. Furthermore, subsequent meta-analysis of 22 randomized, placebo-controlled trials involving over 2300 children with ADHD demonstrated no difference in rates of *de novo* or worsening tics for stimulants compared to placebo (Cohen *et al.*, 2015). The risk of new onset or worsening of tics associated with stimulant treatment was similar to that observed with placebo (risk ratio = 0.99, 95% CI 0.78–1.27) and the type of psychostimulant, dose, duration of treatment, recorder, and participant age did not affect risk of new onset or worsening of tics (Cohen *et al.*, 2015). In sum, methylphenidate offers the greatest and most immediate improvement of ADHD symptoms and typically does not worsen tic symptoms (Bloch *et al.*, 2009). As noted above, alpha-2 agonists can also improve ADHD symptoms although patience is required as the beneficial effects are not immediate (Weisman *et al.*, 2013). Atomoxetine, a selective norepinephrine reuptake inhibitor, has also been found to reduce ADHD symptoms in children with comorbid tics (Bloch *et al.*, 2009). Please refer to Chapter 54 for more details on the treatment of ADHD.

Pharmacotherapy of coexisting obsessive–compulsive disorder

The presence of a comorbid tic disorder may predict a poorer outcome in the acute pharmacological treatment of pediatric-onset OCD. Specifically, children with tic-related OCD tend to be less responsive to SSRI monotherapy to treat their OCD symptoms (Geller *et al.*, 2004; March *et al.*, 2007). In contrast, OCD symptoms in individuals with comorbid tic disorders appear equally responsive to cognitive behavioral therapy (CBT) with exposure and response prevention (ERP) (March *et al.*, 2007) Consequently, children and adolescents with OCD and a comorbid tic disorder should begin treatment with ERP alone or the combination of ERP plus an SSRI. In adult OCD subjects, meta-analysis of placebo-controlled clinical trials have demonstrated that antipsychotic augmentation of SSRI pharmacotherapy may be an effective treatment for OCD, especially in patients with comorbid tic disorders (Bloch *et al.*, 2006a). Despite the relative increased efficacy of antipsychotic augmentation and decreased efficacy of SSRI pharmacotherapy in OCD patients with comorbid tics, it is still recommended to initiate and engage in SSRI pharmacotherapy, similar to other OCD patients, given that many OCD patients with comorbid tics still respond to SSRI pharmacotherapy (albeit slightly less than OCD without tics) and despite the substantially worse side-effect burden of antipsychotics compared to antidepressants. Please refer to Chapter 60 for more details on the treatment of OCD.

Future directions

Along with a deepening appreciation of the clinical phenomenology and natural history, recent progress in genetics, neuroanatomy, systems neuroscience, and functional *in vivo* neuroimaging has set the stage for major advances in our understanding of TS and related NDDs. Many mysteries remain including: (i) Why is there such a high rate of co-occurring NDDs in individuals with TS, particularly those with complex motor and vocal tics, relative to individuals with just chronic motor tics?; (ii) Why are there differences in clinical course in many children with TS?; and (iii) What is the etiological cause, genetically, neurologically, and chemically, of most tics?

The development of CBIT has been a major advance for the field. Now the challenge is to understand the neural mechanisms underlying this treatment and how best to train a sufficient number of practitioners to ensure access to this intervention. Despite these therapeutic advances, we are still in need of ideal anti-tic medications that work quickly, effectively, and with few side effects. For interventions currently in use, it will be important to determine the relative long-term benefits of behavioral interventions when combined with drugs.

Acknowledgments

We are indebted to the Yale Tourette's Syndrome; Obsessive–Compulsive Disorder; and Trichotillomania Research Group. We are also indebted to our patients, as well as the participants in research studies of Tourette syndrome who have taught us about this condition.

Dr. Bloch has received grant or research support from Therapix Biosciences, Emalex Biosciences, Neurocrine Biosciences, Janssen Pharmaceuticals, Bionomics Pharmaceuticals, NIH (R01MH125203, T32MH018268), Lesbian Health Fund, and the Yale Foundation for Lesbian and Gay Studies (FLAGS). He has served as associate editor of *The Journal of Child Psychology and Psychiatry* and on the editorial boards of the *Journal of Child and Adolescent Psychopharmacology* and the *Journal of the American Academy of Child and Adolescent Psychiatry*. He has received royalties from Wolters Kluwer for *Lewis's Child and Adolescent Psychiatry: A Comprehensive Textbook*, 5th edition. He has received moonlighting pay from the Veteran's Administration. He serves on the Scientific Advisory Board of the Tourette Association of America and the TLC Foundation for Body-Focused Repetitive Behaviors.

References

Abdallah, S.B. & Fernandez, T.V. (2022) Genetic susceptibility in Tourette syndrome. In: *Tourette Syndrome*. (eds D. Martino & J.F. Leckman), 2nd edn. Oxford University Press, New York. pp. 125–136.

Albin, R.L. & Mink, J.W. (2006) Recent advances in Tourette syndrome research. *Trends in Neurosciences* **29**(3), 175–182.

American Psychiatric Association (2022) *Diagnostic and Statistical Manual of Mental Disorders*, 5th edn, text revision (DSM-5-TR). American Psychiatric Association, Washington, DC.

Anderson, S. *et al.* (2022) Tourette syndrome support organizations around the world. In: *Tourette Syndrome*. (eds D. Martino & J.F. Leckman), 2nd edn. Oxford University Press, New York. pp. 537–548.

Artukoglu, B.B. *et al.* (2020) Pharmacologic treatment of tardive dyskinesia: a meta-analysis and systematic review. *The Journal of Clinical Psychiatry* **81**(4).

Baron-Cohen, S. *et al.* (1999) The prevalence of Gilles de la Tourette's syndrome in children and adolescents with autism. *Journal of Child Psychology and Psychiatry* **40**(2), 213–218.

Bawden, H.N. *et al.* (1998) Peer relationship problems in children with Tourette's disorder or diabetes mellitus. *Journal of Child Psychology and Psychiatry* **39**(5), 663–668.

Behling, E. *et al.* (2022) Meta-analysis: efficacy and tolerability of vesicular monoamine transporter type 2 inhibitors in the treatment of tic disorders. *Movement Disorders* **37**(4), 684–693.

Berg, L. *et al.* (2022) Sudden onset tic and tic-like presentations in older adolescents and adults. *Current Developmental Disorders Reports* **9**(4), 146–155.

Black, K.J. *et al.* (2021) Course of tic disorders over the lifespan. *Current Developmental Disorders Reports* **8**(2), 121–132.

Bloch, M.H. (2022) Clinical course and adulthood outcome in Tourette syndrome. In: *Tourette Syndrome*. (eds D. Martino & J.F. Leckman), 2nd edn. Oxford University Press, New York. pp. 95–104.

Bloch, M.H. & Leckman, J.F. (2009) Clinical course of Tourette syndrome. *Journal of Psychosomatic Research* **67**(6), 497–501.

Bloch, M.H. *et al.* (2005) Caudate volumes in childhood predict symptom severity in adults with Tourette syndrome. *Neurology* **65**(8), 1253–1258.

Bloch, M.H. *et al.* (2006a) Fine-motor skill deficits in childhood predict adulthood tic severity and global psychosocial functioning in Tourette's syndrome. *Journal of Child Psychology and Psychiatry* **47**(6), 551–559.

Bloch, M.H. *et al.* (2006b) A systematic review: antipsychotic augmentation with treatment refractory obsessive-compulsive disorder. *Molecular Psychiatry* **11**(7), 622–632.

Bloch, M.H. *et al.* (2006c) Adulthood outcome of tic and obsessive-compulsive symptom severity in children with Tourette syndrome. *Archives of Pediatrics & Adolescent Medicine* **160**(1), 65–69.

Bloch, M.H. *et al.* (2009) Meta-analysis: treatment of attention-deficit/hyperactivity disorder in children with comorbid tic disorders. *Journal of the American Academy of Child & Adolescent Psychiatry* **48**(9), 884–893.

Bohlhalter, S. *et al.* (2006) Neural correlates of tic generation in Tourette syndrome: an event-related functional MRI study. *Brain* **129**(8), 2029–2037.

Brander, G. *et al.* (2018) Perinatal risk factors in Tourette's and chronic tic disorders: a total population sibling comparison study. *Molecular Psychiatry* **23**(5), 1189–1197.

Bronheim, S. (1991) An educator's guide to Tourette syndrome. *Journal of Learning Disabilities* **24**(1), 17–22.

Brown, R.T. *et al.* (2005) Treatment of attention-deficit/hyperactivity disorder: overview of the evidence. *Pediatrics* **115**(6), e749–e757.

Caine, E.D. *et al.* (1988) Tourette's syndrome in Monroe County school children. *Neurology* **38**(3), 472–475.

Caroff, S.N. (2022) A new era in the diagnosis and treatment of tardive dyskinesia. *CNS Spectrums* **28**(4), 4–14.

Carter, A.S. *et al.* (2000) Social and emotional adjustment in children affected with Gilles de la Tourette's syndrome: associations with ADHD and family functioning. Attention deficit hyperactivity disorder. *Journal of Child Psychology and Psychiatry* **41**(2), 215–223.

Cavanna, A.E. (2022) Clinical rating instruments in Tourette syndrome. In: *Tourette Syndrome*. (eds D. Martino & J.F. Leckman), 2nd edn. Oxford University Press, New York. pp. 343–365.

Cavanna, A.E. *et al.* (2012) Predictors during childhood of future health-related quality of life in adults with Gilles de la Tourette syndrome. *European Journal of Paediatric Neurology* **16**(6), 605–612.

Chang, K. *et al.* (2015) Clinical evaluation of youth with pediatric acute-onset neuropsychiatric syndrome (PANS): recommendations from the 2013 PANS Consensus Conference. *Journal of Child and Adolescent Psychopharmacology* **25**(1), 3–13.

Chappell, P.B. *et al.* (1994) Enhanced stress responsivity of Tourette syndrome patients undergoing lumbar puncture. *Biological Psychiatry* **36**(1), 35–43.

Church, J.A. *et al.* (2009) Control networks in paediatric Tourette syndrome show immature and anomalous patterns of functional connectivity. *Brain* **132**(Pt 1), 225–238.

Coffey, B.J. *et al.* (2000) Anxiety disorders and tic severity in juveniles with Tourette's disorder. *Journal of the American Academy of Child and Adolescent Psychiatry* **39**(5), 562–568.

Cohen, D.J. *et al.* (1988) Family functioning and Tourette's syndrome. In: *Tourette's Syndrome and Tic Disorders*. (eds D.J. Cohen, *et al.*). John Wiley and Sons, New York. p. 179.

Cohen, S.C. *et al.* (2015) Meta-analysis: risk of tics associated with psychostimulant use in randomized, placebo-controlled trials. *Journal of the American Academy of Child and Adolescent Psychiatry* **54**(9), 728–736.

Deckersbach, T. *et al.* (2005) Habit reversal versus supportive psychotherapy in Tourette's disorder: a randomized controlled trial and predictors of treatment response. *Behaviour Research and Therapy* **44**(8), 1079–1090.

Dyke, K. *et al.* (2022) Abnormalities of neural microcircuits in Tourette syndrome. In: *Tourette Syndrome*. (eds D. Martino & J.F. Leckman), 2nd edn. Oxford University Press, New York. pp. 184–198.

Dykens, E. *et al.* (1990) Intellectual, academic, and adaptive functioning of Tourette syndrome children with and without attention deficit disorder. *Journal of Abnormal Child Psychology* **18**(6), 607–615.

Ercan-Sencicek, A. *et al.* (2010) L-histidine decarboxylase and Tourette's syndrome. *New England Journal of Medicine* **362**(20), 1901–1908.

Espil, F.M. *et al.* (2022) Long-term outcomes of behavior therapy for youth with Tourette disorder. *Journal of the American Academy of Child & Adolescent Psychiatry* **61**(6), 764–771.

Farhat, L.C. *et al.* (2023) Comparative efficacy, tolerability, and acceptability of pharmacological interventions for the treatment of children, adolescents, and young adults with Tourette's syndrome: a systematic review and network meta-analysis. *The Lancet Child Adolescent Health* **7**(2), 112–126.

Fasching, L. *et al.* (2022) Cellular and molecular pathology in Tourette syndrome. In: *Tourette Syndrome.* (eds D. Martino & J.F. Leckman), 2nd edn. Oxford University Press, New York. pp. 171–183.

Fernandez de la Cruz, L. *et al.* (2017) Suicide in Tourette's and chronic tic disorders. *Biological Psychiatry* **82**(2), 111–118.

Ferrão, Y.A. *et al.* (2022) The phenomenology of obsessive-compulsive symptoms in Tourette syndrome. In: *Tourette Syndrome.* (eds D. Martino & J.F. Leckman), 2nd edn. Oxford University Press, New York. pp. 45–64.

Findley, D.B. *et al.* (2003) Development of the Yale Children's Global Stress Index (YCGSI) and its application in children and adolescents with Tourette's syndrome and obsessive-compulsive disorder. *Journal of the American Academy of Child and Adolescent Psychiatry* **42**(4), 450–457.

Frey, J. *et al.* (2022) TikTok Tourette's: are we witnessing a rise in functional tic-like behavior driven by adolescent social media use? *Psychology Research and Behavior Management* **15**, 3575–3585.

Geller, D.A. *et al.* (2004) Paroxetine treatment in children and adolescents with obsessive-compulsive disorder: a randomized, multicenter, double-blind, placebo-controlled trial. *Journal of the American Academy of Child and Adolescent Psychiatry* **43**(11), 1387–1396.

Gilbert, D.L. (2019) Inflammation in tic disorders and obsessive-compulsive disorder: are PANS and PANDAS a path forward? *Journal of Child Neurology* **34**(10), 598–611.

Gilbert, D.L. *et al.* (2018) Ecopipam, a D1 receptor antagonist, for treatment of Tourette syndrome in children: a randomized, placebo-controlled crossover study. *Movement Disorders* **33**(8), 1272–1280.

Gilbert, D.L. *et al.* (2023) Ecopipam for Tourette syndrome: a randomized trial. *Pediatrics* **151**(2), e2022059574.

Gilles de la Tourette, G. (1885) Étude sur une affection nerveuse caractèrisée par de l'incoordination motrice accompagnée d'écholalie et de copralalie. *Archive Neurologie* **9**(19–42), 158–200.

Gorman, D.A. *et al.* (2010) Psychosocial outcome and psychiatric comorbidity in older adolescents with Tourette syndrome: controlled study. *The British Journal of Psychiatry: the Journal of Mental Science* **197**(1), 36–44.

Graybiel, A.M. & Canales, J.J. (2001) The neurobiology of repetitive behaviors: clues to the neurobiology of Tourette syndrome. *Advances in Neurology* **85**, 123–131.

Greene, D.J. *et al.* (2022) Neurobiology and functional anatomy of tic disorders. In: *Tourette Syndrome.* (eds D. Martino & J.F. Leckman), 2nd edn. Oxford University Press, New York. pp. 199–230.

Hampson, M. *et al.* (2009) Brain areas coactivating with motor cortex during chronic motor tics and intentional movements. *Biological Psychiatry* **65**(7), 594–599.

Hoekstra, P.J. & Dietrich, A. (2022) Perinatal adversities and Tourette syndrome. In: *Tourette Syndrome.* (eds D. Martino & J.F. Leckman), 2nd edn. Oxford University Press, New York. pp. 137–145.

Hollis, C. *et al.* (2021) Therapist-supported online remote behavioural intervention for tics in children and adolescents in England (ORBIT): a multicentre, parallel group, single-blind, randomised controlled trial. *The Lancet Psychiatry* **8**(10), 871–882.

Hounie, A.G. *et al.* (2006) Obsessive-compulsive disorder in Tourette syndrome. *Advances in Neurology* **99**, 22–38.

Hsu, C.J. *et al.* (2021) Immunological dysfunction in Tourette syndrome and related disorders. *International Journal of Molecular Sciences* **22**(2), 853.

Hyde, T.M. *et al.* (1992) Relationship of birth weight to the phenotypic expression of Gilles de la Tourette's syndrome in monozygotic twins. *Neurology* **42**(3 Pt 1), 652–658.

Itard, J.M.G. (1825) Memoire sur quelques fonctions involontaries ses appareils de la locomotion de la prehension et de la voix. *Archives Generales de Medecine* **8**, 385–407.

Jain, P. *et al.* (2023) Polygenic risk score-based phenome-wide association study identifies novel associations for Tourette syndrome. *Translational Psychiatry* **13**(1), 69.

Jankovic, J. *et al.* (2010) A randomised, double-blind, placebo-controlled study of topiramate in the treatment of Tourette syndrome. *Journal of Neurology, Neurosurgery, and Psychiatry* **81**(1), 70–73.

Johnson, K.A. *et al.* (2023) Tourette syndrome: clinical features, pathophysiology, and treatment. *The Lancet Neurology* **22**(2), 147–158.

Kalanithi, P.S. *et al.* (2005) Altered parvalbumin-positive neuron distribution in basal ganglia of individuals with Tourette syndrome. *Proceedings of the National Academy of Sciences of the United States of America* **102**(37), 13307–13312.

Kataoka, Y. *et al.* (2010) Decreased number of parvalbumin and cholinergic interneurons in the striatum of individuals with Tourette syndrome. *The Journal of Comparative Neurology* **518**(3), 277–291.

Khalifa, N. & von Knorring, A.L. (2005) Tourette syndrome and other tic disorders in a total population of children: clinical assessment and background. *Acta Paediatrica* **94**(11), 1608–1614.

King, R.A. & Landeros-Weisenberger, A. (2022) Comprehensive assessment strategies. In: *Tourette Syndrome.* (eds D. Martino & J.F. Leckman), 2nd edn. Oxford University Press, New York. pp. 335–342.

Kurlan, R. *et al.* (1994) Tourette's syndrome in a special education population: a pilot study involving a single school district. *Neurology* **44**(4), 699–702.

LaFaver, K. *et al.* (2021) Treatment of functional neurological disorder: current state, future directions, and a research agenda. *CNS Spectrums* **26**(6), 607–613.

Lebowitz, E.R. & Artukoglu, B.B. (2022) Psychoeducational interventions: what every parent and family member needs to know. In: *Tourette Syndrome.* (eds D. Martino & J.F. Leckman), 2nd edn. Oxford University Press, New York. pp. 407–420.

Leckman, J.F. *et al.* (1984) The pathogenesis of Gilles de la Tourette's syndrome. a review of data and hypothesis. In: *Movement Disorders.* (eds A.B. Shah, *et al.*). Plenum, New York. pp. 257–273.

Leckman, J.F. *et al.* (1989) The Yale Global Tic Severity Scale: initial testing of a clinician-rated scale of tic severity. *Journal of the American Academy of Child and Adolescent Psychiatry* **28**(4), 566–573.

Leckman, J.F. *et al.* (1990) Perinatal factors in the expression of Tourette's syndrome: an exploratory study. *Journal of the American Academy of Child and Adolescent Psychiatry* **29**(2), 220–226.

Leckman, J.F. *et al.* (1993) Premonitory urges in Tourette's syndrome. *The American Journal of Psychiatry* **150**(1), 98–102.

Leckman, J.F. *et al.* (1995) Cerebrospinal fluid biogenic amines in obsessive compulsive disorder, Tourette's syndrome, and healthy controls. *Neuropsychopharmacology* **12**(1), 73–86.

Leckman, J.F. *et al.* (1997) Symptoms of obsessive-compulsive disorder. *The American Journal of Psychiatry* **154**(7), 911–917.

Leckman, J.F. *et al.* (1998) Yale approach to assessment and treatment. In: *Tourette's Syndrome Tics, Obsessions, Compulsions: Developmental Psychopathology and Clinical Care.* (eds J.F. Leckman & D.J. Cohen). John Wiley and Sons, New York. pp. 285–309.

Leckman, J.F. *et al.* (2022) Phenomenology of tics and sensory urges: the self under siege. In: *Tourette Syndrome.* (eds D. Martino & J.F. Leckman), 2nd edn. Oxford University Press, New York. pp. 7–25.

Lennington, J.B. *et al.* (2016) Transcriptome analysis of the human striatum in Tourette syndrome. *Biological Psychiatry* **79**(5), 372–382.

Levine, J.L.S. *et al.* (2019) Meta-analysis: adulthood prevalence of Tourette syndrome. *Progress in Neuro-Psychopharmacology & Biological Psychiatry* **95**, 109675.

Li, Y. *et al.* (2022) Clinical characteristics of pediatric patients with treatment-refractory Tourette syndrome: an evidence-based survey in a Chinese population. *World Journal of Psychiatry* **12**(7), 958–969.

Lin, H. *et al.* (2007) Psychosocial stress predicts future symptom severities in children and adolescents with Tourette syndrome and/or obsessive-compulsive disorder. *Journal of Child Psychology and Psychiatry* **48**(2), 157–166.

Lin, H. *et al.* (2010) Streptococcal upper respiratory tract infections and psychosocial stress predict future tic and obsessive-compulsive symptom severity in children and adolescents with Tourette syndrome and obsessive-compulsive disorder. *Biological Psychiatry* **67**(7), 684–691.

Luo, F. *et al.* (2004) Prospective longitudinal study of children with tic disorders and/or obsessive-compulsive disorder: relationship of symptom exacerbations to newly acquired streptococcal infections. *Pediatrics* **113**(6), e578–e585.

Makki, M.I. *et al.* (2009) Altered fronto-striato-thalamic connectivity in children with Tourette syndrome assessed with diffusion tensor MRI and probabilistic fiber tracking. *Journal of Child Neurology* **24**(6), 669–678.

March, J.S. *et al.* (2007) Tics moderate treatment outcome with sertraline but not cognitive-behavior therapy in pediatric obsessive-compulsive disorder. *Biological Psychiatry* **61**(3), 344–347.

Martino, D. & Hedderly, T. (2019) Tics and stereotypies: a comparative clinical review. *Parkinsonism & Related Disorders* **59**, 117–124.

Martino, D. & Leckman, J.F. (eds) (2022) *Tourette Syndrome*, 2nd edn. Oxford University Press, New York.

Martino, D. *et al.* (2022) Infections and tic disorders. In: *Tourette Syndrome.* (eds D. Martino & J.F. Leckman), 2nd edn. Oxford University Press, New York. pp. 146–167.

Mason, A. *et al.* (1998) The prevalence of Tourette syndrome in a mainstream school population. *Developmental Medicine and Child Neurology* **40**(5), 292–296.

Mataix-Cols, D. *et al.* (2015) Familial risks of Tourette syndrome and chronic tic disorders: a population-based cohort study. *JAMA Psychiatry* **72**(8), 787–793.

McGuire, J.F. *et al.* (2014) A meta-analysis of behavior therapy for Tourette syndrome. *Journal of Psychiatric Research* **50**, 106–112.

McGuire, J.F. *et al.* (2018) A multicenter examination and strategic revisions of the Yale Global Tic Severity Scale. *Neurology* **90**(19), e1711–e1719.

McGuire, J. *et al.* (2022) Behavioral and cognitive-behavioral therapy for Tourette disorder. In: *Tourette Syndrome.* (eds D. Martino & J.F. Leckman), 2nd edn. Oxford University Press, New York. pp. 421–430.

Mell, L.K. *et al.* (2005) Association between streptococcal infection and obsessive-compulsive disorder, Tourette's syndrome, and tic disorder. *Pediatrics* **116**(1), 56–60.

Muller-Vahl, K.R. *et al.* (2022) Stop that! It's not Tourette's but a new type of mass sociogenic illness. *Brain* **145**(2), 476–480.

Oakley, C. *et al.* (2015) Primary complex motor stereotypies in older children and adolescents: clinical features and longitudinal follow-up. *Pediatric Neurology* **52**(4), 398–403 e391.

Peterson, B.S. & Leckman, J.F. (1998) The temporal dynamics of tics in Gilles de la Tourette syndrome. *Biological Psychiatry* **44**(12), 1337–1348.

Peterson, B.S. *et al.* (1998a) A functional magnetic resonance imaging study of tic suppression in Tourette syndrome. *Archives of General Psychiatry* **55**(4), 326–333.

Peterson, B.S. *et al.* (1998b) A double-blind, placebo-controlled, crossover trial of an antiandrogen in the treatment of Tourette's syndrome. *Journal of Clinical Psychopharmacology* **18**(4), 324–331.

Peterson, B.S. *et al.* (2001) Regional brain and ventricular volumes in Tourette syndrome. *Archives of General Psychiatry* **58**(5), 427–440.

Piacentini, J.C. & Chang, S.W. (2006) Behavioral treatments for tic suppression: habit reversal training. *Advances in Neurology* **99**, 227–233.

Piacentini, J. *et al.* (2010) Behavior therapy for children with Tourette disorder: a randomized controlled trial. *JAMA* **303**(19), 1929–1937.

Plessen, K.J. *et al.* (2009) Imaging evidence for anatomical disturbances and neuroplastic compensation in persons with Tourette syndrome. *Journal of Psychosomatic Research* **67**(6), 559–573.

Price, R.A. *et al.* (1985) A twin study of Tourette syndrome. *Archives of General Psychiatry* **42**(8), 815–820.

Pruitt, S.K. & Packer, L.E. (2022) Information and support for educators. In: *Tourette Syndrome.* (eds D. Martino & J.F. Leckman), 2nd edn. Oxford University Press, New York. pp. 521–537.

Rothenberger, A. & Roessner, V. (2022) The phenomenology of attention-deficit/hyperactivity disorder in Tourette syndrome. In: *Tourette Syndrome.* (eds D. Martino & J.F. Leckman), 2nd edn. Oxford University Press, New York. pp. 26–44.

Scahill, L. *et al.* (2006) Disruptive behavior problems in a community sample of children with tic disorders. *Advances in Neurology* **99**, 184–190.

Scahill, L. *et al.* (2014) The prevalence of tic disorders and clinical characteristics in children. *Journal of Obsessive-Compulsive and Related Disorders* **3**(4), 394–400.

Scharf, J.M. *et al.* (2013) Genome-wide association study of Tourette's syndrome. *Molecular Psychiatry* **18**(6), 721–728.

Scharf, J.M. *et al.* (2015) Population prevalence of Tourette syndrome: a systematic review and meta-analysis. *Movement Disorders* **30**(2), 221–228.

Shapiro, A.K. *et al.* (1988) *Gilles de la Tourette Syndrome*, 2nd edn. Raven Press, New York.

Singer, H.S. & Augustine, F. (2022) Tourette syndrome: circuits and neurotransmitters. In: *Tourette Syndrome.* (eds D. Martino & J.F. Leckman), 2nd edn. Oxford University Press, New York. pp. 231–256.

Sowell, E.R. *et al.* (2008) Thinning of sensorimotor cortices in children with Tourette syndrome. *Nature Neuroscience* **11**(6), 637–639.

Stokes, A. *et al.* (1991) Peer problems in Tourette's disorder. *Pediatrics* **87**(6), 936–942.

Sukhodolsky, D.G. *et al.* (2003) Disruptive behavior in children with Tourette's syndrome: association with ADHD comorbidity, tic severity, and functional impairment. *Journal of the American Academy of Child and Adolescent Psychiatry* **42**(1), 98–105.

Sukhodolsky, D.G. *et al.* (2005) Adaptive, emotional, and family functioning of children with obsessive-compulsive disorder and comorbid attention deficit hyperactivity disorder. *The American Journal of Psychiatry* **162**(6), 1125–1132.

Swedo, S.E. *et al.* (1998) Pediatric autoimmune neuropsychiatric disorders associated with streptococcal infections: clinical description of the first 50 cases. *The American Journal of Psychiatry* **155**(2), 264–271.

Swedo, S.E. *et al.* (2017) Overview of treatment of pediatric acute-onset neuropsychiatric syndrome. *Journal of Child and Adolescent Psychopharmacology* **27**(7), 562–565.

Swerdlow, N.R. & Sutherland, A.N. (2006) Preclinical models relevant to Tourette syndrome. *Advances in Neurology* **99**, 69–88.

Swerdlow, N.R. *et al.* (2001) Tactile prepuff inhibition of startle in children with Tourette's syndrome: in search of an "fMRI-friendly" startle paradigm. *Biological Psychiatry* **50**(8), 578–585.

Tourette's Syndrome Study Group (2002) Treatment of ADHD in children with tics: a randomized controlled trial. *Neurology* **58**, 527–536.

Tsetsos, F. *et al.* (2023) Genome-wide association study points to novel locus for Gilles de la Tourette syndrome. *Biological Psychiatry* **96**(2), 114–124.

Weisman, H. *et al.* (2013) Systematic review: pharmacological treatment of tic disorders – efficacy of antipsychotic and alpha-2 adrenergic agonist agents. *Neuroscience and Biobehavioral Reviews* **37**(6), 1162–1171.

Wen, F. *et al.* (2021) Grey matter abnormalities in Tourette syndrome: an activation likelihood estimation meta-analysis. *BMC Psychiatry* **21**(1), 184.

Willsey, A.J. *et al.* (2017) De novo coding variants are strongly associated with Tourette disorder. *Neuron* **94**(3), 486–499.e489.

Woods, D.W. *et al.* (2005) Premonitory urge for tics scale (PUTS): initial psychometric results and examination of the premonitory urge phenomenon in youths with tic disorders. *Journal of Developmental and Behavioral Pediatrics* **26**(6), 397–403.

Worbe, Y. *et al.* (2012) Functional immaturity of cortico-basal ganglia networks in Gilles de la Tourette syndrome. *Brain* **135**(Pt 6), 1937–1946.

World Health Organization (2021) *International Statistical Classification of Diseases and Related Health Problems*, 11th edn. World Health Organization, Geneva, Switzerland.

Xu, M. *et al.* (2015) Targeted ablation of cholinergic interneurons in the dorsolateral striatum produces behavioral manifestations of Tourette syndrome. *Proceedings of the National Academy of Sciences of the United States of America* **112**(3), 893–898.

Yu, D. *et al.* (2019) Interrogating the genetic determinants of Tourette's syndrome and other tic disorders through genome-wide association studies. *The American Journal of Psychiatry* **176**(3), 217–227.

Zheng, Y. *et al.* (2016) A proprietary herbal medicine (5-Ling granule) for Tourette syndrome: a randomized controlled trial. *Journal of Child Psychology and Psychiatry* **57**(1), 74–83.

Ziemann, U. *et al.* (1997) Decreased motor inhibition in Tourette's disorder: evidence from transcranial magnetic stimulation. *The American Journal of Psychiatry* **154**(9), 1277–1284.

CHAPTER 56
Schizophrenia and psychosis

Marinos Kyriakopoulos
[1] 1st Department of Psychiatry, National and Kapodistrian University of Athens, Eginition Hospital, Athens, Greece
[2] Department of Child and Adolescent Psychiatry, Institute of Psychiatry, Psychology and Neuroscience, King's College London, London, UK
[3] Kaleidoscope Child Development Centre, South London and Maudsley NHS Foundation Trust, London, UK

Introduction

Schizophrenia and related disorders are severe mental health conditions most commonly presenting at the end of the second and the third decade of life (Solmi *et al.*, 2022). They manifest with debilitating symptoms of disordered reality testing including hallucinations and delusions, disorganized thinking or behavior, negative or catatonic symptoms, and significant functional impairment. When these symptoms do not arise as part of another mental health, organic, or substance misuse condition, the disorder is classified as primary (American Psychiatric Association, 2013; World Health Organization, 2019). Schizophrenia and other primary psychotic disorders, commonly referred to as schizophrenia spectrum disorders, are serious and frequently long-term or recurrent mental health conditions, commonly co-occurring with a degree of cognitive decline and social communication deficits (Pina-Camacho *et al.*, 2016). Beyond primary psychotic disorders, psychotic symptoms may also be seen in mood disorders (Smith *et al.*, 2017; Jääskeläinen *et al.*, 2018; Carlson & Pataki, 2020), autism spectrum disorders (ASD) (Pina-Camacho *et al.*, 2016), personality disorders (Balaratnasingama *et al.*, 2015), substance misuse (Beckmann *et al.*, 2020), and in neurological and endocrine conditions (Merritt *et al.*, 2020). Psychosis, as a term, applies to such symptoms irrespective of their etiology and is a broader construct compared to schizophrenia.

The characterization of early-onset schizophrenia (EOS), with onset before the age of 18 years, followed to some extent the evolution of schizophrenia during the 20th century but was further complicated by somewhat increased atypicality and rarity of presentation in younger individuals. The description of infantile autism by Leo Kanner in 1943 as a condition separate from schizophrenia cast doubt on the nosological validity of early-onset variants of the disorder. Early versions of the classification systems for mental disorders made no distinction between schizophrenia and autism, with the latter being perceived as the form of psychosis manifesting in childhood. Despite Kanner's distinction between these conditions, several terms, including "infantile autism," "symbiotic psychosis," "dementia preacossima," "dementia infantilis," and "schizophrenic syndrome of childhood," continued to be used to describe the same children (Rutter, 1972). Further work, most notably by Kolvin *et al.* (1971), led to the recognition of childhood schizophrenia as a separate entity to autism. This was reflected in the *International Classification of Diseases*, 9th edition (ICD-9; World Health Organization, 1977). However, the term "psychoses with origin specific to childhood" was kept in reference to infantile autism, childhood disintegrative disorder (CDD), and other atypical or unspecified childhood psychoses. In the *Diagnostic and Statistical Manual of Mental Disorders*, 3rd edition (DSM-III; American Psychiatric Association, 1980) "schizophrenia childhood-type" was placed together with the adult forms of schizophrenia, and "pervasive developmental disorders" (PDD) formed a separate category before being replaced by ASD in DSM-5 (American Psychiatric Association, 2013) and ICD-11 (World Health Organization, 2019). It has been recognized that children and young people (CYP) may develop EOS, which lies in the same continuum with the adult form of the disorder. Throughout this chapter, attention will be called to any differences between adult schizophrenia and EOS, whenever data are available. These differences are also summarized in Table 56.1.

Clinical features

Main symptoms of early-onset schizophrenia

Schizophrenia and psychosis at any age are diagnosed by the presence of psychotic symptoms. No specific distinction applies for younger individuals in the characterization of such symptoms for diagnostic purposes. These include:

Rutter's Child and Adolescent Psychiatry and Psychology, Seventh Edition.
Edited by Anita Thapar, Daniel S. Pine, Samuele Cortese, Cathy Creswell, Tamsin J. Ford, James F. Leckman, and Argyris Stringaris.

Companion website: www.wiley.com/go/thapar/rutterspsych7

Table 56.1 Comparison of early-onset and adult-onset schizophrenia.

	Early-onset schizophrenia (EOS) versus adult-onset schizophrenia
Phenomenology	Similar positive and negative symptoms across all ages. EOS is associated with more insidious onset, more frequent hallucinations in all modalities, more significant negative symptoms, and less well-formed delusions. It is also more difficult to differentiate formal thought disorder from premorbid language abnormalities in EOS compared to adult-onset schizophrenia.
Course and outcome	EOS is associated with a worse course and poorer long-term outcome compared to adult-onset schizophrenia, although there is some evidence that early intervention may be beneficial in these respects.
Premorbid development	EOS is characterized by more severe premorbid deficits in language, social and academic adjustment, and possibly development of motor function.
Neuropsychology	The mean IQ of EOS patients is significantly lower than the pooled mean IQ of patients with adult-onset schizophrenia. Most cognitive domains seem to be similarly affected in EOS compared to adult-onset schizophrenia, except for crystalized knowledge, manual dexterity, and spatial working memory, all of which seem to be more pronounced in EOS, and selective and sustained attention, which are less impaired.
Epidemiology	Only 8.2% of schizophrenia cases present in children and adolescents.
Genetics	There is evidence of stronger familial aggregation of schizophrenia and associated phenotypes in relatives, higher penetrance effects of preliminary reported susceptibility genes, and more frequently identified rare copy number variants (CNVs) in EOS compared to adult-onset schizophrenia.
Environmental risk factors	No clear differential effects of environmental risk factors affecting age of onset have been identified.
Neuroimaging	No clearly different patterns of brain structural and functional changes associated with age of onset have been identified.

Hallucinations

These are sensory perceptions in the absence of external stimuli. Auditory hallucinations are by far the most common type of hallucination in schizophrenia with their content typically being threatening, derogatory, or commanding. Auditory hallucinations are classified according to their form: voices addressing the patient directly (second person); voices discussing or commenting on the patient's actions in the third person (third person or running commentary); and voices speaking the patient's thoughts aloud (thought echo). The characteristics of hallucinations may be different depending on the person's age, but auditory hallucinations are typically present in EOS (Kyriakopoulos & Frangou, 2007). In adolescents diagnosed with childhood-onset schizophrenia (COS), typically characterized by onset before the 13th birthday, the presence of visual, somatic/tactile, and olfactory hallucinations in addition to auditory ones may also be the rule rather than the exception. David *et al.* (2011) examined 117 COS patients with a mean age of 13.6 years and identified 111 of them (94.9%) as having auditory hallucinations, and 94 (80.3%) as having visual hallucinations. Somatic/tactile (60.7%) and olfactory (29.9%) hallucinations occurred almost exclusively in patients who also had visual hallucinations. Visual hallucinations were associated with lower IQ, earlier age of onset, and more severe illness.

Delusions

These are typically described as fixed beliefs that are not amenable to change despite conflicting evidence (American Psychiatric Association, 2013). Paranoid delusions (beliefs that one is persecuted), delusions of reference (beliefs that events or people's behavior refer to oneself), delusions of control (beliefs that one's own thoughts, emotions, or movements are controlled by external forces), and delusional perception (a normal perception invested with a delusional interpretation), are particularly common in schizophrenia. Delusions may also include passivity phenomena like the experience of one's own thoughts being broadcast out loud so that they are available to others (thought broadcast), one's thoughts not being one's own but rather being inserted into one's mind (thought insertion), and the experience of one's thoughts being removed from one's mind (thought withdrawal). As in the case of hallucinations, the characteristics of delusions may depend on the age of the individual. Delusions in EOS may be less well-formed the younger the person is, and unusual beliefs in very young children may be developmentally appropriate and nonpathological (Kyriakopoulos & Frangou, 2007; Driver *et al.*, 2020;). Apparently paranoid interpretations and unusual reactions associated with beliefs can also be seen in other disorders with neurodevelopmental deviance, most notably ASD (Pina-Camacho *et al.*, 2016).

Disordered thinking

This is commonly referred to as formal thought disorder and is inferred from the person's speech. It may present as incoherent speech (loosening of associations),missing the target of an answer (tangentiality), and may lead to complete incomprehensibility (word salad). The person's speech may also include unusual, created words (neologisms) or expressions. In EOS, the identification of formal thought disorder seems to depend on the sample and definition used (Caplan *et al.*, 2000). The age of the young person and comorbidity with neurodevelopmental disorders (NDDs), in particular with those affecting the structure or content of language like disorders of intellectual development and ASD, need to be taken into consideration in the assessment of thought abnormalities. The identification of the premorbid language baseline of the individual is paramount when conclusions are drawn on potential deviance from it.

Grossly disorganized or catatonic behaviors

Such behaviors may impede goal-directed activity due to bizarreness, purposelessness, unpredictability, or inappropriateness, incorporate incongruous emotional responses, and interfere with organization. Catatonic behaviors include restlessness or agitation, posturing, mannerisms, stereotypies, resistance to instructions (negativism), and may amount to complete lack of verbal and motor responses (mutism and stupor). The overlap of such behaviors with other NDDs is substantial (Pina-Camacho *et al.*, 2016).

Negative symptoms

In contrast to the symptoms listed above, which can be seen as representing an excess or distortion of normal function and are commonly termed positive symptoms, negative symptoms are thought to represent a reduction or loss of normal function. These symptoms significantly affect people with schizophrenia and include diminished emotional expression (affective flattening), and reduced motivation in self-initiated purposeful activities (avolition). The content of speech and ideas may appear adversely affected in quantity (poverty of speech, alogia), pleasure from activities is diminished (anhedonia), and interest in social interactions is reduced (asociality). Negative symptoms lead to social withdrawal and isolation and are frequently present in EOS (Stentebjerg-Olesen *et al.*, 2016).

Classification of early-onset schizophrenia and other types of early-onset psychosis

There are some differences in making the diagnosis of schizophrenia between the two main classification systems, which also apply to EOS. Persistent delusions, including experiences of influence, passivity, or control, persistent hallucinations, and thought disorder, are considered core symptoms in both DSM-5 (American Psychiatric Association, 2013) and ICD-11 (World Health Organization, 2019). In accordance with ICD-11, at least one of these symptoms and at least two types of symptoms from all categories in total must have persisted for at least one month in order for a diagnosis of schizophrenia to be made. In DSM-5, the criterion of symptom duration differs and a six-month period of continuous signs of disturbance, which must include at least one month (or less, if successfully treated) of the same group of symptoms, must be present. Other types of psychosis depending on predominance of delusions without prominent hallucinations (delusional disorder), psychotic symptoms associated with mood states (schizoaffective disorder, depressive disorder, or mania with psychotic symptoms), or shorter duration (brief psychotic episode/acute and transient psychotic disorder, schizophreniform disorder) are also described in the classification systems. These symptoms should not be a manifestation of another health condition (e.g. a brain tumor) or due to the effect of a substance or medication on the central nervous system (CNS; e.g. corticosteroids), including withdrawal (e.g. alcohol withdrawal), in which cases different diagnoses are made. Shared psychotic disorders, i.e. psychotic conditions characterized by the development of psychotic symptoms in the context of a close relationship with a person with psychosis, involving CYP, have also been described in the literature (Vigo *et al.*, 2019).

Comorbidities

Comorbid conditions have frequently been observed in children and adolescents with EOS. These can be conceptualized as part of the neurobiological processes underpinning the trajectory leading to schizophrenia or as independently diagnosable conditions forming different aspects of a pan-developmental disturbance. A systematic review evaluating the clinical characteristics of schizophrenia spectrum psychosis in children and adolescents (Stentebjerg-Olesen *et al.*, 2016) estimated the rate of comorbidity with attention deficit hyperactivity disorder (ADHD) and conduct disorders to be 33.5% (range 8–74% in 5 included studies), with PDD to be 12.5% (range 4–25% in 3 studies), and with post-traumatic stress disorders (PTSD) to be 34.3% (range 16–43% in 2 studies). The co-occurrence of substance abuse was also found to be 32% (range 13–68% in 7 studies).

Developmental impairments in early-onset schizophrenia

Language development

Developmental speech and language abnormalities are commonly observed in EOS (Kyriakopoulos & Frangou, 2007; Jerrell & McIntyre, 2016). Several lines of evidence suggest that the earlier the onset, the more likely it is for individuals with schizophrenia to present with such deficits (Kyriakopoulos & Frangou, 2007; Driver *et al.*, 2020). A review of the US National Institute of Mental Health (NIMH) COS cohort in 2012 identified 51% of patients having premorbid language abnormalities (Driver *et al.*, 2020), while in the UK's Maudsley Hospital EOS study, developmental speech and language deficits were present in 19% of adolescents, more commonly in boys (Vourdas *et al.*, 2003). Jerrell and McIntyre (2016) employed a retrospective cohort design using the South Carolina Medicaid claims database for outpatient and inpatient medical services over 15 years and identified significantly more frequent speech, language, and educational disorders in COS compared to adolescent-onset cases. This also points toward more significant developmental deviance in this regard the earlier the onset of the disorder.

Psychomotor development

One of the earliest developmental aberrations in schizophrenia has been identified to be in motor function (Kyriakopoulos & Frangou, 2007). Deficits in motor development seem to have varied in frequency across studies of EOS. Hollis (1995) identified 31% of EOS cases to have premorbid motor abnormalities including restlessness, stereotyped movements, coordination problems, and delayed motor milestones, which were more common in males. In the Maudsley EOS study, there was additional evidence of developmental gross motor deficits, as 3% of the EOS cases could not walk unsupported by the age of two years (Vourdas *et al.*, 2003). In the 2012 update of the NIMH COS cohort, 52/118 children (44%) were found to have premorbid motor impairments (Driver *et al.*, 2020). Fine and gross motor function abnormalities also seem to be more common in youth diagnosed with EOS compared to health controls (Byrial *et al.*, 2022), and although some improvements have been reported at follow-up, these seem to persist to a large extent (Byrial *et al.*, 2023).

Social and academic adjustment

Premorbid deficits in social and academic adjustment seem to be the most common correlates of developmental deviance in EOS. EOS seems to impact social and academic adjustment significantly more in comparison with other disorders in childhood and adolescence (Kyriakopoulos & Frangou, 2007; Paya *et al.*, 2013). Premorbid withdrawal and difficulties in social adjustment, reduced socialization, social isolation, behavioral problems, suboptimal school performance, including failing grades at school, and a need for special educational provision, are not uncommon (Kyriakopoulos & Frangou, 2007). EOS subjects seem to be more affected in comparison to adult-onset cases (Vourdas *et al.*, 2003; Holmén *et al.*, 2012). Premorbid academic impairments were identified in 65/118 children (55%) and premorbid social/behavior impairments in 85/118 children (72%) in the 2012 review of the NIMH COS cohort (Driver *et al.*, 2020). Premorbid academic underachievement seems to be associated with the development of schizophrenia regardless of age of onset (Dickson *et al.*, 2020). Finally, a pattern of deterioration in social and academic adjustment preceding EOS suggests that worsening of global adjustment between childhood and early adolescence may be a marker of vulnerability or transition to psychosis. School adaptation seems to be particularly susceptible to impairment just prior to psychosis onset (Paya *et al.*, 2013).

Neuropsychology of early-onset schizophrenia

The pattern of cognitive deficits

Cognitive deficits are among the core features of schizophrenia, contributing substantially to functional impairments and poor clinical outcomes in the disorder, and have attracted increasing research interest in recent decades (McCutcheon *et al.*, 2023). Such deficits have been identified in general intellectual ability and almost all cognitive domains in EOS, with the mean IQ of EOS patients being significantly lower than the pooled mean IQ of patients with adult-onset schizophrenia (Frangou, 2013). A broad range of impairments has also been reported in different cognitive domains in EOS (Frangou, 2013; Harvey & Isner, 2020). Overall, the identified deficits were of large effect size in general intellectual ability, processing speed, working memory, and verbal memory and learning, of medium effect size in rule discovery and perseveration, and planning and problem-solving, and of minimal effect size in sustained and selective attention (Frangou, 2013). Most cognitive domains seem to be similarly affected in EOS compared to adult-onset schizophrenia with the notable exceptions of crystalized knowledge, manual dexterity and spatial working memory which seem to be more pronounced in EOS, and selective and sustained attention which are less impaired (Harvey & Isner, 2020).

Deficits in social cognition

Social cognition has been defined as the mental operations that underlie social interactions, including perceiving, interpreting, and generating responses to the intentions, dispositions, and behaviors of others (Green *et al.*, 2008). It consists of four core domains including emotion processing (perceiving and employing emotion), social perception (decoding and interpreting social cues in others), theory of mind/mental state attribution (mentalizing/ability to comprehend and represent the mental states of others), and attributional style (explaining or making sense of the cause of social events or interactions) (Harvey & Isner, 2020). EOS spectrum disorders have been associated with deficits in theory of mind (Pilowsky *et al.*, 2000; Bourgou *et al.*, 2016; Li *et al.*, 2017; Sağlam *et al.*, 2022; Tin *et al.*, 2018) and social perception (Jepsen *et al.*, 2022). Furthermore, in adolescents with EOS the sensitivity in discriminating angry faces, as well as the specificity in discriminating sad faces, seemed impaired, with their reaction being fastest on happy faces and slowest on sad and fearful faces (Seiferth *et al.*, 2009). In the two studies also including children and adolescents with ASD, ASD was associated with more pronounced deficits in theory of mind tasks (Pilowsky *et al.*, 2000; Tin *et al.*, 2018).

The course of cognitive deficits

The course of cognitive deficits in EOS has been the subject of considerable investigation alongside population studies exploring premorbid cognitive development in adult-onset schizophrenia (e.g. Reichenberg *et al.*, 2005). Overall, cognitive function in patients with first episode psychosis (FEP) seems to improve over time following a decline during the prodromal stage (Bora & Murray, 2014). Transition from clinical high risk for psychosis (CHR-P) to psychosis may be associated with a deterioration in processing speed compared to baseline (Hedges *et al.*, 2022). A pattern of relative IQ stabilization after an initial decline was demonstrated in several independent samples (Frangou, 2013). In the sample with the longest follow-up period, Øie and colleagues evaluated the cognitive function of young people with EOS at two time points beyond baseline, after 13 years and after 25 years. They identified a period of cognitive stagnation or deterioration between baseline assessment and assessment at 13 years followed by improvement from 13 to 25 years, supporting a stable level of cognitive performance over the whole follow-up period (Øie *et al.*, 2021). In terms of specific areas of cognitive function in EOS, working memory and rule discovery do not seem to be further affected longitudinally, while there is evidence of increasing deviance in verbal memory and learning, attention, and perseverative errors. There is limited or conflicting evidence on progression of deficits in processing speed, planning and problem-solving, and response inhibition (Frangou, 2013).

Prodromal phase of psychosis and at risk mental state

Since the 1990s there has been an exponential rise in research efforts aiming at prediction, prevention, and early identification of psychosis. For most patients, the development of schizophrenia and psychosis is preceded by a long period of nonspecific psychiatric symptoms, attenuated psychotic symptoms, and impaired functioning. It has been argued that the identification of such symptoms is likely to provide opportunities for timely and specific intervention (Nelson & McGorry, 2020). Although the prodromal phase of psychosis, i.e. the early stages of the disorder, can only safely be determined retrospectively due to the nonspecific nature of its symptoms, in practice, different combinations of symptoms have been found to confer specific risk for psychosis and have been conceptualized as "risk states" (Fusar-Poli, 2017; Nelson & McGorry, 2020). Constructs such as the "at risk mental state" (ARMS) and "ultra/clinical high risk for psychosis" (CHR-P) have been developed to facilitate research and early intervention. However, there seems to be substantial heterogeneity in terms of predictive potential within these constructs (Fusar-Poli, 2017; Salazar de Pablo *et al.*, 2021). Nevertheless, primary indicated prevention in individuals at CHR-P has grown exponentially becoming one of the most established preventive approaches in psychiatry (Catalan *et al.*, 2021). This approach targets individuals who accumulate risk factors for psychosis and functional impairment and seek help at specialized mental health clinics. Within this framework, the presence of related symptoms, typically attenuated or brief-limited intermittent psychotic symptoms, or the combination of genetic risk with deterioration syndrome (a drop of at least 30% in the Global Assessment of Functioning score over the past month as compared with 12 months ago), is established, and need-based and preventative interventions are provided (Catalan *et al.*, 2021). The early detection and intervention paradigm is designed to apply across the childhood–adulthood boundary. However, its usefulness in younger ages has been debated based on limited evidence and the premise that there may be developmental aspects differentially affecting individuals' clinical presentation and response to treatment depending on their age (Fusar-Poli & Salazar de Pablo, 2022; Lång *et al.*, 2022; Lång & Kelleher, 2022). Indeed, CYP meeting CHR-P criteria seem to have reduced risk of transition to psychosis compared to adults (9.5% at 1 year, 12.1% at 2 years, and 16.1% at >5 years) which reduces further (to 3.9% at 1 year, 11.6% at 2 years, and 14.3% at >5 years) when only studies with a low risk of bias are considered (Salazar de Pablo *et al.*, 2021; Lång *et al.*, 2022). Psychotic symptoms in CYP have been associated with several other mental health problems (e.g. depression, anxiety, substance misuse disorder, emerging personality disorder) requiring a range of alternative targeted interventions (Hayes & Kyriakopoulos, 2018). In addition, there is no evidence of effective interventions which can prevent psychosis in this age group (Catalan *et al.*, 2021), and the ARMS/CHR-P label, which conveys a future risk of psychosis or schizophrenia, may be perceived as stigmatizing (Lång *et al.*, 2022). Stigmatization related to mental health difficulties in CYP is a significant concern as it affects help-seeking, engagement, and treatment outcomes (Kaushik *et al.*, 2016). This may be even more important in the case of long-term conditions like psychosis, which require ongoing input and medication adherence. As a result, caution should be exercised when using the ARMS methodology for children and adolescents (Lång *et al.*, 2022). Finally, the relationship between early-onset psychosis (EOP) and schizotypal disorder (ICD-11)/schizotypal personality disorder (SPD, DSM-5) has not been fully clarified. The latter is typically characterized by enduring subthreshold psychotic symptoms, which are usually associated with persistent personality features (American Psychiatric Association, 2013—please also refer to Chapter 66). This symptom pattern has been identified premorbidly in young people presenting with EOS and in wider families of children with COS (Kyriakopoulos & Frangou, 2007). Schizotypal traits also seem to overlap with autism traits in adolescents with ASD, 40% of whom met criteria for SPD in one study (Barneveld *et al.*, 2011). Possible transition patterns from SPD to psychosis have not been systematically studied.

Course and long-term outcome

EOS spectrum disorders are generally considered as more severe types of psychosis compared to adult-onset conditions (Kyriakopoulos & Frangou, 2007). Adverse short- and long-term outcomes include high need for inpatient care, low rates of remission and recovery, negative symptoms, adverse educational and occupational outcomes, low rates of independent living and suboptimal psychosocial functioning, significant suicidality and mortality, and overall poor global functioning (Remschmidt *et al.*, 2007; Uggerby *et al.*, 2011; Clemmensen *et al.*, 2012; Remberk *et al.*, 2014; Remberk *et al.*, 2015; Stentebjerg-Olesen *et al.*, 2016; Vernal *et al.*, 2020; Xu *et al.*, 2020). Compared to other severe and complex mental health conditions requiring hospitalization, children with EOS spectrum disorders may have similar short-term functional outcomes despite greater functional deficits on admission (Galitzer *et al.*, 2021). Some EOS studies have also reported similar outcomes to adult-onset schizophrenia at short-term follow-up (e.g. Pencer *et al.*, 2005), while studies from early intervention services suggest that older adolescents with EOS might have an equally good or even better outcome than adult-onset patients associated with these approaches (Schimmelmann *et al.*, 2013). The sample characteristics in different studies, including severity of illness at baseline, referral pathways, treatments offered, and follow-up period are likely to affect their results. At least some of these outcomes may be mediated by longer duration of untreated psychosis (DUP) and worse premorbid functioning in EOS compared to adult-onset schizophrenia, which are factors associated with a poorer outcome regardless of age (Diaz-Caneja *et al.*, 2015; Stentebjerg-Olesen *et al.*, 2016; Driver *et al.*, 2020). It is of note that the mean DUP in EOS was estimated to be almost 3.5 times longer that in adult-onset schizophrenia (Stentebjerg-Olesen *et al.*, 2016). Other factors associated with poorer outcome include lower premorbid intelligence, more insidious onset of symptoms, more severe psychopathology, longer stay in hospital, residual and negative symptoms, and repeated hospitalizations (Clemmensen *et al.*, 2012; Del Rey-Mejías *et al.*, 2015; Diaz-Caneja *et al.*, 2015). In a population-based cohort, younger age at first hospitalization with schizophrenia was associated with a greater likelihood of having a longer first admission, more than one hospital admission, more hospital admissions per year, and more inpatient days per year. The ages of 17 years and 12 years seem to mark cutoff points with the earlier the onset the worse the prognosis (Rabinowitz *et al.*, 2007). However, the effects of age, age of onset, and sex on outcomes within EOS are not totally consistent across studies (Diaz-Caneja *et al.*, 2015). Within EOP, negative symptoms, ASD, older age at first presentation, Black ethnicity, and family history of psychosis have also been associated with multiple treatment failure. This was defined as the initiation of the third novel antipsychotic due to prior insufficient response, intolerable adverse effects, or nonadherence (Downs *et al.*, 2019).

In terms of diagnostic trajectories, Stentebjerg-Olesen *et al.* (2016), who included in their systematic review studies of children and adolescents with at least 50% of participants having nonaffective psychosis, identified 88% of the patients at baseline and 75% at follow-up as having a diagnosis of a schizophrenia spectrum disorder, whereas 12.2% of patients at baseline and 24.5% at follow-up had a diagnosis of an affective disorder. The proportions of diagnosed schizophrenia increased from 31.9% at baseline to 40.2% at follow-up, of bipolar disorder from 8.9% to 14.3%, and of depressive disorder from 1.9% to 4.1%. At the same time, the proportions of diagnosed psychosis not otherwise specified (NOS) decreased from 15.8% to 12.0% and of schizophreniform disorder from 21.3% to 1.1%. These diagnostic shifts did not reach statistical significance, supporting the relative diagnostic stability of these conditions.

Epidemiology

Incidence and prevalence

Psychotic symptoms have very commonly been reported in population-based studies both in adults and in children and adolescents (Kelleher *et al.*, 2012; Maijer *et al.*, 2018). In all ages, their median annual incidence was estimated as 2.5% and the median prevalence as 7.2% (Linscott & Van Os, 2013). The median prevalence of psychotic symptoms seems to be higher in younger ages, 17% in childhood and 7.5% in adolescence (Kelleher *et al.*, 2012). In a more recent review and meta-analysis focusing on auditory hallucinations across the life span, the mean prevalence rates were 12.7% in children, 12.4% in adolescents, 5.8% in adults (18–60 years), and 4.5% in the elderly (>60 years) (Maijer *et al.*, 2018). Most included studies, in both systematic reviews and meta-analyses, employed self-reported measures. In CYP community clinic samples, psychotic symptoms seem to be even more common. Depending on the inclusion criteria and the setting, rates of such symptoms have been found to vary between 43–97.7% (Brandizzi *et al.*, 2014; Kelleher *et al.*, 2014; Gin *et al.*, 2018; Pontillo *et al.*, 2018). The high prevalence of psychotic symptoms, both in population and in clinical studies of children and adolescents, support their lack of specificity in terms of risk for psychosis.

On the other hand, psychotic disorders are extremely rare in children and relatively rare in adolescents. The proportion of EOS is estimated as 8.2% of all schizophrenia cases, while for EOS spectrum disorders the respective proportion was estimated as 12.3% (Solmi *et al.*, 2022). COS incidence is generally accepted to be less than 0.04% (Driver *et al.*, 2020). Surveillance data from the UK suggest that the 1-year incidence of nonaffective psychoses under the age of 14 years is 0.21/100,000 (Tiffin & Kitchen, 2015), much smaller than the estimated 1-year incidence of schizophrenia across all ages at 0.2/1000 (Messias *et al.*, 2007).

Sex differences

The peak age of onset for schizophrenia has been estimated to be at 20.5 years (Solmi *et al.*, 2022) and there is meta-analytic evidence of a lifetime incidence rate ratio (IRR) for males: females of 1.4 : 1 (McGrath *et al.*, 2008). Males seem to have an earlier onset by approximately 1.5 years compared to females (Eranti *et al.*, 2013). In epidemiological samples, by the age of 14 years, schizophrenia has presented in 6% of all male cases and 2.5% of all female cases, and by the age of 18 years in 11.6% and 8.3%, respectively (Solmi *et al.*, 2022). This significant predominance of male sex in younger children, which is attenuated in adolescence, is also reflected in clinical samples (e.g. Kolvin *et al.*, 1971; Hollis, 2000; Vourdas *et al.*, 2003; Stentebjerg-Olesen *et al.*, 2016).

Genetics

The heritability of schizophrenia is estimated as 64–81% in epidemiological studies (Sullivan *et al.*, 2003; Lichtenstein *et al.*, 2009; Wray & Gottesman, 2012; Owen *et al.*, 2016;). Existing genetic data suggest that multiple alleles of varying frequencies (common to rare) and effect sizes contribute to the risk of developing the disorder (Nakamura & Takata, 2023). There is a significant genetic overlap with other mental health disorders and NDDs (see Chapter 21).

Common variants in schizophrenia

The contribution of common variants to the risk for schizophrenia is explored through genome-wide association studies (GWAS; see Chapter 21) of common single nucleotide polymorphisms (SNPs) with small effect sizes (typically with OR < 1.2). To date, the largest GWAS of common SNPs by the Psychiatric Genomics Consortium (Trubetskoy *et al.*, 2022) analyzed data from up to 76,755 schizophrenia cases and 243,649 control individuals, identifying 287 distinct loci with genome-wide significant association. The SNP with the largest effect size (OR 1.23) was the rs140365013 variant on chromosome 6 near the major histocompatibility complex region. Associations were identified in genes that are expressed in excitatory and inhibitory neurons of the CNS and are implicated in neuronal function, including synaptic organization, differentiation, and transmission. Fine-mapped candidates were enriched for genes associated with rare disruptive coding variants in people with schizophrenia, including the glutamate receptor subunit GRIN2A and transcription factor SP4, and were also enriched for genes implicated by such variants in NDDs. The proportion of the variance in schizophrenia liability explained by all SNPs was found to be 24%.

Rare variants in schizophrenia

The contribution of rare variants has received significant support with the discovery of structural variations in the genome (copy number variants—CNVs; see Chapter 21). Rare gene-disrupting mutations typically have much larger effects on individual risk (OR 2–60) but, due to their rarity, make only a small contribution to overall heritability in the population (Singh *et al.*, 2022). Post-zygotic mutations also seem to play a significant role in that respect (Castellani *et al.*, 2017; Bae *et al.*, 2022). Several rare (minor allele frequency < 0.1%), recurrent CNVs have been associated with schizophrenia, the most significant of which are 22q11.2 microdeletions causing velocardiofacial syndrome (Ivanov *et al.*, 2003; Marshall *et al.*, 2017). Such deletions are present in nearly 1% of patients with schizophrenia (Ivanov *et al.*, 2003), and constitute one of its largest individual risk factors (20–25% risk of schizophrenia in this group). In a companion study of rare variants to the GWAS mentioned in the previous section, Singh *et al.* (2022), meta-analyzed the whole exomes of 24,248 schizophrenia cases, 97,322 controls, and 3402 parent–proband trios, and identified ultra-rare coding variants in 10 genes (SETD1A, CUL1, XPO7, TRIO, CACNA1G, SP4, GRIA3, GRIN2A, HERC1, and RB1CC1) as conferring substantial risk for schizophrenia (OR 3–50), and 32 additional genes at a false discovery rate of <5%. These genes are implicated in the formation, structure, and function of the synapse, while the GRIN2A (n-methyl-D-aspartate [NMDA] receptor subunit) and GRIA3 (α-amino-3-hydroxy-5-methyl-4-isoxazolepropionic acid [AMPA] receptor subunit) provide support to the hypothesis of glutamatergic dysfunction in the pathogenesis of schizophrenia (Singh *et al.*, 2022).

Genetic data related to early-onset schizophrenia

Large-scale genetic data exclusive to EOS is limited. There is some evidence suggestive of stronger familial aggregation of schizophrenia and associated phenotypes in relatives of COS probands compared to adults with the disorder and higher penetrance effects of preliminary reported susceptibility genes in COS (Addington & Rapoport, 2009; Forsyth & Asarnow, 2020). In the first GWAS study in EOS, including 2159 cases and 6561 controls in total from populations of Han Chinese ancestry, Guo *et al.* (2021), identified four genome-wide significant risk loci for EOS while polygenic risk score (PRS) analysis revealed substantial genetic overlap between EOS and adult-onset schizophrenia. The functional variant rs1801133, which showed the strongest association with EOS, has previously been implicated in schizophrenia, being associated with age of onset (Vares *et al.*, 2010) and disrupted prefrontal function (Roffman *et al.*, 2008). In the NIMH COS sample (Ahn *et al.*, 2014), 11.9% of COS patients had rare CNVs, one-third of which (4%) were 22q11.2 microdeletions, which was significantly higher than the rate reported for adult-onset cases (0.3–1%). These CNVs were significantly more common among COS patients compared to their siblings and adults with schizophrenia. In general, a number of different CNVs have been implicated in COS but large studies are lacking (Fernandez *et al.*, 2019). In a larger recent study, the prevalence of 47 recurrent CNVs and the functional impact of deletions and duplications genome-wide in 137 children and adolescents with EOP was compared with 5540 individuals with ASD and 16,504 population control subjects (Brownstein *et al.*, 2022). CNV risk scores (CRS), indices reflecting the dosage sensitivity for any gene across the genome within a deletion or duplication, were compared between groups. The study identified higher prevalence of recurrent CNVs in EOP compared to ASD (OR 2.42) and control subjects (OR 5.19). When EOP participants with co-occurring ASD were excluded the difference from ASD was not statistically significant. The EOP and ASD groups also had similar and higher CRS compared with the control group for both deletions and duplications.

Transcriptomic and epigenomic studies

Large transcriptomic and epigenomic analyses have provided new insights into the molecular pathology of schizophrenia and their use is likely to further promote our understanding of transcriptional and epigenetic regulation of genes associated with the disorder (Nakamura & Takata, 2023). No such studies have specifically explored factors associated with earlier age of onset.

Gene–environment interactions

The interplay between environmental and genetic factors is thought to be important in the development of schizophrenia and goes beyond their independent additive effects (Wahbeh & Avramopoulos, 2021). Gene—environment interactions are difficult to detect because of the millions of genetic variants and several combinations of environmental factors which reduce statistical power.

Environmental risk factors

Parental age

Since the first population-based birth cohort study linked advanced paternal age, compared to age 25–29 years, to schizophrenia risk (Malaspina *et al.*, 2001), several studies have replicated this finding using different designs and populations (Khachadourian *et al.*, 2022). This association seems to be present from as early as the mid-to-late 30s with the risk increasing the older the paternal age (McGrath *et al.*, 2014; Khachadourian *et al.*, 2022). Increased risk for schizophrenia also seems to be present in the offspring of younger fathers and mothers (age < 20 years), and to a smaller extent older mothers (Miller *et al.*, 2011; McGrath *et al.*, 2014; Davies *et al.*, 2020). Maternal age 20–29 seems to be a protective factor (OR 0.93 for ages 20–24 years and 0.92 for ages 25–29 years) (Davies *et al.*, 2020). There is only one recent study by Wang *et al.* (2019) specifically studying the relationship between advanced parental age and age of schizophrenia onset. This found that even after directly controlling for both paternal and maternal PRS for schizophrenia, advanced paternal age was significantly associated with an earlier onset of the disorder among sporadic cases. Several hypotheses have been made to explain these findings including *de novo* mutations, inherited effects related to late fatherhood, and molecular and biological factors associated with aging (Khachadourian *et al.*, 2022).

Prenatal and perinatal factors

A recent meta-analysis quantified the risk and protective effects to the later emergence of schizophrenia of all relevant prenatal and perinatal factors (Davies *et al.*, 2020). Risk factors include any maternal (OR 4.60) or paternal (OR 2.73) psychopathology, maternal psychosis (OR 7.61) and affective disorder (OR 2.26), three or more pregnancies (OR 1.30), toxoplasma (OR 1.30), herpes simplex 2 (OR 1.35), maternal infections NOS (OR 1.27), suboptimal number of antenatal visits (OR 1.83), winter (OR 1.05) and winter to spring (OR 1.05) season of birth in the northern hemisphere, maternal stress NOS (OR 2.40), famine (OR 1.61), any famine or nutritional deficits in pregnancy (OR 1.40), maternal hypertension (OR 1.40), hypoxia (OR 1.63), ruptured (OR 1.86) and premature rupture (OR 2.29) of membranes, polyhydramnios (OR 3.05), definite obstetric complications NOS (OR 1.83), birthweights of less than 2000 g (OR 1.84), less than 2500 g (OR 1.53), or 2500–2999 g (OR 1.23), birth length less than 49 cm (OR 1.17), small for gestational age (OR 1.40), premature birth (OR 1.35), and congenital malformations (OR 2.35). Influenza infection during pregnancy has not emerged as a significant risk factor. Significant protective factors, in addition to maternal ages of 20–29, were nulliparity (OR 0.91), and birthweights 3500–3999 g (OR 0.90) or more than 4000 g (OR 0.86). No similar comprehensive work has been conducted in relation to EOS spectrum disorders, but all these factors affect the emergence of schizophrenia across the life span.

Infection and inflammation

In addition to the prenatal and perinatal period, infections during critical periods of neurodevelopment, such as childhood and adolescence, have been associated with schizophrenia. A large meta-analysis of population-based studies identified a more than twofold increase in the risk of adult nonaffective psychosis associated with childhood CNS viral infection (Khandaker *et al.*, 2012). CNS bacterial infections were not found to be associated with such risk in that study (Khandaker *et al.*, 2012). More recent studies have also supported the link between childhood infection and schizophrenia (e.g. Debost *et al.*, 2019, 2022). The relative significance of the direct effect of neuroinvasion and the effects of an associated inflammatory response/immune activation on the developing brain is yet to be fully understood in schizophrenia, although there is evidence that both are relevant to its later emergence (Khandaker *et al.*, 2012; Kulaga & Miller, 2021). In terms of inflammation, interleukin-6 elevations at age 9 were found to correlate with psychotic symptoms at age 18 years in a dose-dependent manner, and higher elevations were associated with psychotic disorder at that age (Khandaker *et al.*, 2014). A longitudinal association between childhood and adolescent C-reactive protein (CRP) levels, and adult schizophrenia diagnosis, has also been found (Metcalf *et al.*, 2017; Müller, 2018). Low-level neuroinflammation has been associated with alterations of dopaminergic, serotonergic, noradrenergic, and glutamatergic neurotransmission which are considered significant factors in the generation of psychotic symptoms (Müller, 2018). Human coronaviruses have also been associated with psychotic disorders; COVID-19 seems to have neuroinvasive properties similar to those of other such viruses and a propensity to generate a massive inflammatory response, which makes it likely for it to also contribute to future psychopathology including psychosis (Kulaga & Miller, 2021).

Cannabis and other psychoactive substances

Psychosis in adolescents is frequently related to the acute effects or withdrawal of psychoactive substances. Many such substances are known to predispose to, induce, or exacerbate psychosis. These include prescribed medication like steroids, methylphenidate, amphetamines, or antibiotics such as fluoroquinolones, or psychoactive substances used recreationally (e.g. cannabinoids, cocaine, hallucinogens, synthetic drugs, and prescribed medication mentioned above diverted for recreational use) (Beckman *et al.*, 2020). Daily tobacco use is also associated with increased risk of psychosis and an earlier estimated age at onset by approximately one year, although the possible causality of this exposure needs further exploration (Gurillo *et al.*, 2015). Cannabis use was associated with a dose-dependent risk of developing psychosis, with an earlier onset of psychotic illness by 2–3 years, with increased relapse rates of psychosis, and with more hospitalizations and pronounced positive symptoms in psychotic patients (Hasan *et al.*, 2020). A systematic synthesis of umbrella reviews identified cannabis as one of the most robust risk factors for nonorganic psychosis with OR 3.90 (Arango *et al.*, 2021). Despite a higher prevalence of substance abuse in men diagnosed with psychotic disorders, the association between substance use and psychosis may be stronger in women (Pence *et al.*, 2022).

Migration, ethnic minority status, urbanicity, and socioeconomic status

Several factors that are related to social adversity and the living environment have been associated with a higher risk of developing nonorganic psychotic disorders (Arango *et al.*, 2021). These include being first- and second-generation immigrant (IRR 2.10 and 1.68, respectively), belonging in an ethnic minority in a high and low ethnic density area (IRR 2.11 and 3.71, respectively), having Black-Caribbean ethnicity in England (IRR 4.87), being a North African immigrant in Europe (IRR 2.22), and living in urban environments (OR 2.19) (Arango *et al.*, 2021). In addition, Kirkbride *et al.* (2017) have demonstrated that the link between migration and psychosis remains for several ethnic minority groups after controlling for important confounders, including socioeconomic status, neighborhood-level population density, and multiple deprivation. In that study, excess risk for psychosis for first-generation immigrants was associated with migration in childhood rather than adolescence or adult life. Growing up in an urban environment and migration may have a stronger association with psychosis risk in men than in women (Pence *et al.*, 2022). The link between psychosocial adversity and psychosis is not totally understood. For migration, adversity at all stages of the process, low ethnic density, social isolation, discrimination, and lack of access to private accommodation and economic opportunities, have been suggested as possible contributing factors. For urbanicity, the roles of greater exposure to prenatal and perinatal infections and complications, cannabis use, social deprivation, income inequality, and social fragmentation have been speculated upon (Stilo & Murray, 2019).

Childhood adversity

Childhood adversity is used to describe a set of experiences including child maltreatment (e.g. sexual abuse, physical abuse, emotional/psychological abuse, and neglect), peer victimization (e.g. bullying), parental loss and separation, witnessing violence, suffering displacement and war, and exposure to traumatic events (Varese *et al.*, 2012; Sideli *et al.*, 2020; Stanton *et al.*, 2020). Childhood adversity is associated with an increased risk of nonorganic psychosis with an overall OR of 2.80 (Arango *et al.*, 2021). An interaction between early and recent adversities and the mediating role of attachment and mood symptoms on the relationship between childhood adversity and psychotic symptoms/disorder have been suggested (Sideli *et al.*, 2020). Physical assault and bullying have been associated with subsequent psychotic experiences in adolescents 13–16 years (Kelleher *et al.*, 2013). A dose–response relationship was observed between severity of bullying and risk for psychotic experiences, with cessation of it in the course of the study predicting cessation of psychotic experiences (Kelleher *et al.*, 2013). Exposure to any trauma up to the age of 17 years has been associated with increased odds of psychotic experiences at age 18 years (OR 2.91) with the population-attributable fraction for such trauma on psychotic experiences at that age being estimated as 45% (Croft *et al.*, 2019). Childhood trauma has also been reported in 86.8% of CHR-P subjects (Kraan *et al.*, 2015) and has been correlated in this population to the severity of perceptual disturbances, general/affective symptoms, and functional impairment in a dose–response fashion (Loewy *et al.*, 2019). However, data on the relationship between childhood adversity and age of onset of diagnosable nonorganic psychotic disorders before adulthood are very limited, with only one small study suggesting higher levels of traumatic experiences in EOS compared to adult-onset schizophrenia (Trovão *et al.*, 2022).

Aggregate environmental risk

It has been recognized that, up until recently, the exploration of environmental factors in schizophrenia involved hypothesis-driven paradigms which have significant limitations as they do not fully account for the dense network of interconnected exposures in the disorder. This led to the development of aggregate environmental risk approaches and related scores aiming to capture the combined effect of different nongenetic exposures in schizophrenia, also taking into account their different weights on outcome (Padmanabhan *et al.*, 2017; Guloksuz *et al.*, 2018; Vassos *et al.*, 2020). Particularly promising is the predictive modeling approach used to construct the exposome score, an aggregated score which considers the interdependency of environmental exposures for schizophrenia and has some evidence of utility in risk prediction and stratification for research purposes (Pries *et al.*, 2019, 2020).

Neurobiology

Schizophrenia is a disorder emerging through the interaction of neurodevelopment with adverse environmental risk factors, most of which act during childhood and adolescence (Murray *et al.*, 2017). This interaction leads to deviant maturational trajectories in brain development, potentiated during critical periods and resulting in aberrant integration of brain regions into functional networks, giving rise to the symptoms of the disorder. Specific neurobiological changes have been associated with this process, although the etiopathogenesis of schizophrenia remains elusive.

Neurochemistry and neuropathology

Schizophrenia affects almost all the major neurotransmitter systems. Extensive evidence strongly supports the implication of dopamine dysfunction in the development of psychotic symptoms (Owen *et al.*, 2016; Murray *et al.*, 2017). Elevated presynaptic striatal dopamine synthesis is associated with psychosis and prodromal states, while dopaminergic hypofunction in the dorsolateral prefrontal cortex has been proposed to account for negative and cognitive symptoms (Murray *et al.*, 2017; Howes *et al.*, 2017a). Postmortem studies identified increased striatal D2 receptor levels, but this finding is limited by the fact that most participants had been on antipsychotic medication (McCutcheon *et al.*, 2020). Positron emission tomography (PET) studies provide little consistent evidence of altered striatal D2/3 receptor levels although consistently identifying a striatal presynaptic hyperdopaminergic state in schizophrenia (McCutcheon *et al.*, 2020). Another neurotransmitter system implicated in schizophrenia and also supported by postmortem, genetic, and neuroimaging studies is the glutamatergic system (McCutcheon *et al.*, 2020; Nakamura & Takata, 2023). An excitatory/inhibitory imbalance may manifest in schizophrenia, potentially associated with excessive pruning of dendritic spines, gamma-aminobutyric acid (GABA)ergic abnormalities, or NMDA hypofunction. Due to the widespread glutamate signaling across the brain and limitations in its study, it is not possible to precisely characterize the nature of this dysfunction (McCutcheon *et al.*, 2020). However, the interaction of these two systems is gaining support as underlying the pathophysiology of schizophrenia. A hypothesis that brings together evidence from all different lines of research implicates synaptic dysfunction through a multihit model. The model incorporates genetic vulnerability to synaptic elimination followed by environmental risk factors, which cause aberrant synapse–microglia interactions, synaptic dysfunction, excess microglia-mediated pruning, and the emergence of symptoms. This may underlie other pathophysiological findings in schizophrenia, including structural and functional brain-imaging results, and dopaminergic dysfunction. It could also explain why schizophrenia is rare in childhood, when synaptogenesis protects against overactive pruning and synaptic dysfunction, and increases in prevalence in adolescence and early adulthood when active synaptic elimination unmasks individual vulnerability to overactive pruning (Howes & Onwordi, 2023). Triggers of synaptic pruning in adolescence may include factors related to immunity like the complement component 4 (Johnson & Stevens, 2018).

Neuroimaging

Several neuroimaging studies have identified brain structural changes in EOS spectrum disorders both cross-sectionally and longitudinally. In the largest neuroimaging dataset to date, including 263 patients with EOP and 359 healthy controls (HC), Gurholt *et al.* (2022) identified significantly lower intracranial and hippocampal volumes, and higher caudate and pallidum volumes in EOP compared to HC. Intracranial volume was lower in both EOS and affective psychosis, and only EOS showed lower hippocampal and higher pallidum volumes compared to HC. The findings showed a similar pattern of brain alterations in EOP as previously reported in adult psychosis (van Erp *et al.*, 2016), but with notably low intracranial volume which may be associated to more severe deviance in the maturational trajectory. In addition, cortical thinning has been noted in widespread brain regions in EOS including frontal, temporal, and occipital regions (Voets *et al.*, 2008; Janssen *et al.*, 2009; Thormodsen *et al.*, 2013; Janssen *et al.*, 2014). White matter integrity, as inferred by diffusion tensor imaging, seems to also be affected in EOS, with changes in frontal, fronto-temporal, and fronto-limbic connections being more commonly reported (Samartzis *et al.*, 2014). In a mega-analysis of 321 adolescents with EOP and 265 HC (Barth *et al.*, 2022), widespread lower fractional anisotropy was found in EOP compared to HC, with the largest effect sizes in the superior longitudinal fasciculus, posterior corona radiata, and superior fronto-occipital fasciculus. These changes were most prominent in male individuals with EOS. Progressive structural brain changes in frontal gray matter and temporal cortical thickness have also been reported in EOP (Fraguas *et al.*, 2016; Pina-Camacho *et al.*, 2022). Taken together, all these studies support the existence of structural dysconnectivity in EOS spectrum disorders.

Similarly, functional magnetic resonance imaging (fMRI) studies have identified brain regions suboptimally recruited during specific cognitive tasks in EOS. A recent meta-analysis of all but resting state fMRI studies (Ioakeimidis *et al.*, 2020) reported reduced brain activation in EOS compared to HC at the right anterior cingulate cortex and the right superior temporal gyrus/temporoparietal junction across all cognitive tasks. It also identified hypoactivation at the left superior parietal cortex/precuneus, the right inferior parietal lobule, and the right supramarginal gyrus/right temporoparietal junction during working memory tasks. It was shown via *post hoc* analysis that the hypoactivating nodes are functionally connected with the salience network. Saliency dysfunction may play a central role in EOS and lead to cognitive symptoms in the disorder, such as poor working memory and goal-directed attention. A review focusing on functional connectivity studies of the default mode network (DMN), the most extensively studied brain network relevant to social cognition, identified 14 DMN studies in EOP, 6 of them reporting DMN hypoconnectivity and 5 reporting both hyper- and hypoconnectivity (Nair *et al.*, 2020). Disrupted DMN connectivity appeared to be associated with social impairments and less so with hallucinations or delusions in EOP. One longitudinal study of adolescents with EOS and HC, exploring working memory neurodevelopmental changes within and between the groups after a four-year period, identified widespread functional reductions in frontotemporal and cingulate brain areas in both groups with no between-group differences (Ioakeimidis *et al.*, 2022).

Diagnostic assessment and differential diagnosis

A thorough diagnostic assessment should be conducted for all children and adolescents with psychotic symptoms or FEP (Figure 56.1). This should include a detailed psychiatric and medical history, family, psychosocial, developmental, and educational history, history of substance use, mental state examination, physical examination, assessment of risk to self or others, and cognitive function if possible (National Institute for Health and Care Excellence, 2016; Pina-Camacho *et al.*, 2016; Merritt *et al.*, 2020; Skikic & Arriola 2020; Tyson *et al.*, 2020) (see

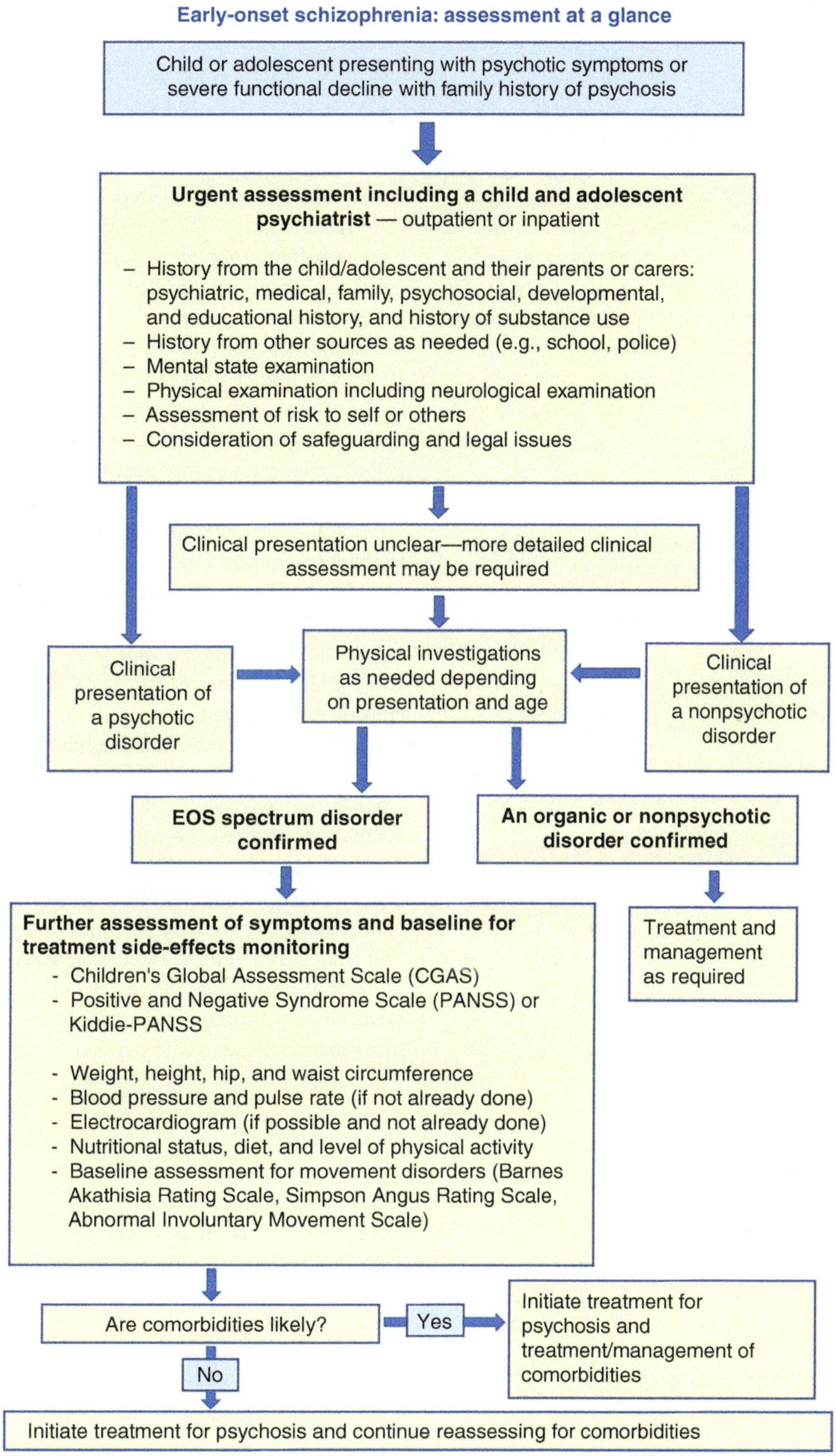

Figure 56.1 Early-onset schizophrenia (EOS) assessment at a glance.

Chapters 2 and 27–30). Neurological, autoimmune, infectious, endocrine, sleep, and metabolic disorders, nutritional deficiencies, chromosomal abnormalities, and psychotropic substances may all cause secondary psychosis (Pina-Camacho *et al.*, 2016; Skikic & Arriola 2020). Investigations to exclude organic causes of psychosis may need to be more extensive in EOP (Table 56.2) and will also depend on the age of onset, with psychosis in children generally warranting a more detailed physical assessment. Rating scales for symptoms associated with psychotic disorders, e.g. the Positive and Negative Syndrome Scale (PANSS; Kay *et al.*, 1987) and the Kiddie-PANSS (Fields *et al.*, 1994), for functional impairment, e.g. the Children's Global Assessment Scale (CGAS; Shaffer *et al.*, 1983), and for movement disorders, e.g. the Barnes Akathisia Rating Scale (Barnes, 1989), the Simpson Angus Rating Scale (Simpson & Angus, 1970), and the Abnormal Involuntary Movement Scale (AIMS; Rapoport *et al.*, 1985), have been extensively used for assessment and monitoring purposes in research and clinical practice.

Table 56.2 Physical investigations to consider in early-onset schizophrenia (EOS) spectrum disorders.

Investigation	Target/rationale
Full blood count	Hematologic abnormalities (e.g. hemolytic anemia), infections
Urea, electrolytes, liver function tests	Renal and hepatic function, endocrine disorders
Fasting glucose, hemoglobin A1c (HbA1c), lipids, and prolactin	Endocrine disorders, baseline of monitoring for metabolic syndrome
Thyroid function tests, bone profile	Thyroid/endocrine abnormalities
Urine drug screen	Psychosis secondary to psychoactive substances
Autoimmune serology (e.g. n-methyl-D-aspartate (NMDA) receptor antibodies, anti-basal ganglia antibodies, anti-thyroid peroxidise antibodies)	Autoimmune disorders/ encephalitis
Investigations for infections (e.g. C-reactive protein (CRP), Lyme serology, toxoplasma serology)	Infections
Heavy metals (e.g. lead)	Exposure to heavy metals, organophosphates
Serum ceruloplasmin, serum and urinary copper	Wilson's disease
Plasma amino acids, white cell enzymes, lactate, ammonia, urinary organic acids, urinary porphyrins	Rare metabolic causes
Vitamins (e.g. B12, folate, vitamin D)	Vitamin/nutritional deficiencies
Brain magnetic resonance imaging (MRI) scan	Space-occupying lesions, brain abnormalities (e.g. demyelination, stroke)
Electroencephalography (EEG)	Epilepsy, abnormal brain electrical activity
Genetic testing (e.g. array comparative genomic hybridization, whole-exome sequencing)	Genetic abnormalities

Distinguishing between EOS and neurodevelopmental or other mental health disorders is paramount. Premorbid ASD, in particular, has been reported in up to 30–50% of COS cases (Rapoport *et al.*, 2009). Negative symptoms, social withdrawal, flattened affect, poor eye contact, communication and reciprocal interaction problems, idiosyncratic beliefs and odd behaviors, and psychomotor abnormalities including catatonia in EOS can sometimes be hard to differentiate from symptoms of ASD. Deficits in higher-order social cognition in ASD may also lead under stress to paranoid or unusual interpretations which may give the impression of delusional thinking. However, in EOS, hallucinations, delusions, and thought disorganization are generally more pronounced and there is often a clear exacerbation of preexisting developmental deviance (Pina-Camacho *et al.*, 2016). Individual diagnostic items from the construct of multiple complex developmental disorder (MCDD), which has been used to describe children presenting with thought disorder, social communication difficulties, and affective dysregulation (Cohen *et al.*, 1986; Buitelaar & van der Gaag, 1998) have allowed the empirical differentiation of ASD into groups with and without psychotic symptoms, with hallucination being significantly more common as an external validator in the former compared to the latter group (Kyriakopoulos *et al.*, 2015). Possible psychotic symptoms may also be more prevalent in CDD compared to ASD although data on this are very limited (Mehra *et al.*, 2019). The detailed evaluation of mood and anxiety, and identification of any traumatic events, alongside the timing of psychotic symptoms in relation to these events, are likely to lead to alternative or additional diagnoses (Hayes & Kyriakopoulos, 2018). Early-onset bipolar disorder, regardless of the polarity of the episode, is likely to be associated with psychotic symptoms (see Chapter 62).

Treatment

Once the diagnosis of EOS has been confirmed, the treatment should start as soon as possible with the aim of preventing a long DUP. This includes antipsychotic medication in conjunction with psychological interventions. Psychological interventions alone should not be encouraged and, if chosen by young people and their families, such a treatment course should be very time limited (National Institute for Health and Care Excellence, 2016) (Figure 56.2).

Antipsychotic medications

Antipsychotic medications are the first-line treatment for EOS spectrum disorders. The choice of antipsychotic should be made by the parents or carers of younger children, or jointly with the young person and their parents or carers, and health care professionals after sufficient information has been provided

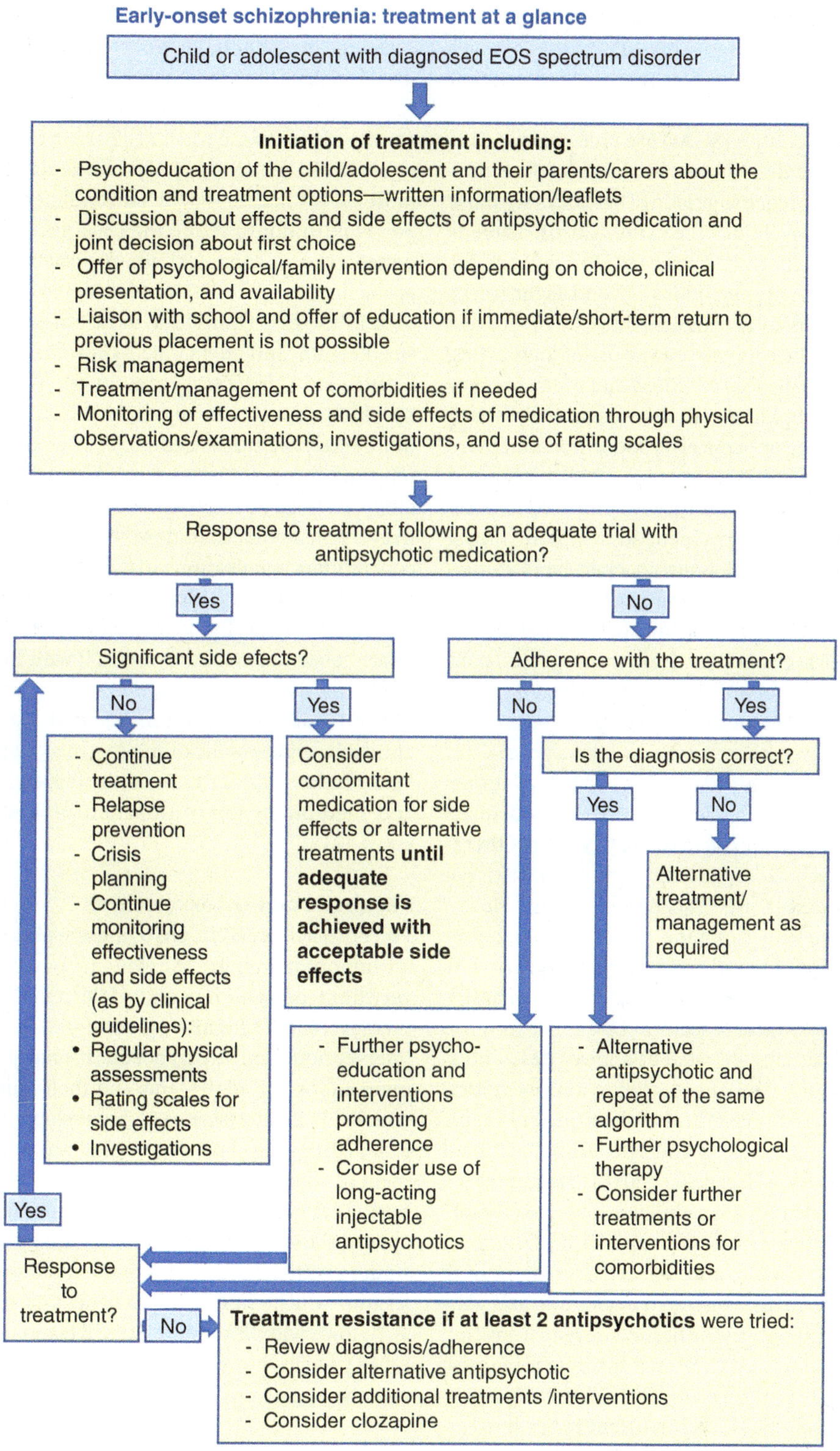

Figure 56.2 Early-onset schizophrenia (EOS) treatment at a glance.

(National Institute for Health and Care Excellence, 2016). While antipsychotic medications are similarly effective in adults and younger individuals, the latter group is thought to experience a higher prevalence of side effects (National Institute for Health and Care Excellence, 2016; Correll *et al.*, 2022;). Meta-analytic evidence supports the effectiveness and safety of antipsychotics including aripiprazole, clozapine, haloperidol, lurasidone, molindone, olanzapine, risperidone, paliperidone, and quetiapine, while asenapine and ziprasidone do not seem superior to placebo (Lopez-Morinigo *et al.*, 2022). Due to delays from evidence base to drug approval, high off-label prescription rates in EOS have been identified (Lopez-Morinigo *et al.*, 2022). Second-generation antipsychotics (SGAs) are preferred for children and adolescents due to their more tolerable side-effect profile, but there is no clear evidence suggesting that SGAs are more effective than typical antipsychotics (Lee *et al.*, 2020). There is very limited randomized controlled trial (RCT) evidence for maintenance treatment on antipsychotics beyond eight weeks (Singapulli *et al.*, 2021), which is complemented by open-label studies (Lee *et al.*, 2020). The evidence on the use of long-acting injectable antipsychotics is also very limited and of low or very low quality in this age group; however, their use has a place in clinical practice when there are concerns about nonadherence (Hayes & Kyriakopoulos, 2018; Lee *et al.*, 2020; Benarous *et al.*, 2022). Clozapine is superior in efficacy compared to other antipsychotics in EOS with improvement in symptoms being maintained during long-term follow-up in open-label studies (Adnan *et al.*, 2022). Although clozapine has not been associated with any fatalities in this age group, due to the possibility of severe side effects requiring specialized monitoring, clinicians may hesitate to initiate this treatment. However, given its effectiveness, clozapine should be considered as an option in EOS patients who do not show good response to adequate trials of two other antipsychotics (Schneider *et al.*, 2014; National Institute for Health and Care Excellence, 2016). An adequate trial is generally defined as lasting at least six weeks on a therapeutic dose of an antipsychotic (Schneider *et al.*, 2014; National Institute for Health and Care Excellence, 2016; Howes *et al.*, 2017b). Treatment with clozapine is usually initiated in inpatient settings in the UK due to the monitoring requirements necessary for its use. In general, the therapeutic doses of antipsychotic medication in adolescents seem to be similar to those for adults. Treatment is usually initiated at a lower dose and is titrated more slowly. In any case of prescribing antipsychotics, there should be careful baseline physical evaluation, and monitoring and recording of effectiveness and side effects (National Institute for Health and Care Excellence, 2016). Treatment for comorbid conditions, such as mood stabilizers for bipolar disorder symptoms and selective serotonin reuptake inhibitors for anxiety and depression, should also be considered in EOP (Hayes & Kyriakopoulos, 2018). Treatment of children and adolescents with CHR-P with antipsychotics to prevent transition to psychosis is not recommended (National Institute for Health and Care Excellence, 2016; Catalan *et al.*, 2021; Lång *et al.*, 2022).

Tolerability of antipsychotics is an important factor in treatment decisions, given the similar effectiveness of first-line options. Relatively common side effects include weight gain, sedation, constipation, prolactin elevation, cardiovascular side effects, movement side effects, and metabolic changes, while rarer and more severe side effects may also be seen (Lee *et al.*, 2020). Severe side effects of clozapine include seizures, cardiac complications, neutropenia/agranulocytosis, and paralytic ileus (Schneider *et al.*, 2014; Adnan *et al.*, 2022). Although the latter has not been reported in EOS, it is important that clinicians are vigilant as it can be fatal in adults (Schneider *et al.*, 2014). The side-effect profile of antipsychotics varies among SGAs (Pagsberg *et al.*, 2017; Krause *et al.*, 2018; Arango *et al.*, 2020; Yee *et al.*, 2022); olanzapine and clozapine are the most likely to cause weight gain and metabolic changes, and aripiprazole and lurasidone the least likely; risperidone, paliperidone and, to some extent, olanzapine are associated with prolactin elevation. Use of olanzapine is generally not encouraged as the first choice due to its potential for more significant weight gain and metabolic syndrome (National Institute for Health and Care Excellence, 2016). The possibility of tardive dyskinesia needs to be regularly assessed; this side effect may be more common in Black ethnicity (Wonodi *et al.*, 2007), has been reported in up to 5.8% of children treated with mostly SGAs after one-year (Garcia-Amador *et al.*, 2015), and is potentially irreversible. Other than dose reduction and medication change, concomitant medications may be used to assist in the management of side effects. Metformin is an important option in that respect having RCT evidence on the reduction of antipsychotic-related overweight/obesity in CYP with EOP, while healthy lifestyle education alone was not sufficient (Correll *et al.*, 2020). Other medication that can be used for side effects includes anticholinergic medications for dystonias and parkinsonism, beta-blockers for akathisia, anticholinergic drops for sialorrhea, and medication for constipation or dyslipidemias (Stroup & Gray, 2018).

Psychosocial interventions

Psychosocial interventions alongside pharmacological treatment are important in EOP. The evidence base for their effectiveness is very limited in children and adolescents. Cognitive remediation therapy (CRT), cognitive behavioral therapy (CBT), a family intervention, and a psychoeducational problem-solving group intervention for adolescents and their families have been tested with RCTs in adolescence (Anagnostopoulou *et al.*, 2019; Müller *et al.*, 2020; Puig *et al.*, 2020). CRT was associated with improvement in cognitive function, while CBT and CRT seem to have a positive effect in psychosocial functioning. Psychotic symptoms appeared to not be significantly improved by treatment in most studies, with the exceptions of the small study by Müller and colleagues which showed some benefit in delusions and negative symptoms with the addition of CBT, and the study by Calvo *et al.* (2014) which showed benefits of the psychoeducational group in negative symptoms.

Early intervention, community rehabilitation, and transition to adult services

The implementation of evidence-based interventions for EOS spectrum disorders requires child and adolescent services organization incorporating early identification, timely treatment, ongoing psychiatric and psychosocial support, and effective transition to adult services. Early intervention in psychosis services have demonstrated evidence of effectiveness in the course and outcomes of psychotic disorders across the life span (Correll *et al.*, 2018) although studies with less positive outcomes have also been published (e.g. Hansen *et al.*, 2023). There is also some evidence specifically in early-onset cases (Thomson *et al.*, 2019). Community rehabilitation recovery-oriented programs for psychosis, including combinations of care coordination, cognitive rehabilitation, supported education and employment, and peer support, also have some evidence of effectiveness in the younger age group (Rouhakhtar & Schiffman, 2020). There seem to be overlaps in different components and overall structure of services supporting young people with early psychosis incorporating elements that have been found effective in adults. However, the need for developmentally appropriate services, tailored to the needs of children and adolescents has been acknowledged. Transition to adult services is associated with its own challenges. These include moving from family-oriented input to approaches where autonomy and self-sufficiency are emphasized, changes in legal frameworks around mental health, reduced resources and suboptimal communication, and less training and experience in managing neurodevelopmental comorbidities which are frequent in EOS (Arango *et al.*, 2022). Early liaison and detailed handover between adolescent and adult services and the devising of individualized care plans agreed with the young person and their family are among the important aspects of the transition.

Conclusions

EOS spectrum disorders are severe variants of the adult-onset conditions associated with greater morbidity and premorbid abnormalities, a higher familial risk, a more severe clinical course, and poorer outcome. Research and clinical management approaches on these conditions have progressed in the last few decades but significant gaps remain. Further research on the pathophysiology of early presentation, treatment approaches, side-effect reduction, and effective psychosocial interventions will promote the most favorable outcomes for affected CYP.

References

Addington, A. & Rapoport, J.L. (2009) The genetics of childhood-onset schizophrenia: when madness strikes the prepubescent. *Current Psychiatry Reports* **11**, 156–161.

Adnan, M. *et al.* (2022) Clozapine for management of childhood and adolescent-onset schizophrenia: a systematic review and meta-analysis. *Journal of Child and Adolescent Psychopharmacology* **32**, 2–11.

Ahn, K. *et al.* (2014) High rate of disease-related copy number variations in childhood onset schizophrenia. *Molecular Psychiatry* **19**, 568–572.

American Psychiatric Association (1980) *Diagnostic and Statistical Manual of Mental Disorders*, 3rd edn. American Psychiatric Association, Washington, DC.

American Psychiatric Association (2013) *Diagnostic and Statistical Manual of Mental Disorders*, 5th edn. American Psychiatric Association, Washington, DC.

Anagnostopoulou, N. *et al.* (2019) Psychological interventions in psychosis in children and adolescents: A systematic review. *European Child and Adolescent Psychiatry* **28**, 735–746.

Arango, C. *et al.* (2020) Lurasidone compared to other atypical antipsychotic monotherapies for adolescent schizophrenia: a systematic literature review and network meta-analysis. *European Child and Adolescent Psychiatry* **29**, 1195–1205.

Arango, C. *et al.* (2021) Risk and protective factors for mental disorders beyond genetics: an evidence-based atlas. *World Psychiatry* **20**, 417–436.

Arango, C. *et al.* (2022) The transition from adolescence to adulthood in patients with schizophrenia: Challenges, opportunities and recommendations. *European Neuropsychopharmacology* **59**, 45–55.

Bae, T. *et al.* (2022) Analysis of somatic mutations in 131 human brains reveals aging-associated hypermutability. *Science* **377**, 511–517.

Balaratnasingama, S. *et al.* (2015) Normal personality, personality disorder and psychosis: Current views and future perspectives. *Current Opinion in Psychiatry* **28**, 30–34.

Barnes, T.R. (1989) A rating scale for drug-induced Akathisia. *British Journal of Psychiatry* **154**, 672–676.

Barneveld, P.S. *et al.* (2011) Overlap of autistic and schizotypal traits in adolescents with autism spectrum disorders. *Schizophrenia Research* **126**, 231–236.

Barth, C. *et al.* (2022) In vivo white matter microstructure in adolescents with early-onset psychosis: a multi-site mega-analysis. *Molecular Psychiatry* **28**, 1159–1169. doi:10.1038/s41380-022-01901-3.

Beckmann, D. *et al.* (2020) Substance-induced psychosis in youth. *Child and Adolescent Psychiatric Clinics of North America* **29**, 131–143.

Benarous, X. *et al.* (2022) Efficacy, tolerability, and acceptance of long-lasting antipsychotics in children and adolescents: a systematic review. *Journal of Child and Adolescent Psychopharmacology* **32**, 312–327.

Bora, E. & Murray, R.M. (2014) Meta-analysis of cognitive deficits in ultra-high risk to psychosis and first-episode psychosis: Do the cognitive deficits progress over, or after, the onset of psychosis? *Schizophrenia Bulletin* **40**, 744–755.

Bourgou, S. *et al.* (2016) Theory of mind in adolescents with early-onset schizophrenia: Correlations with clinical assessment and executive functions. *Acta Neuropsychiatrica* **28**, 232–238.

Brandizzi, M. *et al.* (2014) Self-reported attenuated psychotic-like experiences in help-seeking adolescents and their association with age, functioning and psychopathology. *Schizophrenia Research* **160**, 110–117.

Brownstein, C.A. *et al.* (2022) Similar rates of deleterious copy number variants in early-onset psychosis and autism spectrum disorder. *The American Journal of Psychiatry* **179**, 853–861.

Buitelaar, J.K. & van der Gaag, R.J. (1998) Diagnostic rules for children with PDD-NOS and multiple complex developmental disorder. *Journal of Child Psychology and Psychiatry* **39**, 911–919.

Byrial, P. *et al.* (2022) Motor impairments in early onset schizophrenia. *Early Intervention in Psychiatry* **16**, 481–491.

Byrial, P. *et al.* (2023) Motor function in early onset schizophrenia-a 2-year follow-up study. *Early Intervention in Psychiatry* **17**, 910–920. doi:10.1111/eip.13383.

Calvo, A. *et al.* (2014) Intervention for adolescents with early-onset psychosis and their families: a randomized controlled trial. *Journal of the American Academy of Child and Adolescent Psychiatry* **53**, 688–696.

Caplan, R. *et al.* (2000) Thought disorder in childhood schizophrenia: replication and update of concept. *Journal of the American Academy of Child and Adolescent Psychiatry* **39**, 771–778.

Carlson, G.A. & Pataki, C. (2020) Affective disorders with psychosis in youth: A-an update. *Child and Adolescent Psychiatric Clinics of North America* **29**, 91–102.

Castellani, C.A. *et al.* (2017) Post-zygotic genomic changes in glutamate and dopamine pathway genes may explain discordance of monozygotic twins for schizophrenia. *Clinical and Translational Medicine* **6**, 43.

Catalan, A. *et al.* (2021) Annual research review: prevention of psychosis in adolescents - systematic review and meta-analysis of advances in detection, prognosis and intervention. *Journal of Child Psychology and Psychiatry* **62**, 657–673.

Clemmensen, L. *et al.* (2012) A systematic review of the long-term outcome of early onset schizophrenia. *BMC Psychiatry* **12**, 150.

Cohen, D.J. *et al.* (1986) Issues in the classification of pervasive and other developmental disorders: toward DSM-IV. *Journal of the American Academy of Child and Adolescent Psychiatry* **25**, 213–220.

Correll, C.U. *et al.* (2018) Comparison of early intervention services vs treatment as usual for early-phase psychosis: a systematic review, meta-analysis, and meta-regression. *JAMA Psychiatry* **75**, 555–565.

Correll, C.U. *et al.* (2020) Metformin add-on vs. antipsychotic switch vs. continued antipsychotic treatment plus healthy lifestyle education in overweight or obese youth with severe mental illness: Results from the IMPACT trial. *World Psychiatry* **19**, 69–80.

Correll, C.U. *et al.* (2022) Treatment approaches for first episode and early-phase schizophrenia in adolescents and young adults: a Delphi Consensus Report from Europe. *Neuropsychiatric Disease and Treatment* **18**, 201–219.

Croft, J. *et al.* (2019) Association of trauma type, age of exposure, and frequency in childhood and adolescence with psychotic experiences in early adulthood. *JAMA Psychiatry* **76**, 79–86.

David, C.N. *et al.* (2011) Childhood onset schizophrenia: High rate of visual hallucinations. *Journal of the American Academy of Child and Adolescent Psychiatry* **50**, 681–686.e3.

Davies, C. *et al.* (2020) Prenatal and perinatal risk and protective factors for psychosis: a systematic review and meta-analysis. *The Lancet Psychiatry* **7**, 399–410.

Debost, J.C. *et al.* (2019) Childhood infections and schizophrenia: the impact of parental SES and mental illness, and childhood adversities. *Brain, Behavior, and Immunity* **81**, 341–347.

Debost, J.P.G. *et al.* (2022) Genetic and psychosocial influence on the association between early childhood infections and later psychiatric disorders. *Acta Psychiatrica Scandinavica* **146**, 406–419.

Del Rey-Mejías, Á. *et al.* (2015) Functional deterioration from the premorbid period to 2 years after the first episode of psychosis in early-onset psychosis. *European Child and Adolescent Psychiatry* **24**, 1447–1459.

Díaz-Caneja, C.M. *et al.* (2015) Predictors of outcome in early-onset psychosis: a systematic review. *NPJ Schizophrenia* **1**, 14005.

Dickson, H. *et al.* (2020) Academic achievement and schizophrenia: a systematic meta-analysis. *Psychological Medicine* **50**, 1949–1965.

Downs, J. *et al.* (2019) Negative symptoms in early-onset psychosis and their association with antipsychotic treatment failure. *Schizophrenia Bulletin* **45**, 69–79.

Driver, D.I. *et al.* (2020) Childhood-onset schizophrenia and early-onset schizophrenia spectrum disorders: an update. *Child and Adolescent Psychiatric Clinics of North America* **29**, 71–90.

Eranti, S.V. *et al.* (2013) Gender difference in age at onset of schizophrenia: a meta-analysis. *Psychological Medicine* **43**, 155–167.

Fernandez, A. *et al.* (2019) Childhood-onset schizophrenia: a systematic overview of its genetic heterogeneity from classical studies to the genomic era. *Frontiers in Genetics* **10**, 1137.

Fields, J.H. *et al.* (1994) Assessing positive and negative symptoms in children and adolescents. *American Journal of Psychiatry* **151**, 249–253.

Forsyth, J.K. & Asarnow, R.F. (2020) Genetics of childhood-onset schizophrenia 2019 update. *Child and Adolescent Psychiatric Clinics of North America* **29**, 157–170.

Fraguas, D. *et al.* (2016) Progressive brain changes in children and adolescents with early-onset psychosis: a meta-analysis of longitudinal MRI studies. *Schizophrenia Research* **173**, 132–139. doi:10.1016/j.schres.2014.12.022.

Frangou, S. (2013) Neurocognition in early-onset schizophrenia. *Child and Adolescent Psychiatric Clinics of North America* **22**, 715–726.

Fusar-Poli, P. (2017) The clinical high–risk state for psychosis (CHR–P), version II. *Schizophrenia Bulletin* **43**, 44–47.

Fusar-Poli, P. & Salazar de Pablo, G. (2022) No meta-analytic effect of age on probability of developing psychosis in individuals at clinical high risk. *Journal of the American Academy of Child and Adolescent Psychiatry* **61**, 731–732.

Galitzer, H. *et al.* (2021) Functional outcomes and patient satisfaction following inpatient treatment for childhood-onset schizophrenia spectrum disorders vs non-psychotic disorders in children in the United Kingdom. *Early Intervention in Psychiatry* **15**, 412–419.

Garcia-Amador, M. *et al.* (2015) Neurological adverse effects of antipsychotics in children and adolescents. *Journal of Clinical Psychopharmacology* **35**, 686–693.

Gin, K. *et al.* (2018) Childhood unusual experiences in community child and adolescent mental health services in south east London: prevalence and impact. *Schizophrenia Research* **195**, 93–96.

Green, M.F. *et al.* (2008) Social cognition in schizophrenia: an NIMH workshop on definitions, assessment, and research opportunities. *Schizophrenia Bulletin* **34**, 1211–1220.

Guloksuz, S. *et al.* (2018) The complexities of evaluating the exposome in psychiatry: a data-driven illustration of challenges and some propositions for amendments. *Schizophrenia Bulletin* **44**, 1175–1179.

Guo, S. *et al.* (2021) Genome wide association study identifies four loci for early onset schizophrenia. *Translational Psychiatry* **11**, 248.

Gurholt, T.P. *et al.* (2022) Intracranial and subcortical volumes in adolescents with early-onset psychosis: a multisite mega-analysis from the ENIGMA consortium. *Human Brain Mapping* **43**, 373–384.

Gurillo, P. *et al.* (2015) Does tobacco use cause psychosis? Systematic review and meta-analysis. *The Lancet Psychiatry* **2**, 718–725.

Hansen, H.G. *et al.* (2023) Clinical recovery and long-term association of specialized early intervention services vs treatment as usual among individuals with first-episode schizophrenia spectrum disorder: 20-year follow-up of the OPUS trial. *JAMA Psychiatry* **80**, 371–379.

Harvey, P.D. & Isner, E.C. (2020) Cognition, social cognition, and functional capacity in early-onset schizophrenia. *Child and Adolescent Psychiatric Clinics of North America* **29**, 171–182.

Hasan, A. *et al.* (2020) Cannabis use and psychosis: a review of reviews. *European Archives of Psychiatry and Clinical Neuroscience* **270**, 403–412.

Hayes, D. & Kyriakopoulos, M. (2018) Dilemmas in the treatment of early-onset first-episode psychosis. *Therapeutic Advances in Psychopharmacology* **8**, 231–239.

Hedges, E.P. *et al.* (2022) Meta-analysis of longitudinal neurocognitive performance in people at clinical high-risk for psychosis. *Psychological Medicine* **52**, 2009–2016.

Hollis, C. (1995) Child and adolescent (juvenile onset) schizophrenia: a case control study of premorbid developmental impairments. *British Journal of Psychiatry* **166**, 489–495.

Hollis, C. (2000) Adult outcomes of child- and adolescent-onset schizophrenia: diagnostic stability and predictive validity. *American Journal of Psychiatry* **157**, 1652–1659.

Holmén, A. *et al.* (2012) Executive function in early- and adult-onset schizophrenia. *Schizophrenia Research* **142**, 177–182.

Howes, O. *et al.* (2017b) Treatment-resistant schizophrenia: treatment response and resistance in psychosis (TRRIP) working group consensus guidelines on diagnosis and terminology. *American Journal of Psychiatry* **174**, 216–229.

Howes, O.D. & Onwordi, E.C. (2023) The synaptic hypothesis of schizophrenia version III: A master mechanism. *Molecular Psychiatry* **28**, 1843–1856. doi:10.1038/s41380-023-02043-w.

Howes, O.D. *et al.* (2017a) The role of genes, stress, and dopamine in the development of schizophrenia. *Biological Psychiatry* **81**, 9–20.

Ioakeimidis, V. *et al.* (2020) A meta-analysis of structural and functional brain abnormalities in early-onset schizophrenia. *Schizophrenia Bulletin Open* **1**. doi:10.1093/schizbullopen/sgaa016.

Ioakeimidis, V. *et al.* (2022) Functional neurodevelopment of working memory in early-onset schizophrenia: a longitudinal FMRI study. *Schizophrenia Research Cognition* **30**, 100268.

Ivanov, D. *et al.* (2003) Chromosome 22q11 deletions, velo-cardio-facial syndrome and early-onset psychosis: molecular genetic study. *British Journal of Psychiatry* **183**, 409–413.

Jääskeläinen, E. *et al.* (2018) Epidemiology of psychotic depression - systematic review and meta-analysis. *Psychological Medicine* **48**, 905–918.

Janssen, J. *et al.* (2009) Gyral and sulcal cortical thinning in adolescents with first episode early-onset psychosis. *Biological Psychiatry* **66**, 1047–1054.

Janssen, J. *et al.* (2014) Cortical morphology of adolescents with bipolar disorder and with schizophrenia. *Schizophrenia Research* **158**, 91–99.

Jepsen, J.R.M. *et al.* (2022) Cross–sectional associations between adaptive functioning and social cognitive and neurocognitive functions in adolescents with first-episode, early-onset schizophrenia spectrum disorders. *Development and Psychopathology* **9**, 1–11.

Jerrell, J.M. & McIntyre, R.S. (2016) Factors differentiating childhood-onset and adolescent-onset schizophrenia: a claims database study. *Primary Care Companion for CNS Disorders* **18**. doi:10.4088/PCC.15m01901.

Johnson, M.B. & Stevens, B. (2018) Pruning hypothesis comes of age. *Nature* **554**, 438–439.

Kaushik, A. *et al.* (2016) The stigma of mental illness in children and adolescents: a systematic review. *Psychiatry Research* **243**, 469–494.

Kay, S.R. *et al.* (1987) The positive and negative syndrome scale (PANSS) for schizophrenia. *Schizophrenia Bulletin* **13**, 261–276.

Kelleher, I. *et al.* (2012) Prevalence of psychotic symptoms in childhood and adolescence: a systematic review and meta-analysis of population-based studies. *Psychological Medicine* **42**, 1857–1863.

Kelleher, I. *et al.* (2013) Childhood trauma and psychosis in a prospective cohort study: Cause, effect, and directionality. *The American Journal of Psychiatry* **170**, 734–741.

Kelleher, I. *et al.* (2014) Psychotic experiences in a mental health clinic sample: implications for suicidality, multimorbidity and functioning. *Psychological Medicine* **44**, 1615–1624.

Khachadourian, V. *et al.* (2022) Reprint of: Advanced paternal age and risk of schizophrenia in offspring: review of epidemiological findings and potential mechanisms. *Schizophrenia Research* **247**, 84–91.

Khandaker, G.M. *et al.* (2012) Childhood infection and adult schizophrenia: a meta-analysis of population-based studies. *Schizophrenia Research* **139**, 161–168.

Khandaker, G.M. *et al.* (2014) Association of serum interleukin 6 and C-reactive protein in childhood with depression and psychosis in young adult life: A population-based longitudinal study. *JAMA Psychiatry* **71**, 1121–1128.

Kirkbride, J.B. *et al.* (2017) Ethnic minority status, age-at-immigration and psychosis risk in rural environments: evidence from the SEPEA study. *Schizophrenia Bulletin* **43**, 1251–1261.

Kolvin, I. *et al.* (1971) Studies in the childhood psychoses. II. The phenomenology of childhood psychoses. *British Journal of Psychiatry* **118**, 385–395.

Kraan, T. *et al.* (2015) Trauma and recent life events in individuals at ultra high risk for psychosis: Review and meta-analysis. *Schizophrenia Research* **161**, 143–149.

Krause, M. *et al.* (2018) Efficacy, acceptability, and tolerability of antipsychotics in children and adolescents with schizophrenia: a network meta-analysis. *European Neuropsychopharmacology* **28**, 6596–6574.

Kulaga, S.S. & Miller, C.W.T. (2021) Viral respiratory infections and psychosis: a review of the literature and the implications of COVID-19. *Neuroscience and Biobehavioral Reviews* **127**, 520–530.

Kyriakopoulos, M. & Frangou, S. (2007) Pathophysiology of early onset schizophrenia. *International Review of Psychiatry* **19**, 315–324.

Kyriakopoulos, M. *et al.* (2015) Determination of psychosis-related clinical profiles in children with autism spectrum disorders using latent class analysis. *European Child and Adolescent Psychiatry* **24**, 301–307.

Lång, U. & Kelleher, I. (2022) Dr. Lång *et al.* Reply. *Journal of the American Academy of Child and Adolescent Psychiatry* **61**, 733–734.

Lång, U. *et al.* (2022) Systematic review and meta-analysis: psychosis risk in children and adolescents with an at-risk mental state. *Journal of the American Academy of Child and Adolescent Psychiatry* **61**, 615–625.

Lee, E.S. *et al.* (2020) Psychopharmacologic treatment of schizophrenia in adolescents and children. *Child and Adolescent Psychiatric Clinics of North America* **29**, 183–210.

Li, D. *et al.* (2017) Comparing the ability of cognitive and affective theory of mind in adolescent onset schizophrenia. *Neuropsychiatric Disease and Treatment* **13**, 937–945.

Lichtenstein, P. *et al.* (2009) Common genetic determinants of schizophrenia and bipolar disorder in Swedish families: a population-based study. *The Lancet* **373**, 234–239.

Linscott, R.J. & van Os, J. (2013) An updated and conservative systematic review and meta-analysis of epidemiological evidence on psychotic experiences in children and adults: on the pathway from proneness to persistence to dimensional expression across mental disorders. *Psychological Medicine* **43**, 1133–1149.

Loewy, R.L. *et al.* (2019) Childhood trauma and clinical high risk for psychosis. *Schizophrenia Research* **205**, 10–14.

Lopez-Morinigo, J.D. *et al.* (2022) Pharmacological treatment of early-onset schizophrenia: a critical review, evidence-based clinical guidance and unmet needs. *Pharmacopsychiatry* **55**, 233–245.

Maijer, K. *et al.* (2018) Auditory hallucinations across the lifespan: a systematic review and meta-analysis. *Psychological Medicine* **48**, 879–888.

Malaspina, D. *et al.* (2001) Advancing paternal age and the risk of schizophrenia. *Archives of General Psychiatry* **58**, 361–367.

Marshall, C.R. *et al.* (2017) Contribution of copy number variants to schizophrenia from a genome-wide study of 41,321 subjects. *Nature Genetics* **49**, 27–35.

McCutcheon, R.A. *et al.* (2020) Dopamine and glutamate in schizophrenia: biology, symptoms and treatment. *World Psychiatry* **19**, 15–33.

McCutcheon, R.A. *et al.* (2023) Cognitive impairment in schizophrenia: aetiology, pathophysiology, and treatment. *Molecular Psychiatry* **28**, 1902–1918. doi:10.1038/s41380-023-01949-9.

McGrath, J. *et al.* (2008) Schizophrenia: a concise overview of incidence, prevalence, and mortality. *Epidemiologic Reviews* **30**, 67–76.

McGrath, J.J. *et al.* (2014) A comprehensive assessment of parental age and psychiatric disorders. *JAMA Psychiatry* **71**, 301–309.

Mehra, C. *et al.* (2019) Childhood disintegrative disorder and autism spectrum disorder: a systematic review. *Developmental Medicine and Child Neurology* **61**, 523–534.

Merritt, J. *et al.* (2020) Medical etiologies of secondary psychosis in children and adolescents. *Child and Adolescent Psychiatric Clinics of North America* **29**, 29–42.

Messias, E.L. *et al.* (2007) Epidemiology of schizophrenia: review of findings and myths. *The Psychiatric Clinics of North America* **30**, 323–338.

Metcalf, S.A. *et al.* (2017) Serum C-reactive protein in adolescence and risk of schizophrenia in adulthood: a prospective birth cohort study. *Brain, Behavior, and Immunity* **59**, 253–259.

Miller, B. *et al.* (2011) Meta-analysis of paternal age and schizophrenia risk in male versus female offspring. *Schizophrenia Bulletin* **37**, 1039–1047.

Müller, H. *et al.* (2020) Cognitive behavioral therapy in adolescents with early-onset psychosis: a randomized controlled pilot study. *European Child and Adolescent Psychiatry* **29**, 1011–1022.

Müller, N. (2018) Inflammation in schizophrenia: pathogenetic aspects and therapeutic considerations. *Schizophrenia Bulletin* **44**, 973–982.

Murray, R.M. *et al.* (2017) 30 years on: how the neurodevelopmental hypothesis of schizophrenia morphed into the developmental risk factor model of psychosis. *Schizophrenia Bulletin* **43**, 1190–1196.

Nair, A. *et al.* (2020) A review of default mode network connectivity and its association with social cognition in adolescents with autism spectrum disorder and early-onset psychosis. *Frontiers in Psychiatry* **11**, 614.

Nakamura, T. & Takata, A. (2023) The molecular pathology of schizophrenia: an overview of existing knowledge and new directions for future research. *Molecular Psychiatry* **28**, 1868–1889.

National Institute for Health and Care Excellence (2016) Psychosis and schizophrenia in children and young people: recognition and management: Clinical guideline CG155 NICE 2013; updated: 2016. National Institute for Health and Care Excellence (NICE), London. Available: www.nice.org.uk/guidance/cg155 [19 November 2024].

Nelson, B. & McGorry, P. (2020) The prodrome of psychotic disorders: identification, prediction, and preventive treatment. *Child and Adolescent Psychiatric Clinics of North America* **29**, 57–69.

Øie, M.G. *et al.* (2021) Cognitive performance in early-onset schizophrenia and attention-deficit/hyperactivity disorder: a 25-year follow-up study. *Frontiers in Psychology* **11**, 606365.

Owen, M.J. *et al.* (2016) Schizophrenia. *The Lancet* **388**, 86–97.

Padmanabhan, J.L. *et al.* (2017) The "polyenviromic risk score": aggregating environmental risk factors predicts conversion to psychosis in familial high–risk subjects. *Schizophrenia Research* **181**, 17–22.

Pagsberg, A.K. *et al.* (2017) Acute antipsychotic treatment of children and adolescents with schizophrenia-spectrum disorders: a systematic review and network meta-analysis. *Journal of the American Academy of Child and Adolescent Psychiatry* **56**, 191–202.

Payá, B. *et al.* (2013) Premorbid impairments in early-onset psychosis: differences between patients with schizophrenia and bipolar disorder. *Schizophrenia Research* **146**, 103–110.

Pence, A.Y. *et al.* (2022) Gender differences in the association between environment and psychosis. *Schizophrenia Research* **243**, 120–137.

Pencer, A. *et al.* (2005) Outcome of a first episode of psychosis in adolescence: a 2-year follow-up. *Psychiatry Research* **133**, 35–43.

Pilowsky, T. *et al.* (2000) Theory of mind abilities of children with schizophrenia, children with autism, and normally developing children. *Schizophrenia Research* **42**, 145–155.

Pina-Camacho, L. *et al.* (2016) Autism spectrum disorder and schizophrenia: boundaries and uncertainties. *BJPsych Advances* **22**, 316–324.

Pina-Camacho, L. *et al.* (2022) Cortical thinning over two years after first-episode psychosis depends on age of onset. *Schizophrenia (Heidelb)* **8**, 20.

Pontillo, M. *et al.* (2018) All that glitters is not gold: prevalence and relevance of psychotic-like experiences in clinical sample of children and adolescents aged 8–17 years old. *Early Intervention in Psychiatry* **12**, 702–707.

Pries, L.K. *et al.* (2019) Estimating exposome score for schizophrenia using predictive modeling approach in two independent samples: the results from the EUGEI study. *Schizophrenia Bulletin* **45**, 960–965.

Pries, L.K. *et al.* (2020) Predictive performance of exposome score for schizophrenia in the general population. *Schizophrenia Bulletin* **47**, 277–283.

Puig, O. *et al.* (2020) Early- versus adult-onset schizophrenia as a predictor of response to neuroscience-informed cognitive training. *Journal of Clinical Psychiatry* **81**, 18m12369.

Rabinowitz, J. *et al.* (2007) A population based elaboration of the role of age of onset on the course of schizophrenia. *Schizophrenia Research* **88**, 96–101.

Rapoport, J. *et al.* (2009) Autism spectrum disorders and childhood-onset schizophrenia: clinical and biological contributions to a relation revisited. *Journal of the American Academy of Child and Adolescent Psychiatry* **48**, 10–18.

Rapoport, J.L. *et al.* (1985) Rating scales and assessment instruments for use in paediatric psychopharmacology research. *Psychological Bulletin* **21**, 713–1111.

Reichenberg, A. *et al.* (2005) Elaboration on premorbid intellectual performance in schizophrenia: premorbid intellectual decline and risk for schizophrenia. *Archives of General Psychiatry* **62**, 1297–1304.

Remberk, B. *et al.* (2014) Adolescent insanity revisited: course and outcome in early-onset schizophrenia spectrum psychoses in an 8-year follow-up study. *Comprehensive Psychiatry* **55**, 1174–1181.

Remberk, B. *et al.* (2015) Which aspects of long-term outcome are predicted by positive and negative symptoms in early-onset psychosis? An exploratory eight-year follow-up study. *Psychopathology* **48**, 47–55.

Remschmidt, H. *et al.* (2007) Forty-two-years later: the outcome of childhood-onset schizophrenia. *Journal of Neural Transmission* **114**, 505–512.

Roffman, J.L. *et al.* (2008) MTHFR 677C → T genotype disrupts prefrontal function in schizophrenia through an interaction with COMT 158Val → met. *Proceedings of the National Academy of Sciences of the United States of America* **105**, 17573–17578.

Rouhakhtar, P.R. & Schiffman, J. (2020) Community rehabilitation for youth with psychosis spectrum disorders. *Child and Adolescent Psychiatric Clinics of North America* **29**, 225–239.

Rutter, M. (1972) Childhood schizophrenia reconsidered. *Journal of Autism and Childhood Schizophrenia* **2**, 315–337.

Sağlam, Y. *et al.* (2022) Neurocognitive and social cognitive impairments in remission and symptomatic states of early-onset schizophrenia spectrum disorders. *European Child and Adolescent Psychiatry* **32**, 1621–1631. doi:10.1007/s00787-022-01977-w.

Salazar de Pablo, G. *et al.* (2021) Probability of transition to psychosis in individuals at clinical high risk: an updated meta-analysis. *JAMA Psychiatry* **78**, 970–978.

Samartzis, L. *et al.* (2014) White matter alterations in early stages of schizophrenia: a systematic review of diffusion tensor imaging studies. *Journal of Neuroimaging* **24**, 101–110.

Schimmelmann, B.G. *et al.* (2013) Treatment of adolescents with early-onset schizophrenia spectrum disorders: in search of a rational, evidence-informed approach. *Current Opinion in Psychiatry* **26**, 219–230.

Schneider, C. *et al.* (2014) Systematic review of the efficacy and tolerability of clozapine in the treatment of youth with early onset schizophrenia. *European Psychiatry* **29**, 1–10.

Seiferth, N.Y. *et al.* (2009) Neuronal correlates of facial emotion discrimination in early onset schizophrenia. *Neuropsychopharmacology* **34**, 477–487.

Shaffer, D. *et al.* (1983) A children's global assessment scale (CGAS). *Archives of General Psychiatry* **40**, 1228–1231.

Sideli, L. *et al.* (2020) Childhood adversity and psychosis: a systematic review of bio-psycho-social mediators and moderators. *Psychological Medicine* **50**, 1761–1782.

Simpson, G. & Angus, J.S.W. (1970) A rating scale for extrapyramidal side effects. *Acta Psychiatrica Scandinavica* **212**, 9–11.

Singappuli, P. *et al.* (2021) Antipsychotic long-term treatment in children and young people: a systematic review and meta-analysis of efficacy and tolerability across mental health and neurodevelopmental conditions. *CNS Spectrums* **27**, 570–587.

Singh, T. *et al.* (2022) Rare coding variants in ten genes confer substantial risk for schizophrenia. *Nature* **604**, 509–516.

Skikic, M. & Arriola, J.A. (2020) First episode psychosis medical workup: evidence-informed recommendations and introduction to a clinically guided approach. *Child and Adolescent Psychiatric Clinics of North America* **29**, 15–28.

Smith, L.M. *et al.* (2017) Characterizing the experience of auditory verbal hallucinations and accompanying delusions in individuals with a diagnosis of bipolar disorder: a systematic review. *Bipolar Disorders* **19**, 417–433.

Solmi, M. *et al.* (2022) Age at onset of mental disorders worldwide: large-scale meta-analysis of 192 epidemiological studies. *Molecular Psychiatry* **27**, 281–295.

Stanton, K.J. *et al.* (2020) Childhood trauma and psychosis: an updated review. *Child and Adolescent Psychiatric Clinics of North America* **29**, 115–129.

Stentebjerg-Olesen, M. *et al.* (2016) Clinical characteristics and predictors of outcome of schizophrenia-spectrum psychosis in children and adolescents: a systematic review. *Journal of Child and Adolescent Psychopharmacology* **26**, 410–427.

Stilo, S.A. & Murray, R.M. (2019) Non-genetic factors in schizophrenia. *Current Psychiatry Reports* **21**, 100.

Stroup, T.S. & Gray, N. (2018) Management of common adverse effects of antipsychotic medications. *World Psychiatry* **17**, 341.

Sullivan, P.F. *et al.* (2003) Schizophrenia as a complex trait: Evidence from a meta-analysis of twin studies. *Archives of General Psychiatry* **60**, 1187–1192.

Thomson, A. *et al.* (2019) Treatment outcomes and associations in an adolescent-specific early intervention for psychosis service. *Early Intervention in Psychiatry* **13**, 707–714.

Thormodsen, R. *et al.* (2013) Age-related cortical thickness differences in adolescents with early-onset schizophrenia compared with healthy adolescents. *Psychiatry Research* **214**, 190–196.

Tiffin, P.A. & Kitchen, C.E.W. (2015) Incidence and 12-month outcome of childhood non-affective psychoses: British national surveillance study. *The British Journal of Psychiatry* **206**, 517–518.

Tin, L.N.W. *et al.* (2018) High-functioning autism patients share similar but more severe impairments in verbal theory of mind than schizophrenia patients. *Psychological Medicine* **48**, 1264–1273.

Trovão, L.O. *et al.* (2022) Early trauma and schizophrenia onset: preliminary results of an outpatient cohort in Brazil. *Trends in Psychiatry and Psychotherapy* **44**, e20200024.

Trubetskoy, V. *et al.* (2022) Mapping genomic loci implicates genes and synaptic biology in schizophrenia. *Nature* **604**, 502–508.

Tyson, J.W., Jr. *et al.* (2020) Assessing youth with psychotic experiences: a phenomenological approach. *Child and Adolescent Psychiatric Clinics of North America* **29**, 1–13.

Uggerby, P. *et al.* (2011) Characteristics and predictors of long-term institutionalization in patients with schizophrenia. *Schizophrenia Research* **131**, 120–126.

van Erp, T.G. *et al.* (2016) Subcortical brain volume abnormalities in 2,028 individuals with schizophrenia and 2,540 healthy controls via the ENIGMA consortium. *Molecular Psychiatry* **21**, 585.

Vares, M. *et al.* (2010) Association between methylenetetrahydrofolate reductase (MTHFR) C677T polymorphism and age of onset in schizophrenia. *American Journal of Medical Genetics. Part B, Neuropsychiatric Genetics* **153b**, 610–618.

Varese, F. *et al.* (2012) Childhood adversities increase the risk of psychosis: a meta-analysis of patient-control, prospective- and cross-sectional cohort studies. *Schizophrenia Bulletin* **38**, 661–671.

Vassos, E. *et al.* (2020) The Maudsley environmental risk score for psychosis. *Psychological Medicine* **50**, 2213–2220.

Vernal, D.L. *et al.* (2020) Long-term outcome of early-onset compared to adult-onset schizophrenia: a nationwide Danish register study. *Schizophrenia Research* **220**, 123–129.

Vigo, L. *et al.* (2019) Shared psychotic disorder in children and young people: a systematic review. *European Child and Adolescent Psychiatry* **28**, 1555–1566.

Voets, N.L. *et al.* (2008) Evidence for abnormalities of cortical development in adolescent-onset schizophrenia. *NeuroImage* **43**, 665–675.

Vourdas, A. *et al.* (2003) Increased developmental deviance and premorbid dysfunction in early onset schizophrenia. *Schizophrenia Research* **62**, 13–22.

Wahbeh, M.H. & Avramopoulos, D. (2021) Gene–environment interactions in schizophrenia: a literature review. *Genes (Basel)* **12**, 1850.

Wang, S.H. *et al.* (2019) Advanced paternal age and early onset of schizophrenia in sporadic cases: not confounded by parental polygenic risk for schizophrenia. *Biological Psychiatry* **86**, 56–64.

Wonodi, I. *et al.* (2007) Tardive dyskinesia in children treated with atypical antipsychotic medications. *Movement Disorders* **22**, 1777–1782.

World Health Organization (1977) *Manual of the International Statistical Classification of Diseases, Injuries, and Causes of Death*: based on the recommendations of the ninth revision conference,

1975, and adopted by the Twenty-ninth World Health Assembly, 1975 revision. World Health Organization (WHO), Geneva, Switzerland.

World Health Organization (2019) *International Statistical Classification of Diseases and Related Health*, 11th edn. World Health Organization (WHO), Geneva, Switzerland.

Wray, N.R. & Gottesman, I.I. (2012) Using summary data from the Danish National Registers to estimate heritabilities for schizophrenia, bipolar disorder, and major depressive disorder. *Frontiers in Genetics* **3**, 118.

Xu, L. *et al.* (2020) Predictors of outcome in early onset schizophrenia: a 10-year follow-up study. *BMC Psychiatry* **20**, 67.

Yee, C.S. *et al.* (2022) Comparative efficacy and tolerability of antipsychotics for juvenile psychotic disorders: a systematic review and network meta-analysis. *Journal of Clinical Psychopharmacology* **42**, 198–208.

B: Emotional

CHAPTER 57

Disorders of attachment and social engagement related to deprivation

Julianna Finelli and Charles H. Zeanah
Department of Psychiatry and Behavioral Sciences, Tulane University School of Medicine, New Orleans, LA, USA

Although attachment disorders have been described in the literature since the 1940s and have been defined by specified criteria in psychiatric nosologies since the 1990s, they have been studied systematically only recently. The vast majority of the research related to understanding attachment disorders has appeared since the 2000s. Controversies remain, but there is at least a growing consensus about the manifestations of the disorders in early childhood.

The purpose of this chapter is to review what is known about reactive attachment disorder (RAD) and disinhibited social engagement disorder (DSED), especially in the context of severe deprivation, and in light of emerging research. Although different or more expanded versions of attachment disorders have been proposed by some (Zeanah & Boris, 2000; van IJzendoorn & Bakermans-Kranenburg, 2002; Minnis *et al.*, 2006), these alternative approaches are less well studied, and we have focused our review primarily on the traditional conceptualization of the disorders, as defined in contemporary nosologies.

Definitions

The term "attachment" itself has been used variably to refer to different constructs, and this has led to confusion in the literature. Bowlby, who developed attachment theory, asserted that attachment referred to the young child's strong disposition "to seek proximity to and contact with a specific figure and to do so in certain situations, notably when . . . frightened, tired, or ill. The disposition to behave in this way is an attribute of the child, an attribute which changes only slowly over time and which is unaffected by the situation of the moment" (Bowlby, 1982, p. 371). Therefore, we describe attachment as a tendency for human infants to seek comfort, support, nurturance, and protection preferentially from one or more caregivers. This is sometimes referred to as "focused," "preferred," "selective," or "discriminated" attachment between child and parent. Because the parent–child attachment relationship is asymmetrical, the young child is the seeker and the adult caregiver/parent is the provider of care in the attachment relationship (see also Chapter 6).

The tendency to approach an adult is believed to be stimulated by increased levels of negative arousal, accompanied by emotions such as distress, fear, and frustration. These increase the child's motivation to seek support and comfort from someone they have learned is reliably available to provide it. In attachment terms, the child seeks proximity in order to attain a feeling of security from the physical closeness and emotional availability of a trusted adult caregiver. Attachment behaviors are those that the child displays that are designed to promote physical proximity to attachment figures, such as clinging, reaching for, crawling to, walking to, or crying. Attachment relationships involving caregivers and young children range from healthy to unhealthy and may be different with different caregivers. That is, because attachment is a relationship construct rather than a trait in the child, the qualitative features of the relationship are co-constructed by parent and child through recurrent patterns of interaction over time.

Under species-typical rearing conditions, virtually all children form attachments to their caregivers, so a significant challenge in determining clinical "caseness" is the very ubiquity of attachment in young children. If a child has an established unhealthy attachment to one of their primary caregivers, a diagnosis of relationship-specific disorder of infancy and early childhood can be considered. This disorder is defined in a nosology for early childhood disorders, DC:0-5 (ZERO TO THREE, 2005) that is not recognized in the *Diagnostic and Statistical Manual of Mental Disorders*, 5th edition (DSM-5; American Psychiatric Association, 2013) or the *International*

Rutter's Child and Adolescent Psychiatry and Psychology, Seventh Edition.
Edited by Anita Thapar, Daniel S. Pine, Samuele Cortese, Cathy Creswell, Tamsin J. Ford, James F. Leckman, and Argyris Stringaris.

Companion website: www.wiley.com/go/thapar/rutterspsych7

Box 57.1 Definitions

Attachment
A term that describes an infant/young child's tendency to seek comfort, support, nurturance, and protection selectively from a small number of caregivers (specifically, primary caregivers on whom they have learned they can rely). This tendency is believed to be so strong that only in highly atypical and maladaptive caregiving environments do attachments fail to develop.

Attachment behaviors
Proximity-seeking behaviors that serve to bring the infant/young child closer to their primary caregiver ("attachment figure"). Behaviors can include searching, approaching, reaching, clinging, and following, as well as signaling behaviors such as crying, smiling, and vocalizing. Importantly, attachment behaviors are distinct from "affiliative behavior" or social engagement because they are exhibited when the infant experiences distress.

Attachment classification
Refers to an infant/young child's overall pattern of attachment with a specific caregiver as assessed via Ainsworth's Strange Situation Procedure (SSP). Classifications (including "secure," "avoidant," "ambivalent," and "disorganized") are based on the observed organization of attachment behaviors and the balance between the child's tendency to seek proximity to the attachment figure and to move away and explore. Importantly, classifications are relationship-specific, and are distinct from attachment disorders.

Attachment disorders
Refers to reactive attachment disorder (RAD) and disinhibited social engagement disorder (DSED), two rare and clinically distinct psychiatric disorders described in DSM-5 and ICD-11 that both arise from extremes of insufficient caregiving.

Relationship-specific disorder of infancy/early childhood
A clinical disorder described in DC:0-5 that defines symptomatic behavior in the infant/young child—which can include oppositional behavior, aggression, fearfulness, feeding or sleep problems, self-endangering behavior, and role-inappropriate behavior with a caregiver—that is limited to one relationship context.

Sources: ZERO TO THREE (2005); Finelli *et al.* (2019); American Psychiatric Association (2022).

Classification of Diseases, 11th revision (ICD-11; World Health Organization, 2019). Relationship-specific disorder means the young child is experiencing symptomatology that involves significant distress and/or functional impairment, and that it is confined to one specific relationship (see Box 57.1 for definitions used in this chapter).

Development of attachment

Parents' affiliative feelings for their infants often begin prenatally. Studies have indicated that parents are willing to describe a sense of who the baby is and assert that they have a relationship with the baby even before the baby is born (Zeanah *et al.*, 1985; Benoit *et al.*, 1997). The birth of the infant usually intensifies feelings of affection, and the newborn's physical attributes, called "babyishness" (Lorenz, 1943), are known to draw the attention, interest, and even affection of adults (Stern, 1977).

Although most parents report feeling attached at birth or even before, infants are not born attached to their caregivers. The tendency for selective seeking of comfort is not apparent in the first 6 months after birth. Instead, attachment emerges gradually over the first year of life. By 2–3 months of age, social engagement behaviors emerge, with responsive smiling and cooing and more sustained eye-to-eye contact between infants and adult caregivers. Of note, these behaviors are readily displayed toward both familiar and unfamiliar adults until about 7–8 months of age. Two new infant behaviors become apparent at that point: stranger wariness and separation protest. Stranger wariness describes an apparent discomfort with unfamiliar adults and preferentially turning to those caregivers the child knows and trusts. Separation protest refers to the infant's tendency to protest separation from familiar caregivers. Although individual differences in the intensity and expression of these behaviors are clear, they may be considered universal. When these behaviors appear, the infant is said to be "attached" to one or more caregivers. The phases in the development of attachment that correspond to these behavioral changes, which are modified slightly from Bowlby's (1982) original formulation, are described in Figure 57.1.

From a clinical perspective, we emphasize that two conditions appear to be necessary for infants to form attachments to adult caregivers. First, infants must have a significant amount of interaction on a regular basis with the caregiver. Infants can neither develop nor sustain attachments to adults with whom they have contact for only a few hours a week, although they may have positive connections with those adults, that is, social and/or play relationships with them. Second, they must attain a cognitive age of 7–9 months before the kind of preference seeking that defines attachment is present. By 12 months, infants demonstrate a balance between exploratory and proximity seeking behaviors with their caregivers. Attachment theory postulates that exploration and ventures away from the caregiver represents use of the attachment figure as a secure base from which to venture out and a safe haven to return to when distressed or anxious (Bowlby, 1982).

By the end of the first year of life, it is possible to assess the quality of the young child's attachment to a particular caregiver. Usually, this is accomplished by means of a laboratory paradigm known as the Strange Situation Procedure (SSP; Ainsworth *et al.*, 1978). Alternating episodes of separations and reunions highlight differences between a young child's behavior with a familiar caregiver and an unfamiliar adult or stranger, especially following moderately stressful separation from their caregiver in an unfamiliar setting. Qualitative differences in children's

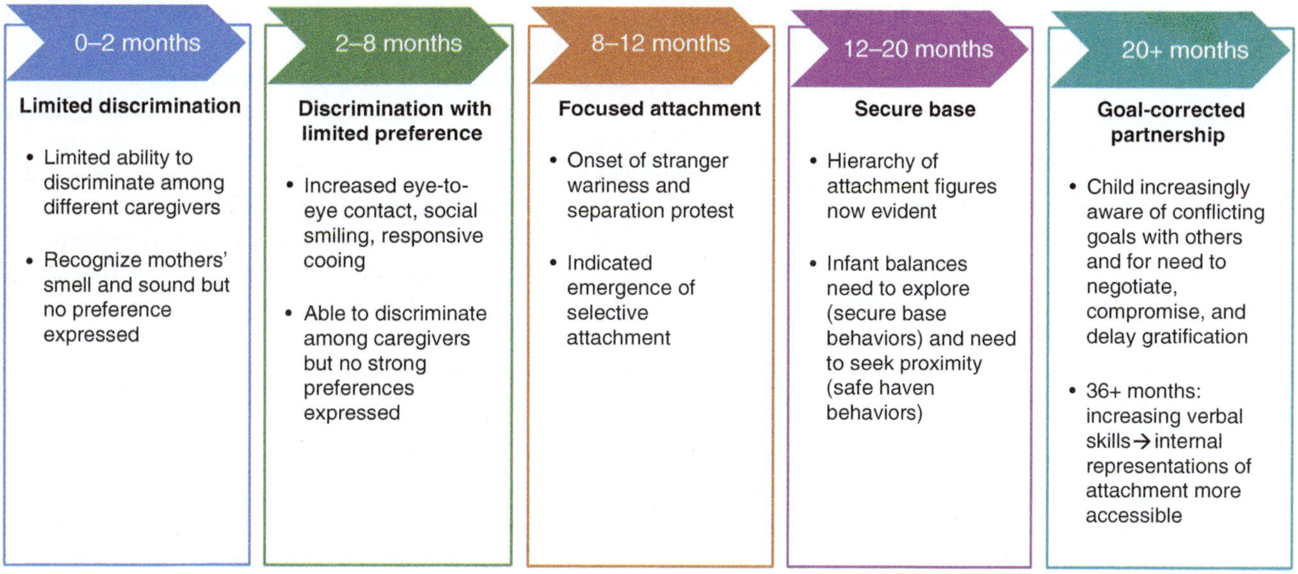

Figure 57.1 Development of attachment.

behavior, especially during reunion episodes, yields one of four classifications of a young child's pattern of attachment to the caregiver with whom they are assessed as secure, insecure/avoidant, insecure/resistant, or disorganized.

Attachment classifications as protective and risk factors

Young children whose attachments are classified as secure seek comfort readily from their caregivers following brief separation and use the caregiver to regulate their distress. Children with secure attachments are more likely to exhibit more adaptive interpersonal qualities subsequently and reduced risk for psychopathology (Carlson *et al.*, 2003). Secure attachments are especially important as protective factors for young children developing in high-risk environments (Feldman *et al.*, 2011; McGoron *et al.*, 2012; Tharner *et al.*, 2012).

By contrast, children with insecure/avoidant attachments to their caregivers show little distress during separation and do not seek comfort during reunions, despite experiencing physiological arousal comparable to secure infants who display frank distress (Sroufe & Waters, 1977). Children with insecure/resistant attachments display distress during separation from their caregivers, but they are not soothed when the attachment figure returns and display difficulties regulating their distress during reunion episodes. Both insecure/avoidant and insecure/resistant attachments to primary caregivers render infants at increased risk of later social and psychological difficulties. Thus, they may be considered risk factors which have their strongest effects in high-risk groups lacking protective factors.

Infant behaviors in the presence of the parent or caregiver suggesting fearfulness, freezing, or other contradictory attachment behaviors (e.g., initial approach followed by avoidance while in close contact with the caregiver) during the SSP are indices of the final attachment classification, disorganized attachment. Although disorganized attachment has a prevalence of 14% in low-risk samples (van IJzendoorn *et al.*, 1999), it is as high as 75–80% in maltreated and institutionalized samples (Carlson *et al.*, 1989; Vorria *et al.*, 2003; Zeanah *et al.*, 2005). Furthermore, disorganized attachment is associated with various disturbances in caregiving behavior, including frightening/frightened behavior, as well as antagonism, role confusion, withdrawal, and contradictory cues (Lyons-Ruth *et al.*, 1999; Schuengel *et al.*, 1999). As some children reach preschool age, disorganization is transformed into controlling/punitive or solicitous/caregiving behaviors directed toward the parent, though in some high-risk preschool samples, disorganized behaviors remain evident (Smyke *et al.*, 2010). Of the various attachment classifications, disorganized attachment has the strongest links to subsequent psychopathology, including social difficulties, role-inappropriate parent–child interactive behavior, peer rejection and poor social adjustment, aggression, and disruptive behavior in middle childhood, in addition to emotional problems, low self-esteem, and dissociative disorders in adolescence (Green & Goldwyn, 2002; Zeanah *et al.*, 2011).

It is important to note that these classifications are not diagnoses and do not represent clinical disorders. First, attachment classifications may vary with different caregivers, unlike disorders of attachment whose clinical presentations are consistent across different relationships. Second, insecure or disorganized attachments may not necessarily be impairing, especially for children in low-risk, well-resourced environments.

Most descriptions of attachment as a clinical disorder have derived from studies of the effects on social and emotional development in young children who have experienced severe deprivation, such as that associated with institutional rearing. Because of that, we turn next to a brief review of the association between institutional care and attachment disorders and consider how studies of institutionalized children informed psychiatric nosologies.

Historical considerations

Institutional care and deprivation

Maternal deprivation and the material deprivation that often accompanies it have long been recognized as important risk factors to development in humans (Chapin, 1915; Spitz, 1945; Bowlby, 1965; Rutter, 1981), primates (Suomi *et al.*, 1976; O'Connor & Cameron, 2006), and rodents (Zhang *et al.*, 2002; Hofer, 2006). Since the 1970s, children raised in institutions have been studied to assess the risks associated with this atypical rearing environment because it has been associated with deprivation. A series of small-scale descriptive studies began to raise questions about the consequences of institutionalization in the 1940s. Early studies focused on behavioral and cognitive manifestations of the effects of poor rearing environments (Goldfarb, 1945; Levy, 1947). In addition to disturbances of growth, cognitive development, and language, these studies also documented that children who had been institutionalized during the first three years of life demonstrated consistently greater levels of problem behaviors, including feeding and sleeping difficulties, aggressive behavior and hyperactivity, and excessive attention-seeking and sociability with strangers, when compared with children in foster care.

A recent resurgence in studies of children adopted or fostered out of Romanian and other institutions has demonstrated some significant problems across a range of outcomes, including disturbed attachment (Chisholm, 1998; Vorria *et al.*, 2003; The St. Petersburg—USA Orphanage Research Team, 2008; Dobrova-Krol *et al.*, 2010; Rutter *et al.*, 2010; Bakermans-Kranenburg *et al.*, 2011; Smyke *et al.*, 2012). These findings have elaborated many important features of the disorders which had been defined descriptively by previous studies of children living in conditions of deprivation.

Tizard's study

Barbara Tizard's (1977) landmark study deconstructed the institutional experience by largely removing the material deprivation often associated with institutional care and focusing selectively on the variable of caregiver–child relationship. She described the cognitive and socioemotional development of a group of children who experienced varying lengths of institutional care in residential nurseries in Great Britain in the early 1970s. Caregiver to child ratios in these nurseries were substantially better than those found in older studies of institutions (Goldfarb, 1945; Provence & Lipton, 1962). Children were maintained in small, mixed-age groups, in a stimulating environment which included books, toys, and instruction (Tizard, 1977).

Three groups of children with histories of early institutional rearing were studied at age 4 years: 24 children who were adopted between 2–4 years of age, 15 children who were returned to their biological families (often despite marked ambivalence on the part of their parents), and 26 children who remained institutionalized between 2–4 years of age (Tizard, 1977). By age 4, this latter group had experienced an average of 50 different caregivers who had cared for the child for at least a week. Of these 26 children who remained in the residential nurseries, 8 had developed a preferred attachment, 8 were withdrawn and unresponsive, and 10 were indiscriminate, attention-seeking, and socially superficial (Tizard & Rees, 1975). The latter two groups displayed behaviors that had been described in some earlier studies and formed the basis of the criteria for RAD and DSED in DSM-5 (American Psychiatric Association, 2013) and ICD-11 (World Health Organization, 2019).

An important contribution of this landmark study is that much of the material and even social privation that is evident in studies of children in other institutional settings (such as the contemporary studies of children raised in Romanian, Ukrainian, or Russian institutions) were not present. Because these residential nurseries were better staffed, had smaller groups of children, and included adequate material resources, this study permitted isolating the effects of the variable of interest for attachment disorders, that is, children's opportunity to form selective attachments to caregivers. Because caregivers were explicitly discouraged from forming attachments to children (or encouraging children to attach to them), the Tizard study showed that this particular caregiving condition was linked clearly to the phenotypes that we now call attachment disorders.

Attachment disorders in current nosologies

Descriptive studies in the mid-20th century of what is now defined as RAD were modified in formal nosologies toward more precisely defined disorders. RAD changed from presentations involving socially aberrant behaviors more generally to absence of attachment behaviors more specifically. DSED, which does involve aberrant behaviors socially, began to be defined distinctly as its own disorder following data demonstrating that DSED symptoms may be present in children who have secure, insecure, disorganized, or no attachments to their caregivers (see Zeanah *et al.*, 2006). There is now a convergence in definitions of these disorders in DSM-5 (American Psychiatric Association, 2013), ICD-11 (World Health Organization, 2019), and DC:0-5 (ZERO TO THREE, 2005). Chapter 7 discusses more generally how classifications of early childhood disorders are made in different nosologies.

Clinical disorders of attachment: the phenotypes

Attachment disorders, which have been assessed both continuously and categorically, describe a constellation of aberrant attachment behaviors and other social behavioral anomalies in early childhood. These are believed to result from the child having limited opportunities to form selected attachments.

Historically, attachment disorders have been linked to deprivation or social neglect. The diagnosis is excluded in the presence of autism spectrum disorder (ASD) to distinguish them from social abnormalities associated with that disorder. Although attachment classifications are relationship-specific for the young child, signs of attachment disorders must be evident across situations and relationships.

Two clinical patterns of attachment disorders have been described:

- An emotionally withdrawn/inhibited pattern, in which the child exhibits limited or absent seeking or responding to comfort when distressed, and a variety of aberrant social and emotional behaviors, such as lack of responsiveness and reciprocity, reduced positive affect, and emotion regulation difficulties. In both ICD-11 and DSM-5, this disorder is RAD. Evidence suggests that this disorder represents absence of preferred attachment in children who are old enough to have formed them. In keeping with this formulation, institutionalized children showed moderately high convergence between observer-rated absence of attachment behaviors with familiar caregivers and caregiver reports of RAD (Zeanah *et al.*, 2005).
- An indiscriminately social/disinhibited pattern, in which the child exhibits lack of expectable selectivity in seeking comfort, support, and nurturance, with lack of social reticence with unfamiliar adults, including a willingness to "go off" with strangers and a violation of expected verbal and social boundaries with relative strangers. In ICD-11 (World Health Organization, 2019) and DSM-5 (American Psychiatric Association, 2013), this disorder is DSED. The essence of this disorder is indiscriminate social behavior in children who are expected developmentally to show some degree of stranger wariness.

Reactive attachment disorder

Core features of RAD include lack of social and emotional responses, an absence or near-absence of attachment behaviors even in times of stress, and serious problems of emotion regulation. In addition, RAD includes a paucity of positive emotional responses and bouts of fear or irritability that are seemingly unprovoked, or at least out of proportion to the situation. Social and emotional reciprocal interactions are absent or at least severely dampened, and interest in interacting with others is limited. Cognitive and language delays, though not core features, are often associated with RAD because the conditions of neglect believed to lead to this pattern of attachment disorder are also associated with developmental delays. These signs have been described in young children with a history of severe neglect (Zeanah *et al.*, 2004; Oosterman & Schuengel, 2007; Bruce *et al.*, 2019) and those being raised in institutions (Smyke *et al.*, 2002; Zeanah *et al.*, 2005; Humphreys *et al.*, 2017a). Interestingly, signs of RAD have not been reported in children adopted out of institutions (Chisholm, 1998; Vorria *et al.*, 2003; Rutter *et al.*, 2010).

Disinhibited social engagement disorder/disinhibited attachment disorder

Core behavioral features of this disorder in young children include inappropriate approach to unfamiliar adults, a lack of wariness of strangers, failure to check back with a caregiver in unfamiliar settings, and a readiness to accompany a stranger, and wander away from a familiar caregiver. Indiscriminate behavior also may be associated with lack of appropriate verbal and physical boundaries, so that children may interact with strangers intrusively and aggressively and may even seek out physical contact (O'Connor & Zeanah, 2003).

For example, some investigators have referred to "indiscriminately friendly" behavior (Chisholm, 1998; Tarullo *et al.*, 2011), but others have suggested that these terms imply more than is actually known about the nature of the child's behavior (O'Connor & Zeanah, 2003). Some children exhibit passive lack of reticence and willingness to accompany a stranger, but this may be quite distinct from children who eagerly accompany a stranger without even checking back with their putative attachment figure. Other behaviors subsumed under this description include lack of initial reticence around unfamiliar adults (e.g., sitting in the lap of an unfamiliar adult at an initial meeting), actively choosing to approach an unfamiliar adult over an attachment figure in times of need, failing to monitor the whereabouts of the attachment figure in unfamiliar settings, displaying inappropriate social boundaries (e.g., making eye contact for too long or asking overly personal questions on initial meeting), or verbally or physically aggressive engagement of unfamiliar adults. These behaviors are not experienced as sociable or friendly by those on the receiving end, and they are not always demonstrated indiscriminately (O'Connor & Zeanah, 2003). Because of this heterogeneity, more precise delineation of behaviors subsumed by this term is indicated.

Still, measurement of the construct has been reasonably consistent across studies. For example, comparing three different caregiver interview measures of indiscriminate behavior, Zeanah *et al.* (2002) showed substantial convergence across measures. Subsequent studies have shown concordance between interviews and observational measures (O'Connor *et al.*, 2003; Gleason *et al.*, 2011a; Oliveira *et al.*, 2012).

Middle childhood and adolescence

Less is known about the measurement of attachment and attachment relationships in middle childhood and adolescence than in early childhood. There is no gold standard in older children for assessment comparable to the SSP, and the observable behaviors used to index attachment are less obviously demonstrable in middle childhood. Since attachment itself is challenging to define in middle childhood and adolescence, defining disorders of attachment in these age groups is especially challenging.

Studies of RAD prior to the publication of DSM-5 (American Psychiatric Association, 2013) often did not differentiate between emotionally withdrawn inhibited behavior and social disinhibition (the two subtypes of RAD), making conclusions about RAD and DSED as we now understand them more difficult. More recent studies have used structured interviews with children who experienced maltreatment to assess RAD in middle childhood. For example, in the Bucharest Early Intervention Project (BEIP), a randomized controlled trial comparing foster care to institutional care in young children, investigators used the same structured interview to assess RAD and found some continuity from early childhood to early adolescence in signs of RAD, especially for children with later age of placement into families and greater percentage time in institutional care (Guyon-Harris *et al.*, 2019). Of course, using the same measure from early childhood to adolescence also complicates interpretation since it assumes homotypic continuity. A newer measure, the Reactive Attachment Disorder (RAD) and Disinhibited Social Engagement Disorder (DSED) Assessment, used factor analysis to lend support for the DSM-5 conceptualization of RAD and DSED as separate dimensions of child psychopathology.

A study of RAD with Norwegian adolescents living in residential care found that dimensional measures of RAD and DSED symptoms were associated with both emotional and behavioral problems in adolescence (Seim *et al.*, 2020). These investigators used the RAD module of the Preschool Age Psychiatric Assessment (PAPA), a measure designed to assess RAD in preschoolers, for reasons that are unclear.

Indiscriminate behavior, on the other hand, has been described and studied in several different populations of children longitudinally from early to middle childhood and has been defined reasonably similarly across studies (Tizard & Hodges, 1978; Bruce *et al.*, 2009; Smyke *et al.*, 2012; Guyon-Harris *et al.*, 2018). The most careful and intentional examination of the DSED phenotype in middle childhood to date was the English and Romanian Adoptees (ERA) Study (Rutter *et al.*, 2007a, 2007b). They used a combination of an examiner-based interview of parents when children were 6 and 11 years old and observed interactions with an unfamiliar adult. A factor analysis suggested that two internally consistent composites best summarized the data: violation of boundaries and physical contact. They found significant convergence in these measures of indiscriminate behavior, suggesting a cohesive construct across middle childhood.

Hodges and Tizard (1989) reported no relationship between indiscriminate behavior with unfamiliar adults at age 8 and age 16 years. However, they did report that children who had shown indiscriminate behavior at age 8, tended to be indiscriminate with peers at age 16. Rutter and colleagues (Kreppner *et al.*, 2010) reported the persistence of what they called "disinhibited attachment" into adolescence as part of their examination of deprivation-specific psychological patterns. They noted the changing clinical picture as they tracked disinhibited attachment from early childhood, where specific behavioral patterns were more clearly defined, to adolescence. They developed measures to assess disinhibited attachment in a way which reflected issues associated with the emerging developmental tasks of adolescence, including difficulties with social boundaries and behaviors which appeared flirtatious to others but were not thought to be so by the previously institutionalized young person. On the other hand, they noted that at times the intrusive and outgoing social style exhibited by some of their subjects had seemed to become a relative social strength in interaction with peers. Nonetheless, symptoms of disinhibited attachment appeared to persist in close to 70% of children who had exhibited these signs earlier on (Kreppner *et al.*, 2010).

Differential diagnosis

RAD shares some features with ASD, including disturbances in emotion regulation and reduced or absent social and emotional reciprocity. In addition, children with either disorder may have cognitive delays or stereotypies. However, children with RAD should not have a selective impairment in pretend play, repetitive preoccupations, or language abnormalities other than delays. Further, they should have a history of seriously adverse caregiving. Because RAD and cognitive delays are associated with severe deprivation, meaning social neglect warranting intervention by child protection or institutional rearing (Zeanah *et al.*, 2006), RAD also may be confused with intellectual disability. Young children with RAD should be distinguishable from children with intellectual disability because the latter group has social and emotional behaviors that are consistent with their developmental age, whereas children with RAD show clear evidence of deviance in their social responsiveness and regulation of emotion. Clearly, both conditions may co-occur. Reduced positive affect and social withdrawal occur both in children with RAD and in children with depression; however, children with depression typically do not display aberrant attachment relationships with caregivers (Gleason *et al.*, 2011a).

DSED may share features of attention deficit hyperactivity disorder (ADHD), particularly impulsivity. Both ADHD and DSED have been reported as sequelae of institutional rearing, and they have both been defined as deprivation-specific behavior patterns in post-institutional children (see Rutter *et al.*, 2010). Roy and colleagues (Roy *et al.*, 2004) found that school-age children with a history of institutional rearing had high levels of both "disinhibited attachment" behavior and inattention/hyperactivity, as well as a strong association between the two. In addition to lack of selectivity in relationships with caregivers, the children also showed lack of selectivity with peers, echoing the findings of Hodges and Tizard (1989) with adolescents who had formerly been indiscriminate with caregivers. Less clear has been whether the social impulsivity of DSED is related to the cognitive and behavioral impulsivity of ADHD. In children with histories of institutional or other challenging rearing environments, impulse control difficulties are apparent in some children who exhibit indiscriminate behavior (Bruce *et al.*, 2009; Pears *et al.*, 2010), but it is clear that DSED and ADHD may be distinguished clinically (Gleason *et al.*, 2011a). A child with

DSED without ADHD will not show inattention/distractibility or restless/overactive behavior in situations demanding quiet and focused behavior. In addition, there is no reason to expect impulsivity beyond social impulsivity in a child with DSED only. For children with ADHD who also demonstrate social impulsivity, both diagnoses may be appropriate if full criteria for DSED are evident. Willingness to accompany unfamiliar adults, on the other hand, is not a part of the ADHD phenotype, unless the child's attention is drawn to some specific activity (e.g., joining a game or throwing a ball).

The shared and unique features of RAD, DSED, ASD, and ADHD are illustrated in Figure 57.2.

Prevalence

There is a consensus that these disorders are rare, even though there have been no careful epidemiological studies of their prevalence in community samples of young children. When diagnostic criteria are applied, both RAD and DSED are unusual in populations attending outpatient clinics and more likely to be detected in extreme populations, that is, in young children who have experienced severe deprivation (Chisholm, 1998; Smyke *et al.*, 2002; O'Connor *et al.*, 2003; Boris *et al.*, 2004; Zeanah *et al.*, 2004). In a sample of 300 children aged 2–5, recruited from pediatric clinics in Durham, North Carolina, US, Egger *et al.* (2006) found no cases of attachment disorders using DSM-IV (American Psychiatric Association, 1994) or the Research Diagnostic Criteria-Preschool Age (RDC-PA) criteria (Boris & Zeanah, 2005). In a similarly designed study in Bucharest, Romania, Gleason and colleagues (Gleason *et al.*, 2011b), also found no cases of RAD or DSED.

Several recent studies of clinic-referred and high-risk children have assessed signs of disordered attachment using structured interviews and observational assessments. These studies have found that, even among maltreated children, few met criteria for attachment disorders, with the exception of some maltreated children in foster care (Boris *et al.*, 2004; Zeanah

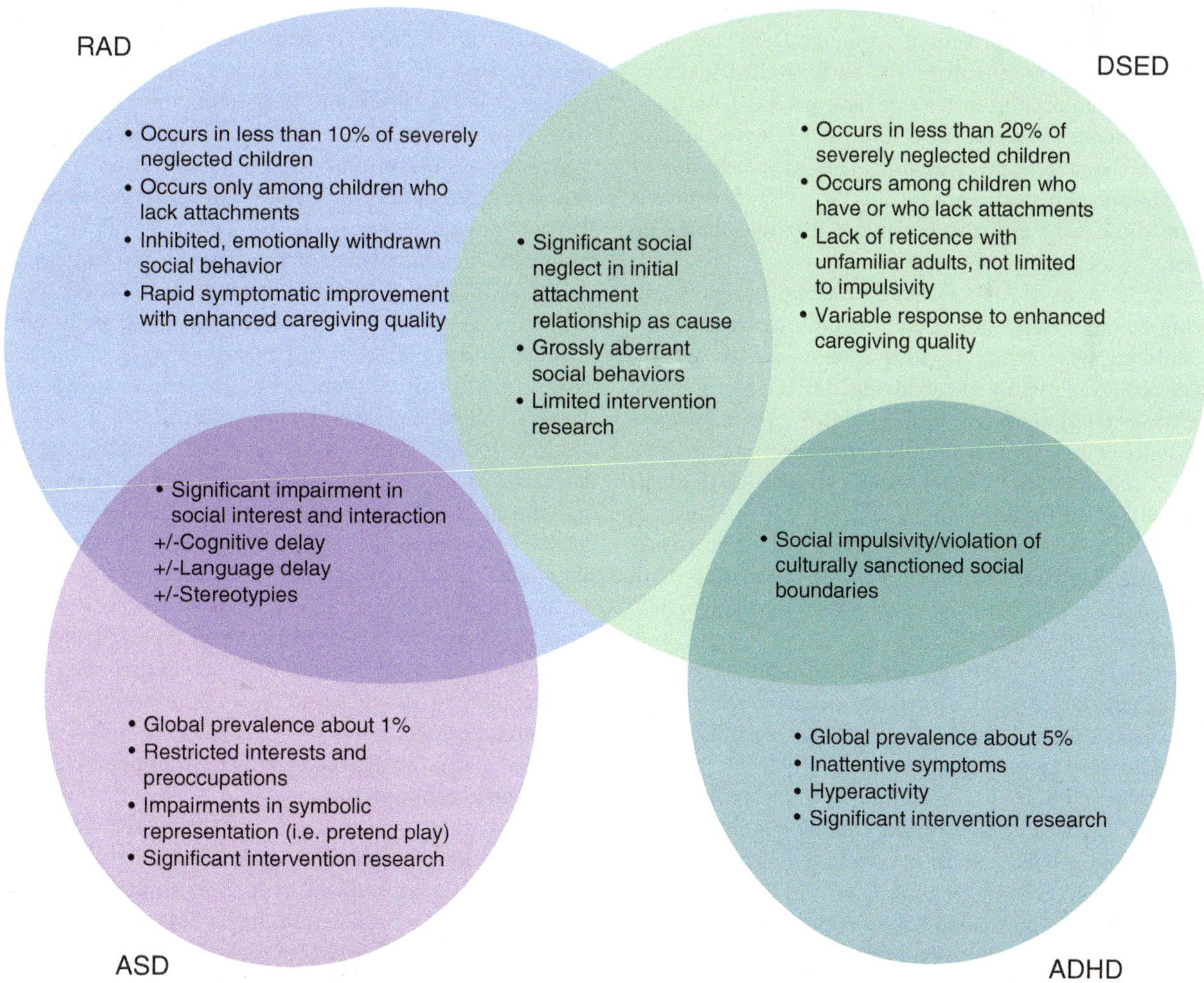

Figure 57.2 Differential diagnosis: attention deficit hyperactivity disorder (ADHD); autism spectrum disorder (ASD); disinhibited social engagement disorder (DSED); reactive attachment disorder (RAD).

et al., 2004; Oosterman & Schuengel, 2007). In a sample of 12–30-month-old children living in institutions in Bucharest, 5–10% met criteria for RAD and 24–30% for DSED (Zeanah *et al.* 2005; Gleason *et al.*, 2011a, 2011b). Thus, although signs of the disorder may be common in extreme populations, a minority of children seem to reach the threshold of disorder.

Etiology

Together with post-traumatic stress disorder (PTSD), RAD and DSED are among the few psychiatric disorders in which the etiology is specified as one of the diagnostic criteria. A requirement of DSM-5 is that the child has experienced extremes of insufficient caregiving, such as serious social neglect or deprivation (i.e., persistent lack of having basic emotional needs for comfort, stimulation, and affection met), repeated changes of primary caregivers that limit opportunities to form stable attachments, or rearing in institutions that limit opportunities to form selective attachments. In ICD-11, "grossly inadequate child care" is illustrated with examples of "severe neglect, maltreatment, institutional deprivation." Although DSED has been described in children with parents who have psychiatric disorders, and many children in foster care have parents with these disorders or serious substance use disorders, we caution against using parent characteristics other than caregiving behavior to identify extremes of insufficient care. It is the seriously deficient caregiving and not the feature associated with it that should be identified.

In the BEIP, signs of RAD assessed by caregiver report and caregiving quality assessed by coding naturalistic interactions when children were living in institutions were compared. Observer ratings of quality of caregiving, defined by caregiver sensitivity, stimulation of development, positive regard toward child, absence of detachment, absence of flat affect, and absence of intrusiveness, were inversely related to signs of RAD (Zeanah *et al.*, 2005). This finding cannot address the direction of effects, but it does illustrate the grossly insufficient care associated with this disorder. For children in the same study with signs of DSED, no relationship with caregiving quality was found (Zeanah *et al.*, 2005).

Understanding the link with grossly insufficient care is especially important for indiscriminate behavior for at least three reasons. First, the boundaries between highly sociable children and children exhibiting pathologically indiscriminate behavior are not completely delineated. Second, some children with ADHD seem to be socially as well as cognitively and behaviorally impulsive, and this makes delimiting what is indiscriminate behavior challenging. Third, children with congenital abnormalities may exhibit high levels of indiscriminate behavior. Children with Williams syndrome, for example, have been reported to show high levels of indiscriminate behavior, even with more than adequate caregiving (Järvinen-Pasley *et al.*, 2010). Williams syndrome is caused by a microdeletion on chromosome 7q11.23, and is characterized by a tendency for affected individuals to approach persons they do not know and interact with them verbally. Parents of young children with Williams syndrome expend much effort to monitor their children's whereabouts and teach them to refrain from approaching strangers. Compared with nonaffected individuals, they are unable to distinguish threatening faces and consider them just as trustworthy as nonthreatening faces (Järvinen-Pasley *et al.*, 2010). Soares *et al.* (2013) proposed that children with exposure to institutional rearing will be most likely to display indiscriminate behavior when they carry specific polymorphisms within the Williams syndrome critical region. However, genetic studies to date lack adequate sample sizes to identify genetic risk variants.

The courses of the disorders

Based upon the results from several longitudinal studies, however, it seems clear that RAD and DSED generally have different courses.

Studies of children adopted out of institutions have not reported evidence of RAD following adoption (Tizard & Hodges, 1978; Chisholm, 1998; O'Connor *et al.*, 2003). Furthermore, in the BEIP, the first randomized controlled trial to evaluate an intervention for attachment disorders, children who were being raised in institutions were assessed between 11–30 months of age for signs of RAD. Half were randomized to a foster care intervention and half to continued institutional rearing (CAU). Follow-ups were conducted at 30, 42, 54, and 96 months of age. Signs of RAD in the group removed from institutions and placed in foster care dropped to the level of never institutionalized children by 30 months and remained low at every subsequent assessment age (Smyke *et al.*, 2012). For children in the CAU group, signs of the disorder slowly decreased over time, but they were always significantly greater than the intervention group. Further, reduced signs of the disorder were accounted for completely by children who were placed in families—either reintegrated with their own biological families or placed into government-sponsored foster care (Smyke *et al.*, 2012). In other words, over a six-year period, there was no significant reduction in signs of RAD for children who remained in institutions. This latter finding is important, as it represents preliminary evidence of persistence of the disorder in children who remain in an adverse caregiving environment. These results indicate that signs of RAD are eliminated by placement of children into families where they receive at least adequate care. In a prospective longitudinal study of RAD in children with a history of institutional rearing, Guyon-Harris and colleagues found both decreasing and stable trajectories of RAD signs from early childhood to adolescence, with a decreasing course associated with early family placement and a stable elevated course associated with more prolonged exposure to institutional care (Guyon-Harris *et al.*, 2019). There is also evidence that even when RAD in early childhood resolves following placement in an enhanced caregiving environment, children with the prior diagnosis are at increased risked for social difficulties in adolescence (Guyon-Harris *et al.*, 2019).

In contrast, there is reasonably clear evidence demonstrating that indiscriminate behavior persists over time—sometimes even after improvements in the caregiving environment. This was demonstrated originally in the work of Tizard and colleagues, who showed that young children who had been indiscriminate with caregivers at age 4 were more likely to have serious peer disturbances at 16 years, including superficial and even indiscriminate behavior with peers (Hodges & Tizard, 1989). Subsequent studies of children adopted into Canada and the UK from Romanian institutions have also demonstrated a tendency for indiscriminate behavior to persist, even after the child forms attachments to the adopted family (Chisholm, 1998; O'Connor *et al.*, 2003). In fact, of those children adopted into the UK from Romanian institutions who had high levels of indiscriminate behavior at age 6, more than half continued to show high levels at age 11 (Rutter *et al.*, 2007a). Furthermore, in the BEIP, indiscriminate behavior persisted in children who had been reared in institutions (Smyke *et al.*, 2012), although elevated or persistent courses were associated with older age at placement into foster care, more time in institutional care, and greater placement disruptions (Guyon-Harris *et al.*, 2018). Pears *et al.* (2010) also found that signs of DSED among children in foster care were related to the number of placement disruptions rather than severity of maltreatment. These findings have important implications for child welfare systems, as early and sustained placements could help decrease signs of DSED into early adolescence.

Box 57.2 Assessment at a glance

- Caregiver interviews:
  - Structured interviews focused on attachment behaviors:
    - Psychiatric Assessment Preschool Age (PAPA) (Egger & Angold, 2004)
    - Diagnostic Infant and Preschool Assessment (DIPA) (Scheeringa & Haslett, 2010)
    - Disturbances of Attachment Interview (DAI) (Smyke & Zeanah, 1999)
- Observed interactions:
  - Naturalistic observations
  - Formal observations:
    - Strange Situation Procedure (SSP) (Ainsworth *et al.*, 1978)
    - Clinical Observation of Attachment (COA) (Boris *et al.*, 2004)
- Differential diagnosis:
  - Reactive attachment disorder (RAD):
    - Autism spectrum disorder (ASD)
    - Intellectual disability/Global developmental delay
    - Depression
  - Disinhibited social engagement disorder (DSED):
    - Attention deficit hyperactivity disorder (ADHD)
    - High sociability (non-impairing)
    - Williams syndrome
    - Fetal alcohol syndrome

Clinical assessment

In keeping with recent trends in the assessment of early childhood psychopathology (del Carmen-Wiggins & Carter, 2004), attachment disorders are best identified through a combination of caregiver interview and observed interactions. In our view, there are no gold standard interviews nor observational paradigms of interactions between parents and children that must be included, but several useful approaches have been described (Box 57.2).

Although our understanding of RAD has continued to deepen through increased systematic research, controversies remain regarding misdiagnosis. Giltaij *et al.* (2017) showed that when an observational measure (Clinical Observation of Attachment [COA]) was added to an interview measure (Disturbances of Attachment Interview [DAI]), fewer children met criteria for RAD than if only the interview measure alone was used. This is important since the majority of studies of RAD have used interviews only. A study by Woolgar and Baldock (2015) found that community practitioners were four times more likely to diagnose children with RAD than those working in a specialty clinic. Allen and Schuengel (2020), using well-validated methods and experienced clinicians to conduct evaluations of 38 children in foster or adoptive care who were diagnosed with RAD by community clinicians, found that none of the 38 children met criteria for RAD. These examples highlight the importance of a comprehensive assessment using both well-validated structured interviews and observational measures (Zeanah *et al.*, 2016;Boris & Renk, 2017; Zeanah & Guyon-Harris, 2020).

Interviews

Structured interviews specifically focused on the child's attachment behaviors and signs of disordered attachment (O'Connor *et al.*, 1999; Smyke *et al.*, 2002; Boris *et al.*, 2004; Zeanah *et al.*, 2005) are more likely to be useful than interviews that are less specifically focused. At least two structured psychiatric interviews, the Psychiatric Assessment Preschool Age (PAPA; Egger & Angold, 2004) and the Diagnostic Infant and Preschool Assessment (DIPA; Scheeringa & Haslett, 2010) include modules on attachment disorders for young children. These approaches are able to characterize attachment disorders both categorically and continuously. The DAI (Smyke *et al.*, 2002), a 12-item semistructured interview that assesses signs of RAD, DSED, and secure base distortions (self-endangering, excessive clinging, hypervigilance with caregiver, role inappropriate behavior), has also been used in many investigations. It has distinguished between children with histories of deprivation and those without (Smyke *et al.*, 2002; Zeanah *et al.*, 2005), as well as those removed from institutions and placed in foster care and those with more prolonged institutional exposure (Smyke *et al.*, 2012; Humphreys *et al.*, 2017b).

Recently, an interview to assess attachment disorders in middle childhood has been developed. Lehman *et al.* (2020) modified the Child and Adolescent Psychiatric Assessment for RAD to update it from DSM-IV to DSM-5 criteria for RAD and DSED, renaming it the RAD and DSED Assessment (RADA). In a sample of adolescents who had experienced maltreatment, foster parents completed the RADA online. Using confirmatory factor analysis, the investigators derived one factor consistent with DSED and two factors consistent with RAD (failure to seek/accept comfort and withdrawal/hypervigilance).

Based on research to date, it seems clear that caregivers of school-age children and adolescents will endorse signs of RAD and DSED in some children at risk for these disorders. What is less clear is what the nature of the clinical phenotype of these disorders is in older children, especially RAD. For example, clinically concerning patterns of failing to seek and respond to comfort are much more challenging to operationalize after early childhood. In addition, lack of social reciprocity is a core symptom of RAD in early childhood—it is unclear how this manifests in middle childhood and adolescence. Clarifying the phenotype is an important area for future research.

Observations

Potentially clinically useful observations of parent and child together include procedures designed specifically to examine attachment behaviors (O'Connor *et al.*, 2003; Boris *et al.*, 2004; Oliveira *et al.*, 2012), or those in which other aspects of parent–child interaction are also assessed (Zeanah *et al.*, 2000). It is generally useful to include in the observation some degree of distress that is likely to activate the child's need for the attachment figure. Conventionally, this has involved brief separations followed by reunions, but other approaches, such as a novel (i.e., scary) toy, have also been used (Boris *et al.*, 2004). Although the SSP was not designed for clinical assessments, in some circumstances it may be helpful (Zeanah *et al.*, 2011). The Circle of Security Intervention, for example, includes review of videotaped recordings of a child's Strange Situation behavior with the parent as a part of the intervention (Hoffman *et al.*, 2006). Although systematic observations of the child's behavior in paradigms designed to elicit attachment behaviors are often clinically valuable, naturalistic observations of a child's attachment behaviors may also yield important data.

Although there are limited data on observational measures to assess RAD symptoms in school-aged children, one study (Zimmerman & Iwanski, 2019) provided support for an observational approach using dyadic social interactions that induced negative emotions in children and activated their need for comfort or social regulation by adults. The authors caution, however, that further validation is needed before these findings can be generalized.

Laboratory assessments of indiscriminate behavior have used modified versions of the SSP (see O'Connor *et al.*, 2003; Lyons-Ruth *et al.*, 2019), but the most compelling laboratory measure of indiscriminate behavior was developed by Lawler *et al.* (2014). They had young children interact with a stranger in the presence of the child's mother and compared the responses of three groups: post-institutionalized adopted children, children adopted internationally from foster care, and nonadopted children. They found that a nonphysical social dimension (e.g., initiations, proximity) was variably distributed across the three groups, whereas displays of close physical contact were significantly less common in nonadopted children compared to the two adopted groups. They concluded that the social dimension reflected sociability whereas the physical dimension was clinically relevant social disinhibition.

One of the only naturalistic observations of indiscriminate behavior was conducted in BEIP. Using a "stranger at the door" procedure, they observed whether 54-month-old children were willing to leave their place of residence with an unfamiliar adult. They found a stepwise increase in willingness to leave with the stranger from never institutionalized (7%) to foster care (24%) to care as usual (42%). In addition, the children's behavior in this procedure was strongly associated with caregiver reports of indiscriminate behavior (Gleason *et al.*, 2014). Those children who left with the stranger were significantly less likely to meet the threshold for competence compared to those children who remained with their caregiver (Guyon-Harris *et al.*, 2019).

Interventions

Studies of interventions for RAD and DSED are limited. Intervention efforts to date have been guided by the principle that enhancing the caregiving environment will ameliorate signs of attachment disorder (Box 57.3). Smyke *et al.* (2002), for example, studied signs of RAD and DSED in young children

Box 57.3 Treatment at a glance

- Reactive attachment disorder (RAD):
  - Enhanced caregiving:
    - Emotionally available attachment figure
    - Sensitive and responsive caregiving
    - Psychological investment in the child
  - Dyadic therapy
    - Focusing on strengths, building trust → processing and reshaping interactions
    - Attachment video-feedback intervention (AVI)
    - Circle of Security Intervention (COS-I)
    - Attachment and biobehavioral catch-up (ABC)
    - Child–parent psychotherapy (CPP)
- Disinhibited social engagement disorder (DSED):
  - Enhanced caregiving environment may be helpful; not as responsive to enhanced caregiving as RAD
  - Consider limiting contacts with noncaregiving adults for several months following a new placement
  - Trauma-focused treatments may be helpful (parent–child interaction therapy [PCIT]; trauma-focused cognitive behavioral therapy [TF-CBT])
  - Consider adjunctive interventions for comorbid oppositional or aggressive behaviors

being raised in a large institution for young children in Bucharest. This institution had implemented a pilot unit designed to reduce the number of caregivers responsible for each child. In fact, compared to the more standard units, which included large numbers of rotating caregivers, on the pilot unit no more than four caregivers were responsible for each child on the day and evening shifts. Caregivers on the pilot unit reported that children had significantly fewer signs of both RAD and DSED. Importantly, this reduction was evident even though the ratio of caregivers to children remained at 1 : 12 on the pilot unit (the same as on the standard units).

Studies of young children adopted out of institutions are also useful to examine because they represent such a dramatic change in caregiving environments. Two longitudinal studies of young children adopted out of Romanian institutions are particularly instructive. A longitudinal study of young children adopted into Canada from Romanian institutions used parent reports of attachment and indiscriminate behavior. They found significant increases in attachment to adoptive parents during the first several years following adoption, although indiscriminate behavior persisted in a minority of children (Chisholm, 1998). The ERA longitudinal study of children adopted from Romanian institutions into families in the UK assessed signs of disordered attachment from parent reports at ages 4, 6, 11, and 15 (O'Connor & Rutter 2000; O'Connor *et al.*, 2003; Rutter *et al.*, 2007a; Rutter *et al.*, 2010). They reported little change in the numbers of children with high levels of indiscriminate behaviors between 4–6 years, but some decline by age 11 years (O'Connor & Rutter, 2000; Rutter *et al.*, 2007a). To date, however, there has been no demonstration that quality of care in adoptive homes is inversely related to signs of indiscriminate behavior in children.

In summary, findings from studies of children living in institutions and those adopted out of institutions suggest that signs of DSED are remediated by enhanced caregiving only in some children. It is unclear whether this represents individual differences among children or partial remediation with persistence in those most severely affected initially. To date, adoption studies have not included assessments of children in the institutions prior to adoption, making it difficult to explain individual differences in response.

The only contemporary intervention study that included assessments of children's attachment prior to removal from institutions and placement in an enhanced caregiving environment is the BEIP. Results of this study indicate that foster care leads to significant and lasting reductions in signs of RAD in young children who had signs of the disorder when they were living in institutions (Smyke *et al.*, 2012; Humphreys *et al.*, 2017b). There was also diminishment of signs of DSED in children randomized to foster care, but the response was less complete (Smyke *et al.*, 2012; Humphreys *et al.*, 2017b).

At this stage, clinicians must be guided by data indicating that secure attachment is fostered by caregivers who are emotionally available and sensitively responsive, who know and value the child as an individual, and who place the needs of the child ahead of their own needs. A responsive caregiving environment is the most important initial intervention with children with RAD and DSED. Preliminary data indicate that psychoeducational approaches involving training parents to respond sensitively to their child (Juffer *et al.*, 2005) and to understand their own and their child's attachment behavior (Hoffman *et al.*, 2006) have been shown to promote attachment security in the child. Though not formally studied in children diagnosed with RAD or DSED, manualized interventions that have been shown to promote secure attachments in high-risk samples include child–parent psychotherapy (CPP) (Lieberman *et al.*, 1991), Circle of Security (Hoffman *et al.*, 2006), attachment video-feedback intervention (AVI) (Moss *et al.*, 2011) video-feedback intervention to promote positive parenting and sensitive discipline (Juffer *et al.*, 2017), and attachment and biobehavioral catch-up (ABC) (Bernard *et al.*, 2012; Chapter 6). These interventions are reasonable starting points for developing an evidence base about intervening in disordered attachments (Zeanah & Gleason, 2015) (see also Chapter 36).

Conclusions

Our understanding of attachment disorders has deepened considerably in the past decade as a result of a number of systematic studies of children with histories of severe neglect or institutional rearing. These studies have affirmed the reliable identification of both RAD and DSED. They also have supported the link between extremes of inadequate caregiving and these disorders. Further, they have demonstrated that the specific "pathogen" is any environment in which young children have limited opportunities to form selective attachments, as happens in cases of severe social neglect or in settings in which the child lacks regular and consistent contact with an emotionally involved caregiver (e.g., institutional settings or frequent changes in foster care).

Although RAD and DSED arise from similar conditions of risk, they have different correlates and different courses. In particular, placement in enhanced caregiving environments seems to lead to rapid and complete elimination of signs of RAD, but DSED remains persistent in some children, apparently for years.

Nevertheless, a number of questions remain to be addressed. First, not enough is known about individual vulnerabilities to the disorder—in particular, why such phenomenologically distinctive syndromes arise from similar conditions of risk. Genetic polymorphisms, temperamental dispositions, and differential caregiving experiences should all be examined. In addition, the relationship between the two disorders—if any—needs to be clarified. Second, why some children with DSED seem to respond to enhanced caregiving and others do not is unclear. Third, the specific components of enhanced caregiving that are crucial for amelioration of signs of the disorders are unclear. This is especially important, given the heterogeneity of outcomes in postadoption studies. Fourth, the putative social cognitive abnormalities that characterize indiscriminate behavior need to be delineated. It seems reasonable that such abnormalities are the most concerning aspect of the disorder from the standpoint of functional impairment. Finally, the underlying neurobiology of these disorders remains to be clarified. The phenomenological similarities and differences between indiscriminate behavior and Williams syndrome may suggest hypotheses about the neural substrate of DSED. Answers to these questions will assist clinicians concerned with helping children recover from the long-term effects of early adversity.

References

Ainsworth, M. *et al.* (1978) *Patterns of Attachment*. Lawrence Erlbaum, Hillsdale, NJ.

Allen, B. & Schuengel, C. (2020) Attachment disorders diagnosed by community practitioners: a replication and extension. *Child Adolescent Mental Health* **25**(1), 4–10.

American Psychiatric Association (1994) *Diagnostic and Statistical Manual of Mental Disorders*, 4th edn. American Psychiatric Association, Washington, DC.

American Psychiatric Association (2013) *Diagnostic and Statistical Manual of Mental Disorders*, 5th edn. American Psychiatric Association, Washington, DC.

American Psychiatric Association (2022) *Diagnostic and Statistical Manual of Mental Disorders*, 5th edn. text revision edn. American Psychiatric Association, Washington, DC.

Bakermans-Kranenburg, M. *et al.* (2011) Attachment and emotional development in institutional care: characteristics and catch-up. In: *Children without Permanent Parental Care: Research, Practice, and Policy*. (eds R.B. McCall, *et al.*), Monographs of the Society for Research in Child Development, Serial No. 301, Vol. 76. pp. 62–91.

Benoit, D. *et al.* (1997) Mothers' representations of their infants assessed prenatally: stability and association with infants' attachment classifications. *Journal of Child Psychology and Psychiatry, and Allied Disciplines* **38**, 307–313.

Bernard, K. *et al.* (2012) Enhancing attachment organization among maltreated children: results of a randomized clinical trial. *Child Development* **83**(2), 623–636.

Boris, N. & Zeanah, C. (2005) Reactive attachment disorder. In: *Kaplan & Sadock's Comprehensive Textbook of Psychiatry*. (eds B.J. Sadock & V.A. Sadock), 8th edn. Williams and Wilkins, Philadelphia, PA. pp. 3248–3254.

Boris, N. *et al.* (2004) Comparing criteria for attachment disorders: establishing reliability and validity in high-risk samples. *Journal of the American Academy of Child and Adolescent Psychiatry* **43**, 568–577.

Boris, N.W. & Renk, K. (2017) Beyond reactive attachment disorder: how might attachment research inform child psychiatry practice? *Child and Adolescent Psychiatric Clinics of North America* **26**(3), 455–476.

Bowlby, J. (1965) *Child Care and the Growth of Love*. Penguin, London.

Bowlby, J. (1982) *Attachment and Loss*, 2nd edn, Vol. 1. Attachment. Basic Books, New York.

Bruce, J. *et al.* (2009) Disinhibited social behavior among internationally adopted children. *Development and Psychopathology* **21**(01), 157–171.

Bruce, M. *et al.* (2019) Reactive attachment disorder in maltreated young children in foster care. *Attachment & Human Development* **21**(2), 152–169.

Carlson, E.A. *et al.* (2003) Implications of attachment theory and research for developmental-behavioral pediatrics. *Journal of Developmental & Behavioral Pediatrics* **24**(5), 364–379.

Carlson, V. *et al.* (1989) Finding order in disorganization: lessons from research on maltreated infants' attachments to their caregivers. In: *Child Maltreatment: Theory and Research on the Causes and Consequences of Child Abuse and Neglect*. (eds D. Cicchetti & V. Carlson). Cambridge University Press, New York. pp. 494–528.

Chapin, H. (1915) Are institutions for infants necessary? *JAMA* **64**, 1–3.

Chisholm, K. (1998) A three year follow-up of attachment and indiscriminate friendliness in children adopted from Romanian orphanages. *Child Development* **69**, 1092–1106.

del Carmen-Wiggins, R. & Carter, A. (2004) *Handbook of Infant, Toddler, and Preschool Mental Health Assessment*. Oxford University Press, New York.

Dobrova-Krol, N. *et al.* (2010) The importance of quality of care: effects of perinatal HIV infection and early institutional rearing on preschoolers' attachment and indiscriminate friendliness. *Journal of Child Psychology and Psychiatry* **51**, 1368–1376.

Egger, H. & Angold, A. (2004) The Preschool Age Psychiatric Assessment (PAPA): a structured parent interview for diagnosing psychiatric disorders in preschool children. In: *Handbook of Infant, Toddler, and Preschool Mental Health Assessment*. (eds R. DelCarmen-Wiggins & A. Carter). Oxford University Press, New York. pp. 223–243.

Egger, H. *et al.* (2006) Test-retest reliability of the Preschool Age Psychiatric Assessment (PAPA). *Journal of the American Academy of Child and Adolescent Psychiatry* **45**, 538–549.

Feldman, R. *et al.* (2011) Mother and infant coordinate heart rhythms through episodes of interaction synchrony. *Infant Behavior and Development* **34**(4), 569–577.

Finelli, J. *et al.* (2019) Attachment disorders in early childhood. In: *Handbook of Infant Mental Health*. (ed C.H. Zeanah), 4th edn. Guilford Press, New York. pp. 452–466.

Giltaij, H.P. *et al.* (2017) Convergence between observations and interviews in clinical diagnosis of reactive attachment disorder and disinhibited social engagement disorder. *Clinical Child Psychology and Psychiatry* **22**(4), 603–619.

Gleason, M. *et al.* (2011a) Validity of evidence-derived criteria for reactive attachment disorder: indiscriminately social/disinhibited and emotionally withdrawn/inhibited types. *Journal of American Academy of Child and Adolescent Psychiatry* **50**, 216–231.

Gleason, M. *et al.* (2011b) Epidemiology of psychiatric disorders in very young children in a Romanian pediatric setting. *European Journal of Child and Adolescent Psychiatry* **20**, 527–535.

Gleason, M. *et al.* (2014) Indiscriminate behaviors in young children with a history of institutional care. *Pediatrics* **133**(3), e657–e665.

Goldfarb, W. (1945) Effects of psychological deprivation in infancy and subsequent stimulation. *American Journal of Psychiatry* **102**, 18–33.

Green, J. & Goldwyn, R. (2002) Annotation: attachment disorganization and psychopathology: new findings in attachment research and their potential implications for developmental psychopathology in childhood. *Journal of Child Psychology and Psychiatry* **43**, 835–846.

Guyon-Harris, K.L. *et al.* (2018) Course of disinhibited social engagement disorder from early childhood to early adolescence. *Journal of the American Academy of Child and Adolescent Psychiatry* **57**(5), 329–335.

Guyon-Harris, K.L. *et al.* (2019) A prospective longitudinal study of reactive attachment disorder following early institutional care: considering variable- and person-centered approaches. *Attachment & Human Development* **21**(2), 95–110.

Hodges, J. & Tizard, B. (1989) Social and family relationships of ex-institutional adolescents. *Journal of Child Psychology and Psychiatry, and Allied Disciplines* **30**, 77–97.

Hofer, M. (2006) Psychobiological roots of early attachment. *Current Directions in Psychological Science* **15**, 84–88.

Hoffman, K. *et al.* (2006) Changing toddlers' and preschoolers' attachment classifications: the Circle of Security Intervention. *Journal of Consulting and Clinical Psychology* **74**, 1017–1026.

Humphreys, K.L. *et al.* (2017a) Psychopathology following severe deprivation: history, research, and implications of Bucharest Early intervention Project. In: *Child Maltreatment in Residential Care: History, Research, and Current Practice.* (eds A.V. Rus, *et al.*). Springer International Publishing/Springer Nature, Cham, Switzerland. pp. 129–148.

Humphreys, K.L. *et al.* (2017b) Signs of reactive attachment disorder and disinhibited social engagement disorder at age 12 years: effects of institutional care history and high-quality foster care. *Development and Psychopathology* **29**, 677–686.

Järvinen-Pasley, A. *et al.* (2010) Affiliative behavior in Williams syndrome: social perception and real-life social behavior. *Neuropsychologia* **48**, 2110–2119.

Juffer, F. *et al.* (2005) Enhancing children's socio-emotional development: A review of intervention studies. In: *Handbook of Research Methods in Developmental Science.* (ed D.M. Teti). Blackwell, Oxford. pp. 213–232.

Juffer, F. *et al.* (2017) Pairing attachment theory and social learning theory in video-feedback intervention to promote positive parenting. *Current Opinion in Psychology* **15**, 189–194.

Kreppner, J. *et al.* (2010) Developmental course of deprivation-specific psychological patterns: early manifestations, persistence to age 15, and clinical features. In: *Deprivation-Specific Psychological Patterns: Effects of Institutional Deprivation.* (eds M. Rutter, *et al.*), Monographs of the Society for Research in Child Development, Serial No. 295, Vol. 75. pp. 79–101.

Lawler, J. *et al.* (2014) Disinhibited social engagement in postinstitutionalized children: differentiating normal from atypical behavior. *Development and Psychopathology* **26**(2), 451–464.

Lehman, S. *et al.* (2020) Development band examination of the reactive attachment disorder and disinhibited social engagement disorder assessment interview. *Assessment* **27**(4), 749–765.

Levy, R. (1947) Effects of institutional vs. boarding home care on a group of infants. *Journal of Personality* **15**, 233–241.

Lieberman, A. *et al.* (1991) Preventive intervention and outcome with anxiously attached dyads. *Child Development* **62**, 199–209.

Lorenz, K. (1943) Die angeborenen Formen möglicher Erfahrung. *Zeitschrift für Tierpsychologie* **5**, 235–409.

Lyons-Ruth, K. *et al.* (1999) Maternal frightened, frightening, or atypical behavior and disorganized attachment patterns. In: *Atypical Attachment in Early Childhood Among Children at Developmental Risk.* (eds K. Lyons-Ruth, *et al.*), Monographs of the Society for Research in Child Development, Serial No. 258, Vol. 64. pp. 67–96.

Lyons-Ruth, K. *et al.* (2019) Disinhibited attachment behavior among infants of mothers with borderline personality disorder, depression, and no diagnosis. *Personality Disorders* **10**(2), 163–172.

McGoron, L. *et al.* (2012) Recovering from early deprivation: Attachment mediates effects of caregiving on psychopathology. *Journal of the American Academy of Child and Adolescent Psychiatry* **51**, 683–693.

Minnis, H. *et al.* (2006) Reactive attachment disorder: a theoretical model beyond attachment. *European Journal of Child and Adolescent Psychiatry* **15**(6), 336–342.

Moss, E. *et al.* (2011) Efficacy of a home-visiting intervention aimed at improving maternal sensitivity, child attachment, and behavioral outcomes for maltreated children: a randomized control trial. *Development and Psychopathology* **23**(1), 195–210.

O'Connor, T. & Cameron, J. (2006) Translating research findings on early experience to prevention: animal and human evidence on early attachment relationships. *American Journal of Prevention Medicine* **31**, S175–S181.

O'Connor, T. & Rutter, M. (2000) Attachment disorder behavior following early severe deprivation: extension and longitudinal follow-up. *Journal of the American Academy of Child and Adolescent Psychiatry* **39**, 703–712.

O'Connor, T. & Zeanah, C. (2003) Assessment strategies and treatment approaches. *Attachment & Human Development* **5**, 223–244.

O'Connor, T. *et al.* (1999) Attachment disturbances and disorders in children exposed to early severe deprivation. *Infant Mental Health Journal* **20**, 10–29.

O'Connor, T. *et al.* (2003) Child-parent attachment following early institutional deprivation. *Development and Psychopathology* **15**, 19–38.

Oliveira, P. *et al.* (2012) Indiscriminate behavior observed in the strange situation among institutionalized toddlers: relations to caregiver report and to early family risk. *Infant Mental Health Journal* **33**, 187–196.

Oosterman, M. & Schuengel, C. (2007) Autonomic reactivity of children to separation and reunion with foster parents. *Journal of the American Academy of Child and Adolescent Psychiatry* **46**, 1196–1203.

Pears, K. *et al.* (2010) Indiscriminate friendliness in maltreated foster children. *Child Maltreatment* **15**, 64–75.

Provence, S. & Lipton, R. (1962) *Infants in Institutions.* International Universities Press, New York.

Roy, P. *et al.* (2004) Institutional care: associations between overactivity and lack of selectivity in social relationships. *Journal of Child Psychology and Psychiatry* **45**, 866–873.

Rutter, M. (1981) *Maternal Deprivation Reassessed*, 2nd edn. Penguin Books, Harmondsworth, UK.

Rutter, M. *et al.* (2007a) Effects of profound early institutional deprivation: an overview of findings from a UK longitudinal study of Romanian adoptees. *European Journal of Developmental Psychology* **4**, 332–350.

Rutter, M. *et al.* (2007b) Early adolescent outcomes for institutionally deprived and non-deprived adoptees. I. Disinhibited attachment. *Journal of Child Psychology and Psychiatry* **48**, 17–30.

Rutter, M. *et al.* (2010) Deprivation-specific psychological patterns: effects of institutional deprivation. *Monographs of the Society for Research in Child Development* serial no. 295 **75**, 48–78.

Scheeringa, M. & Haslett, N. (2010) The reliability and criterion validity of the Diagnostic Infant and Preschool Assessment: a new diagnostic instrument for young children. *Child Psychiatry and Human Development* **41**, 299–312.

Schuengel, C. *et al.* (1999) Frightening maternal behavior linking unresolved loss and disorganized infant attachment. *Journal of Consulting and Clinical Psychology* **67**, 54–63.

Seim, A.R. *et al.* (2020) Validity of reactive attachment disorder and disinhibited social engagement disorder in adolescence. *European Journal of Child and Adolescent Psychiatry* **29**(10), 1465–1476.

Smyke, A. *et al.* (2002) Disturbances of attachment in young children. I. The continuum of caretaking casualty. *Journal of the American Academy of Child and Adolescent Psychiatry* **41**, 972–982.

Smyke, A. *et al.* (2012) A randomized controlled trial comparing foster care and institutional care for children with signs of reactive attachment disorder. *American Journal of Psychiatry* **169**, 508–514.

Smyke A.T. & Zeanah C.H. (1999) Disturbances of Attachment Interview-Revised. Available: https://medicine.tulane.edu/sites/default/files/pictures/DAI%20Revised%207.17.17.pdf [8 January 2025].

Smyke, A.T. *et al.* (2010) Placement in foster care enhances quality of attachment among young institutionalized children. *Child Development* **81**(1), 212–222.

Soares, I. *et al.* (2013) Why do only some institutionalized children become indiscriminately friendly? Insights from the study of Williams syndrome. *Child Development Perspectives* **7**, 1–6.

Spitz, R.A. (1945) Hospitalism: an inquiry into the genesis of psychiatric conditions in early childhood. *Psychoanalytic Study of the Child* **1**, 53–74.

Sroufe, L.A. & Waters, E. (1977) Attachment as an organizational construct. *Child Development* **48**(4), 1184–1199.

Stern, D. (1977) *The First Relationship: Mother and Infant.* Harvard University Press, Cambridge, MA.

Suomi, S. *et al.* (1976) Effects of maternal and peer separation on young monkeys. *Journal of Child Psychology and Psychiatry* **17**, 101–112.

Tarullo, A. *et al.* (2011) Atypical EEG power correlates with indiscriminately friendly behavior in internationally adopted children. *Developmental Psychology* **47**, 417–431.

Tharner, A. *et al.* (2012) Infant attachment, parenting stress, and child emotional and behavioral problems at age 3 years. *Parenting: Science and Practice* **12**(4), 261–281.

The St. Petersburg—USA Orphanage Research Team (2008) The effects of early social-emotional and relationship experience on the development of young orphanage children. *Monographs of the Society for Research in Child Development, Serial No. 291* **73**, vii–295.

Tizard, B. (1977) *Adoption: A Second Chance.* Open Books, London.

Tizard, B. & Hodges, J. (1978) The effect of early institutional rearing on the development of eight year old children. *Journal of Child Psychology and Psychiatry* **19**, 99–118.

Tizard, B. & Rees, J. (1975) The effect of early institutional rearing on the behaviour problems and affectional relationships of four-year-old children. *Journal of Child Psychology and Psychiatry* **16**, 61–73.

van IJzendoorn, M. & Bakermans-Kranenburg, M. (2002) Disorganized attachment and the dysregulation of negative emotions. In: *Emotion Regulation and Developmental Health: Infancy and Early Childhood.* (eds B. Zuckerman, *et al.*). Johnson and Johnson Pediatric Institute, Somerville, NJ. pp. 159–179.

van IJzendoorn, M. *et al.* (1999) Disorganized attachment in early childhood: meta-analysis of precursors, concomitants, and sequelae. *Development and Psychopathology* **11**, 225–249.

Vorria, P. *et al.* (2003) Early experiences and attachment relationships of Greek infants raised in residential group care. *Journal of Child Psychology and Psychiatry* **44**(8), 1208–1220.

Woolgar, M. & Baldock, E. (2015) Attachment disorders versus more common problems in looked after and adopted children: comparing community and expert assessments. *Child and Adolescent Mental Health* **20**, 34–40.

World Health Organization (2019) *International Statistical Classification of Disease and Related Health Problems*, 11th edn. World Health Organization (WHO), Geneva, Switzerland.

Zeanah, C.H. & Boris, N. (2000) Disturbances and disorders of attachment in early childhood. In: *Handbook of Infant Mental Health.* (ed C.H. Zeanah), 2nd edn. Guilford Press, New York. pp. 353–368.

Zeanah, C.H. & Gleason, M.M. (2015) Annual research review: attachment disorders in early childhood—clinical presentation, causes, correlates, and treatment. *Journal of Child Psychology and Psychiatry* **56**, 207–222.

Zeanah, C.H. & Guyon-Harris, K.L. (2020) Commentary: Increasing diagnostic precision in reactive attachment disorder - a commentary on Allen & Schuengel (2019). *Child and Adolescent Mental Health* **25**(1), 11–12.

Zeanah, C.H. *et al.* (1985) Prenatal perception of infant personality: a preliminary investigation. *Journal of the American Academy of Child Psychiatry* **24**, 204–210.

Zeanah, C.H. *et al.* (2000) Infant-parent relationship assessment. In: *Handbook of Infant Mental Health.* (ed C.H. Zeanah), 2nd edn. Guilford Press, New York. pp. 222–235.

Zeanah, C.H. *et al.* (2002) Disturbances of attachment in young children. II. Indiscriminate behavior and institutional care. *Journal of the American Academy of Child and Adolescent Psychiatry* **41**, 983–989.

Zeanah, C.H. *et al.* (2004) Reactive attachment disorder in maltreated toddlers. *Child Abuse and Neglect* **28**, 877–888.

Zeanah, C.H. *et al.* (2005) Attachment in institutionalized and noninstitutionalized Romanian children. *Child Development* **76**, 1015–1028.

Zeanah, C.H. *et al.* (2006) Orphanages as a developmental context for early childhood. In: *Blackwell Handbook of Early Childhood Development.* (eds K. McCartney & D. Phillips). Blackwell Publishing, Malden, MA. pp. 224–254.

Zeanah, C.H. *et al.* (2011) Practitioner review: clinical applications of attachment theory and research for infants and young children. *Journal of Child Psychology and Psychiatry* **52**, 819–833.

Zeanah, C.H. *et al.* (2016) Practice parameters for the assessment and treatment of children and adolescents with reactive attachment disorder of infancy and early childhood and disinhibited social engagement disorder. *Journal of the American Academy of Child and Adolescent Psychiatry* **55**, 990–1003.

ZERO TO THREE (2005) *Diagnostic Classification: 0-3R: The Diagnostic Classification of Mental Health and Developmental Disorders of Infancy and Early Childhood*, revised edn. Zero to Three Press, Washington, DC.

Zhang, L. *et al.* (2002) Maternal deprivation increases cell death in the infant rat brain. *Developmental Brain Research* **133**, 1–11.

Zimmermann, P. & Iwanski, A. (2019) Attachment disorder behavior in early and middle childhood: associations with children's self-concept and observed signs of negative internal working models. *Attachment & Human Development* **21**(2), 170–189.

CHAPTER 58

Post-traumatic stress disorder

Richard Meiser-Stedman[1], Patrick Smith[2] and William Yule[2]

[1] Department of Clinical Psychology & Psychological Therapies, Norwich Medical School, University of East Anglia, Norwich, UK

[2] Department of Psychology, Institute of Psychiatry, Psychology and Neuroscience, King's College London, London, UK

The diagnosis of post-traumatic stress disorder in children and adolescents

Post-traumatic stress disorder (PTSD) first entered the *Diagnostic and Statistical Manual of Mental Disorders*, 3rd edition (DSM-III) in 1980 (American Psychiatric Association, 1980). While people's adverse reactions to traumatic events had been documented and debated before that point (e.g., Andreasen, 2010), the introduction of a formal psychiatric diagnosis facilitated a leap forward in the following decades in the scientific understanding of responses to such experiences, and consequently the assessment, management, and treatment of this disorder. The distinct needs of children and adolescents have been recognized amid this progress, and now a considerable evidence base exists to support the delivery of evidence-based care for PTSD in this population.

Central to the diagnosis of PTSD—regardless of whether the DSM or the *International Classification of Diseases* (ICD) is used—is exposure to a traumatic stressor. The current definitions of trauma for both DSM ("exposure to actual or threatened death, serious injury, or sexual violence") and ICD ("an extremely threatening or horrific event or series of events") have converged in that they recognize the role of threat. This of course presents some issues when working with children and adolescents, but does allow the clinician to acknowledge the central importance of the child's perspective. DSM has additional requirements—the trauma must have been either: directly experienced; witnessed; involve learning about a trauma occurring to a close family member or friend; or involve repeated or extreme exposure to aversive details of the event.

A PTSD diagnosis requires the presence of a range of symptoms in addition to exposure itself. While there are clear commonalities between DSM and ICD conceptualizations of PTSD—with a focus on reexperiencing, avoidance, and current threat or hyperarousal—DSM-5 (American Psychiatric Association, 2013) PTSD has very specific symptom requirements across four clusters, whereas ICD-11 (World Health Organization, 2019) has a less prescribed definition.

The reexperiencing symptoms of PTSD are the most distinctively associated with this disorder. Starting almost immediately, children may be troubled by repetitive, intrusive memories of the event. Such thoughts can occur at any time, but particularly when the children are otherwise quiet, as when they are trying to drop off to sleep. At other times, the thoughts and vivid recollections are triggered off by reminders in their environment. Vivid, dissociative flashbacks may be less common, but certainly occur. In a flashback, the child reports that they are reexperiencing the event, as if it were happening all over again. Nightmares with clear themes relating to the trauma can occur, though sometimes the content of such nightmares can be less obvious. These different forms of reexperiencing may be accompanied by strong physiological sensations (e.g., increased heart rate, sweating, shaking).

Children and adolescents certainly attempt to avoid trauma reminders in a variety of ways—cognitively, they may push memories or thoughts of the trauma out of mind, while behaviorally they make efforts to avoid places, people, or objects reminiscent of the trauma(s). These efforts may become quite automatic, and can be quite sophisticated (e.g., anticipating television programs that may potentially present trauma-related stimuli) or very overgeneral (e.g., avoiding all men; being outside). They may also be supported and encouraged in these processes by families and schools, as people and systems around the child become fearful of causing additional distress.

The hyperarousal symptoms of PTSD can be very disturbing and have a major impact on a child's self-concept and

Rutter's Child and Adolescent Psychiatry and Psychology, Seventh Edition.
Edited by Anita Thapar, Daniel S. Pine, Samuele Cortese, Cathy Creswell, Tamsin J. Ford, James F. Leckman, and Argyris Stringaris.

Companion website: www.wiley.com/go/thapar/rutterspsych7

functioning. Hypervigilance—an excessive monitoring of the environment for potential threats—is common, as is an exaggerated startle response. Many experience difficulties in concentration, especially in schoolwork. Sleep disturbances are common. Greater irritability and anger—and the consequent interference with relationships with others—can be pronounced and highly distressing, as it can add to the perception that they have undergone an enduring personality change.

Numerous other difficulties, not necessary for a diagnosis of PTSD, may also be seen. Not surprisingly, many develop fears associated with specific aspects of their experiences. In addition to nightmares, fears of the dark and waking through the night are widespread (and often manifest outside the developmental age range in which they normally occur). Separation difficulties are frequent, even among teenagers. For the first few days, children may not want to let their parents out of their sight, even reverting to sleeping in the parental bed.

A major difference between the DSM and ICD conceptualizations of PTSD is the inclusion of the complex post-traumatic stress disorder (CPTSD) diagnosis in ICD-11. CPTSD is conceived of as a distinctive form of PTSD that may result from exposure to "prolonged or repetitive events from which escape is difficult or impossible", though may also result from more "simple" trauma. In addition to the core symptom requirements of PTSD, CPTSD requires the presence of problems in affect regulation, beliefs about oneself as diminished, defeated or worthless, and difficulties in sustaining relationships and in feeling close to others. The addition of CPTSD has been welcomed as a positive contribution to the PTSD field, as it specifically recognizes the impact of sustained trauma exposure, which may reflect the particular experiences of many children and adolescents (e.g., different forms of abuse). However, the literature around this construct is still in its infancy, particularly with regards to children and adolescents.

Comorbidity

The presence of comorbid conditions, such as depression, other anxiety disorders, and externalizing conditions, is very common in children and adolescents with PTSD. Data from the large UK Environmental Risk Longitudinal Twin (E-Risk) Study show that in 160 youth with a lifetime history of PTSD, 54.7% had had a major depressive episode in the previous year (Lewis *et al.*, 2019); depression occurred at a significantly greater rate than in trauma exposed youth without a history of PTSD. Youth with a history of PTSD also commonly experienced generalized anxiety disorder (23.8%) and psychotic symptoms (9.4%), at significantly greater rates than trauma-exposed youth without a history of PTSD. In 6132 Chinese adolescents exposed to the 2013 Ya'an earthquake, 13.1% were estimated to have PTSD; of these youth with PTSD, 71.5% reported anxiety, and 49.7% reported depression (i.e., above cutoff on a self-report questionnaire; Tang *et al.*, 2018). PTSD is associated with greater suicidal ideation and substance abuse. Some children may have been bereaved and may develop traumatic grief reactions.

Recognition of the broader impact of trauma on youth mental health and functioning is critical for good care. It is also important to bear in mind that children and adolescents identified as having one disorder (e.g., conduct problems) may have undiagnosed PTSD that is strongly related to their presenting difficulty.

Developmental aspects

There are multiple ways in which children's cognitive immaturity may impact their processing of a traumatic experience, and the risk of developing PTSD (Salmon & Bryant, 2002). However, older children and adolescents seem to experience the full range of PTSD symptoms, and diagnostic frameworks can be applied to these youth without major difficulty. This is borne out by meta-analyses that suggest a very small relationship between being younger and risk of PTSD (Trickey *et al.*, 2012).

In the case of preschool children, however, it is recognized that the typical diagnostic criteria are not appropriate. Since young children are typically less able to describe complicated cognitive and physiological states, assessment is reliant on observable symptoms and interviews with caregivers. Following careful work by Scheeringa *et al.* (2006), DSM-5 (American Psychiatric Association, 2013) includes a preschool PTSD diagnosis, with lower symptom thresholds and the reformulating of other criteria in more developmentally appropriate terms. Both DSM and ICD note how reexperiencing may manifest through play reenactment, that frightening dreams may not comprise content clearly related to the trauma, and the increased presence of temper tantrums; ICD notes several other manifestations of PTSD in preschool children (e.g., inhibited and disinhibited behaviors, separation anxiety, regression in skills [e.g., verbal skills, toileting], exaggerated age-associated fears). The use of such age-appropriate criteria has led to increased detection rates (Woolgar *et al.*, 2022).

Cultural aspects

Research into children's responses to trauma and PTSD has been dominated by a White Western perspective; a recent commentary reported that 84% of first authors of clinical trials in the area of child and adolescent PTSD were White, with the majority of research being conducted in western countries; only 7 out of 61 trials (11%) were published by lead authors who were of color and/or based in a low- or middle-income country (LMIC; Alisic *et al.*, 2021). We raise this to acknowledge the authors' own perspectives, and underline the need for efforts to support a more inclusive and representative field of researchers in this area. This is especially important given youth in LMICs are more likely to experience trauma such as wars and natural disasters.

While recognizing this important limitation about the state of research into child and adolescent PTSD, some features of this disorder might be considered to be universal, given the insights gleaned from studies so far. There is evidence from a number of sources that PTSD presents very similarly in many different cultures, but ways of intervening may need to be modified. For example, very similar stress reactions have been reported in children across all continents where studies have been undertaken (Thabet & Vostanis, 1999; Neuner *et al.*, 2006).

Many studies have used similar self-completed screening questionnaires to assess trauma symptoms. If PTSD transcends cultural barriers, then similar underlying factor structures should be found if they are measuring the same construct. To date, this has been the case in Cambodia (Sack *et al.*, 1997), Bosnia (Smith *et al.*, 2003), and China (Wang *et al.*, 2011), indicating that stress reactions demonstrate cross-cultural validity for children and adolescents.

Impact on functioning and long-term severity

Is PTSD an important condition to assess for in children and adolescents; and when present, does it warrant treatment? A diagnosis of PTSD does imply something more than distress alone; the ICD-11 conceptualization requires impaired functioning, while the DSM-5 (American Psychiatric Association, 2013) diagnosis requires impaired functioning or "clinically significant distress." The importance of taking PTSD seriously is supported by a considerable literature that documents the impact this disorder can have for children and adolescents. PTSD in children and adolescents is associated with worse social functioning and academic attainment (Saigh *et al.*, 1997; McLean *et al.*, 2013). This literature is founded on comparison with youth exposed to trauma but without PTSD (or with less severe PTSD). Moreover, data from the UK E-Risk study show that relative to trauma-exposed youth without PTSD, youth with a history of having PTSD are more likely to experience loneliness, social isolation, not be in education, employment, or training, undertake self-harm or make a suicide attempt, and commit a violent offense (Lewis *et al.*, 2019).

A further key consideration is that PTSD can persist for years or even decades. A significant proportion (17.5%) of the *Jupiter* ferry survivors (the ferry carried many UK schoolchildren and sank in Greek waters in 1988) continued to have PTSD at a five year follow-up assessment (Yule *et al.*, 2000). Long-term follow-up studies of repeated trauma, such as maltreatment, suggest that the risks of PTSD are as high, if not higher (Strathearn *et al.*, 2020).

In summary, PTSD can be a chronic condition in youth, with major implications for wider well-being, functioning, and mental health. The case for viewing PTSD as a significant mental disorder that warrants assessment and treatment, and not just transient distress, is robust.

Epidemiology and course

The prevalence of exposure to trauma

The undeniable tragedy is that exposure to trauma is a common, even ubiquitous, occurrence for children and adolescents. Numerous large-scale surveys, from a variety of countries, indicate the widespread nature of trauma exposure. In high-income countries prevalence rates are typically larger than 40%.

In their survey of over 6,000 Swiss 16-year-olds, Landolt *et al.* (2013) found a trauma prevalence rate of 56%. In the UK E-Risk study, 31% of the 2064 participants reported trauma exposure by age 18 years (Lewis *et al.*, 2019). In over 6,000 13–17-year-old adolescents in the US, an estimate of lifetime exposure to trauma of 61% was obtained (McLaughlin *et al.*, 2013).

Estimates of trauma prevalence rates in LMICs are less available. One recent study utilized responses from over 160,000 12–15-year-olds across 68 LMICs (Han *et al.*, 2019). This analysis suggested a prevalence rate of 35.6% for physical attacks, 36.4% for physical fighting, and 42.9% for serious injuries in the previous 12 months. In their meta-analysis of the global prevalence of child sexual abuse, comprising data from over 9 million child participants across 331 studies, Stoltenborgh *et al.* (2011) reported a *self-reported* prevalence estimate of 12.7%; their *informant* estimate was much lower at 0.4%.

Preschool children are at less risk of exposure to trauma according some large-scale surveys. A UK survey suggested a trauma exposure rate of only 7% (Hitchcock *et al.*, 2021) though it is important to note that this age group are less able to report trauma, and data for this age group are of course based on caregiver report rather than self-report. In the US, certain trauma types (kidnapping, physical abuse by a caregiver) were much more common in early childhood (McLaughlin *et al.*, 2013).

The range of estimates of trauma exposure clearly vary to a large degree, and understanding what factors explain the variation in these estimates—e.g., sampling methods, diagnostic framework used, survey tools used, age group—is an important issue. Nevertheless, the evidence we have underscores the scale of the issue, and the need to see trauma exposure in childhood and adolescence as a major public health issue.

The prevalence of post-traumatic stress disorder

While trauma may be common, it is not the case that all children and adolescents exposed to trauma develop PTSD. Indeed, several systematic reviews suggest that only a minority of trauma-exposed youth develop PTSD. A key clinical concern related to this can be to reassure those caring for youth that their child may not necessarily develop a severe reaction, like PTSD, in response to trauma, while also recognizing that this is a possibility.

In their landmark systematic review and meta-analysis, Alisic *et al.* (2014) pooled data from surveys of trauma-exposed children and adolescents that used gold-standard structured interview assessments. Forty-three samples comprising 3563 children and adolescents were included in the review. The overall estimate was 15.9%. However, both trauma type and sex moderated this result. Noninterpersonal trauma yielded a significantly lower rate of PTSD (9.7%) compared to interpersonal trauma (25.2%), while girls yielded a higher rate (20.8%) than boys (11.1%). The review was predominantly based on studies of youth in high-income countries, however. With respect to trauma-exposed preschool children, Woolgar *et al.* (2022)

obtained a pooled estimate for PTSD of 21.5% in 18 studies (N = 1941).

The alternative approach to considering rates of PTSD is to consider whole communities, rather than trauma-exposed groups exclusively. Most such epidemiological studies have been of older adolescents and adults. Merikangas *et al.* (2010) report a lifetime prevalence of 5% using data collected from over 10,000 US adolescents (up to 18 years old). The UK E-Risk study yielded a lifetime prevalence for PTSD of 7.8% (by age 18; Lewis *et al.*, 2019). In summary, PTSD is a common psychiatric disorder in children and adolescents.

The course of post-traumatic stress disorder

Both DSM and ICD diagnostic systems require that PTSD symptoms be present for several weeks before a formal diagnosis can be made; such systems implicitly assume that an early reaction to trauma is a common response and may not necessarily be pathological or go on to be persistent. Recognizing that this approach left some individuals without a pathway to accessing mental health care, DSM-IV (American Psychiatric Association, 1994) introduced the "acute stress disorder" diagnosis to encapsulate reactions within the first four weeks of a trauma that warrant attention, and also to serve as a means to identify youth at risk of persistent PTSD.

In their systematic review and meta-analysis of the prevalence of acute stress disorder in children and adolescents, Walker *et al.* (2020) obtained an estimate of 16.5% from 17 studies that met their inclusion criteria. This figure is consistent with the review undertaken by Hiller *et al.* (2016). In their meta-analysis of 27 longitudinal studies, a pooled PTSD prevalence rate of 21% was obtained for the acute (1 month) post-trauma phase. However, this rate declined to 15% at 3 months, to 12% at 6 months, and to 11% at 1 year post-trauma. The frequency of recovery is borne out by other large scale longitudinal studies (e.g., Lai *et al.*, 2021). These recent analyses show that a minority of trauma-exposed young people develop PTSD, and that many recover spontaneously; however, the chances of spontaneous recovery after 6 months become slim.

That so many youth can recover over time without formal intervention is a key feature of PTSD in youth that is important for clinicians to consider when planning a response to trauma, particularly when dealing with large numbers of trauma-exposed children and adolescents. Attempting early intervention (e.g., in the first few weeks, post-trauma) is not always feasible, but these studies suggest that early intervention may also be *unnecessary*.

It is important to note that this evidence base is weighted toward high-income countries and noninterpersonal trauma, e.g., accidental injuries that necessitate a visit to a hospital emergency department. Studies of more at-risk populations yield different patterns. For example, Khadr *et al.* (2018) undertook a study of 141 (overwhelmingly female) adolescent victims of sexual assault, recruited from sexual assault referral centers in Greater London. Rates of PTSD were high at baseline (90% scored above the cutoff on the CRIES-13, a widely used questionnaire tool for assessing PTSD in youth) and did not significantly diminish by the time of the 4–5 month follow-up (83%) or the 13–15 month follow-up (87%).

Risk factors and etiology

As outlined above, typically only a minority of trauma-exposed young people will develop persistent PTSD. These findings have prompted much research into understanding these individual differences in outcomes and identifying risk factors for PTSD. Findings from such research have potential for practical clinical application. For example, identification of fixed markers (such as severity of trauma exposure, or gender) may be useful in identifying children most at risk so that services can be directed to them. Identification of causal risk factors may help to refine our understanding of the etiology of PTSD in children and adolescents, and define targets for therapeutic intervention. In this section, we outline different risk factors for PTSD in children and adolescents, and consider how they might inform our understanding of the etiology of PTSD. We summarize the results of meta-analyses relating to specific risk factors, in particular the correlation between different risk factors and PTSD severity, in Table 58.1.

Trauma-related and demographic risk factors for post-traumatic stress disorder

Early studies investigated whether the severity of exposure to trauma was associated with later pathology. There is now good evidence for a significant exposure–response relationship among children exposed to single-event trauma (Pynoos *et al.*, 1987), war (Dyregrov *et al.*, 2000), and mass disaster (La Greca *et al.*, 2010). A meta-analysis (of 96 studies; total N = 74,000) of children exposed to disaster (Furr *et al.*, 2010) found a medium effect size (r = 0.33) for proximity to the event, on PTSD symptoms. In sum, there is a significant relationship between the "objective" level of trauma exposure and later adjustment across a broad range of trauma types. However, the strength of this relationship is generally modest. A robust finding in the literature is that the *type* of trauma exposure is important, with multiple reviews finding that interpersonal trauma is associated with a greater risk of developing PTSD than noninterpersonal trauma (Alisic *et al.*, 2014; Walker *et al.*, 2020; Woolgar *et al.*, 2022).

In this context, researchers have investigated additional factors that may be associated with the development of persistent PTSD. A meta-analysis by Trickey *et al.* (2012) of risk factors provides a helpful and timely account of this rapidly growing area. Using data from 64 studies (N = 32,000 children and adolescents aged 6–18 years) which included a broad range of trauma types, population effect size estimates were derived for 25 potential risk factors for PTSD. Peri- and post-traumatic factors showed larger effect sizes on persistent PTSD than

Table 58.1 Correlates of post-traumatic stress disorder (PTSD) in children and adolescents: a summary of meta-analysis results.

Risk factor	Number of studies	Number of participants	Effect size estimate (r)	95% confidence interval (CI)	Author
Demographic variables					
Age	29	2,940	−0.01[ns]	−0.07, 0.05	Alisic *et al.*(2011)
	18	NR	0.03[ns]	−0.04, 0.10	Trickey *et al.* (2012)
Gender[a]	31	3,195	0.13	0.08, 0.17	Alisic *et al.* (2011)
	29	NR	0.15	0.13, 0.18	Trickey *et al.* (2012)
Minority status	13	1,308	0.09[ns]	−0.05, 0.23	Alisic *et al.* (2011)
	5	NR	0.08	0.04, 0.12	Trickey *et al.* (2012)
Prior mental health difficulty	14	NR	0.15	0.11, 0.20	Trickey *et al.* (2012)
Objective trauma severity					
Injury severity	18	1,381	0.09	0.01, 0.16	Alisic *et al.* (2011)
Trauma severity	41	NR	0.29	0.24, 0.35	Trickey *et al.* (2012)
Social and familial risk factors					
Parent post-traumatic stress disorder (PTSD) symptoms	32	NR	0.31	0.25, 0.37	Morris *et al.* (2012)
Parent depression	9	NR	0.32	0.21, 0.41	Morris *et al.* (2012)
Parent mental health	25	NR	0.29	0.22, 0.36	Trickey *et al.* (2012)
Parenting—negative	14	NR	0.23	0.13, 0.26	Williamson *et al.* (2017)
Parenting—positive[b]	11	NR	0.14	0.04, 0.25	Williamson *et al.* (2017)
Family functioning	7	NR	0.46	0.15, 0.77	Trickey *et al.* (2012)
Social support	41	23,756	−0.12	−0.16, −0.07	Allen *et al.* (2021)
Attachment—secure	20	8,544	−0.16	−0.24, −0.07	Cushing *et al.* (2024)
Attachment—insecure	16	4,019	0.20	0.14, 0.27	Cushing *et al.* (2024)
Attachment—avoidant	9	2,242	0.20	0.11, 0.29	Cushing *et al.* (2024)
Attachment—anxious	7	2,842	0.32	0.26, 0.37	Cushing *et al.* (2024)
Attachment—disorganized	5	214	0.17	0.06, 0.28	Cushing *et al.* (2024)
Cognitive psychological risk factors					
Subjective threat	28	23,744	0.37	0.31, 0.42	Memarzia *et al.* (2021)
Peritraumatic dissociation	5	566	0.17	0.03, 0.29	Memarzia *et al.* (2021)
Anxiety sensitivity	6	1,331	0.56	0.47, 0.64	Chiu *et al.* (2024)
Trauma memory characteristics	11	1,270	0.52	0.31, 0.68	Reed *et al.* (2023)
Negative appraisals	25	9,326	0.59	0.54, 0.64	Gomez de la Cuesta *et al.* (2019)

Note: NR—not reported; ns—nonsignificant; r—pooled correlation coefficient estimate. Correlation coefficients >0.1 are conventionally described as "small", >0.3 are "medium", and >0.5 are "large".

[a] Positive associations indicate that females were associated with more severe PTSD symptoms.

[b] Positive associations indicate that more positive parent behaviors were associated with decreased PTSD severity.

pre-trauma demographic factors and the severity of exposure. Specifically, fixed markers such as age, gender, and ethnicity showed negligible to small effects (r = 0.03–0.15). Objective trauma severity showed a small to medium effect (r = 0.29) but was highly variable. Broadly similar results were found in a meta-analytic review undertaken by Alisic and colleagues (Alisic *et al.*, 2011; see Table 58.1).

Biomarkers and genetic risk factors

In their review of literature concerning the psychophysiological characteristics of PTSD in children and adolescents, Kirsch *et al.* (2011) observed evidence for differential sympathetic nervous system activity. Consistent evidence was found for elevated heart rate (HR) post-trauma in children who go on to develop PTSD, with a stronger relationship the earlier HR is assessed. This is based on studies of children attending emergency departments, particularly following road traffic collisions. The literature they summarized did not show evidence of differences between youth with PTSD and healthy controls during tasks that did not involve trauma-related stressors, but did emerge during exposure to trauma scripts. This finding might be interpreted in multiple ways: elevated heart rate might reflect the acute onset of hyperarousal symptoms, a greater conditioning response, be linked to greater subjective threat, a marker of greater pre-trauma anxiety, or a combination of these processes.

The Kirsch review also found that noradrenaline and adrenaline (based on both urinary and serum samples) were higher in children who develop PTSD. Hypothalamic–pituitary–adrenal axis (HPA axis) differences were consistent across different methods for measuring cortisol (i.e., urinary, salivary, and serum), with cortisol levels higher in the evening and over 24 hours, but lower in the morning. However, the authors note the comparative lack of research into children and adolescents, with a considerable amount of methodological variation between studies. Some efforts have been made to make use of such biomarkers for the identification of youth at-risk of developing PTSD (Winston *et al.*, 2003), but further pragmatic evaluations of such procedures have not been conducted.

Considerable research uses brain-imaging methods in an attempt to identify biomarkers related to trauma exposure or the diagnosis of PTSD. This research is reviewed in Cisler and Herringa (2021); see also Chapters 11 on brain imaging, 12 on systems neuroscience, 20 on biological mechanisms associated with childhood adversity, and 59 on anxiety disorders. Studies in children link the experience of trauma or symptoms of PTSD to the structure and function of brain regions associated with multiple psychological processes. These psychological processes include aspects of executive function, reward processing, and threat responsivity. Moreover, associated brain regions include the prefrontal cortex, amygdala, hippocampus, basal ganglia, and cingulate gyrus. Despite the rapid pace of this research, findings in PTSD parallel those described in other textbook chapters concerning most areas of pediatric psychopathology: brain-imaging research remains at an early stage, with most findings based on small samples without replication.

Genetically informative studies of adults have established that PTSD risk is modestly heritable (Smoller, 2016), but such findings have yet to be reliably replicated in children and adolescents. Adult twin studies find evidence for some degree of heritability of risk for exposure to trauma and PTSD, probably via genetic effects on personality (Stein *et al.*, 2002). Twin studies of adults report heritability estimates of PTSD to be around 30% for males (True *et al.*, 1993), with higher estimates for females (Sartor *et al.*, 2011), and a striking degree of overlap in heritability of PTSD and depression in trauma-exposed adults (Sartor *et al.*, 2012). Molecular genetic perspectives have recently focused on genome-wide association study (GWAS) designs, with some loci identified (Stein *et al.*, 2021). Work continues with such approaches, but there is no evidence of replicability across multiple studies so far, and efforts to build larger datasets are underway (Nievergelt *et al.*, 2018).

Epigenetic research—the study of how gene expression can differ—is a further advance in our understanding of genetic factors. One study found that DNA methylation—which can be used to track epigenetic age acceleration—was associated with direct experience of violence in 101 6–13-year-olds (Jovanovic *et al.*, 2017). The authors speculate that such age acceleration may be adaptive in the short term (e.g., through improved heart rate regulation) but at the cost of long-term harm (e.g., greater risk of cardiovascular disease). Further research with children and adolescents is needed to explore the intricate links between genes and the expression of PTSD.

The role of families, social support, and attachment

Multiple strands of research suggest that a child's social context is related to PTSD. Family functioning and parental mental health post-trauma both show significant associations with children's PTSD symptoms in a number of studies. Numerous studies have established that poor parental mental health (depression, anxiety, and PTSD) correlates with child PTSD symptoms, showing a medium effect size overall (Morris *et al.*, 2012; Trickey *et al.*, 2012).

Aspects of parenting have been shown to be correlated with children's PTSD symptoms following trauma. Williamson *et al.* (2017) demonstrated a small but significant relationship ($r = 0.23$) between negative parenting behaviors (e.g., hostility, overprotection) and child PTSD, as well as a small but significant protective relationship between greater positive parenting behaviors (e.g., support, warmth) and PTSD ($r = 0.14$).

Although there are far fewer studies of family functioning than parental mental health, initial effect size estimates are larger for family functioning than for parental mental health. The mechanisms underlying these familial associations remain unclear. In part, they may derive from a complex interaction between parents and children who can become locked into cycles of not talking about the event for fear of upsetting each other. That is, carers and children may negatively reinforce each other for avoiding processing their traumatic memories, and this is likely to maintain the symptoms of both. Trickey *et al.* (2012) found a moderate association ($r = 0.46$) between family functioning and PTSD severity, but this was based on seven relatively small studies.

Social support has been of increasing interest to researchers. In summarizing the extensive research into social support since the 2000s, Allen *et al.* (2021) found that while a significant effect was present it was only small in size ($r = -0.12$), but broadly similar in strength across peers, families, and teachers.

Attachment has been a topic of considerable interest for considering responses to trauma. In their recent review, Cushing *et al.* (2024) found that secure and insecure attachment were the most common studied forms of attachment, yielding a small negative relationship (r = −0.16) and a small positive relationship (r = 0.20), respectively.

In summary, there are consistent but mostly small relationships between children's PTSD and their social environment.

The role of behavioral and cognitive factors

A key cognitive model in the adult literature, that of Ehlers and Clark (2000), proposes that PTSD becomes persistent as a result of excessively negative appraisals of the trauma and/or its sequelae, and disturbances in the autobiographical memory for the trauma, such that the trauma memories are characterized by poor elaboration and contextualization, and strong associative memory. Moreover, changes in negative appraisals and the trauma memory are thought to be inhibited by maladaptive behavioral and cognitive strategies. Another cognitive theory stresses the role of different memory systems in producing the characteristic symptoms of PTSD (i.e., dual representation theory; Brewin *et al.*, 1996).

An emerging literature supports the relevance of these theories for children and adolescents. A robust relationship exists between subjective threat and the appraisal of threat to life during a trauma, and subsequent risk of developing PTSD, while dissociation during the trauma has also been shown to have a role, even if less powerful (Memarzia *et al.*, 2021). Such processes are thought to be associated with laying down more sensory-based, fragmented memories for trauma, as proposed in cognitive accounts of PTSD. Several studies—albeit typically conducted in high-income countries—have found that children and adolescents reporting more sensory-based and fragmented memories for a given trauma are more likely to report having PTSD symptoms (Reed *et al.*, 2023). Analysis of children's trauma narratives has also found some evidence of a relationship between fragmented accounts and PTSD severity (Salmond *et al.*, 2011) but this has not been replicated (e.g., McGuire *et al.*, 2021).

Children's and adolescents' negative appraisals of trauma—e.g., beliefs that they are vulnerable to harm from others, weak, permanently psychologically damaged, or "going mad"—have been shown to be a consistently strong correlates and predictors of PTSD (Gomez De La Cuesta *et al.*, 2019). Several studies have demonstrated that such appraisals can have an important role for children soon after a trauma (Meiser-Stedman *et al.*, 2019), as well as for children who have been repeatedly maltreated, abused, or neglected (Hiller *et al.*, 2021). Cross-cultural evidence for the role of unhelpful trauma-related appraisals has also been demonstrated, e.g., in Sri Lankan children (Ponnamperuma & Nicolson, 2016).

It is encouraging that some of the largest effects of any correlate or risk factor studied to date have been for processes that can in principle be targeted and modified in therapy. Indeed, multiple randomized control trials (RCTs) of trauma-focused psychological therapies for young people with PTSD (e.g., Smith *et al.*, 2007; Jensen *et al.*, 2018) have found that the effect of therapy was partially mediated by changes in unhelpful appraisals.

Assessment

An overview of the key considerations when conducting an assessment of a trauma-exposed child is provided in Box 58.1.

Assessment of trauma history and journey to the clinic

Taking a good trauma history as part of normal screening procedures should reduce the risk of misidentifying child PTSD as merely intrusive phenomena such as hallucinations. Poor concentration or learning difficulties are common in PTSD but can be misdiagnosed as attention deficit hyperactivity disorder (ADHD). A diagnosis of PTSD is more readily recognized following a single-incident traumatic event than following multiple adverse events. Therefore, unlike many other child mental health complaints, the traumatic event is likely to be well known to parents or others (other than sexual and physical abuse). Thus, on referral, the clinician can gather together considerable details of the incident in the form of publicly available press reports, videos, and plans of where it happened. This can greatly help the child recall details of the experience and place it in context.

A clinically focused assessment that is aimed at understanding a child's needs, particularly the presence and severity of PTSD symptoms, may be very different in nature to a forensic or legal assessment where gathering a child's testimony is the key objective. In the former case, much more attention will be paid to the child's interpretation of events, and ensuring that the child feels that they are being listened to. The latter situation is beyond the scope of the present chapter and may warrant a different approach, according to the requirements of whichever court or other statutory body is involved. In each instance, the role of the assessment needs to be clear.

Child and parent interviews

While psychological help is nowadays often made available shortly after a major incident, there are many individual events whose impact on the child goes unrecognized for some time.

Box 58.1 Assessment at a glance

- When possible, it is helpful to gather information about the traumatic event prior to meeting the young person for assessment.
- Self-report questionnaires have a useful role but should be kept to a minimum during routine assessment.
- Following a joint family meeting, separate interviews with young people allow them to give their own account of what happened and how they reacted.
- Children can be asked directly to tell the interviewer about the traumatic event.
- Assessment provides opportunities to normalize children's traumatic stress reactions as common and well understood.
- In addition to assessing for post-traumatic stress disorder (PTSD) symptoms, comorbidity is the norm, so it is important to enquire about a range of problems.
- Clarity about confidentiality is needed, especially when the assessment is primarily for legal purposes.

Even if recognized, parents and child frequently avoid discussing the event for fear of upsetting each other. Hence, it is important to get the child's own memory of what happened and how they reacted. This can involve considerable tact on behalf of the clinician to ensure separate interviews with child and parents.

It follows that after a brief meeting with child and parents together to outline the assessment procedure, separate interviews are undertaken. Some clinicians prefer to get all parties to complete standardized self-report measures prior to undertaking interviews. It is important that the parental interviews gather a good developmental history, as well as an account of how the child's behavior has changed following the incident. This information can help the assessor to appreciate how preexisting factors may have affected a child's perception of the trauma and their reactions to it, as well as highlighting ongoing problems that may need additional advice or management.

How to conduct interviews and manage distress

However long the gap is between the traumatic event and coming for assessment, various patterns of behavior may well have become entrenched. Family and friends may have tried getting the child to describe the incident, but only succeeded in them avoiding further discussion. The clinician has to show the child that they can listen to the story, as well as indicate that they know how to help. One approach is to say to the child that they know the child has been through a dreadful experience and that they are probably worried about coming to talk about it. However, in order to help, the clinician needs to talk separately to child and parents, so who does the child want them to speak to first? This small question gives the child back some control over what is to happen when previously they may well have felt out of control of events.

Sometimes parents are reluctant to let the child be seen separately. They may be worried that the child will be too upset. At other times, they may be worried about what the child may reveal (especially when legal proceedings are under way). Our experience is that most children respond by asking to be seen first. Even during this brief meeting, every opportunity is taken to listen to the child and normalize their reactions. These are recognized as frequent and well understood, even though they are distressing initially.

Parents can be reassured that the team has experience in helping children through these reactions and that by the end of the assessment session they will pool information and formulate a plan to help.

When a younger child is reluctant to separate from their parents or caregivers, we might spend additional time allowing the child to warm up and get used to being around the interviewer, particularly watching the carers interact with the interviewer. Engaging activities (e.g., drawing, toys) can help to build rapport and trust. Seeing where the parents will be when the child is being interviewed can also help to allay the child's fears.

On seeing the child alone, the clinician settles them down with possibly neutral enquiries about their school or interests, and then approaches the issue of what happened and how they have reacted by asking, "Now tell me about it." These five words usually unleash a torrent of memories. Sometimes, the child has told the story so often that they give a journalistic headlines account. Just take them through gently to get more detail. Often, they will tell you things they have not told their parents so try to get agreement that you are able to share bits that are necessary when the family meet up at the end of the session.

Comorbidity and functioning

It is rare to find a child presenting with only PTSD. Separation anxiety, bereavement reactions, fears, and so on may be present. Thus, it is important to enquire about the whole range of problems. This is where the use of self-completed questionnaires by child and parents separately can speed the assessment process.

Questionnaires

These can have a useful role but should be kept to a minimum during routine assessment and subsequent intervention. The eight-item child version of the original Impact of Event Scale has been found to be useful both for screening and tracking progress (Smith *et al.*, 2003). Brief questionnaires measuring depression or anxiety have a place.

Following multiple traumatic events, questionnaires can help identify children needing help. Pooling all information after interviewing parents and child helps determine what intervention, if any, should be offered. Increasingly, good practice determines that progress is regularly checked during therapy. Again, brief questionnaires can help in this.

Medico-legal aspects

The concept of patient confidentiality has no basis in most jurisdictions. Where the consultation is primarily for a legal purpose, then it is clearer that everything that is said will be accessible by a court. Where the assessment and treatment are part of routine clinical help, it is to be hoped that the standard of information gathering and recording is of equally high standard.

Treatment

The evidence base

Efficacy

Highly efficacious therapies are available for treatment of PTSD in children and young people.

International practice guidelines are consistent in recommending cognitive behavioral therapies with a trauma focus (CBTs-TF) as the first-line treatment. For example, the UK National Institute for Health and Care Excellence (2018) recommends that individually delivered CBTs-TF—including trauma-focused CBT (TF-CBT), cognitive therapy for post-traumatic stress disorder (CT-PTSD), prolonged exposure (PE), cognitive processing therapy (CPT), and narrative exposure therapy (NET)—are offered initially for the treatment of PTSD and/or clinically important symptoms of PTSD; with eye movement desensitization and reprocessing (EMDR) being considered for young people who do not respond to CBTs-TF. Broadly similar recommendations are made by the World Health Organization (2013), the International Society for Traumatic Stress Studies (Forbes *et al.*, 2019), the American Academy for Child and Adolescent Psychiatry (Cohen et al., 2010); and the Australian National Health and Research Guidelines (Phelps *et al.*, 2022).

Findings from several systematic reviews (e.g., Gutermann *et al.*, 2016; Morina *et al.*, 2016) and from more recent network meta-analyses support these recommendations. For example, Mavranezouli *et al.*'s (2020) network meta-analysis of 32 RCTs (N = 2260 participants) of broadly defined psychological and psychosocial interventions found that individual CBTs-TF were the most effective treatments; EMDR was effective, but to a lesser extent, while supportive counseling was not superior to waiting list controls. Similarly, Xiang *et al.*'s (2021) larger network meta-analysis (k = 56 RCTs, N = 5327 participants) found that CPT, PE, individual and group CBTs-TF, and EMDR were all significantly superior to all control conditions.

Trial evidence also demonstrates broad benefits of trauma-focused therapies on comorbid difficulties such as symptoms of anxiety and depression. Improvements after therapy are usually sustained at follow-up (ranging between 3–12 months post-treatment in published trials), and relapse after successful treatment is very rare.

While the majority of trials to date have included older children and adolescents, there is an emerging evidence base for CBTs-TF for young (3–8 year-old) children. In an early-stage RCT, Hitchcock *et al.* (2022) compared a developmentally adapted form of CT-PTSD to treatment as usual (TAU). Most children (85%) lost their PTSD diagnosis after completing CT-PTSD, compared to few (7%) in the TAU arm. This study extends earlier work which demonstrated positive outcomes for developmentally adapted trauma-focused CBT in preschool children (e.g., Scheeringa et al., 2011; Salloum *et al.*, 2016).

Acceptability

Available evidence suggests that trauma-focused therapies are well-tolerated and generally acceptable to children and families. A meta-analysis of 40 RCTs of trauma-focused interventions found an overall dropout rate of around 11% from CBTs-TF and EMDR (Simmons *et al.*, 2021). This was not significantly different to the dropout rate of around 13% from non-trauma-focused treatments and other control arms and is broadly in line with dropout rates from therapy for other disorders such as depression. A large-scale effectiveness-implementation study from Norway (Skar *et al.*, 2022) found a similar dropout rate of 13% from TF-CBT that was delivered in regular community settings. Other reviews have reported higher dropout rates of over 30% for TF-CBT (Wamser-Nanney & Walker, 2023), but the field is complicated by differing definitions of dropout, attrition, and treatment completion. Risk of dropout may be higher for older children, and for children exposed to multiple trauma; and may be lower for children who are treated by intensively trained therapists (Skar *et al.*, 2022; Wamser-Nanney & Walker, 2023). However, few studies have investigated moderators of dropout and completion, and further work is needed. Qualitative studies show that young people find talking about trauma in therapy difficult but helpful (Dittman & Jensen, 2014).

Cognitive behavioral therapies with a trauma focus

Cognitive behavioral therapies with a trauma focus (CBTs-TF) is the broad term (World Health Organization, 2013) for a related set of specific therapy protocols including TF-CBT, CT-PTSD, CPT, NET, and PE. These interventions are based on empirically supported psychological theories of persistent PTSD (see the earlier section "The role of behavioral and cognitive factors") and aim to target and reverse identified maintaining factors. Components of most CBTs-TF are shown in Box 58.2 (also see National Institute for Health and Care Excellence, 2018).

While specific CBTs-TF protocols differ in various ways, there is broad overlap across protocols in the components used. Differences between protocols are apparent in the relative importance placed on particular aspects of intervention. For example, PE emphasizes relaxation and imaginal exposure, while CT-PTSD places relatively more weight on cognitive restructuring and memory updating. However, both approaches share many of the empirically supported components above. CBTs-TF are: structured therapies; usually time-limited, delivered over 10–24 sessions; normally offered as a 1 : 1 therapy (but see later section for group interventions); and will always involve caregivers.

Other evidence-based treatments

EMDR is the only non-CBTs-TF therapy that is recommended in practice guidelines as an evidence-based intervention for children and young people with PTSD (Shapiro, 2001). EMDR lacks an empirically supported psychological model but is based on the idea that negative thoughts, feelings, and behaviors result from unprocessed memories. Treatment follows a detailed and specific protocol that includes deliberate recall of traumatic events while engaging in bilateral stimulation such as repeated

Box 58.2 Cognitive behavioral therapies with a trauma focus components

- psychoeducation about post-traumatic stress disorder (PTSD) and its treatment
- development of a shared treatment rationale
- behavioral activation
- arousal management (e.g., learning relaxation or grounding skills)
- elaboration and processing of trauma memories
- processing of trauma-related emotions such as shame, guilt, loss, and anger
- restructuring and updating of problematic trauma-related meanings and appraisals
- dropping unhelpful cognitive and behavioral avoidance
- planned exposure to trauma reminders and triggers
- work with parents throughout
- completion of between-session homework tasks

lateral eye movements, or alternate tapping. Like CBTs-TF, EMDR is a 1 : 1, time-limited therapy. Unlike CBTs-TF, EMDR does not require detailed spoken or written narratives of traumatic events, does not involve direct challenging of beliefs, and does not employ homework.

Single trauma versus multiple events

PTSD can arise following different types of traumatic events and following exposure to single or multiple traumas: the diagnosis does not differ according to trauma type or frequency. Hoppen *et al.*'s (2023) recent meta-analysis found that psychological interventions can effectively treat PTSD in youth reporting multiple (e.g., sexual abuse), as well as single-event (e.g., traffic collision), trauma exposure. Adaptations to therapy may be needed with young people exposed to multiple traumas, for example, including components to address emotional stabilization and/or comorbidities, and use of a timeline to map out multiple events.

Therapist factors

Therapists from a variety of professional backgrounds can deliver trauma-focused therapies effectively to children and young people. In a meta-analysis of 40 RCTs, Grainger *et al.* (2022) found that PTSD outcomes did not significantly differ according to therapist background or educational attainment. In one effectiveness trial, there was no association between therapist professional background or experience and clinical outcomes (Pfeiffer *et al.*, 2020). These findings suggest that wider dissemination of evidence-based trauma-focused therapies is possible. Nevertheless, many clinicians report a number of barriers to implementing evidence-based interventions, including: lack of training and supervision; lack of confidence; a belief that evidence-based therapy protocols are rigid and inflexible; a fear that trauma-focused therapy will increase clients' distress or retraumatize clients; and a fear that the therapy will be emotionally burdensome and lead to therapist burnout (Finch *et al.*, 2020). In seeking to implement effective therapies more widely, it is vital that therapist-level barriers are understood and addressed.

Early intervention

Given that PTSD has clear onset following exposure to trauma, it should be possible to develop early interventions to prevent persistent PTSD.

Debriefing is a single-session group intervention universally delivered to all trauma-exposed individuals soon after exposure, with the aim of preventing onset of PTSD. Several forms of debriefing have been tested in trials with children and young people, none of which demonstrated effects on preventing PTSD (Kramer & Landolt, 2011). For these reasons, the UK National Institute for Health and Care Excellence guideline for PTSD recommends that debriefing is not offered to young people or adults after trauma exposure (National Institute for Health and Care Excellence, 2018).

Rather than single-session, universally delivered interventions, efforts have been made to develop multisession early interventions that are offered only to children who show early signs of post-traumatic stress symptoms (PTSS). For example, Berkowitz *et al.* (2011) developed a 4-session intervention, the Child and Family Traumatic Stress Intervention (CFTSI), which includes psychoeducation, techniques to improve family communication, and behavioral and cognitive skills teaching. CFTSI is delivered flexibly in the first 2 months post-trauma to children with at least 1 symptom of PTSS, and their parents or carers. An initial RCT reported positive findings for this screen-and-intervene approach for young people (7–17 years old) exposed to a variety of traumatic events, and CFTSI is now widely used in Child Advocacy Centers in the US (Hahn *et al.*, 2016, 2019). More recently, Haag *et al.* (2020) trialed a 2-session CBT-based intervention, Coping with Accident Reactions (CARE), for very young children (1–6 years old) and their carers. The intervention was offered to children who screened positive for PTSD risk 1-week post-trauma. Compared to children who received TAU, children who received the CARE intervention showed a significantly quicker reduction in PTSS severity in the first 3 months post-trauma.

Medication

Medication should not be offered to children and young people for the prevention or treatment of PTSD, according to the UK National Institute for Health and Care Excellence (2018), based on their systematic review of the very small evidence base. The Australian national guideline (Phelps *et al.*, 2022) also states that medication is not recommended for treatment of PTSD in children and adolescents.

Most young people with PTSD also have other comorbid difficulties for which evidence-based treatments include medication. Given the trial evidence on improvements in comorbid difficulties following psychological therapy for PTSD, some practitioners prefer to reevaluate comorbidities after young people have completed a course of trauma-focused therapy before considering pharmacotherapy for comorbidities.

In the US, some child psychiatrists prescribe selective serotonin reuptake inhibitors (SSRIs) for children who suffer from PTSD, despite the absence of RCT evidence to support this practice. In these instances, practitioners feel most justified in doing so when a child remains minimally improved after completing a trial of CBTs-TF. Moreover, practitioners also feel justified in such instances when a child with CBT-refractory PTSD also suffers from a comorbid anxiety disorder, such as generalized anxiety disorder or social anxiety disorder. This is because, for children with one of these comorbid conditions, SSRIs have demonstrated efficacy for the comorbid condition (see Chapter 59 on anxiety disorders).

Complex presentations: complex post-traumatic stress disorder and beyond

The establishment of the new diagnosis of CPTSD (see earlier section "The diagnosis of post-traumatic stress disorder in children and adolescents") raises the question of whether new or modified treatments are needed. In particular, do the CPTSD symptoms of "disturbances in self organization" (DSO) (i.e., problems in affect regulation, relating to others, and self-concept) need to be directly addressed, and if so at what stage in therapy? Early guidelines for adults with CPTSD recommended a phased approach to therapy, with a period of stabilization work to support affect regulation and interpersonal functioning implemented prior to trauma-focused or memory-focused work (Cloitre *et al.*, 2012). Others argued that a phase-based approach runs the risk of delaying all-important memory-focused work (de Jongh *et al.*, 2016), and a recent trial failed to find superiority of a phase-based approach over standard exposure treatment with respect to either clinical outcomes or tolerability of treatment (Oprel *et al.*, 2021). Recent research suggests that if additional therapy components to help adult clients with complexities in presentation are needed, then these may be woven throughout therapy depending on an individual formulation (see Murray and El-Leithy, 2022) and/or using a modular approach (see Karatzias and Cloitre, 2019).

Although developed long before CPTSD was defined, TF-CBT (Cohen *et al.*, 2004) was developed initially for children exposed to multiple repeated interpersonal traumas and sexual abuse, traumatic events which confer high risk for CPTSD; and TF-CBT is intended to address broad-based trauma reactions including, but not restricted to, PTSD symptoms. Sachser *et al.* (2017) directly addressed the question of whether TF-CBT is efficacious for young people with CPTSD. In a secondary analysis of a large trial dataset (Goldbeck *et al.*, 2016), it was found that children who met criteria for CPTSD responded as well to TF-CBT as did children with PTSD. Similarly, in a naturalistic study in community clinics, Jensen *et al.* (2022) found that after completing TF-CBT, young people with a diagnosis of CPTSD showed a steeper decline in PTSD and CPTSD than young people with a diagnosis of PTSD. CPTSD is a relatively new diagnosis, and further work is clearly needed, but existing evidence suggests that wholesale changes to existing evidence-based treatments for children and young people may not be needed.

Contingency and disaster planning

Contingency planning to deal with major civil emergencies is a statutory requirement in most countries, although many countries' plans are underdeveloped and lack specific psychosocial components (Tehrani, 2023). Contingency plans specify actions to be taken at various stages before and after critical incidents by relevant sectors such as public health, primary care, emergency responders, and others—including mental health services for young people.

It is argued that promoting resilience and preparedness before a critical incident can enhance children's coping if a disaster occurs (Houston *et al.*, 2016). Education about risk and disaster are key aspects of disaster preparedness, provided through information campaigns, schools-based activities, and parental guidance. However, evaluations of disaster preparedness programs are largely absent.

After a critical incident, effective cross-sector leadership, communication, and coordination are vital (Tehrani, 2023). The mostly widely used framework implemented in the immediate aftermath of major incidents is psychological first aid (PFA), initially proposed by Hobfoll (2007). While there are now different versions of PFA, at its core are the five principles of safety, calm, connectedness, self-efficacy, and hope. For many children and young people, the natural community in which to implement PFA is their school. A number of agencies have worked with education sectors to plan for implementation of PFA in schools after disasters (Beeke, 2021). For example, the UK Trauma Council makes critical incident resources freely available for schools (https://uktraumacouncil.org/resources/trauma-and-ptsd-working-with-children-and-young-people).

The American Academy for Child and Adolescent Psychiatry practice parameters (Cohen et al., 2010) recommend school-based screening for PTSS and other common trauma reactions, about a month after critical incidents, followed by schools-based, group-delivered interventions for those in need (e.g., Jaycox *et al.*, 2012).

Mass disasters and complex emergencies can occur in LMIC, where resources to provide help may be scarce. The WHO and the UN Inter-Agency Standing Committee (IASC) have produced detailed guidance and resources on how and when to help after disasters (see https://interagencystandingcommittee.org/mental-health-and-psychosocial-support-emergency-settings). Coordination between intergovernmental and nongovernmental organizations (NGOs) is crucial. Encouragingly, when therapies for PTSD have been trialed in LMICs, they have shown medium-to-large effect sizes (Morina *et al.*, 2017). In low-resource settings, the task of delivering psychosocial assistance is often shared with lay workers or peers. Examples of task-sharing approaches to deliver evidence-based cognitive behavioral therapy (CBT) interventions to children after critical incidents in low-resource settings are Teaching Recovery Techniques (TRT) developed by the Children and War Foundation (Yule *et al.*, 2013), and Early Adolescent Skills for Emotion (EASE) developed by the WHO (see Dawson *et al.*, 2019).

Responding to the public health crisis around trauma and post-traumatic stress disorder in young people

Well-established highly efficacious treatments that have demonstrated robust effectiveness in large-scale implementation trials are available. Nonetheless, most young people with PTSD do not receive an evidence-based therapy (Lewis *et al.*, 2019). In an effort to make effective treatment more widely available, alternative methods of delivery and implementation have been developed.

Stepped care and stratified care

Under a stepped care approach, a step-one, low-intensity intervention is delivered to all young people in need of treatment, followed by a step-two, high-intensity intervention delivered only to those who fail to respond to the initial step. Step one uses a task-sharing approach whereby the intervention is delivered to children by their parents with guidance from a clinician; step two is delivered by a trained clinician as usual. The intention is to allow more children to engage with the intervention by making step one more accessible, and to relieve the burden and cost on services by offering a high-intensity intervention only to those who need it.

In the largest trial to date, that compared stepped care to standard TF-CBT for 183 4–12-year-old children (Salloum *et al.*, 2022a, 2022b), 47% responded to step one alone, and stepped care was noninferior to TF-CBT at post-treatment and at 6- and 12-month follow-ups. Costs of stepped care were again lower than costs of standard TF-CBT. Evidence on treatment response predictors may help to refine delivery of stepped care in the future. For example, step one outcomes were worse if parents were depressed and/or if children showed angry outbursts (Salloum *et al.*, 2022b).

Group interventions

Individual treatment is effective but is resource-intensive and costly. Group treatment has potential to increase the capacity of services to deliver interventions efficiently at scale, if clinical effectiveness is maintained. All of the evidence-based interventions above (CBTs-TF and EMDR) have been adapted for group delivery. A recent meta-analysis (Davis *et al.*, 2023) included 42 RCTs (N = 5998 children) of group-delivered PTSD interventions, most of which were CBT-based (N = 37) and carried out in schools (N = 25). Children randomized to group-delivered interventions had significantly lower PTSS and depression compared to controls at post-treatment and at follow-up. Effect sizes for PTSS ranged from medium to large although there was considerable variability between study outcomes. It is notable that many of the RCTs in this meta-analysis were conducted in complex emergencies (e.g., post-war and post-disaster), with groups led by trained lay workers; however, the majority of the included trials comprised youth who were all exposed to the same trauma, possibly limiting the utility of this approach in more general clinical contexts where experiences may be very varied. Nevertheless, group interventions, especially CBT-based groups, can offer a valuable and effective clinical resource.

Digital therapy

Delivery of therapy via the Internet has enormous potential for increasing the availability and accessibility of effective treatments (see Chapter 49). A number of digital guided-self-help interventions show promise for treating PTSD in adults (see Siddaway *et al.*, 2022), but few have been developed or tested for young people with PTSD. An Internet-delivered self-help tool to enhance support for trauma-exposed youth showed encouraging preliminary outcomes in a schools-based trial (Jaycox *et al.*, 2019). A digital intervention for preventing PTSD symptoms in injured children was shown to be feasible and clinically promising (Kassam-Adams *et al.*, 2016). A large-scale evaluation following a tornado (Ruggiero *et al.*, 2015) found that use of a web-based psychoeducation intervention was associated with improvements in PTSD symptoms in trauma-exposed adolescents. Young people themselves are positive about the potential of digital health interventions in general (National Collaborating Centre for Mental Health, 2014). Outcomes for digital therapy for depression or anxiety tend to be better when young people are supported or guided by a therapist (Hollis *et al.*, 2017), and this principle is likely to hold true for digital therapy for PTSD. To maximize engagement, it is important that young people are involved as key stakeholders when designing and producing new digital interventions. No studies have yet reported on the development or evaluation of digital CBTs-TF for PTSD in young people, but at least two trials are ongoing (Schulte *et al.*, 2022; Smith *et al.*, 2022).

Next steps for research

Enormous strides have been made in understanding reactions of young people to trauma, and in developing effective interventions. Future steps include development of evidence-informed implementation strategies to make such interventions more broadly and equitably accessible. Further work on evaluating interventions for very young children is needed. There has been surprisingly little work on early or preventative interventions, and this may become a focus for future research. The growing field of transdiagnostic interventions is likely to see trauma center-stage, and future research complexity in PTSD will be of huge benefit. Agenda setting for future research strategies should ideally include young people themselves and their families, including those from historically underrepresented communities (Alisic *et al.*, 2021).

Post-traumatic stress disorder and the COVID-19 pandemic

Since the onset of the COVID-19 pandemic, concerns have been raised about its potential impact on the mental health of children and adolescents. Widespread protracted exposure to major stressors combined with reductions in health and education services led to early predictions of significant and lasting effects on children's mental health. Some three years later, empirical findings shed some light on the issue.

Longitudinal studies of large representative cohorts were running before the pandemic, some of which have reported on changes to depression anxiety and general well-being during the pandemic. Caution is needed in inferring causal effects of the pandemic on observed changes, especially given a likely preexisting trend toward increases in prevalence of youth mental health problems in the years before the pandemic (Sadler *et al.*, 2018). Findings are mixed but some consistent patterns are emerging. Many primary-school-age children appeared to show increases in emotional and behavioral difficulties during times of lockdown, especially children with preexisting vulnerabilities (Adegboye *et al.*, 2021; Creswell *et al.*, 2021). Although most adolescents did not report significant persistent worsening of mental health during the pandemic (Bouter *et al.*, 2022), some specific adolescent subpopulations seem to be more affected, including those with preexisting individual vulnerabilities, such as anxiety (Waite *et al.*, 2021) or neurodevelopmental difficulties (Houghton *et al.*, 2022), and those from low-income or overcrowded households (Knowles *et al.*, 2022). COVID-19 has potential for family-wide effects, and there is some evidence that effects on children's well-being are partially mediated via effects on parents (Lengua *et al.*,2022).

In relation to PTSD specifically, a number of aspects of the pandemic are relevant. First, the pandemic was associated with increased rates of exposure to potentially traumatic events such as witnessing or learning about life-threatening illnesses in others, sudden bereavements, and increases in domestic violence during lockdown. Second, contextual factors that are known to confer resilience were reduced as a consequence of public health measures such as lockdown and school closures: for example, children had less peer support, less day-to-day structure, less activity and exercise, and much less certainty about the future. Third, the capacity of mental health services was reduced; practically, many clinics were closed for face-to-face appointments, and the mental health workforce was itself impacted by illness.

In this context, elevated rates of COVID-related PTSD or PTSS might be expected. However, reliable empirical data is so far sparse. Cross-sectional questionnaire surveys from around the globe have reported a wide range of probable PTSD prevalence in the community, with an early meta-analysis (Yang *et al.*, 2022) reporting a combined rate of 28% from 10 studies (N = 17,385). Pfefferbaum (2022) notes some methodological limitations to studies published so far (including convenience sampling, lack of evidence of COVID-related trauma exposure, unclear use of adapted scales, and failure to assess the full constellation of PTSD symptoms or impairments in functioning), and therefore cautions against overdiagnosis. Importantly, to further our understanding of the impact of this and future pandemics, Pfefferbaum (2022) also calls for reflection on Criterion A of the DSM-5 PTSD diagnosis to clarify which pandemic-related experiences should qualify as trauma exposure.

It is hoped that future studies will help us to understand the various trajectories of pandemic-related youth mental health problems including PTSD, and their determinants. Meanwhile, initiatives are underway to provide evidence-based interventions for young people and their families who have been affected by the pandemic. These include parenting apps, remotely delivered programs for anxiety, and online resources codeveloped with adolescents (see Creswell, 2023).

Conclusion

In our experience, the presence of PTSD in a child or adolescent is a cause for some trepidation in many clinicians. There may be concern that efforts to discuss the child's traumatic experience or experiences may be overwhelming and even harmful. We hope that in this chapter we have outlined the wealth of understanding that now exists around children's responses to trauma. While undeniably a serious condition, PTSD is also a condition that is both explicable and responsive to psychological treatment. Cognitive behavioral models for the treatment of PTSD have proved to be particularly effectual, with the evidence for the mechanism of its effect documented.

Several issues warrant further research. Young children's responses to trauma require further investigation, as do issues around comorbidity and the treatment of CPTSD. A central challenge is that of dissemination; given the prevalence of PTSD in youth, providing evidence-based therapies for such numbers will require both committed health policy and a large degree of innovation.

References

Adegboye, D. *et al.* (2021) Understanding why the COVID-19 pandemic-related lockdown increases mental health difficulties in vulnerable young children. *JCPP Advances* **1**, e12005. doi:10.1111/jcv2.12005.

Alisic, E. *et al.* (2011) Building child trauma theory from longitudinal studies: a meta-analysis. *Clinical Psychology Review* **31**, 736–747.

Alisic, E. *et al.* (2014) Rates of post-traumatic stress disorder in trauma-exposed children and adolescents: meta-analysis. *The British Journal of Psychiatry* **204**, 335–340.

Alisic, E. *et al.* (2021) Working towards inclusive and equitable trauma treatment guidelines: a child-centered reflection. *European Journal of Psychotraumatology* **11**. doi:10.1080/20008198.2020.1833657.

Allen, L. *et al.* (2021) The correlation between social support and post-traumatic stress disorder in children and adolescents: a meta-analysis. *Journal of Affective Disorders* **294**, 543–557.

American Psychiatric Association (1980) *Diagnostic and Statistical Manual of Mental Disorders*, 3rd edn. American Psychiatric Association, Washington DC.

American Psychiatric Association (1994) *Diagnostic and Statistical Manual of Mental Disorders*, 4th edn. American Psychiatric Association, Washington DC.

American Psychiatric Association (2013) *Diagnostic and Statistical Manual of Mental Disorders*, 5th edn. American Psychiatric Association, Washington DC.

Andreasen, N.C. (2010) Posttraumatic stress disorder: a history and a critique. *Annals of the New York Academy of Sciences* **1208**, 67–71.

Beeke, M. (2021) Towards a co-ordinated framework for critical incident response in school communities: a review of current evidence. *Educational and Child Psychology* **38**(1), 75–86.

Berkowitz, S.J. *et al.* (2011) The child and family traumatic stress intervention: secondary prevention for youth at risk of developing PTSD. *Journal of Child Psychology & Psychiatry* **52**(6), 676–685.

Bouter, D.C. *et al.* (2022) A longitudinal study of mental health in at-risk adolescents before and during the COVID-19 pandemic. *European Child and Adolescent Psychiatry* **32**, 1109–1117. doi:10.1007/s00787-021-01935-y.

Brewin, C.R. *et al.* (1996) A dual representation theory of posttraumatic stress disorder. *Psychological Review* **103**, 670–686.

Chiu, H.T.C. *et al.* (2024) Relationship between anxiety sensitivity and post-traumatic stress symptoms in trauma-exposed children and adolescents: a meta-analysis. *Cognitive Therapy and Research* **103**, 102857.

Cisler, J.M. & Herringa, R.J. (2021) Posttraumatic stress disorder and the developing adolescent brain. *Biological Psychiatry* **89**(2), 144–151.

Cloitre, M. *et al.* (2012) The ISTSS Expert Consensus Treatment Guidelines for Complex PTSD in Adults International Society for Traumatic Stress Studies, Brentwood, TN. Available: https://terrorvictimresponse.ca/wp-content/uploads/ISTSS-Expert-Concesnsus-Guidelines-for-Complex-PTSD-Updated-060315.pdf [9 December 2024].

Cohen, J. & The Workgroup on Quality Issues (2010) Practice parameter for the assessment and treatment of children and adolescents with posttraumatic stress disorder. *Journal of the American Association of Child & Adolescent Psychiatry* **49**(4), 414–430.

Cohen, J.A. *et al.* (2004) A multisite, randomized controlled trial for children with sexual abuse-related PTSD symptoms. *Journal of the American Association of Child & Adolescent Psychiatry* **43**, 393–402.

Creswell, C. (2023) Editorial perspective: rapid responses to understand and address children and young people's mental health in the context of COVID-19. *Journal of Child Psychology & Psychiatry* **64**(1), 209–211.

Creswell, C. *et al.* (2021) Young people's mental health during the COVID-19 pandemic. *The Lancet Child & Adolescent Health* **5**, 535–537.

Cushing, T. *et al.* (2024) The relationship between attachment and post-traumatic stress in children and adolescents: a meta-analytic review. *Development and Psychopathology* **36**(3), 1055–1069.

Davis, R.S. *et al.* (2023) Systematic review and meta-analysis: group-based interventions for treating posttraumatic stress symptoms in children and adolescents. *Journal of the American Academy of Child & Adolescent Psychiatry* **62**(11), 1217–1232. doi:10.1016/j.jaac.2023.02.013.

Dawson, K. *et al.* (2019) Improving access to evidence-based interventions for young adolescents: Early Adolescent Skills for Emotions (EASE). *World Psychiatry* **18**(1), 105–107.

de Jongh, A. *et al.* (2016) Critical analysis of the current treatment guidelines for complex PTSD in adults. *Depression and Anxiety* **33**(5), 359–369. doi:10.1002/da.22469.

Dittman, I. & Jensen, T. (2014) Giving a voice to traumatized youth: experiences with trauma-focused cognitive behavioral therapy. *Child Abuse and Neglect* **38**, 1221–1230.

Dyregrov, A. *et al.* (2000) Trauma exposure and psychological reactions to genocide among Rwandan children. *Journal of Traumatic Stress* **13**, 3–21.

Ehlers, A. & Clark, D.M. (2000) A cognitive model of posttraumatic stress disorder. *Behaviour Research and Therapy* **38**, 319–345.

Finch, J. *et al.* (2020) A survey of evidence-based practice, training, supervision and clinician confidence relating to post-traumatic stress disorder (PTSD) therapies in UK child and adolescent mental health professionals. *European Journal of Psychotraumatology* **11**(1), 1815281.

Forbes, D. *et al.* (eds) (2019) *Effective Treatments for PTSD: Practice Guidelines from the International Society for Traumatic Stress Studies*, 3rd edn. Guilford Press, New York.

Furr, J.M. *et al.* (2010) Disasters and youth: a meta-analytic examination of posttraumatic stress. *Journal of Consulting and Clinical Psychology* **78**, 765.

Goldbeck, L. *et al.* (2016) Effectiveness of trauma-focused cognitive behavioral therapy for children and adolescents: a randomized controlled trial in eight German mental health clinics. *Psychotherapy and Psychosomatics* **85**, 159–170.

Gomez De La Cuesta, G. *et al.* (2019) The relationship between maladaptive appraisals and posttraumatic stress disorder: a meta-analysis. *European Journal of Psychotraumatology* **10(1), 1620084**.

Grainger, L. *et al.* (2022) Associations between therapist factors and treatment efficacy in randomized controlled trials of trauma-focused cognitive behavioral therapy for children and youth: a systematic review and meta-analysis. *Journal of Traumatic Stress* **35**(5), 1405–1419.

Gutermann, J. *et al.* (2016) Psychological treatments for symptoms of posttraumatic stress disorder in children, adolescents, and young adults: a meta-analysis. *Clinical Child and Family Psychology Review* **19**(2), 77–93. doi:10.1007/s10567-016-0202-5.

Haag, A.-C. *et al.* (2020) Preventive intervention for trauma reactions in young injured children: results of a multi-site randomised controlled trial. *Journal of Child Psychology and Psychiatry* **61**(9), 988–997.

Hahn, H. *et al.* (2016) Findings of an early intervention to address Children's traumatic stress implemented in the Child Advocacy Center setting following sexual abuse. *Journal of Child and Adolescent Trauma* **9**(1), 55–66.

Hahn, H. *et al.* (2019) Child and Family Traumatic Stress Intervention (CFTSI) reduces parental posttraumatic stress symptoms: a multi-site meta-analysis (MSMA). *Child Abuse and Neglect* **92**, 106–115.

Han, L. *et al.* (2019) Unintentional injuries and violence among adolescents aged 12–15 years in 68 low-income and middle-income countries: a secondary analysis of data from the Global School-based Student Health Survey. *The Lancet Child & Adolescent Health* **3**, 616–626.

Hiller, R.M. *et al.* (2016) Research review: changes in the prevalence and symptom severity of child posttraumatic stress disorder in the year following trauma - a meta-analytic study. *Journal of Child Psychology and Psychiatry* **57**, 884–898.

Hiller, R.M. *et al.* (2021) A longitudinal study of cognitive predictors of (complex) post-traumatic stress in young people in out-of-home care. *Journal of Child Psychology and Psychiatry* **62**, 48–57.

Hitchcock, C. *et al.* (2021) Population prevalence of the posttraumatic stress disorder subtype for young children in nationwide surveys of the British general population and of children-in-care. *Journal of the American Academy of Child and Adolescent Psychiatry* **60**, 1278–1287.

Hitchcock, C. *et al.* (2022) The early course and treatment of posttraumatic stress disorder in very young children: diagnostic prevalence and predictors in hospital-attending children and a randomized controlled proof-of-concept trial of trauma-focused cognitive therapy, for 3- to 8-year-olds. *Journal of Child Psychology and Psychiatry* **63**(1), 58–67.

Hobfoll, S. *et al.* (2007) Five essential elements of immediate and mid-term mass trauma intervention: empirical evidence. *Psychiatry* **70**(4), 283–315.

Hollis, C. *et al.* (2017) Annual research review: digital health interventions for children and young people with mental health problems—a systematic and meta-review. *Journal of Child Psychology and Psychiatry* **58**(4), 474–503.

Hoppen, T. *et al.* (2023) Efficacy of psychological interventions for post-traumatic stress disorder in children and adolescents exposed to single versus multiple traumas: metaanalysis of randomised controlled trials. *British Journal of Psychiatry* **222** (5), 196–203. doi:10.1192/bjp.2023.24.

Houghton, S. *et al.* (2022) Longitudinal trajectories of mental health and loneliness for Australian adolescents with-or-without neurodevelopmental disorders: the impact of COVID-19 school lockdowns. *Journal of Child Psychology and Psychiatry* **63**(11), 1332–1243.

Houston, J.B. *et al.* (2016) Public disaster communication and child and family disaster mental health: a review of theoretical frameworks and empirical evidence. *Current Psychiatry Reports* **18**(6), 1–9.

Jaycox, J. *et al.* (2012) Cognitive behavioral intervention for trauma in schools. *Journal of Applied School Psychology* **28**(3), 239–255.

Jaycox, L. *et al.* (2019) Development and preliminary evaluation of a self-guided, internet-based tool for coping with stress and trauma: life improvement for teens (LIFT). *Psychological Services* **16**(1), 85–94.

Jensen, T. *et al.* (2022) Complex PTSD and treatment outcomes in TF-CBT for youth: a naturalistic study. *European Journal of Psychotraumatology* **13**(2), 2114630.

Jensen, T.K. *et al.* (2018) Change in post-traumatic cognitions mediates treatment effects for traumatized youth: a randomized controlled trial. *Journal of Counseling Psychology* **65**, 166.

Jovanovic, T. *et al.* (2017) Exposure to violence accelerates epigenetic aging in children. *Scientific Reports* **7**, 8962.

Karatzias, T. & Cloitre, M. (2019) Treating adults with complex PTSD (CPTSD) using a modular approach to treatment: rationale, evidence, and directions for future research. *Journal of Traumatic Stress* **32**(6), 870–876.

Kassam-Adams, N. *et al.* (2016) Pilot randomized controlled trial of a novel web-based intervention to prevent posttraumatic stress in children following medical events. *Journal of Pediatric Psychology* **41**(1), 138–148.

Khadr, S. *et al.* (2018) Mental and sexual health outcomes following sexual assault in adolescents: a prospective cohort study. *The Lancet Child & Adolescent Health* **2**, 654–665.

Kirsch, V. *et al.* (2011) Psychophysiological characteristics of PTSD in children and adolescents: a review of the literature. *Journal of Traumatic Stress* **24**, 146–154.

Knowles, G. *et al.* (2022) Covid-19, social restrictions, and mental distress among young people: a UK longitudinal, population-based study. *Journal of Child Psychology and Psychiatry* **63**(11), 1392–1404.

Kramer, D.N. & Landolt, M.A. (2011) Characteristics and efficacy of early psychological interventions in children and adolescents after single trauma: a meta-analysis. *European Journal of Psychotraumatology* **2**(1), 7858.

La Greca, A.M. *et al.* (2010) Hurricane-related exposure experiences and stressors, other life events, and social support: concurrent and prospective impact on children's persistent posttraumatic stress symptoms. *Journal of Consulting and Clinical Psychology* **78**, 794.

Lai, B.S. *et al.* (2021) Trajectories of posttraumatic stress in youths after natural disasters. *JAMA Network Open* **4**, e2036682.

Landolt, M.A. *et al.* (2013) Trauma exposure and posttraumatic stress disorder in adolescents: A national survey in Switzerland. *Journal of Traumatic Stress* **26**, 209–216.

Lengua, L. *et al.* (2022) Maternal mental health mediates the effects of pandemic-related stressors on adolescent psychopathology during COVID-19. *Journal of Child Psychology and Psychiatry* **63**(12), 1544–1552.

Lewis, S.J. *et al.* (2019) The epidemiology of trauma and post-traumatic stress disorder in a representative cohort of young people in England and Wales. *The Lancet Psychiatry* **6**, 247–256.

Mavranezouli, I. *et al.* (2020) Research review: psychological and psychosocial treatments for children and young people with post-traumatic stress disorder: a network meta-analysis. *Journal of Child Psychology and Psychiatry* **61**(1), 18–29.

McGuire, R. *et al.* (2021) A longitudinal investigation of children's trauma memory characteristics and their relationship with posttraumatic stress disorder symptoms. *Research on Child and Adolescent Psychopathology* **49**, 807–816.

McLaughlin, K.A. *et al.* (2013) Trauma exposure and posttraumatic stress disorder in a National Sample of adolescents. *Journal of the American Academy of Child & Adolescent Psychiatry* **52**, 815–830.e14.

McLean, C.P. *et al.* (2013) Social and academic functioning in adolescents with child sexual abuse-related PTSD. *Child Abuse & Neglect* **37**, 675–678.

Meiser-Stedman, R. *et al.* (2019) A core role for cognitive processes in the acute onset and maintenance of post-traumatic stress in children and adolescents. *Journal of Child Psychology and Psychiatry* **60**, 875–884.

Memarzia, J. *et al.* (2021) Psychological peritraumatic risk factors for post-traumatic stress disorder in children and adolescents: a meta-analytic review. *Journal of Affective Disorders* **282**, 1036–1047.

Merikangas, K.R. *et al.* (2010) Lifetime prevalence of mental disorders in US adolescents: results from the National Comorbidity Survey Replication–Adolescent Supplement (NCS-A). *Journal of the American Academy of Child & Adolescent Psychiatry* **49**, 980–989.

Morina, N. *et al.* (2016) Interventions for children and adolescents with posttraumatic stress disorder: a meta-analysis of comparative outcome studies. *Clinical Psychology Review* **47**, 41–54.

Morina, N. *et al.* (2017) Psychological interventions for post-traumatic stress disorder and depression in young survivors of mass violence in low-and middle-income countries: meta-analysis. *The British Journal of Psychiatry* **210**, 247–254.

Morris, A. *et al.* (2012) The association between parent PTSD/depression symptoms and child PTSD symptoms: a meta-analysis. *Journal of Pediatric Psychology* **37**, 1076–1088.

Murray, H. & El-Leithy, S. (2022) *Working with Complexity in PTSD: A Cognitive Therapy Approach*. Routledge, New York.

National Collaborating Centre for Mental Health (2014) *E-therapies Systematic Review for Children and Young People with Mental Health Problems*. The British Psychological Society and The Royal College of Psychiatrists, London/Leicester, UK. Available: www.rcpsych.ac.uk/docs/default-source/improving-care/nccmh/nccmh-etherapies-full-review.pdf?sfvrsn=3947b9df_2 [22 November 2024].

National Institute for Health and Care Excellence (2018) *Post-Traumatic Stress Disorder (update): Guideline Consultation*. National Institute for Health and Care Excellence (NICE), London.

Neuner, F. *et al.* (2006) Post-tsunami stress: a study of posttraumatic stress disorder in children living in three severely affected regions in Sri Lanka. *Journal of Traumatic Stress* **19**, 339–347.

Nievergelt, C.M. *et al.* (2018) Genomic approaches to posttraumatic stress disorder: the Psychiatric Genomic Consortium Initiative. *Biological Psychiatry* **83**, 831–839.

Oprel, D. *et al.* (2021) Effect of prolonged exposure, intensified prolonged exposure and STAIR+prolonged exposure in patients with PTSD related to childhood abuse: a randomized controlled trial. *European Journal of Psychotraumatology* **61**(8). doi:10.1080/20008198.2020.1851511.

Pfefferbaum, B. (2022) Posttraumatic stress disorder in children in the context of the COVID-19 pandemic. *Journal of the American Academy of Child and Adolescent Psychiatry* **61**(8), 957–959.

Pfeiffer, E. *et al.* (2020) Does the therapist matter? Therapist characteristics and their relation to outcome in trauma-focused cognitive behavioral therapy for children and adolescents. *European Journal of Psychotraumatology* **11**, 1776048.

Phelps, A. *et al.* (2022) Australian guidelines for the prevention and treatment of posttraumatic stress disorder: updates in the third edition. *The Australian and New Zealand Journal of Psychiatry* **56**(3), 230–247.

Ponnamperuma, T. & Nicolson, N.A. (2016) Negative trauma appraisals and PTSD symptoms in Sri Lankan adolescents. *Journal of Abnormal Child Psychology* **44**, 245–255.

Pynoos, R.S. *et al.* (1987) Life threat and posttraumatic stress in school-age children. *Archives of General Psychiatry* **44**, 1057–1063.

Reed, J. *et al.* (2023) Associations between the Trauma Memory Quality Questionnaire and posttraumatic stress symptoms in youth: a systematic review and meta-analysis. *Journal of Traumatic Stress* **36**, 31–43.

Ruggiero, K. *et al.* (2015) Web intervention for adolescents affected by disaster: population-based randomized controlled trial. *Journal of the American Academy of Child and Adolescent Psychiatry* **54**(9), 709–717.

Sachser, C. *et al.* (2017) Complex PTSD as proposed for ICD-11: validation of a new disorder in children and adolescents and their response to trauma-focused cognitive behavioral therapy. *Journal of Child Psychology and Psychiatry* **58**(2), 160–168. doi:10.1111/jcpp.12640.

Sack, W.H. *et al.* (1997) Does PTSD transcend cultural barriers? A study from the Khmer adolescent refugee project. *Journal of the American Academy of Child & Adolescent Psychiatry* **36**, 49–54.

Sadler, K. *et al.* (2018) *The Mental Health of Children and Young People in England 2017: Trends and Characteristics.* Health and Social Care Information Centre, London.

Saigh, P.A. *et al.* (1997) Scholastic impairments among traumatized adolescents. *Behaviour Research and Therapy* **35**, 429–436.

Salloum, A. *et al.* (2016) Stepped care versus standard trauma-focused cognitive behavioral therapy for young children. *Journal of Child Psychology and Psychiatry* **57**, 614–622.

Salloum, A. *et al.* (2022a) Exploring treatment response predictors of a parent-led therapist-assisted treatment for childhood trauma. *Research on Social Work Practice*, 1–14.

Salloum, A. *et al.* (2022b) Stepped care versus standard care for children after trauma: a randomized non-inferiority clinical trial. *Journal of the American Academy of Child and Adolescent Psychiatry* **61**(8), 1010–1022.

Salmon, K. & Bryant, R.A. (2002) Posttraumatic stress disorder in children: the influence of developmental factors. *Clinical Psychology Review* **22**, 163–188.

Salmond, C.H. *et al.* (2011) The nature of trauma memories in acute stress disorder in children and adolescents. *Journal of Child Psychology and Psychiatry* **52**, 560–570.

Sartor, C.E. *et al.* (2011) Common genetic and environmental contributions to post-traumatic stress disorder and alcohol dependence in young women. *Psychological Medicine* **41**, 1497–1505.

Sartor, C.E. *et al.* (2012) Common heritable contributions to low-risk trauma, high-risk trauma, posttraumatic stress disorder, and major depression. *Archives of General Psychiatry* **69**, 293–299.

Scheeringa, M.S. *et al.* (2006) Factors affecting the diagnosis and prediction of PTSD symptomatology in children and adolescents. *The American Journal of Psychiatry* **163**, 644–651.

Scheeringa, M.S. *et al.* (2011) Trauma-focused cognitive behavioural therapy for posttraumatic stress disorder in three through six year old children: a randomized clinical trial. *Journal of Child Psychology and Psychiatry* **52**, 853–860.

Schulte, C. *et al.* (2022) Internet- and mobile-based trauma-focused intervention for adolescents and young adults with posttraumatic stress disorder: a study protocol of a proof-of-concept feasibility study. *European Journal of Psychotraumatology* **13**(2), 2101345.

Shapiro, F. (2001) *Eye Movement Desensitization and Reprocessing: Basic Principles, Protocols, and Procedures.* Guilford Press, New York.

Siddaway, A. *et al.* (2022) Trauma-focused guided self-help interventions for posttraumatic stress disorder: a meta-analysis of randomized controlled trials. *Depression and Anxiety* **39**(10–11), 675–685.

Simmons, C. *et al.* (2021) A meta-analysis of dropout from evidence-based psychological treatment for post-traumatic stress disorder (PTSD) in children and young people. *European Journal of Psychotraumatology* **12**(1), 1947570.

Skar, A.-M. *et al.* (2022) Predictors of nonresponse and drop-out among children and adolescents receiving TF-CBT: investigation of client-, therapist- and implementation factors. *BMC Health Services Research* **22**, 1212.

Smith, P. *et al.* (2003) Principal components analysis of the impact of event scale with children in war. *Personality and Individual Differences* **34**, 315–322.

Smith, P. *et al.* (2007) Cognitive-behavioral therapy for PTSD in children and adolescents: A preliminary randomized controlled trial. *Journal of the American Academy of Child and Adolescent Psychiatry* **46**, 1051–1061.

Smith, P. *et al.* (2022) Therapist-supported online cognitive therapy for post-traumatic stress disorder (PTSD) in young people: protocol for an early-stage, parallel-group, randomised controlled study (OPTYC trial). *BMJ Open* **12**(3), e054852.

Smoller, J.W. (2016) The genetics of stress-related disorders: PTSD, depression, and anxiety disorders. *Neuropsychopharmacology* **41**, 297–319.

Stein, M.B. *et al.* (2002) Genetic and environmental influences on trauma exposure and posttraumatic stress disorder symptoms: a twin study. *American Journal of Psychiatry* **159**, 1675–1681.

Stein, M.B. *et al.* (2021) Genome-wide association analyses of post-traumatic stress disorder and its symptom subdomains in the million veteran program. *Nature Genetics* **53**(2), 174–184.

Stoltenborgh, M. *et al.* (2011) A global perspective on child sexual abuse: Meta-analysis of prevalence around the world. *Child Maltreatment* **16**, 79–101.

Strathearn, L. *et al.* (2020) Long-term cognitive, psychological, and health outcomes associated with child abuse and neglect. *Pediatrics* **146**, 1–15.

Tang, W. *et al.* (2018) Post-traumatic stress disorder, anxiety and depression symptoms among adolescent earthquake victims: comorbidity and associated sleep-disturbing factors. *Social Psychiatry and Psychiatric Epidemiology* **53**, 1241–1251.

Tehrani, N. (2023) Early psycho-social interventions for individuals and groups affected by disasters. Oxford Research Encyclopaedia of Psychology. Available: https://oxfordre.com/psychology/display/10.1093/acrefore/9780190236557.001.0001/acrefore-9780190236557-e-104 [22 November 2024].

Thabet, A.A. & Vostanis, P. (1999) Post-traumatic stress reactions in children of war. *Journal of Child Psychology and Psychiatry* **40**, 385–391.

Trickey, D. *et al.* (2012) A meta-analysis of risk factors for post-traumatic stress disorder in children and adolescents. *Clinical Psychology Review* **32**, 122–138.

True, W.R. *et al.* (1993) A twin study of genetic and environmental contributions to liability for posttraumatic stress symptoms. *Archives of General Psychiatry* **50**, 257–264.

Waite, P. *et al.* (2021) How did the mental health symptoms of children and adolescents change over early lockdown during the COVID-19 pandemic in the UK? *JCPP Advances* **1**, e12009.

Walker, J. *et al.* (2020) Acute stress disorder in children and adolescents: a systematic review and meta-analysis of prevalence following exposure to a traumatic event. *Journal of Affective Disorders Reports* **2**.

Wamser-Nanney, R. & Walker, H. (2023) Attrition from pediatric trauma-focused cognitive behavioral therapy: a meta-analysis. *Journal of Traumatic Stress* **36**, 17–30.

Wang, L. *et al.* (2011) Posttraumatic stress disorder symptom structure in Chinese adolescents exposed to a deadly earthquake. *Journal of Abnormal Child Psychology* **39**, 749–758.

Williamson, V. *et al.* (2017) The role of parenting behaviors in childhood post-traumatic stress disorder: a meta-analytic review. *Clinical Psychology Review* **53**, 1–13.

Winston, F.K. *et al.* (2003) Screening for risk of persistent posttraumatic stress in injured children and their parents. *JAMA* **290**, 643–649.

Woolgar, F. *et al.* (2022) Systematic review and meta-analysis: prevalence of posttraumatic stress disorder (PTSD) in trauma-exposed preschool-aged children. *Journal of the American Academy of Child and Adolescent Psychiatry* **61**, 366–377.

World Health Organization (2013) Guidelines for the Management of Conditions Specifically Related to Stress. World Health Organization (WHO), Geneva, Switzerland.

World Health Organization (2019) *International Classification of Disease and Related Health Problems*, 11th revision. World Health Organization (WHO), Geneva, Switzerland.

Xiang, Y. *et al.* (2021) Comparative efficacy and acceptability of psychotherapies for post-traumatic stress disorder in children and adolescents: a systematic review and network meta-analysis. *BMJ Evidence Based Mental Health* **24**, 153–160.

Yang, F. *et al.* (2022) Prevalence and related factors of child posttraumatic stress disorder during COVID-19 pandemic: a systematic review and meta-analysis. *European Psychiatry* **65**(1), e37.

Yule, W. *et al.* (2000) The long-term psychological effects of a disaster experienced in adolescence: I: The incidence and course of PTSD. *Journal of Child Psychology and Psychiatry, and Allied Disciplines* **41**, 503–511.

Yule, W. *et al.* (2013) Children and war: the work of the Children and War Foundation. *European Journal of Psychotraumatology* **4**, 18424.

CHAPTER 59

Anxiety disorders

Daniel S. Pine

Section on Development and Affective Neuroscience, National Institute of Mental Health (NIMH) Intramural Research Program, Bethesda, MD, USA

Introduction

The chapter reviews six anxiety disorders: specific phobias, separation anxiety disorder, social anxiety disorder, generalized anxiety disorder, panic disorder, and agoraphobia. The first four are unique in at least one respect: features that define them represent typical aspects of development. This raises difficult questions on the boundary separating children and adolescents' expected expressions of anxiety and anxiety disorders.

While different scholars proffer different definitions of fear and anxiety, the current chapter defines *fear* as a brain state elicited by immediately present threats, which are stimuli capable of harming the organism. Based on this view, some authors categorize phobias as prototypical "fear" disorders. *Anxiety* occurs in situations that are not acutely dangerous, but which are experienced as dangerous, due to signs suggesting the presence of a distal threat. Based on this view, some authors categorize generalized anxiety disorder as a prototypical "anxiety" disorder. Fear and anxiety represent examples of emotions, defined as brain states with features that yield adaptive advantages. This includes helping animals avoid threats when the emotion is fear or anxiety.

Chapter 5 provides an extensive discussion on the definition of emotions. Briefly summarized, emotions are evoked by reinforcers, stimuli that animals will exert effort to either approach or avoid, and emotions can be differentiated from reflexes based on many parameters (Anderson & Adolphs, 2014; LeDoux & Pine, 2016; Pine *et al.*, 2021). Emotional brain states can occur in people or other organisms in the absence of alterations in conscious experience. Thus, organisms can manifest emotions through changes in their behavior and physiology without subjective experiences of distress. The subjective experiences of distress associated with fear and anxiety are defined in neuroscience using the term *feelings*. Feelings powerfully relate to anxiety symptoms. Although adaptive, fear and anxiety represent features of a disorder when they are provoked by stimuli loosely tied to threats or when they limit function.

The chapter begins by discussing aspects of diagnosis, assessment, and epidemiology. This is followed by a review of data on longitudinal course and risk. The chapter closes with sections on pathophysiology and treatment. Overall, the chapter provides clinicians with a guide for recognizing, understanding, and treating key features of pediatric anxiety disorders.

Diagnosis

The boundaries distinguishing anxiety disorders from other anxiety states remain incompletely specified, without clear markers that allow clinicians to easily distinguish among these states. When severe, anxiety disorders are readily recognized in the same way that extreme intellectual disability is readily distinguished from conditions that allow children to work on or above grade levels. For milder expressions, decisions can be difficult because anxiety is adaptive in some contexts and in some developmental periods. Clinicians face dilemmas because anxiety disorders require treatment, but inappropriate application of a diagnosis can bring stigma. Identifying anxiety disorders requires the clinician to recognize a departure from anxiety's adaptive role based on judgments about avoidance or distress.

At any age, an anxiety disorder is present when it interferes with adaptive behavior. Parents and clinicians are often quick to recognize markedly impairing anxiety, as occurs in children unable to attend school due to fear or anxiety. More difficulty arises in children experiencing only distress, without obvious impairment. In this context, evaluating a child's ability to recover and remain anxiety-free when provoking circumstances disappear is informative; failure to adapt to changing circumstances is a hallmark of an anxiety disorder.

Rutter's Child and Adolescent Psychiatry and Psychology, Seventh Edition.
Edited by Anita Thapar, Daniel S. Pine, Samuele Cortese, Cathy Creswell, Tamsin J. Ford, James F. Leckman, and Argyris Stringaris.

Companion website: www.wiley.com/go/thapar/ruttерspsych7

Nosology

The 1980 publication of the *Diagnostic and Statistical Manual for Mental Disorders*, 3rd edition (DSM-III) signaled a major switch, which introduced several unique anxiety disorders, with distinct clinical features. The current nosology in DSM-5-TR (2022) and the *International Classification for Diseases*, 11th revision (ICD-11; 2019) reflects this legacy. Concerns remain with the number of anxiety disorders in nosology, which can be recognized as unique but usually co-occur in clinical settings. In the future, boundaries will hopefully more strongly reflect data on outcome, genetics, biology, and treatment (Beesdo *et al.*, 2009a; Smoller *et al.*, 2019; Strawn *et al.*, 2021). As compared to DSM-III, significant differences in DSM-5-TR and ICD-11 involve the placement of obsessive-compulsive disorder (OCD) and post-traumatic stress disorder (PTSD). Both fall outside the anxiety disorders.

Specific conditions

Specific phobia

This diagnosis is defined by marked, unreasonable fear of specific objects or situations that do not pose actual danger, such as various animals or environmental settings, like high places. Although unreasonable fears are common, they are diagnosable only when they cause clinically significant distress or avoidance, severe enough to interfere with normal activities. Phobic disorders may begin at any age, but onset is typically in childhood, though most childhood phobias remit by adulthood (Fyer, 1998; Pine et al., 1998).

Separation anxiety disorder

Relative to other anxiety disorders, separation anxiety disorder has an unusually skewed age distribution, typically occurring before the age of 18 and often remitting before adulthood. Separation anxiety as a normal early-childhood experience must be distinguished from separation anxiety disorder, which typically involves impairment, where children avoid activities that require ordinary separation from caretakers. Clinical descriptions of "school phobia" typically do not, strictly speaking, identify children with a phobia. Such children often suffer from an extreme form of separation anxiety. Severe separation anxiety may develop in children without prior concerns about separation.

Social anxiety disorder

Social anxiety disorder typically involves concerns about being perceived as acting foolish, either expressed by report or through behavior. At a behavioral level, the diagnosis is based on observations about children's avoidance, refusal to speak, or self-consciousness in social settings. These symptoms commonly occur around unfamiliar adults, but they must also manifest with peers.

Though many children with social anxiety disorder appear to speak without difficulty, some children with the disorder either speak hesitantly or refrain from speaking in contexts that evoke fear. Others only report being afraid in the absence of concomitant behaviors. Features of social anxiety disorder related to outcome and treatment described in the current chapter apply to selective mutism, which has been studied less extensively than social anxiety disorder. For a small number of children, selective mutism can relate to language or learning problems, as well as problems with disruptive behavior. Material in chapters 37, 51, 52, and 65 can guide readers seeking information on these problems.

Selective mutism

Selective mutism appears in DSM-5-TR as an anxiety disorder. This convention reflects the fact that children with selective mutism often show severe social anxiety associated with marked hesitation in speaking, which can also occur in social anxiety disorder.

Both selective mutism and social anxiety must be differentiated from mental disorders involving impaired capacity for socialization, a cardinal feature of autism spectrum disorders (ASDs). This aspect of classification can complicate diagnosis, as children who meet criteria for ASD may also meet criteria for social anxiety disorder or selective mutism, provided their anxiety can be distinguished from the dysfunction they exhibit due to impaired socialization.

Generalized anxiety disorder

Generalized anxiety disorder manifests as recurrent worry, often about one's ability to succeed, perform schoolwork, or experience failure. The age of onset is incompletely understood, but available evidence places peak onset in late adolescence or early adulthood (Beesdo *et al.*, 2009a; Beesdo *et al.*, 2010; Beesdo-Baum *et al.*, 2011). Relative to other anxiety disorders, generalized anxiety disorder is more likely to occur with other psychopathology, particularly depressive disorders, to the point where the disorder rarely occurs on its own, particularly in clinical settings (Costello *et al.*, 2002; Rapee *et al.*, 2023).

Panic disorder

Panic disorder manifests as repeated episodes of unprovoked, spontaneous panic attacks, accompanied by physical symptoms, in addition to persistent worry about additional attacks or changes in behavior due to the attacks. Panic disorder is rare before puberty. Typically, the disorder begins with an initial spontaneous panic attack, occurring around late adolescence. Most individuals suffer only a few such attacks, and progression to recurring attacks is the exception, but when it happens, this typically occurs by early adulthood (Pine *et al.*, 1998).

Agoraphobia

Agoraphobia refers to extreme fear and avoidance of open spaces. While agoraphobia relates closely to panic disorder, it can also be diagnosed as an isolated condition. Since panic disorder rarely occurs before puberty, minimal work examines pediatric agoraphobia, which is rare and easily confused with other diagnoses. Children with separation anxiety disorder, for example, may fear traveling on their own, and children with social anxiety disorder may avoid open spaces where people congregate. When avoidance of open spaces is age-inappropriate and pervasive, it is appropriate to consider the diagnosis, particularly in a child without another anxiety disorder.

Boundary conditions

As discussed in the section on nosology, PTSD (see Chapter 58) and OCD (see Chapter 60) were classified as anxiety disorders in DSM-III. Both conditions involve high levels of anxiety, frequently co-occur with anxiety disorders, and resemble anxiety disorders in course and treatment. Like differentiations among anxiety disorders, clinical features distinguish anxiety disorders from OCD and PTSD. Definitive insights on relations among these conditions await advanced understanding of pathophysiology. Similarly, many children with an ASD present with high levels of anxiety, particularly concerning social settings. As noted above, it is important to differentiate social anxiety from a lack of social skills, so that the clinician can select the appropriate treatment for the presenting problems.

Developmental fluctuations

Children in many cultures display fears and anxiety that may be a core developmental feature (Ollendick *et al.*, 1996; Ingman *et al.*, 1999). Developmental risk for anxiety may manifest as temperamental variations displayed in the first two years of life. At later phases, beginning in preschool, the onsets of anxiety disorders mimic features of typical development. For example, fears of animals begin during this period, a time shortly before specific phobias often develop. Fears of separation also first manifest in early childhood, and separation anxiety disorder exhibits a particular high prevalence only a few years later (Pine *et al.*, 1998; Beesdo *et al.*, 2009a). Finally, social concerns typically emerge as part of adolescence (Ollendick & Hirshfeld-Becker, 2002), when incidence of social anxiety disorder rises (Beesdo *et al.*, 2007; Beesdo *et al.*, 2009a). Changing rates of anxiety disorders across development may reflect children's changing cognitive capacities, changing exposures to social contexts, or changes in biology, such as those that occur at puberty.

Comorbidity

Because greater dysfunction typically occurs in patients with multiple disorders, clinicians should monitor comorbidity in patients with anxiety disorders. Rates of comorbidity vary across studies, but high comorbidity among anxiety disorders, as well as with OCD and PTSD, occurs in most studies (Rapee *et al.*, 2023). This raises questions about the distinctiveness of anxiety disorders. Comorbidity is also important because it affects treatment. This includes instances where anxiety co-occurs with a medical disorder discussed in the section on risk factors. Comorbidity with either psychiatric or medical disorders complicates treatment where therapies for each disorder can either influence the other therapy or expressions of the illness. Therapeutic complications from comorbidities with psychiatric disorders are discussed in the final chapter section.

Major depression in adolescence is highly comorbid with anxiety disorders, with anxiety typically preceding the mood disorder (Angold *et al.*, 1999; Strawn *et al.*, 2021; Rapee *et al.*, 2023). The strength of this relation rivals most in developmental psychopathology. Since major depression is rarer than anxiety disorders, especially before adolescence, it stands to reason that rates of anxiety disorders in patients with depression exceed rates of depression in patients with anxiety disorders, especially in young children. Some clinical studies report comorbidity between anxiety disorders and attention deficit hyperactivity disorder (ADHD), but population-based studies suggest relations are weaker than with other conditions, particularly depression and other anxiety disorders (Angold *et al.*, 1999; Rapee *et al.*, 2023). While some have reported comorbidity between current anxiety disorders and substance abuse or conduct disorder, these associations also are relatively weak (Kaplow *et al.*, 2001; Rutter *et al.*, 2006). Interestingly, naturalistic studies suggest that symptoms of social anxiety disorder may predict better outcome in conduct problems (Pine *et al.*, 2000). Although few studies have linked anxiety disorders to learning disorders in children, it behooves clinicians to rule out learning problems, particularly in children who present with school-based anxiety. Finally, social anxiety symptoms frequently occur in children who meet criteria for ASD.

Assessment

Many instruments exist for assessing anxiety. Chapter 28 and other reviews summarize features of these instruments (Brooks & Kutcher, 2003; Seligman *et al.*, 2004; Silverman & Ollendick, 2005; Creswell *et al.*, 2020). Only an overview is provided in this chapter.

Rating scales

As discussed in Chapter 28, rating scales can be useful for screening or research. Some scales assess anxiety symptoms as part of broader psychopathology domains; others specifically target anxiety symptoms. Assessments can be made by many informants, whose ratings often poorly correlate. This complicates treatment decisions, especially when children's and other informants' ratings correlate poorly with ratings from clinicians (Rupp, 2003). Clinicians must work with children and families so that agreement can be reached on the need for treatment and on the targets to be monitored.

Scales may provide overall estimates of anxiety levels. The Multidimensional Anxiety Scale for Children (MASC) (March *et al.*, 1997; March and Sullivan, 1999) and the Screen for Child Anxiety Related Emotional Disorders (SCARED) (Birmaher *et al.*, 1997) have been used for these purposes, including across many cultures (Hale *et al.*, 2011). They possess strong psychometrics and can be sensitive to treatment effects, rendering them useful in clinical monitoring. The Pediatric Anxiety Rating Scale (PARS) is a clinician-rated scale used in important comparative efficacy studies (Rupp, 2003). Further discussion of these and other scales can be found in Chapter 28 and in a recent review emphasizing the importance of measuring both interference and features of symptoms (Creswell *et al.*, 2021).

Diagnostic interviews

Chapter 28 describes multiple interviews that serve different purposes. This includes highly structured interviews where support for clinical utility is mixed. The Kiddie-Schedule for Affective Disorder and Schizophrenia (K-SADS) was developed for use by clinicians, and most of the many versions allow full latitude of inquiry for use in clinical studies. However, one recently developed version used in an important large-scale community-based study, is designed for lay interviewers and operates more similarly to other lay-interviewer measures described in Chapter 28 (Mennies *et al.*, 2021). Like the K-SADS, the Anxiety Disorders Interview Schedule for Children (ADISC) was designed for clinicians, and it provides a particularly in-depth assessment of anxiety disorders, which can be especially useful in treatment studies (Silverman *et al.*, 2001). This has led many clinical and treatment studies to utilize the ADISC (Creswell *et al.*, 2020; Rapee *et al.*, 2023) and has led other studies to combine versions of the K-SADS and ADISC to maximize each interview's strengths (White *et al.*, 2017). Each interview demonstrates adequate psychometrics, with one major factor informing selection being the availability of clinicians for implementation and regular monitoring.

Epidemiology

Prevalence

Epidemiology studies find anxiety disorders to be common, with prevalence approximating 5–10% (Table 59.1). Studies have followed children over extended periods to identify typical ages of onsets and incidence (Costello *et al.*, 2004; Costello *et al.*, 2005; Copeland *et al.*, 2009; Beesdo *et al.*, 2010; Copeland *et al.*, 2011; Polanczyk *et al.*, 2015). In childhood, phobias and separation anxiety disorder are most prevalent, diminishing in adolescence, when incidence of social anxiety disorder rises. Rates of generalized anxiety disorder increase later in adolescence, and panic disorder is rare before this period (Beesdo *et al.*, 2009a).

The current chapter highlights data from studies that estimate prevalence in representative samples, assessed with structured psychiatric interviews, where rates vary widely (Table 59.1). Prospective studies and studies of lifetime prevalence find much higher rates than studies using a single assessment (Angold *et al.*, 1996; Costello *et al.*, 2003; Jaffee *et al.*, 2005; Copeland *et al.*, 2011; NHS, 2018; Mennies *et al.*, 2021). This reflects the episodic nature of anxiety disorders and methodologic differences across studies.

Table 59.1 highlights features impacting prevalence. Developmental factors may explain some cross-study differences: studies finding relatively high rates of separation anxiety disorder tend to include young children, whereas those that include older children find high rates of social anxiety disorder. Studies in Table 59.1 conducted in the same country but using different methods also vary in prevalence estimates. Here, different approaches for combining informant reports are important, given the low rates of informant agreement. Two recent studies (Dalsgaard *et al.*, 2020; Mennies *et al.*, 2021) report overall rates of anxiety disorders in aggregate as opposed to rates of specific diagnoses, such as separation anxiety disorder or social anxiety disorder. This convention may reflect the above-noted disagreements on the meaningfulness of narrowly defined anxiety disorders.

Finally, some scholars suggest that secular changes affect data in Table 59.1, and recent data on rates during the COVID-19 pandemic hint at this possibility. While findings remain inconsistent (Zeytinoglu *et al.*, 2021), data tend to suggest increased symptoms manifested during the pandemic (Racine *et al.*, 2021). Chapter 18 provides further discussion of these important issues.

Longitudinal outcome

High rates in epidemiological studies raise concerns about the long-term consequences of pediatric anxiety disorders. As highlighted in Chapter 28, the modest test–retest reliability of some measures suggests that available data provide only lower-bound estimates of stability. While frank anxiety disorders have an earlier onset than other emotional disorders, such as major depression, the preclinical antecedents of anxiety can be detected even earlier.

Inhibited temperament and psychopathology

Kagan (1994) and Kagan *et al.* (2001) first described a type of temperamental variation in the first three years of life that predicts risk for anxiety disorders in childhood and adolescence. Of note, only a narrow subset of research on temperament targets relations with anxiety disorders. Chapter 8 describes the many ways to conceptualize temperamental variation and its relation to psychopathology. Young children with the temperament of behavioral inhibition tend to cease activity and refrain from speaking in the face of novel stimuli, scenarios, and people, presented in standard laboratory paradigms. Studies of associations with psychopathology have been conducted in thousands of children (Rosenbaum *et al.*, 1993; Clauss & Blackford, 2012; Fox & Kalin, 2014; Tang *et al.*, 2020). Inhibited temperament has been consistently linked to anxiety disorders, including separation anxiety, social anxiety, and phobias. Research demonstrates a developmental progression, which begins as behavioral inhibition, followed by various anxiety disorders in childhood and then social anxiety disorder in early adolescence (Clauss &

Table 59.1 Prevalence (%) of anxiety disorders in children, adolescents, and adults followed prospectively.

Location	Authors	N	Age in Years	Interview	Time frame	Rates (%)					
						Any	SiPh	SAD	OAD/GAD[a]	SoPh	PD
New Zealand											
Dunedin	Anderson *et al.* (1987)[b]	785	11	DISC-C[c]	12 months[d]	1.8–7.5	0–2.4	0.06–3.5	0.05–2.9	0–0.9	–
				DISC-P	12 months[e]	3.6[f]	1.7	1.9	2.5	0.4	–
	McGee *et al.* (1990)[b]	943	15	DISC-C	12 months[g]	10.7	3.6	2.0	5.9	1.1	–
	Kim-Cohen *et al.* (2003)[b]	976	26	DISC	12 months[g]	26.1	7.1	–	5.5[a]	10.7	3.9
Christchurch	Fergusson *et al.* (1993)	986	15	DISC-P	12 months[g]	3.9	1.3	0.1	0.6	0.7	–
		965	15	DISC-C	12 months[g]	10.8	5.1	0.5	2.1	1.7	–
	Goodwin *et al.* (2004)	969	16–18	M-CIDI[h,i]	12 months[g]	18.4	9.6	–	2.7[a]	7.5	–
		957	18–21	M-CIDI[h,i]	12 months[g]	14.6	6.5	–	1.8[a]	6.7	–
Germany											
Mannheim	Esser *et al.* (1990)	191	13	Graham/Rutter parent/child[j,k,l]	6 months	5.8	–	–		–	–
Munich	Reed and Wittchen (1998)[b]	3021	14–24	M-CIDI[m,n]	12 months	–	–	–	–	–	0.6
					Lifetime	–	–	–	–	–	0.8
	Wittchen *et al.* (1999)[b]	925	14–17	M-CIDI[m,n]	12 months	–	–	–	–	3.0	–
					Lifetime	–	–	–	–	4.0	–
Bremen	Essau *et al.* (1999)	1035	12–17	M-CIDI[m,n]	Lifetime	–	–	–	–	1.6	–
England											
London[m]	Kramer and Garralda (1998)	131	13–17	K-SADS[o,p]	12 months	5.3	–	–	3.1	1.5	0.8
England	NHS (2018)	18,029	5–19	DAWBA[q]	1 month	7.2	0.8	0.7	1.5[a]	0.8	1.1
Denmark	Dalsgaard *et al.* (2020)	1.3 million	Birth–18	Patient register	Lifetime	2.6	–	–	–	–	–
Netherlands	Verhulst *et al.* (1997)	312/780[r]	13–18	DISC-C	6 months	10.5	4.5	1.4	1.8	3.7	0.2
				DISC-P		16.5	9.2	0.6	1.5	6.3	0.3
				DISC[s]		23.5	12.7	1.8	3.1	9.2	0.4
				DISC[l]		5.3	–	–	–	–	–
						4.4	–	–	–	–	–
Puerto Rico	Bird *et al.* (1988)	386/777[n]	4–16	DISC[l]	6 months	7.0	2.6	4.7	–	–	–
							1.3	2.1	–	–	–
USA											
Pennsylvania	Costello *et al.* (1988)[b]	300/789[r]	7–11	DISC-C	12 months	10.5	6.7	4.1	2.0	1.0	–
				DISC-P	12 months	6.5	3.0	0.4	2.8	0	–
	Benjamin *et al.* (1990)[b]	300/789[q]	7–11	DISC[g]	12 months	15.4	9.1	4.1	4.6	1.0	–
New York State	Pine *et al.* (1998)	776	9–18	DISC[g]	12 months	–	11.6	8.6	14.3	8.4	0.0
		760	11–20	DISC[g]	12 months	–	5.9	3.7	8.0	9.9	0.0
		716	17–26	DISC[g]	12 months	–	22.1	–	5.0[a]	5.6	0.1
Nationwide	Kessler *et al.* (2012)	10,148	13–17	CIDI[i]	12 months	24.9	15.8	1.6	1.1[a]	8.2	1.9

Nationwide	Magee *et al.* (1996)	1765	15–24	CIDI[h,i]	Lifetime	–	10.8	–	–	14.9	–
Nationwide	Merikangas *et al.* (2010)	3042	8–15	DISC[c]	12 months	0.7	–	–	0.3[a]	–	0.4
Nationwide	Mennies *et al.* (2021)	11,875	9–10	K-SADS[f]	Lifetime	37.1	–	–	–	–	–
North Carolina	Costello *et al.* (1996)	1015	9, 11, 13	CAPA[s,u]	3 months	5.7	0.3	3.5	1.4	0.6	0.03
	Costellos *et al.* (2003)	1420	9–16	CAPA[o,u]	3 months	2.4	–	–	–	–	–
Georgia	Shaffer *et al.* (1996)	1285	9–17	DISC-P[v,w]	6 months	21.0	11.7	2.5	4.3	7.9	–
New Haven				DISC-C[w]		23.7	11.2	3.1	5.4	8.5	–
New York				DISC[l]		18.5	9.5	4.1	8.0	8.2	–
						13.9	6.8	3.5	6.5	6.6	–
Puerto Rico				DISC		20.5	3.3	5.8	7.7	7.6	–
Oregon	Lewinsohn *et al.* (1998)	1709	15.5	K-SADS	12 months	2.8	1.3	0.2	0.5	0.9	0.3
Virginia	Simonoff *et al.* (1997)	2762, (twins)	8–16	CAPA[a,t]	3 months	–	21.2	7.2	10.8	8.4	–
						–	4.4	1.5	4.4	2.5	–

Note: SiPh—simple phobia; SAD—separation anxiety disorder; OAD—overanxious disorder; GAD—generalized anxiety disorder; SoPh—social phobia; PD—panic disorder.

[a] Wherever superscript appears, rate is for GAD

[b] Same cohort within site

[c] DISC-C and DISC-P—Diagnostic Interview Schedule for Children, child and parent version, respectively (Costello *et al.*, 1988)

[d] Rates vary depending on diagnostic criteria based on DISC-C, and parent and teacher ratings, e.g., diagnostic criteria met: (i) by two of three sources or by one source and symptoms confirmed by at least one other source; (ii) by one source but no other source confirms symptoms; (iii) by combining symptoms from all three sources.

[e] Percent meeting diagnostic criteria applying same standards as at age 15 in McGee *et al.* (1990)

[f] Rates calculated from papers

[g] Percent meeting criteria based on DISC-C plus parent ratings

[h] Diagnosis based on interview with adolescent

[i] CIDI—Composite International Diagnostic Interview (Wittchen *et al.*, 1999)

[j] Interview by Graham and Rutter

[k] Includes anxiety and mood disorders

[l] Top line: percent meeting diagnostic criteria on parent OR child interview and had a Children's Global Assessment Scale (CGAS) <61 (Shaffer *et al.*, 1985). Bottom line: percent meeting diagnostic criteria on parent OR child interview and had a CGAS between 61–70.

[m] Adolescents in primary care clinics

[n] M-CIDI—Munich modification of CIDI (Wittchen *et al.*, 1999)

[o] K-SADS—Kiddie Schedule for Affective Disorders and Schizophrenia

[p] DAWBA—Development and Well-being Assessment

[q] Two-stage study: N in Stage 2/N in Stage 1

[r] Percent meeting diagnostic criteria based on interview with parent OR child

[s] K-SADS: performed by lay interviewer, only based on parent

[t] CAPA—Child and Adolescent Psychiatric Assessment (Angold & Costello, 2000).

[u] DISC Version 2.3 (Shaffer *et al.*, 1996)

[v] Percent meeting diagnostic criteria only for symptom number, age of onset, and duration

[w] DICA—Diagnostic Interview for Children and Adolescents

[x] Top line: percent meeting diagnostic criteria. Bottom line: percent meeting diagnostic criteria and impairment criteria.

Blackford, 2012; Fox & Kalin, 2014). Finally, as these children reach adulthood, outcomes appear to further diversify, where behavioral inhibition predicts generalized anxiety disorders and major depressive disorder in addition to social anxiety (Caspi *et al.*, 1996; Fox & Kalin, 2014; Tang *et al.*, 2020).

Stability of anxiety disorders

The clearest information about diagnostic stability of frank anxiety disorders emerges from community-based studies. Such studies are free of biases that plague some studies and avoid complications related to treatment delivery in other studies. The best information derives from studies obtaining multiple assessments across development. Many such studies exist, and virtually all find pediatric anxiety disorders predict increased risk for later anxiety disorders (Pine *et al.*, 1998; Kim-Cohen *et al.*, 2003; Beesdo *et al.*, 2009a; Beesdo *et al.*, 2009b; Copeland *et al.*, 2014). However, particular aspects of the longitudinal data appear inconsistent. For example, different studies find distinct anxiety disorders to show unique associations with each other and mood disorders. Similarly, some studies find greater stability in girls (Costello *et al.*, 1999; Rueter *et al.*, 1999), whereas other studies find no such sex differences (Pine *et al.*, 1998; Beesdo *et al.*, 2009a).

Beyond community-based studies, investigations using other designs also find that anxiety in childhood predicts risk for anxiety disorders at various points in time. This includes studies using family-based (Weissman *et al.*, 1997), clinical (Aschenbrand *et al.*, 2003), and treatment designs (Ginsburg *et al.*, 2018). Overall, as compared to epidemiological studies, reports based in treatment-seeking samples tend to find higher rates of persistence. Nevertheless, even in studies of clinical samples that follow severe cases, many affected children appear unaffected by anxiety disorders when assessed many years after study entry. Interestingly, despite this fact, most adults with anxiety disorders, as well as adults with mood disorders, will have had a childhood history of anxiety disorders. Hence, for a significant minority of children, anxiety disorders begin a pattern of chronic suffering that can be expressed in many ways clinically throughout life.

Risk factors

Due to referral biases, epidemiological studies provide the best information about risk. Perhaps the most consistent findings are for sex differences: girls have higher rates than boys for most anxiety disorders with odds ratios in the range of 2.0 (Lewinsohn *et al.*, 1998; Beesdo *et al.*, 2009a). Some data suggests that sex differences become more prominent as children enter adolescence (NHS, 2018). No other risk factors relate as strongly to anxiety disorders, possibly because risk factors interact as part of complex causal webs across development. Accordingly, Figure 59.1 depicts such a risk model whereupon multiple risk factors accumulate to shape risk.

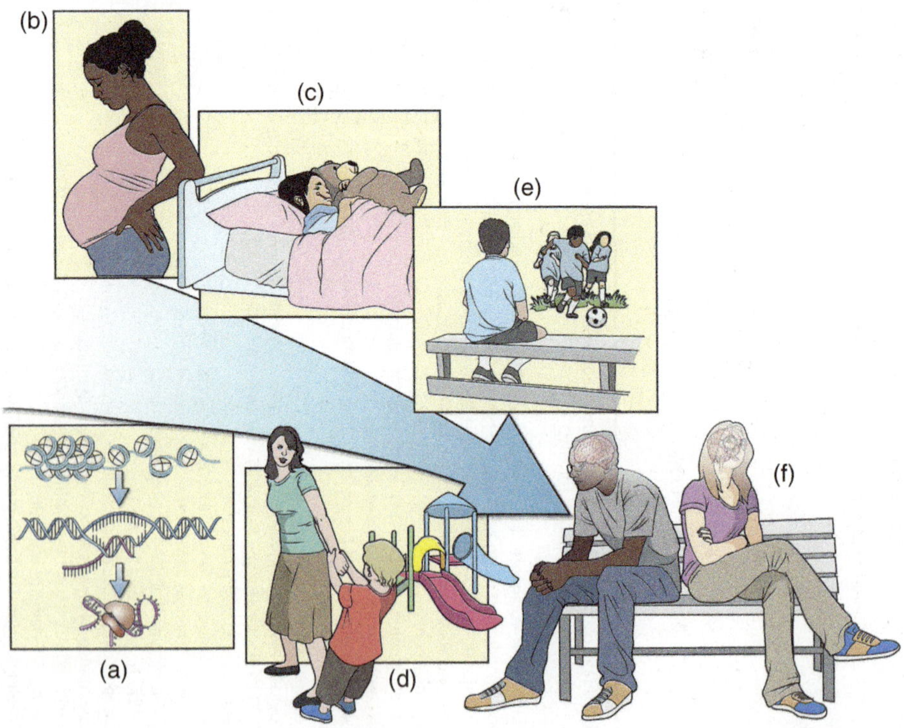

Figure 59.1 The figure shows cascading sets of interacting risk factors. Cascades shape risk across development in the brains of the two adolescents depicted on the bench on the figure's right side (f). Risks include genetics (a), perinatal factors (b), illnesses (c), aspects of parent–child interactions (d), and stress from various events, including peer exclusion (e).

Stress exposure

Considered in the aggregate, stress exposure increases risk for anxiety, but disagreements exist concerning how this aggregate risk accrues from specific stressors. Stressors include economic disadvantage, family dysfunction, single-parent households, and low parental education, where relations with these and other individual risks rarely appear strong (Beesdo *et al.*, 2009b; Beesdo *et al.*, 2010; Penninx *et al.*, 2021; Strawn *et al.*, 2021; Rapee *et al.*, 2023;). In this context, an odds ratio of at least 2.0 can be viewed as "strong." Some factors, like economic disadvantage, can be described as "distal" because they operate indirectly on many children by influencing children's level of exposure to other, "proximal" risk factors. Such proximal factors, like stressful peer relationships, more directly influence individual children through unique experiences faced by each child (Rapee *et al.*, 2023). Figure 59.1 depicts an instance of peer exclusion where a boy silently watches his peers play sports, which is a form of stress that can occur as part of bullying.

Inconsistent findings on stress exposure are notable in anxiety. Relative to anxiety disorders, some forms of social stress relate more consistently to other mental disorders, including disruptive behavior disorders, as described in Chapter 65 on oppositional and conduct disorders, as well as in Chapter 33 on parenting relations with psychopathology. Consistent with such observations, one notable multiwave study used a quasi-experimental design to show stronger and more consistent associations between poverty and its associated stresses with children's disruptive behavior problems than anxiety symptoms (Costello *et al.*, 2010). Nevertheless, when these same children were seen as adults, poverty in childhood did relate to both adult anxiety and adult disruptive behavior problems, despite the more specific relations in childhood (Copeland *et al.*, 2022). Thus, different stresses may relate to distinct forms of child and adult psychopathology.

While epidemiological studies minimize referral biases, they typically include few children with severe disorders. As a result, it is also helpful to consider data from other samples. Data on social factors, such as parenting practices, in these samples yield mixed results. Moreover, variable findings should remind clinicians to avoid blaming parents for the problems faced by their children. Anxiety relates to various parenting practices, including harsh, punitive parenting and excessive accommodation of children's demands, but associations with overprotective parenting appear particularly consistent (Beesdo *et al.*, 2009a; Frenkel *et al.*, 2015; Strawn *et al.*, 2021). Figure 59.1 also illustrates a parent–child interaction, where a child pulls a parent in a way that could lead the parent to accommodate the child's wish to avoid a feared scenario. Studies of overprotective parenting quantify the threshold that different parents use when choosing to limit their child's exposure to mild threats, such as joining a party attended by many unfamiliar children.

The weight of the evidence suggests that many parenting practices represent nonspecific risk factors. As described in Chapter 65, relations manifest with many conditions, including not only anxiety but also mood and behavior disorders (Wood *et al.*, 2003). Particular interest focuses on the role of family accommodation, which can contribute to multiple aspects of pediatric anxiety disorders (Etkin *et al.*, 2022). Moreover, parenting behaviors may have indirect effects, through interactions with genetic influences and children's temperament (Lewis-Morrarty *et al.*, 2012; Zeytinoglu *et al.*, 2022), which complicates attempts to relate specific parenting behavior to children's anxiety in an attempt to inform prevention efforts. Finally, clinicians should monitor their own attitudes when working with parents. When helping parents change their behavior to help their children, a nonjudgmental clinical approach is essential, one that supports rather than blames parents. In many scenarios, parental behaviors involve difficult-to-avoid compromises that parents make to cope with extremely trying circumstances. The clinician's role is to help parents manage in the most effective way possible in such situations.

Despite lack of uniform findings, interest in environmental influences persists for at least two reasons. First, basic research demonstrates strong developmental plasticity through effects of experience on brain systems that respond to threats (Gross & Hen, 2004). Such findings generate interest concerning relations between social experiences and human brain development. Second, from a clinical perspective, anxiety disorders commonly occur after trauma (Steinberg & Avenevoli, 2000; Pine & Cohen, 2002; Penninx *et al.*, 2021; Rapee *et al.*, 2023). Nevertheless, clinicians should avoid assuming that children with anxiety disorders experience trauma, as anxiety disorders often also occur in the absence of trauma. Relations that different types of stress show with multiple disorders could reflect dimensional associations where various clinical problems show different thresholds for occurring after varying levels of stress.

Some studies relate anxiety to an overall tally of adverse events (Eley & Stevenson, 2000; Hankin & Abramson, 2001; Williamson *et al.*, 2005). This includes research linking such a tally during adolescence to risk for anxiety four years later, especially generalized anxiety disorder in females (Pine *et al.*, 2002). Temperament and prestress anxiety, in addition to varieties of stress exposure, may interact in complicated ways, as suggested by research examining anxiety during the pandemic (Zeytinoglu *et al.*, 2021). Children's anxiety symptoms may have increased during the COVID-19 pandemic at least partially through effects of stress on risk for anxiety.

Stress reactivity

Children manifest tremendous variability in their response to stress, which can be quantified using physiological indices (Rapee *et al.*, 2023). This includes heart rate (Kassam-Adams *et al.*, 2005), amalgamations of many physiologic variables (Obradovic *et al.*, 2011), and startle reactivity (Penninx *et al.*, 2021; Beatty *et al.*, 2023; Nelson *et al.*, 2022). This work links altered physiologic measures to later anxiety. Nevertheless, given the multiple differences across studies, consensus views remain elusive. Moreover, the magnitude of effect sizes is not large, rarely exceeding one-half standard deviation differences between anxious and healthy groups, with stronger associations in concurrent versus prospective research (Penninx *et al.*, 2021).

Vulnerability to stress can also be quantified with questionnaires and personality inventories, where links exist with symptomatic measures of anxiety disorders among children followed longitudinally (Pine *et al.*, 2001). Some perspectives view measures of vulnerability assessed with questionnaires as opposed to physiologic variables as lying within a matrix that might inform clinical utility (Kozak & Cuthbert, 2016). This matrix separates risk factors based on the level at which they operate, from molecular levels within cells, through levels of structures composed of many cells in the brain, through functions operating on a whole-person level, and extending up to the level of the society.

Medical conditions

Epidemiological studies establish links between anxiety disorders and multiple medical conditions, as depicted in Figure 59.1 by a pregnant mother in one picture and a child in a bed with a teddy bear in another picture. While evidence documents a range of associations, none are large, with effect sizes from individual studies rarely exceeding an odds ratio of 2.0.

During the perinatal period, risk factors include overt neurological injury, febrile seizures, preterm birth, low birthweight, exposure to toxins, and minor neurological soft signs (Shaffer *et al.*, 1985; Breslau, 1995; Whitaker *et al.*, 1997; Breslau & Chilcoat, 2000; Breslau *et al.*, 2000; Vasa *et al.*, 2002). Recent studies also consider associations in both perinatal and later developmental epochs with a range of specific environmental exposures neglected in past research. This includes air pollution, various toxicants, and potentially harmful aspects of diet. In general, these studies find that exposures associated with various indicators of poor physical health also show relations with indicators of poor mental health, including anxiety (Penninx *et al.*, 2021; Strawn *et al.*, 2021). However, as with exposure to social stress and stress reactivity, all such factors operate with many interacting factors shaping risk for anxiety (Shaffer *et al.*, 1985; Penninx *et al.*, 2021; Strawn *et al.*, 2021). Moreover, as with studies of social risk factors, some medical risks, such as some brain injuries, show stronger and more consistent associations with disruptive behavior than anxiety symptoms, with some injuries even showing protective relations with anxiety symptoms (Vasa *et al.*, 2004; Koenigs *et al.*, 2008).

Medical conditions influencing respiration represent another interesting risk factor, where some level of specificity may exist. Relations with anxiety are found with asthma with relative consistency (Goodwin *et al.*, 2003). Similarly, anxiety's link to smoking may reflect smoking's deleterious effects on pulmonary function (Johnson *et al.*, 2000). Nevertheless, anxiety disorders show relatively strong associations with a range of other medical conditions, which suggests multiple risk pathways (Penninx *et al.*, 2021). For example, as reviewed elsewhere in the textbook, considerable research links immunological factors, including infections with Group-A-beta-hemolytic streptococcus, to anxiety, particularly when accompanied by tics or OCD (see Chapters 55 and 60). Multiple factors could account for such an association. This could include direct medical influences, such as tissue-specific effects from antibodies cross-reacting with neurons, or nonspecific effects from inflammatory proteins produced during an infection. This could also include indirect influences, such as effects from disruption in social support systems or combinations of these factors. Effects from multiple interacting risk factors appear most plausible, based on other research linking risk factors to anxiety disorders.

The COVID-19 pandemic provided an unusual opportunity to study stress. This is because the pandemic simultaneously stressed medical, social, economic, and other systems, each of which had been shown previously to markedly influence risk for anxiety disorders. This allowed the events surrounding the pandemic to create potential synergy among risk factors for anxiety. Research generated two main conclusions related to anxiety. First, levels of anxiety symptoms appeared to increase during the pandemic (Racine *et al.*, 2021). While not unexpected, it is important to document levels of symptoms; given the resilient nature of children, high levels of anxiety symptoms were not preordained. Second, marked variation in symptom levels existed, possibly reflecting the multiple ways in which risk factors interact. Some children experienced a worsening of preexisting anxiety; others developed new problems, and still other children saw improvements in their anxiety (Zeytinoglu *et al.*, 2021). Complex interactions likely influenced these expressions for individual children (Racine *et al.*, 2021). Such complexities exerted particularly profound effects where resources were limited and where an unmet need for appropriate services had existed prior to the pandemic's onset, emphasizing the need to identify children most in need.

Pathophysiology

Genetics

Studies use various methods to affirm the influences of genetic factors on anxiety disorders. Clear conclusions follow from research using family and twin studies, but more tentative insights arise from molecular genetics (Smoller *et al.*, 2019; Purves *et al.*, 2020).

Behavioral genetics research firmly establishes the familial nature of pediatric anxiety disorders (Lee *et al.*, 2021; Penninx *et al.*, 2021; Zeytinoglu *et al.*, 2021; Rapee *et al.*, 2023). In anxiety disorders, twin studies generally find stronger contributions to such familial aggregation from the environment, particularly the so-called "non-shared environment," than from genetics (Smoller *et al.*, 2019). Moreover, nonspecificity exists: a broad risk for anxiety and depression, as opposed to a risk specifically for anxiety, might be transmitted within families (Middeldorp *et al.*, 2005; Waszczuk *et al.*, 2014; Lewis &

Plomin, 2015; Penninx *et al.*, 2021). Twin studies that have longitudinally followed children find multiple forms of genetic risk (Waszczuk *et al.*, 2014; Lewis & Plomin, 2015). One form may influence risk primarily in childhood; another may only operate in adolescence or adulthood; and a final form may shape risk at many ages.

Recent molecular studies have changed views on genetic aspects of anxiety. Scholars initially considered data from so-called "candidate gene studies" (see Chapter 21 on genetics), but current views eschew such data in favor of results from genome-wide association studies (GWAS). For virtually all psychiatric disorders, GWAS consistently finds very small risk associated with individual genes (Smoller *et al.*, 2019). Moreover, these studies suggest that risk is transmitted for relatively broad categories of disorders, as opposed to more narrow categories, such as anxiety disorders in general, let alone specific anxiety disorders in DSM-5-TR. Given the modest contribution of genetics to anxiety in behavioral studies, fewer GWAS studies examine anxiety disorders as compared to disorders, such as ADHD, where behavioral data find strong heritability. Early positive GWAS results in adult anxiety are appearing (Purves *et al.*, 2020), but efforts thus far have been less successful in youth (Jami *et al.*, 2022). Finally, the poor correspondence between findings in GWAS and DSM-5-TR groupings has led investigators to consider codifying risk using alternative phenotypes that might mediate the genetic connection to clinical measures. These alternative phenotypes include measures of temperament, laboratory measures such as responsivity to respiratory stimulation, or measures derived from brain imaging.

Psychobiology

Basic science suggests that anxiety states arise from the engagement of specific neural circuits (Gross & Hen, 2004; LeDoux & Pine, 2016; LeDoux & Daw, 2018; Penninx *et al.*, 2021). Development shapes these circuits in ways that can begin early in life, with placental programming. Figure 59.2 depicts the mammalian threat-responsive circuitry. Subcortical structures include the bed nucleus of the stria terminalis (BNST) appearing in green and the amygdala appearing in red. The hippocampus appears in aqua, and the caudate nucleus appears in blue (Kovner *et al.*, 2020). Threat-responsive circuitry also includes the prefrontal cortex (PFC) and insula, which appears in pink in Figure 59.2 (Penninx *et al.*, 2021; Kenwood *et al.*, 2022). Subcortical structures support threat-responsive behavior in both rodents and primates, whereas some PFC structures evolutionarily arose after the last common rodent–primate ancestor (Pine *et al.*, 2021).

Studies use peripheral measures as indirect indicators of threat-responsive brain circuitry function. This includes measures of attention and physiologic responding. Research in rodents and nonhuman primates shows the capacity of threats to influence attention (Pine & Fox, 2015; Abend *et al.*, 2018;Pagliaccio *et al.*, 2019). Moreover, children with anxiety disorders tend to allocate more attention to mild threats than children without anxiety disorders (Abend *et al.*, 2018), a pattern that may provide targets for novel treatment (Shechner *et al.*, 2014; White *et al.*, 2017).

Some research uses physiologic indices to examine response to threat. Most studies find patients with anxiety disorders, relative to healthy individuals, manifest enhanced responding in

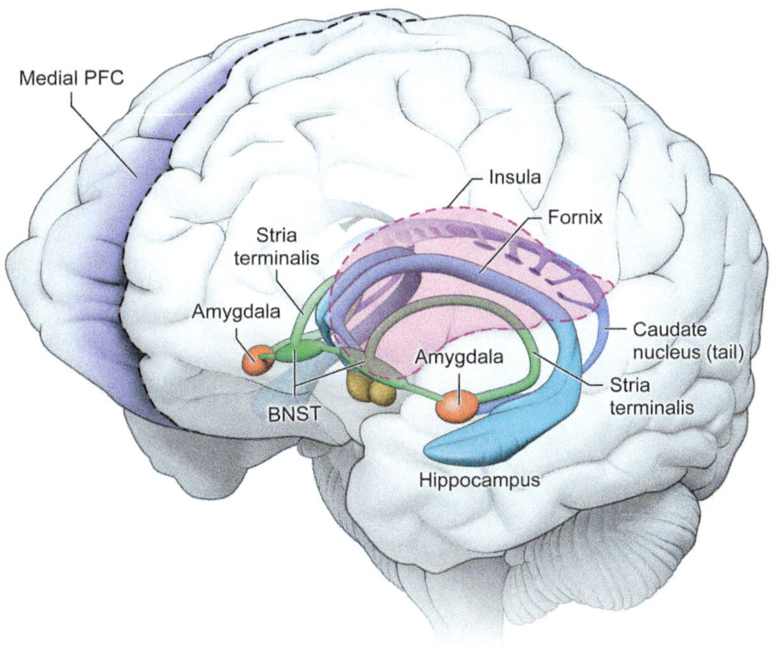

Figure 59.2 The figure illustrates threat-responsive brain areas. Subcortical structures appear in color. BNST bed nucleus of the stria terminalis; PFC = , prefrontal cortex.

the context of threat-learning experiments (Duits *et al.*, 2015; Dvir *et al.*, 2019; Abend *et al.*, 2020) or when exposed to an acute threat (Kujawa *et al.*, 2015; Abend *et al.*, 2020; Penninx *et al.*, 2021; Nelson *et al.*, 2022). This includes work examining multiple forms of threat and diverse biological parameters (Penninx *et al.*, 2021; Rapee *et al.*, 2023). Nevertheless, healthy and anxiety groups typically do not differ in their tendency to learn about aspects of threats.

Imaging studies quantify brain structure and function in a more direct manner than studies of attention or physiologic responding. Here, few consistent findings exist (Penninx *et al.*, 2021). Results from studies of brain function generally appear more promising than studies of brain structure (Linke *et al.*, 2021), with the most promising research examining PFC function.

To examine PFC function, some studies use imaging paradigms derived from techniques used to study peripheral physiology. For example, studies examining lateral PFC function tend to extend past research on attention, as illustrated in Figure 59.3 for the behavior and section of the PFC shaded in green (White *et al.*, 2017). These studies relate lateral PFC function to anxiety in the context of attention capture by a distracting threat, such as the snake in the picture. Studies examining functioning of the medial PFC tend to extend past research on threat learning, as illustrated in Figure 59.3 for a procedure used to study rodents and a section of the PFC shaded in blue

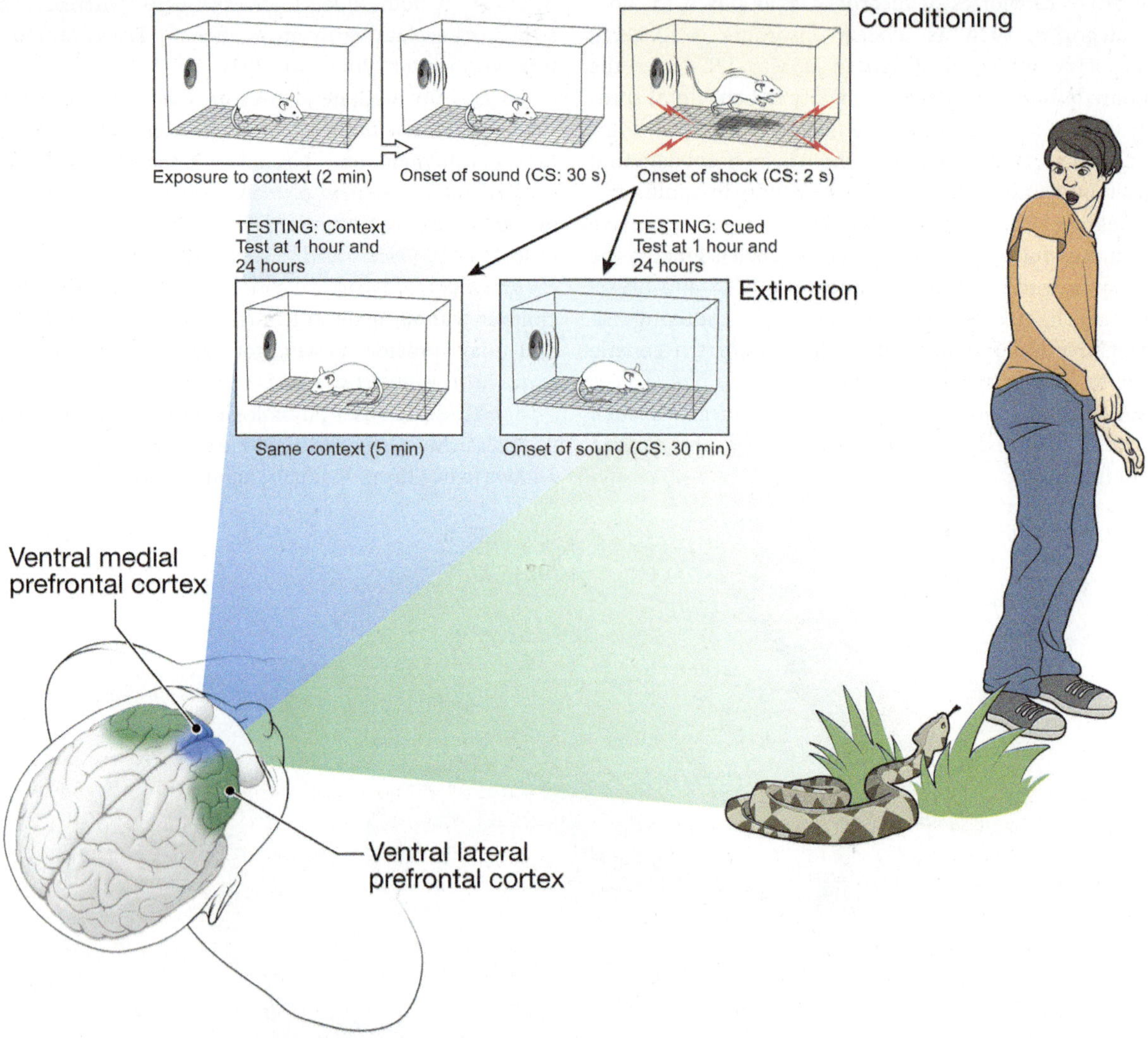

Figure 59.3 The figure depicts two sets of behaviors that have been studied in animals and extended through brain-imaging research with children. These behaviors relate to different sections of the prefrontal cortex (PFC). One of these behaviors involves threat learning, which appears above the blue shading in the figure. Threat learning includes conditioning, when the neutral sound in the picture is paired with a shock, and extinction, where the conditioned sound (CS) is then presented without the shock. Maintaining memory of extinction requires engagement of the medial PFC, which is shaded in blue. The other behavior involves the bottom-up capture of attention, which appears to the right of the green shading in the figure and relates to the ventral lateral PFC. Capture of attention occurs when a task-irrelevant threat, such as the snake in the picture, engages the focus of an individual, as shown in the boy's reaction in the figure.

(Gold *et al.*, 2020). These studies relate medial PFC function to anxiety in the context of memory for an extinguished threat cue that ceases to predict the occurrence of a loud sound. Such studies find unique medial PFC function in healthy youth compared to youth with anxiety disorders.

Immaturity in methods leads to inconsistent brain-imaging findings (Marek *et al.*, 2022). At least for mood and anxiety disorders, the most recent findings from structural brain-imaging studies suggest that, prior to the last few years, findings in patients likely reflect Type I errors (Bas-Hoogendam *et al.*, 2022). More recent large-scale studies generally fail to detect replicable structural correlates of pediatric anxiety symptoms (Marek *et al.*, 2022). Moreover, while findings from studies of PFC function appear more promising (Gold *et al.*, 2020), some research suggests that PFC function may primarily relate to overall levels of psychopathology. For example, functional brain-imaging studies in adults, where more data exist, find that both anxiety disorders and other conditions manifest similar threat hypersensitivity (McTeague *et al.*, 2020).

Research on the neural correlates of cognitive control represent a promising relatively new area for studies of the PFC (Penninx *et al.*, 2021). Cognitive control occurs when children must suppress inappropriate habitual actions so that they can correctly make difficult choices. Considerable recent work links pediatric anxiety to difficulty responding to task rules in high-conflict scenarios, findings linked to functioning in the dorsal regions of the frontal and parietal cortex (Cardinale *et al.*, 2023). As with threat-responsiveness, this pattern may be nonspecific, as it occurs in many disorders besides pediatric anxiety disorders (McTeague *et al.*, 2017). A more anxiety-specific pattern may arise for studies of error sensitivity, where anxiety disorders appear relatively unique in showing neural hypersensitivity to errors. The most consistent findings arise for a measure known as the error-related negativity (ERN), which manifests in the electroencephalographic response to errors (Penninx *et al.*, 2021).

Treatment

Evidence of suffering and long-term effects on functioning highlight the need to examine treatments in large-scale, controlled studies. Several therapies effectively treat pediatric anxiety disorders. This conclusion derives from the results of large-scale studies that include children with either generalized anxiety disorder, separation anxiety disorder, or social anxiety disorder. Treatment guidelines reflecting findings from these studies appear in Box 59.1—a "treatment-at-a-glance" textbox that orients readers considering treatments for a child with an anxiety disorder.

Some interventions, such as cognitive behavioral therapy (CBT), were originally implemented based on theory; others, such as selective serotonin reuptake inhibitor (SSRI) medications, followed data in adults. However, for both, decisions on clinical utility ultimately rest on results of well-conducted randomized controlled trials. Differences exist in attitudes toward treatment across multiple settings for both families and clinicians. For example, psychopharmacology is more widely accepted in the United States than some countries, but even in the United States, some families are uneasy with the prospect of medication treatment. Chapters 31 and 39 review some of the issues that affect such thinking, including safety, tolerability, and factors affecting acceptability. Since pharmacology involves the ingestion of a substance, many families are more uneasy with pharmacologic than psychological treatments. This is particularly true for anxiety disorders, where features overlap with facets of typical child development and where strong data exist for CBT. While more research on medication is needed, at the current time, little data support serious safety concerns when treating children with severe forms of anxiety disorders.

Box 59.1 Treatment at a glance

- Careful assessment to establish diagnosis and complete formulation is the first step of providing comprehensive care. Clinicians should attend to the presence of comorbidity and other complicating factors.
- Cognitive behavioral therapy (CBT) is the first-line treatment in most scenarios, particularly for uncomplicated cases.
- Comorbidity is a common complicating factor; a comorbid condition may need treatment at the same time that treatment is required for an anxiety disorder. Attention deficit hyperactivity disorder (ADHD), mood disorders, and autism spectrum disorder (ASD) represent particularly common comorbidities that affect treatment.
- When CBT is not available or patients fail to respond, a selective serotonin reuptake inhibitor (SSRI) is recommended. Typically, escitalopram, fluoxetine, fluvoxamine, or sertraline are acceptable first-line agents.
- For patients who fail to respond to one SSRI, a second SSRI, or a serotonin-norepinephrine reuptake inhibitor (SNRI) is recommended.

Psychotherapy

CBT is the best-studied psychotherapy, as discussed in greater depth in Chapter 34. Moreover, Chapter 49 describes how digital technology influences many psychotherapies, including CBT. CBT seeks to replace a child's negative beliefs with realistic, neutral thoughts, and it focuses heavily on changing behavior to reduce avoidance. Much research shows that when children can be assisted to confront their fears and no longer avoid them, many children learn to overcome them. As discussed in Chapter 34, CBT contains both cognitive and behavioral components, with the behavioral component sometimes being termed "exposure therapy." While debate persists on the utility of specific cognitive and behavioral components, the forms of CBT used in most comparative efficacy research studies involve both components. In such approaches, CBT implements gradual exposure to feared situations, seen as a behavioral intervention. At the same time, such approaches also typically contain cognitive components. This includes psychoeducation about anxiety and other features, such as the teaching of cognitive strategies for coping and cognitive restructuring.

In anxiety disorders, the success of the therapy rests on a range of features that can be applied specifically to successful treatment of anxiety disorders. For a specific discussion of psychotherapy in anxiety, Chapter 34 describes aspects of CBT that are important for achieving success. This chapter also considers important facets when treating both patients with anxiety disorders and patients with many other mental health conditions.

Only some CBT treatments explicitly dictate the details of family involvement. In some instances, such involvement focuses on reducing family accommodation; excessive accommodation can facilitate avoidance by the child and contribute to poor treatment outcomes (Etkin *et al.*, 2022). Parents are a vital influence on children; hence, active involvement of families is expected in virtually all forms of CBT, as is discussed in depth in Chapter 34.

Studies have compared CBT to various other scenarios, most often a no-treatment or waitlist control. Meta-analyses demonstrate strong overall evidence of efficacy with moderate effect sizes (James *et al.*, 2020). Because waitlist controls are inadequate, results using other designs are important. One study found that CBT was superior to a pill placebo and that CBT might increase efficacy over SSRI monotherapy (Walkup *et al.*, 2008). Moreover, the effect of CBT alone was generally comparable to the effect of SSRI monotherapy. However, when evaluating the benefits of SSRI/CBT combined treatment, the study possessed problematic blinding, and a subsequent report that controlled for blinding found similar efficacy between CBT monotherapy and combined SSRI/CBT treatment (Hudson *et al.*, 2021). Taken together, the data suggest that both SSRIs and CBT are effective, reasonable treatments, with roughly comparable effect sizes, in the moderate range. When concerns with safety exist, CBT is a good first-line choice, and for children who fail to respond to CBT, addition of an SSRI is also reasonable.

CBT has been examined for potential preventative effects. Some studies target children already affected with mild anxiety or with behavioral inhibition, a potential precursor of more severe anxiety. Results are promising (Rapee *et al.*, 2005; Rapee *et al.*, 2023). Other work considers the utility of CBT in low-resource settings, where evidence of efficacy suggests the possible benefit for low- and middle-income countries (LMICs). This possibility is notable, since LMICs and underserved sectors of high-income countries experience a disproportionate lack of needed services. Chapter 46 provides extensive discussions on approaches to increasing availability of treatments in such settings.

Increasing the portability of CBT into these low-resource settings is a worthy goal, given the strength of the data from developed countries documenting its efficacy for pediatric anxiety disorders. Studies are beginning to explore the circumstances that might address the need for more services by increasing access using various approaches. Some evidence appears promising in this area, though not all studies agree (Jeppesen *et al.*, 2021; Sharifi *et al.*, 2023). This suggests the need for more research on service delivery to both increase access to care and to tailor treatments to children most likely to benefit from the treatments. Moreover, greater access is needed in virtually all societies. In most settings around the world, children with anxiety disorders need greater access to CBT (Rapee *et al.*, 2023).

Finally, as noted above, CBT also provides a strong avenue for prevention, by targeting children at risk for developing anxiety disorders. This provides one of the better opportunities to impact risk for mental disorders in children before they manifest clinical problems related to various risk factors. Such groups at risk include the offspring of parents with mental disorders, children with subthreshold anxiety symptoms, children with temperaments that place them at risk, or children exposed to various stressors and other risk factors in the environment. In many such groups, clinical trials demonstrate effective prevention for treatments based on principles of CBT (Rapee *et al.*, 2023). More in depth discussions of these issues can be found in Chapter 8 on temperament and Chapter 32 on the prevention of mental disorders.

Pharmacotherapy

SSRIs have extensive documentation of safety and efficacy in adult anxiety disorders, though specific phobias are the exceptions where strong evidence of efficacy is absent. In children, SSRIs are highly effective in social anxiety, separation anxiety, and generalized anxiety disorders. This conclusion reflects effect sizes in the moderate range from clinical trials comparing anxiety outcomes in children randomized to an SSRI relative to placebo (Locher *et al.*, 2017). The largest multisite study demonstrated efficacy for sertraline with an effect size in this range (Walkup *et al.*, 2008), and more than 12 additional trials find efficacy for other SSRIs and serotonin and norepinephrine reuptake inhibitors (SNRIs), such as duloxetine (Locher *et al.*, 2017; Strawn *et al.*, 2023).

When choosing a medication, some clinicians select Lexapro (escitalopram) or Cymbalta (duloxetine), based on US Food and Drug Administration (FDA) approval for use in pediatric anxiety disorders in the United States. However, meta-analyses suggest overall stronger response in SSRIs than SNRIs (Locher *et al.*, 2017). Therefore, other clinicians begin with an SSRI, such as escitalopram, rather than an SNRI, such as duloxetine. Beyond escitalopram, strong justification also exists for selecting fluoxetine, fluvoxamine, and sertraline, three other SSRIs, as these medications have been used in many pediatric clinical trials, for both anxiety and other disorders.

Each SSRI has similar side effect profiles, the most troublesome being behavioral disinhibition, that can lead a child to become impulsive or oppositional. This is part of a broader series of effects on behavior that can be troublesome, though most of such effects arise more rarely than disinhibition. One of the most concerning effects involves thoughts or possible acts related to suicide, which is more common when children take either SSRIs or SNRIs, compared to when they take placebo.

Nevertheless, this side effect is rare, generally thought to occur in fewer than 5% of children initiating SSRI treatment. Other, even rarer, adverse effects include the precipitation of a manic episode, which is mostly a concern among children with a history of bipolar disorder in a first-degree relative. In situations where concerns with such effects are high, it seems wise to initiate treatment with a short-acting SSRI, and possibly switch to a long-acting formulation, if indicated, such as when compliance is deficient or when the clinician has concerns about potential withdrawal effects.

Other treatment considerations

While the utility of CBT and SSRIs has been the focus of considerable research for many years, other important treatment issues have received less attention. One such issue has concerned the development of novel treatments. Given cross-species conservation in some neural architecture supporting defensive behavior, some scientists have attempted to utilize insights from neuroscience to develop novel treatments. This includes novel medications, brain stimulation techniques, and cognitive training approaches designed to correct presumed problems associated with pediatric anxiety disorders. While none of these treatments are ready for routine clinical use, promising findings with some approaches raise hopes of an expanding treatment toolkit in coming years.

Beyond the need for novel treatments, another issue confronting clinicians has concerned the influence of comorbidity on treatment. Three scenarios commonly arise that present dilemmas for the clinician. Because none of these scenarios has been studied in large clinical trials, only tentative recommendations can be made for clinical approaches. One scenario involves adolescents who present with a comorbid mood and anxiety disorder. This typically requires medication treatment for the mood disorder using an agent also shown to be effective in anxiety disorders, coupled with psychotherapy potentially targeting both disorders, as discussed in Chapters 31 or 34 on issues in psychotherapy or Chapters 63 on mood disorders. A second scenario involves children who present with comorbid ADHD and an anxiety disorder. This typically requires medication treatment for ADHD, sometimes with an agent other than a psychostimulant due to side-effect burdens, coupled with CBT for the anxiety disorder. This issue also is discussed in Chapter 54 on ADHD. A final scenario involves children who present with comorbid ASDs and an anxiety disorder. Here, again, CBT is often the first line for the anxiety disorder, due to the possible higher rate of side effects and lower efficacy of SSRIs in children with this clinical presentation. In fact, an impressive array of clinical trials documents efficacy of CBT in this scenario (Sharma *et al.*, 2021), providing further justification for considering this to be the first-line treatment. In all three scenarios, as well as in many other scenarios, parent accommodation can contribute to anxiety persistence. Novel therapies exist that directly target parental accommodation. This and other key issues also are discussed in Chapter 50.

Summary

Multiple findings demonstrate the clinical importance of anxiety disorders. These include their: relatively high prevalence; associated impairment; and relations with long-term outcome, including continuity with anxiety disorders in adulthood. Epidemiological data generate high prevalence, with girls being overrepresented. Long-term stability has been found for anxiety disorders as a group, but limited evidence of differential outcomes has emerged for anxiety disorders. Importantly, childhood anxiety disorders have generally not been found to predict adult psychopathology other than anxiety and depression.

Identifying antecedents facilitates prevention. Early inhibited temperament is one of the few replicated antecedents. A modest influence for genetic transmission has been found. Non-shared environmental factors appear to play a relatively large role, but their nature and mechanism of action remain poorly understood. As a result, there is little promise in the targeting of environmental factors for prevention or clinical management.

Models of brain circuits in multiple species informs brain-imaging research. However, the cross-sectional nature of most studies limits their clinical utility. Treatment of anxiety disorders encompasses psychotherapeutic and psychopharmacological interventions, specifically CBT and SSRIs. Extensive research with both treatments documents safety and efficacy.

Acknowledgement

The work for this chapter was supported by projects ZIA-MH002781 and ZIA-MH002782 in the Intramural Research Program of the National Institute of Mental Health.

References

Abend, R. *et al.* (2018) Association between attention bias to threat and anxiety symptoms in children and adolescents. *Depression and Anxiety* **35**, 229–238.

Abend, R. *et al.* (2020) Anticipatory threat responding: associations with anxiety, development, and brain structure. *Biological Psychiatry* **87**, 916–925.

Anderson, D.J. & Adolphs, R. (2014) A framework for studying emotions across species. *Cell* **157**, 187–200.

Anderson, J. *et al.* (1987) DSM-III disorders in preadolescent children: prevalence in a large sample from the general population. *Archives of General Psychiatry* **44**, 69–76.

Angold, A. & Costello, E.J. (2000) The Child and Adolescent Psychiatric Assessment (CAPA). *Journal for the American Academy of Child and Adolescent Psychiatry* **39**(1), 39–48.

Angold, A. *et al.* (1996) Precision, reliability and accuracy in the dating of symptom onsets in child and adolescent psychopathology. *Journal of Child Psychology and Psychiatry* **37**, 657–664.

Angold, A. *et al.* (1999) Comorbidity. *Journal of Child Psychology and Psychiatry* **40**, 57–87.

Aschenbrand, S.G. *et al.* (2003) Is childhood separation anxiety disorder a predictor of adult panic disorder and agoraphobia? A seven-year longitudinal study. *Journal of the American Academy of Child and Adolescent Psychiatry* **42**, 1478–1485.

Bas-Hoogendam, J.M. *et al.* (2022) ENIGMA-anxiety working group: rationale for and organization of large-scale neuroimaging studies of anxiety disorders. *Human Brain Mapping* **43**, 83–112.

Beatty, C.C. *et al.* (2023) Neurobiological sensitivity to unpredictable threat and familial risk for the internalizing and externalizing spectra in adolescents. *Psychological Medicine* **53**, 5395–5404.

Beesdo, K. *et al.* (2007) Incidence of social anxiety disorder and the consistent risk for secondary depression in the first three decades of life. *Archives of General Psychiatry* **64**, 903–912.

Beesdo, K. *et al.* (2009a) Anxiety and anxiety disorders in children and adolescents: developmental issues and implications for DSM-V. *Psychiatric Clinics of North America* **32**, 483–524.

Beesdo, K. *et al.* (2009b) Anxiety and anxiety disorders in children and adolescents: developmental issues and implications for DSM-V. *The Psychiatric Clinics of North America* **32**, 483–524.

Beesdo, K. *et al.* (2010) Incidence and risk patterns of anxiety and depressive disorders and categorization of generalized anxiety disorder. *Archives of General Psychiatry* **67**, 47–57.

Beesdo-Baum, K. *et al.* (2011) The diagnostic threshold of generalized anxiety disorder in the community: a developmental perspective. *Journal of Psychiatric Research* **45**, 962–972.

Benjamin, R.S. *et al.* (1990) Anxiety disorders in a pediatric sample. *Journal of Anxiety Disorders* **4**, 293–316.

Bird, H. *et al.* (1988) Estimates of the prevalence of childhood maladjustment in a community survey in Puerto Rico: the use of combined measures. *Archives of General Psychiatry* **45**, 1120–1126.

Birmaher, B. *et al.* (1997) The Screen for Child Anxiety Related Emotional Disorders (SCARED): scale construction and psychometric characteristics. *Journal of the American Academy of Child and Adolescent Psychiatry* **36**, 545–553.

Breslau, N. (1995) Psychiatric sequelae of low birth weight. *Epidemiologic Reviews* **17**, 96–106.

Breslau, N. & Chilcoat, H.D. (2000) Psychiatric sequelae of low birth weight at 11 years of age. *Biological Psychiatry* **47**, 1005–1011.

Breslau, N. *et al.* (2000) Neurologic soft signs and low birthweight: their association and neuropsychiatric implications. *Biological Psychiatry* **47**, 71–79.

Brooks, S.J. & Kutcher, S. (2003) Diagnosis and measurement of anxiety disorder in adolescents: a review of commonly used instruments. *Journal of Child and Adolescent Psychopharmacology* **13**, 351–400.

Cardinale, E.M. *et al.* (2023) Cross-sectional and longitudinal associations of anxiety and irritability with adolescents' neural responses to cognitive conflict. *Biological Psychiatry: Cognitive Neuroscience and Neuroimaging* **8**, 436–444.

Caspi, A. *et al.* (1996) Behavioural observations at age 3 years predict adult psychiatric disorders: longitudinal evidence from a birth cohort. *Archives of General Psychiatry* **53**, 1033–1039.

Clauss, J.A. & Blackford, J.U. (2012) Behavioural inhibition and risk for developing social anxiety disorder: a meta-analytic study. *Journal of the American Academy of Child and Adolescent Psychiatry* **51**, 1066–1075 e1.

Copeland, W. *et al.* (2011) Cumulative prevalence of psychiatric disorders by young adulthood: a prospective cohort analysis from the Great Smoky Mountains study. *Journal of the American Academy of Child and Adolescent Psychiatry* **50**, 252–261.

Copeland, W.E. *et al.* (2009) Childhood and adolescent psychiatric disorders as predictors of young adult disorders. *Archives of General Psychiatry* **66**, 764–772.

Copeland, W.E. *et al.* (2014) Longitudinal patterns of anxiety from childhood to adulthood: the Great Smoky Mountains study. *Journal of the American Academy of Child and Adolescent Psychiatry* **53**, 21–33.

Copeland, W.E. *et al.* (2022) Long-term outcomes of childhood family income supplements on adult functioning. *JAMA Pediatrics* **176**, 1020–1026.

Costello, E. *et al.* (1988) Psychiatric disorders in pediatric primary care: prevalence and risk factors. *Archives of General Psychiatry* **45**, 1107–1116.

Costello, E. *et al.* (1996) The Great Smoky Mountains study of youth: functional impairment and serious emotional disturbance. *Archives of General Psychiatry* **53**, 1137–1143.

Costello, E.J. *et al.* (1999) Adolescent outcomes of childhood disorders: the consequences of severity and impairment. *Journal of the American Academy of Child and Adolescent Psychiatry* **38**, 121–128.

Costello, E.J. *et al.* (2002) Development and natural history of mood disorders. *Biological Psychiatry* **52**, 529–542.

Costello, E.J. *et al.* (2003) Prevalence and development of psychiatric disorders in childhood and adolescence. *Archives of General Psychiatry* **60**, 837–844.

Costello, E.J. *et al.* (2004) Developmental epidemiology of anxiety disorders. In: *Phobic and Anxiety Disorders in Children and Adolescents.* (eds T.H. Ollendick & J. March). Oxford University Press, New York.

Costello, E.J. *et al.* (2005) The developmental epidemiology of anxiety disorders: phenomenology, prevalence, and comorbidity. *Child and Adolescent Psychiatric Clinics of North America* **14**, 631–648.

Costello, E.J. *et al.* (2010) Association of family income supplements in adolescence with development of psychiatric and substance use disorders in adulthood among an American Indian population. *JAMA* **303**, 1954–1960.

Creswell, C. *et al.* (2020) Practitioner review: anxiety disorders in children and young people - assessment and treatment. *Journal of Child Psychology and Psychiatry* **61**, 628–643.

Creswell, C. *et al.* (2021) Research review: recommendations for reporting on treatment trials for child and adolescent anxiety disorders - an international consensus statement. *Journal of Child Psychology and Psychiatry* **62**, 255–269.

Dalsgaard, S. *et al.* (2020) Incidence rates and cumulative incidences of the full spectrum of diagnosed mental disorders in childhood and adolescence. *JAMA Psychiatry* **77**, 155–164.

Duits, P. *et al.* (2015) Updated meta-analysis of classical fear conditioning in the anxiety disorders. *Depression and Anxiety* **32**, 239–253.

Dvir, M. *et al.* (2019) Fear conditioning and extinction in anxious and non-anxious youth: A meta-analysis. *Behaviour Research and Therapy* **120**, 103431.

Eley, T.C. & Stevenson, J. (2000) Specific life events and chronic experiences differentially associated with depression and anxiety in young twins. *Journal of Abnormal Child Psychology* **28**, 383–394.

Essau, C. *et al.* (1999) Frequency and comorbidity of social phobia and social fears in adolescents. *Behaviour Research and Therapy* **37**, 831–843.

Esser, G. *et al.* (1990) Epidemiology and course of psychiatric disorders in school-age children: results of a longitudinal study. *Journal of Child Psychology and Psychiatry* **31**, 243–263.

Etkin, R.G. *et al.* (2022) Clinical update: the role of family accommodation in youth anxiety treatment outcomes. *Evidence-Based Practice in Child and Adolescent Mental Health* **7**, 295–305.

Fergusson, D.M. *et al.* (1993) Prevalence and comorbidity of DSM-III-R diagnoses in a birth cohort of 15 year olds. *Journal of the American Academy of Child & Adolescent Psychiatry* **32**, 1127–1134.

Fox, A.S. & Kalin, N.H. (2014) A translational neuroscience approach to understanding the development of social anxiety disorder and its pathophysiology. *The American Journal of Psychiatry* **171**, 1162–1173.

Frenkel, T.I. *et al.* (2015) Early childhood behavioural inhibition, adult psychopathology and the buffering effects of adolescent social networks: a twenty-year prospective study. *Journal of Child Psychology and Psychiatry* **56**, 1065–1073.

Fyer, A.J. (1998) Current approaches to etiology and pathophysiology of specific phobia. *Biological Psychiatry* **44**, 1295–1304.

Ginsburg, G.S. *et al.* (2018) Results from the child/adolescent anxiety multimodal extended long-term study (CAMELS): primary anxiety outcomes. *Journal of the American Academy of Child and Adolescent Psychiatry* **57**, 471–480.

Gold, A.L. *et al.* (2020) Age differences in the neural correlates of anxiety disorders: an fMRI study of response to learned threat. *The American Journal of Psychiatry* **177**, 454–463.

Goodwin, R.D. *et al.* (2003) Asthma and panic attacks among youth in the community. *The Journal of Asthma* **40**, 139–145.

Goodwin, R.D. *et al.* (2004) Association between anxiety disorders and substance use disorders among young persons: results of a 21-year longitudinal study. *Journal of Psychiatric Research* **38**, 295–304.

Gross, C. & Hen, R. (2004) The developmental origins of anxiety. *Nature Reviews Neuroscience* **5**, 545–552.

Hale, W.W., 3rd *et al.* (2011) A meta-analysis of the cross-cultural psychometric properties of the Screen for Child Anxiety Related Emotional Disorders (SCARED). *Journal of Child Psychology and Psychiatry* **52**, 80–90.

Hankin, B.L. & Abramson, L.Y. (2001) Development of gender differences in depression: an elaborated cognitive vulnerability-transactional stress theory. *Psychological Bulletin* **127**, 773–796.

Hudson, J.L. *et al.* (2021) Combining CBT and sertraline does not enhance outcomes for anxious youth: a double-blind randomised controlled trial. *Psychological Medicine* **53**, 1–9.

Ingman, K.A. *et al.* (1999) Cross-cultural aspects of fears in African children and adolescents. *Behaviour Research and Therapy* **37**, 337–345.

Jaffee, S.R. *et al.* (2005) Cumulative prevalence of psychiatric disorder in youths. *Journal of the American Academy of Child and Adolescent Psychiatry* **44**, 406–407.

James, A.C. *et al.* (2020) Cognitive behavioural therapy for anxiety disorders in children and adolescents. *Cochrane Database of Systematic Reviews* **11**, CD013162.

Jami, E.S. *et al.* (2022) Genome-wide association meta-analysis of childhood and adolescent internalizing symptoms. *Journal of the American Academy of Child and Adolescent Psychiatry* **61**, 934–945.

Jeppesen, P. *et al.* (2021) Effectiveness of transdiagnostic cognitive-behavioural psychotherapy compared with management as usual for youth with common mental health problems: a randomized clinical trial. *JAMA Psychiatry* **78**, 250–260.

Johnson, J.G. *et al.* (2000) Association between cigarette smoking and anxiety disorders during adolescence and early adulthood. *JAMA* **284**, 2348–2351.

Kagan, J. (1994) *Galen's Prophecy*. Basic Books, New York.

Kagan, J. *et al.* (2001) Temperamental contributions to the affect family of anxiety. *The Psychiatric Clinics of North America* **24**, 677–688.

Kaplow, J.B. *et al.* (2001) The prospective relation between dimensions of anxiety and the initiation of adolescent alcohol use. *Journal of Clinical Child Psychology* **30**, 316–326.

Kassam-Adams, N. *et al.* (2005) Heart rate and posttraumatic stress in injured children. *Archives of General Psychiatry* **62**, 335–340.

Kenwood, M.M. *et al.* (2022) The prefrontal cortex, pathological anxiety, and anxiety disorders. *Neuropsychopharmacology* **47**, 260–275.

Kessler, R.C. *et al.* (2012) Composite international diagnostic interview screening scales for DSM-IV anxiety and mood disorders. In: *Psychological Medicine*, Vol. 43. pp. 1625–1637.

Kim-Cohen, J. *et al.* (2003) Prior juvenile diagnoses in adults with mental disorder: developmental follow-back of a prospective-longitudinal cohort. *Archives of General Psychiatry* **60**, 709–717.

Koenigs, M. *et al.* (2008) Focal brain damage protects against post-traumatic stress disorder in combat veterans. *Nature Neuroscience* **11**, 232–237.

Kovner, R. *et al.* (2020) Transcriptional profiling of primate central nucleus of the amygdala neurons to understand the molecular underpinnings of early-life anxious temperament. *Biological Psychiatry* **88**, 638–648.

Kozak, M.J. & Cuthbert, B.N. (2016) The NIMH research domain criteria initiative: background, issues, and pragmatics. *Psychophysiology* **53**, 286–297.

Kramer, T. & Garralda, M.E. (1998) Psychiatric disorders in adolescents in primary care. *The British Journal of Psychiatry* **173**, 508–513.

Kujawa, A. *et al.* (2015) Affective modulation of the startle response among children at high and low risk for anxiety disorders. *Psychological Medicine* **45**, 2647–2656.

LeDoux, J. & Daw, N.D. (2018) Surviving threats: neural circuit and computational implications of a new taxonomy of defensive behaviour. *Nature Reviews Neuroscience* **19**, 269–282.

LeDoux, J.E. & Pine, D.S. (2016) Using neuroscience to help understand fear and anxiety: a two-system framework. *The American Journal of Psychiatry* **173**, 1083–1093.

Lee, P.H. *et al.* (2021) Pleiotropy and cross-disorder genetics among psychiatric disorders. *Biological Psychiatry* **89**, 20–31.

Lewinsohn, P.M. *et al.* (1998) Gender differences in anxiety disorders and anxiety symptoms in adolescents. *Journal of Abnormal Psychology* **107**, 109–117.

Lewis, G.J. & Plomin, R. (2015) Heritable influences on behavioural problems from early childhood to mid-adolescence: evidence for genetic stability and innovation. *Psychological Medicine* **45**, 2171–2179.

Lewis-Morrarty, E. *et al.* (2012) Maternal over-control moderates the association between early childhood behavioural inhibition and adolescent social anxiety symptoms. *Journal of Abnormal Child Psychology* **40**, 1363–1373.

Linke, J.O. *et al.* (2021) Shared and anxiety-specific pediatric psychopathology dimensions manifest distributed neural correlates. *Biological Psychiatry* **89**, 579–587.

Locher, C. *et al.* (2017) Efficacy and safety of selective serotonin reuptake inhibitors, serotonin-norepinephrine reuptake inhibitors, and placebo for common psychiatric disorders among children and adolescents: a systematic review and meta-analysis. *JAMA Psychiatry* **74**, 1011–1020.

Magee, W. *et al.* (1996) Agoraphobia, simple phobia, and social phobia in the national comorbidity survey. *Archives of General Psychiatry* **53**, 159–168.

March, J.S. & Sullivan, K. (1999) Test-retest reliability of the multidimensional anxiety scale for children. *Journal of Anxiety Disorders* **13**, 349–358.

March, J.S. *et al.* (1997) The Multidimensional Anxiety Scale for Children (MASC): factor structure, reliability, and validity. *Journal of the American Academy of Child and Adolescent Psychiatry* **36**, 554–565.

Marek, S. *et al.* (2022) Reproducible brain-wide association studies require thousands of individuals. *Nature* **603**, 654–660.

McGee, R.O.B. *et al.* (1990) DSM-III disorders in a large sample of adolescents. *Journal of the American Academy of Child & Adolescent Psychiatry* **29**, 611–619.

McTeague, L.M. *et al.* (2017) Identification of common neural circuit disruptions in cognitive control across psychiatric disorders. *The American Journal of Psychiatry* **174**, 676–685.

McTeague, L.M. *et al.* (2020) Identification of common neural circuit disruptions in emotional processing across psychiatric disorders. *The American Journal of Psychiatry* **177**, 411–421.

Mennies, R.J. *et al.* (2021) The main and interactive associations between demographic factors and psychopathology and treatment utilization in youth: a test of intersectionality in the ABCD study. *Research on Child and Adolescent Psychopathology* **49**, 5–17.

Merikangas, K.R. *et al.* (2010) Prevalence and treatment of mental disorders among US children in the 2001–2004 NHANES. *Pediatrics* **125**, 75–81.

Middeldorp, C.M. *et al.* (2005) The co-morbidity of anxiety and depression in the perspective of genetic epidemiology: a review of twin and family studies. *Psychological Medicine* **35**, 611–624.

Nelson, B.W. *et al.* (2022) Concurrent and prospective associations between fitbit wearable-derived RDoC arousal and regulatory constructs and adolescent internalizing symptoms. *Journal of Child Psychology and Psychiatry* **63**, 282–295.

NHS (2018) *Mental Health of Children and Young People in England, 2017*, National Health Service (NHS), UK. [Online]. Available: https://digital.nhs.uk/data-and-information/publications/statistical/mental-health-of-children-and-young-people-in-england/2017/2017 [25 November 2024].

Obradovic, J. *et al.* (2011) The interactive effect of marital conflict and stress reactivity on externalizing and internalizing symptoms: the role of laboratory stressors. *Development and Psychopathology* **23**, 101–114.

Ollendick, T.H. & Hirshfeld-Becker, D.R. (2002) The developmental psychopathology of social anxiety disorder. *Biological Psychiatry* **51**, 44–58.

Ollendick, T.H. *et al.* (1996) Fears in American, Australian, Chinese, and Nigerian children and adolescents: a cross-cultural study. *Journal of Child Psychology and Psychiatry* **37**, 213–220.

Pagliaccio, D. *et al.* (2019) Cross-species convergence in pupillary response: understanding human anxiety via non-human primate amygdala lesion. *Social Cognitive and Affective Neuroscience* **14**, 591–599.

Penninx, B.W. *et al.* (2021) Anxiety disorders. *The Lancet* **397**, 914–927.

Pine, D.S. & Cohen, J.A. (2002) Trauma in children and adolescents: risk and treatment of psychiatric sequelae. *Biological Psychiatry* **51**, 519–531.

Pine, D.S. & Fox, N.A. (2015) Childhood antecedents and risk for adult mental disorders. *Annual Review of Psychology* **66**, 459–485.

Pine, D.S. *et al.* (1998) The risk for early-adulthood anxiety and depressive disorders in adolescents with anxiety and depressive disorders. *Archives of General Psychiatry* **55**, 56–64.

Pine, D.S. *et al.* (2000) Social phobia and the persistence of conduct problems. *Journal of Child Psychology and Psychiatry* **41**, 657–665.

Pine, D.S. *et al.* (2001) Adolescent fears as predictors of depression. *Biological Psychiatry* **50**, 721–724.

Pine, D.S. *et al.* (2002) Adolescent life events as predictors of adult depression. *Journal of Affective Disorders* **68**, 49–57.

Pine, D.S. *et al.* (2021) Evolution, emotion, and episodic engagement. *The American Journal of Psychiatry* **178**, 701–714.

Polanczyk, G.V. *et al.* (2015) Annual research review: a meta-analysis of the worldwide prevalence of mental disorders in children and adolescents. *Journal of Child Psychology and Psychiatry* **56**, 345–365.

Purves, K.L. *et al.* (2020) A major role for common genetic variation in anxiety disorders. *Molecular Psychiatry* **25**, 3292–3303.

Racine, N. *et al.* (2021) Global prevalence of depressive and anxiety symptoms in children and adolescents during COVID-19: a meta-analysis. *JAMA Pediatrics* **175**, 1142–1150.

Rapee, R.M. *et al.* (2005) Prevention and early intervention of anxiety disorders in inhibited preschool children. *Journal of Consulting and Clinical Psychology* **73**, 488–497.

Rapee, R.M. *et al.* (2023) Anxiety disorders in children and adolescents: A summary and overview of the literature. *Behaviour Research and Therapy* **168**, 104376.

Reed, V. & Wittchen, H.U. (1998) DSM-IV panic attacks and panic disorder in a community sample of adolescents and young adults: how specific are panic attacks? *Journal of Psychiatric Research* **32**, 335–345.

Rosenbaum, J.F. *et al.* (1993) Behavioural inhibition in childhood: a risk factor for anxiety disorders. *Harvard Review of Psychiatry* **1**, 2–16.

Rueter, M.A. *et al.* (1999) First onset of depressive or anxiety disorders predicted by the longitudinal course of internalizing symptoms and parent-adolescent disagreements. *Archives of General Psychiatry* **56**, 726–732.

Rupp, A.S.G. (2003) The Pediatric Anxiety Rating Scale (PARS): development and psychometric properties. *Journal of the American Academy of Child and Adolescent Psychiatry* **42**, 13–21.

Rutter, M. *et al.* (2006) Continuities and discontinuities in psychopathology between childhood and adult life. *Journal of Child Psychology and Psychiatry* **47**, 276–295.

Seligman, L.D. *et al.* (2004) The utility of measures of child and adolescent anxiety: a meta-analytic review of the Revised Children's Manifest Anxiety Scale, the State-Trait Anxiety Inventory for Children, and the Child Behaviour Checklist. *Journal of Clinical Child and Adolescent Psychology* **33**, 557–565.

Shaffer, D. *et al.* (1985) Neurological soft signs: their relationship to psychiatric disorder and intelligence in childhood and adolescence. *Archives of General Psychiatry* **42**, 342–351.

Shaffer, D. *et al.* (1996) The NIMH Diagnostic Interview Schedule for Children version 2.3 (DISC-2.3): description, acceptability, prevalence rates, and performance in the MECA Study. *Journal of the American Academy of Child & Adolescent Psychiatry* **35**, 865–877.

Sharifi, V. *et al.* (2023) Effect of general practitioner training in a collaborative child mental health care program on Children's mental health outcomes in a low-resource setting: a cluster randomized trial. *JAMA Psychiatry* **80**, 22–30.

Sharma, S. *et al.* (2021) Cognitive behavioural therapy for anxiety in children and young people on the autism spectrum: a systematic review and meta-analysis. *BMC Psychology* **9**, 151.

Shechner, T. *et al.* (2014) Attention bias modification treatment augmenting effects on cognitive behavioural therapy in children with anxiety: randomized controlled trial. *Journal of the American Academy of Child and Adolescent Psychiatry* **53**, 61–71.

Silverman, W.K. & Ollendick, T.H. (2005) Evidence-based assessment of anxiety and its disorders in children and adolescents. *Journal of Clinical Child and Adolescent Psychology* **34**, 380–411.

Silverman, W.K. *et al.* (2001) Test-retest reliability of anxiety symptoms and diagnoses with the Anxiety Disorders Interview Schedule for DSM-IV: child and parent versions. *Journal of the American Academy of Child and Adolescent Psychiatry* **40**, 937–944.

Simonoff, E. *et al.* (1997) The Virginia twin study of adolescent behavioral development: influences of age, sex, and impairment on rates of disorder. *Archives of General Psychiatry* **54**(9), 801–808.

Smoller, J.W. *et al.* (2019) Psychiatric genetics and the structure of psychopathology. *Molecular Psychiatry* **24**, 409–420.

Steinberg, L. & Avenevoli, S. (2000) The role of context in the development of psychopathology: a conceptual framework and some speculative propositions. *Child Development* **71**, 66–74.

Strawn, J.R. *et al.* (2021) Research review: pediatric anxiety disorders - what have we learnt in the last 10 years? *Journal of Child Psychology and Psychiatry* **62**, 114–139.

Strawn, J.R. *et al.* (2023) A multicenter double-blind, placebo-controlled trial of escitalopram in children and adolescents with generalized anxiety disorder. *Journal of Child and Adolescent Psychopharmacology* **33**, 91–100.

Tang, A. *et al.* (2020) Infant behavioural inhibition predicts personality and social outcomes three decades later. *Proceedings of the National Academy of Sciences of the United States of America* **117**, 9800–9807.

Vasa, R.A. *et al.* (2002) Anxiety after severe pediatric closed head injury. *Journal of the American Academy of Child and Adolescent Psychiatry* **41**, 148–156.

Vasa, R.A. *et al.* (2004) Neuroimaging correlates of anxiety after pediatric traumatic brain injury. *Biological Psychiatry* **55**, 208–216.

Verhulst, F.C. *et al.* (1997) The prevalence of DSM-III-R diagnoses in a national sample of Dutch adolescents. *Archives of General Psychiatry* **54**(4), 329–336.

Walkup, J.T. *et al.* (2008) Cognitive behavioural therapy, sertraline, or a combination in childhood anxiety. *The New England Journal of Medicine* **359**, 2753–2766.

Waszczuk, M.A. *et al.* (2014) The phenotypic and genetic structure of depression and anxiety disorder symptoms in childhood, adolescence, and young adulthood. *JAMA Psychiatry* **71**, 905–916.

Weissman, M.M. *et al.* (1997) Offspring of depressed parents: 10 years later. *Archives of General Psychiatry* **54**, 932–940.

Whitaker, A.H. *et al.* (1997) Psychiatric outcomes in low-birth-weight children at age 6 years: relation to neonatal cranial ultrasound abnormalities. *Archives of General Psychiatry* **54**, 847–856.

White, L.K. *et al.* (2017) Complementary features of attention Bias modification therapy and cognitive-Behavioural therapy in pediatric anxiety disorders. *The American Journal of Psychiatry* **174**, 775–784.

Williamson, D.E. *et al.* (2005) Stressful life events in anxious and depressed children. *Journal of Child and Adolescent Psychopharmacology* **15**, 571–580.

Wittchen, H.-U. *et al.* (1999) Social fears and social phobia in a community sample of adolescents and young adults: prevalence, risk factors and co-morbidity. *Psychological Medicine* **29**, 309–323.

Wood, J.J. *et al.* (2003) Parenting and childhood anxiety: theory, empirical findings, and future directions. *Journal of Child Psychology and Psychiatry* **44**, 134–151.

Zeytinoglu, S. *et al.* (2021) A developmental pathway from early behavioural inhibition to young adults' anxiety during the COVID-19 pandemic. *Journal of the American Academy of Child and Adolescent Psychiatry* **60**, 1300–1308.

Zeytinoglu, S. *et al.* (2022) Pathways from maternal shyness to adolescent social anxiety. *Journal of Child Psychology and Psychiatry* **63**, 342–349.

CHAPTER 60

Obsessive–compulsive disorder

Philip Shaw[1] and Judith L. Rapoport[2]

[1]King's Maudsley Partnership for Children and Young People, Department of Child and Adolescent Psychiatry, Institute of Psychiatry, Psychology and Neuroscience, King's College London, London, UK
[2]National Institute of Mental Health (NIMH) Intramural Research Program, Bethesda, MD, USA

Characteristics and definitions: phenomenology

Once considered rare in childhood, obsessive–compulsive disorder (OCD) is now well-recognized as a common cause of distress for children and adolescents. Obsessions are unwanted, intrusive thoughts that are repetitive and persistent, and usually evoke anxiety and distress. Compulsions are unnecessary repetitive behaviors or mental activities, often conducted in response to an obsession to relieve anxiety, attain a sense of "completeness" or to avoid an imagined, dreaded event. The behaviors or mental acts are excessive in the amount of time each day they can occupy and are "irrational" as the acts will not realistically forestall any adverse outcomes. Obsessions and compulsions are common phenomena in many young people but become a disorder (OCD) when they cause impairment across multiple settings: at home with the family, at school interfering with learning, or with peers during leisure time.

Obsessive and compulsive symptoms tend to fall in clusters, with analyses of symptoms in children suggesting five domains: mental rituals/touching/ordering; cleaning/contamination; superstitions; obsessions/checking/confessing; and somatic concerns (Ivarsson & Valderhaug, 2006). A large community-based study of young adolescents found females more frequently reported compulsions and males more commonly reported obsessions (Valleni-Basile *et al.*, 1994). The most common compulsions were arranging (56%), counting (41%), washing (17%), and checking (12%). A more recent study, using data on 10,000 youth, approximating the diversity of the US childhood population (the Adolescent Brain and Cognitive Development Cohort), similarly found thoughts and acts around ordering or checking things in a certain manner were common (between 2.7–4.8% of 9–10-year-olds), with recurrent thoughts about contamination, harming others, and other taboo ideations all occurring in around or less than 1%. In short, obsessions on the themes of symmetry, order, contamination, danger to self or others (such as fears that parents will be harmed), or moral issues are common; typical compulsions include ordering, washing, checking, and repeating—particularly until the child experiences a feeling of "getting it just right." Most children have a combination of obsessions and rituals, and pure obsessives are rare compared with the more frequent pure ritualizers.

The clinical course of the disorder indicates some developmental influence on symptoms over time. In a clinic sample, sensitivity to developmental stage was found first in symptom profile, with the presenting obsessions and compulsions changing over time in 90% of the National Institute of Mental Health (NIMH) pediatric patients (Rettew *et al.*, 1992). Most children began with a single obsession or compulsion and continued with this for months to years, and then gradually acquired different obsessions or rituals. Although the primary symptom would change (e.g., from counting to washing and then checking), some earlier symptoms often remained problematic, although to a lesser degree. The nature of the compulsive rituals also changed over time. A study of adolescents demonstrated that counting and symmetry were most prominent during grade school years, but were replaced by washing rituals during early and mid-adolescence (Maina *et al.*, 1999).

The presentation of OCD in children is moderated by the level of developmental maturity. Children with an onset below age 6 usually begin their rituals or obsessions in an easily recognizable fashion, such as excessive handwashing or ritualized checking and repeating. In some cases, however, the clinical presentation is altered by immaturity. For example, one 6-year-old boy, who was compelled to draw zeros repetitively, had started at age 3 to circle manhole covers on city streets. His tantrums when the circling was interrupted, his subjective distress during the behavior, and his lack of other psychosocial abnormalities or disorders (such as autism or pervasive

Rutter's Child and Adolescent Psychiatry and Psychology, Seventh Edition.
Edited by Anita Thapar, Daniel S. Pine, Samuele Cortese, Cathy Creswell, Tamsin J. Ford, James F. Leckman, and Argyris Stringaris.

Companion website: www.wiley.com/go/thapar/rutterspsych7

developmental disorder) led to the diagnosis of OCD. Another child, who presented at age 7 with clinically significant checking compulsions, had been evaluated previously at 3 years of age when he developed a "compulsion" to walk only on the edges of the floor tiles. Cleaning rituals in children too young to reach the water faucet can present as excessive hand-wiping or licking.

Approximately one-third of pediatric patients report that certain stimuli trigger their rituals and that avoidance of the trigger "protects" them from the obsessive–compulsive symptoms (Swedo *et al.*, 1989). For example, a 16-year-old girl with elaborate front door touching and stepping rituals would "sneak" into her house by a side door, avoiding the sight of the front door and successfully averting the compulsion. Several children avoided looking at certain parts of a room (e.g., "corners of the ceiling") that set off various gaze rituals. These phenomena have been viewed from an ethological perspective, with the compulsions conceptualized as "fixed action patterns" released by key environmental stimuli (Modell *et al.*, 1989). These triggers are of particular interest for treatment as they often determine the key approach during behavioral desensitization, namely, exposure with response prevention—vignettes appear in Boxes 60.1 and 60.2. As these cases will highlight, the symptoms of OCD unfold in, and can be moderated by multiple contextual factors, particularly the family. A child can sometimes attempt to impose rules, rituals, or prohibition on other family members, who may accommodate to these demands, often mistakenly thinking that they will help ease the distress of the child but instead may reinforce the maladaptive behaviors.

Box 60.1 The development of obsessive–compulsive disorder symptoms

A 14-year-old boy, whose symptoms had begun gradually, recalls at a very early age having to wash his hands repetitively. He was unable to associate an obsessive thought with this ritual, but he felt compelled to perform it. By age 6, he had developed an obsessive fear of tornadoes. He would repeatedly check the sky for clouds, listen to all weather reports and query his mother about approaching storms. The tornado obsession faded over time and was replaced by a generalized fear of harm coming to himself or his family. He responded with extensive rituals to protect himself and his family. Particularly at times of separating, such as bedtime or leaving for school, the patient would be compelled to repeat actions perfectly or to check repetitively. When asked how many times he would have to repeat an action, he replied, "It depends. The number is not always the same, I just have to do it right." When asked how he knew when it was right, he said, "I do not know, it just feels right." As the patient entered puberty, he became obsessed with acquired immunodeficiency syndrome (AIDS) and was convinced he would acquire it thorough his mouth. He began spitting to cleanse his mouth and would spit every 15–20 seconds. In addition, he began extensive washing rituals. Despite these cleansing and washing compulsions, his personal appearance was slovenly and dirty. He never tied his shoelaces because they had touched the ground and were "contaminated"; if he tied them, his hands would be "dirty" and he would have to wash until they were "clean" again. Remarkably, although his family was aware that "something had been wrong for a long time," most of the content of his obsessions was kept secret. This case illustrates the contamination concerns common to adolescents, as well as the variety and evolution of obsessive–compulsive symptoms during development.

Box 60.2 Obsessive–compulsive disorder symptoms in adolescence

A 16-year-old girl had symptoms that began abruptly, shortly after the onset of menses. She called herself "a prisoner of my own mind." Her obsessions centered around a fear of harm to her parents. She was plagued by recurrent thoughts of her mother dying in a car accident, her father being killed by an intruder, or both her parents dying of burns received in a house fire. Always a light sleeper, she began to get up during the night to check. She spent hours checking that the doors were locked, that the coffee pot was unplugged, and that the family dog was safely ensconced in the garage. Despite her obsessions about fire, however, she did not check the smoke detector, an excellent example of the irrationality of this superficially rational disorder. This patient involved her family in her rituals. Her mother made a checklist that the daughter carried to school, and both parents had to check the 24 items on the list, signing that they had done so. At night she would wake her father to help her check. The family involvement was so profound that behavioral treatment could only take place after a period of family counseling in which the parents were helped to separate from their daughter's illness.

Differences between childhood and adult presentations

While clinical experience suggests that the adult criteria can be applied to childhood cases, there are several important caveats. Both the *Diagnostic and Statistical Manual of Mental Disorder*, 5th edition (DMS-5; American Psychiatric Association, 2013) and the *International Classification of Diseases*, 11th revision (ICD-11; World Health Organization, 2019) state that compulsions are designed to neutralize or prevent some dreaded event according to rules that must be applied rigidly. The concept of "rules applied rigidly" is particularly useful for childhood OCD. While some children may not be willing or able to verbalize their obsessive thoughts, long-term contact has demonstrated that about 40% of children do not in fact have obsessive thoughts; they steadfastly report the presence of only compulsive rituals (dictated by rigid rules) accompanied by a vague sense of discomfort if the rituals are not carried out (Swedo *et al.*, 1989). The degree of insight needed for the diagnosis is also in dispute as some patients, at least some of the time, "believe" their obsessive thoughts. It is probable that for both children and adolescents and particularly in severe cases, diagnostic criteria should allow some partial "belief" in the necessity for these thoughts/behaviors. This degree of insight can now be added as a specifier in DSM-5.

As noted above, symptom clusters seen in children overlap with those identified in adults, which indicate clusters of: symmetry/ordering, contamination/cleaning, harm-related (thought and checking), and unacceptability-related symptoms (e.g., sexual, aggressive thoughts and neutralizing mental rituals) (Mataix-Cols *et al.*, 2005). There are some differences between childhood and adult symptom profiles, such as the absence of a hoarding subgroup in children, as well as the prominence of a "superstition" symptom cluster in children characterized by magical thinking. In adults, the dimensions tend to be stable across time within the person, although this may not be the case for youth (Mataix-Cols *et al.*, 2005).

Such developmental considerations lead to the question as to whether OCD with very early onset represents an important subtype of the disorder. There is growing evidence that at the very least, early age of onset represents a more familial form of the disorder, particularly for pediatric cases with ordering compulsions (Leckman *et al.*, 2009). By contrast, in one study, no patient with adult onset of OCD had a first-degree relative with OCD (Nestadt *et al.*, 2000). Additionally, very early onset OCD is more frequently associated with tics and/or Tourette syndrome (Chabane *et al.*, 2004). Moreover, family studies have found that tic disorders are more likely to occur in patients who have relatives with OCD than in patients who lack a familial loading for OCD (Pauls *et al.*, 1995).

Evolution of concept and controversies

It is surprising to recall that until the 1980s, OCD was unfamiliar to most child psychiatrists for several reasons. As obsessive–compulsive thoughts and rituals are usually recognized by the child as nonsensical, they are often kept hidden for as long as possible from both parents and practitioners, and such secrecy may have contributed to the widespread lack of recognition. Nonetheless, there are descriptions of childhood onset OCD in the literature—albeit few and far between. Freud (1906) speculated about the similarity between obsessive–compulsive phenomena, children's games, and religious rites. Although psychoanalytic theory is empirically unproved and has not been shown to be effective in the treatment of OCD, the broad questions raised by Freud about continuity and discontinuity within individual development and OCD, as well as about secular and religious rituals, and cross-cultural studies linking cleanliness and "purity," remain fascinating issues. The recognition of childhood OCD stemmed from a recognition that the disorder was more common in adults than previously believed, along with retrospective reports that one-half to one-third of adult subjects had their onset in childhood or adolescence (Karno *et al.*, 1988). Such data focused the attention of the child psychiatric community on this chronic and often disabling disorder

Cultural and contemporary issues

The similarity of symptoms of OCD across cultures is more striking than the differences. While culture undoubtably influences the content of obsessions (for example, the nature of a feared infection will likely vary by country) at a more abstract level, symptoms still tend to fall within the general dimensions noted above (Lewis-Fernández *et al.*, 2011). The COVID-19 pandemic raised concerns that the necessary focus on handwashing, hygiene measures, and the general stress of the pandemic could exacerbate OCD symptoms in youth (Guzick *et al.*, 2021). Such concerns have been supported by most but not all studies, and as the pandemic switches to its endemic phase it will be important to assess for any lingering exacerbations.

Classification in ICD-11 and DSM-5

DMS-5 reconceptualized OCD as lying at the heart of obsessive–compulsive and a set of related disorders, which all share the theme of overfocused concerns and maladaptive behaviors. The "related" disorders, which are grouped with OCD in DSM-5, include body dysmorphic disorder (see Chapter 61), trichotillomania (a prior impulse control disorder), and the new disorders of hoarding and excoriation (e.g., skin picking). ICD-11 adds to the group of OCD and related disorders the following: Tourette syndrome, hypochondriasis (excessive worry over serious illness in the absence of objective evidence), and olfactory reference syndrome (the erroneous belief that the body is emitting an unpleasant odor, leading to distress and behaviors such as frequent cleansing).

The relationship between OCD and these other, related disorders is complex. There are some clear phenomenological similarities (see Chapters 59 and 61). For example, like OCD, body dysmorphic disorder and skin picking are characterized by overfocused ideation and anxiety arousing concerns. The diagnosis of OCD is only given if symptoms are not accounted for by these spectrum disorders. A neurobiological overlap with OCD is suggested by the increased rate of subclinical OCD features in relatives of those with spectrum disorder and clinical comorbidity of these spectrum disorders for OCD probands (Bienvenu *et al.*, 2012). However, most spectrum disorder patients do not have comorbid OCD (Philips et al. 2010), and body dysmorphic disorder is only comorbid with OCD in about one-third of patients, and their insight is more limited. Hoarding disorder is a new diagnosis for DSM-5 and is only comorbid with OCD in 20% of adults, and the extent to which hoarding is a clinical problem in childhood is unclear.

DSM-5 and ICD-11 both include specifiers for the degree of insight ranging for good, through fair to poor. In children, the specifier of poor insight may help prevent the obsession which the child believes to be valid and true from being misclassified as a delusion, triggering an inappropriate treatment chain (Leckman *et al.*, 2010). The specifier of having tics in DSM-5 both alerts the clinician to assess motor behavior and may impact treatment planning.

Impact of disorder on functioning

OCD can be highly impairing. The National Comorbidity Replication study in the US found that about two-thirds of those with OCD had severe impairment in key roles in life, particularly in social relationships (Ruscio *et al.*, 2010). Considerable evidence indicates significant psychological distress, impaired global functioning, and poorer quality of life in individuals with OCD compared to unaffected controls, with the disorder ranked sixth among all psychiatric conditions in terms of disability-adjusted life years (Hollander *et al.*, 2016). Similarly, a meta-analysis considering studies of impact of childhood OCD on quality of life report a large, clinically meaningful impact across most domains, particularly in young males with more severe symptoms (Coluccia *et al.*, 2017). The impact of OCD is not confined to the affected young person but can extend to the family, with significant increases within families of measure of "burden" and lowered quality of life (Cicek *et al.*, 2013). In OCD, as with many other disorders, functional impairment—meaning a reduced ability to meet demands of life due to psychiatric symptoms—can be distinct from the severity of OCD symptoms per se. This has been charted in a clinic-based cohort of youth followed over three years. While most youth in this cohort improved with treatment and maintained low levels of impairment, a subgroup remained at pretreatment levels of high impairment throughout, even when core OCD symptoms improved (Smárason *et al.*, 2023).

Comorbidity

As in nearly all child psychiatry, comorbidity is the rule rather than the exception, likely reflecting shared transdiagnostic dimensions of underlying cognitive, neural, and genetic differences. In one national survey, around 90% met criteria for another lifetime disorder, most commonly anxiety disorders (75.8%), followed by mood disorders (63.3%), impulse-control disorders (55.9%), and substance use disorders (38.6%). In children, there is an overlap with attention deficit hyperactivity disorder (ADHD), with rates of around 11.8–25% in youth with OCD (Masi *et al.*, 2010). While symptoms of OCD are extremely common in those with autism spectrum disorder (ASD), the full diagnosis is present in around 11–37%. A meta-analysis of 30 studies found a moderate to high association between OCD and suicidality—both ideation and attempts (Angelakis *et al.*, 2015), accentuated by severity of the disorder itself along with comorbid anxiety and depressive symptoms. The high rates of comorbid disorders should be remembered during assessment and treatment planning. Research bears out the clinical intuition that those with comorbid OCD will require more intensive treatment settings and medication than those without comorbidity (Ortiz *et al.*, 2016).

Assessment

The pillars of assessment are shown in Figure 60.1. The informant is paramount as secrecy appears to be a hallmark of

- **Informants**: Child/parent or caregiver/teachers
- Consider **semistructured interviews** (e.g., K-SADS)
- Consider **questionnaires**

SCALE	Completed by	Format
Children,s Yale–Brown Obsessive–Compulsive Scale (C-YOBCS)	Clinician-rated inventory with parent/child	Semistructured interview: presence and severity of obsessions and compul sions over the past week in children. It is comprised of a Symptom Checklist and a 10-item Severity Scale. The 5-item Obsession Severity and Compulsion Severity subscales are summed to produce a Total Severity score. Has a self-report version also (58-item symptom checklist and 10-item severity scale).
Obsessive Compulsive Inventory-Revised (OCI-R)	Self-report	18-item symptom checklist: severity and impairment- time occupied, interfer ence, distress, resistance, and degree of control.
Florida Obsessive–Compulsive Inventory	Self-report	20-item symptom checklist covering the past month. Endorsed symptoms receive a value of 1 (range: 0–20). Endorsed symptoms are rated on a 5-item Severity Scale that measures severity and impairment and summed to produce a Severity score (range: 0–25).

- **Mental state and physical examination**

Component	Examples
Appearance and behavior	Compulsive touching, counting, ordering; skin marks from excoriation; dry, cracked hands from washing. Tics (vocal, motor). Choreiform movements (sudden jerks)
Speech	Usually typical
Mood/affect	Often distressed by obsessions. Affect can be guarded to limit disclosure of distressing information. High emotional expression when experiencing acute anxiety.
Thought process	Obsessions = thoughts/urges/images that are recurrent/intrusive/undesired and cause distress/anxiety. Compulsions = repetitive behaviors/mental rituals often in response to obsessions, aimed to reduce anxiety.
Safety	Obsessional thoughts of self-harm or harming others. Assess safety: degree of planning; previous acts.
Perception	Intrusive imagery, but in internal space
Cognition	Usually intact
Insights	Often egodystonic; but can have poor or no insight.
Additional features	For a SUDDEN onset of symptoms, check for signs and symptoms of infectious processes (e.g., fever, temperature, pulse, sore throat, lymphadenopathy, tender, red joints, small painless bumps under skin, rarely cardiac murmurs)

Figure 60.1 Assessment at a glance.

childhood onset OCD. It is vital to talk to both the affected child and the primary caregivers. The affected child will often recognize that their symptoms are nonsensical and are embarrassed by them, so they go to great lengths to hide them, even from parents. Handwashing might be disguised as more frequent voiding and rituals are carried out in private, so that children are often symptomatic for months before their parents are aware of a problem. As with Tourette syndrome, children may expend effort controlling their behaviors in public and "let go" when at home. This partial voluntary control of symptoms often baffles and angers parents. Because of the variable degree and timing of control of symptoms, the nature of the informant has particularly important influence on recognition and diagnosis of OCD. Indeed, in one study (Rapoport *et al.*, 2000), only 0.3% of cases were identified by parents while 2.5% were identified through self-report from the child, with only one overlapping case. Thus, both the parent and the child are needed as informants. In addition, assessment of the family is needed to assess if there is familial accommodation, which can take the form of helping the child avoid anxiety or aiding in the completion of the ritual. In addition, the impact of OCD frequently extends to school, and it is often helpful with consent to have the teacher act as an informant.

The gold standard for diagnosis is an interview that elicits the cardinal symptoms of OCD, conducted by an experienced, trained clinician with both the parents and the affected young person. In this setting, semistructured interviews, such as the Schedule for Affective Disorder and Schizophrenia for School-Age Children (Kaufman *et al.*, 1997), or the Mini International Neuropsychiatric Interview for Children and Adolescents (Sheehan *et al.*, 2010), can be particularly helpful. The questions in these interview schedules cover all the criteria needed for diagnosis and ensure that comorbid disorders, expected in most children, are also assessed. It should be noted that the suggested questions can be modified as an experienced clinicians feels to be appropriate. In standard clinical practice a less structured interview is more common but nonetheless should enquire about all cardinal features of OCD. The assessment of impairment is critical and can be captured by considering time spent on the obsessions or compulsions, as well as the magnitude and pervasiveness of any impairment. In the diagnosis for DSM-5, a diagnostic hierarchy is applied so that OCD is only diagnosed if symptoms are not better explained by another disorder (which we consider below in the differential diagnosis) nor due to substances, including medications.

The age and nature of onset of symptoms should be determined. For those with very abrupt onset, the possibility of pediatric acute-onset neuropsychiatric syndrome should be considered (Swedo *et al.*, 2012). Here the child also presents with sudden onset of food restriction, anxiety, emotional lability, depression, behavioral regression with deterioration in school performance, sensorimotor anomalies, and somatic features such as disrupted sleep or enuresis. These features should not be better explained by another medical or neurological disorder (e.g., autoimmune encephalitis). Often, these children will appear extremely ill, prompting appropriate referral to pediatric colleagues.

Rating scales, completed by the parent or young person can also be helpful, particularly at the baseline assessment and in assessing the response to treatment. Among the most widely used are the: Children's Yale-Brown Obsessive–Compulsive Scale (C-YBOCS)/Dimensional Yale-Brown Obsessive–Compulsive Scale; Florida Obsessive–Compulsive Inventory; and parent and self-report of the Obsessional Compulsive Inventory. The Family Accommodation Scale can help determine the degree to which families may need guidance in stopping their participation in their child's OCD. Screening for suicidality is necessary (and can be conducted quickly using tools such as an ASQ (ask suicide-screening questions)). Sensory phenomena, such as getting things "just right," have been a valid and reliable auxiliary measure for OCD using the Sao Paulo Sensory Phenomena Scale (Rosario *et al.*, 2009).

Key features in mental state and physical examination are given in Figure 60.1 below.

Routine bloods are unnecessary unless otherwise indicated (e.g., in an extremely ill child with a very abrupt onset of OCD, in which case the child should be jointly assessed with a colleague in general pediatrics) (Chang *et al.*, 2015). Neuroimaging is rarely if ever needed, and genetic tests are not indicated, with the possible exception of OCD occurring in the context of ASD.

Differential diagnosis

OCD can be a challenging diagnosis to make—as is illustrated in Figure 60.2. OCD is defined in both ICD-11 and DSM-5 as repetitive intrusive thoughts and/or rituals that are unwanted, and which interfere significantly with function or cause marked distress. The severity criteria avoid confusion of OCD with many childhood habits that are part of normal development. Both the content and relative insight into the unreasonableness of the thoughts/behaviors differentiates OCD from other disorders.

Boundary with typical development

At one end, OCD merges in the typical intrusive thoughts and repetitive behaviors that many typically developing youth show. Individual "habits" that are reminiscent of the core symptoms of OCD are extremely common across populations. For example, in one Israeli study, only 18% of the sample endorsed no obsessive–compulsive symptoms at all, while a longitudinal population study found 21–25% of children and adults endorsed specific obsessions or compulsions (Fullana *et al.*, 2009). Moreover, many ritualistic and "magical" behaviors are part of normal development (Leonard, 1989). Indeed, one population-based study found that more intense perfectionism and intolerance of uncertainty at age 11 were tied to more severe symptoms of OCD a year later (Pozza *et al.*, 2019). These symptoms become a disorder when they entail persistent impairment, particularly across multiple domains, and occupy over an hour a

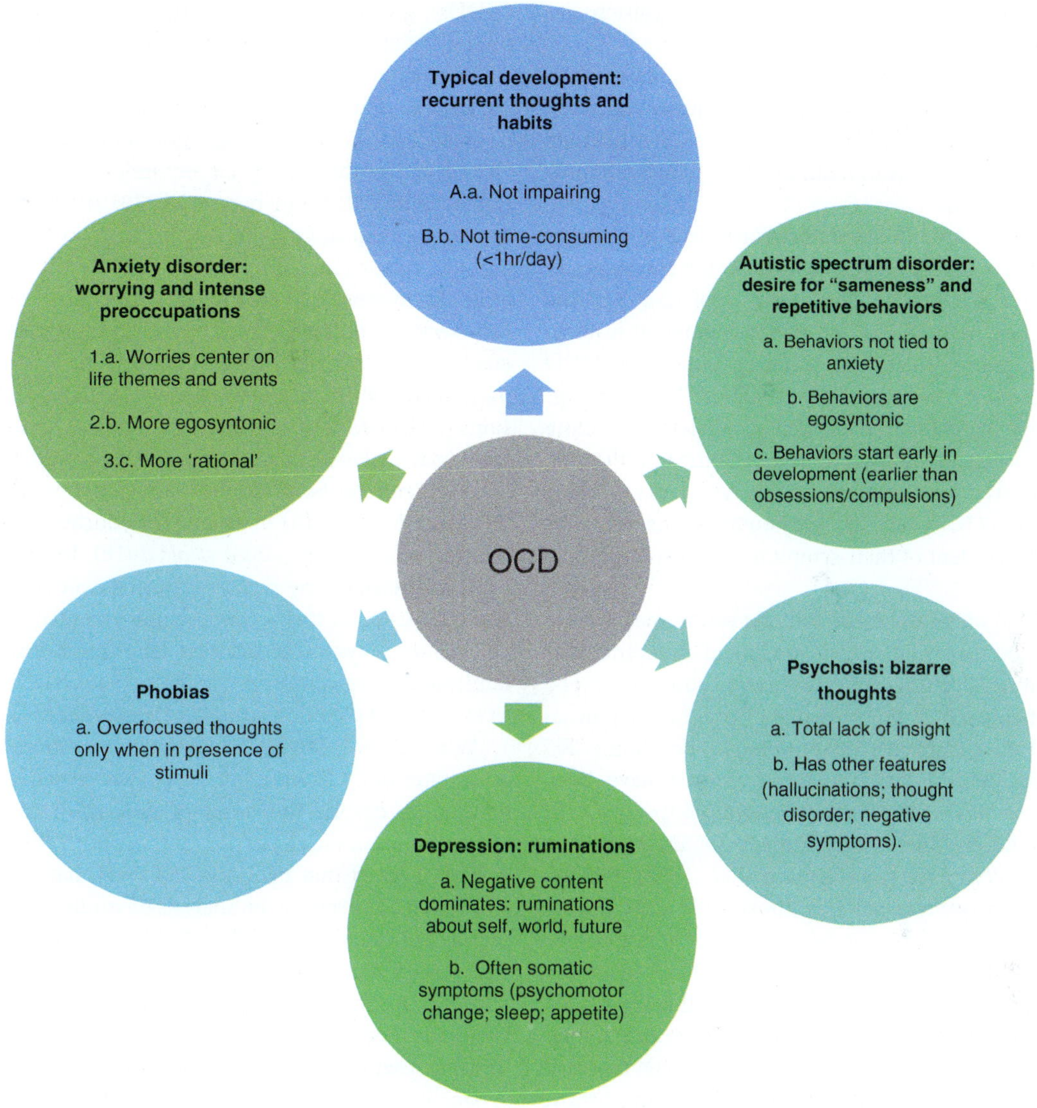

Figure 60.2 Differential diagnosis of obsessive–compulsive disorder.

day. Obsessions have an intensity and persistence that fleeting concerns lack. Etiologically, the "blurred" boundary with typical development makes sense as family genetic studies indicate that the heritability of obsessive–compulsive symptoms may extend across the entire range of severity, and, similarly, twin studies support the model of OCD as the extreme of a continuously distributed trait with biological continuity between normal and abnormal behaviors (Jonnal *et al.*, 2000).

Boundaries with other mental disorders

The diagnosis of OCD must be made only if the "obsessive worries" are true obsessions, rather than symptoms of another disorder such as depressive ruminations or phobic avoidance. For example, when OCD is comorbid with bulimia or anorexia, the content of the obsessions or compulsions must be typical for OCD, e.g., washing, arranging, counting, and repeating, and not be solely overfocused ideas about food or diet. Depressive ruminations and psychotic preoccupations are also distinguished by the negative content (e.g., everyone dislikes me, I fail at everything). Phobic disorders are not only distinguished by the content of the preoccupation (more often heights, spiders, the dark, etc.), but also by the absence of discomfort when the patient is not confronted with the phobic object. Disorders such as anorexia nervosa, pyromania, pathological gambling disorder and substance abuse disorder overlap with OCD principally in that their symptoms involve overfocused ideation but are neither comorbid for OCD probands nor is there increase in their families (Bienvenu *et al.*, 2012).

The boundary between OCD and the worries and ruminations that are found in anxiety disorders can be hard to delineate sharply. Among the useful differentiating features is that worries tend to center on life-related themes, are less egodystonic and lack the "irrationality" that characterizes obsessions. Compulsions are not characteristic of either anxiety or depression.

At its extreme, severe obsessional thought, particularly when accompanied by a lack of insights into their nature, can seem delusional. However, OCD will lack many of the other features of psychotic disorder, such as thought disorder, negative symptoms, and hallucinations.

OCD shares with ASD the symptoms of restricted interests and repetitive behaviors. However, OCD lacks the challenges in social communication that are characteristics of ASD, and the two disorders have markedly different developmental history: while ASD symptoms stem from infancy, childhood OCD mostly has later onset. Additionally, in OCD the "neutralizing" compulsive behavior can often be tied to anxiety-provoking obsessions, a feature that can be less salient in those with ASD. The compulsive need for sameness seen in ASD lacks many of the features seen in OCD, such as egodystonicity (the individual's sense that the content of their symptoms is alien and unlike their normal self).

The differential diagnosis from Tourette syndrome can also be challenging and the two disorders are linked by several neurobiological features. Distinguishing between a compulsion or a tic may be difficult, given the presence of premonitory urges before tics and the complexity of some motor tics. Some 20–80% of patients with clear Tourette syndrome have been reported to have obsessive–compulsive symptoms or OCD, while 24–67% of children with primary OCD have been observed to have comorbid tics (Leonard *et al.*, 1992). Tics are seen most often in younger patients, those with acute illness, and in males. Preliminary impressions are that compulsions associated with Tourette syndrome may be more likely to involve symmetry, rubbing, touching, or staring and blinking rituals, than washing and cleaning (Leckman *et al.*, 1994). Additionally, aggressive and/or sexual thoughts or rituals have been reported as more frequent in patients with tics and OCD than in those with OCD alone (Masi *et al.*, 2005). However, although some features distinguish the two disorders, the overlapping clinical profiles and family studies provide partial support for the speculation that some cases of OCD and Tourette syndrome may be alternate forms of the same disorder, both underpinned by basal ganglia-frontal circuitry dysfunction.

Epidemiology

OCD has a lifetime prevalence rate of 2–3%, and affects around 1% of the population (~3.3 million in the United States) each year (Ruscio *et al.*, 2010). More than half of OCD cases arise before the age of 18 years (Dell'Osso *et al.*, 2016), and even when diagnostic criteria are first met in adulthood, obsessions and compulsions often have their roots in childhood subdiagnostic obsessive–compulsive symptoms (Fullana *et al.*, 2009). Childhood-onset OCD may represent a disorder subtype, associated with comorbid tic and neurodevelopmental disorders (NDDs), greater familial clustering, male preponderance, and poorer insight (Ruscio *et al.*, 2010; Dell'Osso *et al.*, 2016).

The majority of youths identified as meeting criteria for OCD in epidemiological surveys had not been diagnosed with or treated for OCD, and the duration of untreated illness for OCD is one of the highest for any serious psychiatric condition (James *et al.*, 2017; Fineberg *et al.*, 2019). Underdiagnosis and undertreatment of OCD likely results in part from health care provider factors, including missed or incorrect diagnosis or lack of access to treatment resources (James *et al.*, 2017). However, help-seeking is often delayed due to concealment of obsessions and compulsions from loved ones and health care providers, particularly in the case of aggressive, sexual, or religious obsessions (Dell'Osso *et al.*, 2016; Fineberg *et al.*, 2019).

Of particular relevance to pediatric populations, academic achievement can be profoundly impacted, with children with OCD less likely to finish secondary education or enter higher level education (Pérez-Vigil *et al.*, 2018). In the United States, costs to the economy resulting from direct costs of treatment and indirect costs such as underemployment, academic underachievement, days lost to sickness, labor market marginalization, family and caregiver impact, and mortality, have been estimated to exceed US$10 billion annually (Hollander *et al.*, 2016).

While OCD is held to be a chronic condition, similar prevalence rates of OCD have been reported in both childhood and adulthood, despite the onset of new adult cases, suggesting remission occurs for a portion of those with childhood OCD. It is often argued that pediatric cases will have a more chronic course, and a recent meta-analysis of studies based on 16 independent samples (521 OCD participants) followed for a mean of 11.2 years indicated earlier age of onset to be a poor prognosis factor, along with comorbid psychiatric illness and poor initial treatment response (Stewart *et al.*, 2004). Overall, there was a 41% persistence for full and 60% for full or subthreshold OCD. A small study in which 45 of 62 pediatric OCD cases were recontacted a mean of 9 years later in early adulthood found 44% remitted in agreement with earlier studies (Bloch *et al.*, 2009). Worse outcome was associated with absence of tics, more severe baseline symptoms, and female gender, as well as poor visuospatial and fine motor skills. The pathways determining clinical outcome are complex, and any single developmental variable, such as age of onset, is likely to account for only a modest amount of the overall variance in outcome. OCD patients with comorbid tics or Tourette syndrome have a waxing and waning course (Bloch *et al.*, 2006). In patients with comorbid Tourette syndrome and OCD, tics generally start to improve around age 10, while the obsessive–compulsive symptoms typically continue for several more years. Pediatric autoimmune neuropsychiatric disorder associated with streptococcal infections (PANDAS) is also characterized as relapsing/remitting in relation to streptococcal infection (Leonard *et al.*, 1999). However, many of these estimates are based on data from clinical cohorts of typically moderate to severe cases, often in national specialist or inpatient clinics, with most participants receiving treatment for the disorder. More work is therefore needed in epidemiological cohorts to estimate rates of remission for community cases of the disorder. As with other disorders, community-based samples of those with OCD tend to have more favorable outcomes, possibly due to less severe baseline presentations compared to clinic-ascertained cohorts.

Risk factors

Genomics of obsessive–compulsive disorder

OCD is a heritable disorder, with twin studies suggesting that 45–65% of variance in the disorder can be explained by inherited genetic factors (Pauls, 2022). Heritability may be higher for those with early onset OCD, particularly when accompanied by tics. The disorder clusters in families, with between 6–55% of first-degree relatives of an affected youth showing lifetime OCD. The familial aggregation may also be greater for childhood onset OCD: in one study the prevalence of OCD in relatives of probands with an early onset was 13.8%, compared to 0% in probands with later onset (Bienvenu *et al.*, 2000).

Most of this heritability is unexplained. As in all psychiatric genomics, a focus on specific genes thought to be strong candidates, such as serotoninergic genes targeted by effective medication, has not yielded replicable results. Looking across the entire genome for common genetic variants tied to the disorder (identified through genome-wide association studies [GWAS]) has proved a more fruitful approach in other psychiatric disorders, and such studies are underway in OCD. A preliminary report contrasting 14,140 OCD cases against over 500,000 unaffected controls found a single variant to be significantly associated with OCD, after appropriate adjustment for the number of tests. This single variant lay within a gene-rich part of the genome that contains genes previously associated with schizophrenia and neuroticism (Strom *et al.*, 2021). Additionally, in this study, two genes emerged as strong candidate for OCD, Telomere Replication Complex Component 1 gene (*CTC1*) and Transmembrane Protein 107 gene (T*MEM107*), and both were in the same locus on chromosome 17. Combined, all the common genetic variants associated with OCD explained about 16% of its heritability. Another GWAS examined obsessive–compulsive symptoms. It assessed 33,943 individuals and pointed to set of genes involved in dysregulated insulin signaling, which has previously shown genetic overlap with obsessive–compulsive symptoms in children (Strom *et al.*, 2022). Unsurprisingly, the common genetic variants associated with obsessive–compulsive symptoms overlap greatly with those tied to the disorder. As in other areas of psychiatry, there has been considerable interest in the possible clinical translation of such findings. When summed across the genome, the OCD-associated variants provide give a "polygenic risk score" for the disorder. However, a current major barrier to clinical translation is the lack of ancestral diversity in genetic studies, with most prior GWAS being confined to those of European ancestry, thus limiting the applicability of any derived polygenic risk scores.

Looking at rare genetic variants, there have been reports of large gene deletions or duplication (copy number variants [CNVs]) in genes that have been linked to other NDDs, particularly Tourette syndrome and ASD (Saraiva *et al.*, 2020). These CNVs also appear to impact genes involved in basic neurodevelopmental processes. Sequencing of the exome (the gene coding portion of the genome) in parent-affected child trios has found that rare variants, present in the affected child but not parents, contributed risk to OCD in 22% of the cases (Cappi *et al.*, 2020). As with CNVs, these rare "point mutations" impacted genes that are involved in neurodevelopmental processes. Initial examinations of the postmortem brain from those who had lifetime histories of OCD suggests altered expression of genes relating to synaptic processes and the brain's major excitatory transmitter, glutamate (Piantadosi *et al.*, 2021).

Given the striking overlap between OCD and other disorders it is perhaps unsurprising that there is often a marked overlap between the disorder in genetic risk factors. The transdiagnostic genetic correlations are highest between OCD and anorexia nervosa (at 0.5), but high correlations are also found for Tourette syndrome, bipolar affective disorder, and schizophrenia (Lee *et al.*, 2019). Interestingly, despite the high comorbidity between OCD and both ASD and ADHD, initial studies suggest that the genetic overlap is not as striking.

Environmental risk factors

Twin studies also emphasize the importance of the environment in the etiology of OCD, with around 42–55% of the variance of obsessive–compulsive symptoms being explained by nonshared environmental factors (Hudziak *et al.*, 2004). Many of the environmental risk factors that are associated with an increased risk of OCD also confer risk for many other childhood psychiatric disorders. The most robust evidence from meta-analyses points to a role for perinatal, reproductive, and stressful life events, but all lack a clear demonstration of a causal role (Brander *et al.*, 2016). The family environment may also contribute to OCD, particularly the ways in which family members take part in the performance of rituals and help relatives avoid anxiety-provoking situations. Such familial accommodation is associated with symptom severity and its reduction is associated with symptom improvement, a point we will return to as we consider treatment (Lebowitz *et al.*, 2012).

Neurological trauma

A small literature documents the onset of OCD subsequent to processes that damage the basal ganglia, including encephalitis lethargica stemming from influenza, Sydenham's chorea, and neuroacanthocytosis (Laplane *et al.*, 1989). The postulation of a postinfectious subgroup of pediatric OCD came about because of early reports of the association of OCD with Sydenham's chorea. This supported converging evidence of basal ganglia involvement in the etiology and/or maintenance of OCD (Wise & Rapoport, 1989).

One example of a postinfectious subgroup has been identified by research at the NIMH which identified a group of pediatric patients in whom symptom onset or exacerbations are triggered by streptococcal infections; the subgroup is identified by the acronym PANDAS (Swedo *et al.*, 2004). The disorder is thought to arise through a process of molecular mimicry, with the group A ß-hemolytic streptococcus (*Streptococcus pyogenes*) (GABHS) evoking antibodies that are capable of cross-reacting with specific areas of the human brain (e.g., the basal ganglia) to produce neuropsychiatric and behavioral symptoms. Moreover, some initial evidence found that this group showed some response to immunotherapy (Perlmutter *et al.*, 1999)., though this finding bears replication in larger, multisite studies and has not been replicated. This concept has been broadened to the category of pediatric acute-onset neuropsychiatric syndrome or PANS (Swedo *et al.*, 2012). A mainly US-based working group proposed PANS to be defined by its abrupt onset rather than etiology and it must include OCD or food restriction and other concurrent psychiatric symptoms (Murphy *et al.*, 2014), such as lability, depression, behavioral regression with deterioration in school performance, sensorimotor anomalies, and somatic features such as disrupted sleep or enuresis. These features should not be better explained by another medical or neurological disorder (e.g., autoimmune encephalitis). PANS is characterized by a "sawtooth" course, in that symptoms may remit between acute episodes, but patients often fail to return to baseline functioning even during remission (Calaprice *et al.*, 2018). This concept is not without controversy. It has been argued that given the high community prevalence of both streptococcal infections and OCD, chance temporal associations are highly likely (reviewed in Gilbert, 2019). Furthermore, there are concerns around the accurate detection of acute, rather than previous, streptococcal infections. Additionally, PANDAS/PANS is tied to inflammatory neural processes, which are usually associated with a more severe clinical manifestations such as seizures, delirium, and abnormal motor behaviors, rather than the arguably narrow symptom profile of PANDAS.

It has also been suggested that prenatal infections may predispose to later OCD. A large population register study found that while OCD and Tourette syndrome were increased among those exposed to maternal (but not paternal) prenatal infection, this association did not hold in analyses that considered siblings. This suggests that unmeasured familial confounding largely explains the associations found in the population-level analyses Zhang *et al.*, (2023). Meta-analyses also point to childhood trauma as a potent risk factor for both the severity of OC symptoms and OCD itself (Destrée *et al.*, 2021)

Pathology/Processes

OCD is remarkable in the consistency of support for a conceptual model which links a disorder characterized by endless, repetitive thoughts and actions with uncontrolled activity of parallel, discrete loops within the brain. These loops connect the basal ganglia, prefrontal cortex (PFC)—particularly the orbitofrontal and anterior cingulate regions—and thalamus, the so-called cortico-striato-thalamo-cortical (CSTC) loops, see Figure 60.3 (Alexander *et al.*, 1986; Saxena *et al.*, 2001). Within each loop, direct, bottom-up, excitatory pathways mediate the initiation and continuation of thoughts and behaviors, while indirect inhibitory pathways are responsible for inhibiting and flexibly switching between thoughts and behaviors in a goal-directed fashion. Classical neurobiological models of OCD thus attribute obsessive–compulsive symptoms to imbalances of these antagonistic pathways within CSTC loops, with a relative dominance of direct excitatory pathways underlying the inflexible thought and behavior patterns that characterize obsessions and compulsions (van den Heuvel *et al.*, 2016).

A striking feature of OCD is that compulsive behaviors are often performed even when patients can report them as unwanted, unnecessary, and even absurd. Compulsions are thus deemed "egodystonic," as they appear to represent internal conflicts between instinctive behavioral responses and what individuals with OCD know and desire. Recent reformulations of the classical CSTC model therefore propose an imbalance between loops involved in bottom-up, habitual, stimulus-driven responses and loops responsible for implementing more adaptive, goal-directed control over behavior (Gillan *et al.*, 2016). In support of this, some groups find that trained behaviors persist in both children and adults with OCD following removal of stimulus–response–outcome associations ("devaluation") (Gillan & Sahakian, 2015). For example, following explicit and immediate devaluation via removal of a shock-pad from the wrist of the participant, adults with OCD showed an increased tendency to continue button-pressing to avoid mild shocks. In other words, individuals with OCD continue to perform stimulus-driven behaviors, despite intact explicit knowledge that they are no longer necessary (Gillan *et al.*, 2015).

Other evidence for a role of CSTC loops in the pathophysiology of OCD comes from case reports in which insults to the basal ganglia produced OCD-like symptoms (Cheyette & Cummings, 1995). Using positron emission tomography (PET) and single-photon emission computed tomography, early neuroimaging work reported resting-state hypermetabolism across CSTC regions, particularly within the caudate and orbitofrontal cortex, which normalized with pharmacological and psychological treatment (Saxena & Rauch, 2000). Consistent with the habit model, functional magnetic resonance imaging (fMRI) studies point to functional overactivation within the same set of brain regions during symptom provocation and habit-responding (Gillan et al., 2015), but underactivation during goal-directed functions such as inhibitory control and reward processing (Norman *et al.*, 2018; Norman *et al.*, 2019). Recent large-scale structural neuroimaging studies also provide partial support for the CSTC model. Results from Enhancing Neuroimaging Genetics Through Meta-Analysis (ENIGMA) consortium indicated enlarged volume within the pallidum, a structure forming part of the basal ganglia, in adults with OCD on medication relative to controls ($N = 2967$; $d = 0.29$), as well

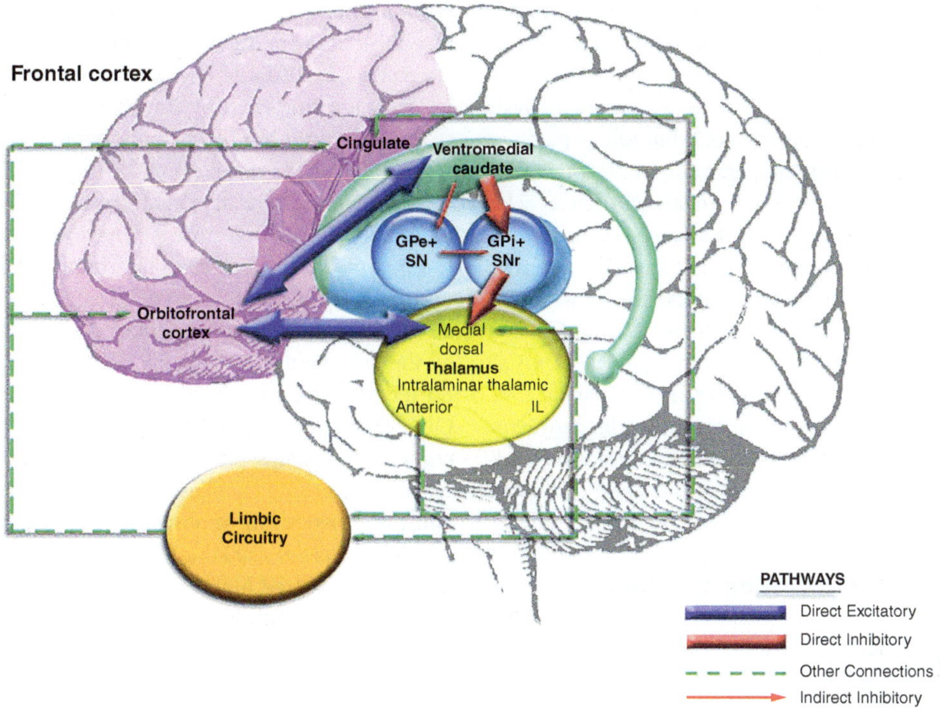

Figure 60.3 The direct and indirect circuitry thought to underlie the pathogenesis of obsessive–compulsive disorder (OCD). In the DIRECT pathway (thick arrows), the frontal cortex projects to the ventromedial caudate and then to the GPi/SNr complex which provides the main output of the basal ganglia. This, in turn, projects to the thalamus and finally back to the frontal cortex. The pathway has two excitatory and two inhibitory projections and thus is a net positive feedback loop. This circuit is balanced by the INDIRECT pathway (in thin arrows) which has a net inhibitory effect. This differs in its projection from the caudate to the GPe/SN complex (which also receives direct frontal input) before relaying onto the output station of the basal ganglia (the GPi/SNr complex). Interactions with the limbic system occur at several points and have been increasingly recognized in view of deficits in emotional processing and the anxiety prominent in OCD. *Note*: GPe—globus pallidus pars externa; GPi—globus pallidus pars interna, SNr—substantia nigra pars reticulata.

as enlarged thalamus in unmedicated OCD youth relative to age-matched peers (N = 622; d = 0.38) (Boedhoe *et al.*, 2017, 2020,). In addition, adults with OCD showed a smaller hippocampus (d = −0.13) particularly if they had an adult onset of OCD, a lifetime history of comorbid depression, and were on medication. These morphological alterations were not shared with individuals with ADHD and ASD though all were of small effect, and many tied to medication exposure. Findings of enlarged thalamic volume in youth with OCD were replicated in a large Dutch childhood cohort (Weeland *et al.*, 2022).

Studies of direct modulation of CSTC functioning in humans and animals also supports its role in OCD. First, deep brain stimulation within the ventral striatum and subthalamic nucleus has been reported to provide therapeutic benefit for adult patients with severe refractory OCD, along with accompanying normalization of heightened CSTC connectivity and metabolism at rest, and a normalization of CSTC underactivation during reward processing and inhibitory control (Suetens *et al.*, 2014; Figee *et al.*, 2017). Second, noninvasive transcranial magnetic stimulation (TMS) of medial frontal CSTC sites has received US Food and Drug Administration (FDA) approval as a therapy for treatment-resistant OCD in adults (Carmi et al., 2019). This followed a randomized controlled trial (RCT) in which response rates (30% reduction in Y-BOCS) were 38% in the active group compared with 11% in the sham condition (Voelker, 2018). Preliminary neuroimaging evidence also supports that TMS therapy for OCD acts via a normalization of CSTC functioning, which correlates with individual differences in symptom improvement (Dunlop *et al.*, 2016). In animals, an influential study by Ahmari and colleagues (Ahmari *et al.*, 2013) showed that repeated activation of CSTC circuitry in mice via optogenetics induced compulsion-like grooming behaviors, which persisted after stimulation ceased (although this finding has not always replicated; see de Oliveira *et al.* (2021) for discussion). Thus, converging lines of clinical and preclinical evidence support the role of CSTC circuitry in the genesis of OCD symptoms.

Beyond the traditional CSTC framework, a second classical, "cybernetic" model of OCD views the disorder as the result of overactivation of a system designed to monitor performance completion leading to a constant feeling that an action is "not just right" (obsessions), which thus creates a need to correct perceived mistakes (compulsions) (Pitman, 1987). In support of this, a recent cross-disorder meta-analysis of N = 97 published electrophysiological studies reported heightened feedback and error-related negativity in individuals with OCD (d ~ 0.5) relative to controls, which was shared with Tourette syndrome but not with other childhood onset disorders including ADHD and ASD (Bellato *et al.*, 2021). Similarly, a voxel-wise meta-analysis of 10 fMRI studies reported modest (d ~ 0.2) but robust patterns of overactivation within anterior cingulate and fronto-opercular regions during error processing in individuals with OCD relative to controls (Norman *et al.*, 2019). Enhanced error-related negativity is observed even in individuals with lifetime OCD following remission, as well as in asymptomatic first-degree OCD family members, countering the claim that heightened error processing is an epiphenomenal consequence of OCD symptoms (Riesel, 2019). Since the first report by Gehring *et al.* (2000), more than 30 studies have reported heightened error processing in OCD, making it one of the most replicated findings in the psychiatric neuroscience literature (Gillan *et al.*, 2017).

Obsessive–compulsive disorder: the doubting disorder

Modern psychological theories have also centralized the role of uncertainty and doubt in the generation of OCD symptoms (Fradkin *et al.* 2020; Loosen & Hauser, 2020). Specifically, individuals with OCD appear to be less able to use internal models of the environment as a reliable source of information, meaning that they need to keep acting via repeated checking, mental reconstruction, and requests for external validation or reassurance to reduce uncertainty. Supporting these accounts, individuals with OCD show prolonged evidence gathering in information sampling tasks, and rate themselves as relatively uncertain even when given enough information for the outcome to be objectively certain (Stern *et al.*, 2013). Relatedly, multiple studies indicate that individuals with OCD rate themselves as and behave as less certain in their perception and memory abilities (Cougle *et al.*, 2007). Such accounts may provide alternative explanations for other observed neurobehavioral differences associated with OCD. For instance, prolonged performance of habit behaviors may result from a relative lack of confidence in the memory or mental model for the devaluation occurring (Fradkin *et al.*, 2020). Furthermore, contemporary computational models propose that individuals who are less confident in their internal models of the world and their actions within it will give more weight to incoming evidence from the environment (Fradkin *et al.*, 2020). Under such circumstances, larger error mismatch signals are expected, as have been observed in individuals with OCD. Efforts to formalize the role of uncertainty reduction in OCD symptom generation via testable computational models, and to link them with established neurobiological alterations within CSTC loops, are a new and important area of ongoing research.

Monoaminergic neurotransmitters which extensively project from the brain stem to regions within the fronto-striato-thalamic circuitry may contribute to the pathogenesis of OCD. OCD symptoms are frequently exacerbated by serotonin agonists (such as meta-chlorophenylpiperazine), and the serotonin reuptake inhibitors are the most effective therapeutic agents (Gross-Isseroff *et al.*, 2004). Abnormalities of serotonergic transmission in OCD are suggested by imaging studies of central serotonin receptors using specific ligands, which have demonstrated a reduction in 5-HT synthesis in the ventral PFC and caudate in 11 treatment-naïve pediatric subjects, which partially normalized following successful treatment (Simpson *et al.*, 2003). Inconsistent findings on the levels of central serotonin transporter availability may be partly attributable to developmental effects, as reports of an increase of central serotonin transporter availability (indexed by the binding profiles of a ligand thought to bind to the transporter) were found only in those with child, but not adult, onset OCD (Pogarell *et al.*, 2003; Simpson *et al.*, 2003). There are less consistent findings for the dopaminergic system, with mixed results concerning changes in peripheral dopaminergic markers and the provocation of obsessive symptoms by dopamine agonists (Denys *et al.*, 2004b). PET neuroimaging studies, however, have demonstrated higher caudate dopamine transporter densities in tandem with lower concentrations of the dopamine D2 receptor, consistent with receptor down-regulation resulting from higher synaptic concentrations of striatal dopamine in adults with OCD (Denys *et al.*, 2004a). Glutamate is the major excitatory neurotransmitter in the fronto-striatal circuitry, and magnetic resonance spectroscopy has demonstrated elevation in levels of glutamate and glutamine in the thalamus of treatment-naïve children with OCD, with a reduction in symptoms occurring in tandem with normalization of the glutamatergic marker (Rosenberg *et al.*, 2000). A decrease in glutamate levels in the anterior cingulate has also been found, although this may not be specific to OCD as it was also seen in children with major depression (Rosenberg *et al.*, 2004). There is, thus, some direct support for anomalous serotonergic neurotransmission and more indirect and somewhat inconsistent evidence of abnormal dopaminergic and glutamatergic signaling.

Nonhuman animal models

The understanding of OCD has benefited from nonhuman animal models of the disorder (reviewed in Chamberlain & Ahmari, 2021). This initially included the early observation of compulsive-like behaviors such as acral lick dermatitis in dogs. This is a naturally occurring disorder in which excessive licking of paws or flank can produce ulcers and is reversed by selective serotonin reuptake inhibitors (SSRIs). More recently, there has been a focus on transgenic animal models, such as the "compulsive" (or repetitive) behaviors seen in mice that have had "knockouts" of certain genes. These transgenic models include the *Sapap-3* gene knockout mouse, which shows excessive grooming behaviors, impaired reversal learning, and habit formation, all of which are reversed by SSRIs. In turn, these behaviors have been tied to neural anomalies that mimic those seen in humans with OCD, such as decreased synapse formations between the orbitofrontal cortex and striatum. Other researchers have used highly targeted alterations of key neurocircuitry, such as the use of toxins to ablate key neuronal subpopulations, to simulate compulsive behaviors. Such experimental manipulations allow for causal pathways to be mapped, although such work is inherently limited by phenomenological differences, such as the inability to model obsessional thinking in animals.

Treatment

The first stage of any treatment program is education around OCD and the engagement of the child and family in therapy—see Figure 60.4. Prior to contact with mental health services the family and young person can access a wealth of helpful and reliable information on websites from organizations such as the International OCD Foundation (https://iocdf.org). Engagement of the child in therapy is usually accomplished by a thorough assessment, followed by psychoeducation on OCD, aimed in large part at reducing any stigma or feelings of shame around symptoms. The "therapeutic team" should be assembled and at a minimum will include the family, child, and therapist. The school often needs to be involved at an early stage if symptoms are impairing in that setting.

The cornerstone of psychological therapies for children is cognitive behavioral therapy (CBT) that is based on exposure

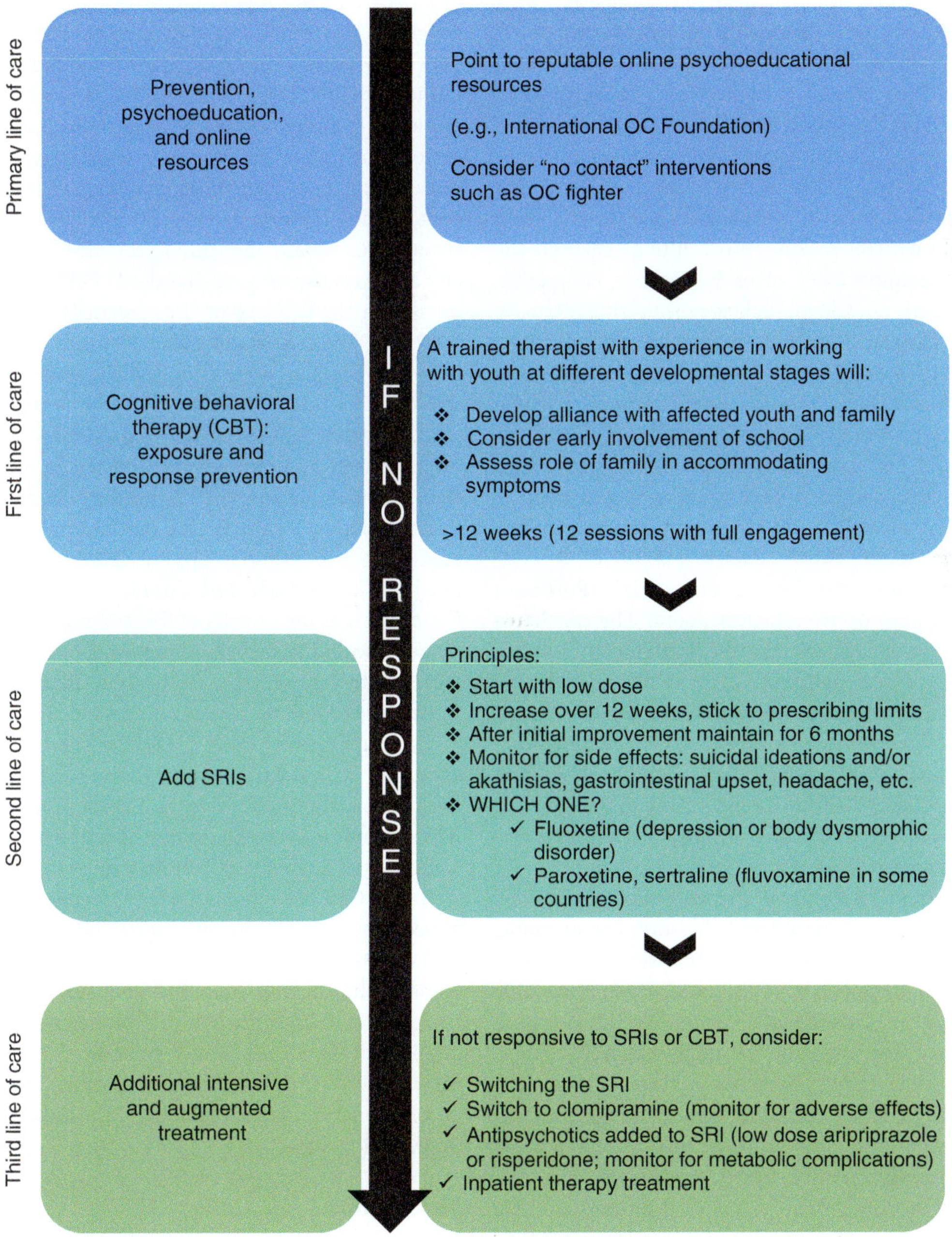

Figure 60.4 Treatment at a glance.

and response prevention (ERP). The efficacy of this approach is captured by a meta-analysis of 20 CBT trials, which found a large benefit for treatment, with an effect size of 1.21 (McGuire *et al.*, 2015). Overall, the number needed to treat (NNT) was three for treatment response and symptom/diagnostic remission (that is three children would have to receive treatment for one to show benefit). This meta-analysis also demonstrated the superiority of CBT over medication, as medication had only a moderate treatment effect ($g = 0.50$), and the NNT was five.

In CBT-ERP, a hierarchy of increasingly intense anxiety-provoking situations that trigger obsessional thinking is constructed, and subjects are exposed gradually to these situations and encouraged to refrain from engaging in compulsive behaviors (March & Mulle, 1998). Gradually, the patient progresses through the hierarchy so that situations can be tolerated with minimal anxiety, thus attaining an ever-decreasing urge to engage in compulsions. In clinical practice, and in all controlled studies, ERP is usually combined with other behavioral techniques, such as anxiety management training and extinction (e.g., instructing parents not to give reassurance when a child compulsively seeks it). This makes it difficult to disentangle the relative therapeutic importance of each element. Frequently, cognitive components are added, such as normalizing intrusive thoughts and reappraising notions of personal responsibility. Again, the necessity of these cognitive components is unclear in children as there are no controlled trials comparing these approaches. Tailoring therapy to the symptom profile of the child may be helpful. For example, ERP may be ideal for younger children as it has been shown to be effective in those under 11 and may be particularly helpful for symptoms such as contamination fears and symmetry rituals (Barrett *et al.*, 2003). By contrast, cognitive approaches may be more suited to the child with obsessional moral guilt or pathological doubt. The treatment should be delivered by an experienced therapist, for a minimum of 10–20 sessions. The benefits of CBT extend beyond core symptoms and improvement in depressive and anxiety symptoms is also often found (Rozenman *et al.*, 2019). Pre- and post-treatment assessments of symptom severity, using tools such as the CY-BOCS, are very helpful in measuring response, and evidence-based optimal cutoffs indicating remission for these tools have been reported (Farhat *et al.*, 2022).

The involvement of the family in treatment is essential. The family can sometimes accommodate behaviors. For example, siblings and parents might engage in excessive cleaning to reduce the fears of infection of a child; others may provide excessive reassurance. Psychoeducation can help the family to avoid both punitive responses and the family accommodation that can occur if the family becomes enmeshed in rituals. Coercive and disruptive behaviors, and attacks of rage are associated with family accommodation. These disruptive behaviors are often associated with family attempts to limit OCD symptom expression. Behavioral management of these episodes can be critical to successful treatment. There is a particularly strong evidence base for the Supportive Parenting for Anxious Childhood Emotions program (SPACE), a parent-based intervention that focuses on changing parental (not child) accommodating behaviors (Lebowitz *et al.*, 2016).

The most efficient and efficacious method of providing ERP for children is unclear. A randomized controlled study demonstrated that such family-based CBT may be equally efficacious when conducted either with individual families or in a group setting (Barrett *et al.*, 2004). The degree of personal contact with the therapist continues to be an important issue given the cost of more intense programs. At one extreme lies computer-based delivery systems including web camera-based treatment with minimal therapist contact time (Kenwright *et al.*, 2005); at the other extreme are highly intensive day or inpatient treatment programs. Only one trial has directly compared once weekly with daily therapy; no significant differences in outcome were found, although this study was not randomized and thus conclusions are limited (Franklin *et al.*, 1998). A meta-analysis suggested that while more therapist-intensive approaches were more efficacious, even those involving relatively little therapist contact time (less than 10 hours) were also effective (National Institute for Health and Care Excellence, 2005). Given the scarcity and expense of "gold standard" CBT, there is considerable interest in the delivery of "low-intensity" CBT, usually via the Internet. This consists of either web-based CBT (mainly web-based CBT material with limited therapist contact) or guided self-help (written web-based materials, with no therapist contact). Evidence for the efficacy of these approaches is mixed and no large-scale randomized study has focused on youth. There is also considerable interest in the development of technology-assisted therapy—such as CBT mobile applications (apps) delivered on smartphones/laptops but demonstrations of efficacy are needed (Gershkovich *et al.*, 2021).

In practice, the severity of the symptom profile, the complexity of comorbidity, and resources available within the family and local health care services are likely to determine the treatment intensity. Barriers to access include a paucity of trained therapists, geographic obstacles, and the significant time and cost associated with the treatment. Given the many barriers to effective treatment, it is important to alert families to self-help groups which provide a valuable source of support and information, as well as act as advocates for those living with the disorder.

While CBT is a robust frontline treatment overall, about 30% of pediatric populations have little or no response. Poor response is associated with diminished insight, family accommodation, comorbidity (depression, Tourette syndrome, and cognitive deficits Storch *et al.*, 2010). In nonresponders, it is worthwhile starting afresh with a new formulation of the symptoms and their causes, with a particular focus of the possibility of familial accommodation, often overlooked in initial treatment focused on the child alone.

Medication

While usually a second-line treatment, there are some instances in which it is appropriate to consider medication as a first-line option. These include when CBT is unavailable, when the young person or family declines CBT, when there was a previous robust response to medication, or when the child is so impaired by symptoms that they cannot engage in CBT.

There is an abundance of RCTs demonstrating the efficacy of selective serotonin reuptake inhibitors (SSRIs; sertraline, fluoxetine, paroxetine, and fluvoxamine) in the acute phase treatment of childhood OCD (for an excellent overview see Marazziti & Pozza, 2022). A recent meta-analysis found that SSRIs were superior to placebo but the magnitude of improvement was small (effect size is small [SMD = −0.43], which converts to a 3.5-point reduction in the CY-BOCS score—which is of marginal clinical significance) (Kotapati *et al.*, 2019). There was no additional benefit of combination treatment over CBT alone, but CBT added substantial benefit to SSRI monotherapy. Fluoxetine and sertraline appear to be superior to fluvoxamine (which has been removed from some markets due to other safety concerns). This meta-analysis thus gave a different result from the largest single RCT, which directly compared sertraline against CBT, combined treatment, and placebo (recruiting 112 children for 12 weeks) (POTS, 2004). This RCT found all active treatments were superior to pill placebo. Combined treatment also proved superior to CBT alone and to sertraline alone, which did not differ from each other. Site differences emerged for CBT and sertraline but not for combined treatment, suggesting that combined treatment is less susceptible to setting-specific variations, and, given this generalizability, combined treatment may be the option of choice. Notably, there was no evidence of treatment-emergent suicidality. In short, the meta-analyses support the primacy of CBT as a first-line treatment, although, in some cases, CBT is not possible to implement without concomitant medication, not available, or not accepted by the young person.

Which SRI should be used? The choice of SRI will be influenced partly by local licensing, with medications having different approvals in different countries. Some choices can be informed by comorbidity. For example, fluoxetine is a good choice when there is comorbid major depression and/or when there are body dysmorphic symptoms. In children, low initial doses with slow upward titration are the rule. In adults, higher doses are clearly associated with improved treatment efficacy without significant increase in adverse events, but this has not been systematically studied for pediatric populations. Thus, medication should be given above the recommended upper limits. Patients should be made aware of the common side effects, particularly the possibility of increases in suicidal thoughts, and the need for a 12-week treatment trial. Partial or complete failure to respond to the first SRI should prompt reevaluation, combination with CBT (if not already in place), and consideration of another SRI or clomipramine, as discussed in the following section.

Augmenting strategies for partial/non responders

Up to 50% of children will show only a partial response to initial SRI treatment (Geller *et al.*, 1998). There are several options to consider. First, after ensuring that the initial trial of an SRI was adequate a second SRI could be considered. After a second SRI (or in some cases, instead of), a trial of clomipramine should be considered given its solid evidence base. An early meta-analysis of 12 studies of SRIs and clomipramine found all medications to be superior to placebo and found that clomipramine showed superiority over all the SRIs which did not differ from one another (Geller *et al.*, 2003). While clomipramine is effective, it has a troublesome side-effect profile, such as sedation, dry mouth, constipation, and potential arrhythmogenic effects, and thus is no longer considered a first-line option. When used, it requires careful monitoring, ideally under specialist clinics.

Augmentation of SRIs with antipsychotics is another option. There is some evidence supporting the use of risperidone or aripiprazole among children (McDougle *et al.*, 2000; Ardic *et al.*, 2017). The principles of prescribing are to use the antipsychotic as an augmenting agent (combined with the best response SRI), to use low doses, and to monitor closely for adverse side effects (particularly metabolic side effects). A double-blind trial of d-cycloserine augmentation of CBT in 30 pediatric OCD subjects did not reach significance from placebo, but indicated a small-to-moderate effect supporting other studies in adults showing potentiation of antianxiety CBT with this agent (Storch *et al.*, 2010).

While there is no role in youth for neurosurgical procedures, such as deep brain stimulation, there is understandable interest in noninvasive neuromodulation. This uses techniques such as transcranial direct or alternating cranial stimulation or TMS on all targeted areas such as the supplementary motor areas, medial and dorsolateral PFC. Studies have been conducted almost exclusively in adults, with some promising proof-of-concept findings, but have yet to be conducted systematically in youth with intractable OCD.

Maintenance treatment

OCD is frequently a chronic disorder and long-term maintenance therapy should be anticipated, with the current recommendation being a minimum treatment period of 6 months following full remission. The need for such maintenance was illustrated by an 8-month study of 26 children and adolescents with severe OCD who had received clomipramine for a mean of 17 months; a 2-month double-blind desipramine-substitution phase resulted in 89% of the substituted (versus 18% of the non-substituted) subjects relapsing during the substitution phase (Leonard *et al.*, 1991).

Other treatments

For children who meet criteria for PANS, consensus treatment guidelines have been issued (Swedo *et al.*, 2017). The first step is to alleviate symptoms through standard CBT and SRIs (perhaps at lower doses). The remaining steps should only be conducted in close consultation with tertiary level/specialist services. For those with persisting symptoms, some may benefit from non-steroidal anti-inflammatory drugs and/or short oral corticosteroid bursts. For even more severe symptoms, stepping up to intravenous corticosteroids may be indicated, and some authorities recommend intravenous immunoglobulin for such extreme presentations. In exceptionally rare life-threatening presentations, therapeutic plasma exchange is the first-line therapy, given either alone or in combination with intravenous immunoglobulins, high-dose intravenous corticosteroids, and/or rituximab. This treatment should only be conducted in highly specialized centers. There is less robust evidence in support of prophylactic measures such as tonsillectomy. Youth with a history of PANS should be closely monitored for infections following acute presentations (pharyngitis, dermatitis flares in the child or close contacts), and treated promptly with standard antibiotic regimens. Above all, for the general child and adolescent psychiatrist, when seeing a child with a very sudden onset of OCD, the treatment approach should be standard, but retaining an awareness of when to refer onto specialist services.

Conclusions

Public awareness of OCD has increased greatly over recent years, allowing this once "secret" disorder to be more readily recognized both by families and mental health professionals. The etiology of the disorder is a complex mix of common and rare genetic variants, that unfold against the context of environmental risk factors. The strides in understanding the neurobiology and neurocognitive features of the disorder are thus matched by definitive demonstrations of treatment efficacy in children. For the clinician, it is gratifying to see how children respond well and robustly to CBT, which can be boosted by a judicious use of SRI medications. While the management of those with more difficult-to-treat symptoms remains challenging, the strides being made in adult OCD promise the option of noninvasive neuromodulation for some youth. The efficacy of treatments makes it more important that children, parents, and health care professionals remain aware of the disorder and the availability of effective treatments.

References

Ahmari, S.E. *et al.* (2013) Repeated cortico-striatal stimulation generates persistent OCD-like behavior. *Science* **340**(6137), 1234–1239.

Alexander, G. *et al.* (1986) Parallel organization of functionally segregated circuits linking basal ganglia and cortex. *Annual Review of Neuroscience* **9**, 357–381.

American Psychiatric Association (2013) *Diagnostic and Statistical Manual of Mental Disorders*, 5th edn. American Psychiatric Association, Washington, DC.

Angelakis, I. *et al.* (2015) Suicidality in obsessive compulsive disorder (OCD): A systematic review and meta-analysis. *Clinical Psychology Review* **39**, 1–15.

Ardic, U.A. *et al.* (2017) Successful treatment response with aripiprazole augmentation of SSRIs in refractory obsessive–compulsive disorder in childhood. *Child Psychiatry & Human Development* **48**, 699–704.

Barrett, P. *et al.* (2003) Behavioral avoidance test for childhood obsessive-compulsive disorder: a home-based observation. *American Journal of Psychotherapy* **57**(1), 80–100.

Barrett, P. *et al.* (2004) Cognitive-behavioral family treatment of childhood obsessive-compulsive disorder: a controlled trial. *Journal of the American Academy of Child & Adolescent Psychiatry* **43**(1), 46–62.

Bellato, A. *et al.* (2021) A systematic review and meta-analysis of altered electrophysiological markers of performance monitoring in obsessive-compulsive disorder (OCD), Gilles de la Tourette syndrome (GTS), attention-deficit/hyperactivity disorder (ADHD) and autism. *Neuroscience & Biobehavioral Reviews* **131**, 964–987.

Bienvenu, O.J. *et al.* (2000) The relationship of obsessive-compulsive disorder to possible spectrum disorders: results from a family study. *Biological Psychiatry* **48**(4), 287–293.

Bienvenu, O. *et al.* (2012) Is obsessive-compulsive disorder an anxiety disorder, and what, if any, are spectrum conditions? A family study perspective. *Psychological Medicine* **42**(1), 1.

Bloch, M. *et al.* (2006) Adult outcome of tic and obsessive-compulsive severity in children with Tourette syndrome. *Archives of Pediatric and Adolescent Medicine* **160**, 65–69.

Bloch, M.H. *et al.* (2009) Predictors of early adult outcomes in pediatric-onset obsessive-compulsive disorder. *Pediatrics* **124**(4), 1085–1093.

Boedhoe, P.S.W. *et al.* (2017) Distinct subcortical volume alterations in pediatric and adult OCD: a worldwide meta-and mega-analysis. *American Journal of Psychiatry* **174**(1), 60–69.

Boedhoe, P.S. *et al.* (2020) Subcortical brain volume, regional cortical thickness, and cortical surface area across disorders: findings from the ENIGMA ADHD, ASD, and OCD working groups. *American Journal of Psychiatry* **177**(9), 834–843.

Brander, G. *et al.* (2016) Systematic review of environmental risk factors for obsessive-compulsive disorder: a proposed roadmap from association to causation. *Neuroscience & Biobehavioral Reviews* **65**, 36–62.

Calaprice, D. *et al.* (2018) Treatment of pediatric acute-onset neuropsychiatric disorder in a large survey population. *Journal of Child and Adolescent Psychopharmacology* **28**(2), 92–103.

Cappi, C. *et al.* (2020) De novo damaging DNA coding mutations are associated with obsessive-compulsive disorder and overlap with Tourette's disorder and autism. *Biological Psychiatry* **87**(12), 1035–1044.

Carmi, L. *et al.* (2019) Efficacy and safety of deep Transcranial magnetic stimulation for obsessive-compulsive disorder: a prospective multicenter randomized double-blind placebo-controlled trial. *The American Journal of Psychiatry* **176**(11), 931–938.

Chabane, N. *et al.* (2004) Early-onset obsessive-compulsive disorder: a subgroup with a specific clinical and familial pattern? *Journal of Child Psychology and Psychiatry* **46**, 881–887.

Chamberlain, B.L. & Ahmari, S.E. (2021) Animal models for OCD research. In: *The Neurobiology and Treatment of OCD: Accelerating Progress.* (eds N.A. Fineberg & T.W. Robbins). Springer, Cham, Switzerland. pp. 55–96.

Chang, K. *et al.* (2015) Clinical evaluation of youth with pediatric acute-onset neuropsychiatric syndrome (PANS): recommendations from the 2013 PANS consensus conference. *Journal of Child and Adolescent Psychopharmacology* **25**(1), 3–13.

Cheyette, S.R. & Cummings, J.L. (1995) Encephalitis lethargica: lessons for contemporary neuropsychiatry. *The Journal of Neuropsychiatry and Clinical Neurosciences* **7**(2), 125–134.

Cicek, E. *et al.* (2013) Quality of life, family burden and associated factors in relatives with obsessive–compulsive disorder. *General Hospital Psychiatry* **35**(3), 253–258.

Coluccia, A. *et al.* (2017) Quality of life in children and adolescents with obsessive–compulsive disorder: a systematic review and meta-analysis. *Neuropsychiatric Disease and Treatment* **13**, 597–608.

Cougle, J.R. *et al.* (2007) Perception of memory ability and confidence in recollections in obsessive-compulsive checking. *Journal of Anxiety Disorders* **21**(1), 118–130.

de Oliveira, A.R. *et al.* (2021) Lost in translation: no effect of repeated optogenetic cortico-striatal stimulation on compulsivity in rats. *Translational Psychiatry* **11**(1), 315.

Dell'Osso, B. *et al.* (2016) Childhood, adolescent and adult age at onset and related clinical correlates in obsessive–compulsive disorder: a report from the International College of Obsessive–Compulsive Spectrum Disorders (ICOCS). *International Journal of Psychiatry in Clinical Practice* **20**(4), 210–217.

Denys, D. *et al.* (2004a) Low level of dopaminergic D2 receptor binding in obsessive-compulsive disorder. *Biological Psychiatry* **55**(10), 1041–1045.

Denys, D. *et al.* (2004b) The role of dopamine in obsessive-compulsive disorder: preclinical and clinical evidence. *Journal of Clinical Psychiatry* **65**(Suppl 14), 11–17.

Destrée, L. *et al.* (2021) The effect of childhood trauma on the severity of obsessive-compulsive symptoms: a systematic review. *Journal of Psychiatric Research* **142**, 345–360.

Dunlop, K. *et al.* (2016) Reductions in cortico-striatal hyperconnectivity accompany successful treatment of obsessive-compulsive disorder with dorsomedial prefrontal rTMS. *Neuropsychopharmacology* **41**(5), 1395–1403.

Farhat, L.C. *et al.* (2022) Systematic review and meta-analysis: an empirical approach to defining treatment response and remission in pediatric obsessive-compulsive disorder. *Journal of the American Academy of Child and Adolescent Psychiatry* **61**(4), 495–507.

Figee, M. *et al.* (2017) 235. Deep brain stimulation modulates frontostriatal inhibitory control in obsessive-compulsive disorder. *Biological Psychiatry* **81**(10), S96–S97.

Fineberg, N.A. *et al.* (2019) Early intervention for obsessive compulsive disorder: an expert consensus statement. *European Neuropsychopharmacology* **29**(4), 549–565.

Fradkin, I. *et al.* (2020) Searching for an anchor in an unpredictable world: a computational model of obsessive compulsive disorder. *Psychological Review* **127**(5), 672.

Franklin, M.E. *et al.* (1998) Cognitive-behavioral treatment of pediatric obsessive-compulsive disorder: an open clinical trial. *Journal of the American Academy of Child & Adolescent Psychiatry* **37**(4), 412–419.

Freud, S. (1906) Obsessive actions and religious practices. In: *The Standard Edition of the Complete Psychological Works of Sigmund Freud.* (ed J.A. Strachey), Vol. 9. Hogarth Press, London. pp. 117–127.

Fullana, M. *et al.* (2009) Obsessions and compulsions in the community: prevalence, interference, help-seeking, developmental stability, and co-occurring psychiatric conditions. *American Journal of Psychiatry* **166**(3), 329–336.

Gehring, W.J. *et al.* (2000) Action-monitoring dysfunction in obsessive-compulsive disorder. *Psychological Science* **11**(1), 1–6.

Geller, D.A. *et al.* (1998) Obsessive-compulsive disorder in children and adolescents: a review. *Harvard Review of Psychiatry* **5**(5), 260–273.

Geller, D.A. *et al.* (2003) Which SSRI? A meta-analysis of pharmacotherapy trials in pediatric obsessive-compulsive disorder. *American Journal of Psychiatry* **160**(11), 1919–1928.

Gershkovich, M. *et al.* (2021) Integrating exposure and response prevention with a mobile app to treat obsessive-compulsive disorder: feasibility, acceptability, and preliminary effects. *Behavior Therapy* **52**(2), 394–405.

Gilbert, D.L. (2019) Inflammation in tic disorders and obsessive-compulsive disorder: are PANS and PANDAS a path forward? *Journal of Child Neurology* **34**(10), 598–611.

Gillan, C.M. & Sahakian, B.J. (2015) Which is the driver, the obsessions or the compulsions, in OCD? *Neuropsychopharmacology* **40**(1), 247.

Gillan, C.M. *et al.* (2015) Functional neuroimaging of avoidance habits in obsessive-compulsive disorder. *American Journal of Psychiatry* **172**(3), 284–293.

Gillan, C.M. *et al.* (2016) The role of habit in compulsivity. *European Neuropsychopharmacology* **26**(5), 828–840.

Gillan, C.M. *et al.* (2017) A trans-diagnostic perspective on obsessive-compulsive disorder. *Psychological Medicine* **47**(9), 1528–1548.

Gross-Isseroff, R. *et al.* (2004) Serotonergic dissection of obsessive compulsive symptoms: a challenge study with m-chlorophenylpiperazine and sumatriptan. *Neuropsychobiology* **50**(3), 200–205.

Guzick, A.G. *et al.* (2021) Obsessive–compulsive disorder during the COVID-19 pandemic: a systematic review. *Current Psychiatry Reports* **23**, 1–10.

Hollander, E. *et al.* (2016) The cost and impact of compulsivity: a research perspective. *European Neuropsychopharmacology* **26**(5), 800–809.

Hudziak, J.J. *et al.* (2004) Genetic and environmental contributions to the Child Behavior Checklist Obsessive-Compulsive Scale: a cross-cultural twin study. *Archives of General Psychiatry* **61**(6), 608.

Ivarsson, T. & Valderhaug, R. (2006) Symptom patterns in children and adolescents with obsessive-compulsive disorder (OCD). *Behaviour Research and Therapy* **44**(8), 1105–1116.

James, S.C. *et al.* (2017) Description and prevalence of OCD in children and adolescents. In: *The Wiley Handbook of Obsessive Compulsive Disorders.* (eds J.S. Abramowitz, *et al.*), Vol. 1. Wiley Blackwell, Oxford, UK. pp. 5–23.

Jonnal, A.H. *et al.* (2000) Obsessive and compulsive symptoms in a general population sample of female twins. *American Journal of Medical Genetics* **96**(6), 791–796.

Karno, M. *et al.* (1988) The epidemiology of obsessive-compulsive disorder in five US communities. *Archives of General Psychiatry* **45**, 1094–1099.

Kaufman, J. *et al.* (1997) Schedule for Affective Disorders and Schizophrenia for School-Age Children-Present and Lifetime Version (K-SADS-PL): initial reliability and validity data. *Journal of the American Academy of Child and Adolescent Psychiatry* **36**, 980–988.

Kenwright, M. *et al.* (2005) Brief scheduled phone support from a clinician to enhance computer-aided self-help for obsessive-compulsive disorder: randomized controlled trial. *Journal of Clinical Psychology* **61**(12), 1499–1508.

Kotapati, V.P. *et al.* (2019) The effectiveness of selective serotonin reuptake inhibitors for treatment of obsessive-compulsive disorder in adolescents and children: a systematic review and meta-analysis. *Frontiers in Psychiatry* **10**, 523.

Laplane, D. *et al.* (1989) Obsessive-compulsive and other behavioural changes with bilateral basal ganglia lesions: a neuropsychological, magnetic resonance imaging and positron tomography study. *Brain* **112**(3), 699–725.

Lebowitz, E.R. *et al.* (2012) Family accommodation in obsessive-compulsive disorder. *Expert Review of Neurotherapeutics* **12**(2), 229–238.

Lebowitz, E.R. *et al.* (2016) Family accommodation in obsessive-compulsive and anxiety disorders: a five-year update. *Expert Review of Neurotherapeutics* **16**(1), 45–53.

Leckman, J.F. *et al.* (1994) Tic-related vs. non-tic-related obsessive compulsive disorder. *Anxiety* **1**(5), 208–215.

Leckman, J.F. *et al.* (2009) Symptom dimensions and subtypes of obsessive-compulsive disorder: a developmental perspective. *Dialogues in Clinical Neuroscience* **11**(1), 21.

Leckman, J.F. *et al.* (2010) Obsessive–compulsive disorder: a review of the diagnostic criteria and possible subtypes and dimensional specifiers for DSM-V. *Depression and Anxiety* **27**(6), 507–527.

Lee, P.H. *et al.* (2019) Genomic relationships, novel loci, and pleiotropic mechanisms across eight psychiatric disorders. *Cell* **179**(7), 1469–1482. e1411

Leonard, H.L. (1989) Childhood rituals and superstitions: developmental and cultural perspective. In: *Obsessive-Compulsive Disorder in Children & Adolescents.* (ed J.L. Rapoport). American Psychiatric Press, Washington, DC. pp. 289–309.

Leonard, H.L. *et al.* (1991) A double-blind desipramine substitution during long-term clomipramine treatment in children and adolescents with obsessive-compulsive disorder. *Archives of General Psychiatry* **48**(10), 922–927.

Leonard, H.L. *et al.* (1992) Tics and Tourette's disorder: a 2- to 7-year follow-up of 54 obsessive-compulsive children. *The American Journal of Psychiatry* **149**(9), 1244–1251.

Leonard, H.L. *et al.* (1999) Postinfectious and other forms of obsessive-compulsive disorder. *Child and Adolescent Psychiatric Clinics of North America* **8**(3), 497–511.

Lewis-Fernández, R. *et al.* (2011) Culture and the anxiety disorders: recommendations for DSM-V. *Focus* **9**(3), 351–368.

Loosen, A.M. & Hauser, T.U. (2020) Towards a computational psychiatry of juvenile obsessive-compulsive disorder. *Neuroscience & Biobehavioral Reviews* **118**, 631–642.

Maina, G. *et al.* (1999) Obsessive-compulsive syndromes in older adolescents. *Acta Psychiatrica Scandinavica* **100**(6), 447–450.

Marazziti, D. & Pozza, A. (2022) An overview of the pharmacological options for pediatric obsessive-compulsive disorder. *Expert Opinion on Pharmacotherapy* **23**(16), 1793–1800.

March, J.S. & Mulle, K. (1998) *OCD in Children and Adolescents: A Cognitive-Behavioral Treatment Manual.* Guilford Press, New York.

Masi, G. *et al.* (2005) A naturalistic study of referred children and adolescents with obsessive-compulsive disorder. *Journal of the American Academy of Child and Adolescent Psychiatry* **44**(7), 673–681.

Masi, G. *et al.* (2010) A naturalistic exploratory study of the impact of demographic, phenotypic and comorbid features in pediatric obsessive-compulsive disorder. *Psychopathology* **43**(2), 69–78.

Mataix-Cols, D. *et al.* (2005) A multidimensional model of obsessive-compulsive disorder. *The American Journal of Psychiatry* **162**(2), 228–238.

McDougle, C.J. *et al.* (2000) A double-blind, placebo-controlled study of risperidone addition in serotonin reuptake inhibitor–refractory obsessive-compulsive disorder. *Archives of General Psychiatry* **57**(8), 794–801.

McGuire, J.F. *et al.* (2015) A meta-analysis of cognitive behavior therapy and medication for child obsessive–compulsive disorder: moderators of treatment efficacy, response, and remission. *Depression and Anxiety* **32**(8), 580–593.

Modell, J.G. *et al.* (1989) Neurophysiologic dysfunction in basal ganglia/limbic striatal and thalamocortical circuits as a pathogenetic mechanism of obsessive-compulsive disorder. *The Journal of Neuropsychiatry and Clinical Neurosciences* **1**, 27–36.

Murphy, T.K. *et al.* (2014) Pediatric acute-onset neuropsychiatric syndrome. *Psychiatric Clinics* **37**(3), 353–374.

National Institute of Health and Care Excellence (2005) *Obsessive-Compulsive Disorder and Body Dysmorphic Disorder: Treatment.* Clinical guideline CG31. National Institute for Health and Care Excellence (NICE), London.

Nestadt, G. *et al.* (2000) A family study of obsessive-compulsive disorder. *Archives of General Psychiatry* **57**(4), 358–363.

Norman, L.J. *et al.* (2018) Frontostriatal dysfunction during decision making in attention-deficit/hyperactivity disorder and obsessive-compulsive disorder. *Biological Psychiatry: Cognitive Neuroscience and Neuroimaging* **3**(8), 694–703.

Norman, L.J. *et al.* (2019) Error processing and inhibitory control in obsessive-compulsive disorder: a meta-analysis using statistical parametric maps. *Biological Psychiatry* **85**(9), 713–725.

Ortiz, A. *et al.* (2016) Clinical significance of psychiatric comorbidity in children and adolescents with obsessive–compulsive disorder: subtyping a complex disorder. *European Archives of Psychiatry and Clinical Neuroscience* **266**, 199–208.

Pauls, D.L. (2022) The genetics of obsessive-compulsive disorder: a review. *Dialogues in Clinical Neuroscience* **12**(2), 149–163.

Pauls, D.L. *et al.* (1995) A family study of obsessive-compulsive disorder. *The American Journal of Psychiatry* **152**(1), 76–84.

Pérez-Vigil, A. *et al.* (2018) Association of obsessive-compulsive disorder with objective indicators of educational attainment: a nationwide register-based sibling control study. *JAMA Psychiatry* **75**(1), 47–55.

Perlmutter, S.J. *et al.* (1999) Therapeutic plasma exchange and intravenous immunoglobulin for obsessive-compulsive disorder and tic disorders in childhood. *The Lancet* **354**(9185), 1153–1158.

Piantadosi, S.C. *et al.* (2021) Transcriptome alterations are enriched for synapse-associated genes in the striatum of subjects with obsessive-compulsive disorder. *Translational Psychiatry* **11**(1), 171.

Pitman, R.K. (1987) A cybernetic model of obsessive-compulsive psychopathology. *Comprehensive Psychiatry* **28**(4), 334–343.

Pogarell, O. *et al.* (2003) Elevated brain serotonin transporter availability in patients with obsessive-compulsive disorder. *Biological Psychiatry* **54**(12), 1406–1413.

POTS (2004) Cognitive-behavior therapy, sertraline, and their combination for children and adolescents with obsessive-compulsive disorder: the Pediatric OCD Treatment Study (POTS) randomized controlled trial. *JAMA* **292**(16), 1969–1976.

Pozza, A. *et al.* (2019) Perfectionism and intolerance of uncertainty are predictors of OCD symptoms in children and early adolescents: a prospective, cohort, one-year, follow-up study. *Clinical Neuropsychiatry* **16**(1), 53.

Rapoport, J.L. *et al.* (2000) Childhood obsessive-compulsive disorder in the NIMH MECA study: parent versus child identification of cases. Methods for the epidemiology of child and adolescent mental disorders. *Journal of Anxiety Disorders* **14**(6), 535–548.

Rettew, D.C. *et al.* (1992) Obsessions and compulsions across time in 79 children and adolescents with obsessive-compulsive disorder. *Journal of the American Academy of Child and Adolescent Psychiatry* **31**(6), 1050–1056.

Riesel, A. (2019) The erring brain: error-related negativity as an endophenotype for OCD—a review and meta-analysis. *Psychophysiology* **56**(4), e13348.

Rosario, M.C. *et al.* (2009) Validation of the University of Sao Paulo sensory phenomena scale: initial psychometric properties. *CNS Spectrums* **14**(6), 315–323.

Rosenberg, D.R. *et al.* (2000) Decrease in caudate glutamatergic concentrations in pediatric obsessive-compulsive disorder patients taking paroxetine. *Journal of the American Academy of Child & Adolescent Psychiatry* **39**(9), 1096–1103.

Rosenberg, D.R. *et al.* (2004) Reduced anterior cingulate glutamatergic concentrations in childhood OCD and major depression versus healthy controls. *Journal of the American Academy of Child & Adolescent Psychiatry* **43**(9), 1146–1153.

Rozenman, M. *et al.* (2019) Improvement in anxiety and depression symptoms following cognitive behavior therapy for pediatric obsessive compulsive disorder. *Psychiatry Research* **276**, 115–123.

Ruscio, A.M. *et al.* (2010) The epidemiology of obsessive-compulsive disorder in the National Comorbidity Survey Replication. *Molecular Psychiatry* **15**(1), 53–63.

Saraiva, L.C. *et al.* (2020) Cutting-edge genetics in obsessive-compulsive disorder. *Faculty Reviews* **9**, 30.

Saxena, S. & Rauch, S.L. (2000) Functional neuroimaging and the neuroanatomy of obsessive-compulsive disorder. *Psychiatric Clinics of North America* **23**(3), 563–586.

Saxena, S. *et al.* (2001) Brain-behavior relationships in obsessive-compulsive disorder. *Seminars in Clinical Neuropsychiatry* **6**(2), 82–101.

Sheehan, D.V. *et al.* (2010) Reliability and validity of the mini international neuropsychiatric interview for children and adolescents (MINI-KID). *The Journal of Clinical Psychiatry* **71**(3), 17393.

Simpson, H.B. *et al.* (2003) Serotonin transporters in obsessive-compulsive disorder: A positron emission tomography study with [(11)C]McN 5652. *Biological Psychiatry* **54**(12), 1414–1421.

Smárason, O. *et al.* (2023) Long-term functional impairment in pediatric OCD after and during treatment: an analysis of distinct trajectories. *Psychiatry Research* **324**, 115223.

Stern, E.R. *et al.* (2013) Subjective uncertainty and limbic hyperactivation in obsessive-compulsive disorder. *Human Brain Mapping* **34**(8), 1956–1970.

Stewart, S.E. *et al.* (2004) Long-term outcome of pediatric obsessive-compulsive disorder: a meta-analysis and qualitative review of the literature. *Acta Psychiatrica Scandinavica* **110**(1), 4–13.

Storch, E.A. *et al.* (2010) A preliminary study of D-cycloserine augmentation of cognitive-behavioral therapy in pediatric obsessive-compulsive disorder. *Biological Psychiatry* **68**(11), 1073.

Strom, N.I. *et al.* (2021) Genome-wide association study identifies new locus associated with OCD. *medRxiv* 2021.2010. 2013.21261078.

Strom, N.I. *et al.* (2022) Genome-wide association study of obsessive-compulsive symptoms including 33,943 individuals from the general population. *medRxiv* 2022.2011. 2030.22282898.

Suetens, K. *et al.* (2014) Differences in metabolic network modulation between capsulotomy and deep-brain stimulation for refractory obsessive-compulsive disorder. *Journal of Nuclear Medicine* **55**(6), 951–959.

Swedo, S. *et al.* (1989) Obsessive-compulsive disorder in children and adolescents: Clinical phenomenology of 70 consecutive cases. *Archives of General Psychiatry* **46**(4), 335–341.

Swedo, S. *et al.* (2004) The pediatric autoimmune neuropsychiatric disorders associated with streptococcal infection (PANDAS) subgroup: Separating fact from fiction. *Pediatrics* **113**(4), 907–911.

Swedo, S. *et al.* (2012) From research subgroup to clinical syndrome: modifying the PANDAS criteria to describe PANS (pediatric acute-onset neuropsychiatric syndrome). *Pediatrics & Therapeutics* **2**(2).

Swedo, S.E. *et al.* (2017) Overview of treatment of pediatric acute-onset neuropsychiatric syndrome. *Journal of Child and Adolescent Psychopharmacology* **27**(7), 562–565.

Valleni-Basile, L.A. *et al.* (1994) Frequency of obsessive-compulsive disorder in a community sample of young adolescents. *Journal of the American Academy of Child & Adolescent Psychiatry* **33**(6), 782–791.

van den Heuvel, O.A. *et al.* (2016) Brain circuitry of compulsivity. *European Neuropsychopharmacology* **26**(5), 810–827.

Voelker, R. (2018) Brain stimulation approved for obsessive-compulsive disorder. JAMA 320(11), 1098.

Weeland, C.J. *et al.* (2022) Thalamic subregions and obsessive-compulsive symptoms in 2,500 children from the general population. *Journal of the American Academy of Child & Adolescent Psychiatry* **61**(2), 321–330.

Wise, S.P. & Rapoport, J.L. (1989) Obsessive compulsive disorder: Is it a basal ganglia dysfunction? In: *Obsessive-Compulsive Disorder in Children and Adolescents*. (ed J.L. Rapoport). American Psychiatric Press, New York. pp. 327–344.

World Health Organization (2019) *International Statistical Classification of Disease and Related Health Problems*, 11th edn, World Health Organization (WHO), Geneva, Switzerland.

Zhang, T. *et al.* (2023) Prenatal and early childhood infections and subsequent risk of obsessive-compulsive disorder and tic disorders: a nationwide, sibling-controlled study. *Biological Psychiatry* **93**(11), 1023–1030.

CHAPTER 61

Body dysmorphic disorder

Georgina Krebs[1,2] and David Mataix-Cols[3,4,5]

[1] Research Department of Clinical, Educational and Health Psychology, University College London, London, UK

[2] Anxiety, self-Image and Mood (AIM) Clinic, North London NHS Foundation Trust, London, UK

[3] Centre for Psychiatry Research, Department of Clinical Neuroscience, Karolinska Institutet, Stockholm, Sweden

[4] Stockholm Health Care Services, Region Stockholm, CAP Research Centre, Stockholm, Sweden

[5] Department of Clinical Sciences, Lund University, Lund, Sweden

Introduction

Body dysmorphic disorder (BDD) is a strikingly underresearched disorder, particularly among young people. However, it is increasingly being recognized as a relatively common condition that can have a profoundly negative impact on young people's lives. In recent years, BDD has received increased empirical attention, leading to a better understanding of the phenomenology, epidemiology, and treatment of this condition in youth. This chapter aims to provide an overview of current knowledge regarding the characteristics of BDD in youth, its epidemiology, and its etiology. In addition, guidance is provided to aid the clinical assessment and treatment of BDD in young people. Last, key knowledge gaps are identified and areas for future research are proposed.

Characteristics and diagnosis of body dysmorphic disorder

Core features

The cardinal feature of BDD is an excessive preoccupation with perceived flaws in physical appearance, which are not visible to other people or appear as very minor. For example, a person with BDD might be excessively worried that their nose is deformed, when in fact it appears "normal" to others. Appearance concerns in BDD can relate to any body part, but facial features are the most common focus (Box 61.1 and Figure 61.1). Most people with BDD have multiple appearance concerns, and typically describe themselves as looking "ugly," "hideous," "deformed," "abnormal," or even "inhuman."

In an effort to cope with their appearance concerns, young people with BDD typically engage in time-consuming, repetitive behaviors, which are often aimed at checking, concealing, or correcting perceived flaws in their physical appearance (Box 61.1 and Figure 61.2). For example, a young person with BDD might spend hours every day checking their appearance in the mirror or other reflective surfaces. They may try to conceal their perceived flaws, for example, with excessive makeup or clothing, and they may try to correct their perceived flaws with excessive use of cosmetic products and procedures.

Another striking feature of BDD is that insight is often poor. Some young people have good insight and recognize that their appearance beliefs may be unreasonable or excessive. However, approximately half of young people with BDD have poor or absent insight, and are convinced that they have a physical defect in their appearance (Rautio *et al.*, 2022b). Not only does insight vary between individuals, but it is also a dynamic construct and can fluctuate considerably over relatively short periods of time (Schulte *et al.*, 2021).

Impact of body dysmorphic disorder

BDD can have a profound and pervasive impact on young people's lives. In extreme cases, young people can withdraw completely and become housebound. A substantial proportion of young people with BDD (as high as 44% in treatment-seeking samples) experience psychiatric inpatient admission (Phillips *et al.*, 2006). Although BDD can affect all aspects of a young person's life, research has indicated that the greatest functional impairment is typically in school and social activities (Rautio *et al.*, 2022b). Clinical studies have found that approximately one-quarter to one-third of young people with BDD drop out of school because of their BDD (Phillips *et al.*, 2006; Rautio *et al.*, 2022b). Social functioning is often negatively affected by BDD because sufferers are fearful of being judged negatively by

Rutter's Child and Adolescent Psychiatry and Psychology, Seventh Edition.

Edited by Anita Thapar, Daniel S. Pine, Samuele Cortese, Cathy Creswell, Tamsin J. Ford, James F. Leckman, and Argyris Stringaris.

Companion website: www.wiley.com/go/thapar/ruttерspsych7

Box 61.1 Prototypical case examples of body dysmorphic disorder in youth

Case example 1

Saskia (pseudonym) is a 15-year-old Black British girl, with a history of anorexia nervosa, for which she had received treatment. Her weight had been restored to the normal range and she was eating a healthy diet. She had some residual concerns about her body weight and shape, but these were no longer preoccupying or impacting on her day-to-day life. However, she disclosed to her therapist that she continued to feel very worried about her appearance and felt "ugly." In particular, she worried that her lips were too big, her eyes were too small, and her nose was too broad. Upon clinical examination, these features appeared to be within the normal range of variation. She was spending up to two hours every day applying heavy contouring make up and mascara, and would frequently check her appearance using her phone. Consequentially, she was struggling to get to school on time and often missing lessons. She was also withdrawing from social activities and spending large amounts of time in her bedroom researching rhinoplasty and other cosmetic procedures online, and comparing her appearance to others on social media. She expressed being "200%" convinced that there was something very wrong with her appearance. She felt that the only solution to her problems would be surgery and was hesitant attending child and adolescent mental health services (CAMHS).

Commentary

Although Saskia had some residual body image disturbance related to her prior eating disorder, she had several other appearance concerns that were clearly distinct (i.e., related to her face, not body weight or body shape). She met diagnostic criteria for body dysmorphic disorder (BDD) because these appearance concerns were associated with repetitive behaviors and avoidance, and resulted in impairment in education and social functioning. Her insight was deemed to be poor to absent, given her reluctance to consider the idea that her concerns may be emotional in origin.

Case example 2

Dhilan (pseudonym) is a 17-year-old Asian British boy, who had become increasingly withdrawn over the last year. He had previously been very sociable but no longer met up with friends outside school, and instead was spending several hours every day exercising, particularly weightlifting. His dietary habits had also changed, and he was eating large quantities of eggs and meat. His parents also noticed that he had started to wear many layers of clothing, regardless of the weather. On a recent family holiday, Dhilan avoided the swimming pool and spent most of his time indoors. His parents became very concerned about Dhilan when he told them he had experienced low mood and thoughts that his life was not worth living. Dhilan attended a mental health assessment, where he disclosed that he felt very self-conscious and distressed about his body build, and believed that he looked "puny." Upon questioning, he also described excessive concern about his skin looking oily and his teeth being crooked. After some discussion, he was able to admit that these concerns were excessive, and that other people probably do not see him as puny.

Commentary

Dhilan met diagnostic criteria for BDD, with good insight and muscle dysmorphia. The muscle dysmorphia specifier is characterized by a concern about lacking adequate muscularity, and behaviors aimed at increasing muscle bulk (e.g., excessive weightlifting and a high protein diet) or creating an illusion of a bigger build (wearing excessive layers). Dhilan's social functioning was substantially impaired and he was experiencing low mood and suicidal ideation as a consequence of his appearance concerns.

others. Consequently, young people tend to avoid social situations and may withdraw partially or completely from friendships and/or romantic relationships.

Most young people with BDD experience psychiatric comorbidity, with data from clinical and epidemiology samples showing that approximately 70% meet criteria for at least one additional diagnosis (Rautio *et al.*, 2022b; Krebs *et al.*, 2023a). Comorbid anxiety and mood disorders (e.g., major depressive disorder [MDD], social anxiety disorder) are particularly common, but attention deficit hyperactivity disorder (ADHD) and disruptive behaviors disorders (e.g., oppositional defiant disorder and conduct disorder) are not atypical and occur in approximately 10–20% of young people with BDD (Rautio *et al.*, 2022b; Krebs *et al.*, 2023a). Autism spectrum disorder (ASD) has been reported in approximately 16% of young people seen in specialist BDD clinics (Rautio *et al.*, 2022b).

Suicidality is also common among young people with BDD. In clinical samples, it has been reported that 11–44% have a history of attempted suicide (Phillips *et al.*, 2006; Rautio *et al.*, 2022b). To our knowledge, no studies on the prevalence of death by suicide have been published in either adults or young people with BDD.

Diagnostic classification

The earliest descriptions of BDD date back to 1891 (Morselli, 1891), but BDD was not included in the *Diagnostic and Statistical Manual of Mental Disorders* (DSM) until 1980 (DSM-III; American Psychiatric Association, 1980), or the *International Classification of Diseases* (ICD) until 1992 (ICD-10; World Health Organization, 1992). In these editions, BDD was classified as a somatoform disorder because of the focus on bodily concerns, and because very little was known about BDD with respect to patterns of comorbidity, etiology, or treatment options.

A major change in the field was the reclassification of BDD as an "obsessive–compulsive related disorder" in DSM-5 (American Psychiatric Association, 2013), along with obsessive–compulsive disorder (OCD), trichotillomania (hair-pulling disorder), excoriation (skin picking) disorder, and hoarding disorder. A few years later, ICD-11 followed suit (World Health Organization, 2019) and included BDD as a separate diagnostic category within a new obsessive–compulsive and related disorders chapter. The grouping of these disorders in the same chapter was largely based on that fact that they are all characterized by repetitive thoughts and behaviors that are believed to have certain commonalities with respect to etiology (e.g., shared genetic influences) and involve similar neurocircuitry (Phillips *et al.*, 2010; Marras *et al.*, 2016).

The reclassification of BDD has been widely considered as positive, primarily because specialist OCD clinics could easily justify treating BDD patients who would otherwise not have been eligible to receive specialist treatment. Nevertheless, there is ongoing debate regarding its classification (Abramowitz &

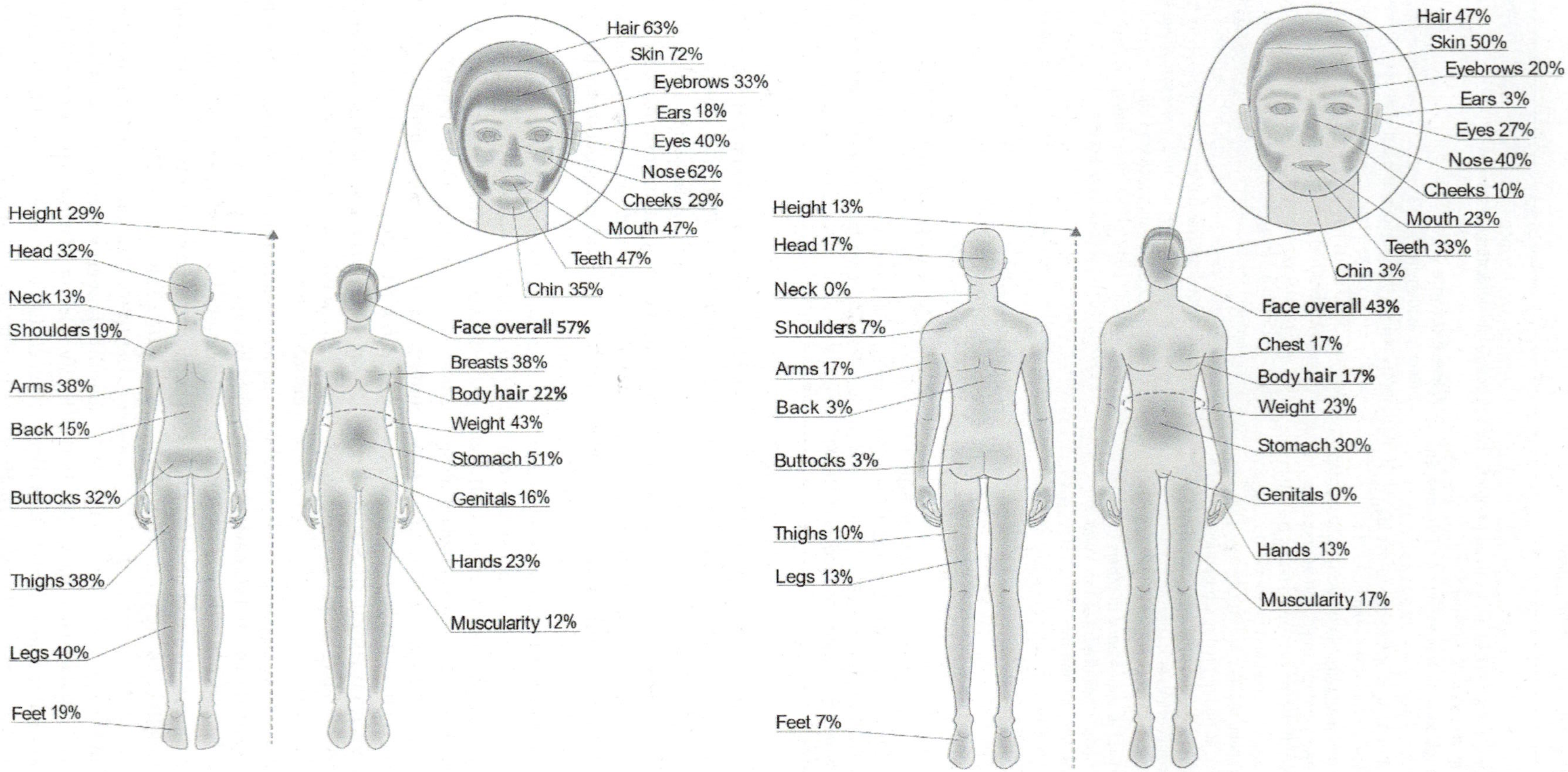

Figure 61.1 The focus of preoccupation among girls (left; $n = 129$) versus boys (right; $n = 30$) with body dysmorphic disorder (BDD). *Source:* Data are taken from Rautio *et al.* (2022b). Figure produced by Lily Wood.

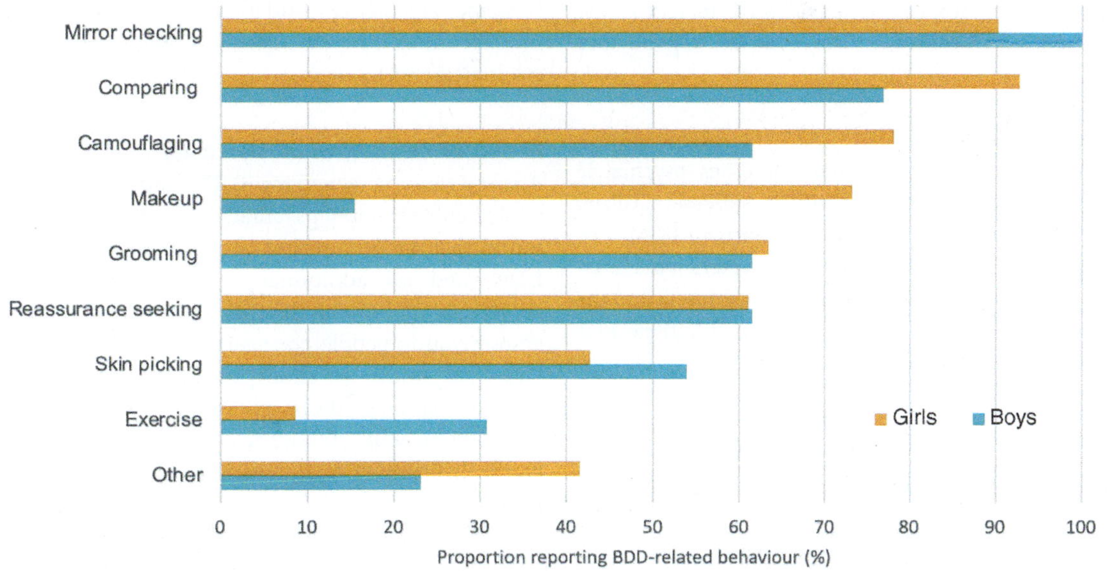

Figure 61.2 Body dysmorphic disorder (BDD)-related behaviors in girls ($n = 74$) versus boys ($n = 13$) with BDD. *Note*: "Other" includes, for example, searching information on cosmetic procedures on the Internet and taking pictures of oneself. *Source:* Data are taken from Rautio *et al.* (2022b).

Jacoby, 2015; Schneider *et al.*, 2018a; Hartmann *et al.*, 2020). For example, it has been suggested that BDD is better viewed as a body image disorder, along with eating disorders (Hartmann *et al.*, 2020). It has also been noted that BDD has commonalities with depression (Hartmann *et al.*, 2020) and social anxiety disorder (Kelly *et al.*, 2013).

Diagnostic criteria

The diagnostic criteria for BDD, as set out in DSM-5 (American Psychiatric Association, 2013) are:

- Criterion A: Preoccupation with one or more perceived defects or flaws in physical appearance that are not observable or appear slight to others.
- Criterion B: At some point during the course of the disorder, the individual has performed repetitive behaviors (e.g., mirror checking, excessive grooming, skin picking, reassurance seeking) or mental acts (e.g., comparing his or her appearance with that of others) in response to the appearance concerns.
- Criterion C: The preoccupation causes clinically significant distress or impairment in social, occupational, or other areas of functioning.
- Criterion D: The appearance preoccupation is not better explained by concerns with body fat or weight in an individual whose symptoms meet diagnostic criteria for an eating disorder.

DSM-5 also includes two specifiers for the diagnosis of BDD. The first is for muscle dysmorphia, which indicates that the individual is concerned about being too slight or lacking sufficient muscularity. Muscle dysmorphia is more common in boys than girls and is often associated with changes in dietary intake (e.g., eating a high-protein diet and taking protein supplements), excessive weightlifting, and anabolic-androgenic steroid use (Mitchison *et al.*, 2022; Rautio *et al.*, 2022b). Importantly, the DSM-5 muscle dysmorphia specifier can be assigned even if other appearance concerns are also present, which is in fact common. The second specifier relates to insight. Clinicians can indicate whether the individual's level of insight into their BDD-related beliefs is: (i) good or fair (they recognize that their beliefs may not be true or are definitely not true); (ii) poor (they think that their beliefs are probably true); and (iii) absent (they are completely convinced that their beliefs are true). BDD with poor/absent insight was previously viewed as a psychotic phenomenon, and in DSM-IV (American Psychiatric Association, 1994) a diagnosis of delusional disorder could be assigned in addition to BDD. This approach has been replaced by the insight specifier in DSM-5, partly to discourage clinicians from attempting to treat BDD with antipsychotic medications. Importantly, even young people with poor insight can benefit from evidence-based BDD treatment (Rautio *et al.*, 2022a).

The BDD diagnostic criteria set out in ICD-11 (World Health Organization, 2019) are broadly similar to DSM-5, but there are several differences. First, in addition to having *preoccupation* about perceived flaws in appearance, ICD-11 also require the presence of excessive *self-consciousness* about the perceived flaw(s). It is noted that this often includes a conviction that other people are taking notice, judging, or talking about the perceived flaws. Second, while DSM-5 highlights BDD-related repetitive behaviors as a necessary feature of the disorder in Criterion B, ICD-11 is broader and states that any of the following must be present: repetitive behaviors (e.g., mirror checking); attempts to camouflage or alter the perceived flaws (e.g., through cosmetic procedures); or marked avoidance of social or other situations. Third, insight is the only specifier in ICD-11, with two categories: fair to good; and poor to absent.

Differential diagnosis

BDD has similar features to a number of other psychiatric disorders (e.g., OCD, social anxiety disorder, depression, eating disorders) and conditions (e.g., gender dysphoria in DSM-5 or gender incongruence in ICD-11), which can present a diagnostic challenge. This can lead to BDD being misdiagnosed, and the delivery of inappropriate and ineffective treatment. Table 61.1 outlines the key similarities and differentiating features of BDD versus other conditions.

Epidemiology and longitudinal outcomes

Prevalence in community-based studies

There have been five nationwide studies examining the point prevalence of BDD in representative, population-based sample of adults in Germany (Rief, 2006; Buhlmann *et al.*, 2010; Schieber *et al.*, 2015), Sweden (Brohede *et al.*, 2015), and the United States (US) (Koran *et al.*, 2008). These have found prevalence estimates ranging between 1.7–3.2% among adults. Fewer studies have examined the prevalence of BDD in community samples of young people. The majority of these have been conducted in schools or colleges and estimated the point prevalence of probable BDD to be 1.7–3.6% (Schneider *et al.*, 2016; Möllmann *et al.*, 2017). In a larger study, the prevalence of clinically significant BDD symptoms was examined in a twin sample in Sweden, and estimated to be 1.0% among 15-year-olds (n = 6,968) and 2.0% among 18-year-olds (n = 3,738) (Enander *et al.*, 2018). However, it is important to note that these studies have all relied on brief self-report questionnaires to assess BDD symptoms, which may not correspond to clinical diagnostic assessments.

Recently, the prevalence of BDD has been examined in a large, representative, population-based sample of children and young people (CYP) aged 5–19 years in England (N = 7, 654). In this study, BDD and a wide range of other psychiatric disorders were assessed using a clinician-rated standardized diagnostic assessment. The overall point prevalence of DSM-5 BDD was estimated as 1.0%. Importantly, this study found substantial effects of age on BDD prevalence. BDD was relatively rare in children under 12 years of age (0.1%), but was significantly more common among adolescents (1.9%). There were also striking sex effects, with BDD affecting 3.4% of adolescent girls versus 0.4% of adolescent boys. This finding is consistent with a number of previous studies that have also shown BDD to be more common among girls than boys in community and clinical samples of young people (Mataix-Cols *et al.*, 2015; Enander *et al.*, 2018; Rautio *et al.*, 2022b). Interestingly, there is some indication that sex differences in the prevalence of BDD might reduce in early adulthood (Enander *et al.*, 2018), and it has been suggested that this may indicate later age of onset in males and/or sex-specific etiological mechanisms.

Prevalence in clinical settings

A study which screened for BDD symptoms in a sample of 208 adolescents receiving psychiatric inpatient treatment in the US found that 4.8% of young people met diagnostic criteria for BDD, and an additional 1.9% had possible BDD (Dyl *et al.*, 2006). Little is known about the frequency of BDD among young people accessing *outpatient* mental health services, but studies in adult populations indicate that BDD is common among those seeking treatment for depression (Nierenberg *et al.*, 2002), social anxiety (Wilhelm *et al.*, 1997), eating disorders (Dingemans *et al.*, 2012), and OCD (Wilhelm *et al.*, 1997).

BDD has also been shown to be common among individuals accessing cosmetic medical services. For example, a meta-analysis found the weighted prevalence of BDD to be approximately 11% in dermatology and 20% in rhinoplasty clinics (Veale *et al.*, 2016). However, all these studies are based on adult samples. To our knowledge, there have not been any studies examining the frequency of BDD among young people seeking cosmetic interventions, such as dermatology or orthognathic surgery, although this has been highlighted as an important clinical issue (Dennin & Lee, 2018).

Body dysmorphic disorder in specific population subgroups

An important question is whether the clinical presentation of BDD varies across different subgroups of the population, as such knowledge could assist in improving detection and diagnosis of the condition. For example, does BDD present differently in children versus adolescents, or boys versus girls? Few studies of BDD in youth have had large enough samples to enable comparisons of subgroups. The largest study of BDD in young people to date involved 136 girls and 32 boys attending specialist BDD clinics, of whom 43 were aged 10–14 years and 129 were aged 15–19 years (Rautio *et al.*, 2022b). In this study, the clinical presentation of BDD was largely similar across the younger and older age group, although the older group had more severe compulsive behaviors and were more likely to report a desire for cosmetic procedures. Similarly, the characteristics of BDD were broadly similarly across sexes, but with some notable differences (Figures 61.1 and 61.2). Girls reported significantly more areas of appearance concern. Furthermore, girls more frequently reported preoccupation with weight, while boys more frequently reported preoccupation with muscularity (referred to as "muscle dysmorphia").

Little is known about whether the phenomenology of BDD varies across different countries and ethnic groups. Available evidence suggests that there are likely to be more similarities than differences, but there is some suggestion that the focus of

Table 61.1 Differential diagnosis of body dysmorphic disorder (BDD).

Diagnosis	Similarities with body dysmorphic disorder (BDD)	Key differentiating features
Obsessive–compulsive disorder (OCD)	Time-consuming, repetitive behaviors which can include grooming rituals.	Unlike in BDD, grooming rituals in OCD are not driven by an attempt to correct perceived appearance flaws. They may instead be driven by contamination fears, "just right" urges, or a need for symmetry.
Social anxiety disorder	Fear of negative evaluation by others. Avoidance of and/or distress in social situations.	Social anxiety disorder involves a fear of saying or doing something to embarrass oneself. BDD involves anxiety that others will negatively judge and/or reject them based on their appearance.
Depression	Negative self-concept, which can include beliefs about being ugly.	Concerns about appearance are not the primary preoccupation in depression and are not associated with significant distress and impairment in their own right. They are not typically associated with the repetitive behaviors that are characteristic of BDD (e.g., mirror checking, grooming).
Eating disorders	Distressing and impairing preoccupation with appearance	Appearance preoccupation in eating disorders is focused on body weight and shape, leading to dysfunctional eating behaviors in an attempt to lose weight.
Excoriation disorder	Repetitive skin picking	Skin picking in excoriation disorder is not driven by an attempt to improve appearance, whereas skin picking in BDD is intended to improve the appearance of perceived defects in the skin.
Trichotillomania	Repetitive hair pulling	Hair pulling in trichotillomania is not driven by an attempt to improve appearance, whereas hair pulling in BDD is intended to improve the appearance (e.g., by removing facial or body hair, or specific hairs that are viewed as unattractive).
Gender dysphoria	Distressing and impairing preoccupation with body parts that are sex signifiers (e.g., breasts, genitalia). Often seeking surgery or other medical interventions to change appearance.	Gender dysphoria is typically associated with concerns about physical features being "not right," rather than ugly per se. The goal is generally removal of sex signifiers and rather than "correcting" flaws in appearance.
Psychotic disorders	Delusional beliefs	Unlike psychotic disorders, BDD involves prominent appearance preoccupations and associated repetitive behaviors. Disorganized behavior, hallucinations, and other psychotic symptoms are not features of BDD.

appearance concerns may relate to culturally defined standards for beauty. For example, one study in the US found that adults with BDD who were of Asian heritage were more likely to be preoccupied with concerns about their skin being too dark or their hair being too straight, compared to those who were White (Marques *et al.*, 2011a). Conversely, in the same study the White group were more likely to endorse concerns about their stomach, hips, waist, and buttocks than the Asian-American group. To our knowledge, there has not been any research examining the characteristics of BDD across ethnic groups in young people.

Age at onset of body dysmorphic disorder

BDD often has an insidious onset, with many patients reporting some concerns about their appearance dating back to childhood. Most commonly, appearance concerns start to become impairing and distressing, and eventually meet the threshold for a diagnosis of BDD, during adolescence. This is perhaps not surprising, given that adolescence is a period when young people experience substantial puberty-related body changes, as well as increased self-referential processing (Moses-Payne *et al.*, 2022) and heightened social sensitivity (Foulkes & Blakemore, 2016).

Among adults with BDD, approximately two-thirds retrospectively report onset before 18 years of age, with a mean age of 16.7 years (Bjornsson *et al.*, 2013). However, the most *common* (i.e., modal) age at BDD onset retrospectively by adults is 12–13 years (Bjornsson *et al.*, 2013). This aligns with the age of onset observed in clinical samples of young people with BDD. For example, among young people attending specialist BDD clinics, the mean age at onset was 12.5 years (Rautio *et al.*, 2022a). There is some evidence that earlier onset BDD (prior to 18 years) is associated with poorer outcomes in adulthood including greater psychiatric comorbidity, higher rates of suicidality, and poorer insight (Bjornsson *et al.*, 2013), highlighting the importance of early detection and diagnosis.

Course and long-term outcomes

Strikingly little is known about the natural course of BDD. To our knowledge, no long-term follow-up data from *untreated* individuals exist. However, the small number of existing studies that have examined long-term outcomes (Phillips *et al.*, 2013), and expert clinical consensus, suggest that the disorder is likely to follow a chronic course if left untreated.

Long-term follow-up data of *treated* young people with BDD are exceedingly rare but converge to suggest reasonable outcomes. In a follow-up study of adolescents ($N = 26$) who received cognitive behavioral therapy (CBT) for BDD as part of a clinical trial, gains were found to be maintained over a 12-month period (Krebs *et al.*, 2017b). At 12-month follow-up, 50% of participants were classified as responders and 23% as remitters according to empirically derived cutoffs (Fernández de la Cruz *et al.*, 2021). In a larger, naturalistic study of young people ($N = 140$) who received CBT for BDD with or without pharmacotherapy, 83% were classified as responders and 68% as full or partial remitters at 12-month follow-up (Rautio *et al.*, 2022a). Thus, the current evidence indicates that the prognosis of young people with BDD is reasonably positive when managed within a specialist multidisciplinary setting.

Time trends

It has been suggested that increasing sociocultural pressures relating to appearance, narrowly defined beauty ideals, and the rapid surge of image-based social media may have increased vulnerability to BDD and other body image problems, particularly among youth. To our knowledge, no studies to date have explored secular trends in BDD. There is preliminary evidence that appearance concerns in the broader sense have increased in recent years. For example, the Understanding Society survey has assessed happiness with appearance among young people in the United Kingdom (UK) on a yearly basis, and has shown that happiness with appearance significantly decreased between 2009 and 2020 among 10–15-year-olds (The Children's Society, 2022). However, it should be noted that happiness scores also decreased in other domains (namely, friendships, school, and life overall), suggesting a nonspecific effect.

Risk factors and pathological processes

The etiology of BDD is poorly understood, although research has started to shed light on possible mechanisms.

Genetic influences

The diathesis-stress model of BDD (Fang *et al.*, 2014) suggests that the disorder arises as a result of a complex interplay between biological predisposing factors, such as a genetic liability, and environmental stressors. Consistent with this, twin studies have confirmed both genetic and environmental factors account for variance in BDD symptoms (Monzani *et al.*, 2014; Lopez-Sola *et al.*, 2016; Enander *et al.*, 2018). The first twin study of BDD symptoms was conducted with a sample of adult, female twins in the UK ($N = 3{,}544$) (Monzani *et al.*, 2012a). This study found genetic factors to account for approximately 44% of the variance in BDD symptoms, with nonshared environmental factors accounting for the remaining 56% of variance (Monzani *et al.*, 2012a). Nonshared environmental factors are defined as environmental experiences that differ between members of a twin pair and give rise to phenotypic differences. This could include experiences within the family (e.g., differential experiences of parenting) or outside the family (e.g., bullying). Similar BDD heritability estimates have been obtained in independent twin cohorts in Australia (López-Solà *et al.*, 2014) and Sweden (Enander *et al.*, 2018), the latter of which included adolescents.

Of note, while the first twin study of BDD symptoms included females only (Monzani *et al.*, 2012a), both the Swedish and Australian studies have included both males and females (López-Solà *et al.*, 2014; Lopez-Sola *et al.*, 2016; Enander *et al.*, 2018).

The Australian twin study found a trend toward qualitative sex differences in genetic influences. If replicated, this could suggest that different biological processes underpin BDD symptoms in males versus females (López-Solà *et al.*, 2014).

Multivariate twin studies have also been conducted to examine the etiological relationship between BDD symptoms and psychiatric symptoms. These studies have shown that there is some overlap in the genetic factors that influence symptoms of BDD and other obsessive–compulsive-related disorders (OCD, hoarding disorder, trichotillomania, and skin-picking disorder) (Monzani *et al.*, 2014), and anxiety disorders (panic disorder, generalized anxiety disorder, and social anxiety disorder) (Lopez-Sola *et al.*, 2016). However, these studies also show *distinct* genetic influences on BDD, and in fact *most* (approximately 65%) of the genetic risk for BDD is not shared with other obsessive–compulsive-related disorders or anxiety disorders (Monzani *et al.*, 2014; Lopez-Sola *et al.*, 2016).

It is important to note that the twin studies described above all assessed BDD symptoms using the Dysmorphic Concerns Questionnaire (DCQ), a seven-item self-report questionnaire. Although the DCQ has been shown to be a valid and reliable measure of BDD symptoms (Oosthuizen *et al.*, 1998), it does not correspond directly to BDD diagnostic criteria (e.g., it does not explicitly ask about distress and impairment). The DCQ may also capture broader body dissatisfaction (e.g., body weight and shape concerns that might be associated with eating disorder psychopathology) and concerns relating to bodily dysfunction (e.g., body odor). An additional limitation of current genetic research on BDD is that there have not been any genomic studies (e.g., genome-wide association studies [GWAS]) to date, and therefore the specific genetic variants that may underpin BDD symptoms remain unknown.

Environmental influences

The twin studies described above demonstrate that the risk for developing BDD is not only due to genetic factors, and in fact nonshared environmental experiences might play an even bigger role in the development of the disorder. Identifying and understanding these environmental factors is crucial, since they may be modifiable and therefore indicate potential targets for prevention or early intervention.

Currently, little is known about the specific aspects of an individual's environment that may confer risk for BDD. Several putative environmental risk factors have been highlighted including peer victimization and childhood trauma (e.g., abuse and neglect). In a recent meta-analysis, BDD symptoms were found to have a small association with childhood abuse ($r = 0.22$) and experiences of bullying ($r = 0.28$), and a moderate association with experiences of teasing ($r = 0.42$) (Longobardi *et al.*, 2022). However, studies to date have major limitations including: (i) overreliance on retrospective and cross-sectional designs, meaning that the direction of effects cannot be inferred; (ii) use of convenience samples which may be biased and not representative; and (iii) failure to control for key potential confounders, including genetic influences. Genetic confounding is important because research has shown that experiences such as exposure to trauma and bullying are not purely "environmental," but also under some genetic influence (i.e., gene–environment correlation) (Knafo & Jaffee, 2013). If some of these genetic influences also play a role in the development of BDD, this could confound the association between the exposure to trauma/bullying/teasing and BDD.

There is much speculation about the role of sociocultural influences on BDD. It has been suggested that exposure to narrowly defined beauty standards may predispose individuals to develop body image problems, such as BDD. Similarly, growing up in an appearance-focused culture where young people are frequently exposed to highly curated and enhanced images, for example, through social media, may be a risk factor for developing appearance-related anxiety. There has been strikingly little research of sociocultural factors in relation to BDD. Existing evidence is limited to correlational studies showing an association of BDD symptoms with sociocultural attitudes toward appearance, perceived media pressure, and use of image-based social media use (Ahmadpanah *et al.*, 2019; Alsaidan *et al.*, 2020; Ryding & Kuss, 2020). Prospective and experimental studies are needed to determine where there is a causal effect of these environmental factors on BDD.

Assessment

BDD is strikingly underdetected and underdiagnosed in clinical settings. For example, in one study 122 adult and adolescent psychiatric inpatients were systematically screened for BDD, and although 13% met diagnostic criteria for BDD, none had received this diagnosis as part of their routine clinical care (Grant *et al.*, 2001). The reasons that BDD often goes undetected are likely to be multifaceted, and may include: a tendency for individuals with BDD to desire and seek cosmetic procedures rather than mental health support; limited awareness and knowledge of BDD among some mental health clinicians; dismissing BDD-related appearance concerns as being a normal adolescent phase; and reluctance of people with BDD to disclose their symptoms. Young people with BDD are often hesitant to disclose their symptoms due to embarrassment or a fear of sounding vain. In addition, they may be concerned that if they tell a clinician about their appearance concerns, it will attract attention to their perceived flaws (e.g., if they say they are worried about having a crooked nose, the clinician's attention will automatically be drawn to their nose). This means that even when young people with BDD do present to mental health services, they often describe their distress and functional impairment, rather than their core appearance concerns and related behaviors, which may lead to misdiagnosis (e.g., depression, social anxiety).

Encouragingly, although young people with BDD rarely disclose their appearance concerns *spontaneously*, the majority will *if directly asked*. For example, one study found that 97% of young people with

BDD positively endorsed a brief BDD screening item, asking about appearance worries (Buckley *et al.*, 2018). Of course, a broad screening question such as this will result in "false positives" and therefore requires follow-up with more detailed assessment.

Given that BDD often goes undiagnosed, it is important that clinicians are vigilant to signs and "clues" of BDD. Some clues, such as social avoidance and high levels of self-criticism, are not specific to BDD and could be indicative of other psychiatric disorders. Nevertheless, in such cases, directly asking about appearance concerns is important. Other clues are more BDD-specific, for example, buying or requesting a large quantity of cosmetic products, or expressing a desire for cosmetic procedures. Additionally, many young people with BDD will engage in certain appearance-related compulsive behaviors during a clinical assessment (see section on "Behavioral observations" below).

Overview of body dysmorphic disorder assessment

An initial BDD assessment should involve the key components of a standard mental health assessment for young people (see Chapter 27), and typically involve the young person and at a least one parent or guardian. The clinician should start by obtaining a brief description of the main concerns from both the young person's and parents' perspectives, being aware that these views may differ. Parents may underestimate their child's emotional distress and dismiss appearance concerns as a normal developmental phase. Conversely, parents may be extremely concerned about their child's mental health, while the young person minimizes their symptoms due to embarrassment, shame, or limited insight. Sensitively acknowledging both perspectives and adopting a curious and open-minded stance is key.

After establishing the main concerns, subsequent assessment should include a history of the presenting problem, as well as a developmental, medical, and family history. Clinicians should additionally assess for specific family factors which may perpetuate a young person's BDD. In particular, parents may facilitate avoidance, provide excessive reassurance about appearance, or supply large quantities of cosmetic product in an attempt to reduce their child's distress, but inadvertently fuel BDD (Jassi *et al.*, 2020).

A detailed assessment of the current BDD symptoms should be carried out directly with the young person. This is often best achieved without the parent or guardian present, to minimize embarrassment and anxiety. Examples of questions that can be asked, corresponding to DSM-5 diagnostic criteria for BDD, are shown in Box 61.2. Assessment should additionally involve a mental state examination with special attention given to suicidality and common co-occurring disorders such as MDD, social anxiety disorder, OCD, and eating disorders.

Behavioral observations

Given that young people are often hesitant about disclosing their BDD symptoms, it is important that clinicians are vigilant to behavioral clues during the assessment. These might include:

- wearing a hood, hat, or sunglasses inside
- wearing a coat and/or multiple layers despite the ambient temperature being warm
- covering parts of their face with their hands or an item of clothing (e.g., a scarf pulled up over their mouth)
- wearing heavy or unusual makeup, or tanning product
- sitting in an unusual position
- touching their face, hair, or body repeatedly

Box 61.2 Examples of questions to ask when assessing for body dysmorphic disorder, corresponding to DSM-5 criteria

Criterion A (preoccupation):

- Most people worry about how they look from time to time, but some people have worries about their appearance that take up a lot of their time and really upset them. Does this happen to you?

If yes:

- Can you tell me what aspects of your appearance worry you most?
- Do you think about this a lot? How much is it on your mind during an average day? What's the longest you go without thinking about your appearance?

Criterion B (repetitive behaviors):

- Do you find yourself spending a lot of time doing things to try to hide, change, or check your appearance?
- Do you spend a lot of time doing things in your head, like comparing your appearance to others?

***If yes*:**

How much time in an average day do you spend *[summary of repetitive behavior and mental acts that young person has described]*?

***If no*:**

Has there ever been a period in the past when you spent a lot of time doing things to try to hide, change, check, or compare your appearance?

Criterion C (distress and impairment):

- How much do these worries about your appearance upset you? Do they make you feel very sad, or very anxious?
- Do these worries about your appearance get in the way of day-to-day life?
- Do you avoid anything due to these worries?

Muscle dysmorphia specifier:

- Do you spend a lot of time worrying that your body build is too small or that you are not muscular enough? Do you spend a lot of time trying to build your muscles, e.g., weightlifting at the gym?

Insight specifier:

- You have done really well to explain some of the specific worries that you have about your appearance. If you had to describe your appearance in a single word, what word would you choose?
- How convinced are you that you look *[use young person's descriptor]*? Do you think other people see you the same way?

Note: during the assessment the clinician should additionally assess **Criterion D**, to determine that the appearance concerns are not better accounted for by an eating disorder.

- looking at their reflection in the window or their phone frequently
- taking frequent or long bathroom breaks (to check/adjust their appearance).

Measures for assessing body dysmorphic disorder

Several measures have been developed and validated for assessing BDD symptom severity in young people, and can form an important part of the assessment process and also assist in monitoring progress during treatment. The gold-standard measure is the BDD version of the Yale-Brown Obsessive–Compulsive Scale (BDD-YBOCS). This is a clinician-administered measure of BDD symptom severity, and is widely used in randomized controlled trials (RCTs) as the primary outcome measure (Harrison *et al.*, 2016). The BDD-YBOCS has been adapted for adolescents (BDD-YBOCS-A), although it retains the same format. Both the adult and adolescent versions include 12 items which assess appearance preoccupation, appearance-related compulsive behaviors, insight into appearance beliefs, and avoidance due to BDD symptoms. Each item is rated on a 0–4 scale, producing a total BDD severity score ranging between 0–48, with higher scores reflecting higher symptom severity. The scale has been shown to have good internal consistency, convergent validity, and sensitivity to change over treatment (Monzani *et al.*, 2022).

Although the BDD-YBOCS-A has many advantages, it can be time-consuming to administer (often taking 30–60 minutes), and requires experience and training. It may therefore not be feasible to integrate into clinical assessments in some service settings. Furthermore, as noted above, some young people with BDD are fearful about describing their appearance concerns to another person in case it draws attention to their perceived flaws, and they may report their appearance worries more readily in a questionnaire format. Although a large number of self-report questionnaires have been developed to assess BDD symptoms in adults, only a few questionnaires have been evaluated in young people specifically, namely the Body Image Questionnaire—Child and Adolescent version (BIQ-C) (Schneider *et al.*, 2018b), the Appearance Anxiety Inventory (AAI) (Roberts *et al.*, 2018); and the Multidimensional Youth Body Dysmorphic Inventory (MY BODI) (Roberts *et al.*, 2019). Information about these measures is outlined in Table 61.2. Of note, there are currently no parent-report or teacher-report questionnaires of BDD symptoms in young people.

Challenges and pitfalls

Engaging young people with BDD in a mental health assessment can be challenging, because: (i) anxiety levels are often very high during social interaction, including with professionals; and (ii) insight is often poor and therefore young people may be skeptical about the benefit of attending mental health services. To assist in establishing a good rapport, it is crucial to empathize with and normalize anxiety, and assure the young person that their appearance preoccupation will not be misconstrued as vanity. Additionally, there are several pitfalls that clinicians should hold in mind during the assessment;

- Do not attempt to provide reassurance to the young person about their perceived flaws as this may: (i) provide temporary relief but fuel a counterproductive cycle of reassurance-seeking; or (ii) be interpreted as dismissive or disingenuous.
- Empathize with the young people's experience without colluding with their BDD-related beliefs. This is often best achieved by acknowledging the distress that the young person is experiencing.
- Be cautious about introducing the term "BDD" early in an assessment. Some young people may have prior knowledge of BDD and have decided that they do not identify with the diagnosis because they are convinced that they have a genuine flaw in their appearance. Using terms such as "appearance anxiety" or "worries about appearance" may be more helpful initially.
- When communicating the diagnosis of BDD at the end of the assessment, focus on the distress and impairment as being the main indicators since this is usually the "common ground" between the clinician and young person's perspective. Avoid discussions about whether the perceived flaws are genuine or not.
- If the young person is seeking a cosmetic procedure, share concerns about this not being an effective solution to their problem. Ask if they would be willing to delay plans and try BDD treatment first. Take a "what is there to lose?" approach to discussing BDD treatment.

Differentiating body dysmorphic disorder from normal or "reasonable" appearance concerns

It is well-recognized that appearance concerns are highly prevalent in the general population, particularly among young people. It is important to note that BDD is distinct from normative appearance concerns and can be differentiated according to several criteria. First, BDD is associated with more extreme levels of appearance preoccupation, with most young people with BDD saying that concerns about their appearance are at the forefront of their mind for several hours per day (although there is no specific time requirement in the diagnostic criteria). Second, BDD is defined not just by the presence of appearance concerns but also time-consuming repetitive behaviors (e.g., frequent mirror checking) and/or avoidance (e.g., of social situations). Third, to fulfill diagnostic criteria for BDD, the appearance preoccupation and related behaviors must be causing significant distress and/or impairment in psychosocial functioning. Impairment often occurs in multiple domains, including within school, home, and friendships.

A similar challenge can occur when assessing BDD symptoms in the presence of a genuine, observable difference in appearance. For example, a young person may report

Table 61.2 Summary of body dysmorphic disorder (BDD) symptoms severity measures that are validated for use in young people.

Measure	Key reference	Description	Advantages	Disadvantages
Body dysmorphic disorder (BDD) Yale-Brown Obsessive–Compulsive Scale: adolescent version	Monzani *et al.* (2022)	• Clinician-administered, semistructured • 12 items, scored on 0–4 Likert scale • Total scores range from 0 to 48 • A total score of ≥20 is suggestive of BDD	• Gold-standard measure • Can be used to elicit a detailed description of BDD • Can be an opportunity to establish rapport • Empirically derived criteria for classifying treatment response and remission	• Can take 30–60 min to administer • Requires experience/training • Some young people may find it hard to disclose symptoms in interview format
Body Image Questionnaire: Child and Adolescent version (BIQ-C)	Schneider *et al.* (2018b) Blacker *et al.* (2024)	• Self-report • 9- and 12- item versions (9-item recommended) • Items score on 0–8 Likert scale • Total scores range from 0 to 72 • A total score of ≥40 on 9-item version is suggestive of BDD	• Quick to complete • Captures core features of BDD as per DSM-5 and ICD-11, namely appearance-related preoccupation, behaviors, impairment, and distress	• No validation studies in clinical samples in young people
Appearance Anxiety Inventory (AAI)	Roberts *et al.* (2018) Gumpert *et al.* (2024)	• Self-report • 10 items, scored on 0–4 Likert scale • Total scores range from 0 to 40 • A total score of ≥19 is suggestive of BDD	• Quick to complete • Assesses cognitive and behavioral processes that maintain BDD, and therefore can indicate processes to target in treatment	• Designed as a therapy process measure, not a BDD screening measure • Does not correspond to DSM-5 diagnostic criteria
Multidimensional Youth Body Dysmorphic Inventory (MY BODI)	Roberts *et al.* (2019)	• Self-report • 21 items, scored on a 1–4 Likert scale • Total scores range from 21 to 84	• Developed in line with DSM-5 criteria for BDD	• No validation studies in clinical samples • No clinical cutoffs have been established

Note: Suggested cutoffs are not empirically derived.

preoccupation with the condition of their skin in the context of visible acne, and therefore the concerns may seem "reasonable." In fact, DSM-5 allows for the coding of "Body dysmorphic-like disorder with actual flaws" in the Other Specified Obsessive–Compulsive and Related Disorders section. Key factors to consider here are: whether the preoccupation and distress is disproportionate to the physical problem (in other words, would most other people their age worry as much and feel similar distress if they experienced the same physical condition?); whether the young person is engaging in time-consuming, repetitive behaviors or avoidance in relation to these concerns (a diagnostic criterion for BDD); whether other significant appearance concerns at present (most young people with BDD report multiple appearance concerns); and the associated functional impairment (another diagnostic criterion for BDD). There is a paucity of data but, in practice, these individuals are likely to benefit from the same evidence-based treatments as young people who meet strict criteria for the disorder.

Physical examination

A diagnosis of BDD usually requires direct visual observation of the young person's perceived defect/s in appearance, to inform the clinical judgment about whether their preoccupation and distress is disproportionate to any visible difference in appearance. If a young person's perceived flaw is concealed by clothing, the clinician can encourage the young person to remove the relevant clothing briefly, explaining that this is to help gain a better understanding of their distress. If a young person is too anxious to do this, or if it is not appropriate to ask them because of the nature of their appearance concerns (e.g., concerns about genitalia), then corroborative evidence can be sought, for example, from parents or another professional. Often, young people will have had a physical assessment by a general practitioner, cosmetic surgeon, dermatologist, or orthodontist. In rare cases, the young person may not have revealed their perceived flaw to anyone. In these instances, a physical examination should be arranged where possible (e.g., with their general practitioner).

Risk assessment

Thorough and dynamic risk assessment is crucial in BDD. Key areas of risk assessment include, but are not limited to, self-harm, suicidality, and unwarranted or unsafe cosmetic procedures. The frequency of suicidal ideation and suicide attempts in BDD is highlighted in the earlier section "Impact of body dysmorphic disorder." Self-harm behaviors and cosmetic procedures in BDD are outlined in this section.

Approximately half of young people with BDD report self-harm (Rautio *et al.*, 2022b). Self-harm can be related to low mood or emotional dysregulation, as is seen across many other psychiatric disorders. However, self-harm in BDD can also be specifically related to appearance concerns, and serve as an attempt (albeit counterproductive) to change or improve physical appearance. For example, young people may apply bleach to their skin in an effort to remove freckles, or gouge their skin in an attempt to remove blemishes.

Similarly, approximately half of young people with BDD report a desire for cosmetic procedures (Rautio *et al.*, 2022b), which can include surgical procedures (e.g., rhinoplasty) and nonsurgical cosmetic treatments (e.g., dermatological treatment or dermal fillers). This is concerning because the current weight of evidence (primarily in adults) suggests that psychological outcomes of cosmetic procedures in people with BDD are poor (Bowyer *et al.*, 2016). That is, most people either feel disappointed with the results, which can in turn precipitate a deterioration in mental health, or the focus of their appearance concerns shifts to another feature. Although young people are often unable to access cosmetic treatments in clinical settings, due to age restrictions and/or financial constraints, they may attempt to undertake "treatments" themselves at home. This can involve highly risky behaviors, such as ordering dermal fillers online from unregulated sources and injecting themselves. Similarly, young people with muscle dysmorphia may attempt to order steroids or dietary supplements.

Treatment

An overview of the key recommendations for treatment of BDD in CYP is provided in Box 61.3. The National Institute for Health and Care Excellence (NICE) in the UK published guidelines for the treatment of body dysmorphic disorder across the life span (National Institute for Health and Clinical Excellence, 2005). These guidelines recommend that all young people with BDD should be offered CBT as the first-line treatment. The guidelines further specify that CBT for BDD should: incorporate exposure and response prevention (ERP described in the later section "Format and content of cognitive behavioral

Box 61.3 Treatment at a glance

- The recommended first-line treatment is cognitive behavioral therapy (CBT), specifically tailored for body dysmorphic disorder (BDD).
- CBT for BDD typically involves 12–22 weekly sessions.
- Exposure and response prevention (ERP) is a core component of CBT for BDD. Additional strategies include attention training, mirror retraining, and habit reversal strategies.
- Selective serotonin reuptake inhibitors (SSRIs) are recommended as a second-line treatment for adolescents with moderate-to-severe BDD-related functional impairment who have not had an adequate response to CBT.
- Expert clinical opinion indicates BDD typically requires relatively high doses of SSRIs, although formal dose-finding studies are currently lacking.
- Individuals with BDD typically need to remain on SSRI medication for relatively long periods to reduce the likelihood of relapse occurring.
- When a young person achieves remission from BDD, they should be offered follow-up appointments for 12 months to support maintenance of gains.
- Surgical and nonsurgical procedures are not recommended.

Note: The evidence base is currently limited and primarily based on extrapolation from adult studies, particularly in relation to recommendations about medication.

therapy for body dysmorphic disorder"); involve the family or carers; and be adapted to suit the developmental level of the young person. The NICE guidelines also recommend that SSRIs should be used as a second-line treatment for young people aged 12–18 years who have moderate-to-severe BDD-related functional impairment, and who have not had an adequate response to CBT. However, it has been noted that the 12–18-year age range is relatively arbitrary. It has also been suggested that reserving SSRIs as a second-line treatment may be disadvantageous for young people with more severe symptoms. It should be noted that the NICE guidelines were published in 2005 and at this time the evidence base for BDD treatment in youth was virtually nonexistent, and therefore recommendations were primarily based on extrapolation of data from adult samples and expert clinical opinion.

Evidence base for cognitive behavioral therapy

To date, there have been 10 RCTs of CBT for BDD (Harrison *et al.*, 2016; Wilhelm *et al.*, 2019; Wilhelm *et al.*, 2022; Ritter *et al.*, 2023), primarily in adult samples. Early trials compared CBT with a waitlist control (Rosen *et al.*, 1995; Veale *et al.*, 1996; Rabiei *et al.*, 2012; Wilhelm *et al.*, 2014), while some more recent trials have used credible psychological control interventions such as anxiety management (Veale *et al.*, 2014) and supportive psychotherapy (Enander *et al.*, 2016; Wilhelm *et al.*, 2019) (see Chapter 15 for a detailed discussion of the strengths and limitations of control conditions). A meta-analysis of the 7 RCTs published prior to 2016 found CBT to be efficacious relative to waitlist and psychological control conditions in reducing BDD symptoms (delta = −1.22) (Harrison *et al.*, 2016). Additionally, CBT was associated with a greater improvement in depression and BDD-related insight, compared to control conditions (Harrison *et al.*, 2016).

There has only been one RCT of CBT for adolescent BDD (Mataix-Cols *et al.*, 2015). In this pilot RCT, 30 adolescents with BDD were randomly assigned to receive 14 sessions of specialist CBT for BDD or to a control condition which comprised brief psychoeducation materials and weekly risk monitoring. Overall, CBT was associated with significantly greater reductions in BDD symptoms relative to control, with a large between-group effect size (d = 1.13). CBT was also associated with greater improvements on secondary outcome measures, including insight, depression, and quality of life, and gains were maintained up to a 12-month follow-up (Krebs *et al.*, 2017b). Although encouraging, analysis of individual outcomes indicated that only 40% of adolescents who received CBT met criteria for treatment response. This may be partly due to the severity of the sample and high levels of BDD-related impairment. Nevertheless, these findings highlight that some young people with BDD may require more comprehensive treatment packages, which could include a longer course of CBT, home-based CBT sessions, and/or optimization of medication.

Since the initial RCT of CBT for adolescent BDD, a larger naturalistic study has examined outcomes associated with multimodal treatment among young people accessing specialist BDD services in London and Stockholm (Rautio *et al.*, 2022b). In this study, 140 young people aged 10–18 received specialist CBT for BDD (mean number of sessions = 17.2, range 2–80). The majority (72%) of young people also received concurrent medication, primarily SSRIs. For some young people, medication was stable but for others medication was optimized during the course of CBT. The study found that multimodal treatment was associated with significant reductions in BDD symptoms, with 79% of participants classified as responders and 59% as full or partial remitters by the end of treatment. Improvement in depressive symptoms and psychosocial functioning were also observed, and additional gains were made over the 12-month follow-up period. Interestingly, in this study the presence of comorbidity (e.g., ASD) was not associated with treatment response, suggesting that multimodal treatment can effectively treat BDD symptoms in the context of co-occurring neurodevelopmental and psychiatric disorders.

Engaging young people in cognitive behavioral therapy for body dysmorphic disorder

Often, young people with BDD do not attend services for treatment by choice, and instead are being brought along by concerned parents. Engaging young people with BDD in treatment can be challenging, particularly when insight is poor and the young person views their problem as being a physical one and, therefore, is often seeking a physical solution (e.g., cosmetic treatments). It is important to refrain from polarizing physical and psychological explanations and instead explain that the goal of treatment is to reduce distress, improve quality of life, and/or build self-confidence. Motivational interviewing (Naar & Suarez, 2021) techniques are often used at the start of therapy (and potentially throughout therapy) to increase engagement. For example, eliciting the pros and cons of psychological support for BDD can be a useful exercise for engaging young people at the start of therapy.

Format and content of cognitive behavioral therapy for body dysmorphic disorder

CBT for BDD in young people comprises three main stages: psychoeducation and formulation (typically sessions 1–3; see Figure 61.3 for example formulation); ERP and/or behavioral experiments (typically from session 4 onwards); and relapse prevention (the final two sessions). A typical course of CBT for adolescent BDD comprises 12–22 sessions, usually occurring on a weekly basis (Mataix-Cols *et al.*, 2015; Greenberg *et al.*, 2016). While there are no empirical guidelines for determining the optimal numbers of sessions, it has been noted that in young people with more severe BDD symptoms may require a longer course of CBT. This suggestion is supported by findings from an adult RCT showing that additional improvements occurred after session 12 (Veale *et al.*, 2014), and by a naturalistic study in young people showing that some young people may need a large

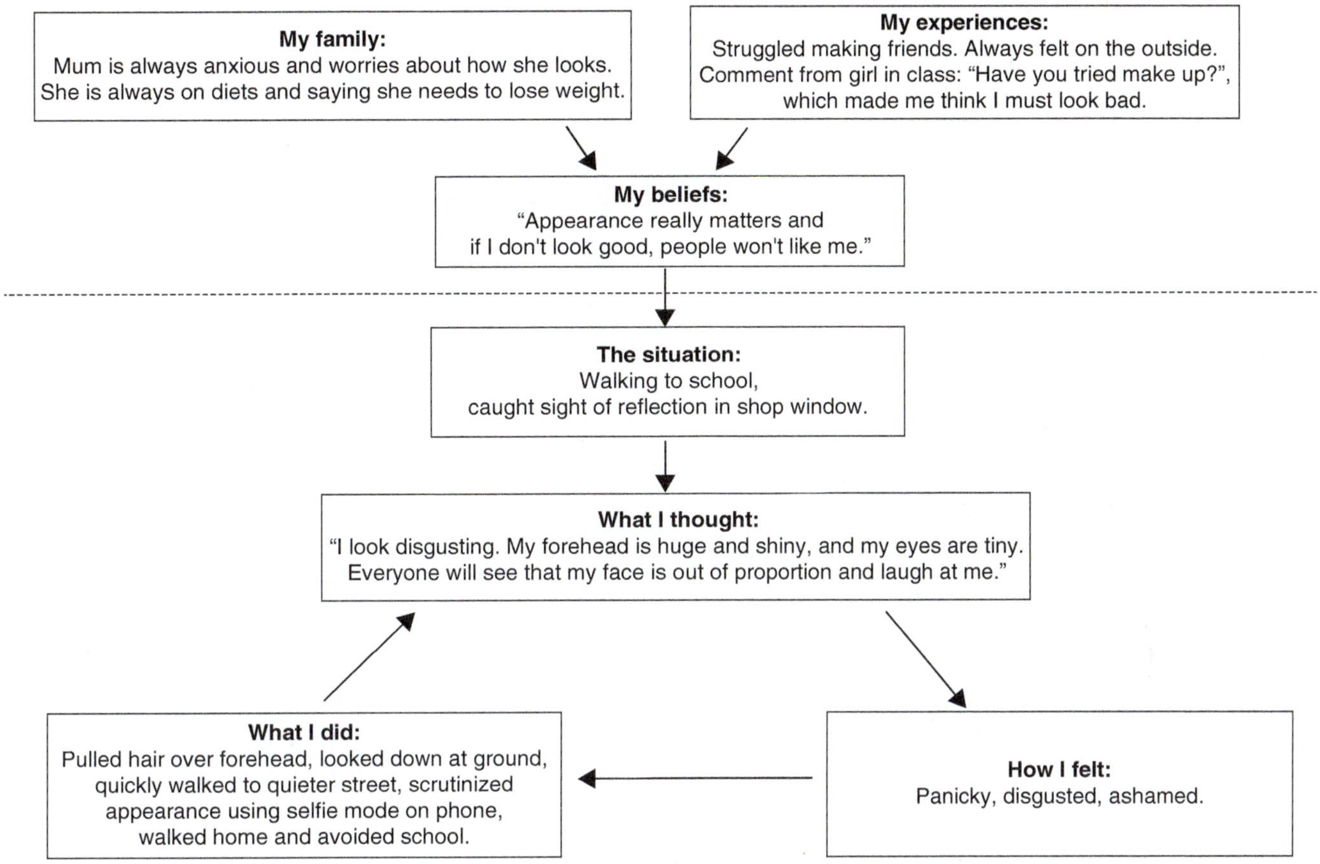

Figure 61.3 Example of a cognitive behavioral formulation. *Note*: Above the dashed line represents vulnerability factors, below the dashed line respresents a specific example.

number of sessions to achieve clinical benefit (Rautio *et al.*, 2022a).

The key components of CBT for BDD are outlined in Table 61.3. There are many similarities between CBT for BDD and CBT for other related disorders, such as OCD (see Chapter 60). Most notably, the main focus of CBT for both BDD and OCD is ERP, which involves encouraging the young person to gradually confront feared or avoided situations, while resisting the urge to engage in compulsive safety behaviors. For example, a girl with concerns about the size and shape of her ears might be encouraged to walk down the street with her hair tied up and without a hat or hood. Behavioral models posit that through doing these tasks, the young person discovers that their initial anxiety subsides over time, and with repeated practice it extinguishes altogether (i.e., anxiety habituation). Of note, inhibitory learning models have challenged the notion that anxiety habituation is the key mechanism underlying exposure-based treatments, and suggest that other processes, such as expectancy violation (violating expectancies regarding the frequency or intensity of aversive outcomes), may be more important (Craske *et al.*, 2014). In this vein, changes in beliefs about appearance, as well as behavioral changes (reducing checking, grooming, and avoidance) have been found to mediate response to CBT for BDD in adults (Fang *et al.*, 2020).

Despite the similarities, there are also key differences between CBT for BDD and OCD. While anxiety is typically the primary emotion associated with OCD, young people with BDD often report other emotions as being more prominent, such as shame or disgust. These emotional responses may not habituate in the same way as anxiety during ERP tasks. In such cases, it is more helpful to frame exposure exercises as behavioral experiments aimed at testing negative beliefs (e.g., "People will stare at my ears and laugh if I do cover them up"). Another important difference between CBT for BDD versus OCD is that BDD treatment often requires the inclusion of a range of techniques in addition to ERP, such as mirror retraining to target visual processing abnormalities, attention training to facilitate reduction of self-focused attention, and habit reversal training to tackle skin picking/hair pulling.

Parental involvement in cognitive behavioral therapy

It is usually beneficial for parents/carers to be included in CBT for BDD in young people. As a minimum, it is suggested that at least one parent is involved in the psychoeducation sessions at

Table 61.3 The key components of cognitive behavioral therapy (CBT) for body dysmorphic disorder (BDD).

Treatment phase	Technique	Overview
Start of treatment	Psychoeducation about body dysmorphic disorder (BDD)	Key concepts include: • Physical appearance versus body image, emphasizing that: (i) the former is objective whereas the latter is subjective; and (ii) the two do not necessarily go hand-in-hand (i.e., desirable physical appearance does not necessarily mean positive body image, and vice versa). • Visual perception. Optical illusions and visual puzzles (e.g., Rubin's vase and Muller-Lyer illusion**)** can be used to illustrate that: (i) people can see things in different ways; (ii) what we see can be a "trick of the mind"; and (iii) what we see can change depending on our focus of attention. • Selective and self-focused attention. Experiential exercises can be used to illustrate that: (i) overfocusing on a stimulus (e.g., a white wall) can distort our visual perception; (ii) overfocusing a stimulus can mean that we miss important information (e.g., the "moonwalking bear" video). This can be related to heightened *self*-focused attention and its consequences.
Start of treatment	Psychoeducation about anxiety	• Anxiety as a normal, protective process (fight or flight). • Developing an idiosyncratic anxiety rating scale. • Anxiety habituation, emphasizing that: (i) when confronting a feared situation anxiety initially increases but subsides over time; and (ii) with repeated practice it extinguishes altogether.
Start of treatment	Constructing a hierarchy	• Young person generates a list of all their BDD-related safety behaviors and avoided situations, and rates how anxious they would feel if they resisted each behavior.
Start of treatment	Cognitive behavioral therapy (CBT) formulation	• Consider how early experiences may have informed beliefs about self and appearance, and how these feed into a cycle of thoughts, behaviors, and feelings that maintain the problem (see Figure 61.3). • Use as opportunity to identify solutions to the problem (i.e., changing avoidance and safety behaviors will break the maintenance cycle). • Crucial that formulation provides a *credible* explanation of the young person's difficulties.
Start of treatment	Goal setting	• Young people should set goals for the short term (next month or so), medium term (by the end of treatment), and longer term. • Goals should be "SMART": Specific, Measurable, Achievable, Relevant, and Time-bound. • Long-term goals may be harder to identify, and can be revisited later in treatment if needed.
Main phase of treatment	Exposure and response prevention (ERP)	• Young person is encouraged to confront feared and avoided situations (e.g., social situations) while resisting the urge to engage in safety behaviors (e.g., covering up their perceived flaw/s), with the goal of experiencing anxiety habituation. • Guided by their hierarchy, generally starting with less anxiety-provoking tasks and building up to more challenging tasks over the course of therapy. However, hierarchy does not need to be followed rigidly; tasks that are most likely to result in functional gains should be prioritized. • ERP tasks should be completed in session with therapist assistance, and in between sessions for homework.
Main phase of treatment	Behavioral experiments	• Often similar to ERP, but the aim is to explicitly test negative beliefs (e.g., "People will sneer at me because I am ugly"). • Often a helpful approach when the young person's primary emotion is shame or disgust, which may not habituate in the same way as anxiety.
Main phase of treatment	Evaluating thoughts	• Young people are encouraged to identify maladaptive thoughts about appearance (e.g., "appearance is all that matters"), consider evidence for and against these beliefs, and develop a more balanced perspective. • Behavioral experiments and surveys can be used to gather evidence as part of this process.
Main phase of treatment (optional)	Mirror retraining	• The goal is to encourage the young person to: (i) process their image as a whole, rather than fixate on specific body parts; and (ii) view themselves in a neutral, nonjudgmental way. • Involves standing in front of a full-length mirror and describing body from head to toe using nonjudgmental language and without ritualizing. • Often helpful for the therapist to model the process first.
Main phase of treatment (optional)	Attention training	• Attention training can be used to develop greater attentional control, and ultimately reduce self-focused attention. • Involves systematic training in focusing attention externally, such as sounds in the room and colors in a picture.
Main phase of treatment (optional)	Habit reversal therapy	• Habit reversal techniques may be used to tackle skin picking or hair pulling that has a habitual quality. • Involves awareness training and use of competing responses, such as making a fist rather than picking or pulling.
End of treatment	Relapse prevention	Involves: • Developing a plan for building on treatment gains. • Identifying potential triggers for a lapse or relapse. • Identifying "warning signs" of relapse. • Action plan for tackling any symptoms that reemerge. • Identifying sources of support if a lapse or relapse were to occur.

the start of treatment, to ensure a shared understanding of BDD and to give parents the opportunity to learn how best to support the child in treatment (Mataix-Cols *et al.*, 2015). The level of parental involvement thereafter will depend on a range of factors including:

- the developmental level of the young person
- the young person's motivation and ability to practice CBT techniques autonomously in between sessions
- the extent to which parents are involved in BDD-related rituals, such as providing reassurance, which may inadvertently fuel BDD
- the presence of other parental behaviors and beliefs that might contribute to the maintenance of BDD (e.g., overvaluing appearance)
- the extent to which parental involvement might inhibit disclosure of symptoms or discussion of relevant experiences (e.g., shaming and humiliating experiences within the family or within an intimate relationship).

Evidence base for selective serotonin reuptake inhibitors

There have been no open trials or RCTs of SSRIs in the treatment of BDD in youth. Nevertheless, in keeping with clinical guidelines and research in adult populations, SSRIs are commonly prescribed to young people with BDD (Rautio *et al.*, 2022a; Krebs *et al.*, 2023b). A range of SSRIs have been used in the treatment of BDD in adults including fluoxetine, fluvoxamine, citalopram, and escitalopram, as well as non-selective serotonin reuptake inhibitors (SRIs) such as clomipramine (Krebs *et al.*, 2017a). Four RCTs have been conducted to formally evaluate the efficacy of these drugs for adults with BDD (Hollander *et al.*, 1999; Phillips *et al.*, 2002; Phillips, 2005; Phillips *et al.*, 2016). Encouragingly, these RCTs have found SSRI/SRIs to be associated with response rates ranging between 53–65% (Hollander et al., 1999; Phillips et al., 2002). There have not been any formal dose-finding studies in BDD, but the available evidence and expert clinical opinion indicates that BDD typically requires relatively high doses of SSRI/SRIs (probably higher than those required to treat depression, for example) (Phillips and Stein, 2015). There is also a suggestion that individuals with BDD need to remain on SSRI/SRI medication for relatively long periods to reduce the likelihood of a relapse occurring (Phillips *et al.*, 2016).

At present, it is unclear whether certain SSRIs are more effective than others in the treatment of BDD, and further research is needed to compare efficacy. There is also a need to further evaluate pharmacological augmentation strategies for BDD patients who do not respond to initial trials of SSRI/SRIs. Clinical guidelines suggest that SSRI/SRI augmentation with an atypical antipsychotic may be considered in CYP (National Institute for Health and Care Excellence, 2005), but this is largely based on clinical experience as opposed to empirical evidence. Only one RCT has been conducted to evaluate the efficacy of augmentation strategies in adults with BDD and it found that pimozide augmentation of fluoxetine was not more effective than placebo (response rates of 18.2% versus 17.6%, respectively) (Phillips, 2005). More recently, new pharmacotherapy strategies have been examined. For example, an open-label trial found promising outcomes of single-dose psilocybin for adults with SSRI-resistant BDD (Schneier *et al.*, 2023), but controlled trials have not yet been undertaken.

Access to evidence-based treatments

There are major barriers to individuals with BDD accessing evidence-based treatment. For example, a survey study conducted in the US found that only 17% of adults who screened positive for BDD had received CBT, and 34% had been prescribed an SSRI medication (Marques *et al.*, 2011b). Similarly, a study conducted in a national and specialist clinic in the UK found that over half of young people with BDD had not received CBT for BDD prior to referral to the specialist clinic (Krebs *et al.*, 2023b), which goes against the NICE guidelines (National Institute for Health and Care Excellence, 2005).

A key obstacle to accessing CBT for BDD is lack of trained therapists. For example, it is notable that BDD is not part of core training curricula for Improving Access to Psychological Therapies (IAPT) or Children and Young People's Improving Access to Psychological Therapies (CYP-IAPT), major providers of mental health treatment in England. There is a clear need to increase BDD training for clinicians working in CAMHS, in order to aid detection and diagnosis and to increase treatment capacity. An additional strategy for improving accessibility to CBT for BDD in youth is the development of digitalized programs which integrate self-help with low-intensity therapist support. Such programs have been developed for adults with BDD and shown in two RCTs to be efficacious relative to waitlist control (Wilhelm *et al.*, 2022) and supportive therapy (Enander *et al.*, 2016). Importantly, these trials involved coaches with no formal clinical qualifications (Wilhelm *et al.*, 2022) or therapists who were clinical psychology trainees (Enander *et al.*, 2016), and in both cases they provided minimal levels of support, highlighting the potential scalability of this approach. Similar programs have been developed for adolescents with BDD, with evaluation under way (e.g., Hartmann *et al.*, 2021; Kuck *et al.*, 2022).

Future research

BDD is an underresearched condition, particularly in children and adolescents. Clear knowledge gaps exist across most areas, including but not limited to prevalence across cultures, etiological factors, long-term consequences, and treatment.

Importantly, all the prevalence studies conducted to date have been done in Europe, the US, or Australia, meaning that little is known about the prevalence of BDD in other parts of the world (Veale *et al.*, 2016). It has been suggested that the incidence of BDD may be increasing due to the pressure from social media on young people (Kaur *et al.*, 2020; Watson & Ban, 2021). While this hypothesis has some face value, supporting evidence is currently lacking. Epidemiological studies including new cohorts of young people evaluated over several years, or even decades, will be needed to address this question.

For a variety of reasons, BDD is severely underdetected and underdiagnosed in CAMHS settings. Due to the lack of awareness among the public and health professionals alike, young people may not seek help for BDD or do so for other reasons, such as low mood or anxiety. A substantial proportion of young people with BDD may instead present to dermatology or plastic surgery clinics, which typically do not have established collaborations with CAMHS. CAMHS professionals are often ill-equipped to screen for the disorder and are unfamiliar with the best evidence-based treatments. More needs to be done to train child psychiatrists, psychologists, and other professionals to identify the symptoms of the disorder. How to best achieve this is an empirical question that can be formally studied (Henrich *et al.*, 2023).

While we know that BDD runs in families and is moderately heritable, very little is known about the specific genetic and environmental risk factors associated with the disorder. Assuming that BDD is similar to OCD, we would expect BDD to be a polygenic disorder, that common genetic variation will contribute to the risk of developing BDD, and that large-scale genomic studies will be required to discover significant genetic loci implicated in the disorder. Similarly, we would also expect rare risk variants (e.g., deletions, duplications) to be implicated in a small proportion of individuals with BDD. However, this remains speculative until enough DNA samples are available for analysis. This will require unprecedented international collaboration. To our knowledge, only two ongoing studies are collecting DNA samples from individuals of all ages with strictly diagnosed BDD, the Nordic OCD and Related Disorders Consortium in Scandinavia (Mataix-Cols *et al.*, 2020) and the LATINO study in the Americas (Crowley *et al.*, 2023). Unfortunately, it may take many years before sufficiently large cohorts of patients with BDD are available for genomic analyses. It may be possible to accelerate genetic discovery by conducting large-scale GWAS of self-assessed body dysmorphic traits in large population-based cohorts, as it has been recently done for obsessive-compulsive (Strom *et al.*, 2022a) and hoarding (Strom *et al.*, 2022b) symptoms, although very large samples are likely needed.

Because BDD and OCD are hypothesized to be genetically close to one another (Monzani *et al.*, 2012b; Monzani *et al.*, 2014), there may be opportunities to learn about the genetics of BDD from the considerable amount of genetic data that are already available for OCD. For example, once DNA is collected from a modest number of individuals with BDD, it may be interesting to calculate polygenic risk scores for OCD in them. If individuals with BDD carry a significantly higher polygenic risk for OCD than matched healthy controls, it would support the hypothesis of close genetic relatedness between these two disorders. A similar approach could be adopted with other disorders that share diagnostic boundaries with BDD, such as mood or eating disorders.

By contrast, evidence from twin studies suggests that environmental (i.e., nongenetic) risk factors involved in BDD are likely to differ from those that are involved in OCD (Monzani *et al.*, 2012b; Monzani *et al.*, 2014). Several environmental risk factors have been suggested, including childhood abuse and appearance-related teasing or bullying (reviewed in the earlier section "Genetic influences") but the strength of the evidence is currently weak and causality has not been established. Longitudinal studies, preferably employing genetically informative designs to adjust for unmeasured familial confounding (e.g., monozygotic twin differences designs) are sorely needed to push the field forward. Hopefully, some of the identified risk factors are modifiable, enabling the rational design of prevention or early intervention efforts.

The long-term adversities associated with adolescent BDD are largely unknown and in need of investigation. The mortality risk of BDD is currently unknown. Is there an association between repeated cosmetic and plastic surgery interventions and premature mortality in BDD? What is the risk of suicide in BDD? Similarly, the short- and long-term socio-economic impacts of the disorder are largely unknown. Is BDD associated with violent victimization? Does BDD impair educational attainment and labor market participation in children and young adults? What are the societal costs of BDD (cost of illness studies)? These and other similar questions would be best addressed in the context of large epidemiological surveys or register-based studies.

Regarding treatment research, several evidence gaps are notable. First, there have been no pharmacological trials in young people with BDD, though clinical experience suggests that SSRIs, which have a reasonable evidence base in adults with the disorder, should be the first drugs of choice. Second, evidence supporting the efficacy of CBT for BDD in children and adolescents is limited to a single RCT ($N = 30$) comparing CBT for BDD with an enhanced waitlist (Mataix-Cols *et al.*, 2015). Larger trials are needed to confirm the efficacy of CBT for BDD, particularly compared to active control conditions, and in preadolescent populations. Third, it will be important to understand the mechanisms of change in CBT for BDD, which may in turn inform the refinement and improvement of existing protocols and ultimately increase efficacy. Fourth, the relative efficacy of SSRIs and CBT for BDD, and their combination, have not been formally investigated in either adults or children with BDD. Fifth, there is also a need to evaluate if CBT can augment the efficacy of SSRIs, and vice versa, in individuals who do not adequately respond to a first treatment trial. Finally, there is a need to evaluate if CBT can be delivered remotely either via the telephone or the Internet without sacrificing efficacy, compared to in-person CBT for BDD. Successful trials in young people with OCD (Aspvall *et al.*, 2021) and related disorders (Hollis *et al.*, 2021), suggest that this may be a viable way to dramatically increase access to evidence-based treatment in a cost-effective manner, as CBT for BDD is a highly specialized treatment that is rarely available.

References

Abramowitz, J.S. & Jacoby, R.J. (2015) Obsessive-compulsive and related disorders: a critical review of the new diagnostic class. *Annual Review of Clinical Psychology* **11**, 165–186.

Ahmadpanah, M. *et al.* (2019) Sociocultural attitudes towards appearance, self-esteem and symptoms of body-dysmorphic disorders among young adults. *International Journal of Environmental Research and Public Health* **16**(21), 4236.

Alsaidan, M.S. *et al.* (2020) The prevalence and determinants of body dysmorphic disorder among young social media users: a cross-sectional study. *Dermatology Reports* **12**(3), 8774.

American Psychiatric Association (1980) *Diagnostic and Statistical Manual of Mental Disorders*, 3rd edn. American Psychiatric Association, Washington, DC.

American Psychiatric Association (1994) *Diagnostic and Statistical Manual of Mental Disorders*, 4th edn. American Psychiatric Association, Washington, DC.

American Psychiatric Association (2013) *Diagnostic and Statistical Manual of Mental Disorders*, 5th edn. American Psychiatric Association, Washington, DC.

Aspvall, K. *et al.* (2021) Effect of an internet-delivered stepped-care program vs in-person cognitive behavioral therapy on obsessive-compulsive disorder symptoms in children and adolescents: a randomized clinical trial. *JAMA* **325**(18), 1863–1873.

Bjornsson, A.S. *et al.* (2013) Age at onset and clinical correlates in body dysmorphic disorder. *Comprehensive Psychiatry* **54**(7), 893–903. doi:10.1016/j.comppsych.2013.03.019.

Blacker, L. *et al.* (2024) A psychometric evaluation of the Body Image Questionnaire Child and Adolescent version. *Child Psychiatry & Human Development*. doi:10.1007/s10578-024-01768-1.

Bowyer, L. *et al.* (2016) A critical review of cosmetic treatment outcomes in body dysmorphic disorder. *Body Image* **19**, 1–8. doi:10.1016/j.bodyim.2016.07.001.

Brohede, S. *et al.* (2015) Prevalence of body dysmorphic disorder among Swedish women: a population-based study. *Comprehensive Psychiatry* **58**, 108–115.

Buckley, V. *et al.* (2018) Innovations in practice: body dysmorphic disorder in youth–using the development and well-being assessment as a tool to improve detection in routine clinical practice. *Child and Adolescent Mental Health* **23**(3), 291–294.

Buhlmann, U. *et al.* (2010) Updates on the prevalence of body dysmorphic disorder: a population-based survey. *Psychiatry Research* **178**(1), 171–175. doi:10.1016/j.psychres.2009.05.002.

Craske, M.G. *et al.* (2014) Maximizing exposure therapy: an inhibitory learning approach. *Behaviour Research and Therapy* **58**, 10–23.

Crowley, J.J. *et al.* (2023) Latin American Trans-ancestry INitiative for OCD genomics (LATINO): study protocol. *medRxiv* 2023. 2002.2023.23286373. doi:10.1101/2023.02.23.23286373.

Dennin, M.H. & Lee, M.S. (2018) Body dysmorphic disorder in pediatric dermatology. *Pediatric Dermatology* **35**(6), 868–874.

Dingemans, A.E. *et al.* (2012) Body dysmorphic disorder in patients with an eating disorder: prevalence and characteristics. *International Journal of Eating Disorders* **45**(4), 562–569.

Dyl, J. *et al.* (2006) Body dysmorphic disorder and other clinically significant body image concerns in adolescent psychiatric inpatients: prevalence and clinical characteristics. *Child Psychiatry and Human Development* **36**(4), 369–382. doi:10.1007/s10578-006-0008-7.

Enander, J. *et al.* (2016) Therapist guided internet based cognitive behavioural therapy for body dysmorphic disorder: single blind randomised controlled trial. *British Medical Journal* **352**. doi:10.1136/bmj.i241.

Enander, J. *et al.* (2018) Prevalence and heritability of body dysmorphic symptoms in adolescents and young adults: a population-based nationwide twin study. *Psychological Medicine* **48**(16), 2740–2747. doi:10.1017/S0033291718000375.

Fang, A. *et al.* (2014) Body dysmorphic disorder. *Psychiatric Clinics of North America* **37**(3), 287–300. doi:10.1016/j.psc.2014.05.003.

Fang, A. *et al.* (2020) Mechanisms of change in cognitive behavioral therapy for body Dysmorphic disorder. *Cognitive Therapy and Research* **44**(3), 596–610.

Fernández de la Cruz, L. *et al.* (2021) Empirically defining treatment response and remission in body dysmorphic disorder. *Psychological Medicine* **51**(1), 83–89.

Foulkes, L. & Blakemore, S.-J. (2016) Is there heightened sensitivity to social reward in adolescence? *Current Opinion in Neurobiology* **40**, 81–85.

Grant, J.E. *et al.* (2001) Prevalence and clinical features of body dysmorphic disorder in adolescent and adult psychiatric inpatients. *The Journal of Clinical Psychiatry* **62**(7), 517–522.

Greenberg, J.L. *et al.* (2016) Cognitive-behavioral therapy for adolescent body dysmorphic disorder: a pilot study. *Behavior Therapy* **47**(2), 213–224.

Gumpert, M. *et al.* (2024) Psychometric evaluation of the appearance anxiety inventory in adolescents with body dysmorphic disorder. *Cognitive Behaviour Therapy* **53**(3), 254–266.

Harrison, A. *et al.* (2016) Cognitive-behavioral therapy for body dysmorphic disorder: a systematic review and meta-analysis of randomized controlled trials. *Clinical Psychology Review* **48**, 43–51. doi:10.1016/j.cpr.2016.05.007.

Hartmann, A.S. *et al.* (2020) An empirically derived recommendation for the classification of body dysmorphic disorder: findings from structural equation modeling. *PLoS One* **15**(6), e0233153.

Hartmann, A.S. *et al.* (2021) Imagin Youth—a therapist-guided internet-based cognitive-behavioral program for adolescents and young adults with body Dysmorphic disorder: study protocol for a two-arm randomized controlled trial. *Frontiers in Psychiatry* **12**, 701.

Henrich, D. *et al.* (2023) Systematic review of training in cognitive-behavioral therapy: summarizing effects, costs and techniques. *Clinical Psychology Review* **101**, 102266.

Hollander, E. *et al.* (1999) Clomipramine vs desipramine crossover trial in body dysmorphic disorder: selective efficacy of a serotonin reuptake inhibitor in imagined ugliness. *Archives of General Psychiatry* **56**(11), 1033–1039.

Hollis, C. *et al.* (2021) Therapist-supported online remote behavioural intervention for tics in children and adolescents in England (ORBIT): a multicentre, parallel group, single-blind, randomised controlled trial. *The Lancet Psychiatry* **8**(10), 871–882.

Jassi, A.D. *et al.* (2020) Family accommodation in pediatric body dysmorphic disorder: a qualitative study. *Bulletin of the Menninger Clinic* **84**(4), 319–336.

Kaur, A. *et al.* (2020) Rising dysmorphia among adolescents: a cause for concern. *Journal of Family Medicine and Primary Care* **9**(2), 567.

Kelly, M.M. *et al.* (2013) A comparison study of body dysmorphic disorder versus social phobia. *Psychiatry Research* **205**(1–2), 109–116.

Knafo, A. & Jaffee, S.R. (2013) Gene–environment correlation in developmental psychopathology. *Development and Psychopathology* **25**(1), 1–6.

Koran, L.M. *et al.* (2008) The prevalence of body dysmorphic disorder in the United States adult population. *CNS Spectrums* **13**(4), 316–322.

Krebs, G. *et al.* (2017a) Recent advances in understanding and managing body dysmorphic disorder. *BMJ Mental Health* **20**(3), 71–75.

Krebs, G. *et al.* (2017b) Long-term outcomes of cognitive-behavioral therapy for adolescent body dysmorphic disorder. *Behavior Therapy* **48**(4), 462–473.

Krebs, G. *et al.* (2023a) Epidemiology of body dysmorphic disorder the youth: prevalence, comorbidity and psychosocial impact. *PsyArXiv.* doi:10.31234/osf.io/zmd2h.

Krebs, G. *et al.* (2023b) Access to evidence-based treatments for young people with body dysmorphic disorder. *Archives of Disease in Childhood* **108**(8), 684–685.

Kuck, N. *et al.* (2022) A smartphone app for the prevention and early intervention of body dysmorphic disorder: development and evaluation of the content, usability, and aesthetics. *Internet Interventions* **28**, 100521.

Longobardi, C. *et al.* (2022) Adverse childhood experiences and body dysmorphic symptoms: a meta-analysis. *Body Image* **40**, 267–284. doi:10.1016/j.bodyim.2022.01.003.

López-Solà, C. *et al.* (2014) Prevalence and heritability of obsessive-compulsive spectrum and anxiety disorder symptoms: a survey of the Australian twin registry. *American Journal of Medical Genetics Part B: Neuropsychiatric Genetics* **165**(4), 314–325.

Lopez-Sola, C. *et al.* (2016) Aetiological overlap between obsessive–compulsive related and anxiety disorder symptoms: Multivariate twin study. *The British Journal of Psychiatry* **208**(1), 26–33.

Marques, L. *et al.* (2011a) Body dysmorphic symptoms: Phenomenology and ethnicity. *Body Image* **8**(2), 163–167.

Marques, L. *et al.* (2011b) Treatment utilization and barriers to treatment engagement among people with body dysmorphic symptoms. *Journal of Psychosomatic Research* **70**(3), 286–293. doi:10.1016/j.jpsychores.2010.10.002.

Marras, A. *et al.* (2016) Obsessive compulsive and related disorders: comparing DSM-5 and ICD-11. *CNS Spectrums* **21**(4), 324–333.

Mataix-Cols, D. *et al.* (2015) A pilot randomized controlled trial of cognitive-behavioral therapy for adolescents with body Dysmorphic disorder. *Journal of the American Academy of Child & Adolescent Psychiatry* **54**(11), 895–904. doi:10.1016/j.jaac.2015.08.011.

Mataix-Cols, D. *et al.* (2020) Nordic OCD & Related Disorders Consortium: Rationale, design, and methods. *American Journal of Medical Genetics Part B: Neuropsychiatric Genetics* **183**(1), 38–50.

Mitchison, D. *et al.* (2022) Prevalence of muscle dysmorphia in adolescents: findings from the EveryBODY study. *Psychological Medicine* **52**(14), 3142–3149.

Möllmann, A. *et al.* (2017) Prevalence of body dysmorphic disorder and associated features in German adolescents: a self-report survey. *Psychiatry Research* **254**, 263–267. doi:10.1016/j.psychres.2017.04.063.

Monzani, B. *et al.* (2012a) A twin study of body dysmorphic concerns. *Psychological Medicine* **42**(9), 1949–1955. doi:10.1017/s0033291711002741.

Monzani, B. *et al.* (2012b) Evidence for a genetic overlap between body dysmorphic concerns and obsessive–compulsive symptoms in an adult female community twin sample. *American Journal of Medical Genetics Part B: Neuropsychiatric Genetics* **159**(4), 376–382. doi:10.1002/ajmg.b.32040.

Monzani, B. *et al.* (2014) The structure of genetic and environmental risk factors for dimensional representations of DSM-5 obsessive-compulsive spectrum disorders. *JAMA Psychiatry* **71**(2), 182–189. doi:10.1001/jamapsychiatry.2013.3524.

Monzani, B. *et al.* (2022) Psychometric evaluation of the Yale-Brown Obsessive-Compulsive Scale modified for body Dysmorphic disorder for adolescents (BDD-YBOCS-A). *Child Psychiatry & Human Development* **54**(3), 1–8.

Morselli, E. (1891) Sulla dismorfofobia e sulla tafefobia. *Bolletinno della R Accademia di Genova* **6**, 110–119.

Moses-Payne, M. *et al.* (2022) Age-related changes in the impact of valence on self-referential processing in female adolescents and young adults. *Cognitive Development* **61**, 101128.

Naar, S. & Suarez, M. (2021) *Motivational Interviewing with Adolescents and Young Adults.* Guilford Press, New York.

National Institute for Health and Care Excellence (2005) *Obsessive-compulsive Disorder: Core Interventions in The Treatment of Obsessive-compulsive Disorder and Body Dysmorphic Disorder.* National Institute for Health and Care Excellence (NICE), London.

Nierenberg, A.A. *et al.* (2002) Body dysmorphic disorder in outpatients with major depression. *Journal of Affective Disorders* **69**(1–3), 141–148.

Oosthuizen, P. *et al.* (1998) Dysmorphic concern: Prevalence and associations with clinical variables. *Australian & New Zealand Journal of Psychiatry* **32**(1), 129–132. doi:10.3109/00048679809062719.

Phillips, K.A. (2005) Placebo-controlled study of Pimozide augmentation of fluoxetine in body Dysmorphic disorder. *American Journal of Psychiatry* **162**(2), 377–379. doi:10.1176/appi.ajp.162.2.377.

Phillips, K.A. & Stein, D.J. (eds) (2015) *Handbook on Obsessive Compulsive and Related Disorders.* American Psychiatric Association, Washington, DC.

Phillips, K.A. *et al.* (2002) A randomized placebo-controlled trial of fluoxetine in body dysmorphic disorder. *Archives of General Psychiatry* **59**(4), 381–388. doi:10.1001/archpsyc.59.4.381.

Phillips, K.A. *et al.* (2006) Clinical features of body dysmorphic disorder in adolescents and adults. *Psychiatry Research* **141**(3), 305–314. doi:10.1016/j.psychres.2005.09.014.

Phillips, K.A. *et al.* (2010) Should an obsessive–compulsive spectrum grouping of disorders be included in DSM-V? *Depression and Anxiety* **27**(6), 528–555.

Phillips, K.A. *et al.* (2013) A 4-year prospective observational follow-up study of course and predictors of course in body dysmorphic disorder. *Psychological Medicine* **43**(5), 1109–1117. doi:10.1017/s0033291712001730.

Phillips, K.A. *et al.* (2016) Pharmacotherapy relapse prevention in body dysmorphic disorder: a double-blind, placebo-controlled trial. *The American Journal of Psychiatry* **173**(9), 887–895. doi:10.1176/appi.ajp.2016.15091243.

Rabiei, M. *et al.* (2012) Metacognitive therapy for body dysmorphic disorder patients in Iran: Acceptability and proof of concept. *Journal of Behavior Therapy and Experimental Psychiatry* **43**(2), 724–729. doi:10.1016/j.jbtep.2011.09.013.

Rautio, D. *et al.* (2022a) Effectiveness of multimodal treatment for young people with body dysmorphic disorder in two specialist clinics. *Behavior Therapy* **53**(5), 1037–1049.

Rautio, D. *et al.* (2022b) Clinical characteristics of 172 children and adolescents with body dysmorphic disorder. *European Child & Adolescent Psychiatry* **31**, 133–144.

Rief, W. *et al.* (2006) The prevalence of body dysmorphic disorder: A population-based survey. *Psychological Medicine* **36**(6), 877–885. doi:10.1017/S0033291706007264.

Ritter, V. *et al.* (2023) Efficacy of cognitive therapy for body dysmorphic disorder: a randomized controlled pilot trial. *Behavior Therapy* **54**(1), 65–76.

Roberts, C. *et al.* (2018) The appearance anxiety inventory: factor structure and associations with appearance-based rejection sensitivity and social anxiety. *Journal of Obsessive-Compulsive and Related Disorders* **19**, 124–130.

Roberts, C. *et al.* (2019) The multidimensional youth body dysmorphic inventory: development and preliminary validation. *Child Psychiatry & Human Development* **50**, 927–939. doi:10.1007/s10578-019-00893-6.

Rosen, J.C. *et al.* (1995) Cognitive-behavioral body image therapy for body dysmorphic disorder. *Journal of Consulting and Clinical Psychology* **63**(2), 263–269. doi:10.1037/0022-006X.63.2.263.

Ryding, F.C. & Kuss, D.J. (2020) The use of social networking sites, body image dissatisfaction, and body dysmorphic disorder: A systematic review of psychological research. *Psychology of Popular Media* **9**(4),412.

Schieber, K. *et al.* (2015) Classification of body dysmorphic disorder. What is the advantage of the new DSM-5 criteria? *Journal of Psychosomatic Research* **78**(3), 223–227. doi:10.1016/j.jpsychores.2015.01.002.

Schneider, S.C. *et al.* (2016) Prevalence and correlates of body dysmorphic disorder in a community sample of adolescents. *Australian & New Zealand Journal of Psychiatry* **51**(6), 595–603. doi:10.1177/0004867416665483.

Schneider, S.C. *et al.* (2018a) The classification of body dysmorphic disorder symptoms in male and female adolescents. *Journal of Affective Disorders* **225**, 429–437.

Schneider, S.C. *et al.* (2018b) Measurement invariance of a body dysmorphic disorder symptom questionnaire across sex: the Body Image Questionnaire–Child and Adolescent version. *Assessment* **25**(8), 1026–1035.

Schneier, F.R. *et al.* (2023) Pilot study of single-dose psilocybin for serotonin reuptake inhibitor-resistant body dysmorphic disorder. *Journal of Psychiatric Research* **161**, 364–370.

Schulte, J. *et al.* (2021) Temporal dynamics of insight in body dysmorphic disorder: an ecological momentary assessment study. *Journal of Abnormal Psychology* **130**(4), 365.

Strom, N.I. *et al.* (2022a) Genome-wide association study of obsessive-compulsive symptoms including 33 943 individuals from the general population. *medRxiv* 2022.2011.2030.22282898. doi:10.1101/2022.11.30.22282898.

Strom, N.I. *et al.* (2022b) Meta-analysis of genome-wide association studies of hoarding symptoms in 27,537 individuals. *Translational Psychiatry* **12**(1), 479.

The Children's Society (2022) *The Good Childhood Report 2022.* The Children's Society, London.

Veale, D. *et al.* (1996) Body dysmorphic disorder: a cognitive behavioural model and pilot randomised controlled trial. *Behaviour Research and Therapy* **34**(9), 717–729. doi:10.1016/0005-7967(96)00025-3.

Veale, D. *et al.* (2014) Efficacy of cognitive behaviour therapy versus anxiety management for body dysmorphic disorder: a randomised controlled trial. *Psychotherapy and Psychosomatics* **83**(6), 341–353. doi:10.1159/000360740.

Veale, D. *et al.* (2016) Body dysmorphic disorder in different settings: a systematic review and estimated weighted prevalence. *Body Image* **18**, 168–186. doi:10.1016/j.bodyim.2016.07.003.

Watson, C. & Ban, S. (2021) Body dysmorphic disorder in children and young people. *British Journal of Nursing* **30**(3), 160–164.

Wilhelm, S. *et al.* (1997) Prevalence of body dysmorphic disorder in patients with anxiety disorders. *Journal of Anxiety Disorders* **11**(5), 499–502.

Wilhelm, S. *et al.* (2014) Modular cognitive-behavioral therapy for body dysmorphic disorder: a randomized controlled trial. *Behavior Therapy* **45**(3), 314–327. doi:10.1016/j.beth.2013.12.007.

Wilhelm, S. *et al.* (2019) Efficacy and posttreatment effects of therapist-delivered cognitive behavioral therapy vs supportive psychotherapy for adults with body dysmorphic disorder: a randomized clinical trial. *JAMA Psychiatry* **76**(4), 363–373.

Wilhelm, S. *et al.* (2022) Efficacy of app-based cognitive behavioral therapy for body dysmorphic disorder with coach support: initial randomized controlled clinical trial. *Psychotherapy and Psychosomatics* **91**(4), 277–285.

World Health Organization (1992) *International Statistical Classification of Disease and Related Health Problems*, 10th revision edn. World Health Organization (WHO), Geneva, Switzerland.

World Health Organization (2019) *International Statistical Classification of Diseases and Related Health Problems, 11th revision.* World Health Organization (WHO), Geneva, Switzerland.

CHAPTER 62

Bipolar disorder in childhood and adolescence

Daniel P. Dickstein[1,2] and Danella M. Hafeman[3]

[1] Simches Division of Child and Adolescent Psychiatry, McLean Hospital, Belmont, MA, USA

[2] Harvard Medical School, Boston, MA, USA

[3] Department of Psychiatry, University of Pittsburgh School of Medicine, Pittsburgh, PA, USA

Introduction

Bipolar disorder (BD) is among the most impairing child or adolescent psychiatric illnesses. Our understanding about early-onset BD has increased greatly since the 2000s.

Here, we first review data on the characteristics and diagnosis of childhood-onset BD, including its phenomenology, distinction from typical development, impact on functioning, and differential diagnosis. Second, we describe assessment of BD, including comorbid psychopathology, such as attention deficit hyperactivity disorder (ADHD). Then, we discuss its epidemiology, longitudinal course, and risk factors, before summarizing recent data about the pathophysiology and treatment. We conclude with future directions for research and clinical care.

Characteristics and diagnosis of the condition

Diagnosis and phenomenology

BD is a mood disorder involving a change from baseline normal mood, known as euthymia, to a manic or hypomanic episode involving elevated, expansive, or irritable mood.

In the *Diagnostic and Statistical Manual of Mental Disorders*, 5th edition (DSM-5; American Psychiatric Association, 2013), a manic episode is defined by a change of mood involving elevated and expansive mood (known as "euphoria") or irritable mood coupled with increased energy and activity level. Importantly, irritable mood is not specific to mania or hypomania, and, correspondingly, if irritability is the only mood change in the episode (without any euphoria) patients must have four associated "B" symptoms, whereas if euphoria is present, only three "B" symptoms are required. These associated "B" symptoms include decreased need for sleep (i.e., not sleeping and not tired, in contrast with insomnia in depression or anxiety), pressured speech (talking faster or louder than typical), increased distractibility, and engaging excessively in activities that are pleasurable but likely to have adverse consequences (i.e., shoplifting, risky sexual activity).

The mood and activity changes need to represent an episode—i.e., change from the child's typical mood. The symptoms are present throughout the day, nearly every day during the episode. Associated features must have appeared (or worsened) during the episode, and do not reflect the child's usual state. Episodicity is therefore an important part of the definition: a manic episode should last for at least a week and may last much longer. A hypomanic episode lasts at least four days.

DSM-5 recognizes five types of BD, based on lifetime history of episode type:

- "BD type I" (BD-I) requires at least one manic episode (no major depressive episode required).
- "BD type II" (BD-II) requires at least one hypomanic episode plus at least one major depressive episode (i.e., a two-week period of depressed mood [or irritable mood for children] lasting most of the day, nearly every day accompanied by additional symptoms, including decreased sleep, interest, and energy; inability to experience pleasure ["anhedonia"]; increased or decreased appetite/eating and physical activity; and suicidal ideation, plans, or attempts).
- Representing a change from previous functioning (see Chapter 63), "cyclothymia" is defined in children as at least one year (in adults two years) of hypomanic symptoms or depressive symptoms not meeting criteria for a major depressive episode without an asymptomatic period of two months or longer.
- "Other Specified BD" has clinically significant impairment from BD symptoms that do not meet the full criteria for types I,

Rutter's Child and Adolescent Psychiatry and Psychology, Seventh Edition.
Edited by Anita Thapar, Daniel S. Pine, Samuele Cortese, Cathy Creswell, Tamsin J. Ford, James F. Leckman, and Argyris Stringaris.

Companion website: www.wiley.com/go/thapar/rutterspsych7

II, or cyclothymia (e.g., hypomanic episodes lasting two to three days plus major depressive episodes).

- "Unspecified BD" involves clinically significant impairment from BD symptoms that do not meet criteria for any of the previous types.

The *International Classification of Diseases*, 11th revision (ICD-11; World Health Organization, 2019) adopts DSM-5's approach with a manic or hypomanic episode requiring euphoric or irritable mood plus increased activity or energy. This may be more conservative than ICD-10 (World Health Organization, 1993) in not requiring activity or energy changes. However, other ICD-11 changes liberalize who receives a BD diagnosis because ICD-11 no longer differentially weighs the number of required associated symptoms (known as "B" symptoms in DSM-5) based on whether the mood is primarily euphoria or irritability (as was done in ICD-10, DSM-IV (American Psychiatric Association, 1994), and DSM-5). Instead, ICD-11 states "several other characteristic symptoms" are required without specifying any minimum number. While DSM-5 requires at least four days for a hypomanic episode, ICD-11 requires a hypomanic episode to last "several days," with "several" associated symptoms not differentially weighted by mood type, and functional impairment "apparent to people who know the individual well." In sum, the use of "several" may lead to more people being diagnosed with BD-I using ICD-11, whereas ICD-10's approach to BD was more conservative (Angst *et al.*, 2020).

Diagnostic considerations, including normal versus pathological

Unlike normal fluctuations in mood and behavior, episodes of mania and depression last longer, are associated with other symptoms (e.g., "B" symptoms of mania or neurovegetative dysfunction in depression), and cause impairment to peer, occupational/educational, and family function.

Three issues make establishing the diagnosis of BD difficult in children: (i) duration of a manic episode, (ii) the role of irritability versus euphoria in defining a manic episode, and (iii) overlap with other illnesses, including ADHD.

Regarding duration, two substantive changes from DSM-IV-TR (American Psychiatric Association, 2000), to DSM-5 increase both the specificity of the diagnosis of a manic episode, and make it easier to distinguish from normal mood and behavior fluctuations. First, DSM-5 now requires the irritable or euphoric mood in mania/hypomania to last "most of the day nearly every day" akin to DSM-IV and DSM-5 specifications of a major depressive episode. Second, the irritable or euphoric mood must be accompanied by increased activity or subjective increase in energy. This language applies regardless of the patient's age—i.e., to children and to adults equally. This change is designed to refute prior assertions that BD in children or adolescents is a chronic illness, with fluctuations between all three mood states often occurring within a single day (e.g., "ultradian cycling") (Geller *et al.*, 1998, Biederman *et al.*, 2004). Instead, this promotes the classical view that BD in both children and adults is an episodic illness, with distinct periods (days to weeks) of mania, depression, and euthymia (Leibenluft *et al.*, 2003, Birmaher *et al.*, 2006).

Second, euphoric mood is unique to mania, but it is not necessary for the diagnosis in DSM-5, which allows irritable mood to fulfill this criterion. In contrast, irritability is an explicit diagnostic criterion not only for mania, but also for several other disorders, including generalized anxiety disorder (GAD), child-specific modified criterion for a major depressive episode, and oppositional defiant disorder (ODD). Irritability is an associated symptom for disorders including autism spectrum disorders (ASD) and ADHD (American Psychiatric Association, 2000). Therefore, DSM-5 is clear that irritability in mania must occur simultaneously with "B" symptom changes (e.g., decreased need for sleep), and irritability and euphoria are weighted differently, so that three associated "B" symptoms are required if the mood is primarily euphoric, and four if the mood is primarily irritable.

The third diagnostic factor leading to potential confusion is the overlap between some of the associated features of mania and those of ADHD. For example, how does one distinguish pressured speech in mania from talking excessively and blurting out answers in ADHD? How to distinguish distractibility in mania from distractibility in ADHD? Unlike DSM-IV, DSM-5 builds on work by Geller *et al.*, who found that five symptoms best distinguished children with BD from those with ADHD ((i) elation, (ii) grandiosity, (iii) hypersexuality, (iv) flight of ideas/increased goal-directed activity, and (iv) decreased need for sleep), to now require that these "B" symptoms only count toward a diagnosis of mania if they are present during the episode of mood and activity/energy change (Geller *et al.*, 2002a, Geller *et al.*, 2002b).

Regarding children or adolescents specifically, the UK's National Institute for Health and Care Excellence (NICE) BD guidelines state BD should only be diagnosed in young people after a period of intensive, prospective longitudinal monitoring by a health care professional or team experienced with the assessment and management of children with BD. NICE guidelines for children or young people require: (i) mania must be present (not just hypomania), (ii) euphoria must be present most days, most of the time for at least seven days, (iii) irritability should not be considered a core diagnostic criterion, and (iv) children or young people themselves meet diagnostic criteria for BD (National Collaborating Centre for Mental Health, 2014).

Differential diagnosis

The differential diagnosis for childhood-onset BD includes any disorder involving euphoria, irritability, depression, or psychosis. This includes substance intoxication and substance-related mood or psychotic disorders, plus primary medical problems including toxidromes (e.g., anticholinergic ingestion resulting in psychosis/mania), thyroid abnormalities (e.g., hypothyroidism/depression, or hyperthyroidism/mania), or seizure disorders (temporal lobe epilepsy).

Disentangling the differential diagnosis of BD in children requires a careful psychiatric history with the child and their primary caretakers; screening for medical or substance-related conditions; collateral sources of information (e.g., teachers, primary care doctor, other mental health providers); and repeat assessments.

Considering this differential diagnosis in children can be particularly challenging regarding disorders involving irritability, because irritability is a diagnostic criteria or associated feature of many psychiatric disorders, including mania, depression (in children), GAD, ADHD, autism, ODD, and the new DSM-5 diagnosis "disruptive mood dysregulation disorder (DMDD)," which was added based on over two decades of research showing youth with chronic nonepisodic irritability have a very different course from those with BD (Leibenluft *et al.*, 2003, Brotman *et al.*, 2006, Copeland *et al.*, 2013). Moreover, patients with BD, whether children or adults, have high rates of co-occurring mental health conditions, including anxiety, ADHD, substance use disorders, and psychosis. So, clinicians may be confronted with not just "either BD or ADHD, etc." but "both BD and ADHD, etc."

Generally, unlike anxiety disorders, irritability in mania is not the result of worry or fear. Distinguishing whether a child has primary BD, primary ADHD, or both is complicated; clinicians should ascertain if behavioral changes are episodic, suggesting BD, or chronic, suggesting ADHD. Although psychosis can accompany either mania or depression, psychosis unaccompanied by mania or depression suggests either schizophrenia or schizoaffective disorder. Patients cannot have BD and DMDD by definition, and, in fact, if they have another clear cause of their irritability, such as major depressive disorder (MDD) or ASD, they cannot have DMDD (see Chapter 63).

Cultural issues

There is a great need for studies evaluating cultural differences in the phenomenology of childhood-onset BD, particularly those examining how culture impacts the definition of aberrant, impairing irritability and euphoria. In one example, Escamilla *et al.* found similar presentation and longitudinal course in Spanish youth diagnosed with BD and followed for two years (Escamilla *et al.*, 2011).

Impact of the disorder on functioning

BD in childhood is associated with significant morbidity and mortality, including high rates of psychiatric inpatient hospitalization (more than 52–74% hospitalized at least once), suicidal ideation (70–85%), and suicide attempts (30–65%) (Algorta *et al.*, 2011; Axelson *et al.*, 2006).

Assessment

Core aspects

Assessing a child for BD requires determining whether a child has had episodes of mania and depression. If episodes are identified, the interviewer must determine if the features associated with mania or depression (e.g., sleep and activity changes, increased distractibility, etc.—associated "B" criteria of DSM-5) occurred concurrent with mood changes. The absence of distinct episodes suggests BD may not be the correct diagnosis (Figure 62.1).

Euphoria should exceed that which a typically developing child (TDC) experiences in a very exciting situation, such as going to an amusement park, and true grandiosity should be distinguished from developmentally appropriate fantasy or oppositional behavior. Grandiosity or euphoria should represent a distinct change from the child's usual level of function, and should occur at the same time as other manic symptoms (e.g., decreased need for sleep, increased goal-directed activity). Decreased need for sleep (e.g., two or more consecutive days of not sleeping and not being tired without compensatory naps) should be differentiated from more typical insomnia (e.g., difficulty falling or staying asleep, but feeling tired or trying to compensate by napping).

When possible, clinicians should see a child when the parent states the child is exhibiting manic behavior. Clinicians must balance concerns about over- and underdiagnosis of BD. While overdiagnosis can lead to overuse of antimanic medications (and side effects), underdiagnosis leads to inappropriate medication choices, poor course, and treatment resistance (Berk *et al.*, 2011). A longitudinal approach is required, because children who initially present with one diagnosis, such as unipolar depression or ADHD, might subsequently develop mania. Data including: (i) prospective mood ratings from children, parents, and other significant caregivers, such as teachers; (ii) smartphone camera recordings of manic or depressive behavior; and (iii) the child seen repeatedly over time, may help clinicians and parents achieve a shared understanding of target behaviors and symptoms.

Comorbid illnesses should be diagnosed only if symptoms are present when the patient is not in an acute mood episode. For example, a child with BD should be diagnosed with ADHD only if ADHD symptoms are present when they are euthymic or subsyndromally ill. Family history of BD in a first-degree relative raises concern about BD in the child, but children should be diagnosed and treated based on their own clinical presentation. At-risk studies show 15–20% of offspring of parents with BD develop bipolar spectrum disorder (compared to <3% of community controls), while a larger percentage develop nonbipolar psychopathology (Axelson *et al.*, 2015).

Common diagnostic challenges and how to proceed

Establishing the history of a hypomanic or manic episode to diagnose someone with BD may have the following challenges. First, for children and adolescents who are chronically depressed, it can be difficult to distinguish hypomania from a return to baseline, especially if they have comorbid conditions (e.g., ADHD) potentially mimicking symptoms of hypomania. Second, in a child with significant chronic behavioral concerns, identifying episodic changes in mood, energy, and other symptoms that exceed the

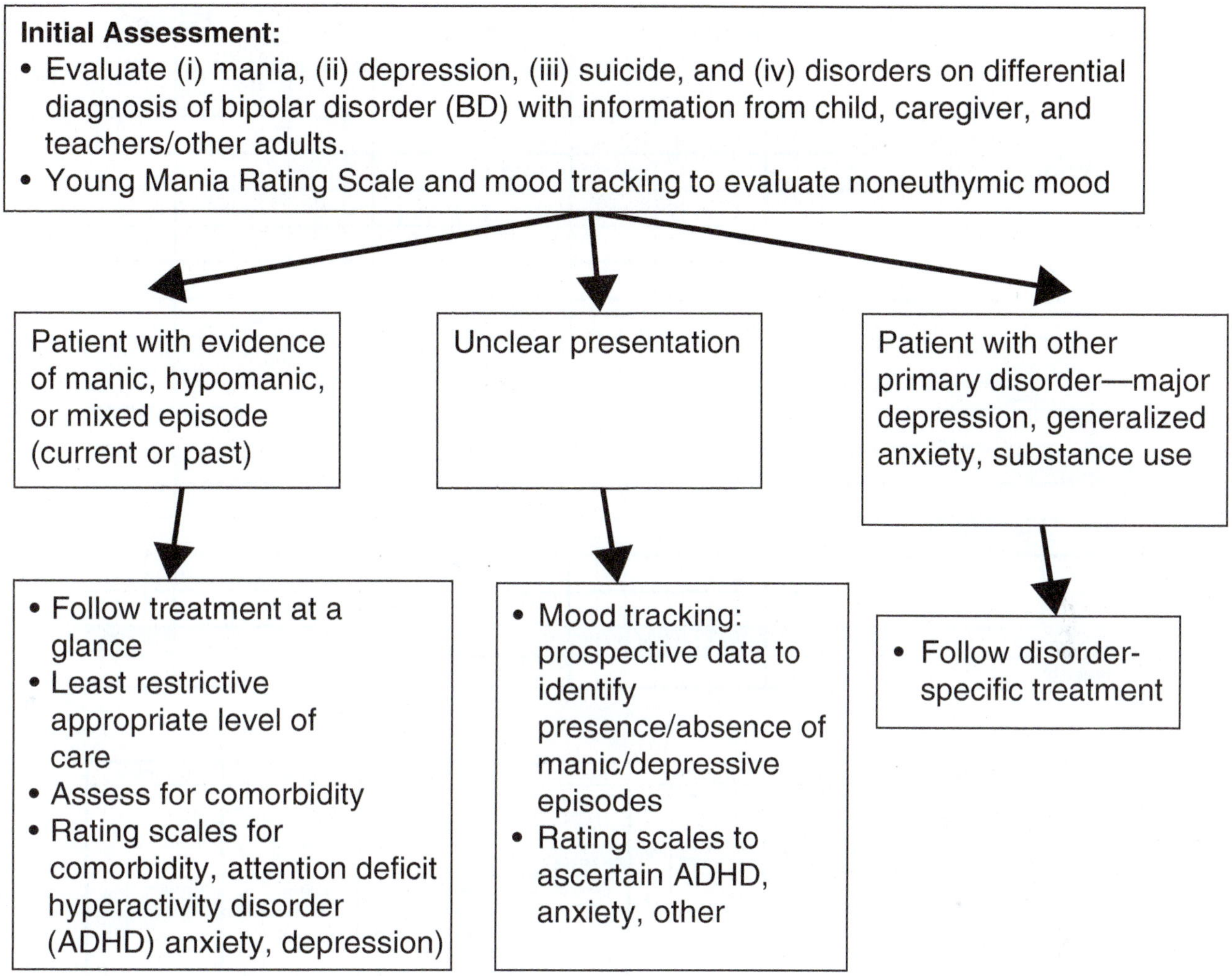

Figure 62.1 Pediatric bipolar disorder (BD) assessment at a glance.

child's baseline may not be easy. For example, in a child with ODD and ADHD, it is important to identify whether there are episodic and concurrent increases in irritability, energy, hyperactivity, distractibility, and talkativeness. Similarly, while an adolescent with borderline personality disorder may have marked affective lability, we would not expect a spontaneous, durable (e.g., > 1 day) period of elevated mood and energy plus decreased need for sleep and goal-directed activity. Third, parent and child informants typically disagree, with one endorsing mania symptoms, and the other not.

A mood-tracking log to visually map the mood timeline may help inquiry about episodic changes in energy and associated symptoms (Figure 62.2). The identification of symptoms more specific to mania (e.g., decreased need for sleep) is vital. Establishing a "baseline" for mood and energy, prior to the onset of mood disorder, is important. Regarding informant disagreement, parent-report of manic symptoms tends to be most reliable, while the child-report of depressive symptoms is most helpful (Youngstrom *et al.*, 2015). However, this can depend on the insight of the child and their caregiver. Even with the most comprehensive assessment, it may not be possible to definitively establish a BD diagnosis cross-sectionally, requiring a provisional working diagnosis, with prospective mood charting used to refine the child's diagnosis over time.

Use of rating scales, diagnostic interviews, and standardized observations

The gold standard for assessment of BD is a clinician interview (Goldstein *et al.*, 2017). For example, the Kiddie Schedule for Affective Disorders and Schizophrenia, Present and Lifetime (K-SADS-PL) is a semistructured interview assessing DSM-5 criteria for mania, depression, and comorbid disorders (Kaufman *et al.*, 1997). Galanter's comparison of six research diagnostic interviews highlights the complexity associated with current standardized assessment tools (Galanter *et al.*, 2012). These authors reported considerable variation in how each interview conceptualized the mood criterion, whether the symptoms had to represent a change from the patient's usual state, and whether B-symptoms had to co-occur with the A (mood) symptoms (Young *et al.*, 1978).

Name________________ Month____________ Year____________ BEAM

	DAYS		1	2	3	4	5	6	7	8	9	10	11	12	13	14	15	16	17	18	19	20	21	22	23	24	25	26	27	28	29	30	31
ELEVATED	Severe	Significant impairment Not able to work																															
	Moderate	Significant impairment Able to work																															
	Mild	Without significant impairment																															
NORMAL																																	
	NORMAL																																
DEPRESSED	Mild	Without significant impairment																															
	Moderate	Significant impairment Able to work																															
	Severe	Significant impairment Not able to work																															
	Anxiety	0=None 1=Mild 2=Moderate 3=Severe																															
	Irritability																																
	Weight on day 28																																
	Hours slept																																

Name: ____________

	Sunday			Monday			Tuesday			Wednesday			Thursday			Friday			Saturday		
Overall Mood Rating	Too good, sky high		10	Too good, sky high		10	Too good, sky high		10	Too good, sky high		10	Too good, sky high		10	Too good, sky high		10	Too good, sky high		10
	The best but not too much		9	The best but not too much		9	The best but not too much		9	The best but not too much		9	The best but not too much		9	The best but not too much		9	The best but not too much		9
Put a STAR for the BEST mood of the day	Excellent, great		8	Excellent, great		8	Excellent, great		8	Excellent, great		8	Excellent, great		8	Excellent, great		8	Excellent, great		8
	Very good		7	Very good		7	Very good		7	Very good		7	Very good		7	Very good		7	Very good		7
	Pretty good		6	Pretty good		6	Pretty good		6	Pretty good		6	Pretty good		6	Pretty good		6	Pretty good		6
Put a CIRCLE for what it was for MOST OF THE DAY	OK		5	OK		5	OK		5	OK		5	OK		5	OK		5	OK		5
	Not so good		4	Not so good		4	Not so good		4	Not so good		4	Not so good		4	Not so good		4	Not so good		4
	Sort of bad		3	Sort of bad		3	Sort of bad		3	Sort of bad		3	Sort of bad		3	Sort of bad		3	Sort of bad		3
Put an X for the WORST mood of the day	Bad		2	Bad		2	Bad		2	Bad		2	Bad		2	Bad		2	Bad		2
	Very bad, terrible		1	Very bad, terrible		1	Very bad, terrible		1	Very bad, terrible		1	Very bad, terrible		1	Very bad, terrible		1	Very bad, terrible		1
	Horrible, the worst		0	Horrible, the worst		0	Horrible, the worst		0	Horrible, the worst		0	Horrible, the worst		0	Horrible, the worst		0	Horrible, the worst		0
Sadness, Down, Depressed	A little	Some	A lot	A little	Some	A lot	A little	Some	A lot	A little	Some	A lot	A little	Some	A lot	A little	Some	A lot	A little	Some	A lot
Angry, Mad, Irritable	A little	Some	A lot	A little	Some	A lot	A little	Some	A lot	A little	Some	A lot	A little	Some	A lot	A little	Some	A lot	A little	Some	A lot
Anxious, Worried, Scared	A little	Some	A lot	A little	Some	A lot	A little	Some	A lot	A little	Some	A lot	A little	Some	A lot	A little	Some	A lot	A little	Some	A lot
Energy Put an X for how you felt today (can use multiple if it changed a lot)	Very low	Low	OK	Very low	Low	OK	Very low	Low	OK	Very low	Low	OK	Very low	Low	OK	Very low	Low	OK	Very low	Low	OK
	Good	High	Too high	Good	High	Too high	Good	High	Too high	Good	High	Too high	Good	High	Too high	Good	High	Too high	Good	High	Too high

Figure 62.2 Examples of mood tracking (top: BEAM; center: mood, energy; bottom: sleep).

Sleep

	Sunday	Monday	Tuesday	Wednesday	Thursday	Friday	Saturday
Time when I went to bed	am pm	am pm	am pm	am pm	am pm	am pm	am pm
Time when I fell asleep	am pm	am pm	am pm	am pm	am pm	am pm	am pm
Number of times I woke up after first falling asleep							
Total time I was awake after first falling asleep (Put an X)	Less than 15 min 15–30 min 31–60 min 1–2 hours More than 2 hours	Less than 15 min 15–30 min 31–60 min 1–2 hours More than 2 hours	Less than 15 min 15–30 min 31–60 min 1–2 hours More than 2 hours	Less than 15 min 15–30 min 31–60 min 1–2 hours More than 2 hours	Less than 15 min 15–30 min 31–60 min 1–2 hours More than 2 hours	Less than 15 min 15–30 min 31–60 min 1–2 hours More than 2 hours	Less than 15 min 15–30 min 31–60 min 1–2 hours More than 2 hours
Time when I woke up for good	am pm	am pm	am pm	am pm	am pm	am pm	am pm
When I woke up, I felt (Put an X)	Very tired A little tired OK Well Rested Tons of Energy	Very tired A little tired OK Well Rested Tons of Energy	Very tired A little tired OK Well Rested Tons of Energy	Very tired A little tired OK Well Rested Tons of Energy	Very tired A little tired OK Well Rested Tons of Energy	Very tired A little tired OK Well Rested Tons of Energy	Very tired A little tired OK Well Rested Tons of Energy
Amount of time napping during the day (hours)							

Figure 62.2 (Continued)

Currently, there are no well-validated rating scales that are sensitive and specific to BD in children, though the following illustrate three examples of relevant research. First, in $n = 2252$ youth, the 10-item version of the Parent-report General Behavior Inventory (PGBI-10M) discriminated childhood-onset BD from other diagnoses better than chance (AUROC = 0.79) (Youngstrom *et al.*, 2020). Nevertheless, the PGBI-10M requires further investigation and should not be used routinely to screen children for mania. Second, the Child Mania Rating Scale-Parent Report (CMRS-P) distinguished BD from healthy controls and ADHD with very good accuracy (AUCs = 0.96 and 0.91, respectively). Yet, without a clinician, it is difficult to ensure reported symptoms on the CMRS-P are episodic and concurrent and to assess functional impairment. Third, some suggested the combination of Child Behavior Checklist (CBCL) T-scores greater than 70 on the attention problems, aggression, and anxiety/depression subscales had acceptable sensitivity and specificity in identifying BD, calling this combination the "CBCL juvenile BD phenotype" (Faraone *et al.*, 2005). However, others have demonstrated the CBCL does not specifically identify BD in youths (Volk & Todd, 2007), with the results leading these researchers to rename this subscale combination as the CBCL "dysregulation profile" (Althoff *et al.*, 2012).

Coexisting problems: attention deficit hyperactivity disorder, anxiety, oppositional defiant disorder/conduct disorder, and learning disabilities

Comorbidity is the rule rather than the exception in childhood BD. Across studies, 60% of children with BD also have ADHD, >50% have at least one anxiety disorder, 47% have ODD, 21% have conduct disorder, and >15% have a substance use disorder (Fahrendorff *et al.*, 2023). Referral bias may affect these data, with clinical samples having sicker children with greater comorbidity. However, the question remains whether these are truly comorbid psychiatric disorders—i.e., fully present in their own right—or whether they represent using a separate label to capture the same symptoms. In clinical and research studies, the truest assessment of comorbid psychopathology comes from examining if symptoms of co-occurring disorders are present during euthymia, when symptoms of mania and/or depression abate.

Family and school context

Families of BD youth struggle with substantial impairment, including decreased family function and maternal warmth, and increased expressed emotion, conflict, and family stress (Miklowitz *et al.*, 2020).

Youth with BD have impaired psychosocial functioning (Goldstein *et al.*, 2009), particularly in school, work, and interpersonal domains. This is worse in mania or depression, but persists even during euthymia (Hower *et al.*, 2019).

Physical investigations

Currently there is no laboratory test or scan to diagnose BD. Selective laboratory studies may help exclude medical conditions from the differential diagnosis, particularly hyperthyroidism and substance intoxication/ingestion.

Epidemiology

Incidence and prevalence

Epidemiological studies demonstrate childhood-onset BD is not so rare, with prevalence being less than ADHD (3.7%), but more than either panic disorder or GAD (0.7%), or eating disorders

(0.1%) (Merikangas *et al.*, 2010). Methodological differences—e.g., whether children alone or children and parents were assessed and/or whether less specific forms of BD (i.e., DSM-IV BD "not otherwise specified" [BD-NOS]) were included or not—may falsely make it appear that most BD cases start in childhood.

A meta-analysis of epidemiological studies of youth with BD published from 1985 to 2007, including 16,222 youths from 6 US and 6 non-US studies, found the overall rate of BD was 1.8% (range 1.1–3.0%). Importantly, they found no significant difference in mean rates between US and non-US studies. However, studies using broad definitions of BD, including BD-NOS, reported the highest prevalence estimates, and US studies had a wider range of rates. Controlling for methodological issues, they did not find a significant increase in rates of childhood-onset BD over time between 1985–2007 (Van Meter *et al.*, 2011).

As expected, the prevalence of BD increases from childhood to adulthood. For example, Merikangas *et al.* conducted a cross-sectional survey of 10,123 US adolescents that showed 2.5% met criteria for lifetime BD-I or BD-II, with a nearly two-fold increase in mania when comparing 13–14-year-olds to 17–18-year-olds. However, this study used a modified version of the Composite International Diagnostic Interview administered to adolescents, without corroboration from parental informants, which may result in overdiagnosis (Merikangas *et al.*, 2012). Lewinsohn's longitudinal studies corroborate this, with 1.1% of adolescents ($n = 1507$) meeting criteria for BD when both parents' and children's reports were assessed, while 2.1% of a subset reassessed using only individual report at age 24 ($n = 893$) did so (Lewinsohn *et al.*, 2000).

These data align with those of prior cross-national epidemiologic studies of adults showing a lifetime prevalence of 1–3% for BD (Weissman *et al.*, 1996, Kessler *et al.*, 2005). Two large epidemiologic studies of BD adults report a median onset age of 18 (Christie *et al.*, 1988) or 25 years (Kessler *et al.*, 2005). The BD age of onset is not distributed normally, with two studies each reporting three peaks of onset age (Bellivier *et al.*, 2003, Lin *et al.*, 2006). Early onset may be familial or associated with a strong family history of BD, though recall bias may influence these retrospective, rather than prospective, recollections of BD onset (Kennedy *et al.*, 2005, Lin *et al.*, 2006).

Global and time variations

Despite the abovementioned meta-analysis by Van Meter *et al.* suggesting similar rates of BD among US and non-US child studies, we know little about global differences in morbidity, mortality, and service utilization among BD youth.

Methodological questions

While epidemiological studies with standardized assessments of BD have shown relative stability in BD among children and adolescents over time, clinical studies suggest increasing numbers of children are being diagnosed with BD. For example, the percentage of minors discharged from psychiatric hospitals in the US with a BD diagnosis has surged from less than 10% in the mid-1990s to more than 20% in the mid-2000s (Blader & Carlson, 2007). Another study demonstrated a 40-fold rise in the incidence of US outpatient visits assigned the diagnosis of BD during a similar period, from 25/100,000 in 1993–1994 to 1003/100,000 in 2002–2003 (Moreno *et al.*, 2007). This phenomenon is not restricted to the US, with rates of under 19-year-olds admitted to German psychiatric hospitals increasing by 68.5% between 2000–2007, an increase which exceeded that for other diagnoses (Holtmann *et al.*, 2010).

Public health implications

From a public health perspective, the inconsistency between epidemiological data suggesting relative stability in rates of youth diagnosed with BD, and clinical data suggesting increasing numbers of youth globally being diagnosed with BD, supports the need for more specific tools clinicians can use to effectively diagnose mania and BD. Without them, we run the risk of over-, under-, and misdiagnosis of youth with BD, potentially resulting in incorrect or suboptimal treatment.

Longitudinal outcome

Methodological factors

Longitudinal studies are critical to determine what happens to children with BD as they become adolescents and, ultimately, adults. Existing longitudinal studies of BD in youth are recruited from clinical samples, which may result in different findings from population studies, as those presenting to clinics are often more severely impaired.

Course and Outcome of Bipolar Youth study

The Course and Outcome of Bipolar Youth (COBY) was a longitudinal study of children meeting DSM-IV criteria for BD-I or BD-II, or criteria for BD-NOS operationalized as: (i) clinically relevant BD symptoms of euphoric or irritable mood lasting a minimum of 4 hours within a 24-hour period; (ii) at least 2 "B" symptoms if the mood was primarily euphoric (3 if primarily irritable); and (iii) at least 4 cumulative lifetime days meeting these criteria. COBY's focus was thus on children with episodes of mania of varying duration and intensity.

The COBY study found at intake, BD-I ($n = 255$), BD-II ($n = 30$), and BD-NOS ($n = 153$) participants did not differ in age of onset, duration of illness, rates of comorbid disorders, suicidal ideation, or manic symptoms during the most serious episode. Elevated and/or expansive mood was found in 91.8% of BD-I and 81.9% of BD-NOS participants. BD-I participants had more severe manic symptoms, greater overall functional impairment, and higher rates of psychiatric hospitalization, psychosis, and suicide attempts than those with BD-NOS (Axelson *et al.*, 2006).

However, 4-year longitudinal follow-up data indicated BD-NOS participants had significantly longer mean time to recovery from the index episode and significantly longer mean time to recurrence; approximately 50% of youth with BD-NOS converted to BD-I or BD-II. Over an average of

8 years of follow-up, latent class analysis identified 4 mood trajectories among COBY participants: predominantly euthymic (24.0%), moderately euthymic (34.6%), ill with improving course (19.1%), and predominantly ill (22.3%) (Birmaher *et al.*, 2014). BD subtype was not associated with class membership. During follow-up, 27% of youth had at least one suicide attempt, and 14% had at least two (Goldstein *et al.*, 2022). Approximately 40% of youth who experienced at least one manic or hypomanic episode during adolescence continued to have manic or hypomanic episodes in adulthood; and this risk did not differ according to age at onset (child versus adolescent) (Hafeman *et al.*, 2021).

Overall, the COBY study demonstrated BD can be reliably diagnosed in children and adolescents, its impairment is similar across BD-I/II/NOS, and longitudinally, progressive numbers of BD-NOS participants develop more distinct episodes consistent with BD-I or BD-II. While many youths improve over time, a substantial subset remain highly symptomatic, and there is continuity between BD in childhood/adolescence and adulthood.

Other longitudinal studies

Another longitudinal BD study was conducted by Barbara Geller MD's group at Washington University in St. Louis. While concerns have been raised about how manic episodes were operationalized with the K-SADS-E (epidemiological) interview allowing double-counting of symptoms, leading to longer duration of mania and depression than other K-SADS versions, their data align with those of the COBY study in indicating mania may start in childhood (mean age of onset = 7.4 ± 3.5) and youth with BD suffer from recurrent manic and/or depressive symptoms (Carlson & Klein, 2014). Specifically, a 4-year study of 86 children with DSM-IV BD-I (manic or mixed), with at least 1 cardinal symptom (elation and/or grandiosity) to ensure differentiation from ADHD, found participants spent 56.9 ± 28.8% of the total weeks with mania or hypomania (unipolar or mixed), and 47.1 ± 30.4% of the total weeks with major or minor depression and dysthymia (unipolar or mixed) (Geller *et al.*, 2004).

Ellen Leibenluft MD's group at the US National Institute of Mental Health (NIMH) also conducted a longitudinal study focusing on two groups of children: (i) narrow-phenotype pediatric BD (NP-BD) and (ii) severe mood dysregulation (SMD). Prospective data showed only 1 of 84 SMD subjects (1.2%) experienced a (hypo)manic or mixed episode during a median 28.7 months of follow-up, whereas 58 of 93 NP-BD participants (62.4%) experienced such a (hypo)manic or mixed episode (Stringaris *et al.*, 2010).

Risk factors

Family studies

First-degree relatives of people with BD have an approximately 10-fold increased risk for BD, versus those without such a history (Mortensen *et al.*, 2003; Smoller & Finn, 2003). However, studies show children whose parents have BD have much higher rates of disorders other than BD, including ADHD, anxiety, and depression (25–65% versus 3% of children whose parents do not have mental health disorders) (Weissman *et al.*, 1984). This is not surprising given those other disorders have higher incidence rates than BD (Hillegers *et al.*, 2005, Mesman *et al.*, 2013).

Twin and adoption studies

Twin studies suggest the heritability of BD in adults has 60–70% concordance for monozygotic twins and 20–30% in dizygotic twins (Smoller & Finn, 2003).

Molecular genetic studies

The genetics of BD are complex and rapidly evolving, but several themes emerge. First, BD is due to multiple genes, not a single gene (Kelsoe, 2003). Second, the genes conferring risk for BD and those implicated in schizophrenia may overlap (Priebe *et al.*, 2012, Craddock & Sklar, 2013).

Recent meta-analyses of genome-wide association studies (GWAS) including up to 40,000 individuals with BD have identified a large number of single nucleotide polymorphisms (SNPs) associated with risk for BD. A weighted average of these findings has helped define a "polygenic risk score" (PRS) for BD (Mullins *et al.*, 2021). PRSs are elevated in youth and adults with BD, and those at family risk for BD (Birmaher *et al.*, 2021). They predict the development of BD in adults with MDD (Musliner *et al.*, 2020). These studies suggest PRSs may explain 5–10% of variance in which offspring have BD, which is less than the estimated 30% explained by parental history of BD (Birmaher *et al.*, 2022). While PRSs are not sufficiently predictive alone, studies are testing how they can be combined with other markers of BD risk for more accurate prediction of who will develop BD.

Clinical prodromes/risk factors

Several longitudinal community-based studies have queried which childhood or adolescent diagnoses are associated with increased risk for later BD. A 10-year longitudinal study suggests progression from symptoms of BD to full-blown BD was predicted by symptom persistence—i.e., the longer symptoms exist, the more they progress (Tijssen *et al.*, 2010). Studies following children with depression into late adolescence or early adulthood find prepubertal MDD is associated with increased risk for BD (Kovacs *et al.*, 1994, Rao *et al.*, 1995, Weissman *et al.*, 1999). However, the prevalence of BD ranged widely, perhaps because of small sample sizes or because of differences in patient characteristics (e.g., inpatients versus outpatients). Positive family history, psychosis, and rapid symptom onset may predict BD (Geller *et al.*, 1994). COBY study data indicate after 5 years of longitudinal follow-up, 45% of BD-NOS patients converted to either BD-I or BD-II, with the strongest predictor of conversion being first- or second-degree family history of mania or hypomania (Axelson *et al.*, 2011). Among offspring of parents with BD, mood lability and subthreshold manic symptoms, particularly in offspring of parents with early BD onset, predict BD onset (Hafeman *et al.*, 2016). Clinic-based follow-up studies of children with ADHD do not consistently support an elevated risk for developing BD by adulthood (Hazell *et al.*, 2003).

Pathophysiology

Brain volume findings: structural magnetic resonance imaging

Studies have found decreased subcortical brain volumes in children with BD, with the most prominent finding being decreased amygdala volume (Pfeifer *et al.*, 2008; Long *et al.*, 2023). Studies have shown decreased cortical thickness in the prefrontal cortex (PFC) (Guo *et al.*, 2021). In the future, it is possible structural magnetic resonance imaging (sMRI) studies of BD youth will be united, either in a consortium or via meta-analysis, as is ongoing for adults with BD via the Enhancing Neuroimaging Genetics through Meta-Analysis (ENIGMA) consortium.

Neurocognitive deficits: computerized behavioral tasks and functional magnetic resonance imaging

Studies using cognitive and emotional tasks, out-of-scanner and with magnetic resonance imaging (MRI) as functional MRI (fMRI), have demonstrated BD youths have aberrant functioning in at least three processes: social cognition including emotional face processing, reward processing including response to frustration via rigged feedback and cognitive flexibility via adaptation to changing rewards and punishments, and response inhibition. Face processing is linked to basic emotional processing. Studies show BD youth make a significantly greater number of errors when categorizing emotional faces versus both healthy controls and those with anxiety disorders (Guyer *et al.*, 2007), and those with primary ADHD (Seymour *et al.*, 2013). FMRI studies show BD youths have abnormal PFC–amygdala–striatal neural activation versus controls when viewing faces with happy, angry, or neutral emotions (Wegbreit *et al.*, 2014). Reward processing is linked to many forms of therapy, including behavior modification. Studies tapping either frustration or cognitive flexibility have shown BD youths are impaired compared to controls and youth with chronic irritability (Dickstein *et al.*, 2004, Dickstein *et al.*, 2007, Rich *et al.*, 2007). FMRI studies have shown BD youths have the opposite PFC–striatal activation during cognitive flexibility tasks versus controls and youth with chronic irritability (Dickstein *et al.*, 2010, Adleman *et al.*, 2011). Response inhibition is linked to distractibility and impulsivity, including risk for substance use and self-harm. Studies show BD youth may either have reduced striatal "error signal" versus controls during failed motor inhibition (Leibenluft *et al.*, 2007) or greater reliance on cognitive control areas to maintain adequate behavioral performance (Singh *et al.*, 2010). Such data are relevant to developing mechanism-targeted treatments and diagnostic approaches.

Neurochemistry: magnetic resonance spectroscopy

Magnetic resonance spectroscopy (MRS) research in BD has focused on N-acetyl aspartate (NAA), an intraneuronal marker whose levels are decreased in neuropathology, and *myo*-Inositol (mI), an intracellular second messenger, thought to be overabundant in mania, whose levels are decreased by lithium (Moore *et al.*, 1999, Silverstone *et al.*, 2002).

Youth with familial BD (Chang *et al.*, 2003), and adults with BD (Winsberg *et al.*, 2000), have significantly decreased NAA in the dorsolateral prefrontal cortex (DLPFC) versus controls. NAA was decreased in PFC regions of youth with BD, but not in unmedicated youth with BD (Tannous *et al.*, 2021). BD youths have increased anterior cingulate cortex (ACC) mI versus controls and youth with intermittent explosive disorder (Davanzo *et al.*, 2003), with mI levels being responsive to lithium treatment (Davanzo *et al.*, 2001). Together, these MRS studies suggest BD youths may be characterized by specific neurochemical alterations that respond to psychopharmacological treatment; future work in this area may ultimately inform such treatment.

With respect to glutamate, a meta-analysis including 40 studies (7 with a pediatric sample) found elevated ACC glutamate adults with BD, but not in children and/or adolescents with BD (Ino *et al.*, 2023).

Diffusion tensor imaging

Diffusion tensor imaging (DTI) studies have shown disrupted white matter integrity in tracts connecting the PFC as indexed by decreased fractional anisotropy among BD versus controls (Adler *et al.*, 2006). However, others have suggested these changes might not be specific to BD, as similar alterations have been shown in youths with primary ADHD (Pavuluri *et al.*, 2009). Radial diffusivity (RD), a marker of abnormal myelination, may be a specific DTI marker for BD. Youth with BD (but not DMDD) showed widespread increased RD (Linke *et al.*, 2019), akin to findings in adults with BD (Lu *et al.*, 2011).

Treatment

General approach

Treating children and adolescents with BD requires a comprehensive approach to focus first on treating the most acute and disabling aspects of BD—e.g., acute mania, depression, psychosis, substance intoxication, and suicidality. Later treatment addresses other problems—e.g., comorbid anxiety, ADHD, substance use disorders, and deficient social skills (Figure 62.3).

Treatment decisions require collaboration among physicians, patients, and families to identify target symptoms, educate about side effects, and evaluate each treatment's efficacy. Daily ratings of target symptoms by parents and/or patients allow treatment to be based upon prospective, rather than retrospective, data. Moreover, patient safety, including functional impairment, suicidal thoughts, and treatment-emergent side

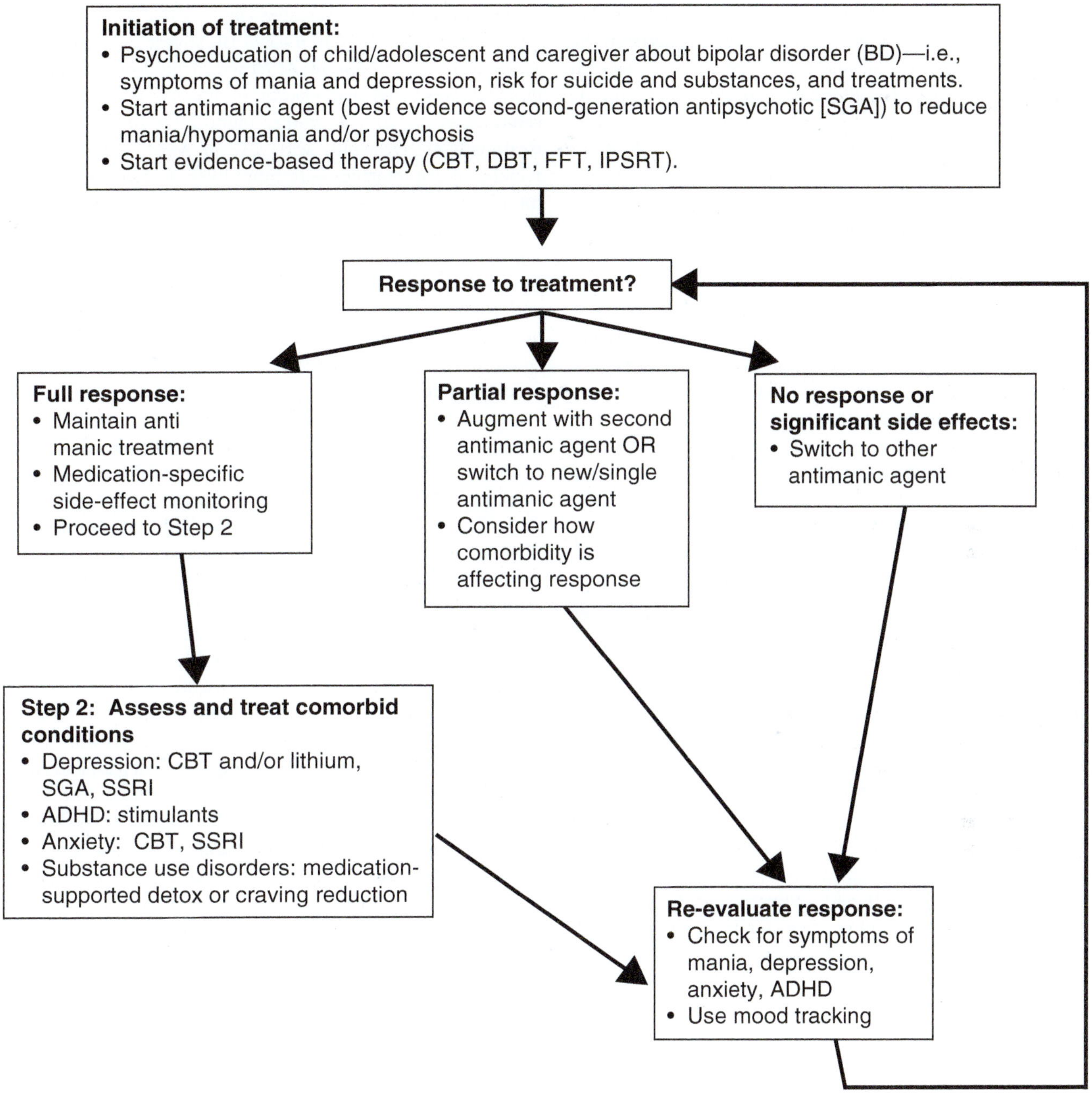

Figure 62.3 Pediatric bipolar disorder (BD) treatment at a glance. *Note*: ADHD: attention deficit hyperactivity disorder; CBT: cognitive behavioral therapy; DBT: dialectical behavioral therapy; FFT: family-focused therapy; IPSRT: interpersonal and social rhythm therapy; SSRI: selective serotonin reuptake inhibitor.

effects, must be evaluated continuously. This includes considerations of the level of care required to manage the patient safely, though there are no universal standards for inpatient versus outpatient care. Here, we emphasize double-blind randomized placebo-controlled trials (RCTs) in children or adolescents where available. We indicate if discussing an adult BD study, because youth may respond differently than adults, for example, as was found with antidepressant medications leading to the US Food and Drug Administration (FDA) black box warning up to age 25 years.

Furthermore, clinicians must consider common issues affecting children and adolescents, including substance use and pregnancy. Most antimanic and antidepressant agents are metabolized by the liver. Thus, any other medication or drug of abuse metabolized by the liver, including alcohol, may influence treatment response and side-effect risk. Regarding pregnancy, certain antimanic agents, including antiepileptic drugs (AEDs, e.g., valproate) and lithium, have known adverse effects on the developing fetus. Thus, clinicians must discuss these risks with their patients, and potential alternatives to medication and the need for contraception.

Ideally, medication trials should last at least six to eight weeks, with one new agent added at a time. However, this approach may not be feasible in acutely manic or psychotic patients. Physicians should regularly assess the need for each medication to avoid adding more and more medications without considering if any can be discontinued or if there is a simpler medication strategy. Moreover, symptoms do not typically resolve on medication alone; rather, comprehensive treatment usually requires both psychopharmacology and psychotherapy. Finally, treatment must address the phase of a child's illness, since acute and maintenance interventions differ.

Psychopharmacology for pediatric bipolar disorder

Pharmacotherapy of mania

Current antimanic medications intended to reduce symptoms of, and to prevent occurrence of, mania or hypomania include: (i) second-generation antipsychotic medications (SGAs, e.g., risperidone, aripiprazole), (ii) lithium, and (iii) AEDs.

Recent RCTs support the following conclusions. First, SGAs are effective, and potentially superior to other antimanic agents, in the treatment of BD. However, such medications are associated with significant side effects, notably impairing weight gain and metabolic abnormalities. Second, lithium's role in BD children is less clear than in BD adults, though further study is warranted given studies showing its efficacy in pediatric patients with extreme aggression. Third, AEDs may be less efficacious than other antimanic agents for children with BD. Thus, the lack of a "silver bullet" or single best antimanic agent complicates efforts to select any one agent as a first-line treatment and again emphasizes the importance of thorough discussions with patients and families. For an individual, a step-wise approach is often needed, involving trying different antimanic agents if initial attempts are unsuccessful. We focus our discussion on efficacy and the most important side effects, but for dosing guidelines and a more thorough discussion of side effects, see Kowatch *et al.* (2005), Correll *et al.* (2006), and Klein *et al.* (2020).

Second-generation antipsychotic medications

SGAs have the strongest efficacy data in BD youths; however, there are concerns about side effects, such as substantial weight gain and metabolic syndrome, and about potential overprescription to children in general (Andrade *et al.*, 2011). Risperidone, aripiprazole, quetiapine, and olanzapine have FDA indications to treat mania or mixed states associated with BD in 10–17-year-olds (13–17 for olanzapine) based on RCTs in BD youth. Additional RCTs in BD youth support the consideration of other SGAs, including ziprasidone and asenapine (Findling *et al.*, 2015b, Findling *et al.*, 2022).

Aripiprazole was evaluated in a 4-week double-blind placebo-controlled RCT of $n = 296$ 10–17 year-olds currently in a mixed or manic episode. At either 10 mg/d or 30 mg/d, aripiprazole was better than placebo in reducing manic symptoms (Findling *et al.*, 2009). Another found after 16 weeks of open treatment, 4–9-year-olds with BD ($n = 96$), randomized to remain on aripiprazole, were more likely to remain without a mood episode versus those switched to placebo ($n = 30$ per group; weeks without mood episode 6.14 ± 11.8 on aripiprazole, 2.29 ± 0.38 on placebo) (Findling *et al.*, 2012).

Studies of risperidone include a study of 10–17 year-olds with BD-I, currently manic or mixed, randomized to receive risperidone 0.5–2.5 mg/d ($n = 50$), 3–6 mg/d ($n = 61$), or placebo ($n = 58$) for 3 weeks. Both risperidone groups showed significant reductions in mania versus placebo (Haas *et al.*, 2009). Others have compared the clinical and neural outcome of BD youths treated with risperidone versus divalproex (Depakote), showing neither treatment was clearly superior, although this may have been a type II error given the small sample size ($n = 24$ total). They did find risperidone may have reduced mania faster (Pavuluri *et al.*, 2010). Studies of quetiapine include a 6-week double-blind RCT of $n = 109$ 10–17-year-olds with BD-I, currently manic or mixed, found 72% of those randomized to 400–600 mg of quetiapine and 49% of those randomized to serum levels of 1.0–1.2 mEq/l of lithium responded (defined as change in Young Mania Rating Scale [YMRS] score), with no difference in remission rate (defined as YMRS < 12) (Patino *et al.*, 2021).

A particular concern is the association of SGAs with "metabolic syndrome"—i.e. extreme and rapid weight gain and endocrine abnormalities, including diabetes mellitus. A study of $n = 338$ children ages 4–19 years old, treated for a median of 10.8 weeks with SGAs, showed weight increased by a mean of 8.5 kg for olanzapine, 6.1 kg with quetiapine, 5.3 kg with risperidone, and 4.4 kg with aripiprazole, versus 0.2 kg in an untreated group. Increases were noted in total cholesterol, triglycerides, and non-high-density lipoprotein (Correll *et al.*, 2009). Children treated with SGAs have a greater risk of developing diabetes (3.23/1000) than those receiving antidepressants (1.86/1000) or no treatment (0.76/1000) (Andrade *et al.*, 2011). Patients should be monitored routinely for weight, height, and body-mass index, and undergo a fasting glucose and lipid panel every six months. Finally, for SGAs, firm conclusions on the risk of tardive dyskinesia are not possible because of the lack of long-term data (Ghaemi *et al.*, 2006).

Lithium

Support for lithium's efficacy in childhood-onset BD is mixed. Efficacy and safety data place it in the middle of the three categories of medications typically used in childhood-onset BD—ahead of AEDs but weaker than SGAs. Moreover, lithium has an FDA indication for the treatment of mania in patients as young as 12 years, but it was "grandfathered" in based on studies of BD adults and prior to the availability of large numbers of RCTs in BD youth. Nevertheless, there is robust evidence for lithium's efficacy in BD adults, including for acute mania (Bowden *et al.*, 2005), long-term prophylaxis (Bowden *et al.*, 2003), and reduction of suicide risk (Cipriani *et al.*, 2005). Thus, it may be reasonable to prescribe lithium for individual BD youths, especially those who do not respond to SGAs.

The largest and most recent dataset about lithium comes from the Treatment of Early Age Mania (TEAM) study of $n = 279$ children aged 6–15 years old with BD-I randomized to receive 8 weeks of either lithium, risperidone, or divalproex sodium. Lithium was not significantly better in treating mania than divalproex, and resulted in a higher discontinuation rate than risperidone (Geller *et al.*, 2012). However, one wonders if atypical features of this sample related to how mania and depression symptoms were double-counted, resulting in reporting longer duration of mania than other studies, may reduce its generalizability to typical childhood-onset BD cases. Other RCTs are equivocal, for example, an 8-week RCT found 7–17 year-olds with BD-I, manic or mixed, treated with lithium ($n = 53$) had significantly greater reduction in YMRS than placebo ($n = 28$) (Findling *et al.*, 2015c), whereas another RCT study failed to find a significant difference between adolescents ($n = 108$) whose acute mania was initially stabilized with open lithium treatment, and who were then randomized to either continue lithium or switch to placebo during a double-blind discontinuation study (Kafantaris *et al.*, 2004).

Adult studies suggest optimal lithium levels are between 0.6–1.0 mEq/l for acute mania and down to 0.4 mEq/l for maintenance treatment, but this has not been tested rigorously in youth (Gelenberg *et al.*, 1989). Interestingly, an MRS study showed BD youth ($n = 9$) had lower brain/serum lithium concentrations than BD adults ($n = 18$) (Moore *et al.*, 2002), suggesting BD youths may require higher doses of lithium to achieve the same brain concentration of lithium than adults. However, the clinical implications of this finding have not been studied systematically.

Antiepileptic drugs

AEDs have the weakest support for efficacy in childhood-onset BD. However, safety data for AEDs (largely gleaned from pediatric epilepsy studies) is generally strong, with the exception of questions regarding acute hepatic or pancreatic failure and possible adverse effects on female gonadal function (see paragraph on valproate below) (de Silva *et al.*, 1996).

RCT data fail to demonstrate benefit from divalproex, lamotrigine, or oxcarbazepine in childhood-onset BD (Wagner *et al.*, 2006, Wagner *et al.*, 2009, Findling *et al.*, 2015a). Open-label trials, most of them small, document some evidence of benefit for carbamazepine, valproate, or lamotrigine, but without a placebo control these studies can provide only weak support for efficacy (Wagner *et al.*, 2002, Chang *et al.*, 2006).

In adults, AEDs have shown efficacy for acute and maintenance antimanic treatment, leading to FDA indications for valproate and a long-acting form of carbamazepine (Pope *et al.*, 1991). Lamotrigine has an FDA indication for BD in adults, although data suggest it is more effective as a maintenance treatment, preventing depressive and manic relapse, than for acute mania (Bowden *et al.*, 2003).

Valproate has a black-box FDA warning due to the possibility of acute, life-threatening hepatic failure and pancreatitis, both of which are more common in those on multiple medications or less than two years old (Grauso-Eby *et al.*, 2003). Therefore, any patient taking valproate who develops the acute onset of nausea, vomiting, or acute abdominal pain should receive prompt medical evaluation. Irregular menses and polycystic ovary syndrome (PCOS; i.e. polycystic ovarian morphology, increased serum testosterone or luteinizing hormone, and irregular menses) may be associated with valproate use, particularly in young women (Grauso-Eby *et al.*, 2003).

Lamotrigine has an FDA black-box warning in children younger than 16 due to potential for two different life-threatening rashes, Stephens-Johnson syndrome, and toxic epidermal necrolysis. More benign rashes are common, and a meta-analysis found increased risk for such rashes was associated with patients age less than 12 years old or co-administration of medications inhibiting hepatic metabolism (e.g. valproate) (Calabrese *et al.*, 2002).

Pharmacotherapy of depression in childhood-onset bipolar disorder

Currently, there are 4 published RCTs of depression in BD-I youth. Detke *et al.* found 10–17 year-olds with a BD-I depressed episode had a greater improvement in Children's Depression Rating Scale (CDRS) score for those randomized to the combination of olanzapine plus fluoxetine ($n = 170$) versus to placebo ($n = 85$) though those taking olanzapine/fluoxetine had significantly greater weight gain (4.4 kg versus 0.5 kg) (Detke *et al.*, 2015). DelBello *et al.* showed depressed BD-I youth had significantly greater CDRS reduction for those randomized to 6 weeks of lurasidone ($n = 175$) versus placebo ($n = 172$) (DelBello *et al.*, 2017). Two RCTs failed to show significant differences between quetiapine versus placebo for depressed BD youth—DelBello *et al.* (2009): quetiapine $n = 17$, placebo $n = 15$; Findling et al. (2014): quetiapine $n = 70$, placebo $n = 74$;.

The lack of RCT data to guide medication treatment of depression or anxiety in BD youths is problematic. Data suggest: (i) BD youths spend a considerable amount of time struggling with depression and/or anxiety; (ii) BD youths often receive selective serotonin reuptake inhibitors (SSRIs) to augment their antimanic treatment without the induction of mania; (iii) there is some suggestion the risk of antidepressant-induced mania is higher in prepubertal children than in older adolescents or adults (Martin *et al.* 2004); and (iv) in adult BD, it is unclear whether SSRI antidepressants or lithium are preferable in the treatment of adult bipolar depression (Thase, 2007). Specifically, Martin *et al.* used nationally representative pharmacy data from 87,920 5–29-year-olds, showing 5.4% ($n = 4781$) experienced manic conversion during a median of 41 weeks of follow-up. This was more common in prepubertal children than older adolescents or adults (number needed to harm = 10 in 10–14-year-olds versus

23 in 15–29 year-olds) and more common after exposure to tricyclic antidepressants than SSRIs (Martin *et al.*, 2004).

Thus, there is considerable need for study of antidepressant/antianxiety medications, including the safety and efficacy of primary serotonergic agents.

Pharmacotherapy of attention disorder hyperactivity disorder in childhood-onset bipolar disorder

There is a similar lack of evidence-based guidance to treat ADHD among children with BD. Although concerns have been raised about the possibility of ADHD-medication-induced mania, myriad studies show these agents are commonly used without such exacerbation (Carlson *et al.*, 2000). One double-blind crossover RCT in children with childhood-onset BD and ADHD found once mania remitted on valproate, amphetamine salts plus valproate was more effective in reducing ADHD symptoms than placebo plus valproate, without exacerbating mania ($n = 30$) (Scheffer *et al.*, 2005). Thus, clinicians treating youth with BD and comorbid ADHD should treat the patient's mania, and then consider psychostimulant treatment.

Psychotherapy for pediatric bipolar disorder

When combined with pharmacotherapy, several types of psychotherapy show promise in treating childhood-onset BD. Family-focused therapy (FFT) includes psychoeducation, communication enhancement, and problem-solving skills. Twenty-one FFT sessions over nine months after an index mood episode resulted in faster recovery and fewer weeks depressed versus those randomized to receive only three family sessions on relapse prevention. However, there was no significant difference in rates of recovery from mania or time to recurrence of mania or depression (Miklowitz *et al.*, 2008). A review of 30 years of FFT research including 8 RCTs in adolescents and adults with BD has shown FFT combined with pharmacotherapy hastens recovery from mood episodes, reduces recurrences, and reduces symptom severity compared to briefer forms of psychoeducation plus pharmacotherapy (Miklowitz & Chung, 2016).

Multifamily psychoeducational groups increase parents' knowledge about BD and ability to obtain services. Multifamily psychoeducational groups administered in eight 90-minute sessions have shown greater reduction in the mood severity index, a combination of the YMRS and CDRS, than those receiving a waitlist control (Fristad *et al.*, 2009).

Cognitive behavioral therapy (CBT) for BD changes dysfunctional thoughts and behaviors associated with noneuthymic mood states. While substantial research demonstrates CBT's role for youth with MDD, results for CBT in youth with BD are less favorable. For example, group CBT was not significantly better than pharmacotherapy in an RCT with $n = 32$ female BD adolescents (Arman *et al.*, 2018).

Dialectical behavioral therapy (DBT) promotes interpersonal effectiveness and emotional regulation. An RCT comparing DBT ($n = 14$) to psychosocial treatment as usual ($n = 7$) for 12–18-year-olds with BD-I/-II/-NOS showed those receiving DBT had less severe depressive symptoms and reduction in suicidal ideation during 1-year of follow-up (Goldstein *et al.*, 2015). More RCTs are needed to document efficacy and of head-to-head comparisons.

Future developments and necessary research

Hopefully, the future will bring greater understanding of the biological and environmental mechanisms, precision of the diagnosis and prognosis, and more effective treatments for childhood-onset BD. We highlight the need for novel assessment tools, risk calculators, and treatments.

Novel assessment tools

Psychiatry currently relies on retrospective cross-sectional reports (i.e., asking patients "how did you feel this past week?" in interviews/rating scales). This approach is inherently biased by recency effects and poor recall that is particularly problematic for BD, where assessment of mood fluctuations and episodes across time is vital. Research examining better ways to prospectively and objectively assess episodic mood symptoms includes:

- Ecological momentary assessment (EMA), which prompts patients to complete mood charting prospectively, rather than retrospectively. A recent study in adults with BD-I and BD-II showed EMA detected symptoms (e.g. worry, agitation) predictive of episode recurrence (Bos *et al.*, 2022).
- Actigraphy, i.e., wearable motion and other physiological sensors that may provide an objective measure of sleep and activity. Studies in adults with BD have begun assessing whether actigraphy can distinguish between mood polarity (Scott *et al.*, 2017) or predict suicidal thoughts and behaviors (Benard *et al.*, 2019).
- Passive sensing, i.e., smartphone data regarding activity, social interaction, and phone activity that is collected all the time without any active input from the patient. Emerging data in adults suggests such parameters (e.g. physical activity, duration and number of calls and texts) may differentiate and potentially predict mood states (Beiwinkel *et al.*, 2016).

None of these tools are validated for clinical use. Ongoing research will test how they may enhance our assessment, monitoring, and, ultimately, treatment of BD in the future.

Risk calculators

Risk calculators (RCs) are mathematical models harnessing known risk factors for a particular condition, and applying this to estimate the risk for a given individual. RCs are used regularly in medicine (e.g. to predict cardiovascular disease; AUCs = 0.7–0.9). RCs are not the standard of care in psychiatry. However, RCs have been developed to predict BD onset (Hafeman *et al.*, 2017), progression from BD-NOS to BD-I/BD-II (Birmaher *et al.*, 2018), recurrence of threshold mood disorder in BD (Birmaher *et al.*, 2020), and suicide (Goldstein *et al.*, 2022). In the future, RCs may inform clinical treatment.

Novel treatments

There is considerable need for novel treatments for BD, given substantial impairment due to BD despite our best treatments. Examples include ketamine, which has evidence for unipolar depression in adolescents and BD depression in adults, though it is untested in adolescents with BD depression. Similarly, transcranial magnetic stimulation (TMS) has shown promise for adults with unipolar depression, but thus far, TMS studies of adolescents with depression have not separated from placebo, and studies of BD depressed adults have shown mixed results. A third example is cognitive remediation, i.e., use of drill-and-practice exercises to address deficits in cognitive or emotional functioning, much as one would do physical exercises to rehabilitate from physical injuries. Cognitive remediation has shown promise in adults with schizophrenia (McGurk *et al.*, 2007), and is being studied in children with ADHD or DMDD (Dickstein *et al.*, 2015, Stoddard *et al.*, 2016).

References

Adleman, N.E. *et al.* (2011) Neural correlates of reversal learning in severe mood dysregulation and pediatric bipolar disorder. *Journal of the American Academy of Child and Adolescent Psychiatry* **50**, 1173–1185. e2

Adler, C.M. *et al.* (2006) Evidence of white matter pathology in bipolar disorder adolescents experiencing their first episode of mania: a diffusion tensor imaging study. *The American Journal of Psychiatry* **163**, 322–324.

Algorta, G.P. *et al.* (2011) Suicidality in pediatric bipolar disorder: predictor or outcome of family processes and mixed mood presentation? *Bipolar Disorders* **13**, 76–86.

Althoff, R.R. *et al.* (2012) Temperamental profiles of dysregulated children. *Child Psychiatry and Human Development* **43**, 511–522.

American Psychiatric Association (1994) *Diagnostic and Statistical Manual of Mental Disorders*, 4th edn. American Psychiatric Association, Washington, DC.

American Psychiatric Association (2000) *Diagnostic and Statistical Manual of Mental Disorders*, 4th edn, text revision. American Psychiatric Association, Washington DC.

American Psychiatric Association (2013) *Diagnostic and Statistical Manual of Mental Disorders*, 5th edn. American Psychiatric Association, Washington, DC.

Andrade, S.E. *et al.* (2011) Antipsychotic medication use among children and risk of diabetes mellitus. *Pediatrics* **128**, 1135–1141.

Angst, J. *et al.* (2020) Bipolar disorders in ICD-11: current status and strengths. *International Journal of Bipolar Disorders* **8**, 3.

Arman, S. *et al.* (2018) Efficacy of group cognitive-behavioral therapy in maintenance treatment and relapse prevention for bipolar adolescents. *Advanced Biomedical Research* **7**, 41.

Axelson, D. *et al.* (2006) Phenomenology of children and adolescents with bipolar spectrum disorders. *Archives of General Psychiatry* **63**, 1139–1148.

Axelson, D. *et al.* (2015) Diagnostic precursors to bipolar disorder in offspring of parents with bipolar disorder: a longitudinal study. *The American Journal of Psychiatry* **172**, 638–646.

Axelson, D.A. *et al.* (2011) Course of subthreshold bipolar disorder in youth: diagnostic progression from bipolar disorder not otherwise specified. *Journal of the American Academy of Child and Adolescent Psychiatry* **50**, 1001–1016.

Beiwinkel, T. *et al.* (2016) Using smartphones to monitor bipolar disorder symptoms: a pilot study. *JMIR Mental Health* **3**, e2.

Bellivier, F. *et al.* (2003) Age at onset in bipolar I affective disorder: further evidence for three subgroups. *The American Journal of Psychiatry* **160**, 999–1001.

Benard, V. *et al.* (2019) Sleep and circadian rhythms as possible trait markers of suicide attempt in bipolar disorders: an actigraphy study. *Journal of Affective Disorders* **244**, 1–8.

Berk, M. *et al.* (2011) Does stage of illness impact treatment response in bipolar disorder? Empirical treatment data and their implication for the staging model and early intervention. *Bipolar Disorders* **13**, 87–98.

Biederman, J. *et al.* (2004) Further evidence of unique developmental phenotypic correlates of pediatric bipolar disorder: findings from a large sample of clinically referred preadolescent children assessed over the last 7 years. *Journal of Affective Disorders* **82**(Suppl 1), S45–S58.

Birmaher, B. *et al.* (2006) Clinical course of children and adolescents with bipolar spectrum disorders. *Archives of General Psychiatry* **63**, 175–183.

Birmaher, B. *et al.* (2014) Longitudinal trajectories and associated baseline predictors in youths with bipolar spectrum disorders. *The American Journal of Psychiatry* **171**, 990–999.

Birmaher, B. *et al.* (2018) A risk calculator to predict the individual risk of conversion from subthreshold bipolar symptoms to bipolar disorder I or II in youth. *Journal of the American Academy of Child and Adolescent Psychiatry* **57**, 755–763. e4

Birmaher, B. *et al.* (2020) Predicting personalized risk of mood recurrences in youths and young adults with bipolar spectrum disorder. *Journal of the American Academy of Child and Adolescent Psychiatry* **59**, 1156–1164.

Birmaher, B. *et al.* (2021) A longitudinal study of psychiatric disorders in offspring of parents with bipolar disorder from preschool to adolescence. *Journal of the American Academy of Child and Adolescent Psychiatry* **60**, 1419–1429.

Birmaher, B. *et al.* (2022) Role of polygenic risk score in the familial transmission of bipolar disorder in youth. *JAMA Psychiatry* **79**, 160–168.

Blader, J.C. & Carlson, G.A. (2007) Increased rates of bipolar disorder diagnoses among U.S. child, adolescent, and adult inpatients, 1996-2004. *Biological Psychiatry* **62**, 107–114.

Bos, F.M. *et al.* (2022) Anticipating manic and depressive transitions in patients with bipolar disorder using early warning signals. *International Journal of Bipolar Disorders* **10**, 12.

Bowden, C.L. *et al.* (2003) A placebo-controlled 18-month trial of lamotrigine and lithium maintenance treatment in recently manic or hypomanic patients with bipolar I disorder. *Archives of General Psychiatry* **60**, 392–400.

Bowden, C.L. *et al.* (2005) A randomized, double-blind, placebo-controlled efficacy and safety study of quetiapine or lithium as monotherapy for mania in bipolar disorder. *The Journal of Clinical Psychiatry* **66**, 111–121.

Brotman, M.A. *et al.* (2006) Prevalence, clinical correlates, and longitudinal course of severe mood dysregulation in children. *Biological Psychiatry* **60**, 991–997.

Calabrese, J.R. *et al.* (2002) Rash in multicenter trials of lamotrigine in mood disorders: clinical relevance and management. *The Journal of Clinical Psychiatry* **63**, 1012–1019.

Carlson, G.A. & Klein, D.N. (2014) How to understand divergent views on bipolar disorder in youth. *Annual Review of Clinical Psychology* **10**, 529–551.

Carlson, G.A. *et al.* (2000) Stimulant treatment in young boys with symptoms suggesting childhood mania: A report from a longitudinal study. *Journal of Child and Adolescent Psychopharmacology* **10**, 175–184.

Chang, K. *et al.* (2003) Decreased N-acetylaspartate in children with familial bipolar disorder. *Biological Psychiatry* **53**, 1059–1065.

Chang, K. *et al.* (2006) An open-label study of lamotrigine adjunct or monotherapy for the treatment of adolescents with bipolar depression. *Journal of the American Academy of Child and Adolescent Psychiatry* **45**, 298–304.

Christie, K.A. *et al.* (1988) Epidemiologic evidence for early onset of mental disorders and higher risk of drug abuse in young adults. *The American Journal of Psychiatry* **145**, 971–975.

Cipriani, A. *et al.* (2005) Lithium in the prevention of suicidal behavior and all-cause mortality in patients with mood disorders: a systematic review of randomized trials. *The American Journal of Psychiatry* **162**, 1805–1819.

Copeland, W.E. *et al.* (2013) Prevalence, comorbidity, and correlates of DSM-5 proposed disruptive mood dysregulation disorder. *The American Journal of Psychiatry* **170**, 173–179.

Correll, C.U. *et al.* (2006) Recognizing and monitoring adverse events of second-generation antipsychotics in children and adolescents. *Child and Adolescent Psychiatric Clinics of North America* **15**, 177–206.

Correll, C.U. *et al.* (2009) Cardiometabolic risk of second-generation antipsychotic medications during first-time use in children and adolescents. *JAMA* **302**, 1765–1773.

Craddock, N. & Sklar, P. (2013) Genetics of bipolar disorder. *The Lancet* **381**, 1654–1662.

Davanzo, P. *et al.* (2001) Decreased anterior cingulate myo-inositol/creatine spectroscopy resonance with lithium treatment in children with bipolar disorder. *Neuropsychopharmacology* **24**, 359–369.

Davanzo, P. *et al.* (2003) Proton magnetic resonance spectroscopy of bipolar disorder versus intermittent explosive disorder in children and adolescents. *The American Journal of Psychiatry* **160**, 1442–1452.

de Silva, M. *et al.* (1996) Randomised comparative monotherapy trial of phenobarbitone, phenytoin, carbamazepine, or sodium valproate for newly diagnosed childhood epilepsy. *The Lancet* **347**, 709–713.

Delbello, M.P. *et al.* (2009) A double-blind, placebo-controlled pilot study of quetiapine for depressed adolescents with bipolar disorder. *Bipolar Disorders* **11**, 483–493.

Delbello, M.P. *et al.* (2017) Efficacy and safety of lurasidone in children and adolescents with bipolar I depression: a double-blind, placebo-controlled study. *Journal of the American Academy of Child and Adolescent Psychiatry* **56**, 1015–1025.

Detke, H.C. *et al.* (2015) Olanzapine/fluoxetine combination in children and adolescents with bipolar I depression: a randomized, double-blind, placebo-controlled trial. *Journal of the American Academy of Child and Adolescent Psychiatry* **54**, 217–224.

Dickstein, D.P. *et al.* (2004) Neuropsychological performance in pediatric bipolar disorder. *Biological Psychiatry* **55**, 32–39.

Dickstein, D.P. *et al.* (2007) Cognitive flexibility in phenotypes of pediatric bipolar disorder. *Journal of the American Academy of Child and Adolescent Psychiatry* **46**, 341–355.

Dickstein, D.P. *et al.* (2010) Altered neural function in pediatric bipolar disorder during reversal learning. *Bipolar Disorders* **12**, 707–719.

Dickstein, D.P. *et al.* (2015) Cognitive remediation: potential novel brain-based treatment for bipolar disorder in children and adolescents. *CNS Spectrums* **20**, 382–390.

Escamilla, I. *et al.* (2011) Pediatric bipolar disorder in a Spanish sample: results after 2.6 years of follow-up. *Journal of Affective Disorders* **132**, 270–274.

Fahrendorff, A.M. *et al.* (2023) Psychiatric comorbidity in patients with pediatric bipolar disorder - a systematic review. *Acta Psychiatrica Scandinavica* **148**, 110–132.

Faraone, S.V. *et al.* (2005) The CBCL predicts DSM bipolar disorder in children: a receiver operating characteristic curve analysis. *Bipolar Disorders* **7**, 518–524.

Findling, R.L. *et al.* (2009) Acute treatment of pediatric bipolar I disorder, manic or mixed episode, with aripiprazole: a randomized, double-blind, placebo-controlled study. *The Journal of Clinical Psychiatry* **70**, 1441–1451.

Findling, R.L. *et al.* (2012) Double-blind, randomized, placebo-controlled long-term maintenance study of aripiprazole in children with bipolar disorder. *The Journal of Clinical Psychiatry* **73**, 57–63.

Findling, R.L. *et al.* (2014) Efficacy and safety of extended-release quetiapine fumarate in youth with bipolar depression: an 8 week, double-blind, placebo-controlled trial. *Journal of Child and Adolescent Psychopharmacology* **24**, 325–335.

Findling, R.L. *et al.* (2015a) Adjunctive maintenance Lamotrigine for pediatric bipolar I disorder: a placebo-controlled, randomized withdrawal study. *Journal of the American Academy of Child and Adolescent Psychiatry* **54**, 1020–1031. e3

Findling, R.L. *et al.* (2015b) Asenapine for the acute treatment of pediatric manic or mixed episode of bipolar I disorder. *Journal of the American Academy of Child and Adolescent Psychiatry* **54**, 1032–1041.

Findling, R.L. *et al.* (2015c) Lithium in the acute treatment of bipolar I disorder: a double-blind, placebo-controlled study. *Pediatrics* **136**, 885–894.

Findling, R.L. *et al.* (2022) Efficacy, safety, and tolerability of flexibly dosed ziprasidone in children and adolescents with mania in bipolar I disorder: a randomized placebo-controlled replication study. *Journal of Child and Adolescent Psychopharmacology* **32**, 143–152.

Fristad, M.A. *et al.* (2009) Impact of multifamily psychoeducational psychotherapy in treating children aged 8 to 12 years with mood disorders. *Archives of General Psychiatry* **66**, 1013–1021.

Galanter, C.A. *et al.* (2012) Variability among research diagnostic interview instruments in the application of DSM-IV-TR criteria for pediatric bipolar disorder. *Journal of the American Academy of Child and Adolescent Psychiatry* **51**, 605–621.

Gelenberg, A.J. *et al.* (1989) Comparison of standard and low serum levels of lithium for maintenance treatment of bipolar disorder. *The New England Journal of Medicine* **321**, 1489–1493.

Geller, B. *et al.* (1994) Rate and predictors of prepubertal bipolarity during follow-up of 6- to 12-year-old depressed children. *Journal of the American Academy of Child and Adolescent Psychiatry* **33**, 461–468.

Geller, B. *et al.* (1998) Prepubertal and early adolescent bipolarity differentiate from ADHD by manic symptoms, grandiose delusions, ultra-rapid or ultradian cycling. *Journal of Affective Disorders* **51**, 81–91.

Geller, B. *et al.* (2002a) DSM-IV mania symptoms in a prepubertal and early adolescent bipolar disorder phenotype compared to attention-deficit hyperactive and normal controls. *Journal of Child and Adolescent Psychopharmacology* **12**, 11–25.

Geller, B. *et al.* (2002b) Phenomenology of prepubertal and early adolescent bipolar disorder: examples of elated mood, grandiose behaviors, decreased need for sleep, racing thoughts and hypersexuality. *Journal of Child and Adolescent Psychopharmacology* **12**, 3–9.

Geller, B. *et al.* (2004) Four-year prospective outcome and natural history of mania in children with a prepubertal and early adolescent bipolar disorder phenotype. *Archives of General Psychiatry* **61**, 459–467.

Geller, B. *et al.* (2012) A randomized controlled trial of risperidone, lithium, or divalproex sodium for initial treatment of bipolar I disorder, manic or mixed phase, in children and adolescents. *Archives of General Psychiatry* **69**, 515–528.

Ghaemi, S.N. *et al.* (2006) Extrapyramidal side effects with atypical neuroleptics in bipolar disorder. *Progress in Neuro-Psychopharmacology & Biological Psychiatry* **30**, 209–213.

Goldstein, B.I. *et al.* (2017) The International Society for Bipolar Disorders Task Force report on pediatric bipolar disorder: knowledge to date and directions for future research. *Bipolar Disorders* **19**, 524–543.

Goldstein, T.R. *et al.* (2009) Psychosocial functioning among bipolar youth. *Journal of Affective Disorders* **114**, 174–183.

Goldstein, T.R. *et al.* (2015) Dialectical behavior therapy for adolescents with bipolar disorder: results from a pilot randomized trial. *Journal of Child and Adolescent Psychopharmacology* **25**, 140–149.

Goldstein, T.R. *et al.* (2022) A risk calculator to predict suicide attempts among individuals with early-onset bipolar disorder. *Bipolar Disorders* **24**, 749–757.

Grauso-Eby, N.L. *et al.* (2003) Acute pancreatitis in children from Valproic acid: case series and review. *Pediatric Neurology* **28**, 145–148.

Guo, Y.B. *et al.* (2021) Shared and specific patterns of structural and functional thalamo-frontal disturbances in manic and euthymic pediatric bipolar disorder. *Brain Imaging and Behavior* **15**, 2671–2680.

Guyer, A.E. *et al.* (2007) Specificity of facial expression labeling deficits in childhood psychopathology. *Journal of Child Psychology and Psychiatry* **48**, 863–871.

Haas, M. *et al.* (2009) Risperidone for the treatment of acute mania in children and adolescents with bipolar disorder: a randomized, double-blind, placebo-controlled study. *Bipolar Disorders* **11**, 687–700.

Hafeman, D.M. *et al.* (2016) Toward the definition of a bipolar Prodrome: dimensional predictors of bipolar spectrum disorders in at-risk youths. *The American Journal of Psychiatry* **173**, 695–704.

Hafeman, D.M. *et al.* (2017) Assessment of a person-level risk calculator to predict new-onset bipolar spectrum disorder in youth at familial risk. *JAMA Psychiatry* **74**, 841–847.

Hafeman, D.M. *et al.* (2021) Prospectively ascertained mania and hypomania among young adults with child- and adolescent-onset bipolar disorder. *Bipolar Disorders* **23**, 463–473.

Hazell, P.L. *et al.* (2003) Manic symptoms in young males with ADHD predict functioning but not diagnosis after 6 years. *Journal of the American Academy of Child and Adolescent Psychiatry* **42**, 552–560.

Hillegers, M.H. *et al.* (2005) Five-year prospective outcome of psychopathology in the adolescent offspring of bipolar parents. *Bipolar Disorders* **7**, 344–350.

Holtmann, M. *et al.* (2010) Bipolar disorder in children and adolescents in Germany: national trends in the rates of inpatients, 2000–2007. *Bipolar Disorders* **12**, 155–163.

Hower, H. *et al.* (2019) Predictors of longitudinal psychosocial functioning in bipolar youth transitioning to adults. *Journal of Affective Disorders* **246**, 578–585.

Ino, H. *et al.* (2023) Glutamatergic neurometabolite levels in bipolar disorder: a systematic review and meta-analysis of proton magnetic resonance spectroscopy studies. *Biological Psychiatry: Cognitive Neuroscience and Neuroimaging* **8**, 140–150.

Kafantaris, V. *et al.* (2004) Lithium treatment of acute mania in adolescents: a placebo-controlled discontinuation study. *Journal of the American Academy of Child and Adolescent Psychiatry* **43**, 984–993.

Kaufman, J. *et al.* (1997) Schedule for affective disorders and schizophrenia for school-age children-present and lifetime version (K-SADS-PL): initial reliability and validity data. *Journal of the American Academy of Child and Adolescent Psychiatry* **36**, 980–988.

Kelsoe, J.R. (2003) Arguments for the genetic basis of the bipolar spectrum. *Journal of Affective Disorders* **73**, 183–197.

Kennedy, N. *et al.* (2005) Incidence and distribution of first-episode mania by age: results from a 35-year study. *Psychological Medicine* **35**, 855–863.

Kessler, R.C. *et al.* (2005) Prevalence, severity, and comorbidity of 12-month DSM-IV disorders in the National Comorbidity Survey Replication. *Archives of General Psychiatry* **62**, 617–627.

Klein, C.C. *et al.* (2020) The importance of second-generation antipsychotic-related weight gain and adherence barriers in youth with bipolar disorders: patient, parent, and provider perspectives. *Journal of Child and Adolescent Psychopharmacology* **30**, 376–380.

Kovacs, M. *et al.* (1994) Childhood-onset dysthymic disorder: clinical features and prospective naturalistic outcome. *Archives of General Psychiatry* **51**, 365–374.

Kowatch, R.A. *et al.* (2005) Treatment guidelines for children and adolescents with bipolar disorder. *Journal of the American Academy of Child and Adolescent Psychiatry* **44**, 213–235.

Leibenluft, E. *et al.* (2003) Defining clinical phenotypes of juvenile mania. *The American Journal of Psychiatry* **160**, 430–437.

Leibenluft, E. *et al.* (2007) Neural circuitry engaged during unsuccessful motor inhibition in pediatric bipolar disorder. *The American Journal of Psychiatry* **164**, 52–60.

Lewinsohn, P.M. *et al.* (2000) Bipolar disorder during adolescence and young adulthood in a community sample. *Bipolar Disorders* **2**, 281–293.

Lin, P.I. *et al.* (2006) Clinical correlates and familial aggregation of age at onset in bipolar disorder. *The American Journal of Psychiatry* **163**, 240–246.

Linke, J.O. *et al.* (2019) White matter microstructure in pediatric bipolar disorder and disruptive mood dysregulation disorder. *Journal of the American Academy of Child and Adolescent Psychiatry.*

Long, X. *et al.* (2023) Gray matter alterations in adolescent major depressive disorder and adolescent bipolar disorder. *Journal of Affective Disorders* **325**, 550–563.

Lu, L.H. *et al.* (2011) White matter microstructure in untreated first episode bipolar disorder with psychosis: Comparison with schizophrenia. *Bipolar Disorders* **13**, 604–613.

Martin, A. *et al.* (2004) Age effects on antidepressant-induced manic conversion. *Archives of Pediatrics & Adolescent Medicine* **158**, 773–780.

McGurk, S.R. *et al.* (2007) A meta-analysis of cognitive remediation in schizophrenia. *The American Journal of Psychiatry* **164**, 1791–1802.

Merikangas, K.R. *et al.* (2010) Prevalence and treatment of mental disorders among US children in the 2001-2004 NHANES. *Pediatrics* **125**, 75–81.

Merikangas, K.R. *et al.* (2012) Mania with and without depression in a community sample of US adolescents. *Archives of General Psychiatry* **69**, 943–951.

Mesman, E. *et al.* (2013) The Dutch bipolar offspring study: 12-year follow-up. *The American Journal of Psychiatry* **170**, 542–549.

Miklowitz, D.J. & Chung, B. (2016) Family-focused therapy for bipolar disorder: reflections on 30 years of research. *Family Process* **55**, 483–499.

Miklowitz, D.J. *et al.* (2008) Family-focused treatment for adolescents with bipolar disorder: results of a 2-year randomized trial. *Archives of General Psychiatry* **65**, 1053–1061.

Miklowitz, D.J. *et al.* (2020) Effects of family-focused therapy vs enhanced usual care for symptomatic youths at high risk for bipolar disorder: a randomized clinical trial. *JAMA Psychiatry* **77**, 455–463.

Moore, C.M. *et al.* (2002) Brain-to-serum lithium ratio and age: an in vivo magnetic resonance spectroscopy study. *The American Journal of Psychiatry* **159**, 1240–1242.

Moore, G.J. *et al.* (1999) Temporal dissociation between lithium-induced changes in frontal lobe myo-inositol and clinical response in manic-depressive illness. *American Journal of Psychiatry* **156**, 1902–1908.

Moreno, C. *et al.* (2007) National trends in the outpatient diagnosis and treatment of bipolar disorder in youth. *Archives of General Psychiatry* **64**, 1032–1039.

Mortensen, P.B. *et al.* (2003) Individual and familial risk factors for bipolar affective disorders in Denmark. *Archives of General Psychiatry* **60**, 1209–1215.

Mullins, N. *et al.* (2021) Genome-wide association study of more than 40,000 bipolar disorder cases provides new insights into the underlying biology. *Nature Genetics* **53**, 817–829.

Musliner, K.L. *et al.* (2020) Polygenic risk and progression to bipolar or psychotic disorders among individuals diagnosed with unipolar depression in early life. *The American Journal of Psychiatry* **177**, 936–943.

National Collaborating Centre for Mental Health (UK) (2014) *Bipolar Disorder: The NICE Guideline on the Assessment and Management of Bipolar Disorder in Adults, Children and Young People in Primary and Secondary Care.* British Psychological Society/The Royal College of Psychiatrists, Leicester/London.

Patino, L.R. *et al.* (2021) A randomized, double-blind, controlled trial of lithium versus quetiapine for the treatment of acute mania in youth with early course bipolar disorder. *Journal of Child and Adolescent Psychopharmacology* **31**, 485–493.

Pavuluri, M.N. *et al.* (2009) Diffusion tensor imaging study of white matter fiber tracts in pediatric bipolar disorder and attention-deficit/hyperactivity disorder. *Biological Psychiatry* **65**, 586–593.

Pavuluri, M.N. *et al.* (2010) Double-blind randomized trial of risperidone versus divalproex in pediatric bipolar disorder. *Bipolar Disorders* **12**(6), 593–605.

Pfeifer, J.C. *et al.* (2008) Meta-analysis of amygdala volumes in children and adolescents with bipolar disorder. *Journal of the American Academy of Child and Adolescent Psychiatry* **47**, 1289–1298.

Pope, H.G., Jr. *et al.* (1991) Valproate in the treatment of acute mania: a placebo-controlled study. *Archives of General Psychiatry* **48**, 62–68.

Priebe, L. *et al.* (2012) Genome-wide survey implicates the influence of copy number variants (CNVs) in the development of early-onset bipolar disorder. *Molecular Psychiatry* **17**, 421–432.

Rao, U. *et al.* (1995) Unipolar depression in adolescents: clinical outcome in adulthood. *Journal of the American Academy of Child and Adolescent Psychiatry* **34**, 566–578.

Rich, B.A. *et al.* (2007) Different psychophysiological and behavioral responses elicited by frustration in pediatric bipolar disorder and severe mood dysregulation. *The American Journal of Psychiatry* **164**, 309–317.

Scheffer, R.E. *et al.* (2005) Randomized, placebo-controlled trial of mixed amphetamine salts for symptoms of comorbid ADHD in pediatric bipolar disorder after mood stabilization with divalproex sodium. *The American Journal of Psychiatry* **162**, 58–64.

Scott, J. *et al.* (2017) A pilot study to determine whether combinations of objectively measured activity parameters can be used to differentiate between mixed states, mania, and bipolar depression. *International Journal of Bipolar Disorders* **5**, 5.

Seymour, K.E. *et al.* (2013) Emotional face identification in youths with primary bipolar disorder or primary attention-deficit/hyperactivity disorder. *Journal of the American Academy of Child and Adolescent Psychiatry* **52**, 537–546. e3

Silverstone, P.H. *et al.* (2002) Chronic treatment with both lithium and sodium valproate may normalize phosphoinositol cycle activity in bipolar patients. *Human Psychopharmacology* **17**, 321–327.

Singh, M.K. *et al.* (2010) Neural correlates of response inhibition in pediatric bipolar disorder. *Journal of Child and Adolescent Psychopharmacology* **20**, 15–24.

Smoller, J.W. & Finn, C.T. (2003) Family, twin, and adoption studies of bipolar disorder. *American Journal of Medical Genetics. Part C, Seminars in Medical Genetics* **123C**, 48–58.

Stoddard, J. *et al.* (2016) An open pilot study of training hostile interpretation bias to treat disruptive mood dysregulation disorder. *Journal of Child and Adolescent Psychopharmacology* **26**, 49–57.

Stringaris, A. *et al.* (2010) Pediatric bipolar disorder versus severe mood dysregulation: risk for manic episodes on follow-up. *Journal of the American Academy of Child and Adolescent Psychiatry* **49**, 397–405.

Tannous, J. *et al.* (2021) Altered neurochemistry in the anterior white matter of bipolar children and adolescents: a multivoxel (1)H MRS study. *Molecular Psychiatry* **26**, 4117–4126.

Thase, M.E. (2007) Step-BD and bipolar depression: what have we learned? *Current Psychiatry Reports* **9**, 497–503.

Tijssen, M.J. *et al.* (2010) Prediction of transition from common adolescent bipolar experiences to bipolar disorder: 10-year study. *The British Journal of Psychiatry* **196**, 102–108.

Van Meter, A.R. *et al.* (2011) Meta-analysis of epidemiologic studies of pediatric bipolar disorder. *The Journal of Clinical Psychiatry* **72**, 1250–1256.

Volk, H.E. & Todd, R.D. (2007) Does the Child Behavior Checklist juvenile bipolar disorder phenotype identify bipolar disorder? *Biological Psychiatry* **62**, 115–120.

Wagner, K.D. *et al.* (2002) An open-label trial of divalproex in children and adolescents with bipolar disorder. *Journal of the American Academy of Child and Adolescent Psychiatry* **41**, 1224–1230.

Wagner, K.D. *et al.* (2006) A double-blind, randomized, placebo-controlled trial of oxcarbazepine in the treatment of bipolar disorder in children and adolescents. *The American Journal of Psychiatry* **163**, 1179–1186.

Wagner, K.D. *et al.* (2009) A double-blind, randomized, placebo-controlled trial of divalproex extended-release in the treatment of bipolar disorder in children and adolescents. *Journal of the American Academy of Child and Adolescent Psychiatry* **48**, 519–532.

Wegbreit, E. *et al.* (2014) Developmental meta-analyses of the functional neural correlates of bipolar disorder. *JAMA Psychiatry* **71**, 926–935.

Weissman, M.M. *et al.* (1984) Psychiatric disorders in the relatives of probands with affective disorders. The Yale University – National Institute of Mental Health collaborative study. *Archives of General Psychiatry* **41**, 13–21.

Weissman, M.M. *et al.* (1996) Cross-national epidemiology of major depression and bipolar disorder. *JAMA* **276**, 293–299.

Weissman, M.M. *et al.* (1999) Children with prepubertal-onset major depressive disorder and anxiety grown up. *Archives of General Psychiatry* **56**, 794–801.

Winsberg, M.E. *et al.* (2000) Decreased dorsolateral prefrontal N-acetyl aspartate in bipolar disorder. *Biological Psychiatry* **47**, 475–481.

World Health Organization (1993) *International Statistical Classification of Disease and Related Health Problems*, 10th revision. In: *World Health Organization (WHO)*, Geneva, Switzerland.

World Health Organization (2019) *International Statistical Classification of Disease and Related Health Problems*, 11th revision. In: *World Health Organization (WHO)*, Geneva, Switzerland.

Young, R.C. *et al.* (1978) A rating scale for mania: reliability, validity and sensitivity. *The British Journal of Psychiatry* **133**, 429–435.

Youngstrom, E.A. *et al.* (2015) Multivariate meta-analysis of the discriminative validity of caregiver, youth, and teacher rating scales for pediatric bipolar disorder: mother knows best about mania. *Archives of Scientific Psychology* **3**, 112–137.

Youngstrom, E.A. *et al.* (2020) Developing and validating short forms of the parent general behavior inventory mania and depression scales for rating youth mood symptoms. *Journal of Clinical Child and Adolescent Psychology* **49**, 162–177.

CHAPTER 63
Depressive disorders in children and adolescents

John T. Walkup[1] and Jeffrey R. Strawn[2]

[1] Pritzker Department of Psychiatry and Behavioral Health, Lurie Children's Hospital of Chicago & Northwestern University Feinberg School of Medicine, Chicago, IL, USA

[2] Department of Psychiatry, College of Medicine, University of Cincinnati, Cincinnati, OH, USA

> . . .many clinical writings on depressive disorders have not taken account of developmental research or theory on affective expression. Similarly, most developmental writings have not considered the clinical distinctions between depressive feelings as an affective phenomenon and depressive disorders as psychopathological conditions.
>
> *Source*: Rutter *et al.* (1986) p. ix.

Introduction—goals of the chapter

This chapter describes depressive disorders as they present in children and adolescents. Children of all ages have the capacity for intense and persistent low moods that can occur in response to life events, social disruptions, or for no apparent reason. Understanding and differentiating normal, expectable but intense, and persistent mood changes triggered by life events from mood changes attributable to depressive illness is a critical skill for clinicians. Major depressive illness is not the same as sadness, demoralization, or depression symptoms. Historically, the key to differentiating low mood associated with depressive illness from normal human sadness or demoralization emphasized the distinctive quality of the low mood of depression as different from sadness or demoralization that one might experience after disappointment, loss, and adversity. Although recent research and current diagnostic approaches do not require such distinctions, it can be useful for clinicians to consider the quality of the mood state as they engage with the patient in understanding their experience of low mood. Yet, low mood is only one feature of depressive illness; major depressive disorder (MDD), as defined by the *Diagnostic and Statistical Manual of Mental Disorders*, 5th edition, text revision (DSM-5-TR; American Psychiatric Association, 2022) and the *International Classification of Diseases*, 11th revision (ICD-11; World Health Organization, 2019), is defined by a constellation of multiple, different symptoms that include loss of interest or enjoyment in activities, and changes in appetite, sleep, and energy, among other features. The presence of these additional features of MDD coming together as a change from what is typical for the young person, including functional impairment, will improve confidence that the complaint of low mood is associated with a depressive disorder. Given the focus of this chapter on children and adolescents we adopt a developmental perspective in the approach to assessment and treatment. DSM-5-TR also groups persistent depressive disorder (dysthymia) and disruptive mood dysregulation disorder (DMDD) as depressive disorders, which is not the case for ICD-11 (with respect to DMDD; also see Chapter 5), and these will not be discussed in this chapter.

Normal human sadness

Sadness is a normal and healthy human emotion important for our survival and interpersonal engagement. It can occur at any time over a lifetime as sad mood is universally triggered by substantive life events (e.g., loss of nutritional, economic, or housing support) or disruption of human attachments (e.g., death or loss of a parent/relative, sibling or friend, pet; breakdown of a romantic relationship). Given the nature of the triggering event, the event's importance to the person, and the duration of the event and its sequelae, low mood can range in severity from mild and manageable to intense and persistent but would be expected to pass as the event passes or loses emotional salience. Thus, the course of normal human sadness is highly dependent on the nature of the event, the capacity of the person experiencing the event to cope or manage, and the resources of support in the environment. Most of those with intense periods of normal human sadness experience their sadness as normal and expectable, as they have had many experiences of sadness over a

Rutter's Child and Adolescent Psychiatry and Psychology, Seventh Edition.
Edited by Anita Thapar, Daniel S. Pine, Samuele Cortese, Cathy Creswell, Tamsin J. Ford, James F. Leckman, and Argyris Stringaris.

Companion website: www.wiley.com/go/thapar/rutterspsych7

lifetime and understand that this mood state will pass, and they will move on.

Demoralization

In contrast, low mood states in response to unremitting stressors can be severe and persistent if there is no actual or perceived "out" or solution to their experience of adversity. Poverty, racism, war, few educational or employment opportunities, or inconsistent nurturing environments can induce an expectable, persistent, and even severe mood state in children. For many youth, the COVID-19 pandemic could be understood as a cause of substantial demoralization secondary to the broad-based effects of quarantine on academic and social engagement (Gohari *et al.*, 2023; see Chapter 18). Similarly, unremitting suffering from psychiatric or neurodevelopmental disorders that are not recognized and/or not treated effectively can also be demoralizing and result in a mood state that may mimic depressive illness.

The course of demoralization is, by definition, chronic as the perceived lack of escape in the presence of ongoing adversity is core to the persistently low mood. Patients experiencing demoralizing circumstances may or may not identify the cause of their distress (e.g., poverty or racism) but will also not necessarily experience their distress as unexpected or disproportional to their life experience or capacity to cope. When made aware, both normal human sadness and demoralization "make sense" to the affected person as these experiences are universal and would be considered to be distinct from the change in mood from depressive illness.

Major depressive disorder

Diagnostic criteria for MDD describe a necessary change in mood state and other symptoms that occur together that are consistent over time and of significant impact to cause a change in functional capacity. Major depression is considered to have a typical age of onset in the mid-teens, and to occur in episodes and be recurrent. Rating scales and diagnostic interviews that capture the nature and extent of depressive symptoms and related impairment are valuable aids as part of assessment (see Chapter 28). Although intense normal human sadness, demoralization, and major depression all have intense low mood in common, a key characteristic of low mood in major depression is the inability to experience pleasure (pervasive anhedonia), which is not present in those with normal human sadness and demoralization where affected individuals can maintain reactivity to positive mood experiences, i.e., support of loved ones after a loss or relief of a demoralizing burden. MDD can range in severity from subsyndromal to mild to severe, psychotic forms can occur, and, for a minority, MDD can represent the first manifestation of bipolar disorder (BD; see Chapter 62).

As a change in mood state is key to the diagnosis of clinical depression, the young person may be in the best position to report their mood. The young person with major depression can often differentiate their low mood from normal human sadness and may be perplexed if there is a lack of an apparent event or circumstance that would explain why they feel the way they do. Some young people with major depression may not recognize their low mood as a unique mood state; they may focus their concern on other aspects of the syndrome, such as irritability, exhaustion, sleep problems, loss of appetite, physical complaints, and inability to focus and concentrate.

That said, some youth are uncomfortable discussing their changing mood state as it may reflect poorly on them to admit a vulnerability or may cause a parent to become overly concerned, emotional, and overinvolved, or the contrary, to be dismissive or invalidating of the youth's experience. While caretakers may not be able to speak to mood state, they are able to identify changes in observable behaviors or functional capacity—change in affect expression, exhaustion, decrease in academic functioning, and loss of interest in pleasurable activities like sports, peer activities, and family events. Similarly, teachers and others involved in a child's life may also be able to provide needed information regarding symptoms and changes in functional capacity.

The challenge for the clinician and the researcher

Differentiating among low mood states may not be as easy, as suggested by the sections above. Historically, reliability challenges related to these distinctions have led to an approach to diagnosis that focuses mainly on a change in mood state, low mood (including irritability) more generally, and associated symptoms, but backing away from attempting to sort by cause or by the distinctive quality of the mood state.

While the ultimate goal of a diagnostic assessment is to consistently differentiate among low mood states in order to match a mood state to an appropriate and effective intervention choice, we are not there yet. Thus, current diagnostic manuals reflect "etiological neutrality" in their criteria and, in DSM-5-TR, extended further to incorporate more dimensional elements to depression diagnosis (Park & Kim, 2019). Hopelessness, which is clearly a feature of demoralization, is now included as a feature of low mood in clinical depression. Similarly, intense low mood related to the death of a loved one, which was an exclusion for major depression, has now been removed.

From a research point of view, the sampling frames for most modern studies have used existing diagnostic schema and thus may include a range of patients with prominent low mood symptoms. This is of concern for all research studies but is of particular concern in treatment studies where high placebo response rates are common, especially in industry-sponsored medication trials and where psychotherapy demonstrates efficacy in some studies but appears to have limited value in others. It is for this reason that UK National Institute for Health and Care Excellence (NICE) guidance suggests "watchful waiting" for two weeks for children and adolescents with mild MDD (National Institute for Health and Care Excellence, 2019). A further complication is that because MDD is a naturally remitting and relapsing disorder, some individuals will show remission regardless of intervention choice.

For the clinician, a key goal in differentiating among mood states is for the clinician, the patient, and the family to develop a shared understanding of factors associated with the patient's low mood, to match evidence-based treatment recommendations to a solid diagnostic formulation (see Chapter 27) to achieve optimal outcomes. Further, our current diagnostic practice, which does not provide guidance about how best to differentiate among low mood states, also impacts the scientific literature. Astute clinicians must read the literature with care, understanding that low mood symptoms as reported in research studies may reflect great heterogeneity. The variability to the assessment of low mood in research studies may account for some of the differing and potentially confusing outcomes among studies, as mood symptoms in one study may be evaluated and measured differently than mood symptoms in another study.

Medical evaluation

Clinicians need to consider whether there are non-psychiatric medical illnesses that could account for an uncharacteristic change in mood (Table 63.1)—diabetes, hypo- or hyperthyroidism, anemia, sleep apnea, vitamin D deficiency, substance misuse, a contribution from medication, etc. (see Chapter 30 on "Physical examination and medical investigation"). However, neurologic, endocrine, and cardiac diseases that mimic depression are relatively uncommon in the pediatric population. Screening for these should be based on history, specific risk factors, vital signs, and physical examination. For example, thyroid stimulating hormone (TSH) levels are routinely evaluated in pediatric patients with depressive and anxiety disorders; however, the yield of such screening is low and, importantly, enhanced when triggered by specific clinical indicators, including recent weight gain/loss, treatment with thyroid-affecting medications, and metromenorrhagia (Luft *et al.*, 2019). Additionally, a thorough history includes reviewing medications while paying particular attention to steroids and antihistamines, among others, as these have been associated with fatigue or other symptoms that overlap with depression. Additional factors that may be considered in working up nonpsychiatric etiologies are shown in Table 63.1 and include the evaluation of vitamin B_{12} and D deficiencies (Misra *et al.*, 2008).

Table 63.1 Nonpsychiatric causes of depression in children and adolescents.

Body system	Condition	Findings on physical examination or history	Possible laboratory findings
Cardiac	Bradyarrhythmias	• bradycardia	decreased heart rate on EKG or holter monitoring
Endocrine	Hypothyroidism	• thyromegaly or palpable nodules • thyroid tenderness on palpation. • lid lag • hypoactivity • cool, dry skin • hyporeflexia • constipation	↑ thyroid stimulating hormone (TSH) concentrations ↓ T_3 and T_4
	Hypo- or hyperparathyroidism	• fatigue • generalized weakness • myalgias • headaches	hypo- or hypercalcemia hypo- or hyperphosphatemia ↓ or ↑ serum parathyroid hormone
Medications	β-antagonists	• bradycardia	
	Corticosteroids	• weight gain • hypertension • Cushingoid features (truncal obesity, buffalo hump, moon facies)	
Neurologic	Migraines Idiopathic hypersomnia	• fatigue • decreased attention	not applicable
Nutritional	Iron deficiency	• pallor • dry or rough skin • atrophic glossitis with loss of tongue papillae • cheilosis koilonychia (spoon nails)	microcytic, hypochromic anemia, ↓ reticulocyte count and iron studies suggestive of iron deficiency
	Vitamin D deficiency		↓ vitamin D • vitamin D sufficiency—20–100 ng/ml • vitamin D insufficiency—12–20 ng/ml • vitamin D deficiency—< 12 ng/ml ↑ alkaline phosphatase and other bone turnover markers
	Vitamin B_{12} deficiency		↓ serum B_{12} macrocytic, hypochromic anemia

Psychiatric evaluation

The evaluation of depression symptoms

The presence of anhedonia and the distinct quality of depressed mood are key to differentiating between normal human sadness, demoralization, and clinical depression (Box 63.1). As noted above, it is possible that patients presenting in distress with low mood may have a variety of reasons for their distress and display symptoms that appear to represent illness. While anhedonia and distinct quality of mood are not required for a diagnosis of clinical depression, they are features that, if present, may help the clinician in parsing among low mood states and may positively inform treatment choices.

Evaluating functional impairment

There is a considerable body of evidence suggesting untreated clinical depression is associated with academic decline and social impairment. As many young people with clinical depression do not come to treatment at their first episode or experience long wait times for specialist assessment, the clinical presentation can include different levels of impairment. Thus, patients with a first onset of major depression may have a different level of impairment than a patient coming to care after repeated episodes of depression, who has associated academic and social decline or has developed maladaptive approaches to coping. Such patients would require different levels of treatment; treatment that focuses not only on the disorder's symptoms, but also treatment that addresses accumulated functional impairment or maladaptive behaviors, such as substance misuse or self-injury and suicidal behavior. It is important to note that treatment studies often require patients to have significant symptoms and impairment, yet study treatments are often only directed at reducing depressive symptomatic distress and may not specifically address or measure the effects of treatments on functional impairment.

Box 63.1 Assessment at a glance

- Screen universally for depression and screen for suicide at all mental health visits.
- Confirm major depressive disorder (MDD) versus normal sadness versus demoralization.
- Exclude nonpsychiatric causes of depressive symptoms, including, as appropriate, those listed in Table 63.1
- Assess comorbidity, including anxiety disorders; attention deficit hyperactivity disorder (ADHD), autism spectrum disorder (ASD), and sleep disorders.
- Assess substance use.
- Evaluate depression-related impairment and function.
- Consider a rating scale to assess symptom severity:
  - Quick Inventory of Depressive Symptoms—Self Report (QIDS-SR)
  - Patient Health Questionnaire-9 (PHQ-9)
- Investigate precipitating and perpetuating factors:
  - school environment (bullying, learning disorders, accommodations)
  - adversity
  - family environment/positive parenting

Evaluating safety and suicidality in children and adolescents

Assessing suicidality and safety is a necessary and routine aspect of assessment in specialist child and adolescent mental health services (CAMHS) and is especially important in the context of youth depression (see Chapter 64). There also are a number of rating scales/measures, such as the Columbia Suicide Severity Rating Scale (Posner *et al.*, 2011) and the Ask Suicide-Screening Question, which have been translated into multiple languages and are available through the US National Institute of Mental Health (NIMH) website (http://www.nimh.nih.gov/research/research-conducted-at-nimh/asq-toolkit-materials) (Horowitz *et al.*, 2012). All measures focus on past and current suicidal ideation and behavior to establish context, and, importantly, if there is evidence of current suicidal ideation or intent, indicate the need for overall risk assessment plus acute risk planning and management. Positive screens require further exploration of potential risk factors and, importantly, potential protective factors, leading to a comprehensive plan.

Standardized assessments of low mood symptoms and clinical depression

Self/parent reports

A full range of standardized measures are available to assess depressive symptoms in youth. The instruments vary in time of implementation, complexity from brief to labor intensive, and from free to costly. Depression screening for youth aged 12 and older is recommended in the US but not elsewhere, including the UK, other than when depression is suspected. Measures commonly used include the self-report Patient Health Questionnaire-9 (PHQ-9; 9 items including suicide screen) (Johnson *et al.*, 2002) or PHQ-2 (2 items and suicide screen) and, more recently, PHQ-A (adolescent version, 9 depression items with 2 suicide items). Historically, the Beck Depression Inventory (21 items) and Children's Depression Inventory 2 (28 items) have been utilized for screening and assessment, but both are proprietary and, even though brief, may be considered too time-intensive for most primary care settings. The Mood and Feelings Questionnaire (MFQ) (Costello & Angold, 1988) is a self-report measure for 6–17-year-olds, which comes in a short (13 items) and long form (33 items). The revised Children's Anxiety and Depression scale is another commonly used measure.

Clinician-administered scales

Three clinician-administered measures have been commonly used: the Children's Depression Rating Scale-Revised (CDRS-R; Poznanski & Mokros, 1996), the Montgomery-Åsberg Depression Rating Scale (Montgomery & Åsberg, 1979), and the Hamilton Depression Rating Scale (HDRS). Of the three, the CDRS-R (adapted from the HDRS), is specifically for youth and is the most used dimensional measure of depression severity in clinical trials. There are two challenges with CDRS-R: (i) the rater must have experience with the symptoms and functional impairment of MDD to correctly attribute the symptoms and impairment to the depression—this is not a trivial challenge;

and (ii) the symptoms and function domains overlap with symptoms of anxiety disorders, and there is no mechanism inherent in the measure to differentiate anxiety with demoralization (which is not associated with pervasive anhedonia) from clinical depression. This differential is critical to both diagnosis and treatment planning.

Diagnostic interviews

Diagnostic interviews come in a variety of formats, including highly structured, semistructured, and now computer-based formats, and are described in Chapter 28. Although used in research studies, routine use in clinical settings is less common. Highly structured, respondent-based interviews yield higher prevalence rates of MDD than less structured, interviewer-based interviews, which require skilled, trained interviewers.

Epidemiology

MDD exhibits a low prevalence in children but significantly increases during adolescence and young adulthood, particularly among females (Kessler *et al.*, 2003, 2005a, 2005b). Globally, the 1-year prevalence of MDD affects around 1 in 100 children and adolescents, although significant heterogeneity is observed across studies. Factors contributing to this variability include sample representativeness, sampling frames, and the diagnostic instruments and thresholds used (Thapar *et al.*, 2022).

Depression is approximately twice as prevalent in girls as compared to boys, and this sex difference emerges peripubertally (Platt *et al.*, 2021), with some studies suggesting that sex steroids may contribute to this prevalence difference during puberty (Stumper & Alloy, 2023). Further, this sex difference in the prevalence of MDD has increased in youth, although not adults, over the past 40 years (Platt *et al.*, 2021).

Although rates of youth depression in clinically referred and population-based samples appear to have increased over time, it is uncertain as to why this is, given the lack of our current diagnostic capacity to differentiate between intense normal human sadness, demoralization, and clinical depression. Readers are cautioned, when assessing the scientific literature on the prevalence of major depression, to appreciate all the potential challenges in epidemiology methods, data analysis, and interpretation,

The epidemiology of treatment-resistant depression (TRD) in adolescents largely focuses on patients who have failed to respond to initial antidepressant therapy, and there has been considerable effort to define TRD in adolescents (Dwyer *et al.*, 2020; Strawn & Croarkin, 2020). In one prospective study, adolescents with treatment-resistant MDD are predominantly female (65%) and frequently have a recurrent illness (78%), with nearly 1 in 5 having been hospitalized for depression (Strawn *et al.*, 2020)

Comorbidity

The presence of co-occurring conditions with depression is more the rule than the exception. Current diagnostic practice focuses on the patient's symptoms and function at a point in time (cross section). Thus, diagnostic assessment captures current symptom patterns but not necessarily the relationship among conditions or an appreciation of how symptom patterns may have evolved, are influenced by the environment, and, importantly, how patients interact with and react to the symptoms of their conditions and individualize the expression of their depressive symptoms (Boyce *et al.*, 2021).

Between 40–90% of youth with depressive disorders have psychiatric and/or neurodevelopmental comorbidities, and these comorbidities may include anxiety, attention deficit hyperactivity disorder (ADHD), autism spectrum disorder (ASD), and substance use disorders. When combined with another disorder, youth with depression have increased symptom severity and impairment (Husky *et al.*, 2012). Further, comorbid conditions may adversely impact treatment response and require separate treatment (Melton *et al.*, 2016). Important to the cross-sectional assessment is the attribution of the symptom picture to depression or a comorbid condition (Box 63.2). For example, a teen with depression who emphasized the impact of their depressive disorder on attention and concentration may be at risk of being misdiagnosed as ADHD rather than as MDD.

Box 63.2 The importance of attribution in depression assessment

> . . .the first point that requires emphasis is that the concept of depression (as a symptom or a syndrome) is not synonymous with sadness and unhappiness.
>
> . . .although sadness is a common component of the dysphoric mood associated with depression, it is by no means a universal feature.
>
> . . .the negative mood of depression may be more represented by loss of interest or pleasure, an emotional emptiness, and a lack of responsiveness. . .
>
> *Source*: Rutter *et al.* (1986) referencing Hamilton (1982).

Anxiety disorders

Early anxiety disorders serve as risk factors for later clinical depression (Stein *et al.*, 2001; Goodwin *et al.*, 2004; Beesdo *et al.*, 2007). Unpacking this relationship is critical to conceptualizing the relationship between conditions and treatment planning. Anxiety disorders as a group are earlier in the age of onset risk than clinical depression (Beesdo-Baum & Knappe, 2012; Wehry, *et al.*, 2015). Thus, an anxiety disorder may be a risk factor for later depression or secondary demoralization, which, when chronic and severe, could potentially be confused with clinical depression. Similarly, those experiencing clinical depression may express distress and anxiety related to the change in mood state and the loss of capacity to function as previously. Anxiety in reaction to experiencing depression may be substantial and expected, and thus not a pathological comorbidity per se.

Attention deficit hyperactivity disorder and autism spectrum disorder

ADHD and ASD, like anxiety disorders, have a prepubertal age of onset (Solmi *et al.*, 2022), before the typical age of onset for clinical depression. The literature suggests that ADHD and ASD are associated with heightened risk for later clinical depression (Riglin *et al.*, 2021). The diagnostic challenge is similar to the anxiety disorders. For clinicians, deciding whether ADHD or ASD is resulting in demoralization or whether the low mood symptoms reflect a depressive disorder (and a true comorbidity) is key to treatment planning. For example, a young person with a neurodevelopmental disorder (see Chapters 50 and 54), as well as MDD, would require treatments that address both conditions. Psychological therapies, whether for depression or demoralization, also may have to be adjusted for neurodivergent young people.

Sleep disorders and disordered sleep

Three in four depressed children and 9 in 10 depressed adolescents report sleep disturbances, including initial, middle, and terminal insomnia, as well as hypersomnia (Roberts & Duong, 2013) (see Chapter 68). Importantly, disrupted sleep in pediatric patients with MDD may be moderated by the patient's biological sex (Emslie *et al.*, 1994). Successful treatment of depression fails to relieve dyssomnia in 10% of children, although, on average, it is associated with improvement (Reynolds *et al.*, 2020). However, sleep problems that persist after successfully treating the depressive episode may increase the risk of having another depressive episode (Alfano *et al.*, 2009), which emphasizes the importance of addressing sleep aggressively in depressed children and adolescents (Hamill Skoch *et al.*, 2021). When considering sleep problems, particularly initial insomnia, it is prudent to consider a broad differential, including anxiety disorders and neurodevelopmental disorders, and, importantly, poor sleep hygiene.

Youth at risk of developing bipolar disorder

Recent studies have also evaluated youth who present with depression and are at risk of developing BD (Wals *et al.*, 2001; Faedda *et al.*, 2019; De la Serna *et al.*, 2021). Many individuals diagnosed with BD during adolescence or early adulthood often had prior anxiety disorders, significant depressive symptoms, and heightened sensitivity to stressors. In most cases, the initial mood episode in bipolar disorder is depressive, occurring years before the first manic episode (Faedda *et al.*, 2019). However, a switch to mania in the majority of young people with MDD is rare apart from data in highly selected samples. Episodic mood lability (rather than chronic irritability) before the onset of BD may represent a precursor to syndromic (hypo)mania. Also, the presence of co-occurring hypomanic features in an adolescent with MDD increases the risk of developing bipolar compared to a depressive disorder without these features. Recurrent or persistent hypomanic symptoms, especially when combined with other predictors of BD, significantly elevate the risk.

Taken together, these findings suggest that in youth with depressive symptoms and a family history of BD, episodic mood lability (irritability/euphoria) may represent a clinical prodrome leading to (hypo)mania. These symptoms are important because they are inherent to BD but not adequately covered by diagnostic criteria. However, affective instability (and irritability) is very common in other mood and anxiety disorders in adolescents, making accurate diagnosis challenging. Despite this, depressive symptoms are more often linked to depressive episodes or mixed states in patients without a family history of BD (Faedda *et al.*, 2019).

Etiology, mechanisms, and risk factors

Neurobiology of depression in youth

The complex neurobiology of depression in youth involves many brain structures (Kerestes *et al.*, 2014). Accumulating data from task-based functional magnetic resonance imaging (fMRI) studies suggest that emotional stimuli trigger an amplified amygdala response in depressed adolescents, potentially impeding the development of cognitive control mechanisms and contributing to heightened emotional and social reactivity (Li & Wang, 2021; Willinger *et al.*, 2022). In parallel, resting-state functional connectivity studies reveal altered connectivity between the amygdala and the subgenual anterior cingulate cortex (sgACC), a structure involved in emotional processing and decision-making. In depressed adolescents, connectivity among the amygdala, hippocampus, and ventrolateral prefrontal cortex (VLPFC) may also be altered along with structure and function in the striatum.

Beyond functional differences, data from structural examinations reveal decreased gray matter volume in the prefrontal cortex (PFC), hippocampus, amygdala, anterior cingulate cortex (ACC), and dorsolateral prefrontal cortex (DLPFC) (Seewoo *et al.*, 2022). Cortical thickness studies reveal thinning in key regions, including the DLPFC, the VLPFC, the ACC, the medial PFC, and the orbitofrontal cortex. Thinning in these regions could relate to a number of developmental factors or risk factors and could reveal alterations in pruning or synaptogenesis, and related alterations in neurotropic factors or neuroinflammation. Regardless of the processes underlying altered cortical thickness in youth with depression, structural derangements may parallel functional alterations related to emotional regulation, cognitive control, memory processing, and selective attention (Sylvester *et al.*, 2012).

Taken together, neuroimaging studies reveal alterations in structures subserving threat processing and striatum-based neurocircuitry that may contribute to reward processing and motivation. Finally, as we consider the neurobiology of depression, particularly in adolescents, it is essential to note that adolescents (depressed, anxious, or healthy) have incomplete PFC development (Casey *et al.*, 2005a, 2005b), which may contribute to an increased risk of depression due to impaired emotion regulation and impulse control.

Genetics and family history

Our understanding of the specific genetic loci associated with depression in youth is limited (see Chapter 21). Family and adoption studies, as well as twin studies, consistently find that early-onset MDD (in youth) is the most strongly familial subtype of depression and that genetic factors play a more substantial role when onset is early, with contributions potentially exceeding 50%.

Having a parent with recurrent MDD is one of the most potent risk factors for youth MDD. However cross-generational designs also highlight that environmental, as well as genetic, factors contribute. Furthermore, genetic liability to depression is correlated with environmental risk exposures (e.g., life events, maltreatment). Thus, those with genetic liability are more likely to experience the "double whammy" risk effects of higher genetic loading and greater environmental adversity (Thapar *et al.*, 2022). Genetic designs also suggest that adversities (e.g., life events) have causal effects on MDD with associations not purely explained by shared genetic liability. Molecular genetic discovery studies (genome-wide association) have focused on adults with MDD and much broader definitions of depression. More than 100 common genetic loci, each of small effect size, have been discovered (see Chapter 21). Composite measures of these common gene variants (polygenic scores) predict youth and adult depression symptom scores. However, these loci, like those for all psychiatric disorders, are nonspecific in that they strongly overlap (pleiotropy) with risk loci associated with other psychiatric and neurodevelopmental disorders, as well as many physical health problems.

Taken together, these findings underscore the complex genetic and environmental co-actions and interactions that shape the neurobiology of depression and emphasize the importance of studying these relationships in the context of depression in youth. In addition, accumulating data suggest myriad risk factors for developing depression in children and adolescents, including genetic, family, and environmental factors (Table 63.2).

Table 63.2 Risk factors for depressive disorders in children and adolescents.

Category	Risk factors
Environmental	Childhood adversity (e.g., abuse, neglect, trauma)
	Chronic stress
	Socioeconomic stressors in the family
Family environment	Family dysfunction and instability
	Inadequate parental support and affection
	Parental mental illness or substance abuse
	Parent–child conflict and poor communication
Genetic	Family history of depression
Psychiatric and neurodevelopmental antecedents	Anxiety disorder
	Sleep disorder or disturbed sleep
	Substance abuse
	Other psychiatric disorders, e.g., oppositional defiant disorder Irritability
	Attention deficit hyperactivity disorder (ADHD), autism spectrum disorder (ASD)
Psychological	Low self-esteem
	Negative cognitive style and rumination
	Perfectionism and high self-criticism
Social	Academic stress
	Peer victimization and bullying
	Social isolation and loneliness

Treatment

To fully understand the treatment literature, it is critical to understand how clinical treatment trials are conceptualized and implemented. For both high-quality medication and psychotherapy trials, participants and families are required to provide informed assent/consent to be voluntarily randomized to either a potentially effective or potentially less effective intervention. Study procedures often restrict the sample under study to those who are ill but not too ill, impaired but not too impaired, and are invested in the outcome of the experiment rather than hoping for a positive treatment outcome. Thus, clinical features of patients in treatment studies are relatively consistent in symptoms pattern to identify whether the study intervention is superior to the comparison condition on the single outcome of interest. As a result, trials have historically excluded participants with high-risk behaviors and clinical complexity. The study duration of treatment is limited by the duration a participant can be ethically maintained on what might be considered a less effective treatment (e.g., pill placebo or waitlist or ineffective psychosocial treatment)—thus our literature is largely short, term-controlled trials and any longer-term data likely comes from open, uncontrolled, observational studies. In addition, the choice of a single primary outcome often results in a reduction in depressive symptoms that can be identified within the study's time frame. Outcomes such as remission, functional impairment, and other quality-of-life measures are considered secondary and may actually be lagging indicators of symptom reduction and not identifiable in short-term studies focused specifically on depressive symptom reduction.

Studies are not typically designed or powered to detect adverse event differences. Thus, only those common adverse events that rise to a statistical threshold can be identified and considered attributable to the intervention (Strawn *et al.*, 2023). Events such as suicide attempts and manic reactions are rare in short-term trials and, until recently, have not been systematically collected. Thus, data from older studies regarding suicide risk have primarily focused on suicidal thoughts and have required pooling of multiple studies with varying levels of rigor to identify safety signals. Inferences about the safety of our evidence-based treatments need to be considered carefully, given when and how the data has been collected.

With the caveats noted above, in our review of the literature, two main issues would arise regarding the treatment of depression in children and adolescents: (i) there is a lack of data that treatment can, in the short term, substantially improve quality of life or other measures outside symptoms; and (ii) as most clinical trials have excluded participants with suicidal symptoms, there is limited data on the risk for suicidal behavior attributable to treatment—one of the most significant concerns in clinical practice.

How to start treatment?

Treatment always begins with an evaluation. Guidelines suggest a comprehensive evaluation is considered the best starting point but given the high prevalence and the almost universal lack of mental health providers, early recognition and treatment may, in many countries, take place in primary care or nonspecialist settings rather than in specialist mental health settings. Thus, the initial evaluation of a child may now begin with a screening instrument at school or in the primary care office. Many European countries require that medication should only be initiated for youth by a specialist mental health care provider, which means that any young person with moderate–severe depression or intractable mild depression will require referral. UK NICE guidelines further recommend that medication should not be used for the treatment of mild depression and never without combining a psychological intervention. For mild depression, watchful waiting for two weeks and psychotherapy are recommended. However, specialist mental health care is not possible in many settings (see Chapter 46 "Working in low-resource settings"). While the NICE guidelines are intended to hedge clinicians against overtreatment with medication, it has been argued that given the high prevalence of depression in youth, the lack of specialist mental health resources, and the restrictive nature of the NICE guidelines, there may be a substantial number of depressed teens who will not get the opportunity to benefit from medication treatment (Walkup & Strawn, 2020). While a number of efforts have been made to train primary care providers in the US (REACH, ECHO, [Bechelli *et al.*, 2020; Osei-Twum *et al.*, 2022]), such practice is less common in Europe or low–moderate income communities. At the current time, it is unclear whether existing models of provider training can effectively: (i) take advantage of the long-term relationship community primary care providers have with their patients to provide psychological support consistent with evidence-based approaches; (ii) train non-mental health providers to differentiate clinical depression from demoralization and intense normal human sadness experienced after a significant life event; (iii) use measurement-based care for treatment monitoring and helping patients reach remission; and (iv) how best to identify refractoriness to ensure youth have the best opportunity to fully recover (see Chapter 45). Treatment at a glance is illustrated in Box 63.3.

Box 63.3 Treatment at a glance

- Refer to cognitive behavioral therapy (CBT) or interpersonal psychotherapy for adolescents (IPT-A); however,
- Consider selective serotonin reuptake inhibitors (SSRIs), specifically fluoxetine and escitalopram:
  - Ensure adequate SSRI dosing and attempt to reach goal dose by week 6 of treatment (fluoxetine 40 mg/d in adolescents; escitalopram 10–15 mg/d).
  - Serially assess adherence.
- In SSRI nonresponders, consider a trial of a second SSRI:
  - There is less evidence to support adjunctive psychopharmacologic interventions in children and adolescents, but extended-release bupropion, as well as some adjunctive second-generation antipsychotics, may produce some benefit.
- Optimize psychotherapeutic treatment and attend to factors that may attenuate treatment response:
  - Address session frequency and engagement as well as alliance.
  - Ensure that co-occurring attention deficit hyperactivity disorder (ADHD) is managed.
- During treatment, continue to assess comorbidity, including anxiety disorders, ADHD, autism spectrum disorder (ASD), and sleep disorders, as well as substance use.
- Serially evaluate depression-related impairment and function.
- Serially investigate precipitating and perpetuating factors:
  - school environment (bullying, learning disorders, accommodations)
  - adversity
  - family environment/positive parenting

Psychoeducation

After the evaluation is complete, the first treatment step is psychoeducation of the patient, their caregivers, and others important in the young person's life. Traditional psychoeducation begins in person with the provider who describes the condition, explains how and why the affected young person became depressed, reviews the current symptoms and impairment, describes how and why treatment is expected to be effective, the specific targets of treatment, and what is expected from the youth and family during treatment, and how treatment will be monitored to achieve not only remission but also recovery (Bevan Jones *et al.*, 2018). A comprehensive approach to psychoeducation will also lead to a discussion of prognosis when treatment can be discontinued, and the plan for long-term monitoring. Given the transition in clinical practice to population-based approaches, much of the psychoeducation is done via handouts, brochures, books, websites, and online videos. Reputable professional organizations have built content for providers, patients, and families that can help prepare the patient and family for treatment.

Psychotherapy for pediatric major depression

Psychotherapy has two main components—nonspecific factors common across all psychotherapies and specific factors common to one school of thought or approach (Weersing *et al.*, 2017) (see Chapter 31). Nonspecific factors would include the therapist–patient alliance, and specific factors would include behavioral activation approaches to counteract withdrawal or retardation or cognitive restructuring of depressive cognitions such as hopelessness and helplessness (see Chapters 31–39 on psychological therapies). Historically, cognitive behavioral therapy (CBT) and interpersonal psychotherapy (IPT) have been recommended as evidence-based psychological treatments for major depression. However, positive evidence has now emerged for other psychological interventions, including family therapy and brief psychodynamic therapy. As a result, UK NICE guidance recommends a variety of psychological interventions for depression.

Cognitive behavioral therapy

As psychological theory has evolved from a strictly behavioral focus to include cognitive and emotional factors, treatment models have similarly evolved. Simply stated, CBT posits that depression is the result of negative thought patterns that result in the negative symptoms of depression. Negative views of the self, the world, and the future form the core cognitions of depression and result in the range of symptoms seen in depression. CBT is less focused on where the cognitions come from and more on the here and now, and concentrates on the dominant and problematic cognitions (cognitive distortions) felt to cause depression and, through improving cognitive processes, improve depression. Other forms of CBT focus on improving the regulation of emotions and thus changing behavior and the role of one's mood and behavior in the development of interpersonal problems. Similarly, some CBT focuses more on changes in behavior, such as behavioral activation, with the goal of improving cognition and mood functioning. CBT is considered an evidence-based intervention for depression.

Interpersonal psychotherapy

IPT posits that interpersonal factors and life events interact to cause mood disturbance and that mood disturbance can likewise cause interpersonal problems. It may even result in changes in behavior that impact life trajectory. IPT borrows from both psychodynamic and CBT approaches with an emphasis on relationship roles and life experiences and the here-and-now approaches of CBT. First developed for adults, IPT has been adapted for adolescents and demonstrated efficacy in randomized clinical trials (Mufson *et al.*, 1999, 2004). The treatment protocol typically involves 12–16 sessions, where the therapist works with the adolescent to identify and address specific interpersonal problems, improve communication and conflict resolution skills, and explore and process emotions related to their depression (see Chapter 36).

Psychodynamic psychotherapy

Much of psychotherapy practice in the community is informed by the psychodynamic model. Evidence for the efficacy of these approaches in children or teens has been evaluated in a large comparative trial. The IMPACT study (Goodyer *et al.*, 2007), in addition to retrospective studies and small prospective trials, provides some evidence for the usefulness of these approaches. The IMPACT study, the largest and most recent trial, is a rater-blind, randomized controlled superiority trial conducted at 15 National Health Service CAMHS clinics in the UK. Youth aged 11–17 years with MDD were randomized to three interventions (individual + family sessions/differing durations)—short-term psychoanalytic therapy (28 + 7 sessions/30 weeks), CBT (20 + 4 sessions/30 weeks), or a brief psychological intervention (8 + 4 session/20 weeks). The study used the MFQ as its primary outcome. Depressive symptoms did not significantly differ between CBT or short-term psychoanalytic therapy at 6 months or 1 year leading the authors to conclude that "short-term psychoanalytical therapy is as effective as CBT, for adolescents with moderate to severe depression" (Goodyer *et al.*, 2007). One challenge in interpreting the outcome of this study is that nearly 70% of individuals in all groups had a clinical response to treatment, including the brief psychological intervention group. When all treatment outcomes are similar, particularly at a high rate of response, it is difficult to interpret whether the treatments were all useful, whether there was spontaneous remission, or whether there was bias in reporting symptoms or assessing outcomes. While the data from this study are difficult to interpret, UK NICE guidance in 2019 recommended a much broader array of psychological treatment approaches than previously for youth depression (National Institute for Health and Care Excellence, 2019).

In general, meta-analyses suggest the efficacy of psychodynamic psychotherapy in youth with depression (Abbass *et al.*, 2013; Midgley *et al.*, 2021), and a noninferiority trial further supports its efficacy. This noninferiority trial randomized 272 adolescents aged 15–19 with MDD to Internet-delivered psychodynamic psychotherapy or Internet-delivered CBT and found similar improvement and rates of remission for both treatments (38% for Internet-delivered psychodynamic psychotherapy and 40% for Internet-delivered CBT) (Mechler *et al.*, 2022).

Adaptations of psychotherapy

Most evidence-based therapies are focused on individual treatment and have been manualized for research. A major concern regarding clinical trial data is the need for more generalizability to real-world settings, resulting in efforts to adapt individual to group settings to reach more patients and increasingly focus on family involvement to address some of the here-and-now interactional factors relevant to young people.

Adaptations are also driven by concerns regarding the lack of generalizability of the evidence base to a range of marginalized populations not traditionally represented in clinical studies. While it is unlikely that large-scale clinical trials of individual psychotherapies will be undertaken in the future, treatment trials that use novel mechanisms of recruitment, such as via social media and interactive computer-based interventions to address generalizability and access gaps respectively, may be more feasible and add to the current evidence base. The challenges of digital approaches to psychological care are similar to the challenges of psychotherapeutic treatment more generally. The patient must form "an alliance" with the digital platform, and the intervention's approach and content must be relevant to maintain engagement (see Chapter 49).

Problems with psychotherapeutic treatment

The field has struggled dramatically to disseminate evidence-based practice into the community. To date, the professional organizations that oversee the training of those providing psychotherapy have not necessarily embraced mastery of evidence-based psychotherapy. Even clinical guidelines based on rigorous meta-analyses of ~25 psychotherapy studies suggest the use of psychotherapy but are less clear about their efficacy and whether the benefits outweigh the harms (Walter *et al.*, 2023) In addition, dissemination of evidence-based psychotherapies may be impacted by the fact that they are proprietary (i.e., "branded" psychotherapies), which adds to the cost of training, often means they are of long duration (i.e., multiple sessions over months), which impacts feasibility in the "real world", and reflects "an approach" that may not appear relevant to the clinician's view of the clinical situation. Efforts to address the challenge of "branded" therapies through the packaging of strategies and techniques used in evidence-based treatments and matching those to the patient's needs have effectively availed more "generic" forms of psychotherapy and have the promise of being more relevant to systems of care.

Perhaps the biggest problem facing psychotherapy practice for depression is that the Treatment for Adolescents with Depression Study (TADS) (March *et al.*, 2004), the Adolescent Depression Antidepressant and Psychotherapy Trial (ADAPT) (Goodyer *et al.*, 2007), and the Treatment of Resistant Depression in Adolescents (TORDIA) (Emslie *et al.*, 2015) demonstrated little additional value of psychotherapy above and beyond medication treatment in moderate-to-severe depression. Yet, the marketplace continues to promulgate the notion of the effectiveness of psychotherapy as the initial treatment of clinical depression. Further, a network meta-analysis of 71 trials of psychotherapy, pharmacotherapy, or psychotherapy plus pharmacotherapy in young people with MDD found fluoxetine (alone or in combination with CBT) more efficacious than placebo. However, the efficacy of fluoxetine plus CBT did not differ from the efficacy of fluoxetine alone (−0.22, 95% CI −0.86–0.42) (Zhou *et al.*, 2020).

Psychotherapy is likely highly effective in helping some young people with intense normal human sadness after a significant life event, particularly in a young person with limited coping and adaptation skills and psychosocial support. Psychotherapy in this context can help a young person become aware, build skills, cope effectively, and overcome. Similarly, psychotherapy is likely effective for demoralization in the face of persistent and unalterable life circumstances. Psychotherapy in this context can promote awareness, build skills, promote effective coping, and improve relationship quality and support. Psychotherapy is also likely to help support patients with severe clinical depression who need to maintain engagement in treatment, support an understanding of their experience of severe depression, and prepare them for adherence to all aspects of treatment during the acute and maintenance phases. The literature is less clear on whether psychotherapy can be effective in the core symptoms of severe clinical depression. In severe depression, psychotherapy may even do harm by encouraging a formulation that depressive suffering is amenable to psychological, emotional, or behavioral change.

Psychopharmacologic treatment

Overview—The context of clinical trials of antidepressant medications

Multiple studies have examined the efficacy of various antidepressant agents in the treatment of children and adolescents with depressive disorders, most commonly MDD. Most published studies have been sponsored by the pharmaceutical industry and have followed a typical design—large sample size, large numbers of sites, randomized, double-blind, placebo-controlled trials. A much smaller number of studies have been supported by government organizations such as the US National Institute of Mental Health and Health Technology Assessment Program of the National Institute of Health Research. Of those industry-sponsored trials in the US, a majority were implemented under the 1997 Food and Drug Administration Modernization Act (FDAMA), which financially incentivized pharmaceutical companies to undertake clinical trials of any medication for which there was a lack of pediatric data (Walkup, 2017). The incentivization (6 months of additional patent "exclusivity") was remarkably successful in increasing the pharmaceutical industry's interest in conducting clinical trials for those many medications without pediatric use data (Strawn *et al.*, 2017), including antidepressants. FDAMA required studies to follow the design of studies used for the initial indication in adult populations. FDAMA also requires the studies to be completed before their patent expires, which for some medications was imminent and required the mobilization of significant resources (Sharav, 2003; Califf, 2016). In review, the studies were notable for large numbers of sites with few patients per site, unknown/unlisted investigators, limited clinical (as opposed to operational) training of investigative teams, limited ongoing clinical quality monitoring (data monitoring was high quality), and study populations that included prepubertal children. The industry-sponsored studies have had high placebo response rates with small, if any, differences in response rates between medication and placebo. Given the lack of between-group differences, the many industry-sponsored studies in the literature have been variably reported as not demonstrating efficacy (negative studies) and have been critiqued as *failed* trials due to substantive implementation challenges. Differentiating between a negative and failed trial is critical, as failed studies are not amenable to inclusion in meta-analyses (Strawn & Walkup, 2020). Exploration of the high placebo response in these studies not surprisingly revealed that large numbers of study recruitment sites, prepubertal participants, and mild symptoms at baseline were positively correlated with placebo response (Bridge *et al.*, 2007). These many industry-sponsored studies are to be contrasted with the few government-funded studies that often had expert teams of investigators well-known in the field, fewer sites with adequate Ns per site, extensive clinical training, and ongoing clinical monitoring. These studies, while few, resulted in demonstrated efficacy and low(er) placebo response rates with number needed to treat (NNT) ~4 (Walkup, 2017; Mossman *et al.*, 2021).

Thus, reviewing the extant literature, many industry-sponsored trials were and continue to be associated with a myriad of implementation challenges (large number of sites, few patients per site, unknown/unlisted investigators, poor clinical training and clinical monitoring, and prepubertal patients, to name a few) that increase placebo response (Walkup & Strawn, 2020). Yet, the ongoing effort to meta-analyze data from the many arguably failed trials overwhelms the data from the few high-quality government-sponsored studies, leaving the clinical community and the public with a distorted impression of the efficacy of antidepressants (Walkup & Strawn, 2020).

Evidence for psychopharmacologic interventions in treating depression in children and adolescents

As of January 2025, fluoxetine is the only antidepressant approved by the European Medicines Agency (EMA) for the treatment of major depressive episodes unresponsive to psychotherapy in children and adolescents aged 8–18. In addition to fluoxetine, for the same age range, the FDA has also approved escitalopram for the treatment of major depressive episodes in adolescents aged 12–17 (Cortese *et al.*, 2023b).

In terms of the evidence related to the efficacy and tolerability of antidepressants in children and adolescents with depression, a network meta-analysis analyzed randomized controlled trials (RCTs) of 14 antidepressants in children and adolescents. Only fluoxetine was statistically significantly more efficacious than placebo, with an effect size = 0.51 (but large 95% CI [0.03–0.99] [−0·99 to −0·03]); however, such meta-analyses should be interpreted with caution given the large number of industry-sponsored trials included in them and the related limitations described in the preceding section. Another network meta-analysis focused on new generation antidepressants (Hetrick *et al.*, 2021). Overall, most antidepressants were associated with a small reduction in depression symptoms compared with placebo (high-certainty evidence: paroxetine and desvenlafaxine; moderate-certainty evidence: sertraline, fluoxetine, and escitalopram; low-certainty evidence: duloxetine and vortioxetine; very low certainty evidence for comparisons between other antidepressants and placebo). In relation to the suicidal risk, the analysis found: very uncertain evidence for mirtazapine, duloxetine, vilazodone, desvenlafaxine, citalopram, and vortioxetine on suicide-related outcomes compared with placebo; low-certainty evidence that escitalopram may "at least slightly" reduce odds of suicide-related outcomes compared with placebo; and that fluoxetine, paroxetine, sertraline, and venlafaxine may "at least slightly" increase odds of suicide-related outcomes compared with placebo.

A network meta-analysis including both pharmacological and nonpharmacological interventions (Zhou *et al.*, 2020) showed that fluoxetine plus CBT was more efficacious than CBT alone and psychodynamic therapy, but not more effective than fluoxetine alone, even though there was only one direct comparison of psychotherapy with medication. No pharmacotherapy alone was more effective than psychotherapy alone. Only fluoxetine plus CBT and fluoxetine were significantly more efficacious than pill placebo or psychological controls. Nortriptyline and waiting list were less efficacious than most active interventions.

We will now summarize the most relevant individual RCTs in the field.

TADS (March *et al.*, 2004), one of the largest trials examining selective serotonin reuptake inhibitors (SSRIs) in adolescents with MDD (N = 439), randomized youth to four treatment groups: (i) fluoxetine monotherapy (10–40 mg/d), (ii) CBT, (iii) CBT combined with fluoxetine (10–40 mg/d), or (iv) pill placebo. After 12 weeks of treatment, fluoxetine + CBT and fluoxetine alone were more effective for patients than CBT alone and pill placebo. CBT alone was not found to be more effective than pill placebo. Longer-term data suggest the persistence of symptoms in many patients (Kennard *et al.*, 2006).

ADAPT, in clinical services in England (Goodyer *et al.*, 2007), compared SSRI versus SSRI + CBT in a population of severely depressed 11–17-year-olds (N = 208). After the 12-week acute treatment phase, there was an approximately 50% response rate in both groups with no identified between-group differences on primary or secondary outcome measures.

While TADS was instrumental in establishing the evidence base for interventions in youths with MDD, guidance for clinicians treating SSRI-nonresponders was limited until the completion of the TORDIA study (Brent *et al.*, 2008). In TORDIA, adolescents aged 12–18 years with MDD (N = 334) who did not respond to an adequate dose of an SSRI for at least 8 weeks were randomized to one of four treatments over 12 weeks. Notably, these patients had a more chronic course on average compared to those enrolled in TADS. In TORDIA, patients were randomized to: (i) a different SSRI (paroxetine, citalopram, or fluoxetine), (ii) a different SSRI combined with CBT, (iii) venlafaxine ER, or (iv) venlafaxine ER combined with CBT. Combining CBT with a medication switch (to another SSRI or venlafaxine ER) led to a marked decrease in depressive symptoms compared to solely changing medication. The two arms with CBT plus medication demonstrated a higher response rate (55%) than the medication switch alone (41%). However, in the original analysis, no differences in the outcome were observed between switching to venlafaxine ER versus another SSRI. Still, patients who switched to a second SSRI experienced less suicidal ideation than those treated with venlafaxine and encountered fewer adverse events.

Additionally, when considering the tolerability and efficacy of the SSRIs together, adolescents treated with citalopram and fluoxetine showed better outcomes than those treated with paroxetine. A recent reanalysis of the TORDIA data, utilizing contemporary statistical approaches, revealed that SSRIs produced greater and faster improvement in depressive symptoms compared to venlafaxine ER (Suresh *et al.*, 2020). However, for CBT-treated patients, SSRIs and venlafaxine ER yielded similar improvements in anxiety and depression symptoms.

General principles of psychopharmacologic treatment of depression in children and adolescents

In terms of general principles of psychopharmacologic treatment of depression in children and adolescents, the importance of dose is increasingly appreciated (Strawn *et al.*, 2021), particularly with regard to SSRIs. The most prescribed SSRIs for depression in children and adolescents—fluoxetine and escitalopram—are metabolized by highly polymorphic cytochromes in the liver (specifically CYP2D6 for fluoxetine and CYP2C19 for escitalopram). The time course of treatment response in children and adolescents with depression is logarithmic (Varigonda *et al.*, 2015), meaning that the greatest improvement occurs early during treatment and that treatment effects, over time, plateau. Given this consistent trajectory of improvement observed across studies, clinicians may consider more proactively managing depressive symptoms when the typically expected improvement is absent. As an example, one sequenced intervention trial recently randomized depressed adolescents who had failed to demonstrate expected improvements in early augmentation or late augmentation with either fluoxetine or an increased frequency of interpersonal psychotherapy for adolescents (IPT-A) and found that earlier augmentation within the first four weeks of treatment produced greater remission over time (Gunlicks-Stoessel *et al.*, 2019).

Management of antidepressant side effects

When considering antidepressant tolerability and handling adverse events related to antidepressants, we must consider how each medication's pharmacology contributes to certain side effects and how the risk of specific side effects varies among different antidepressant medications and classes. It is crucial to note that many physical symptoms improve in children and adolescents treated with SSRIs (Strawn *et al.*, 2023)

While, as a class, antidepressants are associated with headaches, nausea, abdominal pain, and dyssomnia, SSRIs are more likely to induce activation, abdominal pain, sedation/drowsiness, and discontinuation due to adverse effects compared to placebo. However, certain side effects manifest early and dissipate quickly, such as activation and gastrointestinal symptoms (Strawn *et al.*, 2023). On the other hand, some side effects emerge later or persist over time, like weight gain or sexual dysfunction. In the case of immediately arising side effects like gastrointestinal symptoms, there may be dynamic physiological mechanisms that alleviate these effects. For instance, nausea, which appears early on, could be linked to acute increases in serotonergic activity that enhances gastrointestinal motility (Baumel *et al.*, 2023). The resolution of these effects might be connected to the desensitization of serotonergic receptors in the gut. It is crucial to discuss the temporal patterns of side effects and differentiate between persistent and transient ones. It is important to ensure that patients are informed not only about the side effects but also about the tendency of certain side effects to be temporary. This information should be incorporated into discussions with patients and their families. For many individuals, knowing that a side effect is likely to be short-lived rather than enduring can significantly impact their anxiety or concerns regarding medication.

In general, early emerging side effects like activation, gastrointestinal symptoms, and sedation can be addressed by adjusting exposure and considering individual variations in medication metabolism (Strawn *et al.*, 2023). However, it is critical to evaluate baseline symptoms before initiating pharmacotherapy for early emerging side effects, as they overlap syndromically with depression.

Managing late-emerging adverse effects, such as weight gain, requires a more nuanced approach (Strawn *et al.*, 2023). Weight gain, particularly with SSRIs, may be influenced by medication metabolism and the specific drug used (Aldrich *et al.*, 2019). In such instances, switching medications, possibly with cross-titration, can be a reasonable strategy (Strawn & Stahl, 2023).

Mania seems less likely to occur than previously thought, yet caution is still warranted when there is a positive family history of BD, prior manic episode, concurrent manic or subsyndromal manic symptoms, or bipolar depression. Yet, clinical guidance varies as to the best approach (McNamara *et al.*, 2012)—whether antidepressant monotherapy is to be avoided or combined with a mood stabilizer or whether combinations of mood stabilizers are optimal.

Several studies have examined pharmacologic and nonpharmacologic strategies for youth presenting with affective/depressive symptoms who are at risk of developing BD (Findling et al., 2008; McNamara et al., 2012; Cotton *et al.*, 2015, 2020). These studies suggest that youth with a parent with BD may not tolerate antidepressant medications as well as their peers without a family history of BD (Findling *et al.*, 2008; Strawn *et al.*, 2014). Moreover, this decreased antidepressant tolerability in youth with depressive symptoms has been associated in some small studies with progression to the development of hypomanic episodes (Nery *et al.*, 2020).

It is important to distinguish treatment-emergent mania from behavioral activation. The International Society for Bipolar Disorders Task Force recommends using the term treatment emergent activated switch (TEAS), instead of antidepressant-induced switch, to emphasize association of (hypo-)manic symptoms when treating with antidepressants without implying causality. In the activation syndrome, symptoms can include impulsivity, insomnia, restlessness, hyperactivity, and irritability, while on the other hand antidepressant-induced manic switch presents with the symptoms of a (hypo-)manic episode. Mild hypomanic symptoms are much more common than manic switching (Cortese *et al.*, 2023a). The treatment for a manic switch includes immediate discontinuation of the antidepressant (and possible use of antimanic agents), whereas a reduction of or discontinuation of antidepressants can be used to address activation symptoms (Wilens *et al.*, 2003; Luft *et al.*, 2018).

Discontinuing antidepressants in children and adolescents with depression

While the optimal duration of antidepressant treatment for youth with MDD remains a topic of debate, the primary goal of treatment is clear: achieving remission (Hathaway *et al.*, 2017). Discussions surrounding treatment discontinuation presuppose that the patient has attained remission of depressive symptoms, indicating both symptom relief and functional recovery (Stimpfl *et al.*, 2025). In cases where remission is not achieved through initial treatment, either with antidepressant monotherapy or a combination of antidepressants and psychotherapy, clinicians should consider switching antidepressants without unnecessary delay, as delayed response to the initial SSRI is unlikely after an initial eight-week treatment period. Switching to a different SSRI among nonresponders has shown beneficial effects, as described earlier. The TORDIA study reinforces the importance of early intervention among nonresponders, as many individuals exhibit signs of eventual remission within the first six weeks following an antidepressant switch. While studies on the way to discontinue antidepressants in children and adolescents have not adequately reported tapering or discontinuation-related adverse effects, emerging data from adults with depressive and anxiety disorders suggest the potential benefits of a slower (Lewis *et al.*, 2021) discontinuation approach (Tint *et al.*, 2008), and this approach has been advocated for youth (Strawn *et al.*, 2023).

To date, four studies have examined relapse following SSRI discontinuation in adolescents (citalopram, escitalopram and fluoxetine), revealing a higher and earlier incidence of relapse among patients who discontinued fluoxetine compared to those who continued SSRI treatment (Emslie *et al.*, 2008; Kennard *et al.*, 2014). Most relapses occurred within the first three months of discontinuation, despite fluoxetine's long half-life (Emslie *et al.*, 2008) and a similar pattern is observed for escitalopram and citalopram (Stimpfl *et al.*, 2025). This finding has significant implications for patient monitoring upon discontinuation of SSRI therapy. Additionally, combining fluoxetine with CBT has reduced the risk of relapse in youth who have received treatment for MDD (Emslie *et al.*, 2015).

When considering discontinuing antidepressants, clinicians should carefully assess the timing, considering the adolescent's psychosocial environment. Shamseddeen *et al.* observed that depressed adolescents who ended treatment during summer vacation had nearly double the likelihood of achieving satisfactory treatment responses (Shamseddeen *et al.*, 2012). Consequently, clinicians should plan antidepressant discontinuation during periods of lower stress while recognizing the significance of non-disorder-related factors, such as school or separation-related events.

Novel and emerging treatments for depression in children and adolescents

A systematic analysis of RCTs on novel compounds tested as antidepressants for children and adolescents in the past 10 years did not identify any compounds for which there were at least two positive trials, with no negative trials. However, among the novel compounds, it is worth mentioning ketamine and esketamine. In one study involving adolescents with TRD, a small proof-of-concept trial with 17 participants found that ketamine (0.5 mg/kg) was more effective than a control infusion (midazolam) in reducing depressive symptoms and was also well tolerated by the participants (Dwyer *et al.*, 2021), and two controlled trials of esketamine in adolescents have demonstrated benefit in adolescents with depression (Zhou *et al.*, 2023).

In parallel to studies in adults with MDD, pediatric studies have increasingly focused on neuromodulation. A meta-analysis of neurostimulation therapies with search conducted up to 2021 did not include any RCT of transcranial magnetic stimulation (TMS) or transcranial direct current stimulation (tDCS) in children/adolescents (Hyde *et al.*, 2022). A subsequent trial of TMS did not demonstrate efficacy in adolescents with TRD (aged 12–21 years) in a randomized, multi-site, sham-controlled trial sponsored by the industry. Interestingly, the sham group showed a response rate (36%), while the response rate in the TMS group was slightly higher (42%) (Croarkin *et al.*, 2021). However, in 2023, the US FDA cleared TMS for the treatment of adolescents with TRD based on registry data. When it comes to electroconvulsive therapy (ECT), research in pediatric populations has been slower compared to studies in adults. This delay is partly due to societal, cultural, and legal concerns surrounding the use of ECT in children and adolescents (Dwyer *et al.*, 2020).

Summary of two key treatment guidelines

National Institute for Health and Care Excellence

The 2019 NICE guidelines recommend not using antidepressants for the initial treatment of children and young people with mild depression (National Institute for Health and Care Excellence, 2019). For 5–11-year-olds with mild depression continuing after 2 weeks of watchful waiting and without significant comorbid problems or active suicidal ideas or plans, the following options should be considered: digital CBT, group CBT, group nondirective supportive therapy, and group IPT. If these options are unsuitable or not preferred by the patient, attachment-based family therapy and individual

CBT should be considered. The same options are recommended for 12–18-year-olds, for a limited period (approximately 2–3 months). For 5–11-year-olds with moderate-to-severe depression, family-based IPT, family therapy, psychodynamic psychotherapy, and individual therapy should be considered. For 12–18-year-olds with moderate-to-severe depression, individual CBT for at least 3 months should be offered, or, if this is not the preferred option, IPT-A, family therapy, brief psychosocial interventions, and psychodynamic psychotherapy.

Combined therapy (fluoxetine and psychological therapy) for initial treatment of moderate-to-severe depression in young people (12–18 years), can be an alternative to psychological therapy followed by combined therapy. Fluoxetine should be offered if moderate-to-severe depression in a young person (12–18 years) is unresponsive to a specific psychological therapy after 4–6 sessions.

Fluoxetine should be considered if moderate-to-severe depression in a child (5–11 years) is unresponsive to a specific psychological therapy after 4–6 sessions, although the evidence for fluoxetine's effectiveness in this age group is not established.

If moderate-to-severe depression in a child or young person is unresponsive to combined treatment with a specific psychological therapy and fluoxetine after a further 6 sessions, an alternative psychological therapy, systemic family therapy, or psychodynamic therapy should be considered.

When a child or young person responds to treatment with fluoxetine, medication should be continued for at least six months. If treatment with fluoxetine is unsuccessful or is not tolerated because of side effects, sertraline or citalopram (off-label) are the recommended second-line treatments.

Paroxetine, venlafaxine, and tricyclic antidepressants are generally not recommended for the treatment of depression in children and young people.

American Academy of Child and Adolescent Psychiatry practice parameters

According to the American Academy of Child and Adolescent Psychiatry (AACAP) clinical practice guideline (Walter *et al.*, 2023), a thorough evaluation is necessary to assess depressive symptoms, associated problems, and potential risk factors. This guidance suggests involving parents or caregivers in the assessment process and considers the cultural context in which the young person lives. The practice guidelines do not provide clear guidance related to the duration of treatment, dosing, and sequencing, which are limited in these clinical practice guidelines. In short, AACAP recommends:

- Cognitive-behavioral and interpersonal therapy could be offered to adolescents and children with depressive disorders.
- SSRIs (except paroxetine), and "preferably fluoxetine," could be offered to youth with depression.
- Combination therapy, specifically CBT plus fluoxetine, could be offered to youth with depression.

Summary

Differentiating normal human sadness, demoralization, and clinical depression is critically important in evaluating and treatment planning and, importantly, understanding the literature on depression in youth where the lack of such differentiation can and has likely impacted the literature from epidemiology to clinical trials. While our current nosology has not taken on this challenge, the clinician who desires to practice at a high level would be advised to consider the range of unhappiness in the office and adjust their approach to treatment accordingly.

References

Abbass, A.A. *et al.* (2013) Psychodynamic psychotherapy for children and adolescents: a meta-analysis of short-term psychodynamic models. *Journal of the American Academy of Child and Adolescent Psychiatry* **52**(8), 863–875. doi:10.1016/j.jaac.2013.05.014.

Aldrich, S.L. *et al.* (2019) Influence of CYP2C19 metabolizer status on escitalopram/citalopram tolerability and response in youth with anxiety and depressive disorders. *Frontiers in Pharmacology* **10**, 99. doi:10.3389/fphar.2019.00099.

Alfano, C.A. *et al.* (2009) Sleep problems and their relation to cognitive factors, anxiety, and depressive symptoms in children and adolescents. *Depression and Anxiety* **26**(6), 503–512. doi:10.1002/da.20443.

American Psychiatric Association (2022) *Diagnostic and Statistical Manual of Mental Disorders*, 5th edn. text revision edn. American Psychiatric Association, Washington, DC.

Baumel, W.T. *et al.* (2023) Gastrointestinal symptoms in pediatric patients with anxiety disorders and their relationship to selective serotonin reuptake inhibitor treatment or placebo. *Child Psychiatry and Human Development*. doi:10.1007/s10578-023-01586-x.

Bechelli, M. *et al.* (2020) 9.1 a systematic review of child psychiatry access program outcomes: preliminary results. *Journal of the American Academy of Child and Adolescent Psychiatry* **59**(10), S172–S173. doi:10.1016/j.jaac.2020.08.138.

Beesdo, K. *et al.* (2007) Incidence of social anxiety disorder and the consistent risk for secondary depression in the first three decades of life. *Archives of General Psychiatry* **64**(8), 903–912. doi:10.1001/archpsyc.64.8.903.

Beesdo-Baum, K. & Knappe, S. (2012) Developmental epidemiology of anxiety disorders. *Child and Adolescent Psychiatric Clinics of North America* **21**, 457–478. doi:10.1016/j.chc.2012.05.001.

Bevan Jones, R. *et al.* (2018) Psychoeducational interventions in adolescent depression: a systematic review. *Patient Education and Counseling* **101**(5), 804–816. doi:10.1016/j.pec.2017.10.015.

Boyce, W.T. *et al.* (2021) Genes, environments, and time: the biology of adversity and resilience. *Pediatrics* **147**(2), e20201651. doi:10.1542/peds.2020-1651.

Brent, D. *et al.* (2008) Switching to another SSRI or to venlafaxine with or without cognitive behavioral therapy for adolescents with SSRI-resistant depression: the TORDIA randomized controlled trial. *JAMA* **299**(8), 901–913. doi:10.1001/jama.299.8.901.

Bridge, J.A. *et al.* (2007) Clinical response and risk for reported suicidal ideation and suicide attempts in pediatric antidepressant treatment: a meta-analysis of randomized controlled trials. *JAMA* **297**(15), 1683–1696. doi:10.1001/jama.297.15.1683.

Califf, R.M. (2016) *Best Pharmaceuticals for Children Act and Pediatric Research Equity Act July 2016 Status Report to Congress.* DHHS-FDA Reports, Food and Drug Administration (FDA), Silver Spring, MD.

Casey, B.J. *et al.* (2005a) Changes in cerebral functional organization during cognitive development. *Current Opinion in Neurobiology* **15**(2), 239–244. doi:10.1016/j.conb.2005.03.012.

Casey, B.J. *et al.* (2005b) Imaging the developing brain: what have we learned about cognitive development? *Trends in Cognitive Sciences* **9**(3), 104–110. doi:10.1016/j.tics.2005.01.011.

Cortese, S. *et al.* (2023a) Common practical questions – And answers – At the British Association for Psychopharmacology Child and Adolescent Psychopharmacology course. *Journal of Psychopharmacology* **37**(2), 119–134. doi:10.1177/02698811221140005.

Cortese, S. *et al.* (2023b) Psychopharmacology in children and adolescents: unmet needs and opportunities. *The Lancet. Psychiatry* **11**(2), 143–154.

Costello, E.J. & Angold, A. (1988) Scales to assess child and adolescent depression: checklists, screens, and nets. *Journal of the American Academy of Child and Adolescent Psychiatry* **27**(6), 726–737. doi:10.1097/00004583-198811000-00011.

Cotton, S. *et al.* (2015) Mindfulness-based cognitive therapy for youth with anxiety disorders at risk for bipolar disorder: a pilot trial. *Early Intervention in Psychiatry* **10**(5), 426–434. doi:10.1111/eip.12216.

Cotton, S. *et al.* (2020) Mindfulness-based cognitive therapy for children and adolescents with anxiety disorders at-risk for bipolar disorder: a psychoeducation waitlist controlled pilot trial. *Early Intervention in Psychiatry* **14**(2), 211–219. doi:10.1111/eip.12848.

Croarkin, P.E. *et al.* (2021) Left prefrontal transcranial magnetic stimulation for treatment-resistant depression in adolescents: a double-blind, randomized, sham-controlled trial. *Neuropsychopharmacology* **46**(2), 462–469. doi:10.1038/s41386-020-00829-y.

De la Serna, E. *et al.* (2021) Lifetime psychopathology in child and adolescent offspring of parents diagnosed with schizophrenia or bipolar disorder: a 2-year follow-up study. *European Child & Adolescent Psychiatry* **30**(1), 117–129. doi:10.1007/s00787-020-01500-z.

Dwyer, J.B. *et al.* (2020) Annual research review: defining and treating pediatric treatment-resistant depression. *Journal of Child Psychology and Psychiatry* **61**(3), 312–332. doi:10.1111/jcpp.13202.

Dwyer, J.B. *et al.* (2021) Efficacy of intravenous ketamine in adolescent treatment-resistant depression: a randomized midazolam-controlled trial. *American Journal of Psychiatry* **178**(4), 352–362. doi:10.1176/appi.ajp.2020.20010018.

Emslie, G.J. *et al.* (1994) Sleep EEG features of adolescents with major depression. *Biological Psychiatry* **36**(9), 573–581. doi:10.1016/0006-3223(94)90067-1.

Emslie, G.J. *et al.* (2008) Fluoxetine versus placebo in preventing relapse of major depression in children and adolescents. *American Journal of Psychiatry* **165**(4), 459–467. doi:10.1176/appi.ajp.2007.07091453.

Emslie, G.J. *et al.* (2015) Continued effectiveness of relapse prevention cognitive-behavioral therapy following fluoxetine treatment in youth with major depressive disorder. *Journal of the American Academy of Child and Adolescent Psychiatry* **54**(12), 991–998. doi:10.1016/j.jaac.2015.09.014.

Faedda, G.L. *et al.* (2019) An International Society of Bipolar Disorders Task Force Report: Precursors and Prodromes of bipolar disorder. *Bipolar Disorders* **21**(8), 720–740. doi:10.1111/bdi.12831.

Findling, R.L. *et al.* (2008) A pilot pharmacotherapy trial for depressed youths at high genetic risk for bipolarity. *Journal of Child and Adolescent Psychopharmacology* **18**, 615–621. doi:10.1089/cap.2008.018.

Gohari, M.R. *et al.* (2023) Adolescents' depression and anxiety symptoms during the COVID-19 pandemic: longitudinal evidence from COMPASS. *Journal of Adolescent Health* **74**(1), 36–43. doi:10.1016/j.jadohealth.2023.07.024.

Goodwin, R.D. *et al.* (2004) Panic attacks and the risk of depression among young adults in the community. *Psychotherapy and Psychosomatics* **73**(3), 158–165. doi:10.1159/000076453.

Goodyer, I. *et al.* (2007) Selective serotonin reuptake inhibitors (SSRIs) and routine specialist care with and without cognitive behaviour therapy in adolescents with major depression: randomised controlled trial. *BMJ* **335**(7611), 142. doi:10.1136/bmj.39224.494340.55.

Gunlicks-Stoessel, M. *et al.* (2019) Critical decision points for augmenting interpersonal psychotherapy for depressed adolescents: a pilot sequential multiple assignment randomized trial. *Journal of the American Academy of Child and Adolescent Psychiatry* **58**(1), 80–91. doi:10.1016/j.jaac.2018.06.032.

Hamill Skoch, S. *et al.* (2021) Pediatric insomnia: assessment and diagnosis. *Current Psychiatry* **20**(12), 9–25.

Hamilton, M. (1982) Symptoms and assessment of depression. In: *Handbook of Affective Disorders.* (ed E.S. Paykel). Churchill Livingstone, London.

Hathaway, E.E. *et al.* (2017) Antidepressant treatment duration in pediatric depressive and anxiety disorders: how long is long enough? *Current Problems in Pediatrics and Adolescent Health Care* **48**(2), 31–39. doi:10.1016/j.cppeds.2017.12.002.

Hetrick, S.E. *et al.* (2021) New generation antidepressants for depression in children and adolescents: a network Meta-analysis. *Cochrane Database of Systematic Reviews* **2021**(5). doi:10.1002/14651858.CD013674.pub2.

Horowitz, L.M. *et al.* (2012) Ask Suicide-Screening Questions (ASQ): a brief instrument for the Pediatric Emergency Department. *Archives of Pediatrics & Adolescent Medicine* **166**(12), 1170–1176. doi:10.1001/archpediatrics.2012.1276.

Husky, M.M. *et al.* (2012) Twelve-month suicidal symptoms and use of services among adolescents: results from the National Comorbidity Survey. *Psychiatric Services* **63**(10), 989–996. doi:10.1176/appi.ps.201200058.

Hyde, J. *et al.* (2022) Efficacy of Neurostimulation across mental disorders: systematic review and meta-analysis of 208 randomized controlled trials. *Molecular Psychiatry* **27**(6), 2709–2719. doi:10.1038/s41380-022-01524-8.

Johnson, J.G. *et al.* (2002) The Patient Health Questionnaire for Adolescents: validation of an instrument for the assessment of mental disorders among adolescent primary care patients. *Journal of Adolescent Health* **30**(3), 196–204. doi:10.1016/S1054-139X(01)00333-0.

Kennard, B. *et al.* (2006) Remission and residual symptoms after short-term treatment in the Treatment of Adolescents with Depression Study (TADS). *Journal of the American Academy of Child and Adolescent Psychiatry* **45**(12), 1404–1411. doi:10.1097/01.chi.0000242228.75516.21.

Kennard, B.D. *et al.* (2014) Sequential treatment with fluoxetine and relapse-prevention CBT to improve outcomes in pediatric depression. *American Journal of Psychiatry* **171**(10), 1083–1090. doi:10.1176/appi.ajp.2014.13111460.

Kerestes, R. *et al.* (2014) Functional brain imaging studies of youth depression: a systematic review. *NeuroImage: Clinical* **4**, 209–231. doi:10.1016/j.nicl.2013.11.009.

Kessler, R.C. *et al.* (2003) The epidemiology of major depressive disorder. *JAMA* **289**(23), 3095. doi:10.1001/jama.289.23.3095.

Kessler, R.C. *et al.* (2005a) Lifetime prevalence and age-of-onset Distributions' of DSM-IV disorders in the National Comorbidity Survey Replication. *Archives of General Psychiatry* **62**, 6, 593–602. doi:10.1001/archpsyc.62.6.593.

Kessler, R.C. *et al.* (2005b) Prevalence, severity, and comorbidity of 12-month DSM-IV disorders in the National Comorbidity Survey Replication. *Archives of General Psychiatry* **62**(6), 617–627. doi:10.1001/archpsyc.62.6.617.

Lewis, G. *et al.* (2021) Maintenance or discontinuation of antidepressants in primary care. *The New England Journal of Medicine* **385**(14), 1257–1267. doi:10.1056/NEJMoa2106356.

Li, X. & Wang, J. (2021) Abnormal neural activities in adults and youths with major depressive disorder during emotional processing: a meta-analysis. *Brain Imaging and Behavior* **15**(2), 1134–1154. doi:10.1007/s11682-020-00299-2.

Luft, M.J. *et al.* (2018) Antidepressant-induced activation in children and adolescents: risk, recognition and management. *Current Problems in Pediatric and Adolescent Health Care* **48**(2). doi:10.1016/j.cppeds.2017.12.001.

Luft, M.J. *et al.* (2019) Thyroid function screening in children and adolescents with mood and anxiety disorders. *Journal of Clinical Psychiatry* **80**(5). doi:10.4088/JCP.18m12626.

March, J. *et al.* (2004) Fluoxetine, cognitive-behavioral therapy, and their combination for adolescents with depression: Treatment for Adolescents with Depression Study (TADS) randomized controlled trial. *JAMA: The Journal of the American Medical Association* **292**(7), 807–820. doi:10.1001/jama.292.7.807.

McNamara, R.K. *et al.* (2012) Interventions for youth at high risk for bipolar disorder and schizophrenia. *Child and Adolescent Psychiatric Clinics of North America* **21**(4), 739–751. doi:10.1016/j.chc.2012.07.009.

Mechler, J. *et al.* (2022) Therapist-guided internet-based psychodynamic therapy versus cognitive behavioural therapy for adolescent depression in Sweden: a randomised, clinical, non-inferiority trial. *The Lancet Digital Health* **4**(8), E594–E603. doi:10.1016/S2589-7500(22)00095-4.

Melton, T.H. *et al.* (2016) Comorbid anxiety and depressive symptoms in children and adolescents: a systematic review and analysis. *Journal of Psychiatric Practice* **22**(2), 84–98. doi:10.1097/PRA.0000000000000132.

Midgley, N. *et al.* (2021) The evidence-base for psychodynamic psychotherapy with children and adolescents: a narrative synthesis. *Frontiers in Psychology* **12**. doi:10.3389/fpsyg.2021.662671.

Misra, M. *et al.* (2008) Vitamin D deficiency in children and its management: review of current knowledge and recommendations. *Pediatrics* **122**(2), 398–417. doi:10.1542/peds.2007-1894.

Montgomery, S.A. & Åsberg, M. (1979) A new depression scale designed to be sensitive to change. *The British Journal of Psychiatry* **134**(4), 382–389.

Mossman, S.A. *et al.* (2021) The impact of failed antidepressant trials on outcomes in children and adolescents with anxiety and depression: a systematic review and meta-analysis. *Journal of Child and Adolescent Psychopharmacology* **31**(4), 259–267. doi:10.1089/cap.2020.0195.

Mufson, L. *et al.* (1999) Efficacy of interpersonal psychotherapy for depressed adolescents. *Archives of General Psychiatry* **56**(6), 573–579. doi:10.1001/archpsyc.56.6.573.

Mufson, L. *et al.* (2004) A randomized effectiveness trial of interpersonal psychotherapy for depressed adolescents. *Archives of General Psychiatry* **61**(6), 577–584. doi:10.1001/archpsyc.61.6.577.

National Institute for Health and Care Excellence (2019) *Depression in Children and Young People: Identification and Management.* NICE Guideline [NG134]. National Institute for Health and Care Excellence (NICE), London.

Nery, F.G. *et al.* (2020) Medication exposure and predictors of first mood episode in offspring of parents with bipolar disorder: a prospective study. *Brazilian Journal of Psychiatry* **42**(5). doi:10.1590/1516-4446-2019-0802.

Osei-Twum, J.A. *et al.* (2022) Impact of project ECHO on patient and community health outcomes: a scoping review. *Academic Medicine* **97**(9), 1393–1402. doi:10.1097/ACM.0000000000004749.

Park, S.C. & Kim, Y.K. (2019) Diagnostic issues of depressive disorders from Kraepelinian dualism to the *Diagnostic and Statistical Manual of Mental Disorders*, fifth edition. *Psychiatry Investigation* **16**(9), 636–644. doi:10.30773/pi.2019.09.07.

Platt, J.M. *et al.* (2021) Is the US gender gap in depression changing over time? A meta-regression. *American Journal of Epidemiology* **190**(7), 1190–1206. doi:10.1093/aje/kwab002.

Posner, K. *et al.* (2011) The Columbia-Suicide Severity Rating Scale: initial validity and internal consistency findings from three multisite studies with adolescents and adults. *The American Journal of Psychiatry* **168**(12), 1266–1277. doi:10.1176/appi.ajp.2011.10111704.

Poznanski, E.O. & Mokros, H.B. (1996) *Children's Depression Rating Scale-Revised (CDRS-R) Manual.* Western Psychological Services, Los Angeles.

Reynolds, S. *et al.* (2020) Do sleep disturbances in depressed adolescents improve following psychological treatment for depression? *Journal of Affective Disorders* **262**, 205–210. doi:10.1016/j.jad.2019.10.029.

Riglin, L. *et al.* (2021) ADHD and depression: investigating a causal explanation. *Psychological Medicine* **51**(11), 1890–1897. doi:10.1017/S0033291720000665.

Roberts, R.E. & Duong, H.T. (2013) Depression and insomnia among adolescents: a prospective perspective. *Journal of Affective Disorders* **148**(1), 66–71. doi:10.1016/j.jad.2012.11.049.

Rutter, M. *et al.* (1986) *Depression in Young People: Developmental and Clinical Perspectives.* Guilford Press, New York.

Seewoo, B.J. *et al.* (2022) Neurostructural differences in adolescents with treatment-resistant depression and treatment effects of transcranial magnetic stimulation. *The International Journal of Neuropsychopharmacology* **25**(8). doi:10.1093/ijnp/pyac007.

Shamseddeen, W. *et al.* (2012) Adjunctive sleep medications and depression outcome in the treatment of serotonin-selective reuptake inhibitor resistant depression in adolescents study. *Journal of Child and Adolescent Psychopharmacology* **22**(1), 29–36. doi:10.1089/cap.2011.0027.

Sharav, V.H. (2003) The impact of the Food and Drug Administration Modernization Act on the recruitment of children for research. *Ethical Human Sciences and Services* **5**(2), 83–108.

Solmi, M. *et al.* (2022) Age at onset of mental disorders worldwide: large-scale meta-analysis of 192 epidemiological studies. *Molecular Psychiatry* **27**(1), 281–295. doi:10.1038/s41380-021-01161-7.

Stein, M.B. *et al.* (2001) Social anxiety disorder and the risk of depression: a prospective community study of adolescents and young adults. *Archives of General Psychiatry* **58**(3), 251–256. doi:10.1001/archpsyc.58.3.251.

Stimpfl, J.N. *et al.* (2025) Deprescribing antidepressants in children and adolescents: a systematic review of discontinuation approaches, cross-titration, and withdrawal symptoms. *J Child Adolesc Psychopharmacol* (in press). doi: 10.1089/cap.2024.0099.

Strawn, J.R. & Croarkin, P.E. (2020) Commentary: Treatment failure and success: a commentary on defining and treating pediatric treatment-resistant depression - reflections on Dwyer *et al.* (2020). *Journal of Child Psychology and Psychiatry* **61**(3), 333–335. doi:10.1111/jcpp.13207.

Strawn, J.R. & Stahl, S.M. (2023, Cambridge, UK) *Case Studies: Stahl's Essential Psychopharmacology: Children and Adolescents*. Cambridge University Press.

Strawn, J.R. & Walkup, J.T. (2020) Identifying the best treatment for young people with depression. *The Lancet Psychiatry* **7**(7), 562–563. doi:10.1016/S2215-0366(20)30236-4.

Strawn, J.R. *et al.* (2014) Antidepressant tolerability in anxious and depressed youth at high risk for bipolar disorder: a prospective naturalistic treatment study. *Bipolar Disorders* **16**(5), 523–530. doi: 10.1111/bdi.12113.

Strawn, J.R. *et al.* (2017) Buspirone in children and adolescents with anxiety: a review and Bayesian analysis of abandoned randomized controlled trials. *Journal of Child and Adolescent Psychopharmacology* **28**(1). doi:10.1089/cap.2017.0060.

Strawn, J.R. *et al.* (2020) Treatment-resistant depression in adolescents: clinical features and measurement of treatment resistance. *Journal of Child and Adolescent Psychopharmacology* **30**(4). doi:10.1089/cap.2020.0008.

Strawn, J.R. *et al.* (2021) Pediatric therapeutic drug monitoring for selective serotonin reuptake inhibitors. *Frontiers in Pharmacology* **12**, 749692. doi:10.3389/fphar.2021.749692.

Strawn, J.R. *et al.* (2023) Adverse effects of antidepressant medications and their management in children and adolescents. *Pharmacotherapy* **43**(7), 675–690. doi:10.1002/phar.2767.

Stumper, A. & Alloy, L.B. (2023) Associations between pubertal stage and depression: a systematic review of the literature. *Child Psychiatry and Human Development* **54**(2), 312–339. doi:10.1007/s10578-021-01244-0.

Suresh, V. *et al.* (2020) What next? A Bayesian hierarchical modeling re-examination of treatments for adolescents with selective serotonin reuptake inhibitor-resistant depression. *Depression and Anxiety* **37**(9), 926–934. doi:10.1002/da.23064.

Sylvester, C.M. *et al.* (2012) Functional network dysfunction in anxiety and anxiety disorders. *Trends in Neurosciences* **35**(9), 527–535. doi:10.1016/j.tins.2012.04.012.

Thapar, A. *et al.* (2022) Depression in young people. *The Lancet* **400**(10352), 617–631.

Tint, A. *et al.* (2008) The effect of rate of antidepressant tapering on the incidence of discontinuation symptoms: a randomised study. *Journal of Psychopharmacology* **22**(3), 330–332. doi:10.1177/0269881107081550.

Varigonda, A.L. *et al.* (2015) Systematic review and meta-analysis: early treatment responses of selective serotonin reuptake inhibitors in pediatric major depressive disorder. *Journal of the American Academy of Child and Adolescent Psychiatry* **54**(7), 557–564. doi:10.1016/j.jaac.2015.05.004.

Walkup, J.T. (2017) Antidepressant efficacy for depression in children and adolescents: industry- and NIMH-funded studies. *American Journal of Psychiatry* **174**(5), 1–8. doi:10.1176/appi.ajp.2017.16091059.

Walkup, J.T. & Strawn, J.R. (2020) High-quality antidepressant prescribing: please consider whether "perfection is the enemy of Progress.". *BMC Medicine* **18**(1), 150. doi:10.1186/s12916-020-01621-x.

Wals, M. *et al.* (2001) Prevalence of psychopathology in children of a bipolar parent. *Journal of the American Academy of Child and Adolescent Psychiatry* **40**(9), 1094–1102. doi:10.1097/00004583-200109000-00019.

Walter, H.J. *et al.* (2023) Clinical practice guideline for the assessment and treatment of children and adolescents with major and persistent depressive disorders. *Journal of the American Academy of Child and Adolescent Psychiatry* **62**(5), 479–502. doi:10.1016/j.jaac.2022.10.001.

Weersing, V.R. *et al.* (2017) Evidence base update of psychosocial treatments for child and adolescent depression. *Journal of Clinical Child and Adolescent Psychology* **46**(1), 11–43. doi:10.1080/15374416.2016.1220310.

Wehry, A.M. *et al.* (2015) Assessment and treatment of anxiety disorders in children and adolescents. *Current Psychiatry Reports* **17**(7), 591. doi:10.1007/s11920-015-0591-z.

Wilens, T.E. *et al.* (2003) A systematic chart review of the nature of psychiatric adverse events in children and adolescents treated with selective serotonin reuptake inhibitors. *Journal of Child and Adolescent Psychopharmacology* **13**(2), 143–152.

Willinger, D. *et al.* (2022) Deficient prefrontal-amygdalar connectivity underlies inefficient face processing in adolescent major depressive disorder. *Psychiatry* **12**(1). doi:10.1038/s41398-022-01955-5.

World Health Organization (2019) *International Statistical Classification of Disease and Related Health Problems*, 11th edn. World Health Association (WHO), Geneva, Switzerland.

Zhou, X. *et al.* (2020) Comparative efficacy and acceptability of antidepressants, psychotherapies, and their combination for acute treatment of children and adolescents with depressive disorder: a systematic review and network meta-analysis. *The Lancet Psychiatry* **7**(7), 581–601. doi:10.1016/S2215-0366(20)30137-1.

Zhou, Y. *et al.* (2023) Effect of repeated intravenous esketamine on adolescents with major depressive disorder and suicidal ideation: a randomized active-placebo-controlled trial. *Journal of the American Academy of Child and Adolescent Psychiatry* **63**(5), 507–518. doi:10.1016/j.jaac.2023.05.031.

CHAPTER 64
Self-harm in young people

Dennis Ougrin[1,2] and Michael Kaess[3,4]

[1] Youth Resilience Unit, Centre for Psychiatry and Mental Health, Wolfson Institute of Population Health, WHO Collaborating Centre for Mental Health Services Development, Queen Mary University of London, London, UK

[2] East London NHS Foundation Trust, London, UK

[3] University Hospital of Child and Adolescent Psychiatry and Psychotherapy, University of Bern, Bern Switzerland

[4] Department of Child and Adolescent Psychiatry, Center for Psychosocial Medicine, University Hospital Heidelberg, Heidelberg, Germany

Overview of the chapter

In this chapter we will provide a comprehensive overview of the definition, clinical characteristics, and diagnostic issues related to self-harm in youth, as well as of the key data on the epidemiology, longitudinal outcomes, related risk factors, and underlying mechanisms. Finally, we will present the evidence base and clinical recommendations in relation to evidence-based treatment and prevention strategies.

Definition, characteristics, and diagnosis of self-harm

Self-harm is defined as self-injury or self-poisoning, irrespective of the presence or absence of suicidal intent (National Institute of Health and Care Excellence, 2022). This encompasses a wide spectrum of behaviors that can be categorized into self-harm with suicidal intent (suicide attempts), self-harm without suicidal intent (nonsuicidal self-injury [NSSI] and nonsuicidal self-poisoning), and self-harm with undetermined intent. However, a key problem in self-harm research remains inconsistent nomenclature and classification of self-harm-related concepts, with some researchers distinguishing NSSI and suicide attempts, and others focusing on broadly defined self-harm, including self-injury or self-poisoning, irrespective of suicidal intent. Many other names depicting self-harm, some historical and some in current use, have been proposed, including parasuicide, self-mutilation, self-injurious behavior, and self-inflicted violence. The prefix "deliberate" was removed from clinical guidance on self-harm in the mid-to-late 2000s for two main reasons. First, concerns were raised about it being judgmental and pejorative in tone (Kapur *et al.*, 2013). The Royal College of Psychiatrists (2020) expressed concerns that it assigns blame to the patient, suggesting that their self-harm is "a calmly planned action rather than the result of emotional anguish or intense distress." Second, it is not always clear whether the behavior is "deliberate" or "intentional" (Kapur *et al.*, 2013).

In this chapter, the term "self-harm" will be used as per the broad definition given above (National Institute of Health and Care Excellence, 2022). This overall term is justified due to the fact that NSSI and suicide attempts often coexist. In addition, many of the risk factors for NSSI, suicide attempts, and suicide overlap; these include psychiatric comorbidities, such as depression and borderline personality disorder (BPD), as well as a personal history of sexual or physical abuse. NSSI itself is also an independent risk factor for future suicide attempts (Brent *et al.*, 2009). In case empirical findings relate to definitions that are more specific regarding the intent to die, we will refer to either suicide attempts or NSSI specifically.

Suicide is the leading or second leading (after accidents) cause of death among young people (Centers for Disease Control and Prevention, 2020) in many regions worldwide, including Western Europe, Eastern Europe, Central Europe, high-income North America, southern Latin America, Australasia, Central Asia, high-income Asia-Pacific, South Asia, and Oceania (Naghavi, 2019). Nearly 80% of all suicides occur in low- and middle-income countries, with India and China alone accounting for about half of all suicides (Knipe *et al.*, 2022). Given the scope of the problem, youth suicide prevention is a global priority, and a priority for many individual nations. In the United Kingdom (UK), United States (US), and other nations, suicide rates have been increasing among adolescents, raising alarm, particularly as other leading causes of death have declined

Rutter's Child and Adolescent Psychiatry and Psychology, Seventh Edition.
Edited by Anita Thapar, Daniel S. Pine, Samuele Cortese, Cathy Creswell, Tamsin J. Ford, James F. Leckman, and Argyris Stringaris.

Companion website: www.wiley.com/go/thapar/rutterspsych7

(World Health Organization, 2020). While not every suicide can be prevented, many suicide deaths are preventable.

Self-harm is one of the strongest known predictors of death by suicide. Self-harm that requires a visit to a hospital emergency department carries a 1% risk of death in the following 10 years, which is associated with a 30-fold increase in mortality risk (Hawton *et al.*, 2020a). Half of this 1% will be confirmed suicides, the rest will include alcohol or drug poisoning, substance use-related disease, traffic accidents, and homicides. Young people presenting to the ER with violent methods of self-harm, such as attempted hanging or asphyxiation, are at a particularly high risk of suicide. Self-harm, therefore, is one of the most promising targets for the prevention of suicide in young people.

Self-harm could occasionally be culturally acceptable, although rarely so in young people. Self-harm for religious reasons has been described, for example, self-flagellation as part of mourning rituals. Self-harm is often accepted in youth subcultures and organized youth criminals. Cultural acceptance of guns and the availability of fertilizers and medications in homes are all major determinants of methods used for self-harm and complete suicide.

The COVID-19 pandemic had a great impact on young people presenting with self-harm to emergency departments (Wong *et al.*, 2023). At the peak of the pandemic, there was a substantial reduction in the number of presentations, especially by young people from the most deprived sections of society (Wong *et al.*, 2022). This was followed by a substantial increase in the presentations, the number surpassing the prepandemic level (Wong *et al.*, 2023). The consequences of the pandemic are likely to influence the field of self-harm for years to come.

Self-harm is described in the *Diagnostic and Statistical Manual of Mental Disorders*, 5th edition, text revision (DSM-5-TR; American Psychiatric Association, 2022) and the eleventh revision of the *International Classification of Diseases* (ICD-11; World Health Organization, 2020). In DSM-5-TR it is a symptom of BPD. It is defined very broadly as recurrent suicidal behavior, suicidal gestures or threats, or self-mutilating behavior. In ICD-11 recurrent episodes of self-harm (e.g., suicide attempts or gestures, self-mutilation) are a criterion of borderline pattern qualifier of personality disorder or personality difficulty. The latter is used to describe personality traits that cause impairment but do not meet the criteria for the diagnosis of personality disorder. NSSI is included in section III of DSM-5-TR as a "condition in need for further study," as is suicidal behavior disorder. Although the diagnosis of BPD can be made in young people under the age of 18, it is important to emphasize that self-harm is a common feature of many disorders (Ghinea *et al.*, 2020) and may occur in young people with no psychiatric disorders.

Assessment

With the increasing prevalence, knowledge of assessment of young people with self-harm is likely to be relevant to a broad range of professionals beyond mental health: primary care workers, ambulance staff and paramedics, ER and general pediatric hospital professionals, social workers, teachers, and criminal justice system workers should all be familiar with these principles.

Current clinical guidelines (National Institute of Health and Care Excellence, 2022) recommend that the assessment of young people with self-harm should:

- be carried out at the earliest opportunity;
- aim at developing a collaborative therapeutic relationship with the person;
- give the person and their family members or carers (as appropriate) information about their condition and diagnosis;
- not be delayed until after medical treatment is completed;
- provide the option to have a health care professional of the same sex carry out the psychosocial assessment; and
- consider the needs of the young person, such as learning difficulties, neurodevelopmental disorders, and cultural needs.

When assessing young people following an episode of self-harm, mental health and allied professionals should ensure that they find a quiet, cool, and well-lit room, that the young person is not hungry or thirsty, that their other basic needs are met, and that the conversation cannot be overheard. A good understanding of how the psychosocial assessment fits with any ongoing physical investigations and treatments is needed. This could also determine which clinicians from the multidisciplinary team should be involved in the assessment. Many jurisdictions recommend joint mental health and social work assessments. Practitioners then need to introduce themselves. This is a very important part, and it is worth practicing, especially for experienced clinicians: professionals should use open and friendly gestures, make the young person and their carers feel comfortable, and acknowledge and validate any concerns, such as delays before the assessment. Practitioners should explain the purpose of the assessment and the likely duration, and inquire how the young person and their carer would like to be addressed and what their pronouns are. Practitioners should explain the limits of confidentiality regarding the information gathered. If it becomes necessary to breach confidentiality, for instance, due to a risk of serious harm to the young person or other people, the young person and their carers should still, as much as possible, be involved with decisions about their care and informed about the course of actions proposed.

Every effort should be made to include family members or carers in the assessment process. Assessment should be informed by any safeguarding concerns, the young person's competence to make decisions, and the consent of the young person. It is important to allow at least some time to interview both the young person and the carer separately.

There are several ways to start the assessment. One way, advocated by practitioners of solution-focused brief therapy, is "When we finish this assessment, how would you know it was useful?" (Bannink, 2007). This could be a difficult question, and the carer may find it easier to answer it than the young person. Professionals might also inquire about the young person's interests or afterschool activities as a potential opening. Another option might be asking several factual questions that the young person will find easy to answer.

As mood problems are very common in young people with self-harm, creating a mood timeline could be an idea. Starting from birth, professionals might ask the young person and the carer to estimate, on a scale from 0 to 10—0 being the worst possible, 10 being the best possible, and 5 being neither good nor bad—what average mood the young person could ascribe to each year of their life. It is worth starting from birth and, if the young person cannot recall, assume it had been a "5" until the young person could recall the first year with a different rating. If there are big changes, inquiries could be made about their causes as perceived by the young person. The year before the assessment could be broken down further into individual months with each month carrying its mood rating. Some young people prefer to think about the past in their school years rather than chronological years. The carer's views could be sought with the caveat to the young person that their mood rating could be very different from how other people might perceive their mood (Figure 64.1).

The assessment should proceed along the lines of the standard mental health assessment (see Chapter 27). It is important to note that asking about self-harm or suicidal thinking does not increase the risk of either (Gould *et al.*, 2005). Specific points are as follows.

Presenting problems

In *presenting problems* focus on the characteristics of the self-harm episode. Inquire about the circumstances and the sequence of events surrounding self-harm. Precipitants for self-harm should be identified. It is most commonly an interpersonal conflict that triggers self-harm but it could also be intrapersonal phenomena such as psychotic experiences, dissociative states, or symptoms of post-traumatic stress disorder (PTSD). Were alcohol or drugs consumed? Was the young person influenced by self-harm in other people including those on social media? What methods of self-harm were used?

The following characteristics of the index episode are of particular importance: suicidal intent, motivation, lethality, and method.

Suicidal intent

When assessing suicidal intent, the following four factors may be considered:

- *The young person's belief about intent.* Did they want to die? Are they relieved that they are still alive? Do they still want to die?
- *Preparation before the suicide attempt.* Was the episode impulsive or planned? Did the young person select a significant date? How long before the event did they decide to self-harm? Had they been drinking or using drugs before self-harm? Did they give their possessions away?
- *Prevention of discovery.* Did they make efforts to avoid discovery? Were they alone? Did they resist help?
- *Communication.* Did the young person communicate their intention to self-harm to others? Did they leave a suicide note? The intent to die is not always clear. Many young people will be ambivalent as to whether they want to live or die.

Motivation

Young people may present a range of motives for self-harm; most of the time they are intrapersonal, most commonly designed for the young person to feel better (Nock *et al.*, 2009).

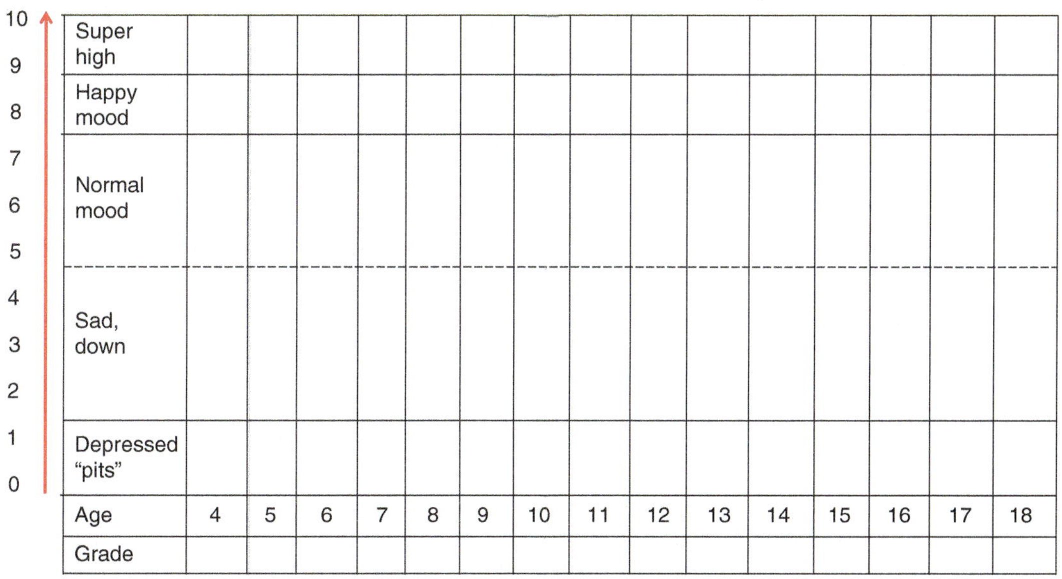

Figure 64.1 Mood chart.

- Intrapersonal motives: to die, to escape thoughts and feelings linked with intolerable distress, to feel less pain, to punish themselves, to reduce tension, or to replace emotional pain with physical pain.
- Interpersonal motives: to get help, to get someone to change their mind.

Lethality

Clinicians should distinguish between objective lethality, that is the actual degree of danger to life, and subjective lethality, the young person's anticipated consequences of self-harm. Did the youth require medical intervention? Did they attend the hospital or their family doctor? Did they think they could die by holding their breath, something that very young children might strongly believe? There is often a low correlation between suicidal intent and objective lethality in children and adolescents, especially in the youngest ones. This low correlation could be moderated by subjective lethality or may reflect a lack of knowledge regarding lethality in children.

Method

This refers to the way or the process that is used by the young person to self-harm. The method is closely linked with objective lethality, ranging from highly lethal behaviors, like shooting and attempted hanging at one extreme, to superficial cutting and scratching on the opposite end of the spectrum. One of the key questions in assessing risk is whether the young person has access to lethal agents like dangerous drugs, sharp objects, or firearms and could they be prevented from accessing these objects when they are at their most vulnerable. Having access to firearms is of particular importance. Young people who live in households with firearms have three to four times the risk of dying by suicide Swanson *et al.*, 2020

Past psychiatric history

In *past psychiatric history*, one should inquire about past episodes of self-harm, paying special attention to whether there is a recent escalation in the objective and subjective lethality of self-harm. Practitioners should inquire about any history of psychiatric disorders, especially mood disorders, autism, attention deficit hyperactivity disorder (ADHD), psychotic disorders, substance misuse, eating disorders, and conduct disorders. It is important to establish what interventions for psychiatric disorders have been tried and to what effect, if the young person is receiving treatment from a mental health service, and whether there is a care plan.

Past medical history

In *past medical history*, professionals should find out about any previous diagnoses, especially chronic and associated with pain, their treatment, medications used, allergies, and over-the-counter remedies used by the young person.

Personal history

In *personal history*, key questions are about bullying, including cyberbullying, abuse and neglect, social work involvement, exposure to self-harm and suicide in a friendship group (including those online), belonging to the lesbian, gay, bisexual, transgender plus (LGBT+) community, and having special educational needs. One way to ask about sexual abuse, typically a difficult subject, is "Has anyone ever touched you in your private parts when they should not have done?"

Family history

In *family history*, practitioners should ask about any history of suicide or self-harm, or any psychiatric or medical disorders and, importantly, what interventions were tried and to what effect. This could be an important guide to how the young person might perceive any intervention offered.

Social history

In *social history*, professionals should focus on social adversity (especially isolation and loneliness), social connections and social support, caring responsibilities, child protection or safeguarding needs, and social interests, including afterschool activities beyond computer games and social media browsing.

Forensic history

In *forensic history*, practitioners should inquire about any contact with the youth justice system, belonging to antisocial groups of young people, and what roles drugs, alcohol, and self-harm play in the young person's circle of friends.

Mental state examination

On *mental state examination* practitioners should observe any scars and how old the scars look, tattoos and piercings, or age-inappropriate clothes. It is also important to observe phenotypical features that may relate to an eating disorder or neurodevelopmental problems. It is important to understand how the young person defines their ethnic background, sexuality, and gender. Comment on how easy it is to establish rapport with the young person. Observe how the young person interacts with their carer. Both objective and subjective assessment of the young person's mood is required. Asking about hopelessness, and suicidal thoughts and plans is very important. One way to inquire about this difficult topic is "Many young people who experience low mood have thoughts about hurting or killing themselves. Do you have these thoughts?" It is important to understand if the young person has a specific plan and access to means of self-harm, and what protective factors there are.

At the end of the assessment, practitioners should thank the young person and their carer for their time and inquire if the initial expectations from the assessment were achieved. This should be followed by a clear plan codesigned with the young person and their carer whenever possible.

Current research cautions against using risk assessment scales and categorizing risk into low, medium, and high (Quinlivan *et al.*, 2016). Instead, a full assessment with a formulation and the establishment of individualized needs and goals, and ensuring the young person's safety is advocated. Nonetheless, rating scales and interviews might be useful as *aides-mémoire* and tools to identify coexisting problems. Examples of self-harm-specific tools are the Self-Injurious Thoughts and Behaviors Interview (SITBI) (Nock *et al.*, 2007) which is clinician-administered, or the young person-reported Self-Harm Questionnaire (used for screening) (Ougrin & Boege, 2013).

In summary, when assessing adolescents with self-harm, clinicians should pay particular attention to the method used and patterns of current and past self-harm and suicidal intent, establishing the presence of psychiatric illnesses, evaluating depressive symptoms, establishing the possible triggers for self-harm, and documenting risk factors and protective factors (Box 64.1).

Box 64.1 Key areas to cover during a psychological assessment of adolescents who have self-harmed

- History or recent difficulties: new onset/deterioration of mental health disorders, insomnia, frequent nightmares, excessive screen time, life stresses (academic, conflict with parents and peers, sexual assault, discharge from inpatient psychiatric unit)
- Circumstances of the index self-harm episode (before, during, and after):
  - Method: violent versus nonviolent
  - Lethality: subjective and objective
  - Alcohol and other drugs consumption at the time of self-harm
  - Motives/reasons for self-harm: intrapersonal versus interpersonal
  - Precipitant
  - Suicidal intent
  - Evidence of preplanning: impulsive versus planned
- Patterns of current and past self-harm: is there an escalation of frequency/lethality?
- Exposure to self-harm/suicide by others including on social media
- Psychiatric history: mood disorders, substance abuse, anxiety, conduct problems, eating disorders, attention deficit hyperactivity disorder (ADHD), autism, and psychosis; treatment with medication that might increase the risk
- Physical health: chronic disorders, poor general health, cigarette smoking, being obese/overweight
- Personal/social history: history of maltreatment; legal problems; being a looked-after child, social deprivation; experiencing discrimination; gender dysphoria, being a member of the LGBTQ+ community, social isolation, and loneliness
- Family psychiatric history, including self-harm and suicide
- Interpersonal relationships:
  - bullying, including cyberbullying
  - peer victimization
  - domestic violence
  - invalidating environment
- Mental state:
  - current suicidal ideation
  - current suicidal plan
  - hopelessness
  - low, anxious, angry, or irritable mood; evidence of emotional dysregulation
  - psychotic symptoms
  - cognitive disturbance, rumination, and impulsiveness
- Access to means
- Protective factors: support from friends and family, good coping skills; spiritual beliefs, being in education, employment, or training; good problem solving, parental self-efficacy
- What help would the family like?
- Availability of support
- Agree to further actions and aftercare

Epidemiology

To date, several meta-analyses on the prevalence of self-harm in young people have increased our knowledge of the magnitude of the problem. However, beneath the estimates of the prevalence of self-harm underlie some uncertainties that are mainly caused by the varying definitions of self-harm available, the variety of different assessment tools (e.g., prevalence estimates are lower in the case of single-item measures compared to measures that assess a variety of different self-harm methods), different informants (e.g., self-report questionnaires, interviews, or parent reports), and different sampling methods of epidemiological studies.

Overall, the lifetime prevalence of any occurrence of self-harm has been estimated to be around 17% (Muehlenkamp *et al.*, 2012; Swannell *et al.*, 2014) among adolescents, with few differences in prevalence rates between the two constructs of self-harm and NSSI. In a large-scale study investigating the prevalence of self-injury (irrespective of suicidal intent) across 11 countries, the mean lifetime prevalence among adolescents was even higher (28%) (Brunner *et al.*, 2014), with considerable heterogeneity between countries. For suicide attempts, recent meta-analyses revealed a pooled lifetime prevalence of 6% among adolescents (Lim *et al.*, 2019) and 3.2% among college students (Swannell *et al.*, 2014; Mortier *et al.*, 2018). For children aged 6–12 years, prevalence rates are lower, with 1.4% for self-harm, and 1.3% for suicide attempts, but a still remarkable rate of 21.9% for NSSI (however, this last finding was only from two studies) (Geoffroy *et al.*, 2022). In another meta-analysis, the combined incidence of NSSI and suicide attempt co-occurrence was 9.6% (Ye *et al.*, 2022).

In child and adolescent psychiatric inpatient settings, the prevalence of self-harm is remarkably high—between 60–80% (Adrian *et al.*, 2011; Kaess *et al.*, 2013). In addition, self-harm accounts for approximately one-quarter of the rising rates of mental health presentations to emergency departments (Hiscock *et al.*, 2018).

Self-harm is associated with an enormous economic burden to society. Hospital costs for the assessment and treatment of self-harm were estimated to be £162 million per year in England (Tsiachristas *et al.*, 2017), while data from Australia suggest that hospital costs represent only a small proportion of the true economic impact of self-harm compared to the major driver of societal costs, namely the loss of productivity (Kinchin *et al.*, 2017).

There are some indicators of a potential rise in self-harm since the late 1990s. However, clear empirical evidence is rare, given that methodologically sound studies using current definitions were hardly available before the 21st century. Some evidence for a potential increase in self-harm over since the late 1990s can be drawn from age differences that have been found for lifetime prevalence rates of self-harm: in a meta-analysis, lifetime prevalence should theoretically increase with age but was found to be 17.2% among adolescents, 13.4% among young adults, and 5.5% among adults (Swannell *et al.*, 2014). These findings could indicate a potential increase of self-harm within generations, however, a recall bias that leads to lower estimates of self-harm with growing age cannot be ruled out at this stage. More evidence for an increase in self-harm comes from a recent study that analyzed data from the Adult Psychiatric Morbidity Survey administered to people aged 16 years or older in the general population of England, Scotland, and Wales in 2000, 2007, and 2014 (Borschmann & Kinner, 2019). Here, the authors found that self-harm increased from 2.4% to 6.4% between 2000–2014, with rises noted across both genders and all age groups. The largest increase was in women and girls aged 16–24 years (from 6.5% in 2000 to 19.7% in 2014). While the study only captures individuals aged 16 years and older, it is quite plausible that the findings may also apply across the whole adolescent population.

Self-harm commonly occurs during early to mid-adolescence with a suggested peak of around 15–16 years of age, and a decline in prevalence toward adulthood (Plener *et al.*, 2015). Sex differences (higher prevalence of both NSSI and suicide attempts in females) can commonly be found for adolescent self-harm (Kaess *et al.*, 2011; Valencia-Agudo *et al.*, 2018), but seem to be nonexistent among children (Geoffroy *et al.*, 2022). In addition to the overall sex differences in prevalence, there are marked differences in the methods of self-harm: there is a female preponderance in cutting the skin, while males tend to hit or burn themselves (Brunner *et al.*, 2014). Sex differences also apply to the methods of suicide attempts, with boys commonly engaging in methods with potentially higher lethality (Jopling *et al.*, 2021)—leading to the so-called "gender paradox" (females tend to harm themselves more frequently, while males are at higher risk of death by suicide).

In summary, self-harm is a frequent phenomenon and an important public health concern among adolescents. This conclusion can be drawn from the increasingly high prevalence of self-harm among young people since the late 1990s, as well as the high economic burden on society.

Longitudinal outcomes

Regarding longitudinal outcomes, we can distinguish between the longitudinal course of self-harm itself, and further health outcomes including mental health, physical health, functioning, and quality of life.

The course of self-harm

Self-harm shows a characteristic rise after puberty and a subsequent decline from mid-to-late adolescence into adulthood. A large longitudinal population-based study from Australia revealed that more than 80% of individuals with self-harm did not continue their behavior into adulthood (Moran *et al.*, 2012). In their systematic review, Plener and colleagues summarized the current (but limited) evidence on the longitudinal course of NSSI (Plener *et al.*, 2015). They found a rise between 11–16 years of age followed by a subsequent decline. Commonly, suicide attempts seem to show a delayed trajectory compared to NSSI (Groschwitz *et al.*, 2015a).

Despite the general tendency for a decline toward adulthood, self-harm comes with a large risk of repetition. Any history of self-harm increases the risk for future nonfatal and even fatal self-harm. Nonfatal self-harm repetition rates have recently been summarized at 15%, 17%, 21%, and 24% during a 0.5-year, 1-year, 2-year, and 3-year follow-up (Liu *et al.*, 2020). Within the spectrum of nonfatal self-harm, NSSI increases the risk of future suicide attempts (Scott *et al.*, 2015), in particular by increasing the likelihood of turning suicidal thoughts into action (Barzilay *et al.*, 2019). Thus, current theories consider NSSI as a potential "gateway to suicide." Likewise, there is also longitudinal evidence that the risk for suicide attempts decreases after cessation of self-injury (Koenig *et al.*, 2017). The high risk of repetition is also reflected in longitudinal studies showing an increased risk of lifetime death from suicide following self-harm in adolescence. The above-mentioned recent study from the UK following children and adolescents over 10–15 years, who had presented with self-harm to a hospital at least once, found that the 12-month incidence of suicide in this cohort was more than 30 times higher than the expected rate in the general population of individuals (Hawton *et al.*, 2020a). In the systematic review by Liu *et al.*, rates of fatal repetition at follow-ups were 0.77%, 1.34%, 1.49%, and 2.46%, respectively (Liu *et al.*, 2020).

A recent meta-analysis identified several predictors for both repetition of self-harm and completed suicide after self-harm. Repetition of self-harm was predicted by female gender and younger age, as well as diagnosis and treatment of a mental disorder, whereas completed suicide after self-harm was predicted by male gender, older age, and physical illness, as well as, again, diagnosis and treatment of a mental disorder (Liu *et al.*, 2022).

Under treatment conditions, reductions in the frequency of self-harm can commonly be achieved in clinical samples (Ougrin *et al.*, 2015). However, despite the mean reduction of the frequency of self-harm under treatment, there seems to be considerable heterogeneity in the treatment response among adolescents with self-harm. A study from Germany investigated 203 adolescents from a specialized outpatient clinic for adolescent self-harm. While 75% of the sample reported a substantial reduction of NSSI frequency after treatment, only one-third of those (25% of the whole sample) achieved full remission. The remaining 25% were considered "nonresponders" who either did not improve or even experienced an exacerbation

(Reichl *et al.*, 2023). In addition, the same study revealed that a clinical follow-up of high-risk adolescents under specialized treatment after a suicide attempt found that the repetition of a suicide attempt occurred in 38% (Rockstroh *et al.*, 2021).

Further health outcomes following self-harm

Besides self-harm being a robust predictor of future suicide risk, several other mental health problems may occur during or following episodes of self-harm. Given that self-harm can be considered a transdiagnostic marker of psychopathology (Ghinea *et al.*, 2020), the likelihood of any mental disorder associated with or following self-harm is increased (Steinhoff *et al.*, 2023), e.g., for depressive disorders in adulthood (Ebert *et al.*, 2019). Frequent self-harm may play a particular role in the prediction of BPD (see Chapter 67). A longer persistence of self-harm during adolescence has repeatedly been associated with the development of BPD (Groschwitz *et al.*, 2015b; Ghinea *et al.*, 2019).

Prospective data in young people also indicate an increased risk for somatic illness in the course of self-harm (Jollant *et al.*, 2022). Since self-harm and depression are very closely associated, added evidence comes from the fact that adolescent depression has been shown to predict a large variety of physical health conditions over the life course (Leone *et al.*, 2021).

One of the most important risks associated with self-harm is the development of severe alcohol or substance misuse. Longitudinal data in adolescents with self-harm suggest that symptom shifts from NSSI to substance abuse are common (Nakar *et al.*, 2016). This view is in line with the substantially increased risk of mortality by drug or alcohol poisoning among individuals who previously engaged in self-harm (Morgan *et al.*, 2017) (see Chapter 66).

Finally, self-harm increases the risk of poor quality of life, as well as reduced psychosocial functioning. This can also be confirmed by the "loss of productivity" that was found in individuals following self-harm (Kinchin *et al.*, 2017). However, the limited data available on this association suggest that it is likely mediated by mental disorders or underlying risk factors (e.g., peer problems) (Ghinea *et al.*, 2021; Gyori *et al.*, 2021), and that there is no direct causal link between self-harm and reduced psychosocial functioning.

Risk factors

Risk factors for self-harm and suicide largely overlap. There are only a few exceptions. As mentioned above, self-harm is more common in females and suicide is more common in males. Self-harm risk increases with increasing levels of deprivation, but suicide risk does not (Cybulski *et al.*, 2022).

When assessing adolescents presenting with self-harm clinicians should consider the following three categories of risk factors: characteristics of the index event (described in the "Assessment" section), proximal risk factors, and distal risk factors.

Proximal risk factors

Proximal risk factors include recent changes in physical or mental state, substance misuse, and recent stressful life events. The latter could include self-harm precipitants like: arguments with a boyfriend/girlfriend or parents; recent losses, for example, bereavement, romantic, or family break-up; school-related stress, for example, exams or being bullied (including cyberbullying); exposure to suicide/self-harm in friends; and pregnancy in self or partner. Adolescents may report a recent episode of abuse (sexual or physical) or have been reminded of past abuse. The subjective meaning attributed to the stressful event may be different from objective reality. For example, some adolescents may feel devastated by relatively innocuous events, and some might self-harm in anticipation of a perceived humiliating punishment.

Recent onset of physical or mental health problems, the escalation of frequency and severity of suicidal thinking and self-harm, and sleep and eating problems have all been linked to increased risk of self-harm. Conditions that decrease the young person's ability to control their behavior (substance misuse, including tobacco smoking, and oppositional-defiant and conduct problems) or increase distress (severe anxiety) are linked with a greater risk of self-harm (Nock *et al.*, 2013). A recent start of treatment or dose escalation of medication could be important, although the risk of self-harm associated with the commencement of antidepressant treatment might be less evident than previously thought (Hetrick *et al.*, 2021) and unlikely to be explained by the initial medication-induced behavioral activation (Vitiello *et al.*, 2009). The increased risk of self-harm appears to be linked with the concurrent use of benzodiazepines and antidepressants (Brent *et al.*, 2009). The "black box" warning about the possible increase in suicide-related events issued in the early 2000s by both American and European regulators resulted in a reduction of young people prescribed selective serotonin reuptake inhibitors (SSRIs) initially. However, this trend has reversed in recent years (Lukmanji *et al.*, 2020). Significant variations in prescribing rates continue to exist in different geographical areas, even those with very similar health care systems (Wesselhoeft *et al.*, 2020). Overall, the use of SSRIs is associated with a greater risk of suicide-related thoughts and behaviors. Based on a network meta-analysis (Hetrick *et al.*, 2021), Table 64.1 summarizes the findings to date:

A recent discharge from inpatient treatment is one of the strongest predictors of both self-harm and suicide in young people and it may occur in clusters (Hawton *et al.*, 2020b). Prolonged inpatient admissions are associated with a higher risk of self-harm compared with briefer admissions followed by intensive community care (Ougrin *et al.*, 2021). The risk of self-harm is also increased in those young people who are transferred to adult services, especially if the transition is poorly managed (Hansen *et al.*, 2023).

Proximal risk factors are of particular importance if they are modifiable, as they could become treatment targets.

Table 64.1 Suicide-related outcomes of psychopharmacological treatment.

Medication	Odds ratio (OR)	95% confidence interval (CI)	Effect on suicide-related outcomes
Mirtazapine	0.50	0.30, 8.04	Uncertain
Duloxetine	1.15	0.72, 1.82	Uncertain
Vilazodone	1.01	0.68, 1.48	Uncertain
Desvenlafaxine	0.94	0.59, 1.52	Uncertain
Citalopram	1.72	0.76, 3.87	Uncertain
Vortioxetine	1.58	0.29, 8.60	Uncertain
Escitalopram	0.89	0.43, 1.84	"At least slightly" reduction
Fluoxetine	1.27	0.87, 1.86	"At least slightly" increase
Paroxetine	1.81	0.85, 3.86	"At least slightly" increase
Sertraline	3.03	0.60, 15.22	"At least slightly" increase
Venlafaxine	13.84	1.79, 106.90	"At least slightly" increase
Venlafaxine versus desvenlafaxine	0.07	0.01, 0.56	Probably increased odds
Venlafaxine versus escitalopram	0.06	0.01, 0.56	Probably increased odds

Note: The table represents the odds ratios and confidence intervals for each medication's effect on suicide-related outcomes compared to placebo. The last two rows compare the odds of suicide-related outcomes between specific medications. Generated by Open AI.

Distal risk factors

There are several known distal risk factors for self-harm. They can be divided into social, demographic, biological, psychiatric, and psychological variables.

Psychiatric, physical, and psychological factors

A history of self-harm is a key predictor of future self-harm (Ougrin *et al.*, 2012). Most psychiatric diagnoses are associated with an increased risk of self-harm and suicide. Neurodevelopmental disorders, including autism and ADHD, personality disorders, substance misuse, disruptive disorders, severe anxiety disorders, mood disorders, eating disorders, body dysmorphic disorders, bipolar disorder, and psychosis, are all associated with an increased risk of self-harm, as are previous psychiatric admissions and substance misuse. High avoidance, perfectionism, trait anger, impulsivity, poor decision-making, hopelessness, neuroticism, rumination, memory biases, subjective reports of loneliness, poor emotional problem-solving, and dichotomous thinking increase the risk of self-harm. Chronic physical problems, especially those associated with pain, are an important risk factor. Cross-diagnostic symptoms might be better predictors of self-harm and suicide than the presence of specific psychiatric disorders (Benton *et al.*, 2021). Emotional dysregulation (Santangelo *et al.*, 2017; Benton *et al.*, 2021) and impulsive aggression (McGirr *et al.*, 2008) are of particular importance.

Social and demographic factors

As mentioned above, females are significantly more likely to self-harm compared with males, though males are more likely to die of suicide. Self-harm often starts in early adolescence and increases toward later teens. Certain ethnic backgrounds, such as Hispanic girls and Native American populations in the US, have been linked with increased rates of self-harm (Centers for Disease Control and Prevention, 2020). A history of physical, emotional, or sexual abuse or neglect, violence, and/or forensic history all seem to increase the risk of self-harm independently. Those who have unstable and poor housing, experienced harsh parenting styles, a history of being bullied, including on social media, recurrent interpersonal problems, and self-harm behavior in friends are all more vulnerable. Likewise, being a child in a single-parent family, being looked after by the local authority, or being in a secure institution is also associated with a greater likelihood of engaging in self-harm. There is also a higher prevalence of self-harm among asylum seekers, those from a more socioeconomically deprived background, or LGBT+ young people. Family history of self-harm or suicide and family psychiatric disorders in general are consistent predictors of self-harm risk. Exposure to self-harm or suicide in family members and other young people, including online exposure is of particular importance. Ultimately, this could lead to clusters of suicide in young people, accounting for 1–2% of all suicides in youth (Niedzwiedz *et al.*, 2014). The role of social media is of particular importance. Most cross-sectional studies (Sedgwick *et al.*, 2019) and, increasingly, longitudinal studies (Lung *et al.*, 2020; Coyne *et al.*, 2021) indicate that heavy social media use is associated with an increased risk of self-harm. However, the direct causality has not yet been established and there may be a differential impact of social media use in girls and boys (Mars *et al.*, 2020).

Biological factors

Genetic and neurobiological factors may play a significant role in the development of self-harm in young people. Suicide tends to cluster within families (Melhem *et al.*, 2007). Epidemiological research suggests that cross-generational transmission of self-harm arises equally from genetic and rearing effects (Kendler *et al.*, 2020), pointing toward both biological and environmental influences. Genetic factors contribute to the familial transmission of suicide attempts, with an estimated heritability of 30–50% (Lutz *et al.*, 2017). While parts of the genetic influence may be independent of other psychiatric conditions, recent studies have also found overlapping genetic risk between suicide and suicidal behavior, and important preceding or comorbid mental disorders (e.g., depression, psychosis, ADHD) (Docherty *et al.*, 2020; Joo *et al.*, 2022). In addition, genetic risk for self-harm is likely mediated by intermediate phenotypes such as impulsive aggression or behavioral disinhibition (Brent & Mann, 2005).

Studies on specific genetic and neurobiological factors associated with suicide in children and adolescents are limited and often based on small sample sizes. However, a few biological underpinnings of self-harm have at least been replicated and may present interesting candidates for biological mechanisms involved in the development of self-harm.

Regarding neural correlates, there is increasing evidence for alterations in fronto-limbic neural systems (Auerbach *et al.*, 2021; Kaess *et al.*, 2021), which are centrally involved in emotion regulation (including stress response), whereas neurobiological evidence for deficits in impulse inhibition or alterations in the reward system remain inconclusive (Kaess *et al.*, 2021).

Regarding peripheral biological correlates, there is increasing evidence for alterations in the biological stress response systems among individuals who self-harm (Miller & Prinstein, 2019; Kaess *et al.*, 2021). An attenuated response of the hypothalamic–pituitary–adrenal axis to stress, as well as a generally reduced vagal functioning (i.e., lower activity of the parasympathetic nervous system), may represent important underpinnings of both emotional and behavioral dysregulation that increase risk of self-harm.

Another important factor that may contribute to adolescent self-harm is altered pain processing. Alterations in pain sensitivity (i.e., reduced sensitivity to painful stimuli) have been found repeatedly in individuals who self-harm (Koenig *et al.*, 2016), and such alterations may play an important role in ideation-to-action theories of suicide (Klonsky *et al.*, 2018).

In addition, there are promising findings on potential biological alterations largely related to inflammation and immune functioning. Those findings certainly need replication and may or may not come up in future biological models of self-harm. Inflammation markers have emerged as potential biomarkers for self-harm in adults with major depression and bipolar disorder, and increased levels of proinflammatory cytokines have been found in the postmortem brains of teenagers who died from suicide (Pandey *et al.*, 2012). A study has indeed found increased inflammatory markers in adolescents with NSSI (Kindler *et al.*, 2022). In addition, low serum cholesterol levels have been found in child and adolescent psychiatric inpatients who have attempted suicide (Plana *et al.*, 2010).

Protective factors

Protective factors are less well understood. They include having social support, having contact with a caring adult, having an intact family, having a religious or spiritual belief, being able to identify reasons for living, being in education, employment, or training, having self-efficacious parents, having good problem-solving, and having emotion regulation and distress tolerance skills (McEvoy *et al.*, 2023).

Summary

As noted above, risk of completed suicide is strongly increased among individuals who self-harm. Table 64.2 summarizes risk factors that predict completed suicide after a hospital presentation with self-harm, based on nearly 10,000 hospital presentations (Hawton et al., 2020a).

Psychological autopsies

Another source of knowledge for the characteristics of the young people who complete suicide is psychological autopsy studies. Recent studies indicate that a substantial proportion of young people who die by suicide have made no previous suicide attempts, that at least one-third are not known to mental health services, and at least half have no recorded mental health diagnosis (Mérelle *et al.*, 2020; Lyu *et al.*, 2021). The proportion of young people who are known to mental health services has increased substantially since the 1990s (Marttunen *et al.*, 1993), but in many countries, this proportion remains low. In England, of those young people who died by likely suicide, 42% were known, or previously known, to social care. This was higher than the proportion of young people who were known to social care who died of any cause (28%). Sixteen percent were known to mental health services at any time, but, interestingly, 50% (n = 12/24) of children and young people who died as a result of drug poisoning were known to mental health services (National Child Mortality Database, 2023).

Pathological and risk processes

Although our knowledge has greatly increased on many aspects of self-harm, our understanding of the exact mechanisms for the development, engagement, and maintenance of the behavior is still very limited.

Overall, self-harm seems to be driven by a cascade of emotional and cognitive processes that finally form a vicious circle contributing to the repetition of the behavior. This cascade may slightly differ depending on the intent of self-harm (nonsuicidal versus suicidal) but many features can be applied to the overall construct. The cascade includes the following steps that individuals who self-harm commonly go through:

i. intolerable negative emotions;
ii. self-harm incident for immediate relief; and
iii. same (or even more) problems and more negative emotions (e.g., feelings of guilt and shame) after self-harm.

The cognitive and emotional processes within this vicious circle have been investigated in detail during since the 2010s using both experimental and experienced sampling methods that provide *in vitro* and *in vivo* evidence for the cascade listed above. Regarding the underlying neurobiological processes, current research knowledge mainly includes research

Table 64.2 Risk factors for competed suicide following an emergency hospital presentation.

Variable	Individuals (n = 9173)	Suicides (n = 55)	Hazard ratio (95% CI)	p-value	Adjusted hazard ratio (95% CI)	p-value
Age at study entry						
10–15 yrs	3210 (35.0%)	11 (20.0%)	1 (ref)	—	1 (ref)	—
16–18 yrs	5963 (65.0%)	44 (80.0%)	2.04 (1.05–3.96)	0.034	1.82 (0.93–3.54)	0.079
Sex						
Female	6828 (74.4%)	29 (52.7%)	1 (ref)	—	1 (ref)	—
Male	2345 (25.6%)	26 (47.3%)	2.66 (1.57–4.42)	.001	2.50 (1.46–4.26)	0.001
Self-harm method at study entry						
Self-poisoning alone	7109 (77.5%)	35 (63.6%)	1 (ref)	—	1 (ref)	—
Self-injury alone	1615 (17.6%)	18 (32.7%)	2.65 (1.50–4.69)	0.001	2.11 (1.17–3.81)	0.013
Self-poisoning and self-injury	449 (4.9%)	2 (3.6%)	0.96 (0.23–3.99)	0.95	0.86 (0.21–3.61)	0.83
The specific method of self-injury						
Self-poisoning alone	7109 (77.5%)	35 (63.6%)	1 (ref)	—	1 (ref)	—
Self-cutting	1595 (17.4%)	16 (29.1%)	2.23 (1.23–4.03)	0.008	1.83 (1.00–3.37)	0.050
Hanging or asphyxiation	143 (1.6%)	3 (5.5%)	6.04 (1.85–19.71)	0.003	4.90 (1.47–16.39)	0.010
Other self-injury	306 (3.3%)	0	NA	1.0	NA	NA
Unknown subtype of self-injury	20 (0.2%)	1 (1.8%)	10.46 (1.43–76.55)	0.021	11.50 (1.55–86.56)	0.017
Number of episodes of self-harm						
Single episode	6452 (70.3%)	29 (52.7%)	1 (ref)	—	1 (ref)	—
Two or more episodes	2721 (29.7%)	26 (47.3%)	1.94 (1.14–3.29)	0.014	1.87 (1.10–3.20)	0.022

Note: NA: not applicable; (ref): reference group that other groups are compared to, indicates the reference value. Generated by Open AI.

on neurobiological traits that may support or drive the self-harm cascade, and some data from experiments that may give preliminary insights into what is potentially going on before, during, and after a self-harm incident (Kaess *et al.*, 2021).

Intolerable negative emotions

There is strong evidence that individuals who self-harm are suffering from intense negative emotions; this is true for both non-suicidal and suicidal self-harm. Research in adolescents using ecological momentary assessment (EMA) could identify a strong increase in negative emotions that commonly preceded incidents of self-injury (Koenig *et al.*, 2021). The underlying neurobiological mechanisms for this "emotional" vulnerability are not entirely clarified, but there are some well-replicated findings on biological alterations that are likely involved, e.g., alterations in front-limbic neural systems (e.g., overactivation of the amygdala in response to interpersonal stressors), as well as alterations in the peripheral stress response systems (e.g., a reduced cortisol response to stress) and the pain system (e.g., a basal endogenous opioid deficit) (Cummins *et al.*, 2021). In summary, biological vulnerabilities seem to promote intense negative emotional reactions to (often interpersonal) stressors.

Self-harm incidents for immediate relief

For this part of the cascade, the expected relief from intolerable emotions is the most common function of all types of self-harm. However, the idea behind a suicide attempt is to end the intolerable state by dying, whereas the idea of NSSI is to terminate the state by applying pain to oneself, which in turn is expected to alleviate the negative affect. Given that suicide attempts are difficult to simulate within an experiment and also difficult to cover during EMA research, most empirical data on mechanisms during self-harm incidents stem from research on NSSI. Laboratory research among individuals with NSSI identified an interaction of somatosensory neural systems (in response to pain) and front-limbic systems (a decrease of amygdala activity) across the NSSI episode. In addition, such research suggests that NSSI (pain stimulation) may decrease subjective arousal and negative affect alongside an increase in cortisol (Kaess *et al.*, 2021).

More negative emotions (e.g., feelings of guilt and shame) after self-harm

This final component of the "vicious circle of stress and pain" is unfortunately common to most individuals who self-harm. Most patients have reasonable insight into the fact that self-harm does not solve their problems and that it may often make things even worse. EMA research recently revealed that the negative affect is already increased after only one hour in response to an incident of self-harm (Koenig *et al.*, 2021). This indicates that the effects of pain on negative emotional states are likely to last for minutes, making self-harm a very short-acting strategy, and suggesting a certain degree of impulsivity in individuals who self-harm.

Treatment and prevention

Immediate management

The priority in terms of immediate management is to ensure the safety of the youth. There are three possible options for immediate management: discharge to the community, admission to a pediatric or general hospital, and admission to a psychiatric hospital. If the young person is admitted to a pediatric or general hospital, according to the UK National Institute for Health and Clinical Excellence (NICE) guidelines, they need to be assessed by a specialist in child and adolescent mental health and should have access to a liaison service around the clock. Daily joint reviews by the pediatric and mental health professionals are recommended, as is the opportunity for daily access to family members and the need for a multidisciplinary review before discharge.

No rigorous randomized controlled trials (RCTs) show that psychiatric inpatient admissions reduce the risk of self-harm (see Chapter 48). However, common sense and clinical judgment dictate the necessity of admission in some cases, especially when there is a significant risk of death by suicide. That said, some adolescents may increase their self-harm behavior once placed in an inpatient unit, especially if the admission is long (Ougrin *et al.*, 2021). If inpatient care is deemed necessary, then clinicians should be planning for discharge at the point of admission and contingencies should be examined to strengthen reinforcers for alternatives to self-harm. Before discharge to the community, linkage to outpatient treatment should be made, preferably with an appointment within the next 48 hours set up before discharge, and a plan for follow-up to check that the outpatient treatment plan has been followed.

In all cases where the youth is to be cared for in the community, a crisis/safety plan should be developed together with the patient and carers before they leave the initial session. The plan should specifically restrict youths' access to potentially dangerous self-harm means.

Simple safety plan

Establishing a brief and simple safety plan together with the young person (and other support persons, if available) is one of the most effective interventions in individuals who self-harm. Such a safety should include the following components:

- establish the means of self-harm
- recognize the triggers and warning signs of increased distress, further self-harm, or a suicidal crisis
- identify individualized coping strategies, including problem-solving and any factors that may act as a barrier to self-harm
- identify social contacts and social settings as a mean of distraction from thoughts about self-harm
- identify family members or friends to provide support and/or help resolve the crisis

- include contact details for the mental health service, including out-of-hours services and emergency contact details
- keep the environment safe by working collaboratively to remove or restrict lethal means of suicide.

In summary, when formulating immediate risk management, clinicians should consider the least restrictive care environment, which is compatible with the safety of the youth, formulate a safety plan, and ensure effective follow-up arrangements.

Brief interventions and treatment engagement

The studies that both aim to improve engagement and report on self-harm repetition have generally been supportive of the value of brief interventions in improving engagement (Spirito *et al.*, 2002; Hughes & Asarnow, 2013; Ougrin *et al.*, 2013). There is also evidence that offering specific psychological therapy improves engagement with treatment (Yuan *et al.*, 2019). Two examples of brief interventions are discussed in Boxes 64.2 and 64.3.

An RCT of therapeutic assessment (TA) (Box 64.2) for young people with self-harm (Ougrin *et al.*, 2013) replicated the results of a pilot (Ougrin *et al.*, 2008) in significantly improving engagement with follow-up. Young people receiving TA versus usual assessment were significantly more likely to attend the first follow-up appointment, 83% versus 49%, (OR 5.12, 95% CI

Box 64.2 The major components of therapeutic assessment

i. Standard psychosocial history and risk assessment as discussed earlier in the section on risk factors (approximately 1 hour).
ii. A 10-minute break to review the information gathered and to prepare for the rest of the session, followed by a 30-minute intervention covering the next four steps.
iii. Joint construction of a diagram aiming to capture the vicious circles that maintain self-harm. Examples are provided in Figures 64.2 (general principles) and 64.3 (an easy example)
iv. Identification of a target problem.
v. Consideration and enhancement of motivation for change.
vi. Exploration of potential "exits" (i.e., ways of breaking the vicious circles identified).
vii. Description of the diagram and the exits in a "letter of understanding" which the clinician is required to prepare based on the initial assessment.

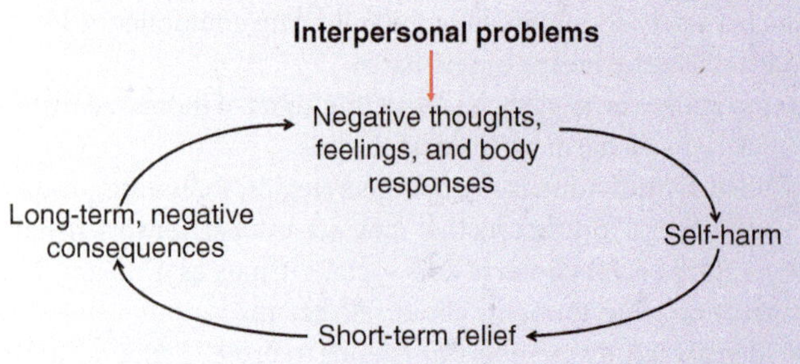

Figure 64.2 Vicious circle—general principles.

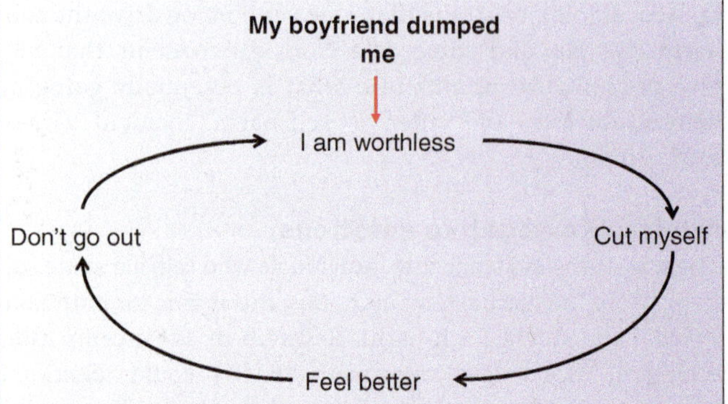

Figure 64.3 Vicious circle—an easy example.

Box 64.3 Family Intervention for Suicide Prevention (FISP)

i. To frame self-harm as a serious problem that must be addressed actively. Psychoeducation emphasizes the importance of linking youths to outpatient mental health treatment, maximizing safety (i.e., restricting access to dangerous suicide attempt methods), and the youth is asked to commit to using a safety plan in future suicidal crises.
ii. To strengthen family support and healthy communication (putative protective factors), young people and family members are encouraged to identify positive attributes in the youth and the family.
iii. To begin linking feelings to a hierarchy of suicide-eliciting situations, an "emotional thermometer" is introduced to assist youths in identifying feelings, their triggers, and associated physiological signals, thoughts, and behaviors.
iv. To develop a "safety plan" that young people could use to reduce "emotional temperature" and risk for suicidality, coping strategies are identified and practiced, including both behavioral strategies (putting a cool washcloth on the forehead, seeking support from parents) and cognitive strategies ("helpful" thoughts).
v. To provide a concrete tool that youths can use at times of acute stress/suicide attempt risk to cue safe/adaptive coping, a "Safety Plan Card" is developed and often supplemented by developing a "Hope Box" filled with reminders of reasons for living and cues/facilitators of the safety plan (coping cards). The crisis therapy session is supplemented by linkage telephone contacts made within the first 48 hours after discharge from the ER/hospital with additional contacts as needed (usually at one, two, and four weeks after discharge). Contacts are structured and focused on enhancing motivation for outpatient treatment, providing referrals, and giving support in addressing treatment barriers.

1.49–17.55), and more likely to attend four or more treatment sessions: 40% versus 11%, (OR 5.19, 95% CI 2.22–12.10).

A second example of a brief intervention associated with improved engagement with follow-up treatment (92% versus 76%; p = 0.004) among young people receiving emergency evaluation for self-harm is the Family Intervention for Suicide Prevention (FISP) based on cognitive behavioral therapy (CBT;

Asarnow *et al.*, 2011). FISP aims to use the emergency visit as a "window of opportunity" to deliver a beneficial intervention and enhance motivation to attend follow-up treatment. The FISP session is also conceptualized as an "imminent risk assessment" with a series of five tasks addressed, and difficulties addressing these tasks conceptualized as behavioral indicators of greater need for further evaluation and/or inpatient hospitalization. Specifically:

In summary, there is growing evidence that brief psychotherapeutic interventions at the point of initial self-harm assessment improve engagement with follow-up treatment. Clinicians should consider gaining training in these interventions and applying them in their practice.

Longer-term management

Current clinical guidelines (National Institute of Health and Care Excellence, 2022) recommend dialectical behavior therapy adapted for adolescents (DBT-A) for young people with significant emotional dysregulation and who have frequent episodes of self-harm (also see Chapters 48 and 67). It is recommended that practitioners delivering DBT-A should be appropriately trained and supervised, that some thought is given to identifying solutions to reduce young people's distress that leads to self-harm, and that transitions to adult services are considered. DBT-A typically lasts for at least six months. It consists of weekly individual and group psychological treatment, therapist consultation groups, and support for carers/parents (McCauley *et al.*, 2018). This is the first time such a recommendation has been made (National Institute of Health and Care Excellence, 2022) and it is based on some evidence, which will be reviewed in the rest of this section.

Up until 2015, there was no evidence that any psychological therapies reduced self-harm. In 2015, for the first time, a meta-analysis established a small but statistically significant advantage of psychological therapies over controls in reducing self-harm (Ougrin *et al.*, 2015). Since then, several further meta-analyses have confirmed these findings (Iyengar *et al.*, 2018; Kothgassner *et al.*, 2020;). However, some have not (Witt *et al.*, 2021).

Of the psychological therapies, DBT-A does stand out. With 4 independent studies (Cooney *et al.*, 2010; McCauley *et al.*, 2018; Mehlum *et al.*, 2019; Santamarina-Perez *et al.*, 2020), it is the only psychological therapy for young people with consistent evidence of a significant reduction of self-harm repetition. Several caveats should be noted. First, the outcome applies in the short term (at 6-month follow-up) but the longer young people are followed up, the smaller the effect. By 12 months, the overall effect in some studies is nonsignificant. It also appears that studies on DBT-A, with the exception of one in Norway (Mehlum *et al.*, 2019), have found that it is likely not cost-effective. All 4 studies had small sample sizes (the total n of all 4 studies = 249), and samples were predominantly female and White (although McCauley *et al.* included a large proportion of Hispanic Whites). Nonetheless, DBT-A remains a clear front-runner in the field with studies done in the US, Norway, New Zealand, and Spain, and more studies under way.

Other psychological therapies with evidence of self-harm reduction at some point in time during RCTs include CBT (Kaess *et al.*, 2020), cognitive analytic therapy (Chanen *et al.*, 2008), and mentalization-based therapy for adolescents (Rossouw & Fonagy, 2012). However, the evidence base for these approaches is significantly weaker than for DBT-A—CBT has very few studies specifically focused on young people.

A long-term follow-up study (King *et al.*, 2019) found that young people who were receiving enhanced social support, despite having no reduction of self-harm at the study's primary endpoints, were nonetheless significantly less likely to die of any cause 11–14 years post-intervention. This might well be the case in other treatments, but few RCTs conduct long-term follow-ups.

We now understand more about the possible key components of effective treatments. A systematic review of 18 RCTs evaluating interventions targeting self-harm in young people identified 27 common elements of both effective and ineffective interventions, dealing with the format, process, and content of these interventions. Compared with unsupported trials (those trials that did not support the effectiveness of the intervention), supported trials shared the following elements: (i) inclusion of therapy for both the youth and family/caregivers; (ii) an emphasis on relationship-building and the therapeutic alliance; (iii) the use of an individualized case conceptualization to guide treatment; (iv) provided skills training (e.g., emotion regulation skills) to both young people and their parents/caregivers; and (v) lethal means restriction counseling as part of self-harm monitoring and safety planning. These components may be incorporated more widely into any interventions offered to young people and their carers.

School-based interventions

With the increasing number of young people who self-harm, more thought should be given to prevention and school-based work (see Chapters 32 and 38). There is good evidence based on a review of eight RCTs (Pierret *et al.*, 2022) that school-based programs are effective in increasing the knowledge, skills, and confidence of school professionals in their approach to students with self-harm. There is also good acceptability and high satisfaction associated with the delivery of these programs.

There is also good evidence provided by the multicenter Saving and Empowering Young Lives in Europe (SEYLE) study that a four-week school-based intervention could reduce suicide attempts. The SEYLE study focused on three conditions:

- Question, Persuade, Refer (QPR)—aimed at all school staff and focused on identifying and appropriately referring pupils at risk.
- Youth Aware of Mental Health program (YAM)—a five-hour intervention targeting all students irrespective of risk or history of self-harm comprising one hour of psychoeducation about mental health, and three hours of role-play sessions on life dilemmas, stress and crises, depression, and suicide, combined with six educational posters and a 32-page booklet that pupils could take home.
- Screening by Professionals (ProfScreen)—focused on health professionals and aimed at creating a clinical pathway for those young people who were screened positive on a self-report questionnaire.

At 12-month follow-up, young people receiving YAM were significantly less likely to attempt suicide (OR 0.45, 95% CI 0.24–0.85; $p = 0.014$) or report suicidal ideation (OR 0.50, 95% CI 0.27–0.92; $p = 0.025$). In a subsequent analysis, YAM was also found to be cost-effective (Ahern *et al.*, 2018). Other programs that have been shown to reduce suicide attempts include Signs of Suicide (SOS) and the Good Behavior Game (Katz *et al.*, 2013).

School-based programs with good evidence of self-harm reduction share the following characteristics:

- universal—targeting all pupils
- clear targets, such as the reduction of suicide attempts
- focus on help-seeking and peer support
- promotion of mental health literacy and life skills
- facilitation of access to health care
- creation of long-term action plans across multiple levels.

Treatment options and treatment decision making are summarised in Box 64.4 and Figure 64.4

Box 64.4 Treatment options for adolescents who self-harm

- Immediate management:
  - discharge to the community
  - admission to a pediatric or general hospital
  - admission to a psychiatric hospital
- Brief interventions and treatment engagement:
  - safety plan
  - therapeutic assessment
  - Family Intervention for Suicide Prevention (FISP)
- Longer-term management:
  - dialectical behavior therapy for adolescents (DBT-A) with multiple and severe self-harm
  - other psychological and physical therapies for associated psychiatric disorders
- School-based interventions
  - Youth Aware of Mental Health (YAM) program
  - Signs of Suicide (SOS) program

Public health measures

Public health measures save lives by allowing young people time to reconsider their decision to end their life. Most young people who are prevented from completing suicide at the moment when they attempt it will live. Evidence from six reviews reported strongly supportive evidence of the effectiveness of structural interventions (restrictions on access to bridges, tall buildings, and railways) and restrictions on access to pharmacological agents, such as paracetamol purchase restrictions. Weakly supportive evidence of effectiveness is available for community-based multilevel programs; restrictions on access to firearms and ligature points in institutional settings (Platt & Niederkrotenthaler, 2020).

Media guidelines on reporting suicide

There is considerable evidence that poor media reporting of suicide and self-harm could be detrimental. Media guidelines, as proposed by the Centers for Disease Control and Prevention, give the following advice:

- Inform the audience without sensationalizing the suicide and minimize prominence.
- Include a hotline logo or local crisis phone numbers.
- Use nonsensational words like "rise" or "higher" when describing recent trends in suicide.
- Most, but not all, people who die by suicide exhibit warning signs. Include the "Warning Signs" and "What to Do" components in the media report.
- If there was a suicide note best to report it as a note from the deceased was found and is being reviewed by the medical examiner.
- Highlight that suicide is a public health issue.
- Involve suicide prevention experts.
- Describe as "died by suicide" or "completed" or "killed him/herself" instead of more emotive language.

Helplines/hotlines designed to prevent suicide and self-harm

A review (Mathieu *et al.*, 2021) identified 11 studies designed to investigate the impact of helplines on self-harm, and specifically on suicide attempts and thinking about suicide. Although observational, these studies tended to report an improvement in the severity of suicidal thinking and intent as the phone calls progressed or as text-based interactions continued. It is at present impossible to determine if helplines reduce self-harm and suicide and well-designed RCTs are an important area of future research in this area.

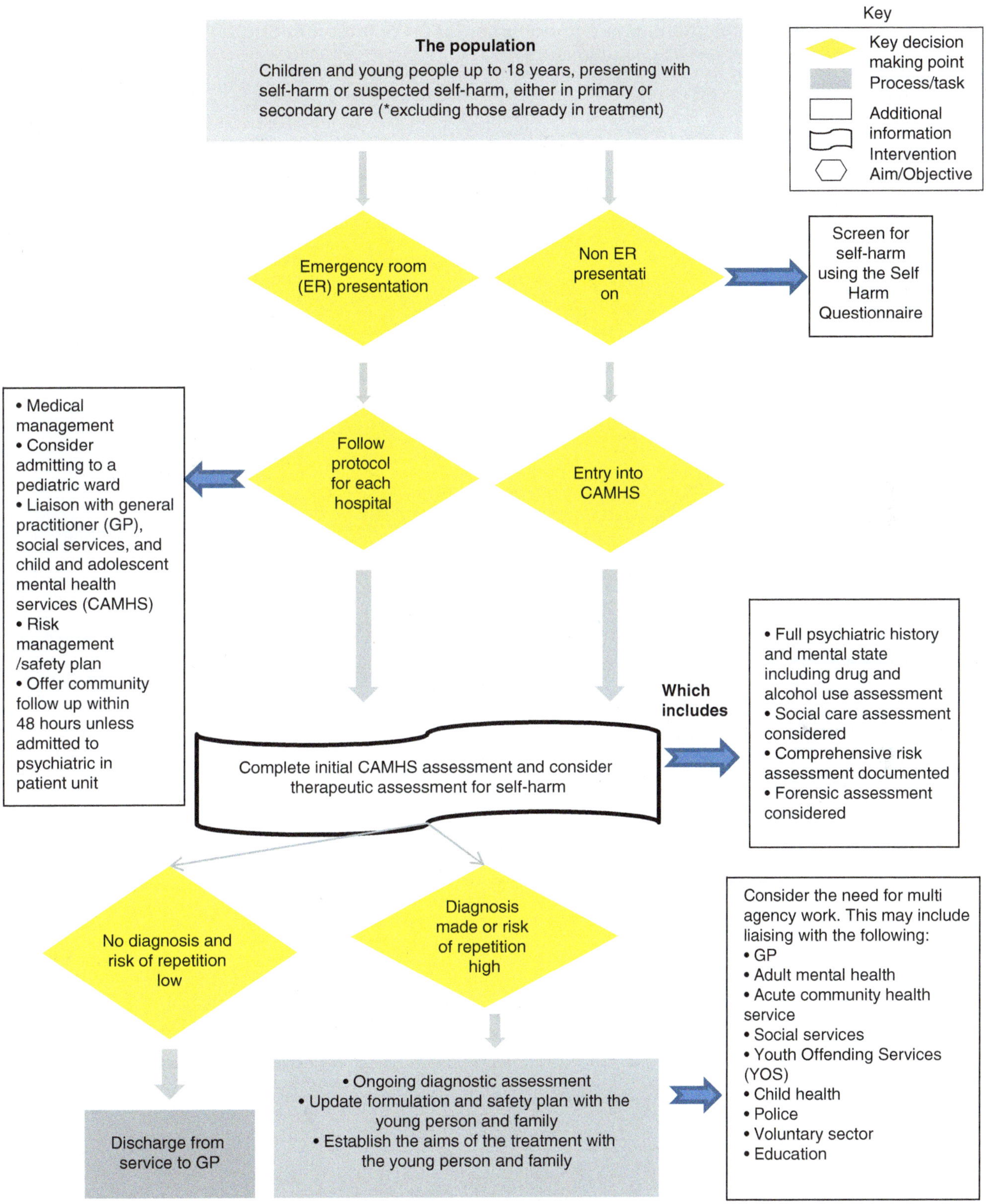

Figure 64.4 Self-harm care pathway.

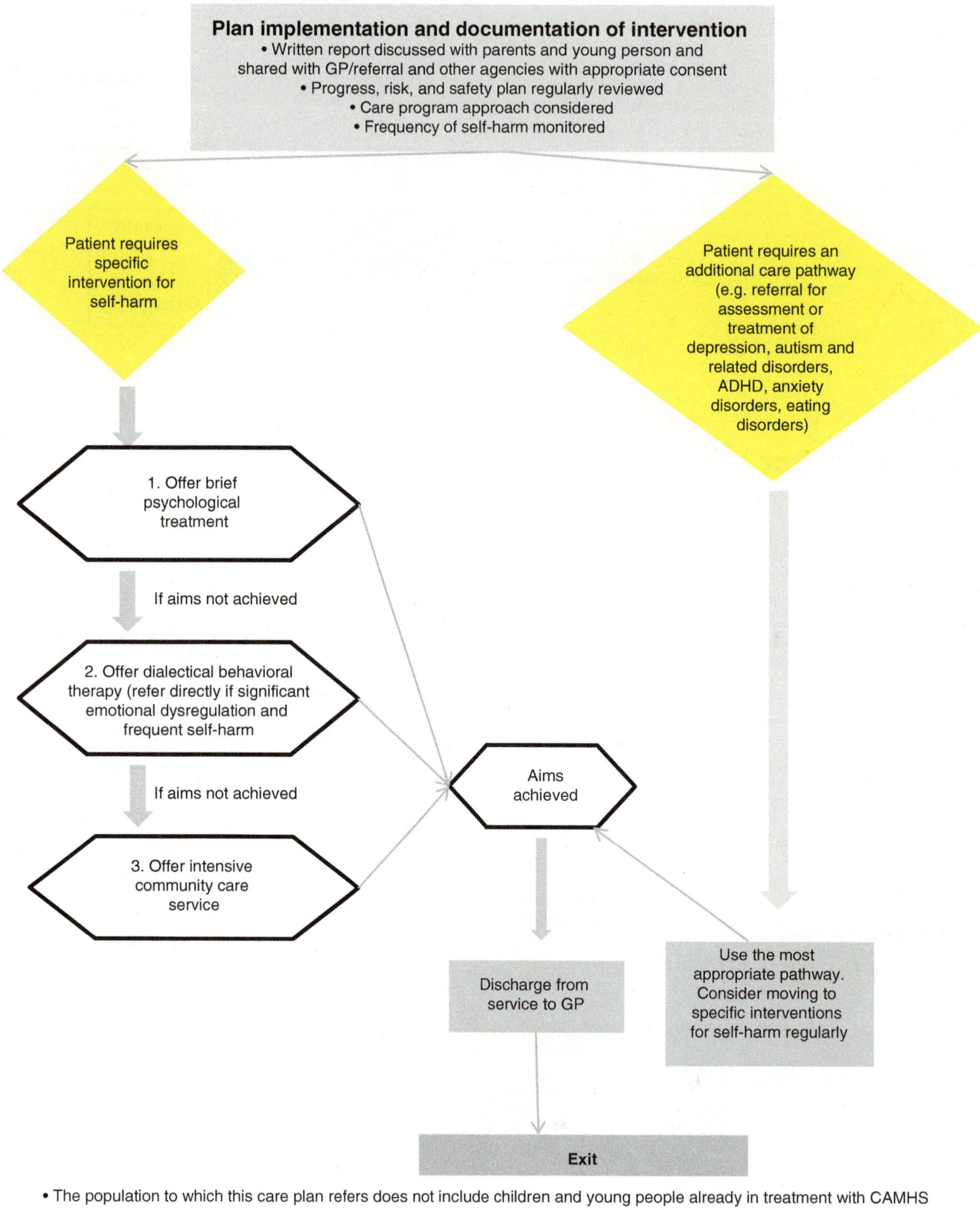

Figure 64.4 (Continued)

Future directions

The field of adolescent self-harm is developing fast; however, much remains to be done:

- Predicting which young people are at the greatest risk of repeating self-harm and dying of suicide. Some promising areas here include the use of big data (Su *et al.*, 2020) and computer-assisted testing where the young people are presented with initial items to determine a provisional estimate of their standing on the risk of suicide attempt, but the follow-up items vary depending on the initial responses to achieve the optimal prediction (King *et al.*, 2021).
- Developing individualized and precise interventions to prevent and treat self-harm, paying particular attention to minoritized groups of young people and their families (McCauley *et al.*, 2018). In particular, more studies are needed to understand the impact of psychological therapies on self-harm in boys and in young people in non-Western countries. Studies investigating the impact of pharmacological agents on self-harm are also needed.
- Understanding the role of social factors in self-harm, especially the role of social media, victimization (Baldwin *et al.*, 2019), and population-level social factors, such as societal and family cohesion. Increasing social support (King *et al.*, 2019) and investigating the role of social prescribing in reducing self-harm both require further studies.

Acknowledgment

The authors would like to acknowledge Miss Martha Fetsyk for her technical assistance in preparing this chapter.

References

Adrian, M. *et al.* (2011) Emotional dysregulation and interpersonal difficulties as risk factors for nonsuicidal self-injury in adolescent girls. *Journal of Abnormal Child Psychology* **39**, 389–400.

Ahern, S. *et al.* (2018) A cost-effectiveness analysis of school-based suicide prevention programmes. *European Child & Adolescent Psychiatry* **27**, 1295–1304.

American Psychiatric Association (2022) *Diagnostic and Statistical Manual of Mental Disorders*, 5th edn. text revision edn. American Psychiatric Association, Washington, DC.

Asarnow, J.R. *et al.* (2011) An emergency department intervention for linking pediatric suicidal patients to follow-up mental health treatment. *Psychiatric Services* **62**, 1303–1309.

Auerbach, R.P. *et al.* (2021) Neural correlates associated with suicide and nonsuicidal self-injury in youth. *Biological Psychiatry* **89**, 119–133.

Baldwin, J.R. *et al.* (2019) Adolescent victimization and self-injurious thoughts and behaviors: a genetically sensitive cohort study. *Journal of the American Academy of Child and Adolescent Psychiatry* **58**, 506–513.

Bannink, F.P. (2007) Solution-focused brief therapy. *Journal of Contemporary Psychotherapy* **37**(2), 87–94.

Barzilay, S. *et al.* (2019) A longitudinal examination of the interpersonal theory of suicide and effects of school-based suicide prevention interventions in a multinational study of adolescents. *Journal of Child Psychology and Psychiatry* **60**, 1104–1111.

Benton, T.D. *et al.* (2021) Dysregulation and suicide in children and adolescents. *Child and Adolescent Psychiatric Clinics of North America* **30**, 389–399.

Borschmann, R. & Kinner, S.A. (2019) Responding to the rising prevalence of self-harm. *The Lancet Psychiatry* **6**, 548–549.

Brent, D.A. & Mann, J.J. (2005) Family genetic studies, suicide, and suicidal behavior. *American Journal of Medical Genetics. Part C, Seminars in Medical Genetics* **133c**, 13–24.

Brent, D.A. *et al.* (2009) Predictors of spontaneous and systematically assessed suicidal adverse events in the treatment of SSRI-resistant depression in adolescents (TORDIA) study. *American Journal of Psychiatry* **166**, 418–426.

Brunner, R. *et al.* (2014) Life-time prevalence and psychosocial correlates of adolescent direct self-injurious behavior: a comparative study of findings in 11 European countries. *Journal of Child Psychology and Psychiatry* **55**, 337–348.

Centers for Disease Control and Prevention (2020) Underlying cause of death, 1999–2019. [Online]. US Department of Health and Human Services, Atlanta, GA. Available: https://wonder.cdc.gov/Deaths-by-Underlying-Cause.html [14 April 2023].

Chanen, A.M. *et al.* (2008) Early intervention for adolescents with borderline personality disorder using cognitive analytic therapy: randomised controlled trial. *British Journal of Psychiatry* **193**, 477–484.

Cooney, E. *et al.* (2010) *Feasibility of Evaluating DBT for Self-harming Adolescents: A Small Randomised Controlled Trial.* Te Pou o Te Whakaaro Nui, Auckland, New Zealand.

Coyne, S.M. *et al.* (2021) Suicide risk in emerging adulthood: associations with screen time over 10 years. *Journal of Youth and Adolescence* **50**, 2324–2338.

Cummins, T.M. *et al.* (2021) Assessment of somatosensory function and self-harm in adolescents. *JAMA Network Open* **4**, e2116853.

Cybulski, L. *et al.* (2022) Risk factors for nonfatal self-harm and suicide among adolescents: two nested case-control studies conducted in the UK Clinical Practice Research Datalink. *Journal of Child Psychology and Psychiatry* **63**, 1078–1088.

Docherty, A.R. *et al.* (2020) Genome-wide association study of suicide death and polygenic prediction of clinical antecedents. *The American Journal of Psychiatry* **177**, 917–927.

Ebert, D.D. *et al.* (2019) Prediction of major depressive disorder onset in college students. *Depression and Anxiety* **36**, 294–304.

Geoffroy, M.-C. *et al.* (2022) Prevalence of Suicidal Ideation and Self-harm Behaviours in Children Aged 12 years and Younger: A Systematic Review and Meta-analysis. *The Lancet Psychiatry* **9**, 703–714.

Ghinea, D. *et al.* (2019) Longitudinal development of risk-taking and self-injurious behavior in association with late adolescent borderline personality disorder symptoms. *Psychiatry Research* **273**, 127–133.

Ghinea, D. *et al.* (2020) Non-suicidal self-injury disorder as a stand-alone diagnosis in a consecutive help-seeking sample of adolescents. *Journal of Affective Disorders* **274**, 1122–1125.

Ghinea, D. *et al.* (2021) Psychosocial functioning in adolescents with non-suicidal self-injury: the roles of childhood maltreatment, borderline personality disorder and depression. *Borderline Personality Disorder and Emotion Dysregulation* **8**, 1–11.

Gould, M.S. *et al.* (2005) Evaluating iatrogenic risk of youth suicide screening programs: a randomized controlled trial. *JAMA* **293**, 1635–1643.

Groschwitz, R.C. *et al.* (2015a) The association of non-suicidal self-injury and suicidal behavior according to DSM-5 in adolescent psychiatric inpatients. *Psychiatry Research* **228**, 454–461.

Groschwitz, R.C. *et al.* (2015b) The situation of former adolescent self-injurers as young adults: a follow-up study. *BMC Psychiatry* **15**, 1–9.

Gyori, D. *et al.* (2021) The association of nonsuicidal self-injury with quality of life and mental disorders in clinical adolescents: a network approach. *International Journal of Environmental Research and Public Health* **18**, 1840.

Hansen, C. *et al.* (2023) Predictors of transfer and prognosis after transfer from child and adolescent mental health services to adult mental health services: a Danish nationwide prospective register-based cohort study. *European Child & Adolescent Psychiatry* **33**, 79–87.

Hawton, K. *et al.* (2020a) Mortality in children and adolescents following presentation to hospital after non-fatal self-harm in the multicentre study of self-harm: a prospective observational cohort study. *The Lancet Child & Adolescent Health* **4**, 111–120.

Hawton, K. *et al.* (2020b) Clustering of suicides in children and adolescents. *The Lancet Child & Adolescent Health* **4**, 58–67.

Hetrick, S.E. *et al.* (2021) New generation antidepressants for depression in children and adolescents: a network meta-analysis. *Cochrane Database of Systematic Reviews* **5**, Cd013674.

Hiscock, H. *et al.* (2018) Paediatric mental and physical health presentations to emergency departments, Victoria, 2008–15. *Medical Journal of Australia* **208**, 343–348.

Hughes, J.L. & Asarnow, J.R. (2013) Enhanced mental health interventions in the emergency department: suicide and suicide attempt prevention. *Clinical Pediatric Emergency Medicine* **14**, 28–34.

Iyengar, U. *et al.* (2018) A further look at therapeutic interventions for suicide attempts and self-harm in adolescents: an updated systematic review of randomized controlled trials. *Frontiers in Psychiatry* **9**, 1–16.

Jollant, F. *et al.* (2022) Self-harm, somatic disorders and mortality in the 3 years following a hospitalisation in psychiatry in adolescents and young adults. *BMJ Mental Health* **25**, 177–184.

Joo, Y.Y. *et al.* (2022) Association of genome-wide polygenic scores for multiple psychiatric and common traits in preadolescent youths at risk of suicide. *JAMA Network Open* **5**, e2148585.

Jopling, E. *et al.* (2021) Potential lethality of suicide attempts in youth. *European Child & Adolescent Psychiatry* **31**, 1–9.

Kaess, M. *et al.* (2011) Explaining gender differences in non-fatal suicidal behaviour among adolescents: a population-based study. *BMC Public Health* **11**, 1–7.

Kaess, M. *et al.* (2013) Adverse childhood experiences and their impact on frequency, severity, and the individual function of nonsuicidal self-injury in youth. *Psychiatry Research* **206**, 265–272.

Kaess, M. *et al.* (2020) Effectiveness of a brief psychotherapeutic intervention compared with treatment as usual for adolescent nonsuicidal self-injury: a single-Centre, randomised controlled trial. *European Child & Adolescent Psychiatry* **29**, 881–891.

Kaess, M. *et al.* (2021) Advancing a temporal framework for understanding the biology of nonsuicidal self- injury: an expert review. *Neuroscience and Biobehavioral Reviews* **130**, 228–239.

Kapur, N. *et al.* (2013) Non-suicidal self-injury v. attempted suicide: new diagnosis or false dichotomy? *British Journal of Psychiatry* **202**, 326–328.

Katz, C. *et al.* (2013) A systematic review of school-based suicide prevention programs. *Depression and Anxiety* **30**, 1030–1045.

Kendler, K.S. *et al.* (2020) The sources of parent-child transmission of risk for suicide attempt and deaths by suicide in Swedish National Samples. *The American Journal of Psychiatry* **177**, 928–935.

Kinchin, I. *et al.* (2017) Understanding the true economic impact of self-harming behaviour. *The Lancet Psychiatry* **4**, 900–901.

Kindler, J. *et al.* (2022) Increased immunological markers in female adolescents with non-suicidal self-injury. *Journal of Affective Disorders* **318**, 191–195.

King, C.A. *et al.* (2019) Association of the Youth-Nominated Support Team Intervention for suicidal adolescents with 11- to 14-year mortality outcomes: secondary analysis of a randomized clinical trial. *JAMA Psychiatry* **76**, 492–498.

King, C.A. *et al.* (2021) Prospective development and validation of the computerized adaptive screen for suicidal youth. *JAMA Psychiatry* **78**, 540–549.

Klonsky, E.D. *et al.* (2018) Ideation-to-action theories of suicide: a conceptual and empirical update. *Current Opinion in Psychology* **22**, 38–43.

Knipe, D. *et al.* (2022) Suicide and self-harm. *The Lancet* **399**, 1903–1916.

Koenig, J. *et al.* (2016) A meta-analysis on pain sensitivity in self-injury. *Psychological Medicine* **46**, 1597–1612.

Koenig, J. *et al.* (2017) Prospective risk for suicidal thoughts and behaviour in adolescents with onset, maintenance or cessation of direct self-injurious behaviour. *European Child & Adolescent Psychiatry* **26**, 345–354.

Koenig, J. *et al.* (2021) High-frequency ecological momentary assessment of emotional and interpersonal states preceding and following self-injury in female adolescents. *European Child & Adolescent Psychiatry* **30**, 1299–1308.

Kothgassner, O.D. *et al.* (2020) Does treatment method matter? A meta-analysis of the past 20 years of research on therapeutic interventions for self-harm and suicidal ideation in adolescents. *Borderline Personality Disorder and Emotion Dysregulation* **7**, 9.

Leone, M. *et al.* (2021) Association of youth depression with subsequent somatic diseases and premature death. *JAMA Psychiatry* **78**, 302–310.

Lim, K.-S. *et al.* (2019) Global lifetime and 12-month prevalence of suicidal behavior, deliberate self-harm and non-suicidal self-injury in children and adolescents between 1989 and 2018: a meta-analysis. *International Journal of Environmental Research and Public Health* **16**, 4581.

Liu, B.-P. *et al.* (2020) The short-term rate of non-fatal and fatal repetition of deliberate self-harm: a systematic review and meta-analysis of longitudinal studies. *Journal of Affective Disorders* **273**, 597–603.

Liu, B.-P. *et al.* (2022) Associating factors of suicide and repetition following self-harm: a systematic review and meta-analysis of longitudinal studies. *Eclinicalmedicine* **49**, 101461.

Lukmanji, A. *et al.* (2020) Antidepressant prescriptions, including tricyclics, continue to increase in Canadian children. *Journal of Child and Adolescent Psychopharmacology* **30**, 381–388.

Lung, F.W. *et al.* (2020) Relationships between internet use, deliberate self-harm, and happiness in adolescents: a Taiwan birth cohort pilot study. *PLoS One* **15**, e0235834.

Lutz, P.E. *et al.* (2017) Neuropathology of suicide: recent findings and future directions. *Molecular Psychiatry* **22**, 1395–1412.

Lyu, J. *et al.* (2021) Relationship and effects of community problems on anxiety and suicide: a case-control psychological autopsy study. *The Journal of Nervous and Mental Disease* **209**, 17–22.

Mars, B. *et al.* (2020) Prospective associations between internet use and poor mental health: a population-based study. *PLoS One* **15**, e0235889.

Marttunen, M.J. *et al.* (1993) Adolescence and suicide: a review of psychological autopsy studies. *European Child & Adolescent Psychiatry* **2**, 10–18.

Mathieu, S.L. *et al.* (2021) Systematic review: the state of research into youth helplines. *Journal of the American Academy of Child & Adolescent Psychiatry* **60**, 1190–1233.

McCauley, E. *et al.* (2018) Efficacy of dialectical behavior therapy for adolescents at high risk for suicide: a randomized clinical trial. *JAMA Psychiatry* **75**, 777–785.

McEvoy, D. *et al.* (2023) Risk and protective factors for self-harm in adolescents and young adults: an umbrella review of systematic reviews. *Journal of Psychiatric Research* **168**, 353–380.

McGirr, A. *et al.* (2008) Impulsive-aggressive behaviours and completed suicide across the life cycle: a predisposition for younger age of suicide. *Psychological Medicine* **38**, 407–417.

Mehlum, L. *et al.* (2019) Long term effectiveness of dialectical behavior therapy versus enhanced usual care for adolescents with self-harming and suicidal behavior. *Journal of Child Psychology & Psychiatry & Allied Disciplines* **60**, 1112–1122.

Melhem, N.M. *et al.* (2007) Familial pathways to early-onset suicidal behavior: familial and individual antecedents of suicidal behavior. *American Journal of Psychiatry* **164**, 1364–1370.

Mérelle, S. *et al.* (2020) A multi-method psychological autopsy study on youth suicides in the Netherlands in 2017: feasibility, main outcomes, and recommendations. *PLoS One* **15**, e0238031.

Miller, A.B. & Prinstein, M.J. (2019) Adolescent suicide as a failure of acute stress-response systems. *Annual Review of Clinical Psychology* **15**, 425–450.

Moran, P. *et al.* (2012) The natural history of self-harm from adolescence to young adulthood: a population-based cohort study. *The Lancet* **379**, 236–243.

Morgan, C. *et al.* (2017) Incidence, clinical management, and mortality risk following self harm among children and adolescents: cohort study in primary care. *BMJ* **359**.

Mortier, P. *et al.* (2018) The prevalence of suicidal thoughts and behaviours among college students: a meta-analysis. *Psychological Medicine* **48**, 554–565.

Muehlenkamp, J.J. *et al.* (2012) International prevalence of adolescent non-suicidal self-injury and deliberate self-harm. *Child and Adolescent Psychiatry and Mental Health* **6**, 10.

Naghavi, M. (2019) Global, regional, and national burden of suicide mortality 1990 to 2016: systematic analysis for the global burden of disease study 2016. *BMJ* **364**, l94.

Nakar, O. *et al.* (2016) Developmental trajectories of self-injurious behavior, suicidal behavior and substance misuse and their association with adolescent borderline personality pathology. *Journal of Affective Disorders* **197**, 231–238.

National Child Mortality Database (2023) Deaths of Children and Young People Due to Traumatic Incidents: Vehicle collisions, Drownings, violence and maltreatment and unintentional injuries. [Online]. National Child Mortality Database, Bristol, UK Available: https://www.ncmd.info/publications/report-child-accident-injury/ [11 December 2024].

National Institute of Health and Care Excellence (2022) *Self-harm: Assessment, Management and Preventing Recurrence.* [Online]. National Institute of Health and Care Excellence (NICE), London. Available: www.nice.org.uk/guidance/ng225/resources/selfharm-assessment-management-and-preventing-recurrence-pdf-66143837346757 [11 December 2024].

Niedzwiedz, C. *et al.* (2014) The definition and epidemiology of clusters of suicidal behavior: a systematic review. *Suicide & Life-Threatening Behavior* **44**, 569–581.

Nock, M.K. *et al.* (2007) Self-injurious thoughts and behaviors interview: development, reliability, and validity in an adolescent sample. *Psychological Assessment* **19**, 309–317.

Nock, M.K. *et al.* (2009) Revealing the form and function of self-injurious thoughts and behaviors: a real-time ecological assessment study among adolescents and young adults. *Journal of Abnormal Psychology* **118**, 816–827.

Nock, M.K. *et al.* (2013) Prevalence, correlates, and treatment of lifetime suicidal behavior among adolescents: results from the National Comorbidity Survey Replication Adolescent Supplement. *JAMA Psychiatry* **70**, 300–310.

Ougrin, D. & Boege, I. (2013) Brief report: the self harm questionnaire: a new tool designed to improve identification of self harm in adolescents. *Journal of Adolescence* **36**, 221–225.

Ougrin, D. *et al.* (2008) Therapeutic assessment based on cognitive-analytic therapy for young people presenting with self-harm: pilot study. *Psychiatric Bulletin* **32**, 423–426.

Ougrin, D. *et al.* (2012) Practitioner review: self-harm in adolescents. *Journal of Child Psychology and Psychiatry* **53**, 337–350.

Ougrin, D. *et al.* (2013) Randomised controlled trial of therapeutic assessment versus usual assessment in adolescents with self-harm: 2-year follow-up. *Archives of Disease in Childhood* **98**, 772–776.

Ougrin, D. *et al.* (2015) Therapeutic interventions for suicide attempts and self-harm in adolescents: systematic review and Meta-analysis. *Journal of the American Academy of Child & Adolescent Psychiatry* **54**, 97–107.e2.

Ougrin, D. *et al.* (2021) Supported discharge service versus inpatient care evaluation (site): a randomised controlled trial comparing effectiveness of an intensive community care service versus inpatient treatment as usual for adolescents with severe psychiatric disorders: self-harm, functional impairment, and educational and clinical outcomes. *European Child & Adolescent Psychiatry* **30**, 1427–1436.

Pandey, G.N. *et al.* (2012) Proinflammatory cytokines in the prefrontal cortex of teenage suicide victims. *Journal of Psychiatric Research* **46**, 57–63.

Pierret, A.C.S. *et al.* (2022) Review: Education and training interventions, and support tools for school staff to adequately respond to young people who disclose self-harm: a systematic literature review of effectiveness, feasibility and acceptability. *Child and Adolescent Mental Health* **27**, 161–172.

Plana, T. *et al.* (2010) Total serum cholesterol levels and suicide attempts in child and adolescent psychiatric inpatients. *European Child & Adolescent Psychiatry* **19**, 615–619.

Platt, S. & Niederkrotenthaler, T. (2020) *Suicide Prevention Programs: Evidence Base and Best Practice. Suicide and Suicide Prevention from a Global Perspective.* Hogrefe, Göttingen, Germany.

Plener, P.L. *et al.* (2015) The longitudinal course of non-suicidal self-injury and deliberate self-harm: a systematic review of the literature. In: *Borderline Personality Disorder and Emotion Dysregulation*, Vol. 2. pp. 1–11.

Quinlivan, L. *et al.* (2016) Which are the most useful scales for predicting repeat self-harm? A systematic review evaluating risk scales using measures of diagnostic accuracy. *BMJ Open* **6**, e009297.

Reichl, C. *et al.* (2023) Frequency and predictors of individual treatment outcomes (response, remission, exacerbation, and relapse) in clinical adolescents with nonsuicidal self-injury. *Psychological Medicine* **282**, 852–857.

Rockstroh, F. *et al.* (2021) Self-rated risk as a predictor of suicide attempts among high-risk adolescents. *Journal of Affective Disorders* **282**, 852–857.

Rossouw, T.I. & Fonagy, P. (2012) Mentalization-based treatment for self-harm in adolescents: a randomized controlled trial. *Journal of the American Academy of Child & Adolescent Psychiatry* **51**, 1304–1313.

Royal College of Psychiatrists (2020). Self harm. Royal College of Psychiatrists, London. Available: https://www.rcpsych.ac.uk/mental-health/problems-disorders/self-harm [30 December 2024].

Santamarina-Perez, P. *et al.* (2020) Adapted dialectical behavior therapy for adolescents with a high risk of suicide in a community clinic: a pragmatic randomized controlled trial. *Suicide & Life Threatening Behavior* **16**, 16.

Santangelo, P.S. *et al.* (2017) Ecological momentary assessment of affective and interpersonal instability in adolescent non-suicidal self-injury. *Journal of Abnormal Child Psychology* **45**, 1429–1438.

Scott, L.N. *et al.* (2015) Non-suicidal self-injury and suicidal ideation as predictors of suicide attempts in adolescent girls: a multi-wave prospective study. *Comprehensive Psychiatry* **58**, 1–10.

Sedgwick, R. *et al.* (2019) Social media, internet use and suicide attempts in adolescents. *Current Opinion in Psychiatry* **32**, 534–541.

Spirito, A. *et al.* (2002) An intervention trial to improve adherence to community treatment by adolescents after a suicide attempt. *Journal of the American Academy of Child & Adolescent Psychiatry* **41**, 435–442.

Steinhoff, A. *et al.* (2023) Self-, other-, and dual-harm during adolescence: a prospective-longitudinal study of childhood risk factors and early adult correlates. *Psychological Medicine* **53**, 3995–4003.

Su, C. *et al.* (2020) Machine learning for suicide risk prediction in children and adolescents with electronic health records. *Translational Psychiatry* **10**, 413.

Swannell, S.V. *et al.* (2014) Prevalence of nonsuicidal self-injury in non-clinical samples: systematic review, meta-analysis and meta-regression. *Suicide and Life-threatening Behavior* **44**, 273–303.

Swanson, S.A. *et al.* (2020) Firearm access and adolescent suicide risk: toward a clearer understanding of effect size. *Injury Prevention* **27**, 264–270.

Tsiachristas, A. *et al.* (2017) General hospital costs in England of medical and psychiatric care for patients who self-harm: a retrospective analysis. *The Lancet Psychiatry* **4**, 759–767.

Valencia-Agudo, F. *et al.* (2018) Nonsuicidal self-injury in community adolescents: a systematic review of prospective predictors, mediators and moderators. *Journal of Adolescence* **65**, 25–38.

Vitiello, B. *et al.* (2009) Suicidal events in the Treatment for Adolescents with Depression Study (TADS). *Journal of Clinical Psychiatry* **70**, 741–747.

Wesselhoeft, R. *et al.* (2020) Trends in antidepressant use among children and adolescents: a Scandinavian drug utilization study. *Acta Psychiatrica Scandinavica* **141**, 34–42.

Witt, K.G. *et al.* (2021) Interventions for self-harm in children and adolescents. *Cochrane Database of Systematic Reviews* **3**, Cd013667.

Wong, B.H.-C. *et al.* (2022) Lockdown stringency and paediatric self-harm presentations during COVID-19 pandemic: Retrospective cohort study. *BJPsych Open* **8**, e75.

Wong, B.H.-C. *et al.* (2023) Self-harm in children and adolescents who presented at emergency units during the COVID-19 pandemic: an international retrospective cohort study. *Journal of the American Academy of Child & Adolescent Psychiatry* **62**, 998–1009.

World Health Organization (2020) *Global Health estimates 2020: Deaths by Cause, Age, Sex, by Country and by Region, 2000-2019*. World Health Organization (WHO), Geneva, Switzerland. Available: https://www.who.int/data/gho/data/themes/mortality-and-global-health-estimates/ghe-leading-causes-of-death [11 December 2024]

Ye, Z. *et al.* (2022) A meta-analysis of co-occurrence of non-suicidal self-injury and suicide attempt: implications for clinical intervention and future diagnosis. *Frontiers in Psychiatry* **13**.

Yuan, S.N.V. *et al.* (2019) Treatment engagement in specific psychological treatment vs. treatment as usual for adolescents with self-harm: systematic review and Meta-analysis. *Frontiers in Psychology* **10**.

C: Behavior

CHAPTER 65

Oppositional defiant and conduct disorders

Stephen Scott[1] and Christian Bachmann[2]

[1] Department of Child and Adolescent Psychiatry, Institute of Psychiatry, Psychology and Neuroscience, King's College London, London, UK

[2] Department of Child and Adolescent Psychiatry, Ulm University Medical Center, Ulm, Germany

Introduction

Oppositional defiant and conduct disorders (ODD/CDs) are characterized by antisocial behaviors outside socially acceptable norms that violate other people's expectations or rights. The behaviors include excessive verbal and physical aggression, temper tantrums, lying and stealing, disobedience, rule breaking, and violence. As adults, many of these individuals continue to act antisocially, with substance misuse and criminality being common. The upset, disruption, and costs inflicted on the family, peer group, school, and wider society are considerable. However, perhaps because these behaviors are present in many children to some extent, are often related to a less than ideal upbringing, and may appear to reflect poor self-control in children who otherwise appear free of psychopathology, ODD/CDs are still considered by some not to be "true" psychiatric disorders but more as character flaws, with the children being seen as "nasty" and "bad."

This is unfortunate for several reasons. First, in recent years there have been many exciting discoveries about what contributes to the development of ODD/CDs, with a substantial biological component involving genetic and brain differences becoming evident, so that in many cases the problems are not just due to poor socialization. Second, different subtypes of conduct problems are now better understood, with, for example, very different life trajectories for those who exhibit early versus later onset, and those who have callous-unemotional (CU) traits, or display marked irritability. Finally, there have been considerable advances in developing effective treatments, especially for prepubertal children.

In this chapter, the term *conduct problems* will be used as a broad overarching dimensional construct, with the term ODD/CD used to refer to the more severe end that meets diagnostic criteria. Occasionally the term *antisocial behavior* will be used as several publications prefer this term. Many medical practitioners, mental health professionals, social workers, teachers, and the general public are not familiar with the terms *oppositional defiant disorder* (ODD) or *conduct disorder* (CD), so using expressions such as antisocial, challenging, or disruptive behavior may improve communication. The term externalizing is not used in this chapter since it connotes that an inner angst is being acted out, for which there is usually no evidence. The term children is used to cover both children and adolescents collectively.

Historical background

Conduct disorders are among the earliest child psychiatric conditions to be described in the scientific literature. The seminal psychiatric textbooks of Hermann Emminghaus (*Die psychischen Störungen des Kindesalters*, 1887) and Henry Maudsley (*The Pathology of Mind*, 1895) both portray a condition in youths labeled "moral insanity," characterized by "a strange perversion of some fundamental instinct that seems to be wilful wickedness." Already back then it was debated whether a psychiatric label for conduct problems in otherwise healthy youths was warranted as it might absolve them from blame. In the following decades diagnostic labels changed (e.g., "anethic psychopathy" (Kramer & von der Leyen, 1934); "moral agenesis" (Karpman, 1947)) until the term "conduct disorder" was established as a diagnostic entity in 1968 (*Diagnostic and Statistical Manual of Mental Disorders*, 2nd edition; DSM-II), followed by the creation of "oppositional-defiant disorder" in 1980 (DSM-III). The place of diagnosis remains disputed (Scott, 2022).

Classification

Introduction

Both the *International Classification of Diseases*, 11th revision (ICD-11, World Health Organization (2019)) and DSM-5-TR (text revision of DSM-5, issued by the (American Psychiatric

Rutter's Child and Adolescent Psychiatry and Psychology, Seventh Edition.
Edited by Anita Thapar, Daniel S. Pine, Samuele Cortese, Cathy Creswell, Tamsin J. Ford, James F. Leckman, and Argyris Stringaris.

Companion website: www.wiley.com/go/thapar/rutterspsych7

Association, 2022), here simply referred to as DSM-5) include oppositional defiant disorder (ODD) and conduct disorder (CD), which are characterized by a repetitive and persistent pattern of antisocial behavior; occasional isolated acts do not qualify. ODD is usually a diagnosis given to younger children, while CD is typically (but not exclusively) a diagnosis given to older children and teenagers. The criteria are similar in the two systems. ICD-11 now uses the term "conduct-dissocial disorder" throughout, but in this chapter we will use the simpler term "conduct disorder." However, a significant difference is that all versions of ICD-11 (clinical and research) now only use general descriptions, whereas previously, in ICD-10, the criteria for research took a menu-driven approach identical to the DSM system.

Oppositional defiant disorder

The ICD-11 criteria for ODD are that a persistent pattern (six months or more) of markedly defiant, disobedient, provocative, or spiteful behavior should be present, that may be manifest in a prevailing, persistently angry or irritable mood, often accompanied by severe temper outbursts or in headstrong, argumentative, or defiant behavior. It should be beyond what is typically observed in same age peers.

The DSM definition of ODD requires four out of eight symptoms from the three following domains to be present for at least six months, in a manner that is outside a range that is developmentally normative: angry and irritable mood, argumentative and defiant behavior, and vindictiveness.

Interestingly, neither DSM nor ICD include physical or verbal aggression, or destruction of property as a criterion for ODD, despite it being a very common characteristic of this pattern of behavior, even in younger children.

Specifiers

ICD-11, but not DSM-5, includes the specifier with (or without) *chronic irritability-anger*, characterized as annoyance and loss of temper out of proportion to any provocation, and may be present with none. In contrast, in DSM-5, this pattern of behavior is categorized as a new, separate diagnosis, disruptive mood dysregulation disorder (DMDD)—see below under differential diagnosis.

The other specifier, in both systems, is with (or without) *limited prosocial emotions*. This is characterized by:

- *limited empathy* or sensitivity to others' feelings or concern for their distress
- *limited remorse*, shame, or guilt about their behavior and relative indifference to the probability of punishment
- *limited concern over poor performance* at school or in other important activities
- *limited or shallow expression of emotions*, particularly loving feelings toward others which may appear shallow, superficial, insincere, or instrumental.

Only DSM-5 ODD includes specifiers for *severity* (mild, moderate, or severe). Both DSM-5 and ICD-11 require an impairment criterion for ODD.

Conduct disorder

ICD-11 defines CD as a repetitive and persistent pattern of behavior in which basic rights of others or major age-appropriate societal norms, rules, or laws are violated, such as aggression toward other people or animals, destruction of property, deceitfulness or theft, and serious violations of rules, for 12 months or more. It should lead to impairment of self or in others.

DSM-5 CD criteria require 3 or more out of 15 criteria from the 3 domains "aggression to people and animals," "destruction of property" (e.g., fire setting), and "serious violations of rules" (e.g., running away from home) to have been manifest in the past 12 months.

Specifiers

Both DSM-5 and ICD-11 include specifiers for *child or adolescent onset*, and for *limited prosocial emotions*. DSM-5, but not ICD-11, specifies severity (mild, moderate, or severe). Unlike for ODD, neither system requires an impairment criterion for CD—arguably, the behaviors almost automatically involve affecting the function of others.

Age

DSM-5 specifically allows both ODD and CD to be diagnosed in adults; they are nested in the section on disruptive disorders. While there is no stated age cutoff in ICD-11, ODD and CD appear in the disorders "with onset usually in childhood or adolescence" suggesting they may be less applicable in adults. Applying a diagnosis in adults would mean that many people with criminal records can be diagnosed with CD, but neither DSM-5 nor ICD-11 make reference to the likely consequences; clinicians, epidemiological surveys, and treatment trials do not usually apply the term to adults. If it were widely applied, then one implication might be that adults displaying this pattern of behavior should have medication or psychological therapy.

One disorder or two?

In ICD-11, ODD is a subtype of CD, whereas in DSM-5 they are separate entities. This reflects a wide-ranging debate. In terms of external validating criteria, there are many similarities between the two conditions, with progression from one to the other being frequent (odds ratio 13 in boys, (Rowe *et al.*, 2002, 2010)), so that on these grounds they can both be seen as age-related progressions of a cluster of symptoms characterized by antisocial behavior. Because many children with CD also have ODD, DSM-IV did not allow both to be diagnosed simultaneously, but this bar has been removed in DSM-5.

Assessment

Before the interview

Because the phenomena of conduct problems are so overt, questionnaires are less essential than in some conditions (such as anxiety and depression, where children may reveal symptoms that the parents are unaware of). However, getting both parent and teacher to fill in questionnaires is helpful for a number of reasons. First, it is important to get the perspective of the school. Second, comorbidity can more easily be picked up if a broad symptomatology questionnaire is used, such as the Strength and Difficulties Questionnaire (SDQ) or the Achenbach System of Empirically Based Assessment (ASEBA). The SDQ is free and shorter, the ASEBA costs and is longer; on the major dimensions they correlate closely (Goodman & Scott, 1999). Domain-specific questionnaires such as the Eyberg Child Behavior Inventory (ECBI) are useful as a baseline from which treatment effects can be monitored. To determine the extent of limited prosocial emotions/callous-unemotional traits, the Inventory of Callous-Unemotional Traits (ICU; Morales-Vives *et al.*, 2019; Ray & Frick, 2020) developed by Frick is widely used. To determine the extent of irritability, the Affective Reactivity Index (Stringaris *et al.*, 2012) is very helpful (see Chapter 28 for more about rating scales).

Children tend to underreport their antisocial behavior, so questionnaires below say the age of 11 are usually unhelpful, but by mid-to-late adolescence self-reports of delinquent acts become more reliable, and typically reveal far more criminal behavior than, for example, is known to official agencies; this is true across ethnic groups and countries (Gomes *et al.*, 2018). A member of the staff at the child's school who knows the child well should be contacted to find out if there are behavioral issues in the classroom and in peer relations, and the latest school report should be requested along with formal examination results and psychometric test reports, if available.

History and examination

A thorough clinical evaluation should be made (see Chapter 27). There may be a litany of complaints from the parents, and it is important to keep a neutral position and show the child or young person that they are also being listened to. The quality of parenting needs to be assessed. Asking about what happens during a typical day and at a typical weekend is often revealing. Detailed blow-by-blow descriptions should be obtained of disciplinary encounters, so that a clear picture is built up of antecedent events, how the parents reacted, and whether any consequences were applied.

An evaluation should be made of how negative the parents are, including whether the child is scapegoated for more of the family's difficulties than appears just, and whether the situation borders on emotional or physical abuse. Coercive cycles and negative reinforcement traps that are maintaining the behavior should be explored. Coercive cycles are present where the parent or child initiates a negative overture, which then in turn elicits a cross response, then the other party gets angrier, and so it continues; they get locked into emotionally charged angry interchanges. Negative reinforcement occurs when the parent asks the child to do something that they do not wish to do, for example, tidy their room, but then, after asking say three times, gives up, thereby inadvertently rewarding the child for their opposition and making it more likely to occur next time. Positive involvement in joint activities, such as play or common interests, needs to be assessed. The clinician should not shy away from asking parents about their own antisocial activities and criminal records, and use of alcohol and drugs, including during pregnancy. The child's strengths should be asked about.

Seeing the young person on their own is crucial. They may reveal emotional concerns including anxiety and depression, and in teenagers, substance and alcohol use that they have withheld from the parent. Gang involvement and witnessing interparental violence should be inquired about. All ages may have experienced cyberbullying and been "canceled" (i.e., excluded from social media; Baumann *et al.*, 2022). Are there positive times with their parents? Do they feel closeness? Can the child seek comfort from them? In young children, what is the quality of attachment to the parent? Because it is easy to become overwhelmed by the saturation of negative events and behavior, it is especially important to ask the young person what they enjoy doing, what they are good at, and their hopes for the future. Are there any positive adults in the child's life? What potential protective factors are operating and how might they be built on? Physical examination (see Chapter 30) should include a check for dysmorphic features including fetal alcohol spectrum disorder.

Investigation

It is important to evaluate the presence of both specific and general learning disabilities in individuals with ODD/CD. Poor school performance can often be attributed to a lazy attitude and failure to complete homework, both of which may be present but may mask an underlying cognitive problem. One-quarter or more of children with ODD/CD also have specific reading retardation (defined as having a reading level two standard deviations below that predicted by their IQ) or dyslexia (see Chapter 52). While this may in part be due to lack of adequate schooling, there is good evidence that the cognitive deficits often precede the behavioral problems. General learning disability (see Chapter 53) is often missed in children with CD unless IQ testing is carried out (see Chapter 29). The rate of CDs rises several-fold as IQ gets below 70 (see Chapter 53).

Differential diagnosis and formulation

Making a diagnosis of ODD or CD is usually straightforward but comorbid conditions are often missed. A particular pitfall is to fail to diagnose comorbid attention deficit hyperactivity disorder (ADHD) despite symptoms being there, because disorganization in the child is attributed to a chaotic or abusive home background, or because there have been several recent disruptive moves of home or school; likewise a disorganized pattern of attachment does not exclude ODD/CD, although there is a vogue at present to label many problems as attributable to attachment and trauma, ignoring the phenomenology. The differential diagnosis may include:

- *ADHD*: Any of the three core symptoms, impulsivity, inattention, and motor overactivity can be misconstrued as antisocial, particularly impulsivity, which is also present in ODD/CD and does not of itself indicate ADHD (see Chapter 54). A careful history of ability to attend and be still both at home and school will usually reveal ADHD if present, in conjunction with a school visit or standardized questionnaire from the teacher. In contrast, conduct problems are not a feature of pure ADHD, but often coexist (see Chapter 54).
- *Depression and bipolar disorder*: Depression can present with irritability and oppositional symptoms but unlike typical ODD/CD, mood is usually clearly low and there are often vegetative features (see Chapter 63). Low self-esteem is the norm in ODD/CD, as is a lack of friends or constructive pastimes. Therefore, it is easy to overlook more pronounced depressive symptoms.
- *Intermittent explosive disorder (IED)*: This exists in both ICD-11 and DSM-5. It refers to regularly occurring severe temper outbursts that are grossly out of proportion in intensity to the provocation. Aggression can be verbal or physical, is not premeditated and is not committed in order to achieve a tangible objective; nonaggressive symptoms, such as lying or stealing, are absent, and general defiance of rules and authority should be absent. Nonetheless the symptoms of IED strongly overlap with ODD with chronic irritability-anger. IED cannot be diagnosed before age six years but unlike DMDD has no upper age limit. Analyses from the National Comorbidity Studies suggest little differentiation from ODD (Radwan & Coccaro, 2020).
- *DMDD*: This only occurs in DSM-5 and was introduced to stop irritable children being prescribed inappropriate powerful medications as often used in bipolar disorder. Onset should be before 10 years old and diagnosis not applied before 6 or after 18. The difference from ODD is that the severe and recurrent temper outbursts occur between episodes of anger or temper tantrums. Nonetheless, the intention to reduce antipsychotic prescribing has not been entirely successful, thus the survey by Findling *et al.* (2022) in the US found that fully 82% of children with DMDD were prescribed antipsychotics.
- *Autistic spectrum disorders (ASD)*: These are often accompanied by marked tantrums or destructiveness, which may be the reason for seeking a referral. As with ODD/CD, a lack of friendships may also be evident. Enquiring about other symptoms of ASD should reveal their presence. In particular, unlike children with ODD/CD who have CU traits, children with ASD fail to understand social situations and accurately judge the emotions of others.
- *Adjustment reaction*: This can be diagnosed when onset occurs soon after exposure to an identifiable psychosocial stressor such as divorce, bereavement, trauma, abuse, or adoption. The onset should be within one month for ICD-11, and three months for DSM-5, and symptoms should not persist for more than six months after the cessation of the stress or its sequelae (see Chapter 22).
- *Subcultural deviance*: Some youths are antisocial and commit crimes but are not particularly aggressive or defiant. They are well adjusted within a deviant peer culture that approves of recreational drug use, shoplifting, etc. Drug and alcohol usage should always be asked about, but often this will fall short of a diagnosable dependence syndrome, both in terms of symptoms and major impairment.

Box 65.1 Assessment at a glance

- assess duration of symptoms
- get teacher report as well as parent account
- elucidate family history of antisocial behavior
- assess cognitive ability, at least through getting reports of performance in school examinations
- assess presence of comorbid attention deficit hyperactivity disorder (ADHD), depression, and post-traumatic stress disorder (PTSD)
- check for callous-unemotional (CU) traits and irritability
- evaluate quality of parenting
- find positive aspects in child
- build a positive alliance with both parents and child

Formulation

The formulation should synthesize all that has been learned from the assessment about the child's predisposing, precipitating, perpetuating, and protective factors in an individualized narrative way, rather than simply impersonally applying a diagnosis. The first assessment session is crucial for engaging the family and identifying strengths that can be worked with to bring about therapeutic change.

Epidemiology

Overall prevalence

The overall prevalence of ODD and CD is around 5%, although this varies according to the methods used and the locality studied. In younger children ODD is more common than CD, in adolescents the opposite holds. Thus, the UK National Health Service (NHS) Digital Survey (NHS Digital, 2018) found a combined prevalence of ODD and CD of 7% in boys between 5–15 years old, but an increase from 3% in girls aged 5–10 up to 5% between 11–16. These rates are similar to the Christchurch (Fergusson *et al.*, 2015) and Dunedin (Caspi *et al.*, 2020) studies in New Zealand, and in four studies from the US (summarized in Merikangas *et al.*, 2022).

While CD is a leading cause of referral to mental health services, it is paradoxically one of the least widely recognized and studied psychiatric disorders (Fairchild *et al.*, 2019), although the more general term of antisocial behavior is more widely researched. The NHS Digital Survey (2018) used the same methods as previous surveys badged as the Office of National Statistics (ONS) and found no increase in ODD or CD over the last two decades.

Variations in prevalence

Gender

Boys outnumber girls by about 2:1 in younger children with ODD, but this ratio goes up for CD in adolescents to between 3:1 and 7:1. This is partly due to using menu-driven approaches, as found in DSM-5 and ICD-10, creating a bias in the conduct recorded, for example, forcing another person to have unwanted sex, using a weapon, and breaking into a house are far more common among boys. When surveys are published using general criteria, as found in ICD-11, behaviors that can be considered toward diagnosis include severe relational aggression, and serious rule breaking with frequent use of alcohol and drugs, so that more girls may get included. However, CD in girls is frequently missed; compared to boys with CD they have more emotional disorders, such as anxiety and depression, and borderline personality traits (Konrad *et al.*, 2022). Girls with CD are twice as likely to exhibit relational aggression, such as demeaning and humiliating other girls (Ackermann *et al.*, 2019).

Socioeconomic status

There is a strong gradient according to socioeconomic status (SES). Thus, for example, in the NHS Digital Survey ODD/CD was four times more common in the lowest SES than the highest (Piotrowska *et al.*, 2023).

Worldwide prevalence

Worldwide, many different rates have been reported, for example, 3.6% for CD and ODD in China (Li *et al.*, 2022), and hugely varying rates in the Middle East, from 0.34% in Iran, using structured interviews, to 33% using questionnaires only (Salmanian *et al.*, 2017). A worldwide pooled prevalence for any disruptive disorder found 5.7% prevalence (Polanczyk *et al.*, 2015).

High-risk populations

Rates of ODD/CD go up considerably in children who have been maltreated (see Chapter 25), who were brought up in residential care, or have been in foster care (see Chapter 42), children with intellectual disability (see Chapter 53), and, unsurprisingly, in young offenders (see Chapter 47).

Long-term outcome

Overall prognosis

Overall, ODD/CD is a condition with markedly poor long-term outcomes, which are summarized in Tables 65.1 and 65.2.

While the precise figures vary from study to study, the elevation in risk is considerable, particularly in cases that start young. Thus, for example, the Christchurch study (Fergusson *et al.*, 2005) found that the 5% most antisocial children (thus equivalent to a diagnosis of ODD/CD) aged 7 years had, at age 26 when compared to those who were not antisocial as children (50% of the sample), the following comparative outcome rates: violent offending 35% versus 3%, heavy drug usage 20% versus 5%, teenage pregnancy 20% versus 4%, leaving school with no exam qualifications 52% versus 6%, receiving state benefits 33% versus 9%. These huge differences in outcome were reduced once controlling for family SES, but still on average carried an increased odds ratio of around three-to-fourfold, an enormous difference.

As individuals with ODD/CD get older, offending reduces considerably in their 40s and 50s. However, this does not mean

Table 65.1 Longitudinal outcome/adult functioning of children who had oppositional defiant disorder/conduct disorder (ODD/CD).

Category	Longitudinal outcome/adult functioning (mean unadjusted odd ratios (OR) from several longitudinal studies included)
Criminal behavior	More violent and nonviolent crimes, e.g., mugging, grievous bodily harm; theft, car crimes, fraud *(OR 6.0)*
Mental health problems	Increased rates of antisocial personality, alcohol and drug abuse, anxiety, depression and somatic complaints, episodes of deliberate self-harm and completed suicide, time in psychiatric hospitals *(OR 5.8)*
Education and training	Poorer examination results, more truancy and early school leaving, fewer vocational qualifications *(OR 7.2)*
Employment	More unemployment, jobs held for shorter time, jobs of lower status with lower income, increased claiming of benefits and welfare *(OR 6.7)*
Social network	Fewer significant friends; friends more likely to be antisocial or in a gang; less constructive joint activities; less emotional confiding; low involvement with relatives, neighbors, clubs, and organizations *(OR 4.7)*
Intimate relationships	Increased rate of short-lived, violent cohabiting relationships including domestic violence; selection of partners who are often also antisocial *(OR 5.2)*
Children	Increased rates of child abuse, conduct problems in offspring, children taken into care *(OR 3.9)*
Health	More medical problems, earlier death by three years or more *(OR 8.1)*

Table 65.2 Factors predicting poor outcome.

Factor	Outcome
Onset	Early onset of severe problems, before age 8
Phenomenology	Antisocial acts which are severe, frequent, and varied; physical aggression; premeditated acts
Comorbidity	Hyperactivity and attention problems; callous-unemotional traits
Intelligence	Lower IQ
Family history	Parental criminality; parental alcoholism
Pregnancy	Heavy alcohol use
Parenting	Harsh, inconsistent parenting, with high criticism, low warmth, low involvement, and low supervision; interparental violence
Wider environment	Low-income family in poor neighborhood with ineffective schools

to say that their lives have become satisfactory. Thus, for example, the Cambridge study of delinquent development found that in the late 40s these individuals showed a high rate of "life failure" defined using multiple indices (Farrington *et al.*, 2023).

Health outcomes are also worse, including increased mortality. Thus, for example, Scott *et al.* (2017) found an almost threefold increase in mortality of individuals who had had ODD/CD in childhood. Langevin *et al.* (2022), using multiple biological indices, found increased biological aging in the early-onset life course persistent group, amounting to 4.3 extra years of biological aging, compared to low-antisocial individuals, by the age of 45.

Figure 65.1 demonstrates the considerable burden of CD. In 2019, in children and adolescents aged 5–14 years, the global rate of disability-adjusted life years (DALYs) caused by CD was about 9-fold higher than that caused by ADHD (262/100,000 versus 29/100,000).

Prognosis of subtypes according to age of onset and longitudinal course

Compared to children and young people who never exhibit antisocial behavior, three distinct patterns have been well replicated. The meta-analysis by Bevilacqua *et al.* (2018) of 13 longitudinal studies compared the three trajectories with high levels of problems against children who had low levels of conduct problems, as shown in Figure 65.2.

The worst outcome is seen in *early onset life-course persistent* (before the age of 8) problems, followed by the *adolescent onset* and, finally, *childhood limited* trajectories. The adolescent onset group tends to have normal neurocognitive profiles but mixes with a delinquent peer group, whereas both of the childhood onset groups have neurocognitive differences, including poorer executive functioning and lower IQ (Dotterer, 2021). While the two childhood onset groups have similar neurocognitive profiles, Odgers *et al.* (2007) found that the early onset life-course persistent trajectory had a strong family history of antisocial

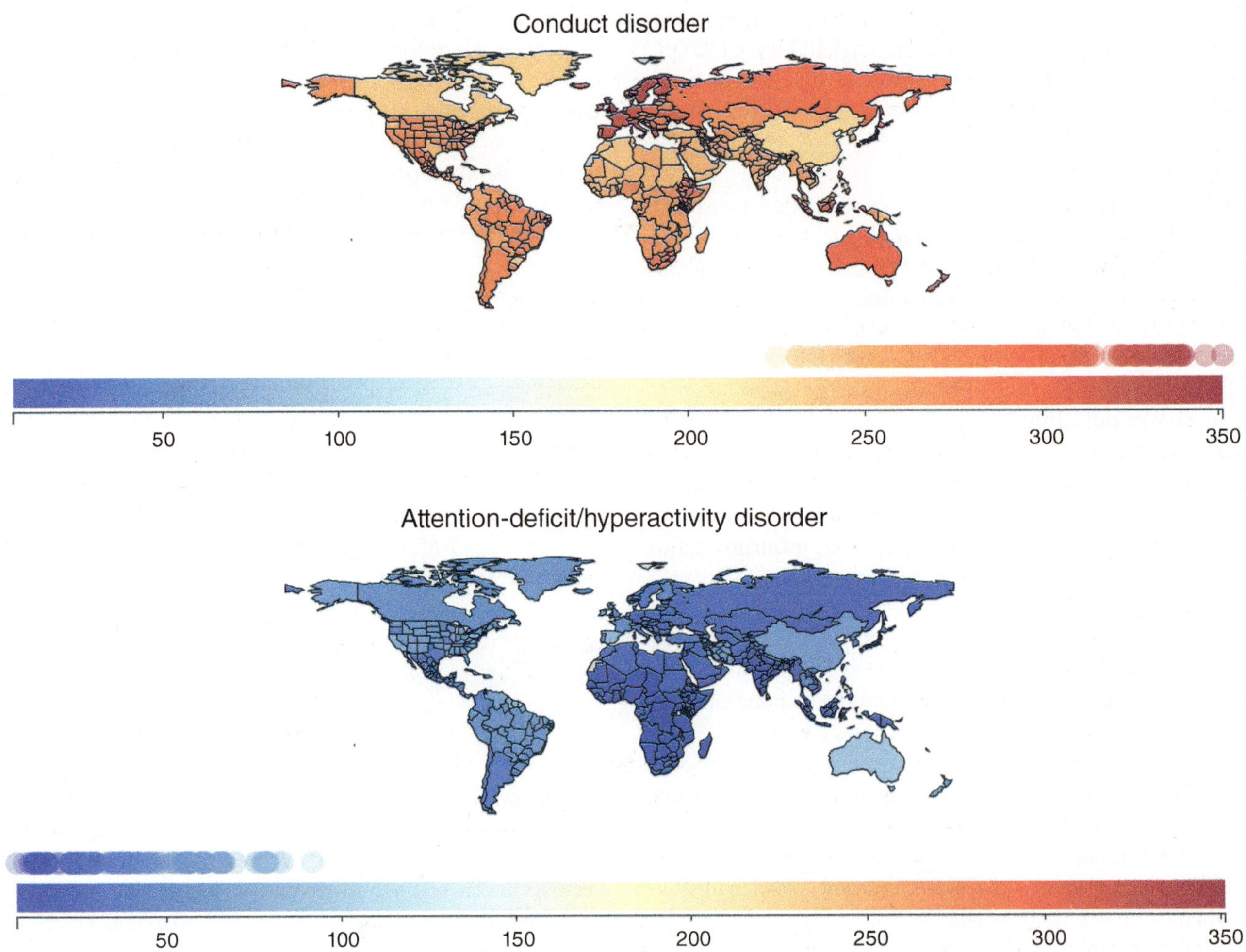

Figure 65.1 Global burden (in disability-adjusted life years [DALYs] per 100,000) of conduct disorder, in comparison to attention deficit hyperactivity disorder (ADHD), in 5–14-year-olds in 2019 (GBD 2019 Mental Disorders Collaborators (2022)). Dark red means high number of DALYs and dark blue means almost no DALYs (© Institute of Health Metrics and Evaluation, 2024).

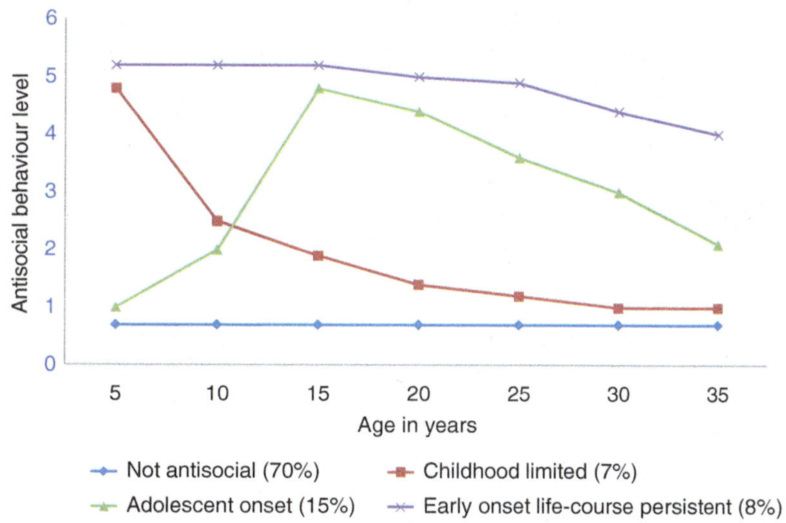

Figure 65.2 Subtypes of antisocial behavior by longitudinal course. The percentage figures in the key are the portions of the total study population.

behavior, and Barker and Maughan (2009) found they had more partner cruelty to the mother, received harsher general parenting, and had higher levels of child undercontrolled temperament.

Prognosis of subtypes according to associated phenomenology

In a classic paper, Stringaris and Goodman (2009) showed that dividing children with ODD into irritable, headstrong, and hurtful predicted different longitudinal outcomes. Those who display more irritable characteristics (angry outbursts and tantrums) were more likely to develop anxiety and depression (but not fears) in the following years, whereas those with headstrong characteristics (defiant and disobedient) were more likely to develop conduct disorder (see Chapters 4 and 5). The hurtful group (characterized by CU traits—see later section "Callous-unemotional traits" and Chapter 67) were more likely to develop aggressive conduct disorder and had a poorer overall prognosis. Both irritability and CU traits have been subject to intense research since the 2010s, see below under "Etiology."

DSM-5 keeps the category of antisocial personality disorder (ASPD). In DSM-5, ASPD cannot be diagnosed under 18, although it requires evidence of CD before 15 years. ICD-11 took the radical step of abolishing separate categories of personality disorder that had been present in ICD-10. Instead of separate categories, ICD-11 has trait domains of which one is "dissociality." ICD-11 has no lower age limit, but the criteria do not appear in the section on childhood disorders and clinicians are usually reluctant to apply the diagnosis outside adulthood (see Chapter 67).

Specifically, DSM-5 conceptualizes personality disorders as a combination of impairment in self/other functioning (Criterion A) and pathological traits (Criterion B). Impairment for ASPD includes egocentricity (identity), absence of prosocial standards (self-direction), lack of concern for others (empathy), and use of dominance to control others (intimacy). Pathological traits required are 6 of 7 traits from the antagonism (manipulativeness, callousness, deceitfulness, and hostility) and disinhibition (i.e., risk taking, impulsivity, and irresponsibility) domains. Additionally, DSM-5 has an alternative model for personality disorders (AMPD) that includes a psychopathy specifier, described by a "lack of anxiety or fear and by a bold interpersonal style that may mask maladaptive behaviors." This has proved quite controversial (Anderson & Kelly, 2022).

Factors that predict progression from ODD/CD to ASPD include early onset, a broad range of symptoms that are severe, ADHD symptoms, and CU traits (Blair *et al.*, 2014). When the majority of these are present, then over 50% of children progress to ASPD.

Follow back studies

A classic follow back study paper from the Dunedin sample looked at prior diagnoses aged 11–15 among adults with a range of disorders (Kim-Cohen *et al.*, 2003). While it might be expected that 60% of adults with ASPD had ODD/CD in childhood, it is perhaps more surprising that the commonest diagnosis in childhood of adults with eating disorders was ODD/CD (almost twice the rate of earlier anxiety), and the leading early diagnosis of adults who turned out to have manic-depressive disorder. Follow forward studies are now needed to see if treatment of ODD/CD in childhood prevents some of these outcomes.

Service use and cost

Both in childhood and in the longer term into adulthood, individuals with ODD/CD are expensive to society. In childhood, they and their families are in contact with multiple agencies. Use of social services is significantly higher than for children with emotional disorders. Over the longer term, by their mid-20s, children in the Inner London Study who had ODD/CD cost an average of ten times as much as controls (Scott *et al.*, 2001); in the Dunedin study, the 9% of children with early antisocial behavior were followed to age 38, and by then they had committed over half of all recorded crime (Rivenbark *et al.*, 2018). Apart from service use, substantial costs fall on the families in terms of lost opportunity to work (Romeo *et al.*, 2006). Rissanen *et al.* (2022) followed up over 5000 children in the Finnish national cohort data and by age 30, on health care and police costs alone, the high conduct problems group (11%) cost over four times more than the low conduct problems group (53%). Koegl and Farrington (2021) found that in Canada, already by age 20, the highest quartile of antisocial youth caught offending cost society on average CA$878,000. Adding in self-reported but undetected crime put the costs up to over CA$3.5 million.

Worldwide, the Global Burden of Disease study (GBD 2019 Mental Disorders Collaborators, 2022) had mental disorders as the seventh most burdensome across all medical conditions, and in children aged 0–14 years CDs were the number one (despite their estimate for prevalence at 0.6%, a serious underestimate).

Predictors of cost and implications

Early severity is the single biggest predictor of lifetime cost. Among children who had early conduct problems, perhaps unsurprisingly boys cost more than girls in all the studies cited above; a further early risk factor is less sensitive parenting, thus Bachmann *et al.* (2022) found that by mid teenage years, children exposed to less sensitive parenting (lowest quartile) between the ages of 4–6 had already cost society £22,000, whereas those in the upper quartile cost only £1,600; these differences were only modestly attenuated after controlling for several potential confounders including demographic variables, exposure to child abuse, IQ, and attachment security. An important mediator variable of these findings is child attachment; as the child grows up they internalize parental styles and values. The same group (Bachmann *et al.*, 2019, 2023a) found that insecurely attached children went on to cost considerably more than those that were securely attached.

Etiology

Below, a number of separate factors are discussed, and at the end of this section it is proposed that these need to be combined and evaluated for their contribution to any individual case, along with recognition that over the life course, different influences may hold different sway (see Chapter 1).

Individual-level influences

Overall genetic effects

It has become clear that for some subtypes, there is a strong genetic contribution. Reviews (e.g., Azeredo *et al.*, 2018; Salvatore & Dick, 2018) of twin and adoption studies have shown substantial genetic influences for those with CU traits, and those with

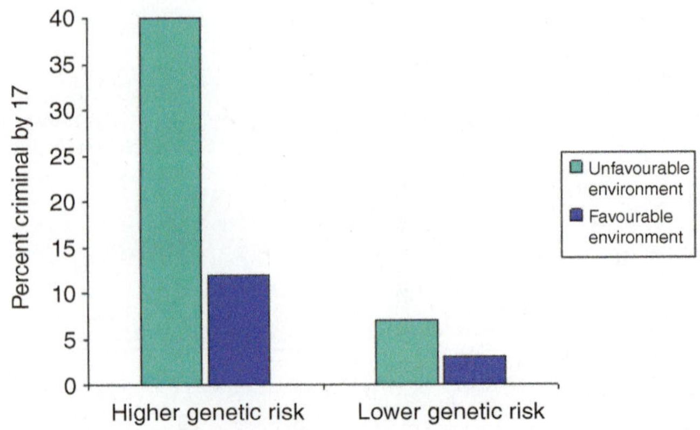

Figure 65.3 Percent of antisocial outcomes of early adopted children according to genetic risk and environmental risk (quality of adopting family).

comorbid ADHD, but environmental (chiefly nonshared) influences prevail where these are absent (see Chapter 21). Isen (2022), in a longitudinal twin study, showed that a persistent high level of antisocial behavior had significant heritability (67%). Adoption studies indicate a strong interaction between high genetic risk and a suboptimal rearing environment. Thus, a classic Swedish adoption study (Bohman, 1996; replicated by Kendler *et al.*, 2014) studied criminal outcome rates (known to police) in 17-year-olds whose biological parents had a criminal record or alcoholism, and whose adoptive parents had similar risk factors, versus these factors being absent. Strikingly, in the low genetic risk and low environmental risk, only 3% had a criminal record; in the low genetic risk and high environmental risk it was 7%; whereas in the high genetic risk and low environmental risk it was 12%, but an incredibly high rate of 40% was found where both were present, showing a strong interaction (Figure 65.3).

Specific genes

The main effects of several particular genotypes for antisocial behavior have been investigated but not reliably replicated (see Chapter 21). Likewise, genome-wide approaches to date have been disappointing for ODD/CD, polygenic risk scores typically accounting for 2% of the variance in the phenomenon (Tielbeek *et al.*, 2022).

Pregnancy and perinatal complications

Several influences during pregnancy have been associated with increased antisocial behavior in children. Thus, heavy maternal alcohol intake during pregnancy can lead to increased antisocial behavior as part of the fetal alcohol syndrome affecting the developing brain (see Chapter 20). Smoking is also associated with increases in antisocial behavior and ADHD, but sensitive designs suggest that this is not causal (Rice *et al.*, 2018).

Temperament

Individual differences in infancy that might contribute to subsequent risk of psychopathology were conceptualized by Thomas *et al.* in terms of temperament (Thomas *et al.*, 1968). Since then, several prospective studies have shown associations between early temperament and later conduct problems, as well as emotional problems (Sayal *et al.*, 2014). Traits usually identified are negative emotionality, poor emotional self-regulation, inattention, and restlessness.

Subtypes according to phenomenology

There have been numerous subdivisions of antisocial behavior using factor analytic techniques on cross-sectional data. They include overt antisocial behavior (tantrums, aggression) versus covert (lying and stealing); proactive aggression (premeditated, predatory attacks) versus reactive aggression (irritable lashing out only when provoked); physical aggression (hitting, biting) versus relational aggression (bullying, scapegoating, verbal insults); and antisocial behavior at home versus antisocial behavior at school. While factor analysis can produce these distinct subtypes, the problem is that often correlations between items across subtypes are as great as those within. Therefore, more robust ways of dividing up different antisocial phenomena are needed that are supported by several independent validating criteria cross-sectionally, such as family history, neuropsychological features, and response to treatment (for more about classification, see Chapter 2), in addition to prediction of longitudinal course. Two sets of characteristics that stand out and affect prognosis, as noted above, are irritability and CU traits.

Irritability

The trait of irritability cuts across diagnostic categories. Where it coexists with conduct problems in children, the longitudinal course makes depression and anxiety, and ADHD, more likely but *not* bipolar disorder. The link seems to be primarily genetic (Vidal-Ribas & Stringaris, 2021) and an underlying psychological process seems to be frustration at not being rewarded (Leibenluft & Kircanski, 2021). For a clinically relevant overview, see Stringaris (2018). Where it coexists in the presence of ADHD, stimulant medication seems to help (de la Cruz *et al.*, 2015 and see brief review by Breaux *et al.*, 2022).

Callous-unemotional traits

CU traits can be reliably identified in middle childhood, have substantial continuity to adulthood, and have a significant genetic contribution to their causation. Thus, in one twin study assessing children at age 7, antisocial children with CU traits had heritability of 81%, whereas in those with antisocial behavior but not CU traits, heritability was only 30% (Viding *et al.*, 2005). The systematic review by Moore *et al.* (2019) found a somewhat lower level of heritability, but, as yet, there have been no identified single genes or polygenic clusters that contribute to the trait. However, benign parenting can reduce the level and impact of the traits as shown by Hyde *et al.* (2016) in an adoption study which thus eliminated gene–environment correlation factors as an explanation for the association. It may be that a different set of genes are associated with initial expression of CU traits, as opposed to their waxing and waning during the life course (Takahashi *et al.*, 2021). A striking and well-replicated finding is that children who have high levels of CU traits have a specific deficit in fear recognition, and this can be detected as early as 5 years of age (White *et al.*, 2016).

Could CU traits be environmentally determined? It is not hard to imagine that a repeatedly abusive upbringing could lead children not to be able to trust in the affection of others or care about their feelings. While there is an association between maltreatment and CU traits, there are not yet sufficient genetically informative studies designed to disentangle whether the maltreatment is a reaction to these often very difficult children, or whether it is primarily causal (see meta-analysis by Todorov *et al.*, 2023). Robertson *et al.* (2023) show how bidirectional effects between antisocial behavior and trauma exposure can lead to the development of CU traits. As noted above in the section on "Prognosis of subtypes according to associated phenomenology," the presence of CU traits considerably increases the risk of progression to ASPD.

Brain function

Systems neuroscience studies (see Chapter 12) and brain-imaging studies (see Chapter 11) have been rather limited for ODD/CD in comparison to ADHD. Findings have often been contradictory or not replicated. Thus, Rogers *et al.* (2019) found white matter alterations in the corpus callosum, Zhou *et al.* (2016) found reduced functional connectivity between the dorsomedial nucleus and other regions, Fairchild *et al.* (2023) found alterations in inferior parietal cortical structure, and Gonzalez-Madruga *et al.* (2020) suggested that sex differences in retrosplenial cingulum connectivity may contribute to sex differences in CD. In a meta-analysis of emotion-processing experiments during functional magnetic resonance imaging (fMRI) in youths with conduct problems, Berluti *et al.* (2023) highlight differences in their brain regions associated with empathic responding, social learning, and facial processing. In a rare study looking at brain changes in response to treatment, Sethi *et al.* (2023) found hypoactivation of the amygdala in children who were resistant to a parenting programme intervention. In conclusion, we need more studies with larger samples to replicate any findings.

Language, IQ, and educational attainment deficits

Low IQ and low school achievement are important predictors of ODD/CD and delinquency. The Christchurch study found the IQ of children with ODD was 86, whereas for those without ODD it was 101 (Fergusson *et al.*, 2015); these findings are typical. In an English epidemiologic study of twins aged 13 years, low IQ of a child predicted conduct problems independently of social class and of the IQ of parents (Goodman *et al.*, 1995). While IQ tests that do not require reading tend not to show any reduction in verbal IQ compared to performance IQ in children with ODD/CD (Hobson *et al.*, 2011), reading and particularly spelling abilities (called by some dyslexia, see Chapter 52) are particularly impaired in around one-quarter of cases with ODD/CD (Visser *et al.*, 2020). Low IQ and reading and spelling problems can contribute to academic difficulties which, in turn, mean that school becomes unrewarding, rather than a source of self-esteem and a sense of achievement; low school attainment further adds to the probability of ODD/CD developing, even after allowing for IQ (Farrington *et al.*, 2023).

Executive dysfunction

Children and adolescents with conduct problems have been shown consistently to have poorer executive functions than typically developing controls. Almost invariably, the diminished executive functioning precedes the manifestations of conduct problems by several years. The meta-analysis by Figueiredo *et al.* (2023) found that effect sizes are significant (typically around 0.3 standard deviations) and domains affected include overall executive functioning, working memory, cognitive inhibition, behavioral inhibition, and cognitive flexibility. Hobson *et al.* (2011) showed that while both "cool" executive functions (motor inhibition, sustained attention, response execution) and "hot" executive functions (risky decision-making) were impaired in both ADHD and ODD/CD, it was only "hot" functioning that was specifically impaired in ODD/CD; these findings were maintained after controlling for IQ. The large study by Kohls *et al.* (2020) further found reduced emotion processing ability in terms of emotion recognition and regulation, with equal deficits among both boys and girls; their finding of impaired punishment learning was confirmed by Elster *et al.* (2024).

Autonomic reactivity and the hypothalamic–pituitary–adrenal axis

A low heart rate has been found consistently to be associated with antisocial behavior, and a meta-analysis of 114 studies suggested it is the best replicated biological correlate of antisocial behavior (Portnoy & Farrington, 2015). Other psychophysiological indicators of slow autonomic system reactivity have also been examined.

Information processing and social cognition

Dodge proposed the leading information-processing model for the genesis of aggressive behaviors within social interactions (Dodge *et al.*, 2022). The model hypothesizes, backed up by good experimental evidence, that children who are prone to aggression focus on threatening aspects of others' actions, interpret hostile intent in the neutral actions of others, and are more likely to select and to favor aggressive solutions to social challenges (Verhoef *et al.*, 2019). This has formed the basis of one form of cognitive therapy using virtual reality (Jo *et al.*, 2022).

Family-level influences

Child-rearing practices

There is ample evidence that ODD/CD is associated with less-than-optimal parenting practices, characterized by harsh, inconsistent discipline, low warmth and involvement, and high criticism (Farrington *et al.*, 2023). Several specific mechanisms operate. First, positive overtures and behaviors by children are ignored and so become extinguished. Second, negative behavior attracts parental attention, which even though it is usually critical and hostile, is nonetheless reinforcing where the overall context is one of being ignored. This is one of the central paradoxes in conduct problem families: parental behaviors that are aversive (and so reduce antisocial behavior) when sparingly applied in the context of plentiful warm interactions, become rewarding and promote oppositional and aggressive behaviors when children receive little other attention. Third, there is what Patterson (1982) called the negative reinforcement trap: a parent responds to mild oppositional behavior by a child with a prohibition to which the child responds by escalating their behavior, and mutual escalation continues until the parent backs off, thus teaching the child that if they get more aggressive, their parents will back off and they will get their way.

In considering the role of coercive processes in the origins or maintenance of conduct problems, we need to consider possible alternative explanations. Regarding common genetic liability, recent studies using genetically sensitive designs have shown that for both genetically related and genetically unrelated parents and children, there was a strong association between parent-to-child hostility and child antisocial behavior, suggesting that the effect is not just due to passive genotype–environment correlation (Klahr *et al.*, 2017). Regarding child effects on parents, there is considerable evidence that children's difficult behaviors do evoke parental negativity. ODD/CD children elicit more negative reactions from all groups of parents than do non-ODD/CD children. Adoption studies have shown that adoptees at genetic risk of antisocial disorders are more likely than low risk children to evoke negative parenting in the adoptive home (Klahr *et al.*, 2017).

The role of the child in influencing parental monitoring has also received attention. The complexity of the relationship was demonstrated in the E-risk longitudinal study by Wertz *et al.* (2016), who confirmed that as young adolescents became more antisocial, partly for genetically mediated reasons, their parents subsequently withdrew; then increased monitoring did not predict lower antisocial behavior later.

The fact that children's behaviors can evoke negative parenting does not, however, mean that negative parenting has no impact on children's behavior. As well as the cross-sectional observational studies mentioned above, several longitudinal studies indicate that it does. For example, the classic E-Risk longitudinal twin study showed that with identical twins, those whose mothers were more critical at 5 had greater antisocial behavior as rated by teachers at age 7, again controlling for initial levels of antisocial behavior (Jaffee *et al.*, 2005).

Attachment insecurity

Even before he had articulated his theory of attachment in detail, John Bowlby's (1944) study of juvenile thieves implicated their attachment to their parents. Insecure attachment patterns, especially disorganization (see Chapter 6), are fairly strongly associated with antisocial behavior. The meta-analysis by Fearon *et al.* (2010) found an effect size of the association of 0.58. Similar findings apply in adolescence (Scott *et al.*, 2011). However, most studies have not been designed to examine whether both attachment insecurity and antisocial behavior are different manifestations of harsh, inconsistent, and frightening parenting. An exception was the study by Scott *et al.* (2011), which examined whether attachment insecurity predicted antisocial behavior once parenting practice had been taken into account; they found that it did. Interestingly, CU traits are not associated with attachment status (Wright *et al.*, 2018), despite being associated with less warm parental behavior (Pauli *et al.*, 2021).

Exposure to interparental conflict and violence

For some time, studies have shown that children exposed to domestic violence between adults are subsequently more likely to become aggressive themselves. Social learning theory suggests that children's aggression may be increased because they imitate aggressive behavior modeled by their parents. More studies are needed however, to see the extent to which interparental conflict adds to child antisocial behavior over and above direct parent–child conflict. While some researchers find an additional effect, others find no extra contribution (Harold & Sellers, 2018).

Maltreatment and trauma

Physical punishment is widely used, and parents of children with conduct problems frequently resort to it out of desperation. Overall, associations between physical abuse and conduct problems are well established (see Chapter 25). Links with conduct problems are not, however, straightforward. The risk for conduct problems does not apply equally to all forms of physical punishment. The E-risk longitudinal twin study was able to compare the effects of corporal punishment (smacking, spanking) versus injurious physical maltreatment using twin-specific reports of both experiences (Jaffee *et al.*, 2005). Results showed that children's genetic endowment accounted for virtually all of the association between their corporal punishment and their conduct problems. This indicated a "child effect," in which children's bad conduct provokes their parents to use more corporal punishment, rather than the reverse. Findings about injurious physical maltreatment were the opposite. There was no child effect provoking maltreatment and, moreover, significant effects of maltreatment on child aggression remained after controlling for any genetic transmission of liability to aggression from antisocial parents.

The meta-analysis by Bernhard *et al.* (2018) found high rates of post-traumatic stress disorder (PTSD) in children with CD and especially young offenders, with a rate of 32% in the latter. Little is known about the possible mechanisms linking maltreatment to conduct problems, although threats to security of attachment, difficulties in affect regulation, distortions of information processing and self-concept, and failure to model and reward prosocial behavior are likely to be relevant. Further, Staginnus *et al.* (2023) found that CD youths with versus without maltreatment differ neurobiologically in their cortical structure. The introduction of the broader term "complex trauma" in ICD-11 has led to even higher rates of association with psychopathology and ODD/CD (Lewis *et al.*, 2021).

Influences beyond the family

Overview of peer effects

Observational studies show that children with ODD/CD have more negative interchanges with other children. Three processes could be at work: the child's individual conduct problems could lead them to have peer problems, or, vice versa, deviant peer relationships could lead to antisocial behavior, or, finally, some common factor could lead to both. Evidence has been found for all three effects.

Peer rejection and deviant peers

There is ample evidence that children with established conduct problems are more likely to have more conflict with peers, to be rejected by nondeviant peers, and to associate with other deviant children (Chen, 2015). Then, deviant youth reinforce each other's antisocial behaviors and attitudes. Antisocial young people who have deviant peers offend more, and increase their rates of antisocial acts and offending after joining a gang, reducing them if they leave the gang (Farrington *et al.*, 2023).

School effects

Children with ODD/CD are far more likely to attend schools with high delinquency rates, that have high levels of distrust between teachers and students, low pupil commitment to the school, and unclear and inconsistently enforced rules. However, it is less clear to what extent the schools themselves influence antisocial behavior, by their organization, climate, and practices, or to what extent the concentration of ODD/CD in certain schools is mainly a function of their intakes. In the Cambridge study, most of the variation between schools in their delinquency rates could be explained by differences in their intakes of troublesome boys (Farrington *et al.*, 2023).

Poverty

That antisocial children come in disproportionate numbers from poor families has been repeatedly confirmed; however, several studies show that the effect is indirect, disappearing after controlling for child-rearing practices. Many longitudinal studies have confirmed this (Farrington *et al.*, 2023). Furthermore, reducing poverty can reduce antisocial behavior, as seen in the "natural experiment" where Native American families in North Carolina, formerly living below the poverty line, benefited from increased income from newly opened casinos. Children's ODD/CD problems decreased (Copeland *et al.*, 2013).

Neighborhood influences

Young people with ODD/CD disproportionately live in inner-city areas characterized by physical deterioration, neighborhood disorganization, and high residential mobility. However, it is difficult to determine to what extent the areas themselves influence antisocial behavior and to what extent it is merely the case that antisocial people tend to live in deprived areas. The relation between community structural characteristics (concentrated poverty, racial heterogeneity, economic resources, and violent crime rate) and individual violence is largely mediated by parenting practices, gang membership, and peer violence (Jennings *et al.*, 2018). Kagawa *et al.* (2019) showed that in the US, children with CD were twice as likely to carry a gun.

Screen time

Nagata *et al.* (2023) found in the ABCD study that higher levels of screen time in 9–11-year-olds (whose mean was already 4 hours per day) were prospectively associated with a higher prevalence of new-onset ODD and CD, with social media especially implicated. However, the study did not control for a number of confounders so the association may not be causal.

Synthesis

The above account has shown that many different factors influence the development of ODD/CD. The question that arises is "How they may operate in the individual case?"; some but not other factors will be present. A number of points can be made. First, a number of these risks are intercorrelated; when measured together, some lose their significance. For example, neighborhood effects and SES are mostly mediated through parenting practices, which repeatedly emerge as a major factor. Second, where there are more highly heritable characteristics, such as inattention/hyperactivity, lower IQ, and CU traits, the prognosis is generally worse. Third, being subject to several risk factors seems to have a cumulative effect so that outcomes exponentially worsen. This seems likely to be due to interactions between child characteristics, such as temperament and the environment, whereby, for example, children with irritable, negative personalities do especially badly when they are brought up in a harsh and inconsistent manner.

Fourth, as antisocial children grow up, they shape their surroundings to some extent, including seeking out more risky environments. Over development, this makes the children more likely to remain in high-risk environments and have restricted opportunities for involvement in more positive relationships and roles. However, the counter of this is that those children and adolescents that have more positive experiences are more likely to desist from delinquency and get qualifications and employment (Farrington *et al.*, 2023). This provides potential optimism for treatment modalities that can provide positive experiences.

Treatment

The next sections will cover treatment; for prevention, please see Chapter 32.

Principles

Personalizing the treatment plan

The treatment plan should follow the assessment and fit the particular needs of the child and family. Intervention needs to be tailored according to the needs and strengths of the family, and be reasonably congruent with their beliefs, otherwise disengagement is particularly likely in this patient group whose lives are often not well organized and who are often suspicious of authority figures such as health professionals.

Engaging the family

Any family coming to a mental health service is likely to have some fears about being judged as bad and possibly mad. Dropout rates in treatment for conduct problem families can be high—the review of 262 studies by Chacko *et al.* (2016) found 25% of families recommended treatment did not enroll in the first place, and then a further 26% began but dropped out prematurely. Practical measures, such as assisting with transport, providing childcare, and holding sessions in the evening or at other times to suit the family help facilitate retention. Forming a good alliance with the family is especially important. Once engaged, the quality of the therapist's alliance with the family affects treatment success, accounting for 10–20% of the variance in outcome, although making a strong alliance is not just a characteristic of the therapist—more compliant families make it easier to plan constructive treatment jointly (Baier *et al.*, 2020).

Encouraging strengths

Identifying strengths of the young person and the family is crucial. This helps engagement, and increases the chances of effective treatment. Encouragement of abilities helps the child spend more time behaving constructively rather than destructively—e.g., more time spent playing football is less time spent hanging round the streets looking for trouble.

Choosing which treatment modality to use

The behavior may predominantly occur in the home, at school, with peers, or in the community; or it may be pervasive. Interventions need to address each context specifically, rather than assuming that successful treatment in one area will generalize to another. Thus, improvements in the home arising from a successful parent training program will not usually lead to fewer conduct problems at school—the meta-analysis by NICE (2013) found that despite a moderate-to-large effect-size (0.6 sd) at home, there was no carry-over at all to school. Therefore, for cases with difficulties that are mainly at home, parent training could be the first line of treatment. If classroom behavior is a problem and a school visit shows that the teacher is not using effective methods, then advice to the teacher and other school staff can be very effective (see later section, "Family interventions"). Where there are pervasive problems, including fights with peers, then individual work on anger management and social skills should be added; on its own, anger management is unlikely to be as successful as when it is combined with other approaches. For most cases, medication is controversial and generally best avoided; possible indications are discussed in the later section "Medication."

Treating comorbid conditions

In clinical referrals, comorbidity is the rule rather than the exception. As noted in earlier section "Differential diagnosis and formulation," common accompaniments are ADHD and depression; a number will have PTSD. In recent years, there has been increasing recognition of the overlap with ASD, where so-called challenging behavior often amounts to ODD (see Chapter 50), and that a minority will have CU traits. Each of these conditions requires appropriate management in their own right.

Promoting social and learning skills

Treatment involves more than the reduction of conduct problems—thus, for example, stopping tantrums and aggressive outbursts, while helpful, will not lead to good functioning if the child lacks the skills to make friends or to negotiate: positive behaviors need to be taught too. Specific learning disabilities such as reading retardation/dyslexia, which is particularly common in these children, require intervention, as do more general difficulties such as planning homework.

Following guidelines

A number of authoritative professional bodies have produced guidelines for the assessment and treatment or ODD/CD, although none in the US since 2007. In the UK, the National Institute for Health and Care Excellence (NICE) published a full guideline on *Antisocial Behavior and Conduct Disorders* in 2013 and updated it in 2017 (National Institute for Health and Care Excellence, 2017). In Germany, the child psychiatrists' professional association has published a similar evidence-based guideline (DGKJP, 2016), as has India (Sagar *et al.*, 2019). The approaches advocated here are consistent with each of these guidelines.

Availability of services

Unfortunately, although ODD/CD is arguably the commonest condition in child and adolescent mental health settings, with a very poor prognosis untreated, and despite the existence of treatments that are as effective as any in the field, the vast majority of children with antisocial behavior/ODD/CD remain neglected and abandoned by services. As Johnston and Burke (2020) put it "Most children with disruptive behavior disorders are neither identified as such nor engaged in treatment." This is reflected in administrative prevalence rates of ODD/CD in child and adolescent mental health services (CAMHS), where data is available. For example, it is 0.1% of the population in Denmark (Bachmann *et al.*, 2023b), and in the majority of UK CAMHS specifically exclude ODD/CD (Coghill, 2013). The review of US services by Ghandour *et al.* (2019) was more encouraging, with around 3.7% of the population getting treatment; in Germany the figure is 3.1% (Bachmann *et al.*, 2023b).

Family interventions

Parenting programs

Parent training programs are the mainstay of treatment of ODD/CD, especially with younger children below the age of about 11 years. They are designed to improve parents' behavior management skills and the quality of the parent–child relationship. Treatment can be delivered in individual parent–child appointments, or in a parenting group. Individual approaches offer the advantages of "*in vivo*" observation of the parent–child dyad and therapist coaching and feedback regarding progress; groups are more cost-effective and enable parents to learn from each other. Parenting programs are discussed in detail in Chapter 33.

The meta-analysis by Beelmann *et al.* (2022) of over 240 randomized controlled trials found that, overall, the mean effect-size for parenting programs was 0.47 for child conduct problems. Long-term effects have been studied. For example, Scott *et al.* (2014) found enduring effects at 8-year follow-up of a clinically referred sample of 4–8-year-olds with ODD reduced from 50% in the control group to 24% in the treated group. CU traits were also significantly reduced, suggesting that the progression to ASPD is less likely. However, parenting programs do not have many effects at school (e.g., Overbeek *et al.*, 2021). To address this, a number of interventions have taught teachers similar methods, getting positive outcomes, for example, in primary-school-age children (Ford *et al.*, 2019), and at secondary school the study by Bonell *et al.* (2018) reduced bullying, although in general school-based interventions are often not well implemented and effects can be weak (Caldwell *et al.*, 2021).

While some clinicians have expressed concerns that the use of time out from positive reinforcement might be harmful for maltreated children or those with attachment problems, Dadds and Tully (2019) have argued cogently that in the context of positive interactions engendered by parenting programs, short periods of time out can help, not hinder, the adjustment of children brought up in adversity. Moreover, the trial by Roach *et al.* (2022) found that a parenting program including time out had rather better outcomes for such children than those without adverse childhood experiences. However, as for most therapies, parent training does not work for all cases and there are few trials of what to do when it has failed. Moving from group to intensive individual work has been advocated, and Scott and Dadds (2009) provide a framework for tackling this in a systematic way by drawing upon attachment theory, family systems, and motivational interviewing. Hawes and Dadds (2021) offer further advice to clinicians where there is resistance to change. A trial is under way of a home-based parenting program for families who have not responded to a group-based approach or have declined to attend one (Senior *et al.*, 2023).

Online programs

Potentially, online programs are cheaper to deliver, with no need for travel, and if therapist involvement is reduced, access can be widened so that parents can engage with the program at a time convenient to themselves, for example, when the children are in bed, at weekends when they are not at work, and so on. Variants include doing live individual coaching but using mobile phones and laptops. This can be notably successful, with effect sizes similar to face-to-face therapy (Baumel *et al.*, 2017;

Engelbrektsson *et al.*, 2023). A number of programs have been transferred to an online platform (e.g., www.triplep.uk.net/uken/what-we-do/triple-p-online; https://parentingmatters.co.uk) and engaging with these can be supported by a therapist, either individually or in groups. Finally, parents can be offered the online program to do entirely on their own. However, the rate of completion in a universal context is only 10% or so (e.g., Dadds 2019). Completion rates are better for parents of children with significant behavior problems (Lintula *et al.*, 2024) when meta-analyses suggest that self-directed usage, without therapist support, can be effective (effect size 0.47 in a meta-analysis by Baumel *et al.*, 2017). However, for parents who are socially disadvantaged, meta-analysis suggests that without therapist support, self-directed programs are ineffective (Harris *et al.*, 2020).

Family systemic therapies for adolescents

Given the strong evidence reviewed above of effectiveness of parenting programs for prepubertal children, one might hope for similar effects among adolescents. However, while the review by von Sydow *et al.* (2013) was encouraging, more in-depth analyses of the two leading interventions cast doubt on their effectiveness outside the US. Functional family therapy (FFT) is a family-based intervention for youth with conduct problems that has been widely implemented in the US and other high-income countries. It is often described as an evidence-based program with consistent, positive effects. However, the Campbell meta-analysis (Littell *et al.*, 2023) found no evidence of effects of FFT compared with other active treatments on any primary outcomes. A more intensive intervention is multisystemic therapy (MST). Therapists engage family members in identifying and changing individual, family, and environmental factors thought to contribute to problem behavior. Rather like FFT, MST is widely considered to be a well-established, evidence-based program. However, the Campbell systematic review and meta-analysis (Littell *et al.*, 2021) found that after 1 year, MST reduced out-of-home placements and arrests in the US (OR 0.52), but not in other countries (OR 1.14). There was no overall evidence of effects on other primary outcomes. At 2.5 years, there was no overall evidence of effects on youth symptoms, substance abuse, peer relations, or school outcomes. Regarding possible "sleeper" effects, i.e., that the intervention might prove to be more effective at later follow-up, the model trial in the UK by Fonagy *et al.* (2020) found no effect on out-of-home placements at 18 months or arrests by police at 5 years.

Why the difference in the US/non-US outcomes? In the US, treatment as usual (TAU) consisted of relatively little contact and few services for youth and families, compared with relatively more robust public health and social services in other high-income countries. This is more likely to be the explanation, rather than investigator independence. Given these rather disheartening results of high-quality interventions delivered by dedicated and skilled staff, why are the findings often negative for adolescents, whereas those for children are much better? One possibility is that by adolescence an antisocial lifestyle has become more deeply ingrained in the character of the youth, and, second, that peer influences are considerably greater, with the young people spending more time with peers, being more concerned to get peer approval, and often being out-of-home and out of the control of their parents. Perhaps in future, peer-based interventions need to be invented and tested.

In the meantime, for adolescents displaying antisocial behavior, in the US the interventions above would be worth trying, whereas in other countries clinicians may wish to try skilled family work and cognitive behavioral therapy (CBT) which has at least some evidence (see next section "Individual child therapies").

Individual child therapies

CBT and social skills therapies for ODD/CD typically aim to: (i) reduce children's aggressive behavior such as shouting, pushing, and arguing; (ii) increase prosocial interactions such as entering a group, starting a conversation, participating in group activities, sharing, cooperating, asking questions politely, listening, and negotiating; (iii) correct the cognitive deficiencies, distortions, and inaccurate self-evaluation; and (iv) ameliorate emotional regulation and self-control problems so as to reduce emotional lability, impulsivity, and explosiveness, enabling the child to be more reflective and able to consider how best to respond in provoking situations.

An example is Lochman's Coping Power Program (Larson & Lochman, 2011). Treatment is delivered in groups of 5–7 children by two therapists. Sessions include imagined scenarios, therapist modeling, role plays with corrective feedback, and assignments to practice outside of sessions. Parent and teacher training components have been developed as adjunctive treatments. Evaluations demonstrate reductions in aggression and substance use, and improved social competence in some trials, many involving the program developers. However, the independent selective meta-analysis of 12 trials by McDaniel *et al.* (2023) found small-to-moderate reductions in antisocial behavior that were not statistically significant. For children with conduct problems, the literature is generally not supportive of the effectiveness of psychodynamic psychotherapy (Midgley *et al.*, 2021), although play therapy may help some antisocial behaviors, but seems less effective for aggression (Parker *et al.*, 2021). Mentalization-based therapy is now popular with adults who have ASPDs, and trials are underway for children with CD (Hauschild *et al.*, 2023). In female adolescents with conduct disorder, START NOW, a cognitive-behavioral, dialectical behavior therapy-oriented skills training program has shown promising results (Stadler *et al.*, 2023).

Medication

There are differing views as to the usefulness of medication in ODD/CD. Prescriptions of medications, particularly antipsychotics such as risperidone, are increasing considerably, especially in the US. In the UK, use of medication would not usually be supported as good practice because well-replicated trials of effectiveness are limited, particularly for children without ADHD, and there is a significant risk of unwanted side effects. Nonetheless, a recent study found that CD was the indication for 6.1% of antipsychotic prescriptions for youths in the UK (Radojčić *et al.*, 2023). The best-studied pharmacological interventions for children with comorbid ADHD and ODD/CD are psychostimulants (methylphenidate and dexamfetamine). In these circumstances, there is good evidence that reduction in hyperactivity/impulsivity also results in reduced conduct problems (see Chapter 54). There is insufficient reliable evidence to decide whether stimulants reduce aggression in the absence of ADHD.

Other pharmacological approaches for conduct problems and antisocial behavior have tended to target reactive aggression and overarousal, primarily in highly aggressive and psychiatrically hospitalized youth. Medications used in these conditions include antipsychotics. The Cochrane Review by Loy *et al.* (2017) found some support for short-term usage, but considerable caution needs to be exercised in using antipsychotics longer term, for example, with risperidone, as well as the side effects of weight gain and lipid metabolism change, tolerance may develop. Aripiprazole is now more often preferred. While medication is prescribed, it is important to continue to work at effective psychological management.

Box 65.2 Treatment at a glance

- form an alliance with parent by being nonblaming and sympathetic to their goals
- treat comorbid attention deficit hyperactivity disorder (ADHD) with stimulants, if possible
- offer group-based parent training if parents willing
- otherwise, offer individual parent training or online training supported by therapist
- consider anger management/cognitive behavioral therapy (CBT), if child willing and capable of engaging
- avoid antipsychotics and inpatient admission

Cost-effectiveness

Because of the high societal cost of ODD/CD, if interventions have enduring effects, they are likely to be highly cost-effective. Observational studies indicate considerable savings from families with better parenting: Bachmann *et al.* (2022) followed up 5-year-olds into adolescence and found the top quartile of parental sensitive responding cost £1,619 in service use, while the lowest quartile cost £21,763, differences that remained significant after controlling for multiple covariates. Chowdry and Fitzsimons (2016) calculated the UK costs of late (or no) intervention for antisocial behavior incidents at £701 million annually. True costs may be larger since there are problems with service use indices of costs, since service use will be low where there are few available services. And pediatric quality-of-life indices stress physical disabilities such as mobility, vision, and hearing, ignoring mental distress and effects on psychosocial functioning (van IJzendoorn & Bakermans-Kranenburg, 2020).

Despite these limitations, Sampaio *et al.* (2017) evaluated the cost-effectiveness of the Triple P parenting program and estimated the cost per DALY averted compared with a "no intervention" scenario in a cohort of 5–9-year-old children followed to age 18 years. They calculated the incremental cost-effectiveness ratio (ICER) at AU$1,013 per DALY averted for group program format and AU$20,498 when delivered in an individual format. Nystrand *et al.* (2019) found similarly positive cost savings across 5 parenting programs. The general reviews by Duncan *et al.* (2017) and Nystrand *et al.* (2020) indicate good cost-effectiveness but point out that families who drop out of studies do not get counted. In future, studies are needed of the cost-effectiveness of online programs, which could potentially be good value.

Conclusions

ODD and CD are prevalent and debilitating conditions worldwide, with poor outcomes for the individual and society if untreated. Exciting advances have been made in understanding factors that contribute to their development, including a much greater emphasis on genetic contributions than in the past; there is good evidence that these interact with suboptimal child-rearing to greatly increase the probability of developing the disorders. Treatment has become well established, especially through parenting programs, although more work is needed to develop effective interventions in adolescence. What is now needed is a recognition across society and by politicians that the quality of life of the families and individuals can be made so much better, while saving society money. In this way, it is to be hoped that treatment will become much more widely available. It may be that the development of online programs will pave the way for more cost-effective interventions. In the meantime, starting treatment before adolescence is far more likely to be effective.

References

Ackermann, K. *et al.* (2019) Relational aggression in adolescents with conduct disorder: sex differences and behavioral correlates. *Journal of Abnormal Child Psychology* **47**, 1625–1637.

American Psychiatric Association (2022) *Diagnostic and Statistical Manual of Mental Disorders*, 5th edn. text revision edn. American Psychiatric Association, Washington, DC.

Anderson, J. & Kelly, S. (2022) Antisocial personality and psychopathy: the AMPD in review. *Personality Disorders* **13**, 397–401.

Azeredo, A. *et al.* (2018) ADHD, CD, and ODD: systematic review of genetic and environmental risk factors. *Research in Developmental Disabilities* **82**, 10–19.

Bachmann, C. *et al.* (2019) The cost of love: financial consequences of insecure attachment in antisocial youth. *Journal of Child Psychology and Psychiatry* **60**, 1343–1350.

Bachmann, C. *et al.* (2022) A good investment: longer-term cost savings of sensitive parenting in childhood. *Journal of Child Psychology and Psychiatry* **63**, 78–87.

Bachmann, C. *et al.* (2023a) Secure attachment predicts lower societal cost amongst adolescents with high levels of antisocial behaviour. *Child and Adolescent Psychiatry and Mental Health* **17**, 56.

Bachmann, C. *et al.* (2023b) Prevalence and treatment of children and adolescents with conduct disorder: a real-world data study from four Western countries. *Child and Adolescent Psychiatry and Mental Health* **18**, 18.

Baier, A. *et al.* (2020) Therapeutic alliance as a mediator of change: a systematic review and evaluation of research. *Clinical Psychology Review* **82**, 101921.

Barker, E. & Maughan, B. (2009) Differentiating early-onset persistent versus childhood-limited conduct problem youth. *The American Journal of Psychiatry* **166**, 900–908.

Baumann, S. *et al.* (2022) Perpetrators and victims of cyberbullying among youth with conduct disorder. *European Child & Adolescent Psychiatry* **32**, 1643–1653.

Baumel, A. *et al.* (2017) Technology -assisted parent training programs for children and adolescents with disruptive behaviours: a systematic review. *Journal of Clinical Psychiatry* **78**, e957–e969.

Beelmann, A. *et al.* (2022) Parent training programs for preventing and treating antisocial behavior in children and adolescents: a comprehensive meta-analysis of international studies. *Aggression and Violent Behavior*, 68, 101798.

Berluti, K. *et al.* (2023) Emotion processing in youths with conduct problems: an fMRI meta-analysis. *Translational Psychiatry* **13**, 105.

Bernhard, A. *et al.* (2018) Association of trauma, posttraumatic stress disorder and conduct disorder: a systematic review and meta-analysis. *Neuroscience and Biobehavioral Reviews* **91**, 153–169.

Bevilacqua, L. *et al.* (2018) Conduct problems trajectories and psychosocial outcomes: a systematic review and meta-analysis. *European Child & Adolescent Psychiatry* **27**, 1239–1260.

Blair, J. *et al.* (2014) Conduct disorder and callous unemotional traits in youth. *The New England Journal of Medicine* **371**, 2207–2216.

Bohman, M. (1996) Predisposition to criminality: Swedish adoption studies in retrospect. In: *Genetics of Criminal and Antisocial Behaviour - Ciba Foundation Symposium 194.* (eds G. Bock & J. Goode). Wiley, Chichester, UK. pp. 99–114.

Bonell, C. *et al.* (2018) Effects of the learning together intervention on bullying and aggression in English secondary schools (INCLUSIVE): a cluster RCT. *The Lancet* **392**(10163), 2452–2464.

Bowlby, J. (1944) Forty-four juvenile thieves: their characters and home-life. *International Journal Psycho-Analysis* **25**, 107–127.

Breaux, R. *et al.* (2022) A mini-review of pharmacological and psychosocial interventions for reducing irritability among youth with ADHD. *Frontiers in Psychiatry* **13**, 794044.

Caldwell, D. *et al.* (2021) *School-based Interventions to Prevent Anxiety, Depression and Conduct Disorder in Children and Young People: A Systematic Review and Network Meta-Analysis.* NIHR Library, Southampton, UK.

Caspi, A. *et al.* (2020) Longitudinal assessment of mental health disorders and comorbidities across 4 decades among participants in the Dunedin birth cohort study. *JAMA Network Open* **3**, e203221.

Chacko, A. *et al.* (2016) Engagement in behavioral parent training: review of the literature and implications for practice. *Clinical Child and Family Psychology Review* **19**, 204–215.

Chen, D. (2015) A developmental perspective on peer rejection, deviant peer affiliation, and conduct problems among youth. *Child Psychiatry and Human Development* **46**, 823–838.

Chowdry, H. & Fitzsimons, P. (2016) *The Cost of Late Intervention: EIF Analysis 2016.* Early Intervention Foundation, London.

Coghill, D. (2013) Do clinical services need to take conduct disorder more seriously? *Journal of Child Psychology and Psychiatry* **54**, 921–923.

Copeland, W. *et al.* (2013) Prevalence, comorbidity, and correlates of DSM-5 proposed disruptive mood dysregulation disorder. *The American Journal of Psychiatry* **170**, 173–179.

Dadds, M. (2019) Keeping parents involved: predicting attrition in a self-directed, online program for childhood conduct problems. *Journal of Clinical Child and Adolescent Psychology* **48**, 881–893.

Dadds, M. & Tully, L. (2019) What is it to discipline a child? A reanalysis of time-out from the perspective of child mental health, attachment, and trauma. *The American Psychologist* **74**, 794–808.

de la Cruz, L. *et al.* (2015) Treatment of children with ADHD and irritability: results from the multimodal treatment study. *Journal of American Academy Child Adolescent Psychiatry* **54**, 62–70.

DGKJP (Deutsche Gesellschaft für Kinder- und Jugendpsychiatrie Psychosomatik und Psychotherapie) (2016) *S3-Leitlinie Störung des Sozialverhaltens.* AWMF, Bonn, Germany.

Dodge, K.A. *et al.* (2022) A defensive mindset: a pattern of social information processing that develops early and predicts life course outcomes. *Child Development* **93**, e357–e378.

Dotterer, H.L. (2021) Neurocognitive abilities associated with antisocial behavior with and without callous-unemotional traits. *Neuropsychology* **35**, 374–387.

Duncan, K. *et al.* (2017) Costs and savings of parenting interventions: systematic review. *Child: Care, Health Development* **43**(6), 797–811.

Elster, E. *et al.* (2024) Impaired punishment learning in conduct disorder. *Journal of the American Academy of Child and Adolescent Psychiatry* **63**(4), 454–463.

Emminghaus, H. (1887) *Die psychischen Störungen des Kindesalters.* Verlag der H. Laupp'schen Buchhandlung, Tübingen, Germany.

Engelbrektsson, J. *et al.* (2023) Parent training via internet or in Group for Disruptive Behaviors: a randomized clinical noninferiority trial. *Journal of the American Academy of Child and Adolescent Psychiatry* **62**(9), 987–997.

Fairchild, G. *et al.* (2019) Conduct disorder. *Nature Reviews Disease Primers* **5**(1), 43.

Fairchild, G. *et al.* (2023) Neuroanatomical markers of familial risk in adolescents with conduct disorder and their unaffected relatives. *Psychological Medicine* **53**, 1721–1731.

Farrington, D.P. *et al.* (2023) *Offending from Childhood to Late Middle Age: Recent Results from the Cambridge Study in Delinquent Development.* Springer Nature, New York.

Fearon, R.P. *et al.* (2010) The significance of insecure attachment and disorganisation in the development of children's externalising behaviour: a meta-analysis. *Child Development* **81**, 435–456.

Fergusson, D. *et al.* (2005) Show me the child at seven: the consequences of conduct problems in childhood for psychosocial functioning in adulthood. *Journal of Child Psychology and Psychiatry* **46**, 837–849.

Fergusson, D. *et al.* (2015) From evidence to policy: findings from the Christchurch health and development study. *Australian & NZ Journal Criminology* **48**, 386–408. doi:10.1177/0004865815589827.

Figueiredo, P. *et al.* (2023) Executive (dys)functions and ODD and CD: a systematic review and meta-analysis. *Neuropsychology* **37**, 133–156.

Findling, R. *et al.* (2022) Diagnostic trends and prescription patterns in disruptive mood dysregulation disorder and bipolar disorder.

Journal of the American Academy of Child and Adolescent Psychiatry **61**, 434–445. doi:10.1016/j.jaac.2021.05.016.

Fonagy, P. *et al.* (2020) Multisystemic therapy versus management as usual in the treatment of adolescent antisocial behaviour (START): 5-year follow-up of a pragmatic RCT. *The Lancet Psychiatry* **7**, 420–430.

Ford, T. *et al.* (2019) The effectiveness and cost-effectiveness of the Incredible Years Teacher Classroom Management programme in primary school children: results of the STARS cluster randomised controlled trial. *Psychological Medicine* **49**(5), 828–842.

GBD 2019 Mental Disorders Collaborators (2022) Global, regional, and national burden of 12 mental disorders in 204 countries and territories, 1990-2019: a systematic analysis. *The Lancet Psychiatry* **9**, 137–150.

Ghandour, R. *et al.* (2019) Prevalence and treatment of depression, anxiety, and conduct problems in US children. *The Journal of Pediatrics* **206**, 256–267.e253.

Gomes, H.S. *et al.* (2018) Measuring offending: self-reports, official records, systematic observation and experimentation. *Crime Psychology Review* **4**(1), 26–44.

González-Madruga, K. *et al.* (2020) White matter microstructure of the extended limbic system in male and female youth with conduct disorder. *Psychological Medicine* **50**, 58–67.

Goodman, R. & Scott, S. (1999) Comparing the Strengths and Difficulties Questionnaire and the Child Behaviour Checklist: Is small beautiful? *Journal of Abnormal Child Psychology* **27**, 17–24.

Goodman, R. *et al.* (1995) The impact of child IQ, parent IQ and sibling IQ on child behavioral-deviance scores. *Journal of Child Psychology and Psychiatry* **36**, 409–425.

Harold, G. & Sellers, R. (2018) Annual research review: Interparental conflict and youth psychopathology: an evidence review and practice focused update. *Journal of Child Psychology and Psychiatry* **59**, 374–402.

Harris, M. *et al.* (2020) Technology-assisted parenting interventions for families experiencing social disadvantage: a meta-analysis. *Prevention Science* **21**, 714–727.

Hauschild, S. *et al.* (2023) Mentalization-based treatment for adolescents with conduct disorder: feasibility study. *European Child & Adolescent Psychiatry* **32**, 2611–2622. doi:10.1007/s00787-022-02113-4.

Hawes, D. & Dadds, M. (2021) Practitioner review: Parenting interventions for child conduct problems: reconceptualising resistance to change. *Journal of Child Psychology and Psychiatry* **62**, 1166–1174.

Hobson, C. *et al.* (2011) Investigation of cool and hot executive function in ODD/CD independently of ADHD. *Journal of Child Psychology and Psychiatry* **52**, 1035–1043.

Hyde, L. *et al.* (2016) Heritable and nonheritable pathways to early callous-unemotional behaviors. *The American Journal of Psychiatry* **173**, 903–910.

Institute for Health Metrics and Evaluation (2024). GBD Compare Data Visualization. Institute for Health Metrics and Evaluation (IHME), University of Washington, Seattle, WA. Available: http://vizhub.healthdata.org/gbd-compare (4 January2025).

Isen, J. (2022) Developmental trajectories of delinquent and aggressive behavior: evidence for differential heritability. *Human Development* **53**, 199–211.

Jaffee, S. *et al.* (2005) Nature x nurture: genetic vulnerabilities interact with physical maltreatment to promote conduct problems. *Development and Psychopathology* **17**, 67–84.

Jennings, W. *et al.* (2018) Conduct disorder and neighborhood effects. *Annual Review of Clinical Psychology* **14**, 317–341.

Jo, H.-J. *et al.* (2022) The applicability of virtual reality-based training for controlling anger in aggressive individuals. *Cyberpsychology, Behavior, and Social Networking* **25**, 278–286.

Johnston, O.G. & Burke, J.D. (2020) Parental problem recognition and help-seeking for disruptive behavior disorders. *The Journal of Behavioral Health Services & Research* **47**, 146–163.

Kagawa, R. *et al.* (2019) Psychiatric disorders and gun carrying among adolescents in the United States. *Journal of Pediatrics* **209**, 198–203. doi:10.1016/j.jpeds.2019.01.010.

Karpman, B. (1947) Moral agenesis. *Psychiatric Quarterly* **21**(3), 361–398.

Kendler, K. *et al.* (2014) A Swedish national adoption study of criminality. *Psychological Medicine* **44**, 1913–1925. doi:10.1017/S0033291713002638.

Kim-Cohen, J. *et al.* (2003) Prior juvenile diagnoses in adults with mental disorder: developmental follow-back of a prospective-longitudinal cohort. *Archives of General Psychiatry* **60**, 709–717.

Klahr, A. *et al.* (2017) Birth and adoptive parent antisocial behavior and parenting: a study of evocative gene–environment correlation. *Child Development* **88**, 505–513.

Koegl, C.J. & Farrington, D.P. (2021) Estimating the monetary cost of risk factors for crime in boys using the EARL-20B. *Psychological Services* **18**(4), 441–453.

Kohls, G. *et al.* (2020) Investigating sex differences in emotion recognition, learning, and regulation among youths with conduct disorder. *Journal of the American Academy of Child and Adolescent Psychiatry* **59**, 263–273.

Konrad, K. *et al.* (2022) Sex differences in psychiatric comorbidity and clinical presentation in youths with conduct disorder. *Journal of Child Psychology and Psychiatry* **63**, 218–228.

Kramer, F. & von der Leyen, R. (1934) Entwicklungsverläufe "anethischer, gemütloser" psychopathischer Kinder. *Zeitschrift für Kinderforschung* **43**, 305–422.

Langevin, S. *et al.* (2022) Life-course persistent antisocial behavior and accelerated biological aging in a longitudinal birth cohort. *International Journal of Environmental Research and Public Health* **19**(21), 14402.

Larson, J. & Lochman, J. (2011) *Helping Schoolchildren Cope with Anger: A Cognitive-behavioral Intervention*, 2nd edn. Guilford Press, New York.

Leibenluft, E. & Kircanski, K. (2021) Chronic irritability in youth: a reprise on challenges and opportunities toward meeting unmet clinical needs. *Child and Adolescent Psychiatric Clinics of North America* **30**, 667–683.

Lewis, S. *et al.* (2021) Unravelling the contribution of complex trauma to psychopathology and cognitive deficits: a cohort study. *The British Journal of Psychiatry* **219**, 448–455.

Li, F. *et al.* (2022) Prevalence of mental disorders in school children and adolescents in China: diagnostic data from detailed clinical assessments of 17,524 individuals. *Journal of Child Psychology and Psychiatry* **63**, 34–46.

Lintula, S. *et al.* (2024) Enrollment and completion rates of a nationwide guided digital parenting program for children with disruptive behavior before and during COVID-19. *European Child & Adolescent Psychiatry.* doi:10.1007/s00787-024-02523-6.

Littell, J.H. *et al.* (2021) Multisystemic therapy® for social, emotional, and behavioural problems in youth age 10 to 17: an updated systematic review and meta-analysis. *Campbell Systematic Reviews* **17**(4), e1158.

Littell, J.H. *et al.* (2023) Functional family therapy for families of youth (age 11-18) with behaviour problems: a systematic review and meta-analysis. *Campbell Systematic Reviews* **19**(3), e1324.

Loy, J.H. *et al.* (2017) Atypical antipsychotics for disruptive behaviour disorders in children and youths. *Cochrane Database of Systematic Reviews* **8**, CD008559.

Maudsley, H. (1895) *The Pathology of Mind*. Macmillan, London.

McDaniel, S. *et al.* (2023) Systematic literature review and meta-analysis of coping power: effects and implications for implementation. *Journal of Applied School Psychology* **39**(4), 1–25.

Merikangas, K. *et al.* (2022) Epidemiology of mental disorders in children and adolescents. *Dialogues of Clinical Neuroscience* **11**(1), 7–20.

Midgley, N. *et al.* (2021) The evidence-base for psychodynamic psychotherapy with children and adolescents: a narrative synthesis. *Frontiers in Psychology* **12**, 662671.

Moore, A. *et al.* (2019) The genetic underpinnings of callous-unemotional traits: a systematic research review. *Neuroscience and Biobehavioral Reviews* **100**, 85–97.

Morales-Vives, F. *et al.* (2019) The inventory of callous-unemotional traits and antisocial behavior (INCA) for young people: development and validation in a community sample. *Frontiers in Psychology* **10**, 713.

Nagata, J. *et al.* (2023) Contemporary screen time modalities and disruptive behavior disorders in children: a prospective cohort study. *Journal of Child Psychology and Psychiatry* **64**(1), 125–135.

National Institute for Health and Care Excellence (2013) Antisocial Behaviour and Conduct Disorders in Children and Young People: Recognition and Management. Clinical guideline, updated 2017 National Institute for Health and Care Excellence (NICE), London.

NHS Digital (2018) *Mental Health of Children and Young People in England, 2017: Behavioural Disorders*. NHS Digital, London.

Nystrand, C. *et al.* (2019) Cost-effectiveness analysis of parenting interventions for the prevention of behaviour problems in children. *PLoS One* **14**(12), e0225503.

Nystrand, C. *et al.* (2020) Economic return on investment of parent training programmes for the prevention of child externalising behaviour problems. *Admininistration and Policy in Mental Health* **47**(2), 300–315.

Odgers, C. *et al.* (2007) Predicting prognosis for the conduct-problem boy: Can family history help? *Journal of the American Academy of Child and Adolescent Psychiatry* **46**, 1240–1249.

Overbeek, G. *et al.* (2021) Longer-term outcomes of the incredible years parenting intervention. *Prevention Science* **22**, 419–431.

Parker, M. *et al.* (2021) Exploring the impact of child-centered play therapy for children exhibiting behavioral problems: a meta-analysis. *International Journal of Play Therapy* **30**, 259–271.

Patterson, G. (1982) *Coercive Family Process*. Castalia, Eugene, OR.

Pauli, R. *et al.* (2021) Positive and negative parenting in conduct disorder with high versus low levels of callous-unemotional traits. *Development and Psychopathology* **33**, 980–991.

Piotrowska, P. *et al.* (2023) Understanding the relationship between family income and conduct problems: findings from the mental health of children and young people survey. *Psychological Medicine* **53**, 3987–3994.

Polanczyk, G. *et al.* (2015) Annual research review: a meta-analysis of the worldwide prevalence of mental disorders in children and adolescents. *Journal of Child Psychology and Psychiatry* **56**, 345–365.

Portnoy, J. & Farrington, D. (2015) Resting heart rate and antisocial behavior: an updated systematic review and meta-analysis. *Aggression and Violent Behavior* **22**, 33–45.

Radojčić, M.R. *et al.* (2023) Trends in antipsychotic prescribing to children and adolescents in England: cohort study using 2000–19 primary care data. *The Lancet Psychiatry* **10**, 119–128.

Radwan, K. & Coccaro, E.F. (2020) Comorbidity of disruptive behavior disorders and intermittent explosive disorder. *Child and Adolescent Psychiatry and Mental Health* **14**, 24.

Ray, J.V. & Frick, P.J. (2020) Assessing callous-unemotional traits using the total score from the inventory of callous-unemotional traits: a meta-analysis. *Journal of Clinical Child & Adolescent Psychology* **49**, 190–199.

Rice, F. *et al.* (2018) Identifying the contribution of prenatal risk factors to offspring development and psychopathology: what designs to use and a critique of literature on maternal smoking and stress in pregnancy. *Development and Psychopathology* **30**(3), 1107–1128.

Rissanen, E. *et al.* (2022) The long-term cost of childhood conduct problems: Finnish Nationwide 1981 birth cohort study. *Journal of Child Psychology and Psychiatry* **63**, 683–692.

Rivenbark, J. *et al.* (2018) The high societal costs of childhood conduct problems: evidence from administrative records up to age 38 in a longitudinal birth cohort. *Journal of Child Psychology and Psychiatry* **59**, 703–710.

Roach, A.C. *et al.* (2022) Using time-out for child conduct problems in the context of trauma and adversity: A nonrandomized controlled trial. *JAMA Network Open* **5**(9), e2229726.

Robertson, E. *et al.* (2023) The bidirectional effects of antisocial behavior, anxiety, and trauma exposure: implications for our understanding of the development of callous-unemotional traits. *Journal of Psychopathology and Clinical Science* **132**, 445–460.

Rogers, J. *et al.* (2019) White matter microstructure in youths with conduct disorder: effects of sex and variation in callous traits. *Journal of the American Academy of Child and Adolescent Psychiatry* **58**(12), 1184–1196.

Romeo, R. *et al.* (2006) The economic cost of severe antisocial behaviour in children, and who for pays it. *The British Journal of Psychiatry* **188**, 547–553.

Rowe, R. *et al.* (2002) The relationship between DSM-IV oppositional defiant disorder and conduct disorder: findings from the Great Smoky Mountains study. *Journal Child Psychology and Psychiatry* **43**, 365–373. doi:10.1111/1469-7610.00027.

Rowe, R. *et al.* (2010) Developmental pathways in oppositional defiant disorder and conduct disorder. *Journal of Abnormal Psychology* **119**, 726–738. doi:10.1037/a0020798.

Sagar, R. *et al.* (2019) Clinical practice guidelines for the management of conduct disorder. *Indian Journal of Psychiatry* **61**(Suppl 2), 270–276.

Salmanian, M. *et al.* (2017) A systematic review on the prevalence of conduct disorder in the Middle East. *Social Psychiatry and Psychiatric Epidemiology* **52**, 1337–1343.

Salvatore, J. & Dick, M. (2018) Genetic influences on conduct disorder. *Neuroscience and Biobehavioral Reviews* **91**, 91–101.

Sampaio, F. *et al.* (2017) Population cost-effectiveness of the Triple P parenting programme for the treatment of conduct disorder: an economic modelling study. *European Child & Adolescent Psychiatry* **27**, 933–944.

Sayal, K. *et al.* (2014) Infant temperament and childhood psychiatric disorder. *Child: Care, Health and Development* **40**, 292–297.

Scott, J. *et al.* (2017) Mortality in individuals with disruptive behavior disorders diagnosed by specialist services: a nationwide cohort study. *Psychiatry Research* **251**, 255–260.

Scott, S. (2022) Debate: 'A rose by any other name would smell as sweet': myths peddled about the ills of diagnosing conduct disorders. *Child and Adolescent Mental Health* **27**, 302–304.

Scott, S. & Dadds, M. (2009) When parent training doesn't work: theory-driven clinical strategies. *Journal of Child Psychology and Psychiatry* **50**, 1441–1450.

Scott, S. *et al.* (2001) Financial cost of social exclusion: Follow up study of antisocial children into adulthood. *BMJ* **323**, 191–194.

Scott, S. *et al.* (2011) Attachment in adolescence: overlap with parenting and unique prediction of behavioural adjustment. *Journal of Child Psychology and Psychiatry* **52**, 1052–1062.

Scott, S. *et al.* (2014) Early prevention of antisocial personality: long-term follow-up of two randomized controlled trials comparing indicated and selective approaches. *The American Journal of Psychiatry* **171**, 649–657.

Senior, R. et al. (2023) Personalised interventions for parents who have children with behaviour problems: registered trial protocol. Available: https://www.isrctn.com/ISRCTN15678369 [12 December 2024].

Sethi, A. *et al.* (2023) Selective amygdala hypoactivity to fear in boys with persistent conduct problems after parent training. *Biological Psychiatry* **94**, 50–56.

Stadler, C. *et al.* (2023) START NOW: a cognitive behavioral skills training for adolescent girls with conduct or oppositional defiant disorder a randomized clinical trial. *Journal of Child Psychology and Psychiatry* **65**(3), 316–327. doi:10.1111/jcpp.13896.

Staginnus, M. *et al.* (2023) Testing the ecophenotype model: cortical structure alterations in conduct disorder with versus without childhood maltreatment. *Biological Psychiatry: Cognitive Neuroscience and Neuroimaging* **8**, 609–619.

Stringaris, A. & Goodman, R. (2009) Longitudinal outcome of youth oppositionality: Irritable, headstrong, and hurtful behaviors. *Journal of the American Academy of Child and Adolescent Psychiatry* **48**, 404–412.

Stringaris, A. *et al.* (2012) The Affective Reactivity Index: a concise irritability scale for clinical and research settings. *Journal of Child Psychology and Psychiatry* **53**, 1109–1117.

Stringaris, A. *et al.* (2018) Practitioner review: definition, recognition, and treatment challenges of irritability in young people. *Journal of Child Psychology and Psychiatry* **59**, 721–739.

Takahashi, Y. *et al.* (2021) Genetic and environmental influences on the developmental trajectory of callous-unemotional traits from childhood to adolescence. *Journal of Child Psychology and Psychiatry* **62**(4), 414–423.

Thomas, A. *et al.* (1968) *Temperament and Behaviour Disorders in Children.* New York University Press, New York.

Tielbeek, J. *et al.* (2022) Uncovering the genetic architecture of broad antisocial behavior through a genome-wide association study meta-analysis. *Molecular Psychiatry* **27**, 4453–4463.

Todorov, J. *et al.* (2023) Association between childhood maltreatment and callous-unemotional traits in youth: a meta-analysis. *Neuroscience and Biobehavioral Reviews* **146**, 105049.

van IJzendoorn, M. & Bakermans-Kranenburg, M. (2020) Problematic cost-utility analysis of interventions for behavior problems in children and adolescents. *New Directions for Child and Adolescent Development* **2020**(172), 89–102.

Verhoef, R. *et al.* (2019) Hostile intent attribution and aggressive behavior in children revisited: a meta-analysis. *Child Development* **90**(5), e525–e547.

Vidal-Ribas, P. & Stringaris, A. (2021) How and why are irritability and depression linked? *Child and Adolescent Psychiatric Clinics of North America* **30**, 401–414.

Viding, E. *et al.* (2005) Evidence for substantial genetic risk for psychopathy in 7-year-olds. *Journal of Child Psychology and Psychiatry* **46**, 592–597.

Visser, L. *et al.* (2020) Comorbidities between specific learning disorders and psychopathology in elementary school children. *Frontiers in Psychiatry* **28**(11), 292. doi:10.3389/fpsyt.2020.00292.

von Sydow, K. *et al.* (2013) The efficacy of systemic therapy for childhood and adolescent externalizing disorders: A systematic review of 47 RCTs. *Family Process* **52**, 576–618.

Wertz, J. *et al.* (2016) Parental monitoring and knowledge: testing bidirectional associations with youths' antisocial behavior. *Development and Psychopathology* **28**, 623–638.

White, S. *et al.* (2016) Can the fear recognition deficits associated with callous-unemotional traits be identified in early childhood? *Journal of Clinical and Experimental Neuropsychology* **38**, 672–684.

World Health Organization (2019) *International Statistical Classification of Disease and Related Health Problems*, 11th edn. World Health Organization (WHO), Geneva, Switzerland.

Wright, N. *et al.* (2018) Maternal sensitivity to distress, attachment and the development of callous-unemotional traits in young children. *Journal of Child Psychology and Psychiatry* **59**(7), 790–800.

Zhou, J. *et al.* (2016) Disrupted default mode network connectivity in male adolescents with conduct disorder. *Brain Imaging and Behavior* **10**, 995–1003.

CHAPTER 66

Substance use and substance use disorder

Eilish Gilvarry

[1] Faculty of Medical Sciences, Newcastle University, Newcastle-upon-Tyne, UK

[2] Addictions Unit, Cumbria, Northumberland, Tyne and Wear NHS Foundation Trust, Newcastle-upon-Tyne, UK

Introduction

Initiation of substance use generally occurs in mid adolescence and often peaks in early adulthood (Degenhardt *et al.*, 2016). Most individuals with substance use disorders (SUDs) initiate use prior to 18 years, with more than 95% initiating use before age 25 years. In adolescence, the pattern of use is often experimental and opportunistic, and sometimes recreational, though some patterns may progress to dependence and daily use. Both genetic and environmental risk factors can increase the risk for continuation and problematic use. Even with experimentation, significant adverse problems can result, for example, related to intoxication and related injury.

There is substantial variation among youth in different countries and cultures in terms of age of onset, types and patterns of use, and amounts used. This demonstrates that young people's use depends on their environment, culture, and social context, which affect drug availability and other factors related to use. Adolescent SUD is associated with adverse consequences; school underachievement, premature mortality, family dysfunction, physical health issues, mental health, and many other problems (Kendler *et al.*, 2020).

Alcohol and drug use contribute substantially to the global burden of disease, through SUDs and from the consequences of use, for example, unintentional injuries, suicide, and multiple medical problems. The global burden of disease related to SUD has increased, with over 5.1% attributable to alcohol as measured by disability-adjusted life years (DALYs) (Degenhardt *et al.*, 2018). Castelpietra *et al.* (2022) reported on the burden in Europe for mental disorders and SUDs from 1990 in those aged 10–24 years. In 2019, per 100,000 population rates were 16,983 for mental disorders and 3,891 for SUDs. Over a 30-year period, there was an increased burden related to drug use disorder (DUD). Lower social economic development was positively associated with mental health disorders and SUDs. The authors advocated mental disorders and SUDs to be a public health priority.

This chapter will discuss classification, prevalence and trends, risk and protective factors, the main substances of abuse and their harms, clinical responses to use and dependence that include public health, psychosocial, and pharmacological interventions, and management of comorbid mental health problems, treatment settings, and models of specialist services.

Classification

The *Diagnostic and Statistical Manual of Mental Disorders,* 5th edition, text revision (DSM-5-TR; American Psychiatric Association, 2022), like DSM-5, uses one category of "SUD". It recognizes disorders resulting from the use of 10 separate classes of drugs and allows clinicians to specify 3 levels of severity—mild, moderate, and severe—reflecting the number of symptoms from a list of 11.

The *International Classification of Disease,* 11th revision (ICD-11) has a new grouping related to substance use—"Disorders due to Substance Use and Addictive Behaviors." Conditions in this group are described as follows: "disorders due to substance use and addictive behaviors are mental and behavioral disorders that develop as a result of the use of predominately psychoactive substances, including medications, or specific repetitive rewarding and reinforcing behaviors" (World Health Organization, 2019). The main changes from ICD-10 include: (i) expanded classes of psychoactive substances; (ii) introduction of single episodes of substance use; (iii) introduction of harmful patterns of substance use; (iv) severity qualifiers for substance intoxication (mild, moderate, or severe); and (v) introduction of the category "Disorders due to addictive behaviors" that includes "Gambling disorder" (previously called habit and impulse disorders) and the new diagnostic category

Rutter's Child and Adolescent Psychiatry and Psychology, Seventh Edition.
Edited by Anita Thapar, Daniel S. Pine, Samuele Cortese, Cathy Creswell, Tamsin J. Ford, James F. Leckman, and Argyris Stringaris.

Companion website: www.wiley.com/go/thapar/rutterspsych7

"Gaming disorder." The section includes two parts, "Disorders due to substance use" and "Disorders due to addictive behaviors." The list of substances has been expanded from 9 in ICD-10 to 14 in ICD-11, reflecting the changes in use of drugs and patterns since the 1990s, such as the addition of synthetic cathinones.

Different professionals select from among many terms to describe the level of problem. These terms include misuse, abuse, hazardous use, and dependent use. Some practitioners may hesitate when assigning diagnoses due to fear of labeling a young person in ways that could be stigmatizing. Moreover, when assigning specific diagnoses concern exists about the need for greater standardization (Degenhardt *et al.*, 2021).

Prevalence and trends

Prevalence

Degenhardt *et al.* reported the global burden of disease related to substance use increases substantially in adolescence and early adulthood (Degenhardt *et al.*, 2016). In young men aged 20–24, alcohol and illicit drugs are responsible for 14% of the total burden.

Worldwide, 26.5% of all 15–19-year-olds are current drinkers, with prevalence rates highest among 15–19-year-olds in the World Health Organization (WHO) European Region (43.8%), followed by the Americas (38.2%), and the Western Pacific Region (37.9%). School surveys indicate that alcohol use often starts before the age of 15 years, with a peak in binge drinking in the 20s (World Health Organization, 2018).

Alcohol is the most used substance among teenagers and young adults. In national surveys in the United States (US), 34% of 12–20 years olds drank at least one drink in their lives, 28% drank in the last year, 15% in the last month, and 1.6% reported heavy alcohol use in the past month. In those aged 12–17, 3.4% met criteria for an alcohol use disorder (AUD) in the past year. For 18–25-year-olds, the percentage was 14.9% (National Center for Drug Abuse Statistics, 2021).

Drug use is a major health concern with at least 1 in 8 US teenagers using an illicit substance in the last year, and 8.3% in the past month, the majority using marijuana, 62% via vaping (National Center for Drug Abuse Statistics, 2021). By 12th grade, 46% had tried an illicit drug and 7% used marijuana daily.

Drug use is highest among youth aged 16–25 years, with 11.2% of overdose deaths occurring in this age group. Among those younger than 21 who initiate heroin use, 80% have abused prescriptions or over-the-counter drugs (Cerda *et al.*, 2015). US high school students who use prescription opioids were 33% more likely to abuse opioids. However, the absolute rate was low: 0.4% of 12th graders had abused heroin, and 2.4% had abused oxycodone. Five percent of 12–17-year-olds had used cocaine in the last year, and 2.2% had met criteria for a DUD in the last year (National Center for Drug Abuse Statistics, 2021). Most (70%) of those who had tried an illegal drug before 13 years of age had developed an SUD within the next 7 years.

In the United Kingdom (UK) approximately 1 in 5 UK youth aged 16–24 years (18.6%) reported drug use in the last year, and 4.7% reported Class A drug use (Office for National Statistics, 2022). In Scotland, 6% of 13-year-olds and 21% of 15-year-olds reported having used drugs, a rate broadly comparable with the US; in Wales, 15% of young people reported having used drugs in their lifetime.

Wide variation exists in the use of conventional cigarettes and e-cigarettes. The European School Survey project on alcohol and drugs (ESPAD Group, 2020) reported 12.4% were current e-cigarette users with variation from 5% in Serbia to 41% in Monaco; 19% were current conventional smokers with a range from 5% in Iceland to 32% in Italy. Compared with non-users, both smokers and e-cigarette users were more likely to be past smokers, early smokers, males, and from less traditional families with poorer parental education, as well as living in countries with fewer tobacco control measures in place (Cerrai *et al.*, 2022).

Trends in use

Global prevalence of drug use remains high. In 2021, 1 in every 17 people aged 15–64 worldwide had used a drug in the past 12 months, a 23% increase from 2011, with cannabis use increasing. In 15–16-year-olds, 5.3% worldwide reported past-year cannabis use. The proportion of adolescents using the drug typically is higher than in the general population aged 15–64 (United Nations Office on Drugs and Crime, 2023). DALYs for cannabis use disorder (CUD) peak at 20–24 years old, with the second-highest subgroup younger than 20 years old (Shao *et al.*, 2023). Opioids make the highest contribution to severe drug-related harm, including fatal overdoses. There is an increase in supply and demand for cocaine worldwide, whereas consumption of methamphetamine in Western and Central Europe stabilized in 2020 and 2021 (United Nations Office on Drugs and Crime, 2023).

Widening availability for new psychoactive substances (NPS), including cannabinoids and ketamine, represents a new trend, with generally higher use among students than in the general population. However, consumption of NPS other than ketamine appears stable or declining among young people (United Nations Office on Drugs and Crime, 2023).

Between 15–20% of UK 15-year-olds (NHS Digital, 2022) and 28% of US 16-year-olds report past-year cannabis use (National Institute on Drug Abuse, 2020b). Globally, CUD incidence increased by 32.3% from 1990 to 2019, with male CUD nearly double that of females.

Surveys document rates of smoking, drinking, and drug use in English secondary school children, aged 11–15 years, every 2 years. They show cigarette use to be declining. NHS Digital reported 12% had smoked, and 3% were current smokers (compared to 16% and 5%, respectively, in 2018). Similarly, drug use has declined: 18% had used, compared to 24% in 2018; 12% in the past year, compared to 17% in 2018; and 6% in the past month, compared to 9% in 2018. Alcohol use at least once a week remained stable at 6% (NHS Digital, 2022).

Vashishtha (2021) reported a decline of adolescent alcohol use since the turn of the Millennium in almost all high-income countries. The decline began in the US, then Northern Europe, with the most marked decline in Northern Europe and the UK and the least in eastern and southern European countries.

The European School Survey Project on Alcohol and Other Drugs (ESPAD) project is a collaborative network across 40 European countries on adolescent substance use. The latest survey (ESPAD Group, 2020) reported decreased trends in smoking and alcohol use. However, concerns remain over use of cannabis and prescription drugs, and new addictive behaviors.

There has been a striking increase of e-cigarette use among young people in North America and Europe (Kapan *et al.*, 2020). From 2014 to 2019, use in Canada nearly tripled from 5.7% to 15% (Nguyen & Mittal, 2022). In the US, more than one-third of high school seniors reported use in 2018 (Miech *et al.*, 2018). Rates of vaping correlate with rates of many mental disorders, including conduct disorder (CD), attention deficit hyperactivity disorder (ADHD), and depression. Although the direction of causality remains uncertain (McArdle *et al.*, 2022), those who vape are more likely to have had past mental health problems, and those with mental health problems appear at greater risk of starting e-cigarette use (Grant *et al.*, 2019). Rates of e-cigarette use also correlate with rates of subsequent cannabis, alcohol, and other drug use. In a systematic review, Chadi (2019) reported the odds of cannabis use among youth using e-cigarettes to be 3.5 times greater than among those not using e-cigarettes. However, use of e-cigarettes and other substances may more fundamentally relate to underlying mental health and behavioral vulnerabilities (McArdle *et al.*, 2022).

The ESPAD Group report (2020) noted the widespread normalization of gambling, the increased use of smartphones for gaming, and greater self-perception of high risk of problems related to social media than gaming activities. Systematic reviews report a global prevalence of internet gaming disorder among adolescents of 8.8%, with much higher figures in males than females. Risk factors include emotional distress, a range of psychiatric symptoms, longer game time, family dysfunction, bullying and being bullied, and poor academic performance (Gao *et al.*, 2022). In a six-year study, Coyne *et al.* (2020) examined the trajectories of adolescent gaming. Approximately 10% showed moderate levels of pathological gaming symptoms at initial assessment, increasing over time with higher levels of depression and anxiety.

Patterns and trends in treatment

In England, the Office for Health Improvement & Disparities (2023) produces an annual report on patterns of drug use and the characteristics of young people under 18 years attending national specialist treatment drug and alcohol services. The most recent report found a greater than 50% reduction in numbers in treatment since 2009. Of those attending, two-thirds were male, with a median age of about 16 years for both males and females. Cannabis remained the most common drug of use (87%), but nearly 50% of clinic attenders reported problems with alcohol, as well as 8% with ecstasy and 8% with powder cocaine. The percentage of attendees with a main problem other than cannabis or alcohol remained steady at 10%.

As expected, from a review of risk factors and vulnerabilities, most patients in treatment have multiple risk factors. Of those in treatment in England, 80% initiated use prior to age 15 years. Females reported more self-harm (46% compared to 17%) than males, and more sexual exploitation (10% compared to 1.5%). More females declared a mental health need, from 32% in 2018, increasing annually in the last 3 years to 46% in 2021–2022; 31% had not had specific treatment. Other vulnerabilities included criminal justice involvement, domestic abuse, and antisocial behavior, which was more common in boys. Chan *et al.* (2009) noted that two-thirds of clients from pooled data of treatment services in the US had co-occurring mental health problems in the year prior to treatment, with young people being most vulnerable to co-occurring problems. Contrary to most studies demonstrating significant correlation of SUD and mental health disorders, Richert *et al.* (2020), in a review in Sweden of young people with SUD, noted there was less severe mental health impairment. They considered this related to the milder presentation of SUD, being seen in an outpatient setting, and having stable home and school environments. Despite its impact, SUD remains severely undertreated. In 2018, only 10% of young adults suffering from SUD received any form of treatment; only 6.3% received treatment at a specialist drug and alcohol facility (Substance Abuse and Mental Health Services Administration, 2019)

In summary, substance use is deeply impairing and potentially lethal. Among those seeking treatment, substance use is enmeshed with trauma and problems of mental health. Trends show shifts from cigarettes to vaping, decreased alcohol use, and increased ketamine use, while cannabis remains a preferred substance.

Risk and protective factors

Substantial cross-country variation manifests in levels, types, and sequences of substance use. These patterns relate to social context, drug availability, and user characteristics (Degenhardt *et al.*, 2016). Many young people who use alcohol and drugs do not progress to SUD, though progression relates to numerous risks and vulnerabilities. Data on modifiable SUD risk factors inform approaches to prevention and treatment.

Multiple risk factors exist. These include person-specific, family, peer-related, and environmental factors, such as childhood adverse events and low socioeconomic status (Santo *et al.*, 2013). In a systematic review, Nawi *et al.* (2021) identify individual, familial, and community risk factors, with protective factors seen as optimism, strong beliefs against substance use, school connectedness, high vigilance of parents, and religious affiliation.

Some individual factors appear similar across countries and cultures. These include early age of initiation, conduct difficulties, poor school performance, and affiliation with like-minded peers. Some environmental risks also appear similar across contexts. These include ready access to substances, perceived tolerance in the environment to drug use, and lower socioeconomic backgrounds. The presence of multiple risk factors might signal particularly high risk. For example, early age of initiation may carry particularly high risks in the context of other risk factors such as behavioral factors and trauma (Moss *et al.*, 2014). As overall levels of alcohol use decline in adolescents, early age of initiation might identify a small, deviant group. This group may be marginalized and express other problems, emphasizing the need for service provision (Caluzzi *et al.*, 2022).

Family history of SUD represents a significant risk factor. Family factors linked to substance-use problems include poor quality of parent–child relationships and parental conflict, as well as parental and sibling drug use. As noted by Hamad *et al.* (2022), such family factors can relate to both genetic and shared environmental risk. Other studies identified adverse childhood experiences (ACEs) as strong risk factors for initiation and continuation of substance use (Grummit *et al.*, 2002). Still other studies highlighted risk associated with sexual and physical abuse, neglect, other traumas, and mental disorders, particularly CD and ADHD (Santo *et al.*, 2022).

Main substances of abuse and their harms

This section will briefly discuss key substances and alcohol, their effects, and related harms. Alcohol and drug use in childhood and youth is associated with many adverse outcomes: acute effects from intoxication such as increased mortality from related accidents and injuries, and unintentional overdose of opioids; and indirect effects related to sharing injecting equipment with increased risk of hepatitis. Drugs taken together may have additive effects. Further, there are long-term risks with increased risks of cancers from tobacco and alcohol, and cardiovascular and respiratory effects.

Access to accurate information helps families and professionals. Websites such as the US National Institute of Drug Abuse (NIDA) (www.nida.com) and a UK-based site, Talktofrank (www.talktofrank.com), provide information for professionals, parents, and children.

Drugs are categorized in different ways; defined in DSM-5 and ICD-11, according to chemical structure or therapeutic factors, or potential for abuse and harm.

See Table 66.1: this outlines the major classifications, and their acute effects.

Alcohol

Ethyl alcohol, more commonly known as alcohol, is a psychoactive drug contained in drinks and widely used for centuries. Effects depend on amount consumed and the strength of the drink. Effects range from reduced feelings of anxiety or, with intoxication, slurred speech, unsteady gait, poor coordination, impaired sleep, and fatalities from poisoning.

Alcohol is a causal factor in over 200 medical and injury conditions, causing early death, disability, and great costs to society and individuals. Worldwide, 5.3% of all deaths involve harmful use of alcohol, and alcohol is the leading risk factor for death, ill-health, and disability among 15–49-year-olds in England. Alcohol impacts health, crime, and families, with over 200,000 children in the UK likely to be living with an alcohol-dependent parent, with many of these parents not being in treatment (Public Health England, 2018). Problems relate to intoxication, excessive use, and dependence, with increased risk of violence, injuries, risky sexual behaviors, self-harm, and suicide. Alcohol use may impact cognitive functioning through effects on the developing brain, which can lead to educational and social problems (Lees *et al.*, 2020).

Cannabis

Cannabis, the principal psychoactive constituent of which is tetrahydrocannabinol (THC), is the most used drug internationally, especially among adolescents. Acute effects vary with the amount and route of use. Symptoms of intoxication include euphoria and relaxation, a heightened sensory perception, increased appetite, and tachycardia. Some experience negative effects such as fear, anxiety and panic, paranoia, and hallucinations. Cannabis use can cause dependence and impair driving.

Hines *et al.* (2020) examined features of high-potency-cannabis use. Epidemiological studies link long-term cannabis use to risk of psychosis and mood disorders, as well as adverse effects on cognitive function and educational attainment (Hall *et al.*, 2020). Ample data link daily use and use of high-potency products to psychosis. However, the mechanism underlying this link remains uncertain, as an "appreciable proportion of the association is not causal" (Gillespie & Kendler, 2020).

Cannabis has been legalized in several countries. In a preliminary review of changes after legalization, Rubin-Kahana *et al.* (2022) noted an increase in cannabis-related hospitalizations, though no major change in driving under the influence, and a significant decrease in cannabis-related criminal offenses among youth. However, a report from the United Nations Office on Drugs and Crime (2023) suggested that legalization had increased daily cannabis use, especially of potent cannabis products associated with risk for psychiatric disorders.

Synthetic cannabinoid receptor agonists (SCRA) (e.g., "Spice"), are chemicals designed to mimic THC, though with more potent effects. They act as a cardiovascular stimulant, can cause respiratory depression, may provoke seizures, increase risk of psychosis, and, with chronic use, create risk for dependence and withdrawal symptoms.

Opioids

Opioids/opiates are narcotic analgesics, classified into three main groups: natural opioids, such as morphine; semisynthetic opioids derived from natural opiates like heroin; and synthetic opioids, such as fentanyl and methadone. They are μ-opioid receptor agonists, usually used as analgesics, and are appropriate when

Table 66.1 Major drug classes and their effects.

Drug class	Major forms	Mechanisms	Acute effects
Cannabis	Marijuana, hashish, hash oil	Agonists for cannabinoid receptors (CB_1, CB_2)	Euphoria, anxiety, tachycardia, impairment of short-term memory, executive functioning, and attention
Opioids	Heroin, morphine, opium, codeine, oxycodone	Agonists for μ, δ, κ neuroreceptors	Euphoria, sedation, respiratory depression, analgesia, suppression of cough reflex, emetic, pupil constriction
Psychostimulants	Methamphetamine (powder, crystal), amphetamine, cocaine (powder, crack, MDMA)	Release, or block, reuptake, of dopamine, noradrenaline, and serotonin	Euphoria, anxiety, delirium, hypertension, vasoconstriction, vasospasm, tachycardia, pupil dilation, psychoses
Hallucinogens	LSD, psilocybin, mescaline	Serotonin agonists (2AR 5HT-mGluR2 receptor families)	Euphoria, hallucinations, delirium
	Dissociative: ketamine, PCP	Dissociative: NMDA receptor antagonists	Dissociation, anesthesia, muscle rigidity, hyperthermia, agitated delirium
New psychoactive substances	Synthetic cannabinoids	Synthetic cannabinoids: agonists for receptors (CB_1, CB_2)	Synthetic cannabinoids: similar to cannabis
	Synthetic opioids, e.g., fentanyl	Agonists for μ, δ, κ neuroreceptors	Similar to opioids
	Synthetic stimulants, e.g., mephedrone, cathinones	Synthetic stimulants: release, or block, reuptake of dopamine, noradrenaline, and serotonin, new hallucinogens are serotonin agonists	Synthetic stimulants: similar to psychostimulants and hallucinogens
	CNS depressants: benzodiazepines, Z drugs, GHB	CNS depressants: GHB, agonist for GHB and GABAa receptors; benzodiazepines, agonist at GABA receptor	GHB: euphoria, respiratory depression; benzodiazepines: sedation, respiratory depression

Source: Darke *et al.* (2019)/Silverback Publishing.

prescribed and monitored. Effects vary depending on speed of action, dose, and potency, with harms particularly related to overdose risk. Acute intoxication effects include euphoria with impaired judgment, and then with significant respiratory depression and death. Dependence and tolerance develop rapidly.

The opioid epidemic is a major public health concern in some countries. In the US, the number of drug overdose deaths increased by nearly 30% from 2019 to 2020 and has quintupled since 1999. Nearly 75% of the drug overdose deaths in 2020 were related to opioids. In the US, the deaths from the 1990s have been related to increased prescribing of opioids (natural and semisynthetic opioids), with increases in heroin-related deaths and, latterly, significant increases in synthetic opioids (fentanyl and illicitly manufactured opioids).

The UK has seen a significant rise in opioid-related deaths with rates increasing every year since 2012, having been relatively stable over the preceding two decades. The fatality rate was 6% higher in 2021 than in 2020, with the overall trend driven by opioid deaths, though there is a rise in cocaine-related deaths, related to the increased prevalence of cocaine (UK Government, 2021).

This has prompted the US and UK to distribute naloxone, with increased availability of training and comprehensive treatments for opioid dependence (National Institute on Drug Abuse, 2021).

Psychostimulants

Cocaine

Cocaine is a stimulant drug, used recreationally. Effects are of rapid onset, with not only tachycardia, alertness, and feelings of increased confidence, but also irritability and paranoid ideation. Harms can include multiple psychological and medical problems, particularly in cardiac and infectious domains.

Amphetamines

Amphetamines are potent central nervous system (CNS) stimulants, used recreationally, though they are prescribed for ADHD and narcolepsy. Effects can include increased alertness, increased energy, agitation, and often panic, with increased risk of a psychotic disorder. Harms can be both acute and chronic, with long-term health harms mainly being cardiovascular, renal, neurological, and gastrointestinal effects. Dependence can occur and withdrawal can be severe in chronic users.

Substituted amphetamines are a group of substances with amphetamine as their parent compound. Examples include, cathinones, 3,4-methylenedioxymethamphetamine (MDMA) and methamphetamine ("crystal meth," "ice"). MDMA has pharmacological differences from amphetamine, and tablets can be contaminated with various psychoactive substances. Methamphetamine is highly addictive and neurotoxic. More potent than amphetamine, methamphetamine dependence is a serious worldwide public health problem. It can be used orally, snorted, or injected and is often taken in a binge pattern. Compared to cocaine, methamphetamine has a much longer duration of action, which leads to prolonged stimulant effects. Significant harms include cardiovascular risks, psychotic symptoms such as paranoia and hallucinations, and neurotoxicity, as well as multiple psychological problems. It can exacerbate existing psychiatric disorders and symptoms.

Hallucinogens

Ketamine is used as an anesthetic and is being evaluated to manage treatment-resistant depression and AUD. Effects occur quickly and include feeling not only detached and happy, but also anxious, with memory loss and a numbness. Of importance, a chemical cystitis, with long-term problematic use, can occur.

New psychoactive substances

NPSs are defined as "a new narcotic or psychotropic drug, substances of abuse, either in pure form or in preparation, that is not controlled by the United Nations drug conventions, but which may pose a public health threat comparable to that posed by substances listed in these conventions." The European Union (EU) Early Warning System, operated by the European Union Drugs Agency (EUDA), plays a central role in supporting national- and EU-level preparedness and responses to NPSs. In the UK, national advisory bodies, such as the Novel Psychoactive Treatment UK Network (NEPTUNE) and the National Poisons Information Service (NPIS), monitor trends of NPSs. Almost 900 were reported by 2018. More recently, the pattern of NPS use has changed with a decrease in the number of new stimulants and synthetic cannabinoids detected, and an increase in new opioids and benzodiazepines available (Shafi *et al.*, 2020). Shafi *et al.* (2020) described an NPS classification system: synthetic stimulants, synthetic cannabinoids, synthetic hallucinogens, and synthetic depressants (which include synthetic opioids and synthetic benzodiazepines). Effects resemble those found with the drugs they mimic, e.g., opioids and synthetic hallucinogens such as phenylcyclohexyl piperidene (PCP) and ketamine.

Synthetic opioids

Synthetic opioids (e.g., carfentanyl) mimic the effects of natural opioids. They are generally more potent at much smaller doses with respiratory depression and death being the most concerning effects. There are growing concerns regarding the nitazenes, otherwise known as benzimidazoles, which are new synthetic opioids on the rise. Many countries have issued alerts due to their increasing availability and presence in counterfeit oxycodone tablets and counterfeit hydromorphone tablets. Of concern is the use of xylazine, a non-opiate sedative analgesic only authorized for veterinary use. Known as "tranq" or "zombie drug," it has been reported in an increasing number of illicit drug mixtures and has an increased presence in overdose fatalities, mainly as an adulterant with fentanyl, heroin, or cocaine (US Drug Enforcement Administration, 2022).

Benzodiazepines

Benzodiazepines are drugs used to treat conditions such as anxiety, sleep difficulties, and seizures. Effects include sedation and decreased alertness, and they may impair driving. Harms relate to risk for dependence and abuse of both prescribed and illicit benzodiazepines, with risk for drug-related deaths particularly when used with opioids and alcohol.

Gamma-hydroxybutyrate and gamma-butyrolactone

Gamma-hydroxybutyrate (GHB) and gamma-butyrolactone (GBL) are CNS depressants, with rapid onset of effects producing euphoria, disinhibition, and impaired judgment. Effects of higher doses include disinhibition, respiratory depression, and overdose risk, and there are increased risks if used with alcohol. Dependence can occur with severe withdrawal syndrome, that may require hospitalization.

Nitrous oxide

Nitrous oxide is clinically used as a dental anesthetic. However, use as a recreational drug, particularly in dance and festival scenes, has increased significantly since the 2010s (European Monitoring Centre for Drugs and Drug Addiction, 2022). It is a colorless gas sold in canisters and inhaled. Effects are dose dependent and include immediate euphoria for a few minutes. A particular harm more often related to the amount used is subacute combined degeneration of the cord, associated with severe B12 deficiency, through inactivation of the vitamin B12 dependent enzyme, methionine synthase (Paris *et al*., 2023). Other harms include severe frostbite or lung injuries due to properties of the gas released from the container. In addition, car accidents involving the gas have increased, particularly in the Netherlands (European Monitoring Centre for Drugs and Drug Addiction, 2022).

Cognitive enhancers

Cognitive enhancers are drugs used to improve memory, and increase alertness and concentration. They are licensed for patients suffering from health conditions, such as dementia and ADHD. Despite media concern, there is little evidence of much abuse of these drugs, although students do report use, obtaining it from colleagues who are prescribed, or online. However, there is little evidence that these drugs significantly improve cognitive function in healthy people (Nicholson *et al*., 2015).

Clinical responses to use and dependence

Public health approaches

This section briefly describes prevention and public health responses before describing clinical approaches. Responses to substance use and SUDs occur at different levels reflecting a continuum-of-care framework: universal prevention approaches aimed at the population; harm reduction through selective and indicated prevention programs targeting vulnerable groups; and treatment approaches such as psychosocial, pharmacological, and recovery interventions (Stockings *et al*., 2016).

Babor *et al*. (2022) reviewed strategies for prevention and reduction of alcohol-related harm. The most effective universal strategies were approaches such as taxation that reduced the affordability and availability of alcohol. Random roadside alcohol testing consistently reduces alcohol-related accidents, as does reducing the alcohol legal limit to drive among young people aged 18–25 years (Martineau *et al*., 2013). In their review, Stockings *et al*. (2016) noted the effectiveness of taxation, restrictions on access and advertising, minimum legal age, decrease in affordability, and diminished availability of alcohol and tobacco. However, these strategies are not available to target illicit drug use. The updated evidence, based on international standards for drug prevention (United Nations Office on Drugs and Crime, 2018), recommended broader prevention strategies that aim to both prevent and reduce risky use and improve quality of life.

Mixed evidence exists on the effectiveness of mass media campaigns and school-based interventions. Das *et al*. (2016) reviewed 46 systematic reviews focused on interventions for substances in adolescents. School-based prevention programs and family-based intensive interventions were effective in reducing smoking. A school-based alcohol prevention intervention with personalized feedback, and brief interventions (BIs), reduced frequency of alcohol use; a small positive effect manifested for family-based interventions. With a focus on drug use, some evidence of efficacy exists for school-based interventions combining social competence and social influence approaches. This small though consistent effect was noted in preventing cannabis use (Faggiano *et al*., 2014). However, approaches based mainly on improving knowledge and awareness of harms have little effect.

Harm reduction is a broad public health approach that refers to a set of interventions and practical strategies that aim to reduce harm associated with use of drugs, without necessarily achieving abstinence. The aim is to reduce risk, prevent escalation of drug use, prevent death, and improve quality of life. While these approaches represent a public health prevention effort, they are also applied at an individual level. The term was introduced in the 1980s in response to the increasing human immunodeficiency virus (HIV) prevalence among drug injectors and with development of needle/syringe exchanges. A harm reduction approach can also address other risk behaviors such as sexual health and risky alcohol use.

Procedures can range from chemical testing of an illicit drug to verify the presence of the actual drug, often at festivals or nightclubs, provision of needle/syringe exchange, and provision of naloxone to individuals and families/friends, as well as information and psychoeducation on the use of drugs and their effects, and vaccination to prevent hepatitis B. Other procedures include low threshold methadone /buprenorphine programs and drug consumption rooms (Harm Reduction International, 2022).

Early interventions aim to identify those at risk of use and reduce risky patterns and harms. Examples of selective approaches include random roadside drug testing, screening and BIs in different contexts, early childhood education, and school policies and culture (United Nations Office on Drugs and Crime, 2018).

Assessment and treatments

This section reviews the approaches to specific substance use treatments; these include psychosocial treatments alone or in combination, such as BIs, motivational approaches, cognitive behavioral therapy, family therapies, recovery, and 12-step approach, and pharmacological approaches. However, treatment begins with an assessment to identify levels of severity and indications for therapy. Accordingly, this section begins by briefly discussing screening and assessment before reviewing the evidence for specific therapies. See Boxes 66.1 and 66.2 for summaries of the key points for assessment and treatment, respectively.

Screening

People can be linked to SUD treatment in many contexts including primary care, emergency departments, and psychiatric services. The main screening tools are the Alcohol Use Disorder Identification Test (AUDIT) (Saunders *et al.*, 1993) and CRAFFT (acronym for: **C**ar, have you ever ridden in a car driven by someone using alcohol or drugs; **R**elax, do you use to relax; **A**lone, do you ever use while alone; **F**orget, do you forget things you do while using; **F**riends, does your family or friends ever say you should cut down; and **T**rouble, have you ever got in trouble while using) (Harris *et al.*, 2014). The full AUDIT is a 10-item questionnaire that takes about two minutes, with the AUDIT-C being the first three questions looking at consumption, and other sections inquiring on potential dependence and experience of alcohol-related harms. Coulton *et al.* (2019) noted that the three-item AUDIT-C was more effective than the AUDIT on screening adolescents for at-risk alcohol use and heavy episodic use, with the full 10 item AUDIT being more effective for identification of alcohol dependence. The CRAFFT is the most widely used screening tool, being validated in a variety of setting and cultures. Training in the use of these tools increases staff confidence in supporting young people.

Box 66.1 Assessment at a glance

- Screening and comprehensive assessment of substance use disorder (SUD), and psychiatric and neurodevelopmental disorders
- Identification of the chronology of alcohol and each drug used: age of initiation, amount, route, frequency, pattern of use (e.g., binge use/daily use/weekend), dependence, social context of use, their direct/indirect consequences, and any past treatment
- Assessment of risk to self and others: significant intoxication, exploitation, self-harm and suicidal ideation, deteriorating mental health, offending (especially with older groups/gangs), violence to self or others, physical risks (e.g., hepatitis B and C, HIV, injuries)
- Physical health assessment/interventions, including diagnostic investigations and hepatitis B vaccination
- Toxicology and monitoring

Box 66.2 Treatment at a glance

Psychosocial interventions—alone or in combination:

- brief interventions
- motivational approaches
- cognitive behavioral therapy (CBT)—individual or group
- adolescent community reinforcement approach (A-CRA)
- family therapies
- relapse prevention—psychological
- recovery-based approaches
- 12-step approach
- mutual aid groups—e.g., Alcoholics Anonymous (AA)
- combinations of the above, e.g., motivational interviewing (MI)/CBT
- promising/commonly used treatments with very little research or evidence base, e.g., solution-focused

Pharmacological interventions:

- detoxification
- stabilization/maintenance
- relapse prevention—pharmacological

Comorbid care and treatment

Assessment

For those with risky alcohol use or SUD, a referral for comprehensive assessment is required. Comorbidities are the rule rather than the exception, with high rates of behavioral problems, anxiety, self-harm, and suicidal ideation. In many young people, especially in underserved populations, such as those who are homeless, pregnant, or involved with criminal justice, drug use may not be the most important issue that they perceive. A trauma-informed assessment approach is helpful with all high-risk youth. Parents should be part of the assessment and ongoing plans, if possible and appropriate. Practitioners need to assess the young person's capacity to give consent and understand all aspects of the proposed treatment interventions. The legalities of consent and refusal of treatment will be different in different countries and for patients of varying ages. Moreover, competence to consent will depend on the maturity of the child and the nature of the proposed treatment; this is important for young people who wish to receive treatment without their parents' knowledge or consent (see Chapter 19, "Legal Issues").

Assessment is a continuing process, with the importance of engagement and building trust essential. For comprehensiveness, it generally requires a team of competent professionals to assess all levels of functioning, as discussed by Bukstein (2005), Perepletchikova *et al.* (2008), and Gilvarry *et al.* (2012). The reader is also referred to Chapters 27, 28, and 30.

On specific assessment of substance use, it is useful to identify the chronology of alcohol and each drug (prescribed, illicit, or over-the-counter) used: age of initiation, amount, route of use, frequency, pattern of use (e.g., binge use), dependence, social context of use, their direct/indirect consequences, and any past treatment. Assessing risk is essential; including the young person's risk to self and the risk to others, related to the need to protect from significant intoxication, exploitation, self-harm, and suicidal ideation. Other risks include deteriorating mental health with psychotic symptoms, offending (especially with older groups/gangs), and violence to self or others. All professionals working with young people may need to share information, with or without consent when necessary, to protect the young person.

Physical health

All youth using alcohol or drugs, or abusing illicit or prescribed drugs, should have their physical health assessed to reduce and prevent health-related consequences. These can include harms from the acute and chronic effects of alcohol or other drugs, and harms related to route of use, such as intravenous (IV) use causing cellulitis or sharing of equipment causing hepatitis B or C. Screening for blood-borne viruses (BBV), such as hepatitis B and C and HIV, is now common within all specialist addictions services and all, with consent, should be screened. Hepatitis B vaccination is useful as a prevention for all young people at risk. Other risky behaviors may need safeguarding. Management of pregnancy and SUDs requires specialist advice with obstetric clinics and specialist addiction services. Physical health assessment and management with psychoeducation on risks can be seen as a broad harm reduction approach to ensure best quality health. Such assessment and psychoeducation should be available for all young people at risk, regardless of what service they attend. Like mental health, physical assessment and review is a dynamic process throughout the contact with the young person.

Toxicology and monitoring

Testing for drugs and alcohol can be helpful if used as part of a comprehensive assessment and ongoing monitoring to support diagnoses, monitor compliance with medication or court-enforced processes, and reinforce motivation. Such testing should not be, or be perceived to be, a punitive process.

The mediums for testing include blood, urine, oral fluid, breathalyzing for alcohol, hair, and occasionally sweat and nails. Urine and oral fluids are more commonly used clinically in detection of drugs. The accuracy and knowledge of these tests is important in making treatment decisions, e.g., urine testing when a person suffers from psychosis, exhibits poor adherence to medication, or there is risk of diversion, e.g., taking prescribed methadone and testing for metabolites. Immunoassays, which use antibodies to detect the presence of specific drugs or metabolites, are the most common method for initial screening. However, false positive results can occur so they require laboratory confirmation. The most sophisticated confirmatory drug testing approach is gas chromatography coupled with mass spectrometry (GC/MS), which is regarded as the gold standard, though inaccuracies can still occur. The timing of detection of illicit drugs varies with the actual substance, the sampling medium, and the accuracy of the test.

Hair testing for alcohol and drugs is generally not used clinically, but is used extensively in court proceedings, especially family courts for parental drug use and if there is any suspicion of use by children. Clinicians need to be aware of these tests and their interpretation.

A breath test for alcohol is useful but limited with timescale of use. Blood tests can be useful but are often indirect markers, such as liver function tests. A direct marker, phosphatidylethanol (PEth), is a minor metabolite of alcohol, and can be administered as a finger-prick blood test. It has the advantage of an extended window of detection and is considered a more sensitive indicator of alcohol use than indirect markers such as carbohydrate-deficient transferrin (CDT), γ-glutamyl transferase (GGT), and mean corpuscular volume (MCV), or a combination of these (Isaksson *et al.*, 2011). These tests are an adjunct to clinical assessment and management. However, it is important that practitioners interpret the results accurately.

Psychosocial treatments for young people

Many psychosocial treatments exist, but data on efficacy is mixed. Hogue *et al.* (2018) reviewed efficacy data, that of recent literature reviews, and meta-analytic studies for BIs, motivational interviewing (MI), individual and group cognitive behavioral therapy (CBT), family therapies, and counseling/12-step facilitation. He concluded that the evidence for BIs was promising and helped identification and access; MI was probably efficacious, CBT and some family therapies well established, and 12-step facilitation possibly efficacious. Some multicomponent treatments, such as CBT/ motivational enhancement therapy (MET), or similar, combined with contingency management, were seen as well-established and probably efficacious. Treatments for those with SUD, however, are often multicomponent and across multiple domains requiring collaboration and coordination across child and family services. Hogue (2018), however, noted that more research was required to determine the impacts of multicomponent therapies and multidomain treatments. Many researched treatments are based on fidelity to manual-based protocols. Those with significant comorbidities are often excluded from research trials. In clinical settings, given the comorbidities that often coexist, integrated approaches may reduce risk of drop out, improve coordination of care across services, and improve the engagement of young people (Brewer *et al.*, 2017).

Brief interventions

Many young people who are using alcohol and/or drugs, or who are at risk, are unlikely to access specialist alcohol services, though they may be in contact with health care staff, and educational and family-based services in different settings.

BIs are an umbrella term for techniques that comprise advice and/or counseling that vary in the number of sessions, on average one to four sessions of short duration. They are structured nonjudgmental therapies, and can be delivered by trained professionals in opportunistic settings (primary care or psychiatric settings) and across substances, age, and ethnocultural groups. While BIs may vary, all share a similar underpinning of health psychology theory, a structure commonly known as FRAMES (Miller & Sanchez, 1994), and are based on a harm reduction paradigm.

Box 66.3 FRAMES

- **F**eedback: provision of personalized and relevant information following screening, highlighting harms and risks, and including harm reduction messages and normative comparisons
- **R**esponsibility: acknowledgment of the individual's responsibility in initiating and maintaining change, "It's up to you to decide what you want to do"
- **A**dvice: provision of clear advice on practical strategies to reduce harm
- **M**enu of options to help achieve behavior change: e.g., ways to change drinking pattern (lower-strength drinks, having drink-free days, taking up other activities); offer ideas if required
- **E**mpathy: discussion in a nonconfrontational, nonjudgmental approach, based on reflective listening
- **S**elf-efficacy: the therapist builds the confidence of the person, enhancing motivation, with recognition that the answer is usually evoked from the person rather than the therapist

The six common elements of BIs are summarized by the acronym FRAMES—Feedback, Responsibility, Advice, Menu for change, Empathy, and enhancing Self-efficacy (Box 66.3).

In one meta-analysis (only studies with comparative conditions included) (Tanner-Smith & Lipsey, 2015), brief alcohol interventions led to reductions in alcohol consumption and alcohol-related problems among adolescents and young adults, with effects persisting for up to one year. However, weaker evidence was noted in other reviews (Hogue *et al.*, 2018). Some modalities appeared to be associated with larger effects than others. The most promising therapies included MI and goal-directed exercises. Although the effects were modest, they were potentially worthwhile given their brevity and low cost. A recent UK trial of screening versus two forms of BI reported no differences in alcohol use by young attenders at emergency settings in the 6- and 12-month follow-ups (DeLuca *et al.*, 2022). However, alcohol use reduced by 30–40% post encounter with the researcher. This could suggest that for some young people screening alone may be an effective tool. Though with quite small effects, because of their brevity, low cost, and potential contribution to enhancing further care, in the US, a comprehensive public health strategy, SBIRT (screening, BI, referral to treatment), advocates the delivery of BIs as treatment for both those with SUD and those at risk. This strategy may also assist with the significant underidentification of young people with SUD (Substance Abuse and Mental Health Services Administration, 2021a).

Motivational approaches

MI and a manual-based adaptation, MET, are designed to enhance motivation to change addictive behaviors (Miller & Rollnick, 1991). They are based on principles of motivational psychology with the assumption that the responsibility and capability for change lies within the person. This treatment strategy seeks to support intrinsic motivation for change, leading the person to initiate, persist in, and comply with behavior change efforts. Miller and Rollnick (1991) described five basic motivational principles underlying the approach: express empathy, develop discrepancy (building awareness and creating a gap in the difference between one's current behavior and a desired different behavior), avoid argumentation, roll with resistance, and support self-efficacy (Miller & Rollnick, 1991). Several meta-analyses indicate strong empirical support for the efficacy of motivational interventions for increasing client retention and decreasing substance use (Project MATCH, 1997; Orford *et al.*, 2005). MI has been shown to be effective in reducing alcohol use and to increase attendance by young people at specialist substance misuse treatment services (Tait *et al.*, 2004). Hogue *et al.* (2018), in a large review of treatment for adolescents' substance use, noted MI to be "probably efficacious."

Cognitive behavioral therapy

CBT, a structured therapy, identifies links among thoughts, feelings, and behaviors (see Chapter 34). By doing so, CBT aims to modify problematic thoughts and behaviors. The UK National Institute for Health and Care Excellence (NICE; 2011) advised that, for children and young people aged 10–17 years who misuse alcohol, individual CBT should be offered for those with limited comorbidities and good social support. Hogue *et al.* (2018) reported the evidence for both individual and group CBT as "well-established" for young people with SUD, with no evidence of iatrogenic effects among group members.

The adolescent community reinforcement approach (A-CRA) is a developmentally appropriate behavioral treatment for young people between 12–24 years of age with SUD. It seeks to increase the family, social, and educational/vocational reinforcers to support recovery. It works with individuals and families, addressing problem-solving and communication skills, and promoting active participation in positive social activities. It appears to be helpful for both SUD and mental health (Godley *et al.*, 2017); those with mental health problems and SUD showing greater improvement than those with SUD alone.

Family therapies

Family therapies and other approaches that engage family members facilitate successful treatment of SUD (see Chapter 35). NICE (2011) reviewed different types of available family therapies and noted the need for further research. For those with significant comorbidities and/or limited social support, multicomponent programs should be offered to young people (National Institute for Health and Care Excellence, 2011). General principles include supporting and engaging the family, as well as the wider social and educational system, identifying maladaptive family practices, problem-solving, and promoting change in specific behaviors within the family.

Relapse prevention: psychosocial

Relapse prevention (RP) is a strategy to reduce the likelihood and severity of relapse following the cessation or reduction of problematic behaviors. It is an umbrella term that incorporates a range of strategies: psychological therapies such as CBT and contingency management, mindfulness-based relapse prevention, medications such as naltrexone, monitoring either with biomarkers or tests for drug use, and peer support such as Alcoholics Anonymous (AA) and Narcotic Anonymous (NA). Generally, a combination of these strategies is more effective.

Recovery

The Substance Abuse and Mental Health Services Administration (SAMHSA) (2020) defined recovery as "a process of change through which individuals improve their health and wellness, live self-directed lives and strive to reach their full potential." Treatment extends beyond achieving a lifestyle of sobriety to also include managing all domains of life and achieving wellness, contentment, and full potential. Adolescents need to be supported to develop their individual and social capital for recovery, e.g., living in collegiate abstinence-only areas, mutual aid self-help groups, reduction of stigma, and peer-based support services.

12-step approach

Twelve-step programs are international mutual aid programs supporting recovery from addictions. The prototype, AA, was founded in the 1930s as a self-help movement. Multiple organizations worldwide adopted the principles, addressing problems of other drugs and addictions such as cocaine, sex, and overeating. The 12 steps incorporate issues such as admitting you are not in control of your addiction, recognizing a "higher power" can give strength, examining past mistakes and making amends, and helping others. The approach envisages a disease model that can be managed with lifelong abstinence and a new way of life.

Adolescent-specific 12-step programs exist, but less research examines this age group than adults (Nash, 2020). Despite some evidence of effectiveness, young people have poor attendance with about 2% in AA and NA being under 21 years, and high dropout rates (Kelly *et al.*, 2008). Possible barriers include the concept of lifelong abstinence, the difficulty relating to some of the "steps," and the spiritual aspects (Kelly & Urbanoski, 2012). Twelve-step attendance predicts greater community capital, more attendance at collegiate programs, and more sustained remission. However, some consider 12-step approaches to be one effective component of a more comprehensive approach to treatment (Fadus *et al.*, 2020).

Self-help groups (mutual aid support groups) provide social and emotional support to group members to maintain recovery. They are an easily accessible (in person or online), important, cost-free resource, often being the only treatment resource available to the individual. Other groups include Cocaine Anonymous (CA) and SMART, which stands for self-management and recovery training, is an international community of peer support groups, based on MI/CBT principles. They are generally attended by people with the same issue but may be attended by their families or friends. While there is much development of mutual aids for young adults, research on effectiveness for adolescents is lacking.

Further interventions

Many of the treatments used in clinical practice are based on principles rather than use of manualized structured treatments. There are treatments commonly used in practice that have not been rigorously researched, including multiple component therapies. These include digital interventions, and new adjunctive treatments such as mindfulness, yoga, exercise-based therapy, recovery-orientated setting, e.g., recovery colleges, and 12-step programs for adolescents. The recovery college or university-provided program includes a supportive environment for a lifestyle of recovery from SUDs within the campus.

Solution-focused brief therapy (SFBT) has been used for decades, though with little research. It is a form of counseling that focuses on working on reliance and the strengths of the person, as well as solutions to problems rather than the problems themselves. Franklin and Hang Hai (2021) reported promising evidence on SFBT's effectiveness in improving substance use behaviors and related psychosocial problems. Five of the nine studies reviewed showed that SFBT could improve both SUD and comorbid mental and psychosocial problems.

Compared to other therapies, digital interventions could be more appealing, more accessible, and more exciting for adolescents, thereby encouraging engagement. Monarque *et al.* (2023) noted the prominence of technologies in providing web-based, game-based, smartphone-based, computer-based, and virtual reality therapies. A personalized feedback approach was the main intervention in young people. Some research suggested that digital BIs and Internet CBT could augment treatment as usual (Kiluk *et al.*, 2016). The interventions reviewed by Monarque *et al.* (2023) more often focused on alcohol, with fewer directed at tobacco and illicit substances, and the focus mainly on early interventions (72%). The authors considered that game-based, and virtual reality-based interventions were underutilized, though further research is needed (see Chapter 49).

Pharmacological interventions

This section reviews the pharmacological interventions (Box 66.4), such as detoxifications and maintenance opiate treatments, as well as drugs, used in RP. All pharmacological treatments should be accompanied by psychosocial interven-

Box 66.4 Pharmacological interventions

- Emergency overdose: use of naloxone—parenteral or nasal
- Harm reduction: naloxone provision to family and person
- Medically managed detoxifications: alcohol, benzodiazepines, opioids
- Stabilization/maintenance: mainly for opioids
- Relapse preventions (RPs): alcohol, opioids, e.g., acamprosate, naltrexone, disulfiram
- Treatment of consequences of dependence/use: acute hepatitis, blood-borne viruses (BBV)
- Treatment of comorbid physical and mental disorder: e.g., respiratory diseases, depression, attention deficit hyperactivity disorder (ADHD)
- Treatment of smoking cessation

tions. As noted below, treatment also relates to acute use of naloxone in overdose, and treatment of its consequences, both physical problems, e.g., hepatitis C and psychiatric conditions, such as depression and anxiety.

There is little specific research on pharmacological interventions for those under 18 years. Generally, if pharmacological interventions such as detoxifications or RP medication are required, the young person will typically have complex comorbid disorders that require concurrent, integrated management.

Pharmacological interventions for SUD, usually alcohol or opioids, may require specialist addiction services and staff such as pediatric staff, children's mental health teams, and primary care, as well as social services (Gilvarry & Britton, 2009; UK Department of Health and Social Care, 2017). For those over 18 years, addiction specialists and/or primary care more often manage the initiation and ongoing pharmacological interventions. Pharmacological interventions require a comprehensive assessment, careful monitoring, and regular review by competent staff with involvement of parents, if appropriate. With the risk of opioid-related overdose and death, services should provide naloxone to patients and families/carers.

Medically assisted withdrawal

Alcohol dependence in people under 18 years is unusual. This diagnosis of dependence needs to be clinically established with any differential diagnoses excluded or managed, such as anxiety disorder or agitation from any other causes, and polysubstance use assessed.

NICE (2011) advised on identification, assessment, and management of AUDs in adults and young people. For young people, the setting for detoxification may vary depending on the severity of dependence, associated social supports, and comorbidities. Inpatient or residential-assisted withdrawal is required for those with severe dependence and multiple physical and mental health difficulties. NICE recommended inpatient care for those requiring assisted withdrawal aged 10–17 years. For those admitted to psychiatric or forensic units, treatment should either be available or transfer to a hospital for detoxification considered. Use of long-acting benzodiazepines, chlordiazepoxide, or diazepam are advised but doses may need to be reduced for young people (National Institute for Health and Care Excellence, 2011).

For patients dependent on illicit opioids, assisted withdrawal may be required with buprenorphine or methadone offered as first line, and use of lofexidine if uncertain of dependence (National Institute for Health and Care Excellence, 2007; Pilling *et al.*, 2007). Clinically, in the UK, lofexidine is not commonly used.

For patients abusing benzodiazepines, withdrawal is very unusual in young people, though there is growing use of illicit benzodiazepines (e.g., etizolam) combined with other drugs. While many will binge use in large doses, it is unusual to elicit withdrawal symptoms. If dependence is present, diazepam is the drug of choice (Lingford-Hughes *et al.*, 2012). There is no evidence for maintenance treatment.

Stabilization/maintenance for opioid management

The US/Europe has seen a significant increase in hospitalizations for overdose of opioids. Early treatment of opioid use disorder (OUD) to prevent death, reduce harm, and maintain in treatment is essential, and should be a priority for treatment providers. Pharmacological treatments are an essential part of a comprehensive treatment paradigm. The prescribing risks of methadone or buprenorphine can be substantially reduced with careful assessment, monitoring, and supervised dispensing from a pharmacist or specialist center.

Considerable evidence exists concerning methadone and buprenorphine therapy in adults with OUD. However, little evidence exists in adolescents; only three randomized controlled trials exist for buprenorphine treatment of young people with OUD (Marsch *et al.*, 2005; Woody *et al.*, 2008; Marsch *et al.*, 2016). Methadone is a synthetic μ-opioid receptor agonist with pharmacological properties resembling morphine. Buprenorphine is a partial μ-opioid receptor agonist treatment, sometimes combined with naloxone. Some suggest buprenorphine +/− naloxone is a preferred option (Woody *et al.*, 2008; Marsch *et al.*, 2016). Buprenorphine is now available as depot medication.

UK guidelines (UK Department of Health and Social Care, 2017) describe issues related to the prescription of opiate medications for young people. The guidelines address the transition to adult services, as well as assessment, initiation, and management of long-term maintenance. For patients dependent on prescription opioids, clinical consensus recommends treatment resembling that for illicit opioids: either reduction of the specific drug if it is a longer-acting drug or transfer to methadone or buprenorphine with careful titration of dose.

Krausz *et al.* (2022), in the development of clinical consensus guidelines noted the lack of access, lack of treatments, and reluctance of practitioners to prescribe for young people with OUD. Many clinicians view prescription of opioid medication as a "last resort" and often wait until a young person has relapsed, encountered much harm, or has aged into adulthood. Clinicians involved in this care need to recognize the continuum of care, from harm reduction to treatment and care of all domains, with crisis responses available and family-based interventions.

Krausz *et al.* (2022) discussed the regulatory boards in the US, noting that buprenorphine was available for those over 16 years and methadone was available for those aged 18 or over, but only for those who had "failed" two 28-day rehabilitation treatments. In the UK and Europe, no such stringent regulation is present. Buprenorphine is licensed for those over 13 years (UK) and methadone is licensed for 16 years and over.

Krausz *et al.* considered that the provision of evidence-based treatments, such as pharmacotherapy for opioid dependence in young people, was more widespread in Europe that in the US. He considered that the lack of youth-focused providers able to prescribe pharmacotherapy, fewer willing to do so or having experience, the dearth of trained youth-focused physicians, and the lack of confidence in prescribing for SUDs, in addition to stigma and unfamiliarity, has led to this limited use of evidence-based treatment options. Feder *et al.* (2017) noted less than 3% of adolescents received pharmacological treatments in the US. With limited access to pharmacological treatment in the US for adolescents, the primary treatment comprises psychosocial interventions alone, or abstinence-based residential treatment, which has high rates of dropout and low retention. This is important, considering the opioid epidemic and related deaths. In the UK, opioid agonist treatment, often buprenorphine, is available and advised, with no specific timescales for treatment length (UK Department of Health and Social Care, 2017).

Hadland *et al.* (2021) noted the position of the Society of Adolescent Health and Medicine; all adolescents with OUD should be offered medications alongside a comprehensive treatment package, with barriers to pharmacological treatment minimized, reduction of associated stigma, and improved training on OUD management for all practitioners.

There is little data available concerning medication treatment for SUD associated with medications other than opioids. No recommended pharmacological interventions exist for treatment of CUD. Cannabis-induced psychosis may need antipsychotic medication if prolonged beyond intoxication. Similarly, no effective or substitute pharmacological medications exist for stimulants. Acute physical effects, such as cardiac effects from cocaine or methamphetamine, may need urgent management. Medications may be required to treat psychosis, prolonged depression, or altered sleep patterns for a short period.

Relapse prevention: pharmacological

The main medications for RP for alcohol include acamprosate, naltrexone, disulfiram, and nalmefene. Naltrexone can be used for opioid use prevention. Acamprosate reduces craving for alcohol, though the mechanism of action is unclear. It has a good safety profile in adults, with few interactions with other prescribed drugs, and does not interact with alcohol, though with need for use multiple times a day adherence can be difficult.

Naltrexone is an opioid antagonist and can be useful for those with AUD and OUD, when abstinent. It is generally safe and well-tolerated, with few drug interactions, though should not be given to those currently prescribed opioids. It is generally taken orally once daily but in some countries is available as a depot injection.

Disulfiram inhibits the metabolism of alcohol, with unpleasant symptoms occurring during the disulfiram–alcohol reaction. The effects can be quite variable, though some severe effects can occur. High levels of monitoring, e.g., supervised consumption to ensure adherence, enhances outcome. Caution is advised in those under 18 years.

For those over 18 years with moderate or severe alcohol dependence, NICE (2011) advises the consideration of acamprosate or oral naltrexone in combination with psychosocial therapies. Disulfiram use is seen as a second-line treatment where the patient must be clearly selected as suitable and it should be ensured that they have adequate knowledge about the risks of using of alcohol and disulfiram. There is limited evidence on the efficacy of RP medications in young people under 18 years. For those over 16 years, NICE (2011) advises use of acamprosate and naltrexone for AUD after careful review of risks and benefits. A comprehensive baseline physical assessment with liver function tests should be routine prior to prescription of these drugs. These drugs can be taken for up to a year as RP if the person continues to progress well; with careful monitoring at least monthly for the first six months.

Nalmefene is recommended by NICE (2014) for adults, though there are no studies in young people. Other drugs with limited research evidence though not recommended in youth are topiramate, MDMA-assisted psychotherapy for AUD, gabapentin, and sodium oxybate (National Institute for Health and Care Excellence, 2011; Lingford-Hughes *et al.*, 2012; UK Department of Health and Care, 2017).

Mental health and comorbid care

This section briefly discusses treatment of comorbid psychiatric disorders and SUDs. Terms such as dual diagnosis or comorbid disorder are often used to describe the co-occurrence of a SUD and another mental disorder. Mental disorders and SUDs can exacerbate or act as risk factors for each other. Comorbidities relate to difficulties in multiple domains, such as physical health problems, behavioral and relationship issues, and educational and safeguarding problems. These complex presentations are more the norm in those with SUD, often leading to multiple barriers to treatment and uncertainty by professionals on how best to treat and when to treat, with fragmented care. There is lack of research or clinical consensus on management, the types of treatment combinations, the specific context, and the settings in which these are provided.

Many adolescents will experiment with alcohol and/or drugs. Practitioners in mental health and health care settings should screen all young people and be able to offer a BI with psychoeducation and motivational approaches. The threshold for referral to a specialist service varies depending on the wishes of the person and their families, frequency of drug use, amount, type of drug and method of use (e.g., cocaine, IV use), and degree of impairment in multiple domains such as decline in physical and mental health, and home and school problems.

These youths have diverse social, behavioral, and educational needs so comprehensive assessment, concurrent treatment, and integrated approaches are crucial. Too often, psychiatric and addiction services work separately and consecutively with an expectation of treating drug use first. However, clinical consensus would advise concurrent and integrated case management. The principle of "no wrong door," with multidisciplinary approaches to co-occurring problems managed simultaneously, apply. Barriers to treatment were thought to be rooted in a fragmented health care system, with different funding arrangements, and the "de-linking" of drug services from other mental health and general health care services (Sterling *et al.*, 2010).

Links between ADHD and early SUD are well recognized. As the age of onset of ADHD is generally much younger than SUD, ADHD appears a significant risk for the development of SUD (Ormel *et al.*, 2015). There is some evidence that early treatment of ADHD with stimulants reduced the risk of later SUD (Young *et al.*, 2023). Further, ADHD and CD may co-occur, a co-occurrence thought to be frequent, and both are likely to predict SUD, with this combination presenting clinical and behavioral challenges in treatment. Those with ADHD and SUD show earlier onset of SUD, a more chronic course, and likely polydrug use. However, while many debate the importance of concurrent treatment of ADHD and SUD, in a meta-analysis of randomized trials Fluyau *et al.* (2021) reported on a range of positive outcomes in those on stimulants: increased abstinence, reduced craving, reduced frequency of ADHD symptoms, and reduction of substance use, though this positive outcome was not always found (Cunill *et al.*, 2015).

Young *et al.* (2023) presented detailed clinical consensus guidelines on treatment of SUD and ADHD, for example: comprehensive assessments with possible training in ADHD and SUD, and/or joint assessments; active pharmacological treatment of SUD and ADHD should be offered subject to appropriate risks, emphasizing that "pharmacological treatment nihilism" was not appropriate; assessment with long-acting stimulant preparations recommended as first line, with concurrent psychoeducation and psychological treatment, e.g., motivational treatments; and interagency working and support networks needed for successful provision of care.

A further consensus (Ozgen *et al.*, 2020) noted the importance of screening for ADHD in those with SUD and screening for SUD in those with ADHD in mental health settings. However, this group could not achieve consensus on whether the requirement of abstinence from substances was critical prior to pharmacological treatment for ADHD, with some against the use of stimulants in those with comorbid SUD regardless of abstinence.

For those aged 14 and upward with severe mental illness and substance misuse, NICE (2016b) considered adaptation of existing specialist services to meet their needs and their wider health. It advised against creating a specialist dual diagnoses service but suggested offering interventions that aimed to improve engagement with all services, support harm reduction, change behavior, and prevent relapse, with advice from specialist addiction services.

There is robust evidence on the association between substance use, self-harm, and suicidality, with this co-occurrence associated with more severe symptoms and poorer outcomes, and with higher rates of perceived service needs (Kaminer *et al.* 2007). Kaminer *et al.* (2007) noted less retention and fewer positive outcomes with piecemeal treatment of depression without any SUD interventions and emphasized the need for coordinated and integrated treatment services.

For the older adolescent, the risk of overdose is significant (Yule *et al.*, 2018). Further, the combination of intoxication and impulsivity may increase behavioral, social, and legal problems and complicate the presentation and the engagement of these young people in treatment. Physical health problems may result from accidents related to intoxication and impulsivity, BBVs such as hepatitis B and C, and HIV, and other infections. Chronic pain can be a difficult clinical problem for those with SUD, as well as patients with chronic pain having a higher prevalence of SUDs (Morasco *et al.* 2011). Further for those with chronic pain, there is higher prevalence of comorbidities such as depression and anxiety disorder, higher suicidal ideation, and relapse from prescription medication abuse and illicit opioid use.

Settings and models of specialist services

For specialist SUD services for youth, considerable guidance on principles of treatment, on differences to adult services, on legal and safeguarding issues, and on transitions to adult services exist.

Some of these principles are (Gilvarry *et al.*, 2012):

- Assessments should be comprehensive.
- Staff need to be competent in assessing developmental needs, parental responsibility, and capacity to consent.
- All decisions made should be in the best interest of the child with awareness of confidentiality and information sharing.
- Treatment should be integrated with all children and young adult services, e.g., mental health, education.
- Services should be collaborative, coordinated, and with shared working protocols.
- Easy access for children and families, e.g., text messages, out of school hours.

The European Monitoring Centre for Drugs and Drug Addiction (EMCDDA) (2022) described similar principles regarding those in the criminal justice system with SUD. They emphasized the importance of evidence-based interventions, demonstration of professional competence, respecting ethical principles, and continuity of care within and between services during care and during transition to adult services. They advised the involvement of young people in design and delivery of services, including use as peer supporters. All services should work to ensure reduction and elimination of stigmatization of young people with SUD, wherever and whenever they access any service.

The US National Institutes of Health (NIH) (National Institute on Drug Abuse, 2014) emphasized the importance of addressing all aspects of need: physical, psychological, and social well-being, as well as education, housing, and family environment. They considered that failure to integrate and simultaneously address all issues could affect the outcome of treatment for substance use.

In the UK, specialist SUD services for young people are normally separate from adult treatment services; preferred because of the differing patterns of alcohol and drug use, and the importance of child-centered services. Such services are more often geared toward prevention, early intervention, and harm reduction to prevent escalation of risk. They are primarily based in community settings, often aligned with adult addiction services, primary care, third-sector integrated services, and criminal justice teams. There is some involvement in schools and with child mental health services.

Residential rehabilitation services in the UK for those under 18 years of age are rare, while older youth may use adult residential facilities. There is some early but minimal development of recovery-specific educational settings, particularly in a few universities, though with little research. These educational settings for recovery are much more developed in the US, with youth noting greater abstinence at six months follow-up (Finch *et al.*, 2018).

Residential treatment in the US is an intense, high level of care, generally for adolescents with severe levels of addiction and comorbidities. Therapeutic communities are a form of long-term residential treatment, are intensive, and use a combination of techniques to "resocialize" the adolescent, enlisting the community, including residents and staff, actively in treatment. Treatment is structured, focused on building personal and social responsibility and developing new coping skills. Such programs may offer a range of family services. They are usually up to 12 months though short-term residential programs also exist (De Andrade *et al.*, 2019, National Institute on Drug Abuse, 2020a).

Mefodeva *et al.* (2022) reviewed the outcomes of young people (aged18–30 years) with polysubstance use who accessed residential or day treatment services for substance use. All had at least moderate mental health symptoms. The authors advocated targeting multiple morbidities in an integrated way. Others report improved outcomes for those with SUD and mental health comorbidities in residential settings that provide integrated treatments (Schoenthaler *et al.* 2017).

Transitions

Within services, there is much variation in access, some provide services up to 18 years, and some up to 24 years, so transition arrangements need to be carefully considered. Often there is lack of clarity for the transition of health care for children and young adults to adult health care services, with the process of transition often fragmented, both within and across specialties (National Confidential Enquiry into Patient Outcome and Death, 2023). NICE (2016a) advised that transitions should be purposeful and planned, and developmentally appropriate, with involvement of the young person and their carer/parents, and clear communications and strong leadership to ensure appropriate treatment and reduce any dropout.

Conclusions

All young people's services should have a philosophy of "no wrong door," to ensure availability and accessibility of treatment (Volkov *et al.*, 2020). Many young people will present with difficulties other than direct drug and alcohol use, such as the consequences of use, e.g., accidents and injuries, overdose, and self-harm. These behaviors and health/mental health issues should be seen as possible risk factors for SUDs. Universal screening for substance use is recommended by SAMHSA (2021a, 2021b). This screening, with BI and referral, is a comprehensive integrated public health approach used to identify those at risk of SUDs.

Every effort should be made by all children's services to improve access to services, and reduce barriers such as stigma and negative perceptions of those who use drugs. Drugs and alcohol use should never be seen as an exclusion to treatment services and all practitioners should ensure a positive approach to engagement.

All services involved in treatments should be coordinated, comprehensive, and collaborative. Having achieved an international consensus on management of high risk youth, Krausz *et al.* (2022) published a number of principles: screening of substance use and mental health should be routine in all settings for all youth; those at risk should receive targeted prevention; all domains of functioning should be assessed in high-risk youth including assessment of trauma; and psychiatric and physical assessment should be routine, and with greater access and more rapid access to treatment.

Especially if problematic drug or alcohol use, many young people will have comorbid disorders, CD and emerging personality issues, neurodevelopmental issues, depression and anxiety, self-harm, and suicidal risk. Working collaboratively and concurrently within a shared care network, with a shared plan involving the young person and their families, is best practice.

References

American Psychiatric Association (2022) *Diagnostic and Statistical Manual of Mental Disorders*, 5th edn. text revision edn. American Psychiatric Association, Washington, DC.

Babor, T. *et al.* (2022) Alcohol: no ordinary commodity, a summary of the third edition. *Addiction* **117**, 3024–3036.

Brewer, S. *et al.* (2017) Treating mental health and substance use disorders in adolescents: What is on the menu. *Current Psychiatry Reports* **19**, 5. doi:10.1007/s11920-017-0755-0.

Bukstein, O. (2005) Practice parameter for the assessment and treatment of children and adolescents with substance use disorders. *Journal of the American Academy of Child and Adolescent Psychiatry* **44**(6), 609–621. doi:10.1097/01.chi.0000159135.33706.37.

Caluzzi, G. *et al.* (2022) Declining drinking among adolescents: Are we seeing a denormalization of drinking and a normalisation of non-drinking. *Addiction* **117**, 1204–1212.

Castelpietra, G. *et al.* (2022) The burden of mental disorders, substance use disorders and self-harm among young people in Europe, 1990-2019: findings from the Global Burden of Disease Study 2019. *The Lancet Regional Health Europe* **16**, 100341. doi:10.1016/j.lanepe.2022.100341.

Cerda, M. *et al.* (2015) Nonmedical prescription opioid use in childhood and early adolescence predicts transitions to heroin use in young adulthood, a national study. *The Journal of Pediatrics* **167**, 605–612.

Cerrai, S. *et al.* (2022) E-cigarette use and conventional cigarette smoking among European students: findings from the 2019 ESPAD survey. *Addiction* **117**, 2918–2932.

Chadi, N. *et al.* (2019) Association between electronic cigarette use and marijuana use among adolescents and young adults: a systemic review and meta-analysis. *JAMA Pediatrics* **173**(10), e192574.

Chan, Y.-F. *et al.* (2009) Prevalence and comorbidity of major internalising and externalising problems among adolescents and adults presenting to substance abuse treatment. *Journal of Substance Abuse Treatment* **34**(1), 14–24.

Coulton, S. *et al.* (2019) Opportunistic screening for alcohol use problems in adolescents attending emergency departments: an evaluation of screening tools. *Journal of Public Health* **41**(1), 1–8.

Coyne, S. *et al.* (2020) Pathological video game symptoms from adolescence to emerging adulthood: a 6-year longitudinal study of trajectories, predictors and outcomes. *Developmental Psychology* **56**(7), 1385–1396.

Cunill, R. *et al.* (2015) Pharmacological treatment of attention deficit hyperactivity disorder with co-morbid drug dependence. *Journal of Psychopharmacology* **29**, 15–23.

Darke, S. *et al.* (eds) (2019) *The Clinicians Guide to Illicit Drugs and Health*. Silverback Publishing, London, UK.

Das, J. *et al.* (2016) Interventions for adolescent substance abuse: an overview of systematic reviews. *Journal of Adolescent Health* **59**(4 Suppl), S61–S75.

De Andrade, D. *et al.* (2019) The effectiveness of residential treatment services for individual s with substance use disorders: a systematic review. *Drug and Alcohol Dependence* **201**, 227–235.

Degenhardt, L. *et al.* (2016) Substance use in young people: 1. The increasing global health priority of substance use in young people. *The Lancet Psychiatry* **3**, 251–264.

Degenhardt, L. *et al.* (2018) The global burden of disease attributable to alcohol and drug use in 195 countries and territories, 1990–2016: a systematic analysis for the global burden of disease study 2016. *The Lancet Psychiatry* **5**, 987–1012.

Degenhardt, L. *et al.* (2021) Concordance between the diagnostic guidelines for alcohol and cannabis use disorders in the draft ICD-11 and other classification systems: analysis of data from the WHO's World Mental Health Surveys. *Addiction* **114**(3), 534–552.

DeLuca, P. *et al.* (2022) Effectiveness and cost-effectiveness of face-to-face and electronic brief interventions versus screening alone to reduce alcohol consumption among high-risk adolescents presenting to emergency departments: three-arm pragmatic randomized trial (SIPS Junior high risk trial). *Addiction* **117**, 2200–2214. doi:10.1111/add.15884.

ESPAD Group (2020) *ESPAD Report 2019: Results from the European School Survey Project on Alcohol and Other Drugs*. EMCDDA Joint Publications, Publications Office of the European Union, Luxembourg.

European Monitoring Centre for Drugs and Drug Addiction (2022) Recreational Use of Nitrous Oxide: A Growing Concern for Europe. European Monitoring Centre for Drugs and Drug Addition (EMCDDA), Lisbon. Available: https://www.euda.europa.eu/publications/rapid-communication/recreational-use-nitrous-oxide-growing-concern-europe_en [15 December 2024].

Fadus, M. *et al.* (2020) Adolescent substance use disorder treatment: an update on evidence-based strategies. *Current Psychiatry Reports* **21**(10), 96. doi:10.1007/s11920-019-1086-0.

Faggiano, F. *et al.* (2014) Universal school-based approaches for illicit drug use. *Cochrane Database of Systematic Reviews* **12**, CD003020.

Feder, K. *et al.* (2017) Medications assisted treatment for adolescents in speciality treatment for opioid use disorder. *The Journal of Adolescent Health* **60**, 747–750.

Finch, A. *et al.* (2018) Recovery high schools: effect of schools supporting recovery from substance use disorders. *The American Journal of Drug and Alcohol Abuse* **44**(2), 175–184. doi:10.1080/00952990.2017.1354378.

Fluyau, D. *et al.* (2021) Systematic review and meta-analysis: treatment of substance use disorder in attention deficit hyperactivity disorder. *The American Journal on Addictions* **30**, 110–121.

Franklin, C. & Hang Hai, A. (2021) Solution focused brief therapy for substance use: a review of the literature heath social work 2021 **46**(2), 103–114.

Gao, Y.-X. *et al.* (2022) The prevalence and possible risk factors of internet gaming disorder among adolescents and young adults: Systematic reviews and meta-analyses. *Journal of Psychiatric Research* **154**, 35–43.

Gillespie, N.&. & Kendler, K. (2020) Use of genetically informed methods to clarify the nature of the association between cannabis use and risk of schizophrenia. *JAMA Psychiatry* **78**(5), 467–468. doi:10.1001/jamapsychiatry.2020.3564.

Gilvarry, E. & Britton, J. (2009) Guidance for the Pharmacological Management of Substance Misuse Among Young People in Secure Environments. UK Department of Health, London. Available: https://www.drugsandalcohol.ie/14428/1/DOH_Guidance_for_pharmacological_management_young_people.pdf [15 December 2024].

Gilvarry, E, et al. (eds) (2012) Practice Standards for Young People with Substance Misuse Problems, publication number CCQI 127. Royal College of Psychiatrists, London.

Godley, M.D. *et al.* (2017) Adolescent community reinforcement approach implementation and treatment outcomes for youth with opioid problem use. *Drug and Alcohol Dependence* **174**, 9–16. doi:10.1016/j.drugalcdep.2016.12.029.

Grant, J.E. *et al.* (2019) E-cigarette (vaping) is associated with illicit drug use, mental health problems and impulsivity in university students. *Annals of Clinical Psychiatry* **31**(1), 27–34.

Grummit, L. *et al.* (2002) An umbrella review of the links between adverse childhood experiences and substance misuse: What, why, and where do we go from here? *Substance Abuse and Rehabilitation* **13**, 83–100.

Hadland, S. *et al.* (2021) Medications for adolescents and young adults with opioid use disorder. *Journal of Adolescent Health* **68**(3), 632–636.

Hall, W. *et al.* (2020) The effects of cannabis use on the development of adolescents and young adults. *Annual Review of Developmental Psychology* **2**(1), 461–483.

Hamad, A. *et al.* (2022) Familial associations in adolescent substance use disorder- a population-based cohort study. *Addiction* **117**, 2720–2729.

Harm Reduction International (2022) *Global State of Harm Reduction 2022*. Harm Reduction International, London.

Harris, S. *et al.* (2014) Screening and brief interventions for alcohol and other abuse. *Adolescent Medicine: State of the Art Reviews* **25**(1), 126–156.

Hines, L. *et al.* (2020) Association of high-potency cannabis use with mental health and substance use in adolescence *JAMA. Psychiatry* **77**(10), 1044–1051. doi:10.1001/jamapsychiatry.2020.1035.

Hogue, A. *et al.* (2018) Evidence base on outpatient behavioural treatment for adolescent substance use 2014–2017. Outcomes, treatment delivery and promising horizons. *Journal of Clinical Child and Adolescent Psychology* **47**(4), 499–526. doi:101.1080/15374416.2018.1466307.

Isaksson, A. *et al.* (2011) Phosphatidylethanol in blood (B-PEth): a marker for alcohol use and abuse. *Drug Testing and Analysis* **3**(4), 195–200. doi:10.1002/dta.278.

Kaminer, Y. *et al.* (2007) Comorbid adolescent substance use and major depressive disorder. *Psychiatry (Edgemont)* **4**(12), 32–43.

Kapan, A. *et al.* (2020) Use of electronic cigarettes in European populations: a narrative review. *International Journal of Environmental Research and Public Health* **17**(6), 1971. doi:10.3390/ijerph17061971.

Kelly, J. & Urbanoski, K. (2012) Youth recovery contexts: the incremental effects of 12-step attendance and involvement on the adolescent outpatient outcomes. *Alcoholism: Clinical and Experimental Research* **36**(7), 1219–1229.

Kelly, J.F. *et al.* (2008) What do adolescents exposed to Alcoholics Anonymous think of the 12 step groups? *Substance Abuse* **29**(2), 53–62.

Kendler, K.S. *et al.* (2020) The risk for drug abuse, alcohol use disorder, and psychosocial dysfunction in off-spring from high-density pedigrees: its moderation by personal, family and community factors. *Molecular Psychiatry* **25**, 1777–1786.

Kiluk, B.,.D. *et al.* (2016) Randomised trial of computerised cognitive behavioural therapy for alcohol use disorders: efficacy as a virtual stand-alone and treatment add-on compared with standard outpatient treatment. *Alcoholism: Clinical and Experimental Research* **40**, 1991–2000.

Krausz, M. *et al.* (2022) Towards an international consensus on the prevention, treatment and management of high-risk substance use and overdose among youth. *Medicina (Kaunas)* **58**(4), 539. doi:10.3390/medicina58040539.

Lees, B. *et al.* (2020) Effect of alcohol use on the adolescent brain and behavior. *Pharmacology Biochemistry and Behaviour* **192**, 172906. doi:10.1016/j.pbb.2020.172906.

Lingford-Hughes, A. *et al.* (2012) British Association of Psychopharmacology (BAP) updated guidelines: evidence-based guidelines for the pharmacological management of substance abuse, harmful use, addiction and comorbidity: Recommendations from BAP. *Journal of Psychopharmacology* **26**(7), 899–952.

Marsch, L.A. *et al.* (2005) Comparison of pharmacological treatments for opioid dependent adolescents: a randomised control trial. *Archives of General Psychiatry* **62**, 1157–1164.

Marsch, L.A. *et al.* (2016) A randomised controlled trial of buprenorphine taper duration among opioid dependent adolescents and young adults. *Addiction* **111**, 1406–1415.

Martineau, F. *et al.* (2013) Population level interventions to reduce alcohol related harm: an overview of systematic reviews. *Preventive Medicine* **57**, 278–296.

McArdle, P. *et al.* (2022) Alcohol misuse among English youth, are harms attributable to alcohol or underlying disinhibitory characteristics? *Alcohol and Alcoholism* **57**, 372–377. doi:10.1093/alcalc/agab077.

Mefodeva, V. *et al.* (2022) Polysubstance use in young people accessing residential and day-treatment services for substance use: substance use profiles, psychotic comorbidity, and treatment completion. *Addiction* **117**(12), 3110, 10.1111/add.16008-3120.

Miech, R.A. *et al.* (2018) *Monitoring the Future: National Survey Results on Drug Use, 1975–2018*. Institute for Social Research, University of Michigan, Ann Arbor, MI. Available: https://monitoringthefuture.org/wp-content/uploads/2022/08/mtf-vol1_2018.pdf [15 December 2024].

Miller, W.R. & Rollnick, S. (1991) *Motivational Interviewing*. Guilford Press, New York.

Miller, W.R. & Sanchez, V.C. (1994) Motivating young adults for treatment and lifestyle change. In: *Issues in Alcohol Use and Misuse in Young Adults*. (ed G. Howard). University of Notre Dame Press, Notre Dame, IN.

Monarque, M. *et al.* (2023) Digital interventions for substance use disorders in young people: rapid review. *Substance Abuse Treatment, Prevention, and Policy* **18**, 13. doi:10.1186/s13011-023-00518-1.

Morasco, B.J. *et al.* (2011) Systematic review of prevalence, correlates, and treatment outcomes for chronic non-cancer pain in patients with comorbid substance use disorder. *Pain* **152**(3), 488–497. doi:10.1016/j.pain.2010.10.009.

Moss, H.B. *et al.* (2014) Early adolescent patterns of alcohol, cigarettes and marijuana polysubstance use and young adult substance use outcomes in a nationally representative sample. *Drug and Alcohol Dependence* **136**, 51–62.

Nash, A. (2020) The twelve steps and adolescent recovery: a concise review. *Substance Abuse* **2020**, 14. doi:10.1177/1178221820904397.

National Center for Drug Abuse Statistics (2021) *Drug Use Among Youth: Facts and Statistics*. National Center for Drug Abuse Statistics (NCDAS) Available: https://drugabusestatistics.org/teen-drug-use/ [15 December 2024].

National Confidential Enquiry into Patient Outcome and Death (2023) *The Inbetweeners*. London.

National Institute for Health and Care Excellence (2007) *Drug Misuse in Over 16s: Opioid Detoxification*. National Institute for Health and Care Excellence (NICE), London. Available: www.nice.org.uk/CG052 [15 December 2024].

National Institute for Health and Care Excellence (2011) *Alcohol-use Disorders: Diagnosis, Assessment and Management of Harmful Drinking (High-Risk Drinking) and Alcohol Dependence*. National Institute for Health and Care Excellence (NICE), London. Available: https://www.nice.org.uk/guidance/cg115 [15 December 2024].

National Institute for Health and Care Excellence (2014) *Nalmefene for Reducing Alcohol Consumption in People with Alcohol Dependence: Technology Appraisal TA325 26/11/2014*. National Institute for Health and Care Excellence (NICE), London. Available: https://www.nice.org.uk/guidance/ta325 [15 December 2024].

National Institute for Health and Care Excellence (2016a) *Transition from Children to Adults' Services for Young People Using Health or Social Care Services: NICE Guideline [NG43]*. National Institute for Health and Care Excellence (NICE), London. Available: https://www.nice.org.uk/guidance/ng43 [15 December 2024].

National Institute for Health and Care Excellence (2016b) *Coexisting Severe Mental Illness and Substance Misuse: Community Health and Social Care Services: NICE Guideline [NG58]*. National Institute for Health and Care Excellence (NICE), London. Available: https://www.nice.org.uk/guidance/ng58 [15 December 2024].

National Institute on Drug Abuse (2014) *Principles of Adolescent Substance Use Disorder Treatment: A Research-Based Guide*. National Institute on Drug Abuse (NIDA), North Bethesda, MD. Available: https://archives.nida.nih.gov/sites/default/files/podat-guide-adolescents-508.pdf [15 December 2024].

National Institute on Drug Abuse (2020a) *Therapeutic Communities Research Report: How Do Therapeutic Communities Treat Populations with Special Needs?* National Institute on Drug Abuse (NIDA), North Bethesda, MD. Available: https://www.scribd.com/document/573386664/LN2-therapeutic-communities-research-report. [15 December 2024].

National Institute on Drug Abuse (2020b) *Monitoring the Future Results Survey 2020*. National Institute on Drug Abuse (NIDA), North Bethesda, MD. Available: https://archives.nida.nih.gov/research-topics/trends-statistics/infographics/monitoring-future-2020-survey-results [15 December 2024].

National Institute on Drug Abuse (2021) Drug Overdose Deaths: Facts and Figures [online]. National Institute on Drug Abuse (NIDA), North Bethesda, MD. Available: https://www.drugabuse.gov/drug-topics/trends-statistics/overdose-death-rates [15 December 2024].

Nawi, A.M. *et al.* (2021) Risk and protective factors of drug abuse among adolescents: q systematic review. *BMC Public Health* **21**, 2088. doi:10.1186/s12889-021-11906-2.

Nguyen, H.V. & Mital, S. (2022) Effects of e-cigarette use on mental health among youths: quasi-experimental evidence from Canada. *Addiction* **117**, 2673–2682.

NHS Digital (2022) Smoking, Drinking and Drug Use Among Young People in England, 2021. NHS Digital, Leeds, UK. Available: https://digital.nhs.uk/data-and-information/publications/statistical/smoking-drinking-and-drug-use-among-young-people-in-england/2021 [15 December 2024].

Nicholson, P.J. *et al.* (2015) *Cognitive Enhancing Drugs and the Workplace*. British Medical Association, London. Available: https://www.bma.org.uk/media/agcf0ol3/bma_cognitive_enhancing_drugs_and_the_workplace_oct_2019.pdf [15 December 2024].

Office for Health Improvement & Disparities (2023) *Young People's Substance Misuse Treatment Statistics 2021-2022: Report*. Office for Health Improvement & Disparities, London.

Office for National Statistics (2022) Drug Misuse in England and Wales: Year Ending June 2022. Office for National Statistics (ONS), Newport, UK.

Orford, J. *et al.* (2005) Effectiveness of treatment for alcohol problems: findings of the randomised UK alcohol treatment trial (UKATT). *BMJ* **331**, 541.

Ormel, J. *et al.* (2015) Mental health in Dutch adolescents: a TRAILS report on prevalence, severity, age of onset, continuity, and comorbidity of DSM disorders. *Psychological Medicine* **45**, 345–360. doi:10.1017/S0033291714001469.

Ozgen, H. *et al.* (2020) International consensus statement for the screening, diagnosis, and treatment of adolescents with concurrent attention-deficit/hyperactivity disorder and substance use disorder. *European Addiction Research* **26**(4–5), 223–232. doi:10.1159/000508385.

Paris, A. *et al.* (2023) Nitrous oxide induced subacute combined degeneration of the cord: diagnosis and treatment. *Practical Neurology* **23**(3). doi:10.1136/pn-2022-003631.

Perepletchikova, F. *et al.* (2008) Practitioner review: Adolescent alcohol use disorders: assessment and treatment issues. *Journal of Child Psychology and Psychiatry* **49**(11), 1131–1154. doi:10.1111/j.1469-7610.2008.01934.x.

Pilling, S. *et al.* (2007) Psychosocial interventions and opioid detoxification for drug misuse: summary of NICE guidance. *BMJ* **335**(7612), 203–205.

Project MATCH (1997) Matching alcoholism treatments to client heterogeneity: Project MATCH posttreatment drinking outcomes. *Journal of Studies on Alcohol* **58**, 7–29.

Public Health England (2018) *Alcohol and Drug Treatment for Adults: Statistics Summary 2017–2018*. Public Health England, London. Available: https://www.gov.uk/government/statistics/substance-misuse-treatment-for-adults-statistics-2017-to-2018/alcohol-and-drug-treatment-for-adults-statistics-summary-2017-to-2018 [16 December 2024].

Richert, T. *et al.* (2020) Mental health problems among young people in substance abuse treatment in Sweden. *Substance Abuse Treatment, Prevention, and Policy* **15**, 43.

Rubin-Kahana, D.S. *et al.* (2022) The impact of cannabis legalization for recreational purposes on youth: a narrative review of the Canadian experience. *Frontiers in Psychiatry* **13**, 984485. doi:10.3389/fpsyt.2022.984485.

Santo, T., Jr. *et al.* (2013) Familial, social and individual factors contributing to risk for adolescent substance use. *Journal of Addiction* **2013**(1), 579310. doi:10.1155/2013/579310.

Santo, T., Jr. *et al.* (2022) Prevalence of mental disorders among people with opioid use disorder: a systematic review and meta-analysis. *Drug and Alcohol Dependence* **238**, 109551. doi:10.1016/j.drugalcdep.2022.109551.

Saunders, J.B. *et al.* (1993) Development of the Alcohol Use Disorder Identification Test (AUDIT): WHO collaborative project on early detection of persons with harmful alcohol consumption. *Addiction* **88**, 791–804.

Schoenthaler, S.J. *et al.* (2017) The effects of residential dual diagnosis treatment on alcohol abuse. *Journal of Systems and Integrative Neuroscience* **2017**, 3. doi:10.15761/JSIN.1000169.

Shafi, A. *et al.* (2020) New psychoactive substances: a review and update. *Therapeutic Advances in Psychopharmacology* **10**, 2045125320967197.

Shao, H. *et al.* (2023) Trends of the Global Burden of Disease attributable to cannabis use disorder in 204 countries and territories, 1990-2019: results from the Disease Burden Study 2019. *International Journal of Mental Health and Addiction* **22**, 2485–2507. doi:10.1007/s11469-022-00999-4.

Sterling, S. *et al.* (2010) Access to treatment for adolescents with substance use and co-occurring disorders: challenges and opportunities. *Journal of the American Academy of Child and Adolescent Psychiatry* **49**(7), 637–726.

Stockings, E. *et al.* (2016) Substance use in young people; prevention, early intervention, harm reduction and treatment of substance use in young people. *Lancet Psychiatry* **3**, 280–296.

Substance Abuse and Mental Health Services Administration (2019) *Key Substance Use and Mental Health Indicators in the United States:*

Results from the 2018 National Survey on Drug Use and Health. Substance Abuse and Mental Health Services Administration (SAMHSA), North Bethesda, MD. Available: https://www.scirp.org/reference/referencespapers?referenceid=2886613 [16 December 2024].

Substance Abuse and Mental Health Services Administration (2020) *Recovery and Recovery Support*. Substance Abuse and Mental Health Services Administration (SAMHSA), North Bethesda, MD. Available: https://www.samhsa.gov/find-help/recovery [16 December 2024].

Substance Abuse and Mental Health Services Administration (2021a) *Screening, Brief Intervention and Referral to Treatment (SBIRT)*. Substance Abuse and Mental Health Services Administration (SAMHSA), North Bethesda, MD. Available: https://www.samhsa.gov/sbirt [16 December 2024].

Substance Abuse and Mental Health Services Administration (2021b) *Screening and Treatment of Substance Use Disorders Among Adolescents*. Advisory Publication Number PEP20-06-04-008. Substance Abuse and Mental Health Services Administration (SAMHSA), North Bethesda, MD. Available: https://store.samhsa.gov/sites/default/files/pep20-06-04-008.pdf [16 December 2024].

Tait, R.J. *et al*. (2004) Effectiveness of a brief intervention and continuity of care in enhancing attendance for treatment by adolescent substance users. *Drug and Alcohol Dependence* **74**, 289–296.

Tanner-Smith, E. & Lipsey, M. (2015) Brief alcohol interventions for adolescents and young adults: a systematic review and meta-analysis. *Journal of Substance Abuse Treatment* **51**, 1–18.

UK Department of Health and Social Care (2017) *Drug Misuse and Dependence: UK Guidelines on Clinical Management*. Department of Health, London.

UK Government (2021) *United Kingdom Drug Situation: Focal Point Annual Report*. UK Government, London. Available: https://www.gov.uk/government/publications/united-kingdom-drug-situation-focal-point-annual-report [13 December 2024].

United Nations Office on Drugs and Crime (2018) *International Standards on Drug Use Prevention*. United Nations Office on Drugs and Crime (UNODC), Vienna, Austria. Available: https://www.unodc.org/documents/prevention/UNODC-WHO_2018_prevention_standards_E.pdf [16 December 2024].

United Nations Office on Drugs and Crime (2023) *World Drug Report 2023*. United Nations Office on Drugs and Crime (UNODC), Vienna, Austria. Available: https://www.unodc.org/unodc/en/data-and-analysis/world-drug-report-2023.html [13 December 2024].

US Drug Enforcement Administration (2022) *The Growing Threat of Xylazine and its Mixture with Illicit Drugs OCTOBER 2022*. US Drug Enforcement Administration (DEA), Arlington County, VA.

Vashishtha, R. *et al*. (2021) Trends in adolescent drinking across 39 high-income countries: exploring the timing and magnitude of decline. *European Journal of Public Health* **31**(2)), 424–431. doi:10.1093/eurpub/ckaa193.

Volkov, N. *et al*. (2020) Managing dual disorders: a statement by the informal scientific network, UN commission on narcotic drugs. *World Psychiatry* **19**(3), 396–397.

Woody, G.E. *et al*. (2008) Extended v short term buprenorphine naloxone for treatment of opioid addicted youth: a randomised trial. *JAMA* **300**, 2003–2011.

World Health Organization (2018) *Global Status Report on Alcohol and Health 2018*. World Health Organization (WHO), Geneva, Switzerland. Available: https://www.who.int/publications/i/item/9789241565639 [16 December 2024].

World Health Organization (WHO) (2019) *International statistical classification of diseases and related health problems*, 11th revision. edn. World Health Organization (WHO, Geneva, Switzerland.

Young, S. *et al*. (2023) Identification and treatment of individuals with attention-deficit/hyperactivity disorder and substance use disorder: an expert consensus statement. *World Journal of Psychiatry* **13**(3), 84–112.

Yule, A.M. *et al*. (2018) Risk factors for overdose in treatment seeking youth with substance use disorders. *The Journal of Clinical Psychiatry* **79**, 17m11678.

CHAPTER 67

Personality disorders

Jonathan Hill[1,2] and Carla Sharp[3]
[1]School of Psychology and Clinical Language Sciences, University of Reading, Reading, UK
[2]Oxford Health NHS Foundation Trust, Oxford, UK
[3]Department of Psychiatry, University of Houston, Houston, TX, USA

Introduction to personality and personality disorder

Personality, personality functioning, personality disorder

Personality refers to a relatively stable set of tendencies in behaviors, cognitions, and emotional patterns, which, together, describe a person's unique character. Personality functioning refers to the way these tendencies contribute to effective performance in different social domains such as in work or school, in romantic relationships and friendships, and to the ways the individual is able to benefit from the resources available in them. Individuals usually have relatively good insight into their own identity and relationships. They understand that the way they behave may impact others and vice versa. This awareness helps individuals make decisions and manage their relationships. In some individuals, however, this insight is limited, and from a psychiatric point of view, such individuals may meet criteria for a diagnosis of personality disorder (Sharp, 2022).

Why is something like the concept of personality disorder needed?

The personality disorders are described within a framework of adult psychiatric diagnoses that makes a distinction between disorders that are episodic, with clear onsets and offsets and circumscribed symptomatology, for example, depression, and disorders that are more enduring, with widespread emotional and behavioral problems. The need for something like the concept of personality disorder arises then in two main ways. First, some individuals have behavioral and emotional problems that precede and extend beyond the confines of episodic disorders. Second, these problems share with personality traits (habitual patterns of behavior, thought, and emotion) the characteristics of being relatively enduring and evident in many situations.

In clinical practice in adolescence the concept is often relevant where the presenting problem can be diagnosed as an episodic disorder, such as depression, but there are additional features that are not accounted for by that diagnosis, nor by an accompanying "comorbid" episodic disorder such as generalized anxiety disorder. Thus, the key is the extensiveness and diversity of the difficulties. In general, consideration of personality disorder will also require that these, or similar, difficulties were present before the onset of the disorder. Furthermore, as the presenting symptoms resolve, those attributed to personality disorder persist. The concept is also relevant where an individual has problems that are severe enough to cause distress to themselves or others, and impair daily functioning, but they do not follow the pattern of episodic disorders. Examples include repeated violence, or self-harm in the absence of diagnosable depression, or difficulties in social role performance, for example, in work or close relationships.

Personality disorder in adolescence: a clinical illustration

The consideration of personality disorder is relatively straightforward when the person is aged 30 years, but suppose they are aged 15 years? Questions are commonly asked as to whether adolescents show the same levels of stability in their behaviors, cognitions, and emotional patterns as adults, and whether difficulties in these areas of their lives are better understood in terms of normal developmental processes than disorder.

We can begin to address these concerns through a summary of the problems which are typical of the young people who are treated in medical and mental health services in Europe and the US. The following example illustrates these problems.

Ellie is a 15-year-old girl who started cutting her arms and legs and overdosing when she was 13. When asked what led to self-harm and overdosing, Ellie said that she feels there is

Rutter's Child and Adolescent Psychiatry and Psychology, Seventh Edition.
Edited by Anita Thapar, Daniel S. Pine, Samuele Cortese, Cathy Creswell, Tamsin J. Ford, James F. Leckman, and Argyris Stringaris.

Companion website: www.wiley.com/go/thapar/ruttersspsych7

"nothing inside" feeling like she is "a thing—not a person" and "might as well be dead because nobody loves me anyway." Although these problems are relatively recent, her behaviors have been a concern for many years. Even as a toddler she would react with strong emotions to minor frustrations or provocations, and during primary school she was diagnosed with attention deficit hyperactivity disorder (ADHD). Increasingly, she has been unable to cope in school because of outbursts of anger and distress, which have also led her friends to avoid her. She has been out of school over the past year, not only spending long hours in her bedroom, but also going missing overnight. She has a sexual relationship with man in his mid-20s who has been violent with her. She has had numerous attendances at the emergency departments of several hospitals, and social services have been concerned for contacts with them. Assessments by child and adolescent mental health services (CAMHS) have established that from time to time she meets diagnostic criteria for major depressive disorder (MDD), but even after recovering from depression most of her difficulties remain—most notably the complex relationships she has with peers whom she texts daily about her feelings of numbness and desire not to live anymore, and who have told her that she is "too much to handle," leading to clingy behavior and continued fears of being alone. Diagnostic assessment established that she does not have autistic spectrum disorder (ASD). Neither psychological treatments, nor a three-month psychiatric admission have led to improvement. Her parents have tried to support her, but they have become angry and demoralized with her, and with the services, which, as they see it, have failed them. They are now considering home schooling.

Validity of personality disorder in adolescence

Clinical pictures such as this illustrate the distinctive emotional, behavioral, and social features of this complex and severe disorder. Nevertheless, for decades, it was considered that personality disorders could not be diagnosed in adolescence because, it was argued, personality is not yet stable enough to warrant any diagnosis and it would be stigmatizing to diagnose young people with personality disorder. However, recent empirical research on borderline personality disorder (BPD), which is the main focus of this chapter, has led to a reconsideration of this view. Perhaps most importantly, this is because the stability of BPD features from adolescence to adult life is no different to stability from one phase of adult life to another (Ferguson, 2010). In both instances, there is not only substantial stability but also considerable change. Further support for the validity of the BPD construct in adolescence, includes that BPD can be separated from other disorders in course and outcome (Wertz *et al.*, 2020), and it is similar to adult BPD with respect to prevalence and risk factors (Stepp *et al.*, 2016). There is also preliminary support for efficacy of treatment for BPD in adolescents (Jørgensen *et al.*, 2021a, 2021b), which is reviewed later in the chapter. Adolescence is a risk period for the onset of personality disorder and advocacy groups have made gains in destigmatizing the disorder in both adults and adolescents, promoting prevention and early intervention (Chanen *et al.*, 2017).

Personality disorder classification

DSM-5 classification of personality disorders

Currently, there are two parallel classification systems for personality disorders in the 5th edition of the *Diagnostic and Statistical Manual of Mental Disorders* (DSM-5; American Psychiatric Association, 2013). Section II, which contains diagnostic criteria and codes for mental disorders, describes ten disorders. There is a list of symptoms for each disorder and a threshold above which an individual is deemed to have the disorder, and below which they do not. This is referred to as a categorical system because it assumes that disorders are either present or absent, and that each disorder is different from another. Ten categorical disorders are described, including paranoid, schizoid, schizotypal, antisocial. borderline, histrionic, narcissistic, avoidant, dependent, and obsessive–compulsive. The predominant features of each personality disorder are summarized in Table 67.1.

It should be borne in mind that descriptions of different personality disorder types have come about through several contrasting routes. Some categories have their origins in empirical observations of the continuities between psychopathological disorders in childhood, and pervasive social malfunction in adult lifestyle. The DSM-5 diagnosis of antisocial personality disorder is the obvious example of this type, with its starting point in the findings of the long-term longitudinal studies pioneered by Robins (1978). By contrast, the DSM-5 BPD diagnosis

Table 67.1 Predominant features of personality disorders as described in Section II of the *Diagnostic and Statistical Manual of Mental Disorders*, 5th edition (DSM-5).

Paranoid	Distrust and suspiciousness such that other's motives are interpreted as malevolent.
Schizoid	Detachment from social relationships and a restricted range of emotional expression.
Schizotypal	Acute discomfort in close relationships, cognitive or perceptual distortions and eccentricities of behavior.
Antisocial	Disregard for, and violation of, the rights of others.
Borderline	Instability in interpersonal relationships, self-image, and affects, and marked impulsivity.
Histrionic	Excessive emotionality and attention-seeking.
Narcissistic	Grandiosity, need for admiration, and lack of empathy.
Avoidant	Social inhibition, feelings of inadequacy, and hypersensitivity to negative evaluation.
Dependent	Submissive and clinging behavior related to an excessive need to be taken care of.
Obsessive–compulsive	Preoccupation with orderliness, perfectionism, and control.

arose from observations made in clinical practice together with psychoanalytic theoretical formulations (Kernberg 1967; Gunderson *et al.*, 1981). A further contrast is provided by schizotypal personality disorder which was informed by genetic findings. The Danish adoption study showed that the biological families of adopted schizophrenic probands included a raised rate of symptoms that seemed to exhibit some features reminiscent of schizophrenia (Kety *et al.*, 1971). This provided the basis for the category of schizotypal personality disorder. There is now substantial support for a genetic relationship between schizotypal personality disorder and schizophrenia based on studies of families, twins, and adoptees (Cannon *et al.*, 2008; Walter *et al.* 2016) and some support for overlapping neurobiological features between the disorders (Ettinger *et al.*, 2014).

The DSM diagnostic system has been criticized because there is no empirical support for there being an absent–present threshold. Rather, there is a continuum of personality disorder symptoms and impaired personality functioning in which variations below and above the arbitrary thresholds are likely to be as important as those which cross them. Furthermore, comorbidity among categories of personality disorders is very common, calling into question their distinctiveness. In addition, studies that have attempted to show that the ten personality disorders each represent a separate entity have not been successful, leading to the conclusion that personality disorder function along a dimension or continuum of severity, rather than a condition that someone has or does not have. Therefore, in Section III of DSM-5, an alternative, dimensional, system for diagnosing personality disorders has been endorsed, as summarized in Table 67.2.

The DSM Alternative Model for Personality Disorders

This system, rather than viewing personality disorders as categorical entities, proposes a combination of categorical and "dimensional" approaches to form a "hybrid" diagnostic scheme. "Dimensional" means that individuals differ in the degree to which they evidence certain personality traits—mild to

Table 67.2 Abbreviated diagnostic criteria for personality disorder adapted from Section III of the *Diagnostic and Statistical Manual of Mental Disorders*, 5th edition (DSM-5) and the *International Classification of Diseases*, 11th revision (ICD-11).

DSM-5 Section III Alternative Model for Personality Disorders	ICD-11
A. Moderate or greater impairment in personality functioning (i.e., self- and interpersonal functioning), rated >2 on a 5-point severity scale (0–4), indicated by at least two of the following four areas of difficulty: 1. Identity 2. Self-direction 3. Empathy 4. Intimacy	A. Impairments in functioning of aspects of the self and interpersonal functioning described in terms of its level of severity: 1. Mild personality disorder 2. Moderate personality disorder 3. Severe personality disorder
B. One or more pathological personality trait domains or trait facets within domains: 1. Negative affectivity 2. Detachment 3. Antagonism 4. Disinhibition 5. Psychoticism (odd, eccentric, or unusual behaviors or cognitions)	B. Personality disorder and personality difficulty can be further described using five trait domain specifiers: 1. Negative affectivity 2. Detachment 3. Dissociality (lack of empathy, callous, mean) 4. Disinhibition 5. Anankastia (obsessive–compulsive)
C. Personality dysfunction and trait expression must be relatively inflexible and pervasive across multiple contexts (i.e., the symptoms do not occur only at home or during certain times)	C. The disturbance has persisted over an extended period of time (e.g., lasting two years or more)
D. Personality dysfunction is stable across time and onset can be traced back to adolescence or early adulthood	D. Manifest in patterns of cognition, emotional experience, emotional expression, and behavior that are maladaptive (e.g., inflexible or poorly regulated)
E. Not better explained by another mental disorder	E. Manifest across a range of personal and social situations, though it may be consistently evoked by particular types of circumstances and not others
F. Not attributable to physiological effects of a substance or another medical condition	F. The symptoms are not due to the direct effects of a medication or substance, including withdrawal effects, and are not better accounted for by another mental disorder, a disease of the nervous system, or another medical condition
G. Impairments are not better understood as normal for an individual's developmental stage or sociocultural environment	G. The disturbance is associated with substantial distress or significant impairment in personal, family, social, educational, occupational, or other important areas of functioning
	H. Personality disorder should not be diagnosed if the patterns of behavior characterizing the personality disturbance are developmentally appropriate or can be explained primarily by social or cultural factors, including sociopolitical conflict

Source: Bohus *et al.* (2021)/with permission of Elsevier.

moderate to severe; and that there are underlying dimensions (constructs) that explain high levels of overlap between personality disorders (Sharp, 2022). For instance, all ten categorical personality disorders share problems in self-regulation and stable relationships, and therefore it makes sense to identify a unifying construct that more parsimoniously diagnoses personality disorder. The Alternative Model for Personality Disorders (AMPD) adopts a stepwise approach in which the clinician first assesses underlying dimensions thought to be shared by all personality disorders: maladaptive self (meaning disordered self-identity and self-direction) and interpersonal functioning (meaning disordered empathy and intimacy). This is referred to as Level of Personality Functioning (Criterion A). Next, the clinician evaluates the severity of five personality traits: negative affectivity, detachment, antagonism, disinhibition, and psychoticism. This is referred to as Criterion B. Thus far the approach is entirely dimensional in terms of severity of impairment and the extent of specific trait abnormalities. In a third step, the clinician has the option to combine ratings of maladaptive self and interpersonal functioning and maladaptive traits to specify one of six discreet personality disorder categories: schizotypal, borderline, narcissistic, antisocial, avoidant, and obsessive–compulsive. The four other disorders (paranoid, schizoid, histrionic, and dependent) were not retained in the AMPD because they lacked sufficient data to validate them as distinct entities.

The ICD-11 diagnostic scheme

The ICD-11 diagnostic scheme for personality disorder (Table 67.2), endorsed by the World Health Organization, is very similar to the AMPD. It requires an initial assessment of criteria of maladaptive self and interpersonal functioning, and of maladaptive trait domains. However, it is more radical than the alternative model, in that the only categorical disorder to have been retained is BPD and this is also expected to be removed in the future.

Borderline personality disorder

While the transition to an alternative model for diagnosing personality disorder is supported by the personality disorder research and clinical community, almost all of the personality disorder research, with adults and with adolescents, has used, or been based on, the existing DSM-5 classification (Sharp & Miller, 2022). In the case of BPD in adolescence, this has been highly informative, providing evidence of a distinctive clinical profile with its own specific risks, and developmental course. Furthermore, the highest quality evidence for various treatments has focused on the needs of young people with BPD. There is also support for the notion that BPD represents features of personality dysfunction that are shared across all manifestations of personality disorder (Sharp *et al.*, 2015), meaning that information on BPD may be relevant to all personality disorders, and therefore the general Level of Personality Functioning. This chapter therefore focuses predominantly on BPD, with perspective provided by the six other categorical disorders that have been retained in the alternative model.

Epidemiology of borderline personality disorder

General population studies of BPD in adults, mainly in the US and Europe, have provided estimates of between 0.7–2.7% (Eaton *et al.*, 2018), similar to prevalence in the general population for other personality disorders. The few studies of adolescent BPD which have been conducted have found similar rates of the disorder. A systematic review has estimated a mean prevalence of BPD of 11.8% for outpatient psychiatric settings and 22.4% for inpatients (Ellison *et al.*, 2018), with some indications of a higher rate in adolescent inpatient settings. The estimate for inpatient settings is likely to vary considerably across and within countries, depending on whether alternatives to admission are available.

Prevalence studies of personality disorders suggest similar rates for men and women in community studies with higher rates for women in clinical psychiatric settings. While most prevalence studies do not show systematic racial or ethnic differences, there are a dearth of studies addressing this issue (Sharp, 2022).

Clinical considerations

Clinical features

The disorder was first included in DSM-III in 1980. In Section II of DSM-5, BPD can be diagnosed when an adult or adolescent meets more than five out of nine diagnostic criteria listed in Table 67.3.

Table 67.3 *Diagnostic and Statistical Manual of Mental Disorders*, 5th edition (DSM-5), Section II: categorically defined borderline personality disorder.

- **A.** A pervasive pattern of instability of interpersonal relationships, self-image, and affects, and marked impulsivity indicated by at least five of the nine following personality traits:
  1. Frantic efforts to avoid abandonment
  2. Unstable and intense interpersonal relationships
  3. Identity disturbance
  4. Impulsivity in at least two areas (e.g., spending, substance abuse, reckless driving, binge eating)
  5. Recurrent suicidal or self-mutilating behavior
  6. Affective instability
  7. Chronic feelings of emptiness
  8. Inappropriate, intense anger or difficulty controlling anger
  9. Transient, stress-related paranoid ideation or severe dissociative symptoms
- **B.** Symptoms must be relatively inflexible and pervasive across multiple contexts (i.e., the symptoms do not occur only at home or during certain times)
- **C.** Symptoms must result in significant distress or impairment in functioning
- **D.** Symptoms or patterns of behavior are stable across time and their onset can be traced back to adolescence or early adulthood
- **E.** Symptoms are not better explained by another mental disorder
- **F.** Symptoms are not attributable to physiological effects of a substance or another medical condition

As illustrated in the clinical example, self-harm and suicidal behaviors are often prominent. As the young person describes in the video (refer to the companion website of this book), the emotional instability can include being triggered by events which would not trouble most other young people, rapid onset of negative emotions, which are highly intense, and take a long time to subside. The interpersonal contexts in which difficulties commonly occur are also clear in the interview. The emotional reactivity is often triggered by perceived rejection, and relationships are often "all or nothing," which can give rise to their instability. Identity disturbance may be subjective, where the young person feels empty or lacking in a coherent or stable sense of self, or observable, for example, when a young person frequently and for short periods of time "tries on" identities with limited success, finding a group or activity where the young person feels they belong.

Assessment

Assessment has six main aims, to assess current risk associated with self-harm or suicidality, to assess personality disorder symptomatology and functioning in detail, to gather enough information to ascertain differential diagnosis and comorbidity, to identify sources of risk or resilience in the young person's network, and to assess involvement with other agencies. The sixth aim, not always seen as part of assessment, but in practice often crucial and, in particular with young people with BPD problems, is to establish a good relationship with the young person and their family. This is central to assessment in numerous ways including that it is likely to increase the young person's readiness to talk about difficult topics, and to enable the clinician to assess the potential for engagement in treatment.

It is essential for assessment to include conversations with the young person, their parents or other caregivers, and other key people who know them, in order to get as full a picture as possible, and also in order to assess differences in knowledge and perceptions across the network. This is of particular importance in relation to disclosure of risky behaviors, and thoughts and plans regarding self-harm or suicide. If the young person has provided partial information to different people, then a comprehensive risk assessment requires information from several sources. The assessment of self-harm and suicidal behaviors is described further in Chapter 64. The diagnostic criteria for personality disorder are assessed through an interview by a clinician, which can be supplemented by semistructured interviews or self-reported measures. Recently, the International Consortium for Health Outcomes Measurement undertook a rigorous consensus process in order to identify the most optimal battery of patient self-reported measures that can be used to assess personality pathology outcomes. This battery of measures is represented in Figure 67.1. Interviews with young people, and with others in their networks, combined with standardized measures, should also be used to assess for disorders which are commonly comorbid, and for those which might better explain the young person's difficulties and so should be considered in the differential diagnosis.

As illustrated in the clinical summary, young people with BPD commonly have conflictual relationships with their parents, they establish relationships which may become a source of risk, and have difficulties in coping in settings such as school or work, which otherwise could be sources of resilience. Such sources of risk may be powerful maintainers of the disorder and hence need to be asked about in planning the intervention.

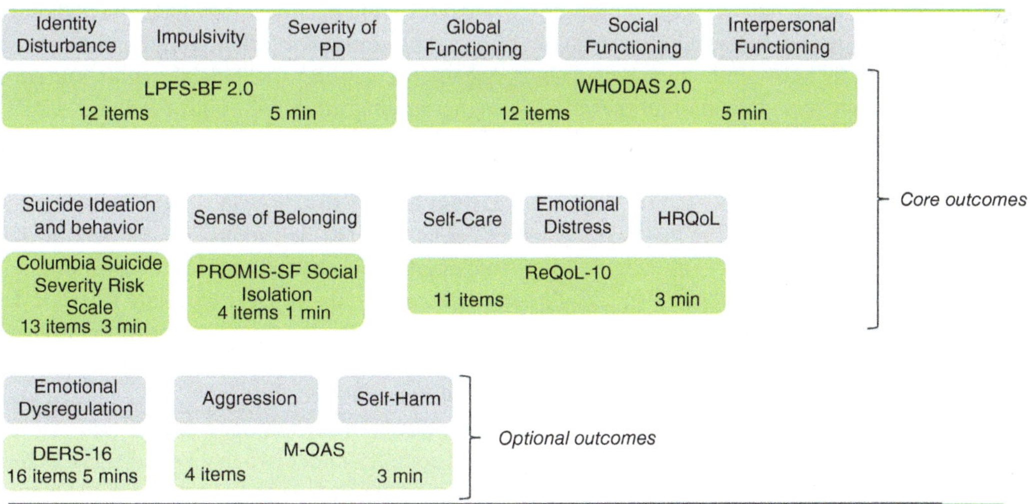

Figure 67.1 Standard set of patient-reported outcomes for personality disorder (PD) (Rupel *et al.*, 2021/US Department of Health and Human Services (HHS)/public domain). *Notes*: LPFS-BF 2.0: Level of Personality Functioning Scale-Brief Form 2.0 (Hutsebaut *et al.*, 2015); WHODAS 2.0: World Health Organization Disability Assessment Schedule 2.0 (Papadopoulou *et al.*, 2020); C-SSRS: Columbia Suicide Severity Risk Scale (Posner *et al.*, 2011); PROMIS-SF Short Form Social Isolation: Patient-Reported Outcomes Measurement Information System (Johnston *et al.*, 2016); ReQoL-10: Recovering Quality of Life (Keetharuth *et al.*, 2018); DERS-16: Difficulties in Emotion Regulation Scale (Bjureberg *et al.*, 2016); M-OAS: Modified Overt Aggression Scale (Ratey and Gutheil, 1991).

Equally in each of these settings, the family, friendships, or romantic partners, and school or work, there may be important sources of support, which may be protective, and crucially may be sustained long after treatment has finished. As outlined later in the chapter, the developmental origins of BPD usually entail a complex interplay between the child's individual characteristics and needs, and their family and wider social environment. This complexity cannot be captured in the time available for most assessments. However, asking parents about their memories of the young person as a child, for example, about how emotionally reactive they were, or how they related to other children, is important in its own right, and can pave the way for a discussion of the challenges of caring for them even when they were very young.

Gathering information from other agencies is important in two ways. First, it provides additional information about the way the young person's difficulties, for example, their difficulties with emotion regulation, their impulsiveness, or their tendency to establish inappropriately intense relationships, may undermine efforts to help. This is essential information for formulation and treatment. Second, it can identify key agencies or professionals who could be important to establishing a coherent therapeutic network. For example, the young person who self-harms regularly may have developed a strong connection to emergency department or pediatric staff, who may continue to be important and influential.

The assessment process often generates a large amount of information which needs to be summarized and focused in a formulation. The aim of the formulation is to identify the key areas in which change is likely to be important, perhaps because of the degree of risk or negative impact on the young person's functioning. Equally, the formulation aims to identify the young person's sources of support or individual strengths or competence. Commonly, it is helpful to draft a formulation to share with the young person, inviting them to comment and contribute, and similarly for parents. Active participation of the young person or their parents in developing the formulation forms part of most evidence-based treatment approaches for personality disorder in young people and can provide a valuable basis for the planning of an intervention.

Box 67.1 Assessment at a glance

- Make use of self-, parent-, and teacher-reports and get information from other involved agencies
- Assess duration of symptoms in the context of emergence of problems in managing self and interpersonal functioning, independent from depression, anxiety, attention deficit hyperactivity disorder (ADHD), post-traumatic stress disorder (PTSD), and/or substance use
- Assess self-harm, suicidal ideation, history of suicide attempts, and current suicide risk
- Assess for symptoms which need to be considered for differential diagnosis
- Ask about the child's early development and experiences
- Assess school and peer functioning
- Assess strengths and protective factors
- Integrate all risk and protective factors into a coherent formulation that can be shared with the young person and their parents

Comorbidity

Comorbidity in medicine refers to the co-occurrence of two or more diseases. While this may arise because they share common risks, as in the case of Type 2 diabetes and coronary artery disease, they are nevertheless different conditions. While co-occurrence of mental disorders is commonly referred to as comorbidity, here its meaning is less clear than in medicine. This is particularly the case for BPD which has high rates of co-occurrence with many other mental disorders. For example, an analysis of data from the National Epidemiologic Survey on Alcohol and Related Conditions study has reported estimates of lifetime co-occurrence with BPD of 84.5% for anxiety disorders, 82.7% for mood disorders, and 78.2% for substance use disorders (Tomko *et al.*, 2014). High rates of post-traumatic stress disorder (PTSD) (30.2%), ADHD (33.7%), bipolar disorder I (21.6%), bipolar disorder II (37.7%), and somatic disorders (30%) and BPD have also been reported (Bohus *et al.*, 2021). This level of co-occurrence, found for BPD and for other mental disorders, has informed a transdiagnostic approach in which "comorbidity" arises from different manifestations of the same underlying processes, for example, emotion dysregulation. The same considerations have motivated the development of the Alternative Model for Personality Disorders outlined earlier in the section "The DSM Alternative Model for Personality Disorders."

Assessing for co-occurring disorders is essential because they may contribute jointly with BPD to suffering and impairment, and they may provide a distinct and tractable target for treatment. This is particularly important because young people with comorbid disorders may have the highest levels of psychiatric symptoms. For example, in a clinical sample, levels of aggression, self-harm, suicidal thoughts, and substance use were higher among those with both BPD and ADHD, compared to either BPD only or ADHD only (Akça *et al.* 2020).

Differential diagnosis

As we outlined earlier, adolescent BPD comprises a distinct profile of emotions, behaviors, social cognitions, and relationships which commonly impacts on many facets of a young person's life, and leads to the involvement of multiple agencies. Where most or all of these features are seen it can be straightforward to establish that the young person does have BPD.

However, determining whether this is the case becomes more complex under two main conditions. In the first, the referral or initial assessment indicates that the young person's most prominent difficulties seem to be related to other disorders such as depression or an eating disorder. This is likely to arise because BPD and other disorders commonly co-occur (Chanen *et al.*, 2016). Inquiry into functioning over time and social context, covering areas described in this chapter is essential. Inquiry over time includes finding out about emotion regulation and social relationships during childhood based on parent and teacher reports. Inquiry by social context in the present needs to document functioning at home, in close friendships, in wider peer interactions, and at school. An examination of the relationship between social impairment and dysregulated mood can be very informative. In disorders such as depression, the impairment can generally be traced to the onset of the symptoms, while BPD difficulties antedate them and may have created a vulnerability, for example, through relationship breakdown or school failure.

In the second condition, behaviors which resemble BPD may be better explained by a different disorder. Bipolar disorder, especially bipolar disorder II characterized by relatively short periods of elation together with depression, may look very similar. In principle, there are substantial differences in that, compared with bipolar disorder, affects are more unstable and triggered by interpersonal events in BPD, and there are characteristic interpersonal problems in BPD not seen in bipolar disorder (Zimmerman *et al.*, 2013). However, where bipolar symptoms have persisted for some time, they may have impacted on interpersonal functioning making the distinction difficult.

ADHD during childhood is strongly associated with adolescent BPD, particularly where ADHD persists. In view of these strong continuities over time and the comorbidity between BPD and ADHD, there has been considerable discussion over whether they are distinct syndromes, much of it focused on impulsivity and emotion dysregulation (Ditrich *et al.*, 2021). According to DSM diagnostic criteria, impulsivity is a key feature of both BPD and ADHD, although the manifestations of the impulsivity are typically different. Impulsive self-harm is characteristic of BPD while impulsive behaviors directed toward others or is more common in ADHD. Impulsive self-harm in BPD, but not in ADHD, is typically stress-related and linked to emotional reactivity. While the evidence for these distinctions is somewhat inconsistent, detailed questioning regarding specific impulsive behaviors and their associations with stressors, may provide support for one rather than another diagnosis, or indeed point to comorbid disorders. According to Section II of the DSM diagnostic criteria, emotional reactivity is a core feature of BPD, but not of ADHD. However, several studies have called this distinction into question, and so even where emotional reactivity is a prominent problem for a young person, systematic enquiry may lead to the diagnosis of ADHD rather than BPD. Moreover, with the reformulation of diagnostic criteria as represented in the DSM-5 AMPD (Section III) and ICD-11 (Table 67.2), the focus has shifted to maladaptive self and interpersonal functioning as the distinguishing features of personality disorder. This reformulation is partly in response to the difficulty of viewing emotion dysregulation as core to personality disorder when emotion dysregulation is a feature of most psychiatric disorders.

Commonly, the question is raised in the clinical setting regarding the role of trauma. As we discussed earlier, rates of child maltreatment are elevated in young people with BPD, but a history of maltreatment is neither necessary nor sufficient for BPD. However, the specific role of trauma has to be considered where the young person has symptoms of PTSD (see Chapter 58). Studies in adults have consistently identified two subgroups of individuals, with PTSD and "complex" (cPTSD) demarcated by whether, in addition to the established PTSD symptoms of intrusive reexperiencing, avoidance of trauma reminders and hyperarousal, they have features of "disturbances of self-organization (DSO)" (Ford *et al.*, 2021). DSO comprise emotional numbing and dysregulation, self-perceptions as a failure or worthless, and emotional detachment in relationships. These resemble, in some respects, features of BPD leading to the question of whether they are the same disorder. The available evidence from a limited number of studies indicates that they commonly co-occur, but they are distinct (Ford & Courtois, 2021). Furthermore, it may be possible to identify differences in the nature of the DSO. In cPTSD, emotion dysregulation involves difficulty in self-calming when distressed, but not the emotional instability and uncontrolled anger found in BPD. Negative self-perceptions in cPTSD tend to involve a stable chronic sense of guilt, shame, and worthlessness, in contrast to the more unstable and fragmented sense of self in BPD (Ford & Courtois, 2021). In cPTSD, relational dysregulation is characterized by avoidance and detachment, rather than the intensity and instability of relationships seen in BPD. Symptoms of BPD that appear to be specific to BPD, compared to both PTSD and cPTSD, are frantic efforts to avoid abandonment, unstable sense of self, unstable and intense interpersonal relationships, and impulsiveness (Cloitre *et al.*, 2014).

Studies of adolescents in the general population and those referred for treatment have also identified distinct PTSD and cPTSD profiles. Daniunate *et al.* (2021) tested the hypothesis that, compared with PTSD, cPTSD would be associated with a greater number of traumatic experiences and found no difference. cPTSD was, however, associated with family problems (such as financial difficulties and conflicts in the home), school problems (bullying and learning difficulties), and lack of social support, underlining that, in common with many other forms of adolescent mental disorder, cPTSD is likely to have multifactorial origins. Thus far, no studies on the differentiation between cPTSD and BPD in adolescents have been published. Importantly, it should be borne in mind that while the role of trauma may be inferred from the symptoms of cPTSD, this is not the case for BPD.

Increasingly, and especially in girls, the possibility is raised as to whether BPD-like symptoms are better explained by ASD (see Chapter 50). This is because there are several apparent overlaps between the symptoms of ASD and BPD (May *et al.*, 2021). Both have impairment in interpersonal relationships and emotion regulation challenges. On the surface, unstable relationships in BPD are similar to the challenges in ASD with forming and maintaining relationships. The extreme emotional distress seen in ASD in response to change or transitions, may resemble the emotional dysregulation seen in BPD. Similar to those with BPD, young people with ASD have elevated rates of self-injurious and suicidal behavior (Hedley & Uljarevic, 2018). Identity concerns, a criterion for BPD, may also be present in some individuals with ASD. For example, autistic preoccupations may relate to religious, political, or gender identity concerns resembling the identity diffusion of BPD (May *et al.*, 2017). Detailed questions about the contexts of emotional dysregulation, relationship breakdown, and self-harm may provide a basis for distinguishing BPD from ASD. This should be done mindful of the limitations in current knowledge. For example, we do not know whether the disorders are in fact distinct, nor whether they co-occur. In practice, it is common to attempt to resolve the problem by conducting a gold-standard ASD assessment such as the Autism Diagnostic Observation Schedule (ADOS). It is important to keep in mind when doing this that studies have yet to be done to establish the validity of an ADOS-based diagnosis in the presence of BPD-like features.

Clinical staging

Given the complexity of the difficulties faced by young people with BPD, and those seeking to care for them, it may be helpful for clinicians to make use of a relatively standardized framework, such as "clinical staging" for assessment and intervention. Clinical staging in mental health (analogous to disease staging in other branches of medicine) was adapted for treatment of psychosis. At its simplest, clinical staging describes progression from Stage 0 (no current symptoms; increased risk of disorder) to Stage 1 (1a, mild or nonspecific symptoms; 1b, moderate but subthreshold symptoms), Stage 2 (full-threshold disorder with moderate-to-severe symptoms), Stage 3 (incomplete remission or relapse), and Stage 4 (severe, unremitting, or refractory illness). A key principle of this model is that assessments should be relevant and interventions should be "proportionate" to the stage of disorder (Chanen *et al.*, 2016). Clinical staging has therefore been viewed as particularly useful for the assessment and treatment of young people, because of its relevance to prevention, help-seeking, and early intervention for mental health needs during this peak period of onset for most of the major mental disorders. As we describe in the next section, for adolescent BPD thus far there are no large scale randomized controlled trials (RCTs), and so we are a long way off having the capacity to test clinical staging as a guide to treatment choice.

Nevertheless, recently published proposals have the potential to offer a systematic framework for assessment. Chanen *et al.* (2016) suggested a clinical staging approach for BPD based on the extent and severity of co-occurring disorders, such as depression, so that the emphasis is on the severity and persistence of symptoms, rather than any one diagnostic profile. The proposals of Hutsebaut *et al.* (2019) and Sharp *et al.* (2018) characterize staging both by the severity of BPD features and the extent of co-occurring mental disorders. Sharp *et al.* link the clinical staging explicitly to the AMPD and ICD-11 (Sharp *et al.*, in press) frameworks described earlier.

Stigma

A departure from a categorical perspective on personality development not only provides a more comprehensive understanding of personality and personality pathology, but is also less stigmatizing because personality functioning (rather than a categorical disorder of being "personality disordered") offers a malleable treatment target (Sharp, 2022). This addresses the final barrier that stands in the way of early intervention and prevention for personality disorder—that is, its stigmatization in mental health settings.

Despite the fact that personality disorder ranks in the top 10 causes of disease burden among young people (Global Burden of Disease, 2017) and despite the substantial accumulated research in support for the diagnosis discussed above, BPD has yet to make the leap from controversial diagnosis to mainstream mental health problem (Chanen, 2021). Many clinicians remain reluctant to assess, diagnose, and treat adolescent personality disorder, with rates of detection 10–20 times lower than that suggested by clinical epidemiological data (Chanen & Nicol, 2021). Despite pleas from both patients and their families (e.g., Baltzersen, 2021), young people living with personality disorder, and those who care for them, have been shown to experience greater stigma than other severe mental disorders, and struggle to be respected and taken seriously (Chanen, 2021). For decades now, individuals with personality disorder are viewed as less worthy of care than individuals with other disorders, especially among health professionals (Chartonas *et al.*, 2017). Lack of training and a "translational research gap" are seen to be driving mistaken beliefs and negative attitudes, with the consequence that care is less likely to be offered to young people with personality disorder and/or early withdrawal from services (Francey *et al.*, 2018). Given this stigma, mental health care professionals often want to protect young people by avoiding the diagnosis of personality disorder. However, this approach could risk colluding with and reinforcing discriminatory beliefs and behaviors, thereby creating further harm, and thus jeopardizing the opportunity for early intervention (Chanen, 2021). Disclosing the diagnosis has been shown to bring relief and instill hope (Klein *et al.*, 2022) for families and young people who, up until a diagnosis of personality disorder, have experienced a revolving door in mental health services, receiving inappropriate treatment targeted at comorbid disorders without addressing the core problem.

In summary, the field has come a long way in establishing the idea that personality is a summary term for the way humans make sense of themselves and others in the context of interpersonal relationships (Sharp & Wall, 2021). This view of personality and personality disorder is most clearly articulated in ICD-11 when it is stated that

> Personality refers to an individual's characteristic way of behaving, experiencing life, and of perceiving and interpreting themselves, other people, events, and situations. Personality Disorder is a marked disturbance in

personality functioning, which is nearly always associated with considerable personal and social disruption. The central manifestations of Personality Disorder are impairments in functioning of aspects of the self (e.g., identity, self-worth, capacity for self-direction) and/or problems in interpersonal functioning (e.g., developing and maintaining close and mutually satisfying relationships, understanding others' perspectives, managing conflict in relationships). Impairments in self-functioning and/or interpersonal functioning are manifested in maladaptive (e.g., inflexible or poorly regulated) patterns of cognition, emotional experience, emotional expressions and behaviors (World Health Organization, 2022, p. 2).

Due to the major developmental tasks of adolescence (consolidation of identity and social reorientation), adolescence constitutes a sensitive period for the development of personality disorder (Sharp & Wall, 2018). There now exist valid and reliable tools to identify young people who diverge from a typical trajectory in their developing capacity to build a representation of self that allows for rewarding and reciprocal interpersonal relationships. Individuals with lived experience, as well as major advocacy groups (National Education Alliance for BPD, Emotions Matter, TARA and Sashbear Foundation), ask that challenges in personality development be addressed early to prevent years of misdiagnosis and mistreatment.

Etiology and mechanisms

Overview

Twin studies have suggested that genetic influences account for around 50% of the risk for BPD. While data on other personality disorders are scarce, some reports suggest moderate heritability (Ma *et al.*, 2016). Environmental influences are equally important and prospective studies have shown that harsh or insensitive parenting, emotional neglect, physical or sexual maltreatment, and victimization by bullying are associated with the development of personality disorder (Stepp *et al.*, 2016).

Theoretical models of the development of personality disorders are based on the view that there are interactions between child characteristics, including those with strong genetic influences, and environmental factors. Consistent with these models, children who show high levels of negative emotionality and who are raised in families in which caregivers struggle to meet their emotional demands, have increased risk for the development of personality disorder (Winsper *et al.*, 2017). The specificity of these risk factors and the role of child temperament in evoking parenting behaviors, is not clear.

Developmental pathways

In relation to adolescent personality disorder, we have some evidence from prospective studies of likely developmental processes for BPD, supporting the role of heightened negative emotionality in infancy (Carlson *et al.*, 2009) and during childhood (Stepp *et al.*, 2014a, 2014b), of ADHD, in increasing the risk. Parental negativity is associated with increased risk (Winsper *et al.*, 2016) and positive aspects of parenting, such as warm sensitive responding, are protective (Brumariu *et al.*, 2020). Very few studies provide insights into the dynamic interplay between developmental processes, and to some extent we have to compile a picture from a range of studies. For example, findings from the large UK general population study, the Avon Longitudinal Study of Parents and Children (ALSPAC), have shown that being bullied during childhood is associated with BPD features at age 11 years after controlling for depressive symptoms (Winsper *et al.*, 2017). Risk for being bullied is not, however, distributed at random across children. Evidence from several large longitudinal studies indicates that bully victims are more likely to have preexisting individual vulnerabilities and to have already experienced family adversities (Winsper *et al.*, 2017; Bowes *et al.*, 2009). Evidence from the E-Risk twin study, shows a protective effect of parental warmth, after controlling for genetic influences, in reducing the risk of adolescent depression among children exposed to bullying. Putting the findings together, it seems plausible to suppose that parental warmth will similarly be protective for BPD features in children exposed to bullying. It is important to bear in mind that, commonly, there are two-way effects, of parental behaviors on young people, and vice versa. For example, transactional effects between dysregulated child behaviors (conduct problems, negative emotionality, hyperactivity) and negative parenting were identified in the ALSPAC study (Winsper *et al.*, 2017) of developmental pathways to BPD. It is possible that once BPD behaviors have become established in adolescence the majority of the effects are on parenting. In the Pittsburgh Girls study of BPD features during adolescence, there were prospective associations between BPD features and subsequent harsh parenting, and low parental warmth, while effects in the opposite direction were not evident (Stepp *et al.*, 2014a, 2014b).

Studies have to take account of quite strong continuities both in child behaviors and family environments over time. Two features of emotional and behavioral problems in childhood and adolescence add complexity to the study of these processes. First, most are moderately correlated, and, second, apparent change may reflect continuity of underlying processes. The extent of the correlation, even among apparently dissimilar emotions and behaviors, means that where we find an association with one set of emotions and behaviors, we can only be confident of its specificity where we account for other possible associations. This is a particularly important issue for BPD features, which in adolescence are moderately to highly correlated with depression. Change over time in emotions and behaviors, which nevertheless reflects a continuity is referred to as heterotypic continuity (see Chapter 1). This may be particularly relevant for BPD which, as we noted earlier, is not seen in its adolescent/adult form during childhood. For example, a low threshold for getting angry, and more prolonged and intense angry responses, is identified as "irritability" in DSM oppositional defiant disorder (ODD), and these externalizing behaviors seen in children are associated with depression in adolescents (Vidal-Ribas *et al.*, 2016). Putting these two points together, the developmental questions would be, Does childhood irritability predict adolescent BPD features, after accounting for its association with depression? and Are there child or environmental characteristics which nudge the pathway toward BPD features?

Increasingly, as peer influences and dating partners become more important they too may create additional risk or provide protection. Young people must integrate multiple perspectives from several sources to begin building a stable and coherent sense of self in order to navigate an increasingly complex social environment as young people get ready to take on adult roles. Doing so relies on strong meta-cognitive and mentalizing abilities, which appear to be impaired in young people with BPD (Sharp, 2014).

Child maltreatment

Many theories of the origins of BPD have proposed a central role for maltreatment, and, in particular, experiences of sexual abuse in childhood. Meta-analyses have confirmed strong associations between child maltreatment and BPD in adults and in adolescents (Winsper *et al.*, 2016). In interpreting these findings five important considerations need to be borne in mind. First, many studies rely on retrospective reporting, which may be open to biases. Second, the prospective study of maltreatment in childhood faces formidable ethical challenges because of the child protection implications of disclosure of abuse. This is likely to result in underreporting of maltreatment or disclosure among particular subgroups of children. This problem has been addressed in studies of children already referred to child protection services, which are, however, unlikely to be representative of children in the general population.

Third, establishing the specificity of one kind of child maltreatment has to take account of other kinds, because children are commonly exposed to more than one form of maltreatment. Fourth, child maltreatment is associated with a wide range of mental health disorders, so that in order to establish specificity for BPD, account has to be taken of other comorbid disorders. Fifth, because of passive gene–environment correlations (see Chapter 21) associations between child maltreatment and BPD cannot be assumed to reflect an influence of one on the other.

Studies rarely address all of these issues, but there are some exceptions. For example, Hecht *et al.* (2014) studied a large sample of 599 children, of whom 314 were known by child protection agencies to have been maltreated. They assessed neglect, emotional maltreatment, physical abuse, or sexual abuse from official records and were therefore able to examine for specificity of maltreatment type. Physical abuse and physical neglect, but not emotional neglect or sexual abuse, were associated with BPD features. They did not, however, control for comorbid disorders, such as depression, which is strongly associated with BPD features (Hill *et al.*, 2023), and so could not establish specificity for BPD. Another large study provided two key contrasts (Belsky *et al.*, 2012). The children were drawn from the general population and they were twins (1,116 pairs), so genetic factors could be accounted for. They showed a genetic contribution to BPD features in young adolescents and an environmental effect of parental physical abuse. However, by comparison with the study by Hecht *et al.*, this study could not account for the full range of child maltreatment, and, for example, did not assess for child sexual abuse. By contrast, in a twin study of young adults, child maltreatment was associated with BPD symptoms, but the association fully accounted for common genetic influences (Bornovalova *et al.*, 2013). Taken together, the evidence indicates that child maltreatment is a factor in adolescent BPD, but equally, the majority of children who suffer from maltreatment do not develop BPD and there are many young people with BPD who have not been maltreated (Wilson *et al.*, 2021). Indeed, a recent meta-analysis (Kleindienst *et al.*, 2021), suggest that 43.9% of individuals with BPD have experienced at least one childhood adverse event; which leaves 56.1% of individuals reporting no childhood adversity of any kind.

Candidate mechanisms in personality disorder

Emotion dysregulation and invalidation

"The inability to sustain positive affect coupled with the pervasive and unremitting distress as experienced by patients with BPD can become a veritable prison to those with the disorder and often as well to those who attempt to treat the individual with BPD" (Putnam & Silk, 2005, p. 900). Borderline individuals commonly have a low threshold for reacting to events, or to anticipated events (such as abandonment), with intense negative emotion. According to Linehan's influential biosocial model of BPD, which forms the basis of dialectical behavioral therapy, one of the evidence-based treatment approaches for BPD, BPD arises from a mismatch between the temperamental characteristics of the child and the perceived "invalidating" aspects of parenting. The child characteristics have been characterized as comprising three components: emotional sensitivity, emotional reactivity, and slow return to baseline arousal, with recent empirical evidence showing support for this (Chapman, 2019). Essentially, this means that individuals with BPD are more likely to notice relevant emotional stimuli in their environment, react more intensely to those stimuli, and take a longer time period to return to their emotional baseline after reacting.

Invalidation is a concept, specific to Linehan's (1993) theory and distinct from other dimensions of positive or negative parenting. It is conceptualized as four kinds of parental behavior which delegitimize a child's emotional experience or expression—often in unintended ways. First, the parent(s) communicates that the child's description and analysis of their own experiences are wrong and/or inaccurate, particularly in their views of what is causing their own emotions, for example, "You aren't sad, you are fine." Second, emotions are seen as an expression of undesirable attitudes, for example, "hostile or manipulative motives." Third, self-reliance is favored over emotional expression, and, fourth, the task of solving life's problems is oversimplified, for example, by "pulling yourself up by the bootstraps." Three key points regarding research in this area should be made. First, many studies have been informed by the concepts, but very few have investigated the specific components (Musser *et al.*, 2018). Second, young people with BPD tend to perceive their parents as invalidating, so that young person reports are likely to reflect one or both of their and their parents' attributions (Bennett *et al.*, 2019). Third, testing the hypothesis poses fearsome methodological challenges because it concerns the moment-by-moment parental responses to a young person's expression of negative emotions.

The study of Vanwoerden *et al.* (2022b) rose to the challenge. They studied 162 young adolescents who were receiving treatment for mood and behavioral problems, and who scored highly on a measure of emotional instability. Using ecological momentary assessment (EMA), young people received prompts on their mobile phones to provide information on BPD symptoms they were experiencing at that moment, and their parents were prompted to report on their behaviors toward their child. Parents' punishing responses to emotional expression in their child were associated with higher BPD features in line with the invalidation hypothesis, but ignoring with lower BPD features, and so contrary to the hypothesis. It may be that the finding of the protective effect of ignoring reflects that the biosocial model does not distinguish between emotions expressed in different parent–child domains, for example, in the contrast of angry opposition, and an expression of sadness or distress (Hill *et al.*, 2003). Ignoring may support emotion regulation in the first, but deprive the child of attachment support in the second.

Fronto-limbic imbalance

Studies of the neurobiology of BPD have focused on impaired behavioral control in the context of intense negative emotions. The main hypothesis is that emotion dysregulation in BPD can be mapped onto an imbalance between limbic structures, representing an emotional response component, and prefrontal structures, representing a regulatory component.

Studies, mostly of adults, have generally asked whether the limbic structure, the amygdala, is more reactive, or prefrontal structures are less active, or the connectivity between limbic and prefrontal structures is reduced, in BPD. There is consistent evidence that individuals with BPD exhibit larger amygdala activity in response to threat-related imagery and to neutral stimuli, and reduced amygdala habituation to repeated negative stimuli than both healthy and depressed samples (Schulze *et al.*, 2019). Whether or not this reflects a causal role for amygdala hyperreactivity in emotion dysregulation BPD is unclear (Sicorello & Schmahl, 2021). In particular, altered amygdala reactivity may simply be a reflection of the increased psychological impact of negative stimuli presented in the scanner on BPD participants, and associations with BPD may be better explained by an association with childhood adversities (Bilek *et al.*, 2019). Findings of reduced prefrontal activation associated with BPD are also reasonably consistent and similarly must be interpreted cautiously. Here, a major concern is that the prefrontal cortex is large, and studies of its role in emotion regulation identify many different nonoverlapping subregions raising the question of whether these are in fact replicated findings (Powers & LaBar, 2019).

Connectivity analyses aim to estimate communication between the limbic and prefrontal cortex, which may potentially be the most direct test of their role in emotion regulation. However, most studies reported so far have examined resting state connectivity, and so do not provide evidence on their role in regulating responses to emotionally challenging situations (Sicorello & Schmahl, 2021).

In summary, the fronto-limbic imbalance hypothesis for BPD is of great potential interest, and in need of further investigation. Most studies have been conducted in adults, so its applicability in adolescence remains to be examined.

Delayed or impaired identity development

Building on long-standing psychodynamic theories of personality (Kernberg, 1967), the AMPD and ICD-11 conceptualizations of personality disorder places self and identity at the center of personality function, which as we have argued earlier, offers a developmentally sensitive application to adolescents (Sharp & Wall, 2021). Research from diverse theoretical backgrounds converge to suggest that a well-functioning identity enables feelings of personal meaning and well-being in addition to rewarding relationships with others (McAdams, 2015). There is also wide consensus that adolescence confers a critical window for the formation of a healthy identity. The flip side of a healthy identity is a diffused or disturbed identity—which has long been suggested to be a hallmark feature of personality pathology. The concept of identity diffusion aims to capture the extent to which a person experiences themselves as an active agent in their lives, contrasted with being a passive recipient of external forces. Measures of identity diffusion include items such as, "Sometimes I feel my interests are not my own but copied from others" and "Sometimes I feel like I disappear in my friendships because I sacrifice my own needs" (Sharp *et al.*, 2022). Since the publication of the AMPD, there is a growing research base supporting identity diffusion as a central feature of personality pathology in adolescence. Several studies have now shown positive associations between borderline features and identity diffusion (Sharp *et al.*, 2022). Like maladaptive personality traits, identity diffusion shows a similar normative increase in adolescents which tracks closely with borderline features (Sharp & Wall, 2021). There is also emerging evidence in support of the prospective relationship between preadolescent maladaptive traits (Criterion B) and the later development of problems in self- and identity function (Criterion A) (Vanwoerden *et al.*, 2022a).

Mentalizing problems

The concept of mentalization, "the capacity to reflect on one's own thoughts and feelings and those of others attributing mental states to others" (Bateman & Fonagy, 2019), is a central concept associated with BPD and forms the basis of the other main evidence-based approach to treating personality disorder (i.e., mentalization-based therapy). Mentalizing has philosophical, psychological, and psychoanalytic origins (Bolton & Hill, 2004; Frith & Frith, 2006). The core idea is that interpreting others' behaviors in terms of their intentions, beliefs, desires, and emotions, is more accurate and quicker than processing the details of those behaviors (Dennett, 1987). Deficits in mentalizing have been shown in autism, schizophrenia, conduct disorder, bipolar disorder, anxiety disorder, depression, and BPD (Frith & Frith, 2006; Bateman & Fonagy, 2019; McLaren *et al.*, 2022). The nature of the deficits in BPD is still uncertain, with evidence both for reduced and for excessive mentalizing (Sharp *et al.*, 2011; Bateman & Fonagy, 2019; Somma *et al.*, 2019).

Some of the more recent evidence in adolescents has indicated that BPD is associated with hypermentalizing (Sharp *et al.*, 2011; Somma *et al.*, 2019), a finding also now well-replicated in adults with BPD. Hypermentalizing is characterized by reading more into the motives for others' behaviors than would be evident to most observers. Many studies reporting this finding have used the Movie for the Assessment of Social Cognition (MASC), which presents study participants with complex emotion-laden social scenarios in a video sequence in which four young adults—two male, two female—meet for dinner. The video is paused 45 times to present subjects with four alternative interpretations of what the participants have said to each other, including a hypermentalizing option.

Sharp and colleagues have proposed that a mutual interaction between hypermentalizing and emotion dysregulation contribute to the emotional and interpersonal instability seen in BPD (Sharp, 2014). In this model, when an individual with BPD is presented with an emotionally intense interpersonal event, heightened mentalizing leads to emotional arousal, which in turn increases errors in interpretation (e.g., rejection), which further dysregulate emotions. Thus, hypermentalizing is seen as the result of a failure to integrate the cognitive and emotional components inherent in most social situations, as well as a failure to integrate mentalizing the other-in-relation-to-self. In many cases, hypermentalizing involves the attribution what is one's own mind to the mind of the other—thinking that others hold the same thoughts and feelings we do. While the link between hypermentalizing and BPD has been replicated several times, recent meta-analyses showed that this association may not be exclusive to BPD (McLaren *et al.*, 2022).

Impaired organization of social domains: "domain disorganization"

According to the social domains hypothesis, effective personality functioning requires a capacity to interpret others' behaviors, and to respond, in accord with widely accepted distinctions between different classes of interaction (Hill *et al.*, 2010). This is seen early in childhood and remains a crucial competence throughout life. Even by the end of the first year of life children show markedly different behaviors with caregivers, seeking them out to share attention or seek comfort, and strangers with whom they are wary (Sroufe, 1977). Similarly, however close they are to peers, children rarely turn to other children for comfort as they do with familiar adults (Rubin *et al.*, 1999; Wright *et al.*, 2023). Adults maintain similar demarcations. For example, within the work setting, most maintain the focus of their interactions on work tasks, and they mentalize within constraints which support efficient completion of those tasks. In romantic relationships, by contrast, in addition to task foci, such as day-to-day household management and financial planning, there are many other areas of mutual concern, including sex, intimacy, fidelity, comfort, shared interests, wider relationships with families, and for many, parenting. Domains, therefore, provide a guide to the scope of mentalizing required for functioning in different kinds of social interaction. This will provide a means for generating rapid accurate social action in interactions with a wide range of people, provided participants share the same framework, and there are mechanisms for detecting that they do not.

The hypothesis that domain organization is a key element in personality development also leads to the prediction that problems in domain organization may be found in personality disorders (Hill *et al.*, 2010). BPD is associated with difficulties in a wide range of relationships in personal and work life, including problems in maintaining distinct boundaries between different relationship domains. A key feature of this "domain disorganization" (Hill *et al.*, 2008) is the presence of features of intimate relationships in social domains where these are not readily accommodated. For example, exclusivity is generally found only in romantic relationships. In a short-term longitudinal study from childhood into early adolescence "friendship exclusivity" was a strong independent predictor of borderline symptoms (Crick *et al.*, 2005).

Hill *et al.* (2023) have proposed that there may be a social domains organization of hypermentalizing in which higher levels of mentalizing, with their attendant mistake-proneness, may be adaptive and accommodated in the establishment and maintenance of romantic relationships, but less appropriate to friendships and social interactions between strangers. They generated hypermentalizing scores for strangers, friends, and romantic interactions, using the MASC, and showed that in a nonclinical sample of adolescents there was a progressive increase in hypermentalizing across the three domains consistent with there being a social domains organization of hypermentalizing. This might therefore be one of the mechanisms for the maintenance of a social domains organization of social behaviors. Furthermore, consistent with the domain disorganization described in adults with BPD, this demarcation was markedly and significantly reduced among young people with high BPD features (Hill *et al.*, 2023).

Treatment

Overview

As illustrated in the clinical vignette at the start of the chapter, many young people with BPD problems become involved with a wide range of agencies, often without apparent benefit. This would suggest that treatment should take a systemic approach, working with all agencies in contact with the young person to devise and deliver a coherent intervention for young people wherever they are in the system. Establishing an RCT to evaluate such an approach would pose major challenges for treatment development, interagency collaboration, and indeed obtaining funding for a study with a large enough sample. No such studies have so far been reported.

There are, however, interventions for young people with BPD referred to specialist treatment centers which have been evaluated in RCTs. These are principally dialectical behavior therapy for adolescents (DBT-A) and mentalization-based therapy for adolescents (MBT-A). Both actively engage with other services with the aim of creating a coherent and consistent wider environment for the young person.

Dialectical behavior therapy for adolescents

The "dialectic" in DBT-A refers to helping the adolescent to change what needs to be changed, while accepting what is a valid response to circumstances. Treatment is delivered by a team, in multifamily skills groups attended by the young people and their parents, where the focus is on acquiring new skills to cope with extremes of emotions and behaviors, and individual therapy, where focus is on the application of the skills to the specific challenges faced by the young person (Rathus & Miller, 2014). Key elements of the approach include, providing information regarding the problem and the solutions, working within a curriculum, and extensive use of handouts, worksheets, and homework. Key activities include discussion of the role of emotions as a guide to action, of the multiple components of emotions (subjective, physiological, and musculoskeletal), and of the links between external events and emotions, and thoughts and emotions. Learning and practicing techniques for managing emotions and impulses are central, for example, using breathing exercises to increase the sense of control through mindfulness, and using tactile senses to increase distress tolerance. "Walking the middle path" is a core technique aiming to avoid extremes of thinking and behaving by generating alternative ways of interpreting events and others' behaviors. Explicit coaching in the application of problem-solutions to the adolescent's real-world situations is designed to increase generalization of skills learned in the program. This may be delivered by between-session skills coaching, by telephone, by case management, or by training family members in the same skills that the adolescents are learning.

Mentalization-based therapy for adolescents

MBT-A aims to increase a young person's capacity to identify mental states in themselves and others (beliefs, wishes, feelings, thoughts). It involves weekly individual MBT-A sessions and monthly mentalization-based therapy for families (MBT-F). The therapist adopts a "mentalizing stance," expressing warmth and respect to the patient and conveying a real interest in them (Rossouw *et al.*, 2021). This requires an ability to adopt a stance of "not knowing" with the aim of communicating a genuine attempt to find out about their mental experience to establish a joint exploration of the patient's mental states. The most frequently used technique in MBT-A is support and empathy. The rationale is that the intense and unpredictable emotions that most young people with BPD experience impairs mentalizing. Support and empathy help to reduce their arousal levels and hence enhance thinking capacities. The focus is on the young person's mind, their thoughts and emotions, and not on their behaviors. Once the therapist has validated the young person's feelings and understood their thoughts, they may go on to explore alternative perspectives as a way of expanding their mentalizing capabilities.

While specialist treatments like DBT-A and MBT-A have shown preliminary effectiveness in 11 treatment trials (see Jørgensen *et al.*, 2021a, 2021b for meta-analysis), specialized treatments may not be feasible in many psychiatric settings given their duration and cost. Therefore, clinical guidelines have been developed to support clinicians in general psychiatric settings who work with young people with BPD (e.g., Hutsebaut *et al.*, 2020; Choi-Kain & Sharp, 2022). These generalist approaches integrate scientific knowledge, professional expertise, and patient experience to design a "good-enough practice" that shares a clinical pathway as illustrated by the framework employed by the guideline-informed treatment for personality disorders (GIT-PD) initiative in the Netherlands (see Figure 67.2).

Treatment effectiveness

There is insufficient evidence from RCTs to support the use of medication in the treatment of adolescent BPD (Chanen, 2015). Psychological interventions are commonly used, although in their systematic review of psychological therapies for adolescents with BPD or BPD features, Jørgensen *et al.* (2021a, 2021b) concluded that the quality of the research so far was low, ". . ..due to high risk of bias, imprecision and inconsistency. . ." Variations across studies include differences in referral routes, in inclusion and exclusion criteria, in treatment offered to control groups, and in outcome measures. Contrasting examples for DBT-A and MBT-A illustrate the points. Mehlum *et al.* (2014), with follow-up at regular intervals up to three years (Mehlum *et al.*, 2019), conducted an RCT with 77 adolescents comparing DBT-A with "enhanced usual care" (EUC). They found that there was a sustained reduction in rates of self-harm in the DBT-A group compared to the EUC group. By contrast, in a study of 173 adolescents with repeat self-harm behaviors comparing DBT-A with individual and group supportive therapy (IGST), there were no statistically significant differences between the groups in self-harm, suicidal ideation, or suicide attempts at one year follow-up (McCauley *et al.*, 2018). There are several possible explanations for the difference in findings. For example, in the

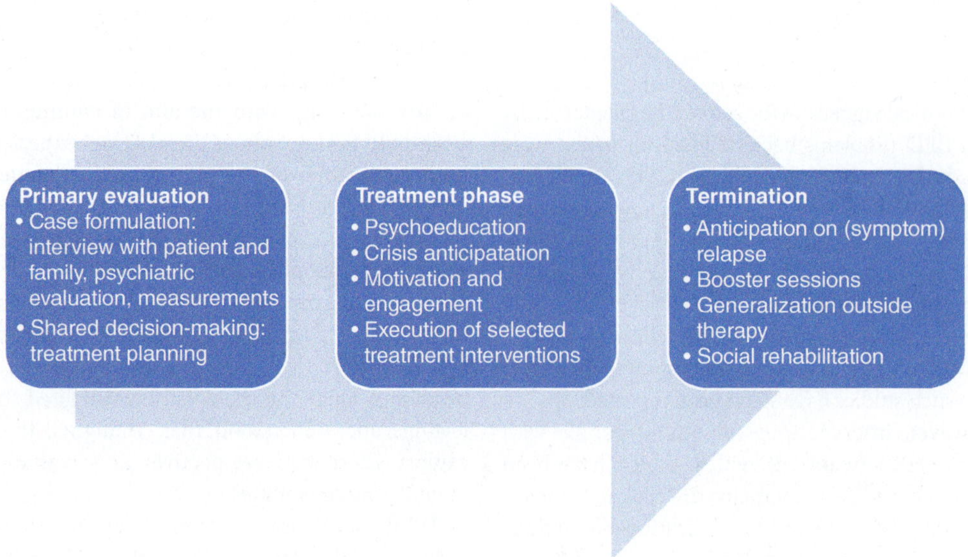

Figure 67.2 Phases of generalist treatment with specific targets for each phase (Hutsebaut *et al.*, 2020/Springer Nature/CC BY 4.0).

Mehlum *et al.* study, the control condition was not manualized nor checked for fidelity, while McCauley *et al.* compared DBT-A with a manualized, supervised treatment, in which adherence was monitored. Inclusion criteria differed between the studies. Mehlum *et al.* required self-harm plus either two BPD symptoms or one plus two subthreshold, while McCauley *et al.* required suicidal behaviors plus three or more BPD symptoms. Part of the explanation may be that compared to McCauley *et al.*, the Mehlum *et al.* study had a therapeutically less effective control condition and participants with less severe disorders.

Rossouw and Fonagy (2012) randomized 80 adolescents consecutively presenting to mental health services with self-harm and comorbid depression, the majority of whom met DSM BPD diagnostic criteria, to either MBT-A or treatment as usual (TAU). At one year follow-up young people treated with MBT-A had lower levels of self-harm than those in the control group. Jørgensen *et al.* (2021b) randomized 111 adolescents of whom all but 5 met DSM criteria for BPD, to MBT-A or TAU and found no differences between the groups at one year follow-up. Once more, several differences in study design may have accounted for the contrasting findings. In particular, in the first study, MBT-A was delivered individually and in the second in groups.

In summary, there has been some progress in the development and evaluation of psychological treatments for adolescent BPD, although we are a long way off from having convincing consistent evidence for treatment effects. Furthermore, the richness of the evidence regarding the key features of the disorder, and our knowledge of developmental pathways, has yet to be translated into measures of treatment outcome. As this chapter describes, the disorder is multifaceted, and impacts multiple aspects of young people's lives, but most trials have focused on self-harm or suicidal behavior. This leaves unanswered, important questions such as whether interventions can assist young people in moving from less to more favorable pathways in the transition to adult life.

Box 67.2 Treatment at a glance

- Treatment should start as early as possible as the disorder becomes more chronic as it progresses
- Provide psychoeducation to the young person and their family about personality disorder; that it is not an intractable disease, but rather a style of interacting with others and challenges in making sense of who one is as a person
- Inform the young person and their family about available specialist treatments, but emphasize that if those treatments are not available, management of personality disorder can be effective
- Define the treatment frame very clearly by providing clear structure and duration of sessions, therapist availability between sessions, procedures for contacts during crisis, and behaviors that could interfere with therapy
- Begin treatment with a focus on strengthening autonomy, enhancing self-esteem, regulating emotion, understanding self and others, and skills to more effectively manage relationships
- Treat comorbid disorders with psychotherapy and/or medication, and communicate to parents that there is no medication for personality disorder itself
- Generalize new skills to psychosocial functioning outside therapy
- Do not excessively focus on suicidality, but treat it the same way as you would in any individual without BPD

Conclusions and future directions

BPD is a distinct entity which can be identified during adolescence with implications for clinical management. Promising treatments have been evaluated but studies have not yet provided consistent evidence of effectiveness. All of the treatments require specialist training and, for the most part, dedicated services. Might inexpensive treatments that require fewer and shorter psychotherapy sessions delivered by less specialized mental health professionals be effective? We do not know. However, the behavioral, psychological, and interpersonal features of BPD which we have discussed can provide valuable starting points for conversations with young people about their struggles, and important pointers to therapeutic targets.

References

Akça, Ö.F. *et al.* (2020) Borderline personality disorder and attention deficit/hyperactivity disorder in adolescence: overlap and differences in a clinical setting. *Borderline Personality Disorder and Emotion Dysregulation* **7**, 1–9.

American Psychiatric Association (2013) *Diagnostic and statistical manual of mental disorders*, 5th edn. American Psychiatric Association, Washington, DC.

Baltzersen, A.L. (2021) Moving forward: closing the gap between research and practice for young people with BPD. *Current Opinion in Psychology* **37**, 77–81. doi:10.1016/j.copsyc.2020.08.008.

Bateman, A. & Fonagy, P. (eds) (2019) *Handbook of Mentalizing in Mental Health Practice.*, 2nd edn. American Psychiatric Association, Washington, DC.

Belsky, D.W. *et al.* (2012) Etiological features of borderline personality related characteristics in a birth cohort of 12-year-old children. *Development and Psychopathology* **24**(1), 251–265. doi:10.1017/S0954579411000812.

Bennett, C. *et al.* (2019) Perceived invalidation in adolescent borderline personality disorder: an investigation of parallel reports of caregiver responses to negative emotions. *Child Psychiatry & Human Development* **50**, 209–221.

Bilek, E. *et al.* (2019) Deficient amygdala habituation to threatening stimuli in borderline personality disorder relates to adverse childhood experiences. *Biological Psychiatry* **86**(12), 930–938.

Bjureberg, J. *et al.* (2016) Development and validation of a brief version of the difficulties in emotion regulation scale: the DERS16. *Journal of Psychopathological and Behavioral Assessment* **38**(2), 284–296.

Bohus, M. *et al.* (2021) Borderline personality disorder. *The Lancet* **398**(10310), 1528–1540.

Bolton, D. & Hill, J. (2004) *Mind, Meaning, and Mental Disorder: The Nature of Causal Explanation in Psychology and Psychiatry.* Oxford University Press, Oxford, UK.

Bornovalova, M.A. *et al.* (2013) Tests of a direct effect of childhood abuse on adult borderline personality disorder traits: a longitudinal discordant twin design. *Journal of Abnormal Psychology* **122**(1), 180–194.

Bowes, L. *et al.* (2009) School, neighborhood, and family factors are associated with children's bullying involvement: a nationally representative longitudinal study. *Journal of the American Academy of Child & Adolescent Psychiatry* **48**(5), 545–553.

Brumariu, L.E. *et al.* (2020) Developmental pathways to BPD-related features in adolescence: infancy to age 15. *Journal of Personality Disorders* **34**(Supplement B), 104–129.

Cannon, T.D. *et al.* (2008) Prediction of psychosis in youth at high clinical risk: a multisite longitudinal study in North America. *Archives of General Psychiatry* **65**(1), 28.

Carlson, E.A. *et al.* (2009) A prospective investigation of the development of borderline personality symptoms. *Development and Psychopathology* **21**(4), 1311–1334.

Chanen, A. *et al.* (2017) Prevention and early intervention for borderline personality disorder: a novel public health priority. *World Psychiatry* **16**(2), 215–216.

Chanen, A.M. (2015) Borderline personality disorder in young people: are we there yet? *Journal of Clinical Psychology* **71**(8), 778–791.

Chanen, A.M. (2021) Bigotry and borderline personality disorder. *Australasian Psychiatry* **29**(6), 579–580. doi:10.1177/10398562211045151.

Chanen, A.M. & Nicol, K. (2021) Five failures and five challenges for prevention and early intervention for personality disorder. *Current Opinion in Psychology* **37**, 134–138. doi:10.1016/j.copsyc.2020.12.005.

Chanen, A.M. *et al.* (2016) Integrating early intervention for borderline personality disorder and mood disorders. *Harvard Review of Psychiatry* **24**(5), 330–341. doi:10.1097/HRP.0000000000000105.

Chapman, A.L. (2019) Borderline personality disorder and emotion dysregulation. *Development and Psychopathology* **31**(3), 1143–1156. doi:10.1017/S0954579419000658.

Chartonas, D. *et al.* (2017) Personality disorder: still the patients psychiatrists dislike? *BJPsych Bulletin* **41**(1), 12–17. doi:10.1192/pb.bp.115.052456.

Cloitre, M. *et al.* (2014) Distinguishing PTSD, complex PTSD, and borderline personality disorder: a latent class analysis. *European Journal of Psychotraumatology* **5**(1), 25097.

Crick, N.R. *et al.* (2005) Borderline personality features in childhood: a short-term longitudinal study. *Development and Psychopathology* **17**(4), 1051–1070.

Daniunaite, I. *et al.* (2021) PTSD and complex PTSD in adolescence: discriminating factors in a population-based cross-sectional study. *European Journal of Psychotraumatology* **12**(1), 1890937.

Dennett, D.C. (1987) *The Intentional Stance.* MIT Press, Cambridge, MA.

Ditrich, I. *et al.* (2021) Borderline personality disorder (BPD) and attention deficit hyperactivity disorder (ADHD) revisited: a review-update on common grounds and subtle distinctions. *Borderline Personality Disorder and Emotion Dysregulation* **8**, 1–12.

Eaton, N. R. & Greene, A. L. (2018). Personality disorders: community prevalence and socio-demographic correlates. *Curr Opin Psychol* **21**, 28–32. doi:10.1016/j.copsyc.2017.09.001.

Ellison, W.D. *et al.* (2018) Community and clinical epidemiology of borderline personality disorder. *The Psychiatric Clinics of North America* **41**(4), 561–573.

Ettinger, U. *et al.* (2014) Genetics, cognition, and neurobiology of schizotypal personality: a review of the overlap with schizophrenia. *Frontiers in Psychiatry* **5**, 18.

Ferguson, C.J. (2010) A meta-analysis of normal and disordered personality across the life span. *Journal of Personality and Social Psychology* **98**(4), 659–667.

Ford, J.D. & Courtois, C.A. (2021) Complex PTSD and borderline personality disorder. *Borderline Personality Disorder and Emotion Dysregulation* **8**(1), 16.

Francey, S.M. *et al.* (2018) Does co-occurring borderline personality disorder influence acute phase treatment for first-episode psychosis? *Early Intervention in Psychiatry* **12**(6), 1166–1172. doi:10.1111/eip.12435.

Frith, C.D. & Frith, U. (2006) The neural basis of mentalizing. *Neuron* **50**(4), 531–534.

Gunderson, J.G. *et al.* (1981) The diagnostic interview for borderline patients. *American Journal of Psychiatry* **138**, 896–903.

Hecht, K.F. *et al.* (2014) Borderline personality features in childhood: the role of subtype, developmental timing, and chronicity of child maltreatment. *Development and Psychopathology* **26**(3), 805–815.

Hedley, D. & Uljarević, M. (2018) Systematic review of suicide in autism spectrum disorder: current trends and implications. *Current Developmental Disorders Reports* **5**, 65–76.

Hill, J. *et al.* (2003) The ecology of attachment in the family. *Family Process* **42**(2), 205–221.

Hill, J. *et al.* (2008) Social domain dysfunction and disorganization in borderline personality disorder. *Psychological Medicine* **38**(1), 135–146.

Hill, J. *et al.* (2010) Social domains, personality and interpersonal functioning. In: *In: Handbook of Interpersonal Psychology: Theory, Research, Assessment, and Therapeutic Interventions.* (eds L.M. Horowitz & S. Strack). John Wiley & Sons, Hoboken, NJ. pp. 281–293.

Hill, J. *et al.* (2023) The social domains organization of mentalizing processes in adolescents: a contribution to the conceptualization of personality function and dysfunction in young people. *Journal of Child Psychology and Psychiatry* **64**(10), 1470–1479.

Hutsebaut, J. *et al.* (2015) Development and preliminary psychometric evaluation of a brief selfreport questionnaire for the assessment of the DSM-5 level of personality functioning scale: The LPFS brief form (LPFS-BF). *Personality Disorder* **7**(2), 192–197.

Hutsebaut, J. et al. (2019) Managing borderline personality disorder from a life course perspective: Clinical staging and health management. *Personality Disorders: Theory, Research and Treatement* **10**(4), 309–316.

Hutsebaut, J. *et al.* (2020) Improving access to and effectiveness of mental health care for personality disorders: the guideline-informed treatment for personality disorders (GIT-PD) initiative in the Netherlands. *Borderline Personality Disorder and Emotion Dysregulation* **7**, 1–7.

Johnston, K. *et al.* (2016) Evaluating PROMIS® instruments and methods for patient-centered outcomes research: patient and provider voices in a substance use treatment setting. *Quality of Life Research* **25**(3), 615–624.

Jørgensen, M.S. *et al.* (2021a) Psychological therapies for adolescents with borderline personality disorder (BPD) or BPD features: a systematic review of randomized clinical trials with meta-analysis and trial sequential analysis. *PLoS One* **16**(1), e0245331.

Jørgensen, M.S. *et al.* (2021b) Mentalization-based treatment in groups for adolescents with borderline personality disorder: 3-and 12-month follow-up of a randomized controlled trial. *European Child & Adolescent Psychiatry* **30**, 699–710.

Keetharuth, A.D. *et al.* (2018) Recovering quality of life (ReQoL): a new generic self-reported outcome measure for use with people experiencing mental health difficulties. *British Journal of Psychiatry* **212**(1), 42–49.

Kernberg, O. (1967) Borderline personality organization. *Journal of the American Psychoanalytic Association* **15**(3), 641–685.

Kety, S.S. *et al.* (1971) Mental illness in the biological and adoptive families of adopted schizophrenics. *American Journal of Psychiatry* **128**, 302–306.

Klein, P. *et al.* (2022) Structural stigma and its impact on healthcare for borderline personality disorder: a scoping review. *International Journal of Mental Health Systems* **16**(1), 48. doi:10.1186/s13033-022-00558-3.

Kleindienst, N. *et al.* (2021) Childhood adversity and borderline personality disorder: analyses complementing the meta-analysis by porter *et al.* (2020). *Acta Psychiatrica Scandinavica* **143**(2), 183–184. doi:10.1111/acps.13256.

Linehan, M.M. (1993) *Cognitive-behavioral Treatment of Borderline Personality Disorder.* Guilford Press, New York.

Ma, G. *et al.* (2016) Genetic and neuroimaging features of personality disorders: state of the art. *Neuroscience Bulletin* **32**(3), 286–306.

May, T. *et al.* (2017) Gender variance in children and adolescents with autism spectrum disorder from the National Database for autism research. *International Journal of Transgenderism* **18**(1), 7–15.

May, T. *et al.* (2021) Overlap of autism spectrum disorder and borderline personality disorder: a systematic review and meta-analysis. *Autism Research* **14**(12), 2688–2710.

McAdams, D.P. (2015) Three lines of personality development: a conceptual itinerary. *European Psychologist* **20**(4), 252–264. doi:10.1027/1016-9040/a000236.

McCauley, E. *et al.* (2018) Efficacy of dialectical behavior therapy for adolescents at high risk for suicide: a randomized clinical trial. *JAMA Psychiatry* **75**(8), 777–785.

McLaren, V. et al. (2022) Hypermentalizing in borderline personality disorder: A meta-analytic review. *Am J Psychotherapy* **75**, 21–31. doi: 10.1176/appi.psychotherapy.20210018.

Mehlum, L. *et al.* (2014) Dialectical behavior therapy for adolescents with repeated suicidal and self-harming behavior: a randomized trial. *Journal of the American Academy of Child & Adolescent Psychiatry* **53**(10), 1082–1091.

Mehlum, L. *et al.* (2019) Long term effectiveness of dialectical behavior therapy versus enhanced usual care for adolescents with self-harming and suicidal behavior. *Journal of Child Psychology and Psychiatry* **60**(10), 1112–1122.

Musser, N. et al. (2018). A systematic review of parenting practices predicting borderline personality disorder: Are we measuring biosocial theory's invalidating environment? *Clinical Psychology Review* **65**, 1–16.

Papadopoulou, M. *et al.* (2020) Psychometric properties of the 12-item world health organization disability assessment schedule (WHODAS 2.0) in adult patients with motor disabilities. *Journal of Developmental and Physical Disabilities* **32**, 801–819.

Posner, K. *et al.* (2011) The Columbia–Suicide Severity Rating Scale: initial validity and internal consistency findings from three multisite studies with adolescents and adults. *American Journal of Psychiatry* **168**(12), 1266–1277.

Powers, J.P. & LaBar, K.S. (2019) Regulating emotion through distancing: a taxonomy, neurocognitive model, and supporting meta-analysis. *Neuroscience & Biobehavioral Reviews* **96**, 155–173.

Putnam, K.M. & Silk, K.R. (2005) Emotion dysregulation and the development of borderline personality disorder. *Development and Psychopathology* **17**(4), 899–926.

Ratey, J.J. & Gutheil, C.M. (1991) The measurement of aggressive behavior: reflections on the use of the overt aggression scale and the modified overt aggression scale. *Journal of Neuropsychiatry and Clinical Neurosciences* **3**(2), S57–S60.

Rathus, J.H. & Miller, A.L. (2014) *DBT Skills Manual for Adolescents.* Guilford Press, New York.

Robins, L.N. (1978) Sturdy childhood predictors of adult antisocial behaviour: replications from longitudinal studies. *Psychological Medicine* **8**, 611–622.

Rossouw, T. *et al.* (eds) (2021) *Mentalization-based Treatment for Adolescents: A Practical Treatment Guide.* Routledge, New York.

Rossouw, T. & Fonagy, P. (2012) Mentalization-based treatment for self-harm in adolescents: a randomized controlled trial. *Journal of the American Academy of Child & Adolescent Psychiatry* **51**(12), 1304–1313.

Rubin, K.H. *et al.* (1999) Peer relationships in childhood. *Developmental Psychology: An Advanced Textbook* **4**, 451–502.

Rupel *et al.* (2021) Standard set of patient-reported outcomes for personality disorder. *Qual Life Research* **30**(12), 3485-3500.

Schulze, L. *et al.* (2019) Neural correlates of affective disturbances: a comparative meta-analysis of negative affect processing in borderline personality disorder, major depressive disorder, and posttraumatic stress disorder. *Biological Psychiatry: Cognitive Neuroscience and Neuroimaging* **4**(3), 220–232.

Sharp, C. (2014) The social-cognitive basis of BPD: A theory of hypermentalizing. In: *Handbook of Borderline Personality Disorder in Children and Adolescents.* (eds C. Sharp & J. Tackett). Springer, New York. pp. 211–228.

Sharp, C. (2022) Personality disorders. *New England Journal of Medicine* **387**(10), 916–923. doi:10.1056/NEJMra2120164.

Sharp, C. & Miller, J.D. (2022) Ten-year retrospective on the DSM-5 Alternative Model of Personality Disorder: seeing the forest for the trees **13**(4), 301–304.

Sharp, C. & Wall, K. (2017) Personality pathology grows up: adolescence as a sensitive period. *Current Opinion in Psychology* **21**, 111–116. doi:10.1016/j.copsyc.2017.11.010.

Sharp, C. & Wall, K. (2021) DSM-5 level of personality functioning: refocusing personality disorder on what it means to be human. *Annual Review of Clinical Psychology* **17**, 313–337. doi:10.1146/annurev-clinpsy-081219-105402.

Sharp, C. *et al.* (2011) Theory of mind and emotion regulation difficulties in adolescents with borderline traits. *Journal of the American Academy of Child and Adolescent Psychiatry* **50**(6), 563.

Sharp, C. *et al.* (2015) The structure of personality pathology: both general ('g') and specific ('s') factors? *Journal of Abnormal Psychology* **124**(2), 387–398.

Sharp, C. *et al.* (2018) Adolescence as a sensitive period for the development of personality pathology. *The Psychiatric Clinics of North America* **41**(4), 669–683.

Sharp, C. *et al.* (2022) The Assessment of Identity Development in Adolescence (AIDA) questionnaire: first psychometric evaluation in two North American samples of young people. *Journal of Personality Assessment* **105**(4), 451–462. doi:10.1080/00223891.2022.2119860.

Sharp, C. *et al.* (In Press) ICD-11 personality disorders: Application to youth. In: *ICD-11 and The Personality Disorders.* (ed B. Bach). Oxford University Press, Oxford, UK.

Sicorello, M. & Schmahl, C. (2021) Emotion dysregulation in borderline personality disorder: a fronto–limbic imbalance? *Current Opinion in Psychology* **37**, 114–120.

Somma, A. *et al.* (2019) Hypermentalizing as a marker of borderline personality disorder in Italian adolescents: a cross-cultural replication of Sharp and colleagues' (2011) findings. *Borderline Personality Disorder and Emotion Dysregulation* **6**, 5. doi:10.1186/s40479-019-0104-5.

Sroufe, L.A. (1977) Wariness of strangers and the study of infant development. *Child Development* **48**(3), 731–746.

Stepp, S.D. *et al.* (2014a) Reciprocal effects of parenting and borderline personality disorder symptoms in adolescent girls. *Development and Psychopathology* **26**(2), 361–378. doi:10.1017/S0954579413001041.

Stepp, S.D. *et al.* (2014b) The impact of childhood temperament on the development of borderline personality disorder symptoms over the course of adolescence. *Borderline Personality Disorder and Emotion Dysregulation* **1**(1), 1–10.

Stepp, S.D. *et al.* (2016) A systematic review of risk factors prospectively associated with borderline personality disorder: taking stock and moving forward. *Personality Disorders* **7**(4), 316–323.

Tomko, R.L. *et al.* (2014) Characteristics of borderline personality disorder in a community sample: comorbidity, treatment utilization, and general functioning. *Journal of Personality Disorders* **28**(5), 734–750.

Vanwoerden, S. *et al.* (2022a) The development of Criterion A personality pathology: the relevance of childhood social functioning for young adult daily self-functioning. *Child Psychiatry and Human Development* **53**(6), 1148–1160. doi:10.1007/s10578-021-01187-6.

Vanwoerden, S. *et al.* (2022b) Momentary borderline personality disorder symptoms in youth as a function of parental invalidation and youth-perceived support. *Journal of Child Psychology and Psychiatry* **63**(2), 178–186.

Vidal-Ribas, P. *et al.* (2016) The status of irritability in psychiatry: a conceptual and quantitative review. *Journal of the American Academy of Child & Adolescent Psychiatry* **55**(7), 556–570.

Walter, E.E. *et al.* (2016) Genetic consideration of schizotypal traits: a review. *Frontiers in Psychology* **7**, 1769.

Wertz, J. *et al.* (2020) Borderline symptoms at age 12 signal risk for poor outcomes during the transition to adulthood: findings from a genetically sensitive longitudinal cohort study. *Journal of the American Academy of Child and Adolescent Psychiatry* **59**(10), 1165–1177 e1162. doi:10.1016/j.jaac.2019.07.005.

Wilson, N. *et al.* (2021) Nature and nurture? A review of the literature on childhood maltreatment and genetic factors in the pathogenesis of borderline personality disorder. *Journal of Psychiatric Research* **137**, 131–146.

Winsper, C. *et al.* (2016) The aetiological and psychopathological validity of borderline personality disorder in youth: a systematic review and meta-analysis. *Clinical Psychology Review* **44**, 13–24.

Winsper, C. *et al.* (2017) Aetiological pathways to borderline personality disorder symptoms in early adolescence: childhood dysregulated behaviour, maladaptive parenting and bully victimisation. *Borderline Personality Disorder and Emotion Dysregulation* **4**, 10. doi:10.1186/s40479-017-0060-x.

World Health Organization (2022) *International Statistical Classification of Diseases and Related Health Problems*, 11th revision. World Health Organization (WHO), Geneva, Switzerland.

Wright, N. *et al.* (2023) Turning to friends in preference to parents for support in early adolescence: does this contribute to the gender difference in depressive symptoms? *Frontiers in Child and Adolescent Psychiatry* **2**, 1150493.

Zimmerman, M. *et al.* (2013) Distinguishing bipolar II depression from major depressive disorder with comorbid borderline personality disorder: demographic, clinical, and family history differences. *Journal of Clinical Psychiatry* **74**(9), 880–886.

D: Somatic/body–brain

CHAPTER 68

Sleep and sleep disorders in children and adolescents

Eleanor L. McGlinchey[1] **and Judith A. Owens**[2]

[1] School of Psychology and Counseling, Fairleigh Dickinson University, Teaneck, NJ, USA

[2] Boston Children's Hospital, Harvard Medical School, Boston, MA, USA

Introduction

Sleep problems are one of the most common complaints brought to professionals working with children by caregivers. At some point during childhood, 25% of all children will experience a sleep problem (Fernandez-Mendoza *et al.*, 2021). These problems range from short-term difficulties in falling asleep to persistent sleep disorders. However, even transient sleep problems can be a source of significant distress for families, particularly if the disrupted sleep in the child results in daytime fatigue and mood disturbances in the caregiver. Relative to other clinical syndromes in child and adolescent psychiatry, sleep problems represent a symptom that is both a risk factor for and a result of almost every other psychiatric syndrome. Hence, the critical need for psychiatrists and pediatricians to work together to reduce the burden of child and adolescent sleep problems. In this chapter we review the basics of sleep regulation in humans and how sleep disturbance contributes to many core problems and symptoms in children and adolescents. We highlight treatments that target sleep disturbances and represent unique opportunities for intervention with potential for a broad range of positive outcomes.

Basics of sleep and sleep regulation

Sleep is a highly complex and intricately regulated phenomenon with neurobiological correlates, that is also influenced by a host of extrinsic factors, ranging from neighborhood, family, and broader sociocultural factors to individual factors, including medical, psychological, and neurodevelopmental elements (Iglowstein *et al.*, 2003; Bathory & Tomopoulos, 2017). Sleep is a biologic imperative, necessary for optimal brain and body functioning (Mason *et al.*, 2021). Sleep is *the* primary activity of the brain during early childhood; for example, by age 2 years, the average child has spent 9500 hours (approximately 13 months) asleep versus 8000 hours awake, and between 2 and 5 years the time asleep is equal to the time awake (Williams *et al.*, 2013; Bathory & Tomopoulos, 2017). Among other effects, sleep impacts include: neuronal "plasticity" or the ability of the brain to change structure/function in response to the environment, neurogenesis, and brain cell protection and repair from stress and injury (Mason *et al.*, 2021).

Sleep has a pervasive impact on physiologic functions that is related to both specific sleep stages and the influence of internal circadian rhythms. These include changes in the autonomic function (sympathetic/parasympathetic) and respiratory/immunologic/endocrine function in the body during sleep (Bathory & Tomopoulos, 2017). For example, growth hormone is released early after sleep onset, cortisol release increases after midnight and peaks in the morning, glucose levels peak during both nocturnal sleep and naps, and core body temperature drops during sleep. Additionally, sleep is associated with risk of obesity and difficulties with weight regulation given that less sleep increases hunger (via the neurohormone ghrelin) and decreases satiety (via the neurohormone leptin) (Boeke *et al.*, 2014; Ferranti *et al.*, 2016). Finally, sleep loss is associated with reduced immune function and with disorders associated with inflammatory processes such as obesity and cardiovascular disease/hypertension (Besedovsky *et al.*, 2019).

The "two-process" model

The concept of *sleep regulation* is based on what is usually referred to as the "two-process model" (Figure 68.1) because it requires the simultaneous operation of two basic, highly coupled processes that govern both sleep and wakefulness. The *homeostatic process* ("Process S" or "sleep drive"), regulates the length and depth of

Rutter's Child and Adolescent Psychiatry and Psychology, Seventh Edition.
Edited by Anita Thapar, Daniel S. Pine, Samuele Cortese, Cathy Creswell, Tamsin J. Ford, James F. Leckman, and Argyris Stringaris.

Companion website: www.wiley.com/go/thapar/rutterspsych7

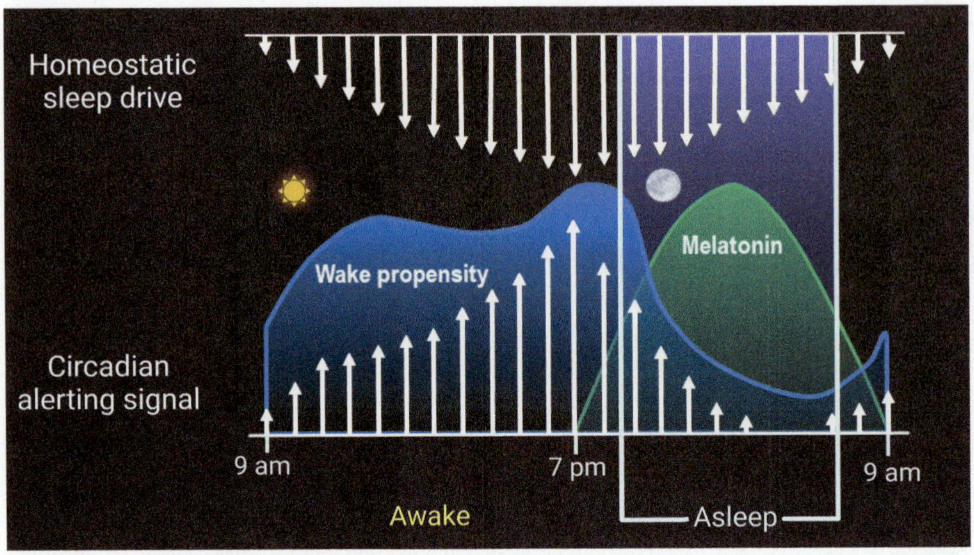

Figure 68.1 The "two process model" of sleep regulation. *Source*: With permission of BioRender.

sleep (Borbély *et al.*, 2016). The sleep drive builds in a fairly linear fashion across the day and appears to build more quickly in infants and young children, thus limiting the duration that wakefulness can be sustained during the day and necessitating periods of daytime sleep (i.e., naps). Process S is thought in part to be related to the accumulation of adenosine, as well as other sleep-promoting chemicals ("somnogens") during normal wake periods during the day. It should be noted that there are both wake-promoting (e.g., histamine, acetylcholine, serotonin) and sleep-promoting (gamma-aminobutyric acid [GABA], galanin) neurotransmitters; this explains the effects of some common pharmacologic agents such as caffeine (reduces adenosine binding and increases acetylcholine, thus disrupting sleep), antihistamines, and selective serotonin reuptake inhibitors (SSRIs) (Saper & Fuller, 2017).

The endogenous *circadian rhythms* ("Process C") influence the internal organization of sleep and the timing and duration of daily sleep–wake cycles, and govern predictable patterns of relative alertness and sleepiness throughout the 24-hour day. The "master circadian clock" or "circadian pacemaker" that controls sleep–wake patterns, of which melatonin secretion is the principal biomarker, is located in the suprachiasmatic nucleus in the anterior hypothalamus (Goel *et al.*, 2013; Baron & Reid, 2014). In addition, "circadian clocks" are now known to be present in virtually every cell in the body, and govern the timing of multiple other physiologic systems (e.g., cardiovascular reactivity, hormone levels, renal and pulmonary functions). Because the human circadian clock is slightly longer than 24 hours, intrinsic circadian rhythms must be synchronized or "entrained" to the 24-hour-day cycle by environmental cues called *zeitgebers*. The dark–light cycle is the most powerful of the zeitgebers; light signals are transmitted to the suprachiasmatic nucleus via the circadian photoreceptor system within the retina (functionally and anatomically separate from the visual system), which switch the pineal gland's production of the hormone melatonin off (light) or on (dark). Importantly, circadian rhythms are also synchronized by other external time cues, such as timing of meals and clock time. A large proportion of our genes are regulated by the biological clock and, consequently, a carefully calibrated circadian rhythm adapts our physiology (metabolism, hormone release, blood pressure, and body temperature) to the different phases of the day.

Sleep propensity is defined as the likelihood of dozing or falling asleep at a given time and under various circumstances, and is both distinct from and often accompanied by fatigue. While sleepiness and fatigue may overlap in their clinical presentation, sleep propensity is characterized by the tendency to fall asleep, particularly under conditions of low stimulation (e.g., riding in the car), while fatigue is often described as a state of low energy, decreased motivation, and "exhaustion." The relative level of sleepiness or alertness experienced at any given time during a 24-hour period is partially determined by the homeostatic *sleep drive*, which in turn depends on the duration and quality of previous sleep and the amount of time awake since the last sleep period. Interacting with this *sleep homeostat* is the 24-hour cyclic pattern or rhythm characterized by clock-dependent periods of maximum sleepiness (*circadian troughs*) and maximum alertness (*circadian nadirs*). There are two periods of maximum sleepiness, one in the late afternoon (approximately 3:00–5:00 p.m.) and one toward the end of the night (around 3:00–5:00 a.m.), and two periods of maximum alertness, one in mid-morning and one in the evening just before the onset of natural sleep, the so-called forbidden zone or second-wind phenomenon, which allows for the maintenance of wakefulness in the face of an accumulated sleep drive. This is a key factor in determining a child's "readiness for sleep." As the name implies, it is often characterized by a surge of alertness and activity level.

A key feature related to the circadian system is the concept of *chronotype*. Or "phase preference," which is the propensity of the individual to sleep or feel most awake at particular times during a 24-hour period (Randler *et al.*, 2017). A morning chronotype or morningness tendency (so-called "morning lark") is defined as a relative preference for an early sleep onset and offset, while "night owls" with an evening chronotype prefer a later fall asleep and wake time. Individuals with chronotype extremes at either end may have a genetic component. However, in general, younger children have a tendency toward a morningness chronotype, and notably, around the onset of puberty, children normally experience a shift in circadian preference to eveningness.

Sleep architecture

Sleep architecture, is defined as the presence and progression of sleep stages across sleep periods (Figure 68.2). It should be recognized that there are three basic states from a sleep perspective: Wake, rapid eye movement (REM), and non-REM sleep, which in turn is divided into light (stages N1 and N2) and deep (N3) sleep (Bathory & Tomopoulos, 2017). *Slow-wave sleep (SWS)* (i.e., N3, delta, or deep sleep) is characterized by a very regular heart and respiratory rate and high arousal threshold. N3 appears to be the most restorative form of sleep and is critical for brain development; it is entered relatively quickly after sleep onset, is preserved in the face of reduced total sleep time, and increases (rebounds) after a night of restricted sleep. *REM* sleep (stage R or "dream" sleep) actually shares active electroencephalogram (EEG) features with wakefulness and is characterized by more irregular breathing and cardiovascular parameters. Most muscle movement (with the exception of the diaphragm and eye movements) are normally suppressed in REM (atonia). REM also appears to be involved in numerous important brain processes, including completion of vital cognitive functions (e.g., consolidation of memory). Sufficient amounts of both of these sleep stages are necessary for optimal cognitive functioning and emotional and behavioral self-regulation.

Definition of deficient sleep

Partial sleep loss (i.e., sleep restriction) on a chronic basis accumulates in a "sleep debt," which, when large enough and not voluntarily repaid by sufficient recovery sleep, may result in periods of sleep propensity (dozing off and unplanned napping) and decreased alertness, recognized as *excessive daytime sleepiness (EDS).* The sleep-restricted individual may also experience very brief (several seconds) repeated daytime microsleeps, of which the individual may be completely unaware, but which nonetheless may result in significant lapses in attention and vigilance. There is also a relationship between the amount of sleep restriction and performance on cognitive tasks, particularly those requiring sustained attention and higher-level cognitive skills or executive functions, with a decay in performance correlating with declines in sleep amounts (Astill *et al.*, 2012).

EDS in children may be recognizable as drowsiness, yawning, and other classic "sleepy behaviors" (Bruni, 2023). EDS may present as difficulty waking spontaneously (i.e., with an alarm or caregiver intervention) in the morning at the desired time and extending sleep when given the opportunity such as on weekends ("if you can sleep more, you need more sleep"). EDS can also manifest as mood disturbance, including complaints of irritability, emotional lability, low frustration tolerance, and depressed or negative mood; fatigue and daytime lethargy, including increased somatic complaints (headaches, gastrointestinal disturbances); cognitive impairment, including problems with memory, attention, concentration, decision-making, and problem solving; daytime behavior problems, including hyperactivity, impulsivity, and noncompliance; and academic problems, including chronic tardiness related to insufficient sleep and school failure resulting from chronic daytime sleepiness (Marten *et al.*, 2023).

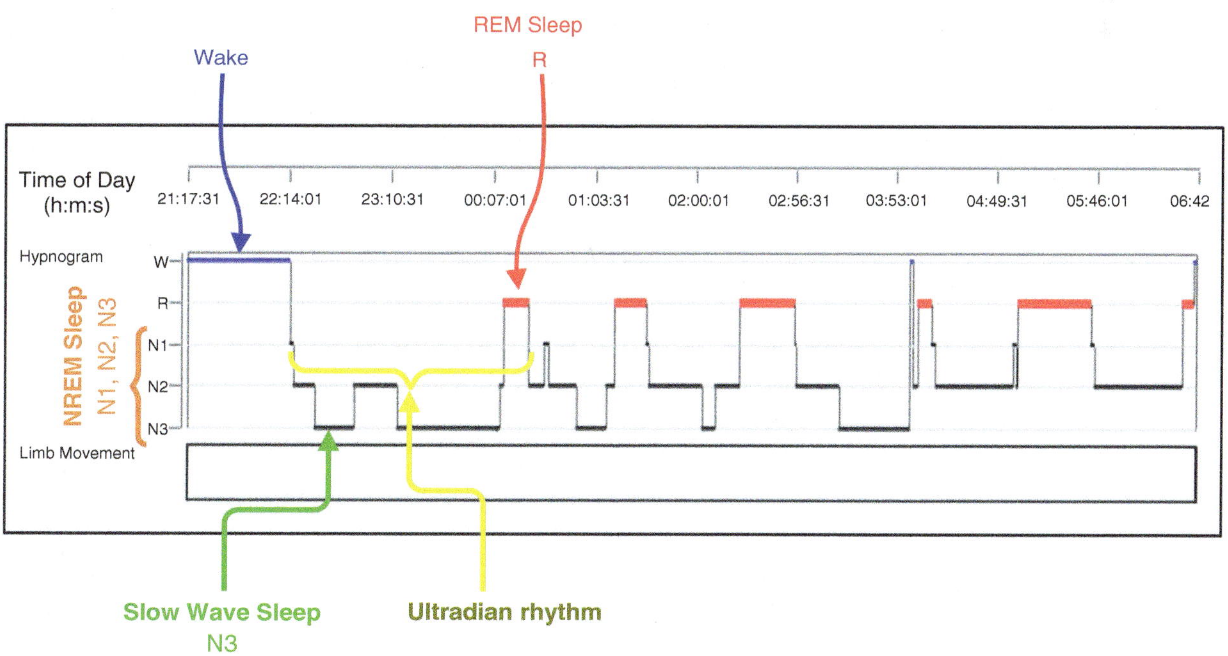

Figure 68.2 Hypnogram illustrating the normal progression and percentages of sleep stages throughout the night. *Source*: With permission of BioRender.

Finally, what may be described as "deficient" sleep involves alterations in both *amount* and *timing* of sleep. While often the focus is on sleep duration, studies have demonstrated that misalignment of intrinsic circadian rhythms with extrinsic societal demands (such as occurs with shift work and early school start times), is associated with deficits in cognitive function and self-regulation, increased emotional and behavioral problems and risk-taking behaviors, and negative impacts on health, such as increased risk of cardiovascular disease, obesity, and metabolic dysfunction (Williams *et al*., 2013; Baron & Reid, 2014). In other words, it's not just *how much* you sleep but *when* you sleep that matters. Thus, insufficient quantity of sleep, mistimed sleep, and poor-quality sleep in children and adolescents (or a combination) can substantially increase the risk of significant negative health, safety, cognitive, mood, behavioral, and performance consequences.

Developmental aspects of sleep across the pediatric age spectrum

Sleep disturbances, as well as many characteristics of sleep itself, have some distinctly different features in children compared to adults. Changes in sleep architecture and the evolution of sleep patterns and behaviors reflect the physiologic, chronobiologic, developmental, and social/environmental changes that are occurring across childhood (Table 68.1). These trends may be summarized as the gradual assumption of more adult sleep patterns as children mature.

There is a gradual decline in the average 24-hour sleep duration from infancy through adolescence, which involves a decrease in both diurnal and nocturnal sleep amounts (Figure 68.3). The variability in total sleep time is highest in the

Table 68.1 Normal developmental changes in children's sleep.

Age category	Sleep duration* and sleep patterns	Additional sleep issues
Newborn (0–2 months)	Total sleep: 10–19 hours per 24 hours (average, 13–14.5 hours), may be higher in premature babies Bottle-fed babies generally sleep for longer periods (2–5-hour bouts) than breastfed babies (1–3-hour bouts) Sleep periods are separated by 1–2 hours awake No established nocturnal–diurnal pattern in first few weeks; sleep is evenly distributed throughout the day and night, averaging 8.5 hours at night and 5.75 hours during the day	American Academy of Pediatrics issued a revised recommendation in 2016 advocating against bed-sharing in the first year of life, instead encouraging proximate but separate sleeping surfaces for mother and infant for at least the first 6 months and preferably the first year of life Safe sleep practices for infants: • Place baby on their back to sleep at night and during nap times • Place baby on a firm mattress with well-fitting sheet in safety-approved crib • Do not use pillows or comforters • Standards require crib bars to be no farther apart than 2 3/8 of an inch • Make sure baby's face and head stay uncovered and clear of blankets and other coverings during sleep
Infant (2–12 months)	Recommended sleep duration (4–12 months) is 12–16 hours (note that there is great individual variability in sleep times during infancy)	Sleep regulation or self-soothing involves the infant's ability to negotiate the sleep–wake transition, both at sleep onset and following normal awakenings throughout the night. The capacity to self-soothe begins to develop in the first 12 weeks of life and is a reflection of both neurodevelopmental maturation and learning. Sleep consolidation, or "sleeping through the night," is usually defined by parents as a continuous sleep episode without the need for parental intervention (e.g., feeding, soothing) from the child's bedtime through the early morning. Infants develop the ability to consolidate sleep between 6 weeks and 3 months.
Toddler (1–2 years)	Recommended sleep amount is 11–14 hours (including naps) Naps decrease from 2 to 1 nap at an average age of 18 months	Cognitive, motor, social, and language developmental issues impact sleep. Nighttime fears develop; transitional objects and bedtime routines are important.
Preschool (3–5 years)	Recommended sleep amount is 10–13 hours (including naps) Overall, 26% of 4-year-olds and just 15% of 5-year-olds nap	Persistent co-sleeping tends to be highly associated with sleep problems in this age group Sleep problems may become chronic
Middle childhood (6–12 years)	Recommended sleep amount is 9–12 hours	School and behavior problems may be related to sleep problems
		Media and electronics, such as television, computer, video games, and the Internet, increasingly compete for sleep time Irregularity of sleep–wake schedules reflects increasing discrepancy between school and nonschool night bedtimes and wake times
Adolescence (13–18 years)	Recommended sleep amount is 8–10 hours Later bedtimes; increased discrepancy between sleep patterns on weekdays and weekends	Puberty-mediated phase delay (later sleep onset and wake times), relative to sleep–wake cycles in middle childhood Earlier required wake times Environmental competing priorities for sleep

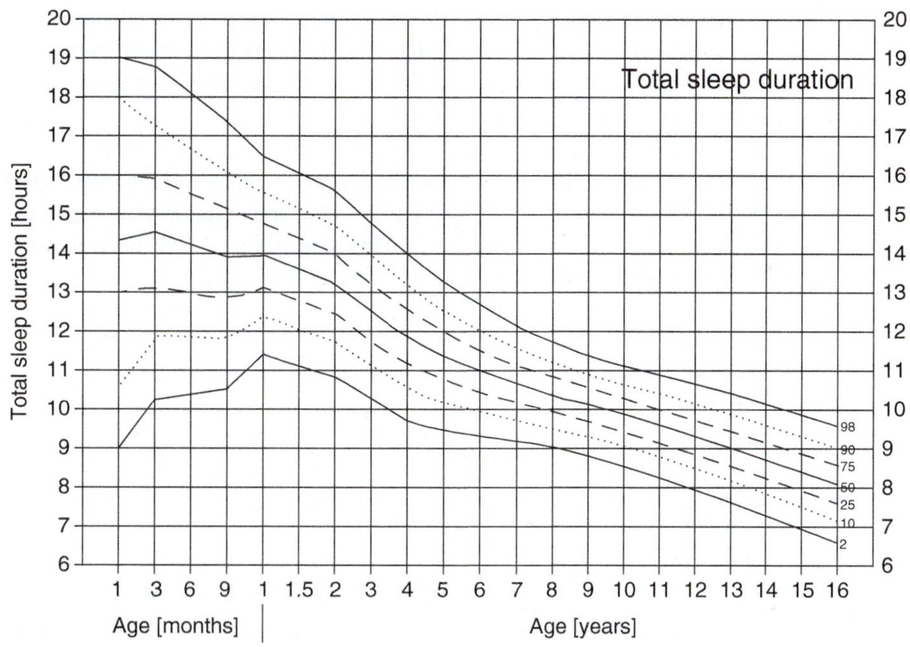

Figure 68.3 Distribution of 24-hour total sleep duration (defined as caregiver-reported time in bed) across the pediatric age range. Percentiles are shown at right-hand end of each line. *Source:* Iglowstein *et al.* (2003)/with permission of the American Academy of Pediatrics.

first year of life and children then tend to follow a "channel" regarding sleep duration percentile, similar to a growth curve (Iglowstein *et al.*, 2003). The decline in daytime sleep (scheduled napping) results in termination of naps typically by age 5, although there is considerable variability in the age at which children cease napping. There is also a gradual continued decrease in nocturnal sleep amounts into late adolescence; however, adolescents still require 8–10 hours of sleep per night (Table 68.2) for optimal sleep (Paruthi *et al.*, 2016).

In addition to reductions in sleep duration, there is also a decline in the relative percentage of REM sleep from birth (50% of sleep) through early childhood into adulthood (25–30%), and a similar initial predominance of SWS that peaks in early childhood, drops off abruptly after puberty (40–60% decline), and then further decreases over the life span (Jenni *et al.*, 2007). This SWS preponderance in early life has clinical significance; for example, the high prevalence of partial arousal parasomnias (sleepwalking and sleep terrors) in preschool and early school-age children is related to the relative increased percentage of SWS in this age group.

Table 68.2 American Academy of Sleep Medicine recommended amount of sleep for pediatric populations (2016).

To promote optimal health, recommended sleep amounts/24 hours on a regular basis:
Infants 4–12 months: 12–16 hours (including naps)
Children 1–2 years of age: 11–14 hours (including naps)
Children 3–5 years of age: 10–13 hours (including naps)
Children 6–12 years of age: 9–12 hours
Teenagers 13–18 years of age: 8–10 hours

Source: Paruthi *et al.* (2016)/American Academy of Sleep Medicine.

Sleep occurs in stages (termed non-REM sleep stages 1-3 and REM sleep) that cycle throughout the night at regular intervals—this cycle is known as the *ultradian cycle*. The within-sleep ultradian cycle lengthens from about 50 minutes in the full-term infant to 90–110 minutes in the school-age child (Bathory & Tomopoulos, 2017). Typically, a brief arousal or awakening occurs during the night at the termination of each ultradian cycle. Thus, as the length of the cycles increase, there is a concomitant decrease in the number of these end-of-cycle arousals (night wakings). This developmental progression can play an important clinical role in that infants and toddlers have a higher frequency and shorter intervals of normal night wakings.

A gradual shift in the circadian sleep–wake rhythm to a delayed (later) sleep onset and offset time, linked to the pubertal stage rather than chronological age, begins with pubertal onset in middle childhood and accelerates in early to mid-adolescence (Randler *et al.*, 2017). This biologic phenomenon often coincides with environmental factors, which further delay bedtime and advance wake time and result in insufficient sleep duration, including exposure to electronic "screens" (television, computer) in the evening, social networking, academic and extracurricular demands, and early (before 8:30 a.m.) high school start times (Touitou *et al.*, 2016). In addition, the accumulation of the homeostatic sleep drive across the day slows, resulting in an increased ability to delay sleep onset, and both sensitivity and exposure to evening light increases (especially blue spectrum light from electronic devices) during adolescence, conspiring to further delay sleep onset.

An increasing irregularity of sleep–wake patterns is typically observed across childhood into adolescence; this is characterized by increasingly larger discrepancies between school night and nonschool night bedtimes and wake times, and increased "weekend oversleep" in an attempt to compensate for chronic weekday sleep insufficiency (Crowley *et al.*, 2018). This phenomenon, often referred to as "social jet lag," not only fails to adequately address performance deficits associated with insufficient sleep on school nights, but also further exacerbates the normal adolescent phase delay and results in additional circadian disruption.

Sleep health may be defined as the absence of sleep disorders that can cause insufficient or poor-quality sleep, or circadian misalignment (such as insomnia, obstructive sleep apnea [OSA], or delayed sleep phase disorder) (Buysse, 2014). A recent approach to sleep health emphasizes its importance to general health: it defines a *positive role* for sleep in the general population and individual health (versus disease impact model), identifies *targets* for health promotion and prevention (Table 68.3), and *metrics* for measuring impact of interventions (versus disease treatment model), provides a *framework* for understanding the role of sleep in various populations (age, gender, race/ethnicity, socioeconomic status [SES]) and identifying health disparities, and emphasizes factors contributing to *resiliency*, as well as vulnerability (Williamson & Mindell, 2019).

Table 68.3 Healthy sleep recommendations.

- Practices promoting sleep regulation (circadian and sleep drive)
  - Maintain an organized and consistent sleep–wake cycle
  - Set and enforce a consistent bedtime on weekdays and weekends
  - Set and enforce a consistent wake time on weekdays and weekends
  - Keep a regular daily schedule of activities, including meals
  - Avoid bright light in the bedroom at bedtime and during the night
  - Increase light exposure in the morning
  - Establish an appropriate napping schedule
- Practices promoting sleep conditioning
  - Establish a regular and consistent bedtime routine
  - Limit activities which promote wakefulness while in bed (watching TV, smartphone use); use the bed for sleep only
  - Do not use bed for punishment (time out)
  - Avoid using staying up late as a reward for good behavior and going to bed as a punishment for undesired behavior
  - Avoid sleeping in environments other than the bedroom (couch, car)
- Practices reducing arousal and promoting relaxation
  - Keep electronics out of the bedroom and limit the use of electronics before bedtime
  - Reduce stimulating play at bedtime
  - Avoid heavy meals and vigorous exercise close to bedtime
  - Reduce cognitive and emotional stimulation before bedtime
  - Eliminate caffeine
  - Include activities in the bedtime routine that are relaxing and calming
- Practices promoting adequate sleep quantity and quality
  - Set an age-appropriate bedtime and wake time to ensure adequate sleep
  - Maintain a safe and comfortable sleeping environment (low noise and light levels, cooler temperatures, age-appropriate bedding and sleeping surface)

Screening for, and clinical assessment of, sleep problems in children and adolescents in mental health settings

There are a number of established tools that are available to screen for the presence and severity of sleep problems in clinical settings. The first approach is based on verbal inquiry. The "BEARS" sleep screen (Table 68.4) was designed as a rapid "first pass" tool to provide a practical and user-friendly vehicle for incorporating a pediatric sleep history into the standard medical history and physical examination in ambulatory settings (Owens & Dalzell, 2005). The "BEARS" instrument is divided into five major sleep domains, which provide a comprehensive screen for the major sleep disorders affecting children in the 2–18-year-old age range. Each sleep domain has a set of age-appropriate "trigger questions" for use in the clinical interview. Use of the BEARS screen has been shown to be more effective in eliciting key sleep concerns for further discussion compared to standard general questions such as "how is your child's sleep"? The Patient-Reported Outcomes Measurement Information System (PROMIS) surveys are available in both 4- and 8-item formats and both parent/caregiver and self-report versions (www.healthmeasures.net) (Yu *et al.*, 2011). The PROMIS measures can also be used as screeners prior to a clinical visit.

Other more comprehensive tools include the Brief Infant Sleep Questionnaire-Revised (BISQ-R; https://www.babysleep.com/bisq) (Mindell *et al.*, 2019), the Children's Sleep Habits Questionnaire (CSHQ; https://njaap.org/wp-content/uploads/2016/04/Childrens-Sleep-Habits-Questionnaire.pdf) for 4–12 year olds (multiple language versions and versions for preschoolers, children with autism, and to screen for behavioral sleep issues only are available) (Markovich *et al.*, 2014), and the Pediatric Sleep Questionnaire (PSQ; https://www.thoracic.org/members/assemblies/assemblies/srn/questionaires/psq.php) for 2–18 year olds.

A systematic and through approach to the clinical evaluation of a child presenting with or screening positive for a sleep problem also involves obtaining a careful history to assess for potential medical causes of sleep disturbances, such as allergies and asthma, concomitant medications, and acute or chronic pain conditions, as well as a complete mental health history that includes symptoms and formal diagnoses of mood, anxiety, attention, and learning disorders, and other mental health conditions. A developmental history is important because of the increased risk of sleep problems in children with neurodevelopmental disorders (NDDs). Assessment of the child's current level of functioning (school, home) is a key part of evaluating the possible mood, behavioral, and neurocognitive sequelae of sleep problems.

It is imperative to compile a list of previous and concurrent use of psychotropic medications, and sleep medications (including melatonin and over-the-counter agents), including dosages, timing and duration of use, efficacy, side effects, and impact on sleep (see the later section "Sleep disturbance as a risk factor for

Table 68.4 The BEARS sleep screen.

	Examples of developmentally appropriate questions (P = parent, C = child):		
	Preschool (2–5 years)	**School-aged (6–12 years)**	**Adolescent (13–18 years)**
1. **B**edtime problems	Does your child have any problems going to bed? Falling asleep?	Does your child have any problems at bedtime? (P) Do you have any problems going to bed? (C)	Do you have any problems falling asleep at bedtime? (C)
2. **E**xcessive daytime sleepiness	Does your child often seem over tired or sleepy during the day? Do they still take naps?	Does your child have difficulty waking in the morning, seem sleepy during the day, or take naps? (P) Do you often feel tired? (C)	Do you often feel sleepy during the day? In school? While driving? (C)
3. **A**wakenings during the night	Does your often child wake up at night?	Does your child often seem to wake up at night? Any sleepwalking or nightmares? (P) Do you often wake up at night? Have trouble getting back to sleep? (C)	Do you often wake up at night? Have trouble getting back to sleep? (C)
4. **R**egularity and duration of sleep	Does your child have a regular bedtime and wake time? What are they?	What time does your child go to bed and get up on school days? Weekends? Do you think they are getting enough sleep? (P)	What time do you usually go to bed on school nights? Weekends? How much sleep do you usually get? (C)
5. **S**leep-disordered breathing	Does your child often snore or have difficulty breathing at night?	Does your child have loud or nightly snoring or any breathing difficulties at night? (P)	Does your teenager snore loudly or nightly? (P)

other psychiatric disorders"). Notably, it is not uncommon to attribute sleep problems to medications such as psychostimulants, when a more careful history may reveal the presence of sleep problems predating the medication trial.

A review of sleep habits, such as bedtime routines, daily caffeine intake, and the sleeping environment (e.g., temperature, noise level, ambient light), may reveal environmental factors that contribute to sleep problems. Use of electronic devices, including laptops and smartphones, and especially highly interactive gaming systems and devices emitting melatonin-suppressing blue spectrum light up to and including bedtime, as well as during the night, is an extremely common contributor to sleep problems, especially delayed sleep onset; it has been shown that even the presence of such devices in the bedroom can disrupt sleep. Spending time in bed engaging in activities other than sleeping (e.g., doing homework, worrying) is also frequently associated with difficulties falling and staying asleep.

A detailed assessment of current sleep patterns, including the usual sleep duration and sleep–wake schedule on both weekdays and weekends, as well as extended nonschool periods, such as the summer vacation, is a mandatory part of the sleep history. Sleep schedules and patterns over time, including habitual bed and wake times, sleep onset latency, and extended periods of wakefulness during the night, are often best assessed prospectively with a *sleep diary or log* (Carney *et al.*, 2012), in which a parent (and/or older child/adolescent) records daily sleep behaviors for an extended period (typically two weeks) (see https://sleepeducation.org/resources/sleep-diary/ for a downloadable sleep diary). Naps should also be recorded on the sleep diary. This helps avoid relying on parent/patient recall of sleep timing, which often reflects "last night" or the "worst case" sleep scenario. Morning wake time evaluation should include when (in relation to desired/required wake time) and how (spontaneous versus need for multiple reminders) the patient wakes on school and nonschool days, and any tardiness or school absences related to difficulty waking. If there is concern about a family's ability to reliably complete a sleep diary or a more in-depth assessment of sleep schedules and patterns is desired, an additional diagnostic tool is an accelerometer type device that resembles a wristwatch and uses data and computerized algorithms regarding body movement to approximate sleep/wake activity over a several week period. While the standard device primarily used in sleep medicine clinics and in research is called an actigraph (Perpétuo *et al.*, 2020), there is mounting evidence that commercial devices, such as FitBit, and especially newer models that include additional sensors measuring heart and respiratory rate, may serve as a reasonable substitute. They also have the advantage of convenience in that many patients already have such devices at home. These devices appear to be most accurate in assessing total sleep time and sleep patterns over time, but are less accurate regarding nocturnal wake periods and sleep onset latency.

Nocturnal symptoms that may be indicative of a medically based sleep disorder, such as OSA (including loud snoring, mouth breathing, breathing pauses, choking or gasping, excessive sweating, and restless sleep) or periodic limb movements (PLMs) (restless sleep, repetitive kicking movements), should also be elicited. Positive symptoms of and risk factors for OSA (see Table 68.5 on sleep-disordered breathing [SDB]) and PLM disorder should be pursued, preferably with an in-lab, all night, attended sleep study or *polysomnogram* (PSG). However, it should be emphasized that even with a history suggestive of a primary medically based sleep disorder, a thorough complete sleep history must be obtained because many patients have more than one sleep disorder (e.g., OSA and sleepwalking, insomnia, and restless legs syndrome).

Home video recording reviewed by a sleep specialist may be helpful in the evaluation of potential parasomnia episodes, as it has the advantage of recording episodic events in real time, as well as the assessment of snoring and increased work of breathing in children with OSA. An overnight sleep study is not routinely indicated in the evaluation of a child or adolescent with sleep problems unless there are symptoms/risk factors suggestive of OSA or PLMs, unusual features of episodic nocturnal events, or unexplained daytime sleepiness.

Common sleep disorders

Childhood sleep problems may be conceptualized as resulting from: (i) inadequate duration of sleep for age and sleep needs (insufficient sleep quantity); (ii) disruption and fragmentation of sleep (poor sleep quality) as a result of frequent, repetitive, and brief arousals during sleep; (iii) misalignment of sleep–wake timing with circadian rhythms; or (iv) central nervous system (CNS)-mediated EDS and increased sleep needs. Insufficient sleep is usually the result of difficulty initiating (*delayed sleep onset*) or maintaining sleep (*prolonged night awakenings*), but especially in older children and adolescents, may also represent a conscious lifestyle decision to sacrifice sleep in favor of competing priorities, such as homework and social activities. The underlying causes of delayed sleep onset/prolonged night awakenings or sleep fragmentation may in turn be related to primarily behavioral factors (e.g., bedtime resistance resulting in shortened sleep duration) or medical causes (e.g., OSA causing frequent, brief arousals).

Certain pediatric populations are relatively more vulnerable to acute or chronic sleep problems (Johnson *et al.*, 2006; Díaz-Román *et al.*, 2018; Marten *et al.*, 2023). These include children with medical problems, such as chronic illnesses or pain conditions (e.g., cystic fibrosis, asthma, idiopathic juvenile arthritis) and acute illnesses (e.g., otitis media); children taking stimulants (e.g., psychostimulants, caffeine), sleep-disrupting medications (e.g., corticosteroids), or daytime-sedating medications (some anticonvulsants, α-agonists); hospitalized children; and children with a variety of psychiatric and NDDs, including attention deficit hyperactivity disorder (ADHD), depression, bipolar disorder, and anxiety disorders. Children with NDDs

Table 68.5 Overview of pediatric sleep disorders.

Disorder	Epidemiology / prevalence	Risk factors	Diagnosis	Prognosis
Insomnia	10–30% of children; 3–39% of teens	Increase with positive family history; other psychiatric disorders; trauma; unrealistic caregiver sleep expectations	Clinical interview assessing difficulty going to bed or staying asleep and is associated with daytime impairment; occurs at least three times per week for at least three months	Good; may resolve with developmental changes, cognitive behavioral therapy (CBT) improves recovery prognosis
Sleep-disordered breathing including obstructive sleep apnea (OSA)	2–4%	Adenotonsillar hypertrophy (ATH); obesity; craniofacial anomalies	In lab overnight polysomnography (PSG)—the "gold standard"	Good; early treatment important to prevent neurobehavioral/cognitive sequelae
Circadian rhythm disorders	2–8%	Inconsistent sleep timing; family history	Examination of sleep timing over at least one week, often through use of sleep diary, actigraphy, or other sleep timing questionnaire	Good; may resolve with developmental changes and/or intervention
Parasomnias	5–20%	Inconsistent sleep timing; unpredictable sleep environment	Clinical interview; video recording of overnight parasomnias	Good; often resolves with developmental changes
Excessive daytime sleepiness (EDS) and central hypersomnias (narcolepsy, idiopathic hypersomnia)	Narcolepsy: 20–50/100,000	Narcolepsy: Positive human leukocyte antigen (HLA)-DQB1*06:02; slight increase with positive family history	Epworth Sleepiness Scale; PSG and multiple sleep onset latency test (MSLT); cerebrospinal fluid (CSF) hypocretin/orexin levels may be helpful	Lifelong disorders; functioning and quality of life (QOL) can be significantly improved with treatment

such as autism, intellectual disability, blindness, and some chromosomal syndromes (e.g., Smith-Magenis syndrome, fragile X syndrome) have especially high rates of sleep disturbances for a wide variety of reasons. They may have comorbid medical issues or may be taking sleep-disrupting medications, could be more prone to nocturnal seizures, are less easily entrained by environmental cues and thus more vulnerable to circadian disruption, and are more likely to have psychiatric and behavioral comorbidities that further predispose them to disrupted sleep. An emerging literature also suggests that children from low socioeconomic households, and racial and ethnic minorities, as well as children in alternative care such as foster placement, are more likely to experience sleep disruption, are less likely to be diagnosed and treated, and are more vulnerable to the negative impact of sleep disorders ranging from chronic insufficient sleep to OSA, resulting in significant sleep health disparities in these pediatric populations (El-Sheikh *et al.*, 2010; Williamson & Mindell, 2019; Hash *et al.*, 2022). In the following sections, we will review the most common pediatric sleep disorders with particular focus on insomnia and OSA. A selection of the following disorders are summarized in Table 68.5.

Insomnia

Insomnia disorder presents differently in children compared to adolescents and adults but is broadly defined across age groups as a persistent difficulty in falling asleep or staying asleep that is associated with daytime impairments such as fatigue, mood complaints or irritability, cognitive difficulties, or general malaise. In children, the complaints are typically observed by the caregiver and may often manifest as bedtime resistance or an inability to sleep without significant caregiver intervention. In the past, pediatric insomnia was referred to as behavioral insomnia of childhood, sleep-onset association disorder, or limit-setting sleep disorder.

Etiology

The guiding model for understanding the etiology of insomnia in adults is known as the three-P model (3P) (Spielman *et al.*, 1987). It is a diathesis-stress model which includes predisposing, precipitating, and perpetuating factors. The predisposing factors can be biological (e.g., regularly elevated cortisol), psychological (e.g., tendency to worry), or social (e.g., school schedule incompatible with sleep schedule). Precipitating factors, such as stressful life events, then trigger the acute onset of sleep problems. Perpetuating factors, such as excessive caregiver intervention or use of screens in bed, can then contribute to the immediate sleep problem developing into a chronic or longer-term disorder. Within this framework, predisposing factors represent a constant vulnerability for sleeping problems. Precipitating factors trigger the acute sleep problem, but the influence of these factors diminishes over time. In contrast, perpetuating factors then come into play and serve to maintain the sleep problems. As such, the perpetuating factors are typically the targets of treatment. Related to perpetuating factors, behavioral insomnia of childhood is presumed to result from improper sleep training or limit-setting by parents or caregiver. Children may become dependent on specific stimulation, objects, or settings for initiating or returning to sleep following an awakening and sleep onset is significantly delayed in the absence of these conditions. Additionally, bedtime stalling or bedtime refusal may result from inadequate limit-setting by a caregiver.

Although the 3P model is a helpful heuristic for clinicians, it does not capture the range of factors that can lead to insomnia in young children. Children can experience fear, as well as other sources of cognitive or emotional arousal, that prevents an overall sense of safety and is likely to be antithetical to sleep. Children and adolescents can get into the habit of mentally reviewing or replaying worrisome thoughts and/or memories from the day. Some youth with stressful memories or specific fears manage to avoid these during the day through distracting activities, but at night—especially when trying to fall asleep—the lack of distracters can result in rumination on these thoughts and overall fear during bedtime.

Idiopathic insomnia may present differently in children. It is characterized by a long-standing complaint of sleep difficulties with onset occurring during infancy or early childhood. Caregivers often describe no discernible cause for the insomnia and find that it persists over time without sustained periods of remission. Given its early onset, stability over time, and often lifelong course, this form of insomnia is thought to result from either genetically determined or congenital aberrations in the sleep-inducing or arousal systems in the brain. However, no consistent genetic markers or neural pathology have been identified among children or adults who report this type of insomnia.

Epidemiology

A sleep problem similar to insomnia is experienced by 25% of all children at some point during childhood (Fernandez-Mendoza *et al.*, 2021). Specific subgroups of children, including those with chronic medical disorders, psychiatric comorbidities, and NDDs such as ADHD and autism spectrum disorder (ASD) have a higher lifetime prevalence of insomnia symptoms (Díaz-Román *et al.*, 2016; Marten *et al.*, 2023). For example, current data suggest that up to 80% of pediatric patients diagnosed with ASD have significant sleep complaints (Díaz-Román *et al.*, 2018).

There are several unique developmental factors that are highly relevant to the conceptualization of insomnia disorder in infants, children, and adolescents. First, insomnia must be understood within the context of sleep norms throughout the developmental trajectory of changes in sleep and circadian biology across the age spectrum. With every passing year of young childhood, there is a gradual decline in the normative duration of nocturnal and daytime sleep. Multiple nighttime awakenings are normal in the first year of life, followed by a decrease in the frequency of normal nighttime awakenings (paralleling the gradual lengthening of the ultradian cycle). As children enter school age, bedtime is progressively delayed, and, by adolescence, circadian and behavioral processes contribute to increased preference for later bedtimes. Sometimes caregivers can unknowingly contribute to insomnia disorder across childhood and adolescence when the caregivers do not or struggle to set limits around sleep and bedtime. However, sometimes a normal developmental process can precipitate difficulties with insomnia that become chronic problems if not addressed in a developmentally appropriate way. For example, developmentally normative separation anxiety and fear of being in the dark may contribute to children requesting the presence of a caregiver in the bedroom, refusing to sleep in their own bed or delaying going to bed. If the caregiver can respond with appropriate concern and limit setting, the child usually resumes sleep quickly. However, maladaptive sleep-onset associations are highly prevalent among young children, and so a diagnosis of chronic insomnia disorder is merited only when both of the following conditions are present: (i) the associations are prolonged, demanding, and typically require caregiver intervention/presence (e.g., extended rocking or car rides), and (ii) in the absence of these specific conditions, sleep onset is significantly prolonged, or night awakenings are extended and disruptive.

Specific developmental factors in adolescence are relevant to chronic insomnia disorder. Adolescents typically seek greater independence from caregivers which may result in resistance to following sleep recommendations and caregivers relinquishing oversight of sleep practices. In comparison to prepubertal children, social factors and changes in chronobiology contribute to a propensity for delaying bedtimes ("eveningness" preference). The timing of sleep may be in conflict with the early rise times dictated by school start times. Thus, if the adolescent tries to fall asleep at an earlier bedtime for more sufficient sleep, repeated unsuccessful attempts at sleep initiation may precipitate a chronic insomnia disorder (which may also be comorbid with a delayed sleep–wake phase disorder).

Diagnosis

The 2023 *International Classification of Sleep Disorders* 3rd edition text revision (ICSD-3-TR; Sateia, 2014) informs the evaluation and management of chronic insomnia disorder in both adults and children. As described, the patient or the patient's caregiver observes difficulty initiating sleep, maintaining sleep, waking too early, resistance to an appropriate schedule, and/or difficulty sleeping without a caregiver presence or intervention. This sleep difficulty is then associated with daytime fatigue/malaise, impaired attention, concentration, and memory, impaired social, family, and academic performance, mood disturbance/irritability, reported daytime sleepiness, behavioral problems (e.g., hyperactivity, impulsivity, aggression), reduced motivation/energy/initiative, proneness for errors/accidents, and/or concerns about sleep. With these criteria, the sleep and daytime concerns cannot be explained by inadequate opportunity or circumstances for sleep (e.g., time allotted for sleep or environmental stimulants). Additionally, these symptoms occur at least three times per week, have been present for at least three months, and are not due to another sleep, medical, or mental disorder. There is considerable overlap between insomnia disorder and other mental health conditions. Readers are referred to chapters 50, 54, and 63 in this volume on ASDs, ADHD, and pediatric depression, respectively.

Obstructive sleep apnea

SDB in children encompasses a spectrum of respiratory disorders that occur exclusively in sleep or that are exacerbated by sleep, including primary snoring, upper airway resistance syndrome, and sleep-related hypoventilation, as well as apnea of prematurity. *OSA*, the most important clinical entity within the SDB spectrum, is characterized by repeated episodes of prolonged upper airway obstruction during sleep despite continued or increased respiratory effort, resulting in reduction (hypopnea) or cessation (apnea) of airflow at the nose and/or mouth, as well as in oxygen desaturations and/or disrupted sleep. Both intermittent hypoxia and the multiple arousals resulting from these obstructive events contribute to significant metabolic, cardiovascular, and neurocognitive-neurobehavioral morbidity (Gulotta *et al.*, 2019). *Primary snoring* is defined as snoring without associated ventilatory abnormalities on an overnight polysomnogram. Increasing evidence suggests that primary snoring in children may also be associated with subtle breathing abnormalities during sleep, including evidence of increased respiratory effort, which in turn may be associated with adverse neurodevelopmental outcomes that may be similar to those associated with OSA.

Etiology

OSA results from an anatomically or functionally narrowed upper airway; this typically involves some combination of decreased upper airway patency (upper airway obstruction and/or decreased upper airway diameter), increased upper airway collapsibility (reduced pharyngeal muscle tone), and decreased drive to breathe in the face of reduced upper airway patency (reduced central ventilatory drive) (Bitners & Arens, 2020). Upper airway obstruction varies in degree and level (i.e., nose, nasopharynx/oropharynx, hypopharynx) and is most frequently caused by adenotonsillar hypertrophy, although tonsillar size does not necessarily correlate with degree of obstruction, especially in older children. Other causes of airway obstruction include allergies associated with chronic rhinitis or nasal obstruction; craniofacial abnormalities, including hypoplasia or displacement of the maxilla and mandible; gastroesophageal reflux; and nasal septal deviation. Reduced upper airway tone may result from neuromuscular diseases, including hypotonic cerebral palsy and muscular dystrophies or hypothyroidism. Reduced central ventilatory drive may be present in some children, such as those with brainstem malformation (e.g., Arnold-Chiari), autonomic dysregulation, and meningomyelocele. In other cases, the etiology is mixed; such as in children with Down syndrome, who are at particularly high risk for OSA, with some estimates of prevalence as high as 70%. Although many children with OSA are of normal weight, an increasingly large percentage are overweight or obese, and there is a significant correlation between weight and the presence of OSA, as well as residual OSA following adenotonsillectomy.

Epidemiology

When defined by parent-reported symptoms, the prevalence of OSA is 4–11% (Gulotta *et al.*, 2019; Bitners & Arens, 2020). The prevalence documented by overnight sleep studies is 1–4% overall. Prevalence is also affected by demographic characteristics such as sex (more common in boys, especially after puberty), race/ethnicity (increased prevalence in African American and Asian children), history of prematurity, and family history of OSA.

Clinical manifestations

The clinical manifestations of OSA may be divided into sleep-related and daytime symptoms (Jones Oguh *et al.*, 2020). The most common nocturnal manifestations of OSA in children and adolescents are loud, frequent, and disruptive snoring; breathing pauses; choking or gasping arousals; restless sleep; and nocturnal diaphoresis. Children with OSA may adopt unusual sleeping positions, keeping their necks hyperextended to maintain airway patency. Frequent arousals associated with obstruction may result in nocturnal awakenings but are more likely to cause fragmented sleep.

Daytime symptoms of OSA include mouth breathing and dry mouth, chronic nasal congestion or rhinorrhea, hyponasal speech, morning headaches, difficulty swallowing, poor appetite, and resumption of bedwetting, as well as an increase in partial arousal parasomnias (sleepwalking and sleep terrors).

One of the most important but frequently overlooked sequelae of OSA in children is the effect on mood, behavior, learning, and academic functioning. The neurobehavioral consequences of OSA in children include daytime sleepiness with drowsiness, difficulty in morning waking, and unplanned napping or dozing off during activities, although evidence of frank hypersomnolence tends to be less common in children compared to adults with OSA (except in very obese children or those with severe disease). Mood changes include increased irritability, mood instability and emotional dysregulation, low frustration tolerance, and depression or anxiety. Behavioral issues include both "internalizing" (i.e., increased somatic complaints and social withdrawal) and "externalizing" behaviors, including aggression, impulsivity, hyperactivity, oppositional behavior, and conduct problems. There is substantial overlap between the clinical impairments associated with OSA and the diagnostic criteria for ADHD, including inattention, poor concentration, and distractibility (Bitners & Arens, 2020). Furthermore, many of the studies that have looked at changes in behavior and neuropsychologic functioning in children after treatment (usually adenotonsillectomy) for OSA have largely documented significant improvement in outcomes, both short-term and long-term, including daytime sleepiness, mood, behavior, academic performance, and quality of life.

Diagnosis

The 2012 revised American Academy of Pediatrics clinical practice guidelines (Marcus *et al.*, 2012) inform the evaluation and management of uncomplicated childhood OSA. Certain physical examination findings, including body mass index (BMI), are consistent with overweight/obesity, evidence of chronic nasal obstruction, enlarged tonsils, and craniofacial features associated with an increased risk of obstruction such as retrognathia and micrognathia, but because no combination of clinical history and physical findings can accurately predict which children with snoring have OSA, the gold standard for diagnosing OSA remains an in-lab, overnight PSG. In addition to these PSG parameters, clinical judgment regarding risk factors for OSA, presence and severity of clinical symptoms, and evidence of daytime sequelae should determine further management.

Parasomnias

Parasomnias occur commonly in young children as sudden, partial awakenings. Parasomnias are often experienced earlier in the night when children are in deep, non-REM sleep. Most children will present in a mixed state with some aspects of being awake and some aspects of being in a deep sleep. Evidence suggests at least two routes to this mixed state: (i) difficulty leaving deep sleep (SWS) at the end of the first sleep cycle, or (ii) a sudden disturbance or disruption during the middle of deep sleep. Parasomnias include sleepwalking, night terrors, and confused partial arousals (some enuretic events can also occur as partial arousals). The intense events (with screaming, agitated flailing, and running) represent the extreme end of a spectrum of partial arousal behaviors that occur in mild forms (such as calm mumbling or a few awkward movements) in many children. The events can last from a few seconds to 20 minutes, with an average duration of about 3 minutes. The termination is usually as sudden as the initiation, with a rapid return to deep sleep. During the parasomnias, the children may seem confused, often not recognizing their parents, being inconsolable, and often appearing incoherent.

Overtiredness can increase or precipitate parasomnias. Any time a child is adjusting to getting less sleep, or has disturbed nighttime sleep, the physiological compensation is to get deeper sleep (especially in the first one to two hours after sleep onset). This deep "recovery" sleep appears to be fertile ground for partial arousal events. When a parasomnia is suspected, the clinical interview should include obtaining a careful history of all sleep-related habits, as well as the characteristics, pattern, and frequency of the events. Occurrence in the first third of the night and an increased frequency corresponding to periods of being overly tired are strongly suggestive of typical parasomnia events.

Delayed sleep phase syndrome

There is evidence that the onset of puberty triggers a change toward a distinct evening preference among approximately 40% of adolescents, which is then exacerbated by various social (e.g., importance of peers, parents less involved in decisions regarding bed and wake times), psychological (e.g., increased pressure at school), and behavioral factors (e.g., use of social media in bed and during the night) (Crowley *et al.*, 2018). Together, these factors can contribute to a tendency toward eveningness or, in the extreme, delayed sleep phase syndrome (DSPS). Problems with delayed sleep in children and adolescents can be further compounded by large differences between weekday and weekend schedules (social jet lag). Often coupled with DSPS and after the onset of puberty and throughout the adolescent period, the most prevalent sleep complaints tend to center on difficulty waking up for school in the morning and the associated difficulties with daytime sleepiness, tiredness, and irritability. It is important to emphasize that there is a broad continuum of severity. This ranges from normative/mild difficulties that appear to affect up to half of all high school students to a much smaller subset of adolescents with severe difficulties with sleep and schedules that result in significant impairments (such as failures in school) and often meet the full criteria for DSPS. It can be difficult to delineate precisely when to diagnose adolescents as having DSPS disorder from the much larger set of youth with mild to moderate problems that include erratic and late sleep schedules. It can also be difficult to recognize DSPS versus insomnia (Baroni, 2019).

In taking a sleep history, it is important to ask specific questions about bedtime schedules. Many families will say the adolescent "usually" goes to bed at a certain time, but when asked for an exact time covering the previous few nights, a much later hour is reported. When assessing the amount of sleep an adolescent is getting, it is important to obtain details of bedtime (such as when the child gets into bed, as well as lights-out time), estimates of how long it takes to fall asleep, nighttime arousals, time of getting up in the morning, difficulty getting up, and the frequency, timing, and duration of daytime naps. It is also essential to get details of sleep/wake schedules on weekends, as well as during the school week.

Excessive daytime sleepiness and central hypersomnias (narcolepsy, idiopathic hypersomnia)

Narcolepsy is characterized by EDS (Tadrous *et al.*, 2021). The classic symptoms include: (i) sleep attacks; (ii) cataplexy (the sudden loss of muscle tone without change of consciousness); (iii) sleep paralysis (inability to move after waking up); and (iv) hypnogogic hallucinations (dream-like imagery before falling asleep). These symptoms do not all occur together or consistently in many cases of narcolepsy. Particularly in younger patients, signs of sleepiness may be the only initial symptom. Cataplexy is typically provoked by laughter, anger, or sudden emotional changes. It may be as subtle as a slight weakness in the legs, or as dramatic as a patient's falling to the floor limp and unable to move.

The diagnosis of narcolepsy requires evaluation in a sleep laboratory. The diagnostic assessment includes tests for human leukocyte antigens (HLAs), and cerebrospinal fluid hypocretin (Hcrt) measurement (Nevsimalova *et al.*, 2009). Notably, narcolepsy is frequently misdiagnosed initially as a psychiatric condition. This can often contribute to a protracted time to accurate diagnosis and intervention. Additionally, there are many psychiatric disorders that are comorbid with narcolepsy. For example, there are possible associations between ADHD and narcolepsy (Modestino & Winchester, 2013).

The differential diagnosis of narcolepsy includes consideration of idiopathic hypersomnia. EDS is common among youth, especially youth with a mood disorder. In addition, during phases of depression patients commonly suffer from periods of hypersomnia. Hypersomnia has adverse consequences for school attendance and performance, relationships, and mood. There is very little existing literature on the mechanisms that contribute to hypersomnia in mood disorder, nor the methods to treat it.

Restless leg syndrome and periodic limb movement disorder

Restless leg syndrome (RLS) is a clinical diagnosis characterized by disagreeable leg sensations that usually occur prior to sleep onset. Periodic limb movement disorder (PLMD) is characterized by periodic episodes of repetitive and highly stereotypic limb movements during sleep with symptoms of insomnia or EDS. PLMD and RLS are distinct entities but can coexist. Most patients with PLMD do not manifest RLS symptoms; however, approximately 80% of patients with RLS have PLMD (Pennestri *et al.*, 2021). PLMD has been described in children with somewhat different clinical presentation. Children with PLMD may present with nonspecific symptoms such as growing pains, restless sleep, and hyperactivity (Crabtree *et al.*, 2003). These symptoms are most often unnoticed by their parents, although a family history of RLS and PLMD is common.

Sleep disturbance as a risk factor for other psychiatric disorders

Untreated sleep problems first presenting in infancy are known to persist during school-aged years and often become chronic (Pollock, 1994). There are complicated interactions between sleep and mental health during the developmental period of childhood and adolescence. Hasler and Pedersen (2020) describe how the well-known sleep and circadian changes that mark the pubertal transition are likely to heighten risk for alcohol abuse. There is also accruing evidence that the timing of adolescent sleep alterations differentially impact risk in female versus male adolescents given the temporal overlap with affective changes that heighten vulnerability for depression in girls (Marver & McGlinchey, 2020). In addition, there is great urgency in better understanding the mechanisms underlying sleep-related problems, and suicidal thoughts and behaviors in adolescents and young adults. Some have suggested adolescent interventions for sleep might serve to prevent internalizing disorders, self-harm, and suicidal behavior in young persons (Blake *et al.*, 2018).

Evidence has steadily accrued indicating that insomnia is an independent risk factor for first and recurrent episodes of depression. There also is substantial evidence that sleep problems emerging during early childhood are independently predictive for the later onset of depression (Gregory *et al.*, 2005). It is possible that chronic activation of the hypo–pituitary–adrenal (HPA) axis via inadequate sleep may create a direct path toward affective vulnerability, although others have argued that a heighted sensitivity to stressful life events, maladaptive cognitive and behavioral responses to stress, and serotoninergic neurotransmission represent shared mechanistic pathways for insomnia and affective disorders.

Multiple large prospective studies with nonclinical adolescents provide evidence that insufficient sleep predicts worse mental health at follow-up, after controlling for baseline levels of functioning (Roberts *et al.*, 2009; Roberts & Duong, 2014). Recent research using data from the National Longitudinal Study of Adolescent Health suggests that insufficient sleep leads to drug use among teens, and that patterns of sleep and drug use are spread via social networks (Mednick *et al.*, 2010). These social network analyses suggest that insufficient sleep mediates the relationship between adolescents' own drug use and the drug use of their friends.

Regarding post-traumatic stress disorder (PTSD), there is evidence that trauma-related sleep disturbances occur in the absence of formal diagnoses, elevating risk for both sleep and other psychiatric disorders. There has been an overall dearth of studies on trauma-related sleep disturbances in youth, calling attention to the lag between adult versus child-focused data, including a lack of validated measures and treatment approaches for use among trauma-exposed youth. Highly relevant to understanding these relationships, findings revealing impaired sleep to hinder consolidation of fear-based memories points toward a potentially vicious cycle whereby trauma memories and sleep disturbance might serve to worsen each other over time (Lewin *et al.*, 2019).

Treatments for sleep disorders

Although treatment research has steadily progressed over the past decades, there remains a great need for it. Behavioral interventions have a strong evidence base for treating insomnia and delayed sleep in children and adolescents, with emerging evidence that these interventions are also effective for improving sleep among children with various comorbidities (e.g., autism, depression, ADHD). Increasingly, there is recognition that there are several advantages to treating sleep problems nonpharmacologically, including that behavioral interventions are: safe (few side effects and no potential for causing adverse interactions with prescribed medications), simple (easy to do), and inexpensive (especially considering that the positive effects have been shown to endure, particularly among infants and young children).

Behavioral treatments for insomnia in young children

Interventions for bedtime problems and night wakings in young children are founded on principles of learning and behavior (e.g., reinforcement, extinction, shaping). Treatments involve training parents with a therapist guiding interventions on how to change their child's problematic sleep habits or sleep-related behaviors. The first of these interventions is "unmodified extinction" and involves having the parents put the child to bed at a designated bedtime and then ignoring any crying, tantrums, or calling out by the child until a set time the next morning (although parents monitor for illness, injury, etc.). The effective use of extinction requires parental consistency. No matter how long the crying lasts, parents must ignore this every night. Otherwise, the child may "learn" to cry longer the next time. The common term used in popular media and self-help books to describe unmodified extinction techniques is the "cry it out" or Ferber approach. The difficulty with the use of unmodified extinction procedures is that it is often perceived as stressful by parents and many are not able to ignore the crying long enough for the procedure to be effective. There is also some concern about child bonding and attachment if infants are crying for long periods of time. An alternative to unmodified extinction is extinction with parental presence. In this variant, the parent stays in the child's room at bedtime but ignores the child and their problematic behavior. For some parents this procedure helps them to be more consistent and is more acceptable to them.

Another intervention based on extinction principals is "graduated extinction." Parents are instructed to ignore bedtime crying and tantrums on a specified schedule of check-ins. The period between check-ins is often tailored with the guidance of a therapist with considerations for the child's age and temperament, and the parents' judgment of how long they can tolerate the child's crying. Parents can also choose to check on their child on a fixed schedule (e.g., every 5 minutes) or with incrementally longer intervals (e.g., 5 minutes, 10 minutes, then 15 minutes). When using incrementally longer intervals, increases across successive checks within the same night or across successive nights can gradually reduce to no check-ins. Parents should only comfort their child for a brief period and no longer than a minute. Through the use of graduated extinction, the goal is for the child to develop "self-soothing" skills so that they fall asleep independently without the parent. In parenting books, this type of intervention is often referred to as "sleep training."

Behavioral interventions can also include powerful methods for increasing the homeostatic drive to sleep, such as developmental adaptations which involve a small amount of sleep restriction that builds the homeostatic process. "Positive routines" is an intervention that involves the parents developing a routine at bedtime that is characterized by quiet and enjoyable activities for the child. Faded bedtime is often used with positive routines and involves taking the child out of bed for predetermined periods of time when the child does not fall asleep. Bedtime is also delayed so that sleep onset occurs quickly, and so that the cues for sleep are paired with the enjoyable activities from the positive routines of bedtime procedure. Once the behavioral chain of events is well established and the child falls asleep more quickly, bedtime is moved earlier by 15–30 minutes over successive nights until an age-appropriate bedtime goal is achieved. In addition, when overnight wakings are the primary problem, scheduled awakenings can be used. This procedure involves the parent awakening and comforting their child approximately 15–30 minutes before a typical awakening. Prior to using this strategy, a baseline of the number and timing of the nighttime awakenings must be established. Preemptive awakenings are then scheduled and can involve rocking or nursing the child back to sleep. Over consecutive nights, scheduled awakenings are faded out, by gradually increasing the time span between awakenings. Scheduled awakenings have been shown to increase the duration of consolidated sleep. Overall, the weight of the evidence from controlled group studies supports behavioral intervention in young children.

Behavioral treatments for insomnia in older children and adolescents

Insomnia is a common complaint among older children and adolescents, particularly sleep-onset insomnia. Cognitive behavioral therapy for insomnia (CBT-I) include a range of powerful behavioral adjustments to sleep. The evidence that CBT-I produces reliable and durable changes in sleep in school-age children and adolescents has been summarized in meta-analyses and excellent review papers (e.g., Dewald-Kaufmann *et al.*, 2022). There is additional evidence that CBT-I for adolescents with comorbid anxiety, depression, and other psychiatric disorders is not only effective at reducing insomnia but also in reducing symptoms of other comorbidities. However, this is a growing area of research. Many of the interventions specific to CBT-I have now been adapted into online and app programs (e.g., Sleepio, SHUTi). There is accumulating evidence that these programs are effective and helpful for teens (de Bruin & Meijer, 2017; Ritvo *et al.*, 2021). Clinical research has also attempted to address common problems of low motivation for treatment, poor treatment adherence, and attrition among adolescent patients by using the school classroom as an alternative arena for sleep intervention. Although promising, low motivation is a concern for adolescents and may require parental and/or clinician assistance in regulating and maintaining healthy sleep schedules.

There are a range of important components of a behavioral intervention for insomnia as described in Table 68.6 and in detail elsewhere (Clarke *et al.*, 2015). Briefly, stimulus control therapy uses the principles of conditioning to reverse the maladaptive association that may be formed with the bed/bedroom/bedtime by limiting sleep incompatible behaviors engaged in within the bedroom environment, thereby decreasing cues for sleep incompatible behaviors while increasing cues for sleep compatible behaviors. The clinician should instruct the following:

- go to bed only when sleepy at night
- use the bed and bedroom only for sleep (i.e., no reading, TV watching, or worrying, either during the day or at night)
- get out of bed and go to another room whenever you are unable to fall asleep or return to sleep within 15–20 minutes and return to bed only when sleepy again
- repeat this last step as often as necessary throughout the night
- arise in the morning at the same time regardless of the amount of sleep obtained on the previous night (Bootzin *et al.*, 1991)
- limited daytime napping (< 1 hour) before 03 : 00 p.m.

There is a growing treatment literature on DSPS in teens, including the use of timed light with teens, as well as practice parameters that indicate evidence for timed light exposure (with a light box) and planned and regular sleep schedules (chronotherapy) in adults. Unfortunately, it can be difficult to motivate teens to use light boxes and to participate in chronotherapy. Traditional chronotherapy involves progressively delaying bedtimes and waketimes until reaching the desired alignment; however, this can tend to be highly disruptive to family and work schedules. Hence, a planned sleep modification protocol derived from circadian principles involving moving bedtimes earlier by 20–30 minutes per week may be preferable for most teens and families. The circadian system can adapt to more rapid changes but it is often better to build a sense of mastery and control over sleep with smaller changes, scaffolded with interventions focused on wind-down bedtimes and gradual wake-ups.

Behavioral interventions for parasomnias and narcolepsy

Given the wide range of intensity of nocturnal partial arousals, the key to behavioral intervention is matching the appropriate intervention to the degree of problem. That is, mild sleepwalking or an occasional night terror in a young child requires only some parental reassurance with general suggestions regarding improved sleep habits and the likelihood that the events will decrease over time. Second, encourage a regular sleep/wake schedule with good sleep habits. The parents should consider an earlier bedtime if there is any evidence that the child is getting inadequate sleep. Finally, more frequent, repetitive, intense, and agitated sleep terrors can be treated effectively through the use of scheduled awakenings.

Table 68.6 Treatment at a glance.

Intervention type	Insomnia	Sleep disorder breathing	Circadian rhythm disorder	Parasomnias	Excessive daytime sleepiness and central hypersomnia	Restless leg syndrome
Behavioral	Stimulus control therapy; sleep restriction therapy (part of cognitive behavioral therapy [CBT])	Weight loss	Bright light therapy; chrono-therapy; gradual changes in sleep timing	Timed awakenings; changes in sleep timing	Psychoeducation of caregivers and patients; scheduled naps; exercise; good nutrition; sleep hygiene	Muscle massage, relaxation; exercise; Sleep hygiene (regular sleep schedule); sufficient sleep
Psychological	CBT; mindfulness cognitive therapy	Continuous positive airway pressure (CPAP) desensitization	Motivational interview; CBT	Guided imagery for nightmares	Treatment for attention deficit hyperactivity disorder (ADHD) / anxiety/depression symptoms (see chapters 54, 59, and 63, respectively, on these disorders)	Mindfulness relaxation (see chapter 36 on relationship-based therapies)
Prevention/ early intervention	Parent training (infants and young children); sleep hygiene; later school start times (teens)	Weight loss; early adenotonsillectomy (AT)	Consistent bed and wake times; later school start times	Parent training to cope with distress and/or safety concerns	Health care provider awareness prevents diagnostic delay	–
Pharmacotherapy	Multiple categories of sedative/ hypnotic agents (Table 68.7)	Nasal steroids, leukotriene esterase inhibitors	Low dose melatonin (0.1–0.5 mg) 2–3 hours before desired bedtime	Rarely needed; benzodiazepines/tricyclic antidepressants (TCAs)	Psychostimulants[a], modafinil; sodium oxybate[a]; pitolisant; solriamfetol	Iron supplements; dopaminergic agents; alpha agonists; gabapentin
Other treatments	Online/ app-based CBT for insomnia (e.g., Sleepio, SHUTi)	Auto-CPAP; oral appliances; myofunctional therapy	–	–	–	Avoid drugs exacerbating symptoms (e.g., selective serotonin reuptake inhibitors [SSRIs], TCAs) Iron supplementation

[a] Approved for pediatric use.

Treatment of restless leg syndrome and periodic limb movement disorder

The guideline from the Standard of Practice Committee of the American Academy of Sleep Medicine states that no specific recommendation can be made regarding treatment of children with RLS or PLMD (Chesson *et al.*, 1999). Other reviews highlight the role of iron deficiency in exacerbating symptoms and explore a potential role for iron supplementation (Picchietti & Picchietti, 2008). Clearly this is an important domain for future research.

Pharmacologic agents for sleep disorders in children and adolescents

We briefly present here some general principles. There have been very few pediatric drug randomized controlled trials (RCTs) conducted and *no* medications approved by the U.S. Food and Drug Administration (FDA) for the treatment of sleep disorders in children, including insomnia, with the one exception of sodium oxybate for cataplexy in type 1 narcolepsy (McDonagh *et al.*, 2019). In general, medication use should *not* be first line in insomnia and should *always* be combined with a behavioral plan. Treatment goals should be realistic, clearly defined, and measurable. Medication type should be based on clinical assessment of the best possible match between the clinical situation and drug properties, as well as the adverse effects profile. Possible interactions with concomitant psychotropic medications should be carefully considered and providers should avoid the practice of adding sedating/hypnotic drugs to offset the side effects of other prescribed medications. Potential dosing modifications should be addressed up front with families, including dose escalation, middle of the night dosing, and nightly versus intermittent use (McDonagh *et al.*, 2019).

A summary of selected hypnotic medications that could be considered for use specifically for insomnia in the pediatric population, is presented in Table 68.7. Several caveats include the following:

- In general, antidepressants are potent REM suppressants and may result in rebound REM upon discontinuation (McCarthy *et al.*, 2016), as well as masking REM-related symptoms of narcolepsy such as cataplexy; they also tend to exacerbate RLS/PLMD (Kolla *et al.*, 2018); use should be considered largely in patients with comorbid mood disorders or anxiety.
- Antipsychotics, such as risperidone, anticonvulsants, and mood stabilizers, have limited use in children due to side effects, unless there is an additional indication besides insomnia (Bruni *et al.*, 2019; Mammarella *et al.*, 2023). Otherwise, antipsychotic medication is inappropriate for the treatment of pediatric sleep disorders.
- Gabapentin has some limited empirical evidence for use in children with neurodevelopmental and psychiatric disorders (Bruni *et al.*, 2019; Williams Buckley *et al.*, 2020).
- Long-term antihistamine use is also inappropriate as an intervention for pediatric sleep (Bruni *et al.*, 2019; McDonagh et al., 2019) because of side effects and limited efficacy beyond when the child has a cold or seasonal allergies.
- Finally, melatonin has become extraordinarily popular as a medication for sleep onset insomnia. A recent meta-analysis of short-term RCTs of melatonin (Salanitro *et al.*, 2022) shows overall good efficacy and tolerability in children with ADHD and autism, or other NDDs. While, in general, short-term side effects are mild, data regarding long-term consequences, such as impact on pubertal development and psychological dependency, are limited. Melatonin is not only used for its sedating properties when given at bedtime, but also as a circadian phase-advancing agent administered in small doses earlier in the evening. Melatonin is primarily indicated for sleep onset and not sleep maintenance insomnia, although a few studies of extended-release formulation have shown efficacy for the latter. Because melatonin is not regulated by the FDA in the U.S., products may be highly variable with regards to actual melatonin content. In the UK and other European countries, melatonin is better regulated. However, use of "pharmaceutical grade" melatonin is recommended regardless of country. Additional clinical recommendations are provided by (Bruni *et al.*, 2015).

Other treatments and cultural considerations

Fortunately, most sleep problems in young children are improved through increased attention to the bedtime routine. For adolescents, there is also increasing recognition that sleep difficulties can largely be addressed through later school start times and reinforcement of bedtime routines by caregivers. However, many will observe that even after changes to bedtime and wake up routines, persistent sleep difficulties remain. Additionally, there is recognition that some of the behavioral treatments outlined above may be inappropriate for some populations of vulnerable children. For example, Hash and colleagues (Hash *et al.*, 2022), highlight the need for trauma-informed treatments for sleep disturbances in children who are involved in institutionalized care and other unpredictable living situations that may or may not involve changes in primary caretakers. It is unclear how exactly these treatments will differ from traditional pediatric sleep interventions but the current recommendations to leave children alone in a cool, dark room may be inappropriate (Hash *et al.*, 2022) and the current practices to prescribe sedative hypnotics or antipsychotic medication, may be unethical (Alfano *et al.*, 2022). Similarly, contextual and cultural issues, including how low- and middle-income countries can effectively treat sleep disturbances among children and caretakers, involves careful knowledge around sleeping practices. For example, for many across the globe, co-sleeping between caretakers and children is common and often seen as best for child health and well-being. Although this is contrary to U.S. and European pediatric sleep recommendations, it may be safer and more effective to discuss ways to ensure co-sleeping is being done safely, rather than forbidding it outright.

Table 68.7 Clinical properties of selected medications used for pediatric insomnia.

Medications	Mechanism of action	Suggested pediatric dosing range (mg/d)[a]	Common side effects	Comments
Benzodiazepine receptor agonists (BzDRA) Example: clonazepam[a]	Bind to central gamma-aminobutyric acid (GABA) receptors	0.5–2.0	Residual daytime sedation, rebound insomnia on discontinuation Psychomotor impairment Anterograde amnesia (dose-dependent); potential respiratory depression Anticonvulsant, anxiolytic, myorelaxant properties	Also (rarely) used to reduce partial arousal parasomnias (sleep terrors, sleepwalking); limited use in pediatrics due to abuse/dependence potential
Non-BzDRA Examples: zolpidem[a] zaleplon[a] zopiclone	Bind to α_1 subunits GABA receptors	5–10	Headache, retrograde amnesia; morning grogginess; reports of complex sleep-related behaviors raise safety concerns (black box warning)	Clinical trial data shows little efficacy; limited clinical experience in children
α Agonists Examples: clonidine guanfacine	α Adrenergic receptor agonists (guanfacine more selective); decrease norepinephrine release	0.05–0.3 0.5–2	Dry mouth, bradycardia, hypotension, possible rebound hypertension on discontinuation; may cause mid-sleep awakenings and exacerbation of partial arousal parasomnias; narrow therapeutic index	Also used in daytime treatment of attention deficit hyperactivity disorder (ADHD)
Atypical antidepressants Example: trazadone	$5\text{-}HT_{2A/C}$ antagonist	25–50	Dizziness, central nervous system (CNS) overstimulation. Cardiac arrhythmias, hypotension, priapism	Main use with comorbid depression
Hormone analog Melatonin (note this is over-the-counter in the U.S. and some other countries)	Main effect suprachiasmatic nucleus; non-selective action at MT_1 and MT_2 receptors	2.5–5 mg (typical clinical pediatric doses) 0.5–10 mg (dosage ranged reported in clinical trials; higher doses may be needed in children with NDDs) Low dose (0.3–0.5 mg) dosed 1–2 hours before desired bedtime in delayed sleep-wake phase disorder (DSWPD)	Headache, nightmares, morning grogginess Possible exacerbation of comorbid autoimmune diseases	Robust empirical evidence for use with children with developmental disabilities, autism, neurologic impairment, blindness; jet lag; DSWPD OTC preparations may be highly variable in actual melatonin content
Novel Mechanism Hypnotics				
Selective histamine receptor antagonist Example: doxepin (Silenor)a	Selective antagonism of the histamine H1 receptor	3–6	Daytime somnolence and residual next-day effect	Used for sleep maintenance insomnia
OTC Medications				
Antihistamines Examples: diphenhydramine (Benadryl) cyproheptadine (Periactin) hydroxyzine (Atarax)	Competitive histamine (H1) receptor blocker in the CNS	25–50 4–8 25–100	Daytime drowsiness, gastrointestinal (appetite loss, vomiting, constipation, dry mouth), paradoxical excitation	Weak soporifics despite high-level parental/practitioner acceptance; short-term use only

[a] US Food and Drug Administration (FDA)-approved medications in adults.

Unfortunately, the cost of treatments currently remains high given the lack of pediatric sleep health training and systemic environmental barriers. For example, many low-income regions are suffering the consequences of climate change, leading to higher temperatures, poor air quality, and increased exposure to environmental toxins, all of which are poor conditions for quality sleep (Altena *et al.*, 2023).

Regarding the impact of electronics, it is important to note that the light-entrainable parts of the brain synchronize networks of subordinate circadian oscillators controlling fluctuations in other brain regions and, in particular, in neural circuitry supporting reward seeking (centered on the ventral striatum) and emotion processing (centered on the amygdala and orbitomedial prefrontal cortex) (Yoo *et al.*, 2007), two circuits highly relevant to risk taking among teens and that continue developing well into the teenage years (Blakemore, 2010). Hence, any intervention to improve sleep must incorporate timed light exposure and inevitably needs to address exposure to sources of both light *and* emotionally salient, rewarding activities in the hour before bed, via the use of smartphones, laptops, social networking, etc. The artificial light exposure suppresses the release of the sleepiness-promoting hormone melatonin, enhances alertness, and shifts circadian rhythms to a later hour. Technology is also highly arousing and engaging and facilitates the much-loved contact with peers. These influences are so potent that it is very difficult for many teens to switch media devices off at night, delaying bedtimes still further. Moreover, smartphones are, too often, a source of sleep disturbance during the night. Clearly, these are modifiable sources of sleep disturbance. However, it is important to note that although technology use at night and sleep disruption are correlated, far less than 90% of the teens polled were experiencing sleep disruptions that could be attributed to technology use. As others have noted, technology use is ubiquitous, does not directly cause sleep disruptions, and can be an opportunity for improving sleep health rather than something to be demonized among teens.

Future developments and needs in research

With all the advances in pediatric sleep research and treatment progress, there remain many opportunities for treatment development and gaps in our current knowledge base. In this chapter we have underscored the evidence for interactions between sleep and the regulation of behavior, emotion, and learning. We have particularly emphasized behavioral principles and behavioral approaches to these problems because we believe that there is great pragmatic and clinical value in understanding and implementing these in many domains of clinical practice.

Unfortunately, knowledge of sleep problems and treatments are not widely disseminated to the public and this may be contributing to the epidemic of sleep deprivation among children and adolescents. As highlighted, the most effective method for "treating" sleep problems is to prevent them before they start. Parent education about normative sleep across the first year of life has been critical in reducing many common sleep problems among infants and young children. However, to our knowledge, this approach has not been utilized among parents of school-age children and teenagers. It is possible that the sleep problems in later childhood and adolescence could be prevented by educating parents about developmental sleep needs, healthy sleep habits, how to set clear limits around technology use at bedtime, and how to *model* healthy sleep to their children. Additionally, teachers, coaches, and health care providers could enhance prevention efforts through receiving education on the common "red flags" of poor sleep among children and teens (e.g., falling asleep in class, snoring). A potential next step may be to introduce prevention programs in schools and primary care clinics aimed at encouraging healthy sleep and providing extra support for children and teens that show early signs of sleep disruption (e.g., excessive sleepiness in class). This type of work has the potential to provide the most economical and time efficient approach to the treatment of pediatric sleep problems. However, equally important to the prevention of pediatric sleep problems is the removal of societal and environmental barriers to healthy sleep. For example, one barrier to healthy sleep among adolescents is early school start times. Indeed, a 30-minute delay in school start time (from 8:00 a.m. to 8:30 a.m.) is associated with significant improvements in measures of adolescent alertness, mood, and health (Owens *et al.*, 2014).

While there is significant evidence that sleep problems predict the development of future physical illness and psychiatric problems and that behavioral interventions for sleep disturbances in childhood and adolescence are effective, there remain several areas requiring future research. First, the risk factors associated with the development of sleep problems need to be better identified and defined. Critically, this has the potential to lead to even more powerful intervention and prevention efforts. Furthermore, the impact of potential moderating variables (e.g., child temperament, household SES) on treatment outcomes needs to be examined with a focus on the potential long-term impact that behavioral interventions may have on the persistence of sleep problems in adulthood. Also important will be the evaluation of behavioral treatments in children with special needs including children with ASDs, mental retardation, neurodevelopmental disabilities, and chronic medical and psychiatric conditions.

Although there is much research and work yet to be done, we have highlighted in this chapter the encouraging evidence that there are few risks—and potentially many benefits—from increasing and enhancing sleep in children and adolescents. Further dissemination of this evidence may offer considerable assistance in providing all children and adolescents with the best opportunities for reaching their physical, educational, and psychological potential via healthy sleep habits.

References

Alfano, C.A. *et al.* (2022) How are the sleep problems of children in the US foster care system addressed? *Journal of Developmental and Behavioral Pediatrics* **43**(8), e525–e532. doi:10.1097/DBP.0000000000001090.

Altena, E. *et al.* (2023) How to deal with sleep problems during heatwaves: Practical recommendations from the European Insomnia Network. *Journal of Sleep Research* **32**(2), e13704. doi:10.1111/jsr.13704.

Astill, R.G. *et al.* (2012) Sleep, cognition, and behavioral problems in school-age children: A century of research meta-analyzed. *Psychological Bulletin* **138**(6), 1109–1138. doi:10.1037/A0028204.

Baron, K.G. & Reid, K.J. (2014) Circadian misalignment and health. *International Review of Psychiatry* **26**(2), 139–154. doi:10.3109/09540261.2014.911149.

Baroni, A. (2019) Teens who can't sleep: insomnia or circadian rhythm disorder? *Journal of the American Academy of Child and Adolescent Psychiatry* **58**(3), 307–312. doi:10.1016/J.JAAC.2018.11.010.

Bathory, E. & Tomopoulos, S. (2017) Sleep regulation, physiology and development, sleep duration and patterns, and sleep hygiene in infants, toddlers, and preschool-age children. *Current Problems in Pediatric and Adolescent Health Care* **47**(2), 29–42. doi:10.1016/j.cppeds.2016.12.001.

Besedovsky, L. *et al.* (2019) The sleep-immune crosstalk in health and disease. *Physiological Reviews* **99**(3), 1325–1380. doi:10.1152/physrev.00010.2018.

Bitners, A.C. & Arens, R. (2020) Evaluation and Management of Children with obstructive sleep apnea syndrome. *Lung* **198**, 257–270. doi:10.1007/s00408-020-00342-5.

Blake, M.J. *et al.* (2018) Mechanisms underlying the association between insomnia, anxiety, and depression in adolescence: Implications for behavioral sleep interventions. *Clinical Psychology Review* **63**, 25–40. doi:10.1016/j.cpr.2018.05.006.

Blakemore, S.J. (2010) The developing social brain: Implications for education. *Neuron* **65**(6), 744–747. doi:10.1016/j.neuron.2010.03.004.

Boeke, C.E. *et al.* (2014) Childhood sleep duration and quality in relation to leptin concentration in two cohort studies. *Sleep* **37**(3), 613–620. doi:10.5665/sleep.3510.

Bootzin, R.R. *et al.* (1991) Stimulus control instructions. In: *Case Studies in Insomnia.* (ed P.J. Hauri). Springer, US, Boston, MA. pp. 19–28.

Borbély, A.A. *et al.* (2016) The two-process model of sleep regulation: a reappraisal. *Journal of Sleep Research* **25**(2), 131–143. doi:10.1111/jsr.12371.

Bruni, O. (2023) Approach to a sleepy child: diagnosis and treatment of excessive daytime sleepiness in children and adolescents. *European Journal of Paediatric Neurology* **42**, 97–109. doi:10.1016/j.ejpn.2022.12.009.

Bruni, O. *et al.* (2015) Current role of melatonin in pediatric neurology: clinical recommendations. *European Journal of Paediatric Neurology* **19**(2), 122–133. doi:10.1016/J.EJPN.2014.12.007.

Bruni, O. *et al.* (2019) Pharmacotherapeutic management of sleep disorders in children with neurodevelopmental disorders. *Expert Opinion on Pharmacotherapy* **20**(18), 2257–2271. doi:10.1080/14656566.2019.1674283.

Buysse, D.J. (2014) Sleep health: Can we define it? Does it matter? *Sleep* **37**(1), 9–17. doi:10.5665/sleep.3298.

Carney, C.E. *et al.* (2012) The consensus sleep diary: standardizing prospective sleep self-monitoring. *Sleep* **35**(2), 287–302. doi:10.5665/sleep.1642.

Chesson, A.L. *et al.* (1999) Practice parameters for the treatment of restless legs syndrome and periodic limb movement disorder. *Sleep* **22**(7), 961–968. doi:10.1093/SLEEP/22.7.961.

Clarke, G. *et al.* (2015) Cognitive-behavioral treatment of insomnia and depression in adolescents: a pilot randomized trial. *Behaviour Research and Therapy* **69**, 111–118. doi:10.1016/j.brat.2015.04.009.

Crabtree, V.M.L. *et al.* (2003) Periodic limb movement disorder of sleep in children. *Journal of Sleep Research* **12**(1), 73–81. doi:10.1046/j.1365-2869.2003.00332.x.

Crowley, S.J. *et al.* (2018) An update on adolescent sleep: New evidence informing the perfect storm model. *Journal of Adolescence* **67**(1), 55--65. doi:10.1016/j.adolescence.2018.06.001.

de Bruin, E.J. & Meijer, A.M. (2017) The impact of online therapeutic feedback on outcome measures in Internet-CBTI for adolescents with insomnia. *Sleep Medicine* **29**, 68–75. doi:10.1016/J.SLEEP.2016.05.017.

Dewald-Kaufmann, J. *et al.* (2022) Cognitive behavioral therapy for insomnia in school-aged children and adolescents. *Sleep Medicine Clinics* **17**(3), 355–365. doi:10.1016/j.jsmc.2022.06.003.

Díaz-Román, A. *et al.* (2016) Sleep characteristics in children with attention deficit hyperactivity disorder: systematic review and meta-analyses. *Journal of Clinical Sleep Medicine* **12**(5), 747–756. doi:10.5664/JCSM.5810.

Díaz-Román, A. *et al.* (2018) Sleep in youth with autism spectrum disorders: systematic review and meta-analysis of subjective and objective studies. *Evidence-Based Mental Health* **21**(4), 146–154. doi:10.1136/EBMENTAL-2018-300037.

El-Sheikh, M. *et al.* (2010) Children's sleep and adjustment over time: the role of socioeconomic context. *Child Development* **81**(3), 870–883. doi:10.1111/j.1467-8624.2010.01439.x.

Fernandez-Mendoza, J. *et al.* (2021) Natural history of insomnia symptoms in the transition from childhood to adolescence: population rates, health disparities, and risk factors. *Sleep* **44**(3). doi:10.1093/sleep/zsaa187.

Ferranti, R. *et al.* (2016) Sleep quality and duration is related with diet and obesity in young adolescent living in Sicily, southern Italy. *Sleep Science* **9**(2), 117–122. doi:10.1016/j.slsci.2016.04.003.

Goel, N. *et al.* (2013) Circadian rhythms, sleep deprivation, and human performance. *Progress in Molecular Biology and Translational Science* **119**, 155–190. doi:10.1016/B978-0-12-396971-2.00007-5.

Gregory, A.M. *et al.* (2005) Prospective longitudinal associations between persistent sleep problems in childhood and anxiety and depression disorders in adulthood. *Journal of Abnormal Child Psychology* **33**(2), 157–163. doi:10.1007/s10802-005-1824-0.

Gulotta, G. *et al.* (2019) Risk factors for obstructive sleep apnea syndrome in children: state of the art. *International Journal of Environmental Research and Public Health* **16**(18), 3235. doi:10.3390/ijerph16183235.

Hash, J.B. *et al.* (2022) Call to action: prioritizing sleep health among US children and youth residing in alternative care settings. *Sleep Health* **8**(1), 23–27. doi:10.1016/J.SLEH.2021.10.002.

Hasler, B.P. & Pedersen, S.L. (2020) Sleep and circadian risk factors for alcohol problems: a brief overview and proposed mechanisms. *Current Opinion in Psychology* **34**, 57–62.

Iglowstein, I. *et al.* (2003) Sleep duration from infancy to adolescence: reference values and generational trends. *Pediatrics* **111**(2), 302–307. doi:10.1542/peds.111.2.302.

Jenni, O.G. *et al.* (2007) Sleep duration from ages 1 to 10 years: Variability and stability in comparison with growth. *Pediatrics* **120**(4), e769–e776. doi:10.1542/peds.2006-3300.

Johnson, E.O. *et al.* (2006) The association of insomnia with anxiety disorders and depression: exploration of the direction of risk. *Journal of Psychiatric Research* **40**(8), 700–708. doi:10.1016/J.JPSYCHIRES.2006.07.008.

Jones Oguh, S. *et al.* (2020) New treatments for obstructive sleep apnea in children. *Paediatric Anaesthesia* **30**(3), 232–240. doi:10.1111/pan.13775.

Kolla, B.P. *et al.* (2018) The influence of antidepressants on restless legs syndrome and periodic limb movements: a systematic review. *Sleep Medicine Reviews* **38**, 131–140. doi:10.1016/j.smrv.2017.06.002.

Lewin, M. *et al.* (2019) Early life trauma has lifelong consequences for sleep and behavior. *Scientific Reports* **9**(1), 16701. doi:10.1038/s41598-019-53241-y.

Mammarella, V. *et al.* (2023) Using pharmacotherapy to address sleep disturbances in autism spectrum disorders. *Expert Review of Neurotherapeutics* 23(12), 1261–1276. doi:10.1080/14737175.2023.2267761.

Marcus, C.L. *et al.* (2012) Diagnosis and management of childhood obstructive sleep apnea syndrome. *Pediatrics* **130**(3), 576–584. doi:10.1542/peds.2012-1671.

Markovich, A.N. *et al.* (2014) Validating the Children's Sleep Habits Questionnaire against polysomnography and actigraphy in school-aged children. *Frontiers in Psychiatry* **5**(JAN). doi:10.3389/FPSYT.2014.00188.

Marten, F. *et al.* (2023) Sleep parameters and problems in adolescents with and without ADHD: a systematic review and meta-analysis. *JCPP Advances* **3**(3), e12151. doi:10.1002/JCV2.12151.

Marver, J.E. & McGlinchey, E.A. (2020) Sex differences in insomnia and risk for psychopathology in adolescence. *Current Opinion in Psychology* **34**, 63–67. doi:10.1016/j.copsyc.2019.09.004.

Mason, G.M. *et al.* (2021) Sleep and human cognitive development. *Sleep Medicine Reviews* **57**, 101472. doi:10.1016/j.smrv.2021.101472.

McCarthy, A. *et al.* (2016) REM sleep homeostasis in the absence of REM sleep: effects of antidepressants. *Neuropharmacology* **108**, 415--425. doi:10.1016/j.neuropharm.2016.04.047.

McDonagh, M.S. *et al.* (2019) Pharmacologic treatments for sleep disorders in children: a systematic review. *Journal of Child Neurology* **34**(5), 237–247. doi:10.1177/0883073818821030.

Mednick, S.C. *et al.* (2010) The spread of sleep loss influences drug use in adolescent social networks. *PLoS One* **5**(3), e9975. doi:10.1371/journal.pone.0009775.

Mindell, J.A. *et al.* (2019) Norm-referenced scoring system for the Brief Infant Sleep Questionnaire – Revised (BISQ-R). *Sleep Medicine* **63**, 106–114. doi:10.1016/j.sleep.2019.05.010.

Modestino, E.J. & Winchester, J. (2013) A retrospective survey of childhood ADHD symptomatology among adult narcoleptics. *Journal of Attention Disorders* **17**(7). doi:10.1177/1087054713480033.

Nevsimalova, S. *et al.* (2009) Does age at the onset of narcolepsy influence the course and severity of the disease? *Sleep Medicine* **10**(9), 967–972. doi:10.1016/j.sleep.2009.01.010.

Owens, J. *et al.* (2014) Insufficient sleep in adolescents and young adults: an update on causes and consequences. *Pediatrics* **134**(3), e921–e932. doi:10.1542/peds.2014-1696.

Owens, J.A. & Dalzell, V. (2005) Use of the "BEARS" sleep screening tool in a pediatric residents' continuity clinic: a pilot study. *Sleep Medicine* **6**, 1, 63–69. doi:10.1016/j.sleep.2004.07.015.

Paruthi, S. *et al.* (2016) Recommended amount of sleep for pediatric populations: a consensus statement of the American Academy of Sleep Medicine. *Journal of Clinical Sleep Medicine* **12**(6), 785–786. doi:10.5664/jcsm.5866.

Pennestri, M.H. *et al.* (2021) Childhood restless legs syndrome: a longitudinal study of prevalence and familial aggregation. *Journal of Sleep Research* **30**(3), e13161. doi:10.1111/jsr.13161.

Perpétuo, C. *et al.* (2020) Comparison between actigraphy records and parental reports of child's sleep. *Frontiers in Pediatrics* **8**, 567390. doi:10.3389/FPED.2020.567390.

Picchietti, M.A. & Picchietti, D.L. (2008) Restless legs syndrome and periodic limb movement disorder in children and adolescents. *Seminars in Pediatric Neurology* **15**(2), 91–99. doi:10.1016/j.spen.2008.03.005.

Pollock, J.I. (1994) Night-waking at five years of age: predictors and prognosis. *Journal of Child Psychology and Psychiatry* **35**(4), 699–708. doi:10.1111/j.1469-7610.1994.tb01215.x.

Randler, C. *et al.* (2017) From lark to owl: developmental changes in morningness-eveningness from new-borns to early adulthood. *Scientific Reports* **7**. doi:10.1038/srep45874.

Ritvo, P. *et al.* (2021) Online mindfulness-based cognitive behavioral therapy intervention for youth with major depressive disorders: randomized controlled trial. *Journal of Medical Internet Research* **23**(3). doi:10.2196/24380.

Roberts, R.E. & Duong, H.T. (2014) The prospective association between sleep deprivation and depression among adolescents. *Sleep* **37**(2), 239–244. doi:10.5665/sleep.3388.

Roberts, R.E. *et al.* (2009) Sleepless in adolescence: Prospective data on sleep deprivation, health and functioning. *Journal of Adolescence* **32**(5), 1045–1057. doi:10.1016/J.ADOLESCENCE.2009.03.007.

Salanitro, M. *et al.* (2022) Efficacy on sleep parameters and tolerability of melatonin in individuals with sleep or mental disorders: A systematic review and meta-analysis. *Neuroscience and Biobehavioral Reviews* **139**, 104723. doi:10.1016/j.neubiorev.2022.104723.

Saper, C.B. & Fuller, P.M. (2017) Wake–sleep circuitry: an overview. *Current Opinion in Neurobiology* **44**, 186–192. doi:10.1016/J.CONB.2017.03.021.

Sateia, M.J. (2014) International classification of sleep disorders. *Chest* **146**(5), 1387–1394.

Spielman, A.J. *et al.* (1987) A behavioral perspective on insomnia treatment. *Psychiatric Clinics of North America* ***10***(4), 541–553.

Tadrous, R. *et al.* (2021) Health-related quality of life in narcolepsy: a systematic review and meta-analysis. *Journal of Sleep Research* **30**(6), e13383. doi:10.1111/jsr.13383.

Touitou, Y. *et al.* (2016) Disruption of adolescents' circadian clock: the vicious circle of media use, exposure to light at night, sleep loss and risk behaviors. *Journal of Physiology Paris* **110**(4B), 467–479. doi:10.1016/j.jphysparis.2017.05.001.

Williams Buckley, A. *et al.* (2020) Practice guideline: treatment for insomnia and disrupted sleep behavior in children and adolescents with autism spectrum disorder. *Neurology* **94**(9), 392–404. doi:10.1212/wnl.0000000000009033.

Williams, J.A. *et al.* (2013) Norms and trends of sleep time among US children and adolescents. *Archives of Pediatrics and Adolescent Medicine* **167**(1), 55–60. doi:10.1001/jamapediatrics.2013.423.

Williamson, A.A. & Mindell, J.A. (2019) Cumulative socio-demographic risk factors and sleep outcomes in early childhood. *Sleep* 43(3), zsz233. doi:10.1093/sleep/zsz233.

Yoo, S.S. *et al.* (2007) The human emotional brain without sleep - a prefrontal amygdala disconnect. *Current Biology* **17**(20), 877–878. doi:10.1016/j.cub.2007.08.007.

Yu, L. *et al.* (2011) Development of short forms from the PROMIS™ sleep disturbance and sleep-related impairment item banks. *Behavioral Sleep Medicine* **10**(1), 6–24. doi:10.1080/15402002.2012.636266.

CHAPTER 69

Feeding and eating disorders

Rachel Bryant-Waugh and Julian Baudinet
Michael Rutter Centre, South London and Maudsley NHS Foundation Trust, London, UK

Introduction

Feeding and eating disorders occur across the age range from childhood to adulthood. Both the American Psychiatric Association's *Diagnostic and Statistical Manual of Mental Disorders*, 5th edition, text revision (DSM-5-TR; American Psychiatric Association, 2022) and the World Health Organization's *International Classification of Diseases*, 11th revision (ICD-11; World Health Organization, 2019) classify these presentations as mental disorders, with both including six main diagnoses within the category of feeding and eating disorders: pica; rumination-regurgitation disorder; avoidant/restrictive food intake disorder (ARFID); anorexia nervosa (AN); bulimia nervosa (BN); and binge eating disorder (BED). Both also include the diagnosis of other specified feeding or eating disorder (OSFED), as well as a residual category of unspecified feeding or eating disorders. All these disorders share the central core feature of the presence of a significant disturbance in eating or eating-related behavior associated with psychosocial and/or physical impairment. All can be serious and damaging conditions irrespective of age at onset or clinical presentation.

Diagnosis and presentation

There have been long-standing inconsistencies in use of terminology to describe the range of eating disturbances seen in clinical practice, and a poor fit with the diagnostic categories available in previous versions of DSM and ICD (Nicholls *et al.*, 2000). This situation has contributed to an unhelpful fragmentation of knowledge and expertise, with associated limited advancement in research findings (Bryant-Waugh *et al.*, 2010). Since the revision of the feeding and eating disorder diagnostic categories in DSM-5-TR (American Psychiatric Association, 2022) and ICD-11 (World Health Organization, 2019), improved fit between clinical presentations and diagnostic definitions has been reported, with a reduction in numbers assigned to "unspecified," "not otherwise specified," or "other" diagnostic categories (Mancuso *et al.*, 2015). Revised criteria have also contributed to an associated increase in research attention, particularly relating to children and young people with ARFID.

Current descriptions of the six main feeding and eating disorders are set out in the sections below with comment on their presenting features. Obesity is not included as there is little evidence to support its conceptualization as a mental disorder (Marcus & Wildes, 2009). Common comorbidities and main differential diagnoses are listed in Table 69.1. Due to underreporting in some populations around the world we cannot be confident that presentations are entirely uniform across all ethnicities and cultures; however, the disorder definitions are consistent and intended for global use.

Pica

Pica is characterized by the eating of nonnutritive substances, which may be nonfood items or raw food ingredients eaten in large amounts. A diagnosis of pica may be given when such behavior is persistent or sufficiently severe to warrant clinical intervention. Pica is not usually diagnosed where the ingestion of nonfood items is part of a culturally sanctioned practice, such as clay eating in some African communities (Chung *et al.*, 2019), or when chronological or developmental age is below two years, as mouthing of objects with some ingestion is not uncommon at this stage. Pica may occur in autistic individuals or those with intellectual disability (ID) but can also occur in the context of typical development. In some young people, oral sensory seeking behavior may play a role, as may stress. Pica can lead to severe medical complications, including poisoning and obstructions or perforations in the gastrointestinal tract. It can be associated with appetite loss, reduced food intake, and weight loss. In extreme cases, pica can be fatal.

Rutter's Child and Adolescent Psychiatry and Psychology, Seventh Edition.
Edited by Anita Thapar, Daniel S. Pine, Samuele Cortese, Cathy Creswell, Tamsin J. Ford, James F. Leckman, and Argyris Stringaris.

Companion website: www.wiley.com/go/thapar/rutterspsych7

Table 69.1 Differential and common comorbid diagnoses.

Feeding and eating disorder	Differential diagnosis	Comorbid disorders
Pica	AN; factitious disorder; nonsuicidal self-harm	Autism spectrum disorder (ASD); intellectual disability (ID); schizophrenia; obsessive–compulsive disorder (OCD); AN; ARFID
Rumination disorder	AN; BN; gastrointestinal conditions (incl. gastroesophageal reflux, vomiting)	Generalized anxiety disorder; depression; ASD; ID
Avoidant/restrictive food intake disorder (ARFID)	AN; reactive attachment disorder; factitious or induced illness; specific phobia; social anxiety disorder; depressive disorder; medical conditions	Anxiety disorders; OCD; attention deficit hyperactivity disorder (ADHD); ASD; ID; gastrointestinal conditions
Anorexia nervosa (AN)	ARFID; BN; body dysmorphic disorder; specific phobia; social anxiety disorder; depressive disorder; medical conditions	Depressive and anxiety disorders; OCD; ASD
Bulimia nervosa (BN)	AN; BED; mood disorder; borderline personality disorder; Klein-Levine syndrome	Mood disorders; anxiety disorders; substance misuse; borderline personality disorder
Binge eating disorder (BED)	BN; Prader-Willi syndrome; Klein-Levine syndrome	Mood disorders; anxiety disorders; substance misuse

Rumination disorder

Rumination disorder, also known as rumination-regurgitation disorder, is characterized by the repeated regurgitation of food that has been swallowed. The regurgitate is then rechewed and reswallowed or spat out. The bringing back up of food occurs without undue effort and is not associated with nausea. Regurgitation should be differentiated from vomiting and gastroesophageal reflux. To warrant diagnosis, this behavior should be frequent, sustained over a period, and not primarily accounted for by an underlying medical condition. In both diagnostic systems, criteria are applicable to anyone aged two years or over. Rumination may have a soothing or calming function, playing a role in anxiety management or emotion or arousal regulation, and so may been seen in the context of high levels of stress or emotional distress. It may also develop in the context of neglect or other forms of trauma, and in some individuals, onset appears to be triggered by an acute illness episode. It may be associated with autism and ID but is also seen in typically developing individuals. It is often a secretive disorder and is typically associated with significant impairment in social development and functioning. Repeated regurgitation can be associated with significant medical problems, including reduced intake with associated weight loss or low weight, malnutrition, dental problems, halitosis, and esophagitis. In extreme cases, rumination disorder can have a fatal outcome. Many clinicians fail to ask questions related to the possible presence of rumination disorder, which can hinder identification and diagnosis (Hartmann *et al.*, 2012)

Avoidant/restrictive food intake disorder

ARFID was introduced as a new diagnostic category, first in DSM-5 (Bryant-Waugh & Kreipe, 2012; American Psychiatric Association, 2013) and later in ICD-11 (Claudino *et al.*, 2019), with criteria applicable across the age range. It is characterized by limited food intake in relation to the range or overall amount of food eaten, or both. The eating disturbance may be maintained by a lack of interest in food and eating, avoidance based on the sensory characteristics of food (e.g., texture, appearance), concern about perceived aversive consequences of eating (e.g., choking, vomiting), or typically a combination of one or more of these. A requirement for diagnosis is that due to the eating behavior, the individual presents with clinically significant impairment to physical development and functioning, psychosocial impairment, or impairment across both these domains. Young people presenting with ARFID might be at a low weight, expected weight, or high weight. There is no formal lower age limit for onset, although many clinicians would not diagnose under the age of two years. There may be significant weight loss, growth faltering, and/or significant nutritional deficiencies or other adverse physical consequences, which can be associated with high risk. The criteria for ARFID allow for the fact that where food refusal is persistent, oral nutritional supplements or enteral feeds may be administered. This means that where an individual with the characteristic eating pattern of avoidance or restriction has become supplement or tube dependent, a diagnosis of ARFID can still be made despite their physical and nutritional needs being met via these routes. Concern about weight and shape or avoidance of weight gain as drivers of the avoidance or restriction of food intake should be ruled out as these features suggest that AN or BN might be more appropriately considered.

Relatively high rates of co-occurring conditions have been noted in ARFID, including autism, attention deficit hyperactivity disorder (ADHD), anxiety disorders, obsessive–compulsive behaviors, diagnosed food allergies and a range of gastrointestinal conditions, as well as a history of prematurity or early enteral feeding. ARFID presentations may also be seen in young people with certain genetic syndromes (e.g., Marfan syndrome), suggesting wider genetic anomalies may increase risk of eating difficulties.

Anorexia nervosa

Anorexia nervosa (AN) is characterized by restriction of food intake leading to failure to meet energy requirements, weight loss, or weight maintenance at a suboptimal level. Self-evaluation is linked with weight and/or shape preoccupation. Despite being low weight there is typically a failure to recognize this, accompanied by persistent efforts to avoid weight gain. Two subtypes are generally recognized, the restricting subtype and the binge–purge subtype. AN is seen clinically from around the age of seven to eight years upwards (Nicholls & Bryant-Waugh, 2009), most commonly in females. There have been some reports of AN in children as young as five years (e.g., Chatoor *et al.*, 2019), although this is not commonly reported. Younger patients tend to present with the restricting subtype of AN, with vomiting and then laxative misuse becoming more common features as age at presentation increases. Persistent undernutrition and rapid weight loss can adversely affect physical development and functioning, and have irreversible effects such as permanent short stature and deficits in bone mineral density, as well as fatal outcome (Katzman, 2005). The mortality risk for AN is among the highest of all mental disorders.

Revisions to criteria in DSM-5-TR included rewording the weight criterion to specify that weight should be less than is minimally expected, or less than might be expected taking the individual's age, sex, stage of development, and physical health into account (Freidl *et al.*, 2012). The judgment of "minimally normal" and whether this is applicable to any one individual lies with the clinician rather than being determined by population norms. This is important as risk is not directly associated with body mass index (BMI) centile or Z score (Peebles *et al.* 2010). In DSM-5-TR, severity of AN is rated based on BMI percentile, adjusted up or down depending on clinical symptoms, functional disability, and the need for supervision (American Psychiatric Association, 2022).

Wording changes have also been made to the cognitive criteria for clarification and to ensure better applicability to younger patients. The previous requirement for the individual to express fear of weight gain or becoming fat has been removed as some individuals may not verbally endorse fear or fatness despite determined food refusal (Bravender *et al.*, 2010). Behavioral indicators and parent/carer report are now accepted as valid sources of information so that the clinician can draw on observation and reports from other informants. This is relevant to cultural variations as observations from non-Western cultures and countries suggest that some individuals give other explanations for restricting their intake and actively avoiding weight gain, such as fullness or abdominal discomfort (also known as nonfat phobic AN, see further Becker *et al.*, 2009). The term "denial" in relation to acknowledging the seriousness of low weight has also been removed and replaced with wording that implies that there may be an inability to appreciate the risks, consistent with the view that younger patients may have a reduced capacity for general risk appraisal (Bravender *et al.*, 2010). Finally, the presence of amenorrhea is no longer included as diagnostic criterion, as this excludes several groups and there was insufficient evidence that this indicates significant clinical difference (Attia & Roberto, 2009).

Bulimia nervosa

BN is characterized by binge eating episodes, defined in DSM-5-TR as recurrent episodes of eating large amounts accompanied by a sense of loss of control. The ICD-11 definition of binge eating emphasizes the aspect of loss of control without specifying that the amount must be large. Binge eating is followed by behaviors intended to compensate for the amounts consumed to prevent weight gain, known as inappropriate compensatory behaviors. These include self-induced vomiting, laxative, or other substance/medication misuse, excessive exercising, and fasting. As in AN, the individual's sense of self-worth is strongly influenced by self-perception of weight or shape. In most instances, individuals with BN tend to be of average or above average weight. Binge eating and purging behaviors tend to be secretive and accompanied by distress and feelings of shame and disgust. There may be a greater tendency to seek help than seen in AN. BN typically first presents in later adolescence or adulthood, more frequently in females than males. Younger patients may be less likely to engage in laxative misuse, with self-induced vomiting being the most common purging behavior in younger adolescents. In some young people, BN may be associated with other behaviors such as self-harm, sexual promiscuity, and drug and alcohol misuse. Purging behaviors can have serious medical consequences such as electrolyte imbalance, cardiac arrhythmias, and dental decay. In extreme cases, repeated purging can have fatal consequences, for example, through cardiac complications or esophageal rupture.

Changes in DSM-5-TR criteria include a reduction in the required frequency criteria for binge eating episodes and compensatory behaviors to once a week over a three-month period (Wilson & Sysko, 2009). A further change has been to abandon the requirement to specify subtypes, previously purging or non-purging BN, given insufficient supporting evidence for this subdivision (van Hoeken *et al.*, 2009). Severity ratings in DSM-5-TR allow the clinician to specify the severity of BN based on the weekly frequency of inappropriate compensatory behaviors (Wolfe *et al.*, 2012).

Binge eating disorder

BED is characterized by recurrent episodes of eating large amounts accompanied by a sense of loss of control, similar to BN, but without the inappropriate compensatory behaviors. The binge eating is associated with marked distress and several specific features, such as continuing to eat when full or eating when not hungry, eating rapidly, avoiding eating with others, and feeling disgusted or guilty. Individuals with BED tend to be at a high weight or obese, which itself is associated with increased health risks.

BED was included as a new diagnostic category in both DSM-5 (American Psychiatric Association, 2013) and ICD-11 based on reviewing data relating to its validity and clinical utility. The frequency criterion for binge eating episodes is specified as a minimum of once a week for three months with the required duration of symptoms being three months, in line with BN.

Severity ratings in BED allow the clinician to specify the severity of the disorder based on the frequency of binge eating episodes per week (De Young *et al.*, 2012).

Other specified and unspecified feeding or eating disorders

Both DSM-5-TR and ICD-11 have two additional diagnostic categories covering presentations that do not fit the above six main categories: OSFED and unspecified feeding or eating disorder. DSM-5-TR includes five examples of OSFED presentations. These are: atypical AN, where despite significant weight loss, the individual's weight may remain at expected or higher than expected levels in population terms; BN and BED of lower frequency and/or more limited duration than specified in the full criteria; purging disorder, where there is recurrent purging to influence weight or shape in the absence of any binge eating; and night eating syndrome, where there are recurrent episodes of eating at night. Studies on purging disorder, where individuals regularly engage in the use of inappropriate compensatory behaviors after eating normal or small amounts of food, have reported average age of onset around 20 years, although sporadic cases have been reported in older adolescents (Keel & Streigel-Moore, 2009). Night eating syndrome is less consistently defined, but most descriptions include three main features: consumption of a significant amount of food in the evening or night; disturbed sleep, often with consumption of food on waking up in the night; and lack of appetite in the morning (Striegel-Moore *et al.*, 2009; Vander Wal, 2012). As with purging disorder, most studies have been conducted with adults, suggesting that this presentation might be only rarely encountered in child and adolescent clinical settings.

The diagnostic category of unspecified feeding or eating disorder is used for disturbances of eating behavior resulting in clinically significant distress or impairment but where full diagnostic criteria for any of the other above categories are not known to be met.

Epidemiology

Interpreting epidemiological data on child and adolescent feeding and eating disorders remains challenging. Studies have used different populations and methods of case detection making results difficult to compare.

Trends over time

A small global increase in eating disorders has been reported throughout the 20th century and into the 21st century (Wu *et al.*, 2020; Global Burden of Disease [GBD] 2019 Mental Disorders Collaborators, 2022). Improved case detection and greater public awareness may account for some of the reported changes in incidence, rather than changes in rates being a true representation of any increase or decrease in occurrence of eating disorders. Notably, there is a reported decline in the incidence of BN over recent decades in some studies (van Eeden *et al.*, 2021), but not all (Qian *et al.*, 2022).

A notable international spike in incidence of eating disorders and the need for inpatient treatment for eating disorders occurred during the recent novel coronavirus (COVID-19) pandemic (Agostino *et al.*, 2021; Asch *et al.*, 2021; Taquet *et al.*, 2022). National referral statistics for eating disorders in England show a doubling of urgent referrals during 2020 and a smaller increase in nonurgent referrals (Ford *et al.*, 2021; NHS England, 2021).

Current knowledge of incidence and prevalence

There are limited epidemiological data for pica in children and adolescents. Some have suggested that pica is most prevalent in children aged two to six years and slightly more common in males compared to females (Leung & Hon, 2019). Current prevalence estimates of pica vary substantially and range from 3% to more than 20% in predominantly Western communities, with culturally sanctioned higher rates of consumption of nonfood substances as high as 77% in some African communities, thus not necessarily diagnosed as a disorder (Leung & Hon, 2019). A study involving three groups of autistic children,[1] those with developmental disorders, and a general population sample, identified rates of 23.2%, 8.4%, and 3.5%, respectively (Fields *et al.*, 2021).

The incidence and prevalence of rumination disorder in children and adolescents is unclear. This is likely to be related to low clinician awareness, variability in diagnostic terminology and practice, and because regurgitation and rumination often occur in secret (Josefsson *et al.*, 2022). A large-scale international survey of adults in 26 countries revealed differences in rates between countries, with prevalence estimates ranging from 1.7–5.5% (Josefsson *et al.*, 2022). A school survey of 2183 Sri Lankan children and adolescents revealed an estimated prevalence rate of 5.1% (Rajindrajith *et al.*, 2021).

Reported rates of ARFID in child and adolescent eating disorder clinical populations range from 5–22.5% and in other clinical settings estimates vary between 1.5–32%, the latter in a pediatric feeding clinic (Archibald & Bryant-Waugh, 2023). Existing point prevalence estimates for ARFID in children and young people in general population studies range between 0.3–15.5% (Dinkler & Bryant-Waugh, 2021). Emerging clinical evidence suggests a more equal sex ratio than seen in AN or BN, with approximately even rates of presentation (Watts *et al.*, 2023).

Prevalence rates of AN, BN, and BED in children and adolescents vary depending on the country and age range studied. Age-standardized prevalence of AN and BN in the recent GBD 2019 were 45.08 (95% Uncertainty Interval [UI]: 29.21–66.82)

[1] Current preferences from autistic people are to use language such as "Autistic," "Person on the Autism Spectrum," and "Autistic Person" (Bury *et al.*, 2023).

and 58.55 (95% UI: 32.15–101.10) per 100,000, respectively (Piao *et al.*, 2022). In a recent systematic review and meta-analysis, BED was reported to be 1.53% (95% CI: 1.00–2.17) (Qian *et al.*, 2022). Prevalence rates are generally reported to be higher for females compared to males, particularly for AN and BN, and for adolescents and young adults compared to other age groups (Galmiche *et al.*, 2019; Martinez-Gonzalez *et al.*, 2020; van Eeden *et al.*, 2021; Qian *et al.*, 2022).

Age-standardized incidence rates per 100,000 for AN and BN reported in GBD 2019 were 23.64 (95% UI: 14.76–34.23) and 192.38 (95% UI: 99.88–330.80), respectively (Piao *et al.*, 2022). Compared to all-age estimates, the incidence of AN is highest between the ages of 10 and 29 years (Martinez-Gonzalez *et al.*, 2020).

Mortality

Strikingly, eating disorders were the only mental health disorder associated with mortality in children and adolescents in GBD 2019 data (Piao *et al.*, 2022). People diagnosed with AN have been estimated to have a five to seven times higher mortality than the general population, especially if they have received inpatient treatment (van Hoeken & Hoek, 2020; Iwajomo *et al.*, 2021; Miskovic-Wheatley *et al.*, 2023). Notably, there are also data suggesting that, despite a lower prevalence and incidence rate, males with AN or BN have a higher mortality risk than females (van Eeden *et al.*, 2021). Mortality rates for pica, rumination disorder, and ARFID are unclear.

Disease burden, quality of life, and economic burden

Recent GBD data from 2019 indicate that the burden of eating disorders remains high and has increased globally, regardless of socioeconomic status (GBD 2019 Mental Disorders Collaborators, 2022; Micali, 2022). Estimated years lived with disability for people with eating disorders was ranked #65 for children and younger adolescents (0–14 years) and #28 for older adolescents and emerging adults (15–24 years). Similarly, disability-adjusted life years (DALYs) were ranked #105 for children and younger adolescents (0–14 years) and #51 for emerging adults (15–24 years) (GBD 2019 Mental Disorders Collaborators, 2022).

Of note, GBD 2019 only included two eating disorders, AN and BN (Santomauro *et al.*, 2021). Santomauro *et al.* (2021) extended GBD 2019 estimates to include a wider range of eating disorder diagnoses and estimated that 41.9 million people (95% UI: 27.9–59.0) with eating disorders were missing from GBD 2019 figures and that BED and OSFED account for the majority of eating disorder cases and DALYs globally. The burden of eating disorders has been found to be highest in high-income countries, but evidence suggests there is a global trend toward increasing burden worldwide, particularly in Asia (Wu *et al.*, 2020).

A recent systematic review of health-related quality of life in children and adolescents with disordered eating found that those with BN, BED, purging disorder, and other eating disorder symptoms had poorer quality of life and poorer psychosocial well-being than healthy peers (Wu *et al.*, 2019). Regarding the economic burden of eating disorders, the annual health care costs for an individual with AN, BN, and BED were reported to be €2,993–€55,270, €888–€18,823, and €1,762–€2,902, respectively, in a recent review (Ágh *et al.*, 2016).

Risk factors and etiology

It is generally accepted that feeding and eating disorders are likely to result from multiple contributing factors and that a biopsychosocial approach to understanding etiology is indicated. Possible contributory factors described in the literature are set out in the sections below.

Biological factors

Genetic factors

There have been significant advances in the study of genetic influences on eating disorders since the early 2000s. Reported genetic influence is generally thought to result from interaction between genetic vulnerability and environmental factors. Evidence from genome-wide association studies (GWAS) studies suggest specific genetic polymorphisms are associated with AN, BN, and BED (Himmerich *et al.*, 2019; Hübel *et al.*, 2020; Manfredi *et al.*, 2021). Historically, the heritability of eating disorders was estimated through family and twin studies, whereas genome-wide data are now much more available and aid direct estimates of illness heritability. Current heritability estimates of AN, BN, and BED from twin studies are 0.28–0.74, 0.55–0.62, and 0.39–0.45, respectively (Bulik *et al.*, 2022). Genetic studies of ARFID are just beginning to appear, with some preliminary estimates of heritability for ARFID, suggesting these may be high (Koomar *et al.*, 2021; Dinkler *et al.*, 2023). Little is known about genetic influences in pica and rumination disorder. Given the complex interplay of biology, environment, and learning, it is becoming increasingly apparent that there is a need to reconceptualize eating disorders, particularly AN, as a metabo-psychiatric disorder (Watson *et al.*, 2019).

Neurobiological factors

Mesocorticolimbic and mesolimbic pathways are now widely thought to influence a range of cognitive, emotional, reward processing, and motivational processes, which may represent transdiagnostic factors underlying AN, BN, and BED (Bulik *et al.*, 2022). Neuroimaging studies have suggested that disordered eating may be a consequence of dysregulated reward systems and/or dysregulated awareness of homeostatic needs. This may be due to enhanced executive ability to inhibit incentive motivational drives, with the symptom expression of restricted eating considered a means of reducing negative mood caused by skewed interactions between serotonin aversive or inhibitory and dopamine reward systems (Frank *et al.*, 2019).

Thomas *et al.* (2017) have proposed a three-dimensional neurobiological model underpinning the etiology of ARFID, taking the three main maintaining mechanisms of low interest, avoidance based on sensory sensitivities, and concern about aversive consequences into account. They suggest that abnormalities in homeostatic appetite, sensory perception, and negative valence systems may underpin the typical disturbances of eating behavior seen in the context of ARFID.

Neuropsychological factors

Several neuropsychological domains have been found to be impaired in those with eating disorders and may increase risk for the development of eating disorders, including attention, memory, visuospatial processing, cognitive flexibility (set-shifting), impulsivity, emotion processing, and decision-making (Donnelly *et al.*, 2018; Schaumberg *et al.*, 2020). Most studies have been conducted with adults and while findings can be contradictory, sample sizes are small, and methodologies differ, some specific, subtle, cognitive impairments are emerging as being implicated in eating disorders (e.g., Miles *et al.*, 2020). Although some impairments resolve with weight restoration, others appear to be more trait-like phenomena, such as deficits in set-shifting (Fuglset, 2019). In children and adolescents, emerging research in these domains is less clear. For example, cognitive flexibility has been found to be comparable in adolescents with AN and healthy comparisons (Miles *et al.*, 2020). Further research in this area is needed before conclusions can be drawn regarding the etiological contribution of neuropsychological factors.

Microbiome and gut factors

There is a growing recognition of the relationship between gastrointestinal microbiota and the regulation of mood, appetite, and body mass (Butler *et al.*, 2021). Diet, infection, stress, and antibiotics are known to impact microbial composition, both directly and indirectly via the gut–brain axis (Herman & Bajaka, 2021). As is common in most eating disorders, periods of severe food restriction are associated with microbial dysbiosis and can lead to delayed gastric emptying, resulting in bloating and feelings of fullness (Norris *et al.*, 2016; Herman & Bajaka, 2021). In turn, this can lead to a specific gastrointestinal environment and a unique microbial profile (Terry *et al.*, 2022). It has been postulated that microbial diversity is correlated with eating disorder psychopathology, although this has not been consistently demonstrated and only empirically explored in AN currently (Terry *et al.*, 2022).

Emerging data indicate that people with eating disorders show notable differences in their microbiome compared to healthy comparisons (Frank *et al.*, 2019; Seitz *et al.*, 2019; Santonicola *et al.*, 2020; Herman & Bajaka, 2021). Emerging data also suggest there are bidirectional interactions between the adipose tissue, microbiome, gut, and brain that may contribute to the development of eating disorders (Smitka *et al.*, 2021).

Sex assigned at birth

It is well documented that eating disorders, particularly AN, and to a lesser extent BN and BED, occur more frequently in people assigned female sex at birth. Estimates of the female to male ratio range from approximately 2 : 1 to 10 : 1 depending on age, pubertal status, and eating disorder diagnosis (Culbert *et al.*, 2021). The greatest disparity between sexes is observed in AN, with incidence in females estimated to be 10 times that of males (van Eeden *et al.*, 2021). Recent estimates of BN sex ratios are reported to be closer to 4 : 1 (Gorrell & Murray, 2019). Emerging data suggest sex-specific genetic and biological mechanisms that might underlie differential risk for eating disorder psychopathology. Some known genetic variants that are associated with eating pathology differ between the sexes and some sex-steroids may play a role in activating genetic risk for eating disorders (Timko *et al.*, 2019). Additionally, ovarian hormones, namely estradiol and progesterone, may increase risk, in varying ways both during and after puberty, for eating disorder pathology (Culbert *et al.*, 2021). Note that sex at birth and gender present different risk, see section "Sociocultural factors" below for a discussion of gender and influence, and feeding and eating disorders.

Perinatal factors

Studies have consistently identified an association between perinatal factors and the later development of eating disorders (Culbert *et al.*, 2021). Such factors are independent of sociodemographic confounders and have been reported to contribute a 3.6% risk for AN (Lindberg & Hjern, 2003). Obstetric complications have been found to be significant independent predictors of AN and BN (Larsen *et al.*, 2021), and the risk of developing AN was found to increase with the total number of obstetric complications (Favaro *et al.*, 2006). Obstetric complications may contribute to or indicate impairment in neurodevelopment which could be implicated in the pathogenesis of eating disorders. Additionally, exposure to testosterone during the prenatal/perinatal periods may be protective in reducing risk of eating pathology in people assigned sex as males at birth, relative to those assigned females (Culbert *et al.*, 2021).

Puberty

Connan *et al.* (2003) proposed a neurodevelopmental model of AN which includes consideration of both the biological changes and the psychosocial transitions faced by young people as they go through puberty. These authors postulate that the rigidity of those vulnerable to AN may be challenged by change, resulting in increased vulnerability to dysregulation in relevant biopsychosocial systems. Research findings suggest that both advanced pubertal development and early pubertal onset are associated with increased rates of eating disorders, although this is less consistent for boys compared to girls (Klump, 2013). A recent narrative review of sex differences in eating disorders reported that activation of testosterone during puberty and in adulthood may be protective for people assigned male at birth (Culbert *et al.*, 2021).

Infection/illness/physical triggers

Mineral deficiencies, in particular iron deficiency, have long been associated with contributing to the onset of pica behaviors (Borgna-Pignatti & Zanella, 2016). Pica has also been described in individuals with specific clinical presentations, such as sickle cell anemia (Ivascu *et al.*, 2001). Pediatric autoimmune neuropsychiatric disorders associated with streptococcal infection (PANDAS), and the broader category of pediatric acute-onset neuropsychiatric syndrome (PANS), have been implicated in triggering restricted eating and, in some cases, AN (Swedo *et al.*, 2012). *In utero* exposure to viral infection has also been suggested as a risk factor for AN, with exposure during the sixth month of pregnancy to chickenpox and rubella infections found to be significantly associated with an increased risk of developing AN in one population study (Favaro *et al.*, 2011). A range of other co-occurring medical conditions including diabetes, diagnosed food allergies, irritable bowel disease, and Crohn's disease, which include a specific focus on dietary limitations, have also been implicated in increased risk for eating disorders. However, a directly causative mechanism between these physical illnesses and eating disorders is unlikely.

Psychosocial factors

Family theories

The notion of family dynamics as a direct etiological mechanism has not been validated and is no longer thought to be appropriate (Eisler, 2005). In recent years, the earlier emphasis on a family etiology has shifted more toward an understanding of how the evolution of the family dynamics, in the context of the development of the eating disorder, may function as a maintenance mechanism (Schmidt & Treasure, 2006; Baudinet *et al.*, 2021b).

Temperament

Certain temperament and personality traits have consistently been associated with eating disorders (Culbert *et al.*, 2015). Children with more emotional temperaments have been found to display more food-avoidant eating behaviors (Haycraft *et al.*, 2011), with higher levels of negative emotionality also having been linked to the development of later eating concerns (Martin *et al.*, 2000). Correlational research suggests that AN and BN are characterized by perfectionism, obsessive–compulsiveness, narcissism, concern with acceptance and approval from others, and autonomy, whereas impulsivity and sensation seeking have been described as more typical in disorders characterized by bingeing (Cassin & von Ranson, 2005). Higher levels of persistence are consistently reported for people with AN and BN, but not BED (Atiye *et al.*, 2014). Some studies support the likelihood that neuroticism and perfectionism are risk factors for eating disorders (Vacca *et al.*, 2021) and emerging data in adolescents suggest eating disorder symptom severity may be associated with increased inflexibility, reduced reward processing, and greater levels of suppression of emotional expression (Baudinet *et al.*, 2020, 2021d). Other temperament and personality traits that characterize eating disorders need further research to confirm their role as risk factors (Lilenfeld, 2011), however, emerging data suggest differences in levels of inhibitory control between AN and BN (Isaksson *et al.*, 2021). Of note, the majority of these data are correlational and derived from cross-sectional studies, with few prospective risk factors consistently identified (Culbert *et al.*, 2015).

Attachment and trauma

There is a consistently reported link between attachment insecurity and risk for an eating disorder (Tasca & Balfour, 2014; Jewell *et al.*, 2016, 2023). Pica occurs worldwide and is observed more commonly in areas of lower socioeconomic status, with traumatic events such as maternal deprivation, neglect, abuse, disorganized family structure, and poor parent–child interaction having been found to differentiate children with and without pica (Leung & Hon, 2019). Early negative childhood experiences, including trauma and abuse, have also been found to be associated with BN and BED (Ericsson *et al.*, 2011; Groleau *et al.*, 2012). A meta-analysis of over 3 million psychiatric cases found that childhood sexual abuse was significantly associated with a lifetime diagnosis of an eating disorder (Chen *et al.*, 2010).

Early feeding behavior

Maternal eating disorders have been found to increase the risk of childhood feeding difficulties, and this association appears to be a direct effect of the maternal eating disorder mediated via maternal distress (Micali *et al.*, 2011). Children of mothers with an eating disorder scored higher on a measure of eating disorder psychopathology than control children, and their eating disturbance was found to be associated with length of exposure to mothers' eating disorder and mother–child mealtime conflict at five years (Stein *et al.*, 2006). Childhood overeating has been found to increase risk of adolescent binge eating and BED, whereas persistent undereating was associated with higher risk of AN in adolescent girls only (Herle *et al.*, 2020). These same authors found that fussy or picky eating was also associated with greater risk for AN.

Sociocultural factors

Cross-cultural research has been dominated by the assumption that Western values regarding thinness are responsible for the development of AN in non-Western contexts, but the empirical research does not corroborate this (Weissman, 2019). Recent reviews indicate there are more similarities than differences in eating disorder incidence and risk across cultures (Cheng *et al.*, 2019). Nevertheless, external media influences have been shown to affect increases in scores on an eating disorder questionnaire measure and increased incidence of self-induced vomiting following prolonged exposure to television in adolescent girls in Fiji (Becker *et al.*, 2002). Further research on both direct and indirect media influence on the development of eating pathology found that social network media exposure was associated with increased eating pathology in adolescent girls in Fiji (Becker *et al.*, 2011).

Elevated dietary restraint, unhealthy weight control behaviors, and pursuit of the thin ideal have consistently been found to increase risk for onset of any eating disorder (Culbert *et al.*, 2015; Stice *et al.*, 2017) and adolescent females who report high dietary restraint have shown elevated risk for onset of threshold or subthreshold BN (Stice *et al.*, 2008). Literature and meta-analytic reviews of risk factors for eating pathology highlight the importance of factors associated with the "dieting domain." These include family and personal history of obesity and critical comments from family members about weight, shape, and eating as being risk factors for the development of BN, but not AN (Stice *et al.*, 2017; Weissman, 2019).

Weight concern as a risk factor for the development of eating disorders has been well-replicated in the literature (Keel & Forney, 2013). Evidence from a prospective study found that body dissatisfaction was a strong predictor for onset of any eating disorder and that this risk was further amplified by higher levels of depressive symptoms (Stice *et al.*, 2011). A recent review reports that females who described greater pursuit of a thin ideal and associated behaviors are at increased risk for binge/purge difficulties, whereas young people who have always been leaner are at greater risk for AN (Stice *et al.*, 2017).

Other wider sociocultural risk factors identified include socioeconomic status, immigration, and identifying as being gay, lesbian, gender nonconforming or belonging to another part of the LGBTQI+ community (Weissman, 2019; Nagata *et al.*, 2020; Parker & Harriger, 2020). Self-identified gender, as opposed to sex assigned at birth, is a distinct risk factor for the development of an eating disorder (Coelho *et al.*, 2019). Body dissatisfaction can be a core part of gender incongruence, which may be further exacerbated by minority stress and discrimination experienced by gender nonconforming youth (Nagata *et al.*, 2020).

A higher level of parental socioeconomic status has been associated with increased AN and other eating disorders (Weissman, 2019). Additionally, food insecurity, a proxy measure of family poverty or deprivation, is associated with bulimic-spectrum disorders (Hazzard *et al.*, 2020). Lastly, social media use might also be a risk factor for eating pathology (Padín *et al.*, 2021).

Assessment

Feeding and eating disorders are unique in that clinicians are required to concurrently assess, identify, and manage both mental and physical health risk. This makes working within a multidisciplinary team essential to effective eating disorder assessment and treatment. Due to the wide range of potential contributory factors and pathways in the development of these disorders, and resulting varying levels and domains of risk, it is important to conduct a comprehensive assessment, with the adoption of a biopsychosocial framework generally regarded as essential. Table 69.2 summarizes the main recommended components of

Table 69.2 The main components of a comprehensive biopsychosocial assessment and their relationship to risk.

Domain	Areas to cover in assessment
History	
Developmental	From birth, milestones, early feeding, speech and language, oral motor, sensory sensitivities, separation, social communication, relationships, play, character traits, behavior patterns
Feeding and eating	Onset of feeding/eating difficulties, relationship to weight/shape concerns, course, duration of current problems, key triggers
Medical	From birth, medical conditions and symptoms, operations, time off school due to illness
Significant events	Major personal and family life events, trauma, events having significant impact on individual
Current	
Feeding/eating behavior	Avoidance, restriction, self-feeding, binge eating, pattern of eating, speed of eating, eating in relation to hunger/satiety, solitary eating, eating nonfood substances
Behaviors associated with eating	Regurgitation, rechewing, spitting out, retching, gagging, vomiting, laxative (or other medication) misuse, exercise, behavior interfering with weight gain
Cognitions/emotions related to eating/weight/shape	Fear (distinguish between fear of weight gain/fat and fear of consequences of eating, e.g., vomiting), disgust related to food and own eating behavior, level of interest in food and eating, importance of shape/weight to self-worth, self-appraisal of body size and shape, understanding of current weight status, level of distress related to eating
Current intake	Range, nutritional breakdown, amounts, overall energy content, taken orally or enterally, intake defined by sensory characteristics (e.g., smooth, uniform color, regular appearance)?
Growth and development status	Weight, height, body mass index (BMI) centile (from BMI charts), weight loss/gain, faltering growth, pubertal delay, amenorrhea
Physical state	Pulse, blood pressure, electrolytes, minerals and full blood count, muscle strength, reflexes, concurrent medical conditions and symptoms. As indicated: dental exam (for enamel erosion due to vomiting), electrocardiogram (ECG), pelvic ultrasound, wrist X-Ray, dual-energy X-ray absorptiometry (DEXA)
Mental state	General mental state exam, comorbid diagnoses (e.g., depression, obsessive–compulsive disorder [OCD], anxiety disorders, autism), insight, motivation to address eating difficulty
General functioning	Current developmental level, family relationships, peer relationships, school attendance and performance, engagement in activities, use of leisure time
Context	
Family/care environment	Family structure, adequacy of food availability, adequacy of appropriate caregiving, child's place of residence, social care involvement
Sociocultural background	Family, social, and cultural practices around food and eating, weight and shape; values and attitudes influencing self esteem

(*Continued*)

Table 69.2 (Continued)

Domain	Areas to cover in assessment
School	Ethos and expectations, mealtime arrangements, pastoral care arrangements, relationship between staff and parents
Main areas of risk	
Physical	Consequences of low weight/rapid weight loss, malnutrition, consequences of repeated rumination or purging behavior, poisoning, abdominal obstructions. *Note*: risk of death must be considered
Psychological	Suicide, self-harm, vulnerability to abuse
Developmental	Growth, bone age and density, puberty, cognitive, social, emotional, educational

assessment to allow consideration of the full range of feeding and eating disorder diagnoses. Figure 69.1 summarizes the main domains of assessment. Assessment should cover salient aspects of the individual's history, detail regarding the eating disturbance, information about current mental and physical state, and information about family, social, and educational context. This breadth of information will also allow ascertainment of the nature and severity of risk across different domains of development and functioning, and prioritization of interventions.

Assessment and diagnosis will usually be based on clinical interview and assessment involving the young person and parents, carers, or other adults (see Chapter 27). Children may not have the cognitive capacity to formulate and express the reasons behind their eating behavior. In AN or BN, the ability to articulate a fear of weight gain or the influence of body shape or weight on self-evaluation may not be present. Adult observation from parents, teachers, or others can be important in providing indirect evidence for weight or shape preoccupation and avoidance of weight gain.

Physical examination and appropriate medical investigations are also important (see Chapter 30); all feeding and eating disorders are associated with significant medical risk and can be life-threatening, with relatively high mortality rates compared to other mental disorders (van Hoeken & Hoek, 2020). Recent guidance developed in the UK, Medical Emergencies in Eating Disorders (MEED; Royal College of Psychiatrists, 2022), indicates the importance of a comprehensive medical assessment for all people with eating disorder across the age range. MEED guidance replaces and extends the previous documents, Management of Really Sick Patients with Anorexia Nervosa (MaRSiPAN) and Junior MaRSiPAN, in covering a wider range of eating disorders. Domains to assess include weight loss, BMI and weight, heart rate and cardiovascular health, hydration status, temperature, muscular function (sit-up, squat, stand test, hand grip, mid

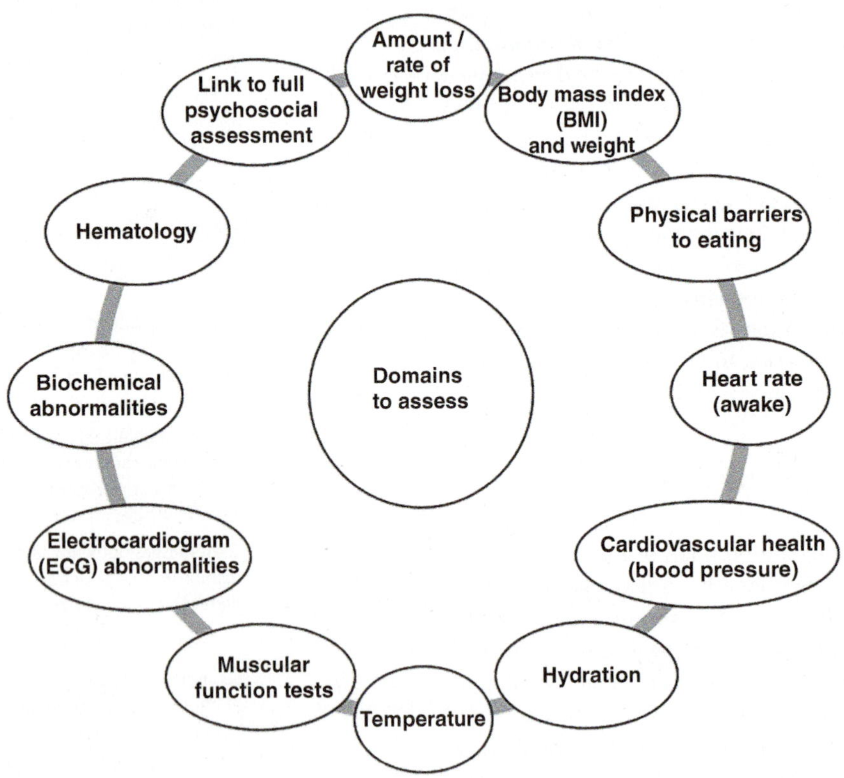

Figure 69.1 Medical risk assessment for youth presenting with eating disorder and related behaviors (e.g., restriction, binging, purging, exercise). *Source*: With permission of Royal College of Psychiatrists (2022).

upper arm circumference), electrocardiogram (ECG) abnormalities, biochemical abnormalities (e.g., hypophosphatemia, hypokalemia, hypoglycemia), hematology, and level of activity and exercise (Royal College of Psychiatrists, 2022). A traffic light system of low, medium, and high-risk status for each of these domains is provided in the MEED guidance (Royal College of Psychiatrists, 2022).

For some presentations, direct observation of eating and mealtime behavior can also be extremely informative. For example, the behavioral component of rumination disorder can often be directly observed. The individual may contract tongue or abdominal muscles, cough, induce a retch or gag, or place a hand over the mouth in the process of regurgitating. Observation of mealtime interactions, aversion to food, fear responses, idiosyncratic eating behavior, and the presence of a sensory component to the presentation can usefully contribute to the clinician's assessment of the nature and severity of the presenting disturbance.

Screening and assessment instruments

There are several standardized assessment measures relevant to the assessment of child and adolescent feeding and eating disorders. These range from diagnostic assessment instruments delivered in an interview format, through self and parent report questionnaires to screening tools used in primary care settings. As with all such measures they vary in terms of strengths and weaknesses, and none comprehensively covers the full range of feeding and eating disorder presentations. Helpful reviews of the screening and assessment measures for use in child and adolescent populations can be found in Micali and House (2011), and Dinkler and Bryant-Waugh (2021). As well as feeding and eating disorder specific measures, the clinician may choose to use broader measures covering multiple diagnoses such as the Structured Clinical Interview for DSM-5-TR Disorders (SCID-5; First *et al.*, 2015), the Diagnostic Interview Schedule for Children (DISC; Shaffer *et al.*, 2000), or the Development and Well-being Assessment (DAWBA; Goodman *et al.*, 2000), all of which include sections on eating behavior. The NHS Access and Waiting Times document (NHS England, 2015) provides guidance on assessment measures recommended in England. The Eating Disorders Examination Questionnaire (Fairburn *et al.*, 2008) is probably the most widely used symptom screen in clinical services currently. See Chapter 28 for further information about assessment and screening tools.

Formulation and treatment planning

Having obtained information relating to the multiple domains described above, the clinician is required to evaluate and synthesize the information to allow diagnosis and appropriate treatment planning. This might include the need to consider the appropriateness of an admission or other high-intensity treatment option (see Chapter 48). Table 69.3 sets out common indicators for the clinician to consider in this respect.

Due to the multifaceted nature of feeding and eating disorders, information about factors that may be maintaining the disorder can be helpfully integrated using a formulation approach. One such model is the widely used "Five Ps approach" (MacNeil *et al.*, 2012), which proposes that information obtained at assessment can be sorted into five sets of factors: presenting issues, predisposing factors, precipitating factors, perpetuating factors, and protective factors. This framework has applied to include context and systemic patterns in individual young people with eating disorders (Baudinet *et al.*, 2021a). Presenting issues and perpetuating factors form a natural focus for intervention, utilizing where possible relevant positive factors. Risk, as discussed above and outlined in Table 69.2, will also be important in prioritizing interventions.

Table 69.3 Common indications for admission/increased intensity of treatment.

Physical
Severe weight loss (either rapid or extremely low weight)
Electrolyte disturbance
Dehydration
Hypothermia
Significant renal function abnormalities
Cardiovascular complications—e.g., hypotension, tachycardia, bradycardia
Intractable vomiting
Psychological
Severe depression, suicidal ideation/intent
Other significant psychiatric disturbance
Other
Parents/carers unable to manage required level of supervision and input
Failed outpatient treatment

Box 69.1 Assessment at a glance (see Table 69.2 for further detail)

History
- developmental factors
- feeding and eating behavior
- medical history
- significant events

Current presentation
- eating behavior
- current nutritional intake
- behaviors associated with eating (e.g., compensatory, regurgitation)
- growth and developmental status
- physical state
- mental state
- general functioning

Context
- family/care environment
- sociocultural background
- school/educational context

Areas of risk
- physical
- mental health
- developmental

Treatment and prevention

Prevention and early intervention

Much of the work on eating disorders prevention has been conducted within school settings, mostly in the form of the evaluation of specific preventative programs delivered in classroom settings. These have delivered mixed findings with no one clearly superior program. The impact of such interventions on incidence of eating disorders is hard to ascertain, and it is generally recognized that such initiatives can only ever form part of a comprehensive preventative approach, which also requires family and societal components, as well as improved understanding of the complex etiological pathways of eating disorders. A recent meta-analysis of randomized controlled trials (RCTs) reported that dissonance-based (designed to reduce psychological discomfort between attitudes and behavior), self-esteem, and healthy lifestyle modification programs are effective at reducing the future onset of eating disorders. However, psychoeducational, cognitive and behavioral, and family-based prevention programs are not (Stice *et al.*, 2021).

Increasingly, there is also a move to develop more effective and accessible early intervention programs, given the recognized unmet need and disparity in treatment access internationally (Allen *et al.*, 2023). It is well documented that longer illness duration can be associated with poorer treatment outcome (Ambwani *et al.*, 2020; Fernandez-Aranda *et al.*, 2021), emphasizing the need to develop and disseminate effective early intervention treatments. Despite the need, research into early intervention for eating disorders remains limited. Self-help and guided self-help models show promise for BN and BED, although little is known of their effectiveness for AN (Yim & Schmidt, 2019), and even less for ARFID, rumination disorder, and pica.

Overview of the current evidence base for psychological treatments

The main recommended treatment for all eating disorders is a form of psychological intervention, provided for the majority in outpatient settings (Hay, 2020). This makes sense as eating disorders are characterized by a core disturbance in eating behavior which in turn leads to physical, nutritional, and psychosocial impairment. Where physical or nutritional risk is high, a period of stabilization may be required before psychological treatment can commence, but, in general, psychological treatment would be commenced early.

There are no published treatment trials relating to pica and rumination disorder in children and young people, although the consensus in the literature is that both disorders can be treated using a behavioral approach (Leung & Hon, 2019), or a cognitive behavioral approach (Murray *et al.*, 2021). Similarly, little is yet known about effective treatment interventions for individuals presenting with ARFID, but the prominent avoidance behaviors characteristic of the disorder indicate that cognitive behavioral, behavioral, or family therapy interventions may be the most promising approaches (Couturier *et al.*, 2020). Where there is an associated emotional disturbance, such as anxiety, cognitive behavioral therapy (CBT) may prove to be an effective intervention (Kenney & Walsh, 2013).

While the evidence base for treatment of children and adolescents with AN is strongest for family interventions, this is still somewhat limited. There are only a small number of RCTs, most of which involved small sample sizes (e.g., Lock *et al.*, 2005; Eisler *et al.*, 2016a; Le Grange *et al.*, 2016). Some, but not all, of these trials suggest that family therapy may be better than individual psychotherapy in terms of physical improvement (weight gain and resumption of menstruation) and reduction of cognitive distortions, particularly in younger patients. While these studies provide the best evidence available for the treatment of AN in adolescents, their sample sizes are generally low. In addition, most of the study participants are adolescents rather than children. Lock *et al.* (2010) conducted an RCT with a larger sample size (n = 121), comparing a version of eating disorder-focused family therapy with adolescent-focused individual therapy in adolescents with AN and found no significant differences in full remission at the end of treatment. However, some differences were found that favored family therapy at 6- and 12-month follow-up. There is also some evidence that adding adjunctive multifamily therapy groups (for families experiencing similar difficulties to share experiences, find support, try new approaches, and learn together) to eating disorder-focused family therapy can improve weight outcomes (Eisler *et al.*, 2016b; Baudinet *et al.*, 2021c).

Three RCTs have compared family therapy with individual interventions in adolescents with BN. Schmidt *et al.* (2007) compared family therapy and CBT-guided self-care and found that CBT-guided self-care was superior to family therapy in reduction of binge eating behavior. Le Grange *et al.* (2007) compared family therapy and supportive psychotherapy (SPT) and found significantly greater early reductions in symptomatic behavior for patients in family therapy than in SPT. In addition, significantly more patients in family therapy than in SPT remitted at end of treatment and at follow-up. A further study compared family therapy to CBT adapted for adolescent BN, finding those who received family therapy reporting higher abstinence rates compared to those who received CBT at end of treatment (Le Grange *et al.*, 2015).

Recent reviews and meta-analyses of family therapy for both AN and BN concluded that family therapy for adolescents with eating disorders is superior to individual therapy at 6–12-month follow-up, although differences at end of treatment are not always observed (Couturier *et al.*, 2013; Jewell *et al.*, 2016; Fisher *et al.*, 2019).

While there is some support for individual CBT approaches in adolescents with BN and other binge eating syndromes (Gorrell & Le Grange, 2019), and more recently for enhanced CBT (CBT-E) in adolescents with AN (Atwood & Friedman, 2020; Le Grange *et al.*, 2022), the evidence base for CBT for AN in adolescents is still emerging. Nevertheless, eating disorders represent a good example of how dysfunctional thoughts and behaviors combine to result in physical and social impairment and thus, in theory, cognitive behavioral approaches could provide an effective strategy for treating these disorders (Dalle Grave & Pike, 2023).

For further detail and discussion of CBT and family-focused interventions for youth see Chapters 34 and 35, respectively.

Physical health monitoring and management during treatment

Ongoing physical health monitoring is an essential component of best practice eating disorder treatment (National Institute for Health and Care Excellence, 2017; Royal College of Psychiatrists, 2022). Attention to physical and nutritional aspects may include pediatric and dietetic reviews, interventions to manage any medical problems resulting from the eating disturbance, and implantation or restoration of a nutritionally adequate oral diet. In cases where the child or adolescent is underweight, restoration and maintenance of a healthy weight will be an important treatment component. Current practice varies widely in relation to rate of expected weight gain; in general, weekly gain of 0.5–1 kg is recommended as an aim of treatment for AN (National Institute for Health and Care Excellence, 2017). In severely malnourished patients, a more gradual increase of energy intake combined with regular physical monitoring to prevent the development of refeeding syndrome (typically characterized by fluid disorders such as edema and electrolyte disturbances, particularly hypophosphatemia) may be indicated. MEED guidelines offer a comprehensive framework of physical health markers to monitor, including a traffic light system to help clinicians describe the level of risk in each domain assessed (Royal College of Psychiatrists, 2022). Typically, medical intervention and reviews are more frequent at the beginning of treatment compared to the later stages. However, mechanisms always need to be in place to increase the frequency of monitoring should symptoms increase.

Pharmacotherapy

Medication has a limited role as first-line treatment for child and adolescent feeding and eating disorders. There is a very limited evidence base supporting the use of any pharmacological interventions with child and adolescent eating disorders (Correll *et al.*, 2021), and caution is needed in view of the physical vulnerability of this group (National Institute for Health and Care Excellence, 2017). Nevertheless, drugs are used, in practice albeit with uncertain effectiveness, most commonly selective serotonin reuptake inhibitors and antipsychotics, with main indications being depression, anxiety, rigidity, and weight concern (Gowers *et al.*, 2010b; Couturier *et al.*, 2019). Increasingly, olanzapine is also being used in clinical settings for children and adolescents with AN; however, evidence to support its effectiveness remains unclear (Han *et al.*, 2022).

Treatment setting and intensity

Most young people who receive treatment for a feeding or eating disorder will do so in an outpatient setting. Historically, inpatient treatment was considered when outpatient treatment was not sufficient. However, outcomes following hospitalization are mixed and the benefit of inpatient care beyond medical stabilization disputed (Gowers *et al.*, 2010a; Madden *et al.*, 2015a, 2015b; Hay *et al.*, 2019).

To better meet the needs of this group of young people, an array of more intensive treatment options has emerged in recent decades that straddle traditional outpatient and inpatient treatment. Options include brief intensive outpatient treatments where young people and families are seen multiple days per week (e.g., Rockwell *et al.*, 2011; Fink *et al.*, 2017), intensive group-based multifamily treatment interventions (see Baudinet *et al.*, 2021c for review), day programs (see Baudinet & Simic, 2021 for review), and residential treatments (Friedman *et al.*, 2016; Peckmezian & Paxton, 2020). Emerging data suggest all can be effective at improving physical health, symptom reduction, quality of life, and general functioning.

There is also an increase in the use of digital and telehealth interventions, which has exponentially increased in recent years related to the COVID-19 pandemic. Emerging data suggest outpatient (Stewart *et al.*, 2021) and day program treatment (Brothwood *et al.*, 2021) is appreciated and helpful for many, although young people, parents, and clinicians initially held reservations (Gorrell *et al.*, 2022).

The multidisciplinary team and interteam working

Increasingly, service context and the importance of having a multidisciplinary team has been acknowledged (Eisler *et al.*, 2022). Evidence suggests that training teams, rather than individuals, is the most effective way of disseminating evidence-based practice (Greenhalgh *et al.*, 2004).

A seminal study in London, UK, investigated the impact of service context on child and adolescent eating disorder outcomes. House *et al.* (2012) compared treatment outcomes for young people who received outpatient treatment in a specialist eating disorder service compared to a generic child and adolescent mental health service. In specialist services, eating disorders were two to three times more likely to be identified, treatment was more consistent and less expensive, and there was significantly less need for inpatient admissions (House *et al.*, 2012). This speaks to the importance of a cohesive, knowledgeable team, with specialist knowledge. It also highlights the importance of future research measuring nontreatment factors (known as "common factors") that may be impacting treatment outcome, independent of the type of treatment provided, techniques used, or adherence to protocols.

Considerations for diverse populations

The field of eating disorders, like many others, has been dominated by a White, Western-centric focus (Halbeisen *et al.*, 2022), with most of the treatments developed by, and evidence reported for, this group. A 20-year review of publications between 2000–2020 involving human participants in the *International*

Journal of Eating Disorders, a leading journal in the field of eating disorders, by Egbert *et al.* (2022), found that only 42.5% reported race/ethnicity data and White participants made up 70% of the data reported. It is increasingly recognized that people from diverse ethnic and gender groups may underreport symptoms, are typically underdiagnosed with eating disorders, and are less likely to seek and access treatment (Ali *et al.*, 2017; Gorrell *et al.*, 2021). It is important, therefore, to consider the way service, staffing, and treatment factors may unintentionally exclude or deter access.

Consent and ethical issues

Eating disorders are potentially life-threatening and may have very serious physical and psychosocial consequences if effective treatment is not provided. Given that young people with eating disorders are often reluctant to seek or accept treatment, practitioners need effective ethical and legal guidelines to make treatment decisions (Foreman, 2006).

All possible attempts should be made to form a therapeutic alliance with the young person, both to achieve consent to treatment on ethical grounds, and because therapeutic alliance is associated with effectiveness of treatment (Werz *et al.*, 2022). In England and Wales, parents, or those with parental authority, may in theory consent on their children's behalf up to the age of 18 but different countries operate different age limits, and a range of factors may need to be considered such as future impact on the parent–child relationship. Assessments of capacity to make decisions and legal frameworks for overriding the young person's stated wishes vary across countries with clinicians advised to adhere to local guidance. While it is desirable to obtain the young person's consent, it is helpful to make a distinction between treatment directed at reducing risk from the physical consequences of the eating disorder and psychological treatment of the eating disorder. The decision to treat against the young person's wishes is usually most likely to arise when hospital admission is indicated, and the young person declines treatment. However, the decision to treat a young person against their will should always be considered a last resort.

See Chapter 19 for wider discussion of legal issues in psychiatric treatment for youth.

Box 69.2 Treatment at a glance: for all feeding and eating disorders

- Monitor and manage the physical health consequences of the eating disturbance and related risks
- Monitor and manage nutritional status (micro- and macronutrient profile and energy needs)
- Offer a form of psychological intervention to address the core eating disturbance; this may include:
  - family therapy (evidence base strongest for anorexia nervosa [AN])
  - individual therapy, for example, cognitive behavioral therapy (CBT; evidence base strongest for bulimia nervosa [BN])
  - Parent- or carer-led interventions, for example, for younger children or those with intellectual disability (ID)

Outcome

Outcome studies can generally be divided into two categories: those that attempt to establish the efficacy of a particular treatment and those that attempt to establish prognostic factors.

Recovery and remission

Despite advances and an increase in treatment options, full remission rates at the end of first-line child and adolescent eating disorder treatment remains relatively modest for adolescent AN (20–50%) and BN (~40%) (Lock & Le Grange, 2019), with less known for BED, ARFID, and other eating disorders. It is often difficult to generalize findings from studies of outcome of eating disorders as there is wide variation in the outcome parameters used across studies.

Longer-term outcomes and prognostic factors

Generally, treatment gains are maintained at short- and long-term follow-up in both clinical and community settings (Eisler *et al.*, 2007; Stewart *et al.*, 2022). A systematic review of relapse, remission, and recovery in AN reported that relapse rates ranged from 9–52%, depending on how relapse was defined and tended to increase with duration of follow-up (Khalsa *et al.*, 2017). In a 22-year follow-up study of 228 people 62.8% of people with AN and 68.2% of people with BN were recovered (Eddy *et al.*, 2017). In the same study, early (9-year) recovery predicted later (22-year) recovery in AN, but not BN. Generally, for every study that identifies a group of prognostic factors, another study will fail to replicate the significance of the group of variables identified. Age at onset, duration of inpatient care, comorbidity, and social problems have all been suggested as potentially important prognostic factors.

Migration between diagnoses

There is some diagnostic instability and migration between feeding and eating disorder diagnoses has been reported. Nevertheless, in a large (N = 9622) Swedish sample, recent data suggests migration between threshold eating disorder diagnoses is infrequent (Schaumberg, 2019). Their data also indicated that eating disorder not otherwise specified (EDNOS) diagnosis was relatively stable and was not a diagnosis that individuals simply "passed through."

Cross-cultural differences in outcomes

There are very little data available regarding the impact of race, ethnicity, and other sociocultural factors on treatment outcome. This has made it difficult for researchers to test whether diverse groups respond differently to current evidence-based treatments (Hamadi & Holliday, 2020). A recent review of meta-analyses found only one meta-analysis examining the impact of race/ethnicity on eating disorders treatment outcomes, which was focused on adult BED (Cougle & Grubaugh, 2022). Regarding treatment and service experience, it is consistently reported that non-White, non-female individuals can experience increased barriers to accessing treatment, and adaptations of evidence-based treatments are only beginning to emerge (Halbeisen *et al*., 2022). Accurso *et al*. (2021) recently published a protocol for the adaptation of family-based treatment for racially diverse and socioeconomically disadvantaged young people; however, this is yet to be tested.

Conclusion

This chapter summarizes current knowledge, understanding, and practice in feeding and eating disorders in children and adolescents. The implications for clinicians and their patients of recent changes in DSM-5-TR and ICD-11 are beginning to become apparent through better fit with clinical presentations in young people and an increase in research interest. There is undoubtedly still a long way to go in improving the quality and consistency of care for children and adolescents with significant eating difficulties. It is unclear whether current approaches to classification in the form of categorical diagnostic groups will prove most useful in the long term as a basis for research endeavors. Developments in cross-cutting dimensional research, such as initiatives attempting to classify psychopathology based on dimensions of observable behavior and neurobiological measures (Cuthbert & Insel, 2013), may in due course result in more meaningful, useful, and effective changes in how we develop and select appropriate treatments for our patients.

References

Accurso, E.C. *et al*. (2021) Adaptation to family-based treatment for Medicaid-insured youth with anorexia nervosa in publicly funded settings: protocol for a mixed methods implementation scale-out pilot study. *Journal of Eating Disorders* **9**, 99.

Ágh, T. *et al*. (2016) A systematic review of the health-related quality of life and economic burdens of anorexia nervosa, bulimia nervosa, and binge eating disorder. *Eating and Weight Disorders* **21**(3), 353–364.

Agostino, H. *et al*. (2021) Trends in the incidence of new-onset anorexia nervosa and atypical anorexia nervosa among youth during the COVID-19 pandemic in Canada. *JAMA Network Open* **4**(12), e2137395.

Ali, K. *et al*. (2017) Perceived barriers and facilitators towards help-seeking for eating disorders: a systematic review. *International Journal of Eating Disorders* **50**(1), 9–21.

Allen, K.L. *et al*. (2023) A framework for conceptualising early intervention for eating disorders. *European Eating Disorders Review* **3**(2), 320–334.

Ambwani, S. *et al*. (2020) A multicentre audit of outpatient care for adult anorexia nervosa: symptom trajectory, service use, and evidence in support of "early stage" versus "severe and enduring" classification. *International Journal of Eating Disorders* **53**(8), 1337–1348.

American Psychiatric Association (2013) *Diagnostic and Statistical Manual of Mental Disorders*, 5th edn. American Psychiatric Association, Washington, DC.

American Psychiatric Association (2022) *Diagnostic and Statistical Manual of Mental Disorders*, 5th edn. text revision edn. American Psychiatric Association, Washington, DC.

Archibald, T. & Bryant-Waugh, R. (2023) Current evidence for avoidant restrictive food intake disorder: implications for clinical practice and future directions. *JCPP Advances* **3**(2), e12160.

Asch, D.A. *et al*. (2021) Trends in US patients receiving care for eating disorders and other common behavioral health conditions before and during the COVID-19 pandemic. *JAMA Network Open* **4**(11), e2134913.

Atiye, M. *et al*. (2014) A meta-analysis of temperament in eating disorders. *European Eating Disorders Review* **23**(2), 89–99.

Attia, E. & Roberto, C. (2009) Should amenorrhea be a diagnostic criterion for AN? *International Journal of Eating Disorders* **42**, 581–589.

Atwood, M.E. & Friedman, A. (2020) A systematic review of enhanced cognitive behavioral therapy (CBT-E) for eating disorders. *International Journal of Eating Disorders* **53**, 311–330.

Baudinet, J. & Simic, M. (2021) Adolescent eating disorder day programme treatment models and outcomes: a systematic scoping review. *Frontiers in Psychiatry* **12**, 539.

Baudinet, J. *et al*. (2020) Targeting maladaptive overcontrol with radically open dialectical behaviour therapy in a day programme for adolescents with restrictive eating disorders. *Journal of Eating Disorders* **8**(1), 68.

Baudinet, J. *et al*. (2021a) Formulation in eating disorder focused family therapy: why, when, and how? *Journal of Eating Disorders* **9**(1), 97.

Baudinet, J. *et al*. (2021b) From treatment models to manuals: Maudsley single- and multi-family therapy for adolescent eating disorders. In: *Systemic Approaches to Therapy Manuals*. (ed M. Mariotti), 1st edn. Springer, Cham, Switzerland. pp. 349–372.

Baudinet, J. *et al*. (2021c) Multi-family therapy for eating disorders: a systematic scoping review of the quantitative and qualitative findings. *International Journal of Eating Disorders* **54**(12), 2095–2120.

Baudinet, J. *et al*. (2021d) Radically open dialectical behaviour therapy for adolescents: a case series. *BMJ Psychiatry* **21**(1), 462.

Becker, A. *et al*. (2002) Eating behaviours and attitudes following prolonged television exposure among ethnic Fijian adolescent girls. *British Journal of Psychiatry* **180**, 509–514.

Becker, A. *et al*. (2009) Should non-fat-phobic AN be included in DSM-V? *International Journal of Eating Disorders* **42**, 620–635.

Becker, A. *et al*. (2011) Social network media exposure and adolescent eating pathology in Fiji. *British Journal of Psychiatry* **198**, 43–50.

Borgna-Pignatti, C. & Zanella, S. (2016) Pica as a manifestation of iron deficiency. *Expert Review of Hematology* **9**(11), 1075–1080.

Bravender, T. *et al*. (2010) Classification of eating disturbance in children and adolescents: proposed changes for the DSM-V. *European Eating Disorders Review* **18**, 79–89.

Brothwood, P.L. *et al*. (2021) Moving online: young people and parents' experiences of adolescent eating disorder day programme treatment during the COVID-19 pandemic. *Journal of Eating Disorders* **9**(1), 62.

Bryant-Waugh, R. & Kreipe, R.E. (2012) Avoidant/restrictive food intake disorder in DSM-5-TR. *Psychiatric Annals* **42**, 402–405.

Bryant-Waugh, R. *et al*. (2010) Feeding and eating disorders in childhood. *International Journal of Eating Disorders* **43**, 98–111.

Bulik, C.M. *et al*. (2022) Genetics and neurobiology of eating disorders. *Nature Neuroscience* **25**(5), 543–554.

Bury, S.M. *et al*. (2023) "It defines who I am" or "It's something I have": what language do [autistic] Australian adults [on the autism spectrum] prefer? *Journal of Autism and Developmental Disorders* **53**, 677–687.

Butler, M.J. *et al.* (2021) The role of the gut microbiome, immunity, and neuroinflammation in the pathophysiology of eating disorders. *Nutrients* **13**(2), 500.

Cassin, S. & von Ranson, K. (2005) Personality and eating disorders: a decade in review. *Clinical Psychology Review* **25**, 895–916.

Chatoor, I. *et al.* (2019) Anorexia nervosa and depression in a 5-year-old girl: treatment with focused family play therapy and medication. *International Journal of Eating Disorders* **52**, 1065–1069.

Chen, L. *et al.* (2010) Sexual abuse and lifetime diagnosis of psychiatric disorders: a systematic review and meta-analysis. *Mayo Clinic Proceedings* **85**, 618–629.

Cheng, Z.H. *et al.* (2019) Ethnic differences in eating disorder prevalence, risk factors, and predictive effects of risk factors among young women. *Eating Behaviors* **32**, 23–30.

Chung, E.O. *et al.* (2019) Characteristics of pica behavior among mothers around Lake Victoria, Kenya: a cross-sectional study. *International Journal of Environmental Research and Public Health* **16**, 2510.

Claudino, A.M. *et al.* (2019) The classification of feeding and eating disorders in the ICD-11: results of a field study comparing proposed ICD-11 guidelines with existing ICD-10 guidelines. *BMC Medicine* **17**, 93.

Coelho, J.S. *et al.* (2019) Eating disorder diagnoses and symptom presentation in transgender youth: a scoping review. *Current Psychiatry Reports* **21**(11), 107.

Connan, F. *et al.* (2003) A neurodevelopmental model for AN. *Physiology and Behaviour* **79**, 13–24.

Correll, C.U. *et al.* (2021) Efficacy and acceptability of pharmacological, psychosocial, and brain stimulation interventions in children and adolescents with mental disorders: an umbrella review. *World Psychiatry* **20**(2), 244–275.

Cougle, J.R. & Grubaugh, A.L. (2022) Do psychosocial treatment outcomes vary by race or ethnicity? A review of meta-analyses. *Clinical Psychology Review* **96**, 102192.

Couturier, J. *et al.* (2013) Efficacy of family-based treatment for adolescents with eating disorders: a systematic review and meta-analysis. *International Journal of Eating Disorders* **46**, 3–11.

Couturier, J. *et al.* (2019) Psychotropic medication for children and adolescents with eating disorders. *Eating Disorders in Child and Adolescent Psychiatry* **28**(4), 583–592.

Couturier, J. *et al.* (2020) Canadian practice guidelines for the treatment of children and adolescents with eating disorders. *Journal of Eating Disorders* **8**, 4.

Culbert, K.M. *et al.* (2015) Research review: What we have learned about the causes of eating disorders: a synthesis of sociocultural, psychological, and biological research. *The Journal of Child Psychology and Psychiatry* **56**, 1141–1164.

Culbert, K.M. *et al.* (2021) A narrative review of sex differences in eating disorders: is there a biological basis? *Clinical Therapeutics* **43**(1), 95–111.

Cuthbert, B.N. & Insel, T.R. (2013) Toward the future of psychiatric diagnosis: the seven pillars of RdoC. *BMC Medicine* **11**, 126.

Dalle Grave, R. & Pike, K. (2023) Cognitive behaviour therapy and eating disorders. In: *Eating Disorders*. (eds P. Robinson, *et al.*). Springer, Cham, Switzerland. pp. 1103–1117.

De Young, K.P. *et al.* (2012) Review of BED and proposal for inclusion in DSM-5-TR. *Psychiatric Annals* **42**, 410–413.

Dinkler, L. & Bryant-Waugh, R. (2021) Assessment of avoidant restrictive food intake disorder, pica and rumination disorder: interview and questionnaire measures. *Current Opinion in Psychiatry* **34**(6), 532–542.

Dinkler, L. *et al.* (2023) Etiology of the broad avoidant restrictive food intake disorder phenotype in Swedish twins aged 6 to 12 years. *JAMA Psychiatry* **80**(3), 260–269.

Donnelly, B. *et al.* (2018) Neuroimaging in bulimia nervosa and binge eating disorder: a systematic review. *Journal of Eating Disorders* **6**, 3.

Eddy, K.T. *et al.* (2017) Recovery from anorexia nervosa and bulimia nervosa at 22-year follow-up. *Journal of Clinical Psychiatry* **78**(2), 84–189.

Egbert, A.H. *et al.* (2022) Reporting racial and ethnic diversity in eating disorder research over the past 20 years. *International Journal of Eating Disorders* **55**(4), 455–462.

Eisler, I. (2005) The empirical and theoretical base of family therapy and multiple family day therapy for adolescent AN. *Journal of Family Therapy* **27**, 104–131.

Eisler, I. *et al.* (2007) A randomised controlled treatment trial of two forms of family therapy in adolescent anorexia nervosa: a five-year follow-up. *Journal of Child Psychology and Psychiatry and Allied Disciplines* **48**(6), 552–560.

Eisler, I. *et al.* (2016a) A pragmatic randomised multi-centre trial of multifamily and single family therapy for adolescent anorexia nervosa. *BMC Psychiatry* **16**(1), 422.

Eisler I. *et al.* (2016b) Maudsley Service Manual for Child and Adolescent Eating Disorders. Available: https://mccaed.slam.nhs.uk/wp-content/uploads/2019/11/Maudsley-Service-Manual-for-Child-and-Adolescent-Eating-Disorders-July-2016.pdf [18 December 2024].

Eisler, I. *et al.* (2022) Implementing service transformation for children and adolescents with eating disorders across England: the theory, politics, and pragmatics of large-scale service reform. *Journal of Eating Disorders* **10**, 146.

Ericsson, N. *et al.* (2011) Parental disorders, childhood abuse and binge eating in a large community sample. *International Journal of Eating Disorders* **45**, 316–325.

Fairburn, C. *et al.* (2008) Eating disorders examination (Edition 16.0D). In: *Cognitive Behavior Therapy and Eating Disorders*. (ed C. Fairburn). Guilford Press, New York. pp. 265–308.

Favaro, A. *et al.* (2006) Perinatal factors and the risk of developing AN and BN. *Archives of General Psychiatry* **63**, 82–88.

Favaro, A. *et al.* (2011) In utero exposure to virus infections and the risk of developing AN. *Psychological Medicine* **41**, 2193–2199.

Fernandez-Aranda, F. *et al.* (2021) The impact of duration of illness on treatment nonresponse and drop-out: exploring the relevance of enduring eating disorder concept. *European Eating Disorders Review* **29**(3), 499–513.

Fields, V.L. *et al.* (2021) Pica, autism, and other disabilities. *Pediatrics* **147**(2), e20200462.

Fink, K. *et al.* (2017) Exploring the effects of a family admissions program for adolescents with anorexia nervosa. *Journal of Eating Disorders* **5**(1), 51.

First, M.B. *et al.* (2015) *Structured Clinical Interview for DSM-5-TR Disorders, (SCID-5)*. American Psychiatric Association, Arlington, VA.

Fisher, C.A. *et al.* (2019) Family therapy approaches for anorexia nervosa. *Cochrane Database of Systematic Reviews* **10**(10), CD0044780.

Ford, T. *et al.* (2021) Mental health of children and young people during pandemic. *BMJ* **372**, n614.

Foreman, D. (2006) The law in relation to children. In: *Seminars in Child and Adolescent Psychiatry.* (ed S.G. Gowers), 2nd edn. Gaskell, London. pp. 99–101.

Frank, G.K.W. *et al.* (2019) The neurobiology of eating disorders. *Child and Adolescent Psychiatric Clinics of North America* **28**(4), 629–640.

Freidl, E.K. *et al.* (2012) AN in DSM-5-TR. *Psychiatric Annals* **42**, 414–417.

Friedman, K. *et al.* (2016) A narrative review of outcome studies for residential and partial hospital-based treatment of eating disorders. *European Eating Disorders Review* **24**(4), 263–276.

Fuglset, T.S. (2019) Set-shifting, central coherence and decision-making in individuals recovered from anorexia nervosa: a systematic review. *Journal of Eating Disorders* **7**(1), 22.

Galmiche, M. *et al.* (2019) Prevalence of eating disorders over the 2000–2018 period: a systematic literature review. *The American Journal of Clinical Nutrition* **109**(5), 1402–1413.

GBD 2019 Mental Disorders Collaborators (2022) Global, regional, and national burden of 12 mental disorders in 204 countries and territories, 1990-2019: a systematic analysis for the global burden of disease study 2019. *The Lancet Psychiatry* **9**(2), 137–150.

Goodman, R. *et al.* (2000) The Development and Well-being Assessment: Description and initial validation of an integrated assessment of child and adolescent psychopathology. *Journal of Child Psychology and Psychiatry* **41**, 645–655.

Gorrell, S. & Le Grange, D. (2019) Update on treatments for adolescent bulimia nervosa. *Child and Adolescent Psychiatric Clinics of North America* **28**(4), 537–547.

Gorrell, S. & Murray, S.B. (2019) Eating disorders in males. *Child and Adolescent Psychiatric Clinics of North America* **28**(4), 641–651.

Gorrell, S. *et al.* (2021) Gender identity, race/ethnicity and eating pathology in a treatment-seeking community sample. *Journal of Behavioral and Cognitive Therapy* **31**(1), 77–89.

Gorrell, S. *et al.* (2022) Use of telehealth in the management of adolescent eating disorders: patient perspectives and future directions suggested from the COVID-19 pandemic. *Adolescent Health, Medicine and Therapeutics* **13**, 45–53.

Gowers, S. *et al.* (2010a) A randomised controlled multicentre trial of treatments for adolescent anorexia nervosa including assessment of cost-effectiveness and patient acceptability: the TOuCAN trial. *Health Technology Assessment* **14**(15), 1–98.

Gowers, S. *et al.* (2010b) Drug prescribing in child and adolescent eating disorder services. *Journal of Child and Adolescent Mental Health* **15**, 18–22.

Greenhalgh, T. *et al.* (2004) Diffusion of innovations in service organizations: systematic review and recommendations. *The Milbank Quarterly* **82**(4), 581–629.

Groleau, P. *et al.* (2012) Childhood emotional abuse and eating symptoms in bulimic disorders: an examination of possible mediating variables. *International Journal of Eating Disorders* **45**, 326–332.

Halbeisen, G. *et al.* (2022) A plea for diversity in eating disorders research. *Frontiers in Psychiatry* **13**, 820043.

Hamadi, L. & Holliday, J. (2020) Moderators and mediators of outcome in treatments for anorexia nervosa and bulimia nervosa in adolescents: a systematic review of randomized controlled trials. *International Journal of Eating Disorders* **53**(1), 3–19.

Han, R. *et al.* (2022) Effectiveness of olanzapine in the treatment of anorexia nervosa: a systematic review and meta-analysis. *Brain and Behavior* **12**(2), e2498.

Hartmann, A.S. *et al.* (2012) Pica and rumination disorder in DSM-5-TR. *Psychiatric Annals* **42**, 426–430.

Hay, P. (2020) Current approach to eating disorders: a clinical update. *Internal Medicine Journal* **50**(1), 24–29.

Hay, P.J. *et al.* (2019) Inpatient versus outpatient care, partial hospitalisation and waiting list for people with eating disorders. *Cochrane Database of Systematic Reviews* **1**.

Haycraft, E. *et al.* (2011) Relationships between temperament and eating behaviours in young children. *Appetite* **56**, 689–692.

Hazzard, V.M. *et al.* (2020) Food insecurity and eating disorders: a review of emerging evidence. *Current Psychiatry Reports* **22**(12), 74.

Herle, M. *et al.* (2020) A longitudinal study of eating behaviours in childhood and later eating disorder behaviours and diagnoses. *British Journal of Psychiatry* **216**(2), 113–119.

Herman, A. & Bajaka, A. (2021) The role of the intestinal microbiota in eating disorders: Bulimia nervosa and binge eating disorder. *Psychiatry Research* **300**, 113923.

Himmerich, H. *et al.* (2019) Genetic risk factors for eating disorders: an update and insights into pathophysiology. *Therapeutic Advances in Psychopharmacology* **9**.

House, J. *et al.* (2012) Comparison of specialist and nonspecialist care pathways for adolescents with anorexia nervosa and related eating disorders. *International Journal of Eating Disorders* **45**(8), 949–956.

Hübel, C. *et al.* (2020) One size does not fit all: genomics differentiates among anorexia nervosa, bulimia nervosa, and binge-eating disorder. *International Journal of Eating Disorders* **54**, 785–793.

Isaksson, M. *et al.* (2021) Overcontrolled, undercontrolled, and resilient personality styles among patients with eating disorders. *Journal of Eating Disorders* **9**, 47.

Ivascu, N.S. *et al.* (2001) Characterization of pica prevalence among patients with sickle cell disease. *Archives of Pediatric and Adolescent Medicine* **155**, 1243–1247.

Iwajomo, T. *et al.* (2021) Excess mortality associated with eating disorders: population-based cohort study. *The British Journal of Psychiatry* **219**(3), 487–493.

Jewell, T. *et al.* (2016) Attachment and mentalization and their association with child and adolescent eating pathology: a systematic review. *International Journal of Eating Disorders* **49**(4), 354–373.

Jewell, T. *et al.* (2023) Attachment in individuals with eating disorders compared to community controls: a systematic review and meta-analysis. *International Journal of Eating Disorders* **56**(5), 888–908.

Josefsson, A. *et al.* (2022) Global prevalence and impact of rumination syndrome. *Gastroenterology* **162**, 731–742.

Katzman, D.K. (2005) Medical complications in adolescents with AN: a review of the literature. *International Journal of Eating Disorders* **37**(Suppl), S52–S59.

Keel, P. & Forney, K. (2013) Psychosocial risk factors for eating disorders. *International Journal of Eating Disorders* **46**, 433–439.

Keel, P.K. & Striegel-Moore, R.H. (2009) The validity and clinical utility of purging disorder. *International Journal of Eating Disorders* **42**, 706–719.

Kenney, L. & Walsh, T. (2013) Avoidant / restrictive food intake disorder. *Eating Disorders Review* **24**, 1–4.

Khalsa, S.S. *et al.* (2017) What happens after treatment? A systematic review of relapse, remission, and recovery in anorexia nervosa. *Journal of Eating Disorders* **5**(1), 20.

Klump, K.L. (2013) Puberty as a critical risk period for eating disorders: a review of human and animal studies. *Hormones and Behavior* **64**(2), 399–410.

Koomar, T. *et al.* (2021) Estimating the prevalence and genetic risk mechanisms of ARFID in a large autism cohort. *Frontiers in Psychiatry* **12**, 668297.

Larsen, J.T. *et al.* (2021) Prenatal and perinatal factors and risk of eating disorders. *Psychological Medicine* **51**, 870–880.

Le Grange, D. *et al.* (2007) A randomized controlled comparison of family based treatment and supportive psychotherapy for adolescent BN. *Archives of General Psychiatry* **64**, 1049–1056.

Le Grange, D. *et al.* (2015) Randomized clinical trial of family-based treatment and cognitive-behavioral therapy for adolescent bulimia nervosa. *Journal of the American Academy of Child and Adolescent Psychiatry* **54**(11), 886–894.

Le Grange, D. *et al.* (2016) Randomized clinical trial of parent-focused treatment and family-based treatment for adolescent anorexia nervosa. *Journal of the American Academy of Child and Adolescent Psychiatry* **55**(8), 683–692.

Le Grange, D. *et al.* (2022) Enhanced cognitive-behavior therapy and family-based treatment for adolescents with an eating disorder: a non-randomized effectiveness trial. *Psychological Medicine* **52**(13), 2520–2530.

Leung, A.K.C. & Hon, K.L. (2019) Pica: a common condition that is commonly missed - an update review. *Current Pediatric Reviews* **15**, 164–169.

Lilenfeld, L. (2011) Personality and temperament in eating disorders. In: *Current Topics in Behavioral Neurosciences*. (eds W.H. Kaye & R. Adan). Springer, New York. pp. 3–16.

Lindberg, L. & Hjern, A. (2003) Risk factors for AN: a national cohort study. *International Journal of Eating Disorders* **34**, 397–408.

Lock, J. & Le Grange, D. (2019) Family-based treatment: where are we and where should we be going to improve recovery in child and adolescent eating disorders. *International Journal of Eating Disorders* **52**(4), 481–487.

Lock, J. *et al.* (2005) A comparison of short- and long-term family therapy for adolescent AN. *Journal of the American Academy of Child and Adolescent Psychiatry* **44**, 632–639.

Lock, J. *et al.* (2010) Randomized clinical trial comparing family-based treatment with adolescent-focused individual therapy for adolescents with eating disorders. *Archives of General Psychiatry* **67**, 1025–1032.

MacNeil, C.A. *et al.* (2012) Is diagnosis enough to guide interventions in mental health? Using case formulation in clinical practice. *BMC Medicine* **10**, 111.

Madden, S. *et al.* (2015a) A randomized controlled trial of in-patient treatment for anorexia nervosa in medically unstable adolescents. *Psychological Medicine* **45**(2), 415–427.

Madden, S. *et al.* (2015b) Systematic review of evidence for different treatment settings in anorexia nervosa. *World Journal of Psychiatry* **5**(1), 147–153.

Mancuso, S.G. *et al.* (2015) Classification of eating disorders: comparison of relative prevalence. *British Journal of Psychiatry* **206**(6), 519–520.

Manfredi, L. *et al.* (2021) A systematic review of genetic polymorphisms associated with binge eating disorder. *Nutrients* **13**(3), 848.

Marcus, M.D. & Wildes, J.E. (2009) Obesity: is it a mental disorder? *International Journal of Eating Disorders* **42**, 739–753.

Martin, G.C. *et al.* (2000) A longitudinal study of the role of childhood temperament in the later development of eating concerns. *International Journal of Eating Disorders* **27**, 150–162.

Martínez-González, L. *et al.* (2020) Incidence of anorexia nervosa in women: a systematic review and meta-analysis. *International Journal of Environmental Research and Public Health* **17**(11), 3824.

Micali, N. (2022) What's weighing us down: closing the gap between the global burden of eating disorders and their representation. *European Child and Adolescent Psychiatry* **31**(11), 1653–1654.

Micali, N. & House, J. (2011) Assessment measures for child and adolescent eating disorders: a review. *Child and Adolescent Mental Health* **16**, 122–127.

Micali, N. *et al.* (2011) Maternal eating disorders and infant feeding difficulties: maternal and child mediators in a longitudinal general population study. *Journal of Child Clinical Psychology and Psychiatry* **52**, 800–807.

Miles, S. *et al.* (2020) Cognitive flexibility in acute anorexia nervosa and after recovery: a systematic review. *Clinical Psychology Review* **81**, 101905.

Miskovic-Wheatley, J. *et al.* (2023) Eating disorder outcomes: findings from a rapid review of over a decade of research. *Journal of Eating Disorders* **11**, 85.

Murray, H.B. *et al.* (2021) Comprehensive cognitive-behavioral interventions augment diaphragmatic breathing for rumination syndrome: a proof-of-concept trial. *Digestive Diseases and Science* **66**(10), 3461–3469.

Nagata, J.M. *et al.* (2020) Emerging trends in eating disorders among sexual and gender minorities. *Current Opinion in Psychiatry* **33**(6), 562–567.

National Institute for Health and Care Excellence (2017) *Eating Disorders: Recognition and Treatment (NICE Guideline NG69).* National Institute for Health and Care Excellence (NICE), London. Available: www.nice.org.uk/guidance/ng69 [19 December 2024].

NHS England (2015) *Access and Waiting Time Standard for Children and Young People with an Eating Disorder: Commissioning Guide (Version 1).* NHS England, Leeds, UK. Available: https://www.england.nhs.uk/statistics/statistical-work-areas/cyped-waiting-times [19 December 2024].

NHS England (2021) Children and Young Persons Eating Disorder ED waiting times series. NHS England, Leeds, UK. Available: https://www.england.nhs.uk/statistics/wp-content/uploads/sites/2/2021/02/CYP-ED-Waiting-Times-Timeseries-Q3-2020-21.xls [19 December 2024].

Nicholls, D. & Bryant-Waugh, R. (2009) Eating disorders of infancy and childhood: definition, symptomatology, epidemiology, and comorbidity. *Child and Adolescent Psychiatric Clinics of North America* **18**, 17–30.

Nicholls, D. *et al.* (2000) Children into DSM don't go: a comparison of classification systems for eating disorders in childhood and early adolescence. *International Journal of Eating Disorders* **28**, 317–324.

Norris, M.L. *et al.* (2016) Gastrointestinal complications associated with anorexia nervosa: a systematic review. *International Journal of Eating Disorders* **49**(3), 216–237.

Padín, P.F. *et al.* (2021) Social media and eating disorder psychopathology: a systematic review. *Cyberpsychology: Journal of Psychosocial Research on Cyberspace* **15**(3).

Parker, L.L. & Harriger, J.A. (2020) Eating disorders and disordered eating behaviors in the LGBT population: a review of the literature. *Journal of Eating Disorders* **8**, 51.

Peckmezian, T. & Paxton, S.J. (2020) A systematic review of outcomes following residential treatment for eating disorders. *European Eating Disorders Review* **28**(3), 246–259.

Peebles, R. *et al.* (2010) Are diagnostic criteria for eating disorders markers of medical severity? *Pediatrics* **125**, 1993–1201.

Piao, J. *et al.* (2022) Alarming changes in the global burden of mental disorders in children and adolescents from 1990 to 2019: a systematic analysis for the Global Burden of Disease study. *European Child and Adolescent Psychiatry* **31**, 1827–1845.

Qian, J. *et al.* (2022) An update on the prevalence of eating disorders in the general population: a systematic review and meta-analysis. *Eating and Weight Disorders - Studies on Anorexia, Bulimia and Obesity* **27**((2)), 415–428.

Rajindrajith, S. *et al.* (2021) Rumination syndrome in children and adolescents: a school survey assessing prevalence and symptomatology. *BMC Gastroenterology* **16**(12), 163.

Rockwell, R.E. *et al.* (2011) An innovative short-term, intensive, family-based treatment for adolescent anorexia nervosa: case series: anorexia nervosa family therapy. *European Eating Disorders Review* **19**(4), 362–367.

Royal College of Psychiatrists (2022) Medical emergencies in eating disorders (MEED): guidance on recognition and management (CR233). Royal College of Psychologists, London. Available: www.rcpsych.ac.uk/improving-care/campaigning-for-better-mental-health-policy/college-reports/2022-college-reports/cr233 [19 December 2024].

Santomauro, D. *et al.* (2021) The hidden burden of eating disorders: an extension of estimates from the Global Burden of Disease Study 2019. *The Lancet Psychiatry* **8**(4), 320–328.

Santonicola, A. *et al.* (2020) Eating disorders and gastrointestinal diseases. *Nutrients **11***, 3038.

Schaumberg, K. (2019) Patterns of diagnostic transition in eating disorders: a longitudinal population study in Sweden. *Psychological Medicine* **49**(5), 819–827.

Schaumberg, K. *et al.* (2020) Prospective associations between childhood neuropsychological profiles and adolescent eating disorders. *European Eating Disorders Review* **28**(2), 156–169.

Schmidt, U. & Treasure, J. (2006) Anorexia nervosa: Valued and visable. A cognitive interpersonal maintenance model and its implications for research and practice. *British Journal of Clinical Psychology* **45**, 343–366.

Schmidt, U. *et al.* (2007) A randomized controlled trial of family therapy and cognitive behavioral therapy guided self-care for adolescents with BN and related disorders. *American Journal of Psychiatry* **164**, 591–598.

Seitz, J. *et al.* (2019) The microbiome and eating disorders. *Psychiatric Clinics of North America* **42**(1), 93–103.

Shaffer, D. *et al.* (2000) NIMH Diagnostic Interview Schedule for Children version IV (NIMH DISC-IV): description, differences from previous versions, and reliability of some common diagnoses. *Journal of the American Academy of Child & Adolescent Psychiatry* **39**, 28–38.

Smitka, K. *et al.* (2021) Current aspects of the role of autoantibodies directed against appetite-regulating hormones and the gut microbiome in eating disorders. *Frontiers in Endocrinology* **12**, 613983.

Stein, A. *et al.* (2006) Eating habits and attitudes among 10-year-old children of mothers with eating disorders. *British Journal of Psychiatry* **189**, 324–329.

Stewart, C. *et al.* (2021) Is this the 'new normal'? A mixed method investigation of young person, parent and clinician experience of online eating disorder treatment during the COVID-19 pandemic. *Journal of Eating Disorders* **9**(1), 78.

Stewart, C. *et al.* (2022) From efficacy to effectiveness: child and adolescent eating disorder treatments in the real world (part 2): 7-year follow-up. *Journal of Eating Disorders* **10**, 14.

Stice, E. *et al.* (2008) Fasting increases risk for onset of binge eating and bulimic pathology: a 5-year prospective study. *Journal of Abnormal Psychology* **117**, 941–946.

Stice, E. *et al.* (2011) Risk factors for onset of eating disorders: evidence of multiple risk pathways from an 8-year prospective study. *Behaviour Research and Therapy* **49**, 622–627.

Stice, E. *et al.* (2017) Risk factors that predict future onset of each DSM-5 eating disorder: predictive specificity in high-risk adolescent females. *Journal of Abnormal Psychology* **126**, 38–51.

Stice, E. *et al.* (2021) A meta-analytic review of trials that tested whether eating disorder prevention programs prevent eating disorder onset. *Clinical Psychology Review* **87**, 102046.

Striegel-Moore, R. *et al.* (2009) The validity and clinical utility of night eating syndrome. *International Journal of Eating Disorders* **42**, 720–738.

Swedo, S. *et al.* (2012) From research subgroup to clinical syndrome: modifying the PANDAS criteria to describe PANS (pediatric acute-onset neuropsychiatric syndrome). *Pediatrics & Therapeutics* **2**, 2.

Taquet, M. *et al.* (2022) Incidence and outcomes of eating disorders during the COVID-19 pandemic. *British Journal of Psychiatry* **220**, 262–264.

Tasca, G.A. & Balfour, L. (2014) Attachment and eating disorders: a review of current research. *International Journal of Eating Disorders* **47**, 710–717.

Terry, S.M. *et al.* (2022) A critical analysis of eating disorders and the gut microbiome. *Journal of Eating Disorders* **10**, 154.

Thomas, J. *et al.* (2017) Avoidant/restrictive food intake disorder: a three-dimensional model of neurobiology with implications for etiology and treatment. *Current Psychiatry Reports* **19**(8), 54.

Timko, C.A. *et al.* (2019) Sex differences in adolescent anorexia and bulimia nervosa: beyond the signs and symptoms. *Current Psychiatry Reports* **21**(1), 1.

Vacca, M. *et al.* (2021) The relationship between perfectionism and eating-related symptoms in adolescents: a systematic review. *European Eating Disorders Review* **29**, 32–51.

van Eeden, A.E. *et al.* (2021) Incidence, prevalence and mortality of anorexia nervosa and bulimia nervosa. *Current Opinion in Psychiatry* **34**(6), 515–524.

van Hoeken, D. & Hoek, H.W. (2020) Review of the burden of eating disorders: mortality, disability, costs, quality of life, and family burden. *Current Opinion in Psychiatry* **33**(6), 521–527.

van Hoeken, D. *et al.* (2009) The validity and utility of subtyping BN. *International Journal of Eating Disorders* **42**, 595–602.

Vander Wal, J.S. (2012) Night eating syndrome: a critical review of the literature. *Clinical Psychology Review* **32**, 49–59.

Watson, H.J. *et al.* (2019) Genome-wide association study identifies eight risk loci and implicates metabo-psychiatric origins for anorexia nervosa. *Nature Genetics* **51**, 1207–1214.

Watts, R. *et al.* (2023) The clinical presentation of avoidant restrictive food intake disorder is largely independent of sex, autism spectrum disorder and anxiety traits. *eClinicalMedicine*. 63, 102190

Weissman, R. (2019) The role of sociocultural factors in the etiology of eating disorders. *Psychiatric Clinics of North America* **42**, 121–144.

Werz, J. *et al.* (2022) Alliance matters: but how much? A systematic review on therapeutic alliance and outcome in patients with anorexia nervosa and bulimia nervosa. *Eating and Weight Disorders - Studies on Anorexia, Bulimia and Obesity* **27**(4), 1279–1295.

Wilson, G.T. & Sysko, R. (2009) Frequency of binge eating episodes in bulimia nervosa and binge eating disorder: diagnostic considerations. *International Journal of Eating Disorders* **42**, 603–610.

Wolfe, B. *et al.* (2012) Bulimia nervosa in DSM-5. *Psychiatric Annals* **42**, 406–409.

World Health Organization (2019) *International Statistical Classification of Diseases and Related Health Problems* (11th revision). World Health Organization (WHO), Geneva, Switzerland.

Wu, X.Y. *et al.* (2019) The association between disordered eating and health-related quality of life among children and adolescents: a systematic review of population-based studies. *PLoS One* **14**(10), e0222777.

Wu, J. *et al.* (2020) Trends in the prevalence and disability-adjusted life years of eating disorders from 1990 to 2017: results from the Global Burden of Disease Study 2017. *Epidemiology and Psychiatric Sciences* **29**, E191.

Yim, S.H. & Schmidt, U. (2019) Self-help treatment of eating disorders. *Psychiatric Clinics* **42**, 231–241.

CHAPTER 70

Somatic symptom and related disorders

Charlotte Ulrikka Rask[1,2], Laura Markley[3,4,5,6] and Eva Szigethy[4,6]

[1]Department for Child and Adolescent Psychiatry, Aarhus University Hospital Psychiatry, Aarhus, Denmark
[2]Department for Clinical Medicine, Aarhus University, Aarhus, Denmark
[3]Department of Pediatrics, Akron Children's Hospital, Akron, OH, USA
[4]Department of Psychiatry and Behavioral Health, Akron Children's Hospital, Akron, OH, USA
[5]Department of Pediatrics, Northeastern Ohio Medical University, Rootstown, OH, USA
[6]Department of Psychiatry, Northeastern Ohio Medical University, Rootstown, OH, USA

Introduction

Somatic symptom and related disorders (SSRD) are common in pediatric medicine. They are characterized by bodily distress with presentation of somatic symptoms or illness worries that are either disproportionate or inconsistent with the history, physical examination, and other objective findings and not better explained by other psychopathology such as anxiety or depression (American Psychiatric Association, 2013). SSRD can be related to any bodily system. In younger children, recurrent abdominal pain is a typical symptom whereas headaches, fatigue, palpitations, and nausea are more frequent in adolescents (Rask *et al.*, 2009; Blake *et al.*, 2018). Neurological symptoms like gait disturbances, sensory loss, or nonepileptic seizures are rarer presentations across the age span (Ani *et al.*, 2013; Raper *et al.*, 2019).

SSRD place substantial psychosocial, educational, and financial strains on children and their families and in young people the associated disability is independent of demographics, comorbid psychological factors, and medical illness (Korterink *et al.*, 2015; Berg *et al.*, 2022). On a societal level, SSRD account for 15–20% of annual health care costs in the United States (US) (Saunders *et al.*, 2020). High cost/resource utilization includes repeated emergency room visits, prolonged hospitalizations, high rates of rehospitalization, excess diagnostic tests, and invasive procedures (Malas *et al.*, 2017). The patient and families often feel dismissed and may fear that a serious medical condition has been overlooked while clinicians may feel frustrated due to lack of knowledge on how to successfully approach SSRD (Hinton & Kirk, 2016).

It is critical that diagnostics and treatment take place in close collaboration with the pediatric/medical setting due to the primary presentation with physical complaints (Kangas *et al.*, 2020). Accurate assessment must include a thorough biopsychosocial formulation providing the basis for a multidisciplinary treatment plan. Since the 2010s, there has been a shift from symptom management to a rehabilitation/recovery model grounded in changing the neurobiology/neuroplasticity underlying symptom perception, mood, cognition, and behavior. Treatment may typically involve psychoeducation, psychological therapies that address the brain–body interface, family interventions, and sometimes pharmacology.

This chapter will describe the diagnostic classification and main clinical presentations of SSRD followed by proposed etiology and epidemiology. We will address assessment and treatment principles and lastly discuss the role of organizational medicine and future research directions. The *Diagnostic and Statistical Manual of Mental Disorders*, 5th edition (DSM-5; American Psychiatric Association, 2013) terminology will primarily be used but it is important to note that in clinical practice and research a variety of terms and diagnoses have been assigned to describe what are here designated as SSRD.

Characteristics and diagnostic classification

Conceptualization

The severity of bodily distress can be regarded on a spectrum, ranging from everyday bodily sensations that reflect temporary and self-limiting physiological changes to conditions with severe chronic and disabling symptoms. Approximately 40–50% of young children presenting unspecific somatic symptoms will have symptom remission within 6 months and only a third will attend primary care due to the symptoms (Rask *et al.*, 2013a).

Rutter's Child and Adolescent Psychiatry and Psychology, Seventh Edition.
Edited by Anita Thapar, Daniel S. Pine, Samuele Cortese, Cathy Creswell, Tamsin J. Ford, James F. Leckman, and Argyris Stringaris.

Companion website: www.wiley.com/go/thapar/rutterspsych7

Between 4–10% will experience recurrent or persistent symptoms with significant impairment (Rask *et al.*, 2009; Janssens *et al.*, 2014a). In the most severe cases, bodily distress is associated with long-lasting school absenteeism, reduced activities (Janssens *et al.*, 2011), and risk of secondary iatrogenic injuries from medical testing (Dunphy *et al.*, 2019). Often the symptoms are accompanied by emotional distress with anxiety and depression (Campo, 2012). Levels of distress, impairment, comorbid psychopathology, and health care use are likely to increase across the bodily distress severity spectrum.

Historically, there has been a dichotomy between "medically explained versus unexplained" and "mental versus physical" in describing SSRD. The current perspective is that these conditions are the product of complex interactions involving multiple biological and psychosocial factors with neurobiological alterations in brain circuits underlying emotions, cognitions, and somatic perceptions (Bègue *et al.*, 2019; Henningsen *et al.*, 2018).

Terminology and diagnostic classification

Classification

Young people with bodily distress often present to pediatric medical services due to the somatic nature of their complaints. In medical health care, depending on the prominent symptom and the medical specialty consulted, a symptom diagnosis like unspecified abdominal pain, nonepileptic seizures, or a functional somatic syndrome (FSS) designation (e.g., chronic widespread pain, irritable bowel syndrome [IBS], or chronic fatigue) may be applied (Kangas *et al.*, 2020). However, research suggests that these syndromes may be overlapping and different permutations of the same underlying phenotype or related phenotypes (Petersen *et al.*, 2020). In parallel, mental health care has its own diagnostic labels for the same group of patients. Severe bodily distress was formerly categorized under somatoform and related disorders in both the *Diagnostic and Statistical Manual of Mental Disorders*, 4th Edition (DSM-IV; American Psychiatric Association, 2000) and the 10th revision of the *International Statistical Classification of Diseases and Health Problems* (ICD-10; World Health Organization, 2004). These classification systems have been criticized for their utility in daily practice (Löwe *et al.*, 2008) and importantly younger children or even adolescents rarely present symptoms sufficiently varied, severe, or disabling enough to qualify for these diagnoses (Schulte & Petermann, 2011). In addition, many clinicians regard the terms "somatoform" and "somatization" as pejorative and overemphasizing a mind–body dualism (Dimsdale *et al.*, 2011).

Changes in classification

Somatoform and related disorders have been renamed and grouped as SSRD in the current DSM-5 (American Psychiatric Association, 2013). These disorders are characterized by the prominence of somatic symptoms associated with significant distress and impairment. The main diagnosis, somatic symptom disorder (SSD), is designed to lump together different DSM-IV somatoform diagnoses (somatization disorder, pain disorder, undifferentiated somatoform disorder, and aspects of hypochondriasis) into a single condition. This category also includes illness anxiety disorder consisting of high levels of illness worries without somatic symptoms, and conversion disorder (functional neurological symptom disorder [FNSD]).

In ICD-11 (World Health Organization, 2019), the new diagnosis bodily distress disorder (BDD) substitutes many of the somatoform disorders and presentations dominated by fatigue, diagnosed as neurasthenia in ICD-10. As opposed to DSM-5, ICD-11 has now placed hypochondriasis within the grouping of obsessive–compulsive and related disorders (World Health Organization, 2019), supported by some evidence that hypochondriasis may respond to the same treatments (Gureje & Reed, 2016). Another difference is that the ICD-11 has functional neurological disorders within the neurology section, though they also remain in the psychiatry section as the separate category of dissociative disorders (Stone *et al.*, 2014).

Suggestion for a new common classification

To provide clarity and a common terminology in describing bodily distress, a new classification system functional somatic disorders (FSD) was recently proposed on behalf of the European research network (EURONET-SOMA; European Network to Improve Diagnostic, Treatment, and Health Care for Patients with Persistent Somatic Symptoms) (Burton *et al.*, 2020). FSD are diagnosed based on symptom patterns as (i) multisystem, (ii) single system, or (iii) single symptoms, depending on the clinical presentation. While additional specifiers may be added to take account of psychological features or co-occurring diseases, neither of these are sufficient nor necessary to make the diagnosis (Table 70.1). However, this diagnostic proposal is currently based on clinical consensus and has yet to prove itself in clinical and scientific practice.

Clinical presentations

A summary of the diagnostic criteria for the three DSM-5 diagnoses (and corresponding ICD-11 diagnoses) of most relevance in clinical practice for youth are listed in Table 70.2 and case vignettes are woven in below to illustrate key presentation features.

Conditions dominated by various persistent physical symptoms

The child's functioning is affected by persistent somatic symptoms causing significant distress and disruption of everyday life, often as school absence and a decrease in social and physical activities. There may be multiple somatic symptoms or only one severe symptom, typically pain. Symptoms can be specific (e.g., pain in the abdomen or headaches) or vaguer (e.g., fatigue). Any part of the body may be involved with multiple symptoms tending to cluster within specific organ systems, including gastrointestinal, cardiorespiratory, musculoskeletal, or fatigue-related

Table 70.1 Comparison of key features of somatic symptom disorder (SSD), bodily distress disorder (BDD), functional somatic syndromes (FSS), and functional somatic disorders (FSD).

Term	Somatic symptom disorder (SSD)	Bodily distress disorder (BDD)	Functional somatic syndromes (FSS)	Functional somatic disorders (FSD)
Classification system	DSM-5	ICD-11	ICD-11 and several specialty-specific classifications	New common classification proposed by EURONET-SOMA
	Mental disorder	Mental disorder	Physical disorder classified according to primary symptom localization	Occupy neutral space within classification systems
Replaces/examples	Largely replaces DSM-IV somatoform disorders; can now also include patients with distressing symptoms attributable to general medical conditions	Largely replaces ICD-10 somatoform disorders; can now also include patients with distressing symptoms attributable to general medical conditions	According to primary symptom localization, e.g., functional abdominal pain/irritable bowel syndrome (IBS); fibromyalgia/chronic widespread pain; tension type headache; chronic fatigue; noncardiac chest pain	Symptoms within one or more body systems: musculoskeletal; gastrointestinal; cardiorespiratory; genito-urinary; nervous system; fatigue-related
Key feature	Excessive, disproportionate, or maladaptive responses to one or more physical symptoms or sensations of any etiology that result in significant distress or impairment	Excessive, disproportionate, or maladaptive responses to one or more physical symptoms or sensations of any etiology that result in significant distress or impairment	Defined by a medical primary symptom or a certain symptom pattern	Persistent and troublesome physical symptoms fitting characteristic symptom patterns
Medically explained or unexplained	Both medically unexplained and medically explained physical symptoms	Both medically unexplained and medically explained physical symptoms	Medically unexplained/poorly explained symptoms	Does not characterize symptoms as medically explained or not but as complex interactions between brain and body
Exclusions/differential diagnoses	Certain psychiatric disorders have to be excluded, general medical diagnoses are not excluded	Does not exclude presence of depression or anxiety, general medical diagnoses are not excluded	Unclear relations to differential diagnoses, multiple FSS diagnoses possible	Other possible and psychological differential diagnoses should be considered
Emotional and behavioral responses required	Yes	Yes	Not required for diagnosis but considered common and may be important for treatment	Not required but can be used as optional specifiers
Severity options	Mild, Moderate, Severe; characterized by emotional or behavioral responses and degree of impairment	Mild, Moderate, Severe; characterized by emotional or behavioral responses and degree of impairment	Not applicable	Single symptom, Single system, Multisystem
Hypothesized cause	Health anxiety and misinterpretation of bodily symptoms	Health anxiety and misinterpretation of bodily symptoms	Malfunction of the central nervous system (CNS) often suggested to be involved (hyperarousal of autonomic nervous system, hypothalamic–pituitary–adrenal [HPA] dysfunction)	Symptoms are the product of complex interactions, involving multiple biological and psychosocial factors

Table 70.2 Summary of the *Diagnostic and Statistical Manual of Mental Disorders*, 5th edition (DSM-5; American Psychiatric Association, 2013) diagnoses corresponding to the most common clinical presentations of severe bodily distress in children and adolescents.

Somatic Symptom Disorder DSM-5 (300.82) *Corresponds to most of F45.x in ICD-10/ Bodily Distress Disorder (DC20) in ICD-11*	**Conversion Disorder (Functional Neurological Symptom Disorder [FNSD]) DSM-5 (300.11)** *Corresponds to dissociative (conversion) motor/ seizure/sensory disorders in ICD-10 (F44.4–7)/ Dissociative Neurological Symptom Disorder (6B60) or functional neurological disorders in the nervous system in ICD-11*	**Illness Anxiety Disorder DSM-5 (300.7)** *Corresponds to hypochondriasis (F45.21) in ICD-10/(6B23) in ICD-11*
I. Physical symptom(s) that are emotionally distressing and functionally impairing. **II.** Excessive thoughts, feelings, and behaviors related to these somatic symptoms or associated health concerns. **III.** Symptoms persistent for >6 months. Specifiers: Predominant pain (previously pain disorder): This category is reserved for individuals presenting predominantly pain complaints who also satisfy criteria II and III.	**I.** Symptom(s) of altered voluntary motor or sensory function. **II.** Clinical findings inconsistent with recognized neurologic or general medical condition. **III.** The symptoms are not better explained by another medical or mental disorder. **IV.** The symptom(s) cause significant distress, functional impairment, or require medical evaluation.	**I.** Preoccupation with having or getting a serious illness. **II.** Somatic symptoms are not present or, if present, are only mild in intensity. If another medical condition is present, the preoccupation is clearly excessive. **III.** There is a high level of anxiety about health. **IV.** There are excessive health-related behaviors (e.g., repeated checks of the body for signs of illness) or exhibition of maladaptive avoidance (e.g., avoids doctor appointments and hospitals). **V.** Illness preoccupation has been present for >6 months. **VI.** The illness-related preoccupation is not better explained by another mental disorder. Specifiers: **1.** Care-seeking type: Medical care, including physician visits or undergoing tests and procedures, is frequently used. **2.** Care-avoidant type: Medical care is rarely used.

Box 70.1 Case vignette: Somatic Symptom Disorder

13-year-old Jim has become increasingly distressed by various physical symptoms over the past years. Since starting school at age six, he has suffered from headaches. Two years ago, he had a flu-like episode. Subsequently, he continued to feel fatigued and developed different and fluctuating physical symptoms. His daily life is now impaired by constant pain in his muscles and joints, headaches, dizziness, and stomachaches with a tendency to constipation. He often stays home from school and spends many hours playing online. During childhood he was described with a fearful temperament and his mother notes he seemed sensitive to life stressors. Both Jim and his parents are very attentive to the symptoms. He has been examined many times by different medical experts. His parents feel that his symptoms are not taken seriously by the doctors and that they think he purposely produces the symptoms for attention. Jim has tried physiotherapy and pain medications but only with short-term effect.

Diagnosis: DSM-5 Somatic Symptom Disorder (SSD), ICD-11 Bodily Distress Disorder (BDD)

symptom clusters. Concurrent anxiety and depression may be present.

Developmental aspects

These conditions tend to present equally among young boys and young girls but are more common among females than males in adolescence (Rask *et al.*, 2009; Münker *et al.*, 2022). Young children usually present with a single prominent symptom such as abdominal pain, whereas older children and adolescents may have more complex presentations with symptoms from several organ systems (see Box 70.1 and Video 70.1). In the youngest age groups, the associated impairment is closely related to parental anxiety and help-seeking behaviors as it is the caregivers who interpret the symptoms and determine the child's symptom-related school absence and medical help seeking (Schulte & Petermann, 2011).

Conditions dominated by neurological symptoms inconsistent with neurological or other medical diseases

The clinical presentation often develops abruptly with symptoms involving apparent deficits in voluntary motor function, e.g., gait disturbances, seizures, weakness or paralysis of limbs, abnormal limb postures, or sensory function, such as loss of sensation in a body part, blindness, or deafness (Raper *et al.*, 2019; see Box 70.2). Speech can also be affected with loss of voice or slurred speech. Some may present with urinary retention. The onset, exacerbation, or maintenance is commonly attributed to psychological stress, but a clear stressor is not always identifiable (Ludwig *et al.*, 2018) and is no longer part of the diagnostic criteria for an FNSD/conversion disorder in DSM-5. Due to the dramatic presentation and serious differential diagnosis, such as epilepsy or a brain tumor, these young persons are often seen in emergency departments and neurological settings. The child or adolescent may appear

Box 70.2 Case vignette: Conversion

Seventeen-year-old Maria started to experience facial numbness one year ago, shortly after starting high school, that she attributed to sleeping with her face against the window during the long school bus drive. The numbness spread to the left side of her upper body and then both her legs. Her mood worsened and she started to isolate herself. She was evaluated in a neurological department where the clinical examination, various blood tests, and brain scans were all normal. Subsequently, she was referred to psychiatry for further assessment.

At the first psychiatric appointment she revealed that one week prior to her first symptoms, her boyfriend broke up with her. Maria was devastated and further exploration revealed it reminded her of feeling helpless when her father abandoned the family when she was five.

Diagnosis: DSM-5 Conversion/Functional Neurological Symptom Disorder (FNSD), ICD-11 Dissociative Disorder

emotionally unaffected despite the severe symptom presentation and associated impairment. However, this so-called "Belle Indifference" is nonspecific and should not be used to establish the diagnosis.

Developmental aspects

Functional neurological symptoms are rarely identified in children under seven years. The incidence increases with age and with a female preponderance (Ani *et al.*, 2013; Hansen *et al.*, 2020). In children, limb weakness, visual disturbances, or seizures are common symptom presentations. More complex and mixed symptoms may become prominent during adolescence (Kozlowska *et al.*, 2007). The clinical presentation of non-epileptic seizures can differ across the age span. In younger children, seizures often present as subtle motor activity such as prolonged staring with unresponsiveness, isolated head shaking, eye fluttering, generalized limpness, and behavioral changes or combativeness. From the age of 13 the semiological features resemble more those seen in adults with prominent motor activity such as generalized arrhythmic jerking or flailing of extremities, side-to-side head movements, and forward pelvic thrusting (Patel *et al.*, 2007).

Conditions dominated by excessive illness worries

If the child or adolescent primarily presents with extensive worries and anxiety about having or developing a serious illness but no or minimal somatic symptoms, it may be more appropriate to consider illness anxiety disorder (DSM-5) or hypochondriasis (ICD-11). The key feature is the cycle of worry and reassurance-seeking regarding health (see Box 70.3), as opposed to a focus on relief of distress caused by somatic symptoms as in SSD.

Developmental aspects

For a long time, it was assumed that severe illness or health anxiety was rare in children and adolescents, but recent research has documented that excessive illness worries can occur at younger

Box 70.3 Case vignette: Illness Anxiety Disorder

Ten-year-old Sara has more and more worries about having heart problems. It started two years ago when she experienced her grandfather having a heart attack. Since then, Sara has become more and more anxious about there being something seriously wrong with her heart, that it will stop beating and that she will die. Her anxiety can be triggered if she hears an ambulance or if she feels dizziness or if she is in pain. She seeks reassurance from her parents many times a day and she has started to involve her teachers in school, for example, by asking them to check her pulse and confirm that she does not look pale. Her parents have taken her to the doctor many times, hoping this could calm her down but it has only become worse. A short time after a medical consultation her anxiety reappears and has led to reduced school performance and social functioning. In infancy, she was described as hypersensitive to sensory and tactile stimuli and at age seven she was diagnosed with attention deficit hyperactivity disorder (ADHD).

Diagnosis: DSM-5 Illness Anxiety Disorder, ICD-11 Hypochondriasis

ages with similar patterns of fears, beliefs, and attitudes as seen in adults (Rask *et al.*, 2016). A developmental issue is that children may not be capable of articulating the content of their fears, or the focus of their apprehension, making it difficult to assess the difference between symptoms of illness anxiety and other types of worries (Caes *et al.*, 2016). The key clinical features with excessive health concerns, and preoccupation with symptoms and illness, might also be difficult to isolate from the beliefs and psychosocial functioning of the parents, especially in young children.

Other symptom presentations

In some cases, it is excessive and seemingly unreasonable parental worries about the child's bodily symptoms, recently conceptualized as health anxiety by proxy (Thorgaard *et al.*, 2017), that lead to unnecessary medical assessments and treatments, risk of iatrogen harm, and may compromise the child's physical and mental health. This is not to be confused with the rarer cases of factitious disorder by proxy (formerly known as "Munchausen Syndrome by Proxy"), where the concerns are an expression of fabricated or induced illness due to the deliberate production or fabrication of somatic symptoms in a child by a parent or caregiver (Glaser, 2020) (see also Chapter 25, "Child abuse and neglect").

Comparatively short-lived episodes with key features of bodily distress may better be diagnosed as an adjustment disorder if they closely follow the experience of a marked and universally stressful event.

Feigned symptoms, i.e., intentional production of either grossly exaggerated or falsely produced symptoms to achieve privileges or attention, are probably rare but should be classified as malingering or factitious disorder. However, a degree of intentionality can also be present and expected across the range of SSRD and should be duly evaluated.

Differential diagnosis and comorbidity

Somatic symptoms and health concerns are often a feature of anxiety and depressive disorders but usually not the primary focus of concern. A depressive disorder should be considered as the primary diagnosis if the young person presents with core depressive symptoms such as low mood and lack of interest, and the somatic symptoms, e.g., tiredness, are not regarded as key or central to distress and impairment. In obsessive—compulsive disorder, a child or adolescent may display distressing illness-related thoughts and behaviors, but the obsessive nature of the thoughts in combination with associated compulsions take the center stage. Likewise, in generalized anxiety disorder the predominant fears are not linked specifically to worries about harboring a serious disease but are about many things (family, peers, school). Nevertheless, anxiety and mood disorders are often comorbid with severe bodily distress and reported to be present in one-third to one-half and even higher numbers of children and adolescents with different clinical presentations of SSRD (Campo, 2012). Also, underlying neurodevelopmental disorders such as autism, attention deficit hyperactivity disorder (ADHD), or learning disabilities have been shown to be common comorbidities (Lipsker *et al.*, 2018).

There is a prominent interplay of post-traumatic stress disorder (PTSD)-related symptoms with SSRD and dissociation where symptoms of hyperarousal in PTSD, particularly physiological reactivation and concentration difficulties, have been shown to be strongly correlated to somatic symptoms (Kratzer *et al.*, 2022) (see also Chapter 58 on PTSD).

Comorbidity of bodily distress and medical disorders is frequent, typically with amplification or expansion of the somatic symptoms related to the medical disorder, e.g., functional gastrointestinal symptoms are reported in up to 30% of children with inflammatory bowel disease in remission (Limbri *et al.*, 2022) and 14% of young people with functional seizures are reported also diagnosed with epilepsy (Hansen *et al.*, 2020) (see Chapter 26, "Neurological disorders and psychopathology").

In rare cases, and mainly in older children and adolescents, the somatic complaints and illness worries can be the expression of an underlying psychotic disorder (Simon *et al.*, 2014). Typically, the health concerns and bodily complaints will be bizarre and fixed. Especially in cases dominated by functional neurological symptoms, rare neurological conditions such as brain tumors or pediatric dementia characterized by chronic global neurocognitive decline (Djafar *et al.*, 2023) must also be considered.

Biopsychosocial explanatory model and risk factors

Current formulations for SSRD suggest that a combination of biological, psychological, and social risk factors in the child, family, and broader environment may bring on individual disabling bodily distress with neurobiological alterations in brain

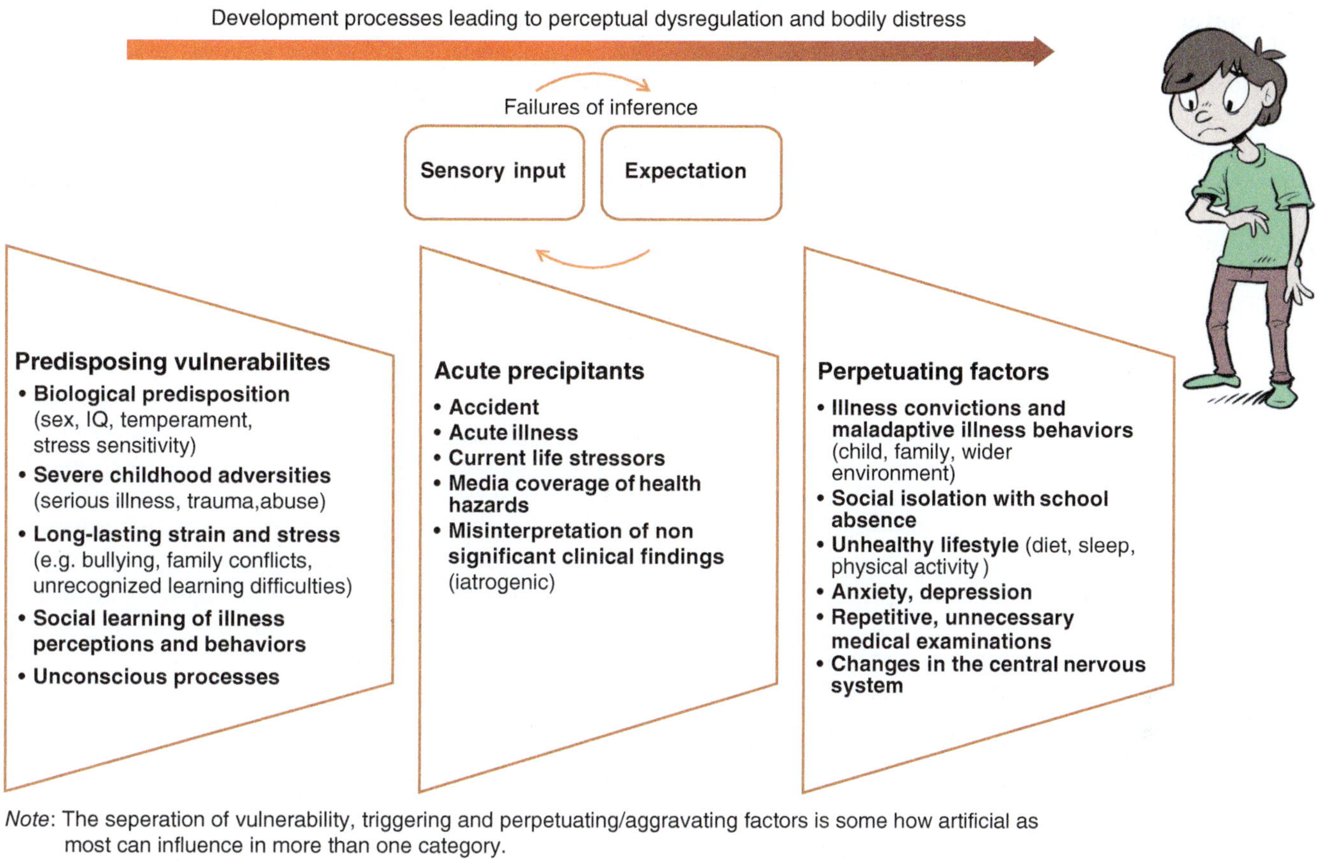

Figure 70.1 Schematic biopsychosocial model for the development of bodily distress within a predictive processing perspective.

circuits underlying emotions, cognitions, and somatic perceptions. These factors are typically categorized as predisposing vulnerabilities, acute precipitants, or perpetuating factors (Figure 70.1). In the following sections, these risk factors are reviewed according to each category, though it should be emphasized that this separation is somewhat artificial as most factors can influence all domains.

Predisposing vulnerabilities

Predisposing factors comprise various innate and acquired vulnerabilities.

Genetic predisposition and personality traits

Although familial clustering is well-established in conditions dominated by bodily distress, such as IBS (Henström & D'Amato, 2016) and chronic fatigue (Dibble *et al.*, 2020), there are only weak genetic associations reported and a lack of evidence to suggest that major genetic factor(s) contribute to pathophysiology.

Females being more at risk than males, especially from puberty onward, is suggested to be due to gender-specific socialization of females to express symptom experiences to a higher degree, and their use of more internalizing or ruminative coping styles compared with boys (Martel, 2013). Sex-based physiological and neurobiological differences associated with puberty may also play a role (Rhee, 2005).

Infants who demonstrate a fearful temperament and problems with hypersensitivity to sensory and tactile stimuli have increased risk of later childhood somatic complaints (Rask *et al.*, 2013b). Insecure attachment styles (Vesterling & Koglin, 2020), and conscientious and perfectionistic personality traits have been described in youth with bodily distress (Bonvanie *et al.*, 2015), as have difficulties with emotional regulation (Buchnik-Daniely *et al.*, 2021), poor awareness of emotional experience (also called alexithymia) and negative affect (Villanueva Badenes *et al.*, 2016; Hadji-Michael *et al.*, 2019). Such lack of emotional competence may lead to difficulty in adaptively handling emotional situations, contributing to prolonged feelings of stress, eventually manifesting as bodily distress. This is further supported by findings of increased stress sensitivity and lesser use of accommodative coping strategies in young people with SSRD (Walker *et al.*, 2007). Also, cognitive difficulties (Kingma *et al.*, 2011), and neurodevelopmental disorders, with impaired social capacity or emotional language to process ongoing stress, have been shown to induce a higher risk of bodily distress (Larsen *et al.*, 2022; Hogendoorn *et al.*, 2023).

Childhood adversities and long-standing stress

Childhood adversity with the exposure to various types of abuse and neglect has long been considered important in the development of bodily distress (Oh *et al.*, 2018). However, several studies also show associations between childhood somatic complaints and broader psychosocial stressors (Undheim & Sund, 2011; Bonvanie *et al.*, 2017a; LaVigne *et al.*, 2020). Likewise, in studies of children with FNSD and chronic/complex pain, antecedent illness or injury, family conflict, and bullying in school, all overwhelming the child's coping resources, have consistently emerged as important antecedents (McInnis *et al.*, 2020). High expectations and peer competition can also contribute to bodily distress in children and adolescents (Bujoreanu *et al.*, 2014). Such exposure to potentially long-lasting traumatic stress, can activate multiple components of the stress system, as well as the brain regions involved in pain, salience detection, arousal, and emotional processing, suggested to cause predisposition to bodily distress (Kozlowska, 2013) (see also Chapters 5, 22, or 59).

Social learning of illness perceptions and behaviors

Intrapersonal child risk factors for bodily distress can be exacerbated by the environment. Higher rates of physical disease have been demonstrated in families of children with somatic complaints (Elliott *et al.*, 2020). These associations can partly be due to genetic predisposition but also due to social learning, i.e., how parents manage their own stress and somatic symptoms, including modeling of adaptive versus maladaptive emotion regulatory strategies, affects how their children cope with somatic symptoms or bodily distress (Levy, 2011). Of more immediate relevance, high parental focus on and involvement with the child's somatic symptoms, as well as overprotective parenting, are associated with the development of bodily distress in young people (Janssens *et al.*, 2009). Thus, growing up with a caregiver with illness anxiety is likely to negatively influence the child's ability to cognitively process body signals.

Unconscious processes

Although psychodynamic principles had their beginnings in theoretical and observational psychology, in more recent years, components of unconscious, such as priming, dissociation, automaticity, and subliminal reactions, have been associated with specific neurobiological pathways (Harvey *et al.*, 2006; Bargh & Morsella, 2008). Although challenging to study, it is plausible that the interplay of biological, environmental, and social priming with developmental windows can predispose to the paradoxical somatic symptoms seen in FNSD, which may more often occur in the context of a stressor or trauma (Kratzer *et al.*, 2022).

Precipitating factors

Precipitating factors cover a broad range of physical and emotional stressors or trauma (acute illness, accidents, and stressful life events) that acutely or more gradually increase the level of overall bodily distress. It has been suggested that precipitating factors can influence which physical symptoms develop. For example, gastroenteritis may trigger recurrent abdominal pain and IBS (Thabane *et al.*, 2010), infection can be followed by persistent fatigue (Katz & Jason, 2013), a bone fracture can induce loss of limb function, or a minor head injury may precede chronic headache and concentration difficulties (Riemann *et al.*, 2021). Wider psychosocial mechanisms, such as media coverage and potentially pathogenic environmental health hazards, can also be precipitating factors. For example, in a post-COVID era, priming of illness anxiety precipitated by an actual viral infection or watching the suffering or death of others from the virus may have left lasting negative impacts on body threat appraisal in youth with preexisting vulnerability to SSRD (Haig-Ferguson *et al.*, 2021; D'Orsi *et al.*, 2025). Iatrogenic factors can also play a significant role. Health care professionals may be motivated to perform extensive medical workups due to fear of overlooking a treatable medical condition (Morabito *et al.*, 2020). Repeated examinations can increase the risk of spurious findings that are wrongly regarded as clinically significant, and thereby induce anxiety and uncertainty, which may further activate bodily distress in the child.

Perpetuating factors

Perpetuating factors include psychosocial factors such as psychiatric comorbidity and factors reinforcing maladaptive illness perceptions and behaviors in the young person.

Illness conviction and maladaptive illness behaviors

Maladaptive illness perceptions and behaviors may be strong maintaining and aggravating factors for bodily distress in young people (Kallesoe *et al.*, 2021a). Negative illness belief examples are catastrophizing that one cannot control the symptoms or that they are signs of serious bodily damage. Maladaptive behaviors, such as an increased focus on bodily sensations and withdrawal from activities, including school absenteeism, due to fear of provoking symptoms (avoidance behavior) or excessive rest (limiting behavior) (Janssens *et al.*, 2014b; Smith *et al.*, 2020), are typically prompted by the negative illness beliefs. Unhealthy lifestyle patterns, such as sleeping problems, may also develop and aggravate the bodily distress (Bonvanie *et al.*, 2016; Christensen *et al.*, 2019).

Reinforcing factors in family and the wider environment

Parents may feel insecure on how to help their child with bodily distress and often report that the disorder can inflict both concern and distress in the family (Hulgaard *et al.*, 2019b). They and others in the close network, (e.g., the school), may unintentionally support the child in maladaptive illness behaviors by encouraging inactivity, withdrawal from normal activities/social events, and school absence, hoping to prevent symptom exacerbation. Demands for excessive medical workup may be rooted in the parents' own excessive and distressing worries about their child's health, and these parents may need help for their own health-related anxiety (Ingeman *et al.*, 2022).

Iatrogenic factors

Often, pediatric and medical services are not well-attuned to identify SSRD in young people (Hinton & Kirk, 2016; Morabito *et al.*, 2020). Physicians can be reluctant to diagnose mental health or behavioral problems, preferring to label bodily distress as a poorly defined disorder with a risk of unjustified therapies (Peri *et al.*, 2019). Furthermore, the increase of medical subspecialization and care fragmentation makes it difficult to consider the whole picture and work within a biopsychosocial illness framework, resulting in doctors excessively pursuing organic explanations, and possibly worsening illness worries and behaviors in the child and family. Therefore, it is important for health care professionals to be aware of the dangers of overinvestigation and increase their proficiency in making a positive diagnosis of SSRD (Cottrell, 2016).

Putative changes in the central and peripheral nervous systems

It may be helpful for clinicians to provide a neurobiological explanation related to brain processes proposed to contribute to somatic symptom perpetuation including attentional biases, unconscious interpretation biases, sensitization, and altered effort perception (van der Schaaf *et al.*, 2018). Both trauma and experience of illness may induce central sensitization with prolonged recovery or symptom recurrence after the traumatic event or illness resolves (De Bellis & Zisk, 2014). This could be due to both a cognitive conditioned response (fearful misinterpretation of and focused attention to physical sensations that amplify symptom perception) but may also involve neuronal sensitivity to further pain sensations due to neuronal memory traces (Price & Inyang, 2015) (see also the later section "A newer explanatory framework: predictive coding theory"). Neuroimaging studies provide emerging evidence for aberrant neurobiological findings in both children and adults with various SSRD, including abnormal activity in cerebral networks and sensorimotor, prefrontal, striatal-thalamic, paralimbic, and limbic structural alterations, i.e., brain areas which are involved in impulse- and self-control, emotion regulation, and sensory discrimination (Bègue *et al.*, 2019).

In terms of the peripheral nervous system, low systemic cortisol after awakening has been associated with overtiredness and musculoskeletal pain and low cortisol during psychosocial stress with gastrointestinal and headache symptoms (Janssens *et al.*, 2012). In adolescents with disabling fatigue, orthostatic anomalies with alterations in hormonal systems controlling osmolality and blood volume have been shown, with improvement associated with better autonomic cardiovascular control (Sulheim *et al.*, 2012).

Protective factors

Less research has focused on protective factors, but factors which reduce stressors and protect against psychopathology in general are also likely to be protective for development of SSRD (Vanderbilt-Adriance & Shaw, 2008). On an individual level, cognitive resources can provide children with a broader range of coping mechanisms, the potential for academic success, self-efficacy, and social standing. In children with chronic abdominal pain accommodative coping (acceptance and self-encouragement) in preference to distress, withdrawal, and acceptance of impairment was associated with less distress and a better long-term outcome (Walker *et al.*, 2005). Intact and/or well-functioning families with good parenting skills and good school and peer supports can similarly decrease stress and facilitate coping, as will a favorable socioeconomic background. Complete recovery has been found to be highly correlated with full parental acceptance of the diagnosis and acknowledgment of a multifactorial illness model (Wiggins *et al.*, 2022). Good channels of communication between health care professionals and schools, with a clear plan for returning to school and how to manage symptoms in the school setting, can be important for faster recovery (Ibeziako & Bujoreanu, 2011). The existence of pediatric liaison teams with experience in the field are also proposed as protective factors (Garralda & Slaveska-Hollis, 2016).

A newer explanatory framework: predictive coding theory

New developments in the conceptualization of how the brain works, emphasizing the predictive nature of the brain, hence known as the predictive coding theory (Friston, 2010; Clark, 2013; Hohwy, 2013), have recently been applied to understand the variable relationship between physiological dysfunction and self-reported symptoms (Henningsen *et al.*, 2018; Pezzulo *et al.*, 2019). This theory proposes that the brain, to construct an adaptive model of the (external and internal) world, uses information from neural activity that is not only triggered by peripheral sensory input, but also by neural activity that is generated by the brain itself (i.e., spontaneous dynamics), reflecting previous experiences. This leads to counterflowing streams of neural activation across several hierarchical levels of the brain where stimulation by peripheral input (called "likelihood" in the context of the statistical method of Bayesian inference) interacts with activations generated by the brain that act as model-based predictions of the input ("priors") within a specific context. These various layers of processing lead to prediction errors, i.e., the brain is constantly generating and updating a mental model of the environment which is used to generate predictions of sensory input that are compared to actual sensory input (Figure 70.2).

According to this view somatic symptoms result from individual prediction models rather than the processing of somatosensory input per se (Ainley *et al.*, 2016). Although predictions ("priors") need not be correct, they can still be given more weight when sensory signals are ambiguous. This means the brain can—as with optical illusions—generate "misinterpretation" of the body's inner state (Van den Bergh *et al.*, 2017). Being critical for symptom perception, this allows and suggests important variability in the relationship between symptom experience and peripheral bodily dysfunction. While this relationship is generally strong in acute monosymptomatic health conditions,

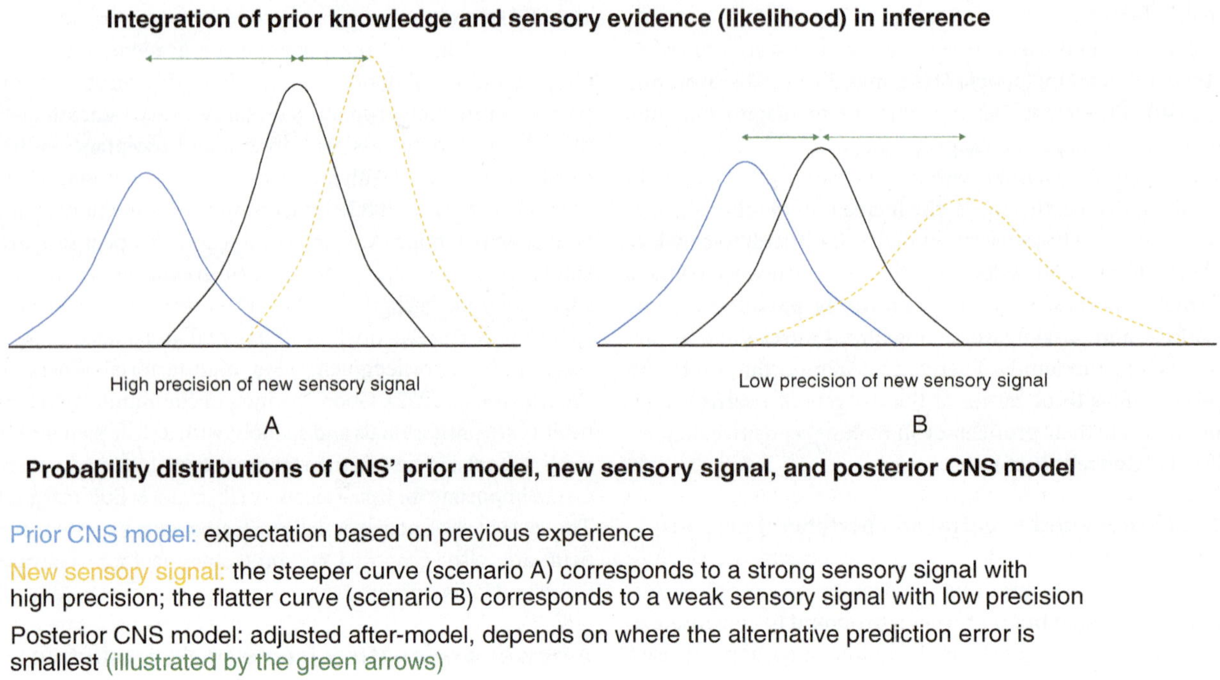

Figure 70.2 The predictive coding model to understand symptom perception. CNS = central nervous system. *Source*: Adapted from Henningsen *et al.* (2018).

it typically becomes much weaker in chronic multisymptomatic conditions, due to factors that may increase the vulnerability for symptom-related learning and memory processes. Bodily distress can thus be regarded as a disorder of perception brought about by the overactivation of symptom representation in memory (Van den Bergh *et al.*, 2017).

Epidemiology

Limitations of existing epidemiological research

There are a multitude of barriers to establishing accurate SSRD epidemiological data. The typically subjective nature of the illness descriptions and assigned diagnoses are often not amenable to operationalized delineation and identification (Kratzer *et al.*, 2022). This is compounded by symptom overlap with other psychological illnesses, primarily anxiety and depression, with limited understanding of how best to categorize associated somatic variances. In pediatrics, the developmental and communicative naivety of patients complicates diagnosis. Furthermore, lack of diagnostic clarity can lead physicians to avoid placing the finding of SSRD in medical records, impacting the overall estimation of affected children and adolescents (Wiggins *et al.*, 2021).

Prevalence and incidence

Despite challenges in determining the epidemiology of SSRD, studies support that these disorders account for a significant amount of morbidity worldwide. The pooled prevalence rate based on 29 studies from various countries has been estimated to be 31.0% for functional somatic symptoms and 3.3% for SSRD (Vesterling *et al.*, 2023). Further, SSRD have been reported to be an underlying diagnosis in 25–50% of all pediatric primary care visits (Malas *et al.*, 2017; Salmon *et al.*, 2022).

Early in the COVID-19 pandemic, a decrease in the prevalence of pediatric chronic pain in the US was reported (Aluko *et al.*, 2023). However, subsequent studies have posited that the multifaceted disruptions of routine, lifestyle, and education caused by COVID-19 may have produced lasting effects on the development, illness awareness, and coping prowess of youth, but that ongoing assessment is necessary (Rider *et al.*, 2021). An increase has been noted in persistent gastrointestinal symptoms and fatigue, even in the absence of concomitant depression and anxiety, among those who had COVID-19 (Noviello *et al.*, 2022), as well as increased risk of anxiety, depression, and somatic symptoms also in youth with minimal symptoms (Meade, 2021).

Sociocultural aspects

Socioeconomic status (SES) impact on SSRD is unclear. Lower SES has been associated with a greater number of adverse childhood events, and for patients with functional seizures it is linked to higher anxiety and lower health care literacy. However, functional seizure patients with high SES were found to have inferior social functioning and increased caregiver burden (Kline *et al.*, 2023).

Racial demographic effects on occurrence and outcome are inconsistent in the literature. Some reports state racial prevalence is consistent with overall population and parallels local populations. Others conclude that non-White adolescents are more likely to report multiple, high-frequency somatic symptoms, but this may be due to evaluator bias, as providers have rated Black pediatric patients as more distressed by pain and with greater pain interference than their White counterparts (Salmon *et al.*, 2022; Kline *et al.*, 2023).

Ethnicity can affect presentation. A study on functional seizures demonstrated that Iranian youth tended to have more severe events than American, Brazilian, Canadian, or Venezuelan youth (Salmon *et al.*, 2022). Furthermore, the same study stated that in Japan, 71% of pediatric patients diagnosed with SSRD reported orthostatic intolerance, i.e., the inability to tolerate the upright posture because of signs, such as hypotension, and symptoms, such as lightheadedness, relieved by lying down (Stewart, 2013), which is a much higher incidence than in other countries (Salmon *et al.*, 2022).

Migratory status appears to be an independent risk for developing an SSRD, which is associated with acculturative stress and experiences with discrimination. Children living in immigration detention housing frequently report somatic symptoms including headaches and abdominal pain (Kline *et al.*, 2023). Maintaining ethnic identity has been found to be protective, whereas acculturative adaptations in children as a source of familial conflict are shown to be associated with increased risk of SSRD. Gender-diverse youth with chronic pain are reported to have a lower quality of life than cisgender youth with pain disorders (Kline *et al.*, 2023).

Longitudinal course

The longitudinal course of pediatric SSRD varies but has in general a more hopeful outlook than the same disorders in adults. Still, childhood SSRD increase the risk for future SSRD, and psychological disorders, such as anxiety and depression (Malas *et al.*, 2017; Jason & Mirin, 2021), but poor patient mental-health follow-up is often the case. This is concerning given that there is an elevated risk of suicidal ideation and attempts in SSRD (Turiaco *et al.*, 2022).

Predictors of a prolonged course include several psychosocial factors, the number of affected organ systems, and also the prominent subtype of SSRD—functional gastrointestinal disorders have prevalent chronicity (60% of affected children will transit to adulthood with symptoms [Hollier *et al.*, 2022]), whereas higher rates of symptom recovery are found in pediatric functional neurological disorders (77% long-term remittance rate [Raper *et al.*, 2019]) and pediatric chronic fatigue (54–94% significant improvement or complete recovery [Collin *et al.*, 2015]). Parental somatic symptoms and/or ill health and the presence of comorbid anxiety and depression in the child have also been reported to potentially worsen prognosis (Malas *et al.*, 2017).

Assessment

Box 70.4 Assessment at a glance

- Review hospital records/illness history with emphasis on medical findings suggesting SSRD, such as negative findings despite thorough medical workup.
- Perform a systematic somatic symptom interview with emphasis on types, patterns, severity, and associated impact of symptoms.
- Obtain a biopsychosocial history focusing on potential predisposing, precipitating, and perpetuating factors.
- Perform a focused physical examination to identify excessive fear of certain movements (kinesiophobia), inconsistent findings, and to judge if further medical evaluation is needed.

An integrative approach

Children and adolescents with transient or mild to moderate symptoms will primarily be assessed by their pediatric doctor. Often, a thorough history and physical examination will, combined with a minimal number of medical tests in parallel with considering potential psychosocial contributors and vulnerabilities, sufficiently clarify the nature of the problem and help shift children and parents toward improvement or a resolution (Cottrell, 2016). The smaller proportion of more complex young patients are usually in need of joint interdisciplinary assessment and care by pediatric and child psychiatry specialties (Ibeziako *et al.*, 2019). Whereas a physical evaluation must be thorough enough to rule out comorbid organic pathophysiology contributing to the somatic symptoms a balance must exist between needed diagnostic evaluation and avoidance of causing undue harm resulting from unnecessary investigations (see Chapter 30 on "physical examination and medical investigation").

Core assessment principles

The core principles of assessment consist of a complete illness history including a thorough review of previous medical records and a screening for typical somatic symptom patterns for SSRD, potential psychosocial stressors, familiar predisposition, and the presence of maladaptive illness beliefs or reinforcing behaviors in a close environment. The possibility of physical or sexual abuse must be carefully explored (Ludwig *et al.*, 2018). The physical examination may reveal that symptoms do not follow known physiological principles or anatomical patterns and may be relieved or disappear under distraction. Also, phenomena such as catastrophic thinking about bodily functions and kinesiophobia, i.e., fear of pain due to certain movements, can be observed. Any comorbid psychiatric disorders must be assessed and diagnosed when suspected.

Whereas the assessment of young children relies primarily on parental information and child/parent interactions, more emphasis will be put on self-report in older children and adolescents. Poor correlation sometimes exists between parental and youth reports of somatic symptoms (Andresen *et al.*, 2011). Therefore, it is critical to obtain both child, family, and other collateral assessments of symptom presentation and severity to

Table 70.3 Selected measures to support assessment for somatic symptom and related disorders (SSRD) in children and adolescents.

Domain	Measure	Age group	No. of items
Somatic symptoms	Children's Somatic Symptom Inventory (CCSI-24) (Walker *et al.*, 2009)	Children and adolescents	24
	Bodily Distress Checklist (BDS-25 Checklist) (Budtz-Lilly *et al.*, 2015)	Adolescents	25
Illness worries	Whiteley-6-R (WI-6) (Carstensen *et al.*, 2020)	Adolescents	6
	Childhood Illness Attitude Scales (CIAS) (Thorisdottir *et al.*, 2017)	Children and adolescents	21
Illness perception	Brief Illness Perceptions Questionnaire (BIPQ) (Broadbent *et al.*, 2006)	Adolescents	8
Illness behavior	Behavioral Responses to Illness Questionnaire (BRIQ) (Spence *et al.*, 2005)	Adolescents	13
	Pain Response Inventory for Children (PRI) (Walker *et al.*,1997)	Children and adolescents	60
Symptom-related interference	Functional Disability Inventory (Walker & Greene, 1991)	Children and adolescents	15
	Limitation index (LI) (Holmstrom *et al.*, 2015)	Children and adolescents	6
Parent's illness response	Adult Responses to Children's Symptoms (ACRS) (protect subscale) (Walker *et al.*, 2006)	Parents	13

gain the fuller picture of the child's symptomatology. Contact with schools to clarify school absence and potential educational and social problems is also important. The combination of (i) certain patterns of somatic symptoms, (ii) the degree of impairment inconsistent with the historical presentation, physical examination, and diagnostic testing, and (iii) the presence of psycho-behavioral factors increases the likelihood of an SSRD diagnosis. Standardized measures that could be helpful in the assessment are summarized in Table 70.3.

Multidisciplinary team

The presented multidisciplinary assessment requires specialized skills in both medical/psychiatric differential diagnoses (see Chapter 43 on pediatric consultation) and skills to help move the families from a purely physical to a biopsychosocial framework, while at the same time avoiding the pitfall of presenting the somatic symptoms in a reductive psychological context (Blake *et al.*, 2018). The medical and psychosocial findings should be presented to the child and the family in a supportive and nonjudgmental manner, and it may also be important to allow room for any prior frustrating experiences with the health care system (Stone & Carson, 2015). Presentation of a chronological timeline can illustrate possible correlations between psychosocial events and symptom debut or exacerbations which can be central to the subsequent rehabilitation process. If the child and family feel understood and met with empathy about the degree of distress the somatic symptoms have produced, they are more likely to be motivated and actively involved in further treatment. Poor communication risks destroying the therapeutic relationship and may cause the child/adolescent and their family to mistrust the whole system approach (Hulgaard *et al.*, 2019b; Hulgaard *et al.*, 2020). This may lead to a renewed search for help, diagnosis, and a cure in the somatic setting or outside the health care system by alternative therapists.

Treatment

Box 70.5 Treatment at a glance

- Psychoeducation on brain–body connectivity with joint consistent messaging from both medical and psychiatric experts.
- Psychological therapies that address the brain–body interface as first line and child and family training as age appropriate, with cognitive behavioral therapy (CBT) having most evidence.
- Temporary pharmacological supplementation for severe somatic symptoms and/or psychiatric comorbidities.
- If there is a concomitant physical disease, help the child foster resilience in symptom self-management.

Treatment approaches

Children with SSRD are most often detected in medical settings either in pediatric outpatient visits, emergency rooms, or for extreme symptoms, during hospitalizations. It is important that across these settings there is a strategic approach that is reinforced by all treatment providers across disciplines. For more moderate to severe presentations, there are societal differences in which clinicians manage SSRD. In Europe, child psychiatrists are much more active in providing both therapy and pharmacological treatment, while in the US, there is a growing trend to treat this population using behavioral therapists embedded in medical clinics to provide education and brief psychological interventions, with the child psychiatrist playing more of a consultant role and/or prescribing medications for comorbid anxiety and depression. For hospitalized youth with SSRD, the use of standardized clinical pathways and tracking psychological outcome metrics as part of routine care has been shown to reduce medical utilization and costs (Ibeziako *et al.*, 2019).

Psychoeducation and psychotherapy are the hallmark in the treatment of all SSRD in children and adolescents. Education of children, adolescents, and their families about the biopsychosocial vulnerability, triggering factors, and maintaining factors covered in this chapter is critical in reducing resistance to the supplementation of medical care with psychotherapy. Such education removes the mind–body dichotomy "demedicalizing" symptoms and helps reset expectations about the condition and its treatment (Kallesøe *et al.*, 2023). Standardization of the information with handouts is helpful.

The remainder of this section will focus on the management of more moderate to severe SSRD. Conceptualizing rehabilitative treatment as three phases is a useful organizational construct with immediate, short-term, and long-term goals (Agarwal *et al.*, 2019). Immediate goals include stopping inappropriate or excessive medical testing and interventions, ensuring the child's safety, and family engagement. Short-term goals include preventing additional unnecessary medical care while maintaining reasonable monitoring and somatic symptom reduction, addressing predisposing and maintaining risk factors, and gradually returning to age-appropriate activities. Longer-term goals are the appropriate use of medical care, further reduction of somatic symptoms, rehabilitation of maladaptive coping habits within the child and family, pharmacological intervention as an adjunct if needed, management of psychosocial stressors, and a return to normal functioning (fostering resilience).

Empirical evidence for psychological therapies that address the brain–body interface

CBT has the most empirical support for treating SSRD in youth and adults. A recent meta-analysis of 27 studies quantified the effectiveness of psychological treatments on symptom load and associated disability, including school absence, in children with bodily distress (Bonvanie *et al.*, 2017b). The most common somatic symptoms were abdominal pain, fatigue, headaches, and musculoskeletal pain. Of the 21 studies with a comparison condition (wait list, treatment as usual, or placebo), the most common intervention was CBT (n = 15) delivered face-to-face or by digitally enhanced means. The active psychological treatments had a greater efficacy in improving somatic symptoms, disability, and school attendance (effect size range; Hedges g -0.42 to -0.61 [moderate effect size]). There was a significant relationship between better outcomes and higher treatment dose but not child age or symptom duration. Psychoeducation, biofeedback, relaxation training, hypnosis, and guided imagery, were also active psychological treatments but with smaller effects compared to CBT. The evidence for effect of CBT on FNSD is weaker, but a small, randomized trial using CBT-based retraining and control therapy (ReACT) for pediatric functional seizures showed a significant improvement in seizure frequency compared to supportive therapy (Fobian *et al.*, 2020). ReACT is based on cognitive behavioral theory to retrain involuntary somatic symptoms by targeting the sense of control over symptoms and catastrophic symptom expectations.

Second and third wave CBT interventions, such as mindfulness- and acceptance-based therapies, have some evidence with modest effects but have primarily targeted teens and with quite small sample sizes (Frostholm & Rask, 2019). Specifically in youth with functional abdominal pain, mindfulness-based therapy (MBT) has shown positive effect (Korterink *et al.*, 2016; Ali *et al.*, 2017). In another study using acceptance-based interoceptive exposure for young children with functional abdominal pain, a 10-week therapy regime was associated with both parent and child reports of reduced pain and emotional reaction to pain over time (Zucker *et al.*, 2017). A group-based version of acceptance and commitment therapy (ACT), AHEAD, showed faster improvement of physical health, symptom severity, and symptom interference, higher treatment satisfaction, and less reported use of pharmacotherapy compared to treatment as usual (Kallesøe *et al.*, 2021b).

Hypnosis is demonstrably effective for IBS in adolescents and young adults, as well as functional abdominal pain in children (Vlieger *et al.*, 2007; Vasant *et al.*, 2021; Gordon *et al.*, 2022), but there is only open trial or case-based support for other SSRD subtypes (Coogle *et al.*, 2021; Chogle *et al.*, 2023). Although less rigorously studied, short-term psychodynamic therapy has shown promise for FNSD, but primarily in adults (Russell *et al.*, 2022). Systemic reviews of physiotherapy (different types of exercise-based and biofeedback interventions) for pediatric conversion disorders are inconclusive in terms of benefit (FitzGerald *et al.*, 2015).

Table 70.4 summarizes the different therapy modalities and ranks them by evidence strength.

Theoretical framework for psychotherapy on brain–body interface

Across SSRD, the social environment can augment somatic sensitivity in children and condition fear reactions, even when somatic symptoms are innocuous (Zucker *et al.*, 2017). Applied to the somatic symptom of pain, the fear avoidance model is a comprehensive framework designed to explain the transition from acute to chronic pain via learning theory. It posits that pain catastrophizing and fear of pain (including avoidance, cognitions, and physiological reactivity) are key antecedents to, and drivers of, pain intensity and disability, in addition to pain-related psychological distress (Rogers & Farris, 2022). This model can be generalized to other somatic symptoms where emotions such as fear being associated with arousal, thoughts, and behaviors in a vicious cycle can perpetuate and amplify the threat of body signal perceptions (Figure 70.3). The psychological techniques described above can be used to recondition/rehabilitate these associations to reduce avoidance and help the child return to optimal functioning. Exposure to interoceptive cues may be a particularly efficacious strategy to facilitate generalization of treatment effects (Hechler, 2021).

These psychological interventions are most effective if delivered in developmentally appropriate ways, using more playful, concrete explanation and application of these techniques with more parental involvement for younger children, and adult-like explanation and *in vivo* skills practice for adolescents. In addition to parental involvement to reinforce the skill acquisition of their child, it is critical that the inadvertent reinforcement of parents or caregivers of sick role behaviors in their children be detected and counterconditioned with education and behavioral skill training (Hulgaard *et al.*, 2019a). Emphasizing habit reversals in parenting and replacing them with positive reinforcement strategies for signs of extinction of somatic distress and acquisition of more adaptive behaviors can powerfully influence their child's return to healthier functioning. Treatment

Table 70.4 Key characteristics of psychotherapies for somatic symptom and related disorders (SSRD).

Modality	Theory	Application	Format	Dose	Strength of evidence
Cognitive behavioral therapy (CBT)	Heightened perception of body signals influenced by negative cognitions and maladaptive behaviors. Therapist as trusted guide/teacher in collaborative, supportive way.	Reduce arousal (relaxation) Reframe negative cognitions Behavioral activation Problem-solving toward goals Reverse avoidance by exposure Primary and secondary control enhancement training Reduce parental reinforcement of sick role behaviors	Individual patient Peer group Parental Digital Self-, coach-, or therapist-guided	8–20 sessions with practice assigned between sessions	Strong to moderate
Mindfulness-based therapy	Utilizes a physiological trance state (change of consciousness) as a vehicle to pay attention to the experiences in the present moment in a nonjudgmental, accepting way. This state buffers secondary negative evaluations of physical sensations (e.g., catastrophizing).	By teaching meditation techniques through experiential learning, the processes of attention regulation, body awareness, emotional regulation, and self-perception are altered.	Individual patient Peer group Self-, coach-, or therapist-guided Digital (audios)	8–12 brief sessions with practice assigned between sessions	Moderate to weak
Acceptance and commitment therapy	By learning psychological flexibility, to stay attentive to present moment regardless of distracting thoughts, emotions, or body sensations, it becomes easier to take actions based on personal values instead of avoiding the inner experience.	Experiential avoidance overcome by combination of mindfulness and behavioral change techniques Anchor breathing (grounding) Cognitive defusion Mindfulness to reduce anxious amplification of body signals Defining value and self as forces greater than physical sensations Committed action toward goals	Individual patient Peer group Therapist-guided	8–20 sessions with practice between sessions	Moderate to weak
Hypnosis	Uses a physiological trance state as vehicle to achieve relative suspension of peripheral awareness, greater inward absorption, dissociation, and suspension of critical thinking, allowing for more susceptibility to suggestions.	This state is achieved by means of induction and allows patients to access internal resources, such as their imagination, to alter relationship between emotions, thoughts, behaviors, and body perceptions.	Individual Peer group Therapist-guided Digital (audios)	1–8 sessions with practice assigned between sessions	Moderate for functional abdominal pain and irritable bowel syndrome (IBS) Weak for other SSRD

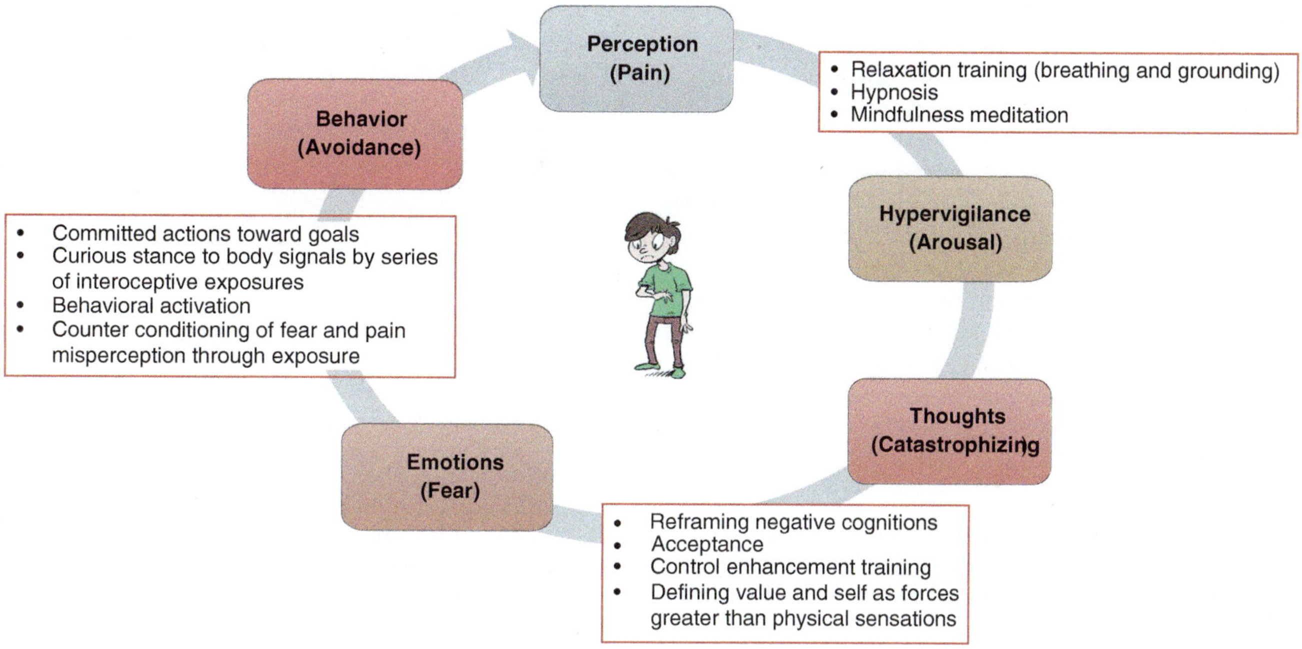

Figure 70.3 Brain–body psychotherapy to rehabilitate the cycle of hypervigilance, thoughts, emotions, behavior, and body perceptions.

of interfering depression and anxiety in caregivers is also important (LaVigne *et al.*, 2020).

Pharmacological treatments

Recent guidelines for adults with SSRD recommend, given the unchanged evidence with regard to risks, adverse effects, and low acceptance by patients, that administration of drugs—particularly psychopharmaceuticals, above all antidepressants—should only be for temporary symptomatic treatment (e.g., of sleep disorders or nervousness), certain types of SSRD dominated by pain (e.g., fibromyalgia), or in the presence of mental comorbidity like anxiety and depression (Roenneberg *et al.*, 2019). Furthermore, a recent network meta-analysis concluded there is no reliable evidence for the long-term efficacy of antidepressants in adults with chronic pain (Birkinshaw *et al.*, 2023).

In children and adolescents, antidepressants targeting serotonergic and noradrenergic neurotransmission (particularly selective serotonin reuptake inhibitors [SSSRIs] and tricyclic antidepressants [TCA]) have largely been utilized to treat pediatric functional abdominal pain but only based on expert reviews (Bonilla & Nurko, 2018). Thus, there is currently no convincing evidence to support the use of drugs to treat this condition or other types of SSRD in young people and well-conducted pediatric randomized controlled trials are needed to evaluate any possible benefits and risks of pharmacological interventions as such (Martin *et al.*, 2017). Drug treatment should therefore be reserved for temporary symptom or pain relief or management of comorbidity like anxiety or depression.

Future development and necessary research

Although the literature on SSRD in children and adolescents has evolved substantially since the 2010s, gaps remain to be addressed. International clinical and research guidelines should be established to promote a common language for diagnostic definition and methodology to be used across the field. More research in aspects regarding cultural awareness and sensitivity in diagnoses will also be important in that respect. Epidemiological studies systematically mapping the extent of SSRD in younger age groups and sociocultural differences, as well as developmental trajectories and early risk factors could help inform further service development and clinical practice. This should include identification of factors that cultivate resilience in SSRD in youth, and also in specific risk groups such as children and adolescents with concurrent chronic medical diseases or neurodevelopmental disorders.

There is growing consensus that a collaborative interdisciplinary approach is warranted when working with youth presenting with SSRD. This calls for more education of care providers in general about appropriate basic principles for formulation, assessment, and first-line treatments of SSRD, as well as systematic development of shared models of care to be implemented across the health care settings. A main area for research in this respect will include interventions aimed at primary care settings, organization of hospital pediatric liaison psychiatry services, and medical–psychiatric inpatient and rehabilitation programs for the most severe cases.

Research into the efficacy and mediating factors in specialized psychotherapy for children and adolescents with SSRD is still scarce. Further research is needed to better understand the proposed role of perceptual dysregulation and thereby identify important psychotherapeutic targets to refine and optimize these therapies. Barriers for providing such types of therapies include shortages of mental health practitioners with relevant expertise, though increasing research has demonstrated the efficacy of delivery of treatment via online platforms. More efficacy studies of psychopharmacological treatment for SSRD and emotional comorbidity would also be beneficial. In addition, research on the role of caregivers in treatment and family therapy-based approaches is still scarce, and future trials could also evaluate if incorporating extended social and school networks would facilitate adherence to and strengthen efficacy of treatments.

References

Agarwal, V. *et al.* (2019) Clinical practice guidelines for the management of somatoform disorders in children and adolescents. *Indian Journal of Psychiatry* **61**, 241–246.

Ainley, V. *et al.* (2016) 'Bodily precision': a predictive coding account of individual differences in interoceptive accuracy. *Philosophical Transactions of the Royal Society of London. Series B, Biological Sciences* **371**, 20160003.

Ali, A. *et al.* (2017) Mindfulness-based stress reduction for adolescents with functional somatic syndromes: a pilot cohort study. *The Journal of Pediatrics* **183**, 184–190.

Aluko, B. *et al.* (2023) Nation-wide decrease in the prevalence of pediatric chronic pain during the COVID-19 pandemic. *Scandinavian Journal of Pain* **23**, 608–612.

American Psychiatric Association (2000) *Diagnostic and Statistical Manual of Mental Disorders* (4th ed., text revised). American Psychiatric Association, Washington, DC.

American Psychiatric Association (2013) *Diagnostic and Statistical Manual of Mental Disorders*, 5th edn. American Psychiatric Association, Washington, DC.

Andresen, J.M. *et al.* (2011) Physical symptoms and psychosocial correlates of somatization in pediatric primary care. *Clinical Pediatrics (Phila)* **50**, 904–909.

Ani, C. *et al.* (2013) Incidence and 12-month outcome of non-transient childhood conversion disorder in the UK and Ireland. *British Journal of Psychiatry* **202**, 413–418.

Bargh, J.A. & Morsella, E. (2008) The unconscious mind. *Perspectives on Psychological Science* **3**, 73–79.

Bègue, I. *et al.* (2019) Structural alterations in functional neurological disorder and related conditions: a software and hardware problem? *NeuroImage: Clinical* **22**, 101798.

Berg, N. *et al.* (2022) Risk factors in adolescence as predictors of trajectories of somatic symptoms over 27 years. *European Journal of Public Health* **32**, 696–702.

Birkinshaw, H. *et al.* (2023) Antidepressants for pain management in adults with chronic pain: a network meta-analysis. *Cochrane Database of Systematic Reviews* **5**, Cd014682.

Blake, L. *et al.* (2018) *Medically Unexplained Symptoms (MUS) in Children and Young People: A Guide to Assessing and Managing Patients Under the Age of 18 Who are Referred To Secondary Care.* Royal College of Psychiatrists, London.

Bonilla, S. & Nurko, S. (2018) Focus on the use of antidepressants to treat pediatric functional abdominal pain: current perspectives. *Clinical and Experimental Gastroenterology* **11**, 365–372.

Bonvanie, I.J. *et al.* (2015) Short report: Functional somatic symptoms are associated with perfectionism in adolescents. *Journal of Psychosomatic Research* **79**, 328–330.

Bonvanie, I.J. *et al.* (2016) Sleep problems and pain: a longitudinal cohort study in emerging adults. *Pain* **157**, 957–963.

Bonvanie, I.J. *et al.* (2017a) Life events and functional somatic symptoms: a population study in older adolescents. *British Journal of Psychology* **108**, 318–333.

Bonvanie, I.J. *et al.* (2017b) Psychological interventions for children with functional somatic symptoms: A systematic review and Meta-analysis. *The Journal of Pediatrics* **187**, 272–281.e17.

Broadbent, E. *et al.* (2006) The Brief Illness Perception Questionnaire. *Journal of Psychosomatic Research* **60**, 631–637.

Buchnik-Daniely, Y. *et al.* (2021) The path to dissociative experiences: a direct comparison of different etiological models. *Clinical Psychology & Psychotherapy* **28**, 1091–1102.

Budtz-Lilly, A. *et al.* (2015) A new questionnaire to identify bodily distress in primary care: the 'BDS Checklist'. *Journal of Psychosomatic Research* **78**, 536–545.

Bujoreanu, S. *et al.* (2014) Characteristics of medically hospitalized pediatric patients with somatoform diagnoses. *Hospital Pediatrics* **4**, 283–290.

Burton, C. *et al.* (2020) Functional somatic disorders: discussion paper for a new common classification for research and clinical use. *BMC Medicine* **18**, 34.

Caes, L. *et al.* (2016) The development of worry throughout childhood: Avon Longitudinal Study of Parents and Children data. *British Journal of Health Psychology* **21**, 389–406.

Campo, J.V. (2012) Annual research review: functional somatic symptoms and associated anxiety and depression--developmental psychopathology in pediatric practice. *Journal of Child Psychology and Psychiatry, and Allied Disciplines* **53**, 575–592.

Carstensen, T.B.W. *et al.* (2020) Detection of illness worry in the general population: a specific item on illness rumination improves the Whiteley index. *Journal of Psychosomatic Research* **138**, 110245.

Chogle, A. *et al.* (2023) Clinical hypnosis for pediatric gastrointestinal disorders: a practical guide for clinicians. *Journal of Pediatric Gastroenterology and Nutrition* **76**, 271–277.

Christensen, J. *et al.* (2019) Neurobiological mechanisms underlying the sleep-pain relationship in adolescence: a review. *Neuroscience and Biobehavioral Reviews* **96**, 401–413.

Clark, A. (2013) Whatever next? Predictive brains, situated agents, and the future of cognitive science. *The Behavioral and Brain Sciences* **36**, 181–204.

Collin, S.M. *et al.* (2015) Chronic fatigue syndrome (CFS) or myalgic encephalomyelitis (ME) is different in children compared to in adults: a study of UK and Dutch clinical cohorts. *BMJ Open* **5**, e008830.

Coogle, J. *et al.* (2021) Hypnosis in the treatment of pediatric functional neurological disorder: the magic glove technique. *Pediatric Neurology* **125**, 20–25.

Cottrell, D.J. (2016) Fifteen-minute consultation: medically unexplained symptoms. *Archives of Disease in Childhood. Education and Practice Edition* **101**, 114–118.

De Bellis, M.D. & Zisk, A. (2014) The biological effects of childhood trauma. *Child and Adolescent Psychiatric Clinics of North America* **23**, 185–222, vii

Dibble, J.J. *et al.* (2020) Genetic risk factors of ME/CFS: a critical review. *Human Molecular Genetics* **29**, R117–R124.

Dimsdale, J. *et al.* (2011) What do physicians think of somatoform disorders? *Psychosomatics* **52**, 154–159.

Djafar, J.V. *et al.* (2023) Childhood dementia: a collective clinical approach to advance therapeutic development and care. *Pediatric Neurology* **139**, 76–85.

D'Orsi, G. *et al.* (2025) A novel analysis of interoceptive underpinnings of anxious psychopathology in COVID-19 survivors. *Behavioural Brain Research* **476**, 115275.

Dunphy, L. *et al.* (2019) Somatic symptom disorder: a diagnostic dilemma. *BML Case Reports* **12**, e231550.

Elliott, L. *et al.* (2020) A systematic review of somatic symptoms in children with a chronically ill family member. *Psychosomatic Medicine* **82**, 366–376.

FitzGerald, T.L. *et al.* (2015) Is physiotherapy effective in the management of child and adolescent conversion disorder? A systematic review. *Journal of Paediatrics and Child Health* **51**, 159–167.

Fobian, A.D. *et al.* (2020) Retraining and control therapy for pediatric psychogenic non-epileptic seizures. *Annals of Clinical Translational Neurology* **7**, 1410–1419.

Friston, K. (2010) The free-energy principle: a unified brain theory? *Nature Reviews Neuroscience* **11**, 127–138.

Frostholm, L. & Rask, C.U. (2019) Third wave treatments for functional somatic syndromes and health anxiety across the age span: a narrative review. *Clinical Psychology in Europe* **1**, 1–13.

Garralda, M.E. & Slaveska-Hollis, K. (2016) What is special about a paediatric liaison child and adolescent mental health service? *Child and Adolescent Mental Health* **21**, 96–101.

Glaser, D. (2020) Fabricated or induced illness: from "Munchausen by proxy" to child and family-oriented action. *Child Abuse & Neglect* **108**, 104649.

Gordon, M. *et al.* (2022) Psychosocial interventions for the treatment of functional abdominal pain disorders in children: a systematic review and Meta-analysis. *JAMA Pediatrics* **176**, 560–568.

Gureje, O. & Reed, G.M. (2016) Bodily distress disorder in ICD-11: Problems and prospects. *World Psychiatry: Official Journal of the World Psychiatric Association* **15**, 291–292.

Hadji-Michael, M. *et al.* (2019) Alexithymia in children with medically unexplained symptoms: a systematic review. *Journal of Psychosomatic Research* **123**, 109736.

Haig-Ferguson, A. *et al.* (2021) Practitioner review: health anxiety in children and young people in the context of the COVID-19 pandemic. *Behavioural and Cognitive Psychotherapy* **49**, 129–143.

Hansen, A.S. *et al.* (2020) Incidence rates and characteristics of pediatric onset psychogenic nonepileptic seizures. *Pediatric Research* **88**, 796–803.

Harvey, S.B. *et al.* (2006) Conversion disorder: towards a neurobiological understanding. *Neuropsychiatric Disease and Treatment* **2**, 13–20.

Hechler, T. (2021) Altered interoception and its role for the co-occurrence of chronic primary pain and mental health problems in children. *Pain* **162**, 665–671.

Henningsen, P. *et al.* (2018) Persistent physical symptoms as perceptual dysregulation: a neuropsychobehavioral model and its clinical implications. *Psychosomatic Medicine* **80**, 422–431.

Henström, M. & D'Amato, M. (2016) Genetics of irritable bowel syndrome. *Molecular and Cellular Pediatrics* **3**, 7.

Hinton, D. & Kirk, S. (2016) Families' and healthcare professionals' perceptions of healthcare services for children and young people with medically unexplained symptoms: a narrative review of the literature. *Health & Social Care in the Community* **24**, 12–26.

Hogendoorn, E. *et al.* (2023) Longitudinal relations between autistic-like features and functional somatic symptoms in adolescence. *Autism* **27**, 1690–1701.

Hohwy, J. (2013) *The Predictive Mind*. Oxford University Press, Oxford, UK.

Hollier, J.M. *et al.* (2022) United States healthcare burden of pediatric functional gastrointestinal pain disorder hospitalizations from 2002 to 2018. *Neurogastroenterology and Motility* **34**, e14288.

Holmstrom, L. *et al.* (2015) Evaluating the statistical properties of the pain interference index in children and adolescents with chronic pain. *Journal of Developmental and Behavioral Pediatrics* **36**, 450–454.

Hulgaard, D. *et al.* (2019a) Family-based interventions for children and adolescents with functional somatic symptoms: a systematic review. *Journal of Family Therapy* **41**, 4–28.

Hulgaard, D.R. *et al.* (2019b) 'I can hardly breathe': exploring the parental experience of having a child with a functional disorder. *Journal of Child Health Care* **24**, 165–179.

Hulgaard, D.R. *et al.* (2020) Illness perceptions of youths with functional disorders and their parents: an interpretative phenomenological analysis study. *Clinical Child Psychology and Psychiatry* **25**, 45–61.

Ibeziako, P. & Bujoreanu, S. (2011) Approach to psychosomatic illness in adolescents. *Current Opinion in Pediatrics* **23**, 384–389.

Ibeziako, P. *et al.* (2019) Developing a clinical pathway for somatic symptom and related disorders in pediatric hospital settings. *Hospital Pediatrics* **9**, 147–155.

Ingeman, K. *et al.* (2022) Health anxiety by proxy: through the eyes of the parents. *Journal of Child Health Care* **28**, 22–36.

Janssens, K.A. *et al.* (2009) Parental overprotection predicts the development of functional somatic symptoms in young adolescents. *The Journal of Pediatrics* **154**, 918–923.e1.

Janssens, K.A. *et al.* (2011) School absenteeism as a perpetuating factor of functional somatic symptoms in adolescents: the TRAILS study. *The Journal of Pediatrics* **159**, 988–993.e1.

Janssens, K.A. *et al.* (2012) Symptom-specific associations between low cortisol responses and functional somatic symptoms: the TRAILS study. *Psychoneuroendocrinology* **37**, 332–340.

Janssens, K.A. *et al.* (2014a) Predictors for persistence of functional somatic symptoms in adolescents. *The Journal of Pediatrics* **164**, 900–905. e2

Janssens, K.A. *et al.* (2014b) An inactive lifestyle and low physical fitness are associated with functional somatic symptoms in adolescents: the TRAILS study. *Journal of Psychosomatic Research* **76**, 454–457.

Jason, L.A. & Mirin, A.A. (2021) Updating the National Academy of medicine ME/CFS prevalence and economic impact figures to account for population growth and inflation. *Fatigue: Biomedicine, Health & Behavior* **9**, 9–13.

Kallesøe, K.H. *et al.* (2021a) Adolescents with functional somatic syndromes: symptom profiles, illness perception, illness worry and attachment orientation. *Journal of Psychosomatic Research* **145**, 110430.

Kallesøe, K.H. *et al.* (2021b) Group-based acceptance and commitment therapy (AHEAD) for adolescents with multiple functional somatic syndromes: a randomised trial. *JCPP Advances* **1**, e12047.

Kallesøe, K.H. *et al.* (2023) Clinical impact of systematic assessment and psychoeducation in specialized treatment of adolescents with severe functional somatic disorders: results from the AHEAD study. *Children* **10**, 1101.

Kangas, M. *et al.* (2020) Functional somatic syndromes (FSS) in children and adolescents. *Zeitschrift für Psychologie* **228**, 81–92.

Katz, B.Z. & Jason, L.A. (2013) Chronic fatigue syndrome following infections in adolescents. *Current Opinion in Pediatrics* **25**, 95–102.

Kingma, E.M. *et al.* (2011) Adolescents with low intelligence are at risk of functional somatic symptoms: the TRAILS study. *The Journal of Adolescent Health* **49**, 621–626.

Kline, C.L. *et al.* (2023) A review of the impact of sociodemographic factors on the assessment and management of pediatric somatic symptom and related disorders. *Journal of the Academy of Consultant Liaison Psychiatry* **64**, 58–64.

Korterink, J.J. *et al.* (2015) Epidemiology of pediatric functional abdominal pain disorders: a meta-analysis. *PLoS One* **10**, e0126982.

Korterink, J.J. *et al.* (2016) Yoga therapy for abdominal pain-related functional gastrointestinal disorders in children: a randomized controlled trial. *Journal of Pediatric Gastroenterology and Nutrition* **63**, 481–487.

Kozlowska, K. (2013) Functional somatic symptoms in childhood and adolescence. *Current Opinion in Psychiatry* **26**, 485–492.

Kozlowska, K. *et al.* (2007) Conversion disorder in Australian pediatric practice. *Journal of the American Academy of Child and Adolescent Psychiatry* **46**, 68–75.

Kratzer, L. *et al.* (2022) Co-occurrence of severe PTSD, somatic symptoms and dissociation in a large sample of childhood trauma inpatients: a network analysis. *European Archives of Psychiatry and Clinical Neuroscience* **272**, 897–908.

Larsen, L.B. *et al.* (2022) Functional somatic symptoms in preschool attention-deficit/hyperactivity disorder: a secondary analysis of data from a randomized controlled trial of parent training. *European Child & Adolescent Psychiatry* **32**, 1979–1988.

LaVigne, T.W. *et al.* (2020) Somatic symptom and related disorders in pediatric patients: associations with parent psychiatric and substance use histories. *Clinical Child Psychology and Psychiatry* **25**, 932–944.

Levy, R.L. (2011) Exploring the intergenerational transmission of illness behavior: From observations to experimental intervention. *Annals of Behavioral Medicine* **41**, 174–182.

Limbri, L.F. *et al.* (2022) Prevalence of irritable bowel syndrome and functional abdominal pain disorders in children with inflammatory bowel disease in remission. *JGH Open* **6**, 818–823.

Lipsker, C.W. *et al.* (2018) Prevalence of autism traits and attention-deficit hyperactivity disorder symptoms in a clinical sample of children and adolescents with chronic pain. *Journal of Pain Research* **11**, 2827–2836.

Löwe, B. *et al.* (2008) Validity of current somatoform disorder diagnoses: perspectives for classification in DSM-V and ICD-11. *Psychopathology* **41**, 4–9.

Ludwig, L. *et al.* (2018) Stressful life events and maltreatment in conversion (functional neurological) disorder: systematic review and meta-analysis of case-control studies. *The Lancet Psychiatry* **5**, 307–320.

Malas, N. *et al.* (2017) Pediatric somatic symptom disorders. *Current Psychiatry Reports* **19**. 12

Martel, M.M. (2013) Sexual selection and sex differences in the prevalence of childhood externalizing and adolescent internalizing disorders. *Psychological Bulletin* **139**, 1221–1259.

Martin, A.E. *et al.* (2017) Pharmacological interventions for recurrent abdominal pain in childhood. *The Cochrane Database of Systematic Reviews* **3**, CD010973.

McInnis, P.M. *et al.* (2020) Stress-system activation in children with chronic pain: a focus for clinical intervention. *Clinical Child Psychology and Psychiatry* **25**, 78–97.

Meade, J. (2021) Mental health effects of the COVID-19 pandemic on children and adolescents: a review of the current research. *Pediatric Clinics of North America* **68**, 945–959.

Morabito, G. *et al.* (2020) The unaware physician's role in perpetuating somatic symptom disorder. *JAMA Pediatrics* **174**, 9–10.

Münker, L. *et al.* (2022) Can the bodily distress syndrome (BDS) concept be used to assess functional somatic symptoms in adolescence? *Journal of Psychosomatic Research* **163**, 111064.

Noviello, D. *et al.* (2022) Functional gastrointestinal and somatoform symptoms five months after SARS-CoV-2 infection: a controlled cohort study. *Neurogastroenterology and Motility* **34**, e14187.

Oh, D.L. *et al.* (2018) Systematic review of pediatric health outcomes associated with childhood adversity. *BMC Pediatrics* **18**, 83.

Patel, H. *et al.* (2007) Nonepileptic seizures in children. *Epilepsia* **48**, 2086–2092.

Peri, F. *et al.* (2019) Somatic symptom disorder should be suspected in children with alleged chronic Lyme disease. *European Journal of Pediatrics* **178**, 1297–1300.

Petersen, M.W. *et al.* (2020) Irritable bowel, chronic widespread pain, chronic fatigue and related syndromes are prevalent and highly overlapping in the general population: DanFunD. *Scientific Reports* **10**, 3273.

Pezzulo, G. *et al.* (2019) Symptom perception from a predictive processing perspective. *Clinical Psychology in Europe* **1**, 1–14.

Price, T.J. & Inyang, K.E. (2015) Commonalities between pain and memory mechanisms and their meaning for understanding chronic pain. *Progress in Molecular Biology and Translational Science* **131**, 409–434.

Raper, J. *et al.* (2019) Long-term outcomes of functional neurological disorder in children. *Archives of Disease in Childhood* **104**, 1155–1160.

Rask, C.U. *et al.* (2009) Functional somatic symptoms and associated impairment in 5-7-year-old children: the Copenhagen child cohort 2000. *European Journal of Epidemiology* **24**, 625–634.

Rask, C.U. *et al.* (2013a) Functional somatic symptoms and consultation patterns in 5- to 7-year-olds. *Pediatrics* **132**, e459–e467.

Rask, C.U. *et al.* (2013b) Infant behaviors are predictive of functional somatic symptoms at ages 5-7 years: results from the Copenhagen Child Cohort CCC2000. *The Journal of Pediatrics* **162**, 335–342.

Rask, C.U. *et al.* (2016) Health anxiety in preadolescence: associated health problems, healthcare expenditure, and continuity in childhood. *Journal of Abnormal Child Psychology* **44**, 823–832.

Rhee, H. (2005) Relationships between physical symptoms and pubertal development. *Journal of Pediatric Health Care* **19**, 95–103.

Rider, E.A. *et al.* (2021) Mental health and wellbeing of children and adolescents during the covid-19 pandemic. *BMJ* **374**, n1730.

Riemann, L. *et al.* (2021) Persistent postconcussive symptoms in children and adolescents with mild traumatic brain injury receiving initial head computed tomography. *Journal of Neurosurgery: Pediatrics* **27**, 538–547.

Roenneberg, C. *et al.* (2019) Functional somatic symptoms. *Deutsches Ärzteblatt International* **116**, 553–560.

Rogers, A.H. & Farris, S.G. (2022) A meta-analysis of the associations of elements of the fear-avoidance model of chronic pain with negative affect, depression, anxiety, pain-related disability and pain intensity. *European Journal of Pain* **26**, 1611–1635.

Russell, L. *et al.* (2022) A review of the treatment of functional neurological disorder with intensive short-term dynamic psychotherapy. *Epilepsy & Behavior* **130**, 108657.

Salmon, M. *et al.* (2022) Systematic review on somatization in a transcultural context among teenagers and young adults: focus on the nosography blur. *Frontiers in Psychiatry* **13**, 897002.

Saunders, N.R. *et al.* (2020) Health care use and costs of children, adolescents, and young adults with somatic symptom and related disorders. *JAMA Network Open* **3**, e2011295.

Schulte, I.E. & Petermann, F. (2011) Somatoform disorders: 30 years of debate about criteria! What about children and adolescents? *Journal of Psychosomatic Research* **70**, 218–228.

Simon, A.E. *et al.* (2014) Cenesthopathy in adolescence: an appraisal of diagnostic overlaps along the anxiety-hypochondriasis-psychosis spectrum. *Comprehensive Psychiatry* **55**, 1122–1129.

Smith, B.M. *et al.* (2020) Relapse of anxiety-related fear and avoidance: conceptual analysis of treatment with acceptance and commitment therapy. *Journal of the Experimental Analysis of Behavior* **113**, 87–104.

Spence, M. *et al.* (2005) The Behavioural Responses to Illness Questionnaire (BRIQ): a new predictive measure of medically unexplained symptoms following acute infection. *Psychological Medicine* **35**, 583–593.

Stewart, J.M. (2013) Common syndromes of orthostatic intolerance. *Pediatrics* **131**, 968–980.

Stone, J. & Carson, A. (2015) Functional neurologic disorders. *Continuum* **21**, 818–837.

Stone, J. *et al.* (2014) Functional disorders in the neurology section of ICD-11: a landmark opportunity. *Neurology* **83**, 2299–2301.

Sulheim, D. *et al.* (2012) Adolescent chronic fatigue syndrome: a follow-up study displays concurrent improvement of circulatory abnormalities and clinical symptoms. *BioPsychoSocial Medicine* **6**, 10.

Thabane, M. *et al.* (2010) An outbreak of acute bacterial gastroenteritis is associated with an increased incidence of irritable bowel syndrome in children. *The American Journal of Gastroenterology* **105**, 933–939.

Thorgaard, M.V. *et al.* (2017) Health anxiety by proxy in women with severe health anxiety: a case control study. *Journal of Anxiety Disorders* **52**, 8–14.

Thorisdottir, A.S. *et al.* (2017) Measurement invariance across genders on the Childhood Illness Attitude Scales (CIAS). *Journal of Psychosomatic Research* **98**, 34–39.

Turiaco, F. *et al.* (2022) Somatic symptom disorder: a narrative review of literature of the last twenty years. *Mediterranean Journal of Clinical Psychology* **10**, 1–27.

Undheim, A.M. & Sund, A.M. (2011) Bullying: a hidden factor behind somatic symptoms? *Acta Paediatrica* **100**, 496–498.

Van Den Bergh, O. *et al.* (2017) Symptoms and the body: taking the inferential leap. *Neuroscience and Biobehavioral Reviews* **74**, 185–203.

Van Der Schaaf, M.E. *et al.* (2018) Fatigue is associated with altered monitoring and preparation of physical effort in patients with chronic fatigue syndrome. *Biological Psychiatry: Cognitive Neuroscience and Neuroimaging* **3**, 392–404.

Vanderbilt-Adriance, E. & Shaw, D.S. (2008) Protective factors and the development of resilience in the context of neighborhood disadvantage. *Journal of Abnormal Child Psychology* **36**, 887–901.

Vasant, D.H. *et al.* (2021) Gut-focused hypnotherapy for children and adolescents with irritable bowel syndrome. *Frontline Gastroenterology* **12**, 570–577.

Vesterling, C. & Koglin, U. (2020) The relationship between attachment and somatoform symptoms in children and adolescents: a systematic review and meta-analysis. *Journal of Psychosomatic Research* **130**, 109932.

Vesterling, C. *et al.* (2023) Epidemiology of somatoform symptoms and disorders in childhood and adolescence: a systematic review and meta-analysis. *Health & Social Care in the Community* **2023**, 6242678.

Villanueva Badenes, L., Prado-Gascó, V., & González Barrón, R. (2016) Emotion awareness, mood and personality as predictors of somatic complaints in children and adults. *Psicothema* **28**, 383–388.

Vlieger, A.M. *et al.* (2007) Hypnotherapy for children with functional abdominal pain or irritable bowel syndrome: a randomized controlled trial. *Gastroenterology* **133**, 1430–1436.

Walker, L.S. & Greene, J.W. (1991) The functional disability inventory: measuring a neglected dimension of child health status. *Journal of Pediatric Psychology* **16**, 39–58.

Walker, L.S. *et al.* (1997) Development and validation of the pain response inventory for children. *Psychological Assessment* **9**, 392–405.

Walker, L.S. *et al.* (2005) Testing a model of pain appraisal and coping in children with chronic abdominal pain. *Health Psychology* **24**, 364–374.

Walker, L.S. *et al.* (2006) Validation of a measure of protective parent responses to children's pain. *The Clinical Journal of Pain* **22**, 712–716.

Walker, L.S. *et al.* (2007) Appraisal and coping with daily stressors by pediatric patients with chronic abdominal pain. *Journal of Pediatric Psychology* **32**, 206–216.

Walker, L.S. *et al.* (2009) Children's somatization inventory: psychometric properties of the revised form (CSI-24). *Journal of Pediatric Psychology* **34**, 430–440.

Wiggins, A. *et al.* (2021) Somatic symptom and related disorders in a tertiary paediatric hospital: prevalence, reach and complexity. *European Journal of Pediatrics* **180**, 1267–1275.

Wiggins, A. *et al.* (2022) Pediatric somatic symptom and related disorders: parent acceptance influences recovery. *The Journal of Pediatrics* **241**, 109–114.

World Health Organization (2004) *International Statistical Classification of Diseases and Related Health Problems* 10th revision. World Health Organization (WHO), Geneva, Switzerland. Available: https://apps.who.int/iris/handle/10665/42980 [20 December 2024].

World Health Organization (2019) ICD-11 for Mortality and Morbidity Statistics. 11th edn. World Health Organization (WHO), Geneva, Switzerland. Available: https://icd.who.int/browse11/l-m/en [20 December 2024].

Zucker, N. *et al.* (2017) Acceptance-based interoceptive exposure for young children with functional abdominal pain. *Behaviour Research and Therapy* **97**, 200–212.

Index

Please Note: entries in *italics* refer to figures, those in **bold**, either tables or boxes.

Rutter's Child and Adolescent Psychiatry and Psychology, Seventh Edition.
Edited by Anita Thapar, Daniel S. Pine, Samuele Cortese, Cathy Creswell, Tamsin J. Ford, James F. Leckman, and Argyris Stringaris.

Companion website: www.wiley.com/go/thapar/rutterspsych7

M